Textbook of Pediatric Gastroenterology, Hepatology and Nutrition

Stefano Guandalini • Anil Dhawan • David Branski†
Editors

Textbook of Pediatric Gastroenterology, Hepatology and Nutrition

A Comprehensive Guide to Practice

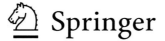 Springer

Editors
Stefano Guandalini
Department of Pediatrics
University of Chicago
Chicago
Illinois
USA

David Branski†
Department of Pediatrics
Hebrew University Hadassah Hospital
Jerusalem
Israel

Anil Dhawan
Professor and Director
Pediatric Liver, GI and Nutrition Center
Clinical Director
Child Health
King's College Hospital
London
United Kingdom

ISBN 978-3-319-17168-5   ISBN 978-3-319-17169-2 (eBook)
DOI 10.1007/978-3-319-17169-2

Library of Congress Control Number: 2015939902

Springer Cham Heidelberg New York Dordrecht London

Springer International Publishing AG Switzerland is part of Springer Science+Business Media (www.springer.com)

Preface

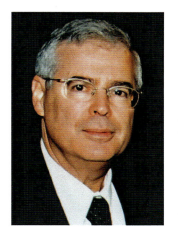

This book would not have seen the light had it not been for David Branski.

It was him who called Stefano asking him if he would consider a second edition of the book 'Textbook of Pediatric Gastroenterology and Nutrition', edited in 2004 by Taylor & Francis, but expanding it to include hepatology. Stefano was reluctant (it takes a huge commitment to edit such a book!), but David had a way of convincing that was hard to resist, and when he brought into the picture Anil as a prospective editor for the liver part, resisting was futile!

The three of us laid out the design of the project together and the enthusiasm about it grew: in fact, David's knowledge, his calm but confident demeanor, his never-ending energy to learn and prolific writing skills were a guarantee of the book's success. Sadly, only few months later, when the details of this book had just been put together, we heard the news of his untimely demise. We debated in panic whether to continue this commitment or abort it, but it did not take us long to agree that we needed to carry this project to completion as a tribute to the doyen of pediatric gastroenterology of our times.

Three sections of this edition, gastroenterology, hepatology and nutrition cover the common disease states with an updated emphasis on pathophysiology and any expected future advances. The chapters are clinically oriented and aim at making easier the decision-making process for trainees in pediatrics and pediatric gastroenterology, pediatricians and nurse practitioners.

The extensive section of gastroenterology covers the main congenital disorders with their newer diagnostic techniques, with chapters specifically dedicated to the term or preterm newborn; common conditions that every pediatric gastroenterologist is likely to face in his/her practice; and conditions that are either relatively new, such as eosinophilic disorders, or in a state of rapidly evolving treatment options like inflammatory bowel diseases. New treatment paradigms (e.g. probiotics or fecal microbial transplantation) are also specifically dealt with.

The chapters on hepatology focus on newer diagnostic techniques, treatment advances and quality of life issues: for instance, the chapter on transition of children with liver disease provides a unique view from a psychologist and adolescent hepatologist on how best to improve the outcome of this group of patients. Some of the chapters like liver transplantation are deliberately longer to give the reader comprehensive information on the state of the art on indications, complications and the management of immunosuppression. Finally, the chapter on the future of hepatology is particularly thought-provoking in that it discusses the role of genomics and other 'omics' in the diagnosis and real options of small molecules, gene therapy and liver cell transplantation in the management of liver disease.

We are humbly but surely confident that David would have loved this book, which we gratefully dedicate to him.

Stefano Guandalini   Anil Dhawan

Acknowledgements

It's hard to summarize in a few lines the gratefulness I feel to so many people whose roles were instrumental in the realization of this book. From the distinguished colleague who picked me and pushed me in the world of pediatric gastroenterology, the late professor Raffaele De Luca, to my splendid mentors at the University of Naples, Salvatore Auricchio and Armido Rubino, to the many, incredibly talented mentees I had the privilege to help as they developed their career in our field, to the many supportive colleagues and friends who wanted me to lead them within ESPGHAN and then FISPGHAN. But above all, had it not been for my wife Greta, who supports and bears me since almost half a century, this work would not have been accomplished. To all of you, and to my patients: thanks.

Stefano Guandalini

I would like to express my sincere thanks to the love of my life, my wife Anita. She has been my friend and a critic who expects excellence only and continues to support me, rather put up with me, to deliver projects like this one, again and again....

My two wonderful sons Atin and Ashish who have been a source of joy and encouragement and I think have forgiven me for not spending much time with them.

To my patients who have helped me to understand the complexity of liver disorders and my personal assistant, Mrs. Kathleen Meader for her hard work that helps me deliver professionally.

Anil Dhawan

Contents

Contributors

Marina Aloi Pediatric Gastroenterology and Liver Unit, Sapienza University of Rome, Rome, Italy

Ruba K. Azzam Section of Gastroenterology, Hepatology and Nutrition, Department of Pediatrics, Comer Children's Hospital, University of Chicago, Chicago, IL, USA

R. Mark Beattie Southampton Children's Hospital, University Hospital Southampton, Southampton, UK

Marc A. Benninga Department of Pediatric Gastroenterology and Nutrition, Emma Children's Hospital, Academic Medical Centre, Amsterdam, The Netherlands

Roberto Berni Canani Department of Translational Medical Science—Section of Pediatrics, University of Naples "Federico II", Naples, Italy

European Laboratory for the Investigation of Food Induced Diseases and CEINGE Advanced Biotechnologies, University of Naples "Federico II", Naples, Italy

European Laboratory for the Investigation of Food Induced Diseases, University of Naples "Federico II", Naples, Italy

Zulfiqar A. Bhutta Division of Women and Child Health, Department of Pediatrics, Aga Khan University, Karachi, Pakistan

SickKids Center for Global Child Health, Hospital for Sick Children, Toronto, ON, Canada

Departments of Pediatrics, Nutritional Sciences and Public Health, SickKids Peter Gilgan Centre for Research and Learning, University of Toronto, Toronto, ON, Canada

Osvaldo Borrelli Division of Neurogastroenterology and Motility, Department of Pediatric Gastroenterology, Great Ormond Street Hospital for Children, NHS Foundation Trust, London, UK

Athos Bousvaros GI Division—Inflammatory Bowel Disease Center, Children's Hospital, Boston, MA, USA

Eugenia Bruzzese Department of Translation Medical Science, Section of Pediatrics, University of Naples "Federico II", Naples, Italy

Vittoria Buccigrossi Department of Translational Medical Science, Section of Pediatrics, University of Naples "Federico II", Naples, Italy

Mike Champion Department of Pediatric Inherited Metabolic Disease, Evelina London Children's Hospital, St Thomas' Hospital, London, UK

Virginie Colomb Department of Pediatric Gastroenterology and Nutrition, Hôpital Necker-Enfants Malades, Paris Cedex 15, France

Corina Gabriela Cotoi   Institute of Liver Studies, Kings College Hospital, London, UK

Tommaso Cozzolino   Department of Translational Medical Science—Section of Pediatrics, University of Naples "Federico II", Naples, Italy

Salvatore Cucchiara   Department of Pediatrics, Pediatric Gastroenterology and Liver Unit, Sapienza University of Rome, Rome, Italy

Lorenzo D'Antiga   Department of Pediatric Hepatology, Gastroenterology and Transplantation, Hospital Papa Giovanni XXIII—Bergamo, Bergamo, Italy

Jai K. Das   Division of Women and Child Health, Department of Pediatrics, Aga Khan University, Karachi, Pakistan

Georges Daube   Département des Sciences des Denrées alimentaires, Faculté de Médecine vétérinaire, Université de Liège, Liège, Belgium

Mark Davenport   Department of Pediatric Surgery, King's College Hospital, London, UK

Nicholas O. Davidson   Department of Medicine, Washington University School of Medicine, St. Louis, MO, USA

Pauline De Bruyne   Department of Pediatrics, Ghent University Hospital, Ghent, Belgium

Ruth De Bruyne   Department of Pediatric Gastroenterology, Hepatology and Nutrition, Ghent University Hospital, Ghent, Belgium

Mario De Curtis   Department of Pediatrics, Neonatology Unit, Policlinico Umberto I, Sapienza University of Rome, Rome, Italy

Annamaria Deganello   Department of Radiology, King's College Hospital, London, UK

Maesha Deheragoda   Institute of Liver Studies, King's College Hospital, London, UK

Ashish P. Desai   Department of Pediatric Surgery, King's College Hospital, London, UK

Niranga Manjuri Devanarayana   Department of Physiology, Faculty of Medicine, University of Kelaniya, Ragama, Sri Lanka

Anil Dhawan   Professor and Director, Pediatric Liver, GI and Nutrition Center, Clinical Director, Child Health, King's College Hospital, London, UK

Margherita Di Costanzo   Department of Translational Medical Science—Section of Pediatrics, University of Naples "Federico II", Naples, Italy

Angelo Di Giorgio   Department of Pediatric Hepatology, Gastroenterology and Transplantation, Hospital Papa Giovanni XXIII—Bergamo, Bergamo, Italy

Giovanni Di Nardo   Department of Pediatrics, Pediatric Gastroenterology and Liver Unit, Sapienza University of Rome, Rome, Italy

Valentina Discepolo   Department of Translational Medical Science—Section of Pediatrics, University of Naples "Federico II", Napoli, Italy

Department of Medicine, University of Chicago, Chicago, IL, USA

Christopher Duggan   Division of Gastroenterology, Hepatology and Nutrition, Boston Children's Hospital, Boston, MA, USA

Christophe Dupont   Department of Pediatric Gastroenterology and Nutrition, Necker—Enfants malades Hospital, Paris Descartes University, AP-HP, Paris, France

Evangelia Farmaki   Pediatric Immunology and Rheumatology Referral Centre, First Dept of Pediatrics, Aristotle University of Thessaloniki, Thessaloniki, Greece

Emer Fitzpatrick Professor and Director, Pediatric Liver, GI and Nutrition Center, Clinical Director, Child Health, King's College Hospital, London, UK

Antonietta Giannattasio Section of Pediatrics, Department of Translational Medical Science, University of Naples "Federico II", Naples, Italy

Francesca Paola Giugliano Section of Pediatrics, Department of Transitional Medical Science, University of Naples "Federico II", Naples, Italy

Praveen S. Goday Division of Gastroenterology, Department of Pediatrics, Medical College of Wisconsin and Children's Hospital of Wisconsin, Milwaukee, WI, USA

Olivier Goulet Department of Pediatric Gastroenterology and Nutrition, Hôpital Necker-Enfants Malades, Paris Cedex, France

Tassos Grammatikopoulos Pediatric Liver, GI and Nutrition Centre, NHS Foundation Trust, King's College Hospital, London, UK

Stefano Guandalini Department of Pediatrics, Section of Gastroenterology, Hepatology and Nutrition, Comer Children's Hospital, University of Chicago, Chicago, IL, USA

Alfredo Guarino Department of Translation Medical Science, Section of Pediatrics, University of Naples "Federico II", Naples, Italy

Section of Pediatrics, Department of Translational Medical Science, University of Naples "Federico II", Naples, Italy

Nedim Hadzic Pediatric Centre for Hepatology, Gastroenterology and Nutrition, King's College Hospital, London, UK

Nigel J. Hall Southampton Children's Hospital, University of Southampton, Southampton, UK

Anna Hames Institute of Liver Studies, King's College Hospital, London, UK

Nigel Heaton King's Health Partners, Institute of Liver Studies, Kings College Hospital FT NHS Trust, London, UK

Margot L. Herman Division of Gastroenterology, Department of Medicine, University of Washington School of Medicine, Seattle, WA, USA

Leslie M Higuchi GI Division—Inflammatory Bowel Disease Center, Children's Hospital, Boston, MA, USA

Susan Hill Department of Gastroenterology, Division of Intestinal Rehabilitation and Nutrition, Great Ormond Street Hospital for Children NHS Foundation Trust, London, UK

Iva Hojsak Referral Center for Pediatric Gastroenterology and Nutrition, Children's Hospital Zagreb, University of Zagreb School of Medicine, Zagreb, Croatia

Geert Huys Laboratory of Microbiology & BCCM/LMG Bacteria Collection, Faculty of Sciences, Ghent University, Ghent, Belgium

Warren Hyer The Polyposis Registry, St Mark's Hospital, Middx, UK

Stacy A. Kahn Section of Gastroenterology, Hepatology and Nutrition, Department of Pediatrics, University of Chicago, Comer Children's Hospital, Chicago, IL, USA

Nicolas Kalach Department of Pediatric Gastroenterology and Nutrition, Necker—Enfants malades Hospital, Paris Descartes University, AP-HP, Paris, France

Department of Pediatrics, Saint Antoine Pediatric Clinic, Saint Vincent de Paul Hospital, Groupement des Hôpitaux de l'Institut Catholique de Lille (GH-ICL), Catholic University, Lille, Nord, France

Deepa Kamat Nutrition and Dietetics Department, King's College Hospital NHS Foundation Trust, London, UK

Binita Maya Kamath Division of Gastroenterology, Hepatology and Nutrition, The Hospital for Sick Children, University of Toronto, Toronto, ON, Canada

Ino Kanavaki Department of Pediatrics, Swiss Center for Liver Disease in Children, University Hospitals Geneva, Geneva, Switzerland

Jess L. Kaplan Division of Pediatric Gastroenterology and Nutrition, MassGeneral Hospital for Children, Boston, MA, USA

Tuomo J. Karttunen Department of Pathology, Oulu University Hospital, Medical Research Center Oulu, University of Oulu, Oulu, Finland

Chayarani Kelgeri Department of Pediatric Gastroenterology, Hepatology and Nutrition, Global Hospital and Health City, Chennai, India

Professor and Director, Pediatric Liver, GI and Nutrition Center, Clinical Director, Child Health, King's College Hospital, London, UK

Barbara S. Kirschner Section of Gastroenterology, Hepatology and Nutrition, Department of Pediatrics, University of Chicago, Comer Children's Hospital, Chicago, IL, USA

Jutta Köglmeier Division of Intestinal Rehabilitation and Nutrition, Department of Gastroenterology, Great Ormond Street Hospital for Children NHS Foundation Trust, London, UK

Hugh Lemonde Department of Pediatric Inherited Metabolic Disease, Evelina London Children's Hospital, St Thomas' Hospital, London, UK

Emile Levy Research Centre, CHU Ste-Justine and Department of Nutrition, Université de Montréal, Montreal, QC, Canada

B U. K. Li Division of Gastroenterology, Hepatology and Nutrition, Medical College of Wisconsin, Milwaukee, WI, USA

Keith J. Lindley Division of Neurogastroenterology and Motility, Department of Gastroenterology, Great Ormond Street Hospital for Children NHS Foundation Trust, London, UK

Department of Pediatric Gastroenterology, Division of Neurogastroenterology and Motility, Great Ormond Street Hospital for Children NHS Foundation Trust, London, UK

Andrea Lo Vecchio Section of Pediatrics, Department of Translational Medical Science, University of Naples "Federico II", Naples, Italy

Alfredo J. Lucendo Department of Gastroenterology, Hospital General de Tomelloso, Tomelloso, Ciudad Real, Spain

Ylenia Maddalena Department of Translational Medical Science—Section of Pediatrics, University of Naples "Federico II", Naples, Italy

Monica Malamisura Department of Translational Medical Science—Section of Pediatrics, University of Naples "Federico II", Naples, Italy

Sara Mancell Nutrition and Dietetics Department, King's College Hospital NHS Foundation Trust, London, UK

Massimo Martinelli Department of Translational Medical Sciences, Section of Pediatrics, University of Naples "Federico II", Naples, Italy

Alisha Mavis   Division of Gastroenterology, Department of Pediatrics, Children's Hospital of Wisconsin, Medical College of Wisconsin, Milwaukee, WI, USA

Valérie McLin   Department of Pediatrics, Swiss Center for Liver Disease in Children, University Hospitals Geneva, Geneva, Switzerland

Erasmo Miele   Section of Pediatrics, Department of Transitional Medical Science, University of Naples "Federico II", Naples, Italy

Giorgina Mieli-Vergani   Pediatric Liver, GI and Nutrition Centre, King's College Hospital, London, UK

Marinita Morelli   Department of Translational Medical Science—Section of Pediatrics, University of Naples "Federico II", Naples, Italy

Natalia Nedelkopoulou   Pediatric Liver, GI and Nutrition Centre, King's College Hospital, London, UK

Agostino Nocerino   Department of Pediatrics, Azienda Ospedaliero-Universitaria "S. Maria della Misericordia" University of Udine, Udine, Italy

Rita Nocerino   Department of Translational Medical Science—Section of Pediatrics, University of Naples "Federico II", Naples, Italy

Lydia O'Sullivan   Department of Pediatric Surgery, King's College Hospital, London, UK

Salvatore Oliva   Department of Pediatrics, Pediatric Gastroenterology and Liver Unit, Sapienza University of Rome, Rome, Italy

Rosemary Pauley-Hunter   Department of Pediatric Gastroenterology, Boys Town National Research Hospital, Boys Town, NE, USA

Vincenza Pezzella   Department of Translational Medical Science—Section of Pediatrics, University of Naples "Federico II", Naples, Italy

Maria Giovanna Puoti   Department of Translational Medical Science—Section of Pediatrics, University of Naples "Federico II", Naples, Italy

Alberto Quaglia   Clinical Lead Liver Pathology, Institute of Liver Studies, King's College Hospital, London, UK

Paolo Quitadamo   Department of Translational Medical Science, Section of Pediatrics, University of Naples "Federico II", Naples, Italy

Shaman Rajindrajith   University Pediatric Unit, Teaching Hospital, Ragama, Sri Lanka

Department of Pediatrics, Faculty of Medicine, University of Kelaniya, Ragama, Sri Lanka

Whitney M. Rassbach   Division of Allergy and Immunology, Department of Pediatrics, The Elliot and Roslyn Jaffe Food Allergy Institute, Kravis Children's Hospital, Icahn School of Medicine at Mount Sinai, New York, NY, USA

Mettu Srinivas Reddy   Institute of Liver Disease and Transplantation, National Foundation for Liver Research, Global Health City, Chennai, India

Brian P Regan   GI Division—Inflammatory Bowel Disease Center, Children's Hospital, Boston, MA, USA

Mohamed Rela   Institute of Liver Disease and Transplantation, National Foundation for Liver Research, Global Health City, Chennai, India

Institute of Liver Studies, King's College Hospital, London, UK

Jacques Rigo CHU de Liege, CHR de la Citadelle, University of Liege, Liege, Belgium

Service Universitaire de Néonatologie, CHU de Liège, University of Liège, CHR de la Citadelle, Liège, Belgium

Nathalie Rock Department of Pediatrics, Swiss Center for Liver Disease in Children, University Hospitals Geneva, Geneva, Switzerland

Véronique Rousseau Department of Pediatric Surgery, Necker—Enfants malades Hospital, Paris Descartes University, AP-HP, Paris, France

Rehana A. Salam Division of Women and Child Health, Department of Pediatrics, Aga Khan University, Karachi, Pakistan

Efstratios Saliakellis Division of Neurogastroenterology and Motility, Department of Pediatric Gastroenterology, Great Ormond Street Hospital for Children, NHS Foundation Trust; UCL Institute of Child Health, London, UK

Marianne Samyn Pediatric Liver, GI and Nutrition Centre, King's College Hospital, London, UK

Maria E. K. Sellars Department of Radiology, King's College Hospital, London, UK

Thibault Senterre CHU de Liege, CHR de la Citadelle, University of Liege, Liege, Belgium

Department of Neonatology, CHU de Liège, Université de Liège, Liège, Belgium

Service Universitaire de Néonatologie, CHR de la Citadelle, Liège, Belgium

Timothy A. Sentongo Department of Pediatrics, Section of Gastroenterology, Hepatology and Nutrition, Comer Children's Hospital, University of Chicago, Chicago, IL, USA

Naresh P. Shanmugam Department of Pediatric Gastroenterology, Hepatology and Nutrition, Global Hospital and Health City, Chennai, India

Pediatric Liver, GI & Nutrition Center, King's College Hospital, London, UK

Department of Pediatric Hepatology, Gastroenterology and Nutrition, Global Hospitals and Health City, Chennai, India

Shailee Sheth Department of Pediatric Surgery, King's College Hospital, London, UK

Scott H. Sicherer Division of Allergy and Immunology, Department of Pediatrics, The Elliot and Roslyn Jaffe Food Allergy Institute, Kravis Children's Hospital, Icahn School of Medicine at Mount Sinai, New York, NY, USA

Piotr Socha Department of Gastroenterology, Hepatology and Nutrition Disorders, The Children's Memorial Health Institute, Warsaw, Poland

Maria Immacolata Spagnuolo Department of Translational Medical Science, Section of Pediatrics, University of Naples "Federico II", Naples, Italy

Annamaria Staiano Section of Pediatrics, Department of Transitional Medical Science, University of Naples "Federico II", Naples, Italy

Department of Translational Medical Sciences, Section of Pediatrics, University of Naples "Federico II", Naples, Italy

Bhanu Sunku Department of Pediatrics, Mount Kisco Medical Group, Mount Kisco, NY, USA

Christina M. Surawicz Division of Gastroenterology, Department of Medicine, University of Washington School of Medicine, Seattle, WA, USA

Stuart Tanner   Academic Unit of Child Health, Sheffield Children's Hospital, University of Sheffield, Sheffield, UK

Marta Tavares   Porto Children's Hospital, Porto, Portugal

Gianluca Terrin   Department of Perinatal Medicine, Neonatology Unit, Sapienza University of Rome, Rome, Italy

Department of Pediatrics, Neonatology Unit, Policlinico Umberto I, Sapienza University of Rome, Rome, Italy

Department of Gynaecology—Obstetrics and Perinatal Medicine, University of Rome "La Sapienza", Rome, Italy

Rakesh Kumar Thakur   Department of Pediatric Surgery, King's College Hospital, London, UK

Nikhil Thapar   Division of Neurogastroenterology and Motility, Department of Pediatric Gastroenterology, Great Ormond Street Hospital for Children, NHS Foundation Trust; UCL Institute of Child Health, London, UK

Richard J. Thompson   Institute of Liver Studies, King's College Hospital, London, UK

Mike Thomson   Department of Gastroenterology, Sheffield Children's Hospital, Sheffield, South Yorkshire, UK

Mark P. Tighe   Department of Pediatrics, Poole Hospital, NHS Foundation Trust, Poole, UK

Sami Turunen   Department of Pediatrics, Oulu University Hospital, Medical Research Center Oulu, University of Oulu, Oulu, Finland

Aliye Uc   Stead Family Department of Pediatrics, University of Iowa Children's Hospital, Iowa City, IA, USA

Babu Vadamalayan   Pediatric Liver, GI and Nutrition Centre, King's College Hospital, London, UK

Yvan Vandenplas   Department of Pediatrics, Universitair Ziekenhuis Brussel, Vrije Universiteit Brussel, Brussels, Belgium

Department of Pediatrics, UZ Brussel, Brussels, Belgium

Jon A. Vanderhoof   Department of Pediatrics, Boston Children's Hospital, Harvard Medical School, Boston, MA, USA

Boys Town National Research Hospital, Boys Town, NE, USA

Diego Vergani   Institute of Liver Studies, King's College Hospital, London, UK

Anita Verma   Institute of Liver Studies, King's College Hospital, NHS, Foundation Trust, London, UK

Steven L. Werlin   Division of Gastroenterology, Department of Pediatrics, Medical College of Wisconsin and Children's Hospital of Wisconsin, Milwaukee, WI, USA

Michael Wilschanski   Pediatric Gastroenterology Unit, Hadassah Hebrew University Medical Center, Jerusalem, Israel

Stefan Wirth   HELIOS Medical Centre, Department of Pediatrics, Witten/Herdecke University, Wuppertal, Germany

Sona Young   Section of Gastroenterology, Hepatology and Nutrition, Department of Pediatrics, Comer Children's Hospital, University of Chicago, Chicago, IL, USA

Elke Zani-Ruttenstock   Department of Pediatric Surgery, King's College Hospital, London, UK

Indre Zaparackaite   Department of Pediatric Surgery, Great Ormond Street Hospital, Brighton, UK

Part I

Gastroenterology and Nutrition

Microvillus Inclusion Disease and Tufting Enteropathy

Agostino Nocerino and Stefano Guandalini

Introduction

The Larger Group of "Intractable Diarrheas of Infancy"

Before focusing on microvillus inclusion disease and tufting enteropathy, we briefly review similarly presenting entities. In 1968 Avery, Villavicencio and Lilly were the first to describe a severe chronic diarrhea in 20 infants and they named it "infantile intractable diarrhea"; according to their description "(it) was prolonged and intractable despite extensive hospital therapy" [1].

This syndrome was defined on the basis of some clinic characteristics, namely: (1) diarrhea of more than 2 weeks duration, (2) age, less than 3 months, (3) three or more stool cultures negative for bacterial pathogens, (4) necessity of intravenous rehydration, and (5) prolonged and intractable diarrhea despite hospital therapy.

The death rate was very high: 9 out of the 20 babies (45 %) in Avery et al.'s record had died; it was even higher in Hyman et al.'s (70 %) record [2].

Heterogeneity and lack of specificity are evident in Avery's original report: different pathologies were grouped in it, some of which with a diagnosis were well defined even at that time. Only autoptic material was available for the first cases, and only after the introduction of total parenteral nutrition (TPN) at the beginning of the 1970s [3] it was possible to study the matter more in depth, thanks to proximal small-intestinal biopsy [4] and later on to the development of endoscopic techniques, which were safe and adequate for the infant as well. It became consequently possible to discriminate different causes for the so-called intractable diarrhea of infancy [5] but its definition superimposes on the definition of "protracted diarrhea of infancy": The latter has duration in common with it, but a failure to gain weight is enough to define the picture [6].

Many cases of "protracted diarrhea of infancy" are diet associated, as a consequence of cow milk or lactose intolerance or malnutrition. Malnutrition causes intestinal atrophy and consequently a malabsorption syndrome and diarrhea, which apparently gets better with fasting. These features have almost disappeared in the developed countries.

The main causes of "intractable diarrhea of infancy," including more severe and longer forms, can thus be summed up (see also Table 1.1):

Autoimmune Enteropathy

This rare disorder mostly occurring in young infants and children (6–18 months old), is characterized by severe diarrhea and small-intestinal mucosal atrophy resulting from immune-mediated injury. It remains a challenging diagnosis because of its clinicopathologic variability. This entity is dealt with in Chap. 2.

Small-Intestinal Enteropathy of Unknown Origin

This entity could be a variation of autoimmune enteropathy, as the increase in inflammatory cells in the lamina propria shows. It appears in less than 12-month-old infants, with a lower death rate compared to those with autoimmune enteropathy, but it can be very severe. Infants can be dependent from TPN [5].

A. Nocerino (✉)
Department of Pediatrics, Azienda Ospedaliero-Universitaria "S. Maria della Misericordia" University of Udine, P.le S. Maria della Misercordia 15, Udine 33100, Italy
e-mail: agostino.nocerino@uniud.it

S. Guandalini
Department of Pediatrics, Section of Gastroenterology, Hepatology and Nutrition, Comer Children's Hospital, University of Chicago, Chicago, 60637, IL, USA
e-mail: sguandalini@peds.bsd.uchicago.edu

© Springer International Publishing Switzerland 2016
S. Guandalini et al. (eds.), *Textbook of Pediatric Gastroenterology, Hepatology and Nutrition*,
DOI 10.1007/978-3-319-17169-2_1

Table 1.1 Main causes of protracted diarrhea in infancy

Small-intestinal enteropathy of unknown origin
Intractable ulcerating enterocolitis of infancy
Congenital enterocyte heparan sulfate deficiency
Congenital intestinal integrin deficiency
Congenital secretory diarrheas
Congenital chloridorrhea
Congenital Na-losing diarrhea
Autoimmune enteropathy
Diseases of the intestinal epithelium
Microvillus inclusion disease
Tufting enteropathy

Intractable Ulcerating Enterocolitis of Infancy

A rare disease initially described in 1991 in five children presenting in the first year of life with intractable diarrhea, ulcerating stomatitis, and large ulcers with overhanging edges throughout the colon within the first year of life [7]. The affected infants can show such a severe colitis that a subtotal colectomy is necessary, even if long-term prognosis is good. It has been suggested that the affected children have a genetically determined primary immune dysregulation [8].

Congenital Enterocyte Heparan Sulfate Deficiency

Described in 1995 in three infants who, within the first weeks of life, presented secretory diarrhea and massive enteric protein loss [9]. The small-intestinal mucosa is normal on light microscopy, but histochemical examinations show a complete absence of enterocyte heparan sulfate. The sulfated glycosaminoglycans of the basocellular membrane are mostly deficient, particularly heparan sulfate, while distribution of vascular and lamina propria glycosaminoglycans is normal [9]. Diarrhea is so severe to make TPN necessary, associated to repeated albumin infusions because of severe protein-losing enteropathy. Studies in men and mice show that heparan sulfate is essential in maintaining intestinal epithelial barrier function [10], and that the specific loss of heparan sulfate proteoglycans from the basolateral surface of intestinal epithelial cells is common to many forms of protein-losing enteropathy [11].

Congenital Intestinal Integrin Deficiency

In 1999, Lachaux et al. described an intractable diarrhea starting from 9 days after birth, associated to pyloric atresia and total epithelial detachment of gastric and intestinal mucosa. Immunofluorescence analysis showed α6β4 integrin deficiency at the intestinal epithelium—lamina propria junction [12].

Mutations in α6 or β4 integrins cause junctional epidermolysis bullosa with pyloric atresia. In 2008, two Kuwaitian brothers with pyloric atresia were described, respectively affected by intractable diarrhea and episodes of protein-losing enteropathy, with a novel mutation in β4 integrin not associated to its reduced expression in tissues [13].

Congenital Secretory Diarrheas

Includes congenital chloridorrhea and congenital sodium diarrhea, dealt with in Chap. 36.

Diseases of the Intestinal Epithelium

Microvillus inclusion disease and tuft enteropathy are the best-known diseases of the intestinal epithelium causing intractable diarrhea of infancy.

In 1994, Girault et al. described eight infants with early-onset severe watery diarrhea associated to facial deformities and unusual tufts of woolly hair with trichorrhexis nodosa. Duodenal biopsies showed moderate to severe villous atrophy, with normal or hypoplastic crypts; colon biopsies were grossly normal. As a consequence, severe malabsorption was present. All patients had no antibody response to immunization antigens; the immunological response to vaccinations was poor. Five children died despite TPN [14]. Two children from the series of Girault et al. had hepatic cirrhosis; six additional patients had signs and symptoms compatible with this new "syndromic diarrhea", associated to hepatic involvement (Tricho-Hepato-Enteric Syndrome, THES) characterized by fibrotic livers with marked hemosiderosis [15–17].

Nine different mutations in *TTC37* gene (5q14.3–5q21.2) were found in 12 children from 11 families with classical features of THES. *TTC37* codes for a protein that has been named thespin (THES ProteIN) [18].

Enlarged platelets with abnormal α-granule secretion can be observed in some patients. The estimated incidence of the syndrome is 1 in 400,000 to 1 in 500,000 live births.

Microvillus Inclusion Disease

In 1978, Davidson et al. described five infants presenting an intractable diarrhea of infancy characterized by secretive diarrhea and malabsorption, starting in the first hours after birth with hypoplastic villous atrophy in the small-intestinal biopsy. Four of these infants had a deceased brother who had presented similar features.

In one of these infants, the electron microscopy identified the presence of a peculiar abnormality of the microvilli of the enterocytes [19] (Fig. 1.1).

Three new cases with the same clinic and histological characteristics of the latter were described in France in 1982,

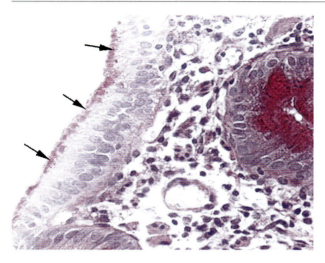

Fig. 1.1 Microvillous in the original label inclusion disease. PAS staining highlights abundant PAS-positive material *(arrows)* in the apical part of the enterocyte cytoplasm. PAS × 260. *PAS* peroidic acid-Schiff (Reprinted from Ref. [20], Fig. 1, with kind permission from Springer Science and Business Media)

and the four of them were grouped in a new disease called congenital microvillus atrophy [21, 22]. Two new cases were described in Great Britain in 1985 [23] and one in Italy in 1986; a subsequently born brother of the latter resulted affected too [24]. A survey completed in 1987 among centers known for their involvement in pediatric gastroenterology identified more than 30 cases worldwide. Additional cases were later published.

In 1989, Cutz et al. proposed the use of the term "microvillus inclusion disease" to highlight the characteristic ultrastructural lesions of the disease [25].

Clinical presentation: case report

First child of parents with no blood relation, A.G. was born after 37 weeks of gestation, the pregnancy having been complicated by a risk of miscarriage in the 5th month. His weight was 3500 g.

The infant was hospitalized when he was 40 days old because of an abundant diarrhea (15–20 evacuations a day of liquid stools), starting on the 6th day of its life and resistant to numerous dietary and pharmacological therapies.

Entering the hospital, the patient weighed 2800 g, it was in severe general conditions with dystrophia and dehydration; a TPN was therefore immediately started. The acid–basic balance showed hyponatremic acidosis (pH 7.2; EB −8,3; Na 128 mEq/l). The secretive nature of diarrhea was confirmed by its entity (about 100 ml/kg/die) with a total absence of oral nutrition and with the persistence of TPN in progress.

Moreover, the typical absence of ionic gap in the stools was present: osmolality 226 mOsm/l, Na 86 mEq/l, K 23.5 mEq/l (gap 7 mOsm/l).

Loperamide and chlorpromazine increased intestinal absorption, but did not change the clinical picture.

Microbiological examinations included an electronic microscope examination of the feces for the identification of viruses and the search for enterotoxigenic bacteria and parasites with specific methods were repeatedly negative.

The abdominal ultrasound showed adrenal hyperplasia associated to hyperaldosteronism (1160 ng/ml, v.n. <125 ng/ml).

Jejunal biopsy showed a picture of villus atrophy with no hyperplastic crypts and periodic acid-Schiff (PAS)-positive material stored in the apical cytoplasm of enterocytes. Electron microscopy was diagnostic for microvillus inclusion disease.

Microvillus Inclusion Disease is a Congenital Secretory Diarrhea Starting in Neonatal Age

Severe diarrhea typically appears in the first days of life, usually within the first 72 h, and it is immediately life threatening. The stools are watery, and the stool output is 100–500 ml/kg/day when the infant is fed, a volume comparable to or higher than that observed in cholera. The diarrhea is of secretory type; therefore, it persists at a stable rate of 50–300 ml/kg/day despite fasting, and the electrolyte content of the stools is increased, without an osmotic gap. However, the mucosal atrophy causes osmotic diarrhea. For this reason, feeding increases the fecal output and oral feeding in nutritionally significant amounts is impossible. Due to the high output, patients can lose up to 30 % of their body weight within 24 h, resulting in profound metabolic acidosis and severe dehydration, unless vigorous intravenous rehydration is started.

In a small percentage of cases (which was in the past considered to be around 20 %, and presently around 5 % of the cases [26]), diarrhea starts later in life, between 1 and 3 months, usually at 6–8 weeks of age. This less severe form has been denominated late-onset microvillus inclusion disease, while the classical form beginning at neonatal age has been denominated early-onset microvillus inclusion disease[27].

The hallmark of the disease is the electron microscopic finding of disrupted enterocytic microvilli (i.e., digitations of the apical membrane of the intestinal epithelial cell protruding into the lumen) and the appearance of characteristic inclusion vacuoles, whose inner surfaces are lined by typical microvilli. Both lesions are seen only with the electronic microscopy.

A few cases have been termed atypical microvillus inclusion disease, in which the onset can be early or late, but the histologic picture is different, particularly for the absence of detectable microvillus inclusions [28].

Therefore, three variants of the disease have been identified: early-onset microvillus inclusion disease, late-onset microvillus inclusion disease, and atypical microvillus inclusion disease. However, because of the sparse distribution of microvillus inclusions, it is not certain that their absence could be limited to the sample.

Microvillus inclusion disease is usually characterized by growth retardation and some developmental delay later in infancy. No other specific findings can be detected. However, the disease can be associated with other abnormalities, indicated in Table 1.2.

Histologic Findings

Findings from duodenal biopsy must not be considered diagnostic. Histologic results of duodenal biopsy samples can range from essentially normal to mildly abnormal, showing the following:
- Thin mucosa caused by hypoplastic villus atrophy
- Diffuse villus atrophy (loss of villus height)
- Crypt hypoplasia

PAS staining of the intestinal biopsy sample does not show the usual linear staining along the brush border, but reveals PAS-positive material in the apical cytoplasm. The PAS staining material corresponds to the increased number of electron dense secretory granules in the epithelium. The abnormal pattern of staining appears in the upper crypt region and continues over the villus [29] (Fig. 1.2).

PAS accumulates in low crypts in atypical microvillus atrophy, in upper crypts in congenital microvillus atrophy, and in low villi in late-onset microvillus atrophy.

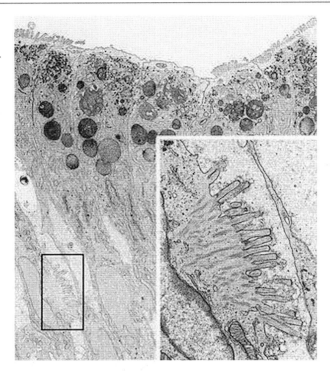

Fig. 1.2 Microvillous in the original label inclusion disease. Villous enterocytes: the *boxed area* shows microvilli on the lateral membrane. *Inset*: Enlargement of the *boxed* area × 6200, *inset* × 22,500. (Reprinted from [20, Fig. 5], with kind permission from Springer Science and Business Media)

Similar results were obtained with anti-CD10 immunohistochemistry: In affected children, the normal linear staining in surface enterocytes is absent, while prominent cytoplasmic reactivity is seen [30]. CD10 is a neutral membrane-associated peptidase; thus, abnormal stain findings with PAS or anti-CD10 immunohistochemistry are expressions of the abnormalities in microvillar structure.

Rectal biopsy findings demonstrate microvillus involutions and an increased number of secretory granules. This test has been proposed as a relatively easy method for making an early diagnosis. Anti-CD10 immunohistochemistry can aid in the diagnosis, because abnormal cytoplasmic CD10 staining of absorptive colonocytes has been observed in microvillus inclusion disease [31].

The diagnosis rests on findings demonstrated by electron microscopy (see Figs. 1.3 and 1.4.). Electron microscopy shows well-preserved crypt epithelium with abundant microvilli. Villus enterocytes are severely abnormal, particularly toward the apices of the short villi. The microvilli are depleted in number, short, and irregularly arranged. Some of the enterocytes contain the typical microvillus involutions, which are intracellular vacuoles where microvilli are observed lining the inner surface. A striking feature is a number of small, membrane-bound vesicles containing electron-dense material (see Figs. 1.3 and 1.4). A few cases have been

Table 1.2 Anomalies described in association to microvillus inclusion disease

Meckel diverticula	Abdominal adhesions
Inguinal hernias	Renal dysplasia
Absent corpus callosum	Hydronephrosis
Mesenteric duct remnants	Craniosynostosis
Abnormal vertebrae	Down syndrome
Aganglionic megacolon	Hematuria
Pneumocystis jiroveci pneumonia	Dihydropyrimidinase deficiency
Autosomal dominant hypochondroplasia	Microcephaly
Renal Fanconi syndrome	Other renal problems
Hypophosphatemic rickets	Diabetes
Cardiac problems	Pulmonary problems
Liver dysfunction	Multiple hepatic adenomas

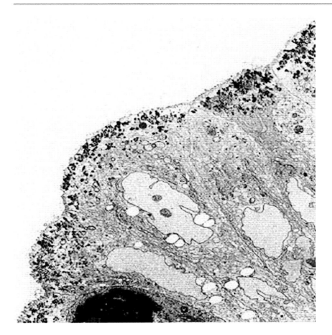

Fig. 1.3 Microvillous in the original label inclusion disease. The apical cytoplasm of villous epithelium shows an increased number of secretory granules associated with microvillus alterations × 2400. (Reprinted from [20, Fig. 4], with kind permission from Springer Science and Business Media)

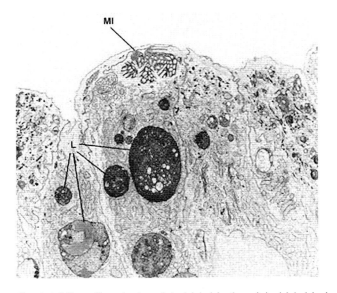

Fig. 1.4 Microvillous in the original label in the original label inclusion disease. The villous enterocytes lack brush-border microvilli, whereas their apical cytoplasm contains a microvillus inclusion *(MI)* and numerous lysosomes *(L)* × 5.500. (Reprinted from [20, Fig. 2], with kind permission from Springer Science and Business Media)

described in which the classic microvillus inclusions are shadowed by other features, such as large aggregates of electron lucent, vermiform membranous vesicles in enterocyte cytoplasm, corresponding to the PAS-positive material [32].

Epidemiology

The cases published or gathered in an online registry were 137 in 2014 [26].

A female preponderance had been observed among the published cases, with a female-to-male ratio of 2:1, but in the total 137 cases there is a 1.54 male to female ratio. A blood relation is present in 41 % of the assessable cases with a genre preference for males. A cluster of cases from the Navajo reservation in northern Arizona suggests an incidence as high as 1 case per 12,000 live births.

Pathophysiology

Due to their alterations, mature enterocytes inefficiently absorb ions and nutrients, causing a malabsorption syndrome; however, the diarrhea is caused mainly by active secretion of water and electrolytes in the intestinal lumen (secretory diarrhea). The pathogenesis of the secretory diarrhea is unknown; it is assumed to result from an imbalance between decreased absorption and unaltered secretion.

Measurement of stool electrolytes and osmolality enables rapid and accurate assessment of the pathogenesis of this chronic diarrhea (osmolar versus secretory) and greatly narrows the differential diagnosis.

Fecal electrolytes demonstrate a typical pattern of secretory diarrhea. Fecal sodium levels are high (approximately 60–120 mEq/l), and no osmotic gap is found. In patients with secretory diarrhea, the following formula applies: 2(Na concentration + K concentration) = stool osmolarity ± 50. In osmotic diarrhea, stool osmolarity exceeds 2(Na concentration + K concentration) by 100 or more.

Secretory diarrhea occurs in the fasting state and is associated with large output losses that cause dehydration and metabolic acidosis.

In osmotic diarrhea, findings on stool microscopy are negative for white blood cells (WBCs), blood (exudative diarrhea), and fat (steatorrhea).

Even if there are data about the anomalies in water and electrolytes transportation in the small intestine, it is not known whether and how the colon mucosa participates to the absorption alterations in the disease.

In one of the Italian cases, we used the technique of rectal perfusion that showed a decrease in sodium absorption, only partially corrected by chlorpromazine administration [33].

Pathogenesis

Severe perturbation of the microvillar cytoskeleton may disrupt the transport of brush border components that have to be assembled at the apical membrane. The postulated abnormality in the cytoskeleton causes a block in exocytosis, mainly of PAS-positive material (e.g., polysaccharides, glycoproteins, glycolipids, neutral mucopolysaccharides). As a consequence, small secretory granules that contain a PAS-positive material accumulate in the apical cytoplasm of epithelial cells.

In 2008, the presence of mutations in the *MYO5B* gene was described in seven patients (out of ten tested), predominantly of Turkish origin [34]. Homozygous mutations in the same gene were subsequently found in seven cases of Navajo origin; five parents were heterozygote [35]. A total of 41 unique *MYO5B* mutations in 40 patients have been identified so far: in more detail 16 different homozygous mutations in 25 patients, and 25 heterozygous mutations in 15 patients [26].

The *MYO5B* gene codifies myosine Vb, an actin-based motor protein which carries the recycling endosomes to the apical plasma membrane along the actin filaments of the microtubules. The functional deficiency of this protein alters the intracellular trafficking of resident apical plasma membrane proteins to the cell surface, and this could be the cause for the impaired apical brush border membrane development [34]. Actually, in microvillus inclusion disease the *MYO5B* mutations associate to a defective myosin Vb expression in enterocytes.

Myosine Vb carries on its action after having bound to a specific small guanosine-5'-triphosphatase (GTPase) rab proteins, such as Rab 11, located on the surface of recycling endosomes [36]. Thanks to this link the recycling endosomes move along the actine filaments (see Fig. 1.5) [37].

When myosine Vb has an altered function, the recycling endosomes are not carried in a normal way: in the enterocytes of the subjects with microvillus inclusion disease, no regular accumulation of myosine Vb and of the recycling endosome-associated proteins (one of these is Rab 11) can be observed close to the apical membrane, and no specific staining pattern is present [38]. Therefore, the Rab 11 distribution in the enterocytes can be a helpful diagnostic tool [39].

Other biochemical mechanisms depending on myosine Vb which can produce alterations in the structure of the microvilli are presently being studied [40].

Myosine Vb is expressed in all the epithelial tissues and, actually, microvillus inclusions in the stomach and colon, in addition to less well-defined inclusions in gallbladder epithelium and in renal tubular epithelial cells, have been reported in some patients with microvillous inclusion disease (MVID). Nevertheless, no extraintestinal symptoms are generally reported. Two children with renal Fanconi syndrome who carried mutation *MYO5B* did not show alterations in the apical brush border morphology and the PAS staining pattern in renal tubular epithelial cells, which makes it unlikely for it to be the cause of proximal tubular renal dysfunction [41].

Recently, Dutch investigators have found [42] that the mild variant of MVID appears to be caused by loss of function of syntaxin 3 (STX3), an apical receptor involved in membrane fusion of apical vesicles in enterocytes. In fact, whole-exome sequencing of DNA from patients with variant MVID revealed homozygous truncating mutations in STX3; and in addition, patient-derived organoid cultures and overexpression of truncated STX3 in CaCo2 cells recapitulated most characteristics of variant MVID.

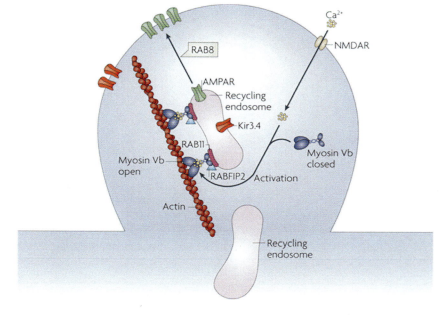

Fig. 1.5 Endocytic recycling. Myosin Vb is a conformation-dependent binding partner of Rab11-FIP2. Activation of myosin Vb induces translocation of recycling endosomes and their cargo. Final transport from the recycling endosome to the cell surface is mediated by Rab8. (Reprinted by permission from Macmillan Publishers Ltd and Nature Publishing Group [37])

Prenatal Diagnosis

Pregnancy and birth are usually normal in individuals with microvillus atrophy, and polyhydramnios is usually absent, in contrast to the clinical picture of patients with other causes of congenital secretory diarrhea [43]. Nevertheless, in some cases, polyhydramnios and bowel dilation in the third trimester have been described [44]. In one case, a high fetal alpha-fetoprotein in the second trimester was observed [45]. Authors have speculated that the fetal alpha-fetoprotein elevation might possibly be caused by in utero body fluid leakage into the amniotic fluid through fetal enteropathy.

Identification of the gene responsible for the disease allows its prenatal diagnosis [46].

Treatment

The prognosis of early-onset microvillus inclusion disease is poor. If patients are untreated, the disease is rapidly fatal because of dehydration and malnutrition.

In late-onset microvillus inclusion disease diarrhea tends to be less severe, and some alimentation is possible.

Medical Care

Agents tentatively given to induce a better growth of the intestinal mucosa (e.g., epithelial growth factor, colostrum) are ineffective. Several drugs (e.g., somatostatin, octreotide, loperamide, chlorpromazine) have been tried to counteract the massive secretory diarrhea in patients with microvillus atrophy; however, none has proven effective.

At present, the only available therapy is TPN. Children with late-onset microvillus inclusion disease usually have less severe diarrhea; with age they can reduce the requirements of TPN to 1–2 per week.

If patients are treated with TPN, their prognosis entirely depends on the complications of this approach. These complications include cholestasis with subsequent liver damage leading to cirrhosis, catheter-related sepsis due to infection with bacterial or fungal agents, and progressive lack of vascular access.

In the observed cases, cholestasis appears worsened by transplant.

The study of eight patients who developed cholestatic liver disease suggests that cholestasis is enhanced by the impairment of the *MYO5B/RAB11A* apical recycling endosome pathway in hepatocytes [47].

Surgical Care

Successful outcomes of small-intestinal transplantation have been reported, and evidence suggests that an early transplant might be beneficial. The limited experience accumulated in a few centers worldwide reflects an overall survival rate of approximately 50% at 5 years after small-bowel transplantation; this is a much better outcome than is seen with other indications for intestinal transplantation [48]. Patients who did not receive colonic transplant weaned later from parenteral nutrition.

The analysis of 16 patients who underwent a small-bowel transplantation shows a lower death rate compared to those who did not (23 versus 37%) after an average observation period of 3.5 years (but variable between 3 months and 14 years). In all of the cases, apart from the first two, colon had been transplanted too [49].

Although only small series have been reported, evidence suggests that early small-bowel transplantation should be performed, at least in children with early-onset microvillus inclusion disease. Patients with late-onset microvillus atrophy appear to have an improved prognosis.

Transplantation appears to be the only option for patients who do not fare well with long-term TPN (e.g., because of sepsis, liver damage, lack of vascular access). For patients in whom transplantation is successful, a gradual return to a normal diet is considered possible.

In the observed cases, TPN-related cholestasis appears worsened by transplant. Therefore, in children with cholestasis, the worsening of this picture after the transplant points to a combined liver-intestinal transplantation.

Tufting Enteropathy (or Intestinal Epithelial Dysplasia)

In 1994, Reifen et al. described two infants less than a month old with protracted diarrhea. The diarrhea was so profuse to make TPN necessary but it improved when enteral nutrition was interrupted. The jejunal biopsies showed a peculiar picture characterized by the presence of focal aggregations of packed enterocytes whose shape resembled of a teardrop, as a consequence of an apical rounding of the plasma membrane. These focal areas resembled a tuft and that is why the term "tufting enteropathy" was coined [50]. Curiously, a case with the same characteristics was identified among those presented by Davidson et al. in the same paper where the first case of microvillus inclusion disease had been described [19].

Clinical Expression

The incidence of the disease has been estimated to be 1:100,000 live births in Western Europe [51], but it seems higher in people of Arabic origin [52].

The picture is a severe secretory diarrhea starting in the first weeks of life. During pregnancy, there is no polyhydramnios, as in the microvillus inclusion disease and differently from congenital sodium diarrhea and congenital chloridorrhea.

The alterations in the enterocytes, in any case, cause an accentuation of the diarrhea with nutrition, including total enteral nutrition, as it had already been observed since the first described cases.

There are two different clinical forms: one is isolated and the other is syndromic, associated to different anomalies, particularly to facial dysmorphism with choanal atresia and superficial punctuated keratitis [53, 54].

Pathophysiology

In 2008, a mutation of the gene for *Epithelial Cell Adhesion Molecule* (EpCAM) was identified in two ill children in the same family, and in three children from unrelated kindreds [55]. EpCAM is a transmembrane protein involved in cell proliferation, differentiation, and adhesion.

In 2010, a mutation in *SPINT2* gene was found in a case affected by a syndromic form of tufted enteropathy. *SPINT2* is a transmembrane protein that seems to be involved in epithelial regeneration [56].

It is interesting to note how mutations in *SPINT2* gene are also present in the syndromic congenital sodium diarrhea, where choanal atresia, hypertelorism, and corneal erosions are particularly frequent and anal atresia can be found in certain cases [57].

Analyzing 57 patients, mutations in the gene for EpCAM were found in 73 % of the cases, all of them presenting an isolated intestinal disease.

But in 21 % of the cases, all showing a syndromic form of the disease, there are mutations the *SPINT2* gene.

According to this study, tufting enteropathy could be separated into at least three genetic classes, each with specific phenotypes [58].

However, it seems impossible at present to discriminate "tufting enteropathy" isolated from the syndromic one, even from a genetic point of view.

Histologic Features

Jejunal biopsy shows a picture of partial villous atrophy associated to crypt hyperplasia. The most characteristic feature, the one which gave the name to the disease, is the presence of "tufts," small focal aggregates of teardrop-shaped enterocytes with an apical rounding (See Fig. 1.6a, b).

The "tufts" are not a characteristic exclusive to intestinal epithelial dysplasia, because they have been observed in other mucosal enteropathies and in normal jejunum. In the latter cases, anyway they were present in <10 % of the epithelial surface, while in "tufting enteropathy" they are present in more than 80 % of the jejunal surface. But the picture is not always so evident in the earliest period of the disease. Attempts at immunohistochemical analysis (including beta-catenin, E-cadherin, desmoglein, laminins) have not been easily applicable [60]. On the contrary, the staining with EpCAM/MOC31 antibody, an EpCAM antibody clone, showed a sensitivity and specificity of 100 % for loss of staining in 15 studied patients [61].

Electronic microscopy shows relatively normal microvilli, and it is not particularly useful for diagnosis, if only to exclude a microvillus inclusion disease.

A mild inflammation of the lamina propria is also present. An infiltration of T lymphocytes within the lamina propria had been observed since the original description, even if inferior to celiac disease, but it sometimes arises suspicion of autoimmune enteropathy [50].

Fig. 1.6 **a** Numerous tufts of enterocytes on the mucosal surface of the duodenum. **b** A characteristic tear-drop-shaped structure *(arrow)* in an epithelial tuft (H&E stain; original magnification: a–x 80; b–x 400). (Reprinted from Ref. [59, Fig. 1], with kind permission from Springer Science and Business Media)

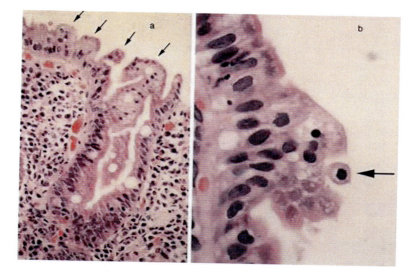

Treatment

Tuft enteropathy is associated to a severe secretory diarrhea, which worsens with nutrition. That is why affected children have to be treated with TPN.

Some cases seem to have a less severe course and they can be given a partial parenteral nutrition [62].

Cases totally dependent on TPN are candidates for intestinal transplantation.

References

1. Avery GB, Villavicencio O, Lilly JR, Randolph JG. Intractable diarrhea in early infancy. Pediatrics 1968;41:712–22
2. Hyman CJ, Reiter J, Rodnan J, Drash AL. Parenteral and oral alimentation in the treatment of the nonspecific protracted diarrheal syndrome of infancy. J Pediatr. 1971;78:17–29.
3. Shwachman H, Filler RM, Khaw KT. A new method of treating malnourished infants with severe chronic diarrhea. Acta Pediatr Scand. 1970;59:446–7.
4. Shwachman H, Lloyd-Still JD, Khaw KT, Antonowicz I. Protracted diarrhea of infancy treated by intravenous alimentation. II: studies of small intestinal biopsy results. Am J Dis Child. 1973;125:365–8.
5. Walker-Smith J A. Intractable diarrhea of infancy. Saudi J Gastroenterol. 1995;1:152–6.
6. Larcher VF, Shepherd R, Francis DE, Harries JT. Protracted diarrhoea in infancy. Analysis of 82 cases with particular reference to diagnosis and management. Arch Dis Child. 1977;52:597–605.
7. Sanderson IR, Risdon RA, Walker-Smith JA. Intractable ulcerating enterocolitis of infancy. Arch Dis Child. 1991;66:295–9.
8. Thapar N, Shah N, Ramsay AD, Lindley KJ, Milla PJ. Long-term outcome of intractable ulcerating enterocolitis of infancy. J Pediatr Gastroenterol Nutr. 2005;40:582–8.
9. Murch SH, Winyard PJ, Koletzko S, Wehner B, Cheema HA, Risdon RA, et al. Congenital enterocyte heparan sulphate deficiency with massive albumin loss, secretory diarrhoea, and malnutrition. Lancet 1996;347:1299–301.
10. Bode L, Salvestrini C, Park PW, Li JP, Esko JD, Yamaguchi Y, et al. Heparan sulfate and syndecan-1 are essential in maintaining murine and human intestinal epithelial barrier function. J Clin Invest. 2008;118:229–38.
11. Bode L, Freeze HH. Applied glycoproteomics–approaches to study genetic-environmental collisions causing protein-losing enteropathy. Biochim Biophys Acta. 2006;1760:547–59.
12. Lachaux A, Bouvier R, Loras-Duclaux I, Chappuis JP, Meneguzzi G, Ortonne JP. Isolated deficient alpha6beta4 integrin expression in the gut associated with intractable diarrhea. J Pediatr Gastroenterol Nutr. 1999;29:395–401.
13. Salvestrini C, McGrath JA, Ozoemena L, Husain K, Buhamrah E, Sabery N, et al. Desquamative enteropathy and pyloric atresia without skin disease caused by a novel intracellular beta4 integrin mutation. J Pediatr Gastroenterol Nutr. 2008;47:585–91.
14. Girault D, Goulet O, Le Deist F, Brousse N, Colomb V, Césarini JP, et al. Intractable infant diarrhea associated with phenotypic abnormalities and immunodeficiency. J Pediatr. 1994;125:36–42.
15. Stankler L, Lloyd D, Pollitt RJ, Gray ES, Thom H, Russell G. Unexplained diarrhoea and failure to thrive in two siblings with unusual facies and abnormal scalp hair shafts: a new syndrome. Arch Dis Child. 1982;57:212–6.
16. Verloes A, Lombet J, Lambert Y, Hubert AF, Deprez M, Fridman V, et al. Tricho-hepato-enteric syndrome: further delineation of a distinct syndrome with neonatal hemochromatosis phenotype, intractable diarrhea, and hair anomalies. Am J Med Genet. 1997;68:391–5.
17. Fabre A, André N, Breton A, Broué P, Badens C, Roquelaure B. Intractable diarrhea with "phenotypic anomalies" and tricho-hepato-enteric syndrome: two names for the same disorder. Am J Med Genet A. 2007;143A:584–8
18. Hartley JL, Zachos NC, Dawood B, Donowitz M, Forman J, Pollitt RJ, et al. Mutations in TTC37 cause trichohepatoenteric syndrome (phenotypic diarrhea of infancy). Gastroenterology 2010;138:2388–98,.e1–2.
19. Davidson GP, Cutz E, Hamilton JR, Gall DG. Familial enteropathy: a syndrome of protracted diarrhea from birth, failure to thrive, and hypoplastic villus atrophy. Gastroenterology 1978;75:783–90.
20. Morroni M, Cangiotti AM, Guarino A, Cinti S. Unusual ultrastructural features in microvillous inclusion disease: a report of two cases. Virchows Arch. 2006;448:805–10.
21. Schmitz J, Ginies JL, Arnaud-Battandier F, et al. Congenital microvillous atrophy, a rare cause of neonatal intractable diarrhoea. Pediatr Res. 1982;16:1014.
22. Goutet JM, Boccon-Gibod L, Chatelet F, Ploussard JP, Navarro J, Polonovski CI. Familial protracted diarrhoea with hypoplastic villous atrophy: report of two cases. Pediatr Res. 1982;16:1045.
23. Phillips AD, Jenkins P, Raafat F, Walker-Smith JA. Congenital microvillous atrophy: specific diagnostic features. Arch Dis Child. 1985;60:135–40.
24. Guarino A, Nocerino A, Cinti S, Berni Canani R, Terracciano L, Raimondi F, Guandalini S. Atrofia congenita dei microvilli intestinali. Riv Ital Ped. 1992;18:150–3.
25. Cutz E, Rhoads JM, Drumm B, Sherman PM, Durie PR, Forstner GG. Microvillus inclusion disease: an inherited defect of brush-border assembly and differentiation. N Engl J Med. 1989;320:646–51.
26. van der Velde KJ, Dhekne HS, Swertz MA, Sirigu S, Ropars V, Vinke PC, et al. An overview and online registry of microvillus inclusion disease patients and their MYO5B mutations. Hum Mutat. 2013;34:1597–605.
27. Phillips AD, Schmitz J. Familial microvillous atrophy: a clinicopathological survey of 23 cases. J Pediatr Gastroenterol Nutr. 1992;14:380–96.
28. Mierau GW, Wills EJ, Wyatt-Ashmead J, Hoffenberg EJ, Cutz E. Microvillous inclusion disease: report of a case with atypical features. Ultrastruct Pathol. 2001;25:517–21.
29. Phillips AD, Szafranski M, Man LY, Wall WJ. Periodic acid-Schiff staining abnormality in microvillous atrophy: photometric and ultrastructural studies. J Pediatr Gastroenterol Nutr. 2000;30:34–42.
30. Groisman GM, Amar M, Livne E. CD10: a valuable tool for the light microscopic diagnosis of microvillous inclusion disease (familial microvillous atrophy). Am J Surg Pathol. 2002;26:902–7.
31. Koepsell SA, Talmon G. Light microscopic diagnosis of microvillus inclusion disease on colorectal specimens using CD10. Am J Surg Pathol. 2010;34:970–2.
32. Weeks DA, Zuppan CW, Malott RL, Mierau GW. Microvillous inclusion disease with abundant vermiform, electron-lucent vesicles. Ultrastruct Pathol. 2003;27:337–40.
33. Guandalini S, Nocerino A, Saitta F, Fasano A, Ascione G, De Curtis M, et al. Valutazione dell'assorbimento di elettroliti ed acqua nel colon di un lattante affetto da atrofia congenita dei microvilli. Riv Ital Pediatr. 1987;13:76
34. Müller T, Hess MW, Schiefermeier N, Pfaller K, Ebner HL, Heinz-Erian P, et al. MYO5B mutations cause microvillus inclusion disease and disrupt epithelial cell polarity. Nat Genet. 2008;40:1163–5.
35. Erickson RP, Larson-Thomé K, Valenzuela RK, Whitaker SE, Shub MD. Navajo microvillous inclusion disease is due to a mutation in MYO5B. Am J Med Genet A. 2008;146A:3117–9.

36. Schafer JC, Baetz NW, Lapierre LA, McRae RE, Roland JT, Goldenring JR. Rab11-FIP2 interaction with *MYO5B* regulates movement of *Rab11a*-containing recycling vesicles. Traffic 2014;15:292–308.

37. Grant BD, Donaldson JG. Pathways and mechanisms of endocytic recycling. Nat Rev Mol Cell Biol. 2009;10:597–608.

38. Szperl AM, Golachowska MR, Bruinenberg M, Prekeris R, Thunnissen AM, Karrenbeld A, et al. Functional characterization of mutations in the myosin Vb gene associated with microvillus inclusion disease. J Pediatr Gastroenterol Nutr. 2011;52:307–13.

39. Talmon G, Holzapfel M, DiMaio DJ, Muirhead D. Rab11 is a useful tool for the diagnosis of microvillous inclusion disease. Int J Surg Pathol. 2012;20:252–6.

40. Dhekne HS, Hsiao NH, Roelofs P, Kumari M, Slim CL, Rings EH, van Ijzendoorn SC. Myosin Vb and *Rab11a* regulate phosphorylation of ezrin in enterocytes. J Cell Sci. 2014; 127(Pt 5):1007–17.

41. Golachowska MR, van Dael CM, Keuning H, Karrenbeld A, Hoekstra D, Gijsbers CF, et al. MYO5B mutations in patients with microvillus inclusion disease presenting with transient renal Fanconi syndrome. J Pediatr Gastroenterol Nutr. 2012;54:491–8.

42. Wiegerinck CL, Janecke AR, Schneeberger K, Vogel GF, van Haaften-Visser DY, Escher JC, et al. Loss of syntaxin 3 causes variant microvillus inclusion disease. Gastroenterology 2014;147:65–8.

43. Ruemmele FM, Schmitz J, Goulet O. Microvillous inclusion disease (microvillous atrophy). Orphanet J Rare Dis. 2006;1:22 (Review).

44. Kennea N, Norbury R, Anderson G, Tekay A. Congenital microvillous inclusion disease presenting as antenatal bowel obstruction. Ultrasound Obstet Gynecol. 2001;17:172–4.

45. Chen CP, Su YN, Chern SR, Wu PC, Wang W. Prenatal diagnosis of microvillus inclusion disease. Taiwan J Obstet Gynecol. 2011;50:399–400.

46. Chen CP, Chiang MC, Wang TH, Hsueh C, Chang SD, Tsai FJ, et al. Microvillus inclusion disease: prenatal ultrasound findings, molecular diagnosis and genetic counseling of congenital diarrhea. Taiwan J Obstet Gynecol. 2010;49:487–94.

47. Girard M, Lacaille F, Verkarre V, Mategot R, Feldmann G, Grodet A, et al. MYO5B and BSEP contribute to cholestatic liver disorder in microvillous inclusion disease. Hepatology 2013;60:301–16.

48. Ruemmele FM, Jan D, Lacaille F, Cézard JP, Canioni D, Phillips AD, et al. New perspectives for children with microvillous inclusion disease: early small bowel transplantation. Transplantation 2004;77:1024–8.

49. Halac U, Lacaille F, Joly F, Hugot JP, Talbotec C, Colomb V, et al. Microvillous inclusion disease: how to improve the prognosis of a severe congenital enterocyte disorder. J Pediatr Gastroenterol Nutr. 2011;52:460–5.

50. Reifen RM, Cutz E, Griffiths AM, Ngan BY, Sherman PM. Tufting enteropathy: a newly recognized clinicopathological entity associated with refractory diarrhea in infants. J Pediatr Gastroenterol Nutr. 1994;18:379–85.

51. Goulet O. Intestinal epithelial dysplasia: a new entity. Arch Pediatr. 1996;3(suppl 1):324s–5s.

52. Goulet O, Salomon J, Ruemmele F, de Serres NP, Brousse N. Intestinal epithelial dysplasia (tufting enteropathy). Orphanet J Rare Dis. 2007;2:20.

53. Bird LM, Sivagnanam M, Taylor S, Newbury RO. A new syndrome of tufting enteropathy and choanal atresia, with ophthalmologic, hematologic and hair abnormalities. Clin Dysmorphol. 2007;16:211–21.

54. Roche O, Putterman M, Salomon J, Lacaille F, Brousse N, Goulet O, Dufier JL. Superficial punctate keratitis and conjunctival erosions associated with congenital tufting enteropathy. Am J Ophthalmol. 2010;150:116-21.e1.

55. Sivagnanam M, Mueller JL, Lee H, Chen Z, Nelson SF, Turner D, et al. Identification of EpCAM as the gene for congenital tufting enteropathy. Gastroenterology. 2008;135:429–37.

56. Sivagnanam M, Janecke AR, Müller T, Heinz-Erian P, Taylor S, Bird LM. Case of syndromic tufting enteropathy harbors SPINT2 mutation seen in congenital sodium diarrhea. Clin Dysmorphol. 2010;19:48.

57. Heinz-Erian P, Müller T, Krabichler B, Schranz M, Becker C, Rüschendorf F, et al. Mutations in SPINT2 cause a syndromic form of congenital sodium diarrhea. Am J Hum Genet. 2009;84:188–96.

58. Salomon J, Goulet O, Canioni D, Brousse N, Lemale J, Tounian P, et al. Genetic characterization of congenital tufting enteropathy: EpCAM associated phenotype and involvement of SPINT2 in the syndromic form. Hum Genet. 2014;133:299–310.

59. El-Matary W, Dalzell AM, Kokai G, Davidson JE. Tufting enteropathy and skeletal dysplasia: is there a link? Eur J Pediatr. 2007;166:265–8.

60. Patey N, Scoazec JY, Cuenod-Jabri B, Canioni D, Kedinger M, Goulet O, Brousse N. Distribution of cell adhesion molecules in infants with intestinal epithelial dysplasia (tufting enteropathy). Gastroenterology 1997;113:833–43.

61. Ranganathan S, Schmitt LA, Sindhi R. Tufting enteropathy revisited: the utility of MOC31 (EpCAM) immunohistochemistry in diagnosis. Am J Surg Pathol. 2014;38:265–72.

62. Lemale J, Coulomb A, Dubern B, Boudjemaa S, Viola S, Josset P, et al. Intractable diarrhea with tufting enteropathy: a favorable outcome is possible. J Pediatr Gastroenterol Nutr. 2011;52:734–9.

The Spectrum of Autoimmune Enteropathy

2

Natalia Nedelkopoulou, Evangelia Farmaki, Maesha Deheragoda and Babu Vadamalayan

Introduction

Chronic, unexplained diarrhea in children younger than 3 months old was first characterized as "intractable diarrhea" [1]. The term "protracted diarrhea" was used later to describe infants with frequent and loose stools severe enough to often require parenteral alimentation as nutritional support [2]. The differential diagnosis of enteropathies in infancy and childhood includes inherited epithelial and congenital transport defects, enzymatic deficiencies and allergic enteropathy (Table 2.1).

The most frequent diagnosis in children with protracted diarrhea is autoimmune enteropathy (AIE) [3, 4]. It is a rare, immune-mediated disorder starting usually within the first months of life. The age of onset is between 1 month and 5 years (median age 17 months) [5], but late-onset adult forms have been also reported [6–9]. The disease was first described by Walker-Smith et al. in 1982 in a male child with clinical features of coeliac disease and villous blunting unresponsive to gluten-free diet [10] and represents a heterogeneous group of disorders rather than a discrete entity. The incidence is estimated at less than 1 in 100,000 infants. The diagnostic criteria are debatable but the presence of circulating anti-enterocyte antibodies and the lack of immunodeficiency have been proposed as the hallmark features of AIE [5, 11]. The latter criterion has been challenged by clinical experience and better understanding of the immunology of autoimmunity and self-tolerance [12].

AIE is characterized by variable clinical expression, ranging from isolated gastrointestinal involvement to severe systemic disease [13, 14]. Patients diagnosed with the disease often exhibit extra-intestinal manifestations of autoimmunity, in contrast to those with tufting enteropathy and microvillus inclusion disease [15]. Based on a genetic approach combined with immunological evaluation, three different forms of AIE have been proposed:

1. A predominately or isolated gastrointestinal form of AIE with typical anti-enterocyte antibodies in both sexes
2. A systemic X-linked form of AIE associated with different endocrinopathies, haematological symptoms and severe eczematous skin disease, known as immune dysregulation, polyendocrinopathy, AIE X-linked syndrome (IPEX) occurring only in males
3. An IPEX-like form, a priori FOXP3 independent occurring in both sexes

IPEX and autoimmune polyendocrinopathy-candidiasis-ectodermal dystrophy (APECED) syndrome (APR-1/autoimmune phenomena, polyendocrinopathy, candidiasis and ectodermal dystrophy) are systemic forms of AIE [16].

Clinical Presentation

Chronic, secretory diarrhea refractory to bowel rest that leads to dehydration, malabsorption and severe weight loss is the typical clinical presentation of AIE. Diarrhea usually begins between 2 and 4 weeks of age and the secretory component can be delayed for a few months [3, 11, 17]. The symptoms are often debilitating and the disease is potentially life threatening. The establishment of the diagnosis is crucial in order to ensure optimal treatment. Patients typically require immunosuppressive therapies and total parenteral

B. Vadamalayan (✉)
Pediatric Liver, GI and Nutrition Centre, King's College Hospital, Denmark Hill, London SE59RS, UK
e-mail: babu.vadamalayan@nhs.net

N. Nedelkopoulou
Pediatric Liver, GI and Nutrition Centre, King's College Hospital, London SE59RS, UK

E. Farmaki
Pediatric Immunology and Rheumatology Referral Centre, First Dept of Pediatrics, Aristotle University of Thessaloniki, Thessaloniki, Greece

M. Deheragoda
Institute of Liver Studies, King's College Hospital, London SE59RS, UK

© Springer International Publishing Switzerland 2016
S. Guandalini et al. (eds.), *Textbook of Pediatric Gastroenterology, Hepatology and Nutrition*,
DOI 10.1007/978-3-319-17169-2_2

13

Table 2.1 Differential diagnosis of diarrhea in infancy and childhood

Transport defects and enzymatic deficiencies	Disaccharidase deficiency
	Sodium–hydrogen exchanger (congenital sodium diarrhea)
	Chloride–bicarbonate exchanger (chloride- losing diarrhea)
	Sodium–glucose cotransporter (glucose–galactose malabsorption)
	Lysinuric protein intolerance
	Chylomicron retention disease
	Abetalipoproteinemia
	Ileal bile acid receptor defect
	Enterokinase deficiency
Inherited epithelial defects and villous atrophy	Autoimmune enteropathy
	IPEX syndrome
	Microvillus inclusion disease
	Tufting enteropathy
	Endocrine cell dysgenesis
Other	Coeliac disease
	Allergic enteropathy
	Eosinophilic enteritis
	Infectious/ post-infectious enteropathy
	Lymphangiectasia
	Acrodermatitis enteropathica
	Metabolic diseases
	Tumours
	Idiopathic

nutrition (TPN) for hydroelectrolytic balance and nutritional support [18, 19].

Despite the fact that the mucosal abnormality is primarily confined to the small intestine, the term "generalized autoimmune gut disorder" has been used to describe the association between AIE and autoimmune colitis [8]. Emerging evidence suggests that AIE can be a manifestation of a more diffuse autoimmune disorder of the gastrointestinal system, which comprises gastritis, colitis, hepatitis and pancreatitis with positivity of a variety of autoantibodies, including anti-parietal, anti-goblet cell and anti-smooth muscle antibodies [6, 20–22].

Furthermore, the involvement of extra-intestinal organs can be present during the course of the disease. Multisystem extra-intestinal manifestations include endocrine, renal, pulmonary, hematologic and musculoskeletal. Hypothyroidism with interstitial fibrosis and lymphocytic infiltration of the thyroid gland, nephrotic, nephritic syndrome and membranous glomerulonephritis, interstitial pneumonopathy, periportal fibrosis and bronchitis, haemolytic anaemia, rheumatoid arthritis and dermatitis/atopic eczema have all been reported [5, 11, 22, 23].

Thymus plays a key role in the deletion of potentially self-reactive clones of T cells. The association between AIE and thymoma has been described in both pediatric and adult patients and provides further evidence about the role of thymoma and the development of autoimmunity [24, 25].

Pathogenesis

The underlying immunologic and molecular mechanisms in AIE have not yet been fully elucidated and are widely debatable. However, it has been established that an autoimmune response is involved in the pathogenesis of the disease. Thymus orchestrates a healthy immune system. The intrathymic maturation of T lymphocytes is crucial for the deletion of potentially self-reactive clones of T cells. The dysfunction of the thymus results in the non-deletion and presence of self-reactive T cells that can induce the expansion of anti-self B cells [11, 26, 27].

In AIE, the gut is the site where the autoimmune reaction takes place and is mediated by the activation of self-reactive T cells locally, resulting in the typical histological lesions. In normal states, the expression of human leukocyte antigen (HLA) class II molecules on the enterocyte surface is crucial in establishing and maintaining the oral tolerance as the epithelial cells present exogenous peptides to the clonotypic T cell receptors. The overexpression of HLA-DR antigens in enterocytes and the inappropriate expression of HLA class II molecules in the crypt epithelium of the proximal small intestine in children with AIE have been reported [15, 28].

An increase in the levels of cluster of differentiation CD4 and CD8 lymphocytes in the lamina propria in subjects affected by AIE provides further evidence that the T cells are involved in the pathogenesis of the disease [29, 30]. The intestinal T lymphocytes cause damage to the enterocytes by exerting direct cytotoxicity, via the production of lymphokines or through an antibody-dependent cytotoxicity resulting in cellular apoptosis [31–33]. The loss of the regulatory function of T lymphocytes and the activation of the immune system are implicated in the pathogenesis of IPEX syndrome, whereas AIE is partly attributed to a humoral immune response with the presence of anti-enterocyte antibodies [34].

A variety of circulating autoantibodies, such as antibodies against gastric parietal cells, pancreatic islets, glutamic acid decarboxylase, insulin, smooth muscle, endoplasmic reticulum, reticulin, gliadin, adrenal cells, nuclear antigens, deoxyribose nucleic acid (DNA), thyroglobulin and thyroid microsomes, has been detected in patients with AIE [7, 18]. The presence of antibodies against goblet cells, enterocytes and colonocytes is supportive of the diagnosis. These antibodies are directed against components of the intestinal brush border membrane, with an increasing intensity from the crypts towards villous tip [5, 13]. However, they are neither diagnostic nor specific for the disease and have been also identified in other disorders such as the cow's milk allergy, inflammatory bowel disease and in adults with human immunodeficiency virus (HIV) infection. Moreover, the appearance of the autoantibodies after the onset of the mucosal damage, the lack of correlation between the titer and the histological severity and their disappearance after treatment, but before the complete mucosal restoration support the hypothesis that these antibodies are most likely a secondary event in the pathogenesis of the disease in response to bowel injury [10, 35–37].

The nature of the gut antigen that elicits the immune response and results in the alteration of the intestinal permeability has been extensively investigated. A 55-kD protein located in both the gut and renal epithelial cells that reacted with serum autoantibodies was first identified by Colletti et al. in 1991 in a patient with complicated presentation of AIE with small bowel and glomerular involvement [38]. A few years later, a 75-kD auto-antigen that is distributed through the whole intestine and the kidney was recognized in patients with X-linked AIE associated with nephropathy [39]. The intestinal auto-antigen in autoimmune polyendo-endocrine syndrome type 1 (APECED) is tryptophan hydroxylase (TPH), which is mainly present in the enterochromaffin cells of the mucosa [40].

Emerging evidence has pointed towards an uncontrolled inflammatory reaction caused by the disturbance of the effector–regulatory T-cell interaction and leading to the production of autoantibodies, such as anti-enterocyte antibodies [41]. The understanding of the underlying molecular mechanism and the identification of the genetic defect in AIE was achieved due to the clinical similarities between scurfy mice and boys with the disease. Scurfy mice are a naturally occurring X-linked mutant that presents with massive lymphoproliferation, diarrhea, intestinal bleeding, scaly skin, anaemia, thrombocytopenia and hypogonadism [42]. Based on the observation that the disease-causing mutation in scurfy mice was on the X chromosome, the human IPEX locus was identified on chromosome Xp11.23-q13.3 and the gene was named *FOXP3*. It comprises 11 exons which encode the FOXP3 protein or scurfin, a 48-kDa protein of the forkhead (FKH)/winged-helix transcription factor family that is predominantly expressed in CD4+CD25+ T cell with regulatory function, at significantly lower levels in CD4+CD25-T cells and not at all in CD8+ or B220+ cells [43–46].

Increasing experimental evidence has shown that scurfin is implicated in the thymic maturation of T cells that are designated to acquire regulatory function. CD4+CD25+ Treg represent a small subset (5–10%) of CD4+ T helper cells in humans and mice. Studies on CD4+CD25+ T cells from IPEX patients with the use of anti-CD127 have shown that FOXP3 plays a crucial role in the generation of functional T regulatory cells (Treg) and intact FOXP3 is indispensable for the development of fully functional Tregs, whereas FOXP3 with amino acid substitutions in the FKH domain is sufficient for the generation of functionally immature Tregs [47].

FOXP3 has DNA-binding activity and due to its structure may serve as nuclear transcription factor and act as a repressor of transcription and regulator of T cell activation [48, 49]. The transcription of a reporter containing a multimeric-FKH-binding site is repressed by intact FOXP3. Such FKH-binding sites are located adjacent to nuclear factor of activated T cells (NFAT), regulatory sites in various cytokine promoters such as interleukin (IL)-2, or granulocyte–macrophage colony-stimulating factor enhancer. Therefore, intact scurfin protein appears to be capable to directly repress NFAT-mediated transcription of the *IL-2* gene in CD4+ cells upon activation [50].

Despite the evidence that FOXP3 plays a key role in the development and function of Treg cells, the underlying mechanisms have not been fully understood. Data from animal models with transgenic induction of FOXP3 have shown that the overexpression of scurfin in normal mice leads to a tremendous suppression of immune functions, whereas the depletion of Tregs in healthy mice results rapidly in the development of different T-cell-mediated autoimmune disorders, similar to scurfy in mice or IPEX in humans that go in complete remission upon reconstitution with Treg cells [51, 52].

The three domains that are crucial for the function of FOXP3 are the C-terminal region, which contains the forkhead domain that directly binds DNA regions, the central domain with a zinc finger and leukine zipper that promotes the oligomerization of the FOXP3 molecule and the repressor domain located in the N-terminal region that binds the NAFT [53, 54]. Genetic screening on X chromosome in patients with AIE revealed that the majority of mutations cluster primarily within the FKH domain and the leukine zipper within the coding region of the *FOXP3* gene causing potentially absent FOXP3 protein expression or a protein product with loss of function [13, 53].

Histopathology

Histologic evaluation of the small bowel in typical AIE reveals partial or total villous blunting/atrophy and crypt hyperplasia. In addition, there is a marked infiltration of the lamina propria by mixed inflammatory cells with a prominence of mononuclear cells, including T lymphocytes [15]. Apoptotic bodies and intraepithelial lymphocytes are present in the crypt epithelia. Most cases show a relative paucity of surface lymphocytosis in contrast to coeliac disease. The lymphocytic infiltration of the intestinal mucosa is constituted by CD4–CD8 T lymphocytes and macrophages. Goblet, Paneth and/or enterochromaffin cells may be reduced in number or absent. Cryptitis and crypt abscesses have been reported in severe AIE. Crypt enterocytes commonly show an increased expression of HLA-A, -B, -C molecules [8, 55, 56]. (See Table 2.2; Fig. 2.1) [12].

AIE primarily involves the small bowel with the histologic lesions being most prominent in the proximal small

Table 2.2 Histological findings in autoimmune enteropathy

Histological findings in autoimmune enteropathy
Partial or total villous blunting/atrophy and crypt hyperplasia
Marked infiltration of mononuclear cells, including activated T lymphocytes in the lamina propria
Apoptotic bodies and intraepithelial lymphocytes present in the crypt/gland epithelia, but relative paucity of surface lymphocytosis
Crypt abscesses in severe autoimmune enteropathy
Increased expression of HLA-A, -B, -C molecules in crypt enterocytes

intestine. However, changes have been also described in the oesophagus, stomach and colon in both pediatric and adult patients supporting the hypothesis for a diffuse disease process involving the entire gastrointestinal tract.

Recent reports describe the infiltration of the squamous epithelium by lymphocytes or eosinophils in the oesophagus. Gastric biopsies can show features of chronic nonspecific gastritis with or without reactivity. Atrophic gastritis, intestinal metaplasia and glandular destruction have been also described. There may be increased apoptosis of glandular epithelium [6, 58]. The colonic morphological lesions vary from diffuse mild active colitis with inflammatory cell infiltration to severe active chronic colitis with goblet cell depletion, Paneth cell metaplasia, distortion of crypt architecture and crypt abscess formation. An increase in intraepithelial lymphocytes has also been described [21, 58].

Diagnosis

The diagnostic criteria for AIE were originally proposed by Unsworth and Walker-Smith et al. and included (a) protracted diarrhea and severe enteropathy with small intestinal villous atrophy, (b) no response to exclusion diets, (c) evidence of predisposition to autoimmune disease (presence of circulating enterocyte antibodies or associated autoimmune disease) and (d) no severe immunodeficiency [18]. A more recent adult study proposed the updated criteria and now the diagnosis is established when all of the criteria are present (Table 2.3). The disease should be considered in the differential diagnosis in all patients presenting with severe, unexplained diarrhea requiring parenteral nutritional support particularly in infants, since AIE is the most common cause of protracted diarrhea in infancy [3]. The endoscopic examination with small bowel biopsy is the cornerstone of investigations.

The diagnostic work up should also include information regarding the birth and family history and the time of onset of diarrhea. The disease is characterized by secretory diarrhea, nonresponsive to bowel rest. Most of the affected infants have no history of gluten ingestion at the time of presentation. Furthermore, the lack of response to a gluten-free diet points towards AIE [5, 11, 59].

Serum immunoglobulin assays show normal immunoglobulin (Ig) M and decreased IgG attributed to protein-losing enteropathy. IgA is often within normal range, but

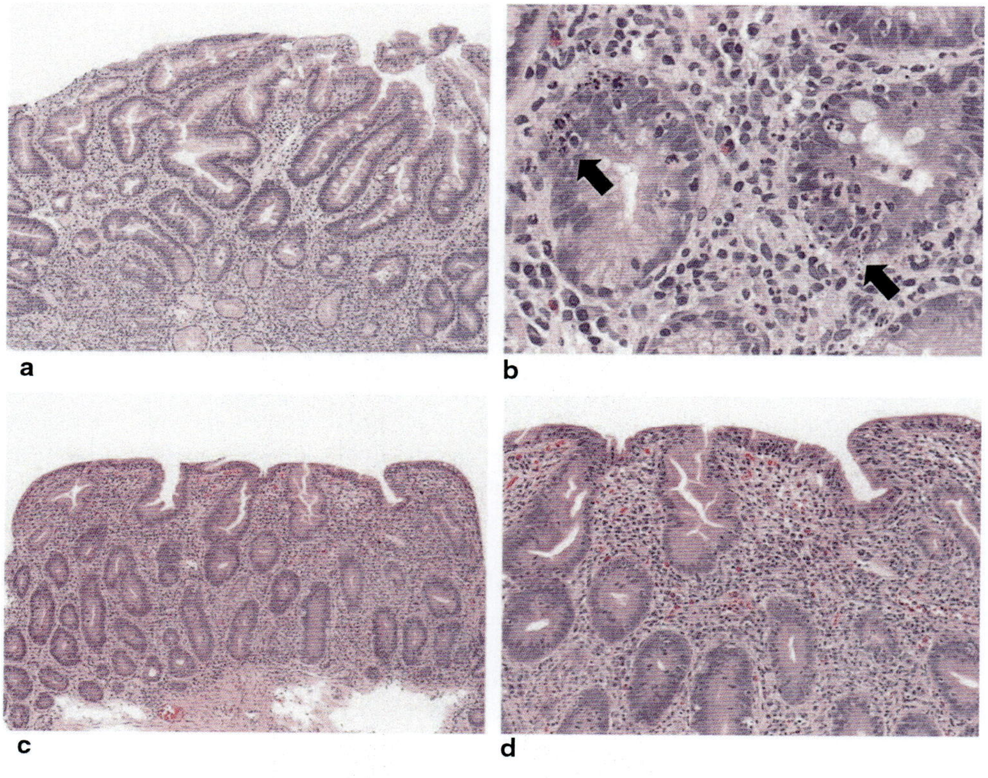

Fig. 2.1 a, b Low and high magnifications, respectively. In some cases of pediatric autoimmune enteropathy, the small intestinal biopsies show cryptitis and crypt abscesses that may obscure the salient finding of autoimmune enteropathy, crypt apoptosis *(arrows)*. There is also an absence of Paneth cells. **c, d** As described in adult patients, small intestinal biopsies can demonstrate a combination of both autoimmune enteropathy and sprue-like histologic findings, characterized by severe villous blunting, marked intraepithelial lymphocytosis, diffuse mononuclear inflammatory infiltrate and prominent crypt apoptosis. Of note, goblet cells are lacking within this specimen [12]. (Reprinted by permission from Macmillan Publishers Ltd, Nature Publishing Group: Ref. [57])

Table 2.3 Diagnostic criteria for AIE [14, 18]

Diagnostic criteria for AIE by Unsworth and Walker-Smith [18]	Updated diagnostic criteria for AIE by Akram et al. [14]
Protracted diarrhea and severe enteropathy with small intestinal villous atrophy	Chronic diarrhea (>6 weeks)
No response to exclusion diets	Malabsorption
Evidence of predisposition to autoimmune disease (presence of circulating enterocyte antibodies or associated autoimmune disease)	Small bowel histology showing partial or complete villous blunting, deep crypt lymphocytosis, increased apoptotic bodies, minimal intraepithelial lymphocytosis
No severe immunodeficiency	Exclusion of other causes of villous atrophy, including coeliac disease, refractory sprue and intestinal lymphoma
	Presence of anti-enterocyte and/or anti-goblet cell antibody supports the diagnosis and sometimes correlates with disease improvement, but is not required to make the diagnosis

AIE autoimmune enteropathy

IgA deficiency associated with villous atrophy has been also reported in AIE. T and B cell function tests, the lymphocytic subsets and polymorphonuclear cell counts are generally normal. Anti-smooth muscle, anti-nuclear and anti-thyroid microsomal autoantibodies have been identified in the course of the disease [5, 8, 22, 60].

Determination of faecal inflammatory markers, like faecal calprotectin, is a simple method that is helpful in distinguishing constitutive intestinal epithelial disorders, such as microvillus atrophy and epithelial dysplasia from immune-inflammatory etiologies such as AIE and inflammatory colitis. It has been proposed that the dramatically increased levels of faecal calprotectin in neonates and infants with immune-inflammatory disorder can distinguish these disorders from constitutive epithelial disorders with 100 % specificity [61].

Treatment

Early recognition and accurate diagnosis of AIE are mandatory to ensure the optimal treatment. The disease is characterized by life-threatening diarrhea often nonresponsive to bowel rest. TPN represents an important step in the management of AIE for nutritional support, adequate rehydration and optimal growth [11, 14, 62]. However, the pediatric patients are not always TPN dependent during the course of the disease [19]. When the gastrointestinal involvement is less severe, elemental or low-carbohydrate-containing formula is recommended to promote enteral delivery of nutrients and calories. The potential tolerance to enteral feeds and the

concomitant inflammatory changes affecting the colon make small bowel transplantation not an ideal treatment option for AIE [17, 63].

Long-term immunosuppression is the mainstay of treatment for the disease. Standard immunosuppressive therapies include corticosteroids, cyclosporine, azathioprine and 6-mercaptopurine. Steroids in the form of prednisolone or budesonide are often needed to induce remission. However, the disease can be refractory to steroids or diarrhea recurs when they are tapered [64].

Since the early 1990s, pediatric patients with AIE have been successfully treated with oral cyclosporine A. Studies have shown that a relatively low drug level (50 ng/mL) led to improvement in growth, intestinal carbohydrate absorption and small bowel histology. However, a number of patients do not respond to the medication and a possible reason is the inefficient absorption of the oral compound due to the underlying chronic enteropathy [65, 66].

Tacrolimus has been used as a therapeutic treatment option with beneficial effects in a variety of autoimmune diseases, including autoimmune hepatitis, primary sclerosing cholangitis and steroid-refractory nephrotic syndrome. Its mechanism of action is similar to cyclosporine. Both drugs block the gene activation for cytokine production by inhibiting the antigenic response of helper T lymphocytes, suppressing IL and interferon-γ [17]. Bousvaros et al. first used tacrolimus as an alternative therapy for AIE and concluded that it can be efficacious if other immunosuppressive regimens fail. Clinical improvement occurred between 1 and 4 months once therapeutic levels were achieved, and serum drug levels were obtained between 5 and 15 ng/mL. Tacrolimus' absorption is less dependent on mucosal integrity compared to cyclosporine; however, mucosal healing improves its absorption, and the dosage should be adjusted to achieve the desired blood levels of the drug. The need for long term or lifelong treatment with tacrolimus in AIE necessitates baseline and frequent monitoring in order to prevent its potential complications, including nephrotoxicity, neurotoxicity, increased predisposition to infections and lymphoproliferative disease [67].

The combination of tacrolimus and infliximab has been proven successful in controlling the inflammation in severe AIE in both pediatric and adult patients. The synergistic effect of these agents is based on the different aspects of the immune system on which they act. Emerging evidence supports that infliximab itself is a highly effective tool for achieving clinical remission and restoring small bowel villous architecture in AIE. The drug has been introduced because of its tumour necrosis factor (TNF)-α antagonistic effect since high levels of this cytokine are being produced by intestinal intraepithelial T lymphocytes of patients with AIE. The response to infliximab is usually rapid and the quality of life of the patients improves dramatically. However, it has been recognized that aggressive immunosuppressive treatment carries a potential risk of life-threatening hypersensitivity reactions and malignancies that should be also considered [17, 68, 69].

Additional immunosuppressive therapies have been used in AIE. Cyclophosphamide is an alkylating agent related to nitrogen mustard and is a potent immunosuppressive agent used in bone marrow transplantation (BMT) conditioning regimens [70]. Low dose of oral cyclophosphamide led to resolution of the intestinal symptoms in a teenage boy with total villous atrophy, selective IgA deficiency and anti-epithelial cell antibodies [71]. However, the use of cyclophosphamide in doses up to 3 mg/kg/d has not always been successful in the management of the disease [38, 72]. Remission of symptoms and improvement of intestinal histopathology was reported in an infant with severe AIE with a single course of high-dose intravenous cyclophosphamide, approximately 20 times greater than those previously used [73].

Mycophenolate mofetil (MMF) has been proposed as an alternative therapeutic option after the successful induction of remission and the improvement of the intestinal absorption and linear growth in an infant with AIE and concomitant factor V Leiden defect [74].

IPEX Syndrome

IPEX is a rare disease and represents a systemic form of AIE characterized by immune dysfunction, polyendocrinopathy, enteropathy and X-linked inheritance. The prevalence of the syndrome remains unknown. Even though the severity of symptoms is variable, the most common feature of IPEX is the involvement of pancreas and thyroid with an early onset. Glucose intolerance can be present at birth and insulin-dependent diabetes mellitus begins often during the first year of life as a result of the complete inflammatory destruction of the pancreatic islet cells prior to the intestinal symptoms [75]. Thyroiditis presents either in the form of hyperthyroidism, or most commonly as hypothyroidism requiring substitutive therapy [13, 61].

The gastrointestinal involvement in children with IPEX syndrome includes severe, secretory diarrhea that can be bloody or mucousy and generally worsens after the breastfeeding is changed to formula [76, 77]. Protein-losing enteropathy with hypoalbuminaemia and a markedly increased clearance of a-1 antitrypsin are indicators of a poor prognosis [41]. Diarrhea often persists despite bowel rest, and TPN is required for nutritional support.

In addition to the endocrinopathies and the gastrointestinal involvement, the basic triad of IPEX syndrome includes chronic dermatitis, most commonly in the form of eczema. In addition, other immune-mediated dermatological disorders like alopecia, pemphigoid nodularis, psoriasiform der-

Table 2.4 Multisystemic disorders in IPEX sydrome

IPEX syndrome
Endocrine: glucose intolerance, insulin-dependent diabetes mellitus, hypo/hyperthyroidism
Gastrointestinal: secretory diarrhea, protein-losing enteropathy, autoimmune hepatitis
Skin: eczema, alopecia, pemphigoid nodularis, psoriasiform dermatitis
Haematologic disorders: autoimmune haemolytic anaemia, neutropenia, thrombocytopenia
Renal: glomerulonephritis, tubulopathy, nephrotic syndrome
Neurological manifestations: seizures, developmental delay
Other: susceptibility to infections, reactions to vaccines

matitis or resembling onychomycosis have been described [76, 78, 79]. The majority of boys with classical IPEX syndrome develop autoimmune hematologic disorders, such as Coombs-—positive haemolytic anaemia, neutropenia or thrombocytopenia with anti-platelet antibodies. Renal involvement affects approximately 30 % of the cases and presents as tubulopathy, nephrotic syndrome or glomerulonephritis. Autoimmune hepatitis is also common. The clinical spectrum of the syndrome includes neurological manifestations, such as seizures and developmental delay. Reactions to vaccines and increased susceptibility to infections can be attributed either to neutropenia and the immunosuppressive therapy or to the altered skin/gut barrier (Table 2.4) [61].

FOXP3 mutations can lead to different phenotypes of IPEX syndrome in terms of symptoms and severity. Genetic analysis for FOXP3 mutations is recommended in all patients with symptoms indicative of IPEX syndrome [80]. However, despite the typical clinical presentation of IPEX syndrome in some patients, no mutations were identified within the coding regions of FOXP3, supporting the hypothesis that conditional or regulatory mutations may occur outside FOXP3 [44, 49, 76]. A mutation in the polyadenylation signal following the final coding exon of FOXP3 that results in a decreased FOXP3 messenger RNA (mRNA) expression has been reported [81]. Furthermore, the fact that females heterozygous for FOXP3 mutation remain completely asymptomatic provides evidence that FOXP3-independent forms of AIE exist. It is likely that these independent forms of IPEX or AIE affecting both boys and girls are transmitted either with X-chromosomal or an autosomatic trait. A marked CD25 deficiency on CD4+ cells caused by an autosomal recessive mutation resulted in the IPEX-like clinical presentation in a patient with normal *FOXP3* gene analysis and pointed towards the implication of IL-2 and its high-affinity receptor CD25 in the pathogenesis of FOXP3-independent forms [82]. These findings need to be confirmed by future studies.

The small bowel histopathology of pediatric subjects with IPEX syndrome can range from a graft-versus-host disease-like pattern with complete villous atrophy, mild inflammation of the lamina propria, apoptotic bodies, crypt abscesses and loss of goblet cells (as described above) to a more coeliac-disease-like pattern with partial villous atrophy, moderate inflammation of the lamina propria, an increase in intraepithelial lymphocytes and crypt hyperplasia. Moreover, a patient with anti-goblet cell antibodies demonstrated partial villous atrophy, moderate inflammation of the lamina propria, an increase in intraepithelial lymphocytosis and complete lack of goblet cells [83]. Depending on the organs involved in IPEX syndrome, the typical lymphocytic infiltration can be also present in thyroid, liver, skin, brain or pancreas with complete destruction of islet cells [62, 84].

The syndrome should be considered in young males presenting with protracted diarrhea with villous atrophy and failure to thrive combined with diabetes mellitus and/or hypothyroidism and skin manifestations. The definite diagnosis is based on genetic studies and mutation analysis of the *FOXP3* gene [85]. Immunocytochemical staining of FOXP3 molecule in bowel biopsies has been proposed as a potential screening test [86].

Given the serious side effects, the toxicity and the limited efficacy for long-term remission of immunosuppressive medication, there is a need for new therapeutic approaches for IPEX and AIE. The most promising is in the form of BMT. Baud and Wildin et al. reported three boys with IPEX syndrome who received BMT as ultimate treatment. Even though BMT was initially successful, lethal complications occurred months to years post transplantation. The authors concluded that BMT is potentially successful in treating resistant IPEX, but further experience must be gained before it is recommended as a rescue therapy for AIE.

Interestingly, the conditioning regimen was itself effective in controlling symptoms in some patients [48, 87] and a reduced-intensity-conditioning regimen prior to engraftment resulted in more FOXP3 T regulatory cells than more aggressive conditioning [88]. Beneficial effect on the pancreatic function and recovery of diabetes mellitus was obtained in some cases; however, the islet damage is often permanent at the time of BMT [86]. Insulin for diabetes and haematic transfusions are often needed for the symptomatic management of IPEX syndrome.

Clinical improvement in patients with IPEX syndrome was also reported after submyeloablative cord blood transplantation [89]. The efficacy of bone marrow-derived mesenchymal stem cells (MSC) in a mutli-organ autoimmunity model caused by a deficiency in T cells led to an MSC-specific improvement in the histopathology of the distal ileum of treated mice. This observation necessitates future investigations into the use of MSCs for the treatment of autoimmune disorders [90]. It was also shown that the direct transduction of T cells with FOXP3-expressing vectors could overtake bone marrow gene therapy and provided evidence that gene therapy of autologous cells could potentially be a future therapeutic approach for IPEX syndrome [91].

APECED Syndrome

APECED, also known as autoimmune polyendocrine syndrome type 1 (APS-1) is a rare, autosomal recessive disease. The understanding of the underlying pathophysiology of this monogenic disease has provided important information on the pathogenesis of organ-specific autoimmunity and T cell selection. The syndrome is characterized immunologically by destruction of the target organs by a cellular- and/or antibody-mediated attack [92, 93]. It has been reported at a relatively higher prevalence in genetically isolated populations like Finns, Sardinians and Iranian Jews [94–97]. The classical triad of APECED consists of Addison's disease, hypoparathyroidism and chronic mucocutaneous candidiasis, and two of them are required for the diagnosis. However, several other endocrine and non-endocrine manifestations accompany the pathognomonic triad.

The onset of APECED is usually in childhood with the first symptoms occurring on average at the age of 5 [98]. The wide spectrum of the clinical manifestations is attributed to a variable pattern of destructive autoimmune reaction mediated by specific antibodies that can attack any tissue or organ [99, 100]. TPH is an enzyme involved in the synthesis of neurotransmitters in the nervous system and in the gastrointestinal endocrine cells. The presence of autoantibodies against this enzyme is associated with AIE in APECED [101–104]. The gastrointestinal involvement also includes diarrhea, constipation, autoimmune hepatitis, chronic atrophic gastritis or autoimmune gastritis with pernicious anaemia [105]. Exocrine pancreatic failure results in malabsorption and steatorrhoea in a small subgroup of patients [98].

Children within large Old Order Amish kindred presented with developmental delay, dysmorphic features, failure to thrive, organomegaly and multisystem autoimmune diseases, including AIE. Human ITCH E3 ubiquitin ligase deficiency was recognized as the underlying cause of this syndromic multisystem autoimmune disease. ITCH deficiency results in abnormal T helper cell differentiation and failure of T cell anergy induction. Genetic mapping in patients revealed a truncating mutation in the *ITCH* gene [106, 107].

In autoimmune polyendoscrinopathy-candidiasis-ectodermal dystrophy, the mutations have been identified in the autoimmune regulatory gene (AIRE) that modulates the transcription of peripheral self-antigens in the thymus presented by HLA molecules to maturing T cells [108]. Patients affected by at least two illnesses among chronic mucocutaneous candidiasis usually starting soon after birth, autoimmune hypoparathyroidism and Addison's disease, especially from populations such as Finns, Sardinians and Iranian Jews should be investigated for APECED syndrome. The identification of mutations on AIRE gene is recommended to confirm the diagnosis [98].

The treatment of APECED syndrome is challenging and is mainly based on parenteral nutritional support. Immunosuppressive treatment includes high doses of intravenous steroids and methotrexate, which is well tolerated in children. Systemic chemotherapy against Candida infection and hormone replacement therapy are also required. Patients with APECED should be closely monitored for new components of the syndrome [109].

Prognosis

AIE is a potentially life-threatening disease. Both intestinal and extra-intestinal manifestations can lead to debilitating symptoms requiring a complex therapeutic approach. The disease itself has not been linked to the development of intestinal malignancies; however, the intensity of immunosuppressive therapy and the increasing longevity of patients potentially increase the risk of malignancy [17]. AIE is now considered as a systemic disease, and, in its most severe form, IPEX syndrome, is often characterized by unresponsiveness to treatment with a high mortality rate [67]. Malnutrition in infants and infections at a later age are the most frequent causes of death. Given the immunologic nature of IPEX syndrome, early BMT currently seems the most promising treatment of choice. However, more experience is needed to ensure that this therapeutic approach leads to permanent remission [48, 87]. Finally, the great variability of the clinical expression and the absence of a clear genotype–phenotype correlation in APECED syndrome create the need for the identification of potential disease-modifying genes that are involved in the clinical expressivity of organ-specific autoimmunity.

References

1. Avery GB, Villavincencio O, Lilly JR, et al. Intractable diarrhea in early infancy. Pediatrics 1968;41:712–22.
2. Anonymous. Chronic diarrhea in children: a nutritional disease. Lancet 1987;329:143–4.
3. Catassi C, Fabiani E, Spagnuolo MI, et al. Severe and protracted diarrhea: results of the 3-year SIGEP multicenter survey. Working Group of the Italian Society of Paediatric Gastroetnerology and Hepatology (SIGEP). J Pediatr Gastroenterol Nutr. 1999;29:63–8.
4. Goulet OJ, Brousse N, Canioni D, et al. Syndrome of intractable diarrhea with persistent villous atrophy in early childhood: a clinicopathological survey of 47 cases. J Pediatr Gastroenterol Nutr. 1998;26:151–61.
5. Russo PA, Brochu P, Seidman EG, Roy CC. Autoimmune enteropathy. Pediatr Dev Pathol. 1999;2:65–71.
6. Mitomi H, Tanabe S, Igarashi M, Katsumata T, Arai N, Kikuchi S, et al. Autoimmune enteropathy with severe atrophic gastritis and colitis in an adult: proposal of a generalized autoimmune disorder of the alimentary tract. Scand J Gastroenterol. 1998;33:716–20.
7. Corazza GR, Biagi F, Volta U, Andreani ML, De Franceschi L, et al. Autoimmune enteropathy and villous atrophy in adults. Lancet 1997;350:106–9.
8. Leon F, Olivencia P, Rodriguez-Pena R, Sanchez L, Redondo C, et al. Clinical and immunological features of adult-onset generalized autoimmune gut disorder. Am J Gastroenterol. 2004;99:1563–71.
9. Daum S, Sahin E, Jansen A, Heine B, et al. Adult autoimmune enteropathy treated successfully with tacrolimus. Digestion 2003;68:86–90.
10. Walker- Smith JA, Unsworth DJ, Hurchins P, et al. Autoantibodies against gut epithelium in a child with small intestinal enteropathy. Lancet 1982;319:566–7.
11. Montalto M, D'Onofrio F, Santoro L, et al. Autoimmune enteropathy in children and adults. Scand J Gastroenterol. 2009;44:1029–36.
12. Singhi AD, Goyal AL Davison JM, Regueiro MD, et al. Pediatric autoimmune enteropathy: an entity frequently associated with immunodeficiency disorders. Modern Pathol. 2014;27(4):543–53. doi: 10.1038/modpathol.2013.150. Epub 2013 Sep 20.
13. Ruemmele FM, Brousse N, Goulet O. Autoimmune enteropathy-molecular concepts. Curr Opin Gastroenterol. 2004;20:587–91.
14. Akram S, Murray JA, Pardi DS, et al. Adult autoimmune enteropathy: Mayo clinic Rochester experience. Clin Gastroenterol Hepatol. 2007;5:1282–90.
15. Cuenod B, Brousse N, Goulet O, et al. Classification of intractable diarrhea in infancy using clinical and immunohistological criteria. Gastroenterology 1990;99:1037–43.
16. Ruemmele FM, Brousse N, Goulet O. Autoimmune—Enteropathy and IPEX syndrome (Chap. 16.3). In: Walker WA et al. editors Pediatric Gastrointestinal disease. 5th ed. People's Medical Publisher House(PMPH); 2008.
17. Vanderhoof JA, Young RJ. Autoimmune enteropathy in a child: response to infliximab therapy. J Ped Gastroenterol Nutr. 2002;34:312–6.
18. Unsworth DJ, Walker-Smith JA. Autoimmunity in diarrheal disease. J Pediatr Gastroenterol Nutr. 1985;4:375–80.
19. Cambarara M, Bracci F, Diamanti A, Ambrosini MI, Pietrobattista A, et al. Long-term parenteral nutrition in pediatric autoimmune enteropahties. Transplant Proc. 2005;37:2270–1.
20. Carroccio A, Volta U, Di Prima L, Petrolini N, Florena AM, Averna MR, et al. Autoimmune enteropathy and colitis in an adult patient. Dig Dis Sci. 2003;48:1600–6.
21. Hill SM, Milla PJ, Bottazzo GF, Mirakian R. Autoimmune enteropathy and colitis: is there a generalized autoimmune gut disorder? Gut 1991;32:36–42.
22. Lachaux A. Autoimmune enteropathy. Arch Pediatr. 1996;3:261–6.
23. Volta U, De Angelis GI, Granito A, et al. Autoimmune enteropathy and rheumatoid arthritis: a new association in the field of autoimmunity. Dig Liver Dis. 2006;38:926–9.
24. Mais DD, Mullhall BP, Adolphson KR, Yamamoto K. Thymoma-associated autoimmune enteropathy. A report of two cases. Am J Clin Pathol. 1999;112:810–5.
25. Elwing JE, Clouse RE. Adult-onset autoimmune enteropathy in the setting of thymoma successfully treated with infliximab. Dig Dis Sci. 2005;50:928–32.
26. Martin-Villa JM, Requeiro JR, De Juan D, Perez-Aciego P, Perez Blas M, Manzanares J, et al. T–lymphocyte dysfunction occurring together with apical gut epithelial cell autoantibodies. Gastroenterology 1991;101:390–7.
27. Pullen AM, Marrack P, Kappler JW. The T cell repertoire is heavily influenced by tolerance to polymorphic self-antigens. Nature 1988;335:796–801.
28. Mirakian R, Hill S, Richardson A, Milla PJ, Walker-Smith JA, et al. HLA product expression and lymphocyte subpopulation in jejenum biopsies of children with idiopathic protracted diarrhea and enterocyte autoantibodies. J Autoimmun. 1988;1:263–77.
29. Lachaux A, Loras-Duclaux I, Bouvier R. Autoimmune enteropathy in infants:pathological study of the disease in two familial cases. Virchows Arch. 1998;433:481–5.

30. Yamamoto H, Sugiyama K, Nomura T, Taki M, Okazaki T. A case of intractable diarrhea firmly suspected to have autoimmune enteropahty. Acta Paediatr Jpn. 1994;36:97–103.

31. Ciccocioppo R, D'Alo S, Di Sabatino A, Parroni R, Rossi M, et al. Mechanisms of villous atrophy in autoimmune enteropathy and coeliac disease. Clin Exp Immunol. 2002;128:88–93.

32. Mowat A McI, Borland A, Parrott DMV. Hypersensitivity reactions in the small intestine. VII Induction of the intestinal phase of murine graft-versus-host reactions by lyt.2- T cells activated Ia alloantigens. Transplantation 1986;41:192–7.

33. Guy-Grand D, Vassalli P. Gut injury in mouse graft-versus-host reaction. Study of its occurrence and mechanisms. J Clin Invest. 1986;77:1584–95.

34. Bishu S, Arsenescu V, Lee EY, et al. Autoimmune enteropathy with a CD8 + CD7- T cell small bowel intraepithelial lymphocytosis: case report and literature review. BMC Gastroenterol. 2011;11:131.

35. Skogh T, Heuman R, Tagesson C. Anti-brush border antibodies (ABBA) in Crohn's disease. J Clin Lab Immunol. 1982;9:147–50.

36. Unsworth J, Hutchins P, Mitchell J, et al. Flat small intestinal mucosa and autoantibodies against the gut epithelium. J Pediatr Gastroenterol Nutr. 1982;1:503–13.

37. Martin–Villa JM, Camblor S, Costa R, Arnaiz-Villema A, et al. Gut epithelial cell autoantibodies in AIDS pathogenesis. Lancet 1993;342:380.

38. Colletti RB, Guillot AP, Rosen S, Bhan AK, Hobson CD, et al. Autoimmune enteropathy and nephropathy with circulating anti-epithelial cell antibodies. J Pediatr. 1991;118:858–64.

39. Kobayashi I, Imamura K, Yamada M, Okano M, Yara A, et al. A 75-kD autoantigen recognized by sera from patients with X-linked autoimmune enteropathy associated with nephropathy. Clin Exp Immunol. 1998;111:527–31.

40. Enkwall O, Hedstrand H, Grimelius L, Haavik J, et al. Identification of tryptophan hydroxylase as an intestinal autoantigen. Lancet 1998;352:279–83.

41. Ruemmele FM, Moes N, Patey-Mariaud de Serre N, Rieux-Laucat F, Goulet O. Clinical and molecular aspects of autoimmune enteropathy and immune dysregulation, polyendocrinopathy, autoimmune enteropathy X-linked syndrome. Curr Opin Gastrenterol. 2008;24:742–8.

42. Clark LB, et al. Cellular and molecular characterization of the scurfy mouse mutant. J Immunol. 1999;162:2546–54.

43. Wildin ES, et al. X-linked neonatal diabetes mellitus, enteropathy and endocrinopathy syndrome is the human equivalent of mouse scurfy. Nat Genet. 2001;27:18–20.

44. Brunkow ME, et al. Disruption of a new forhead/winged-helix protein, scurfin, results in the fatal lymphoproliferative disorder of the scurfy mouse. Nat Genet. 2001;27:68–73.

45. Bennett CL, et al. The immune dysregulation, polyendoxrinopathy, enteropathy X-linked syndrome (IPEX) is caused by mutations of FOXP3. Nat Genet. 2001;27:20–1.

46. Hori S, Nomura T, Sakaguchi S. Control of regulatory Tcell development by the transcription factor Foxp3. Science 2003;299:1057–61.

47. Otsubo K, Kanegane H, Kamachi Y, Kobayashi I, et al. Identification of FOXP3-negative regulatory T-like (CD4 + CD25 + CD127low) cells in patients with immune dysregulation, polyendocrinopathy, enteropathy, X-linked syndrome. Clin Immunol. 2011;141:111–20.

48. Wildin RS, Smyk-Oearsin SM, Filipovitch AH, et al. Clinical and molecular features of the immunodysregulation, polyendocrinopathy, enteropathy, X-linked (IPEX) syndrome. J Med Genet. 2002;9:537–45.

49. Sakaguchi S. The origin of FOXP3-expressing CD4 + regulatory T cells: thymus or periphery. J Clin Invest. 2003;112:1310–2.

50. Schubert LA, et al. Scurfin (FOXP3) acts as a repressor of transcription and regulates T cell activation. J Biol Chem. 2001;276:37672–27679.

51. Sakaguchi S, Sakaguchi N, Shimizu J, et al. Immunologic tolerance maintained by CD25 + CD4 + regulatory T cells: their common role in controlling autoimmunity, tumor immunity, and transplantation tolerance. Immunol Rev. 2001;182:18–32.

52. Khattri R, Kasprowich D, Cox T, et al. The amount of scurfin protein determined peripheral T cell number and responsiveness. J Immunol. 2001;167:6312–20.

53. Li B, Samanta A, Song X, Iacono KT, Brennan P, et al. FOXP3 is a homo-oligomer and a component of a supramolecular regulatory complex disabled in the human XLAAD/ IPEX autoimmune disease. Int Immunol. 2007;19:825–35.

54. Lopes JE, Torgerson TR, Schubert LA, Anover SD, Ocheltree EL, et al. Analysis of FOXPE reveals multiple domains requires for its function as a transcriptional repressor. J Immunol. 2006;177:3133–42.

55. Murch SH, Fertleman CR, Rodriques C, et al. Autoimmune enteropathy with distinct mucosal features in T-cell activation deficiency: the contribution of T cells to the mucosal lesions. J Pediatric Gastroenterol Nutr. 1999;28:393–9.

56. Hartfiled D, Turner J, Huynh H, et al. The role of histopathology in diagnosing protracted diarrhea of infancy. Fetal Pediatr Pathol. 2010;29:144–57.

57. Singhi AD, Goyal A, Davison JM, Regueiro MD, Roche RL, Ranganathan S. Pediatric autoimmune enteropathy: an entity frequently associated with immunodeficiency disorders. Mod Pathol. 2013;27(4):543–53.

58. Masia R, Peyton S, Lauwers G, Brown I. Gastrointestinal biopsy findings of autoimmune enteropathy. Am J Surg Pathol. 2014;38:1319–29.

59. Cutz E, Sherman PM, Davidson GP. Enteropathies associated with protracted diarrhea in infancy: clinicopathological features, cellular and molecular mechanisms. Pediatr Pathol Lab Med. 1997;17:335–68.

60. Catassi C, Mirakian R, Natalizi G, Sbarbati A, et al. Unresponsive enteropathy associated with circulation autoantibodies in a boy with common variable hypogammaglobulinaemia and type I diabetes. J PEediatr Gastroenterol Nutr. 1988;7:608–13.

61. Kapel N, Roman C, Caldari D, et al. Fecal Tumor necrosis factor-a and calprotectin as differential diagnostic markers for severe diarrhea of small infants. J Pediatr Gastroenterol Nutr. 2005;41:396–400.

62. Quiros BA, Sanz AE, Ordiz BD, Adrados GJA. From autoimmune enteropathy to the IPEX syndrome Allergol Immunopathol. 2009;37(4):208–15.

63. Lifschitz CH, Carazza F. Effect of formula carbohydrate concentration on tolerance and macronutrient in infants with severe, chronic diarrhea. J Pediatr. 1990;117:378–91.

64. Gentile NM, Murray JA, Pardi DS. Autoimmune enteropathy: a review and update of clinical management. Curr Gastroenterol Rep. 2012;14:380–5.

65. Sanderson IR, Philips AS, Spencer J, Walker-Smith JA. Response to autoimmune enteropathy to cyclosporine A therapy. Gut 1991;32:1421–25.

66. Seidman EG, Lacaille F, Russo P, et al. Successful treatment of autoimmune enteropathy with cyclosporine. J Pediatr 1990:117:929–32.

67. Bousvaros A, Leichtner AM, Book L, Shigeoka A, et al. Treatment of pediatric autoimmune enteropathy with tacrolimus (FK506). Gastroenterology 1996;111:237–43.

68. Von Hahn T, Stopik D, Koch M, et al. Management of severe refractory adult autoimmune enteropathy with infliximab and tacrolimus. Digestion 2005;71(3):141–4.

69. Valitutti F, Barbato M, Aloi M, et al. Autoimmune enteropathy in a 13-year old celiac girl successfully treated with infliximab. J Clin Gastroenterol. 2014;48(3):264–6.

70. Brodsky RA, Petri M, Smith BD, et al. High-dose cyclophosphamide for aplastic anemia and autoimmunity. Curr Opin Oncol. 2002;14:143–6.

71. McCarthy DM, Katz SI, Gazze L, et al. Selective IgA deficiency associated with total villous atrophy of the small intestine and an organ-specific-anti-epithelial cell antibody. J Immunol. 1978;120:932–8.

72. Savilahti E, Pelkonen P, Holmberg C, et al. Fatal unresponsive villous atrophy of the jejunum, coneective tissue disease and diabetes in a girl woth intestinal cell antibody. Acta Pediatr Scan. 1985;74:472–6.

73. Oliva-Hemker MM, Loeb DM, Abraham SC, Lederman H. Remission of severe autoimmune enteropathy afer treatment with high-dose cyclophosphamide. J Pediatr Gastroentrol Nutr. 2003;36:639–43.

74. Baud O, Goulet O, Canioni D, et al. Treatment of immune dysregulation, polyendocrinopahty, enteropathy, X-linked syndrome (IPEX) by allogeneic bone marrow transplantation. N Engl J Med. 2001;344:1758–62.

75. Levy-Lahad E, Wildin RS. Neonatal diabetes mellitus, enteropathy, thrombocytopenia and endocrinopathy: further evidence for an X-linked lethal syndrome. J Pediatr. 2001;138:677–580.

76. Torgerson TR, Linane A, Moes N, Anover S, et al. Severe food allergy as a variant of IPEX syndrome caused by deletion in a noncoding region of the FOXP3 gene. Gastroenterology 2007;132:1705–17.

77. Marabelle A, Meyer M, Demeocq F, Lachaux A. De l' Ipex a foxp3: une nouvelle contribution de la pediatrie a la comprehension du systeme immunitaire. Arch Pediatr. 2008;15:55–63.

78. McLucas P, Fulchiero Jr GJ, Fernandez E, Miller JJ, Zaengelin AL. Norwegian scabies mimicking onychomycosis and scalp dermatitis in a child with IPEX syndrome J Am Acad Dermatol. 2007;56:S48–9.

79. Mc Ginness JL, Bivens MM, Greer KE, Paterson JW, Saulsbury FT. Immune dysregultation, polyendocrinopathy, enteropathy, X-linked syndrome (IPEX) associated with pemphigoid nodularis: a case report and review of the literature. J Am Acad Dermatol. 2006;55:143–8.

80. Gambineri E, Perroni L, Passerini L, Bianchi L, Doglioni C, et al. Clinical and molecular profile of a new series of patients with immune dysregulation, polyendocrinopathy, enteropathy, X-linked syndrome: inconsistent correlation between forkhead box protein 3 expression and disease severity. J Allergy Clin Immunol. 2008;122(6):1105–12.

81. Bennett CL, Brunkow ME, Ramsdell F, et al. A rare polyadenylation signal mutation of the FOXP3 gene leads to the IPEX syndrome. Immunogenetics 2001;53:435–9.

82. Caudy AA, Reddy ST, Chatila T, et al. CD25 deficiency causes an immune dysregulation, polyendocrinopathy, enteropathy, X-linked-like syndrome and defective IL-10 expression from CD4 lymphocytes. J Allergy Clinc Immunol. 2007;119:482–7.

83. Patey-Mariaud de Serre N, Canioni D, Ganousse S, et al. Digestive histopathological presentation of IPEX syndrome. Mod Pathol. 2009;22:95–102.

84. Bennett CL, Ochs HD. IPEX is a unique X-linked syndrome characterized by immune dysfunction, polyendoscrinopathy, enteropathy and a variety of autoimmune phenomena. Curr Opin Pediatr. 2001;13:533–8.

85. Torgerson TR, Ochs HD. Immune dysregulation, polyendocrinopathy, enteropathy, X-linked: forkhead box protein 3 mutations and lack of regulatory T cells. J Allergy Clin Immunol. 2007;120:744–50.

86. Heltzer ML, Choi JK, Ochs HD, et al. A potential screening tool for IPEX syndrome. Pediatr Dev Pathol. 2007;10:98–105.

87. Quiros-Tejeira R, Ament ME, Vargas J. Induction of remission in a child with autoimmune enteropathy using Mycophenolate Mofetil. J Pediatr Gastroenterol Nutr. 2001;36:482–5.

88. Rao A, Kamani N, Filipovich A, et al. Successful bone marrow transplantation for IPEX syndrome after reduced-intensity conditioning. Blood 2007;109:383–5.

89. Lucas KG, Ungar D, Comito M, et al. Submyeloablative cord blood transplantation corrects clinical defects seen in IPEX syndrome. Bone Marrow Transplant. 2007;39:55–6.

90. Parekkadan B, Tilles A, Yarmush I. Bone marrow-derived mesenchymal stem cells ameliorate autoimmune enteropathy independently of regulatory T cells. Stem Cells. 2008;26:1913–9.

91. Yagi H, Nomura T, Nakamura K, et al. Crucial role of FOXP3 in the development and function of human CD25 + CD4 + regulatory cells. Int Immunol. 2004;16:1643–56.

92. Mathis D, Benoist C. Aire. Annu Rev Immunol. 2009;27:287–312.

93. Husebye ES, Perheentupa J, Rautemaa R, Kampe O. Clinical manifestations and management of patients with autoimmune polyendocrine syndrome type I. J Intern Med. 2009;265:514–29.

94. Ahonen P, Myllarniemi S, Sipila I, Perheentupa J. Clinical variation of autoimmune polyendocrinopathy-candidiasis-ectodermal dystrophy (APECED) in a series of 68 patients. N Engl J Med. 1990;322(26):1829–3610.

95. Aaltonen J, Bjorses P, Sandkuijl L, Perheentupa J, Peltonen L. An autosomal locus causing autoimmune disease: autoimmune polyglandular disease type I assigned to chromosome 21. Nat Genet. 1994;8:83–710.

96. Rosatelli MC, Meloni A, Meloni A, Devoto M, Cao A, Scott HS, et al. A common mutation in Sardinian autoimmune polyendocrinopathy-candidiasis-ectodermal dystrophy spatients. Hum Genet. 1998;103:428–34.

97. Zlotogora J, Shapiro MS. Polyglandular autoimmune syndrome type I among Iranian Jews. J Med Genet. 1992;29:824–6.

98. Perheentupa J. Autoimmune polyendocrinopathy-candidiasis-ectodermal dystrophy. J Clin Endocrinol Metab. 2006;91:2843–50.

99. Capalbo D, Improda N, Esposito A, De Martino L, Barbieri F, Betterle C, et al. Autoimmune polyendocrinopathy-candidiasis-ectodermal dystrophy from the pediatric perspective. J Endocrinol Invest. 2013 Nov;36:903–12.

100. Betterle C, Greggio NA, Volpato M. Autoimmune polyglandular syndrome type 1. J Clin Endocr Metab. 1998;83(4):1049–55.

101. Ekwall O, Hedstrand H, Grimelius L, Haavik J, Perheentupa J, Gustafsson J, et al. Identification of tryptophan hydroxylase as an intestinal autoantigen. Lancet 1998;352:279–83.

102. Scarpa R, Alaggio R, Norberto L, Furmaniak J, Chen S, Smith BR, et al. Tryptophan hydroxylase autoantibodies as markers of a distinct autoimmune gastrointestinal component of autoimmune polyendocrine syndrome type 1. J Clin Endocrinol Metab. 2013;98:704–12.

103. Dal Pra C, Chen S, Betterle C, Zanchetta R, McGrath V, Furmaniak J, et al. Autoantibodies to human tryptophan hydroxylase and aromatic l-amino acid decarboxylase. Eur J Endocrinol. 2004;150:313–21.

104. Gianani R, Eisenbarth GS. Autoimmunity to gastrointestinal endocrine cells in autoimmune polyendocrine syndrome type I. J Clin Endocrinol Metab. 2003;88:1442–4.

105. Capalbo D, De Martino L, Giardino G, Di Mase R, Di Donato I, Parenti G, et al. Autoimmune polyendocrinopathy candidiasis ectodermal dystrophy: insights into genotype-phenotype correlation. Int J Endocrinol. 2012;2012:353250. doi:10.1155/2012/353250.

106. Lohr NJ, Molleston JP, Strauss KA, et al. Human ITCH E3 ubiquitin legase deficiency causes syndromic multisystem autoimmune disease. Am J Hum Genet. 2010;86:447–53.

107. Su J, Liu YC. FOXP3 positive regulatory T cells: a functional regulation by the E3 ubiquitin ligase Itch. Semin Immunopathol. 2010;32:149–56.

108. Michels AW, Gottlieb PA. Autoimmune polyglandular syndromes. Nat Rev Endocrinol. 2010;6:270–7.

109. Perheentupa J. APS-I/APECEC: the clinical disease and therapy. Endocrinol Metab Clin North Am. 2002;31:295–32.

Congenital Problems of the Gastrointestinal Tract

Nigel J. Hall

Introduction

Congenital abnormalities of the gastrointestinal tract (GIT) are relatively common. Owing to their nature, they frequently require surgical correction, and on occasion this must be undertaken as a matter of emergency in order to avoid catastrophic intestinal ischemia and necrosis resulting in loss of bowel or damage to a secondary organ system. This chapter provides an overview of the most common conditions encountered and those which require intervention as a matter of urgency. It is not possible within the space available to describe in detail all of the variants of congenital GIT abnormalities that may be encountered and the precise nature of the treatment options available. For ease of understanding, we commence with the upper GIT and continue in a caudal direction.

Conditions Affecting the Upper Gastrointestinal Tract

Esophageal Atresia and Trache-esophageal Fistula

This complex group of anomalies with an incidence of 1 in 2440–4500 live births [1, 2] results from failure of correct division of the tracheal primordium from the esophagus during early embryonic development. The precise etiology is unknown with a number of embryological theories proposed to explain the different variants of this anomaly. There is a high incidence of coexisting abnormalities including the VACTERL (Vertebral column, Anorectal, Cardiac, Tracheal, Esophageal, Renal, and Limbs) syndrome, CHARGE (Coloboma of the eye, Heart defects, Atresia of the nasal choanae, Retardation of growth and/or development, Genital and/or urinary abnormalities, and Ear abnormalities and deafness) association, and isolated cardiovascular anomalies [3].

Classification
A number of classification systems have been proposed over the years. Table 3.1 describes the most commonly encountered anatomical variants (Fig. 3.1), and the Spitz classification (Table 3.2) [3] incorporating birth weight and presence of major congenital heart disease status may be useful in predicting survival.

Clinical Features
EA is commonly associated with maternal polyhydramnios, and with increasing frequency, the diagnosis is being made antenatally particularly if there is no TEF. In the postnatal period, symptoms associated with the condition include excessive salivation, feeding difficulties, respiratory distress, and cyanotic episodes. Cases of EA (with the exception of the rare EA with double fistula) can be confirmed by failure of passage of a nasogastric tube into the stomach. Cases of TEF in the absence of EA (i.e., H-type fistula) may present later, usually with recurrent episodes of respiratory distress or pneumonia.

Treatment
The overall aim of surgical correction is early division of any fistula with the respiratory tract to protect the lungs and airway, and restoration and maintenance of esophageal continuity to allow normal feeding. Following diagnosis, a Replogle tube is placed in the upper esophageal pouch which allows suction of secretions and minimizes the risk of pulmonary aspiration. Surgical repair involves ligation and division of any fistula and primary anastomosis of the two ends of the esophagus where possible. Infants who are too unstable to tolerate primary esophageal repair, typically preterm infants with respiratory distress, may be treated with ligation of the fistula only followed by delayed esophageal anastomosis once a period of cardiorespiratory stability can be achieved.

N. J. Hall (✉)
Southampton Children's Hospital, University of Southampton, Tremona Road, Southampton SO16 6YD, UK
e-mail: n.j.hall@soton.ac.uk

© Springer International Publishing Switzerland 2016
S. Guandalini et al. (eds.), *Textbook of Pediatric Gastroenterology, Hepatology and Nutrition,*
DOI 10.1007/978-3-319-17169-2_3

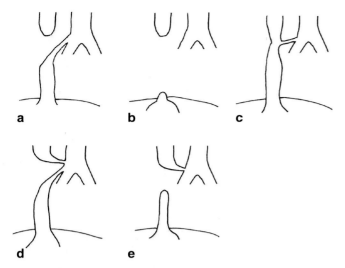

Fig. 3.1 Common anatomical variants of EA/TEF anomalies. **a** EA with distal TEF, **b** isolated EA with no TEF, **c** H-type TEF, **d** proximal and distal TEF, **e** EA with proximal TEF. (Reprinted with permission from [4], Fig. 2.1. *EA* esophageal atresia, *TEF* trache-esophageal fistula)

Most infants with "pure EA," that is, EA without TEF, and some infants with EA with TEF have a gap between the two ends of the esophagus that is too wide for primary anastomosis to be achieved. This group poses a particular surgical challenge. These infants are typically fed by gastrostomy initially, and the esophageal anastomosis is re-attempted after a period of growth (typically at least 6 weeks) during which the esophageal ends often grow closer together permitting anastomosis. If attempts at anastomosis remain unsuccessful, esophageal replacement such as by gastric transposition is considered.

Outcome

The majority of patients do well following anastomosis, but a number of complications may occur, and they require recurrent procedures. The most common surgical complication is anastomotic stricture. Strictures frequently require dilatation, and balloon dilatation is the preferred technique. Other complications include anastomotic leakage, recurrent TEF, gastroesophageal reflux, and disordered peristalsis. The combination of poor esophageal motility and gastroesophageal reflux with or without anastomotic stricture may lead to long-term feeding difficulties.

The Stomach

The most common abnormality of the stomach in the neonatal period is hypertrophic pyloric stenosis. Whether this is truly a congenital abnormality or an acquired disorder is questionable. It is further discussed in Chap. 4.

Other congenital conditions affecting the stomach including congenital microgastria, gastric volvulus, and congenital gastric outlet obstruction due to a pyloric web or atresia are all extremely rare and are mentioned only for completeness.

Obstructive Lesions of the Duodenum, Jejunum, and Ileum

The most common congenital conditions affecting the duodenum, jejunum, and ileum all result in partial or complete gastrointestinal obstruction. The presenting features and investigations recommended to diagnose the underlying abnormality are similar for all conditions. The clinical features and investigations of these conditions are therefore presented first followed by a description of each type of abnormality and the recommended treatment options.

Table 3.1 Classification of EA/TEF anomalies and frequency. (Reprinted with permission from [4], Table 2.1, and [3], Table 2 and 3, with permission from Elsevier)

Type of lesion	Frequency (%)
EA and distal TEF	88.8
Isolated EA	7.3
H-type fistula	4.2
Distal and proximal TEF	2.8
Proximal TEF	1.1

EA esophageal atresia, *TEF* trache-esophageal fistula

Table 3.2 Spitz classification of EA/TEF anomalies and outcome. (Reprinted with permission from [4], Table 2.2, and [3], Tables 2 and 3, with permission from Elsevier)

Group	Clinical features	Survival (%)
I	BW ≥ 1500 g with no major CHD	97
II	BW < 1500 g or major CHD	59
III	BW < 1500 g and major CHD	22

EA esophageal atresia, *TEF* trache-esophageal fistula, *CHD* congenital heart disease, *BW birth weight*

Clinical Features

Obstructive lesions of the small intestine from the pylorus down to the ileocecal valve may give rise to polyhydramnios in the antenatal period which is detectable by antenatal ultrasonography. As a general rule, the more proximal the lesion the more severe the degree of polyhydramnios, and distal ileal lesions may be present in the absence of polyhydramnios [5]. The list of differential diagnoses giving rise to polyhydramnios is however extensive. Another feature that may be seen on antenatal ultrasonography is the presence if dilated loops of intestine with or without echogenic bowel. While the combination of echogenic and dilated loops of bowel is often a sign of some form of intestinal abnormality, the precise nature of any problem is rarely identified before birth. One exception to this is a diagnosis of congenital duodenal obstruction in which case the appearance of a double bubble on antenatal ultrasonography has high sensitivity and specificity.

Following birth, the most common and important clinical manifestation of obstructive lesions of the GIT is bile-stained vomiting. Vomiting with truly bilious staining is always abnormal in the neonatal period and always requires investigation. Lesions in the duodenum and jejunum usually result in bilious vomiting within hours. In addition, the abdomen may appear empty or even scaphoid, and visible gastric peristalsis may be observed. Lesions lower in the ileum result in a distended abdomen if the obstruction is complete, and there may be failure to pass meconium. Obstructive lesions may also give rise to intestinal perforation in the neonatal period and occasionally antenatally. In all cases of neonatal intestinal obstruction, infants become progressively hypovolemic and are prone to circulatory and respiratory collapse. They require fluid resuscitation and may require ventilatory support. GIT obstruction should therefore be considered in any infant who is dehydrated especially if there is a history of vomiting.

Stenotic lesions of the small bowel in which the obstruction is incomplete may give rise to increased diagnostic difficulty. Affected infants may present with intermittent vomiting and episodes of partial obstruction. They eventually fail to thrive or develop complete obstruction at which stage they are fully investigated and the diagnosis becomes apparent.

Intestinal malrotation is considered separately as it may present with a spectrum of clinical scenarios depending on the degree of intestinal obstruction or midgut volvulus or both. The clinical pictures of all types of abnormal rotation are those of acute or chronic intestinal obstruction and/ or acute or chronic abdominal pain suggestive of intestinal ischemia. True malrotation typically presents in the first year of life with symptoms of upper GIT obstruction including vomiting which is usually bile-stained. A coexisting volvulus may be suspected by abdominal pain, peritonitis, and hypovolemic shock associated with intestinal ischemia. However, these signs may be relatively nonspecific in the young infant. Malrotation may also present later in life.

Investigations

The aim of investigating cases of suspected obstruction of the small intestine is twofold. First to identify the nature and anatomical location of the lesion to allow for planning of correct treatment and second to identify cases of malrotation in whom there is a risk of midgut volvulus and intestinal ischemia. These cases require urgent surgical intervention to reduce the risk of potentially catastrophic intestinal necrosis. The history and examination may give clues as to the location of the lesion as described above. An abdominal X-ray may simply confirm the presence of dilated intestinal loops but may also give further clues in some cases. A double bubble appearance on abdominal X-ray with a lack of air in the distal intestine (Fig. 3.2) is characteristic of duodenal obstruction. Multiple air-filled loops of proximal bowel often with air-fluid levels along with a paucity or complete absence of gas in the distal bowel is highly suggestive of obstruction of the ileum. Intestinal perforation if present will usually be apparent on abdominal X-ray, and in the rare cases of antenatal perforation, there may be widespread or localized flecks of calcification representing calcified meconium within the peritoneum.

In cases in which the diagnosis is not clear on abdominal X-ray or in which midgut malrotation or volvulus is suspected, a limited upper gastrointestinal contrast study is indicated. The classical finding in cases of malrotation is that the duodenojejunal flexure lies to the right side of the spine

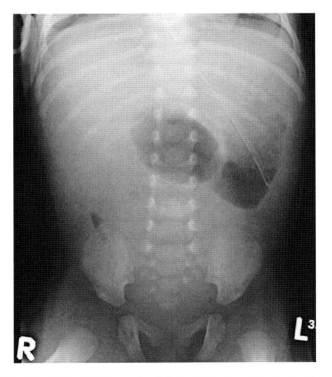

Fig. 3.2 Abdominal X-ray of an infant with duodenal atresia showing the "double-bubble" appearance characteristic of duodenal obstruction. (Reprinted with permission from [4], Fig. 2.2)

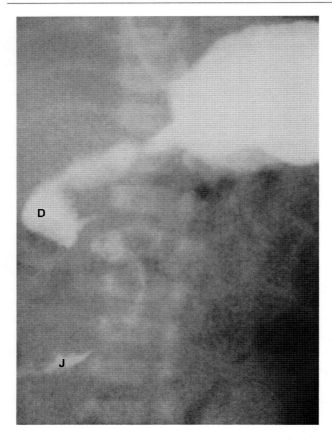

Fig. 3.3 Upper gastrointestinal contrast study of a case of malrotation. The contrast is seen within the duodenum (*D*) and flowing into the upper jejunum (*J*) both of which lie completely to the *right* of the midline. (Reprinted with permission from [4], Fig. 2.3)

instead of its normal left-sided position (Fig. 3.3). This finding should prompt urgent surgical treatment due to the risk of coexisting midgut volvulus. The contrast study may also identify the presence of a stenotic segment or complete obstruction.

Cases of lower ileal stenosis or atresia are often more difficult to diagnose, and a contrast enema is invaluable in distinguishing between ileal and colonic obstruction and could be therapeutic in cases of meconium ileus (see below).

Conditions Affecting the Duodenum

Duodenal atresia and duodenal stenosis both of which may be associated with an annular pancreas are the commonest congenital conditions to affect the duodenum. Both are capable of giving rise to duodenal obstruction. The incidence is reported to be between 1 in 5000 and 10,000 live births [6].

Explanations of the etiology of duodenal atresias are not universally accepted. Unlike atresias of the ileum, they are not thought to be due to vascular accidents, and the most widely accepted explanation is that of failure of recanalization of the intestinal lumen during early embryonic development.

Classification

There are four basic types of duodenal obstruction (Fig. 3.4). In type 1, there is a stenosis of the duodenum resulting from a diaphragm or web partially or totally occluding the lumen. Due to the incomplete nature of the obstruction, cases may present in childhood rather than in the neonatal period. In type 2 duodenal atresia, the proximal and distal segments end blindly but remain connected by a fibrous cord. There is complete separation of the bowel segments in type 3 and type 4 comprises an atretic segment with an annular pancreas. Multiple atresias are said to occur in up to 15 % of cases [7].

Treatment

The principles of treatment are to restore intestinal continuity while avoiding interference with the ductal system draining the pancreas and biliary tree. This is best achieved using a duodenostomy in which the obstructed segment is bypassed by joining the proximal segment directly to the distal segment. Following surgery, the long-term gastrointestinal results are good [8].

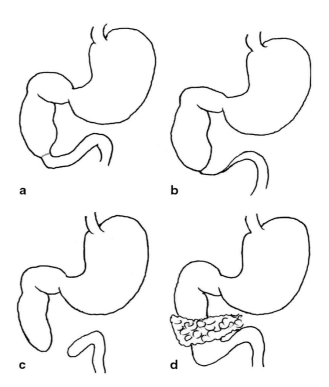

Fig. 3.4 Variants of duodenal atresia. **a** type 1 atresia due to an internal diaphragm, **b** type 2 atresia with blind-ending loops remaining connected by a fibrous cord, **c** type 3 atresia with blind ends completely separated, **d** type 4 duodenal obstruction with an annular pancreas. (Reprinted with permission from [4], Fig. 2.4)

Conditions Affecting the Ileum and Jejunum

The main congenital problems directly affecting the small intestine from the duodenojejunal flexure down to the cecum are atresia and stenosis. Jejunoileal atresia occurs more commonly than its duodenal counterpart with an incidence of varying from 1 in 330 to 3000 live births [9]. Such lesions are one of the most common causes of neonatal intestinal obstruction. The major difference between atresias of the ileojejunum and those of the duodenum is in their etiology. It is postulated that atresia or stenosis of the jejunum and ileum is the result of a localized vascular accident during intrauterine life. Subsequent ischemic necrosis and reabsorption of the affected segment or segments result in a contracted scarred bowel wall leading to stenosis at one end of the spectrum to a complete intestinal and mesenteric defect at the other. Fetal animal experiments have confirmed at least in part this hypothesis [10], and the absence of other congenital abnormalities found in association with jejunoileal stenoses and atresias supports the localized vascular accident theory.

Classification

Morphological classification of these lesions allows different surgeons and centers to compare outcomes, and it is also of therapeutic and prognostic value. The most commonly accepted system is that proposed by Louw [11] and modified by Grosfeld [12]. Whether the lesion is classified as ileal or jejunal is determined by the most proximal affected segment (Fig. 3.5).

Stenosis is a localized narrowing of the lumen without any break in the continuity or mesenteric defect. The intestinal wall may be thickened and rigid at the stenotic site, and there is a small, often minute lumen. The overall intestinal length is not shortened. Type I atresia is the result of a membranous web occluding the lumen with no mesenteric defect and no intestinal shortening. The lumen is usually completely occluded, and the proximal bowel therefore dilated but remaining in continuity with the collapsed distal segment. Type II atresia arises from a complete obliteration of the intestinal segment into a fibrous cord which joins two blind ends and runs in the free edge of the mesentery. There is no mesenteric defect, and once again, the total bowel length is usually normal. In both type III(a) and III(b) atresia, the intestine is likely to be shortened, and this may have significant clinical consequences. Type III(a) atresia consists of blind-ending proximal and distal bowel with no connection and an often large mesenteric defect. The blind ends are often physiologically abnormal with decreased or absent peristaltic activity which may give rise to torsion, distension, or perforation. Type III(b) atresia, also known as apple-peel atresia because of its gross morphology, may involve massive intestinal loss. It consists of intestinal atresia near the ligament of Treitz, obliteration of the superior mesenteric artery (SMA) beyond

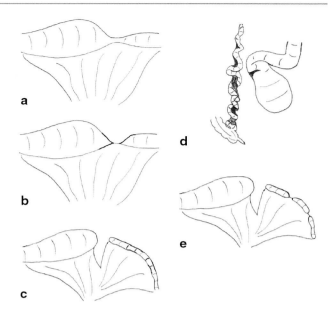

Fig. 3.5 Variants of ileal atresia. **a** type I due to an internal web (not shown) with no mesenteric defect, **b** type II atresia with blind ends joined by a fibrous cord, **c** type III(a)—blind ends separated with a mesenteric defect, **d** type III(b) in which the ileum is coiled like an "apple peel" around a single vessel and completely separated from the proximal dilated jejunum, **e** type IV or multiple atresias. (Reprinted with permission from [4], Fig. 2.5)

the origin of the middle colic branch, and the absence of the dorsal mesentery. The remaining intestine is coiled helically (like an apple peel) around a single perfusing vessel, often has impaired vascularity, and is almost inevitably short. Furthermore, there may be additional segments of type I or II atresia within the apple-peel segment. Such a configuration most likely arises from occlusion of the SMA due to thrombus, embolus, or strangulation as part of a midgut volvulus. In type IV atresia, there are multiple atretic segments, and the intestine may resemble a string of sausages. Overall, bowel length is usually shortened, and the intestine grossly dilated. It has been proposed that the etiology of type IV atresia may be due to failure of recanalization of solid epithelialization throughout the length of the intestine rather than from multiple single vascular events.

While it is generally accepted that stenosis and atresia of types I, II, and III(b) are the result of intrauterine vascular accidents, a genetic component has been suggested in type III(b) and IV.

Treatment

The mainstay of surgical treatment for this type of lesion is resection of the atretic or stenotic segment and primary anastomosis with closure of the mesenteric defect. The proximal intestinal segment is usually dilated and functionally abnormal with absent or ineffective peristalsis. This dilated proximal segment is excised along with a short segment distal to the stenosis or atresia. It is essential to establish patency of the distal bowel by irrigation or wash out intestine, and subsequently, a primary anastomosis is performed. There is a balance to be struck between the length of dilated proximal segment resected and the risk of leaving the infant with a short length of small bowel. As such, it is almost inevitable that the caliber of proximal bowel will be greater than that of the distal intestine, and a number of techniques exist to assist construction of the anastomosis in such circumstances.

Outcome following intestinal atresia is dependent primarily on the length of remaining intestine and the presence of the ileocecal valve. Short bowel syndrome has been defined as the presence of less than 75 cm of the small intestine or 30 % of the predicted intestinal length in a premature infant [13, 14]. Outcomes following short bowel syndrome vary, and there is a high level of dependence on parenteral nutrition. However, intestinal adaptation can occur such that more than 80 % of babies with short bowel syndrome do eventually become entirely enterally nourished [15].

Intestinal Malrotation

The incidence of intestinal malrotation is difficult to truly establish as not all affected patients develop symptoms, but autopsy studies estimate the incidence at approximately 1 in 500.

The traditional embryological basis for disorders of intestinal rotation is that of abnormal positioning of the intestinal loops in relation to one another as they return to the abdominal cavity from the yolk sac. During normal development, the midgut rotates through 270° so that the duodenum lies posterior to the colon, and the duodenojejunal flexure is to the left of the midline. A consistent finding in cases of malrotation is abnormal positioning of the duodenojejunal flexure. However, an alternative hypothesis has been proposed based on animal studies [16]. Kluth proposes that malrotation is the result of failure of localized growth of the duodenal loop rather than a disorder of rotation.

The term "malrotation" covers a spectrum of anatomical abnormalities. In non-rotation, the duodenojejunal flexure lies to the right of the spine along with most of the small intestine. The cecum and colon are typically on the left side of the abdominal cavity. Adhesions formed between loops of bowel or the intestine and abdominal wall are usually responsible for obstructive symptoms at presentation. In malrotation, the distribution of intestinal contents within the abdominal cavity is such that the duodenum again lies to the right of the spine with the cecum anterior to it. Adhesions between these two structures (Ladd's bands) are often present and may result in partial or total occlusion of the second part of the duodenum. In addition, the mesenteric attachment to the posterior aspect of the abdominal cavity is typically very short, and there is a risk of volvulus with ensuing intes-

tinal ischemia. Other forms of abnormal intestinal rotation (inversed rotation, malrotation with mesocolic hernia, and malposition of the cecum) are all rare.

Treatment

There are two aspects to this disorder which require surgical intervention. The first and most important aspect is that of midgut volvulus. Any infant in whom malrotation is suspected based on clinical findings and radiological investigations should undergo laparotomy as a matter of urgency in order to minimize the risk of intestinal ischemia due to a volvulus. At laparotomy, blood-stained peritoneal fluid may indicate the presence of ischemic intestine. Any volvulus should be derotated (usually in clockwise direction), and the intestine examined for viability. Nonviable bowel is resected, and a primary anastomosis performed. If there is doubt about the viability of remaining intestine, a second-look laparotomy can be performed after 24 h.

In cases of malrotation not complicated by volvulus, the procedure of choice for most surgeons is the Ladd's procedure. This involves division of all adhesions or adhesive bands between the cecum, duodenum, and parietal peritoneum, broadening of the mesenteric base around the SMA and repositioning of the intestine within the abdominal cavity such that the duodenum is on the right and the cecum lies in the left upper quadrant. Some surgeons recommend performing an appendicectomy due to the difficulties of diagnosis should appendicitis develop later in life.

Meconium Ileus

Meconium ileus is a common cause of neonatal intestinal obstruction and the commonest cause of antenatal intestinal perforation [17]. It should be included in the differential diagnosis of infants presenting with GIT obstruction. In approximately 80 % of cases, it is associated with cystic fibrosis, [18–20] an autosomal recessive disease affecting predominantly the lungs and pancreas. The underlying defect in cystic fibrosis, an abnormality in a transmembrane chloride channel, results in the production of abnormally viscid and sticky meconium. This meconium sticks to the intestinal mucosa causing intestinal obstruction usually occurring late in gestation. Why some infants with cystic fibrosis do not develop meconium ileus is unclear. Meconium ileus can be classified as: (1) "uncomplicated" when is limited to intraluminal obstruction caused by the abnormal meconium or (2) "complicated" when is associated with intestinal atresia, volvulus, or meconium peritonitis.

Clinical Features

In cases of uncomplicated meconium ileus, the infant usually presents shortly after birth with symptoms of lower gastrointestinal obstruction including abdominal distension and vomiting which may or may not be bile stained. The rectum may appear empty and narrow on plain radiograph, and the infant does not pass meconium. If meconium ileus is complicated by volvulus, intestinal ischemia, or perforation, the infant can be systemically unwell with acidosis and hypovolemic shock and may require ventilatory support. Abdominal X-ray showing dilated intestinal loops and occasionally abundance of meconium in the right lower quadrant are supportive of the diagnosis as is a gastrografin contrast enema revealing a small collapsed colon (microcolon) and often inspissated pellets of meconium in the right lower quadrant.

Treatment

In some cases, the gastrografin enema mentioned above may relieve the obstruction sufficiently to be curative. However, a number of uncomplicated cases and all complicated cases require surgery. The procedure performed depends on the findings during laparotomy. Atretic or grossly dilated segments of bowel may be resected, the inspissated meconium removed from the intestinal lumen, and the distal bowel flushed through. Occasionally, a stoma is formed to allow intestinal decompression. Outcome of surgical treatment is generally good, and gastrointestinal complications are of lesser significance than the pulmonary disease caused by the underlying cystic fibrosis.

Meckel's Diverticulum

Meckel's diverticulum is the commonest omphalomesenteric remnant with a reported incidence of approximately 2%. Of these, only a small proportion become clinically significant. The diverticulum originates from incomplete obliteration of the omphalomesenteric duct and exists as a free lying diverticulum on the anti-mesenteric border of the ileum.

Clinical Features

There are a variety of disease entities attributed to a Meckel's diverticulum including gastrointestinal hemorrhage, intussusception, diverticulitis, and perforation. The commonest presenting symptom is that of gastrointestinal bleeding due to excessive acid and pepsin production from ectopic gastric mucosa which may be present within the diverticulum. Bloody diarrhea in the absence of abdominal pain is the classical presenting picture. Other complications of Meckel's diverticulum are intussusception in which the diverticulum acts as a lead point, diverticulitis with symptoms similar to those of appendicitis, and perforation.

Treatment

Management of all clinically significant cases of Meckel's diverticulum is resection of the diverticulum after adequate preoperative resuscitation. At operation, the diverticulum and a wedge of ileum are resected. The ileal wedge is included as ectopic tissue may not be entirely confined to the diverticulum. Following surgical excision outcome is good.

Congenital Hepatic, Pancreatic, and Biliary Abnormalities

Abnormalities of the hepato-pancreato-biliary system are all quite rare. They are included here as knowledge of their existence is important as they form part of the differential diagnosis for infants with jaundice, malabsorption, and hypoglycemia.

The commonest lesions of the biliary tree are biliary atresia and congenital biliary dilatation. In biliary atresia, the biliary tree is obliterated either completely or partially. Congenital biliary dilatation describes a variety of abnormalities of the biliary tree in which the dilated segment may be either intrahepatic or extrahepatic and either fusiform or cystic in nature. Dilatations of the extrahepatic biliary ducts are commonly known as choledochal cysts. The dilated bile duct is both anatomically and functionally abnormal resulting in cholestasis. Infants with biliary atresia and severe cholestasis associated with biliary dilatation present in the neonatal period with prolonged jaundice due to accumulation of conjugated bilirubin. When the degree of obstruction to the biliary tree is not so severe, congenital biliary dilatation may present later in life with malabsorption, intermittent jaundice, abdominal pain, or even pancreatitis. In addition, a choledochal cyst may present as an upper abdominal mass. Treatment of these lesions is based on allowing drainage of the biliary tree into the intestine, and the surgery involved is often complex. The operation of choice for biliary atresia is the Kasai porto-enterostomy [21]. The atretic remnants of the extrahepatic biliary ducts are removed, and the porta hepatis is anastomosed to a defunctioned loop of jejunum. The timing of surgery is of paramount importance to avoid hepatocellular damage, but even with prompt diagnosis and early surgical intervention, infants with biliary atresia often have residual hepatic impairment due to intrauterine cholestasis. In cases of choledochal cysts, the dilated portion of the extrahepatic ducts is removed together with the gallbladder, and the common hepatic duct is anastomosed to the duodenum or a defunctioned loop of jejunum.

There are a number of congenital hepatic anomalies which give rise to structural and/or functional abnormalities of the liver parenchyma or the intrahepatic biliary tree. These include infantile and adult-type polycystic disease, congenital hepatic fibrosis, biliary hypoplasia, and congenital tumors of the liver such as hamartomas and hemangiomas. Presentation is usually with one of hepatomegaly, portal hypertension, or cholangitis. Treatment is that of resection of suitable lesions and prevention or treatment of hepatic disease.

Congenital lesions involving the pancreas are rare, the commonest being annular pancreas (see section on the duodenum). Other anatomical anomalies are seen including pancreatic ductal anomalies, pancreatic cysts, and very rarely pancreatic agenesis. There are a group of infants who present in the neonatal period with hypoglycemia who are found to have inappropriately high levels of circulating insulin. The condition hyperinsulinemic hypoglycemia (previously commonly referred to as "nesidioblastosis") is characterized by inappropriate endogenous insulin secretion in the presence of low blood glucose. It may result from an insulin-secreting tumor in the pancreas (a so-called insulinoma), but more commonly, no tumor is identified and the disease is a result of a genetic defect in a membrane channel controlling insulin secretion. Infants require high glucose intake to maintain normoglycemia while investigated for the presence of an isolated secretory tumor. Treatment is by surgical excision of the tumor if present; otherwise, a 90–95 % subtotal pancreatectomy is performed.

Conditions Affecting the Lower Gastrointestinal Tract

Hirschsprung Disease

Hirschsprung disease is the commonest congenital malformation of the enteric nervous system with an incidence of approximately 1 in 5000 live births [22–24]. While most cases are sporadic, a positive familial occurrence exists in 3.6–7.8 % of cases [25], and the presence of coexisting abnormalities including trisomy 21 suggests a genetic involvement. The condition is fully addressed elsewhere (see Chap. 22).

Anorectal Anomalies

Congenital abnormalities of the anorectal region occur with an incidence of 1 in 4000–5000 live births [26–28]. A very small minority may be familial with the majority being isolated findings or part of a congenital syndrome such as the VACTERL syndrome. There are a number of different types of anorectal anomalies resulting from the complex embryological development of the anorectal region involving differentiation of the cloaca. The Wingspread classification [29] divides them into high, intermediate, or low based on the relationship of the terminal bowel or any fistula arising from the bowel to the pelvic diaphragm. Precise definition of the abnormal anatomy is of paramount importance when planning corrective surgical treatment.

Clinical Features

Abnormalities of the anorectal region are usually diagnosed on inspection during the newborn period, but surprisingly, this is not always the case. In many cases, the anus will be absent, and meconium may be seen to originate from an abnormal site including a mucocutaneous fistula, the urethra in males, or the vaginal vestibule in females. Anomalies in which the anus is present but abnormally sited or stenosed may be more difficult to diagnose in the absence of adequate experience. The most complex abnormality in females is represented by the cloaca which is represented by a single opening in the perineum with rectum, vagina, and urethra joining a single channel.

Treatment

Treatment is aimed at preventing complications associated with the anomaly including urinary tract infection and lower gastrointestinal obstruction and subsequently restoring the anatomy to as near to normal functional and cosmetic state as possible. In the majority of cases, the initial surgery involves forming a colostomy in the descending or sigmoid colon to allow intestinal drainage and avoid dilatation of the lower bowel [30]. Following assessment, planning of surgery and growth of the infant reconstructive surgery is undertaken most commonly by the posterior sagittal approach [31]. Some anomalies also require a laparotomy to divide a high recto-vesical fistula. Surgery of these cases and particularly of cloaca is complex and should be performed by an experienced surgeon.

Outcome

In similarity to patients with Hirschsprung disease, incontinence and constipation are the most significant long-term complications of anorectal anomalies and often have a significant impact on quality of life. In one large series, soiling occurred in 57 % of 387 cases. The incidence of fecal incontinence was 25 % and constipation 43 % [31]. Ongoing medical and on occasion surgical treatment is necessary to minimize disruption to a normal lifestyle.

Conditions Which May Occur at Any Point in the Gastrointestinal Tract

Gastrointestinal Duplications

Duplication cysts of the GIT are rare congenital abnormalities. They can occur at any point in the GIT from mouth to anus, although they are most commonly found around the ileocecal region. Duplication cysts are defined according to strict criteria as devised by Ladd and Gross; they are closely attached to some part of the GIT, have a smooth muscle coat, and have an epithelial lining which resembles some part of the alimentary canal [32]. Duplications may be spherical or tubular in macroscopic appearance, those that are tubular accounting for 10–20 % and often having a communication with the bowel.

Clinical Features

Between 25 and 30% present in the neonatal period and most have presented by the age of 10 years. Clinical features at presentation depend on anatomical site, size, and secondary effects and include an oropharyngeal, abdominal or rectal mass, respiratory distress, gastrointestinal bleeding, obstruction, and intussusception. Duplication cysts may also be found as incidental findings at laparotomy, and some lesions have been detected on antenatal ultrasound [33, 34].

Treatment

The recommended management of duplication cysts is complete surgical excision wherever possible in order to prevent recurrence and complications secondary to ectopic gastric mucosa. When complete excision is not possible, it is essential to remove the mucosal lining.

Conditions Affecting the Walls of the Abdominal Cavity

While not truly conditions of the GIT, there are a number of conditions which cause the abdominal contents to develop outside the abdominal cavity. These conditions are included as they have secondary effects which may significantly affect the GIT and be a cause of gastrointestinal dysfunction.

Congenital Diaphragmatic Hernia

The incidence of congenital diaphragmatic hernia (CDH) varies from 1 in 3500 to 1 in 5000 live births [35]. Its etiology is unknown although is probably multifactorial. The essential anatomical defect is a breach in the continuity of the diaphragm which allows herniation of the abdominal viscera into the thoracic cavity. This has a secondary effect of impeding development of the lungs during intrauterine life. The resulting hypoplastic lungs are a cause of significant morbidity and mortality in this condition. Compression by misplaced abdominal contents does not explain the severity of lung disease seen, and it is well recognized that lung development is markedly abnormal in infants with CDH.

Classification

A number of different defects can occur owing to the complex development of the diaphragm. The majority of cases are of the Bochdalek type in which the defect is posterolateral and most commonly on the left side. The defect can range in size from a small slit to involve almost the entire hemidiaphragm. Defects in the central tendon of the diaphragm result in Morgagni hernias which are retrosternal in nature and most commonly on the right side. Finally, agenesis of the diaphragm may occur which is usually left sided and extremely rare.

Clinical Features

In the current era, diaphragmatic hernia is often diagnosed during prenatal ultrasound scanning. The advantage of prenatal diagnosis is that delivery can be planned to take place in a unit with appropriate pediatric surgical and intensive care facilities. For those infants who avoid prenatal diagnosis for whatever reason, the clinical features depend on the volume of abdominal contents within the thoracic cavity and the degree of lung hypoplasia. In the most severe cases, there will be severe respiratory distress and cyanosis from shortly after birth. At the other end of the spectrum are infants who have minimal if any respiratory symptoms or signs and in whom intestinal loops are noted to be in the abdomen on chest X-ray (Fig. 3.6).

Treatment

While the definitive treatment of diaphragmatic hernia is surgical closure, the timing of this is not of paramount importance and should be undertaken once the infant is stable from a cardiovascular and respiratory point of view. The respiratory management of these infants can be problematic due to the severe lung hypoplasia and associated pulmonary hypertension. Most require conventional ventilatory support as a minimum, and many require high-frequency oscillatory ventilation (HFOV) to ensure adequate oxygenation. Other measures to reduce pulmonary hypertension including inhaled nitric oxide, adenosine, or sildenafil may be effective. Resistant cases may be candidates for extracorporeal membrane oxygenation (ECMO), during which the infant is placed on a life support system in the hope that the lungs and in particular the pulmonary vasculature will mature. Various criteria for ECMO exist [36] with the aim of reserving it for those who have the most severe respiratory failure and those

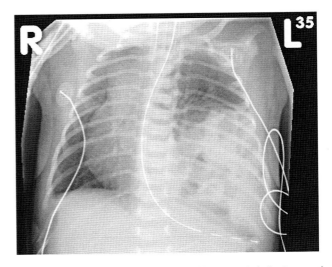

Fig. 3.6 Chest radiograph of an infant with congenital diaphragmatic hernia. Loops of intestine are clearly seen within the *left* hemithorax, and there is mediastinal shift to the *right*. (Reprinted with permission from [4], Fig. 2.7)

who are most likely to benefit. There remain unfortunately a number of infants with CDH whose lung disease presents too great a challenge, and they do not survive.

Surgery

The principles of surgical repair are to return the abdominal contents to the abdominal cavity and repair the diaphragmatic defect. It may be possible to repair the defect by simply suturing the edges together. However, if the defect is large, a patch repair may be undertaken using prosthetic material. The long-term outcome of CDH is dependent primarily on the degree of pulmonary hypoplasia. The main gastrointestinal consequence appears to be gastroesophageal reflux seen in up to 62 % of cases [37].

Anterior Abdominal Wall Defects

Although separate clinical entities, the two conditions exomphalos and gastroschisis which comprise anterior abdominal wall, defects are grouped together due to similarity in their clinical appearance and the recommended course of management. In both conditions, some portion of the viscera lies outside the abdominal cavity extruding through a defect in the anterior abdominal wall.

Exomphalos

The defect on the anterior abdominal wall in cases of exomphalos lies in the midline. Viscera herniate through this defect but remain contained within an avascular hernial sac consisted of peritoneum and amniotic membrane (Fig. 3.7). The size of the defect and hence the size of the sac may vary in size from a small swelling at the base of the umbilical cord (exomphalos minor) to a much larger sac containing liver and

a large proportion of the small intestine (exomphalos major). The embryological origins of exomphalos are believed to be failure of complete closure of the anterior abdominal wall around a persistent body stalk. Visceral contents continue to develop within this body stalk and thus remain outside the abdominal cavity. While the precise etiology of exomphalos is not clear, it is well recognized that exomphalos often coexists with a number of other congenital abnormalities, and this may suggest at least in part a genetic component. Associated abnormalities include Beckwith–Wiedermann syndrome, the trisomies 13, 18, and 21, and the upper and lower midline associations.

Gastroschisis

The anterior abdominal wall defect in cases of gastroschisis is full thickness and typically to the right of the umbilical cord. Unlike exomphalos, there is no sac covering the eviscerated intestine which is usually dilated and inflamed (Fig. 3.8). The liver is not herniated. The precise embryological basis of gastroschisis is unclear, and a number of hypotheses have been proposed. The fact that gastroschisis is rarely associated with any other congenital abnormalities—with the exception of intestinal atresias and malrotation—suggests that the events resulting in exomphalos are likely to have a separate embryological basis.

Treatment

It is now usual for these two abnormalities to be detected in the antenatal period, and delivery in a specialist center with pediatric surgical facilities is recommended. In gastroschisis, there is no convincing evidence to suggest that preterm or caesarean section delivery confers any distinct advantage [38–40] but delivery is commonly induced at around 37 weeks gestation to avoid late gestation fetal death. What is

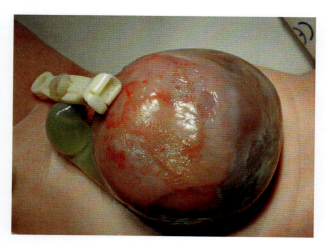

Fig. 3.7 Clinical appearance of an infant with exomphalos. The abdominal contents are enclosed within an avascular hernial sac. (Reprinted with permission from [4], Fig. 2.8)

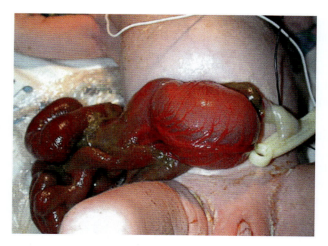

Fig. 3.8 Clinical appearance of an infant with gastroschisis. There is no sac enclosing the herniated intestine which is thickened and inflamed. (Reprinted with permission from [4], Fig. 2.9)

of paramount importance is protection of the intestine and prevention of fluid loss in cases of gastroschisis from the moment of delivery. The eviscerated intestine is wrapped in clingfilm and adequate support provided to prevent fluid loss and ischemic damage to the bowel. For exompahalos vaginal delivery is possible except in cases of exomphalos major. The hernial sac in exomphalos provides protection to the underlying bowel and surgical intervention is usually not emergent. However, cases of exomphalos in which the hernial sac ruptures during delivery should subsequently be treated as for gastroschisis.

Surgical Closure

The aim of surgery in both conditions is the return of abdominal contents to the abdominal cavity and closure of the overlying skin. In some cases, this can be achieved in one surgical procedure (primary closure), but in many instances, the abdominal cavity is not of sufficient volume to accommodate the eviscerated organs. In these cases, a staged closure is performed in which a "silo" is attached under the fascia around the base of the defect and completely encloses the eviscerated abdominal contents. This gives the intestine protection from dehydration and contains the bowel within a manageable sac reducing the risk of intestinal damage. Recently some surgeons have been preferentially using a silo for all cases of gastroschisis at least in part due to the belief that a more gradual return of the bowel to the abdomen may result in favourable outcomes [41–43]. The silo is gradually reduced in size as the abdominal cavity allows and the skin closed either in a final operation or using a technique of non-operative closure. In cases of exomphalos major, some surgeons elect not to reduce the viscera to the abdominal cavity in the newborn period but to allow the sac to epitheliase and perform fascial repair during childhood. Following abdominal wall closure there is a period of intestinal dysmotility which is much more pronounced in infants with gastroschisis. During this period nutrition is maintained using parenteral nutrition. The overall prognosis for infants with both these conditions in the absence of coexisting abnormalities is good.

References

1. Kyyronen P, Himminki K. Gastro-intestinal atresia in Finland in 1970–1979, indicating time-place clustering. J Epidemiol Community Health. 1988;42:257–65.
2. Myers NA. Esophageal atresia: the epitome of modern surgery. Ann R Coll Surg Engl. 1974;54(6):277–87.
3. Spitz L, Kiely EM, Morecroft JA, Drake DP. Oesophageal atresia: at-risk groups for the 1990s. J Pediatr Surg. 1994;29(6):723–5.
4. Hall N, Pierro A. Congenital problems of the gastrointestinal tract. In: Guandalini S, editor. Textbook of pediatric gastroenterology and nutrition. London: Taylor & Francis; 2004. pp. 13–28.
5. Pierro A, Cozzi F, Colarossi G, Irving IM, Pierce AM, Lister J. Does fetal gut obstruction cause hydramnios and growth retardation? J Pediatr Surg. 1987;22(5):454–7.
6. Sweed Y. Duodenal obstruction. In: Puri P, editor. Newborn surgery. 2nd ed. New York: Arnold; 2003. pp. 423–33.
7. Menardi G. Duodenal atresia, stenosis and annular pancreas. In: Freeman NV, Burge DM, Griffiths DM, Malone PSJ, editors. Surgery of the newborn. 1st ed. Edinburgh: Churchill Livingstone; 1994. pp. 107–15.
8. Stauffer UG, Irving I. Duodenal atresia and stenosis–long-term results. Prog Pediatr Surg. 1977;10:49–60.
9. Rode H, Millar AJW. Jejuno-ileal atresia and stenosis. In: Puri P, editor. Newborn surgery. 2nd ed. New York: Arnold; 2003. pp. 445–56.
10. Louw JH, Barnard CN. Congenital intestinal atresia: observations on its origin. Lancet 1955;2:1065.
11. Louw JH. Congenital intestinal atresia and stenosis in the newborn. Observations on its pathogenesis and treatment. Ann R Coll Surg Engl. 1959;25:209.
12. Grosfeld JL, Ballantine TV, Shoemaker R. Operative mangement of intestinal atresia and stenosis based on pathologic findings. J Pediatr Surg. 1979;14(3):368–75.
13. Rickham PP. Massive small intestinal resection in newborn infants. Hunterian Lecture delivered at the Royal College of Surgeons of England on 13th April 1967. Ann R Coll Surg Engl. 1967;41(6):480–92.
14. Touloukian RJ, Smith GJ. Normal intestinal length in preterm infants. J Pediatr Surg. 1983;18(6):720–3.
15. Hollwarth ME. Short bowel syndrome and surgical techniques for the baby with short intestines. In: Puri P, editor. Newborn surgery. 2nd ed. New York: Arnold; 2003. pp. 569–76.
16. Kluth D, Kaestner M, Tibboel D, Lambrecht W. Rotation of the gut: fact or fantasy? J Pediatr Surg. 1995;30(3):448–53.
17. Farber SJ. The relation of pancreatic achylia to meconium ileus. J Pediatr. 1944;24:387–92.
18. Del Pin CA, Czyrko C, Ziegler MM, Scanlin TF, Bishop HC. Management and survival of meconium ileus. A 30-year review. Ann Surg. 1992;215(2):179–85.
19. Fakhoury K, Durie PR, Levison H, Canny GJ. Meconium ileus in the absence of cystic fibrosis. Arch Dis Child. 1992;67(10 Spec No):1204–6.
20. Murshed R, Spitz L, Kiely E, Drake D. Meconium ileus: a ten-year review of thirty-six patients. Eur J Pediatr Surg. 1997;7(5):275–7.
21. Kasai M. Treatment of biliary atresia with special reference to hepatic porto-enterostomy and its modifications. Prog Pediatr Surg. 1974;6:5–52.
22. Passarge E. The genetics of Hirschsprung's disease. Evidence for heterogeneous etiology and a study of sixty-three families. N Engl J Med. 1967;276(3):138–43.
23. Orr JD, Scobie WG. Presentation and incidence of Hirschsprung's disease. Br Med J (Clin Res Ed). 1983;287(6406):1671.
24. Spouge D, Baird PA. Hirschsprung's disease in large birth cohort. Teratology. 1985;32:171–7.
25. Puri P. Hirschsprung's disease. In: Oldham TO, Colombani PM, Foglia RP, editors. Surgery of infants and children: scientific principles and practice. New York: Lippincott-Raven; 1997. pp. 1277–99.
26. Brenner EC. Congenital defects of the anus and rectum. Surg Gynecol Obstet. 1915;20:579–88.
27. Santulli TV. Treatment of imperforate anus and associated fistulas. Surg Gynecol Obstet. 1952;95:601–14.
28. Trusler GA, Wilkinson RH. Imperforate anus: a review of 147 cases. Can J Surg. 1962;5:169–77.
29. Stephens FD, Smith ED. Classification, identification and assessment of surgical treatment of anorectal anomalies. Pediatr Surg Int. 1986;1:200–5.

30. Patwardhan N, Kiely EM, Drake DP, Spitz L, Pierro A. Colostomy for anorectal anomalies: high incidence of complications. J Pediatr Surg. 2001;36(5):795–8.

31. Pena A. Anorectal anomalies. In Puri P, editor. Newborn surgery. 2nd ed. New York: Arnold; 2003. pp. 535–52.

32. Ladd WE, Gross RE. Surgical treatment of duplication of the alimentary tract; enterogenous cysts, enteric cysts, or ileum duplex. Surg Gynecol Obstet. 1940;70:295–307.

33. Duncan BW, Adzick NS, Eraklis A. Retroperitoneal alimentary tract duplications detected in utero. J Pediatr Surg. 1992;27(9):1231–3.

34. Goyert GL, Blitz D, Gibson P, Seabolt L, Olszewski M, Wright DJ, et al. Prenatal diagnosis of duplication cyst of the pylorus. Prenat Diagn. 1991;11(7):483–6.

35. Robert E, Kallen B, Harris J. The epidemiology of diaphragmatic hernia. Eur J Epidemiol. 1997;13(6):665–73.

36. UK Collaborative ECMO Trail Group. UK collaborative randomised trial of neonatal extracorporeal membrane oxygenation. Lancet 1996;348(9020):75–82.

37. Kieffer J, Sapin E, Berg A, Beaudoin S, Bargy F, Helardot PG. Gastresophageal reflux after repair of congenital diaphragmatic hernia. J Pediatr Surg. 1995;30(9):1330–3.

38. Quirk JG, Jr., Fortney J, Collins HB, West J, Hassad SJ, Wagner C. Outcomes of newborns with gastroschisis: the effects of mode of delivery, site of delivery, and interval from birth to surgery. Am J Obstet Gynecol. 1996;174(4):1134–8.

39. Dunn JC, Fonkalsrud EW, Atkinson JB. The influence of gestational age and mode of delivery on infants with gastroschisis. J Pediatr Surg. 1999;34(9):1393–5.

40. Sheth NP. Preterm and particularly, pre-labour cesarean section to avoid complications of gastroschisis. Pediatr Surg Int. 2000;16(3):229.

41. Jona JZ. The 'gentle touch' technique in the treatment of gastroschisis. J Pediatr Surg. 2003;38(7):1036–8.

42. Kidd JN, Jr., Jackson RJ, Smith SD, Wagner CW. Evolution of staged versus primary closure of gastroschisis. Ann Surg. 2003;237(6):759–64.

43. Schlatter M, Norris K, Uitvlugt N, Decou J, Connors R. Improved outcomes in the treatment of gastroschisis using a preformed silo and delayed repair approach. J Pediatr Surg. 2003;38(3):459–64.

Pyloric Stenosis

Shailee Sheth and Ashish P. Desai

Introduction

Pyloric stenosis is a common pediatric surgery emergency. It involves both narrowing and lengthening of the pylorus due to hypertrophy of the pylorus muscle. As this diagnosis is most often found in the first few months of life, it is often referred to as infantile hypertrophic pyloric stenosis (IHPS).

Hirschsprung first clinically described IHPS in 1888; however, it was much earlier in 1717 that Blair actually reported findings of pyloric stenosis following an autopsy [1]. In 1912, Ramstedt incidentally developed pyloromyotomy, which has remained the standard procedure for the treatment for more than a century.

Incidence

Incidence of IHPS is approximately 4/1000 live births, with a higher prevalence amongst the Caucasian population. Males appear to be affected much more commonly than females, at a 4:1 ratio. The condition is commonly seen between 3 and 12 weeks [2] and is rarely seen in babies over 6 months of age.

Anatomy

The pylorus is a muscle, which forms an anatomical connection between the stomach and the duodenum. It consists of two parts: the pyloric antrum and the pyloric canal, which connect to the body of the stomach and the initial part of the duodenum, respectively, allowing the passage of nutrients from the stomach to the small intestine, aiding the digestive process. Before the pyloric antrum, a pre-pyloric sphincter is positioned, which can constrict allowing the stomach to be shut as a private entity from the small intestine for brief seconds during peristaltic waves of activity. Additionally, at the end of the pyloric canal, a pyloric sphincter is located, which is fundamental to allow food to be digested from the stomach to the small intestine. The main function of the pylorus is to prevent food from re-entering the stomach once it has passed into the small intestine acting as a muscular valve.

The pyloric sphincter consists of circular smooth muscle, allowing the sphincters to contract and relax as required. As the content of the duodenum increases, this causes an increase in pressure, closing the pyloric sphincter, thus controlling the amount of food that is digested at any one time. A mucosal membrane underlines this sphincter, allowing gastric secretions to enter the pylorus further aiding digestion. As a general rule, the pylorus mainly refers to the pyloric sphincter, and therefore IHPS refers to a narrowing of the sphincter due to hypertrophy of the circular muscle. As hypertrophy occurs, this also causes the pyloric canal to lengthen and leads to a gastric outlet obstruction.

Histology

Under normal conditions, the pylorus, when viewed under a microscope, contains a number of features that allow for successful digestion. These include gastric pits and parietal cells, secreting gastric acid, as well as neuroendocrine cells to allow communication between the brain and gastrointestinal tract, enabling efficient contraction and secretion. Furthermore, Auerbach's plexus is implicated to play an important role in gut motility, by providing sympathetic and parasympathetic innervation to the muscular layers of the gut. However, during IHPS, it has been found that there is a degeneration of intramuscular ganglion cells in Auerbach's plexus, along with the accretion of lysosomes and cytoplasmic bodies in many of the axons [2]. Additionally, the ganglion cells appear reduced in number and smaller [3]. Cameron [4] has suggested that due to both the degeneration

A. P. Desai (✉) · S. Sheth
Department of Pediatric Surgery, King's College Hospital,
Denmark Hill London, SE5 9RS, UK
e-mail: ashishdesai@nhs.net

and consequent reduction in ganglia cells, Auerbach's plexus is ineffective, causing a reduction in neural activity, leading to asynchronous contraction of the pyloric muscle. As contractions are asynchronous, they increase in an attempt to produce a successful contraction, which is thought to lead to hypertrophy of the circular muscle, and hence IHPS.

Etiology and Risk Factors

Etio-Pathogenesis of pyloric stenosis is still not clearly understood. It is thought to be multifactorial with both environmental and genetic factors contributing towards the disease manifestation.

Genetic Factors

There appears to be a familial link for pyloric stenosis, but the specific genetic factors involved have not yet been identified. In a study conducted in Denmark in 2010, 1,999,738 children were studied in their first year of life, with findings of 3362 having IHPS. From the study, it was identified that, for a singleton, the incidence rate for IHPS was 1.8/1000, compared to 3.1/1000 live births in twins. Additionally, the rate ratio was 182 for monozygotic twins, compared to only 29.4 for dizygotic twins, illustrating a strong genetic link for IHPS. Overall, a heritability of 87 % for IHPS was found [5].

Nitric oxide synthase gene (NOS1) could be a susceptibility locus for IHPS [6]. As nitric oxide (NO) is involved in smooth muscle relaxation, NOS must catalyze the production of NO, to allow the pylorus muscle to relax. It is suggested that reduced levels of NOS lead to a reduction in NO and hence diminish smooth muscle relaxation. As a result, increased muscular contraction occurs, leading to hypertrophy. In further support of this theory, Huang et al. [7] generated mice lacking NOS. These mice were found to have enlarged stomachs and hypertrophy of the pyloric sphincter. These findings could have great implications for future non-surgical treatment of IHPS, as early interventions to increase NO production could lead to management, if not prevention, of the disease.

Other factors implying genetic component are male preponderance as well as four times increased risk of a child of a mother who had IHPS to be diagnosed with the condition, compared to the child of a father who had IHPS.

Environmental Factors

In addition to genetic factors, a number of environmental factors have been implicated as risk factors for IHPS. De-

spite the higher incidence in males and the familial heritability pointing to a genetic cause, the decreasing prevalence in some countries such as Denmark points to environmental factors also playing a role in the development of IHPS [4]. Maternal smoking leads to infants having an increased likelihood of developing pyloric stenosis, probably due to interference with mitochondrial oxidative phosphorylation and increase in the concentration of calcium in pylorus muscle, via an unknown mechanism, leading to increased contraction [8]. Nonetheless, more research into the causal mechanisms is still needed. Furthermore, it could be argued that the decrease in incidence of pyloric stenosis in Denmark (from 1.4/1000 to 1.1/1000 live births) may be related to a possible decrease in consumption of cigarettes in Denmark due to increased health warnings in the media.

A further environmental factor that has received plenty of research and promising results is that of feeding methods for babies. It has been implied that babies who are bottle-fed (with formula) are more likely to develop IHPS compared to those that are breast-fed.

Interestingly, Krogh et al. [9] conducted a study to compare feeding practices and identify their relationships, if any, with IHPS; 70,148 infants were involved in the study, and of that 65 had IHPS, 29 of which were bottle-fed for the first 4 months of life. When looking at the odds ratio, for those who were bottle-fed compared to breast-fed it was 4.62, indicating that babies who were bottle-fed were 4.62 times more likely to suffer from IHPS compared to those who were breast-fed. Furthermore, when comparing babies who were both breast- and bottle-fed to those who were never breast-fed, those who were never breast-fed had a higher risk of developing IHPS. Additionally, McAteer et al. [10], very recently found that, in a state in Washington, the incidence of pyloric stenosis had decreased from 14/10,000 to 9/10,000 whilst the likelihood of breast feeding had increased from 80 to 94 %, therefore, supporting the findings of Krogh et al. [11]. The exact reasons for this are unknown; however, it has been argued that breast milk contains a number of peptide hormones that relax the pylorus, such as vasoactive intestinal peptide (VIP), whereas formula milk has a higher gastrin content, which is thought to be involved in promoting smooth muscle contractions and could therefore be involved in pyloric muscle hypertrophy. However, these theories are still very tentative.

Other risk factors for pyloric stenosis are the first-born children (76.3 % risk if first child, 19.6 % if second), older maternal age, preterm delivery and caesarean section, amongst others [11]. Interestingly, it was also found that if these risk factors were reduced, it also reduced the incidence of pyloric stenosis occurring in males and made the prevalence between males and females much more similar.

Metabolic Changes in Pyloric Stenosis

A fluid electrolyte imbalance is usually present in individuals with IHPS. Classically, child presents with hypochloremic, hyponatremic metabolic alkalosis. Hydrochloric acid is lost, resulting in metabolic alkalosis due to the loss of hydrogen and chloride ions via vomiting (chloride-responsive metabolic alkalosis). Usually, the parietal cells of the stomach secrete H^+ ions via carbonic acid, which cross the lumen membrane to enter the stomach. These are then transported to the duodenum via the spasmodic contraction of the pyloric muscle. However, in pyloric stenosis, this passage of ions from the stomach to the duodenum is not possible due to the anatomical changes, consequently preventing the duodenum from secreting pancreatic bicarbonate that is usually stimulated by the hydrogen ions. This lack of hydrogen ions further adds to the metabolic alkalosis [12]. Selective absorption of H^+ ions in the renal tubules due to metabolic alkalosis leads to loss of Na^+ & HCO_3^- further increasing hypokalemia and hyponatremia.

In children with prolonged fluid loss and vomiting due to delayed diagnosis, kidneys try to compensate for the fluid loss by reducing urine output. However, the kidneys also prevent the loss of potassium ions initially followed by that of sodium ions, at the expense of hydrogen ions, due to a cation exchange. This causes a paradoxical aciduria. Hence, paradoxical aciduria is a sign of prolonged dehydration.

Clinical Features and Differential Diagnosis

The main symptom of this condition, distinguishing it from other gastrointestinal conditions, is that of non-bilious, projectile vomiting after feeding which progressively worsens. Milk often changes from being white to becoming an off-white, pale yellow colour, as it becomes curdled due to mixing with stomach acids whilst it remains stagnant in the stomach. The vomiting causes the metabolic changes of pyloric stenosis to manifest.

Additionally, infants with pyloric stenosis report feeling very hungry immediately after vomiting. Further symptoms relating to the inefficient digestion include a change in stools, with very small, insignificant stools being produced. The reduced intake of food and nutrients inevitably leads to severe weight loss.

The longer the condition progresses, the more severe the symptoms become. If not treated in time, infant is severely dehydrated and has decreased urine output.

Differential diagnosis of pyloric stenosis should include medical conditions like gastro-oesophageal reflux, sepsis, raised intracranial pressure, gastroenteritis and other metabolic conditions. Surgical conditions mimicking symptoms of pyloric stenosis are rare and include pyloric web and pyloric atresia.

Investigations and Diagnosis

A diagnosis of pyloric stenosis is made clinically based on the symptoms and metabolic changes at presentation. A test feed is the common term used for the process of diagnosis. This involves examination of the abdomen, whereby a small 'olive-sized' mass may be palpable in the epigastric region. This mass is the hypertrophic pylorus muscle, indicative of IHPS. Additionally, visible peristalsis in epigastrium is often present due to increased muscular contraction of the stomach and duodenum in an attempt to push food from the stomach to duodenum.

Imaging studies to confirm pyloric stenosis will most often include an ultrasound investigation to assess the level of thickening of the pylorus. On most occasions, a muscle wall thickness of more than 3 mm (usually between 3 and 8 mm) on ultrasound investigation is diagnostic of pyloric stenosis with an average of 5 mm thickness in most cases [13]. Furthermore, a pyloric canal length of more than 14 mm and pyloric diameter of more than 12 mm are set as the parameters for diagnosing IHPS [14] (Figs. 4.1 and 4.2).

However, in a recent article published in *the Permanente Journal,* it was inferred that these parameters can be misleading as both the height and weight of infants can alter the pyloric thickness, although the thickness may be less than 3 mm for an infant of lower than average weight pyloric stenosis may still be present. This study clearly illustrates the importance of taking all factors into account when making a diagnosis, rather than relying solely on imaging techniques. A positive correlation can be seen between both age and weight of the infant with thickness of pyloric muscle [15].

Occasionally, a barium swallow is done, in which a characteristic 'string sign' is found, illustrating the narrowing of the pylorus allowing very limited barium to travel from the stomach to the duodenum. Other signs present on a barium swallow include the 'shoulder sign' which occurs when the hypertrophied pyloric muscle indents into the pyloric antrum and the 'mushroom sign' in which the hypertrophied pyloric muscle indents into the initial part of the duodenum.

Treatment

Preoperative Management

On suspicion of pyloric stenosis, the child should be kept nil by mouth. A nasogastric tube should be inserted and kept on free drainage. All fluid losses should be replaced using normal saline with 10 mmol/l potassium.

Fig. 4.1 Pyloric stenosis ultrasound transverse view

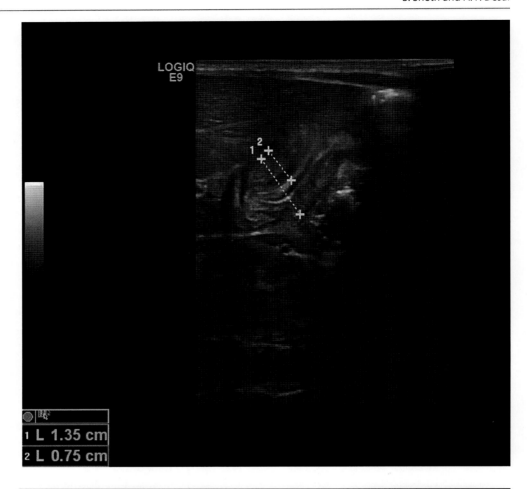

Fig. 4.2 Pyloric stenosis ultrasound longitudinal view

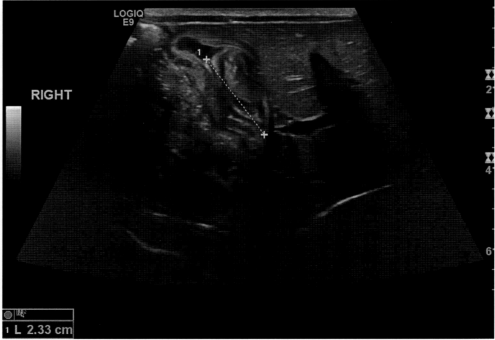

Fluid resuscitation usually using 5% dextrose with 0.45% saline should be used. The amount should be adjusted after assessing the amount of dehydration. Once urine output is established, 20 mmol/l of potassium should be added to IV fluid.

Surgical Treatment

Once the child is fully resuscitated, pyloromyotomy is the treatment of choice.

A pyloromyotomy is a simple procedure during which the hypertrophied pyloric muscle is cut longitudinally and then separated with the pyloric spreader. This releases the tension in the thick hypertrophied muscle and consequently allows the muscle to relax, relieving the stenosed muscle. This procedure is known as the Ramstedt's pyloromyotomy, as he initiated this technique of just spreading the muscle rather than doing pyloromyotomy.

Surgical approaches could be either by right upper transverse abdominal incision or the transumbilical pyloromyotomy, which involves a supraumbilical skinfold incision. Laparoscopic approach is also increasingly utilised. A number of studies have been conducted to establish the differences, if any, between the two. Nonetheless, most studies have suggested that both are effective, with different studies giving contradicting evidence on what form of procedure is more superior. In one study, it was suggested, however, that laparoscopic surgery is slightly superior in that babies are able to have a full feed in a shorter duration of time compared to open pyloromyotomy (18.5 versus 23.9 h), as well as having a shorter duration of stay in hospital [16]. However, in a study by Lemoine et al. in 2011 [17], it has been suggested that a transumbilical pyloromyotomy is associated with increased postoperative pain compared to the laparoscopic approach.

Complications

Most common complications of surgery include inadvertent opening of the mucosa and incomplete myotomy. Other complications include wound infection and self-resolving vomiting.

Complications of surgery are minimal, and in most cases, a pyloromyotomy is said to be very effective. Hulka et al. [18] reviewed 901 pyloromyotomies to assess for both intra- and postoperative complications, with findings that only 4 % of individuals had complications during surgery. The main complication was duodenal perforation. Further, 6 % of individuals had postoperative complications, which most often included vomiting, resolving itself within 5 days. As with many surgeries, wound infection is a further possible complication. An incomplete pyloromyotomy can also be listed as a complication.

Outcome

The death rate for pyloromyotomy is extremely low, at only 0.1 %. It usually does not have any long-term consequences.

References

1. Molenaar JC, Tibboel D, van der Kamp AW, Meijers JH. Diagnosis of innervation-related motility disorders of the gut and basic aspects of enteric nervous system development. Prog Pediatr Surg. 1989;24:173–85.

2. Dieler R, Schroder JM. Myenteric plexus neuropathy in infantile hypertrophic pyloric stenosis. Acta Neuropathol. 1989;78(6):649–61.

3. Nielsen JP, Haahr P, Haahr J. Infantile hypertrophic pyloric stenosis. Decreasing incidence. Dan Med Bull. 2000;47(3):223–5.

4. Cameron HC. Lumleian Lectures ON SOME FORMS OF VOMITING IN INFANCY: delivered before the Royal College of Physicians of London, March–April, 1925. Br Med J. 1925;1(3357):815–20.

5. Krogh C, Fischer TK, Skotte L, Biggar RJ, Oyen N, Skytthe A, et al. Familial aggregation and heritability of pyloric stenosis. JAMA 2010;303(23):2393–9.

6. Svenningsson A, Sodenhall C, Persson S, et al. Genome-wide linkage analysis in families with infantile hypertropic pyloric stenosis indicates novel susceptibility loci. J Hum Genet. 2012;57(2):115–121

7. Huang PL, Dawson TM, Bredt DS, Snyder SH, Fishman MC. Targeted disruption of the neuronal nitric oxide synthase gene. Cell 1993;75(7):1273–86.

8. Sorensen HT, Norgard B, Pedersen L, Larsen H, Johnsen SP. Maternal smoking and risk of hypertrophic infantile pyloric stenosis: 10 year population based cohort study. Br Med J. 2002;325(7371):1011–2.

9. Krogh C, Biggar RJ, Fischer TK, Lindholm M, Wohlfahrt J, Melbye M. Bottle-feeding and the risk of pyloric stenosis. Pediatrics 2012;130(4):943–9.

10. McAteer JP, Ledbetter DJ, Goldin AB. Role of bottle feeding in the etiology of hypertrophic pyloric stenosis. JAMA Pediatr. 2013;167(12):1143–9.

11. Krogh C, Gortz S, Wohlfahrt J, Biggar RJ, Melbye M, Fischer TK. Pre- and perinatal risk factors for pyloric stenosis and their influence on the male predominance. Am J Epidemiol. 2012;176(1):24–31.

12. Rose BD. Clinical Physiology of acid-base and electrolyte disorders. New York: McGraw Hill, 1994;94.

13. Rohrschneider WK, Mittnacht H, Darge K, Troger J. Pyloric muscle in asymptomatic infants: sonographic evaluation and discrimination from idiopathic hypertrophic pyloric stenosis. Pediatr Radiol. 1998;28(6):429–34.

14. Hussain M. Sonographic diagnosis of infantile hypertrophic pyloric stenosis- use of simultaneous grey-scale & colour doppler examination. Int J Health Sci (Qassim). 2008;2(2):134–40.

15. Said M, Shaul DB, Fujimoto M, Radner G, Sydorak RM, Applebaum H. Ultrasound measurements in hypertrophic pyloric stenosis: don't let the numbers fool you. Perm J. 2012;16(3):25–7.

16. Hall NJ, Pacilli M, Eaton S, Reblock K, Gaines BA, Pastor A, et al. Recovery after open versus laparoscopic pyloromyotomy for pyloric stenosis: a double-blind multicentre randomised controlled trial. Lancet 2009;373(9661):390–8.

17. Lemoine C, Paris C, Morris M, Vali K, Beaunoyer M, Aspirot A. Open transumbilical pyloromyotomy: is it more painful than the laparoscopic approach? J Pediatr Surg. 2011;46(5):870–3.

18. Hulka F, Harrison MW, Campbell TJ, Campbell JR. Complications of pyloromyotomy for infantile hypertrophic pyloric stenosis. Am J Surg. 1997;173(5):450–2.

Christophe Dupont, Nicolas Kalach and Véronique Rousseau

Abbreviations

GER	Gastroesophageal reflux
GERD	Gastroesophageal reflux disease
NEC	Necrotizing enterocolitis
GI	Gastrointestinal
VLBW	Very low birth weight
GA	Gestational age
PPI	proton pump inhibitors
SIDs	Sudden infant deaths
DIC	Disseminated intravascular coagulation
SBS	Short bowel syndrome
NICU	Neonatal intensive care unit
MI	Meconium ileus
CF	Cystic fibrosis
EA	Esophageal atresia
TEF	Tracheoesophageal fistula

Gastrointestinal Problems of Term Babies

Normal feeding is essential to the growth and development of newborns: They are able to eat, digest food, and absorb nutrients, with normal bowel movements after being fed. Difficulties may occur, meaning a temporary adjustment or suggesting a more serious problem. Symptoms indicating gastrointestinal (GI) problems need to be recognized.

C. Dupont (✉) · N. Kalach
Department of Pediatric Gastroenterology and Nutrition,
Necker—Enfants malades Hospital, Paris Descartes University,
AP-HP, 149, rue de Sèvres, Paris 75015, France
e-mail: christophe.dupont@nck.aphp.fr

N. Kalach
Department of Pediatrics, Saint Antoine Pediatric Clinic, Saint Vincent de Paul Hospital, Groupement des Hôpitaux de l'Institut Catholique de Lille (GH-ICL), Catholic University, Lille, Nord, France

V. Rousseau
Department of Pediatric Surgery, Necker—Enfants malades Hospital, Paris Descartes University, AP-HP, Paris, France

Difficult Feeding

The clinical evaluation of a neonate with complex issues related to feeding and swallowing includes a physical examination and feeding observation. Instrumental assessments of swallowing may be needed when concerns are noted regarding pharyngeal phase physiology and risks for aspiration with oral feeding. An interdisciplinary approach is often needed. Feeding difficulties may herald more severe and general disorders, listed in Table 5.1 [1]. Some diseases need urgent treatment. Hypothyroidism is diagnosed through a blood sample (low T3 and T4 and high TSH). Prader–Willi syndrome is characterized by hypotonia in an otherwise normal child and may require tube feeding at the beginning. Among a variety of craniofacial syndromes, Pierre Robin syndrome is characterized by retrognathism, glossoptosis, and sometimes cleft palate, with difficulties in breathing and swallowing which need immediate prevention measures such as lying in prone position and tube feeding [1].

Gastroesophageal Reflux

Gastroesophageal reflux (GER) occurs when stomach contents backs up into the esophagus.

GER is most of the time benign, due to high volume inside the stomach and/or temporary cardial insufficiency, and manifested only by regurgitations, spitting up, and dribbling milk with burps or after feedings, without any other symptoms, especially pain. This situation characterizes the "happy spitters." These babies may be helped with feeding of smaller amounts and more frequent, burping the baby often during the feedings, holding the baby in an upright position for about 30 min after feeding, and making sure that the baby's diaper is not too tight. When the child is not breast-fed, using an infant formula enriched with food thickeners may also help [2].

GER may also be more severe. Several symptoms can be related to neonatal gastroesophageal reflux disease (GERD), Table 5.2. After feeding, there may be forceful or projectile

© Springer International Publishing Switzerland 2016
S. Guandalini et al. (eds.), *Textbook of Pediatric Gastroenterology, Hepatology and Nutrition,*
DOI 10.1007/978-3-319-17169-2_5

Table 5.1 Disorders that affect hunger/appetite, food-seeking behavior, and ingestion in newborn infants

Anatomic abnormalities of the oropharynx
Anatomic/congenital abnormalities of the larynx and trachea
Anatomic abnormalities of the esophagus
Disorders affecting suck–swallow–breathing coordination
Disorders affecting neuromuscular coordination of swallowing
Disorders affecting esophageal peristalsis
Mucosal infections and inflammatory disorders causing dysphagia
Other miscellaneous disorders associated with feeding and swallowing difficulties, for example, xerostomia, hypothyroidism, trisomy 18 and 21, Prader–Willi syndrome, allergies, lipid and lipoprotein metabolism disorders, and a variety of craniofacial syndromes

Table 5.2 Symptoms of neonatal gastroesophageal reflux disease (GERD)

Typical or atypical crying and/or irritability
Sleep disturbances
Apnea and/or bradycardia
Poor appetite; weight loss or poor growth (failure to thrive)
Apparent life-threatening event
Vomiting
Hematemesis and/or melena
Recurrent pneumonitis and/or pulmonary atelectasis
Severe laryngomalacia

vomiting or spitting up of large amounts of milk. Reflux may also lead to esophageal irritation by the stomach contents, that is, esophagitis. When the stomach content reaches the pharyngeal regions, it can be aspirated into the lungs, a phenomenon recognized by "rattling," heard and felt in the baby's chest and back. Babies may also gag and choke during feedings.

GERD may be primary, related to several mechanisms mainly of motor origin [2]. Variations during sleep and wakefulness suggest the involvement of autonomic nervous activity changes [3]. Signs and symptoms of GERD traditionally attributed to acidic reflux in neonates do not seem to be significantly altered by proton pump inhibitors (PPI) treatment. In a study, esomeprazole was well tolerated and reduced esophageal acid exposure and the number of acidic reflux events in neonates [4].

GERD may also be secondary, related to either medical of surgical disorders, Table 5.3. Food allergy dominates, especially for milk, to which the child may react either in infant formulas or in breast milk [5, 6]. Diagnosis is based on elimination diets using milk-free infant formulas or cow's milk elimination in mother's diet, since allergy testing is rarely positive at this age [5, 6]. The neonatal period remains a critical period for diagnosing conditions leading to vomiting, such as neonatal medical or surgical conditions. The latter must be kept in mind despite the wide use of prenatal diagnosis.

Table 5.3 Secondary neonatal gastroesophageal reflux disease (GERD)

Medical disorder:
Milk allergy, in formula-fed infants or to milk ingested by mothers in breast-fed children
Other food allergy
Surgical conditions:
Esophageal atresia
Hiatal hernia
Diaphragmatic hernia
Omphalocele
Gastroschisis
Other rare causes of neonatal intestinal obstructions

Diarrhea

In a newborn, the first bowel movements expel meconium, a sticky, greenish-black substance that forms in the intestines during fetal life. Yellow stools appear after the first few days. In breast-fed babies, stools tend to be soft, seedy, yellow-green, often as every few hours with feedings and at least several times a day. In formula-fed babies, stools are yellow and formed and occur once or twice a day.

In a baby with diarrhea, stools are watery, very loose, and occur very frequently. Signs of cramping are absent or difficult to perceive. Different causes may be considered, as indicated in Table 5.4 [7]. Diarrhea may reveal neonatal-onset Crohn's disease and intractable ulcerating enterocolitis [8] or neonatal enteropathies [9]. Several viral infections may be responsible, such as cytomegalovirus even in immuno-competent babies [10]. Other viruses may be involved [11], such as adenoviruses [12], parechoviruses [13], rotavirus, norovirus, astrovirus, and some infections being potentially associated with necrotizing enterocolitis (NEC) [11].

Diarrhea in a newborn can quickly lead to severe dehydration and thus needs immediate oral rehydration. The European Society for Pediatric Gastroenterology, Hepatology, and Nutrition (ESPGHAN) solution contains 60 mOsm/L of Na and is recommended for children of Europe, but it seems to be effective in children living in developing countries

Table 5.4 Frequency, etiology, and current management strategies for diarrhea in newborn infants [7]

Food allergy (20.5%)
Gastrointestinal infections (17.9%)
Antibiotic-associated diarrhea (12.8%)
Congenital defects of ion transport (5.1%)
Withdrawal syndrome (5.1%)
Hirschsprung's disease (2.5%) and parenteral diarrhea (2.5%)
Cystic fibrosis (2.5%)
Metabolic disorders (2.5%)
Incidence 6.72 per 1000 hospitalized child, 39 cases of diarrhea (36 acute, 3 chronic); 3 patients died

[14]. Maintenance of breast feeding in breast-fed infants is always recommended.

Constipation

Constipation is characterized by rare bowel movements, less than once a day, sometimes less than once every 3 or more days. Generally, stools are very compact and free from moisture, appearing as hard balls or pebbles. Signs of discomfort or pain are frequent, quick drawing up of the legs, accompanied by a red-faced grunting as baby attempts to have a bowel movement. Examination of a constipated newborn needs checking the quality of feeding, the presence of abdominal distension, and gently analyzing the anal region.

Delay in passing meconium, abdominal distension, and low weight gain suggest or are associated with organic disturbances, such as Hirschsprung's disease, often requiring a specific surgical procedure. Other severe presentations may need medical treatment such as meconium ileus (MI) (see below) [15].

Functional constipation is the more likely. Breast-feeding newborn babies may pass 3–4 bowel movements per day within the first 2 weeks. The bowel movements of bottle-fed babies may be a bit less frequent. Apply a small dab of lubricating gel on baby's anus to protect the sensitive area and allow stool to pass a bit easier. Avoid using mineral oil as a lubricant.

Anal fissures are possible even in neonates, in the form a small tear in the anus. When limited, anal fissures may occur from baby forcing the passage of hard stool, usually with recurrent straining. Anal fissures may be associated with milk allergy [16]. What appears as a larger anal fissure may be an anomaly of the anal regions participating in the process of anorectal malformations and requiring a surgical procedure.

Colic

Colic is a problem that affects many babies during the first 3–4 months of life, starting typically by 3 weeks of age but sometimes much earlier. It is defined as prolonged or excessive crying in an infant whose examination is normal, often associated with gas, irritability, and sleeping disorders. The crying can be very loud, can last for several hours a day, and predisposes to the shaken baby syndrome [17], hence the necessity for appropriate handling. What causes colic is still unclear. Studies show an increased fecal content of calprotectin [18] a marker of an intestinal inflammation, thereby suggesting a physiological inflammation during the first months of life. Another possible reason for excessive crying in babies might be that they are oversensitive to gas in the intestine, similarly to what is observed in older children

during irritable bowel syndrome, although this disorder is lacking evidence-based approaches [19]. Milk allergy is also possible, thus leading to a trial elimination diet using cow's milk protein hydrolysates [6].

GI Problems of Preterm Infants

Feeding Difficulties

Digestive tolerance of preterm infants is one of the major problems of neonatal wards. Preterm infants have the paradoxical situation of a considerable demand in nutrients contrasting with a low digestive tolerance, owing to immaturity of the digestive tract, low oral sucking, and swallowing maturity, and with the need to interrupt as soon as possible parenteral feeding to reduce the infectious and metabolic risks and to introduce progressively enteral feeding to enhance the digestive tube maturity [20]. Although incompletely understood, difficulties that preterm infants face in the neonatal intensive care unit (NICU) may be related to the potential consequences of an immature intestinal barrier defense and bacterial colonization disturbances [21]. What is at stake in this age range is the need to increase as far and as rapidly as possible the rate of enteral feeding with the constant need to avoid GI signs of bad tolerance, especially trying to avoid NEC.

Progressive Increment of Oral Feeding in Premature Infants

Premature infants of gestational age (GA) >34 weeks are usually able to coordinate sucking, swallowing, and breathing, and so establish breast or bottle feeding. In less mature infants, oral feeding may not be safe or possible because of neurological immaturity or respiratory compromise [20]. In these infants, milk can be given as a continuous infusion or as an intermittent bolus through a fine feeding catheter passed via the nose or the mouth to the stomach [22]. In older babies, around 34 weeks of GA, the infant begins to suckle, and the bottle progressively replaces the tube feeding.

Several Cochrane reviews [23–26] confirm that the introduction of enteral feeding for very preterm infants, that is, less than 32 weeks of GA or very low birth weight (VLBW) <1500 g infants, is often delayed due to the bad clinical tolerance of early enteral introduction and may increase the risk of developing NEC. However, the available trial data suggest that introducing progressive enteral feeding before 4 days after birth and advancing the rate of feed quantities at more than 24 ml/kg/day do not increase the risk of NEC in very preterm infants and VLBW infants [23–26]. In contrast, prolonged enteral fasting may diminish the functional adaptation of the immature GI tract and extend the need for parenteral nutrition with its attendant infectious and metabolic risks [26]. Also, delayed introduction or slow advancement of enteral feeding results in several days of delay in the time taken to regain birth weight and establish full enteral feeds [26]. Trophic feeding, giving preterm infants very small quantities of adapted preterm milk formulas to promote intestinal maturation, may enhance feeding tolerance and decrease the time taken to reach full enteral feeding independently of parenteral nutrition [23–26]. Although it is well agreed that oral feeding should be initiated slowly first by the help of nasogastric tube and then progressively followed by oral feeding, the way in which the preterm infants are introduced and advanced varies widely. The use of dilute formula in preterm or VLBW infants might leads to an important reduction in the time taken for those infants to achieve an adequate daily energy intake [27]. Uncertainty also exists about the risk–benefit balance of different enteral feeding strategies in human milk-fed versus formula-fed very preterm or VLBW infants as the trials and reviews did not contain sufficient data for subgroup analyses [26].

Gastroesophageal Reflux

GER is very common among preterm infants, due to several physiological mechanisms. Its real frequency in preterm and VLBW infants is not well established. The responsibility of GER is suspected in the occurrence of apnea, bradycardia, pallor, cyanosis with or without oxygen desaturation, severe malaise, feeding difficulties with weight loss or poor growth (failure to thrive), crying, hematemesis, melena, and finally sudden infant deaths (SIDs) [2], although GER could be diagnosed for extra-digestive manifestations by 24-h pH-metry monitoring and for digestive manifestations by upper GI endoscopy with specific neonatal endoscopes [28].

The therapeutic management of GER still represents a controversial issue among neonatologists. Overtreatment, often unuseful and potentially harmful, is increasingly widespread. Hence, a stepwise approach, firstly promoting conservative strategies such as body positioning (the best position is the ventral decubitus associated with a 30° of orthostatism position under continuous monitoring in the NICU) or changes of feeding modalities, should be considered the most advisable choice in preterm infants with GER [2]. Non-pharmacological management of GER might represent a useful tool for neonatologists to reduce the use of anti-reflux medications, that is, prokinetics and anti-H2 blockers or PPI, which should be limited, due to their side effects, to selected cases of severe symptomatic infants [29].

Enteropathy

In neonatal units, there is a tendency to assume that any acutely sick infant with gastrointestinal symptoms has NEC. All digestive issues however are not related to as a matter of fact; a better definition of enteropathy in preterm neonates and their risk factors need to be done. Neonatal enteropathy is considered in the presence of feeding difficulties, increased gastric residual, abdominal distension associated with sensitive and/or surgical abdominal examination, and rectal bleeding with bloody stool (hemorrhagic recto-colitis). Sometimes, preterm infants present with sub-occlusion (transient) or complete permanent occlusion syndrome.

In a prospective study by Suc et al. [30], 351 preterm infants admitted to a neonatal ward were fed similarly, depending on their maturation, GA, and GI status; 53 developed GI symptoms: 23 transient obstructions, 6 NEC, and 24 hemorrhagic colitis. Ten risk factors were found to be significantly correlated with GI disturbances: umbilical venous catheter, benzodiazepines, birth weight <1.500 g, patent ductus arteriosus, ventilatory assistance, abnormal amniotic fluid, GA <32 weeks, early antibiotic treatment, passage of meconium >48 h, and episodes of apnea and/or bradycardia. GI problems might thus be separated into three groups: (1) isolated intestinal obstruction, seen in the most immature babies during the first week of life with the risk of developing NEC; (2) frank blood in the stool, indicating colitis and possibly minor forms of NEC; (3) combined obstructive and hemorrhagic symptoms, typical of NEC.

The diagnosis of enteropathy relies on clinical examination associated with biological parameters (complete blood count, C-reactive protein, and bacteriological cultures) and radiological exploration (abdominal X-ray and/or ultrasonography).

Specific treatment is offered according to diagnostic work-up analysis, that is, enteral and/or parenteral nutritional assistance as well as antibiotics treatment and sometimes acute life-threatening events supports.

Necrotizing Enterocolitis

Background of Prematurity and NEC

NEC is a devastating GI disease dominating in preterm infants. The pathogenesis, likely multifactorial, is incompletely understood. At this age, infants experience multiple perturbations to normal postnatal intestinal and immune development, all of which increase their vulnerability to NEC. The prevalence is increased in formula-fed infants, suggesting protection by the bioactive compounds of breast milk. The intestinal microbiota profiles observed during NEC as compared to control infants, suggests a lack of benefits from commensal bacteria and an increased risk of intestinal inflammation and bacterial translocation by pathogenic bacteria [31]. NEC incidence also seems reduced by prebiotics and probiotics and increased after prolonged antibiotics exposure use leading to delayed bacterial colonization, with preference for pathogenic microorganisms. H2-blocker or PPI, decreasing gastric acidity, might dampen one component of the first-line defense against pathogenic antigens provided by intestinal tract [32].

The role of Toll-like receptor-4 (TLR4) is likely to be critical in the postnatal susceptibility to NEC of preterm infants [33]. In animal models, the absence of TLR4, such as in TLR4 knockout mouse, prevented the development of NEC [34]. Downregulation of TLR4 suppresses downstream pro-inflammatory signaling, such as observed with postnatal intestinal bacterial colonization by commensal organisms, whereas TLR4 activation increases pro-inflammatory signaling. TLR4 activation might also mediate other downstream pathways and reduce the epithelial cells capacity for regeneration and proliferation [35].

Signs and Symptoms

NEC affects typically premature infants, with a timing of onset generally inversely proportional to the GA of the child. Initial symptoms include feeding intolerance, increased gastric residuals, abdominal distension, and bloody stools. Symptoms may progress rapidly to abdominal discoloration with intestinal perforation and peritonitis and systemic hypotension requiring intensive medical support [36].

Diagnosis

The diagnosis is usually suspected clinically but often requires the aid of diagnostic imaging modalities. Radiographic signs of NEC include dilated bowel loops, paucity of gas, a "fixed loop" (unaltered gas-filled loop of bowel), pneumatosis intestinalis, portal venous gas, and pneumoperitoneum (extra-luminal or "free air" outside the bowel within the abdomen). More recently, ultrasonography has proven to be useful as it may detect signs and complications of NEC before they are evident on radiographs [37]. Recently, fecal biomarkers, such as fecal calprotectin, have been tested as noninvasive markers for diagnosis and follow-up [38, 39].

Three stages exist:

Stage 1: Apnea, bradycardia, lethargy, abdominal distension, and vomiting

Stage 2: Pneumatosis intestinalis and the above features

Stage 3: Low blood pressure, bradycardia, acidosis, disseminated intravascular coagulation (DIC), and anuria

Treatment

Primary treatment consists of supportive care. Bowel rest is obtained by stopping enteral feeds, intermittent suction to obtain gastric decompression, fluid repletion to correct electrolyte abnormalities and third space losses, adapted support for blood pressure, parenteral nutrition, and prompt antibiotic therapy. Monitoring is clinical, although serial supine and left lateral decubitus abdominal roentgenograms should be performed every 6 h. Where the disease is not halted through medical treatment alone, or when the bowel perforates, immediate emergency surgery to remove the dead bowel is generally required. Surgery may require a colostomy, which may be able to be reversed at a later time. Some children may suffer later as a result of short bowel syndrome (SBS) if extensive portions of the bowel had to be removed.

Prevention

The American Academy of Pediatrics, in a 2012 policy statement, recommended feeding preterm infants human milk, finding "significant short- and long-term beneficial effects," including lower rates of NEC. Meta-analyses of four randomized clinical trials performed over the period 1983–2005 support the conclusion that feeding preterm infants human milk is associated with a significant reduction (58%) in the incidence of NEC. A more recent study of preterm infants fed an exclusive human milk diet compared with those fed human milk supplemented with cow-milk-based infant formula products noted a 77% reduction in NEC [40].

A study demonstrated that using a higher rate of lipid (fats and/or oils), infusion for preterm or VLBW infants in the first week of life resulted in zero infants developing NEC in the experimental group, compared with 14% with NEC in the control group [41].

Neonatologists from NICU reported on the importance of providing small amounts of trophic oral feeds of human milk starting, while the infant is being primarily fed intravenously, to prime the immature gut to mature and become ready to receive greater oral intake [40]. Human milk from a milk bank or donor can be used if mother's milk is unavailable [40]. Finally, probiotic and prebiotic supplementation is a promising approach for the prevention of NEC in preterm and VLBW infants [42].

Typical recovery from NEC if medical, nonsurgical treatment succeeds includes 10–14 days or more without oral intake and then demonstrated ability to resume feedings and gain weight. Recovery from NEC alone may be compromised by comorbid conditions that frequently accompany prematurity. Long-term complications of medical NEC include bowel obstruction, anemia, and SBS.

Meconium Ileus

Definition and Etiology

MI results from an intra-luminal intestinal obstruction produced by thick inspissated meconium. Most patients have cystic fibrosis (CF) disease (90% of cases), others having a history of isolated simple MI. The abnormal meconium is very dry, contains higher-than-usual concentrations of protein, and adheres firmly to the mucosal surface of the distal small bowel, creating an intra-luminal obstruction [43]. This leads to poor intestinal motility, low-grade obstruction, distended loops without air fluid levels. Associated risk factors are severe prematurity and low birth weight, caesarean delivery, maternal MgSO$_4$ therapy, and maternal diabetes. The incidence of MI has shown to increase while its management continues to be challenging and controversial for the risk of complicated obstruction and perforation [44].

Diagnosis

MI is usually manifested by intestinal obstruction. This situation is more common in the very preterm and VLBW infants than preterm infants more than 32-week GA. Clinically, in an otherwise healthy-appearing infant, abdominal distension is visible in the first 12–24 h of life, without meconium elimination in the first 48 h. Physical examination reveals firm palpable masses throughout the abdomen without real surgical signs. There may be feeding difficulties with increased gastric residuals but without vomiting.

MI may be complicated in utero by volvulus, atresia, perforation, and meconium peritonitis, in 30–50% of the cases. When infants born with those complications, infants appear sicker, with often vomiting and signs of neonatal sepsis and more marked abdominal distension causing respiratory distress.

Radiological examination shows dilated bowel loops, and the viscous nature of meconium produces a "ground-glass" appearance. Perforation after birth results in free intraperitoneal air. Newborns suspected of MI or any other distal bowel obstruction are diagnosed with a contrast enema study.

All newborns with MI need to be assessed for CF with the sweat chloride test and the genetic assessment of the several mutations of Cystic fibrosis transmembrane conductance regulator gene (CFTR gene) [43].

Treatment

In case of simple MI, approximately 60% of infants have their obstruction successfully relieved by diagnostic contrast enema, ideally using a water-soluble contrast agent [43]. Failure of the contrast to dislodge the inspissated meconium after two attempts is an indication for surgical intervention and for enterotomy with acetylcysteine irrigation and immediate closure. When the enema fails, acetylcysteine, 5 ml every 6 h, may be given via a nasogastric tube to help complete the clean-out. Complicated MI always requires surgical interventions, and the choice of operations depends on the pathologic findings [43].

Congenital Anomalies

Esophageal Atresia

Definition

Esophageal atresia (EA) is a congenital anomaly of the tracheoesophageal separation where the development of the midst esophagus is lacking and that occurs either rarely isolated or frequently associated with tracheoesophageal fistula (TEF). In the most frequent case (85%), the TEF is located in the distal esophagus (see Table 5.5).

Table 5.5 Classification of esophageal atresia (EA) [45–47]

Gross et al. [45]	Vogt et al. [46]	Ladd et al. [47]	Names	Description	Frequency
	Type 1		Esophageal agenesis	Very rare complete absence of the esophagus, not included in classification by Gross or Ladd	N/A
Type A	Type 2	I	"Long gap," "pure," or "isolated" esophageal atresia	Characterized by the presence of a "gap" between the two esophageal blind pouches with no fistula present	7%
Type B	Type 3A	II	Esophageal atresia with proximal tracheoesophageal fistula (TEF)	The upper esophageal pouch connects abnormally to the trachea. The lower esophageal pouch ends blindly	1%
Type C	Type 3B	III, IV	Esophageal atresia with distal TEF	The lower esophageal pouch connects abnormally to the trachea. The upper esophageal pouch ends blindly	86%
Type D	Type 3C	V	Esophageal atresia with both proximal and distal TEFs	The upper and lower esophageal pouches make an abnormal connection with the trachea in two separate, isolated places	2%
Type E	Type 4		TEF only with no esophageal atresia, H-type	Esophagus fully intact and capable of its normal functions, however	4%
Type F			Congenital esophageal stenosis	A congenital form of esophageal stricture. Esophagus is fully intact and connected to the stomach, however, the esophagus gradually narrows, causing food and saliva to become "caught" in the esophagus. On occasion, this type can go undiagnosed until adulthood. Not included in classification by Vogt or Ladd	N/A

N/A not known

The incidence of EA varies from 1 in 3000 to 1 in 4000 live births, with a slight predominance in male and in preterm infants. The role of genetic remains unclear.

Diagnosis

In approximately one third of pregnancies with EA, the presence of polyhydramnios, due to the inability of the fetus to swallow amniotic fluids, may suggest the disease. Antenatal ultrasound then may show, after about 26 weeks of gestation, an absent or small stomach, which, in the setting of polyhydramnios, strongly suggests EA. The upper neck pouch sign is another sign that may helps antenatal diagnosis.

In almost all types of EA, a feeding tube will not pass through the esophagus at the first neonatal examination in the delivery room. Within first hours, the newborn will present oral secretion followed by severe cough and choking episodes. The infant may become cyanotic and may even stop breathing as the overflow of fluid from the blind pouch is aspirated the trachea. If cyanosis results in laryngospasm (basically a protective mechanism to prevent aspiration into the trachea), a severe respiratory distress will rapidly develop.

Digestive symptoms occur immediately. Infants vomit when they are fed, and owing to the passage of air through the distal TEF, abdominal distension develops. A flat or a gasless abdomen suggests an EA without fistula. The most dramatic presentation of the TEF occurs with a proximal fistula. Affected infants develop life-threatening respiratory failure from aspiration almost immediately after birth. In contrast, with the so-called H-type, infants usually do not develop any symptom in the neonatal period, but present later on with a history of recurrent mild respiratory distress related to feeding or pneumonia.

Other birth defects may coexist in other organs, such as in the VACTERL (Vertebral column, Anorectal, Cardiac, Tracheal, Esophageal, Renal, and Limbs) association involving other organs.

If any of the above signs/symptoms or malformation is noticed, it is mandatory to pass a catheter into the esophagus to check, prompting other tests to confirm the diagnosis if a resistance is noted. This can be done with a catheter visible on a regular X-ray film, demonstrating the blind pouch ending. A small amount of barium placed through the mouth may help.

Treatment

If EA or TEF is suspected, all oral feedings are stopped and replaced by intravenous fluids. Appropriate positioning will help the infant draining the secretions and decrease the risk of aspiration. A tube with a continuous aspiration placed into the proximal esophagus pouch can minimize the aspiration of saliva. Also, minimizing positive pressure ventilation approximately minimizes gastric distension and reflux. The use of systemic anti-H2 or PPI can reduce the toxicity of acid secretion on the lung and the distal esophagus pouch, but reflux in itself might help the development of the lower pouch. If gastric distension occurs progressively, surgery becomes an emergency.

Surgery to fix EA is a semi-emergency. Once the baby is in condition, surgery is made by thoracotomy, thoracoscopy, and robot surgery. The esophagus can usually be sewn together. Following surgery, the baby may be hospitalized for a variable length of time depending mainly on associated malformations. Care for each infant is individualized [47]. Long-term follow-up is mandatory, owing to the risk of chronic reflux (see Table 5.3).

Imperforate Anus

Definition

Anorectal anomalies occur in 1 out of 2500–5000 births, slightly more commonly in males and with associated anomalies in more than half of affected infants. These are vertebral, genitourinary tract, and GI malformations. Imperforate anus may actually occur in the setting of the VACTERL association. The anatomical variability of these anomalies renders genetic analysis complex, so that genetic factors are clearly associated with anorectal anomalies in only 8% of patients. In infants with trisomy 21 and 18, 95% of those with anorectal malformations have imperforate anus without fistula, as opposed to only 5% of all patients with anorectal anomalies.

Imperforate anus is the most common anomaly, but other forms of anorectal malformations may occur, such as anterior ectopic anus [48]. This form is more commonly seen in females and presents with constipation [49].

Diagnosis

Anorectal malformations have been classified according to the level of the rectal pouch, that is, "high," above the elevator sling; "low," below the elevator sling; or "intermediate" and to the presence or the absence of an associated fistula. The latter is present in 95% of cases, either externally as an ano-cutaneous fistula or internally as a recto-urinary tract fistula [50].

Diagnosis relies on clinical examination of the perineal region at birth, completed with X-ray studies in cases of diagnostic uncertainty and for the assessment of the associated malformations.

Females may pass meconium through a perineal, vestibular, or vaginal fistula. Infants with a "low" defect may have cutaneous fistulas, meconium present at the perineum, a bulging anal membrane, and well-formed buttocks. Males with a "low" defect may have a bucket-handle malformation or cutaneous fistulas along the midline raphe toward the penis, discharging meconium drops. Finding meconium in the urine or air in the bladder may identify the presence of an internal fistula [50].

Plain abdominal X-ray may show progressive distal bowel obstruction. To identify the distance between the rectal pouch and the skin, a cross-table prone film is obtained with the pelvis elevated, after the first 24 h of life, during which the gap may appear falsely increased. Perineal ultrasound examination may prove to be more accurate than plain films. Abdominal ultrasound, cardiac echography, and skeletal films may be required to rule out other associated anomalies.

Treatment

Several procedures aim at restoring the anorectal canal in "low" defects, by cut-back of a cutaneous fistula, anal transposition, or limited posterior sagittal ano-rectoplasty.

"High" and so-called intermediate defects require an immediate colostomy, followed by elective repair of the localized fistula. Several approaches to the definitive correction of the anorectal anomalies have been described; the aim is always to close all fistulas and then tunnel the rectal pouch through the anatomic sphincter muscle to the anoderm. Actually, a posterior sagittal ano-rectoplasty is often the choice.

Children born with "low" defects often will be constipated, whereas incontinence may occur in one third of patients with "high" defects. Quality of life correlates closely with whether continence can be established. Nevertheless, a majority of those infants can be rendered functionally continent through a bowel management program with medical laxative treatment, anal enema, and anorectal biofeedback rehabilitation program.

Abdominal Wall Problems

Umbilical Hernia

Umbilical hernia is in infants and is manifested by the intestine protruding through an opening in the abdominal muscles in the navel region. In an infant, it may be hernia may be especially evident when the infant cries, causing the baby's bellybutton to protrude. Many umbilical hernias close on their own by age 1, though some take longer to heal. Surgical repair to prevent complications is needed only when umbilical hernias do not disappear by age 3.

Omphalocele

An omphalocele is an abdominal wall defect where the intestines, liver, and also other organs remain in a sac outside of the abdomen because of a defect in the development of the muscles of the abdominal wall. Omphalocele occurs in 2.5/10,000 births and has a high rate of mortality (25 %)

and of association with other severe malformations, cardiac anomalies (50 %), and neural tube defect (40 %) and may be associated with pulmonary hypoplasia. The digestive omphalocele can be associated with Beckwith–Wiedemann syndrome. Chromosomal abnormalities are seen in approximately 15 % of live-born-affected infants, such as trisomy 13 or 18. Long-term complications include parenteral nutrition dependence, GER, parenteral-nutrition-related liver disease, feeding intolerance, and neurodevelopmental delay, owing to the difficulties encountered during intensive care and long-lasting stay in the hospital [51]. Omphalocele is usually detected during routine ultrasonographic surveillance, during an investigation of a disparity of uterine size with time from conception or during an evaluation of an increased maternal serum alpha-fetoprotein level. Death rate amounts to 15 % of cases and in giant malformations including liver.

Gastroschisis

Gastroschisis is a congenital defect of the anterior abdominal wall, usually less than 4 cm, almost always to the right of the umbilicus, through which the abdominal contents freely, protrude. There is no overlying sac as opposed to omphalocele (which involves the umbilical cord itself and where the organs remain enclosed in visceral peritoneum). The defect may be due to a disruption of the blood supply of the abdominal wall in the first weeks after conception. Antenatal ultrasound examination has made the detection of gastroschisis possible in the first trimester of pregnancy. Surgical management at the birth is an emergency and depends on the presence of perivisceritis. It may require numerous surgical procedures. The neonatal management needs to be careful and done by trained specialists early minimal enteral feeding and gradual enteral nutrition increment and progressive refeeding considerably improve the prognosis [52].

Prune Belly Syndrome

Prune belly syndrome is a group of birth defects that involve three main problems, a poor development of the abdominal muscles, causing the skin of the belly area to wrinkle like a prune, cryptorchidism, and urinary tract problems. The latter are the most common issue in the long-term outcome of affected patients.

Inguinal Hernia

Inguinal hernia occurs when the contents of abdominal cavity protrude through the inguinal canal. Inguinal hernia is very frequent, affecting predominantly male infants, especially premature infants. Inguinal hernia repair in infants is a routine surgical procedure. However, numerous issues, including timing of the repair, the need to explore the contralateral groin, use of laparoscopy, and anesthetic approach, remain unsettled [53].

Omphalomesentéric Band

The omphalomesenteric cord (band) represents the distal residual of the omphalomesenteric duct and may be an origin of obstruction in early infancy with various radiographic presentations, including intermittent obstruction [54]. The treatment requires surgery.

Upper and Lower Endoscopy

Upper Digestive Neonatal Endoscopy

Endoscopy is usually performed at the practitioner's request, upon clinical symptoms that may be considered symptomatic of endoscopic lesions, affecting the sole esophagus or also the stomach, Fig. 5.1. These are mainly hematemesis, of course, but also retching, regurgitation, increased crying, anorexia, difficult feeding and/or failure to thrive, and malaise. In a multicentric study [55], a large range of symptoms led to endoscopy, hematemesis (55.5 %), malaise-like sudden pallor, bradycardia or cyanosis with or without hypotonia (39.4 %), feeding problems, and vomiting (53.3 %).

Upper bleeding is considered to usually affect sick premature infants and to be unusual in term healthy newborns. In 100 infants treated in a NICU [56], 20 % showed GI bleeding and mechanical ventilation was the only risk factor. Several studies described healthy full-term neonates who, after an uneventful delivery, had with more or less profuse bleeding in the first 48 h of life. In a case–control study comprising 5180 newborn babies, 64 (1.23 %) suffered from upper GI bleeding [57]. In the case–control study recently published in neonates with upper gastrointestinal bleeding [57], esophageal damage

was observed in 24/53 patients. Esophageal lesions were isolated in nine cases and occurred jointly with gastric or duodenal damage, respectively, in 14 and 1 cases. Gastric lesions were seen in 43/52 patients, and duodenal ones in 1/52. There were 17 gastric ulcers and 1 duodenal ulcer [57]. Massive bleeding with life-threatening proportions in the first 24 h of life may allow discovering hemorrhagic gastritis, profuse upper GI bleeding, and duodenal ulcers. Antenatal bleeding seems also possible, with esophagitis and gastritis revealed by a bloody amniotic fluid [58]. Fatalities during the first day of life resulting from bleeding due to gastric ulceration have also been described [59]. However, the exact incidence of endoscopic lesions in newborns still remains debatable. Endoscopic examination of newborns is rarely readily available, and even severe lesions in the upper GI tract probably often remain undiagnosed or are not detected until the condition of the patient deteriorates because of perforation or hemodynamically significant bleeding. Also, owing to the abovementioned lesions, already well known by neonatologist, the use of PPI or anti-H2 drugs in neonates at risk may have considerably reduced the actual occurrence of these lesions.

Endoscopy may also be prompted by severe general symptoms, in the form of apparent life-threatening events (ALTEs) led to discovery of severe lesions of esophagus and stomach in two different neonatal cases [60, 61]. If severe esophagogastritis lesions are shown, an antacid treatment is able to control the symptoms and be perhaps lifesaving. In addition, the disease has a spontaneously favorable outcome ruling out the need for home monitoring and alleviating considerably the strain on the family. In the presence of neonatal ALTEs, upper digestive endoscopy might be proposed as part of the initial work-up, along with other mandatory investigations, such as diagnosis of the cardiac rhythm anomaly long QT syndrome, detected by electrocardiogram (ECG). This does not preclude the use of other means of investigation of GER, such as pH-metric esophageal recording.

Mucosal lesions seen at endoscopy may affect the esophagus, in the form of severe esophagitis appearing as ulcers covered with fibrinous material, occupying the whole perimeter of the esophagus and up to 1/3 or 2/3 of its distal part. The cardial orifice is usually constantly open with a frequent local inflammation. Gastric lesions usually appear in the form of petechiae or aphthous ulcers, associated or not to blood in the lumen. Duodenal lesions are limited to erythema and mucosal ulcers being rare. In the group with esophagitis and gastritis, severe mucosal lesions could be found following minor symptoms.

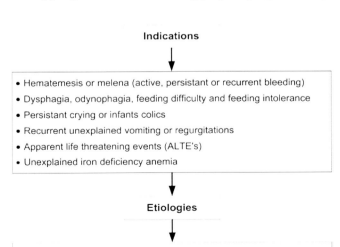

Indications

↓

- Hematemesis or melena (active, persistant or recurrent bleeding)
- Dysphagia, odynophagia, feeding difficulty and feeding intolerance
- Persistant crying or infants colics
- Recurrent unexplained vomiting or regurgitations
- Apparent life threatening events (ALTE's)
- Unexplained iron deficiency anemia

↓

Etiologies

↓

- Neonatal esogastroduodenitis
- Neonatal traumatic upper digestive tract ulceration
- Upper digestive tract lesions after oral drug intake
- Intestinal malabsorption
- Food allergy
- *Helicobacter pylori* infection (exceptional)

Fig. 5.1 Indications and etiologies of upper digestive endoscopy in the neonate

Lower Digestive Neonatal Endoscopy Findings (Colonoscopy)

In infants, rectal bleeding may be confusing when it is due to swallowed maternal blood during delivery or during

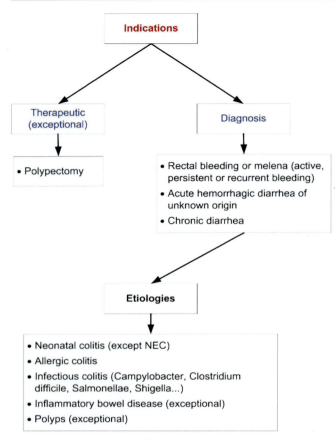

Fig. 5.2 Indications and etiologies of lower digestive endoscopy in the neonate. *NEC* necrotizing enterocolitis

breast-feeding (Fig. 5.2). The stool may be black or bright red, and the infant may be without symptoms. The Apt–Downey test distinguishes fetal from maternal hemoglobin and helps distinguishing the source of bleeding. Hemorrhagic disease of the neonate is now uncommon after prophylactic administration of vitamin K at delivery. Finally, maternal drug such aspirin, phenytoin, cephalothin, and phenobarbital may interfere with clothing function and cause hemorrhage [62]. Anal fissures are regarded as the most common cause. Giacoia and Williams [63] report two cases in which the presence of an anal fissure delayed the diagnosis of nonspecific colitis in premature infants. It is the authors' experience that the aspect of anal fissure in the term or preterm neonate is often the exteriorization of a rectal inflamed mucosa and that such a diagnosis should probably prompt the systematic search for an underlying condition, such as colitis [28].

Rectal bleeding in the neonatal period is nonetheless an alarming event that suggests possible NEC, the latter being associated with a string of other clinical features which may render the diagnosis likely and the need for urgent hospital care and investigation. Early reports, which lack reliability in the absence of endoscopy, had already addressed the issue of rectal bleeding and NEC. In a 1979, survey of 69 infants referred to hospital for rectal bleeding in the first month of life, in which NEC accounted for only 3 % of cases [64]. Six infants born at term and had normal perinatal courses developed an inflammatory proctocolitis in the first month of life while being exclusively breast-fed and had sigmoidoscopy showing focal ulcerations, edema, and increased friability [65]. A personal study [66] aimed at a better appraisal of unexplained neonatal rectal bleeding using rectosigmoidoscopy. Mucosal alterations were ecchymotic patches, either in the form of one or several longitudinally stretched ecchymotic stripes on an otherwise normal mucosa or in the form of shapeless ecchymosis irregularly dispersed on a friable and congestive mucosa. In 18 neonates with rectal bleeding, colonoscopy revealed a colitis characterized endoscopically by ecchymotic mucosal lesions, the so-called ecchymotic colitis [67].

Colonoscopic changes during the neonatal period may involve NEC, Campylobacter infection, Clostridium difficile, and dietary protein intolerance [28]. Rectal bleeding and/or colonoscopic changes have also largely been associated with blood transfusion or exchange transfusion [28]. Ulcerative colitis, a rare condition during infancy [28], may be recognized on the association to rectal bleeding and colonoscopic lesions of a severe and progressively worsening alteration of the general condition (see Fig. 5.2).

References

1. Arvedson JC. Categories of causes of swallowing and feeding disorders. Swallowing and feeding in infants and young children GI motility online; 2006. doi:10.1038/gimo17. Published 16 May 2006.
2. Vandenplas Y, Colin DR, Di Lorenzo C, Hassall E, Liptak G, Mazur L, Sondheimer J, et al. Pediatric gastroesophageal reflux clinical practice guidelines: joint recommendations of the North American Society of Pediatric Gastroenterology, Hepatology, and Nutrition and the European Society of Pediatric Gastroenterology, Hepatology, and Nutrition. J Pediatr Gastroenterol Nutr. 2009;49:498–547.
3. Djeddi DD, Kongolo G, Stéphan-Blanchard E, Ammari M, Léké A, Delanaud S, et al. Involvement of autonomic nervous activity changes in gastroesophageal reflux in neonates during sleep and wakefulness. PLoS One. 2013;8(12):e83464.
4. Davidson G, Wenzl TG, Thomson M, Omari T, Barker P, Lundborg P, et al. Efficacy and safety of once-daily esomeprazole for the treatment of gastro esophageal reflux disease in neonatal patients. J Pediatr. 2013;163:692–8.
5. Vandenplas Y, Koletzko S, Isolauri E, Hill D, Oranje AP, Brueton M, et al. Guidelines for the diagnosis and management of cows' milk protein allergy in infants. Arch Dis Child. 2007;92:902–8.
6. Koletzko S, Niggemann B, Arato A, Dias JA, Heuschkel R, Husby S, et al. Diagnostic approach and management of cow's-milk protein allergy in infants and children: ESPGHAN GI Committee practical guidelines. J Pediatr Gastroenterol Nutr. 2012;55:221–29.
7. Passariello A, Terrin G, Baldassarre ME, De Curtis M, Paludetto R, Canani BR. Diarrhea in neonatal intensive care unit. World J Gastroenterol. 2010;16:2664–68.

8. Shim JO, Hwang S, Yang HR, Moon JS, Chang JY, Ko JS, Park SS, Kang GH, Kim WS, Seo JK. Interleukin-10 receptor mutations in children with neonatal-onset Crohn's disease and intractable ulcerating enterocolitis. Eur J Gastroenterol Hepatol. 2013;25:1235–40.

9. Sherman PM, Mitchell DJ, Cutz E. Neonatal enteropathies: defining the causes of protracted diarrhea of infancy. J Pediatr Gastroenterol Nutr. 2004;38:16–26.

10. Gupta AK, Maria A, Goyal D, Verma A. Intractable diarrhoea caused by cytomegalovirus enterocolitis in an immunocompetent term neonate. J Trop Pediatr. 2013;59:509–11.

11. Bagci S, Eis-Hübinger AM, Yassin AF, Simon A, Bartmann P, Franz AR, et al. Clinical characteristics of viral intestinal infection in preterm and term neonates. Eur J Clin Microbiol Infect Dis. 2010;29:1079–84.

12. Ronchi A, Doern C, Brock E, Pugni L, Sánchez PJ. Neonatal adenoviral infection: a seventeen year experience and review of the literature. J Pediatr. 2014;164:529–35. e1–4.

13. Eyssette-Guerreau S, Boize P, Thibault M, Sarda H. Neonatal parechovirus infection, fever, irritability and myositis. Arch Pediatr. 2013;20:772–4 [Article in French].

14. Guarino A, Albano F, Ashkenazi S, Gendrel D, Hoekstra JH, Shamir R, et al. ESPGHAN/ESPID guidelines for the management of acute gastroenteritis in children in Europe. J Pediatr Gastroenterol Nutr. 2008;46:s1–22.

15. Tabbers MM, Di Lorenzo C, Berger MY, Faure C, Langendam MW, Nurko S, et al. Evaluation and treatment of functional constipation in infants and children: evidence-based recommendations from ESPGHAN and NASPGHAN. J Pediatr Gastroenterol Nutr. 2014;58:258–74.

16. Carroccio A, Mansueto P, Morfino G, D'Alcamo A, Di Paola V, Iacono G, et al. Oligo-antigenic diet in the treatment of chronic anal fissures. Evidence for a relationship between food hypersensitivity and anal fissures. Am J Gastroenterol. 2013;108:825–3.

17. Barr RG, Paterson JA, MacMartin LM, Lehtonen L, Young SN. Prolonged and unsoothable crying bouts in infants with and without colic. J Dev Behav Pediatr. 2005;26:14–23.

18. Rhoads JM, Fatheree NY, Norori J, Liu Y, Lucke JF, Tyson JE, et al. Altered fecal microflora and increased fecal calprotectin in infants with colic. J Pediatr. 2009;155:823–28.

19. Snyder J, Brown P. Complementary and alternative medicine in children: an analysis of the recent literature. Curr Opin Pediatr. 2012;24:539–46.

20. Martin CR, Walker WA. Innate and mucosal immunity in the developing gastrointestinal tract: relationship to early and later disease. In: Gleason CA, Devaskar SU, editors. Avery's diseases of the newborn. 9th ed. Philadelphia: Elsevier; 2012, pp. 994–1006.

21. Martin CR, Walker WA. Intestinal immune defences and the inflammatory response in necrotizing enterocolitis. Semin Fetal Neonatal Med. 2006;11:369–71.

22. McGuire W, Henderson G, Fowlie PW. Feeding the preterm infant. Br Med J. 2004;329:1227–30.

23. Morgan J, Bombell S, McGuire W. Early trophic feeding versus enteral fasting for very preterm or very low birth weight infants. Cochrane Database Syst Rev. 2013;3:CD000504. doi:10.1002/14651858.CD000504.pub4.

24. Morgan J, Young L, McGuire W. Slow advancement of enteral feed volumes to prevent necrotizing enterocolitis in very low birth weight infants (VLBW). Cochrane Database Syst Rev. 2013;3:CD001241. doi:10.1002/14651858.CD001241.pub4.

25. Morgan J, Young L, McGuire W. Delayed introduction of progressive enteral feeds to prevent necrotizing enterocolitis in very low birth weight infants. Cochrane Database Syst Rev. 2013;5:CD001970. pib4.

26. SIFT Investigators group, Abbot J, Berrington JE, Boyle E, Dorling JS, Embleton NE, Jusszczak E, et al. Early enteral feeding strategies for very preterm infants: current evidence from Cochrane reviews. Arch Dis Child Fetal Neonatal Ed. 2013;98:F470–2.

27. Basuki F, Hadiati DR, Turner T, McDonald S, Hakimi M. Dilute versus full strength formula in exclusively formula-fed preterm or low birth weight infants. Cochrane Database Syst Rev. 2013;11:CD007263. doi:10.1002/14651858.CD007263.pub2.

28. Dupont C, Kalach N, de Boissieu D, Barbet JP, Benhamou PH. Digestive endoscopy in neonates. J Pediatr Gastroenterol Nutr. 2005;40:406–20.

29. Corvaglia L, Martini S, Aceti A, Arcuri S, Rossini R, Faldella G. Nonpharmacological management of gastroesophageal reflux in preterm infants. Biomed Res Int. 2013;2013:141967. doi:10.1155/2013/141967. Epub 2013 Sept 1.

30. Suc AL, Blond MH, Gold F, Maurage C, Saliba E, Guerois M, et al. Enteropathy in premature newborn infants. Prospective study over one year. Arch Pediatr. 1992;49:869–73 [Article in French].

31. Wang Y, Hoenig JD, Malin KJ, Qamar S, Petrof EO, Sun J, et al. 16S rRNA gene-based analysis of fecal microbiota from preterm infants with and without necrotizing enterocolitis. ISME J. 2009;3:944–54.

32. Cotten CM, Taylor S, Stoll B, Goldberg RN, Hansen NI, Sánchez PJ, et al. NICHD Neonatal Research Network. Prolonged duration of initial empirical antibiotic treatment is associated with increased rates of necrotizing enterocolitis and death for extremely low birth weight infants. Pediatrics. 2009;123:58–66.

33. Abreu MT. Toll-like receptor signalling in the intestinal epithelium: how bacterial recognition shapes intestinal function. Nat Rev Immunol. 2010;10:131–44.

34. Leaphart CL, Cavallo J, Gribar SC, Cetin S, Li J, Branca MF, et al. A critical role for TLR4 in the pathogenesis of necrotizing enterocolitis by modulating intestinal injury and repair. J Immunol. 2007;179:4808–20.

35. Sodhi CP, Shi XH, Richardson WM, Grant ZS, Shapiro RA, Prindle T, Jr, et al. Toll-like receptor-4 inhibits enterocyte proliferation via impaired beta-catenin signaling in necrotizing enterocolitis. Gastroenterology. 2010;138:185–96.

36. Lin PW, Stoll BJ. Necrotising enterocolitis. Lancet. 2006;7;368:1271–83.

37. Muchantef K, Epelman M, Darge K, Kirpalani H, Laje P, Anupindi SA. Sonographic and radiographic imaging features of the neonate with necrotizing enterocolitis: correlating findings with outcomes. Pediatr Radiol. 2013;43:1444–52.

38. Aydemir G, Cekmez F, Tanju IA, Canpolat FE, Genc FA, Yitdirim S, et al. Increased fecal calprotectine in preterm infants with necrotizing enterocolitis. Clin Lab. 2012; 58:841–4.

39. Young C, Sharma R, Handfield M, et al. Biomarkers for infants at risk for necrotizing enterocolitis: clues to prevention? Pediatr Res. 2009;65:91R–7R.

40. American Academy of Pediatrics. Breastfeeding and the use of human milk. Pediatrics. 2012;129:e827–41.

41. Heird WC, Gomez MR. Total parenteral nutrition in necrotizing enterocolitis. Clin Perinatol. 1994;21:389–409.

42. Caplan MS. Probiotic and prebiotic supplementation for the prevention of neonatal necrotizing enterocolitis. J Perinatol. 2009;29(Suppl 2):S2–6.

43. Garza-Cox S, Keeney SE, Angel CA, Thompson LL, Swischuk LE. Meconium obstruction in the very low birth weight premature infant. Pediatrics. 2004;114:285–90.

44. Paradiso VF, Briganti V, Oriolo L, Coletta R, Calisti A. Meconium obstruction in absence of cyctic fibrosis in low birth weight infants: an emerging challenge from increasing survival. Ital J Pediatr. 2011;37:55–61.

45. Gross, RE. The surgery of infancy and childhood. Philadelphia: WB Saunders; 1953.

46. Vogt EC. Congenital esophageal atresia. Am J Roentgenol. 1929;22:463–65.

47. Ladd WE. The surgical treatment of esophageal atresia and tracheoesophageal fistulas. N Engl J Med. 1944;230:625–37.

48. Bill AH, Jr, Johnson RJ, Foster RA. Anteriorly placed rectal opening in the perineum ectopic anus; a report of 30 cases. Ann Surg. 1958;147:173–9.

49. Leape LL, Ramenofsky ML. Anterior ectopic anus: a common cause of constipation in children. J Pediatr Surg. 1978;13:627–30.

50. Pena A. Advances in ano-rectal malformations. Semin Pediatr Surg. 1997;6:165–69.

51. McNair C, Hawes J, Urquhart H. Caring for the newborn with an oomphalocele. Neonatal Netw. 2006;25:319–27.

52. Walter-Nicolet E, Rousseau V, Kieffer F, Fusarp F, Bourdaud N, Oucherif S, et al. Neonatal outcome of gastroschisis is mainly influenced by nutritional management. J Pediatr Gastroenterol Nutr. 2009;48:612–7.

53. Wang KS, The Committee on Fetus and Newborn and Section on Surgery. Assessment and management of inguinal hernia in infants. Pediatrics. 2012;130:768–73.

54. Gaisie G, Curnes JT, Scatliff JH, Croom RD, Vanderzalm T. Neonatal intestinal obustruction from omphalomesenteric duct remnants. AJR. 1985;144:109–12.

55. Benhamou PH, Francoual C, Glangeaud MC, Barette A, Dupont C, Breart G. Risk factors for severe esophageal and gastric lesions in term neonates: a case-control study. Groupe Francophone d'Hepato-Gastroenterologie et Nutrition Pediatrique. J Pediatr Gastroenterol Nutr. 2000;31:377–80.

56. Kuusela AL, Maki M, Karikoski R, et al. Stress-induced gastric findings in critically ill newborn infants: frequency and risk factors. Intensive Care Med. 2000;26:1501–6.

57. Lazzaroni M, Petrillo M, Tornaghi R, Massironi E, Sainaghi M, Principi N, Porro GB. Upper GI bleeding in healthy full-term infants: a case-control study. Am J Gastroenterol. 2002;97:89–94.

58. Bedu A, Faure C, Sibony O, Vuillard E, Mougenot JF, Aujard Y. Prenatal gastrointestinal bleeding caused by esophagitis and gastritis. J Pediatr. 1994;125:465–7.

59. Pugh RJ, Newton RW, Piercy DM. Fatal bleeding from gastric ulceration during first day of life-possible association with social stress. Arch Dis Child. 1979;54:146–8.

60. Skinner S, Naqvi M, Biskinis EK. Gastric ulcer presenting as gastroesophageal reflux and apnea in a term neonate. Tex Med. 1998;94:57–8.

61. Dupont C, Berg A, Lagueunie G, de Boissieu D, Benhamou PH. Apparent life-threatening events in a neonate with severe lesions of esophagus and stomach. J Pediatr Gastroenterol Nutr. 2000;31:170–2.

62. Steffen RM, Wyllie R, Sivak MV, Michener WM, Caulfield ME. Colonoscopy in the pediatric patient. J Pediatr. 1989;115:507–14.

63. Giacoia GP, Williams GP. Rectal bleeding due to nonspecific colitis in premature infants. South Med J. 1995;88:789–91.

64. Levene Ml. Rectal bleeding in the first month of life. Post Grad Med J. 1979;55:22–23.

65. Lake AM, Whitington PF, Hamilton SR. Dietary-protein induced colitis in breast-fed infants. J Pediatr. 1982;101:906–10.

66. Dupont C, Badoual J, Le Luyer B, Le Bourgeois C, Barbet JP, Voyer M. Rectosigmoidoscopic findings during isolated rectal bleeding in the neonate. J Pediatr Gastroenterol Nutr. 1987;6:257–64.

67. Canioni D, Pauliat S, Gaillard JL, Mougenot JF, Bompard Y, Berche P, Schmitz J, Brousse N. Histopathology and microbiology of isolated rectal bleeding in neonates: the so-called 'ecchymotic colitis'. Histopathology. 1997;30:472–7.

Enteral Nutrition in Preterm Neonates

Gianluca Terrin, Thibault Senterre, Jacques Rigo
and Mario De Curtis

Introduction

In the past decades, there has been a significant increase in the survival rate of preterm infants, especially very-low-birth-weight (VLBW, <1500 g) neonates. The nutritional problems of preterm babies have become particularly relevant, as numerous studies have underlined the importance of early feeding on short- and long-term development [1]. The gastrointestinal (GI) tract of preterm infants and especially of VLBW infants is immature at birth and initially incapable of receiving full enteral feeding [2]. Retard in maturation of GI motility manifests itself in so-called "neonatal feeding intolerance" which is characterized by delayed gastric emptying, abdominal distension, and constipation. This paraphysiologic condition may evolve in necrotizing enterocolitis (NEC), a major GI emergency in preterm newborn. NEC almost always occurred in infants who received enteral nutrition and who show sign of feeding intolerance. For these reasons, the introduction of feeding was frequently delayed, often for prolonged periods, increasing the risk of malnutrition.

Nutrition Objectives in Premature Neonates

The vast majority of infants born at a gestational age lower than 29 weeks do not achieve the median birth weight of the reference fetus at theoretical term or 40 weeks postmenstrual age (PMA) [3, 4]. At discharge, the estimates of growth failure range from 30 to 67%. To reduce the risk of cumulative nutritional deficit and malnutrition, enteral nutrition should be introduced appropriately. However, it remains unclear which postnatal artificial feeding regimens are more appropriate to support postnatal growth adequately [1]. Age of life and clinical conditions influence modalities of enteral nutrition administration. We can differentiate neonatal period in two phase: (i) the early adaptive period of clinical instability (from birth to approximately day 7) and (ii) the intermediate stable growing period (from approximately day 7 to near term/discharge). Recommended intakes and modalities of enteral feeding during these two different phases are reported below.

Enteral Nutrition During the Early Adaptive Period

The main goal of neonatal nutrition during this phase is to provide immediately the recommended intakes in order to limit the cumulative deficit and to reach a positive nitrogen balance since the first days of life [1, 3–5]. Despite many studies enrolling VLBW infants demonstrated that early-optimized nutritional support significantly reduces growth restriction during the first days after birth, it might be difficult to satisfy all nutritional needs. In this period, total fluid intake should be limited in order to prevent neonatal complications (i.e., persistent ductus arteriosus and broncho-pulmonary dysplasia). Parenteral nutrition must be started immediately after birth in all VLBW neonates to maintain adequate fluid, electrolytes, and nutrients intake, until full enteral feeding (120 kcal/kg/day) is reached. In this phase, small amounts of enteral feeding (also called "minimal enteral feeding (MEF)," "GI priming," "trophic feeding," and

M. De Curtis (✉)
Department of Pediatrics, Neonatology Unit, Policlinico Umberto I, Sapienza University of Rome, Viale del Policlinico 155, 00161 Rome, Italy
e-mail: mario.decurtis@uniroma1.it

G. Terrin
Department of Perinatal Medicine, Neonatology Unit, Sapienza University of Rome, Rome, Italy

Department of Gynaecology—Obstetrics and Perinatal Medicine, Rome, Italy

T. Senterre · J. Rigo
CHU de Liege, CHR de la Citadelle, University of Liege, Liege, Belgium

© Springer International Publishing Switzerland 2016
S. Guandalini et al. (eds.), *Textbook of Pediatric Gastroenterology, Hepatology and Nutrition*,
DOI 10.1007/978-3-319-17169-2_6

"hypocaloric feeding") could improve the maturation of the GI tract, digestive hormone release, and gut motility. On the other hand, receiving nothing by enteral route predisposes neonates to the consequences of starvation (i.e., GI atrophy, malnutrition, infections). Thus, MEF should be started possibly in the first 24–48 h of life, if the patient is stable, at a minimal volume of 10–30 ml/kg of body weight, and it could be increased by 20–30 ml/kg of body weight per day when clinical conditions remain stable and feeding intolerance does not occur (Fig. 6.1). In the VLBW infant with prenatal history of blood uteroplacental flow alterations, a delayed onset of MEF could be considered. Measurement of flow in mesenteric vessels, by ultrasonography, could be useful in deciding if starting MEF is safe, in particular for these neonates. [6]. Results of clinical trials in premature infants support the opinion that MEF, preferentially by human milk, has some clinical benefits such as reducing the time to reach full enteral feeding and length of hospitalization without increasing the risk of NEC [7]. MEF could be adopted not only early in life to start enteral feeding but also during the periods of feeding intolerance. When signs of feeding intolerance are neither specific nor systemic (Fig. 6.1), MEF

could be continued in order to reduce the duration of parenteral nutrition and to limit the risk of infections [8]. MEF mainly serves as trophic gut feeding. Therefore, should not be considered in the total energy intakes during total parenteral nutrition (see Chap. 7).

Nutrition During the Intermediate and Stable Growing Period

During this period, parenteral fluid is progressively reduced and, thus, interrupted as soon as 120 ml/kg/day (100 kcal/kg/day) by enteral route is well tolerated, Subsequently, enteral feeding can be slightly increased, up to 140–180 ml/kg/day (115–135 kcal/kg/day), according to nutritional requirements and type of formula used. During any phase of nutritiona approach, protein to energy ratio (PER) should be conserved and parenteral nutrition adjusted in relation to nutrients given by enteral route. Human milk is the preferred feed for preterm infants during the intermediate and stable growing period. Weaning period from parenteral nutrition may be at high risk of relative malnutrition, contributing to

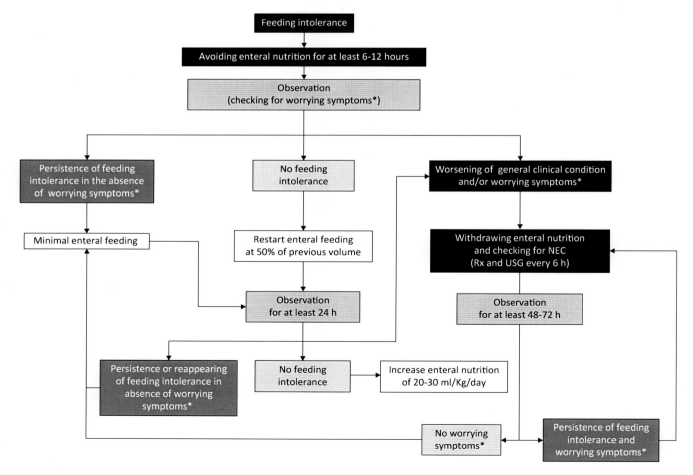

Fig. 6.1 Flow diagram for the management of preterm newborns with feeding intolerance. Note: *Erythematic abdominal wall, absence of bowel sounds, blood in the stools or in aspirates, bile in the aspirate, or radiological or ultrasonographic markers of NEC Bell's stage >I

cumulative nutritional deficit and postnatal growth restriction [9]. It is commonly accepted that human milk needs to be fortified to meet the nutrient needs of the preterm infant. Fortified human milk feeding regime significantly improves growth. Fortification provides adequate intakes when the composition of human milk plus fortifier reaches 2.5 g protein/100 ml with a PER of 3.2 g/100 kcal [1]. Measuring the composition of human milk feeds prior to fortification and targeting the fortification according to individual needs of each infant would be ideal [9]. When human milk is unavailable, preterm formula is used for feeding very preterm infants. All preterm formulas are protein and energy enriched (~80 kcal/dl, PER 3.0–3.6 g/100 kcal), have low osmolarity (325 mmol/kg H_2O), and typically contain added whey protein, glucose polymers, medium-chain triglycerides (MCT), a source of long-chain polyunsaturated fatty acids (LCPUFAs), calcium, phosphorus, electrolytes, folate, and fat-soluble vitamins. Upper limits of recommended nutritional intake are met when preterm formula is fed at rates approaching 160 ml/kg/day [5].

Feeding Mode

Bolus or (Semi-) Continuous Feeding

Bolus feeding results in a significant increase in blood flow to the portal-drained viscera (i.e., stomach, spleen, intestine, and pancreas). There is a surge in GI hormones, which is higher than when neonates are fed continuously. It has been also suggested that in preterm infants fed with fortified human milk, continuous feeding leads to important nutrients' loss on nasogastric tube walls (i.e. fat and calcium). However, it has been demonstrated better tolerance with continuous milk feeding in preterm neonates [10, 11]. Bolus feeding may result in apnea, deteriorating respiratory mechanics with decreased tidal volumes, and transient presence of blocking materials of the nostrils, such as nasogastric tubes, or noninvasive respiratory support devices. However, a large randomized controlled trial showed that even extremely-low-birth-weight (ELBW, <1000 g) infants may tolerate bolus feeding well [10, 11]. In conclusion, there is still not enough evidence to recommend either bolus or (semi-) continuous feeding as the preferred method, but the change from one to another can be justified when feeding intolerance persists in smaller neonates.

Oral Feeding

Oral feeding is possible when an infant is capable of an adequate suck–swallow reflex. In the term infant, the full, complex, integrated mechanism of swallowing, with the movement of the bolus of milk into the stomach, protection of the airway, inhibition of respiration, and appropriate relaxation of the esophageal sphincter and gastric fundus is achieved within 2 days of life. The swallow function is present from 16 weeks of gestational age, and GI motor activity, in small bursts, from 24 weeks onwards [2]. Organized motility is present from around 30 weeks of gestation and nutritive and swallowing function from 32 weeks. Enteral nutrition promotes postnatal maturation of intestinal motor activity. It follows that oral feeding is only possible from 32 weeks onwards, but Nonnutritive sucking can start earlier. The very preterm infant (<32 weeks) may be put on the breast but the likelihood that the infant will ingest a significant volume of milk is very small. However, it may offer the mother a considerable psychological benefit and should therefore be strongly encouraged.

Intragastric Feeding

As oral feeding is not possible in VLBW infants, most frequently gastric tubes are used [11]. Either nasogastric or orogastric tubes can be installed, both checked in the right position (i.e., fundus) by measuring external distance (i.e., distance from nose or mouth to ear plus distance from umbilicus and xiphoid process), and checking the aspirate for acidity with litmus paper. Correct position should be confirmed at the first radiographic examination performed for such reasons and reported in the clinical chart. The nasogastric tube has the advantage of easier fixation but has the disadvantage of (partially) blocking one nostril. With the use of some respiratory devices, only the orogastric tube is possible. Finally, tubes and syringes may lead to loss of nutrients such as lipids and calcium that may not reach the infant [11].

Transpyloric Feeding

Although transpyloric feeding is frequently used in pediatric intensive care, no proven benefits in tolerance, growth, or in aspiration rates have been reported in neonates. Additionally, such evidences showed that mortality rates increase in neonates receiving transpyloric feeding [1, 5].

Start, Check the Tolerance and Increments of Enteral Feeding

Enteral nutrition is started at 10–30 ml/kg of body weight per day. Feeds could be given by gavage or with a continuous infusion pump and increased by 20–30 ml/kg/day according to feeding tolerance. [12]. Feeding intolerance may sometimes be obvious when severe GI manifestations are identified (emesis, vomiting, severe abdominal distension, ileus with visible intestinal loops, blood in the stools) or when GI symptoms are associated with systemic disorders like apnea, bradycardia, poor perfusion, and/or hemodynamic instabilities. However, intermediate situations are frequent in VLBW infants. In particular, abdominal distension is frequently observed during noninvasive ventilation and antegrade peristalsis with bilious gastric aspirates is also commonly described during the first week of life in VLBW infants.

The aspiration of gastric residuals is common practice while tube-feeding infants and aspirate usually need to be reinfused to reduce the loss of enzymes and electrolytes. Most clinical studies demonstrated little if any predictive value of gastric residuals >3–4 ml/kg or >30–50% of the previous feed and of bilious-stained feed [12]. Therefore, in the absence of significant clinical signs or symptoms, the presence of gastric residuals <4 ml/kg or <50% of 3-h previous feed is not a valid reason to interrupt or reduce enteral feeding [12]. Maintaining sufficient enteral feeding can in fact improve GI maturation and feeding tolerance. If enteral feeding has been interrupted but clinical evolution rules out a significant disease, enteral feeding need to be restarted as soon as possible to promote intestinal maturation.

In the absence of signs of feeding intolerance, the volume of enteral nutrition could be daily increased. The ideal rate of progression of milk volume given to VLBW infants is controversial. Cochrane Review has concluded that a rapid rate of advancing feeds was not associated with a higher risk of NEC [13]. Although additional studies are needed, a small progressive increment of 20 ml/kg/day after a few days of stabilization can be suggested. (Fig. 6.1). In the presence of erythematic abdominal wall, absence of bowel sounds, blood in the stools or in aspirates, enteral nutrition should be discontinued and serial abdominal ultrasounds and radiological examinations should be started in order to early identify NEC [8, 12, 14].

Nutrient Needs in Enterally fed Neonates

Protein

Protein Requirements
The optimal quantity of dietary protein for preterm infant formulas is still a matter of debate. Dietary protein needs for preterm infants were calculated through two different methods [15]. The first, the empirical approach, measures biochemical or physiological responses to graded intakes. The second method, the factorial approach, considers the requirements as the sum of the essential losses (e.g., urine, feces, skin), plus the amount incorporated into newly formed tissues accounting theoretical fetal accretion at the same PMA. The empirical approach evaluates physiological and

biochemical variables to determine minimum and maximum protein needs in the growing preterm infant.

In the factorial approach, compositional analysis of fetal tissues has been a valuable source of data for our understanding of the nutrient needs of the fetus and, by extension, those of the growing preterm infant. Fetal accretion rates have been obtained from compositional analyses of aborted fetuses or stillborn infants. From these data, the protein increment for growth has been estimated as approximately 2.5 g/kg/day [5]. Protein requirement is thus calculated by adding to this value the obligatory losses, and the amount needed for the additional catch-up growth. In a large population of preterm infants receiving a controlled energy intake, the minimal protein supply necessary to obtain a zero nitrogen balance (to cover all nitrogen losses) was calculated to be 2 g/kg/day. A similar value was estimated to cover the need for catch-up growth. Thus, the protein requirements of premature infants are between 3.5 and 4.0 g/kg/day (Fig. 6.2) [5].

Protein intake must be sufficient to achieve normal growth without negative effects such as acidosis, uremia, and elevated levels of circulating amino acids [1, 15, 17]. A recent Cochrane analysis aimed to determine whether higher (≥3.0 g/kg/day) versus lower (<3.0 g/kg/day) protein intake during the initial hospital stay of formula-fed preterm infants or LBW infants (<2500 g) results in improved growth and neurodevelopmental outcomes without evidence of short- and long-term morbidity [17]. Five studies comparing low versus high protein intake were included. Improved weight gain and higher nitrogen accretion were demonstrated in infants receiving formula with higher protein content while other nutrients were kept constant. No significant differences were seen in rates of NEC, sepsis, or diarrhea. One study compared high (3 g/kg/day) versus very high (>4 g/kg/day) protein intake during and after an initial hospital stay [18].

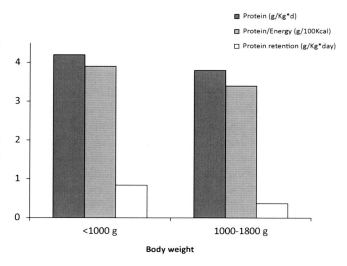

Fig. 6.2 Recommended protein intake and protein to energy ratio for preterm infants to obtain optimal protein retention [5, 16]

Very high protein intake improved gain in length at term, but differences did not remain significant at 12 weeks corrected age. Three of the 24 infants receiving very high protein intake developed uremia, defined as serum urea nitrogen level greater than 6 mM/ml. Formula with higher protein content improves all growth parameters and neurodevelopment [19, 20]. However, available evidence is not adequate to permit specific recommendations regarding the provision of very high protein intake (≥4.5 g/kg/day) from formula during the initial hospital stay or after discharge.

Enteral Nutrition Protein Composition

Nitrogen absorption rate (absorbed/intake) differs significantly according to the feeding regimen (Fig. 6.3) [21]. It is higher with powder whey-predominant protein preterm formulas than with human milk supplemented with fortifiers powder protein hydrolyzed formulas or ready-to-use liquid whey-predominant preterm formulas. These differences result from the nature of the various types of protein supply. Also net protein utilization is higher for preterm formulas compared with human milk, with or without protein supplementation. Technical processes (i.e., hydrolysis) may alter macronutrient concentrations of formula and the pasteurization of human milk before delivery to newborn also cause a reduction in the protein concentration of about 4 % [22].

The whey/casein ratio significantly influences individual amino acid intakes and plasma amino acid concentrations. Plasma threonine increases and tryptophan relatively decreases in infants fed a whey-predominant formula, whereas methionine and aromatic amino acids increase in those fed a casein-predominant formula [23]. The high plasma threonine concentration observed in preterm infants fed whey-predominant formulas is related to the glycomacropeptide obtained from casein by enzymatic casein precipitation of cow's milk proteins. Acidic precipitation, by contrast, removes the glycomacropeptide rich in threonine from the soluble phase [23]. In preterm infants receiving either an enzymatic or an acidic whey-predominant formula, a significant reduction in plasma threonine concentration was observed in acidic whey protein formula-fed infants, compared to those receiving conventional enzymatic whey protein formulas. All other plasma amino acid concentrations were similar, with the exception of valine, which was slightly reduced in acidic whey protein formula-fed infants [15, 24].

The relative percentage of α-lactalbumin depends on the cow's milk protein content [25]. This protein fraction is naturally rich in tryptophan and helps normalize the low levels of this amino acid frequently observed in whey-predominant formula-fed infants. The use of a higher percentage of whey in protein-hydrolyzed formulas may worsen the plasma amino acid pattern by increasing threonine and decreasing aromatic amino acid concentrations [25]. Moreover, a significant decrease of plasma histidine and tryptophan concentrations, probably due to a relative reduction in amino acid bioavailability, could be also observed. Using a more appropriate technology, these formulas have been corrected for the threonine content and supplemented with histidine and tryptophan.

An interesting observation is the relatively lower absorption rate of ready-to-use liquid preterm formulas or protein hydrolyzed preterm formulas, where the technical process seems to impair nitrogen absorption in relation to heat treatment—inducing some Maillard reaction—or to preliminary

Fig. 6.3 Nitrogen balances according to feeding regimen in preterm infants [21]

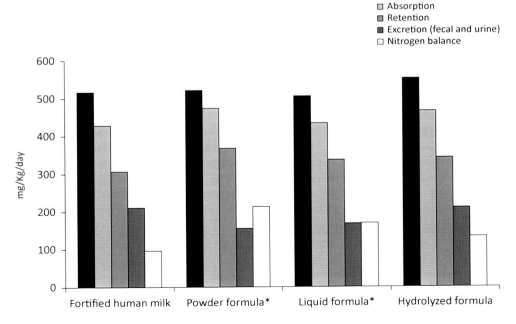

hydrolysis, altering the physiological absorption process in the lumen or at the border of the GI tract. Formulas based on hydrolyzed proteins have been recently proposed for the feeding of preterm infants to reduce GI problems such as delayed gastric emptying, abdominal distension, hard stools, and feeding intolerance [26]. The technological processes of hydrolysis may modify the amino acid content and/or amino acid bioavailability [27]. The efficiency of protein differs also according to non-protein nitrogen contentof different feeding regimens. The highest values were obtained in preterm infants fed powder and liquid preterm formulas. It was significantly lower in those fed protein-hydrolyzed formulas and fortified human milk. The lower value obtained with fortified human milk may be related to nonprotein nitrogen content, which represents 20–25 % of total nitrogen content of human milk, but still 13.5–17 % of total nitrogen content of fortified human milk. The contribution of nonprotein nitrogen fraction of fortified human milk to protein gain is lower than that of the α-lactalbumin or the casein content of human milk [1, 15, 23, 24]. Due to its biological activities, the nonprotein nitrogen of human milk may not be included in protein intakes when human milk is compared to formulas. This may explain why we still frequently observe differences between infants fed human milk or PTF with theoretical similar nitrogen content.

Formulas do not contain any of the biologically active immune proteins nor enzymes, hormones, or growth factors are found in human milk [2]. The long-term implications of this deficiency have not been completely determined. Further long-term randomized studies with higher number of patients, and standardized supplemental amounts and experimental conditions are needed to establish the efficacy of non-nutritional compounds, such as nucleotides, polyamines, and growth factors supplementation in preterm formula [1, 5].

Energy

The energy demands for preterm infants depend on many factors including PMA, genetically determined metabolic rate, thermal environment, activity, sleep status, nutritional status, nutrient intake, body composition, and occurrence of illness [1]. Energy expenditure, measured by indirect calorimetry, increases with postnatal age and varies from 45 to 55 kcal/kg/day. The energy cost for a postnatal weight gain of 17–20 g/kg/day with adequate lean body mass (LBM) accretion vary widely from 50 to 70 kcal/kg/day in premature infants [5, 15, 28]. Energy absorption from enteral nutrition, in healthy growing premature neonates after the first 2–3 days of life, is about 80–90 % of the energy intake. The remainder is lost in stool and a small quantity as urea in the urine. Energy absorbed is in part stored in tissues, mainly as fat but also as protein, and in part spent by the metabolism (energy ex-

penditure). Energy intakes less than or equal to 100 kcal/kg/day may not meet the needs of some preterm infants before discharge. Where PER are adequate (3.2–3.6 g/100 kcal) in a formula providing well-absorbed nutrients, an energy intake around 120 kcal/kg/day is generally appropriate and may result in a fat mass deposition close to intrauterine references. Small-for-gestational-age (SGA) infants, in particular if they experienced intrauterine malnutrition, may need higher energy intake than appropriate-for-gestational-age (AGA) infants [1]. Energy intake recommended for preterm infants is 115–135 kcal/kg/day [5]. All recommendations are related to preterm formula, but energy requirement could differ in preterm receiving human milk in contrast to those fed with preterm formula [22, 28–30].

Protein:Energy ratio

Protein intake and PER are the main determinants of weight gain [17]. Protein intake is the only determinant of LBM gain in contrast to fat mass gain, which is positively related to energy intake and negatively to PER. Protein and energy needs are reciprocally limiting, the intake of one affecting the ability of the infant to assimilate the other [29, 30]. A suboptimal range of the PER leads to untoward consequences [1]. If energy intake is inadequate, proteins are used as an energy source and the nitrogen balance becomes less positive. Increasing the caloric intake will spare protein loss and improve nitrogen retention. If there is a surfeit of energy with limited protein intake, the protein retention reaches a plateau and the energy excess is used for excessive fat deposition. Thus, an adequate PER should be respected at all PMA, with adequate partition of energy intake between fat and carbohydrates. This crucial point should be respected particularly in the period of clinical instability, when nutritional regimens in a significant part depend on parenteral nutrition [16]. Recommended intakes for preterm infants at 26–30 weeks' PMA should be 3.8–4.2 g of protein/kg per day with a high PER above 3.2 g/100 kcal and ideally around 3.6 g/100 kcal [5]. A recent experts panel has recommended 3.6–4.1 g/100 kcal in VLBW infants while the European Society for Pediatric Gastroenterology Hepatology and Nutrition (ESPGHAN) have recommended 3.6–4.1 g/100 kcal in ELBW infants and 3.2–3.6 g/100 kcal for other preterm infants < 1800 g [5, 16].

Fat

Fat Requirements

Fat provides the major source of energy in growing preterm infants. Recommended fat intake is 4.8–6.6 g/kg/day [5]. Although some infants with restricted fluid may need high fat content in their feeds to meet energy needs, 4.4–6.0 g/100 kcal is a reasonable range for most preterm infants [16]. Lipid availability by enteral route depends more on digestion and absorption capability than on enteral nutrition content and composition. Digestion of lipids is not fully developed in premature infants [2]. Lipid malabsorption is the result of low levels of pancreatic lipase and bile salts. The bile acid pool is only half the size of that of a full-term infant. Human milk provides additional lipases: lipoprotein lipase and bile salt-stimulated lipase, which contribute to intestinal lipolysis. However, additional fat should be also provided to human milk because of the possible reduction of fat content in expressed human milk, especially when various processes are applied to human milk prior to delivery to neonates [19, 20].

Enteral Nutrition Fat Composition

Fats represent approximately 50% of the nonprotein energy content of human or formula milk. Fat could be provided in different form with different nutritional power.

Medium Chain Triglycerides MCTs are hydrolyzed more readily than long-chain triglycerides (LCT) and fatty acids with more double bonds are absorbed more efficiently [16]. In order to improve fat absorption, commercial formulas contain a significant quantity of MCTs that are more easily absorbed than LCTs and transported directly to the liver via the portal vein as nonesterified fatty acids. The use of MCTs instead of LCTs in preterm infant formulas can reduce the formation of calcium and magnesium soaps with unabsorbed long-chain saturated fatty acids and, thereby, increase calcium and magnesium absorption. However, it needs to be stressed that the energy content of MCTs corresponds only to 85% of that of LCTs, the use of MCTs in formulas induces an increase in plasma ketones as well as in urinary excretion of dicarboxylic acids, suggesting that MCT metabolism could be slightly limited in preterm neonates [16]. Moreover, since MCTs do not contain essential fatty acids, a high MCT intake can reduce the availability of the essential long-chain fatty acids. For these reasons, it is recommended to limit the maximum MCT intake in preterm formula at 40% of the total fat content [5, 31].

Long-Chain Triglycerides Because humans cannot insert double bonds at the n-3 and n-6 positions, fatty acids with double bonds in these positions cannot be synthesized endogenously. Therefore, either specific *n*-3 and *n*-6 fatty acids or the precursor of each series such as linoleic acid (LA; 18:3n-3) and α-linolenic acid (ALA; 18:2n-6) must be provided as a component of the diet [5, 15]. Both LA and ALA acid are metabolized by a series of desaturation and elongation reactions to more unsaturated longer-chain fatty acids. Important metabolites of these two fatty acids include 20:5n-3 eicosapentaenoic acid (EPA), 22:6n-3 docosahexaenoic acid (DHA), and 20:4n-6 arachidonic acid (AA) [32–34].

Recent studies have repoKrted outcome data in preterm infants fed milk with a DHA content two to three times higher than the current concentration in infant formulas. Overall, these studies show that providing larger amounts of DHA supplements, especially to the smallest infants, is associated with better neurologic outcomes in early life [34]. DHA intakes of 55–60 mg/kg/day from the time of preterm birth to expected term have been tested and appear to be safe, to promote normal DHA status, and to improve visual and neurocognitive functions. These values are likely to represent an adequate intake for very preterm infants, but further research is needed to confirm that they represent adequate intake for other infants subgroups (i.e., extremely, very, and moderately preterm infants, with or without intrauterine growth restriction, and males and females). Because the maximum DHA content of human milk is 84 mg/kg/day (equivalent of 1.5% of fatty acids), and because no studies with such a high intake in preterm infants have been reported, no upper limit can be set with certainty.

Synthesis of long-chain LCPUFAs is limited in preterm infants, thus, these molecules are considered as semi-essential or essential. Several studies have suggested that the LCPUFAs supply in preterm infants has a beneficial effect on growth, visual, and cognitive function, as well as on the immune system. Although some methodological issues in these studies do not allow definitive conclusions to be drawn, most of the formulas in Europe and the USA are currently supplemented with LCPUFAs [32–34].

Recommended intakes are 12–30 mg/kg/day or 11–27 mg/100 kcal for DHA and 18–42 mg/kg/day or 16–39 mg/100 kcal for AA [5]. The ratio of AA to DHA should be in the range of 1.0–2.0 to 1 (wt/wt), and EPA supply should not exceed 30% of the DHA supply [5, 34]. Recently, an experts panel has recommended (18-) 55–60 mg/kg/day or (16.4-) 50–55 mg/100 kcal for DHA and (18-) 35–45 mg/kg/day or (16.4-) 32–41 mg/100 kcal for AA [16].

Fat Composition of Human Milk Human milk composition of fat is highly variable and is affected within hours and to a large extent by maternal nutrition intake. Gestation, lactation, parity, milk volume, caloric, and carbohydrate intake, and weight changes are among the maternal factors that can alter the fat content and composition of human breast milk. The lengths of both gestation and lactation affect the lipids that constitute the milk fat globule membrane. Total phospholipid and cholesterol level is higher in colostrum and transitional milk than in mature milk. The period of colostrum lasts less than 10 days, but during this short time the higher lipid levels are beneficial in such processes as neonatal cell membrane production needed for growth, brain development, and bile salt synthesis. Preterm milk may contain a slightly higher proportion of medium- and intermediate chain fatty acids than term milk, which may be advantageous for fat and calcium absorption in preterm infants. LCPUFA are higher in preterm and transitional milk and remain high for the first 6 months in women who deliver preterm. In term milk, on the other hand, LCPUFA declines throughout the first 6–12 months of lactation. Fatty acids rise with a high-carbohydrate maternal diet. Palmitic acid content of breast milk increases in a low-caloric diet. Weight gain during pregnancy is positively associated with higher milk fat content. Milk fat content changes during each feeding. During feedings, foremilk has less fat content than hind milk. Also, the higher the volume of breast milk, the lower the milk fat concentration. Modalities of human milk collection and storage may also influence fat composition. The estimated mean fat content in banked human milk is around 3.2 g/100 ml, somewhat lower than the generally accepted value for mature human milk [35]. This may be related to inadequate emptying of the breast during pumping or to processes applied before delivery bank human milk to neonates.

Pasteurization and storage of banked human milk induces lipolysis, inactivates bile salt-stimulated lipase and lipoprotein lipase, reduces fats, and increases the absolute amount of free fatty acids in pooled samples. Holder pasteurization involves a modification of the biological activity of a large number of enzymes, including lipases [19, 20]. These effects alter the integrity of human milk and may contribute to slower growth in preterm infants fed banked milk versus their mothers' own milk. On the basis of these evidences, a further supplementation with specific fatty acids could be considered for these infants [34–36].

Carbohydrates

Carbohydrates Requirements

Carbohydrates are essential to provide adequate energy supply and they represent a major source of dietary energy. Based on carbohydrate equivalents of total energy expenditure, the experts have recommended a minimum of 10.5 g/100 kcal and a maximum of 12.0 g/100 kcal [5, 16]. Carbohydrates are essential to provide adequate energy supply. Additionally, carbohydrates promote epithelial cell proliferation, insulin secretion, and calcium absorption [5, 16]. Thus, they are also essential to the overall health of the GI tract other than the fulfillment of energy requirements.

Enteral Nutrition Carbohydrates Composition

The predominant carbohydrate in mammalian milk and in term infant formula is lactose. After digestion by lactase, lactose is absorbed as glucose and galactose, which utilize the same carrier mechanism. In the human fetus, intestinal lactase activity is measurable by 10–12 weeks of gestation [37]. There is a gradual increase in lactase activity with advancing gesta-

tion, although the activity remains low until about 36 weeks of gestation, when it reaches the levels seen in full-term neonates [37]. Based on the low lactase activity in early gestation and the estimated length of the bowel, it was calculated that a preterm infant weighing 1300–1400 g might be expected to absorb only 30–50% of the ingested lactose. The lactose that is not fully digested serves as a source of nutrition for bacterial flora in the colon, where it is transformed into short fatty acids and then absorbed [2]. Through the process of fermentation, this not only facilitates colonic water and electrolytes absorption but also stimulates cell turnover of both the colon and the small intestine. After lactose, oligosaccharides are the largest other carbohydrates component in mature human milk. They represent the third largest solute load of the diet after lactose and fat [37]. Oligosaccharides are hydrolyzed by salivary, pancreatic, and intestinal amylase and maltase to free glucose, which is rapidly absorbed. Many of the protective effects of human milk (i.e., against diarrheal diseases, respiratory, and ear infections) have been attributed to oligosaccharides. A further advantage of oligosaccharides for preterm infant formulas includes the improved gastric emptying [38, 39]. Oligosaccharides may be considered as prebiotics. There are some reports that such prebiotics have beneficial effects on various markers of health. For example, primary prevention trials in infants have provided promising data on prevention of infections and atopic dermatitis. However, additional well-designed prospective clinical trials and mechanistic studies are needed to advance knowledge further in this promising field.

Fluids and Electrolytes

The goal of fluid administration is to replace water loss, maintain water and electrolyte homeostasis to provide extra water and electrolytes to build up new tissues. Total fluid intake is related to ingested caloric and protein intake as well as to the renal solute load [40–44]. Randomized controlled trials on enteral fluid intake of preterm infants are lacking as are studies comparing different fluid volumes providing identical nutrient intakes. From data of combined parenteral/enteral regimens, and assuming full enteral absorption, it follows that fluid volumes between 96 and 200 ml/kg/day are tolerated, and that these values may serve as lower and upper limits [5]. When exclusively enteral feeding is reached, a rate of 150–180 ml/kg/day by standard formula or fortified breast milk should be provided to meet nutrient requirements. Some infants may need higher volumes to meet higher requirements of substrates other than fluid. Preterm infants of less than 35 weeks gestation have obligate high renal and intestinal sodium losses during the first 2 weeks of life, leading to cumulative negative sodium balance in most and hyponatremia in many. It has been demonstrated that increasing dietary sodium intake to 4 mmol/kg/day for infants born at 31–34 weeks, and to 5 mmol/kg/day for those born before 31 completed weeks, prevent the negative sodium balance and hyponatremia and led to more rapid weight gain and earlier discharge from hospital [42, 43]. Premature infants require a higher sodium intake in the first 2 weeks of postnatal life than those born at or near at term, and failure to provide such an intake may predispose to poor neurodevelopmental outcome [43]. Due to the rapid rate of growth and the requirements for intracellular potassium in LBM accretion, potassium intakes are estimated around 2–3 mmol/kg/day and are also high in very preterm infants, like for protein [5, 16].

Calcium and Phosphorus

Calcium and Phosphorus Requirements

Several nutrients cause a reduction of calcium bioavailability [45–47]. Various factors affect calcium absorption: vitamin D status, solubility of calcium salts, and the quality and quantity of fat intake. In preterm infants, the vitamin D body stores at birth depend mainly on maternal vitamin D status. In the USA, where dairy products are routinely supplemented with vitamin D, a daily additional intake of 400 IU in the formula may sometimes be sufficient to maintain an adequate plasma concentration of 25-OH and 1–25(OH)2 vitamin D. By contrast, in most parts of Europe, cord blood concentration of 25-OH vitamin D of premature infants is frequently less than 10 μg/ml; in this case, up to 1000 IU/day of vitamin D are recommended [5]. The increased needs of premature infants could be partly due to a relative malabsorption of vitamin D, resulting from a low secretion of bile acids [48]. A calcium retention close to 90 mg/kg/day could currently be expected in preterm infants fed preterm formula with a highly soluble calcium content. These values are still lower than the estimated fetal accretion during the last trimester of gestation (100–120 mg/kg/day). However, there are dramatic physiological changes in bone metabolism resulting from various factors after birth: disruption in maternal mineral supply, stimulation of calciotropic hormone secretion, change in hormonal environment, and relative reduction in mechanical stress. These events stimulate the remodeling process leading to an increase in endosteal bone resorption and a decrease in bone density. In preterm infants, these adaptation processes modify the mineral requirement, since, by itself, the increased remodeling and bone turnover provides a part of the mineral requirement necessary for postnatal bone growth [46].

Phosphate is one of the main intracellular ions present in the cytoplasm. The provision of adequate amounts of nitrogen, potassium, and phosphorus is the condition required to obtain adequate LBM accretion and rapid cell growth. The phosphorus to nitrogen ratio in the cells is not stable and it is increased in the rapidly growing tissues. A large amount of phosphorus is also deposited in the bone in a fixed proportion with calcium and can act as minerals reservoir. In fact, regardless of the proper bone metabolic status, phosphorus consumption by the cell metabolism is privileged in the growing newborn and phosphorus may be released into circulation from the bone if necessary for cellular requirements. In the case of insufficient phosphorus intakes, hypophosphatemia occurs due to cells metabolism requirements. Afterwards, and due to bone phosphorus mobilization from the bone, bone calcium release induces hypercalcemia and hypercalciuria [45]. The strict relationship among amino acid, calcium, and phosphorus intakes is not specific to the first days of life of parenterally fed neonates. This phenomenon of phosphorus deprivation may also be observed in preterm infants enterally fed when a supplementation of protein was not accompanied by a modification of the Ca/P ratio. Calcium retention level ranging from 60 to 90 mg/kg/day assures appropriate mineralization, it decreases the risk of fracture and it diminishes the clinical symptoms of osteopenia. An intake of 100–160 mg/kg/day of highly bioavailable calcium salts, 60–90 mg/kg/day of phosphorus, and 800–1000 IU of vitamin D per day is recommended [5].

Calcium and Phosphorus Composition in Enteral Nutrition

In preterm infants fed human milk, calcium absorption range from 60 to 70 % depending on the calcium salts and intake. Calcium retention is mainly related to phosphorus supply, which is frequently the limiting factor of bone mineralization. Supplementation of human milk with phosphorus alone improves calcium retention from 25 to 35 mg/kg/day. When calcium and phosphorus are provided together or as human milk fortifiers, calcium retention may reach 60 mg/kg/day. Recent use of human milk fortifiers containing highly soluble calcium glycerophosphate has improved calcium retention up to 90 mg/kg/day at intake of 140 mg/kg/day [47]. In formula-fed infants, calcium absorption is usually less than with human milk, ranging from 35 to 60 % of intake. Calcium absorption is related to calcium, fat intakes, and techniques of milk preparation [19, 20]. With ready-to-use liquid formulas, calcium absorption is usually lower than with powder formulas. With the use of formulas with a well-absorbed fat blend of about 85 %, the formation of calcium soap is of minimal interest in clinical practice. Finally, owing to the poor solubility of calcium salts, especially calcium phosphate, the calcium content measured in the formula could be significantly lower than the claimed value, and additional loss due to precipitation may occur before feeding.

Iron

Preterm infants require iron for erythropoiesis, brain development, muscle function, and cardiac function. The symptoms of iron deficiency are not due to anemia only but are also due to tissue losses of iron containing enzymes and iron–sulfur proteins. It has been estimated that, in the absence of iron supplementation, a VLBW preterm infant has enough iron stores to last 2 months [49]. However, due their growth requirements and blood samples, preterm infants need supplemental iron after 2 weeks of age. Enteral dose of iron for the preterm infant ranges from 2 to 4 mg/kg/day, depending on the degree of prematurity and the amount of phlebotomy. The introduction of erythropoietin puts a greater stress on iron balance, forcing the infant to mobilize endogenous iron stores at a faster rate. For infants receiving this medication, an enteral dose of 6 mg/kg/day is recommended. No study has demonstrated oxidative toxicity from enteral iron given at conventional doses in preterm infants. Iron needs of preterm infants remain greater than those of term infants because of their more rapid relative rate of growth and therefore blood volume expansion. Given their lower endogenous iron stores, it would be prudent in preterm to monitor the presence of anemia earlier than in term infants.

Trace Elements

Trace elements contribute less than 0.01 % of the total body weight. They function as constituents of metalloenzymes, cofactors for metal ion-activated enzymes, or components of vitamins, hormones, and proteins. Because the fetus accumulates important stores of trace elements during the third trimester of pregnancy, premature infants have low stores at birth and are at high risk of developing mineral deficiencies if intakes are inadequate for their growth requirements. Trace minerals with established physiological importance in humans include zinc, copper, selenium, manganese, chromium, molybdenum, and iodine. Recently, it has been suggested that dose of zinc higher than those recommended by the ESPGHAN may reduce morbidity and mortality in preterm neonates [5, 50].

Oral Vitamin Requirements

Vitamins are organic compounds that are essential for metabolic reactions but are not synthesized by the body [1, 5, 28]. Vitamins are classified as water soluble or fat soluble, based on the biochemical structure and function of the compound. Water-soluble vitamins cannot be formed by precursors (with the exception of niacin from tryptophan) and do not accumulate in the body (with the exception of vitamin B12).

They include B complex vitamins and vitamin C. They serve as prosthetic groups for enzymes involved in amino acid metabolism, energy production, and nucleic acid synthesis. A daily intake is required to prevent deficiency. Excretion occurs in the urine and bile. Altered urinary losses due to renal immaturity during the first week of life predispose a preterm infant to vitamin deficiency or excess [1]. Fat-soluble vitamins include vitamin A, D, E, and K. Fat-soluble vitamins require carrier systems, usually lipoproteins, for solubility in blood, and intestinal absorption depends on fat absorption capability [5].

Breast Milk

Benefit of Breast Milk

Since 20 years, the American Academy of Pediatrics (AAP) has acknowledged the advantages of human milk feeding with the statement that it is the preferred feeding for all infants, including those born preterm [51]. The benefits of human milk for host defense, GI function, and neurodevelopmental outcome are briefly reported in Table 6.1. Preterm infants fed human milk have fewer infections than those fed on formula. This advantage has been observed with both fresh and pasteurized human milk [52, 53]. There are studies showing a protective effect of breast milk on the incidence of NEC [53–55]. Feeding with donor human milk was also associated with a significantly reduced risk of NEC [54]. The recent development of human-milk-based human milk fortifier suggest a possibility to decrease the risk of NEC compared with the use of conventional bovine milk fortifier or preterm formula [55, 56]. However, the significant reduction of the cases of NEC may depend on high basal incidence of NEC ($> 15\%$) observed only in several settings. This aspect limits the generalization of the data to other clinical setting with lower incidence of NEC. The protective effect of human milk has been attributed to several factors, such as macrophages, lymphocytes, sIgA, lysozyme, lactoferrin, oligosaccharides, nucleotides, cytokines, growth factors, and enzymes present in breast milk. Immune defense can be provided by an interaction between these factors [2]. Breast milk enhances the growth, motility, and maturity of the GI tract compared to formulas. It also induces faster gastric emptying. The mother's presence in the neonatal nursery combined with breast milk expression, particularly the premature infant's skin-to-skin contact with the mother, may reduce the risk of infections by nosocomial pathogens by passive immunization [57]. Preterm infants fed human milk during hospitalization showed better neurological development and a higher intelligence quotient compared to those formula fed, even after controlling for the mother's educa-

Table 6.1 Benefits and limits of human milk and formula for preterm neonates

	Nutritional power	Effects on infectious diseases	Effects on the risk of necrotizing enterocolitis (NEC)
Human milk			
Fresh	Risk of nutrient deficiencies and slower neonatal growth compared to fortified human milk and preterm formula	Reduced risk of infection (sepsis and urinary tract infection) compared to preterm formula feeding Risk of transmission of CMV infection	Reduced risk of NEC compared to preterm formula feeding
Holder pasteurization	Minimal reduction in fat and energy content compared to fresh human milk Partial reduction in nutritional and biological quality compared to fresh human milk	Reduced risk of infection compared to preterm formula feeding. Similar rate of sepsis compared to fresh human milk No risk of transmission of CMV infection compared to fresh human milk	Reduced risk of NEC compared to preterm formula feeding
Short-term heat pasteurization (5 s at 72°C)	No evidences available	No risk of transmission of CMV infection compared to fresh human milk	No evidences available
Freezing (−20 °C)	Preserve nutritional and biological quality of human milk	Higher risk of transmission of CMV infection compared to holder pasteurized human milk, but reduced compared to fresh human milk	No evidences available
Human fortified milk			
Fortified with bovine milk-based fortifiers	Improvements in growth (weight, length, and head circumference) during hospital stay compared to not-fortified human milkNutrient availability and properties of human milk may be changed by fortification Lower growth compared to preterm formula feeding Improved growth using target fortification	Lower risk of sepsis compared to preterm formula feeding	Lower risk of NEC compared to preterm formula feeding No significantly increased risk of NEC compared to not fortified human milk
Fortified with human milk-based fortifiers	Similar rate of growth compared to human milk fortified with bovine-based products	Similar rate of sepsis compared to human milk fortified with bovine-based product	Reduced risk of NEC compared to feeding with preterm formula or human milk fortified with bovine-based product
Preterm formula			
Powdered	Improvement of fat absorption, nitrogen retention, bone mineralization, and growth compared to pooled human milk	Higher risk of sepsis compared to human milk feeding Risk of *Enterobacter sakazakii* infection	Higher risk of NEC compared to human milk feeding
Liquid	Improvement of fat absorption, nitrogen retention, bone mineralization, and growth compared to pooled human milk Reduced bioavailability of various nutrients (proteins, calcium, or copper) compared to powdered formulation due to precipitation or heat treatment	Higher risk of sepsis compared to human milk feeding	Higher risk of NEC compared to human milk feeding

CMV cytomegalovirus

tion and social class [58–61]. Higher mental developmental index scores were reported in VLBW infants at 18 months of age who received human milk compared to those who never received human milk in hospital [59]. At 16 years follow-up, the percentage of expressed breast milk in the neonatal diet correlated significantly with verbal IQ and white-matter volume in males [60]. Potential factors of human milk that might contribute to neurodevelopment are net protein utilization, amino acids and fat composition, other than hormone, growth factor, and micronutrients [2].

Limits of Breast Milk

Despite many benefits, human milk and its nutrients content are not sufficient to cover the greater needs of VLBW infants. Breast milk composition depends on the gestational age at delivery, collection methods (e.g., drip method vs. expression with a pump), and whether pooled milk or the infant's own mother's milk is used [53]. Greater concentrations of nitrogen, immune proteins, total lipids, medium-chain fatty acids, energy, vitamins, some minerals (calcium and phosphorus), and trace elements in milk from mothers who give birth prematurely (preterm milk) compared with milk of mothers giving birth at term (term milk) have been observed [53]. The higher concentrations of these nutrients tend to decline as lactation progresses, so exclusive feeding of mature preterm milk from 2 weeks postnatally may lead to nutrient deficiencies in the rapidly growing preterm infant [35]. The reason for the difference in nutrient density between preterm and term milk is not well known. Early interruption of pregnancy might induce an incomplete maturation of mammary glands leading to paracellular leakage of serum proteins and ions through junctions that have not completely closed. Also, a different hormonal profile in women who deliver prematurely compared with those who deliver at term could be responsible for a different milk composition. The greater nutrient density in preterm milk could also be related to the higher concentration of nutrients in a lower volume of milk. In fact, the main limits of human milk for preterm infants is its production. Mothers of preterm infants, for several reasons (stress, poor maternal health, delayed initiation of lactation), frequently produce an insufficient quantity of milk [57]. The difficulties faced by mothers trying to provide milk for their preterm infant must not be underestimated. They may need to express milk for a period of weeks or months in the absence of significant suckling stimulus and in the presence of a great deal stress. Increasing the frequency of expression, kangaroo care or skin-to-skin contact, relaxation tapes may improve milk volume produced by mothers. Moreover, a restriction of fluid intake in VLBW infants could reduce the volume of human milk given, and thus not offer a sufficient quantity of nutrients.

Breast Milk Fortification

Human milk fortifiers have been produced to increase the nutritional content of human milk in order to meet the nutritional requirements of VLBW infants and to preserve the benefits of human milk [61]. The protein content of human milk is too low to permit a weight gain similar to the intrauterine fetus. The low sodium level may lead to hyponatremia. The amounts of calcium and phosphorus are widely below the intake needed to achieve adequate bone mineral accretion and to avoid severe osteopenia. Through a process of human milk lacto-engineering, human milk can be fortified with skim and cream components derived from heat-treated, lyophilized mature donor human milk to produce a "'human milk formula." This method of fortification avoids cow's milk proteins but it is impractical for most neonatal units, since it involves a complex and costly process and requires a large supply of donor milk. Preterm human milk, fortified with protein of bovine origin, has become the standard practice in most neonatal units. The composition of several fortifiers expressed per gram of protein varies both qualitatively and quantitatively [61]. In general, they contain bovine whey protein (intact or hydrolyzed), carbohydrates (mainly or exclusively glucose polymers or maltodextrins), minerals, and electrolytes such as sodium, calcium, phosphorus, and magnesium, and some also contain micronutrients and vitamins. The properties of human milk may be changed by nutrient fortification. Fortification may influence nutrient availability and may alter some biological properties of human milk. This is the result of the osmotic content of the fortifier but also of the rapid and continuous activity of human milk amylase on the dextrin content of fortifiers. High osmolality may induce abdominal discomfort and delayed gastric emptying. Recently, in order to avoid these problems, fortifiers with whole proteins, reduced carbohydrate content and fat supplementation have been proposed [61, 62]. The presence of fat in fortifiers has the advantage of increasing the energy intake of human milk without increasing osmolality values [62].

A review for the Cochrane collaboration concluded that the use of multinutrient fortifiers is associated with short-term improvements in weight gain and increments in both length and head circumference growth during hospital stay [62]. Although the fortification of human milk improves the general growth of preterm infants, growth of specific parameters such as LBM, fat mass, and bone mineral content is significantly lower in fortified human milk-fed infants than in those fed preterm formula [63]. These differences could be related to the lower protein content of human milk compared with hypothetic values used to establish fortification. Indeed, the variability in expressed human milk with respect to its protein and energy content is high. This variability may result in undernutrition after standard fortification method. A recent trial demonstrated that individualized fortification may optimize protein and energy intake [9]. Compared with standard fortification, individual fortification significantly reduces the variability in nutritional intakes, allowing the maintenance of protein intake and the PER in the range of the current recommendations. Further studies are advocated to verify the long-term effects of individualized fortification method.

When compared with premature infants fed preterm formula, infants fed exclusively fortified human milk had a significantly lower incidence of NEC and/or sepsis, had fewer positive blood cultures, and required less antibiotic administration [61]. When fortified human milk was evaluated under simulated nursery conditions, bacterial colony counts were not significantly different after 20 h of storage at refrigerator temperature, but increased from 20 to 24 h when maintained at incubator temperature [61, 64]. In conclusion, early use of a human milk fortifier up to 1.3 g of protein per 100 ml may be recommended for more immature or smaller preterm infants, beginning from the time when they are able to tolerate 60–80 ml/kg/day of milk [12].

Expressed Donor Milk

Expressed donor milk can be foremilk or hind milk. These two types of milk, respectively, have lower or higher fat and energy contents than milk received by the breastfed infant [64]. Mature donor milk will have a lower protein sodium, zinc, and copper content than that of milk produced in early lactation. Feeding donor breast milk is classically associated with poor weight gain and growth restriction. However, analysis of available evidences revealed that most of the studies considered were 20–30 years old and from an era when donor breast milk was fed without fortification or mineral supplements, often as the sole diet. It is not clear whether similar effects would be seen when supplementation with fortifiers is adopted. Additionally, infant fed donor breast milk had a significantly reduced risk of NEC [52–54].

Treatment of donor breast milk (i.e., collection, store, froze, pasteurization, exposition to light,) may induce qualitative alteration [21, 22]. Breast milk in human milk banks is stored at low temperatures and subjected to thermal processing to guarantee its microbiological safety. Holder pasteurization (heating at 62.5 °C for 30 min and subsequent fast cooling) is the most frequent. Such pasteurization has been mainly assessed in terms of reduction in the activity of proteins of major biological relevance, such as immunoglobulins, lactoferrin, lysozyme, and GI enzymes such as lipase. It decreases fat and energy content of human milk [65]. Frozen storage at -20 °C of pasteurized milk further reduces fat, lactose, and energy content of human milk [21, 22]. These aspects may influence macronutrients and energy intake and may affect growth and neurodevelopment.

Breast milk transmission of human immunodeficiency virus (HIV) is considered an important mode of neonatal infection. Despite this fact, many researchers have observed that corresponding to the volume of milk consumed by the infant, maternal transmission via breast milk is still comparatively low. Some have noted the long latency period of breast milk HIV transmission with evidence of numerous anti-HIV factors in breast milk [66]. The presence of HIV or of other viruses in maternal milk seems to be a requisite to spur immunological defenses to optimize necessary protection to the infant. Because the only intervention to completely prevent HIV transmission via human milk is not to breast-feed, the AAP recommends that HIV-infected mothers not breastfeed their infants regardless of maternal viral load and antiretroviral therapy. Despite the use of human breast milk from HIV-infected mother is not recommended in industrialized countries, an HIV-infected woman receiving effective antiretroviral therapy with repeatedly undetectable HIV viral loads may choose to breastfeed in particular circumstances. This rare condition generally does not constitute grounds for an automatic referral to child protective services agencies. Infant HIV infection status should be monitored by nucleic acid amplification testing throughout lactation and at 1, 3, and 6 months after weaning.

Some concerns about CMV infection in preterm infants receiving breast milk from seropositive mothers exist because CMV is excreted in breast milk in most lactating mother after a few weeks [67]. Differences in CMV acquisition from fresh or frozen milk have been suggested. Short-term high-temperature pasteurization techniques were found to prevent CMV transmission more effectively than freezing [68]. Cryotreatment preserves the nutritional quality of human milk, but unfortunately does not cancel the risk of CMV transmission. In contrast, compared with freezing, holder pasteurization and short-term heat inactivation for 5 s at 72 °C partially destroy the activity of some digestive enzymes, but contemporarily eliminates viral infectivity in milk in each stage of lactation [69]. Decisions about breastfeeding of VLBW infants by mothers known to be CMV-seropositive should be made with consideration of the potential benefits of human milk versus the risk of CMV transmission.

Preterm Formulas

When human milk is not available or limited, cow's-milk-based formulas for preterm infants must be used. Over the past 20 years, there has been a significant improvement in the nutrient composition of preterm formulas in order to meet the high nutritional needs of growing preterm infants. VLBW infants fed these formulas showed an improvement of fat absorption, nitrogen retention, bone mineralization, and weight gain, when compared to VLBW infants fed standard term formulas or pooled human milk [1]. Although numerous consensus conferences have been organized, the optimal formula for VLBW infants has not yet been designed. European preterm formulas present several differences in the nutrient composition when compared to American formulas [1, 5, 28]. The latter have a higher MCT and a lower LCPU-FA content, provide less lactose, and have a higher mineral intake. Nevertheless, according to more recent data, a general profile in macronutrients could probably be suggested. Energy content could be slightly higher than at present. Current recommendation for energy intakes are 110–135 kcal/kg/day for the ESPGHAN 2010 and 110–130 kcal/kg/day for experts' panel. According to the protein requirements, the protein content would represent 3.2–3.6 g/100 kcal, that is, 2.4–3.2 g/100 ml [5]. Whey-predominant protein with reduced glycomacropeptide and α-lactalbumin enrichment could be used to optimize the amino acid profile [14, 21]. Up to now, the use of protein-hydrolyzed formulas has not been recommended [26, 70]. The partition of the nonprotein energy supply would favor the carbohydrate content up to 50–60% in view of its suggested benefits in sparing protein oxidation, enhancing growth and protein accretion as well as improving quiet sleep and influencing the distribution of behavioral activity states in VLBW infants. The remaining energy supply would be covered by fat with a fat blend carefully designed to reduce the long-chain saturated fatty acids content, and provide the essential fatty acids (LA and ALA) in an appropriate ratio as well as the LCPUFAs such as DHA and AA [34]. MCT could be used with a maximum of 30–40% of lipids content [5]. Highly metabolizable (50–60% absorption rate) calcium content would be limited to 100–120 mg/100 ml. According to the expected nitrogen and calcium retention, the phosphorus content of this formula would represent 55–65 mg/100 ml, considering phosphorus absorption close to 90%. Preterm formulas are available as powder or liquid in glass bottles or cans. Liquid formulas have the advantage that they provide sterile feeding thereby reducing possible infections reported in preterm infants fed powder formulas, such as by *Enterobacter sakazakii* [71]. Nevertheless, it worth remembering that with liquid formulas, there is frequent discordance between claimed and available content of several nutrients. For instance, part of the calcium content of liquid formula may precipitate on the wall of the receptacle reducing the calcium truly available to the preterm infants. In addition, the heat treatment necessary to sterilize the liquid formulas reduces the bioavailability of various nutrients such as proteins, calcium, or copper. In consequence, when human milk is not available, powder formulas allowing adaptation of nutrient density and being of higher nutritional value remain the formulas of choice for the feeding of VLBW infants.

Side Effects and Complications of Enteral Nutrition

Enteral nutrition could present side effects and complications including the risk of NEC and problems associated with the use of tube support for feeding. The risk of NEC could be reduced by employment of breast milk, early introduction of enteral nutrition, slow advancement (maximum 25–30 ml/kg/day), and careful check of the appearance of the first clinical and radiological signs of disease [12]. Contemporarily, the use of MEF in the VLBW newborns with the suspected signs of feeding intolerance may reduce the risk of

prolonged total parenteral nutrition and sepsis without additional risk for NEC [8].

Monitoring Effects of Artificial Nutrition on Growth

Anthropometric Measurements

Overall growth is monitored by anthropometry: measurement of body weight, length, head circumference, and, to a lesser extent, skinfold and arm circumference [73]. Anthropometric method to monitor growth and assess nutritional status in infants is rapid, inexpensive, and noninvasive. Body weight comprises the total mass of the infant's lean tissue, fat, and extracellular and intracellular fluid compartments. Weight gain or loss, reflects also changes in body composition. In utero, the fetus experiences a decrease in extracellular fluid volume and an increase in lean tissue and fat mass as gestational age increases. The initial postnatal weight loss is attributed to contraction of body water compartments and catabolism of endogenous glycogen, fat stores, and lean tissue in the absence of adequate energy and nutrients. Physiologic postnatal weight loss is 5–10% of total body weight. Maximum initial weight loss usually reaches its nadir by the 3–6 day of life and birth weight is usually regained by 7–10 days of age. Body weight should be measured daily to assess growth and fluid and electrolytes status in order to define optimal management. Once birth weight is regained, subsequent weight gain of 17–20 g/kg/day is desirable for infants up to 32 weeks PMA. Weight gain should be evaluated weekly to identify infants with average weight gains of <15 or >25 g/kg/day. Unfortunately, poor weight gain is common in infants with extreme prematurity or pathological conditions (chronic lung disease, severe intraventricular hemorrhage, NEC, and late-onset sepsis). Postnatal growth restriction is mainly due to insufficient nutritional support and can be avoided in most VLBW infants if they received recommended nutritional intakes [73].

Anthropometric measurements should be plotted on percentile growth curves for comparison against established reference data. Plotting weight on classic intrauterine growth charts can determine whether an infant is SGA (weight <10th percentile or <2 standard deviation score), AGA, or large for gestational age (LGA weight >90th percentile or >2 standard deviation score). Serial measures of growth and nutritional status are helpful in assessing response to nutrition support in hospitalized VLBW infants and to define if they develop a growth restriction. Growth restriction is usually defined for infants who cross (decrease) the percentile curves, when their standard deviation score decrease by more than 0.6 or 1.0, or if they become SGA. Using the growth chart, optimal weight for length is identified by finding the weight, which is approximately on the same percentile as the infant's length measurement. Current weight expressed as a percentage of optimal weight for length can be used to identify infants at risk for under- or overnutrition [72]. Term neonates use to accumulate significant fat mass during the first months of life, and it is not known whether preterm neonates need to accumulate the same amount of fat mass during their first months of life, which would be significantly different from fetuses of the same PMA. Despite most experts agree that low weight-for-length status correspond to growth restriction, it is not known what is the optimal weight-for-length status for preterm infant when they are plotted on intrauterine growth charts.

Neonates with a history of intrauterine growth restriction may have growth delays in weight, length, or head circumference. With symmetric or proportionate growth restriction, all parameters are affected, resulting in a greater risk of neonatal morbidity, future growth problems, and neurodevelopmental delay. In asymmetric growth restriction, only one parameter displays impaired growth. If weight is low compared with length and head circumference, catch-up growth may be expected. When head circumference is low compared with weight and length, neurological or developmental impairment may occur.

The type of growth charts used to assess anthropometric measures may influence these evaluations [72, 74–76]. The use of charts based on fetal growth until term (intrauterine curves) or on observed postnatal growth of preterm infants (longitudinal curves) should lead to different interpretations. The first describes how fetuses grow and a possible standard. The second represents how preterm infants actually grow and usually describes a postnatal growth restriction. In addition and after 36 weeks PMA, intrauterine charts usually demonstrate slower weight gain due to progressive placental insufficiency (late intrauterine growth restriction). Preterm infants do not describe similar weight gain at theoretical term that term neonate do with their initial physiologic weight loss. Therefore, it is not easy to monitor and to interpret preterm infants' growth after plotting anthropometric data on charts. To address these issues, the Fenton's charts were designed to commence monitoring infants at 22 weeks' PMA and continue for 10 weeks post term according to gender [74]. In particular, the use of gender-related growth charts reduces the false detection of intrauterine growth retardation in girls [75].

It is not easy to assess LBM and fat mass with classic anthropometric measurements, especially when edema or dehydration is present. Many tools have been tested to define better body composition. Regional anthropometry, triceps skinfold, and mid-arm circumference, or the ratios and formulae derived from these measurements, have been proposed as predictors of infant body composition. Standards are available for infants between 24 and 41 weeks gestation and can be used to compare those of an individual infant with reference values or to assess individual changes over time

[76]. However, intra- and inter-examiner measurement technique variability, critical illness, hydration status, and positioning of infants can contribute to measurement of errors. In addition, the use of calipers to measure triceps skinfold may not be feasible in extremely immature infants who have delicate, easily punctured skin. For these reasons, regional anthropometry is not routinely assessed.

Laboratory and Biomedical Tools

Serum nutrient levels can be used as markers of nutritional status in VLBW infants, but many factors not related to nutrition can alter laboratory results and must be considered when interpreting biological data. Technical factors, such as storage and processing of the specimen, type of laboratory method used, and technician accuracy, may affect the validity of laboratory tests. Blood urea nitrogen (BUN), a by-product of protein degradation, is frequently used to monitor protein intake in premature infant fed human milk after the first month of life [77]. However, BUN does not measure protein nutritional status but reflects dietary intakes, hydration status, renal function, and the presence of catabolism. Serum concentrations of transport proteins albumin, transferrin, prealbumin (transthyretin), and retinol-binding protein (RBP) have also been proposed as indicators of protein nutritional status [78]. Both albumin and transferrin have a longer half-life than prealbumin or RBP, thus serum concentrations of different transport proteins reflect different nutritional intake at different time periods. Prealbumin and RBP concentrations appear to correlate better with nitrogen balance during artificial nutritional therapy. Serum transferrin and RBP levels may be influenced by suboptimal iron, zinc, or vitamin A status. Low values of these proteins are usually described in premature infants during the first 3 months of life when compared to term infants suggesting insufficient nutritional support in premature infants. However, if transport protein concentrations are normal but growth is poor, nutritional supply needs to be increased to meet the nutritional demands of VLBW infants.

Alkaline phosphatase (ALP) is an enzyme predominantly produced in liver and bone. It may be elevated during normal growth conditions, liver diseases, or bone diseases. In preterm neonates an increase of ALP may suggest the presence of an osteopenia of prematurity secondary to calcium, phosphorous, magnesium, or vitamin D deficiencies [79]. As previously discussed, hypophosphatemia and hypercalciuria should also be regularly ruled out to avoid severe osteopenia.

Iron deficiency is frequent in premature infants and typically occurs after 4–8 weeks. Serum ferritin may be use as a good marker of iron store and values above 116 μg/l are advised. Indeed, iron deficiency anemia and low ferritin stores below 75 μg/l have been associated with nonoptimal developmental outcomes. Classical prevention strategy of iron deficiency in preterm infants are delayed (30–120 s) cord clamping at birth and systematic 2–3 mg/kg/day supplementation from the 3rd week of life. On another side, excessive iron intakes may be toxic leading to some oxidative stress, increased risk of infection and retinopathy, and poor growth without any advantages on developmental outcomes. High ferritin concentration above 400 µg/l might be considered as iron overload, and iron intakes should be decreased [80].

Despite premature infants are at high risk for developing complications from deficiencies of zinc, vitamin B12, folate, vitamin E, and copper, laboratory tests used for diagnosis of vitamin deficiency are expensive and should be reserved to the infants at high risk of deficiencies such as malabsorptive diseases and long-term (>3 weeks) parenteral nutrition [81].

Advances in imaging techniques have allowed more direct in vivo measurement of body composition. Dual-energy X-ray absorptiometry (DEXA), requiring minimum radiation exposure (<0.3 mrem), has been successfully used for measurement of lean mass, fat mass, and bone mineral content in newborns. DEXA remains the most widely used method for the in vivo measurement of whole-body composition in humans. However, there are concerns on the accuracy in VLBW infants, especially in regard to determination of fat mass. In particular, the diagnostic power of this method for body composition determination depends on model of device, software, and scanning mode. These aspects limit the possibility to use DEXA reference ranges for preterm neonates. Nowadays, air displacement plethysmography has recently emerged as a noninvasive technique to determine body fat mass and fat-free mass in preterm infants [81, 82]. It is based on the measurement of body volume using gas laws, and several studies have confirmed the reliability and accuracy of air displacement plethysmography in animals, infants, and neonates [81]. Further validation of these techniques is advocated for routine use.

Post-discharge Nutrition in Preterm Infants

In most neonatal units, the discharge of VLBW infants usually occurs when premature infants reach 35–36 weeks PMA and/or a weight of about 1800–2100 g. By that time, they have frequently accumulated energy, protein, and mineral deficits and have developed a growth restriction. Additionally, they still present higher nutrient requirements than healthy term infants and premature infants born at the same PMA [83–85]. Protein- and mineral-enriched formulas have been proposed to feed preterm infants after discharge with the aim of minimizing as much as possible, postnatal growth restriction during the early weeks of life, inducing early catch-up growth and reducing the adverse effects of early malnutrition [83–85]. Energy intakes are the main determinant of milk volume intakes. Compared to regular (standard) formula, a simple increase in energy density without changes

in nutrients proportion had no influence on nutrients supply except in infants with limiting feeding self-sufficiency, not able to drink their quantity for several reason (bronchopulmonary dysplasia, cardiac insufficiency, neurologic insufficiency, "quickly tired" infants) [86]. In contrast, an increase in protein density with high PER influences protein intake and protein metabolism and a positive effect of growth parameters was not observed in all studies [83–85]. The benefit of the nutrient-enriched formula on VLBW infants' growth was mainly seen during the early post-discharge period, between discharge and theoretical term (40 weeks PMA). This increased growth rate is observed in all preterm infants, even in those without postnatal growth deficit at the time of discharge. Additionally, there is a strong gender influence on the result of diet manipulation during the post-discharge period and the main positive results are more obvious in boys [87].

Considerable attention should be focused on specific nutrients, particularly calcium, phosphorus, iron, LCPUFAs, and vitamin A. Feeding post-discharge preterm infants formulas or human milk with greater concentrations of calcium and phosphorus than those contained in term formula improves bone mineralization, particularly if the special formulas used during hospitalization are continued after hospital discharge [88]. However, the relative osteopenia of VLBW infants observed at the time of hospital discharge usually improves spontaneously in most VLBW infants after discharge, in a manner similar to that induced by the acceleration of growth at the first stage of adolescence. Therefore, provision of large amounts of calcium and phosphorous for long periods may not be necessary. With regard to vitamin D intake, there is no evidence that preterm infants should receive greater doses than term infants to maintain a normal plasma vitamin D concentration after discharge [89]. Body iron stores are highly variable at discharge, so it is important to screen for iron deficiency at discharge and during the first year of life [49]. Scientific Societies recommend that preterm infants receive iron supplements for up to 1 year after discharge [49]. Preterm infants fed human milk should receive an iron supplement of 2 mg/kg/day by 1 month of age, and this should be continued at least until the infant is weaned to iron-fortified formula or begins eating complementary foods that supply 2 mg/kg/day of iron. Infants who have received iron loads from multiple transfusions of packed red blood cells may not require supplements. LCPUFAs need to be added in VLBW infants' feeds to improve brain development and the retina in particular [83–85]. Vitamin A status may be suboptimal in formula-fed VLBW infants for many months after discharge. Contrasting data exist regarding the utility of aggressive enteral supplementation with vitamin A (3000 IU/day) after discharge. At the moment, additional studies are needed to determine the dose and duration of vitamin A supplementation that allows infants to reach full repletion values [83–85].

Growth at 4 and 12 months and mineralization at 4 months after discharge are better in VLBW infants fed preterm formula during the first 2 months after discharge than in those fed term formula [83–85]. Protein and nutrient-enriched formula provided after term seems to improve the quality of growth in preterm infants. Infants fed nutrient-enriched formula have lower fat mass, corrected for body size at 6 months' corrected age, than infants fed standard formula or human milk. Preterm infants fed nutrient-enriched formula after discharge exhibit an increase in LBM and peripheral fat mass but not central adiposity compared with infants fed term formula. These data indicate that nutrient-enriched formulas do not promote central adiposity in preterm infants, a feature that is associated with metabolic syndrome later in life.

Even if low protein intakes and poor growth during initial hospitalization in VLBW infants has been associated with poor adverse developmental outcomes, the safety of prolonged high-protein intake in preterm infants after discharge has not been completely established [27]. Thus, further studies are necessary to address this crucial safety aspect. Since early nutrition should not only be considered simply in terms of weight gain but also for the biological effects with possibly lasting or lifelong significance, it seems prudent to suggest an enriched formula only in infants at risk of future growth failure.

Among the preterm infants, not all are at similar risk of later growth failure and adverse developmental outcomes after discharge. SGA infants and preterm infants who have developed a postnatal growth restriction seem to be the population at higher risk, boys in particular. In these infants, breastfeeding should always be promoted with or without a transient fortification of expressed-human milk up to 40–52 weeks PMA. If breastfeeding is not possible, a preterm formula or a special post-discharge formula that contains more protein, minerals, trace elements, and LCPUFAs should be preferred to a standard term formula until the preterm infant reaches between 40 and 52 weeks PMA to improve catch-up growth. AGA infants without growth restriction at the time of discharge from the hospital usually continue to maintain appropriate growth. In these infants, exclusive breastfeeding should be encouraged at discharge and if not possible, a term infant formula with relatively low protein density (2.2 g/100 kcal) should be provided with particular attention to its LCPUFAs, mineral and trace element content.

In conclusion, breastfeeding should always be encouraged in all preterm infants after discharge. In those with high risk of longitudinal growth restriction, fortified human milk or enriched formula (protein, energy, LCPUFA, micronutrients) may also be add to breastfeeding in order to improve the nutrient supply and to promote catch-up growth [83–85]. Immediately discharge, growth should be monitored weekly to adapt feeding and to avoid growth failure, especially in VLBW infants.

References

1. De Curtis M, Rigo J. The nutrition of preterm infants. Early Hum Dev. 2012;88:S5–7.
2. Berni Canani R, Passariello A, Buccigrossi V, Terrin G, Guarino A. The nutritional modulation of the evolving intestine. J Clin Gastroenterol. 2008;42(Suppl 3):S197–200.
3. Corpeleijn WE, Kouwenhoven SM, van Goudoever JB. Optimal growth of preterm infants. World Rev Nutr Diet. 2013;106:149–55.
4. De Curtis M, Rigo J. Extrauterine growth restriction in very-low-birthweight infants. Acta Paediatr. 2004;93:1563–8.
5. Agostoni C, Buonocore G, Carnielli VP, et al. Enteral nutrient supply for preterm infants: commentary from the European Society for Paediatric Gastroenterology, Hepatology, and Nutrition Committee on Nutrition. J Pediatr Gastroenterol Nutr. 2010;50:85–91.
6. Karagianni P, Briana DD, Mitsiakos G, Elias A, Theodoridis T, Chatziioannidis E, Kyriakidou M, Nikolaidis N. Early versus delayed minimal enteral feeding and risk for necrotizing enterocolitis in preterm growth-restricted infants with abnormal antenatal Doppler results. Am J Perinatol. 2010;27:367–73.
7. Morgan J, Bombell S, McGuire W. Early trophic feeding versus enteral fasting for very preterm or very low birth weight infants. Cochrane Database Syst Rev. 2013;3:CD000504.
8. Terrin G, Passariello A, Canani RB, et al. Minimal enteral feeding reduces the risk of sepsis in feed-intolerant very low birth weight newborns. Acta Paediatr. 2009;98:31–5.
9. de Halleux V, Rigo J. Variability in human milk composition: benefit of individualized fortification in very-low-birth-weight infants. Am J Clin Nutr. 2013;98:529S–35S.
10. Dawson JA, Summan R, Badawi N, Foster JP. Push versus gravity for intermittent bolus gavage tube feeding of premature and low birth weight infants. Cochrane Database Syst Rev. 2012;11:CD005249
11. SIFT Investigators Group. Early enteral feeding strategies for very preterm infants: current evidence from Cochrane reviews. Arch Dis Child Fetal Neonatal Ed. 2013;98:F470–2.
12. Senterre T. Practice of enteral nutrition in very low birth weight and extremely low birth weight infants. World Rev Nutr Diet. 2014;110:201–14.
13. Morgan J, Young L, McGuire W. Slow advancement of enteral feed volumes to prevent necrotising enterocolitis in very low birth weight infants. Cochrane Database Syst Rev. 2013;3:CD001241.
14. Lucchini R, Bizzarri B, Giampietro S, De Curtis M. Feeding intolerance in preterm infants. How to understand the warning signs. J Matern Fetal Neonatal Med. 2011;24(Suppl 1):72–4.
15. Rigo J. Protein, amino acid and other nitrogen compounds. In: Tsang RC, Uauy R, Koletzko B, Zlotkin SH, editors. Nutritional of the preterm infant. Cincinnati: Digital Education; 2005. pp. 45–80.
16. Koletzko B, Poindexter B, Uauy R. Recommended nutrient intake levels for stable, fully enterally fed very low birth weight infants. World Rev Nutr Diet. 2014;110:297–9.
17. Fenton TR, Premji SS, Al-Wassia H, Sauve RS. Higher versus lower protein intake in formula-fed low birth weight infants. Cochrane Database Syst Rev. 2014;4:CD003959.
18. Embleton ND, Cooke RJ. Protein requirements in preterm infants: effect of different levels of protein intake on growth and body composition. Pediatr Res. 2005;58:855–60.
19. Young L, Morgan J, McCormick FM, McGuire W. Nutrient-enriched formula versus standard term formula for preterm infants following hospital discharge. Cochrane Database Syst Rev. 2012;14(3):CD004696.
20. Goldman HI, Goldman JS, Kaufman I, Liebman OB. Late effects of early dietary protein intake on low-birth-weight infants. J Pediatr. 1974;85:764–9.
21. Rigo J, Senterre J. Nutritional needs of premature infants: current issues. J Pediatr. 2006;149:s80–8.

22. García-Lara NR, Vieco DE, De la Cruz-Bértolo J, Lora-Pablos D, Velasco NU, Pallás-Alonso CR. Effect of Holder pasteurization and frozen storage on macronutrients and energy content of breast milk. J Pediatr Gastroenterol Nutr. 2013;57(3):377–82.

23. Rigo J, Boehm G, Georgi G et al. An infant formula free of glyco-macropeptide prevents hyperthreoninemia in formula-fed preterm infants. J Pediatr Gastroenterol Nutr. 2001;32:127–30.

24. Fleddermann M, Demmelmair H, Grote V, Nikolic T, Trisic B, Koletzko B. Infant formula composition affects energetic efficiency for growth: the BeMIM study, a randomized controlled trial. Clin Nutr. 2013. pii:S0261-5614(13)00330-0. doi:10.1016/j.clnu.2013.12.007.

25. Sandström O, Lönnerdal B, Graverholt G, Hernell O. Effects of alpha-lactalbumin-enriched formula containing different concentrations of glycomacropeptide on infant nutrition. Am J Clin Nutr. 2008;87(4):921–8.

26. Mihatsh WA, Hogel J, Pohlandt F. Hydrolysed protein accelerates the gastrointestinal transport of formula in preterm infants. Acta Paediatr. 2001;90:196–8.

27. Michaelsen KF, Greer FR. Protein needs early in life and long-term health. Am J Clin Nutr. 2014;99(3):718S–22S. doi:10.3945/ajcn.113.072603. Epub 2014 Jan 22.

28. Ziegler EE. Meeting the nutritional needs of the low-birth-weight infant. Ann Nutr Metab. 2011;58(Suppl 1):8–18. doi:10.1159/000323381. Epub 2011 Jun 21. Review. PubMed PMID: 21701163.

29. Denne SC. Protein and energy requirements in preterm infants. Semin Neonatol. 2001;6:377–82.

30. De Curtis M, Brooke OG. Energy and nitrogen balances in very low birth weight infants. Arch Dis Child. 1987;62:830–2.

31. Koletzko BV, Innis SM. Lipids. In: Tsang RC, editor. Nutritional needs of the preterm infant. Baltimore: Williams & Wilkins; 2003

32. Innis SM. The role of dietary n-6 and n-3 fatty acids in the developing brain. Dev Neurosci. 2000;22:474–80.

33. Koletzko B, Agostoni C, Carlson SE, et al. Long chain polyunsaturated fatty acids (LC-PUFA) and perinatal development. Acta Paediatr. 2001;90:460–4.

34. Lapillonne A, Groh-Wargo S, Gonzalez CH, Uauy R. Lipid needs of preterm infants: updated recommendations. J Pediatr. 2013;162(Suppl 3):S37–47. doi:10.1016/j.jpeds.2012.11.052. PubMed PMID: 23445847.

36. Verger J. Nutrition in the pediatric population in the intensive care unit. Crit Care Nurs Clin North Am. 201426(2):199–215. doi:10.1016/j.ccell.2014.02.005. Review. PubMed PMID: 24878206.

35. Bhatia J. Human milk and the premature infant. Ann Nutr Metab. 2013;62(Suppl 3):8–14. doi:10.1159/000351537. Epub 2013 Aug 19. Review. PubMed PMID: 23970211.

37. Brand Miller J, McVeagh P. Human milk oligosaccharides: 130 reasons to breast-feed. Br J Nutr. 1999;82:333–5.

38. Siegel M, Kranz B, Lebenthal E. Effect of fat and carbohydrate composition on the gastric emptying of isocaloric feedings in premature infants. Gastroenterology 1985;89:785–90.

39. Modi N, Uthaya S, Fell J, Kulinskaya E. A randomized, double-blind, controlled trial of the effect of prebiotic oligosaccharides on enteral tolerance in preterm infants (ISRCTN77444690). Pediatr Res. 2010;68(5):440–5.

40. Davies ID, Avner ED. Fluid and electrolyte management. In: Fanaroff AA, Martin RJ, editors. Neonatal–perinatal medicine. 7th ed. St Louis: Mosby; 2002. pp. 619–27.

41. De Curtis M, Senterre J, Rigo J. Renal solute load in preterm infants. Arch Dis Child. 1990;65:357–60.

42. De Curtis M, Rigo J. Nutrition and kidney in preterm infant. J Matern Fetal Neonatal Med. 2012;25(Suppl 1):55–9.

43. Al-Dahhan J, Jannoun L, Haycock GB. Effect of salt supplementation of newborn premature infants on neurodevelopmental outcome at 10–13 years of age. Arch Dis Child Fetal Neonatal Ed. 2002;86(2):F120–3. PubMed PMID: 11882555; PubMed Central PMCID: PMC1721384.

44. Chow JM, Douglas D. Fluid and electrolyte management in the premature infant. Neonatal Netw. 2008;27(6):379–86.

45. Rigo J, De Curtis M, Salle BL, et al. Bone mineral metabolism in the micropremie. Clin Perinatol. 2000;27:147–70.

46. Rigo J, Pieltain C, Salle B, Senterre J. Enteral calcium, phosphate and vitamin D requirements and bone mineralization in preterm infants. Acta Paediatr. 2007;96(7):969–74.

47. Abrams SA. Committee on nutrition. Calcium and vitamin D requirements of enterally fed preterm infants. Pediatrics. 2013;131(5):e1676–83. doi:10.1542/peds.2013-0420. Epub 2013 Apr 29. Review. PubMed PMID: 23629620.

48. Makishima M, Lu TT, Xie W, Whitfield GK, Domoto H, Evans RM, Haussler MR, Mangelsdorf DJ. Vitamin D receptor as an intestinal bile acid sensor. Science. 2002;296(5571):1313–6.

49. Domellöf M. Iron and other micronutrient deficiencies in low-birth-weight infants. Nestle Nutr Inst Workshop Ser. 2013;74:197–206.

50. Terrin G, Canani BR, Passariello A. Zinc supplementation reduces morbidity and mortality in very low birth weight preterm neonates: a hospital based randomized, placebo-controlled trial in an industrialized country. Am J Clin Nutr. 2013;98(6):1468–74.

51. American Academy of Pediatrics, Work Group on Breast-feeding. Breastfeeding and the use of human milk. Pediatrics. 1997;100:1035–9.

52. Quigley M, McGuire W. Formula versus donor breast milk for feeding preterm or low birth weight infants. Cochrane Database Syst Rev. 2014;4:CD002971.

53. Underwood MA. Human milk for the premature infant. Pediatr Clin North Am. 2013;60:189–207.

54. Sullivan S, Schanler RJ, Kim JH, Patel AL, Trawöger R, Kiechl-Kohlendorfer U, Chan GM, Blanco CL, Abrams S, Cotten CM, Laroia N, Ehrenkranz RA, Dudell G, Cristofalo EA, Meier P, Lee ML, Rechtman DJ, Lucas A. An exclusively human milk-based diet is associated with a lower rate of necrotizing enterocolitis than a diet of human milk and bovine milk-based products. J Pediatr. 2010;156:562–7.

55. Ramani M, Ambalavanan N. Feeding practices and necrotizing enterocolitis. Clin Perinatol. 2013;40:1–10.

56. Cristofalo EA, Schanler RJ, Blanco CL, Sullivan S, Trawoeger R Kiechl-Kohlendorfer U, Dudell G, Rechtman DJ, Lee ML, Lucas A, Abrams S. Randomized trial of exclusive human milk versus preterm formula diets in extremely premature infants. J Pediatr. 2013;163:1592–5. e1. doi:10.1016/j.jpeds.2013.07.011. Epub 2013 Aug 20. PubMed PMID: 23968744.

57. Moore ER, Anderson GC, Bergman N, Dowswell T. Early skin-to-skin contact for mothers and their healthy newborn infants. Cochrane Database Syst Rev. 2012;5:CD003519.

58. Morley R, Fewtrell MS, Abbott RA, Stephenson T, MacFadyen U, Lucas A. Neurodevelopment in children born small for gestational age: a randomized trial of nutrient-enriched versus standard formula and comparison with a reference breastfed group. Pediatrics. 2004;113:515–21.

59. Lucas A, Morley R, Cole TJ, Lister G, Leeson-Payne C. Breast milk and subsequent intelligence quotient in children born preterm. Lancet. 1992;339:261–4.

60. Isaacs EB, Fischl BR, Quinn BT, Chong WK, Gadian DG, Lucas A. Impact of breast milk on intelligence quotient, brain size, and white matter development. Pediatr Res. 2010;67:357–62.

61. Arslanoglu S, Moro GE, Ziegler EE. The WAPM working group on nutrition: optimization of human milk fortification for preterm infants: new concept and recommendations. J Perinatal Med. 2010;38:233–8.

62. Kuschel CA, Harding JE. Multicomponent fortified human milk for promoting growth in preterm infants. Cochrane Database Syst Rev. 2004; (1):CD000343.

63. Henderson G, Anthony MY, McGuire W. Formula milk versus maternal breast milk for feeding preterm or low birth weight infants. Cochrane Database Syst Rev. 2007;(4):CD002972.

64. ESPGHAN Committee on Nutrition, Arslanoglu S, Corpeleijn W, Moro G, Braegger C, Campoy C, Colomb V, Decsi T, Domellöf M, Fewtrell M, Hojsak I, Mihatsch W, Mølgaard C, Shamir R, Turck D, van Goudoever J. Donor human milk for preterm infants: current evidence and research directions. J Pediatr Gastroenterol Nutr. 2013;57:535–42.

65. Vieira AA, Soares FV, Pimenta HP, Abranches AD, Moreira ME. Analysis of the influence of pasteurization, freezing/thawing, and offer processes on human milk's macronutrient concentrations. Early Hum Dev. 2011;87:577–80.

66. Prameela KK. HIV transmission through breastmilk: the science behind the understanding of current trends and future research. Med J Malaysia. 2012;67:644–51.

67. Lanzieri TM, Dollard SC, Josephson CD, Schmid DS, Bialek SR. Breast milk-acquired cytomegalovirus infection and disease in VLBW and premature infants. Pediatrics. 2013;131:e1937–4.

68. Hamprecht K, Maschmann J, Jahn G, Poets CF, Goelz R. Cytomegalovirus transmission to preterm infants during lactation. J Clin Virol. 2008;41:198–205.

69. Goelz R, Hihn E, Hamprecht K, Dietz K, Jahn G, Poets C, Elmlinger M. Effects of different CMV-heat-inactivation-methods on growth factors in human breast milk. Pediatr Res. 2009;65:458–61.

70. Mihatsch WA, Franz AR, Högel J, Pohlandt F. Hydrolyzed protein accelerates feeding advancement in very low birth weight infants. Pediatrics. 2002;110:1199–203.

71. Bar-Oz B, Preminger A, Peleg O, et al. Enterobacter sakazakii infection in the newborn. Acta Paediatr. 2001;90:356–8.

73. Senterre T, Rigo J. Optimizing early nutritional support based on recent recommendations in VLBW infants and postnatal growth restriction. J Pediatr Gastroenterol Nutr. 2011;53:536–42.

72. Bhatia J. Growth curves: how to best measure growth of the preterm infant. J Pediatr. 2013;162(Suppl 3):S2–6.

74. Fenton TR, Kim JH. A systematic review and meta-analysis to revise the Fenton growth chart for preterm infants. BMC Pediatr. 2013;13:59.

75. Niklasson A, Albertsson-Wikland K. Continuous growth reference from 24th week of gestation to 24 months by gender. BMC Pediatr. 2008;8:8.

76. Catalano P, Thomas A, Avallone D, Amini SB. Anthropometric estimation of neonatal body composition. Am J Obstet Gynecol. 1995;173:1176–81.

77. te Braake F, van den Akker C, Wattimena D, Huijmans J, van Goudoever J. Amino acid administration to premature infants directly after birth. J Pediatr. 2005;147:457–61.

78. Ambalavanan N, Ross AC, Carlo WA. Retinol-binding protein, transthyretin, and C-reactive protein in extremely low birth weight (ELBW) infants. J Perinatol. 2005;25:714–9.

79. Pieltain C, de Halleux V, Senterre T, Rigo J. Prematurity and bone health. World Rev Nutr Diet. 2013;106:181–8.

80. Domellof M. Nutritional care of premature infants: microminerals. World Rev Nutr Diet. 2014;110:121–39.

81. Frondas-Chauty A, Loveau L, Le Huerou-Luron, Rozè JC, Darmaun D. Air-displacement plethysmography for determining body composition in neonates: validation using live piglets. Pediatr Res. 2012;72:26–31.

82. Simon L, Frondas-Chauty A, Senterre T, Flamant C, Darmaun D, Rose JC. Determination of body composition in preterm infants at the time of hospital discharge. Am J Clin Nutr. 2014;100:98–104.

83. Lapillonne A, O'Connor DL, Wang D, Rigo J. Nutritional recommendations for the late-preterm infant and the preterm infant after hospital discharge. J Pediatr. 2013;162:S90–100.

84. D, Weaver LT. Feeding preterm infants after hospital discharge: a commentary by the ESPGHAN committee on nutrition. J Pediatr Gastroenterol Nutr. 2006;42:596–603.

85. Lapillonne A. Feeding the preterm infant after discharge. World Rev Nutr Diet. 2014;110:264–77.

86. Biniwale MA, Ehrenkranz RA. The role of nutrition in the prevention and management of bronchopulmonary dysplasia. Semin Perinatol. 2006;30:200–8.

87. Lucas A, Fewtrell MS, Morley R, Singhal A, Abbott RA, Isaacs E, Stephenson T, MacFadyen UM, Clements H. Randomized trial of nutrient-enriched formula versus standard formula for postdischarge preterm infants. Pediatrics. 2001;108:703–11.

88. Demarini S. Calcium and phosphorus nutrition in preterm infants. Acta Paediatr Suppl. 2005;94(449):87–92.

89. Fewtrell MS. Growth and nutrition after discharge. Semin Neonatol. 2003;8:169–76.

Parenteral Nutrition in Premature Infants

7

Thibault Senterre, Gianluca Terrin, Mario De Curtis
and Jacques Rigo

Introduction

Major improvements have been made in neonatal care during the past decade leading to a dramatic decrease in neonatal mortality [1]. The impact of perinatal undernutrition on growth and brain development has been well known for years from both human and animal studies [2–5]. In premature infants, reports also suggest that postnatal protein and energy malnutrition increase the severity of postnatal diseases and induce postnatal growth restriction, inadequate brain development, and poor neurodevelopmental outcomes [3, 6–12].

During the early days or weeks of life, parenteral nutrition (PN) is frequently required in premature infants, especially in very low birth weight (VLBW, <1500 g) infants, due to the immaturity of their gastrointestinal tract. Despite recent recommendations from scientific experts, PN practices are currently nonoptimal [13–15]. A recent survey in the UK observed a high variability in PN composition, supply, and administration in the health-care organization and in the quality assurance [15]. A "good standard of care" was only observed in 24 % of cases with frequent delay in recognizing the need for PN (28 %), delay in the administration of PN (17 %), inadequate intakes for needs (37 %), inadequate monitoring

(19 %), and few multidisciplinary nutritional team [15]. In addition, Lapillonne et al. [14] recently demonstrated that neonatal unit PN protocols were rarely compliant with international guidelines, particularly during the first days of life. Such practices lead to severe cumulative nutritional deficits and postnatal growth restriction that may be considered as iatrogenic malnutrition [13].

Several recent reports have evaluated how to optimize PN support in premature infants [16–24]. This chapter discusses the most important features regarding PN in premature infants, outlining most recent practical aspects and guidelines.

The Standard for Premature Infants Growth

Optimal growth for premature infants is generally defined as similar to that of the fetus of similar gestational age (GA) up to the due date and similar to that of the breast-fed term infant afterwards [25–27]. Fetal growth rate is extremely high during the third trimester of gestation and much greater than during any other periods of life (Fig. 7.1). If the mean fetal weight gain during the last trimester of gestation is around 15 g/kg/day, it must be emphasized that fetal weight gain usually decreases from ~20 g/kg/day at 24–28 weeks of gestation to ~10 g/kg/day at 39–40 weeks [27]. The body weight composition also changes during the last trimester of pregnancy explaining why nutritional requirements also vary in relation to postmenstrual age. Even if these concepts are well accepted, they are not easy to apply in clinical practice due to the major differences observed between the intrauterine and the extrauterine physiology. Postnatal growth is physiologically associated with an increase in fat-mass deposition. Therefore, it has been suggested that lean body mass (LBM) gain should be regarded as the gold standard reference for growth in premature infants [28, 29].

T. Senterre (✉) · J. Rigo
Service Universitaire de Néonatologie, CHU de Liège,
University of Liège, CHR de la Citadelle, Boulevard du
Douzième de Ligne, 1, 4000 Liège, Belgium
e-mail: Thibault.Senterre@chu.ulg.ac.be

G. Terrin · M. De Curtis
Department of Pediatrics, Neonatology Unit, Policlinico Umberto I,
Sapienza University of Rome, Viale del Policlinico 155,
00161 Rome, Italy

G. Terrin
Department of Gynaecology—Obstetrics and Perinatal
Medicine, Rome, Italy

© Springer International Publishing Switzerland 2016
S. Guandalini et al. (eds.), *Textbook of Pediatric Gastroenterology, Hepatology and Nutrition*,
DOI 10.1007/978-3-319-17169-2_7

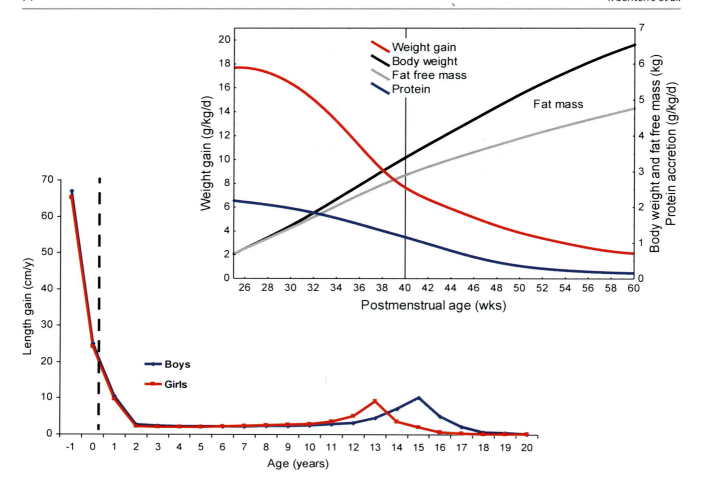

Fig. 7.1 Perinatal growth and changes in weight gain, body composition, and protein accretion

Nutritional Support in Premature Infants

Nutrition of VLBW infants may be divided into two distinct periods: the immediate adaptive or "transitional" period during the first 3–7 days of life and a stable "growing" period up to discharge from the neonatal intensive care unit (NICU). Depending on birth weight (BW) and GA, the transitional period including the immediate postnatal adaptation of the premature newborn to the extrauterine environment may be prolonged, particularly in the more vulnerable infants with major clinical disorders. The more premature a neonate is the more challenging is the influence of the immaturity and the accompanying morbidity on the nutritional supply [13, 14, 30, 31]. During this period, most of these infants require PN as their major source of nutrients despite frequent initiation of enteral nutrition. Recently, several studies have highlighted the importance of reducing the transitional period by rapidly providing sufficient intakes to promote anabolism and to reach stable-growing requirements [16–18, 20, 21].

Energy

Postnatal Energy Metabolism

The Atwater's factors are usually used to calculate the metabolizable energy contents and intakes both in PN and enteral nutrition. However, the energy available from macronutrients is not exactly similar. The gross energy content of 1 g of amino acid (AA, ~4.75 kcal/g) is about 10 % lower than that of 1 g of protein (~5.25 kcal/g). By contrast, the energy provided after oxidation of AA in urea is ~3.75 kcal/g, whereas the energy of AA stored in protein is ~4.75 kcal/g, a value identical to gross energy. Gross and metabolizable energy content of glucose (~3.75 kcal/g) is less than that of more complex carbohydrate (~4 kcal/g). For intravenous lipid emulsions (IVLE), metabolizable energy content is also similar to gross energy (~10 kcal/g including glycerol energy content) but could be lower in IVLE containing medium-chain triglycerides (MCT) [32, 33]. These differ-

Table 7.1 Advisable nutritional intakes for premature infants requiring parenteral nutrition

	Initial dose after birth	Target dose
Amino acids (g/kg/day)	2–3	3–4
		3.5–4.5 (VLBW)
Glucose (g/kg/day)	6–7	12–17
Lipids (g/kg/day)	1–2	3–4
Energy (kcal/kg/day)	40–60	95–125
Water (mL/kg/day)	60–90	120–180
	80–100 (ELBW)	
Sodium (mmol/kg/day)	0–1	3–5
		3–7 (VLBW)
Potassium (mmol/kg/day)	0–1	2–3
Chloride (mmol/kg/day)	0–1	3–5
Calcium (mmol/kg/day)	0.6–1	1.6–2.5
Phosphorus (mmol/kg/day)	0.6–1	1.6–2.5
Magnesium (mmol/kgday)	0.1–0.2	0.2–0.4

ELBW extremely low birth weight infants (< 1000 g), *VLBW* very low birth weight infants (< 1500 g)

ences are not easy to incorporate into practice. This explains why energy requirements in PN are close to that in enteral nutrition when the Atwater's factors are used.

The energy requirements for premature infants correspond to the sum of total energy expenditure plus the energy stored in the new tissue with growth. Energy expenditure measured by indirect calorimetry increases slightly with postnatal age and varies from 45 to 55 kcal/kg/day. The energy cost of growth implies making allowance for fetal LBM accretion, postnatal fat deposition, and the cost of tissue deposition. The energy cost for a postnatal weight gain of 17–20 g/kg/day with adequate LBM accretion vary from 50 to 70 kcal/kg/day in premature infants. Therefore, metabolizable energy requirements for premature infants on PN are estimated to be between 95 and 125 kcal/kg/day [32, 34, 35]. Taking into account the potential need for a prior energy deficit and for catch-up growth, 120 kcal/kg/day is required for most premature infants.

Recommendations for Energy Supply During Total P N

Current recommendations suggest providing a minimum of 40–60 kcal/kg/day on the first day of life followed by a rapid increase of energy intakes up to 95–125 kcal/kg/day within the first week of life. This needs to be adjusted according to growth and metabolism during the stable growing period (Table 7.1).

Recommendations for Energy Supply During Partial PN

Nutritional recommendations include early introduction of enteral feeding in premature infants [36]. However, minimal feeding below 25 mL/kg/day mainly serves as trophic gut feeding. It may not be well absorbed, and therefore, it should not be considered in the total energy intakes. Thereafter, when feeding increases above 40 mL/kg/day, total energy intakes would be calculated as the sum of the parenteral and the enteral intakes taking into account an energy absorption rate of 80 % with human milk and 90 % with preterm formula [16, 33].

Amino Acids

Intravenous AA Solutions

Considerable improvements in intravenous AA solutions have been achieved since the 1960s. Specific pediatric AA solutions were designed in the early 1990s with high essential and conditionally essential AA content for use in premature infants [28]. Three different standards of AA profile have been suggested for premature infants: umbilical fetal cord blood AA during last trimester of gestation, healthy breast-fed term infant's plasma AA, and human milk AA composition. Due to the poor solubility of tyrosine and cystine, current AA solutions have some relative AA imbalance compared to enteral nutrition. The ideal intravenous AA mixture for PN in premature infants is still a matter of debate. Nevertheless, biochemical tolerance and nitrogen utilization in infants do not change significantly despite the different compositions of current pediatric intravenous AA solutions [28, 37, 38].

Postnatal AA Requirements

Fetal protein accretion is estimated around 2–2.5 g/kg/day during the last trimester of gestation [39]. Isotope studies in animals and in human fetuses have demonstrated that fetal AA not only are used for protein synthesis but also serve as an energy source by oxidation [40]. The fetal AA uptake during the last trimester of gestation has been estimated to be between 3.5 and 4.5 g/kg/day up to term [41, 42]. Similarly, Postnatal nitrogen balances in premature infants on PN have shown that an AA intake above 1.5–2.0 g/kg/day from the first day of life allows the infants to avoid a negative nitrogen balance. Thereafter, during the stable growing period, AA intake between 3.5 and 4.5 g/kg/day enables infants to obtain a nitrogen retention between 360 and 400 mg/kg/day, similar to fetal accretion [16, 32, 39, 43, 44]. In addition, an AA intake as high as 2.5–3.5 g/kg/day from the first day of life with current available intravenous AA solutions improves nitrogen retention, protein synthesis, insulin secretion, glucose tolerance, and early postnatal growth without inducing metabolic disturbances and adverse effects [20, 45–50]. In a recent cohort study, Senterre and Rigo demonstrated that providing such AA intakes with a well-balanced PN solution from the first day of life was not only feasible but also improved electrolyte and minerals homeostasis during the first 2 weeks of life, thereby reducing postnatal cumulative nutritional deficits, and may abolish postnatal growth restriction at discharge [17, 21, 47, 51].

Despite any evidence, several concerns persist about potential toxicities of such high AA intakes. The association that has been described between PN and metabolic acidosis is not related to early high AA intakes but is mainly due to imbalance in the electrolyte content in PN solutions [49, 52–54]. Uremia, or blood urea nitrogen (BUN), is frequently used to evaluate the adequacy of protein intakes in infants considering that BUN reflects protein degradation and AA oxidation. However, in VLBW infants during the first 2 weeks of life, BUN is poorly related with AA intakes and mainly reflects renal immaturity and hydration status [48, 55]. Indeed, BUN is highly correlated with plasma creatinine concentration and postnatal increase of BUN is inversely related to GA and BW and normalizes progressively during the first month of life [48, 56]. Therefore, high BUN cannot be used as a marker of protein or AA overload during the first week of life in premature infants.

Recommendations for AA Supply

Practical recommendations for premature infants on PN are to provide 2–3 g/kg/day of AA on the first day of life and to rapidly increase AA intake up to 3–4 g/kg/day within 2–3 days in moderately premature infants and to 3.5–4.5 g/kg/day in VLBW infants (Table 7.1).

Carbohydrates

Intravenous Carbohydrates Solutions

Glucose is the only intravenous carbohydrate used for nutritional support with the exception of the glycerol content in IVLE. Early provision of carbohydrate supply is required to prevent hypoglycemia in premature infants. Glucose is readily available for brain metabolism and represents its main source of energy during PN.

Postnatal Glucose Metabolism

Early postnatal glucose infusion is essential in VLBW infants and an intake of 6–7 g/kg/day (4.2–4.9 mg/kg/min) is necessary to prevent early postnatal hypoglycemia resulting from the interruption of the materno-foetal glucose transfer and the low glycogen reserves of premature infants [34, 57, 58].

After birth, glucose metabolism is frequently impaired and VLBW infants are not only at risk of early hypoglycemia but are also prone to hyperglycemia, in particular during PN. The incidence of hyperglycemia increases with prematurity and has been associated with insulin resistance, persistence of glucose production, and clinical disorders like sepsis or pain. In VLBW infants, the mechanisms for glucose homeostasis are still immature. The endogenous glucose production is not completely suppressed by glucose intakes and the maximal glucose oxidation rate is generally limited to 17 g/kg/day (11.8 mg/kg/min) or less in critically ill VLBW infants [34, 42, 58, 59].

Hypo- and Hyperglycemia in Premature Infants

The definition of hypo- and hyperglycemia, as well as long-term consequences of glucose metabolism disorders, remains controversial in neonates. Reference plasma glucose concentrations are generally defined between 2.6 mmol/L (0.47 g/L) and 6.6 mmol/L (1.2 g/L). In premature infants, hypoglycemia is always a metabolic emergency that needs to be rapidly corrected with 200 mg/kg glucose slow bolus infusion (2 mL/kg of 10% glucose solution) and by increasing the nutritional intakes.

In contrast, while on PN and due to the continuous glucose infusion rate, the highest reference plasma glucose concentrations needs to be adjusted. A plasma glucose concentration up to 10 mmol/L (1.8 g/L) is usually well tolerated without significant adverse effects. When faced with high plasma glucose concentrations, the first step is to evaluate the various contributing factors and to try to correct them (high glucose and energy intakes, hypophosphatemia, stress, sepsis, pain, dehydration, and steroid treatment). Glycosuria also needs to be ruled out to avoid osmotic diuresis, dehydration, and plasma hyperosmolarity [57, 59].

In the case of persistent hyperglycemia during the early transitional and the stable-growing periods, glucose intakes might be initially reduced by 10–15% for a transient period of time. Nevertheless, high AA intakes and high protein to energy ratio are important contributing factor to improve glucose tolerance and decrease the incidence of hyperglycemia. Additionally, considering that adequate protein and energy intakes need to be maintained to avoid nutritional deficits and postnatal growth restriction, insulin treatment could be required when hyperglycemia persists above 10 mmol/L

(1.8 g/l) or if it occurs with glucose intakes below 12–14 g/kg/day (8.3–9.7 mg/kg/min) during the stable-growing period. The initial dosage should be between 0.02 and 0.05 IU/kg/h and needs to be adjusted to avoid hypoglycemia. To adapt insulin infusion rate, the time necessary to adjust the plasma insulin concentration needs to be factored in during the correction of glycemic perturbations, in particular, to avoid any iatrogenic hypoglycemia [59, 60].

Recommendations for Glucose Supply

In premature newborns and especially in VLBW infants, 6–7 g/kg/day (4.2–4.9 mg/kg/min) glucose infusion should be started as soon as possible to avoid hypoglycemia. Afterwards, intakes may be gradually increased during the transitional period up to 12–17 g/kg/day (8.5–11.8 mg/kg/min) according to tolerance in order to provide adequate energy intakes (Table 7.1). The maximum glucose intake should not exceed the maximum glucose oxidation rate and more than 60–75% of the nonprotein energy intakes.

Lipids

Intravenous Lipid Emulsions

IVLE are important constituents of PN because they are the only source of essential fatty acids: linoleic acid (LA, C18:2n-6) and alpha-linolenic acid (ALA, C18:3n-3). IVLE also represent a high-density energy substrate that can be readily utilized. They are isotonic and can be easily infused in peripheral veins [34].

Initially, IVLE were only based on soybean oil which contained about 45–55% LA, 6–9% ALA, and very little saturated or monounsaturated fatty acids. Although apparently safe, experimental reports and clinical studies indicate that these purely soybean-based IVLE could exert an oxidative stress, a negative influence on immunological functions, and a role in PN-associated liver disease. These findings were related to its absolute high polyunsaturated fatty acids (PUFA) content favoring lipid peroxidation and the relative excess of n-6 PUFA favoring pro-inflammatory effects [10].

Newer IVLE have been developed and differ by their fatty acids content and sources: soy, safflower, coconut, olive, and/or fish oil [10, 61, 62]. Composition of IVLE available for clinical use is shown in Table 7.2. These new IVLE have a smaller proportion of soybean oil. MCT are frequently added as they may be preferentially metabolized even if they provide less energy than long-chain triglycerides (LCT). Indeed, structured MCT/LCT emulsions formulated from a random combination of triglycerides synthesized on the same glycerol carbon chain have a less tendency to accumulate in the reticuloendothelial system and are cleared faster from blood in moderately catabolic patients. The addition of olive oil provides derived n-9 monounsaturated fatty acids that are less immunosuppressive and inhibits pro-inflammatory cytokine's release. Olive oil is also less susceptible to peroxidation and well tolerated in critically ill neonates. Fish oil provides predominantly n-3 PUFA and improves PN-associated liver disease. However, it lacks some essential fatty acids and needs to be used as a supplement or manufactured as physical oils mixture (10% fish, 40% soy, and 50% MCT or 30% soy, 30% MCT, 25% olive oil, and 15% fish) [10, 61–63].

Direct comparisons between purely soybean-based IVLE to some of the more recent IVLE have shown several disadvantages for purely soybean-based IVLE [10, 62–64]. A recent systematic review suggests that these IVLE are deleterious to VLBW infants by increasing the incidence of sepsis [62]. Therefore, it seems logical that the routine use of purely soy-based IVLE for VLBW infants should be abandoned [62–64]. Recent studies comparing IVLE containing fish oils to exclusive soybean IVLE have demonstrated several benefits from increasing n-3 PUFA intakes, which include a reduction of oxidative stress, liver diseases, and severity of retinopathy of prematurity [63, 65–68]. Although promising, more research is required to determine the advantages of these newer IVLE with fish oil compared to other mixed IVLE and the safety of providing as much eicosapentaenoic acid as docosahexaenoic acid and no arachidonic acid in premature infants [63].

Postnatal Lipid Metabolism

Lipid oxidation depends on lipid intakes, energy intakes, and energy needs for metabolism. During PN, lipid oxidation is inversely related to glucose intakes that promote lipid storage. Carbon dioxide production is lowered when a part of energy intakes is provided by IVLE instead of a high proportion of glucose. Maximum lipid oxidation in neonates usually occurs when IVLE intakes provide 40% of nonprotein energy intakes, corresponding to 1 g of lipid for 3.6 g of glucose. Additionally, it has been suggested that nitrogen retention could also be improved by adding IVLE to PN [34].

Table 7.2 Commercially manufactured intravenous lipid emulsions

Product	Soybean	Coconut	Olive	Fish
Intralipid®	100	0	0	0
Lipofundin MCT/LCT®	50	50	0	0
Structolipid®	64	36	0	0
ClinOleic®	20	0	80	0
LipoPlus®	40	50	0	10
SMOFlipid®	30	30	25	15
Omegaven®	0	0	0	100

MCT medium-chain triglycerides, *LCT* long-chain triglycerides

In the past, many pediatricians have expressed concerns about IVLE in neonates due to perceived potential adverse effects. However, recent studies do not support these concerns, especially with the most recent IVLE, which can be used from the first days of life [18, 34, 62, 69]. Continuous lipid infusion is generally preferred in neonates, and plasma triglyceride levels need to be monitored to avoid hyperlipidemia, particularly in VLBW infants, in small for gestational age (SGA) infants, and in neonates with high lipid intakes, hyperglycemia, sepsis, hypoxemia, or severe hyperbilirubinemia. Even if there are some controversies about the level of maximal plasma triglycerides tolerance in premature infants because high concentration may be deleterious, there is general consensus that lipid intakes should be reduced when plasma triglycerides concentrations exceed 2.85 mmol/L (250 mg/dL) during continuous IVLE infusion [34].

The use of carnitine supplementation during PN in premature infants is still controversial. Carnitine is necessary for the transportation of long-chain fatty acids through the mitochondrial membranes and the lipids metabolism. Its synthesis and storage are insufficiently developed at birth particularly in premature infants and carnitine is not available through commercial intravenous solutions. In parenterally fed infants, plasma and tissue carnitine levels decline with postnatal age suggesting that carnitine supplementation could be necessary [70]. However, a meta-analysis based on 14 randomized controlled studies showed no effect of carnitine supplementation on lipid metabolism, lipogenesis, or weight gain suggesting that up to now, there is no evidence to support the systematic addition of carnitine supplementation during short-term (<3 weeks) PN in preterm infants. In newborns who require prolonged PN of more than 2 weeks, carnitine supplementation at a dose of 10–20 mg/kg/day could be suggested [63, 71].

Recommendations for Lipid Supply

Lipid intakes during PN should represent 25–40% of non-protein energy intakes in order to promote lipid oxidation and to reduce lipid deposition in fat mass. Current recommendations encourage the provision of IVLE as soon as possible after birth in all premature infants at dosage of 1–2 g/kg/day. Thereafter, IVLE need to increase by 0.5–1 g/kg/day up to 3–4 g/kg/day during the transitional postnatal period according to metabolic tolerance (Table 7.1).

Fluids and Electrolytes

Postnatal Fluid and Electrolytes Metabolism

Birth is associated with major changes in fluid and electrolytes homeostasis. Water as part of the body composition significantly decreases. This is due to physiological contraction of the extracellular compartment. It leads to the so-called postnatal physiological weight loss of the newborn [72].

Compared to term infants, premature infants are characterized by higher transcutaneous and insensible water losses. Due to their renal immaturity, urine output and fractional sodium excretion might also be deregulated. Therefore, fluid and electrolytes disturbances are frequently observed and are associated with increased morbidity, mortality, and adverse developmental outcomes, especially in VLBW infants [54, 73–75]. In particular, dehydration (weight loss above 10%) combined with or without inadvertent increase sodium intake frequently induces severe hypernatremia above 150 mmol/L and brain injuries [54, 74, 76–78]. On the other hand, excessive water intake and relative hyponatriemia below 130 mmol/L might also compromise cardio-respiratory functions and induce brain injuries in premature infants. Fluid overload is associated with patent ductus arterisosus, bronchopulmonary dysplasia, necrotizing enterocolitis, and long-term adverse outcomes [34, 79].

Catabolic state induced by insufficient protein and energy intakes during the first week of life can also induce non-oliguric hyperkalemia. Hyperkalemia can also be potentiated by dehydration, renal failure, and postnatal use of nonsteroidal anti-inflammatory drugs (indomethacin, ibuprofen) to treat patent ductus arteriosus [80, 81].

In order to reduce the occurrence of fluid and electrolytes disorders, previous recommendations were to provide 90–120 mL/kg/day of water on the first day of life and to progressively increase intakes up to 140–180 mL during the stable-growing period [34, 58, 74]. In addition, it was also advised to postpone sodium and potassium supplementation until after 48 h of life or after the increase of urinary output over 1.5 mL/kg/h [34, 58, 74].

Recent studies, however, suggest that optimizing early PN intakes from the first hour of life positively influences postnatal fluid and electrolytes homeostasis [47, 82, 83]. By optimizing early AA and energy intakes combined with early electrolytes supplies from the first day of life with a reduction of insensible water losses, it is possible to limit postnatal weight loss to 6–7% and to regain BW after 7 days on average in both VLBW and extremely low birth-weight (ELBW, <1000 g) infants, [21, 51]. Such strategy also improves the electrolyte homeostasis during the first 2 weeks of life decreasing dramatically the incidence of hypernatremia and non-oliguric hyperkalemia in VLBW infants [47, 82, 83]. As a result of early induction of an anabolic status, the new strategy could induce a "new" metabolic disorder during the first days of life, especially in SGA and VLBW infants, in the form of hypophosphatemia and hypokalemia and sometimes hyponatremia and hypercalcemia [19, 47, 84–88]. These studies suggest that actual optimized PN strategy needs to be accompanied by an increase in early electrolyte and mineral intakes during the first days of life to ensure a complete balanced PN solution from the first day of life in VLBW infants [16, 21, 47, 89].

Chloride homeostasis is also important in premature infants because imbalance between sodium, potassium, and chloride intakes may promote metabolic acidosis or alkalosis [49, 47, 72]. Chloride requirements are generally considered similar to sodium requirements and pediatricians frequently do not control chloride intakes transferring chloride content in PN to the authority of the pharmacist. Hidden chloride intakes are frequent and combined with many other intakes like sodium, potassium, calcium, AA, and also in some drugs like dopamine and dobutamine. Therefore, as a result of the poor ability of the premature kidney to eliminate acid load, an excessive chloride intake frequently induces metabolic acidosis. Thus, limiting chloride intakes and providing sodium and potassium intakes as organic phosphate or as sodium or potassium acetate/citrate in PN preparation might prevent hyperchloridemic metabolic acidosis [49, 47, 54, 72, 90–94].

Postnatal Fluid and Electrolytes Monitoring

Rigorous monitoring of fluid and electrolyte homeostasis is required during the first week of life for all premature infants, especially VLBW and ELBW infants with high insensible water losses. The idea is the close assessment of fluid and electrolyte balance every 6–12 h during the first days of life to monitor intakes, urinary output, and body weight. Prevention of excessive insensible water losses is essential to maintaining fluid and electrolyte homeostasis. Insensible water losses can be easily estimated by subtracting from the total fluid intakes the weight change and the urinary output in order to adapt fluid intakes. Additionally, excessive urine output above 5 mL/kg/h needs to be rapidly compensated volume for volume with 0.45 % sodium chloride infusion to balance water and sodium losses. Excessive sodium intakes from medications should be controlled to avoid any sodium overload and hypernatremia [54, 76–78]. In VLBW infants, urine sodium fractional excretion is high due to immature kidney functions. Regular determination of plasma and urine electrolyte concentrations may also be helpful to adjust intakes.

Recommendations for Fluid and Electrolytes Supply

Current recommendations advocating for revisions are based on the most recent publications. Our suggestion is to provide an initial fluid supply on the first day of life at 60–80 mL/kg/day in VLBW infants and 80–100 mL/kg/day in ELBW infants combined with double wall incubator and high-humidity environment. Then, fluid supply should be increased progressively with careful monitoring of hydration, allowing for a weight loss of 5–10 % during the first 3 days of life. A target fluid intake of between 120 and 160 mL/kg/day is estimated to maintain adequate fluid and electrolyte homeostasis and an appropriate weight gain (Table 7.1).

For sodium and potassium, an initial intake of around 1 mmol/kg/day is currently recommended on the first day of life to match an optimized high protein and energy intake from birth. Thereafter, intakes should be increased up to 3–5 mmol/kg/day for sodium (up to 7 mmol/kg/day in VLBW infants) and 2–3 mmol/kg/day for potassium in order to meet requirements for growth (Table 7.1).

For chloride, an intake of around 1 mmol/kg/day is recommended on the first day of life, then 3–5 mmol/kg/day afterwards assuming the maintenance of a positive difference of 1–2 mmol/kg/day between the sum of sodium and potassium intakes and chloride intakes (Na + K–Cl = 1–2 mmol/kg/day). The use of acetate or lactate (1–2 mmol/kg/day) instead of chloride in PN could be helpful to prevent hyperchloridemia and metabolic acidosis (Table 7.1).

Minerals: Calcium, Phosphorus, and Magnesium

Minerals Sources

In contrast to enteral nutrition, calcium and phosphorus in PN are directly available for metabolism. Calcium may be provided in the form of calcium gluconate, calcium chloride, or calcium glycerophosphate. Due to aluminum contamination, calcium gluconate is now being progressively faced out by the industry to meet the rule of <5 μg/kg/day of aluminum exposure in infants but it still remains frequently used in homemade hospital pharmacy preparations [95, 96]. Calcium chloride is easy to use but its high chloride content needs to be considered in the electrolytes balance of the PN solution. Calcium glycerophosphate with one to one calcium to phosphorus ratio (mmol/mmol) is an adequate source but is not registered for use in PN and need to be prescribed from powdered anhydrous calcium glycerophosphate.

Phosphorus may be provided in the form of inorganic (sodium and potassium phosphate) or organic salts (glucose 1 phosphate, fructose 1–6 diphosphate, sodium glycerophosphate). Thus, phosphorus intake is also associated with sodium or potassium intake. Inorganic potassium phosphate induces a risk of precipitation that limits its use in PN. Organic phosphorus salts and especially disodium glucose-1-phosphate are widely used in PN solutions. However, their sodium content limits their utilization for premature infants, especially during the first days of life. Frequently, potassium salts could be preferred to sodium salts and used as the unique source of potassium in the PN solution.

Magnesium is generally provided as magnesium sulfate because magnesium chloride could induce anionic–cationic imbalance with the risk of metabolic acidosis.

Postnatal Mineral Metabolism

Calcium and phosphorus fetal retention is high during the last trimester of gestation: 2.3–3.2 mmol/kg/day (90–130 mg/kg/day) and 2.4–2.7 mmol/kg/day (65–75 mg/kg/day), respectively. Magnesium fetal accretion is lower at 0.12–0.20 mmol/kg/day (2.9–4.8 mg/kg/day). Due to the interruption of placental transfer at birth and the high metabolic demand, a decrease in blood minerals concentrations may be rapidly observed. In particular, it is well known that early hypocalcemia may rapidly occur during the first days of life due to the relative immaturity of hormonal control [97]. Therefore, minerals need to be provided from the first day of life [97, 98].

In addition to its implication in bone metabolism, phosphorus also plays a critical role in energy metabolism and severe deficiency may induce several clinical disorders including muscle weakness, delay in weaning from respiratory support, glucose intolerance, and nosocomial infections [88, 97, 98]. VLBW infants and SGA premature infants are particularly at risk for early hypophosphatemia due to their limited store and their high needs for growth. Recently, it has been shown that severe hypophosphatemia is frequently observed in VLBW infants and is potentiated by optimized AA intakes. These observations linking hypophosphatemia and hypokalemia have been interpreted as resulting from a potential refeeding-like syndrome [19, 47].

Reference values for hypophosphatemia differ in adults (1.0 mmol/L, 3 mg/dL) and in preterm infants (1.6 mmol/L, 5 mg/dL) [97]. Unfortunately, most pediatricians are unaware that most laboratories use adult reference of plasma phosphate concentration in VLBW infants. Therefore, the diagnosis of hypophosphatemia may be easily missed with the risk of hypercalcemia, hypercalciuria, osteopenia, and nephrocalcinosis [97, 98].

Optimal calcium to phosphorus ratio differs in parenteral and enteral nutrition due to the bypass of the gastrointestinal tract with PN. Phosphorus retention is related to not only bone mineralization with a 1.7 calcium to phosphorus ratio (mmol/mmol) but also LBM accretion with the deposition of nearly 0.3 mmol (10 mg) of phosphorus for 1 g of protein accretion [97, 98]. Therefore, considering the high phosphorus requirements for LBM accretion when optimizing growth with high protein and energy intakes, early provision of calcium and phosphorus are necessary from the first day of life and the optimal calcium to phosphorus ratio on PN is probably between 0.8 and 1.0 (1–1.3 w/w) [16, 17, 47, 85].

Optimal magnesium requirements are not well defined for preterm infants on PN, and little attention is generally focused on postnatal magnesium homeostasis in neonates unless hypomagnesemia below 0.66 mmol/L (1.6 mg/dL) occurs in association with persistent and refractory hypocalcemia. Until recently, plasma magnesium determination was rarely included in the routine biochemical evaluation of premature infants on PN. Like for phosphorus, reference values of serum magnesium provided by laboratories are frequently the adult reference values (0.6–1.0 mmol/L). Recent studies in premature infants during the first 2 weeks of life showed that their reference values are significantly higher than adult reference values and are estimated to be between 0.75 and 1.5 mmol/L. These studies also suggest that plasma magnesium concentrations are related to magnesium intakes, BW, and GA. Magnesium concentrations are also increased in cases of relative renal failure and in infants of mothers that have received magnesium sulfate before delivery. Some other studies have shown that antenatal magnesium sulfate administration prior to delivery might be neuroprotective for premature infants [99, 100]. In those infants, the postnatal magnesium concentrations are higher than that of controls and are frequently between 1.4 and 1.8 mmol/L without demonstrating any adverse effects. This finding tends to suggest that such a level could not be considered as deleterious when renal function is normal. In fact, clinical symptoms with central nervous system depression and hypotonia are generally not observed with a magnesium concentration below 2.0–2.5 mmol/L [97].

Current recommendations for magnesium intakes are based on fetal accretion and on enteral metabolic balance studies suggesting that magnesium retention accounted for 60–70 % of the absorbed magnesium. With such data, magnesium requirement for premature infants on PN is estimated between 0.2 and 0.3 mmol/kg/day in several international recommendations [34, 58]. Besides, some other authors have suggested that higher intake of between 0.3 and 0.4 mmol/kg/day may be needed [101–103]. Additional studies are required to better define magnesium requirements in VLBW infants.

Recommendation for Mineral Supply

With the most recent data on VLBW infants receiving optimized PN, on the first day of life, we recommend providing 0.6–1 mmol/kg/day of calcium (25–40 mg/kg/day) and phosphorus (18–31 mg/kg/day) and 0.1–0.2 mmol/kg/day of magnesium (2.4 mg/kg/day). Afterwards, intakes should increase progressively with macronutrients up to 1.6–2.5 mmol/kg/day for calcium (65–100 mg/kg/day) and phosphorus (50–78 mg/kg/day) and 0.2–0.4 mmol/kg/day for magnesium (5–7.5 mg/kg/day). Such mineral intakes are lower than fetal accretion but are usually higher than the retention observed with enteral nutrition (Table 7.1).

Table 7.3 Reasonable trace elements intakes for premature infants on parenteral nutrition

Iron	100–250 µg/kg/day
Zinc[a]	400–500 µg/kg/day
Copper[b]	20–40 µg/kg/day
Selenium	5–7 µg/kg/day
Chromium	0.05–0.2 µg/kg/day
Molybdenum	0.01–0.25 µg/kg/day
Manganese[b]	0.5–1.0 µg/kg/day
Iodine	1–10 µg/kg/day

[a] Zinc to copper ratio should not exceed 20
[b] Copper and manganese intakes should be decreased in cholestatic liver disease

Table 7.4 Reasonable vitamins supply for premature infants on parenteral nutrition

Hydrosoluble vitamins	
Thiamin (vitamin B1)	350–500 µg/kg/day
Riboflavin (vitamin B2)	150–200 µg/kg/day
Niacin	4–6.8 mg/kg/day
Pyridoxine (vitamin B6)	150–200 µg/kg/day
Folic acid	56 µg/kg/day
Cobalamin (vitamin B12)	0.3 µg/kg/day
Panthotenic acid	1–2 mg/kg/day
Biotin	5–8 µg/kg/day
Ascorbic acid (vitamin C)	15–25 mg/kg/day
Liposoluble vitamins	
Vitamin A	700–1500 IU/kg/day
Vitamin D	40–160 IU/kg/day
Vitamin E[a]	2.8–3.5 IU/kg/day
Vitamin K[b]	10 µg/kg/day

1 mg niacin = 1 niacin equivalent (NE) = 60 mg tryptophan; 1 µg retinol equivalent = 3.33 IU vitamin A; 1 µg vitamin D (cholecalciferol) = 40 IU vitamin D (cholecalciferol); 1 mg tocopherol = 1 IU vitamin E
[a] Vitamin E need may be increased when using DHA and ARA parenterally
[b] 0.5–1.0 mg vitamin K need to be given at birth

Trace Elements

Trace elements are essential micronutrients involved in many metabolic processes. Their needs in premature infants during PN are not well defined and Table 7.3 summarizes recent recommendations [34, 58, 104]. There are few trace element solutions available and designed for neonates. Commercial mixtures usually do not provide iron, but supplements can usually be postponed during short-term PN (<3 weeks). Chromium frequently contaminates PN solution during preparation and additional supplementation is rarely necessary. Micronutrient deficits are rare with current preparations of trace elements, except for zinc, which usually requires supplements, even during short-term PN. In the case of long-term PN (>4 weeks), plasma levels of trace elements should be monitored. Excessive intakes are rare with current neonatal preparations, but in the case of cholestasic liver disease, copper, and manganese toxicity may occur.

Vitamins

Vitamins are essential organic substances that humans cannot synthesize. Neonates have small vitamin stores and deficiencies may occur rapidly if not provided, especially in premature infants with high nutritional requirements and high metabolic rates. The optimal intake of vitamins for premature infants on PN is not well defined, and most studies were undertaken with commercial mixtures. Table 7.4 summarizes most recent recommendations [34, 58, 105].

There are few vitamin preparations designed for neonates on PN available on the market. They distinguish water-soluble and fat-soluble vitamins. Most pediatric vitamin formulations that are currently used in neonatal units are not designed for VLBW infants. Recent data suggest that additional intakes of fat-soluble vitamins A and E may provide some value for VLBW infants [106–109]. For premature infants, vitamin deficiencies are usually defined as below 200 µg/L for vitamin A and below 1 mg/dL for vitamin E, but for vitamin E a ratio below 0.8 mg/g of total lipid is usually

preferred. However, biological assessment of premature infant's vitamins status is only required in the case of long-term PN [34, 58, 105].

Fat-soluble vitamins are generally prepared in a 10% IVLE, and water-soluble vitamins are usually presented as powder that needs to be dissolved by addition to IVLE, sterile water, or glucose solution. Several vitamins are light sensitive and need to be protected from light even if significant clinical consequences are not obvious in premature infants [110]. Therefore, dilution of water- and lipo-soluble vitamins in IVLE should be done to increase vitamin stability and to reduce peroxide load.

Individualized and Standardized PN Solutions

PN solutions can be prescribed using either of two formats: individualized or standardized [111–113]. Individualized solutions are formulated specifically to meet the daily nutritional requirements of each patient, whereas standardized solutions are designed to provide a formulation that may meet most of the nutritional needs while maintaining these infants in stable biochemical and metabolic parameters. Both of these methods have advantages and disadvantages associated with their use.

Individualized solutions are based on the principle that no single standardized solutions can be ideal for all patients, for a wide variety of pathological processes, for all age groups, or for the same patient during a single disease course. The main advantage of individualized solutions is their flexibility. Each solution is formulated for one individual patient and they can be modified when the patient's nutritional needs and metabolic, electrolytes or clinical status change. The disadvantage of these solutions is linked to the expertise and the time required for prescription and the time involved in daily preparation, which may be reduced with the use of specific computer programs. These solutions should be prepared every day with strict aseptic techniques, in the pharmacy, not in the ward, and stored in a refrigerator at 4 °C. They are stable for 96 h and should be rewarmed slowly up to room temperature before infusion [114].

Standardized solutions contain fixed amounts of each component per unit volume. In some hospitals, there are few types of fixed standardized solutions to cover the nutritional requirements of premature infants. The advantage of these solutions is that they include all the essential nutrients in fixed amounts, which eliminates the chances of inadvertent omission or overload. The disadvantage of standardized solutions is their lack of patient specificity and the persistent need for some minimal adjustments, particularly during the first days of life [114]. Some recent surveys suggest that the availability of a unique well-balanced standardized PN solution helps improve nutritional support, postnatal growth, and biological homeostasis in VLBW infants [21, 22, 24, 47, 51, 83].

The development of ready-to-use industrially manufactured multi-chamber bags containing the three macro-nutrient solutions (amino acids, glucose, and lipids) in separate chambers of a single closed plastic system represents a major technological advances for PN in adults [115, 116]. It assures sterility, longer shelf life, and it also minimizes the risks of inadvertent contamination during compounding and storage [116]. It may also contribute to reduced nosocomial infection, especially by reducing lipid manipulations. Recently, an all-in-one standardized PN solution has been evaluated in premature infants [113]. It demonstrated the ease of use of such a system with intakes in the range of recommended doses. Most importantly, it facilitates the prevention of early malnutrition and the promotion of postnatal growth in premature infants [113].

Conclusion

Prematurity occurs during a critical period of development, and optimal nutritional support represents a major challenge for pediatricians. PN plays a major role for all premature infants who cannot be enterally fed from the first day of life and sometimes for a prolonged period. Recent studies demonstrate that optimizing early nutritional support from birth allows reducing or abolishing postnatal cumulative nutritional deficit and postnatal growth restriction in VLBW infants. However, they also highlight the need to upgrade the current recommendations for PN to improve the electrolyte and mineral homeostasis, especially during the first 2 weeks of life.

In summary, the following guidelines could be useful in the management of premature infants requiring PN, especially VLBW infants.

- Well-balanced PN solutions should be available at all the times for any premature infant who cannot be totally fed enterally within a few days. In VLBW infants, PN should be initiated in the first hour of life.
- Nutritional supply during the first days of life requires consideration of the clinical conditions and biochemical homeostasis. After a short transitional period, all premature infants should receive appropriate nutritional intakes in order to maintain biological homeostasis and promote optimal growth and development.
- Amino acid intakes should be initiated at a starting dose of 2–3 g/kg/day to induce positive nitrogen balance and anabolism. Thereafter, amino acids intakes should be progressively increased to 3.5–4.5 g/kg/day by the end of the first week of life.
- Energy intakes should cover the energy expenditure and be above 40 kcal/kg/day from the first day of life and progressively increased to 95–125 kcal/kg/day by the end of the first week of life.
- Glucose intakes should be initiated with 6–7 g/kg/day (4.2–4.7 mg/kg/min) and increased progressively to a maximum of 17 g/kg/day (12 mg/kg/min) as tolerated. All plasma glucose concentrations above 10 mmol/L (180 mg/dL) require the evaluation of the contributing factors and their correction (infection, pain, stress, dehydration, high intakes, hypophosphatemia, and steroid treatment). The initial treatment of hyperglycemia is a 10–15 % reduction of the glucose infusion rate. Continuous insulin infusion with a strict blood glucose monitoring is mandatory in persistent hyperglycemia while maintaining protein and energy intakes within recommendations.
- Most recent lipid emulsions need to be use in premature infants. A initial lipid intake of 1–2 g/kg/day is recommended from the first day of life. Thereafter, intakes should be progressively increased to 3–4 g/kg/day and adjusted to maintain a plasma triglyceride concentration below 250–300 mg/dL during continuous lipid infusion.
- After birth, initial fluid intake should be 60–80 mL/kg/day and need to be adjusted to postnatal weight evolution to allow for an initial weight loss of 5–10 % of BW during the first 3–4 days of life. Fluid intake should be increased when daily weight loss is above 5 %, total weight loss above 10 %, or plasma sodium concentration above 145 mmol/L but also in premature infants on a radiant warmer or during phototherapy. In contrast, fluid intake should be reduced if initial daily weight loss is below 2 % or if plasma sodium concentration is below 135 mmol/L.

- The use of a relatively concentrated PN solution to provide all the nutritional intakes with 120–140 mL/kg/day could facilitate the fluid control without impairment of the nutritional requirement.
- Electrolyte intake should be initiated on the first day of life with about 1 mmol/kg/day of sodium, potassium, and chloride; this will allow early provision of phosphorus and the development of LBM gain. Thereafter, electrolyte intake may then be progressively increased to 3–7 mmol/kg/day for sodium, 2–3 mmol/kg/day for potassium, 2–5 mmol/kg/day for chloride. Careful monitoring of hydration, plasma electrolytes concentrations, and urinary excretions is necessary to adjust the intakes and to improve electrolyte homeostasis. The anion gap (Na + K−Cl) in the PN solution should be maintained between 1 and 2 mmol/kg/day to maintain adequate acid–base homeostasis.
- Mineral intake should be initiated on the first day of life with 0.6–1 mmol/kg/day of calcium and phosphorus and a balanced calcium to phosphorus ratio of 0.8–1.0 to avoid hypocalcemia and hypophosphatemia. Initial magnesium intake should be 0.1–0.2 mmol/kg/day. Thereafter, mineral intake should be progressively increased up to 2.0–2.5 mmol/kg/day for calcium and phosphorus and 0.2–0.4 mmol for magnesium. Careful monitoring of the plasma concentrations and of urinary excretion of minerals is necessary to ensure appropriate intake and to avoid the development of nephrocalcinosis.

References

1. Fellman V, Hellstrom-Westas L, Norman M, Westgren M, Kallen K, Lagercrantz H, et al. One-year survival of extremely preterm infants after active perinatal care in Sweden. JAMA. 2009;301(21):2225–33.
2. Winick M, Rosso P. The effect of severe early malnutrition on cellular growth of human brain. Pediatr Res. 1969;3(2):181–4.
3. Embleton NE, Pang N, Cooke RJ. Postnatal malnutrition and growth retardation: an inevitable consequence of current recommendations in preterm infants? Pediatrics. 2001;107(2):270–3.
4. Widdowson EM, McCance RA. The effect of finite periods of undernutrition at different ages on the composition and subsequent development of the rat. Proc R Soc Lond B Biol Sci. 1963;158:329–42.
5. McCance RA, Widdowson EM. The effects of chronic undernutrition and of total starvation on growing and adult rats. Br J Nutr. 1956;10(4):363–73.
6. Stephens BE, Walden RV, Gargus RA, Tucker R, McKinley L, Mance M, et al. First-week protein and energy intakes are associated with 18-month developmental outcomes in extremely low birth weight infants. Pediatrics. 2009;123(5):1337–43.
7. Ehrenkranz RA, Das A, Wrage LA, Poindexter BB, Higgins RD, Stoll BJ, et al. Early nutrition mediates the influence of severity of illness on extremely LBW infants. Pediatr Res. 2011;69(6):522–9.
8. Lucas A, Morley R, Cole TJ. Randomised trial of early diet in preterm babies and later intelligence quotient. BMJ. 1998;317(7171):1481–7.
9. Isaacs EB, Gadian DG, Sabatini S, Chong WK, Quinn BT, Fischl BR, et al. The effect of early human diet on caudate volumes and IQ. Pediatr Res. 2008;63(3):308–14.
10. Lapillonne A, Groh-Wargo S, Gonzalez CH, Uauy R. Lipid needs of preterm infants: updated recommendations. J Pediatr. 2013;162(3 Suppl):S37–47.
11. Latal-Hajnal B, von Siebenthal K, Kovari H, Bucher HU, Largo RH. Postnatal growth in VLBW infants: significant association with neurodevelopmental outcome. J Pediatr. 2003;143(2):163–70.
12. De Curtis M, Rigo J. Extrauterine growth restriction in very-low-birthweight infants. Acta Paediatr. 2004;93(12):1563–8.
13. Grover A, Khashu M, Mukherjee A, Kairamkonda V. Iatrogenic malnutrition in neonatal intensive care units: urgent need to modify practice. J Parenter Enteral Nutr. 2008;32(2):140–4.
14. Lapillonne A, Carnielli VP, Embleton ND, Mihatsch W. Quality of newborn care: adherence to guidelines for parenteral nutrition in preterm infants in four European countries. BMJ Open. 2013;3(9):e003478.
15. Stewart JAD, Mason DG, Smith N, Protopapa R, Mason M. A mixed bag: an enquiry into the care of hospital patients receiving parenteral nutrition: a report by the national confidential enquiry into patient outcome and death. 2010.
16. Senterre T, Rigo J. Parenteral nutrition in premature infants: Practical aspects to optimize postnatal growth and development. Arch Pediatr. 2013;20(9):986–93.
17. Senterre T. Optimization of nutritional support abolishes cumulative energy and protein deficits and improves postnatal growth in very low birth weight infants. [Medical Science Thesis (Ph.D.)]. Liège: University of Liège; 2012.
18. Vlaardingerbroek H, Vermeulen MJ, Rook D, van den Akker CH, Dorst K, Wattimena JL, et al. Safety and efficacy of early parenteral lipid and high-dose amino acid administration to very low birth weight infants. J Pediatr. 2013;163(3):638–44. e1–5.
19. Bonsante F, Iacobelli S, Latorre G, Rigo J, De Felice C, Robillard PY, et al. Initial amino acid intake influences phosphorus and calcium homeostasis in preterm infants–it is time to change the composition of the early parenteral nutrition. PLoS One. 2013;8(8):e72880.
20. te Braake FW, van den Akker CH, Wattimena DJ, Huijmans JG, van Goudoever JB. Amino acid administration to premature infants directly after birth. J Pediatr. 2005;147(4):457–61.
21. Senterre T, Rigo J. Optimizing early nutritional support based on recent recommendations in VLBW infants and postnatal growth restriction. J Pediatr Gastroenterol Nutr. 2011;53(5):536–42.
22. Embleton ND, Simmer K. Practice of parenteral nutrition in VLBW and ELBW infants. World Rev Nutr Diet. 2014;110:177–89.
23. Morgan C, Herwitker S, Badhawi I, Hart A, Tan M, Mayes K, et al. SCAMP: standardised, concentrated, additional macronutrients, parenteral nutrition in very preterm infants: a phase IV randomised, controlled exploratory study of macronutrient intake, growth and other aspects of neonatal care. BMC Pediatr. 2011;11:53.
24. Doublet J, Vialet R, Nicaise C, Loundou A, Martin C, Michel F. Achieving parenteral nutrition goals in the critically ill newborns: standardized better than individualized formulations? Minerva Pediatr. 2013;65(5):497–504.
25. Agostoni C, Buonocore G, Carnielli VP, De Curtis M, Darmaun D, Decsi T, et al. Enteral nutrient supply for preterm infants: commentary from the European society of paediatric gastroenterology, hepatology and nutrition committee on nutrition. J Pediatr Gastroenterol Nutr. 2010;50(1):85–91.
26. Cole TJ, Wright CM, Williams AF. Designing the new UK-WHO growth charts to enhance assessment of growth around birth. Arch Dis Child Fetal Neonatal Ed. 2012;97(3):F219–22.
27. Fenton TR, Kim JH. A systematic review and meta-analysis to revise the Fenton growth chart for preterm infants. BMC Pediatr. 2013;13:59.

28. Rigo J. Protein, amino acids and other nitrogen compounds. In: Tsang RC, Uauy R, Koletzko B, Zlotkin SH, editors. Nutrition of the preterm infant. Cincinnati: Digital Educating; 2005. pp. 45–80.

29. Simon L, Frondas-Chauty A, Senterre T, Flamant C, Darmaun D, Roze JC. Determinants of body composition in preterm infants at the time of hospital discharge. Am J Clin Nutr. 2014 ;100(1):98–104.

30. Ehrenkranz RA, Younes N, Lemons JA, Fanaroff AA, Donovan EF, Wright LL, et al. Longitudinal growth of hospitalized very low birth weight infants. Pediatrics. 1999; 104(2 Pt 1):280–9.

31. Martin CR, Brown YF, Ehrenkranz RA, O'Shea TM, Allred EN, Belfort MB, et al. Nutritional practices and growth velocity in the first month of life in extremely premature infants. Pediatrics. 2009;124(2):649–57.

32. Rigo J, Senterre T. Parenteral nutrition. In: Buenocore G, Bracci R, Weindling M, editors. Neonatology a practical approach to neonatal diseases. Italia: Springer-Verlag; 2012. pp. 311–9.

33. De Curtis M, Senterre J, Rigo J. Estimated and measured energy content of infant formulas. J Pediatr Gastroenterol Nutr. 1986;5(5):746–9.

34. Koletzko B, Goulet O, Hunt J, Krohn K, Shamir R. Guidelines on paediatric parenteral nutrition of the European society of paediatric gastroenterology, hepatology and nutrition (ESPGHAN) and the European society for clinical nutrition and metabolism (ESPEN), supported by the European society of paediatric research (ESPR). J Pediatr Gastroenterol Nutr. 2005;41(Suppl 2):S1–87.

35. Leitch CA, Denne SC. Energy. In: Tsang RC, Uauy R, Koletzko B, Zlotkin SH, editors. Nutrition of the preterm infant. Cincinnati: Digital Educating; 2005. pp. 23–44.

36. Senterre T. Practice of enteral nutrition in very low birth weight and extremely low birth weight infants. World Rev Nutr Diet. 2014;110:201–14.

37. Van Goudoever JB, Sulkers EJ, Timmerman M, Huijmans JG, Langer K, Carnielli VP, et al. Amino acid solutions for premature neonates during the first week of life: the role of N-acetyl-L-cysteine and N-acetyl-L-tyrosine. J Parenter Enteral Nutr. 1994;18(5):404–8.

38. Tubman TR, Thompson SW, McGuire W. Glutamine supplementation to prevent morbidity and mortality in preterm infants. Cochrane Database Syst Rev. 2008;23(1):CD001457.

39. Ziegler EE. Meeting the nutritional needs of the low-birth-weight infant. Ann Nutr Metab. 2011;58(Suppl 1):8–18.

40. Van den Akker CH, Van Goudoever JB. Recent advances in our understanding of protein and amino acid metabolism in the human fetus. Curr Opin Clin Nutr Metab Care. 2009;13(1):75–80.

41. te Braake FW, van den Akker CH, Riedijk MA, van Goudoever JB. Parenteral amino acid and energy administration to premature infants in early life. Semin Fetal Neonatal Med. 2007;12(1):11–8.

42. Yeung MY. Glucose intolerance and insulin resistance in extremely premature newborns, and implications for nutritional management. Acta Paediatr. 2006;95(12):1540–7.

43. Denne SC. Protein and energy requirements in preterm infants. Semin Neonatol. 2001;6(5):377–82.

44. Thureen PJ. Early aggressive nutrition in very preterm infants. Nestle Nutr Workshop Ser Pediatr Program. 2007;59:193–204; discussion -8.

45. Thureen PJ, Melara D, Fennessey PV, Hay WW, Jr. Effect of low versus high intravenous amino acid intake on very low birth weight infants in the early neonatal period. Pediatr Res. 2003;53(1):24–32.

46. Ibrahim HM, Jeroudi MA, Baier RJ, Dhanireddy R, Krouskop RW. Aggressive early total parental nutrition in low-birth-weight infants. J Perinatol. 2004;24(8):482–6.

47. Senterre T, Abu Zahirah I, Pieltain C, de Halleux V, Rigo J. Electrolyte and mineral homeostasis after optimizing early macronutrient intakes in VLBW infants on parenteral nutrition. J Pediatr Gastroenterol Nutr. 20 May 2015. [Epub ahead of print].

48. Senterre T, Rigo J. Blood urea nitrogen during the first 2 weeks of life in VLBW infants receiving high protein intakes. Pediatr Res. 2011;70 (S5):767.

49. Senterre T, Rigo J. Metabolic acidosis during the first 2 weeks of life in VLBW infants receiving high protein intakes. Intensive Care Med. 2011;37(S2):S397.

50. Wilson DC, Cairns P, Halliday HL, Reid M, McClure G, Dodge JA. Randomised controlled trial of an aggressive nutritional regimen in sick very low birthweight infants. Arch Dis Child Fetal Neonatal Ed. 1997;77(1):F4–11.

51. Senterre T, Rigo J. Reduction in postnatal cumulative nutritional deficit and improvement of growth in extremely preterm infants. Acta Paediatr. 2012;101(2):e64–70.

52. Heird WC, Dell RB, Driscoll JM, Jr., Grebin B, Winters RW. Metabolic acidosis resulting from intravenous alimentation mixtures containing synthetic amino acids. N Engl J Med. 1972;287(19):943–8.

53. Jadhav P, Parimi PS, Kalhan SC. Parenteral amino acid and metabolic acidosis in premature infants. J Parenter Enteral Nutr. 2007;31(4):278–83.

54. Kermorvant-Duchemin E, Iacobelli S, Eleni-Dit-Trolli S, Bonsante F, Kermorvant C, Sarfati G, et al. Early chloride intake does not parallel that of sodium in extremely-low-birth-weight infants and may impair neonatal outcomes. J Pediatr Gastroenterol Nutr. 2012;54(5):613–9.

55. Ridout E, Melara D, Rottinghaus S, Thureen PJ. Blood urea nitrogen concentration as a marker of amino-acid intolerance in neonates with birthweight less than 1250 g. J Perinatol. 2005;25(2):130–3.

56. George I, Mekahli D, Rayyan M, Levtchenko E, Allegaert K. Postnatal trends in creatinemia and its covariates in extremely low birth weight (ELBW) neonates. Pediatr Nephrol. 2011;26(10):1843–9.

57. Mitanchez D. Glucose regulation in preterm newborn infants. Horm Res. 2007;68(6):265–71.

58. Tsang RC, Uauy R, Koletzko B, Zlotkin SH. Summary of reasonnable nutrient intakes for preterm infants. In: Tsang RC, Uauy R, Koletzko B, Zlotkin SH, editors. Nutrition of the preterm infant. Cincinnati: Digital Educating; 2005. pp. 415–8.

59. Ogilvy-Stuart AL, Beardsall K. Management of hyperglycaemia in the preterm infant. Arch Dis Child Fetal Neonatal Ed. 2010;95(2):F126–31.

60. Rigo J, Senterre T. Parenteral nutrition. In: Buenocore G, Bracci R, Weindling M, editors. Neonatology a practical approach to neonatal diseases. Italia: Springer-Verlag; 2011. pp. 311–9.

61. Waitzberg DL, Torrinhas RS, Jacintho TM. New parenteral lipid emulsions for clinical use. J Parenter Enteral Nutr. 2006;30(4):351–67.

62. Vlaardingerbroek H, Veldhorst MA, Spronk S, van den Akker CH, van Goudoever JB. Parenteral lipid administration to very-low-birth-weight infants–early introduction of lipids and use of new lipid emulsions: a systematic review and meta-analysis. Am J Clin Nutr. 2012;96(2):255–68.

63. Lapillonne A. Enteral and parenteral lipid requirements of preterm infants. World Rev Nutr Diet. 2014;110:82–98.

64. Koletzko B. Intravenous lipid emulsions for infants: when and which? Am J Clin Nutr. 2012;96(2):225–6.

65. D'Ascenzo R, D'Egidio S, Angelini L, Bellagamba MP, Manna M, Pompilio A, et al. Parenteral nutrition of preterm infants with a lipid emulsion containing 10 % fish oil: effect on plasma lipids and long-chain polyunsaturated fatty acids. J Pediatr. 2011;159(1):33–8. e1.

66. Pawlik D, Lauterbach R, Turyk E. Fish-oil fat emulsion supplementation may reduce the risk of severe retinopathy in VLBW infants. Pediatrics. 2011;127(2):223–8.

67. Skouroliakou M, Konstantinou D, Koutri K, Kakavelaki C, Stathopoulou M, Antoniadi M, et al. A double-blind, randomized clinical trial of the effect of omega-3 fatty acids on the oxidative stress of preterm neonates fed through parenteral nutrition. Eur J Clin Nutr. 2010;64(9):940–7.

68. Tomsits E, Pataki M, Tolgyesi A, Fekete G, Rischak K, Szollar L. Safety and efficacy of a lipid emulsion containing a mixture of soybean oil, medium-chain triglycerides, olive oil, and fish oil: a randomised, double-blind clinical trial in premature infants requiring parenteral nutrition. J Pediatr Gastroenterol Nutr. 2010;51(4):514–21.

69. Lapillonne A, Fellous L, Kermorvant-Duchemin E. Use of parenteral lipid emulsions in French neonatal ICUs. Nutr Clin Pract. 2011;26(6):672–80.

70. Borum PR. Carnitine in parenteral nutrition. Gastroenterology. 2009;137(5 Suppl):S129–34.

71. Cairns PA, Stalker DJ. Carnitine supplementation of parenterally fed neonates. Cochrane Database Syst Rev. 2000;4(4):CD000950.

72. Fusch C, Jochum F. Water, sodium, potassium and chloride. In: Tsang RC, Uauy R, Koletzko B, Zlotkin SH, editors. Nutrition of the preterm infant. Cincinnati: Digital Educating; 2005. pp. 201–44.

73. Blanco CL, Falck A, Green BK, Cornell JE, Gong AK. Metabolic responses to early and high protein supplementation in a randomized trial evaluating the prevention of hyperkalemia in extremely low birth weight infants. J Pediatr. 2008;153(4):535–40.

74. MacRae Dell K. Fluids, electrolytes, and acid-bas homeostasis. In: Martin RR, Fanaroff AA, Walsh MC, editors. Fanaroff and martin's neonatal-perinatal medicine. 9th ed. St. Louis: Elsevier Mosby; 2011. pp. 669–708.

75. Baraton L, Ancel PY, Flamant C, Orsonneau JL, Darmaun D, Roze JC. Impact of changes in serum sodium levels on 2-year neurologic outcomes for very preterm neonates. Pediatrics. 2009;124(4):e655–61.

76. Barnette AR, Myers BJ, Berg CS, Inder TE. Sodium intake and intraventricular hemorrhage in the preterm infant. Ann Neurol. 2011;67(6):817–23.

77. Gawlowski Z, Aladangady N, Coen PG. Hypernatraemia in preterm infants born at less than 27 weeks gestation. J Paediatr Child Health. 2006;42(12):771–4.

78. Lim WH, Lien R, Chiang MC, Fu RH, Lin JJ, Chu SM, et al. Hypernatremia and grade III/IV intraventricular hemorrhage among extremely low birth weight infants. J Perinatol. 2011;31(3):193–8.

79. Bell EF, Acarregui MJ. Restricted versus liberal water intake for preventing morbidity and mortality in preterm infants. Cochrane Database Syst Rev. 2008;12(1):CD000503.

80. Gruskay J, Costarino AT, Polin RA, Baumgart S. Nonoliguric hyperkalemia in the premature infant weighing less than 1000 grams. J Pediatr. 1988;113(2):381–6.

81. Mildenberger E, Versmold HT. Pathogenesis and therapy of non-oliguric hyperkalaemia of the premature infant. Eur J Pediatr. 2002;161(8):415–22.

82. Bonsante F, Iacobelli S, Chantegret C, Martin D, Gouyon JB. The effect of parenteral nitrogen and energy intake on electrolyte balance in the preterm infant. Eur J Clin Nutr. 2011;65(10):1088–93.

83. Iacobelli S, Bonsante F, Vintejoux A, Gouyon JB. Standardized parenteral nutrition in preterm infants: early impact on fluid and electrolyte balance. Neonatology. 2010;98(1):84–90.

84. Ichikawa G, Watabe Y, Suzumura H, Sairenchi T, Muto T, Arisaka O. Hypophosphatemia in small for gestational age extremely low birth weight infants receiving parenteral nutrition in the first week after birth. J Pediatr Endocrinol Metab. 2012;25(3–4):317–21.

85. Pieltain C, Rigo J. Early mineral metabolism in very-low-birth-weight infants. J Pediatr Gastroenterol Nutr. 2014;58(4):393.

86. Mizumoto H, Mikami M, Oda H, Hata D. Refeeding syndrome in a small-for-dates micro-preemie receiving early parenteral nutrition. Pediatr Int. 2012;54(5):715–7.

87. Christmann V, de Grauw AM, Visser R, Matthijsse RP, van Goudoever JB, van Heijst AF. Early postnatal calcium and phosphorus metabolism in preterm infants. J Pediatr Gastroenterol Nutr. 2014;58(4):398–403.

88. Moltu SJ, Strommen K, Blakstad EW, Almaas AN, Westerberg AC, Braekke K, et al. Enhanced feeding in very-low-birth-weight infants may cause electrolyte disturbances and septicemia–a randomized, controlled trial. Clin Nutr. 2012;32(2):207–12.

89. Rigo J, Senterre T. Intrauterine-like growth rates can be achieved with premixed parenteral nutrition solution in preterm infants. J Nutr. 2013;143(12 Suppl):2066S–2070S.

90. Ekblad H, Kero P, Takala J. Slow sodium acetate infusion in the correction of metabolic acidosis in premature infants. Am J Dis Child. 1985;139(7):708–10.

91. McCague A, Dermendjieva M, Hutchinson R, Wong DT, Dao N. Sodium acetate infusion in critically ill trauma patients for hyperchloremic acidosis. Scand J Trauma Resusc Emerg Med. 2011;19:24.

92. Kalhoff H, Diekmann L, Kunz C, Stock GJ, Manz F. Alkali therapy versus sodium chloride supplement in low birthweight infants with incipient late metabolic acidosis. Acta Paediatr. 1997;86(1):96–101.

93. Peters O, Ryan S, Matthew L, Cheng K, Lunn J. Randomised controlled trial of acetate in preterm neonates receiving parenteral nutrition. Arch Dis Child Fetal Neonatal Ed. 1997;77(1):F12–5.

94. Richards CE, Drayton M, Jenkins H, Peters TJ. Effect of different chloride infusion rates on plasma base excess during neonatal parenteral nutrition. Acta Paediatr. 1993;82(8):678–82.

95. Bohrer D, Oliveira SM, Garcia SC, Nascimento PC, Carvalho LM. Aluminum loading in preterm neonates revisited. J Pediatr Gastroenterol Nutr. 2010;51(2):237–41.

96. Poole RL, Hintz SR, Mackenzie NI, Kerner JA, Jr. Aluminum exposure from pediatric parenteral nutrition: meeting the new FDA regulation. J Parenter Enteral Nutr. 2008;32(3):242–6.

97. Rigo J, Mohamed MW, de Curtis M. Disorders of calcium, phosphorus, and magnesium metabolism. In: Martin RJ, Fanaroff AA, Walsh MC, editors. Fanaroff and martin neonatal-perinatal medicine. 9th ed. St. Louis: Elsevier Mosby; 2011. pp. 1523–55.

98. Pieltain C, de Halleux V, Senterre T, Rigo J. Prematurity and bone health. World Rev Nutr Diet. 2013;106:181–8.

99. Chollat C, Enser M, Houivet E, Provost D, Benichou J, Marpeau L, et al. School-age outcomes following a randomized controlled trial of magnesium sulfate for neuroprotection of preterm infants. J Pediatr. 2014;165(2):398–400.

100. Rouse DJ, Gibbins KJ. Magnesium sulfate for cerebral palsy prevention. Semin Perinatol. 2013;37(6):414–6.

101. Greene HL, Hambidge KM, Schanler R, Tsang RC. Guidelines for the use of vitamins, trace elements, calcium, magnesium, and phosphorus in infants and children receiving total parenteral nutrition: report of the subcommittee on pediatric parenteral nutrient requirements from the committee on clinical practice issues of the American society for clinical nutrition. Am J Clin Nutr. 1988;48(5):1324–42.

102. Mimouni FB, Mandel D, Lubetzky R, Senterre T. Calcium, phosphorus, magnesium and vitamin d requirements of the preterm infant. World Rev Nutr Diet. 2014;110:140–51.

103. Schanler RJ, Shulman RJ, Prestridge LL. Parenteral nutrient needs of very low birth weight infants. J Pediatr. 1994;125(6 Pt 1):961–8.

104. Domellof M. Nutritional care of premature infants: microminerals. World Rev Nutr Diet. 2014;110:121–39.

105. Leaf A, Lansdowne Z. Vitamins–conventional uses and new insights. World Rev Nutr Diet. 2014;110:152–66.

106. Darlow BA, Graham PJ. Vitamin A supplementation to prevent mortality and short- and long-term morbidity in very low birthweight infants. Cochrane Database Syst Rev. 2011;10(10):CD000501.

107. Bell EF, Hansen NI, Brion LP, Ehrenkranz RA, Kennedy KA, Walsh MC, et al. Serum tocopherol levels in very preterm infants after a single dose of vitamin E at birth. Pediatrics. 2013;132(6):e1626–33.

108. Kositamongkol S, Suthutvoravut U, Chongviriyaphan N, Feung-pean B, Nuntnarumit P. Vitamin A and E status in very low birth weight infants. J Perinatol. 2011;31(7):471–6.

109. Meyer S, Gortner L. Early postnatal additional high-dose oral vitamin A supplementation versus placebo for 28 days for preventing bronchopulmonary dysplasia or death in extremely low birth weight infants. Neonatology. 2014;105(3):182–8.

110. Laborie S, Denis A, Dassieu G, Bedu A, Tourneux P, Pinquier D, et al. Shielding parenteral nutrition solutions from light: a randomized controlled trial. J Parenter Enteral Nutr. 2014 doi: 0148607114537523. [Epub ahead of print].

111. Lapillonne A, Fellous L, Mokthari M, Kermorvant-Duchemin E. Parenteral nutrition objectives for very low birth weight infants: results of a national survey. J Pediatr Gastroenterol Nutr. 2009;48(5):618–26.

112. Poole RL, Kerner JA. Practical steps in prescribing intravenous feeding. In: Yu VYH, MacMahon RA, editors. Itravenous feeding of the neonates. Edward Arnold, London; 1992. pp. 259–64.

113. Rigo J, Marlowe ML, Bonnot D, Senterre T, Lapillonne A, Kermorvant-Duchemin E, et al. Benefits of a new pediatric triple-chamber bag for parenteral nutrition in preterm infants. J Pediatr Gastroenterol Nutr. 2012;54(2):210–7.

114. Riskin A, Shiff Y, Shamir R. Parenteral nutrition in neonatology—to standardize or individualize? Isr Med Assoc J. 2006;8(9):641–5.

115. Bischoff SC, Kester L, Meier R, et al. Organisation, regulations, preparation and logistics of parenteral nutrition in hospitals and homes; the role of the nutrition support team. Ger Med Sci. 2009; 7: Doc20, 1–8.

116. Muhlebach S, Franken C, Stanga Z. Practical handling of AIO admixtures. Ger Med Sci. 2009; 7: Doc18, 1–8.

Infectious Esophagitis

Salvatore Cucchiara, Giovanni Di Nardo and Salvatore Oliva

Introduction

Infectious esophagitis is relatively rare in an immunocompetent host and usually is an indicator of a primary or secondary immunodeficiency. In immunocompetent children, infectious esophagitis frequently is associated with conditions that compromise esophageal defence mechanisms [1–3]. The spectrum of esophageal infections has changed over the past few decades. Infectious esophagitis was rare before the advent of acquired immune deficiency syndrome (AIDS) and post-transplant immunosuppressive treatment regimens [1].

Though immunosuppression, in general, can result in infectious esophagitis, infections are most likely to occur in children with HIV infection, during chemoradiotherapy for hematologic malignancies and after solid organ and hematopoietic stem cell transplantation [3–7]. Infectious esophagitis has also been reported in 3 % of patients with ataxia-telangiectasia [8].

The risk of opportunistic infectious esophagitis in HIV is related to the CD4 count with patients noncompliant to highly active retroviral therapy (HAART) more likely to be infected [9]. Chemotherapy and radiation may predispose to esophageal infections due to the immunosuppression as well as the direct cytotoxic effects on the mucosal barrier. Hematological malignancies are more likely to be associated with infectious esophagitis than solid tumors, though the risk is attenuated with routine antimicrobial prophylaxis [10]. The risk of esophageal infections in bone marrow transplantation is higher in allogeneic than autologous transplants.

In an immunocompetent individual, impaired esophageal clearance of swallowed organisms may foster a permissive environment for the development of esophageal infections. These would include impaired saliva production, altered esophageal motility contributing to stasis, and gastric hypochlorhydria. Injury to the esophageal mucosa either from inflammation or endoscopic procedures may facilitate infection in certain instances [3, 4].

Clinical Features

The clinical approach to evaluate a suspected infectious esophagitis is guided by the presence of any underlying immunosuppression, the presenting symptoms, and the physical findings. Pathologic gastroesophageal reflux is the most common cause of esophagitis in children. In previously healthy children, esophageal symptoms are likely to be caused by reflux esophagitis, whereas in immunocompromised patients, the physician needs to rule out infectious esophagitis. Secondary bacterial or fungal infections can be present in reflux esophagitis and Chagas disease, especially with severe inflammation and obstruction. Absence of reflux symptoms (long-standing heartburn, a water brash taste in the mouth, vomiting, spitting up in infants, pillow wetting, or coughing) does exclude reflux esophagitis. Achalasia, diffuse esophageal spasm, foreign body impaction, and mediastinal or retropharyngeal abscesses can cause esophageal symptoms and may result in secondary infection [2].

Patients with infectious esophagitis can present with esophageal, abdominal, or systemic symptoms. Odynophagia and dysphagia are the most common symptoms of esophagitis, but they may not be apparent in small children [5]. In adults, only 59–79 % of patients with documented infectious esophagitis had these symptoms [4]. Odynophagia is usually indicative of underlying esophageal ulceration. The absolute CD4 count stratifies the risk of an opportunistic infection in HIV and coinfections may occur, especially with profound immunosuppression [11].

S. Cucchiara (✉) · G. Di Nardo · S. Oliva
Department of Pediatrics, Pediatric Gastroenterology and Liver Unit, Sapienza University of Rome, University Hospital Umberto I, Viale Regina Elena 324, 00161 Rome, Italy
e-mail: salvatore.cucchiara@uniroma1.it

© Springer International Publishing Switzerland 2016
S. Guandalini et al. (eds.), *Textbook of Pediatric Gastroenterology, Hepatology and Nutrition*,
DOI 10.1007/978-3-319-17169-2_8

Diagnosis

Establishing a specific diagnosis is essential for managing of infectious esophagitis, particularly because fungal and bacterial superinfections occur commonly in viral esophagitis.

A key diagnostic challenge in infectious esophagitis is ascertaining the role of an isolated microorganism in disease causation as many purported pathogens are commensals that may be found even in healthy individuals [1]. Colonization of the oral cavity facilitates colonization of the esophagus following deglutition. Hence diagnosis of infection requires corroborative endoscopic and histological findings. The use of viral culture and polymerase chain reaction (PCR) may increase the diagnostic yield, however decreasing specificity partly due to contamination from latently infected cells. Serologic testing has little role in the evaluation of esophageal infection [1–3].

Esophagoscopy, Biopsy, and Brushing

The technique for performing endoscopy with videoendoscopes miniaturized to a diameter of 4.8 mm has made the procedure far more tolerable in immunocompromised patients, requiring less sedation and anesthesia and allowing the procedure to be performed even in newborns. These new instruments have biopsy capabilities comparable to older, wider endoscopes [2].

Characteristic macroscopic lesions are associated with some infectious agents. Macroscopic appearances overlap considerably, however, and histopathologic or immunohistochemical analysis (or both) of endoscopic and brush biopsy specimens is essential for diagnosis.

Endoscopic biopsy specimens should be obtained from the edge and the base of the lesions. In cytomegalovirus (CMV) infection, specimens from the edge do not yield diagnostic information [12]. The pathologist should be alerted to the possibility of fungal, viral, and polymicrobial infection. Appropriate fixatives should be used for routine hematoxylin and eosin stain, Gram stain, and special stains for fungi and bacteria such as *Mycobacterium.* Immunohistochemical studies and DNA hybridization techniques often are required to establish the diagnosis [1].

Fungal Esophagitis

Candida

Candida is the most common cause of infective esophagitis [13] and immunosuppressed patients are prone to this infection. Candida esophagitis is common in human immunodeficiency virus (HIV)-infected patients, in whom it tends to occur when CD4 counts fall below 200 µl. Treatments with broad-spectrum antibiotics, acid-suppressive therapy and inhaled corticosteroids are also risk factors [14–16]. In apparently immunocompetent individuals, predisposing medical conditions or risk factors are often identified [17, 18]. The causative organism is almost always *Candida albicans,* although other species are occasionally found [19].

Patients present with dysphagia, odynophagia, and/or retrosternal chest pain. Esophageal candidiasis may be the initial presentation of disseminated disease in an immunocompromised patient. The majority of patients, particularly those who are immunocompromised, also have concomitant oropharyngeal candidiasis [19, 20]. Nearly all patients with AIDS and oral candidiasis and odynophagia have endoscopic evidence of esophageal candidiasis [5, 21, 22]. However, some of these patients ultimately proven to have esophagitis have no signs or symptoms at presentation. Children who develop esophageal candidiasis, despite being treated with HAART, are less likely to have typical symptoms (e.g., odynophagia and retrosternal pain) or to have concomitant oropharyngeal candidiasis [11].

A specific etiological diagnosis is established by endoscopy with or without biopsy or brushings. Endoscopy reveals the presence of characteristic confluent yellow-white plaques overlying and adherent to an erythematous mucosa. Remarkably, the presence of ulceration is unusual and should prompt further evaluation for an alternative etiology. Endoscopic findings without biopsy have been reported to have a sensitivity and specificity of 100 and 83 %, respectively, for a diagnosis of candida esophagitis [23].

The histological examination shows active esophagitis with budding spores and pseudohyphae within squamous debris, ulcer slough, and fibrino-purulent exudate. Invasion of mucosal and submucosal blood vessels is sometimes a prominent feature of invasive candidiasis [24]. Candida species are commensal organisms of the gastrointestinal tract, and colonize the esophagus in about one-fifth of healthy adults, making histological evidence of fungal invasion into tissue or ulcer slough important [15]. Parakeratosis with neutrophils may call attention to the presence of Candida.

Brushings may be obtained and stained with Gomori silver or periodic acid-Schiff stains. Fungal culture is not performed routinely as it is generally not useful except in defining the species and drug sensitivities, especially in treatment resistant cases [24].

Candida can colonize preexisting ulcers or damaged mucosa of any etiology, and the pathologist should consider the possibility of dual pathology.

Expert consensus guidelines recommend systemic therapy with newer azole medications (fluconazole, itraconazole solution, or voriconazole) for esophageal candidiasis. Topical therapy may produce an initial response, but early treatment failures are common. Oral fluconazole 200–400 mg (3–6 mg/kg) daily for 14–21 days is recommended. If oral therapy cannot be tolerated, intravenous fluconazole 400 mg daily, amphotericin B, or an echinocandin, such as caspofungin, micafungin, or anidulafungin may be used [25–27]. Oral fluconazole and itraconazole suspension seem comparable in efficacy for initial therapy, and some patients whose disease fails to respond to fluconazole may see improvement with subsequent itraconazole therapy [28]. Although voriconazole has efficacy similar to that of fluconazole, it is associated with a higher rate of adverse events [29].

Other Causes of Fungal Esophagitis

Cases of esophagitis caused by *Aspergillus, Blastomyces, Cryptococcus,* and *Histoplasma* spp. have been described. Unlike Candida, these are not commensals and are acquired by significantly immunocompromised individuals from the environment. Primary infection of the esophagus is very unusual and has been described in immunocompromised patients. Aspergillus infection occurs as a result of contiguous spread from mediastinal infection [30, 31]. Blastomyces and Histoplasma infect the esophagus from a concomitant pulmonary infection or from disseminated infection [1]. Mediastinal fibrosis with esophageal obstruction and esophageal fistula may occur with histoplasmosis [31].

Optimal therapy has not been established, but systemic therapy, as for other manifestations of invasive infection with these organisms, has been successful. Currently, this approach would involve intravenous or oral azole agents or an amphotericin B preparation. Echinocandins (micafungin, caspofungin, or anidulafungin) may be useful for *Aspergillus* or *Histoplasma* infections, but they have no activity against cryptococci.

Viral Esophagitis

Herpes Simplex Virus

Herpes Simplex Virus (HSV) esophagitis is primarily a disease of immunocompromised patients and occurs most commonly in patients with solid organ and bone marrow transplants [32–34]. These patients may have life-threatening disseminated infection at the time of diagnosis [32]. It has also been reported in the setting of acute rejection [34]. In contrast to transplant recipients, it accounts for only 3–5% of esophagitis in HIV patients [35–37]. Most infections in immunocompromised patients probably represent viral reactivation as these patients have higher baseline seroprevalence rates. HSV esophagitis can occasionally occur in subjects with normal immune function, who usually have a self-limiting infection that resolves spontaneously within 1–2 weeks [38, 39].

Although the esophagus is the most frequent site of gastrointestinal involvement, HSV esophagitis is uncommon. The vast majority of documented cases are due to HSV-1, though HSV-2 esophagitis from heterosexual orogenital contact in an immunocompetent patient has been described [40].

Symptoms are similar in both immunocompetent and immunocompromised patients. HSV in the immunocompetent is characterized by the acute onset of odynophagia, while 60–76% of patients exhibit retrosternal chest pain or heartburn [38, 41]. This may be associated with fever and systemic manifestations. Unlike in *Candida,* where oral disease is present in the majority of patients, coexisting herpes labialis and oropharyngeal ulcers are only seen in about one-fourth of patients [4, 38]. Symptoms may be more severe in immunocompromised patients with bleeding, perforation, tracheoesophageal fistula, and necrotizing esophagitis having been reported [42–46].

Endoscopic findings include nonspecific erosive esophagitis and discrete or coalescent superficial ulcers with an exudate. Vesicles that are the earliest manifestations are rarely seen. They coalesce to form ulcers often with normal intervening mucosa. Multiple esophageal ulcers are the commonest endoscopic finding seen in 59–86% of HSV patients, but these are nonspecific [38, 41]. The ulcers are usually small and discrete or occasionally confluent. The ulcers are "volcano-like" in appearance, in contrast to CMV ulcers which are linear or longitudinal and deeper. In addition to ulcers, friable mucosa and white exudates are commonly seen on endoscopy in HSV esophagitis. The distal esophagus is the commonest site of involvement; the entire esophagus may be involved in 15% of patients [38].

The diagnosis is usually based on a combination of histological findings and viral isolation from culture. Biopsies from the edge of the ulcers provide the highest diagnostic yield as the base of the ulcers often lack epithelial cells. Ulceration with neutrophils and an inflammatory exudate may be seen. Squamous cells may show viral cytopathic effects, including multinucleation, groundglass nuclei, and dense eosinophilic inclusions with a thickened nuclear membrane and a clear halo (Cowdry type A inclusion bodies). However, viral inclusions and multinucleated cells are not always identifiable in endoscopic biopsies [32] and may also be seen in other viral infections such as those caused by CMV and Varicella-zoster Virus (VZV). Aggregates of macrophages with convoluted nuclei have been identified adjacent to infected epithelium and may make the pathologist suspect herpes virus infection and prompt further investigation [47]. HSV isolation in the absence of histological findings is of questionable significance as it may represent asymptomatic viral shedding.

Acyclovir for 14–21 days has been advocated in the treatment of immunocompromised individuals with the use of intravenous preparations in those unable to swallow. In contrast to immunocompromised patients, HSV esophagitis in the immunocompetent is an indolent but usually self-limiting disease. The value of treatment with acyclovir is uncertain [41]. While case reports suggest therapeutic benefit in hastening illness resolution [39], the relative rarity of the condition precludes any randomized controlled trials, and spontaneous resolution usually occurs within 1–2 weeks. A search should be made for any underlying immunosuppressive illness in patients presenting with HSV esophagitis.

CMV

CMV is a significant pathogen in the immunocompromised subject, usually occurring in patients with AIDS [23], transplant recipients, malignancies, and those receiving immunosuppressive medications. These patients frequently have multiorgan involvement, while CMV infection is usually subclinical and asymptomatic in immunocompetent patients [48]. Indeed, serious symptomatic CMV esophagitis in immunocompetent patients is rare [49].

Patients with CMV esophagitis clinically present with dysphagia, odynophagia, or nonspecific symptoms such as nausea, vomiting, abdominal pain, anorexia, and fever that reflect multiorgan or systemic involvement. Thrombocytopenia and leucopenia may be present but are not invariable.

Endoscopy may reveal variable findings from esophageal erosions to deep ulcers, located in the mid or distal esophagus with a halo of edema. In the setting of hematopoietic stem cell transplantation, they may be macroscopically confused with graft-versus-host disease. Stricture formation is relatively uncommon despite the occurrence of deep CMV ulceration [50, 51].

Diagnosis needs a combination of histology and of demonstration of CMV in tissue specimens. The histological hallmark of CMV is the presence of cytomegalic cells on hematoxylin and eosin staining of mucosal biopsy. The infected cells are enlarged and contain Cowdry type A intranuclear inclusions with a surrounding halo ("owl's eye" inclusions). Hematoxylin and eosin staining has comparable sensitivity and specificity to immunohistochemical staining with monoclonal antibodies but at a lower cost [52]. Since CMV has a predilection for fibroblasts and not squamous epithelial cells, biopsies should be obtained from the base of ulcers. The use of CMV DNA PCR on mucosal biopsy specimens increases the detection of CMV, but only a fraction of these patients have typical histological changes [53]: noticeably, this increased yield with PCR may be due to contamination from latently infected cells. Likewise, the late CMV antigen assay has 89–100 % sensitivity for CMV viremia but are not pre-dictive for CMV disease [54, 55]. Conversely, CMV disease as detected on histology may be present even in the absence of CMV detection in the blood.

IV ganciclovir is the treatment of choice for CMV disease. Oral Valganciclovir has been shown to be non-inferior to IV ganciclovir for treating CMV in certain solid organ transplantation recipients [56]. However, IV ganciclovir is preferred in patients who do not tolerate oral treatment and those with life-threatening CMV disease. The use of foscarnet has been limited by its nephrotoxicity. The role of maintenance treatment is not well defined. Reduction in immunosuppression should be individualized but considered in transplant recipients with CMV disease.

Other Viral Infections

VZV is rarely associated with esophagitis in severely immunocompromised patients. The typical cutaneous vesicular eruptions are usually present when esophagitis occurs. Esophageal VZV may be a harbinger of disseminated VZV [57]. The endoscopic appearance may be variable with vesicles and ulcers seen [58]. Esophago-bronchial fistula has been reported to occur in VZV infection in an AIDS patient [59]. Biopsies reveal ballooning degeneration, multinucleated giant cells, and intranuclear inclusion bodies similar to HSV, and viral culture is needed to distinguish the two viruses. Though VZV esophagitis is self-limited in immunocompetent patients, it is typically treated with acyclovir for routine and foscarnet for resistant cases.

Esophageal ulcerations have been very rarely reported in Epstein-Barr virus infection in both immunocompetent and immunocompromised patients [60]. The ulcers are deep, linear, and involve the mid-esophagus. Koilocytosis, epithelial thickening, and cell multinucleation are seen on biopsy. The number of patients is too small to draw any firm conclusion on treatment indications [61].

Bacterial Esophagitis

Bacterial infection is a rare cause of esophagitis. It typically occurs in immunocompromised hosts such as those with hematologic malignancies with neutropenia, bone marrow transplantation, diabetic ketoacidosis, and steroid therapy [62, 63]. It is usually polymicrobial and derived from oral flora (i.e., *Streptococcus viridians, Staphylococci*, and *Bacillus* spp). Esophagitis in frequently associated with bacteremia; hence, blood cultures always should be performed.

The diagnosis is made by demonstrating bacterial clusters on Gram stain with evidence of subepithelial bacterial invasion on endoscopic biopsies [64]. Treatment is with broad-spectrum antibiotics. Lack of response to appropriate therapy may indicate concomitant superinfection by other organisms or resistance to the drugs used. Repeat endoscopy is indicated for documenting eradication of infection.

References

1. Namasivayam V, Murray JA. Infectious Esophagitis. In: Shaker R, et al., editors. Principles of deglutition: a multidisciplinary text for swallowing and its disorders. Springer Science+Business Media; 2013.
2. Krogstad P, Ament ME. Esophagitis. In:Cherry JD, Harrison GJ, Kaplan SL, et al., editors. Feigin and Cherry's textbook of pediatric infectious diseases. 7th ed. Philadelphia: Elsevier Saunders; 2014.
3. Nassar NN, Gregg CR. Esophageal infections. Curr Treat Options Gastroenterol. 1998;1:56–63.
4. Baehr PH, McDonald GB. Esophageal infections: risk factors, presentation, diagnosis, and treatment. Gastroenterology. 1994;106:509–32.
5. Chiou CC, Groll AH, Gonzalez CE, et al. Esophageal candidiasis in pediatric acquired immunodeficiency syndrome: clinical manifestations and risk factors. Pediatr Infect Dis J. 2000;19:729–34.
6. Ylitalo N, Brogly S, Hughes MD, et al. Risk factors for opportunistic illnesses in children with human immunodeficiency virus in the era of highly active antiretroviral therapy. Arch Pediatr Adolesc Med. 2006;160:778–87.
7. Brouillette DE, Alexander J, Yoo YK, et al. T-cell populations in liver and renal transplant recipients with infectious esophagitis. Dig Dis Sci. 1989;34:92–6.
8. Nowak-Wegrzyn A, Crawford TO, Winkelstein JA, et al. Immunodeficiency and infections in ataxia-telangiectasia. J Pediatr. 2004;144:505–11.
9. Monkemuller KE, Lazenby AJ, Lee DH, Loudon R, Wilcox CM. Occurrence of gastrointestinal opportunistic disorders in AIDS despite the use of highly active antiretroviral therapy. Dig Dis Sci. 2005;50:230–4.
10. Eid AJ, Razonable RR. New developments in the management of cytomegalovirus infection after solid organ transplantation. Drugs. 2010;70:965–81.
11. Chiou CC, Groll AH, Mavrogiorgos N, et al. Esophageal candidiasis in human immunodeficiency virus-infected pediatric patients after the introduction of highly active antiretroviral therapy. Pediatr Infect Dis J. 2002;21:388–92.
12. Theise ND, Rotterdam H, Dieterich D. Cytomegalovirus esophagitis in AIDS: diagnosis by endoscopic biopsy. Am J Gastroenterol. 1991;86:1123–6.
13. Lamps LW. Infectious disorders of the upper gastrointestinal tract (excluding Helicobacter pylori). Diagn Histopathol. 2008;14:427–36.
14. Karmeli Y, Stalnikowitz R, Eliakim R, Rahav G. Conventional dose of omeprazole alters gastric flora. Dig Dis Sci. 1995;40:2070–3.
15. Simon MR, Houser WL, Smith KA, Long PM. Esophageal candidiasis as a complication of inhaled corticosteroids. Ann Allergy Asthma Immunol. 1997;79:333–8.
16. Larner AJ, Lendrum R. Oesophageal candidiasis after omeprazole therapy. Gut. 1992;33:860–1.
17. Wilcox CM, Karowe MW. Esophageal infections: etiology, diagnosis and management. Gastroenterologist. 1994;2:188–206.
18. Underwood JA, Williams JW, Keate RF. Clinical findings and risk factors for Candida esophagitis in outpatients. Dis Esophagus. 2003;16:66–9.
19. Samonis G, Skordilis P, Maraki S et al. Oropharyngeal candidiasis as a marker for esophageal candidiasis in patients with cancer. Clin Infect Dis. 1998;27:283–6.
20. Wilcox CM, Straub RF, Clark WS. Prospective evaluation of oropharyngeal findings in human immunodeficiency virusinfected patients with esophageal ulceration. Am J Gastroenterol. 1995;90:1938–41.
21. Bonacini M, Laine L, Gal AA, et al. Prospective evaluation of blind brushing of the esophagus for Candida esophagitis in patients with human immunodeficiency virus infection. Am J Gastroenterol. 1990;85:385–9.
22. Tavitian A, Raufman JP, Rosenthal LE. Oral candidiasis as a marker for esophageal candidiasis in the acquired immunodeficiency syndrome. Ann Intern Med. 1986;104:54–5.
23. Werneck-Silva AL, Prado IB. Role of upper endoscopy in diagnosing opportunistic infections in human immunodeficiency virus-infected patients. World J Gastroenterol. 2009;15:1050–6.
24. Maguire A, Sheahan K. Pathology of esophagitis. Hystopahology. 2012;60:864–79.
25. Pappas PG, Kauffman CA, Andes D, et al. Clinical practice guidelines for the management of candidiasis: 2009 update by the infectious diseases society of America. Clin Infect Dis. 2009;48:503–35.
26. Mofenson LM, Oleske J, Serchuck L, et al. Treating opportunistic infections among HIV-exposed and infected children: recommendations from CDC, the national institutes of health, and the infectious diseases society of America. Clin Infect Dis. 2005; 40(Suppl. 1):S1–84.
27. Lake DE, Kunzweiler J, Beer M, et al. Fluconazole versus amphotericin B in the treatment of esophageal candidiasis in cancer patients. Chemotherapy. 1996;42:308–14.
28. Saag MS, Fessel WJ, Kaufman CA, et al. Treatment of fluconazole-refractory oropharyngeal candidiasis with itraconazole oral solution in HIV-positive patients. AIDS Res Hum Retrovir. 1999;15:1413–7.
29. Ally R, Schurmann D, Kreisel W, et al. A randomized, double-blind, double-dummy, multicenter trial of voriconazole and fluconazole in the treatment of esophageal candidiasis in immunocompromised patients. Clin Infect Dis. 2001;33:1447–54.
30. Lee JH, Neumann DA, Welsh JD. Disseminated histoplasmosis presenting with esophageal symptomatology. Am J Dig Dis. 1977;22:831–4.
31. Obrecht WF, Jr, Richter JE, Olympio GA, et al. Tracheoesophageal fistula: a serious complication of infectious esophagitis. Gastroenterology. 1984;87:1174–9.
32. McBane RD, Gross JB, Jr. Herpes esophagitis: clinical syndrome, endoscopic appearance, and diagnosis in 23 patients. Gastrointest Endosc. 1991;37:600–3.
33. Eisen HJ, Kobashigawa J, Keogh A, et al. Three-year results of a randomized, double-blind, controlled trial of mycophenolate mofetil versus azathioprine in cardiac transplant recipients. J Heart Lung Transplant. 2005;24:517–25.
34. Mosimann F, Cuenoud PF, Steinhauslin F, Wauters JP. Herpes simplex esophagitis after renal transplantation. Transplant Int. 1994;7:79–82.
35. Wilcox CM, Schwartz DA, Clark WS. Esophageal ulceration in human immunodeficiency virus infection. Causes, response to therapy, and longterm outcome. Ann Intern Med. 1995;123:143–9.
36. Bini EJ, Micale PL, Weinshel EH. Natural history of HIV-associated esophageal disease in the era of protease inhibitor therapy. Dig Dis Sci. 2000;45(7):1301–7.
37. Bonacini M, Young T, Laine L. The causes of esophageal symptoms in human immunodeficiency virus infection. A prospective study of 110 patients. Arch Intern Med. 1991;151(8):1567–72.
38. Canalejo E, Garcia Duran F, Cabello N, Garcia Martinez J. Herpes esophagitis in healthy adults and adolescents: report of 3 cases and review of the literature. Medicine. 2010;89;204–10.

39. Rodrigues F, Brandao N, Duque V, et al. Herpes simplex virus esophagitis in immunocompetent children. J Pediatr Gastroenterol Nutr. 2004;39:560–3.

40. Wishingrad M. Sexually transmitted esophagitis: primary herpes simplex virus type 2 infection in a healthy man. Gastrointest Endosc. 1999;50:845–6.

41. Ramanathan J, Rammouni M, Baran J, Jr, Khatib R. Herpes simplex virus esophagitis in the immunocompetent host: an overview. Am J Gastroenterol. 2000;95:2171–6.

42. Dieckhaus KD, Hill DR. Boerhaave's syndrome due to herpes simplex virus type 1 esophagitis in a patient with AIDS. Clin Infect Dis. 1998;26:1244–5.

43. Cirillo NW, Lyon DT, Schuller AM. Tracheoesophageal fistula complicating herpes esophagitis in AIDS. Am J Gastroenterol. 1993;88:587–9.

44. Nagri S, Hwang R, Anand S, Kurz J. Herpes simplex esophagitis presenting as acute necrotizing esophagitis ("black esophagus") in an immunocompetent patient. Endoscopy. 2007;39(Suppl 1):E169.

45. Cattan P, Cuillerier E, Cellier C, Carnot F, Landi B, Dusoleil A, et al. Black esophagus associated with herpes esophagitis. Gastrointest Endosc. 1999;49:105–7.

46. Gurvits GE, Robilotti JG. Isolated proximal black esophagus: etiology and the role of tissue biopsy. Gastrointest Endosc. 2010;71:658.

47. Greenson JK, Beschorner WE, Boitnott JK, Yardley JH. Prominent mononuclear cell infiltrate is characteristic of herpes esophagitis. Hum Pathol. 1991;22:541–9.

48. Buckner FS, Pomeroy C. Cytomegalovirus disease of the gastrointestinal tract in patients without AIDS. Clin Infect Dis. 1993;17:644–56.

49. Weile J, Streeck J, Muck J, et al. Severe cytomegalovirus-associated esophagitis in an immunocompetent patient after shortterm steroid therapy. J Clin Microbiol. 2009;47:3031–33.

50. Wilcox CM. Esophageal strictures complicating ulcerative esophagitis in patients with AIDS. Am J Gastroenterol. 1999;94:339–43.

51. Goodgame RW, Ross PG, Kim HS, Hook AG, Sutton FM. Esophageal stricture after cytomegalovirus ulcer treated with ganciclovir. J Clin Gastroenterol. 1991;13:678–81.

52. Monkemuller KE, Bussian AH, Lazenby AJ, Wilcox CM. Special histologic stains are rarely beneficial for the evaluation of HIV-related gastrointestinal infections. Am J Clin Pathol. 2000;114:387–94.

53. Peter A, Telkes G, Varga M, Sarvary E, Kovalszky I. Endoscopic diagnosis of cytomegalovirus infection of upper gastrointestinal tract in solid organ transplant recipients: Hungarian single-center experience. Clin Transplant. 2004;18:580–4.

54. Rowshani AT, Bemelman FJ, van Leeuwen EM, van Lier RA, ten Berge IJ. Clinical and immunologic aspects of cytomegalovirus infection in solid organ transplant recipients. Transplantation. 2005;79:381–6.

55. Koskinen PK, Nieminen MS, Mattila SP, Hayry PJ, Lautenschlager IT. The correlation between symptomatic CMV infection and CMV antigenemia in heart allograft recipients. Transplantation. 1993;55:547–51.

56. Asberg A, Humar A, Rollag H, Jardine AG, Mouas H, Pescovitz MD, et al. Oral valganciclovir is noninferior to intravenous ganciclovir for the treatment of cytomegalovirus disease in solid organ transplant recipients. Am J Transplant. 2007;7:2106–13.

57. Miliauskas JR, Webber BL. Disseminated varicella at autopsy in children with cancer. Cancer. 1984;53:1518–25.

58. Gill RA, Gebhard RL, Dozeman RL, Sumner HW. Shingles esophagitis: endoscopic diagnosis in two patients. Gastrointest Endosc. 1984;30:26–7.

59. Moretti F, Uberti-Foppa C, Quiros-Roldan E, Fanti L, Lillo F, Lazzarin A. Oesophagobronchial fistula caused by varicella zoster virus in a patient with AIDS: a unique case. J Clin Pathol. 2002;55:397–8.

60. Kranz B, Vester U, Becker J, et al. Unusual manifestation of post-transplant lymphoproliferative disorder in the esophagus. Transplant Proc. 2006;38:693–6.

61. Kitchen VS, Helbert M, Francis ND, et al. Epstein-Barr virus associated oesophageal ulcers in AIDS. Gut. 1990;31:1223–5.

62. Richert SM, Orchard JL. Bacterial esophagitis associated with CD4 + T-lymphocytopenia without HIV infection. Possible role of corticosteroid treatment. Dig Dis Sci. 1995;40:183–5.

63. Ezzell JH, Jr, Bremer J, Adamec TA. Bacterial esophagitis: an often forgotten cause of odynophagia. Am J Gastroenterol. 1990;85:296–8.

64. Walsh TJ, Belitsos NJ, Hamilton SR. Bacterial esophagitis in immunocompromised patients. Arch Intern Med. 1986;146:1345–8.

Eosinophilic Esophagitis

9

Natalia Nedelkopoulou, Alberto Quaglia and Babu Vadamalayan

Introduction

In normal states, the esophagus, unlike all other segments of the gastrointestinal tract, is devoid of eosinophils. In healthy subjects, its surface contains a few lymphocytes, but no other leukocytes [1, 2]. The presence of any eosinophils in the esophageal epithelium is considered by definition as esophageal eosinophilia [3], which is only a histologic finding, not specific for a certain disease, and the differential diagnosis is relatively broad. Gastroesophageal reflux disease (GERD), eosinophilic esophagitis (EoE), and proton-pump inhibitor-responsive esophageal eosinophilia (PPI-REE) are the three most common conditions characterized by infiltration of eosinophils in the esophageal epithelium. Furthermore, a number of other clinical conditions have been associated with the esophageal eosinophilia (Table 9.1). Eosinophilic gastroenteropathy was first described by Kaijser in 1937 as a chronic condition characterized by an eosinophilic inflammatory infiltration of the gastro intestinal tract. Attwood et al. first reported EoE in the literature much later, as a unique entity in 1993 [4]. Over the past 15 years, interest in EoE has grown, and once thought to be a rare condition has lot of interests with more clinical experience and research studies. Improved recognition of this condition has also raised number of questions about the definition, diagnosis, treatment, prognosis, and surveillance.

EoE is defined as a clinicopathologic immune and/or allergen-mediated disorder characterized by symptoms of esophageal dysfunction and a marked eosinophilic infiltrate on esophageal biopsy. Symptoms of esophageal dysfunction may mimic like GORD and this may coexist with EoE,

which make it difficult for this condition to be differentiated from EoE. But treatment of GORD alone does not improve EoE. EoE represents the first cause of food impaction in young males and the second most common cause of chronic esophagitis (after GORD) [5] Currently, the gold standard for the diagnosis of EoE is the endoscopy with esophageal biopsies showing esophageal eosinophilia. A recent consensus document has proposed the presence of > 15 eosinophils (peak value) in at least one microscopic high-power field (HPF) of one or more esophageal biopsy specimens stained with hematoxylin and eosin after a course of PPI as necessary for establishing the diagnosis [6]. It is important to note, however, that the histological appearance of EoE can overlap with that of other conditions (Table 9.1) and that the diagnosis should rest on clinicopathological correlation rather than on a simple eosinophil count in isolation.

Since EoE was recognized as a distinct clinicopathologic syndrome, it has been described in industrialized countries, such as Europe, North America, and Australia [7]. Studies in the pediatric population have shown that the incidence of the disease is estimated at 4.4–9.5 cases per 100,000 person/year [8, 9] and the prevalence at 42.9–91 per 100,000 [10–13]. Over the past decade, emerging evidence confirm that the incidence of EoE has raised dramatically and has already approached that of pediatric inflammatory bowel disease [14, 15]. It remains to be clarified whether this is a true rise or it reflects the improved recognition and ascertainment of the disease.

EoE can present at any age, but it is more prevalent in childhood or during the third and fourth decade of life. Males (male to female ratio of 3:1), Caucasians, and patients with other associated atopic disorders are more prone to the disease [16]. Furthermore, it has been shown that familial predisposition can play an important role [17–19]. The estimated sibling risk recurrence ratio (RR) is approximately 80, which is much higher compared to other atopic diseases with inheritance patterns, as asthma [2, 20].

The symptomatology of EoE varies according to the age of presentation and can mimic GORD. Feeding difficulties, feed

B. Vadamalayan (✉) · N. Nedelkopoulou
Pediatric Liver, GI and Nutrition Centre, King's College Hospital, Denmark Hill, London SE5 9RS, UK
e-mail: babu.vadamalayan@nhs.net

A. Quaglia
Clinical Lead Liver Pathology, Institute of Liver Studies,
King's College Hospital, Denmark Hill, London SE5 9RS, UK

© Springer International Publishing Switzerland 2016
S. Guandalini et al. (eds.), *Textbook of Pediatric Gastroenterology, Hepatology and Nutrition,*
DOI 10.1007/978-3-319-17169-2_9

Table 9.1 Differential diagnosis of esophageal eosinophilia

Diseases associated with esophageal eosinophilia
Eosinophilic gastrointestinal disorders
Gastroesophageal reflux disease
PPI-responsive esophageal eosinophilia
Crohn's disease
Infection (parasitic)
Celiac disease
Hypereosinophilic syndrome
Drug hypersensitivity
Achalasia
Vasculitis
Connective tissue disorder (scleroderma, dermatomyositis, polymysitis)
Pemphigus
Graft versus host disease

PPI proton-pump inhibitor

refusal, vomiting, and regurgitation, which can result in poor weight gain are usually the presenting symptoms in infants and toddlers. During childhood and adolescence, the disease presents with upper abdominal or retrosternal pain, dysphagia, and food impaction. Symptoms can rarely vary through the year, reflecting the seasonality of the allergen, when the allergy reaction is most likely directed to aeroallergens [21].

Over the past two decades, numerous studies have contributed to the understanding of the mechanisms of its pathogenesis. However, there are still fundamental questions to be answered. Research needs to shed light on whether EoE consists of one or more discrete subtypes or if it is a single condition with changes in expression over time [22]. Given our current understanding, the most likely driving factor for the process of the disease is an immune reaction to food or inhaled antigens. Taken this into account, elimination diets led to histological improvement and resolution of the eosinophilic eosinophilia and are considered as an effective treatment option [23–25]. However, not every patient's clinical course suggests a causative food allergen [26].

Another question that has been posed in the literature is whether pediatric and adult EoE are two distinct disorders or the manifestation of a single entity. Many similarities and differences regarding the clinical presentation, the endoscopic findings, the response to treatment and the progression of the disease have been reported [27]. Adults most commonly present with dysphagia and have esophageal rings and strictures requiring dilation, whereas children tend to have plaques, furrows, and decreased vascularity on endoscopy [28]. To make things more complicated, it has been proposed that different phenotypes of the disease could result in divergent clinical presentation and outcomes [29–31]. However, given the current knowledge, pediatric and adult EoE share a common pathogenesis, similar histopathologic features, and constitute a single disease [5].

Pathophysiology

In terms of its pathophysiology, EoE has been characterized as a bulk of mysteries. Even though symptoms may differ among children and adults, it is well recognized that in both populations, food and aeroallergen sensitization and allergy have been associated with the pathogenesis of the disease. A history of atopy is documented in 50–60 % of all patients, and 40–93 % of pediatric subjects have been previously diagnosed with another allergic disease [9, 32, 33]. The immune process implicated in OE is most likely a combination of immunoglobulin E (IgE)- and non IgE-mediated reaction to allergens. Peripheral eosinophilia occurs in 50 % of the cases and increased levels of IgE are documented in three fourth of the patients [6]. However, remission of the disease cannot always be easily achieved by eliminating specific food for which patients test positive with skin prick tests (SPTs) and food specific-IgE antibodies. On the contrary, patients who exhibited negative allergy tests have shown a good response to elimination diets [34, 35]. The existing data point only an association between EoE and allergy, and the first is not definitely considered as an allergic condition.

Esophageal eosinophilia is not pathognomonic for the disease, but a nonspecific finding that reflects a state of injury [36]. Eosinophils are multifunctional cells and secrete a variety of cytokines, chemokines, inflammatory mediators, neuromediators, and cytotoxic granule proteins when activated [37]. These cells tend to accumulate in the apical strata, but can be also distributed diffusely throughout the mucosal membrane in EoE [38]. Microabscesses formed by coalesced eosinophils, the extracellular deposition of eosinophilic proteins, and the deposition of major basic proteins (MBP) are specific findings of the disease, not commonly seen in gastroesophageal reflux [39, 40]. The main question to be answered is which is the driving force for the presence of eosinophils in the esophageal squamous epithelium.

Emerging evidence suggests that a Th2-type immune response with systemic and local Th2-cytokine overproduction plays a key role in the pathogenesis and onset of the disease [41]. Studies in murine models have demonstrated that eosinophilic and collagen deposition is interleukin (IL) 5 dependent [42–44]. IL-5, IL-4, and IL-13 act as chemoattractants for eosinophils that leave the vascular space by diapedesis and enter the esophageal mucosa. Subsequently, the expression of the beta-integrin very late antigen (VLA)-4 on the eosinophilic surface and its counter ligand, the vascular endothelial adhesion molecule, VCAM-1 on endothelia is induced. Further studies in murine models and ex vivo analysis of human esophageal cells support the key role for IL-15 in the generation and the perpetuation of esophageal inflammation. IL-15 is a cytokine with the ability to potentiate activated T cell responses. Following IL-15 stimulation, an increase in eotaxins has been identified [45, 46].

The eotaxin proteins (eotaxin-1, -2, and -3), also known as chemokine cysteine–cysteine motif ligand (CCL) 11, CCL24, and CCL26 respectively, are highly potent eosinophilic chemoattractants. Many studies have investigated the role of eotaxin-3 in EoE. Genome-wide microarray analysis on esophageal biopsies from pediatric subjects revealed an increase in eotaxin-3 (messenger ribonucleic acid (mRNA) and protein), which is mainly produced by esophageal epithelial cells, and correlated with the eosinophilic counts. A single-nucleotide polymorphism in the untranslated region of the eotaxin-3 has been associated with increased disease susceptibility [47]. This conserved gene profile, with the increased expression of eotaxin-3, distinguishes between EoE and gastroesophageal reflux disease [48]. Furthermore, the expression of cysteine–cysteine motif containing chemokine receptor 3 (CCR3) that receives signals from eotaxins and CCL5 was found increased and correlated positively with the number of esophageal eosinophilic and biopsy eotaxin message [49]. On the contrary, in murine models, mice deficient in the chemokine receptor CCR3 were protected from EoE [47, 50].

A better understanding of the immunomicroenvironment of the disease has revealed the implication of mast cells. In normal states, mast cells reside at the basement membrane and in the lamina propria of the esophageal mucosa [51]. Even though the exact mechanism of the underlying esophageal mastocytosis in EoE has not yet been clarified, immunohistochemical staining has shown the increased number of intraepithelial mast cells compared to healthy controls and gastroesophageal disease [38, 52–54]. The tryptase-positive mast cell quantification may have diagnostic utility in EoE, particularly in differentiating the disease from gastroesophageal reflux [55]. Taken into consideration that carboxypeptidase A3 has the strongest relation to mast cell number and degranulation, the upregulation of carboxypeptidase A3 gene, specifically seen in EoE, highlights the importance of mast cells in the pathogenesis of the disease [47, 54]. Furthermore, IL-9 is known to promote esophageal mastocytosis and the expression of the IL-9 transcript is increased in the esophagus of patients with EoE [45, 56]. Following treatment with anti-IL-5, the esophageal epithelium of pediatric patients had significantly fewer mast cells, IL-9, and mast cell-eosinophilic couplet [57].

Both eosinophils and mast cells with their secretory products contribute to tissue remodeling and fibrosis in EoE. A complex interplay between eosinophils, mast cells, and fibroblasts has been documented. Tumor growth factor (TGF)-β1 is produced mainly by monocytes and macrophages, and also by eosinophils and mast cells. This pro-fibrotic molecule increases smooth muscle cell hyperplasia, is a potent activator of fibroblasts, and is a strong inducer of epithelial-mesenchymal transition (EMT), the process where epithelial cells assume morphological and phenotypical properties of fibroblasts [58]. Evidence of EMT was seen in esophageal mucosal biopsies from patients with EoE [59]. Increased vimentin expression in the esophageal epithelial cells combined with decreased expression of E-cadherin also indicates the possible presence of EMT in EoE tissues [60].

In a pediatric study, an increased expression of TGF-β1 and its signaling molecule phosphorylated SMAD2/3 (phosphor-SMAD2/3) was documented. The esophageal biopsies also demonstrated remodeling of the esophageal mucosa, especially the lamina propria, as well as increased vascular density and increased expression of the vascular endothelial adhesion molecule, VCAM-1. Increased level of esophageal fibrosis was documented in children with EoE. TGF-β1, VCAM-1, SMAD2/3 seem to contribute to the loss of elasticity of the esophageal wall and the formation of strictures [61, 62]. Basal cell hyperplasia correlates with the intraepithelial eosinophils and the number of mast cells [47]. Furthermore, MBP, released by eosinophils, lead to increased gene expression of fibroblast growth factor (FGF)-9, a cytokine implicated in the proliferate response to eosinophilic inflammation in esophagitis [63]. The role of periostin, a cell adhesion protein with the ability to bind to integrins in the cell membrane and trigger cell proliferation, migration, adhesion, and differentiation, has also been studied. In gene arrays, periostin is highly overexpressed in the esophagus of patients with EoE, it is second in upregulation magnitude only to eotaxin-3 gene and it correlates with the eosinophilic number [47, 64]. Interestingly, tumor necrosis factor (TNF)-a is also highly expressed by epithelial cells in EoE, but it remains to be clarified whether it exerts direct pro-fibrotic effect [65].

Genome-wide association studies that investigate the association between common genetic variants across the genome and the disease have identified various single-nucleotide polymorphisms (SNP) in a discrete region on the long arm of chromosome five associated with the thymic stromal lymphopoietin (TSLP) in patients with EoE. Esophageal biopsies of pediatric patients showed TSLP overexpression compared to unaffected controls and TSLP expression levels correlated significantly with the disease-related rs3806932 SNP [66, 67].

In conclusion, despite the advances in our understanding, the pathogenesis of EoE is yet not fully understood. An interplay between predisposed genetic background with environmental factors seems crucial for the onset of the disease. There is strong evidence that cell types other than eosinophils are also implicated. However, the current challenge is to elucidate the complex cellular and molecular mechanisms of the disease.

Clinical Presentation

EoE can affect any age, but the symptomatology varies according to age. Substantial differences have been described between pediatric and adult patients (Table 9.2); however, it

Table 9.2 Clinical manifestations of eosinophilic esophagitis in children, adolescents, and adult patients

Children	Adolescents and adults
Chest pain or heartburn	Dysphagia
Abdominal pain	Retrosternal pain
Coughing	Food impaction
Dysphagia	–
Food refusal	–
Decreased appetite	–
Choking/gagging/vomiting	–
Nausea	–
Regurgitation	–
Throat pain	–
Sleeping difficulties	–

remains unclear whether this variation could be attributed to the ability to enunciate discomfort or to the different stages of the disease [68].

A broad range of symptoms, affecting the upper gastro-intestinal tract and the respiratory system, has been reported in the pediatric population. Symptoms can attenuate or spontaneously fluctuate, even when histology reveals persistent esophageal eosinophilic infiltrates [69]. In general, the most common symptoms can be divided to GERD-like symptoms and dysphagia, possibly representing two discrete disease phenotypes [70]. In infants and toddlers, the disease presents with nonspecific symptoms, like feeding difficulties, regurgitation, vomiting, and feed refusal, which can result in poor weight gain.

Older children and adolescents complain of upper abdominal and retrosternal pain, heartburn, dysphagia, and food impaction. Furthermore, pediatric patients can experience choking on liquids or solids, the inability to tolerate feeds beyond certain tastes or textures, avoidance of specific solid foods, such as bread, rice, meat, and the need to drink water to assist swallowing during meals as an adaptive behavior to esophageal dysfunction [20, 71]. Acute symptoms are due to intermittent esophageal spasm, most likely related to smooth muscle contraction, whereas the chronicity of dysphagia denotes long-standing esophageal remodeling [72, 73]. Interestingly, the seasonality of symptoms points the implication of aeroallergens [74].

Association with Other Diseases

The relationship between EoE and gastroesophageal reflux disease is complex and the role of acid reflux in the EoE is a matter of debate [68]. Impedance and pH studies are helpful in distinguishing the two entities; however, conflicting data exist about the presence of acid and nonacid reflux in children with EoE [75, 76]. It is postulated that the erosions and ulceration seen in gastroesophageal reflux disease can result in the impairment of the mucosal barrier function and increase the risk for food sensitization. Furthermore, the ineffective esophageal peristalsis in EoE can lead to an impairment of the clearance of the esophagus after gastroesophageal reflux episodes [77, 78]. Emerging evidence shows that the two distinct entities can possibly coexist and exacerbate each other.

The recent identification of PPI-REE that was first described in a series of pediatric patients complicated further the diagnostic algorithms of esophageal eosinophilia [79]. PPI-REE accounts for at least one third of children and adults with esophageal eosinophilia [80–82], but it has not been yet elucidated if this is a new separate entity, a subtype of gastroesophageal reflux disease or a phenotype of EoE. Given the current state of knowledge, the clinical, endoscopic, and histological features cannot differentiate it from EoE, and there is no predictor to show which patient will respond to the PPI trial [83]. According to the most recent guidelines, in order to identify children with PPI-REE and to avoid unnecessary eliminations diets and drug treatment, an 8-week trial of PPIs is recommended, before the diagnosis of EoE is established [80].

Celiac disease and EoE both affect the upper gastrointestinal tract, and they are two clinically, anatomically, and histologically distinct entities. However, recently a clinical association between these two disorders has been proposed. A higher than expected prevalence of EoE in pediatric patients with coeliac disease has been documented, and the estimated risk of each condition is increased 50–75-fold in those pediatric patients diagnosed with the alternative condition. This phenomenon is shown to be limited only to the pediatric population [84–90]. The lack of a genetic connection between EoE and coeliac disease necessitates further prospective studies to shed light to this association and to clarify the underlying mechanisms that justify the coexistence.

The implication of TGF-β1 in the pathogenesis of EoE led to the hypothesis that the disease could be also associated to connective tissue disorders (CTDs) that are known to be caused by genetic variants in TGF-β binding proteins and TGF-β receptors, like Marfan syndrome and Loeys–Dietz syndrome, respectively [91, 92]. In addition, patients diagnosed with the above disorder can exhibit gastrointestinal symptoms, including dysphagia, which is a typical presenting symptom of EoE [93–95]. Taken this into consideration, a new syndrome has been described (EoE-CTD), involving EoE in association with inherited CTDs that represents a new class of this gastrointestinal disorder. There is evidence showing that the dysregulation of collagen transcription in patients with EoE-CTD is distinct from that seen in typical patients with EoE or healthy subjects, and that these patients might be at greater risk for more diffuse eosinophilic extra-esophageal gastrointestinal disease than their peers with EoE without evidence of CTDs [96, 97].

Table 9.3 Diagnostic criteria, macroscopic, and histological findings of eosinophilic esophagitis

Diagnosis	–
Macroscopic findings	Thickened/pale mucosa Linear furrows Trachealization (esophageal rings) Mucosal friability White exudates Luminal strictures
Histological characteristics	Esophageal eosinophilia: After antireflux therapy High eosinophilic count in the most affected area (> 15 eosinophils/HPF as proposed by consensus panel [6]) Eosinophilia affecting lower, mid, and upper esophageal samples Other associated features: Eosinophilic microabcesses Superficial layering Extracellular eosinophilic granules Basal cell hyperplasia Papillary elongation Lamina propria fibrosis Dilated intracellular spaces No parasites or fungi present

HPF high-power field

Diagnosis and Assessment

The presence of eosinophils in the esophageal epithelium should be reported as esophageal eosinophilia. Consensus recommendations have proposed a threshold of 15 eosinophils or more per HPF in at least one endoscopic esophageal mucosal biopsy sample taken at upper gastrointestinal endoscopy. Other microscopic features which often accompany EoE include eosinophilic microabscesses, superficial layering, extracellular eosinophilic granules, the basal cell hyperplasia, papillary elongation, lamina propria fibrosis, and dilatation of intercellular spaces (Table 9.3) [6]. It is important to note that none of these individual histological features are specific, and they should not be used in isolation to differentiate EoE from other conditions associated with esophageal eosinophilia (Table 9.1). Inclusion in the routine staining panel of stains such as diastase-periodic acid-Schiff (PAS) ensures that fungal organisms are not easily overlooked. Even if eosinophilic esophagits is suspected clinically, sampling should include gastric and duodenal mucosa, as presence or absence of gastroduodenal changes may be helpful in the differentiating EoE from other conditions.

In the particular context of differentiating EoE from gastroesophageal reflux, the presence of esophageal eosinophilia in biopsy samples from the mid and upper esophagus is a very useful feature in support of EoE as these sites are rarely affected by reflux. Multiple biopsy samples should always be taken as the eosinophilic infiltrate can be patchy in distribution. In terms of diagnostic sensitivity, this has been reported to range from 55% when one specimen is examined to 100% when five specimens are examined [98]. See (Fig. 9.1). It has been proposed that diagnosis can be achieved in 97% of the patients by at least three biopsies form different parts of the esophagus [99]. It is therefore recommended two to four biopsies to be taken from the proximal and distal esophagus regardless its appearance [6]. EoE cannot be excluded even if esophagus has a normal appearance at endoscopy. However, the characteristic macroscopic findings include thickened, pale mucosa with linear furrows, trachealization (fixed esophageal rings), mucosal friability, white exudates, and less frequently luminal strictures (Table 9.3) [100].

The role of repeat endoscopy and biopsies in order to reassess the disease and the effect of the treatment has not yet been validated. Some centers suggest regular upper endoscopy to ensure maintenance of histological remission, but currently the long-term follow-up management for asymptomatic patients is poorly defined [78]. Upper gastrointestinal (GI) contrast radiography is helpful in identifying esophageal strictures or long-segment narrowing, although the findings are not always confirmed at endoscopy, suggesting transient contractions [101, 102]. Deeper esophageal strictures have been also assessed with the use of endoscopic ultrasound, and data from a pediatric series suggest a significant thickening of the esophageal wall with the involvement of the submucosa and the muscularis propria apart from the mucosa [103].

The most common manometric disorder in EoE is the ineffective peristalsis of the esophagus. High-resolution manometry can reveal pan-esophageal pressurization, the uniform esophageal pressurization form the upper esophageal sphincter to the esophagogastric junction with pressures over 30 mmHg [77]. Pediatric patients have shown significantly more ineffective esophageal peristalsis during fasting and meals than those with gastroesophageal reflux disease and controls [104]. A novel imaging probe, the endolumenal functional lumen imaging probe (endoFLIP), used in adult patients determined that patients with EoE also exhibit significantly reduced distensibility compared to normal controls.

An ideal biomarker for EoE should correlate with disease activity, have high sensitivity and specificity, reflect changes with therapy, be reproducible, noninvasive and cost-effective [105, 106]. Currently, there is no available biomarker to confirm or monitor the disease. Peripheral eosinophilia is not always present, and even when identified, it can be indicative of other diseases. However, the combination of peripheral eosinophilia with elevated serum levels of eotaxin-3 (CCL26) and eosinophil-derived neurotoxin significantly correlated with esophageal eosinophilic density [107]. Furthermore, the Th2 induction implicated in EoE results in cytokine pattern variation in eosinophilic and normal subjects. A cytokine panel scoring system for predicting the

Fig. 9.1 a Twelve-year-old child. Esophageal squamous epithelium from upper esophagus infiltrated by a high number of eosinophils, well in excess of 15 per HPF. H&E 400 × magnification (40 × objective). **b** Twelve-year-old child. Same child as picture (**a**). Esophageal sample from mid esophagus. The heavy eosinophilic infiltrate includes a microabscess (*arrow*)

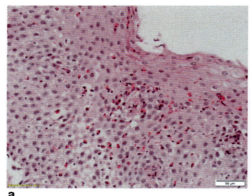

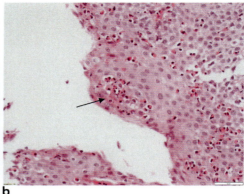

a   b

Table 9.4 Management of eosinophilic esophagitis

Dietary approach	Amino-acid-based formula
	Skin test-directed elimination diet
	Empiric elimination diet
Pharmacological approach	Topical steroids (fluticasone proprionate, oral viscous budesonide)
	Systemic steroids (oral, IV)
Esophageal dilatation	Combined with pharmacological therapy

diagnosis of EoE has been proposed and identified that IL-13 as one of the eight cytokines whose blood levels retrospectively distinguished patients from healthy controls with 100 % specificity and sensitivity. Serum and tissue expression levels of IL-13 is one of the most promising candidate biomarkers for the disease [45, 108].

Mast cell density, the extracellular MBP content, and the presence of fibrosis may serve as potential biomarkers in establishing the diagnosis of EoE [109]. Recently, the use of a minimally invasive test, the esophageal string test (EST), in pediatric patients was shown to have the potential to significantly improve the evaluation and treatment of the disease by measuring the eosinophil-derived proteins in luminal secretions which reflect the state of mucosal inflammation [110].

Treatment

In order to avoid unnecessary elimination diets and drug therapy and to differentiate PPI-REE and EoE, the diagnosis of the latter is established when esophageal eosinophilia does not respond to an 8-week course of PPIs at repeat endoscopy. According to the most recent guidelines, the end points of the treatment should include the combination of clinical remission with histological resolution of the esophageal eosinophilic inflammation [3, 78]. Two different treatment approaches have been proven to be effective in the management of the disease, the elimination diets, and the pharmacological therapy. (Table 9.4)

Dietary Management of EoE

The success of elimination diets in EoE provides strong evidence for the implication of food sensitization as the cause of esophageal inflammation in many cases [74]. The observation that some patients exhibit allergen sensitivity while others do not, points the possibility that the disease may exhibit different phenotypes [111]. Atopy patch test (APT), SPT, and serum IgE tests may be adjunctive in identifying a causative food in EoE, and, for that reason, gastroenterologists should consider consultation with an allergist. However, a food trigger can only be identified when the elimination of the specific food results in disease remission, followed by relapse upon reintroduction [6].

The dietary management of EoE includes the diet based on amino-acid formula, the skin test-directed elimination diet, and the empiric exclusion diet, with the elimination of six foods. The decision as to which of these three dietary approaches to be suggested should be individualized according to the patient's specific needs and family circumstances. Important foods that are excluded from a child's diet should be substituted appropriately and the input of an experienced dietitian in pediatric nutrition is crucial to ensure a balanced nutritional plan, to minimize non-adherence, and to avoid cross-reactive antigens [78, 112].

The efficacy of an amino-acid-based formula for the treatment of EoE in children was first described in 1995 [113]. Since then, several studies have shown the successful use of the elemental formula that seems to achieve clinical and histological remission in less time compared to the other two elimination diets [24, 114–116]. A 4-week trial of amino-acid-based formula is recommended in patients with multiple food allergies, failure to thrive, or those unable to respond or to follow a highly restricted diet [78]. However, the clinical use of this dietary approach is limited by the acceptability that often requires tube feeding (nasogastric or gastrostomy) and the significant cost. Generally, it is better accepted and tolerated in infants [114].

The dietary restriction based on allergy testing has been proposed to be a successful alternative treatment option, but the use of allergy testing to identify causative foods in EoE is controversial. Resolution of both symptoms and histological abnormalities in children with EoE was reported following an elimination diet based on a combination of SPTs and patch tests [117] and even though the follow-up data showed a lower level of response, this was further increased if the elimination of foods identified on allergy testing was combined with the empiric elimination of cow's milk [23]. The poor predictive value of SPTs and radioallergosorbent tests (RASTs) to identify specific food that induce inflammation is the major limitations of this dietary approach. Furthermore, the local production of IgE in patients with EoE probably explains the absence of a relationship between positive allergy test and actual food triggers for the disease. However, targeted elimination diet for 8–12 weeks is recommended if allergy to specific foods is strongly suspected by history and sensitization is supported by allergy testing [78].

The third recommended dietary approach for the treatment of EoE is the elimination of the six foods that are considered to be most allergenic: cow's milk, egg, wheat, soya, peanut, and fish/shellfish (six food exclusion). In a series of 35 pediatric patients, the removal of these food allergens from their diets for 6 weeks regardless of sensitization led to clinical and pathological remission in 74% of the cases [118]. Subsequently, this dietary strategy can be used for 8–12 weeks in the absence of specific food sensitization.

Following remission, the excluded foods should be gradually reintroduced. Based on the available evidence, it is recommended the least allergenic food to be reintroduced first, and the most allergenic to be left as last [119]. This would suggest reintroduction of seafood/nuts first, followed sequentially by soy, wheat, egg, and finally milk for pediatric patients with EoE. Repeat endoscopy after the reintroduction of each food has been used in some centers to ensure the histological remission and to identify specific food antigens under endoscopic and biopsic monitoring; however, further prospective studies need to validate the clinical value of this treatment strategy. In any case, food antigens that have been proven to act as disease triggers should be eliminated indefinitely.

Pharmacological Therapy

The drug therapy for EoE can be used when the dietary management fails or the patient cannot accept or tolerate the dietary restrictions. It is also considered a better option for patients whose symptoms exhibit a seasonal variability. In practice, combined management strategies including both elimination diets and medicines are often employed.

Proton-Pump Inhibitors

Prior to the establishment of the diagnosis and the initiation of treatment for EoE, an 8-week trial of PPI is recommended in order to differentiate the disease from PPI-responsive eosinophilic eosinophilia. PPIs exert their effect on esophageal eosinophilia not only by suppressing the gastric acid, but by modulating the inflammatory process as well [120]. The decision as to whether these medication should be continued as co-therapy in EoE should be individualized, taken into consideration their role on inhibiting the production of proinflammatory cytokines, the increased expression of vascular adhesion molecules and the activation of neutrophils [121]. In addition, in esophageal cells from patients with EoE, PPIs have been shown to inhibit IL-4-stimulated eotaxin-3 expression and block STAT6 binding to the promoter [122].

Corticosteroids

Topical corticosteroids are the first-line pharmaceutical treatment for EoE, and they have been proven to be effective not only at achieving clinical and histological remission but also at reversing tissue fibrosis as well [123–126] The most frequently employed topical steroid is fluticasone proprionate at a dose ranging from 88 to 440 mcg 2–4 times daily for children. Fluticasone is administered by metered-dose inhaler and patients should be instructed to puff the medication into the mouth during a breath hold and then swallow it, in order the drug to coat esophagus and to minimize pulmonary deposition [3]. Avoidance of food and drinks for 30 min after the ingestion of fluticasone is also recommended.

Difficulties in administering fluticasone in pediatric subjects can be overcome with oral viscous budesonide, a successful alternative treatment option. Even though the optimal dose of budesonide in children with EoE has not been formally assessed, the recommended starting dose is 1 mg daily for children younger than 10 years and 2 mg daily for older children split into 2 divided doses [6]. If necessary, the dose can be gradually increased to 2.8 and 4 mg, respectively [127]. The oral viscous budesonide preparation mixed with sucralose covers the entire esophagus and improves the delivery of the steroid [128, 129].

Despite their efficacy, when the treatment with oral steroids is discontinued, relapse of the disease is common. Furthermore, mouthwash after each use of topical steroids is recommended for the prevention of mouth and oral candidiasis [21, 130]. The use of topical steroids has not been associated with systemic side effects, but long-term safety data is not available in the literature.

Oral systemic steroids have similar efficacy to oral topical steroids in the treatment of EoE. Oral prednisolone has been shown to have a better effect on the resolution of histological abnormalities in pediatric patients [131]. The adverse effects of systemic steroids limit their use, and they are reserved as a treatment option when other approaches fail or rapid relief of symptoms is required. The recommended dose of oral prednisolone is 1–2 mg/kg (max 40 mg and then to be weaned down gradually). Careful monitoring for evidence of side effects, such as growth inhibition, bone demineralization, acne, diabetes, and mood disturbances, is essential. Intravenous methylprednisolone can also be considered, when oral medications cannot be tolerated.

Other Medications

Leukotriene receptor antagonist and sodium cromoglycate have been also used in pediatric and adult patients [70, 132, 133], but based on the existing evidence, they are inefficient in inducing and maintaining clinical and histological remission, and they are not recommended for the treatment of EoE. Azathioprine and 6 MP act as immunomodulatory drugs and could possibly decrease inflammation by impeding esophageal lymphocyte recruitment, but there are no data supporting their use in pediatric patients. Monoclonal antibodies against IL-5 and IL-13, the cytokines that orchestrate the Th2 pathway, are being currently investigated and represent a promising area for future therapies [134, 135]. Limited data from adult patients support the use of glucagon in relieving esophageal food impaction in EoE [136].

Esophageal Dilatation

Strictures or long segment narrowing of the esophagus may require mechanical dilatation. This approach provides an immediate relief of symptoms, but has no effect on the underlying inflammation. It also carries a risk of complications, like deep mucosal tears, perforation, hemorrhage, and severe pain. Esophageal dilatation should be considered in selected cases in combination with the pharmacological therapy, when the narrowing persists despite the treatment [20, 68, 78].

Quality of Life

Adherence to the dietary and pharmacological treatment variably influences the quality of life. Dietary restrictions can affect psychosocial functioning (school, parties, dating). The feeling of being different from their family and peers has been reported by pediatric subjects. Disease anxiety and worry about symptoms are common in children and adults. Newly developed quality-of-life tools evaluate the symptoms, the histological findings and parent-proxy outcomes, in an attempt to capture the whole impact of the disease on children [137–140].

Natural History

EoE is characterized by chronicity and dependency on nutrition and medical management. Upon discontinuation of the treatment, the recurrence of symptoms is common and only a small percentage of patients develops tolerance to the food allergens. Delay in diagnosis and untreated disease increases the risk for structural esophageal abnormalities and stricture formation. However, the disease has not been associated with an increased risk of progressing into generalized gastrointestinal disorders or malignancy. Furthermore, it does not affect the life expectancy [29, 141–143]. EoE is an emerging disease and many unresolved issues need to be clarified in the future in terms of its pathogenesis, the different phenotypes, the monitoring of the patients, and the long-term effects of the treatment.

References

1. Kato M, Kephart GM, Talley NJ, et al. Eosinophil infiltration and degranulation in normal human tissue. Anat Rec. 1998;252:418–25.
2. Blanchard C, Wang N, Rothenberg ME. Eosinophilic aophagitis: pathogenesis, genetics and therapy. J Allergy Clinc Immunol. 2006;118:1054–9.
3. Dellon ES, Gonsalves N, Hirano I, Futura GT, et al. ACG clinical guideline: evidence based approach to the diagnosis and management of esophageal eosinophilia and eosinophilic esophagitis (EoE). Am J Gastroenterol. 2013;108:679–92.
4. Attwood SE, Smyrk TC, Demeester TR, et al. Esophageal eosinophilia with dysphagia. A distinct clinicopathologic syndrome. Dig Dis Sci. 1993;38:109–16.
5. Lucendo AJ, Sanchez-Cazalilla M. Adult versus pediatric eosinophilic esophagitis: important diferrenced and similarities for the clinician to understand. Expert Rev Clin Immunol. 2012;8(8):733–45.
6. Liacouras CA, Futura GT, Hirano I, et al. Eosinophilic esophagitis: updated consensus recommendations for children and adults. J Allergy Clin Immunol. 2011;128:3–20.e6.
7. Futura GT, Liacouras C, Collins MH, Gupta S, Justinich C, Putnam P, et al. Eosinophilic esophagitis in children and adults: a systematic review and consensus recommendations for diagnosis and treatment. Gastroenterology. 2007;133:1342–63.
8. Hruz P, Straumann A, Bussmann C, Heer P, Simon HU, et al. Escalating incidence of eosinophilic sophagitis:a 20-year prospective, population-based study in Olten County, Switzarland. J Allergy Clinc Imuunol. 2011;128(6):1349–50.e1345.
9. Prasad GA, Alexander JA, Schleck CD, Zinsmeister AR, Smyrk TC, Elias RM, et al. Epidemiology of eosinophilic esophagitis over three decades in Olmsted County, Minesota. Clin Gastroenterol Hepatol. 2009;7(10):1055–61.
10. Noel RJ, Putnam PE, Rothenberg ME. Eosinophilic esophagitis. N Eng J Med. 351:940–1
11. Cherian S, Smith NM, Forbes DA. Rapidly increasing prevalence of eosinophilic esophagitis in Western Australia. Arch Dis Child. 2006;91:1000–4
12. Gill R, Durst P, Rewalt M, et al. Eosinophilic esophagitis disease in children from West Virginia: a review of the last decade (1995–2004). Am J Gastroenterol. 2007;102:2281–5.
13. Buckmeier BK, Rothenberg ME, Collins MH. The incidence and prevalence of eosinophilic esophagitis. J Allergy Clin Immunol. 2008;121(suppl 2):S71. (AB271).

14. Dellon ES, Jensen ET, Martin CF, Shaheen NJ, Kappelman MD. Prevalence of eosinophilic esophagitis in the United States. Clin Gastroenterol Hepatol. 2014. doi:10/1016/j.cgh.2013.09.008.org/.

15. Kapel RC, Miller JK, Torres C, Aksoy S, Lash R, Katzka DA. Eosinophilic esophagitis: a prevalent disease in the United Sttes that affects all age groups. Gastroenterology. 2008;134:1316–21.

16. Dellon ES. Diagnosis and management of eosinophilic esophagitis. Clin Gastroenterol Hepatol. 2012;10:1066–78.

17. Zink DA, Amin M, Gebara S, Desai TK. Familial dysphagia and eosinophilia. Gastrointest Endosc. 2007;65:330–4.

18. Meyer GW. Eosinophilic esophagitis in a father and a daughter. Gastrointest Endosc. 2005;61:932.

19. Patel SM, Falchuk KR. Three brothers with dysphagia caused by eosinophilic esophagitis. Gastrointest Endosc. 2005;61:165–7.

20. Weinbrand- Goichberg Jenny, Segal I, Ovadia A, Levine A, Dalal I. Eosinophilic esophagitis: an immune –mediated esophageal disease. Immunol Res. 2013;56:249–60.

21. Fell JME. Recognition, assessment and management of eosinophilic oesophagitis. Arch Dis Child. 2013;98:702–6.

22. Dellon ES, Kim HP, Sperry SLW, Rybnicek DA, Woosley JT. A phenotypic analysis shows that eosinophilic esophagitis is a ptogressive fibrostenotic disease. Gastrointestinal Endosc. 2013 (in press). doi.org/10.1016/j.gie.2013.10.027.

23. Spergel JM, Brown-Whitehorn TF, Cianferoni A, et al. Identification of causative foods in children with eosinophilic esophagitis treated with an elimination diet. J Allergy Clin Immunol. 2012;130(2):461–7.e5.

24. Henderson CJ, Abonia JP, Kings EC, et al. Comparative dietery therapy effectiveness in remission of pediatric eosinophilic esophagitis. J Allergy Immunol. 2012;129(6):1570–8.

25. Gonsalves N, Yang GY, Doerfler B, Ritz S, Ditto AM, Hirano I. Elimination diet effectively treats eosinophilic esophagitis in adults;food reintroduction identifies causative factors. Gastroenterology. 2012;142(7):1451–9.

26. Fox VL, Nurko S, Futura GT. Eosinophilic esophagitis: it's not just kid's stuff. Gastrointest Endosc. 2002;56:260–70.

27. Straumann A, Aceves SS, Blanchard C, et al. Paediatric and adult eosinophilic esophagitis: similarities and differences. Allergy. 2012;67(4):477–90.

28. Kim HP, Vance RB, Shaheen NJ, et al. The prevalence and diagnostic utility of endoscopic features of eosinophilic esophagitis: a meta-analysis. Clin Gastroenterolo Hepatol. 2012;10:988–96.e5.

29. Spergel JM, Brown–Whitehorn TF, Beausoleil JL, et al. 14 years of eosinophilic esophagitis:clinical features and prognosis. J Paed Gastroenterol Nutr. 2009;48:30–6.

30. Roy- Ghanta S, Larosa DF, Katzka DA. Atopic characteristics of adult patients with eosinophilic esophagitis. Clin Gastroenterol Hepatol. 2008;6:531–5.

31. Penfield JD, Lang DM, Goldblum JR, et al. The role of allergy evaluation in adults with eosinophilic esophagitis. J Clin Gastroenterol. 2010;44:22–7.

32. Almansa C, Krishna M, Buchner AM, Ghabril MS, Talley N, et al. Seasonal distribution in newly diagnosed cases of eosinophilic esophagitis in adults. Am J Gastroenterol. 2009;104:828–33.

33. Assa'ad A. Eosinophilic esophagitis: association with allergic disorders. Gastrointest Endosc Clin N Am. 2008;18:119–21;x.

34. Simon D, Marti H, Heer P, Simon HU, Baathen LR, Straumann A. Eosinophilic esophagitis is frequently associated with IgE- mediated allergic airway diseases. J Allergy Immunol. 2005;115(5):1090–92.

35. Gonzalez-Cervera J, Angueira T, Rodriguez-Dominguez B, Arias A, et al. Successful food elimination therapy in adult eosinophilic esophagitis: not all patients are the same. J Clin Gastroentetol. 2012:46(10):855–8.

36. Atkins D, Futura GT. Mucosal immunology, eosinophilic esophagitis and other intestinal inflammatory diseases. J Allergy Clin Immunol. 2010;125(2):255–61.

37. Rothenberg ME, Hogan SP. The eosinophil. Annu Rev Immunol. 2006;24:147–74.

38. Lucendo AJ, Navarro M, Comas C, Pascual JM, et al. Immunophenotypic characterization and quantification of the epithelial inflammatory infiltrate in eosinophilic esophagitis through stereology: an analysis of the cellular mechanisms of the disease and the immunologic capacity of the esophagus. Am J Surg Pathol. 2007;31:598–606.

39. Collins MH. Histolpathology associated with eosinophilic gastrointestinal disease. Immunol Allergy Clin North Am. 2009;29:109–17.

40. Orlando RC. Pathophysiology of gastroesophageal reflux disease. J Clin Gastroenterol. 2008;42:584–8.

41. Blanchard C, Rothenberg M E. Basics pathogenesis of eosinophilic esophagitis. Gastrointest Endosc Clin N Am. 2008;18(1):133–43.

42. Mishra A, et al. Esophageal remodeling develops as a consequence of tissue-specific IL -5-induced eosinophilia. Gastrenterology. 2008;134:204–14.

43. Mishra A, Hogan SP, Brandt EB, Rothenberg ME. IL-5 promotes eosinophil trafficking to the esophagus. J Immunol. 2002;168:2464–69.

44. Mishra A, Rothenberg ME. Intratracheal IL-13 induces eosinophilic esophagitis by an IL-5, eotaxin-1 and STAT6-dependent mechanism. Gastroenterology. 2003;125:1419–27.

45. Blanchard C, Stucke EM, Rodriguez-Jimenez B, et al. A striking local esophageal cytokine profile in esophageal esophagitis. J Allergy Clin Immunol. 2011;127:208–17.

46. Zhu X, Wang W, Mavi P, et al. Interleukin-15 expression is increased in human eosinophilic esophagitis and mediated pathogenesis in mice. Gastroenterology. 2010;139:182–93.

47. Blanchard C, et al. Eotaxin-3 and a uniquely conserved gene expression profile in eosinophilic esophagitis. J Clin Invest. 2006;116:536–47.

48. Bhattacharya B, et al. Increased expression of eotaxin-3 distinguishes between eosinophilic esophagitis and gastroesophageal reflux disease. Hum Pathol. 2007;48:1744–53.

49. Bullock JZ, et al. Interplay of adaptive Th2 immunity with eotaxin-3/C-C chemokine receptor 3 in eosinophilic esophagitis. J Pediatr Gastroenterol Nutr. 2007;45:22–31.

50. Rayapudi M, et al. Indoor insect allergens are potent inducers of experimental eosinophilic esophagitis in mice. J Leukoc Biol. 2010;88:337–46.

51. Collins MH. Histopathologic features of eosinophilic esophagitis. Gastrointesy Endosc Clin N Am. 2008;18:59–71.

52. Kirsch R, Bokhary R, Marcon MA, Cutz E. Activated mucosal mast cells differentiate eosinophilic(allergic]esophagitis from gastroesophageal disease. J Paed Gastroenterol Nutr. 2007;44:20–6.

53. Gupta SK, Fitzgerald JF, Kondratyuk T, Hogen Esch H. Cytokine expression in normal and inflamed esophageal mucosa: a study into the pathogenesis of the allergic eosinophilic esophagitis. 2006;42:22–6.

54. Abonia JP, Blanchard C, Butz BB, et al. Involvement of mast cells in eosinophilic esophagitis. J Allergy Clin Immunol. 2010;126:140–9.

55. Dellon ES, Chen X, Miller CR, et al. Tryptase stining of mast cells may differentiate eosinophilic esophagitis from gastroesophageal reflux disease. Am J Gastroenterol. 2011;106:264–71.

56. Whang YH, Hogan SP, Fulkerson PC, et al. Expanding the paradigm of eosinophilic esophagitis: mast cells and IL-9. J Allergy Clin Immunol. 2013;131(6):1583–5.

57. Otani IM, Anikumar AA, Newbury RO, et al. Anti-IL-5 therapy reduces mast cell and IL-9 cell numbers in paediatric patients with eosinophilic esophagitis. J Allergy Clin Immunol. 2013;131(6):1578–82.

58. Kalluri R, Neilson EG. Epithelial –mesenchymal transition and its implications for fibrosis. J Clin Invest. 2003;112:1776–84.

59. Abdulnour-Nakhoul AM, Al-Tawil y, Gyftopoulos AA, et al. Alterations in junctional proteins, inflammatory mediators and extracellular matrix molecules in eosinophilic esophagitis. Clin Immunol. 2013;148:265–78.

60. Kagalwalla AF, Akhtar N, Woodruff SA, Rea BA, et al. Eosinophilic esophagitis: epithelial mesenchymal transition contributes to esophageal remodeling and reverses with treatment. J Allergy Clin Immunol. 2012;129:1387–96.

61. Aceves SS, Newbury RO, Dohil R, Bastian JF, Broide DH. Esophageal remodeling in paediatric eosinophilic esophagitis. J Allergy Clin Immunol. 2007;119(1):206–12.

62. Chehade M, Sampson HA, Moriotu RA, Magid MS. Esophageal subepithelial fibrosis in children with eosinophilic esophagitis. J Paediatr Gastroenterol Nutr. 2007;45:319–28.

63. Mudler DJ, Pacheco I, Hurlbut DJ, et al. FGF-9-induced proliferative response to eosinophilic inflammation in oesophagitis. Gut. 2009;58(2):166–73.

64. Blanchard C, Mingler MK, McBride M, et al. Periostin facilitates eosinophil tissue infiltration in allergic lung and esophageal responses. Mucosal Immunol. 2008;1(4):289–96.

65. Straumann A, Bauer M, Fischer B, Blaser K, et al. Idiopathic eosinophilic esophagitis is associated with T(H)2-type allergic inflammation response. J Allergy Clin Immunol. 2001;108:954–61.

66. Hardy J, Singlton A. Genome wide association studies and human disease. N Engl J Med. 2009;360:1759–68.

67. Rothenberg ME, Spergel JM, Sherrill JD, et al. Common variants at 5q22 associate with pediatric eosinophilic esophagitis. Nat Genet. 2010;42:289–91.

68. Atkins D, Kramer R, Capocelli K, Lovel M, Futura GT. Eosinophilic esophagitis: the newest esophageal inflammatory disease. Nat Rev Gastroenterol Hepatol. 2009;6:267–78.

69. Moreno-Borque R, Gisbert JP, Sestander C. Pathophysioloical bases of eosinophilic esophagitis therapy. Inflamm Allergy-Drug Targets. 2013;12:46–53.

70. Liacouras C, et al. Eosinophilic esophagitis: a 10-year experience in 381 children. Clin Gastroenterol Hepatol. 2005;3:1198–206.

71. Haas A, Creskoff-Naune N. Feeding dysfunction in children with eosinophilic esophagitis. Immunol Allergy Clinc AM (in press).

72. Nurko S, Rosen R. Esophageal dysmotility in patients who have eosinophilic esophagitis. Gastrointest Endoscop Clin N Am. 2008;18:73–69.

73. Lucendo AJ, et al. Endoscopic, bioptic and manometric findings in eosinophilic esophagitis before and after steroid therapy: a case series. Endoscopy. 2007;39:765–71.

74. Fell JME. Recognition, assessment and management of eosinophilic esophagitis. Arch Dis Child. 2013;98:702–6.

75. Rosen R, Futura G, Fritz j, Donovan K, Nurko S. Role of acid and non acid reflux in children with eosinophilic esophagitis compared with patinets with gastroesophagel reflux and control patients. J Pediatr Gastroenterol Nutr. 2008;46:520–3.

76. Sant'Anna AM, Rolland S, Fournet JC, Yazbeck S, Drouin E. Eosinophilic esophagitis in children: symptoms, histology and ph probes results. J Pediatr Gastroenterol Nutr. 2004;39:272–377.

77. Martin Martin L, Santander C, Espinoza-Rios J, et al. Esophageal motor abnormalitiesin eosinophilic esophagitis identified by high-resolution manometry. J Gastroenterol Hepatol. 2011;26:1447–50.

78. Papadopoulou A, Koletzko S, Heuschkel R, et al. Management guidelines of eosinophilic esophagitis in childhood. JPGN. 2014;58:107–18.

79. Ngo P, Futura GT, Antonioli DA, et al. Eosinophils in the esophagus-peptic or allergic eosinophilic esophagitis? Case series of three patients with esophageal eosinophilia. Am J Gastroenterol. 2006;101:1666–70.

80. Molina- Infante J, Ferrando-Lamana L, Ripoll C, et al. Esophageal eosinophilic infiltration responds to proton pump inhibition in most adults. Clin Gastroenterol Hepatol. 2011;9:110–7.

81. Sayej WN, Patel R, Baker RD, et al. Treatment with high-dose proton pump inhibitos helps distinguish eosinophilic esophagitis from noneosinophilic esophagitis. J Pediatr Gastroenterol Nutr. 2009;49:393–9.

82. Schroeder S, Capocelli KE, Masterson JC, et al. Effect of proton pump inhibitor on esophageal eosinophilia. J Pediatr Gastroenterol Nutr. 2013;56:166–72.

83. Dellon EV, Speck Olga, Woodward K, Gebhart JH, et al. Clinical and endoscopic characteristics do not reliably differentiate PPR-responsive esophageal eosinophilia and eosinophilic esophagitis in patients undergoing upper endoscopy: a prospective cohort study.

84. Stewart M, Shaffer A, Urbanski AT, Beck PL, Storr MA. The association between celiac disease and eosinophilic esophagitis in children and adults. BMC Gastroenterol. 2013;13:96.

85. Kagalwalla AF, Shah A, Ritz S, et al. Cow's milk protein-induced eosinophilic esophagitis in a child with gluten-sensitive enteropathy. J Paediatr Gastroenterol Nutr. 2007;44(3):386–8.

86. Quaglietta L, Coccorullo P, Miele E, et al. Eosinophilic esophagitis and coeliac disease: is there an association? Aliment Pharmacol Ther. 2007;26(3):487–93.

87. Verzegnassi F, Bua F, De Angelis P, et al. Eosinophilic esophagitis and coeliac disease: is it just a casual association? Gut. 2007;56(7):1029–30.

88. Shah A, Mc Greal N, Li B, et al. Celiac disease in association with eosinophilic esophagitis: case series of six patients from two centers. JPGN. 2006;43:E24.

89. Ooi CY, Day AS, Jackson R, et al. Eosinophilic esophagitis in children with celiac disease. J Gastroenterol Hepatol. 2008;23:1144–8.

90. Leslie C, Mews C, Charles A, Ravikumara M. Celiac disease and eosinophilic esophagitis: a true association. J Paed Gastroenterol Nutr. 2010;50(4):397–9.

91. Thompson JS, Lebwohl B, Reilly NR, et al. Increased incidence of eosinophilic esophagitis in children and adults with celiac disease. J Clin Gastroenterol. 2012;46:6–11.

92. Lindsay ME, Shepers D, Bolar NA, et al. Loss- of function mutations in TGFB2cause syndromic presentation of thoracic aortic aneurysm. Nat Genet. 2012;44:922–7.

93. Neptune ER, Frischmeyer PA, Arking DE, et al. Dysregulation of TGF-beta activation contributes to pathogenesis in Marfan syndrome. Nat Genet. 2003;33:407–11.

94. Buchman AL, Wolf D, Gramlich T. Eosinophilic gastrojejunitis with connective tissue disease. South Med J. 1996;89:327–30.

95. Reis ED, Martinet OD, Mosimann F. Spontaneous rupture of the esophagus in an adolescent with type IV Ehlers-Danlos syndrome. Ehlers-Danlos and spontaneous esophageal rupture. Eur J Surg. 1998;164:313–6.

96. Eliashar R, Sichel JY, Biron A, Dano I. Multiple gastrointestinal complications in Marfan syndrome. Postgrad Med J. 1998;74:495–7.

97. Abonia JP, Wen T, Stucke E, et al. High prevalence of eosinophilic esophagitis in patients with inherited connective tissue disorders. J Allergy Clin Immunol. 2013;132(2):378–86.

98. Gonzales N, Policarpio-Nicolas M, Zhang Q, et al. Histolpathologic variability and endoscopic correlates in adults with eosinophilic esophagitis. Gastrointest Endosc. 2006;64:313.

99. Shah A, Kagalwalla AF, Gonzales N, et al. Histopathologic variability in children with eosinophilic esophagitis. Am J Gastroenterol. 2009;104:716–21.

100. Prasad GA, Talley NJ, Romeno Y, et al. Prevalence and predictive factors of eosinophilic esophagitis in patients presenting with dysphagia: a prospective study. Am J Gastroenterol. 2007;102:2627–32.

101. Nurko S, et al. Esophageal motor abnormalitiesin patients with allergic esophagitis. A study with prolonged esophageal ph/manometry. J Paediatr Gastroenterol Nutr Abstr. 2001;33:417.

102. Vasilopoulos S, et al. The small-caliber esophagus: an unappreciated cause of dysphagia for solids in patients with eosinophilic esophagitis. Gastrointest Endosc. 2002;55:99–106.

103. Fox VL, Nurko S, Teitelbaum JE, et al. High resolution EUS in children with eosinophilic "allergic" esophagitis. Gastrointest Endosc. 2003;57:30–6.

104. Nurko S, Rosen R, Futura GT. Esophageal dysmotility in children with eosinophilic esophagitis: a study using prolonged esophageal manometry. Am J Gastroenterol. 2009;104:3050–7.

105. Kwiatek MA, Hirano I, Kahrilas PJ, et al. Mechanical properties of the esophagus in eosinophilic esophagitis. Gastroenterology. 2011;140:82–90.

106. Gupta SK. Noninvesive markers of eosinophilic esophagitis. Gastrointest Endosc Clin North Am. 2008;18:157–67.

107. Konikoff MR, et al. Potential of blood eosinophils, eosinophil-derived neyrotoxin and eotaxin-3 as biomarkers of eosinophilic esophagtitis. Clin Gastroenterol Hepatol. 2006;4:1328–36.

108. Bhardwaj N, Ghaffari G. Biomarkers for eosinophilic esophagitis: a review. Ann Allergy Asthma Immunol. 2012;109:155–9.

109. Colombo JM, Neilan NA, Schurman JV, Friesen CA. Validation of methods to assess potential biomarkers in padiatric patients with esophageal eosinophilia. World J Gastrointest Pharmacol Ther. 2013;4:113–9.

110. Futura GT, Kagalwalla AF, Lee JJ, et al. The esophageal string test: a novel, minimally invasive method measures mucosal inflammation in eosinophilic oesophagitis. Gut. 2013;62:1395–405.

111. Rodrigues Mariano de Almeida Rezende, et al. Clinical characteristics and sensitivity to food and inhalants among children with eosinophilic esophagitis. BMC Res Notes. 2014;7:47.

112. Davis BP, Rothenberg ME. Emerging concepts of dietary therapy for pediatric and adult eosinophilic esophagitis. Expert Rev. Clin Immunol. 2013;9(4):285–7.

113. Kelly KJ, Lazenby AJ, Rowe PC, et al. Eosinophilic esophagitis attributed to gastroesophageal reflux: Improvement with an amino acid-based formula. Gastroenterology. 1995;109:1503–12.

114. Markowitz JE, Spergel JM, Ruchelli E, et al. Elemental diet is an effective treatment for eosinophilic esophagitis in children and adolescents. Am J Gastroenterol. 2003;98:777–82.

115. Peterson K, Clayton F, Vinson LA, et al. Utility of an elemental diet in adult eosinophilic esophagitis. Gastroenterology. 2011;140 (suppl 1):AB180.

116. Gonzales N, Yang GY, Doerfler B, Ritz S, Ditto AM, et al. Elimination diet effectively treats eosinophilic esophagitis in adults; food reintroduction identifies causative factors. Gastroenterology. 2012;142:1451–9.

117. Spergel JM, Andrews T, Brown-Whitehorn TF et al. Treatment of eosinophilic esophagitis with specific food elimination diet directed by a combination of skin prick and patch tests. Ann Allergy Asthma Immunol. 2005;95:336–43.

118. Kagalwalla AF, Sentongo TA, Ritz S et al. Effect of six-food elimination diet on clinical and histologic outcomes in eosinophilic eso- phagitis. Clin Gastroenterol Hepatol. 2006;4:1097–102.

119. Spergel JM, Shuker M. Nutritional management of eosinophilic esophagitis. Gastrointest Endosc Clin N Am. 2008;18:179–94.

120. Yoshida N, Yoshikawa T, Tanaka Y, et al. A new mechanism for anti- inflammatory actions of proton pump inhibitors–inhibitory effects on neutrophil-endothelial cell interactions. Aliment Pharmacol Ther. 2000;14:74–81.

121. Handa O, Yoshida N, Fujita N, et al. Molecular mechanisms involved in anti-inflammatory effects of proton pump inhibitors. Inflamm Res. 2006;55:476–80.

122. Zhang X, Cheng E, Huo X, et al. Omeprazole blocks STAT6 binding to the eotaxin-3 promoter in eosinophilic esophagitis cells. PLoS One. 2012;7:e50037.

123. Noel RJ, Putnam PE, Collins MH, et al. Clinical and immunopathologic effects of swallowed fluticasone for eosinophilic esophagitis. Clin Gastroenterol Hepatol. 2004;2:568–75.

124. Aceves SS, Newbury RO, Chen D, et al. Resolution of remodeling in eosinophilic esophagitis correlates with epithelial response to topical corticosteroids. Allergy. 2010;65:109–16.

125. Faubion WA, et al. Treatment of eosinophilic esophagitis with inhaled corticosteroids. J Pediatr Gastroenterol Nutr. 1998;27:90–3.

126. Konikoff MR. A randomized, double-blind, placebo-controlled trial of fluticasone proprionate for pediatric eosinophilic esophagitis. Gastroenterology. 2006;131:1381–91.

127. Gupta SK, Collins MH, Lewis JD et al. Efficacy and safety of oral budesonide suspension (OBS) in pediatric subjects with eosinophilic esophagitis (EoE): results from the double-blind, placebo-controlled PEER study. Gastroenterology. 2011;140:S179.

128. Aceves SS, Dohil R, Newbury RO, Bastian JF. Topical viscous budesonide suspension for treatment of eosinophilic esophagitis. J Allergy Clin Immunol. 2005;116:705–6.

129. Aceves SS, et al. Oral viscous budesonide: a potential new therapy for eosinophilic esophagitis in children. Am J Gastroenterol. 2007;102:2217–9.

130. Straumann A, Conus S, Degen L, et al. Long-term budesonide maintenance treatment is partially effective in patients with eosinophilic esophagitis. Clin Gastroenterol Hepatol. 2011;9:400–9.

131. Schafer ET, Fitzgerald JF, Molleston JP, et al. Comparison of oral prednisolone and topical fluticasone in the treatment of eosinophilic esophagitis: a randomized trial in children. Clin Gastroenterol Hepatol. 2008;6:165–73.

132. Gupta SK, Peters-Golden M, Fitzgerald JF et al. Cysteinylleukotriene levels in esophageal mucosal biopsies of children with eosinophilic inflammation: are they all the same? Am J Gastroenterol. 2006;101:1125–8.

133. Lucendo AJ, DeRezende LC, Jimenez-Contreras S et al. Montelukast was inefficient in maintaining steroid-induced remission in adult eosinophilic esophagitis. Dig Dis Sci. 2011;56:3551–8.

134. Open –Label Extension Study of Reslizumab in Pediatric Subjects with Eosinophilic Esophagitis. ClinicalTrialsgov. National Library of Medicine (US), Bethesda (MD);2000. http://clinicaltrials.gov/ct2/show/NCT00635089?term?/span>=Eosinophilic+Esophagitis+and+reslizumab&rank=2.

135. Efficacy and safety of QAX576 in patients with eosinophilic esophagitis. ClinicalTrialsgov. National Library of Medicine (US), Bethesda (MD);2000. http://clinicaltrials.gov/ct2/show/NCT01022970?term?/span>=Eosinophilic+Esophagitis+IL-13&rank=2.

136. Thimmapuram J, Oosterveen S, Grim R. Use of hlucagon in relieving esophageal food bolus impaction in the era of eosinophilic esophageal infiltration. Dysphagia. 2013;28:212–6.

137. Franciosi JP, Hommel KA, DeBrosse CW, et al. Quality of life in paediatric eosinophilic esophagitis:what is important to patients? Chil Care Health Dev. 2012;38(4):477–83.

138. DeBrosse CW, Franciosi JP, King EC, et al. Long-term outcomes in pediatric-onset esophageal eosinophilia. J Allergy Clin Immunol. 2011;128:132–8.

139. Franciosi JP, et al. Peds QL eosinophilic esophagitis module: feasibility, reliability and validity. Gastroenterology. 2013;57:57–66.

140. Franciosi JP, Hommel KA, DeBrosse CW, et al. Development of a validated patient-report symptom metric for pediatric eosinophilic esophagitis: qualitative methods. BMC Gastroenterol. 2011;11:126.

141. Schoepfer AM, Safroneeva E, Bussmann C, et al. Delay in diagnosis of eosinophilic esophagitis increased risk for stricture formation in a time-dependent manner. Gastroenterol. 2013;145(6):1230–6. e1–2.

142. Manard-Katcher P, Marks KL, Liacouras CA, et al. The natural history of eosinophilic esophagitis in the transition from childhood to adulthood. Aliment Pharmacol Ther. 2013;37(1):114–21.

143. Straumann A. The natural history and complications of eosinophilic esophagitis. Thorac Surg Clin. 2011;21(4):575–87.

Gastroesophageal Reflux

Yvan Vandenplas

Abbreviations

BAL	Bronchoalveolar liquid
CMPA	Cow's milk protein allergy
ENT	Ear–nose–throat
GER(D]	Gastroesophageal reflux (disease]
H2 RA	H2 receptor antagonist
LES	Lower esophageal sphincter
LLM	Lipid laden macrophages
NERD	Non-erosive reflux disease
PPI	Proton pump inhibitor
TLESR	Transient lower esophageal sphincter relaxation

Introduction

Exhaustive consensus documents on the definition, diagnosis, and management of gastroesophageal reflux disease (GERD) have been published in 2009 [1, 2]. These have been confirmed and approved by the American Academy of Pediatrics in 2013 [3]. However, it has recently been shown that neither pediatric gastroenterologists nor family pediatricians apply these guidelines, simply because they are not aware they exist [4]. There is a trend to overdiagnose GERD. Between 2000 and 2005, the annual incidence of GERD and acid-related conditions among infants (age ≤1 year) more than tripled (from 3.4 to 12.3 %) and increased by 30–50 % in other age groups [5].

Labeling an otherwise healthy infant as having a "disease" increased parents' interest in medicating their infant when they were told that medications are ineffective [6]. These findings suggest that use of disease labels may promote overtreatment by causing people to believe that ineffective medications are both useful and necessary [6].

Definitions

Gastroesophageal reflux (GER) is the involuntary passage of gastric contents into the esophagus and is a normal physiological process occurring several times per day in every human, particularly after meals [1, 2, 7]. Most reflux episodes are of short duration, asymptomatic, and limited to the distal esophagus. Typically, a reflux episode is the consequence of a transient relaxation of the lower esophageal sphincter (TRLES), unaccompanied by swallowing. A minority of reflux episodes occur as a consequence of a chronically reduced lower esophageal sphincter (LES) esophageal and extraesophageal pressure. "Physiologic GER" is the consequence of increased abdominal pressure not accompanied by an increase of the LES pressure or when GER is associated with absence of symptoms, or during the first months of life accompanied with regurgitation, and occasionally with vomiting [1, 2]. Healthy and sick individuals do not differ in the presence or absence of GER, but in the frequency, duration, and intensity of GER and in its association with symptoms or complications. Physiologic reflux becomes pathologic if esophageal clearance is insufficient, if acid buffering is insufficient, if gastric emptying is delayed, if abnormalities in epithelial restitution or repair occur, if there are anatomical abnormalities such as hiatal hernia, etc. Both in children and adults, GERD is present when reflux of gastric contents is the cause of troublesome symptoms and/or complications [2, 7]. GERD is reflux associated with esophageal and extraesophageal symptoms severe enough to impair quality of life or mucosal damage. Most patients with GERD show no abnormalities on endoscopy or histology from esophageal biopsies, and suffer nonerosive reflux disease (NERD). To be defined as GERD, reflux symptoms must be troublesome to the infant, child, or adolescent and not simply be troublesome to the caregiver [2]. However, it may be difficult to define when symptoms become troublesome in young children, because they cannot adequately report symptoms [8, 9]

Regurgitation, spitting up, poseting, and spilling are synonyms, and are defined as the passage of refluxed gastric

Y. Vandenplas (✉)
Department of Pediatrics, Universitair Ziekenhuis Brussel,
Vrije Universiteit Brussel, Laarbeeklaan 101, 1090 Brussels, Belgium
e-mail: yvan.vandenplas@uzbrussel.be

© Springer International Publishing Switzerland 2016
S. Guandalini et al. (eds.), *Textbook of Pediatric Gastroenterology, Hepatology and Nutrition*,
DOI 10.1007/978-3-319-17169-2_10

contents into the pharynx, mouth, and sometimes expelled out of the mouth [1]. Although regurgitation is mainly effortless, it may sometimes be forceful. Only a minority of physiologic reflux episodes are accompanied by regurgitation. Regurgitation is a characteristic symptom of reflux in infants, but is neither necessary nor sufficient for a diagnosis of GERD, because it is not sensitive or specific [2]. Up to 50% of all infants under the age of 4 months present at least one to several episodes of spilling per day [10–12]. Regurgitation is distinguished from vomiting by the absence of a central nervous system emetic reflex, retrograde upper intestinal contractions, nausea, and retching. "Vomiting" is defined as expulsion with force of the refluxed gastric contents from the mouth [1, 2]. Vomiting is a coordinated autonomic and voluntary motor response, causing forceful expulsion of gastric contents [1]. Vomiting associated with reflux is likely the result of the stimulation of pharyngeal sensory afferents by refluxed gastric contents. Bilious vomiting should not be diagnosed as GERD. Otherwise, healthy infants and children with reflux symptoms who are not troublesome and are without complications should not be diagnosed with GERD [2]. In adults, heartburn (or pyrosis) and regurgitation are the two most typical symptoms of GERD [7]. However, some adult patients complaining of heartburn do not have GERD, they have a syndrome called functional heartburn [13]. Since heartburn causes distress and pain, crying in infants is often considered as the manifestation of heartburn in infants. However, there is no evidence to sustain this hypothesis [14, 15].

"Rumination" is characterized by a voluntary contraction of the abdominal muscles resulting in the habitual regurgitation of recently ingested food that is subsequently spitted up or reswallowed. Gagging, regurgitation, mouthing, and swallowing of refluxed material is identified as rumination.

Prevalence, Environmental, and Genetic Factors

Determining the exact prevalence of GER and GERD at any age is virtually impossible for many reasons: Most reflux episodes are asymptomatic, symptoms and signs are nonspecific and self-treatment is common. Alcohol, smoking, drugs, food components, excessive intake, and weight are GER-inducing variables. In adults, over-the-counter use of low-dose aspirin and nonsteroidal anti-inflammatory drugs favors GERD [16]. Also in adults, race, sex, body mass index, and age are independently associated with hiatus hernia and esophagitis, race being the most important risk factor [17]. In adults living in developed countries, the prevalence of GERD (defined as symptoms of acid regurgitation, heartburn, or both, at least once a week) is 10–20%, whereas in Asia the prevalence is roughly less than 5% [7, 18, 19]. Pediatricians often discuss the tendency to overdiagnose and overtreat reflux-associated symptoms in infants presenting

with frequent regurgitation, since epidemiologic data suggest that about 20% of all infants regurgitate more than four times a day, and that 20% of the mothers consider this as troublesome [10–12]. However, epidemiological data suggest that troublesome reflux occurs in about 20% of the infants and adults, with a drop in prevalence in between [20, 21]. French data report a prevalence of GER in 10% and of GERD in 6% of all children 0–17 years old [21]. According to data obtained by the Health Improvement Network Incidence, the incidence of GERD in children is 0.84/1000 person-years [20]. The incidence decreases with age from 1.48/1000 person-years among 1-year-old children until the age of 12 years, whereupon it again increases to a maximum at 16–17 years of 2.26/1000 person-years for girls and 1.75/1000 person-years for boys [20]. According to these epidemiologic data, children with GERD had double the risk of an extraesophageal condition such as asthma, pneumonia, cough, or chest pain compared with children and adolescents with no diagnosis of GERD [20].

The rising prevalence of GERD seems to be related to the rapidly increasing prevalence of obesity [7]. Total and abdominal obesity are risk factors for the development of GERD symptoms in children [22]. The risk of GERD symptoms rises progressively with the increase in both body mass index and waist circumference, even in normal weight children [22].

An autosomal dominant inheritance of hiatal hernia was described by discovering familial hiatal hernia in five generations of a large family, but without demonstrating the link to GERD. The genetic influence on GERD is supported by increased GER symptoms in relatives of GERD patients. GERD is associated with GNB3 C825T [23]. The results for GERD subgroups support the hypothesis that enhanced perception of reflux events, as a consequence of the increased signal transduction upon G-protein-coupled receptor (GPCR) activation associated with the 825T allele, underlies this association [23]. The concordance for GER is higher in monozygotic than dizygotic twins [24]. Genes in question have been localized to chromosomes 9 and 13. A locus on chromosome 13q, between microsatellite D13S171 and D13S263, has been linked with severe GERD in five multiple-affected families [25]. This could not be confirmed in another five families, probably due to genetic heterogeneity of GERD and different clinical presentation of patients [26]. The relevance of these findings for the general population remains unclear.

Pathophysiology

TLESRs are the most important pathophysiologic mechanism causing GER at any age, from prematurity into adulthood [1, 7, 27]. TLESRs are a neural reflex, triggered mainly by the distention of the proximal stomach and organized in the brainstem, with efferent and afferent pathways travelling in the vagal nerve, activating an intramural inhibitory neuron which releases nitric oxide to relax the LES.

GER is influenced by genetic, environmental (e.g., diet smoking), anatomic, hormonal, and neurogenic factors (Fig. 10.1) [27]. Three major tiers of defense serve to limit the degree of GER and minimize the risk of reflux-induced injury to the esophagus. The first line of defense is the "anti-reflux barrier," consisting of the LES and the diaphragmatic pinchcock and angle of His. When this line of defense fails, the second, esophageal clearance, assumes greater importance and limits the duration of contact between luminal contents and the esophageal epithelium. Gravity and esopha-

geal peristalsis serve to remove volume from the esophageal lumen, while salivary and esophageal secretions from esophageal submucosal glands serve to neutralize acid. The third line of defense, tissue or esophageal mucosal resistance, becomes relevant when (acid) contact time is prolonged [27]. Esophageal mucosa defense can be divided in pre-epithelial (protective factors in saliva and esophageal secretions containing bicarbonate, mucin, prostaglandin E2, epidermal growth factor, transforming growth factor), epithelial (tight junctions, intercellular glycoprotein material), and post-epithelial factors [27]. There is a very important interindividual variation of reflux perception suggesting different esophageal-sensitive thresholds. Capsaicin levels and the transient receptor potential vanilloid receptor-1 play a role in the sen-

Fig. 10.1 Pathophysiologic mechanisms for GER. (Reproduced from Ref. [29], with permission from John Wiley and Sons)

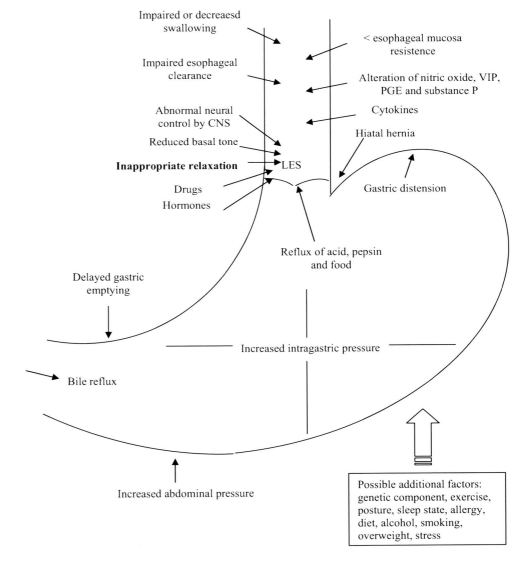

Legend: CNS = central nervous system; LES =lower oesophageal sphincter; PGE = prostaglandin E; VIP = vasoactive intestinal peptide. Inappropriate relaxation is typed in blood as it represents the most important pathophysiological mechanism in GOR

sation of heartburn [28]. The esophageal mucosa contains acid, temperature, and volume-sensitive receptors. A widening of the intercellular spaces is reported in patients with esophagitis and in patients with endoscopy-negative disease. Esophageal sensitivity to acid decreases when the esophagitis has healed. The presence of fat in the duodenum increases the sensitivity to reflux. Hyposensitivity that occurs in patients with Barrett's esophagus is a secondary phenomenon.

GER occurs during episodes of TLESR or inadequate adaptation of the sphincter tone to changes in abdominal pressure. All the factors responsible for maintaining LES tone are not yet determined, but nitric oxide likely plays an important role. Infants have a short intra-abdominal esophagus.

Infants ingest more than twice the volume than adults per kilogram bodyweight (100–150 ml/kg/day compared to 30–50 ml/kg/day), causing more gastric distention and as a consequence more TLESRs. Feeding frequency is higher in infants than in adults, resulting in more postprandial periods during which TLESRs are more common. When investigated in supine position, the frequency of TLESRs in healthy adults and those with acid GERD does not differ. In healthy adults, only 30% of the TLSERs are accompanied by acid reflux, but, in patients with GERD, reflux occurs in 65% of the TLESRs. Thus, in adults, controls and GERD patients have the same number of TLESRs, but in patients with GERD, these TLESRs are more than twice as frequently accompanied with acid GER [30]. Older studies performed in adults in the recumbent position may be more relevant to understand the pathophysiologic mechanisms of acid reflux in infants. Normal individuals rarely experience TLESRs during sleep. Supine position removes all the beneficial gravitational effects of the erect position. Noxious materials, rather than air, are positioned at the cardia, available to move into the esophagus during TLESRs. A reflux is more likely to reach the pharynx in the recumbent than in the upright position. Both salivation and swallowing are markedly reduced during sleep, further impairing clearance. The upper esophageal sphincter is atonic during sleep, allowing reflux almost free to access the airways.

Delayed gastric emptying may increase postprandial reflux possibly by increasing the rate of TLESRs. Delayed gastric emptying has been documented in infants and children with symptomatic GER, particularly those with neurologic disorders. Abnormal gastric accommodation to a meal and prolonged postprandial fundic relaxation has been described in patients with GERD (M30 21). Esophageal acid exposure in patients with GERD is directly correlated with the emptying time of the proximal stomach. GERD was classically considered to be an acid peptic disease. But as a group, the majority of patients with reflux disease do not have a significant increase in gastric acid secretion. Recent analysis of postprandial acidity in the area of the gastroesophageal (GE) junction suggests that local acid distribution ("the gas-

tric acid pocket") rather than total gastric secretion might be more relevant to the pathogenesis of GERD. Differences may exist in the degree of mixing of fundic contents leading to different distributions of acid in the stomach. Studies using pH monitoring, scintigraphy and gastric magnetic resonance suggest that gastric mixing can be incomplete. Different layers of viscosity within the stomach might therefore influence the distribution of the gastric contents. A collection of acid in the gastric part of the esophageal junction was shown in adults in supine position, even in the postprandial period when stomach content was neutralized by the meal [31].

Hiatal hernia increases the number of reflux episodes and delays esophageal clearance by promoting retrograde flow across the esophagogastric junction when the LES relaxes after a swallow. This mechanism underlies the so-called re-reflux phenomenon (acid reflux when the pH is still below 4).

The majority of the studies on pathophysiologic mechanisms have been performed in adults and did not consider weakly acid and nonacid reflux. The refluxed material can be acid, weakly acid, or nonacid. Reflux may be a mix of gas and liquid or pure liquid, and it may or may not contain bile. More than half of the acid and weakly acid reflux episodes are associated with reflux of gas [30]. Weakly acid reflux also occurs predominantly during TLESRs. With liquid meals, patients with GERD had a similar total rate of reflux episodes but a higher proportion of acid reflux events than controls [32]. Weakly acid reflux may be responsible for the remaining symptoms in patients under antisecretory treatment. Components contributing to the noxiousness of refluxate are pepsin, bile acids and salts, and trypsin. The latter two depend on duodenogastric reflux preceding GER and are implicated in the genesis of strictures and Barrett's esophagus. Acid is emptied from the esophagus with one or two sequences of primary peristalsis, and then the residual acidity is neutralized by swallowed saliva. Secondary peristalsis is the response to esophageal distension with air or water, and is more important during sleep when peristalsis is reduced. Patients may have normal primary peristalsis but abnormal secondary peristalsis. Thus, nonacid reflux that occurs in the postprandial period may be inefficiently cleared and cause prolonged esophageal distension, and thus cause symptoms of discomfort. Esophageal clearance modulates the duration of reflux episodes, while mucosal resistance modulates the noxiousness of the components of refluxate. Reflux may cause respiratory symptoms through different pathways, such as (micro-)aspiration or vagally mediated GER (Fig. 10.2).

Helicobacter pylori infection, or eradication of *H. pylori*, does not cause GER. Anyway, because of the decrease of *H. pylori* infection, this issue has become less relevant. Improvement in epigastric pain is significantly correlated with the improvement in GER symptoms but not with eradication of *H. pylori* [33].

Fig. 10.2 Pathophysiologic mechanisms of GER causing respiratory disease. *GER* gastro-esophageal reflux orig

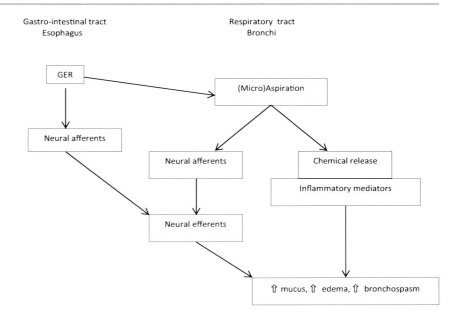

The role of the upper esophageal sphincter in GERD and chronic respiratory disease, laryngitis, hoarseness, coughing, etc., has been insufficiently studied. The upper esophageal sphincter relaxes in response to esophageal body distention by gas, in contract to its contractile response to esophageal body distention by fluid. Symptom presentation has not been linked to different pathophysiologic mechanisms. Children presenting with upper airway disease or ear–nose–throat (ENT) manifestations may rather suffer from an insufficient upper esophageal sphincter, while patients with esophagitis may have more noxious reflux, insufficient clearing mechanisms or a poor esophageal mucosal resistance.

Symptoms and Signs

In normal 3–4-month-old infants, 3–4 episodes of GER are detectable during 5 min of intermittent fluoroscopic evaluation [34]. Normal ranges of esophageal pH monitoring report up to 31 ± 21 acid reflux episodes recorded within a 24-h period (but sample frequency, data handling by the recording device and program do determine this incidence) [35]. Attempts have been made to establish normal ranges in the pediatric age for esophageal impedance [36, 37]. However, for ethical reasons, these investigations were performed in symptomatic children.

While reflux does occur physiologically at all ages, there is also a continuum between physiologic GER and GERD at all ages leading to significant symptoms, signs, and complications (Tables 10.1 and 10.2). GERD is a spectrum of a disease that can best be defined as manifestations of esophageal or adjacent organ injury secondary to the reflux

Table 10.1 Symptoms and signs that may be associated with gastro-esophageal reflux. (Reproduced from Ref. [1], with permission from Lippincott Williams & Wilkins)

Symptoms	
	Recurrent regurgitation with/without vomiting
	Weight loss or poor weight gain
	Irritability in infants
	Ruminative behavior
	Heartburn or chest pain
	Hematemesis
	Dysphagia, odynophagia
	Wheezing
	Stridor
	Cough
	Hoarseness
Signs	
	Esophagitis
	Esophageal stricture
	Barrett's esophagus
	Laryngeal/pharyngeal inflammation
	Recurrent pneumonia
	Anemia
	Dental erosion
	Feeding refusal
	Dystonic neck posturing (Sandifer syndrome)
	Apnea spells
	Apparent life-threatening events (ALTE)

of gastric contents into the esophagus or, beyond, into the oral cavity or airways. The presenting symptoms of GERD differ according to age (Table 10.3). The list of most frequent differential diagnoses of vomiting in infants and children is listed in Table 10.4.

Table 10.2 Warning signals requiring investigation in infants with regurgitation or vomiting. (Reproduced from Ref. [1], with permission from Lippincott Williams & Wilkins)

Bilious vomiting
GI bleeding
Hematemesis
Hematochezia
Consistently forceful vomiting
Onset of vomiting after 6 months of life
Failure to thrive
Diarrhea
Constipation
Fever
Lethargy
Hepatosplenomegaly
Bulging fontanelle
Macro/microcephaly
Seizures
Abdominal tenderness or distension
Documented or suspected genetic/metabolic syndrome

GI gastrointestinal

Table 10.3 Symptoms according to age. (Reproduced from Ref. [29], with permission from John Wiley and Sons)

Manifestations	Infants	Children	Adults
Impaired quality of life	a	a	a
Regurgitation	a	c	c
Excessive crying/irritability	a	c	e
Vomiting	b	b	c
Food refusal/feeding disturbances/anorexia	b	c	c
Persisting hiccups	b	c	c
Failure to thrive	b	c	e
Abnormal posturing/Sandifer's syndrome	b	c	e
Esophagitis	c	b	a
Persistent cough/aspiration pneumonia	c	b	c
Wheezing/laryngitis/ear problems	c	b	c
Laryngomalacia/stridor/croup	c	b	e
Sleeping disturbances	c	c	c
Anemia/melena/hematemesis	c	c	c
Apnea/ALTE/desaturation	c	e	e
Bradycardia	c	f	f
Heartburn/pyrosis	f	b	a
Epigastric pain	f	c	b
Chest pain	f	c	b
Dysphagia	f	c	b
Dental erosions/water brush	f	c	c
Hoarseness/globus pharynges	f	c	c
Chronic asthma/sinusitis	e	b	c
Laryngostenosis/vocal nodules problems	e	c	c
Stenosis	e	d	c
Barrett's esophageal adenocarcinoma	e	d	c

[a] very common
[b] common
[c] possible
[d] rare
[e] absent
[f] unknown
ALTE apparent life-threatening events

Table 10.4 Differential diagnosis of vomiting in infants and children. (Reproduced from Ref. [1], with permission from Lippincott Williams & Wilkins)

GI obstruction	Pyloric stenosis
	Malrotation with intermittent volvulus
	Intestinal duplication
	Hirschsprung disease
	Antral/duodenal web
	Foreign body
	Incarcerated hernia
Other GI disorders	Achalasia
	Gastroparesis
	Peptic ulcer
	Eosinophilic esophagitis/gastroenteritis
	Food allergy
	Inflammatory bowel disease
	Pancreatitis
	Appendicitis
Neurologic	Hydrocephaly
	Subdural hematoma
	Intracranial hemorrhage
	Intracranial mass
	Infant migraine
	Chiari malformation
Infectious	Gastroenteritis
	Sepsis
	Meningitis
	Urinary tract infection
	Pneumonia
	Otitis media
	Hepatitis
Metabolic/endocrine	Galactosemia
	Hereditary fructose intolerance
	Urea cycle defects
	Amino and organic acidemias
	Congenital adrenal hyperplasia
Renal	Obstructive uropathy
	Renal insufficiency
Toxic	Lead
	Iron
	Vitamin A and D
	Medications—ipecac, digoxin, theophylline, etc.
Cardiac	Congestive heart failure
	Vascular ring
Others	Pediatric falsification disorder (Munchausen syndrome by proxy)
	Child neglect or abuse
	Self-induced vomiting (rumination syndrome)
	Cyclic vomiting syndrome
	Autonomic dysfunction

GI gastrointestinal

Belching or eructation occurs during transient relaxation of the LES, and is an important method of venting air from the stomach. Hiccups are involuntary reflex contractions of the diaphragm followed by laryngeal closure. In some cases, hiccups cause GER.

Atypical symptoms such as epigastric pain, nausea, flatulence, hiccups, chronic cough, asthma, chest pain, and hoarseness account for 30–60% of the presentations of GERD [1, 38] (Table 10.1). Possible associations exist between GERD and asthma, pneumonia, bronchiectasis, acute life-threatening event (ALTE), laryngotracheitis, sinusitis, and dental erosion, but causality or temporal association were not established [38]. The paucity of studies, small sample sizes, and varying disease definitions did not allow firm conclusions to be drawn [38]. Less than 10% of infants and children have (acid and troublesome) GERD [35].

The clinician needs to be aware that not all regurgitation and vomiting in infants and young children is GER (disease). Bilious vomiting, gastrointestinal (GI) bleeding, consistently forceful vomiting, weight loss or failure to thrive, diarrhea, constipation, fever, lethargy, hepatosplenomegaly, and abdominal tenderness or distension should raise the possibility of an alternate diagnosis. Bulging fontanelle, macro- and/or microcephaly, and seizures raise the possibility of genetic and/or metabolic syndromes.

GER and Uncomplicated Regurgitation

Regurgitation is the most common presentation of infantile GER, with occasional projectile vomiting.

About 70% of the healthy infants have regurgitation that is physiologic, resolving without intervention in 95% of the individuals by 12–14 months of age [10–12] (Fig. 10.3). Daily regurgitation occurs more frequently in infants during the first 6 months of life than in older infants and children. Frequent regurgitation, defined as >three times per day,

occurs in about 25% of the infants during the first months of life. About 20–25% of the parents seek medical advice because of frequent infantile regurgitation, which corresponds to at least four episodes of regurgitation a day [10–12].

A prospective follow-up reported disappearance of regurgitation in all subjects before 12 months, although an increased prevalence of feeding refusal, duration of meals, parental feeding-related distress, and impaired quality of life were observed, even after the disappearance of symptoms [12]. Regurgitation occurs more frequent in infants than in adults because of the large liquid volume intake, the limited capacity of the esophagus (10 ml in newborn infants), the horizontal position of infants, etc. "Excessive regurgitation" is one of the symptoms of GERD, but the terms regurgitation and GERD should not be used as synonyms.

Although most studies report a comparable incidence of regurgitation in unselected populations of formula versus breastfed infants, Hegar et al. reported a higher incidence in formula-fed infants [10]. This observation fits with the knowledge that GER and symptoms of GERD may be indistinguishable from those of food allergy [1, 2]. The incidence of cow's milk protein allergy (CMPA) is five to ten times higher in formula fed than in breastfed infants [39].

Regurgitation is a characteristic symptom of reflux in infants, but is neither necessary nor sufficient for a diagnosis of GERD, because regurgitation is neither sensitive nor specific. The physician's challenge is to separate regurgitation and vomiting caused by reflux from numerous other disorders provoking the same manifestations. Although the "happy spitter" certainly exists (and is not rare), many infants show some symptoms of distress and discomfort when regurgitating. Irritability may accompany regurgitation and vomiting; however, in the absence of other warning symptoms, it is not an indication for extensive testing [1]. But in fact, parental carrying capacity or anxiousness ("parental coping") will determine if a physician is contacted or not. Infant regurgitation is a benign condition with

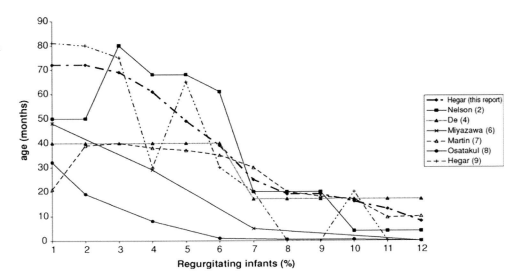

Fig. 10.3 Natural evolution of physiologic regurgitation. (Reproduced from Ref. [10], with permission from John Wiley and Sons)

a good prognosis, needing no other intervention than parental education and anticipatory guidance, and intervention on feeding composition may contribute to parental reassurance. Overfeeding exacerbates recurrent regurgitation. Thickened or anti-regurgitation formula decreases overt regurgitation [1].

GER(D), Recurrent Regurgitation, and Poor Weight Gain

If poor weight gain is documented, it is obvious that the infant is not a happy spitter. Poor weight gain is a crucial warning sign that necessitates clinical management. These infants need a complete diagnostic workup, starting with a dietary history to evaluate caloric intake. Hospitalization of these infants may be needed. Although usually regurgitation causes little more than a nuisance, important regurgitation produces also caloric insufficiency and malnutrition in a minority of infants. There may be abnormal sucking and swallowing, and weight gain may be poor. These infants have no apparent malformations, and may be diagnosed as suffering "nonorganic failure to thrive," a "disorder" that sometimes is attributed to social/sensory deprivation, socioeconomic or primary maternal–child problems. GERD is only one of the many etiologies of "feeding problems" in infancy. Poor weight gain, feeding refusal, back arching, irritability, and sleep disturbances have been reported to be related as well as unrelated to GERD [1, 2, 40].

GER(D) and Cow's Milk Allergy

Guidelines on the symptoms and management of cow's milk allergy unanimously report that persistent regurgitation and vomiting are manifestations of CMPA (Table 10.5: overlapping symptoms between GER(D) and CMPA) [41]. The positive response to cow's milk protein elimination from the diet and relapse of the symptoms is often proposed as a proof of CMPA. An association between GERD and cow milk hypersensitivity was observed in both infants and children with severe GERD [43]. Simultaneous cow milk challenge and pH monitoring had limited value as a method to identify this subgroup. Impedance has shown that the incidence of nonacid postprandial reflux is decreased after a feeding with an amino acid-based formula compared to standard infants' formula [44]. However, since amino acids or extensive hydrolysates have much more rapid gastric emptying than standard infants formula with entire cow milk proteins [45, 46], it is not possible to know if the decrease in GER is due to the enhanced gastric emptying or an immune mechanism.

Table 10.5 Symptoms attributed to GER and CMA. (Reproduced with permission from Ref. [42] by the AAP)

GER	GER+/−CMA	CMA
Dysphagia	Crying	Diarrhea
Hematemesis	Irritability	Bloody stools
Melena	Colic	Rhinitis
Rumination	Parental anxiety	Nasal congestion
Nausea/belching	Feeding refusal	Anaphylaxis
Arching	Failure to thrive	Constipation
Bradycardia	Vomiting	Eczema/dermatitis
Hiccups	Constipation[a]	Angioedema
Sandifer's syndrome	Regurgitation	Lip swelling
Aspiration	Sideropenic anemia	Urticaria/itching
Laryngitis/stridor	Wheezing	
Respiratory infections	Apnea/ALTE/SIDS	
Hoarseness	Sleep disturbances	

[a] Constipation is more towards the CMA symptoms than the GER symptoms

GER gastroesophageal reflux, *ALTE* apparent life-threatening events, *SIDS* sudden infant death syndrome

GERD and Esophagitis

Esophagitis is defined as visible breaks of the esophageal mucosa [1]. Histology is recommended to rule out complications (Barrett's esophagus] or other causes of esophagitis (EoE). Reflux esophagitis is reported to occur in 2–5% of the population. Children with GER symptoms present with esophagitis in 15–62%, Barrett's esophagus in 0.1–3%, and refractory GERD requiring surgery in 6–13% [1, 47]. Erosive esophagitis in 0–17-year-old children with GERD symptoms was reported to be 12.4% and increasing with age 48. The median age of the group with erosive esophagitis was 12.7 ± 4.9 years vs. 10.0 ± 5.1 years in those without erosive esophagitis [48]. The incidence of erosive esophagitis was only 5.5% in those younger than 1 year [48]. This finding is in sharp contrast with the extremely high incidence (24.8%) of anti-reflux medication prescribed in extremely low-birth-weight infants at the moment of discharge [49]. The huge differences in incidence of esophagitis are determined by patient recruitment, differences of definition of esophagitis, and availability of self-treatment. Hiatal hernia is more frequent in children with erosive esophagitis than without (7.7 vs. 2.5%) [48].

The primary symptom of an esophageal stricture is dysphagia. Barrett's esophagus is not rare in adolescents with chronic GERD [1]. In adults, hospital discharges and mortality rates due to gastric cancer, gastric ulcer, and duodenal ulcer have declined during the past three decades, while those of esophageal adenocarcinoma and GERD have markedly risen [50].

Esophagitis, identified by histology, occurs in 61–83% of infants with reflux symptoms severe enough to perform endoscopy. Although esophagitis may present with pain, it can also be asymptomatic. The group with asymptomatic esophagitis is in some ways the most problematic. Even severe esophagitis may remain asymptomatic as demonstrated by children who present with peptic strictures without having experienced any discomfort attributable to esophagitis. Typical substernal burning pain ("heartburn," pyrosis) occurs in many children suffering from esophagitis. Odynophagia, which is pain on swallowing, usually represents esophageal inflammation. In nonverbal infants, behaviors suggesting esophagitis include crying, irritability, sleep disturbance, and "colic". Infants frequently also appear very hungry for the bottle until their first swallows and then become irritable, and refuse to drink. Dysphagia ("typical" for Eosinophilic esophagitis; EoE) has also been linked to esophagitis.

GER(D) and Eosinophilic Esophagitis

The impressive rise in prevalence of EoE is still poorly understood [51], and difficulty in distinguishing EoE from reflux esophagitis may be encountered. In reflux esophagitis, the distal and lower eosinophilic infiltrate is limited to less than 5/per high-power field (HPF) with 85 % positive response to GER treatment, compared to primary EoE with >20 eosinophils per HPF. More recent, failure of proton pump inhibitor (PPI) treatment as a condition to diagnose EoE brought reflux esophagitis back in the picture of EoE [52]. EoE necessitates proper treatment (hypo-allergenic feeding, corticoids, montelukast, etc.). Patients with allergic esophagitis are younger and have atopic features (allergic symptoms or positive allergic tests), but have no specific symptoms. Atopic features are reported in more than 90 % and peripheral eosinophilia in 50 % of patients. At endoscopy, a pale, granular, furrowed, and occasional ringed esophageal mucosa may appear (Ml 1). EoE is becoming more and more important [53]. While symptoms in older children are more oriented to dysphagia for solids, symptoms in infants are more reflux like [53, 54]. Repeated endoscopy with esophageal histology in combination with response to treatment may in some cases be the only way out to separate reflux esophagitis from EoE in young children. An in-depth discussion on EoE is included in Chap. 9.

GER(D), Heartburn, and Infant Crying

While the verbal child can communicate pain, descriptions of the intensity, location, and severity may be unreliable until the age of at least 8 years, and sometimes later [2]. In adults, adolescents, and older children, heartburn and regurgitation are the characteristic symptoms of GERD [7]. GERD in adolescents is more adult like. Heartburn is a symptom of GERD with or without esophagitis. Heartburn is a predominant GER symptom in adults, occurring weekly in 15–20 % and daily in 5–10 % of subjects. Diagnosis and management of GERD in older children (>12 years) and adolescents follows the recommendations for adults [1]. According to parents, heartburn is present in 1.8 % of 3–9-year-old healthy children and 3.5 % of 10–17-year-old adolescents; regurgitation is said to occur in 2.3 and 1.4 %, respectively, and 0.5 and 1.9 % need antiacid medication [12]. In self-reports, adolescents complain about heartburn in 5.2 % and regurgitation in up to 8.2 %, while antiacids are taken by 2.3 % and histamine receptor antagonists (H_2RA) by 1.3 %, suggesting that symptoms of GER are not rare during childhood and are underreported by parents or overestimated by adolescents [12]. In infants, the issue is more complicated. As per definition "heartburn" suggests that the individual with heartburn feels a burning retrosternal pain, parents, and health-care providers almost automatically hypothesize that a "crying baby" or a "baby with colic" is likely to suffer from heartburn or "occult GER." Therefore, acid-reducing medication is often prescribed in infants [49, 55]. Several randomized controlled trials were performed in this indication, and for once all results indicate the same conclusion: PPIs are useless to decrease crying and distressed behavior in newborns and infants [56–59]. Heine and coworkers showed the absence of any relation between crying duration and result of pH monitoring [15].

A symptom-based diagnosis of GERD in infants and young children remains difficult. The reason for the differences in presentation of GERD according to age remains unclear. The persistence of symptoms and progression to complications are unpredictable for a group of patients and for the individual patient. Overall, the correlation between symptoms, results of pH monitoring, acid perfusion test, and histology is poor.

GER(D) and Distressed Behavior

This group of patients is much more difficult to deal with than the infant with poor weight gain. The same amount of distress and crying may be evaluated by some parents as easily acceptable, while the same amount of crying will be unbearable for other parents. In fact, the degree of "coping" capacity of the parents decides if medical help is looked for. Many factors, such as tobacco smoke, may cause infant irritability. CMPA is another well-identified cause of infant irritability. There is substantial individual variability and some healthy infants may cry up to 6 h a day [1].

The concept that infant irritability and sleep disturbances are manifestations of GER is largely derived from adult data [1]. Although this hypothesis seems an acceptable extrapolation, we should be aware that there are not many data on this topic. GERD affects quality of life significantly in adults and probably also in children (and their parents); although, quality of life is more difficult to evaluate in infants and young children. The developing nervous system of infants exposed to acid seems susceptible to pain hypersensitivity despite the absence of tissue damage. In adults, NERD is a general accepted entity. Again in adults, impaired quality of life, notably regarding pain, mental health, and social function, has been demonstrated in patients with GERD, regardless of the presence of esophagitis [60]. In an unselected population, 28% of the adults report heartburn, almost half of them weekly, with a significant impact on the quality of life in 76%, especially if the symptoms are frequent and long lasting. Despite that, only half of the heartburn complainers seek medical help, although 60% takes medications. Thus, some adults "learn to live with their symptoms," and acquire tolerance to long-lasting symptoms, while others accept to live with an impaired quality of life. In infancy and young children, verbal expression of symptoms is often vague or impossible and persistent crying, irritability, back arching, feeding, and sleeping difficulties have been proposed as possible equivalents of adult heartburn. Infants with GERD learn to associate eating with discomfort and thus subsequently tend to avoid eating and develop an aversive behavior around feeds, although behavioral feeding difficulties are also common in control toddlers [61]. Esophageal pain and behaviors perceived by the caregiver (usually the mother) to represent pain (e.g., crying and retching) potentially affect the response of the infant to visceral stimuli and the ability to cope with these sensations, both painful and nonpainful. A placebo-controlled randomized trial with PPI in distressed infants showed an equal decrease in distressed behavior in the treatment and the placebo group [56]. To date, there is no evidence that acid-suppressive therapy is effective in infants who present solely with inconsolable crying. In infants and toddlers, there is no symptom or group of symptoms that can reliably diagnose GERD or predict treatment response. A pilot study suggested that a 40°supine position in a specially developed "Multicare Anti-Regurgitation (AR)-Bed" decreased regurgitation and infant irritability significantly [62].

GER(D), Dysphagia, Odynophagia, and Food Refusal

Dysphagia is the difficulty of swallowing; odynophagia is pain caused by swallowing. Although GERD is frequently mentioned as a cause of dysphagia or odynophagia, there are no pediatric data showing this relation. Dysphagia is a prominent symptom in patients with EoE. Feeding difficulty and/or refusal are often used to describe uncoordinated sucking and swallowing, gagging, vomiting, and irritability during

feeding. A relation between GER, GERD, and feeding refusal has not been established. In case of feeding difficulties, achalasia and foreign body should be among the list of possible differential diagnoses.

GER(D) and Extraesophageal Manifestations

Although evidence is sufficient to support an association between extraesophageal symptoms and GER, establishing that an individual patient's extraesophageal symptoms are caused by reflux is difficult. Pulmonary microaspiration as demonstrated by pepsin detection in bronchoalveolar liquid (BAL) fluid is common in children with chronic lung diseases, suggesting that GER may contribute significantly to the disease pathogenesis [63]. BAL pepsin concentration correlates positively with the number of proximal reflux events [63]. Protein oxidation in BAL is higher in children with extensive proximal acidic reflux, suggesting that pulmonary microaspirations contribute to lung damage [63].

GER(D) and Reactive Airway Disease

An etiologic role for GER in reactive airway disease has not been demonstrated. Different pathophysiologic mechanisms are proposed: direct aspiration, vagal-mediated bronchial and laryngeal spasm, and neural-mediated inflammation. Esophageal acidification in infants with wheezing can produce airway hyperresponsiveness and airflow obstruction [64]. Few studies tempted to evaluate the opposite: the impact of asthma on the severity of GERD. Chronic hyperinflation that occurs in asthma favors many GER mechanisms. An association between asthma and reflux measured by pH or impedance probe has been reported in many studies (M7, M37). Wheezing appears more related to GERD if it is nocturnal. A recent study reports a high prevalence of GER in children and adolescents with persistent asthma, equally distributed in the supine (nocturnal) and upright positions [65]. But, there was no correlation between the result of the pH-metry and pulmonary function tests [65]. There are no studies that help in selecting patients in whom reflux treatment may result in a reduction of asthma medication, if there are such patients at all (M1, M37).

Very few prospective, randomized, and blinded treatment studies have been performed in children. In a series of 46 children with persistent moderate asthma despite bronchodilators, inhaled corticosteroids, and leukotriene antagonists, 59% (27/46) had an abnormal pH-metry [66]. Reflux treatment did result in a significant reduction in asthma medication. Patients with a normal pH-metry were randomized to placebo or reflux treatment: 25% (two of only eight children) of the treated patients could reduce their asthma medication, while this was not possible in any patient on placebo [66]. Another study found omeprazole ineffective in improving asthma symptoms and parameters in children with asthma [67]. Overall, although there seems to be an association between GER and asthma, the causal role of GER has not been demonstrated. There is no association between asthma control status and laryngo-pharyngeal reflux and GER [68]. Current evidence does not support the routine use of anti-GERD medication in the treatment of poorly controlled asthma of childhood [69].

GER(D) and Recurrent Pneumonia

The reported mechanisms are similar to those for reactive airway disease. Direct aspiration during swallowing may be more relevant in this group. No test can determine whether reflux is causing recurrent pneumonia. Upper esophageal and pharyngeal pH and impedance recordings provided contradictory information. Today, it is not yet clear if recording in the upper esophagus or pharynx will help in making therapeutic decisions [70, 71]. A new technique to record pharyngeal reflux has been developed (Restech®) [71]. However, recent results could not confirm that the technique is reliable if compared to esophageal impedance [72].

Lipid-laden macrophages have been used as an indicator of aspiration, but their sensitivity and specificity for GER is poor. One study evaluating nuclear scintigraphy with late imaging reported that 50% of the patients with a variety of respiratory symptoms had pulmonary aspiration after 24 h [73]. However, later studies failed to reproduce these findings [74]. Aspiration also occurs in healthy subjects, especially during sleep [1].

The role of reflux in patients with bronchopulmonary dysplasia and other chronic respiratory disorders is not clear. Today, the clinician has frequently no other option than to make management decisions based on inconclusive diagnostic studies with no certainty regarding outcome [1]. As in reactive airway disease, it is very likely (although not evidence based proven) that (not all) reflux needs to be acid to cause airway manifestations. However, today, medical treatment options are limited to acid-reducing medication.

GER(D) and Cystic Fibrosis

The role of GER in adults and children with cystic fibrosis (CF) has been studied before and after transplant [75, 76]. Acid reflux exists in the majority of CF patients [1]. A high prevalence of acid GER was reported in very young CF infants even before respiratory symptoms developed [75]. CF patients also suffer from duodeno-gastroesophageal reflux of bile acids [77]. It is possible that the acid and bile reflux are aggravating the respiratory symptoms, and that the respiratory symptoms aggravate the reflux. Aggressive medical and surgical reflux treatment in this patient group seems reasonable. In children with CF, a better weight gain was reported during PPI treatment (whether this is due a reduction of acid reflux or better buffering of acid gastric content in the intestine is not clear).

GER(D) and ENT Manifestations

Both acid and weakly acid GER may precede cough in children with unexplained cough, but cough does not induce GER [78]. Objective cough recording improves symptom association analysis (M75 ZCC). Several studies revealed the presence of pepsin in the middle-ear fluid, but with a huge variation in incidence (14–73%) [1, 79]. Also bile acids have been detected in middle-ear liquid, in higher concentrations than in serum [80]. The presence of pepsin and bile in middle ear fluid might as well be the consequence of reflux (and vomiting) at the moment of the acute middle ear infection than an argument to hypothesize that chronic GER may be at the origin of the chronic middle ear problem. However, several epidemiologic studies suggest a low incidence of reflux symptoms in patients with recurrent middle ear infections.

Data suggesting a causal relation between reflux and upper airway disease in children are limited. Data from several placebo-controlled studies and meta-analyses uniformly have shown no effect of anti-reflux therapy on upper airway symptoms or signs [1]. Well designed, prospective, placebo-controlled, blinded studies are needed. Another bias might be the selection of patients: These studies are frequently setup in tertiary care centers in highly selected patient populations. The question is how representative these patients are for the bulk of children with upper respiratory and/or ENT manifestations.

GER(D) and Dental Erosions

Young children and children with neurologic impairment appear to be at greatest risk to have dental erosions caused by GER. Juice drinking, bulimia, and racial and genetic factors that affect dental enamel and saliva might be confounding variables that have been insufficiently considered [1]. Recently, a positive correlation between GERD and dental erosion has been as well confirmed as refuted [81, 82]. There are no long-term (intervention) follow-up studies in high-risk populations.

GER(D) and Sandifer Syndrome

Sandifer syndrome (spasmodic torsional dystonia with arching of the back and opisthotonic posturing, mainly involving the neck and back) is an uncommon but specific manifestation of GERD.

GER(D) and Neurologic Impairment

Children with neurologic impairment have more frequent, more severe, and more difficult to treat GERD than neurologically normal children. Neurologically impaired children accumulate many risk factors for severe GERD: spasticity or hypotonicity, supine position, constipation, etc. Diagnosis of reflux disease in these children is often difficult because of their underlying conditions. Whether this group of patients has more severe reflux disease, or has less effective defense mechanisms, or presents with more severe symptoms because of the inability to express and/or recognize symptoms remains open for debate. Response to treatment, both medical and surgical, is poor in the neurologically impaired child compared to the neurologically normal child.

GER(D) and Apnea, ALTE and SIDS

Literature can best be summarized as follows: series fail most of the time to show a temporal association between GER and pathologic apnea, ALTE, and bradycardia [1, 83]. However, a relation between GER and short, physiologic apnea has been shown [84]. GER is a frequent cause of interrupting sleep in infants, and nonacid GER is equally important as acid GER for causing arousals and awakenings in infants [85]. Discomfort is significantly associated with reflux events and does not differ between weakly acidic and acid refluxes [86]. There are well-selected cases or small series that demonstrate that pathologic apnea can occur as a consequence of GER. However, in general, GER is not related to pathologic apnea, significant bradycardia, ALTE, and sudden infant death syndrome (SIDS) [83].

GER(D) and Other Risk Groups

Symptomatic GER is extremely frequent in patients treated for esophageal atresia and/or tracheoesophageal fistula because of serious structural and functional deficiencies [87]. It is refractory to medical treatment and often requires anti-reflux surgery. However, the high rates of wrap failure invite close follow-up in all cases and reoperation or other measures whenever necessary [87]. Children with congenital abnormalities or after major thoracic or abdominal surgery are at risk for developing severe GERD. Children with anatomic abnormalities such as hiatal hernia, repaired esophageal atresia and malrotation have frequently severe GERD. There are no data in the literature that preterm babies have more (severe) reflux than term-born babies, although many preterms are treated for reflux.

GERD and Complications

Barrett's esophagus, strictures, and esophageal adenocarcinoma are complications of chronic severe GERD. Barrett's esophagus is a premalignant condition in which metaplastic specialized columnar epithelium with goblet cells is present in the tubular esophagus. Differences in esophageal mucosal resistance and genetic factors may partially explain the diversity of lesions and symptoms.

More than 50 years ago, in the absence of reflux treatment, esophageal strictures were reported in about 5 % of the children with reflux symptoms [88]. Currently, esophageal stenosis and ulceration in children have become rare. In a series including 402 children with GERD without neurological or congenital anomalies, no case of Barrett's esophagus was detected [47]. In another series including 103 children with long-lasting GERD, and not previously treated with a H_2RA or a PPIs, Barrett's esophagus was detected in 13 %. An esophageal stricture was present in 5 of the 13 patients with Barrett's esophagus (38 %) [89]. Reflux symptoms during childhood were not different in adults without than in adults with Barrett's esophagus[90]. Barrett's esophagus has a male predominance and increases with age. Patients with short segments of columnar-lined esophagus and intestinal metaplasia have similar esophageal acid exposure but significantly higher frequency of abnormal bilirubin exposure and longer median duration of reflux symptoms than patients without intestinal metaplasia [91]. There is a genetic predisposition in families in patients with Barrett's esophagus and esophageal carcinoma [1].

Children with neurological impairment, chronic lung disease (especially CF), esophageal atresia, and chemotherapy have the most severe pathologic reflux and are at high risk for the development of complications of GERD [1].

Peptic ulcer, esophageal and gastric neoplastic changes in children are extremely seldom. In adults, over the past 30 years, a decreased prevalence of gastric cancer and peptic ulcer with an opposite increase of esophageal adenocarcinoma and GERD has been noted. This has been attributed to independent factors among which changes in dietary habits such as a higher fat intake, an increased incidence of obesity and a decreased incidence of *H. pylori* infection. Recent data suggest obesity does not play a major role [92] The incidence of noninvasive in situ cancer has actually declined after 2003 [93]. Frequency, severity, and duration of reflux symptoms are related to the risk to develop esophageal cancer. Among adults with long-standing and severe reflux, the odds ratios are 43.5 for esophageal adenocarcinoma and 4.4 for adenocarcinoma at the cardia [94]. It is unknown whether mild esophagitis or GER symptoms persisting from childhood is related to an increased risk for severe complications in adults. However, Barrett's esophageal adenocarcinoma affects young individuals [95].

Diagnosis

Diagnostic procedures are not discussed in full detail. Detailed information regarding indications and pitfalls of radiologic contrast studies, nuclear reflux scintigraphy, ultrasound, pH-metry, intraluminal impedance, endoscopy, manometry, gastric emptying tests, and electrogastrography can be found in previous review papers and guidelines [1].

In adults, diagnosis of GER disease is mainly based on clinical history. However, history in children is difficult and considered poorly reliable up to the age of minimally 8 or even 12 years old. Therefore, questionnaires have been developed trying to improve history reliability. Orenstein developed the "infant GER questionnaire" [96]. The questionnaire results in an objective, validated, and repeatable quantification of symptoms suggestions GERD. The I-GER was revised (the "I-GERQ-R") in 185 patients and 93 controls, resulting in an internal consistency reliability from 0.86 to 0.87, and test-retest reliability was 0.85 [97]. However, Aggarwal and coworkers showed that the I-GER-Q had a sensitivity of only 43% and a specificity of 79% [98]. Moreover, pH-metry results were not different according to a "positive" or "negative" score of the I-GER-Q [98]. Our group showed that not one question was found to be significantly predictive for the presence of esophagitis. In our hands, the Orenstein I-GERQ cut-off score failed to identify 26% of the infants with GERD (according to pH-metry results or presence of esophagitis), but was positive in 81% of the infants with a normal histology of esophageal biopsies and normal pH-metry [99]. Deal et al. developed two different questionnaires, one for infants and one for older children, and showed that the score was higher in symptomatic than in asymptomatic children [100]. In other words, the correlation between the results of history obtained by questionnaires and of reflux investigations is poor.

Barium contrast radiography, nuclear scintiscanning, and ultrasound are techniques evaluating postprandial reflux and provide limited information on gastric emptying. Normal ranges are not established for any of these procedures. Barium studies are not recommended as first-line investigation to diagnose GERD, but are of importance to diagnose anatomic abnormalities such as malrotation, duodenal web,

stenosis, and may suggest functional abnormalities such as achalasia, etc. Nuclear scintigraphy may show pulmonary aspiration [73]. Also, aspiration of saliva and gastric contents occurs during sleep in healthy adults [101]. Scintigraphy also can estimate gastric emptying. But the 13C-octanoic acid (for solids) and 13C-acetate (for liquids) breath tests are more appropriate to measure gastric emptying. The role of delayed gastric emptying in GER(D) remains controversial. Ultrasound provides morphological and functional data with high sensitivity and positive predictive value for the diagnosis of GER [102]. Sonographic assessment of findings such as abdominal esophageal length, esophageal diameter, esophageal wall thickness, and gastroesophageal angle provide important diagnostic indicators of reflux and related to the degree of GER [102]. However, there is a need for standardization of the procedure and for defining diagnostic criteria [102]. The results of ultrasound are investigator dependent, and a relation between reflux seen on ultrasound and symptoms has not been established [1]. There is no indication for electrogastrography in the diagnostic work up of a patient suspected of GERD.

Modern endoscopes are so much miniaturized that endoscopy of preterm infants of less than 1000 g has become technically easy. Operator experience is an important component of interobserver reliability [1]. Endoscopy allows direct visual examination of the esophageal mucosa. Macroscopic lesions associated with GERD include esophagitis, erosions, exudate, ulcers, structures, hiatal hernia, etc. Redness of the distal esophagus in young infants is a normal observation because of the increased number of small blood vessels at the cardiac region. Endoscopy may also show a "sliding hernia," the stomach that is protruding in the esophagus during burping. Recent consensus guidelines define reflux esophagitis as the presence of endoscopically visible breaks in the esophageal mucosa at or immediately above the GE junction [1, 2]. Endoscopy-negative reflux disease is common. There is a poor correlation between the severity of symptoms and presence and absence of esophagitis. There is insufficient evidence to support the use of histology to diagnose or exclude GERD. Biopsies of duodenal, gastric, and esophageal mucosa are mandatory to exclude other diseases [1]. More detailed information on pros and cons of histology can be found in the recent consensus papers [1, 2].

Intraluminal esophageal acid perfusion provoking chest pain (Bernstein test) or using other endpoints has found expanded use in practice and research in the USA, but was never popular in Europe. Ambulatory 24-h esophageal pH monitoring measures the incidence and duration of acid reflux, while impedance measures all reflux episodes. Esophageal pH-metry is the best method to measure acid in the esophagus, but not all reflux-causing symptoms are acid and not all acid reflux are causing symptoms. Esophageal pH-metry is useful in evaluating the effect of a therapeutic intervention on reducing esophageal acid exposure. Medical treatment is nowadays focusing on the reduction of gastric acid secretion; the technique offers the possibility to measure intragastric and esophageal recording of pH simultaneously. Both hardware (electrodes, devices) and software influence the results [1]. Normal ranges have been established for pH-metry. However, normal ranges depend also on the hard- and software used and are of limited value for reflux-causing extraesophageal manifestations. It becomes more and more obvious that the major indication of long-term recording of pH and/or impedance is the demonstration of an association between reflux and symptoms.

Manometry does not demonstrate reflux, but is of interest to analyze pathophysiologic mechanisms causing the reflux, mainly by visualizing and measuring TLESRs, and is indicated in the diagnosis of specific conditions such as achalasia. Ambulatory 24-h esophageal manometry, in combination with pH-metry and/or impedance recording, is nowadays technically feasible. This technique is mainly used in (clinical) research, and allows the objective demonstration of reflux-symptom association (e.g., in patients presenting with chronic cough).

Intraluminal impedance measures electrical potential differences. As a consequence, the detection of reflux by impedance is not pH-dependent, but in combination with pH-metry it allows detection of acid (pH < 4.0), weakly acid (pH 4.0–7.0) and alkaline reflux (pH > 7). Experience has shown that impedance needs to be performed in combination with pH-metry, since pH-only events occur (mainly during the night and mainly in young infants). Also gas reflux can be measured, since liquid reflux causes a drop in impedance and gas reflux an increase. Interpretation of the recording is still laborious and necessitates sufficient experience, since the automatic analysis is not standardized and not adequate in (young) children and infants. Impedance seems especially of interest in patients with symptoms suggesting reflux but not esophagitis. Obviously, "more" reflux episodes are detected with impedance pH-metry than with pH-metry alone, but the question remains at this moment unanswered if "more is always necessary or better." The major clinical interest of impedance seems to be demonstration of symptom association, but normal data and validation of symptom association parameters in children are missing. Given the high cost of equipment, electrodes, the time needed for analysis, and interpretation of impedance, the pros and cons in comparison to pH-metry are still debated. Impedance in combination with pH-metry definitively measures more reflux episodes than pH-metry alone. Interestingly, pH-only episodes or reflux episodes detected with pH-metry but not with imped-

ance (drop in pH without bolus movement) occur in young children [103].

Experience in children with spectrophotometric esophageal probes to detect bilirubin is still very limited. Orel and coworkers showed that some children with esophagitis suffer bile reflux [104].

Indirect techniques have been developed, mainly to diagnose GER(D) in patients with extraesophageal manifestations. Accumulation of evidence regarding the determination of lipid-laden macrophages (LLM) in BAL resulted in the conclusion that this method lacks sensitivity and specificity [1]. More recent data show the presence of pepsin in BAL and middle ear fluid [1, 74]. Also, bile salts are detected in middle ear fluid [80]. However, epidemiological data suggest a "protective" role of middle ear infection for the prevalence of GERD [1]. There is no prospective, double-blind, placebo-controlled study treating reflux and evaluating the ENT outcome as primary endpoint.

All GER investigation techniques test different aspects of reflux. Therefore, it is not unexpected that the correlation between the results of the different techniques is poor. There is no "always-best" investigation technique to diagnose GER(D) because the clinical situation of each individual patients differs. "Logic interpretation" (but not evidence-based medicine) suggests that if the question asked is: "does this patient have esophagitis," that endoscopy with biopsy is the best technique. If it is in the interest of the patient to measure acid GER episodes, 24-h pH-metry is the preferred technique. But if quantification of all GER episodes is needed, impedance is likely to be the best. Impedance measures also weakly acid and alkaline reflux. However, postprandial reflux is mainly weakly acid or alkaline, and postprandial reflux was in general considered to be not really relevant, since the techniques measuring postprandial reflux (barium swallow, ultrasound, scintiscanning) are not recommended for this reason. Therapeutic options are mainly limited to acid-reducing medication. As a consequence, it can be questioned if it is really relevant to measure weakly acid and alkaline reflux.

Therapeutic Options

Physiologic GER and regurgitation do not need medical treatment, although they frequently cause parental distress and anxiousness. Any therapeutic intervention should always be a balance between intended improvement of symptoms and risk for side effects. Therapeutic options vary from reassurance, nutritional and positional treatment, prokinetics, and acid-reducing medications to surgery (Table 10.6).

Table 10.6 Schematic therapeutic approach in 2014. (Efficacy and safety data in infants and children for most anti-GER medication are limited)

Phase 1	Parental reassurance, observation, life-style changes, exclude overfeeding
Phase 2	Dietary treatment (to decrease regurgitation and infant distress)
	Thickened formula, thickening agents, (thickened) extensive hydrolysates or amino acid-based formula in cow's milk allergy
	Positional treatment[a]
Phase 3	For immediate symptom relief: alginates (some efficacy in moderate GERD); antacids only in older children
Phase 5	Prokinetics in NERD (but not one product available on the market in 2014 has been shown to be effective)
Phase 4	Proton pump inhibitors (PPIs) in ERD (drug of choice if esophagitis; more safety data needed)
	H$_2$ receptor antagonists less effective than PPIs, but easier to administer if PPI-liquid form does not exist
Phase 6	Laparoscopic surgery

[a] limited data on 40° supine sleeping position in infants

GERD gastroesophageal reflux disease, *NERD* non-erosive reflux disease

Complications of Non-intervention

Although reviews on the natural evolution of regurgitation are available [10–12], there are only limited data on the natural history of GERD in infants and children because most patients do receive treatment at some point.

Traditionally, the impact of regurgitation on the long-term quality of life is trivialized since regurgitation is transitory in the vast majority of infants. However, recent data suggest a decreased quality of life in a number of parents of infants presenting with frequent regurgitation, even if the regurgitation has disappeared [61]. Infants spilling during 90 days or more during the first 2 years of life are at a greater risk for GER symptoms at 9 years [11]. Frequent versus infrequent infant spitting is related to a relative risk at 9 years of 2.3 (95 % CI 1.3–4.0) for at least one GER symptom, of 4.6 (95 % CI 1.5–13.8) for heartburn, of 2.7 (95 % CI 1.4–5.5) for vomiting, and of 4.7 (95 % CI 1.6–14.0) acid regurgitation [10, 11]. It is unclear if regurgitation is less frequent in breastfed than in formula-fed infants, since data are contradictory [10, 11]. Gender is not a confounding factor, but smoking is [24]. Although symptoms improve in more than half of the infants with reflux esophagitis followed longitudinally for 1 year without pharmacotherapy, histology remains abnormal in all [105]. But, it is not known if treatment of regurgitation, GER and GERD during infancy changes the outcome in adults.

In Conclusion Although there is consensus that regurgitation and physiologic GER do not need medical treatment, some data suggest that nonintervention may have in some families a negative impact on the quality of life. Limited data suggest that frequent regurgitation may predispose to develop GER-symptoms later in life.

Nonpharmacological and Nonsurgical Therapies for GER

The most common reason to seek medical help for young infants with suspected GERD is frequent troublesome regurgitation and infant distress. Because infants with physiologic but troublesome regurgitation are difficult to distinguish from infants with mild-to-moderate GERD symptoms, nonpharmacologic treatment (reassurance, dietary, and positional treatment) is recommended as an appropriate first approach. The difference between "physiologic" and "pathologic" GER should not be regarded as a clear delineation, but as a continuum where "at some point" "normal" stops and "disease" begins. Parental coping plays a major factor in this process.

In many situations, reassurance means observation of feeding and handling of the child during and after feeding (Fig. 10.4: Practical algorithm for the management of infant regurgitation). A "reduction of the ingested volume" per feed is a classic recommendation that can be found in all overviews and guidelines or recommendations [1, 3, 106]. However, there are no data that relate ingested volume to frequency and volume of regurgitation, although it seems logical to hypothesize that feeding of large volumes favors regurgitations since it will increase TLESRs. Reassurance while showing compassion for the impaired quality of life is of importance [1,3, 106, 107].

Recent data suggest that parental reports during a first consultation may be inaccurate and overestimate the incidence of regurgitation [107], similar to what is well known regarding crying infants or infant colic. The inclusion criterion for a multicenter French study was more than five episodes of regurgitation per day since more than 1 week [107]. The study started with a 3-day baseline diary, and only 75 % of the infants said initially to regurgitate more than five times did effectively so when the frequency of regurgitation

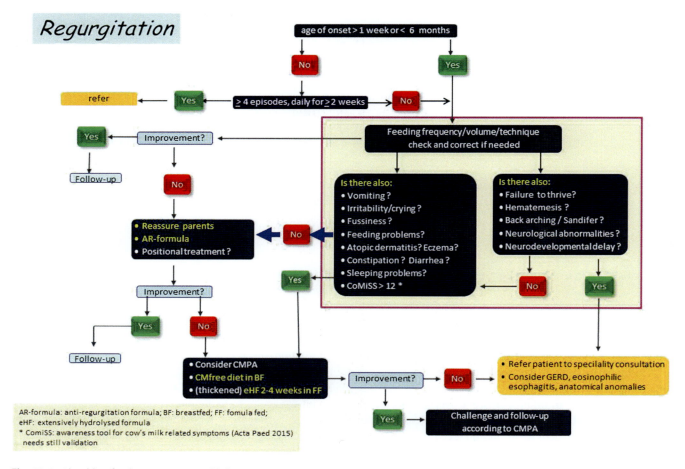

Fig. 10.4 Algorithm for the management of infant regurgitation. *CMPA* cow's milk protein allergy, *BF* breastfed, *CM* cow's milk

was recorded prospectively [107]. These findings question the efficacy of "reassurance and guidance" which in most studies turns around 20%. If the data of this French study are confirmed, the efficacy of "nonintervention" seems to be nothing else than "bring the observations back to reality". Nevertheless, this information illustrates that prospective registration of the so-called problem will help to bring a solution in about one patient/family in four.

Horvath et al. performed a meta-analysis of 14 studies on anti-regurgitation (AR)-formula and concluded that AR-formula decreases the number of episodes of regurgitation and increases the number of infants that do not regurgitate [108]. Thus, a thickened commercialized AR-formula meets up to its expectations, as it decreases visual regurgitation, but not systematically decreases (acid) reflux [109]. AR-formula is "anti-regurgitation" formula and not an "anti-reflux" formula. Thickened formula reduces regurgitation more and faster than the natural evolution [110]. Commercialized thickened formula is preferred to thickening agents added to formula at home because the nutritional content of the thickening agent and its effect on osmolarity has been taken in account in the global composition of the commercialized formula [1, 106].

However, data from three independent studies suggest acid reflux is actually reduced with cornstarch-thickened formula [108]. A French survey reported a significant ($p < 0.05$) greater use of volume reduction or milk thickeners and dorsal positioning in infants with GERD than in infants with physiological GER [21].

At a certain moment, nutritional safety concerns have been raised based on the findings from an in vitro model that bean gum may hamper the absorption of micronutrients [111, 112]. However, in vivo data have contradicted this fear [113]. Therefore, NASPGHAN and ESPGHAN recommend the use of AR formula, irrespective of the thickening agent, for which clinical efficacy has been demonstrated [1]. Recent data suggest that the efficacy may be improved by changing the protein source to a partial or extensive hydrolysate [1, 109]. Partial hydrolysates may be more effective because they have a better digestibility than native protein and an enhanced gastric emptying [114]. Dietary protein allergy may be a cause of reflux, regurgitation, and vomiting and is often accompanied by a distressed behavior [1, 46]. Whether the efficacy of hydrolysates on reducing regurgitation, vomiting, and GER should be regarded as a proof of

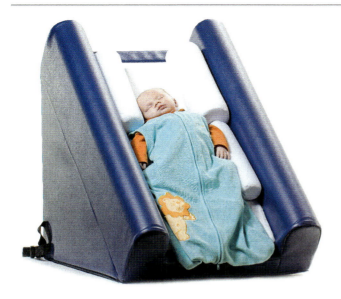

Fig. 10.5 The Multicare AR bed

(non-IgE-mediated) CMPA or whether the efficacy should be considered as an effect of the more rapid gastric emptying of an extensive hydrolysate than native protein is a matter of debate. The fact that postprandial weak acid reflux is increased after a cow milk challenge if compared to an extensive hydrolysate [44], may as well be consecutive to allergy as to a slower gastric emptying, and thus does not contribute to solve this dilemma. Since vomiting, regurgitation, and reflux are also manifestations of CMPA, thickened extensive hydrolysates may be considered since they treat both regurgitation (reflux) and CMPA. Ongoing studies suggest promising results with thickened extensive hydrolysates [115].

Sleeping positions that have been suggested to reduce GER include prone, immediate right side with later left side after feeding, and supine 40° anti-Trendelenburg [62, 116]. Prone position is considered obsolete in infants because of the increased risk forSID. Van Wijk et al. concluded that the biggest benefit was achieved with a strategy of right lateral positioning for the first postprandial hour with a position change to the left thereafter to promote gastric emptying and reduce liquid GER in the late postprandial period [62]. However, at least two independent studies reported a significantly increased risk of SID in the side compared to the supine sleeping position [117, 118]. The results of a pilot study with the "Multicare-AR Bed®" suggest that a specially made bed that nurses the infant in a 40°degree supine body position reduces regurgitation, acid reflux (measured with pH monitoring) and reflux-associated symptoms (evaluated with the I-GERQ; Fig. 10.5) [62].

In Conclusion Labeling an otherwise healthy infant as having a "disease" increases parents' interest in medicating their infant [6]. The use of disease labels may promote overtreat-

ment by causing people to believe that ineffective medications are both useful and necessary [6]. For noncomplicated reflux, no medical intervention is required for most infants. Reassurance and dietary treatment in formula-fed infants are the best therapeutic approach of infant regurgitation. Dietary treatment does not treat GERD. Parental reassurance and education regarding regurgitation and lifestyle changes such as the use of thickened formula are usually sufficient to manage infant noncomplicated reflux and regurgitation [1, 2, 119]. Recent, limited data seem to suggest that the protein source (hydrolysate) may also be effective in reducing regurgitation. Data on the efficacy of positional treatment are limited but encouraging.

Pharmacological and Nonsurgical Therapies for GER

Pharmacotherapeutic agents used to treat GERD encompass antisecretory agents, antacids, surface barrier agents, and prokinetics.

Prokinetics and Other Nonacid Reducing/Blocking Medication

From the pathophysiologic point of view, prokinetics are the most logic therapeutic approach to treat NERD in infants, since acid plays only a minor role in GERD in this age group. However, there is no effective and safe prokinetic agent on the market. Cisapride was probably the prokinetic for which efficacy data were the strongest, although only a decrease of the reflux index (% time pH was <4.0) has been shown: Cisapride significantly reduced the reflux index (weighted mean difference −6.49; 95 % CI −10.13 to −2.85; $P = 0.0005$) [120]. But cisapride was taken off the market in the beginning of this century by the American and European authorities because of its cardiac adverse effects such as QT prolongation and torsades de pointes.

Other prokinetics are metoclopramide and domperidone. The efficacy studies with metoclopramide are limited and outdated [121]. The seven metoclopramide studies performed in children under the age of 2 years are all from before 1990 and used a variety of outcomes (345). Compared to placebo, metoclopramide appears to reduce daily symptoms (SMD −0.73; 95 % CI −1.16 to −0.30), and to reduce the reflux index (WMD −2.80 %; 95 % CI −5.58 to −0.01) [121]. Metoclopramide has a high incidence of side effects such as lethargy, irritability, gynecomastia, galactorrhea, and extrapyramidal reactions and has caused permanent tardive dyskinesia [122–125]. There is no evidence to recommend the use of metoclopramide in GERD [126]. A systematic review of studies on domperidone identified only four randomized controlled trials in children, none providing "robust evidence" for efficacy in pediatric GERD [127]. Domperidone occasionally causes extrapyramidal central nervous system side effects [49]. Recently, the cardiac side effects of domperidone have been highlighted and are reported to be comparable to those of cisapride [128–130]. It is not possible to support the use of domperidone in the treatment of uncomplicated GER in infancy [131]. Governmental agencies should be consequent: If the cardiac risk for cisapride was sufficient to withdraw that molecule from the market, despite the weak evidence of efficacy, the same decision should be taken for domperidone since the cardiac risks seem similar and efficacy was not demonstrated [130, 132].

Other prokinetic molecules, such a mosapride, itopride, prucalopride, and renzapirde, have not or insufficiently been studied in children.

Bethanechol, a direct cholinergic agonist, is studied in a few controlled trials and has uncertain efficacy and a high incidence of side effects in children with GERD [1]. Baclofen is a gamma-aminobutyric acid (GABA)-B receptor agonist used to reduce spasticity in neurologically impaired patients. Baclofen was shown to reduce the number of TLSERs and acid GER during a 2-h test period and accelerate gastric emptying [133]. Baclofen can be used as a supplemental therapy to PPIs in children with refractory GER, although failure rate is around 33 % [134]. The data on baclofen are very limited, and the high incidence of adverse events does not justify its widespread use. Also baclofen did not fulfill its promises. M0003 (Shire) is a "next-generation gastrokinetic," but clinical studies have been postponed. M0003 is a specific and high-affinity 5-HT4 agonist for the treatment of upper GI disorders, focusing initially on severe gastroparesis and pediatric reflux.

In Conclusion Although the prokinetic concept is of interest, there is no effective prokinetic (or nonacid-reducing anti-reflux drug) on the market. Moreover, all have a high incidence of adverse effects. Currently, the NASPGHAN and ESPGHAN practice guidelines concluded that there is insufficient evidence to justify the routine use of prokinetic agents [1]. This viewpoint was recently endorsed by the American Academy of Pediatrics [3].

Alginate (-Antacids) and Mucosaprotectors

Alginate (-antacids) have mainly been validated in adults. Their key therapeutic advantage is their rapid onset of action, within minutes from ingestion. However, there are no convincing efficacy data in pediatrics. Results showed a marginal but significant difference between Gaviscon Infant and placebo in average reflux height (being better for placebo!), and raise questions regarding any perceived clinical benefit of its use [135]. Data on compliance in infants and children (these products have a poor taste) and side effects (many antacids have a high aluminum content) are missing [1].

Extrapolating from adult data, one may conclude that it is unlikely that mucosaprotectors would be effective in children.

In Conclusion Based on expert opinion, there may be a transitory place for alginates in patients with GERD in whom rapid symptom resolution is required, but there is no evidence for this recommendation.

H²-Receptor Antagonists and Proton Pump Inhibitors

Since PPIs are more effective in acid suppression than H^2RAs, PPIs are considered the preferred option for treatment of (acid) GERD in children and adults [136]. Some infants presenting with symptoms assumed to be causing GER and to be acid related fail to respond to acid suppression with ranitidine, either because they need better acid suppression or because the symptoms are not acid related [137]. It has been shown in adults and children that PPIs do not reduce the incidence of reflux episodes [138, 139]: They only change the pH of the reflux from acid to nonacid or weakly acid. Because PPIs in liquid formulation are only available in a very limited number of countries, H^2RA-sirup remains popular since it is available worldwide, making it easier to administer in infants and young children. When compared with H^2RA-initiated patients, PPIs are associated with 30 % less discontinuation, 90 % less therapy switching in the first month, a higher comorbidity burden and pretreatment total health care cost [140].

The prescription rates of antiacid medications such as PPI and H^2RAs are still on the increase [55]. Between 2002 and 2009, there was an 11-fold increase of the use of PPI in the USA [57]. In 2010, lansoprazole was the 9th and ranitidine the 14th most prescribed drug in children under 2 years of age in the USA [55].

Since gastrin release after a meal is one of the most potent activators of H^+-K^+-adenosine triphosphateae (ATPase), PPI should be administered long enough before a meal to be absorbed, but not eliminated, by the time the proton pump is activated [141]. It may be preferred to administer PPI once a day before breakfast because young children eat frequently during the day. PPI must be protected from gastric acid by enteric coating; the granules and tablets should not be crushed, chewed, or dissolved as gastric acid secretion may alter the drug. If the microgranules are enteric coated, the capsules can be opened and administered orally or via a feeding tube, in suspension in an acidic medium such as fruit juice, yogurt, or apple sauce. A "home-made" liquid formulation, produced by dissolving the granula, not the microgranula, in 8.4 % bicarbonate solution has been developed [1].

Omeprazole is approved in the USA and Europe for use in children older than 1 year of age; in the USA, lansoprazole is approved as well. Esomeprazole is now approved in the USA for short-term treatment of GERD with erosive esophagitis in infants aged from 1 to 12 months [119]. In Europe, approval for esomeprazole is identical to the approval of omeprazole. Pharmacodynamics and -kinetics have been studied for many PPI molecules in different age groups. In children aged 6–16 years with GERD, currently available pantoprazole delayed-release tablets can be used to provide systemic exposure similar to that in adults [142]. Simulations indicated that the 1.2-mg/kg dose provides the best comparison to adults [143]. Pantoprazole is generally well tolerated in infants and children aged 1 month through <6 years; compared with adults receiving pantoprazole 40 mg, exposure obtained with the 1.2-mg/kg dose was similar [144]. In neonates, preterm infants, and infants aged 1 through 11 months, pantoprazole (high dose) improved pH-metry parameters after ≥5 consecutive daily doses, and it was generally well tolerated for ≤6 weeks [145]. In preterm infants and neonates, pantoprazole granules are generally well tolerated; mean exposures with pantoprazole 2.5 mg were slightly higher than that in adults who received 40 mg [146]. While the half-life was longer, accumulation did not occur [146]. After 5 days of open-label administration, lansoprazole was well tolerated and increased intragastric pH in pediatric subjects <1 year of age [147]. When PPIs need to be administered through a nasogastric tube, the most satisfactory results were obtained with lansoprazole orally disintegrating tablet [148]. A 5-ml volume of water diluent for suspension and a 10-ml volume of flush-through water made it possible to deliver the full lansoprazole dose administered [148].

Authorities seem to approve PPIs in neonates, infants, and children rather on pharmacologic studies than on effectiveness in the treatment of GERD [57, 141]. Indeed, most studies evaluating the efficacy of PPI in newborns and infants are negative, while efficacy is well established in older children (Table 10.7). Reasons that have been proposed for this discrepancy are complex, ranging from GERD not occurring in this population to a lack of histologic identification of esophagitis related to GERD to questions about the validity of symptom-scoring systems to identify esophagitis when it occurs in infants [141].

For unclear reasons, the belief that many infants do present with (excessive) crying because of (excessive) esophageal acid exposure has become extremely popular over the past 10 years. Many infants have periods of unsettledness, or irritability, over the first months of life. Spilling (or posseting) due to reflux of gastric contents is also seen very frequently. Almost universally, these are normal patterns of infancy that resolve with the passage of time. In recent years, these normal developmental processes have increasingly been ascribed to pathology and treated with medical therapies, including acid suppressants [162]. GERD may cause excessive crying in infants [40]. The concept that infant irritability and sleep disturbances are manifestations of GER is largely extrapolated from adult descriptions of heartburn and sleep disturbances that improve with antacid therapy

Table 10.7 Studies evaluating the efficacy of PPI in newborns, infants, and children (published between 2007 and 2013). (*OA* original article, *rev* review)

Author year	Paper (ref)	Age	Result
Baker (2010)	OA [149]	1–5 year	Pantoprazole effective in GERD with esophageal symptoms
Davidson (2013)	OA [57]	Neonates	PPIs are not effective
Higginbotham (2010)	Rev [150]	Infants and children	PPIs are not effective in common infant GERD-associated symptoms
Lee (2011)	OA [151]	4–18 years	PPIs are effective
Terrin (2012)	OA [152]	Preterm	H²RA not effective; associated with infections, necrotizing enterocolitis and fatal outcome
Tjon (2013)	Rev [153]		RCTs and systematic reviews: lack of efficacy of PPIs, specifically in young infants
Tolia (2010)	OA [154]	1–11 year	Esomeprazole heals macroscopic and microscopic erosive esophagitis
Ummarino (201)	OA [155]	1–181 month	PPI > H²RA for respiratory symptoms
Van der Pol (2011)	Rev [156]	Infants	PPIs not effective in reducing GERD symptoms
Wheatley (2009)	OA [157]	Preterm	H²RA: no effect on bradycardia
Winter (2010)	OA [158]	1–11 month	During double-blind treatment, there were no significant differences between pantoprazole and placebo in withdrawal rates due to lack of efficacy
Winter (2012)	OA [56]	1–11 month	During double-blind treatment, there were no significant differences between esomeprazole and placebo in withdrawal rates due to lack of efficacy
Gilger (2008)	OA [159]	1–11 years	Symptom improvement
Gold (2007)	OA [160]	12–17 years	Symptom improvement
Shashidhar (2013)	Rev [161]	0–18 years	PPIs are effective in healing reflux esophagitis in children of all ages but do not improve GER-related symptoms in infants

The table is not exhaustive but lists the papers on Pubmed between 2007 and 2013 with "proton pump inhibitor infant" and "proton pump inhibitor pediatric" as search terms and illustrates the differences in outcome according to age of the patients

PPI proton pump inhibitor, *H²RA* histamine receptor antagonists, *RCTs* randomized controlled trials, *GERD* gastroesophageal reflux disease

[1]. However, there is no evidence for this hypothesis. In the paper by Heine et al., all infants with pathological GER presented with frequent vomiting, and "silent" pathological reflux did not occur [40]. Poor weight gain, feeding refusal, back arching, and sleep disturbance were not significantly associated with pathological GER [40]. These observations suggest that pathological GER is an unlikely cause of infant irritability under the age of 3 months [40]. Several placebo-controlled prospective trials with PPIs in infants presenting with "excessive crying and reflux-like symptoms" have been performed and show negative results, with an increased incidence of adverse events in the PPI group sometimes as being the only difference in outcome [56–58].

Antiacid medications are among the most commonly prescribed medications in neonatal intensive care units in the USA because they are administered to treat clinical signs thought to be caused by GER, such as apnea, bradycardia, or feeding intolerance, despite the lack of evidence of efficacy in this population [55, 140]. Use of anti-reflux medications at the time of discharge seems to be common for extremely low-birth-weight infants, especially those discharged at postmenstrual age of >42 weeks [49]. In some neonatal centers, nearly 50 % of the infants discharged at postmenstrual age of >42 weeks are discharged with anti-reflux medications [49]. The lack of evidence of PPI in neonates seems not to determine the beliefs of physicians [163]. With no agreed-on standard of care in the setting of widespread use of anti-reflux medications, greater understanding is needed about the ways physicians form clinical impressions, access and process medical evidence, and apply it to patient care [163]. The extreme variability among the centers in use patterns of PPI, H²RAs, and metoclopramide suggests lack of an adequate evidence base to guide practice and indicates that case controlled studies or random controlled trials are needed to devise a consistent evidence-based approach [164].

Prolonged treatment of pediatric patients with PPIs has not caused cancer or significant abnormalities [141]. There are different categories of adverse effects related to PPI: idiosyncratic reactions, drug–drug interactions, drug-induced hypergastrinemia, and drug-induced hypochlorhydria [1]. Idiosyncratic reactions occur in up to 12–14 % of children taking PPIs: headache, diarrhea, constipation, and nausea [1]. Acid suppression or hypochlorhydria causes abnormal GI flora and bacterial overgrowth [165]. As a consequence, the prevalence of infectious respiratory and GI tract infections are increased [1, 166, 167]. PPIs are associated with an increased risk of colonization and infection with *Clostridium difficile* [168, 169]. PPIs, particularly if administered for <30 days or in a high dose, showed an association with community-acquired pneumonia [170]. Hypomagnesemia is reported as a rare but severe complication [171]. Whether or not PPI are associated with an impairment of bone mineralization remains open for debate [172]. Gastric acid suppression predisposes patients to develop food allergy [173–175]. Antiacid medication during pregnancy was reported to increase the risk to develop asthma in the offspring [176].

In Conclusion If acid-reducing medication is indicated, PPI are more effective than H²RAs. PPIs are effective in healing reflux esophagitis in children of all ages but do not improve GER-related symptoms in infants [161]. PPIs have been shown to be very effective to reduce acid GER-related symptoms in older children and adolescents. However, these drugs are overused in newborns, infants, and young children. Several pharmacological studies have shown that PPIs are well tolerated and effectively reduce gastric acid secretion in newborns, infants, and young children. However, the vast majority of the clinical trials evaluating the therapeutic efficacy of PPIs in newborns and infants are negative. Adverse effects of PPIs such as the increased risk for gastroenteritis and respiratory tract infections are more relevant in infants, especially when clinical efficacy could not be demonstrated.

Surgery and Therapeutic Endoscopic Procedures

Different anti-reflux surgical approaches do exist. In general, experience seems to be the best guidance for choosing the preferred technique. Most of the literature on surgical therapy in children with GERD consists of retrospective case series in which documentation of the diagnosis of GERD and details of previous medical therapy are deficient, making it difficult to assess the indications for and responses to surgery [1]. The use of anti-reflux surgery has evolved during the laparoscopic era, with a decreasing percentage of neurologically impaired children undergoing this procedure [161]. Anti-reflux procedures were performed predominantly for infants, most of whom were neurologically normal [177]. Anti-reflux procedures in the USA are reported to be most commonly performed in children during a period of life when regurgitation is normal and physiologic and objective measures of GERD are difficult to interpret [178] In contrast, in Europe, anti-reflux surgery is considered as a treatment of last resort in children with GERD refractory to pharmacological therapies [179]. Recent data suggest that the selection of patients who will benefit from surgery might be enhanced by automated impedance manometry pressure-flow analysis, which relates bolus movement and pressure generation within the esophageal lumen [179].

Adult series report that between 37 and 62 % of the patients are taking PPI (again) a few years after the surgery [180, 181]. Fundoplication in children reduces GER without altering esophageal motility [182]. Since laparoscopic anti-reflux surgery is much less invasive than open surgery, causing less operative pain, faster recovery, shorter hospital stay, and a better cosmetic result, only laparoscopic surgery should be performed. Long-term outcome of open and laparoscopic interventions are similar. While anti-reflux surgery in certain groups of children may be of considerable benefit, a failure rate of up to 22 % has been reported [1]. Long-term follow-up after laparoscopic fundoplication produces a good clinical result and a good quality of life [183]. Surgery for GER patients have a significant improvement in their quality of life, not only by the reduction of their symptoms but also in enhancing from the nutritional status [184]. Patients with respiratory symptoms have a higher satisfaction after surgical treatment than those with GI symptoms [184]. Anti-reflux surgery in children shows a good overall success rate (median 86 %) in terms of complete relief of symptoms [185]. Efficacy of anti-reflux surgery in neurologically impaired children may be similar to normally developed children [185]. The outcome of anti-reflux surgery does not seem to be influenced by different surgical techniques, although postoperative dysphagia may occur less after partial fundoplication [185]. Failure of Nissen fundoplication is particularly frequent in patients previously operated upon for esophageal atresia or congenital diaphragmatic hernia and can be predicted preoperatively [186]. A redo-Nissen is indicated if symptoms of GER recur, but the proportion of failure is even higher [186]. These conclusions are bound by the lack of high-quality prospective studies on pediatric anti-reflux surgery [185].

Children with underlying conditions predisposing to the most severe GERD comprise a large percentage of many surgical series. The robot-assisted Nissen fundoplication in children is a safe alternative to conventional laparoscopic surgery [187]. No data support the need for case selection to one of these two minimally invasive procedures [187]. Cardiaplication results in an increase in cardia yield pressure in young pigs. This procedure may be an alternative anti-reflux operation for infants [188].

Therapeutic endoscopic procedures are rarely indicated and should only be performed in units where there is evidence of experience [189]. The transoral incision-less fundoplication procedure can complement the current surgically and medically available options for children with GERD, especially in complicated patients such as those with neurological impairment [190]. However, complications including hemorrhage emphasize the potential risk of the procedure [190]. Total esophagogastric dissociation is an operative procedure that is useful in selected children with neurologic impairment or other conditions causing life-threatening aspiration during oral feedings.

In Conclusion Surgery in indicated when symptoms are life-threatening or when a child beyond the age of 2–3 years is depending on chronic treatment with antiacid medications such as H²RAs or PPIs. In neurologically impaired children, the risk and benefit of a surgical intervention should be well balanced. Although Nissen fundoplication is now well established as a treatment option in selected cases of GERD in children, its role in neonates and young infants is unclear, and is only reserved for selective infants who did not respond to medical therapy and have life-threatening complications of GERD [119]. Experience with a given surgical procedure seems the best outcome predictor.

References

1. Vandenplas Y, Rudolph CD, Di Lorenzo C, Hassall E, Liptak G, Mazur L, et al. Pediatric Gastroesophageal reflux clinical practice guidelines: joint recommendations of the north american society of pediatric gastroenterology, hepatology, and nutrition and the european society of pediatric gastroenterology, hepatology, and nutrition. J Pediatr Gastroenterol Nutr. 2009;49:498–547.
2. Sherman PM, Hassall E, Fagundes-Neto U, Gold BD, Kato S, Koletzko S, et al. A global, evidence-based consensus on the definition of on the definition of gastroesophageal reflux disease in the pediatric population. Am J Gastroenterol. 2009;104:1278–95.
3. Lightdale JR, Gremse DA, Section on gastroenterology, hepatology, and nutrition. Gastroesophageal reflux: management guidance for the pediatrician. Pediatrics 2013;131:e1684–95.
4. Quitadamo P, Papadopoulou A, Wenzl T, Urbonas V, Kneepkens F, Roman E, et al. European pediatricians' approach to children with GER symptoms: survey on the implementation of 2009 NASP-GHAN-ESPGHAN Guidelines. J Pediatr Gastroenterol Nutr. 2013 (in press).
5. Nelson SP, Kothari S, Wu EQ, Beaulieu N, McHale JM, Dabbous OH. Pediatric gastroesophageal reflux disease and acid-related conditions: trends in incidence of diagnosis and acid suppression therapy. J Med Econ. 2009;12:348–55.
6. Scherer LD, Zikmund-Fisher BJ, Fagerlin A, Tarini BA. Influence of "GERD" label on parents' decision to medicate infants. Pediatrics. 2013;131:839–45.
7. Bredenoord AJ, Pandolfino JE, Smout AJPM. Gastro-oesophageal reflux disease. Lancet 2013;381:933–42.
8. Stanford EA, Chambers CT, Craig KD. The role of developmental factors in predicting young children's use of a self-report scale for pain. Pain 2006;120:16–23.
9. von Baeyer CL, Spagrud LJ. Systematic review of observational (behavioral) measures of pain for children and adolescents aged 3 to 18 years. Pain 2007;127:140–50.
10. Hegar B, Dewanti NR, Kadim M, Alatas S, Firmansyah A, Vandenplas Y. Natural evolution of regurgitation in healthy infants. Acta Paediatr. 2009;98:1189–93. (Article first published online: 21 APR 2009). doi:10.1111/j.1651–2227.2009.01306.x
11. Martin AJ, Pratt N, Kennedy JD, Ryan P, Ruffin RE, Miles H, Marley J. Natural history and familial relationships of infant spilling to 9 years of age. Pediatrics 2002;109:1061–7.
12. Nelson SP, Chen EH, Syniar GM, Christoffel KK. Prevalence of symptoms of gastroesophageal reflux during childhood. Arch Pediatr Adolescent Med. 2000;154:150–4.
13. Galmiche JP, Clouse RE, Balint A. Functional esophageal disorders. Gastroenterology 2006;130:1459–65.
14. Vandenplas Y. Management of paediatric gastro-esophageal reflux disease. Nat Rev Gastroenterol Hepatol. 2013 (in press).
15. Heine RG, Jordan B, Lubitz L, Meehan M, Catto-Smith AG. Clinical predictors of pathological gastro-oesophageal reflux in infants with persistent distress. J Paediatr Child Health. 2006;42:134–9.
16. Kim SL, Hunter JG, Wo JM, Davis LP, Waring JP. NSAIDs, aspirin, and esophageal strictures: are over-the-counter medications harmful to the esophagus? J Clin Gastroenterol. 1999;29:32–4.

17. Kang JY, Ho KY. Different prevalences of reflux oesophagitis and hiatus hernia among dyspeptic patients in England and Singapore. Eur J Gastroenterol Hepatol. 1999;11:845–50.

18. El-Serag H, Hill C, Jones R. Systematic review: the epidemiology of gastro-esophageal reflux disease in primary care, using the UK General Practice Data Base? Aliment Pharmacol Ther. 2009;29:470–80.

19. Dent J, El-Serag H, Wallander MA, Johansson S. Epidemiology of gastro-oesophageal reflux disease: a systematic review. Gut 2005;54:710–7.

20. Ruigómez A, Wallander MA, Lundborg P, Johansson S, Rodriguez LA. Gastroesophageal reflux disease in children and adolescents in primary care. Scand J Gastroenterol. 2010;45:139–46.

21. Martigne L, Delaage PH, Thomas-Delecourt F, Bonnelye G, Barthélémy P, Gottrand F. Prevalence and management of gastroesophageal reflux disease in children and adolescents: a nationwide cross-sectional observational study. Eur J Pediatr. 2012;171:1767–73.

22. Quitadamo P, BuonavolontÃ R, Miele E, Masi P, Coccorullo P, Staiano A. Total and abdominal obesity are risk factors for gastroesophageal reflux symptoms in children. J Pediatr Gastroenterol Nutr. 2012;55:72–5.

23. de Vries DR, ter Linde JJ, van Herwaarden MA, Smout AJ, Samsom M. Gastroesophageal reflux disease is associated with the C825T polymorphism in the G-protein beta3 subunit gene (GNB3). Am J Gastroenterol. 2009;104:281–5.

24. Cameron AJ, Lagergren J, Henriksson C. Gastroesophageal reflux disease in monozygotic and dizygotic twins. Gastroenterology 2002;122:55–9.

25. Hu FZ, Preston RA, Post JC. Mapping of a gene for severe pediatric gastroesophageal reflux to chromosome 13q14. JAMA. 2000;284:325–34.

26. Orenstein SR, Shalaby TM, Barmada MM, Whitcomb DC. Genetics of gastroesophageal reflux disease: a review. J Pediatr Gastroenterol Nutr. 2002;34:506–10.

27. Vandenplas Y, Hassall E. Mechanisms of gastroesophageal reflux and gastroesophageal reflux disease. J Pediatr Gastroenterol Nutr. 2002;35:119–36.

28. Kindt S, Vos R, Blondeau K, Tack J. Influence of intra-oesophageal capsaicin instillation on heartburn induction and oesophageal sensitivity in man. Neurogastroenterol Motil. 2009 21:1032–e82.

29. Salvatore S, Hauser B, Vandenplas Y. The natural course of gastro-oesophageal reflux. Acta Paediatrica. 2004;93(8):1063–1069. (Article first published online: 2 JAN 2007). doi:10.1111/j.1651–2227.2004.tb02719.x.

30. Sifrim D, Holloway R, Silny J, Zhang X, Tack J, Lerut A, Janssens J. Acid, non-acid and gas reflux in patients with gastroesophageal reflux disease during 24 hr ambulatory pH-impedance recordings. Gastroenterology 2001;120:1588–98.

31. Kuiken S, Van Den Elzen B, Tytgat G, Bennink R, Boeckxstaens G Evidence for pooling of gastric secretions in the proximal stomach in humans using single photon computed tomography. Gastroenterology 2002;123:2157–8.

32. Sifrim D, Holloway R. Transient lower esophageal sphincter relaxations: how many or how harmful? Am J Gastroenterol. 2001;96:2529–32.

33. Levine A, Milo T, Broide E, Wine E, Dalal I, Boaz M, Avni Y, Shirin H. Influence of Helicobacter pylori eradication on gastroesophageal reflux symptoms and epigastric pain in children and adolescents. Pediatrics 2004;113:54–8.

34. Cleveland RH. Kushner DC, Schwartz AN. Gastroesophageal reflux in children: results of a standardized fluoroscopic approach. Am J Roentgenol. 1983;141:53–6.

35. Vandenplas Y, Goyvaerts H, Helven R. Gastroesophageal reflux, as measured by 24-hours pH-monitoring, in 509 healthy infants screened for risk of sudden infants death syndrome. Pediatrics 1991;88:834–40.

36. Pilic D, Fröhlich T, Nöh F, Pappas A, Schmidt-Choudhury A, Köhler H, et al. Detection of gastroesophageal reflux in children using combined multichannel intraluminal impedance and pH measurement: data from the German Pediatric Impedance Group. J Pediatr. 2011;158:650–4.e1.

37. Di Pace MR, Caruso AM, Catalano P, Casuccio A, De Grazia E. Evaluation of esophageal motility using multichannel intraluminal impedance in healthy children and children with gastroesophageal reflux. J Pediatr Gastroenterol Nutr. 2011;52:26–30.

38. Tolia V, Vandenplas Y. Systematic review: the extra-oesophageal symptoms of gastro-oesophageal reflux disease in children. Aliment Pharmacol Ther. 2009;29:258–72.

39. Vandenplas Y, Koletzko S, Isolauri E, Hill D, Oranje AP, Brueton M, Staiano A, Dupont C. Guidelines for the diagnosis and management of cow's milk protein allergy in infants. Arch Dis Child. 2007;92:902–8.

40. Heine RG, Jaquiery A, Lubitz L, Cameron DJ, Catto-Smith AG. Role of gastro-oesophageal reflux in infant irritability. Arch Dis Child. 1995;73:121–5.

41. Koletzko S, Niggemann B, Arato A, Dias JA, Heuschkel R, Husby S, et al. European Society of pediatric gastroenterology, hepatology, and nutrition. Diagnostic approach and management of cow's-milk protein allergy in infants and children: ESPGHAN GI Committee practical guidelines. J Pediatr Gastroenterol Nutr. 2012;55:221–9.

42. Salvatore S, Vandenplas Y. Gastroesophageal reflux and cow milk allergy: is there a link? Pediatrics/AAP. 2002;110(5):972–84.

43. Nielsen RG, Bindslev-Jensen C, Kruse-Andersen S, Husby S. Severe gastroesophageal reflux disease and cow milk hypersensitivity in infants and children: disease association and evaluation of a new challenge procedure. J Pediatr Gastroenterol Nutr. 2004;39:383–91.

44. Borrelli O, Mancini V, Thapar N, Giorgio V, Elawad M, Hill S, et al. Cow's milk challenge increases weakly acidic reflux in children with cow's milk allergy and gastroesophageal reflux disease. J Pediatr. 2012;161:476–81.

45. Garzi A, Messina M, Frati F, Carfagna L, Zagordo L, Belcastro M, et al. An extensively hydrolysed cow's milk formula improves clinical symptoms of gastroesophageal reflux and reduces the gastric emptying time in infants. Allergol Immunopathol (Madr). 2002;30:36–41.

46. Vandenplas Y, Gottrand F, Veereman-Wauters G, De Greef E, Devreker T, Hauser B, et al. Gastrointestinal manifestations of cow's milk protein allergy and gastrointestinal motility. Acta Paediatr. 2012;101:1105–9.

47. El-Serag HB, Bailey NR, Gilger M, Rabeneck L. Endoscopic manifestations of gastroesophageal reflux disease in patients between 18 months and 25 years without neurological deficits. Am J Gastroenterol. 2002;97:1635–9.

48. Gilger MA, El-Serag HB, Gold BD, Dietrich CL, Tsou V, McDuffie A, Shub MD. Prevalence of endoscopic findings of erosive esophagitis in children: a population-based study. J Pediatr Gastroenterol Nutr. 2008;47:141–6.

49. Malcolm WF, Gantz M, Martin RJ, Goldstein RF, Goldberg RN, Cotten CM, National Institute of Child Health and Human Development Neonatal Research Network. Use of medications for gastroesophageal reflux at discharge among extremely low birth weight infants. Pediatrics 2008;121:22–7.

50. Sonnenberg A, El-Serag HB. Clinical epidemiology and natural history of gastroesophageal reflux disease. Yale J Biol Med. 1999;72:81–92.

51. Spergel JM, Brown-Whitehorn TF, Beausoleil JL, Franciosi J, Suker M, Verma R, Liacouras CA. 14 years of eosinophilic esophagitis: clinical features and prognosis. J Pediatr Gastroenterol Nutr. 2009;48:30–6.

52. Furuta GT, Liacouras CA, Collins MH, Gupta SK, Justinich C, Putnam PE, et al. First International Gastrointestinal Eosinophil

Research Symposium (FIGERS] Subcommittees. Eosinophilic esophagitis in children and adults: a systematic review and consensus recommendations for diagnosis and treatment. Gastroenterology 2007;133:1342–63.

53. Papadopoulou A, Koletzko S, Heuschkel R, Dias JA, Allen KJ, Murch S, et al. Management guidelines of eosinophilic esophagitis in childhood: a position paper of the Eosinophilic Esophagitis Working Group and the Gastroenterology Committee of ESPGHAN. J Pediatr Gastroenterol Nutr (in press).

54. Dellon ES, Gonsalves N, Hirano I, Furuta GT, Liacouras CA, Katzka DA, American College of Gastroenterology. ACG clinical guideline: evidenced based approach to the diagnosis and management of esophageal eosinophilia and eosinophilic esophagitis (EoE). Am J Gastroenterol. 2013;108:679–92.

55. Chai G, Governale L, McMahon AW, Trinidad JP, Staffa J, Murphy D. Trends of outpatient prescription drug utilization in US children, 2002–2010. Pediatrics 2012;130:23–31.

56. Orenstein SR, Hassall E, Furmaga-Jablonska W, Atkinson S, Raanan M. Multicenter, double-blind, randomized, placebo-controlled trial assessing the efficacy and safety of proton pump inhibitor lansoprazole in infants with symptoms of gastroesophageal reflux disease. J Pediatr. 2009;154:514–20.

57. Chen IL, Gao WY, Johnson AP, Niak A, Troiani J, Korvick J, et al. Proton pump inhibitor use in infants: FDA reviewer experience. J Pediatr Gastroenterol Nutr. 2012;54:8–14.

58. Winter H, Gunasekaran T, Tolia V, Gottrand F, Barker PN, Illueca M. Esomeprazole for the treatment of GERD in infants ages 1–11 months. J Pediatr Gastroenterol Nutr. 2012;55:14–20.

59. Davidson G, Wenzl TG, Thomson M, Omari T, Barker P, Lundborg P, Illueca M. Efficacy and safety of once-daily esomeprazole for the treatment of gastroesophagealtReflux disease in neonatal patients. J Pediatr. 2013;163:692–8.

60. Nandurkar S, Talley NJ. Epidemiology and natural history of reflux disease. Bailliere's Clin Gastroenterol. 2000;14:743–57.

61. Nelson SP, Chen EH, Syniar GM. One year follow-up of symptoms of gastroesophageal reflux during infancy. Pediatrics 1998;102:e67.

62. Vandenplas Y, De Schepper J, Verheyden S, Franckx J, Devreker T, Peelman M, et al. A preliminary report on the efficacy of the "Multicare AR-Bed®" in 3 weeks—3 month old infants on regurgitation, associated symptoms and acid reflux. Arch Dis Child. 2010;95:26–30.

63. Starosta V, Kitz R, Hartl D, Marcos V, Reinhardt D, Griese M. Bronchoalveolar pepsin, bile acids, oxidation, and inflammation in children with gastroesophageal reflux disease. Chest 2007;132:1557–64.

64. Sheikh S, Stephen T, Howell L, Eid N. Gastroesophageal reflux in infants with wheezing. Pediatr Pulmonol. 1999;28:181–6.

65. Molle LD, Goldani HA, Fagondes SC, Vieira VG, Barros SG, Silva PS, Silveira TR. Nocturnal reflux in children and adolescents with persistent asthma and gastroesophageal reflux. J Asthma. 2009;46:347–50.

66. Khoshoo V, Le T, Haydel RM Jr, Landry L, Nelson C. Role of gastro-esophageal reflux in older children with persistent asthma. Chest. 2003;123:1008–13.

67. Stordal K Johannesdottir GB, Bentsen BS, Knudsen PK, Carlsen KC, Closs O, et al. Acid suppression does not change respiratory symptoms in children with asthma and gastro-oesophageal reflux disease. Arch Dis Child. 2005;90:956–60.

68. Kilic M, Ozturk F, Kirmemis O, Atmaca S, Guner SN, Caltepe G, et al. Impact of laryngopharyngeal reflux and gastro-esophageal reflux on asthma control in children. Int J Pediatr Otorhinolaryngol. 2013;77:341–5.

69. Blake K, Teague WG. Gastroesophageal reflux disease and childhood asthma. Curr Opin Pulm Med. 2013;19:24–9.

70. Ramaiah RN, Stevenson M, McCallion WA. Hypopharyngeal and distal esophageal pH monitoring in children with gastroesophageal reflux and respiratory symptoms. J Pediatr Surg. 2005;40:1557–61.

71. Ayazi S, Lipham JC, Hagen JA, Tang AL, Zehetner J, Leers JM, et al. A new technique for measurement of pharyngeal pH: normal values and discriminating pH threshold. J Gastrointest Surg. 2009;13:1422–9.

72. Ummarino D, Vandermeulen L, Roosens B, Urbain D, Hauser B, Vandenplas Y. Gastroesophageal reflux evaluation in patients affected by chronic cough: restech versus multichannel intraluminal impedance/pH metry. Laryngoscope. 2013;123:980–4.

73. Ravelli AM, Panarotto MB, Verdoni L, Consolati V, Bolognini S. Pulmonary aspiration shown by scintigraphy in gastroesophageal reflux-related respiratory disease. Chest 2006;130:1520–6.

74. Morigeri C, Bhattacharya A, Mukhopadhyay K, Narang A, Mittal BR. Radionuclide scintigraphy in the evaluation of gastroesophageal reflux in symptomatic and asymptomatic pre-term infants. Eur J Nucl Med Mol Imaging. 2008;35:1659–65.

75. Blondeau K, Pauwels A, Dupont L, Mertens V, Proesmans M, Orel R, et al. Characteristics of gastroesophageal reflux and potential risk of gastric content aspiration in children with cystic fibrosis. J Pediatr Gastroenterol Nutr. 2010;50:161–6.

76. Button BM, Roberts S, Kotsimbos TC, Levvey BJ, Williams TJ, Bailey M, et al. Gastroesophageal reflux (symptomatic and silent): a potentially significant problem in patients with cystic fibrosis before and after lung transplantation. J Heart Lung Transplant. 2005;24:1522–9.

77. Pauwels A, Decraene A, Blondeau K, Mertens V, Farre R, Proesmans M, et al. Bile acids in sputum and increased airway inflammation in patients with cystic fibrosis. Chest 2012;141:1568–74.

78. Blondeau K, Mertens V, Dupont L, Pauwels A, Farré R, Malfroot A, et al. The relationship between gastroesophageal reflux and cough in children with chronic unexplained cough using combined impedance-pH-manometry recordings. Pediatr Pulmonol. 2011;46:286–94.

79. Abdel-aziz MM, El-Fattah AM, Abdalla AF. Clinical evaluation of pepsin for laryngopharyngeal reflux in children with otitis media with effusion. Int J Pediatr Otorhinolaryngol. 2013;77:1765–70.

80. Klokkenburg JJ, Hoeve HL, Francke J, Wieringa MH, Borgstein J, Feenstra L. Bile acids identified in middle ear effusions of children with otitis media with effusion. Laryngoscope. 2009;119:396–400.

81. Farahmand F, Sabbaghian M, Ghodousi S, Seddighoraee N, Abbasi M. Gastroesophageal reflux disease and tooth erosion: a cross-sectional observational study. Gut Liver. 2013;7:278–81.

82. Marsicano JA, de Moura-Grec PG, Bonato RC, Sales-Peres Mde C, Sales-Peres A, Sales-Peres SH. Gastroesophageal reflux, dental erosion, and halitosis in epidemiological surveys: a systematic review. Eur J Gastroenterol Hepatol. 2013;25:135–41.

83. Zimbric G, Bonkowsky JL, Jackson WD, Maloney CG, Srivastava R. Adverse outcomes associated with gastroesophageal reflux disease are rare following an apparent life-threatening event. J Hosp Med. 2012;7:476–81.

84. Wenzl TG, Schenke S, Peschgens T, Silny J, Heimann G, Skopnik H. Association of apnea and nonacid gastroesophageal reflux in infants: investigations with the intraluminal impedance technique. Pediatr Pulmonol. 2001;31:144–9.

85. Machado R, Woodley FW, Skaggs B, Di Lorenzo C, Splaingard M, Mousa H. Gastroesophageal reflux causing sleep interruptions in infants. J Pediatr Gastroenterol Nutr. 2013;56:431–5.

86. Cresi F, Castagno E, Storm H, Silvestro L, Miniero R, Savino F. Combined esophageal intraluminal impedance, pH and skin conductance monitoring to detect discomfort in GERD infants. PLoS One. 2012;7:e43476.

87. Tovar JA, Fragoso AC. Gastroesophageal reflux after repair of esophageal atresia. Eur J Pediatr Surg. 2013;23:175–81.

88. Carre I. The natural history of the partial thoracic stomach ("hiatal hernia"] in children. Arch Dis Child. 1959;34:344–53.

89. Krug E, Bergmeijer JH, Dees J. Gastroesophageal reflux and Barrett's esophagus in adults born with esophageal atresia. Am J Gastroenterol. 1999;94:2825–8.

90. Hassall E. Barrett's esophagus: new definitions and approaches in children. J Pediatr Gastroenterol Nutr. 1993;16:345–64.

91. Oberg S, Peters JH, DeMeester TR, Lord RV, Johansson J, DeMeester SR, Hagen JA. Determinants of intestinal metaplasia within the columnar-lined esophagus. Arch Surg. 2000;135:651–6.

92. Kroep S, Lansdorp-Vogelaar I, Rubenstein JH, Lemmens VE, van Heijningen EB, Aragonés N, et al. Comparing trends in esophageal adenocarcinoma incidence and lifestyle factors between the United States, Spain, and The Netherlands. Am J Gastroenterol. 2013 (Epub ahead of print).

93. Dubecz A, Solymosi N, Stadlhuber RJ, Schweigert M, Stein HJ, Peters JH. Does the incidence of adenocarcinoma of the esophagus and gastric cardia continue to rise in the twenty-first century?-a SEER database analysis. J Gastrointest Surg. 2013 (Epub ahead of print).

94. Lagergren J, Bergstrom R, Lindgren A, Nyrén O. Symptomatic gastroesophageal reflux as a risk factor for esophageal adenocarcinoma. N Engl J Med. 1999;340:825–31.

95. Riegler M, Asari R, Schoppmann SF. Face Barrett's: esophageal adenocarcinoma affects the young. J Gastrointest Surg. 2013.

96. Orenstein SR, Cohn JF, Shalaby T. Reliability and validity of an infant gastroesophageal questionnaire. Clin Pediatrics. 1993;32:472–84.

97. Kleinman L, Rothman M, Strauss R, Orenstein SR, Nelson S, Vandenplas Y, et al. The infant gastroesophageal reflux questionnaire revised: development and validation as an evaluative instrument. Clin Gastroenterol Hepatol. 2006;4:588–96.

98. Aggarwal S, Mittal SK, Kalra KK, Rajeshwari K, Gondal R. Infant gastroesophageal reflux disease score: reproducibility and validity in a developing country. Trop Gastroenterol. 2004;25:96–8.

99. Salvatore S, Hauser B, Vandemaele K, Novario R, Vandenplas Y. Gastroesophageal reflux disease in infants: how much is predictable with questionnaires, pH-metry, endoscopy and histology? J Pediatr Gastroenterol Nutr. 2005;40:210–5.

100. Deal L, Gold BD, Gremse DA, Winter HS, Peters SB, Fraga PD, et al. Age-specific questionnaires distinguish GERD symptom frequency and severity in infants and young children: development and initial validation. J Pediatr Gastroenterol Nutr. 2005;41:178–85.

101. Gleeson K, Eggli DF, Maxwell SL. Quantitative aspiration during sleep in normal subjects. Chest 1997;111:1266–72.

102. Savino A, Cecamore C, Matronola MF, Verrotti A, Mohn A, Chiarelli F, Pelliccia P. US in the diagnosis of gastroesophageal reflux in children. Pediatr Radiol. 2012;42:515–24.

103. Rosen R, Lord C, Nurko S. The sensitivity of multichannel intraluminal impedance and the pH probe in the evaluation of gastroesophageal reflux in children. Clin Gastroenterol Hepatol. 2006;4:167–72.

104. Orel R, Brecelj J, Homan M, Heuschkel R. Treatment of oesophageal bile reflux in children: the results of a prospective study with omeprazole. J Pediatr Gastroenterol Nutr. 2006;42:376–83.

105. Orenstein SR, Shalaby TM, Kelsey SF, Frankel E. Natural history of infant reflux esophagitis: symptoms and morphometric histology during one year without pharmacotherapy. Am J Gastroenterol. 2006;101:628–40.

106. Vandenplas Y, Gutierrez-Castrellon P, Velasco-Benitez C, Palacios J, Jaen D, Ribeiro H, Shek PC, Lee BW, Alarcon P. Practical algorithms for managing common gastrointestinal symptoms in infants. Nutrition 2013;29:184–94.

107. Vandenplas Y, Leluyer B, Cazaubiel M, Housez B, Bocquet A. Double-blind comparative trial with two anti-regurgitation formulae. J Pediatr Gastroenterol Nutr. 2013;57:389–93.

108. Horvath A, Dziechciarz P, Szajewska H. The effect of thickened-feed interventions on gastroesophageal reflux in infants: systematic review and meta-analysis of randomized, controlled trials. Pediatrics. 2008;122:e1268–77.

109. Vandenplas Y. Thickened infant formula does what it has to do: decrease regurgitation. Pediatrics 2009;123:e549–50.

110. Hegar B, Rantos R, Firmansyah A, De Schepper J, Vandenplas Y. Natural evolution of infantile regurgitation versus the efficacy of thickened formula. J Pediatr Gastroenterol Nutr. 2008;47:26–30.

111. Bosscher D, Van Caillie-Bertrand M, Deelstra H. Do thickening properties of locust bean gum affect the amount of calcium, iron and zinc available for absorption from infant formula? In vitro studies. Int J Food Sci Nutr. 2003;54:261–8.

112. Bosscher D, van Caillie-Bertrand M, van Dyck K. Thickening of infant formula with digestible and indigestible carbohydrate availability of calcium, iron and zinc in vitro. J Pediatr Gastroenterol Nutr. 2000;30:373–8.

113. Levtchenko E, Hauser B, Vandenplas Y. Nutritional value of an "anti-regurgitation" formula. Acta Gastroenterol Belg. 1998;61:285–7.

114. Shergill-Bonner R. Infantile colic: practicalities of management, including dietary aspects. J Fam Health Care. 2010;20:206–9.

115. Vandenplas Y, Devreker T, Hauser B. A pilot trial on acceptability, tolerance, and efficacy of a thickened extensive casein hydrolysate (Allernova AR®). Proceedings of the Belgium Society of Pediatrics, March 2010.

116. van Wijk MP, Benninga MA, Dent J, Lontis R, Goodchild L, McCall LM, et al. Effect of body position changes on postprandial gastroesophageal reflux and gastric emptying in the healthy premature neonate. J Pediatr. 2007;151:585–90.

117. Mitchell EA, Tuohy PG, Brunt JM, Thompson JM, Clements MS, Stewart AW, et al. Risk factors for sudden infant death syndrome following the prevention campaign in New Zealand: a prospective study. Pediatrics. 1997;100:835–40.

118. Scragg RK, Mitchell EA. Side sleeping position and bed sharing in the sudden infant death syndrome. Ann Med. 1998;30:345–9.

119. Czinn SJ, Blanchard S. Gastroesophageal reflux disease in neonates and infants: when and how to treat. Paediatr Drugs. 2013;15:19–27.

120. Maclennan S, Augood C, Cash-Gibson L, Logan S, Gilbert RE. Cisapride treatment for gastro-oesophageal reflux in children. Cochrane Database Syst Rev. 2010;(4):CD002300.

121. Craig WR, Hanlon-Dearman A, Sinclair C, Taback S, Moffatt M. Metoclopramide, thickened feedings, and positioning for gastro-oesophageal reflux in children under two years. Cochrane Database Syst Rev. 2004:CD003502.

122. Putnam PE, Orenstein SR, Wessel HB, Stowe RM. Tardive dyskinesia associated with use of metoclopramide in a child. J Pediatr. 1992;121:983–5.

123. Madani S, Tolia V. Gynecomastia with metoclopramide use in pediatric patients. J Clin Gastroenterol. 1997;24:79–81.

124. Machida HM, Forbes DA, Gall DG, Scott RB. Metoclopramide in gastroesophageal reflux of infancy. J Pediatr. 1988;112:483–7.

125. Shafrir Y, Levy Y, Beharab A, Nitzam M, Steinherz R. Acute dystonic reaction to bethanechol–a direct acetylcholine receptor agonist. Dev Med Child Neurol. 1986;28:646–8OO35.

126. Hibbs AM, Lorch SA. Metoclopramide for the treatment of gastroesophageal reflux disease in infants: a systematic review. Pediatrics. 2006;118:746–52.

127. Pritchard DS, Baber N, Stephenson T. Should domperidone be used for the treatment of gastro-oesophageal reflux in children? Systematic review of randomized controlled trials in children aged 1 month to 11 years old. Br J Clin Pharmacol. 2005;59:725–9.

128. Hegar B, Alatas S, Advani N, Firmansyah A, Vandenplas Y. Domperidone versus cisapride in the treatment of infant regurgitation and increased acid gastro-oesophageal reflux: a pilot study. Acta Paediatr. 2009;98:750–5.

129. Vieira MC, Miyague NI, Van Steen K, Salvatore S, Vandenplas Y. Effects of domperidone on QTc interval in infants. Acta Paediatr. 2012;101:494–6.

130. Michaud V, Turgeon J. Domperidone and sudden cardiac death: how much longer should we wait? J Cardiovasc Pharmacol. 2013;61:215–7

131. Scott B. Question 2. How effective is domperidone at reducing symptoms of gastro-oesophageal reflux in infants? Arch Dis Child. 2012;97:752–5.

132. Hondeghem LM. Domperidone: limited benefits with significant risk for sudden cardiac death. J Cardiovasc Pharmacol. 2013;61:218–25.

133. Omari TI, Benninga MA, Sansom L, Butler RN, Dent J, Davidson GP. Effect of baclofen on esophagogastric motility and gastroesophageal reflux in children with gastroesophageal reflux disease: a randomized controlled trial. J Pediatr. 2006;149:468–74.

134. Vadlamudi NB, Hitch MC, Dimmitt RA, Thame KA. Baclofen for the treatment of pediatric GERD. J Pediatr Gastroenterol Nutr. 2013;57:808–12.

135. Del Buono R, Wenzl TG, Ball G, Keady S, Thomson M. Effect of Gaviscon Infant on gastro-oesophageal reflux in infants assessed by combined intraluminal impedance/pH. Arch Dis Child. 2005;90:460–3.

136. Sigterman KE, van Pinxteren B, Bonis PA, Lau J, Numans ME. Short-term treatment with proton pump inhibitors, H2-receptor antagonists and prokinetics for gastro-oesophageal reflux disease-like symptoms and endoscopy negative reflux disease. Cochrane Database Syst Rev. 2013;5:CD002095.

137. Salvatore S, Hauser B, Salvatoni A, Vandenplas Y. Oral ranitidine and duration of gastric pH > 4.0 in infants with persisting reflux symptoms. Acta Paediatr. 2006;95:176–81.

138. Hemmink GJ, Bredenoord AJ, Weusten BL, Monkelbaan JF, Timmer R, Smout AJ. Esophageal pH-impedance monitoring in patients with therapy-resistant reflux symptoms: 'on' or 'off' proton pump inhibitor? Am J Gastroenterol. 2008;103:2446–53.

139. Turk H, Hauser B, Brecelj J, Vandenplas Y, Orel R. Effect of proton pump inhibition on acid, weakly acid and weakly alkaline gastro-esophageal reflux in children. World J Pediatr. 2013;9:36–41.

140. Malcolm WF, Cotten CM. Metoclopramide, H2 blockers, and proton pump inhibitors: pharmacotherapy for gastroesophageal reflux in neonates. Clin Perinatol. 2012;39:99–109.

141. Ward RM, Kearns GL. Proton pump inhibitors in pediatrics: mechanism of action, pharmacokinetics, pharmacogenetics, and pharmacodynamics. Paediatr Drugs. 2013;15:119–31.

142. Ward RM, Kearns GL, Tammara B, Bishop P, O'Gorman MA, James LP, et al. A multicenter, randomized, open-label, pharmacokinetics and safety study of pantoprazole tablets in children and adolescents aged 6 through 16 years with gastroesophageal reflux disease. J Clin Pharmacol. 2011;51:876–87.

143. Knebel W, Tammara B, Udata C, Comer G, Gastonguay MR, Meng X. Population pharmacokinetic modeling of pantoprazole in pediatric patients from birth to 16 years. J Clin Pharmacol. 2011;51:333–45.

144. Tammara BK, Sullivan JE, Adcock KG, Kierkus J, Giblin J, Rath N, et al. Randomized, open-label, multicentre pharmacokinetic studies of two dose levels of pantoprazole granules in infants and children aged 1 month through < 6 years with gastro-oesophageal reflux disease. Clin Pharmacokinet. 2011;50:541–50.

145. Kierkus J, Furmaga-Jablonska W, Sullivan JE, David ES, Stewart DL, Rath N, et al. Pharmacodynamics and safety of pantoprazole in neonates, preterm infants, and infants aged 1 through 11 months with a clinical diagnosis of gastroesophageal reflux disease. Dig Dis Sci. 2011;56:425–34.

146. Ward RM, Tammara B, Sullivan SE, Stewart DL, Rath N, Meng X, et al. Single-dose, multiple-dose, and population pharmacokinetics of pantoprazole in neonates and preterm infants with a clinical diagnosis of gastroesophageal reflux disease (GERD). Eur J Clin Pharmacol. 2010;66:555–61.

147. Springer M, Atkinson S, North J, Raanan M. Safety and pharmacodynamics of lansoprazole in patients with gas-troesophageal reflux disease aged < 1 year. Paediatr Drugs. 2008;10:255–63.

148. Ponrouch MP, Sautou-Miranda V, Boyer A, Bourdeaux D, Montagner A, Chopineau J. Proton pump inhibitor administration via nasogastric tube in pediatric practice: comparative analysis with protocol optimization. Int J Pharm. 2010;390:160–4.

149. Baker R, Tsou VM, Tung J, Baker SS, Li H, Wang W, et al. Clinical results from a randomized, double-blind, dose-ranging study of pantoprazole in children aged 1 through 5 years with symptomatic histologic or erosive esophagitis. Clin Pediatr (Phila). 2010;49:852–65.

150. Higginbotham TW. Effectiveness and safety of proton pump inhibitors in infantile gastroesophageal reflux disease. Ann Pharmacother. 2010;44:572–6.

151. Lee JH, Kim MJ, Lee JS, Choe YH. The effects of three alternative treatment strategies after 8 weeks of proton pump inhibitor therapy for GERD in children. Arch Dis Child. 2011;96:9–13.

152. Terrin G, Canani RB, Passariello A, Caoci S, De Curtis M. Inhibitors of gastric acid secretion drugs increase neonatal morbidity and mortality. J Matern Fetal Neonatal Med. 2012;25 Suppl 4:85–7.

153. Tjon JA, Pe M, Soscia J, Mahant S. Efficacy and safety of proton pump inhibitors in the management of pediatric gastroesophageal reflux disease. Pharmacotherapy. 2013 (in press).

154. Tolia V, Youssef NN, Gilger MA, Traxler B, Illueca M. Esomeprazole for the treatment of erosive esophagitis in children: an international, multicenter, randomized, parallel-group, double-blind (for dose) study. BMC Pediatr. 2010;10:41.

155. Ummarino D, Miele E, Masi P, Tramontano A, Staiano A, Vandenplas Y. Impact of antisecretory treatment on respiratory symptoms of gastroesophageal reflux disease in children. Dis Esophagus. 2012;25:671–7.

156. van der Pol RJ, Smits MJ, van Wijk MP, Omari TI, Tabbers MM, Benninga MA. Efficacy of proton-pump inhibitors in children with gastroesophageal reflux disease: a systematic review. Pediatrics 2011;127:925–35.

157. Wheatley E, Kennedy KA. Cross-over trial of treatment for bradycardia attributed to gastroesophageal reflux in preterm infants. J Pediatr. 2009;155:516–21.

158. Winter H, Kum-Nji P, Mahomedy SH, Kierkus J, Hinz M, Li H, et al. Efficacy and safety of pantoprazole delayed-release granules for oral suspension in a placebo-controlled treatment-withdrawal study in infants 1–11 months old with symptomatic GERD. J Pediatr Gastroenterol Nutr. 2010;50:609–18.

159. Gilger MA, Tolia V, Vandenplas Y, Youssef NN, Traxler B, Illueca M. Safety and tolerability of esomeprazole in children with gastroesophageal reflux disease. J Pediatr Gastroenterol Nutr. 2008;46:524–33.

160. Gold BD, Gunasekaran T, Tolia V, Wetzler G, Conter H, Traxler B, Illueca M. Safety and symptom improvement with esomeprazole in adolescents with gastroesophageal reflux disease. J Pediatr Gastroenterol Nutr. 2007;45:520–9.

161. Shashidhar H, Tolia V. Esophagitis in children: an update on current pharmacotherapy. Expert Opin Pharmacother. 2013;14:2475–87.

162. Hudson B, Alderton A, Doocey C, Nicholson D, Toop L, Day AS. Crying and spilling–time to stop the overmedicalisation of normal infant behaviour. N Z Med J. 2012;125:119–26.

163. Golski CA, Rome ES, Martin RJ, Frank SH, Worley S, Sun Z, Hibbs AM. Pediatric specialists' beliefs about gastroesophageal reflux disease in premature infants. Pediatrics. 2010;125:96–104.

164. Barney CK, Baer VL, Scoffield SH, Lambert DK, Cook M, Christensen RD. Lansoprazole, ranitidine, and metoclopramide: comparison of practice patterns at 4 level III NICUs within one healthcare system. Adv Neonatal Care. 2009;9:129–31.

165. Williams C, McColl KE. Review article: proton pump inhibitors and bacterial overgrowth. Aliment Pharmacol Ther. 2006;23:3–10.

166. Canani RB, Cirillo P, Roggero P, Romano C, Malamisura B, Terrin G, et al. Therapy with gastric acidity inhibitors increases the risk of acute gastroenteritis and community-acquired pneumonia in children. Pediatrics. 2006;117:e817–20.

167. Garcia Rodriguez LA, Ruigomez A, Panes J. Use of acid-suppressing drugs and the risk of bacterial gastroenteritis. Clin Gastroenterol Hepatol. 2007;5:1418–23.

168. Dial S, Delaney JA, Barkun AN, Suissa S. Use of gastric acid-suppressive agents and the risk of community-acquired Clostridium difficile-associated disease. JAMA. 2005;294:2989–95.

169. Schutze GE, Willoughby RE, Committee on Infectious Diseases; American Academy of Pediatrics. Clostridium difficile infection in infants and children. Pediatrics. 2013;131:196–200.

170. Giuliano C, Wilhelm SM, Kale-Pradhan PB. Are proton pump inhibitors associated with the development of community-acquired pneumonia? A meta-analysis. Expert Rev Clin Pharmacol. 2012;5:337–44.

171. Danziger J, William JH, Scott DJ, Lee J, Lehman LW, Mark RG, et al. Proton-pump inhibitor use is associated with low serum magnesium concentrations. Kidney Int. 2013;83:692–9.

172. Targownik LE, Leslie WD, Davison KS, Goltzman D, Jamal SA, Kreiger N, CaMos Research Group, et al. The relationship between proton pump inhibitor use and longitudinal change in bone mineral density: a population-based study from the Canadian Multicentre Osteoporosis Study (CaMos). Am J Gastroenterol. 2012;107:1361–9.

173. Untersmayr E, Bakos N, Schöll I, Kundi M, Roth-Walter F, Szalai K, et al. Anti-ulcer drugs promote IgE formation toward dietary antigens in adult patients. FASEB J. 2005;19:656–8.

174. Untersmayr E, Jensen-Jarolim E. The role of protein digestibility and antacids on food allergy outcomes. J Allergy Clin Immunol. 2008;121:1301–8.

175. Trikha A, Baillargeon JG, Kuo YF, Tan A, Pierson K, Sharma G, et al. Development of food allergies in patients with gastroesophageal reflux disease treated with gastric acid suppressive medications. Pediatr Allergy Immunol. 2013;24:582–8.

176. Andersen AB, Erichsen R, Farkas DK, Mehnert F, Ehrenstein V, Sørensen HT. Prenatal exposure to acid-suppressive drugs and the risk of childhood asthma: a population-based Danish cohort study. Aliment Pharmacol Ther. 2012;35:1190–8.

177. Lasser MS, Liao JG, Burd RS. National trends in the use of antireflux procedures for children. Pediatrics 2006;118:1828–35.

178. McAteer J, Larison C, Lariviere C, Garrison MM, Goldin AB. Antireflux procedures for gastroesophageal reflux disease in children: influence of patient age on surgical management. JAMA Surg. 2013 (in press).

179. Smits MJ, Loots CM, Benninga MA, Omari TI, van Wijk MP. New insights in gastroesophageal reflux, esophageal function and gastric emptying in relation to dysphagia before and after antireflux surgery in children. Curr Gastroenterol Rep. 2013;15:351.

180. Spechler SJ, Lee E, Ahnen D, Goyal RK, Hirano I, Ramirez F, et al. Long-term outcome of medical and surgical therapies for gastroesophageal reflux disease: follow-up of a randomized controlled trial. JAMA. 2001;285:2331–8.

181. Wijnhoven BP, Lally CJ, Kelly JJ, Myers JC, Watson DI. Use of antireflux medication after antireflux surgery. J Gastrointest Surg. 2008;12:510–7.

182. Loots CM, van Herwaarden MY, Benninga MA, VanderZee DC, van Wijk MP, Omari TI. Gastroesophageal reflux, esophageal function, gastric emptying, and the relationship to dysphagia before and after antireflux surgery in children. J Pediatr. 2013;162:566–73.

183. Esposito C, De Luca C, Alicchio F, Giurin I, Miele E, Staiano AM, Settimi A. Long-term outcome of laparoscopic Nissen procedure in pediatric patients with gastroesophageal reflux disease measured using the modified QPSG Roma III European Society for Pediatric Gastroenterology Hepatology and Nutrition's questionnaire. J Laparoendosc Adv Surg Tech A. 2012;22:937–40.

184. Granero Cendón R, Ruiz Hierro C, Garrido Pérez JI, Vargas Cruz V, Lasso Betancor CE, Paredes Esteban RM. Evaluation of quality of life in patients operated on for gastroesophageal reflux in the pediatric age. Cir Pediatr. 2012;25:82–6.

185. Mauritz FA, van Herwaarden-Lindeboom MY, Stomp W, Zwaveling S, Fischer K, Houwen RH, et al. The effects and efficacy of antireflux surgery in children with gastroesophageal reflux disease: a systematic review. J Gastrointest Surg. 2011;15:1872–8.

186. Lopez-Fernandez S, Hernandez F, Hernandez-Martin S, Dominguez E, Ortiz R, Torre CD, et al. Failed Nissen fundoplication in children: causes and management. Eur J Pediatr Surg. 2013 (Epub ahead of print).

187. Hambraeus M, Arnbjörnsson E, Anderberg M. A literature review of the outcomes after robot-assisted laparoscopic and conventional laparoscopic Nissen fundoplication for gastro-esophageal reflux disease in children. Int J Med Robot. 2013 (in press).

188. Hill SJ, Wulkan ML. Cardiaplication as a novel antireflux procedure for infants: a proof of concept in an infant porcine model. J Laparoendosc Adv Surg Tech A. 2013;23:74–7.

189. Thomson M, Antao B, Hall S, Afzal N, Hurlstone P, Swain CP, Fritscher-Ravens A. Medium-term outcome of endoluminal gastroplication with the EndoCinch device in children. J Pediatr Gastroenterol Nutr. 2008;46:172–7.

190. Chen S, Jarboe MD, Teitelbaum DH. Effectiveness of a transluminal endoscopic fundoplication for the treatment of pediatric gastroesophageal reflux disease. Pediatr Surg Int. 2012;28:229–34.

Esophageal Achalasia

Efstratios Saliakellis, Keith J. Lindley and Osvaldo Borrelli

Introduction

Achalasia literally denotes the inability to relax (from the Greek words α- "not," χάλασις "relaxation"). Sir Thomas Willis first described the classical symptomatology of achalasia in a patient with dysphagia to liquid food in 1672 [1]. He treated this individual by dilating the esophagus using a sponge attached to the tip of a whalebone. The term achalasia was first introduced in 1924 by Hurst in an attempt to describe the inability of the lower esophageal sphincter (LES) to relax in affected individuals [2]. Despite the lack of a clear explanation of the etiopathogenesis of the disease, an effective surgical treatment was proposed by Heller in 1913 [3].

Esophageal achalasia is a primary motility disorder of the esophagus. It is clinically characterized by various degrees of dysphagia to solids and liquids in the absence of other conditions that could possibly cause the same clinical symptoms (e.g., esophageal stricture, eosinophilic esophagitis). The radiological cardinal features consist of abnormal esophageal peristalsis, dilation of the esophageal body, and "bird beak" appearance at the level of the LES with concomitant delayed emptying of the contrast material from the esophagus. Endoscopically, this condition is generally characterized by esophageal dilation, presence of saliva or undigested food within the esophagus and resistance in passing the endoscope through the LES. Manometrically, this clinical entity is defined by the presence of variable impairment of esophageal peristalsis and inability of the LES to relax following swallowing [4]. Primary or idiopathic achalasia is the appropriate term to be used when there is no clear etiology for the disease, whereas in secondary achalasia the cause is by definition known [5].

Epidemiology

There are relatively limited data regarding the incidence of esophageal achalasia in children. It is however a rare disease [6] and according to two more recent studies its incidence in the pediatric population has been estimated between 0.1 and 0.3 cases annually per 100,000 children [7, 8]. This clinical entity can be encountered at any age; however, it seldom occurs in infancy as only 6% of the diagnoses have been made in this age group [9]. The peak incidence of the disease occurs between 30 and 60 years of age [10, 11]. Although there are data in adult population revealing equal gender distribution, childhood achalasia is more frequent in males than females [9]. Available data do not support any racial predilection among affected individuals [4].

Heredity

The majority of patients with achalasia are sporadic cases. Familial achalasia is less frequent [9] and is more commonly encountered among monozygotic twins and offspring of consanguineous parents. The latter may be suggestive of an autosomal recessive inheritance [12–14].

Etiopathogenesis

Despite the fact that achalasia was described more than 300 years ago, its etiopathogenesis remains largely enigmatic [15]. This condition is likely to be multifactorial in origin [5]. It has been postulated that host genetic factors, autoimmunity, and environmental influences contribute to the initiation of an inflammatory neurodegenerative process. The end result is a reduction in the number of the ganglion cells in the myenteric plexus of both esophageal body and LES [16]. During the initial stage of the disease, the neurodegenerative process affects the inhibitory neurons and their neurotransmitter nitric oxide (NO) more than the excitatory neurons and

O. Borrelli (✉) · E. Saliakellis · K. J. Lindley
Division of Neurogastroenterology and Motility, Department of Pediatric Gastroenterology, Great Ormond Street Hospital for Children, NHS Foundation Trust; UCL Institute of Child Health, 30 Guilford Street, WC1N 3JH London, UK
e-mail: osvaldo.borrelli@gosh.nhs.uk

© Springer International Publishing Switzerland 2016
S. Guandalini et al. (eds.), *Textbook of Pediatric Gastroenterology, Hepatology and Nutrition,*
DOI 10.1007/978-3-319-17169-2_11

Table 11.1 Pathologies associated with achalasia-like esophageal dysmotility

Chagas disease
Tumors (e.g., leiomyoma, Hodgkin's disease, gastric carcinoma; "pseudoachalasia")
Sarcoidosis
Hereditary cerebellar ataxia
Eosinophilic esophagitis
Hirschsprung's disease
Chronic idiopathic intestinal pseudo-obstruction
Multiple endocrine neoplasia type 2b
Miscellaneous (e.g., juvenile Sjogren's syndrome, moyamoya disease, Ondine's curse, autism)

Table 11.2 Chief complaints in childhood achalasia

Chief complaints in childhood achalasia	Frequency (%)
Regurgitation/vomiting	80
Dysphagia	76
Loss of body weight	61
Respiratory tract symptoms	44
Thoracic pain	38
Faltering growth	31
Regurgitation at nighttime	21

neurotransmitters, such as acetylcholine, resulting in both high-amplitude non-propagative contractions of the esophageal body and non-relaxing LES, which is described by the term "vigorous achalasia" [16–19]. The disease gradually progresses and cholinergic neurons are affected as well leading to "classical achalasia," which is characterized by very low amplitude esophageal body contractions or aperistalsis in addition to an inability of the LES to relax in response to deglutition [20–23]. There are data suggesting that neurodegeneration might not be limited to the esophagus only as abnormalities (Wallerian degeneration) have been also demonstrated in the vagus nerve of affected humans and experimental animal models [24, 25]. Furthermore, abnormal findings in the brainstem (Lewy bodies), prolonged gastric emptying time and disturbed response of gastric secretions to hypoglycemia have also been also reported in achalasic patients [26–28].

Despite many advances in our understanding of achalasia [29], the triggers of the neurodegeneration are poorly defined. Infections by various agents (e.g., measles, varicella-zoster virus, herpes simplex viruses type 1, 2, 6, human herpes virus 6, Epstein Barr virus, human papilloma viruses) have all been implicated in the pathogenetic process [30, 31]. However, the role of these viruses has been questioned by other authors [32, 33]. Thus, with the exception of Chagas disease caused by *Trypanosoma cruzi*, there is inadequate evidence to support a definitive causative association between infections and esophageal achalasia [34]. Autoimmunity has also been proposed as a key factor in the pathogenesis of esophageal achalasia. The latter was postulated by the identification of inflammatory cells in specimens from patients diagnosed with achalasia [20, 35, 36]. Moreover, the identification of specific human leucocyte antigen (HLA) class II histocompatibility antigens [37, 38] in combination with the presence of antimyenteric autoantibodies further strengthened the hypothesis of the autoimmunity involvement in the disease's pathophysiology. However, these finding have not been confirmed by subsequent studies [39, 40]. In conclusion, current evidence suggests that there may be an element of autoimmune predisposition to achalasia for certain individuals but the available data do not support a definition of achalasia as an autoimmune disease.

Certain reports of achalasia in siblings, monozygotic twins along with familial cases [41–44] raised the possibility of a potential genetic hereditary influence. The latter is particularly true for the cases of achalasia in the context of Allgrove syndrome in which a correlation has been identified between the esophageal dysmotility and the ALADIN gene [45, 46]. The potential genetic basis of this clinical entity is further highlighted by the association of achalasia with other diseases with proven genetic influence (Trisomy 21, Parkinson disease, Rozycki syndrome) [47–49]. Moreover, specific polymorphisms in the genes of NO synthase (NOS), vasoactive peptide (VIPR1), interleukin-23 receptor (IL-23R), interleukin-10 (IL-10) promoter, and protein tyrosine phosphatase non-receptor 22 (PTPN22) may be associated with achalasia providing additional data regarding the pathophysiology of idiopathic achalasia. However, more studies are required to further elucidate the details of the downstream responses that ultimately impair the esophageal body motility and render the LES incapable of relaxation [50–54].

In contrast to idiopathic achalasia in which the cause remains largely unknown, in secondary achalasia, the causative factor can be identified. Table 11.1 depicts certain pathologies which are associated with achalasia-like motility disorders [55–68].

Clinical Presentation

The clinical picture of achalasia depends on the duration of symptoms and the age of the child at the time of the diagnosis [69]. It has been reported that childhood achalasia is more common in males and is largely occurring in school-age children (7–12 years). However, achalasia may occur also in early infancy. Cases have been also reported in premature neonates as young as 29 weeks of gestation and as small as 900 g [70, 71]. The mean duration of symptoms prior to diagnosis was less than 3 years in 80% of the children, and the chief complaints are represented by dysphagia and emesis [9]. Table 11.2 summarizes the clinical symptoms of the children reported in the literature [72]. Noteworthily, children younger than 5 years of age present more frequently

Table 11.3 Differential diagnosis of esophageal achalasia

Gastroesophageal reflux disease
Esophageal stricture
Eosinophilic esophagitis
Asthma
Tumors (pseudoachalasia)
Rumination syndrome
Eating disorders
Chagas disease
Miscellaneous

with vomiting, whereas dysphagia is the predominant complaint in older children [69].

Dysphagia is progressive and initially confined to solids, and in later stages to both solid and liquid. The child usually reports a sensation of food getting "stuck" in the esophagus ("chest") which is usually relieved by multiple swallowing efforts or by washing the food bolus down with liquids. The troublesome deglutition leads to limited oral intake (food refusal) and subsequently in suboptimal weight gain (failure to thrive) or weight loss. As the disease progresses, the esophagus becomes dilated and the patient may experience regurgitation of undigested food or saliva that accumulates at nighttime while the child is asleep, leading also to episodes of recurrent coughing and chocking. The latter may predispose the child to a significant risk of chest infections or even sudden death due to aspiration of esophageal contents [73].

Diagnostic Approach

Diagnosis is often delayed due to several factors, including its low incidence, and the inability of younger children to report the symptoms, which are often nonspecific. Moreover, most of the related symptoms and signs, such as emesis, respiratory involvement, and failure to thrive are commonly attributed to gastroesophageal reflux (GER) disease. Therefore, a detailed history and a careful clinical examination are paramount as they can expedite the diagnostic process by guiding the physician in the correct choice of investigations which will eventually establish the diagnosis. Some individuals will have associated alacrima and adrenal insufficiency (AAA syndrome) and may have dermal hyperpigmentation secondary to high blood adrenocorticotropic hormone (ACTH) concentrations. Radiological, endoscopic, and manometric procedures represent the diagnostic arsenal and are the recommended modalities for the diagnosis of achalasia [4]. Esophageal achalasia needs to be distinguished from other conditions that present with regurgitation, vomiting, and dysphagia. Table 11.3 presents the entities that physicians should include in the differential diagnosis of esophageal achalasia [4, 63, 74–82].

Radiology

Upper gastrointestinal (GI) contrast series (esophagography/ esophagogram/barium swallow) provide a convenient way to assess the anatomy of the upper GI tract. They are usually readily available and as a result can expedite the diagnostic assessment or confirm the diagnosis in many of the suspected cases of achalasia. In spite of its undisputed usefulness, reports from adult studies showed that esophagogram can be nondiagnostic in up to one third of cases [83]. These data however were not substantiated in the pediatric population where 92 % of the studies demonstrated abnormal findings [9].

The esophagogram usually reveals various degree of esophageal body dysmotility with or without esophageal dilation, narrowing of the lumen at the level of esophagogastric junction (EGJ; "bird-beak" or "rat-tail" appearance), poor emptying of the contrast material into the stomach, and prominent tertiary contractions in the case of vigorous achalasia [9, 84–87]. (Figs. 11.1, 11.2, 11.3) Esophagography supports the diagnosis in the case of an equivocal manometry and can also demonstrate findings of end-stage achalasia (e.g., tortuosity and angulation of the esophageal body, megaesophagus) which may modify the clinical decision regarding the most appropriate therapeutic approach [4, 88–92]. Additionally, radiology can be used as an objective tool to evaluate the response to treatment (the so-called timed barium esophagogram (TBE), which measures the height of the barium column in the upright position after an ingestion of a large barium bolus) [93, 94], and as a predictor of treatment's efficacy [95–97].

Upper GI Endoscopy

Endoscopy has an important role in the diagnosis of achalasia as it rules out clinical entities that can mimic achalasia, such as eosinophilic esophagitis and other causes of pseudoachalasia. It can also alter the initial working diagnosis for patients erroneously treated for GER [4, 98, 99]. The major endoscopic findings raising a high index of suspicion for achalasia include esophageal dilation, presence of retained saliva or food along with resistance while negotiating the LES. Mucosal abnormalities detected during endoscopic examination may be due to food stasis and candida infections. However, it is not unusual to witness an unremarkable upper GI endoscopy in the early stages of the disease [4].

Of significant note, an increased number of eosinophils has been reported in the esophageal biopsies of achalasia patients [100]. While the interplay among achalasia and esophageal eosinophilic infiltration needs to be further elucidated, it has been suggested that the latter does not represent a distinct clinical entity. Thus, the presence of esophageal eosinophils in patients complaining of dysphagia may warrant further diagnostic work-up to rule out other

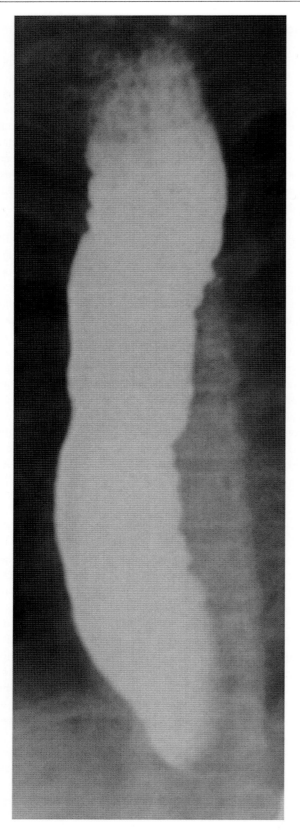

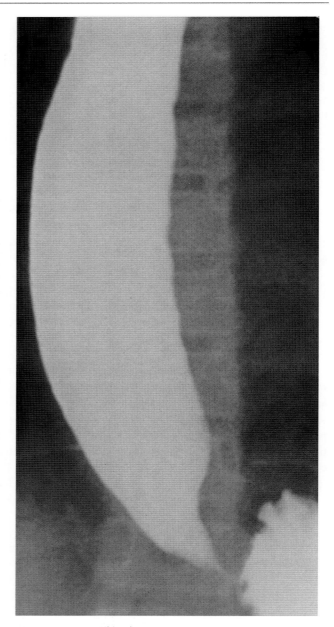

Fig. 11.2 Image of lower esophagus from barium esophagram in 11-year-old female with achalasia. The lower esophagus is dilated; there is tapered ("beak-like") narrowing of the gastroesophageal junction

potential etiologies, including achalasia [101]. High-resolution manometry (HRM) is considered an invaluable tool for discriminating these two entities as they generally have distinctive motor patterns [102–104].

Manometry

Esophageal manometry provides a highly sensitive and specific method for defining the esophageal motility

Fig. 11.1 Image of esophagus from barium esophagram in 11-year-old female with achalasia. There is food residue in the upper esophagus. The esophagus is dilated and shows numerous irregular contraction waves (tertiary contractions)

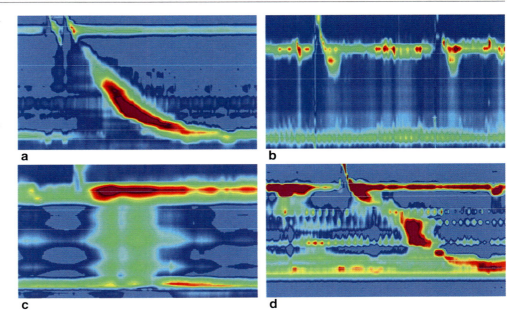

Fig. 11.3 High-resolution esophageal manometry in a healthy (**a**) and three achalasic children. Type I (**b**) is characterized by absence of distal pressurization to greater than 30 mmHg. In type II (**c**), pressurization to greater than 30 mmHg occurs in at least two of ten test swallows, whereas patients with type III (**d**) disease have spastic contractions with or without periods of compartmentalized pressurization

pattern [105]. This is especially true for the combined high-resolution esophageal impedance manometry [106]. Pediatric patients are assessed with a standardized protocol that involves single and multiple rapid wet swallows and solid swallows [104]. The esophageal motor abnormalities found in patients with achalasia are classified in the three subtypes of achalasia according to recently introduced Chicago classification [107]. All three subtypes are characterized by elevated integrated relaxation pressure (IRP—a variable which quantifies residual LES pressure): type I is defined by completely failed esophageal body peristalsis (Fig. 11.3b), in type II there is abnormal peristalsis accompanied by panesophageal pressurization in more than 20 % of the test swallows (Fig. 11.3c), and type III also demonstrates an impaired contractile pattern with fragmental preservation of distal peristalsis or presence of premature (spastic) contractions in more than 20 % of the swallows (Fig. 11.3d) [107]. The recently published results of the "European achalasia trial" demonstrated that HRM may facilitate clinical decision regarding the most appropriate initial treatment according to the manometric subtype [108]. The importance of HRM is highlighted by the fact that it can detect subtle changes in the esophageal motility dynamics and thereby aid in adding an organic element to conditions presenting with dysphagia and previously described as functional in nature [109]. Furthermore, some data suggest that intraoperative HRM along with the novel imaging tool "EndoFLIP" are safe and useful techniques in determining the adequacy of Heller's myotomy, and therefore decreasing potential future recurrence of symptoms [110–113].

Lastly, dysfunction of the upper esophageal sphincter (UES), such as an increased resting pressure, shorter relaxation after swallowing, and shorter interval to pharyngeal contractions after UES relaxation, has been demonstrated in achalasia patients. The clinical significance of such findings is still not well understood [114, 115].

Management

The therapeutic management of achalasia includes pharmacological, interventional, and surgical options. None are curative but they aim in providing symptomatic relief of the EGJ obstruction without addressing the esophageal body dysmotility. However, there is some evidence suggesting potential improvement of the esophageal motility after surgical treatment for achalasia [116]. A simplified management approach is reported in Fig. 11.4.

Pharmacological Therapy

Oral pharmacological treatment is the least effective in managing achalasia [117]. Isosorbide dinitrate and nifedipine act by relaxing the smooth muscles and by blocking the calcium channels, respectively; both reduce the LES pressure [118, 119]. They are administered prior to meals and are considered a temporary measure until a more definitive treatment, either dilatation or surgery, is provided. Oral pharmacotherapy alone is recommended in adult patients who are not willing or eligible for dilatation or surgery and in whom endoscopic botulinum toxin injection (EBTI) has previously failed [4].

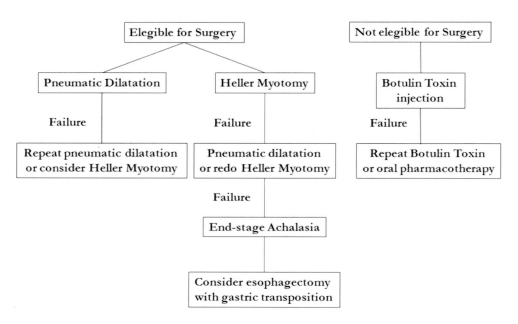

Fig. 11.4 Suggested therapeutic algorithm for children with achalasia

Endoscopic Botulinum Toxin Injection

Intrasphincteric botulinum toxin injection blocks the presynaptic cholinergic terminals in the LES and therefore inhibits the secretion of acetylcholine at the neuromuscular junction. The latter results in chemical denervation with consequent opposition of the excitatory effect of acetylcholine and disruption of the relentless contraction of LES [4]. The experience of EBTI in the treatment of childhood achalasia is relatively limited. The method involves the endoscopic injection of 25 units of botulinum toxin in each one of the four LES quadrants (100 units in total) [69]. Similar to pharmacotherapy, EBTI offers a short-term symptom relief, as pneumatic dilatation (PD) or Heller myotomy (HM) will be eventually required for a more sustained clinical improvement [120, 121]

Pneumatic Dilatation

The goal of performing a forceful esophageal dilatation is to stretch and disrupt the LES fibers to such an extent that it alleviates EGJ obstruction without inducing GER [4, 122]. The procedure is performed under general anesthesia, and patients undergoing dilatation need to be eligible for surgery in the unfortunate event of esophageal perforation [4]. A balloon dilator is inserted with fluoroscopic or endoscopic guidance [67, 123]. The non-radiopaque polyethylene balloon dilators are preferred over the bougienage or the standard balloon dilators as the latter are not effective enough in rupturing the LES fibers and achieving

adequate symptoms' control. The modern dilators are of graded size (3.0, 3.5, 4.0 cm); however, for technical reasons PD is usually performed only in children older than 6 years of age or those weighing over 20 kg [4, 67]. After the correct position is confirmed, the balloon is distended for 60 s with pressures that vary among institutions from 2–12 psi [67, 123]. Balloon distention until obliteration of its waist while under fluoroscopy is more important for achieving symptom control than balloon distention time [4]. It is advisable that all patients are observed for a certain period of time prior to discharge home, and if symptomatic, they need to be assessed with a gastrografin esophagogram to exclude potential esophageal perforation. The incidence of esophageal perforation in adults who underwent PD for achalasia was reported between 4–12% [123]. No cases of post-PD esophageal perforations were documented in recent pediatric studies [67, 123–125]. Small asymptomatic perforations are managed conservatively (intravenous antibiotics, total parenteral nutrition) whereas immediate surgical intervention is mandated for free perforations [126, 127]. The majority of perforations occur during the first dilatation most probably due to inaccurate placement and distention of the dilator; GER has been reported in 15–35% of the patients who underwent dilatation for achalasia treatment [73, 128]. The latter is of important significance as recurrence of symptoms in post-PD patients may be due to reflux-related distal esophageal stricture. Thus, treatment with proton pump inhibitors (PPI) is warranted in post-PD patients complaining of GER symptoms. Other potential post-PD complications include aspiration pneumonia and pain that may require prolonged hospitalization [124].

PD achieves adequate control of symptoms ranging from 67% after the first dilatation to 87.5% after subsequent procedures [67, 123]. Available data suggest that although PD achieves immediate symptom relief, it bears a significant likelihood of symptoms' recurrence that will require subsequent interventions in the form of either repeat PD or surgery [69, 124, 125, 129]. It is worth mentioning that minimally invasive surgical techniques have challenged the role of PD as the first-line treatment in childhood achalasia, and the recently published data question the efficacy of PD as HM was proven to be significantly superior to dilatation [69, 124, 125, 130].

Surgery

The mainstay of surgical treatment for achalasia is Heller's myotomy, which was first described in 1913 [131]. Over the past decades, HM has evolved from the open thoracotomy to the minimally invasive laparoscopic technique, which has become the procedure of choice among surgeons due to its high efficacy, faster recovery, and minimum morbidity rate [124, 129, 130, 132]. The resolution of symptoms after HM largely depends on the length of the myotomy; this should be long enough to diminish the EGJ obstruction but not excessively long so that it induces postoperative GER. The optimal length of HM in children of different age groups has not been established yet. A recent report advocates an incision length between 4–6 cm that ends 5 mm distally to EGJ along with minimal mobilization of the adjacent anatomical structures [133]. The role of both "EndoFLIP" and intraoperative manometry appears to be very promising in determining the optimal myotomy length [110–113].

The addition of a fundoplication after HM and also the type of the anti-reflux procedure are still a matter of debate. An anti-reflux procedure reduces the risk of postoperative GER but at the same time increases the likelihood of dysphagia, as it creates a high pressure zone to an esophageal body with an already impaired motility [134–136]. An anti-reflux procedure may be warranted when a wide mobilization of the esophagus is inevitable in order to technically facilitate the myotomy [133]. Regarding the most appropriate type of the anti-reflux procedure there are data revealing that a loose Nissen, Toupet, Dor, or Thal fundoplication along with HM fundoplication are safe and result in good outcomes in the treatment of childhood achalasia [90, 125, 130, 137, 138]. The American College of Gastroenterology advocates PPI treatment in achalasia adult patients complaining of heartburn post-HM in spite of the presence of a fundoplication [4].

Patients who have developed "end-stage" achalasia and failed myotomy are candidates for esophagectomy with gastric transposition [4, 90, 124, 125]. However, esophagectomy bears greater morbidity and mortality compared to laparoscopic HM; dysphagia requiring PD can still recur up to 50% of the adult patients that underwent esophagectomy for "end-stage" achalasia [139].

Emerging Treatments

POEM is an acronym for "peroral esophageal myotomy": it is a novel technique developed in Japan [140, 141], whereby the endoscopist performs an LES myotomy by creating a submucosal tunnel using a forward-viewing endoscope. The overall success in adult studies has been more than 80% at 12-month follow-up [141]. There are limited data regarding the applicability, safety, and efficacy of this method in childhood achalasia. Experience from a case report and a small case series reveals excellent outcomes regarding its safety and efficacy at 12-month follow-up assessment [142, 143].

Other techniques for treating achalasia such as removable self-expanding metallic stents offer promising results; however, there is a paucity of studies in children to evaluate the safety and efficacy of these modalities [144, 145].

Follow-Up and Surveillance

Currently, there is a lack of consensus regarding the optimal short- and long-term follow-up of children treated for esophageal achalasia. It is however advisable that pediatric patients receive regular follow-up assessment to ensure reduction of symptom severity (Eckardt score) [146]; evaluation of the esophageal emptying with a barium esophagogram may be also considered [4].

Patients treated for achalasia have a normal life expectancy [147]. Despite an increased risk of esophageal carcinoma in patients with achalasia [148, 149], there are limited data to support regular screening for cancer. Thus, the American College of Gastroenterology and the American Society for Gastrointestinal Endoscopy do not advocate routine endoscopic surveillance for achalasia patients [4, 150]. Nevertheless, radiological or endoscopic surveillance is recommended by numerous authorities for the assessment of adult patients treated for achalasia as they are in an increased risk for developing end-stage disease with megaesophagus. This approach with regular evaluation in 3-year intervals is particularly proposed if the disease has been diagnosed for more than 10 to 15 years [151]. Clearly, more data are required for the implementation of such recommendations in childhood achalasia.

Conclusion

Childhood esophageal achalasia is an enigmatic disease. Contemporary diagnostic modalities (upper GI contrast series, endoscopy, HRM) offer rapid and accurate diagnosis.

Current data suggest that laparoscopic HM combined or not with an anti-reflux procedure seems to be the therapeutic procedure that offers the most durable and sustained long-term symptom relief.

References

1. Willis T. Pharmaceutice rationalis sive diatriba do medicamentorum operationibus in humano corpore. London: Hagae Comitis; 1674.
2. Hurst AF, Rowlands RP. Case of achalasia of the cardia relieved by operation. Proc R Soc Med. 1924;17:45–6.
3. Kun L, Herbella FA, Dubecz A. 1913: annus mirabilis of esophageal surgery. Thorac Cardiovasc Surg. 2013;61:460–3.
4. Vaezi MF, Pandolfino JE, Vela MF. ACG clinical guideline: diagnosis and management of achalasia. Am J Gastroenterol. 2013;108:1238–49, quiz 50.
5. Ghoshal UC, Daschakraborty SB, Singh R. Pathogenesis of achalasia cardia. World J Gastroenterol. 2012;18:3050–7.
6. Azizkhan RG, Tapper D, Eraklis A. Achalasia in childhood: a 20-year experience. J Pediatr Surg. 1980;15:452–6.
7. Mayberry JF, Mayell MJ. Epidemiological study of achalasia in children. Gut. 1988;29:90–3.
8. Marlais M, Fishman JR, Fell JM, et al. UK incidence of achalasia: an 11-year national epidemiological study. Arch Dis Child. 2011;96:192–4.
9. Myers NA, Jolley SG, Taylor R. Achalasia of the cardia in children: a worldwide survey. J Pediatr Surg. 1994;29:1375–9.
10. Vaezi MF, Richter JE. Diagnosis and management of achalasia. American college of gastroenterology practice parameter committee. Am J Gastroenterol. 1999;94:3406–12.
11. Francis DL, Katzka DA. Achalasia: update on the disease and its treatment. Gastroenterology. 2010;139:369–74.
12. Dayalan N, Chettur L, Ramakrishnan MS. Achalasia of the cardia in sibs. Arch Dis Child. 1972;47:115–8.
13. Hernandez A, Reynoso MC, Soto F, et al. Achalasia microcephaly syndrome in a patient with consanguineous parents: support for a.m. being a distinct autosomal recessive condition. Clin Genet. 1989;36:456–8.
14. Mayberry JF, Atkinson M. A study of swallowing difficulties in first degree relatives of patients with achalasia. Thorax. 1985;40:391–3.
15. Bohl J, Gockel I, Sultanov F, et al. Childhood achalasia: a separate entity? Z Gastroenterol. 2007;45:1273–80.
16. Park W, Vaezi MF. Etiology and pathogenesis of achalasia: the current understanding. Am J Gastroenterol. 2005;100:1404–14.
17. Crist J, Gidda JS, Goyal RK. Intramural mechanism of esophageal peristalsis: roles of cholinergic and noncholinergic nerves. Proc Natl Acad Sci U S A. 1984;81:3595–9.
18. Sivarao DV, Mashimo HL, Thatte HS, et al. Lower esophageal sphincter is achalasic in nNOS(−/−) and hypotensive in W/W(v) mutant mice. Gastroenterology. 2001;121:34–42.
19. Goyal RK, Chaudhury A. Physiology of normal esophageal motility. J Clin Gastroenterol. 2008;42:610–9.
20. Goldblum JR, Rice TW, Richter JE. Histopathologic features in esophagomyotomy specimens from patients with achalasia. Gastroenterology. 1996;111:648–54.
21. Csendes A, Smok G, Braghetto I, et al. Gastroesophageal sphincter pressure and histological changes in distal esophagus in patients with achalasia of the esophagus. Dig Dis Sci. 1985;30:941–5.
22. Csendes A, Smok G, Braghetto I, et al. Histological studies of Auerbach's plexuses of the oesophagus, stomach, jejunum, and colon in patients with achalasia of the oesophagus: correlation with gastric acid secretion, presence of parietal cells and gastric emptying of solids. Gut. 1992;33:150–4.
23. Wattchow DA, Costa M. Distribution of peptide-containing nerve fibres in achalasia of the oesophagus. J Gastroenterol Hepatol. 1996;11:478–85.
24. Cassella RR, Brown AL Jr, Sayre GP, et al. Achalasia of the esophagus: pathologic and etiologic considerations. Ann Surg. 1964;160:474–87.
25. Khajanchee YS, VanAndel R, Jobe BA, et al. Electrical stimulation of the vagus nerve restores motility in an animal model of achalasia. J Gastrointest Surg. 2003;7:843–9, discussion 9.
26. Qualman SJ, Haupt HM, Yang P, et al. Esophageal Lewy bodies associated with ganglion cell loss in achalasia. Similarity to Parkinson's disease. Gastroenterology. 1984;87:848–56.
27. Eckardt VF, Krause J, Bolle D. Gastrointestinal transit and gastric acid secretion in patients with achalasia. Dig Dis Sci. 1989;34:665–71.
28. Atkinson M, Ogilvie AL, Robertson CS, et al. Vagal function in achalasia of the cardia. Q J Med. 1987;63:297–303.
29. Kahrilas PJ, Boeckxstaens G. The spectrum of achalasia: lessons from studies of pathophysiology and high-resolution manometry. Gastroenterology. 2013;145:954–65.
30. Jones DB, Mayberry JF, Rhodes J, et al. Preliminary report of an association between measles virus and achalasia. J Clin Pathol. 1983;36:655–7.
31. Robertson CS, Martin BA, Atkinson M. Varicella-zoster virus DNA in the oesophageal myenteric plexus in achalasia. Gut. 1993;34:299–302.
32. Niwamoto H, Okamoto E, Fujimoto J, et al. Are human herpes viruses or measles virus associated with esophageal achalasia? Dig Dis Sci. 1995;40:859–64.
33. Birgisson S, Galinski MS, Goldblum JR, et al. Achalasia is not associated with measles or known herpes and human papilloma viruses. Dig Dis Sci. 1997;42:300–6.
34. Dantas RO, Alves LM, Nascimento WV. Effect of bolus volume on proximal esophageal contractions of patients with Chagas' disease and patients with idiopathic achalasia. Dis Esophagus. 2010;23:670–4.
35. Clark SB, Rice TW, Tubbs RR, et al. The nature of the myenteric infiltrate in achalasia: an immunohistochemical analysis. Am J Surg Pathol. 2000;24:1153–8.
36. Raymond L, Lach B, Shamji FM. Inflammatory aetiology of primary oesophageal achalasia: an immunohistochemical and ultrastructural study of Auerbach's plexus. Histopathology. 1999;35:445–53.
37. Verne GN, Hahn AB, Pineau BC, et al. Association of HLA-DR and -DQ alleles with idiopathic achalasia. Gastroenterology. 1999;117:26–31.
38. Wong RK, Maydonovitch CL, Metz SJ, et al. Significant DQw1 association in achalasia. Dig Dis Sci. 1989;34:349–52.
39. Latiano A, De Giorgio R, Volta U, et al. HLA and enteric anti-neuronal antibodies in patients with achalasia. Neurogastroenterol Motil. 2006;18:520–5.
40. Goin JC, Sterin-Borda L, Bilder CR, et al. Functional implications of circulating muscarinic cholinergic receptor autoantibodies in chagasic patients with achalasia. Gastroenterology. 1999;117:798–805.
41. Zilberstein B, de Cleva R, Gabriel AG, et al. Congenital achalasia: facts and fantasies. Dis Esophagus. 2005;18:335–7.
42. Rao PS, Vijaykumar Rao PL. Achalasia in siblings in infancy. Indian J Pediatr. 2001;68:887–8.
43. Senocak ME, Hicsonmez A, Buyukpamukcu N. Familial childhood achalasia. Z Kinderchir. 1990;45:111–3.
44. Tryhus MR, Davis M, Griffith JK, et al. Familial achalasia in two siblings: significance of possible hereditary role. J Pediatr Surg. 1989;24:292–5.

45. Di Nardo G, Tullio-Pelet A, Annese V, et al. Idiopathic achalasia is not allelic to alacrima achalasia adrenal insufficiency syndrome at the ALADIN locus. Dig Liver Dis. 2005;37:312–5.

46. Jung KW, Yoon IJ, Kim do H, et al. Genetic evaluation of ALADIN gene in early-onset achalasia and alacrima patients. J Neurogastroenterol Motil. 2011;17:169–73.

47. Nihoul-Fekete C, Bawab F, Lortat-Jacob S, et al. Achalasia of the esophagus in childhood. Surgical treatment in 35 cases, with special reference to familial cases and glucocorticoid deficiency association. Hepatogastroenterol. 1991;38:510–3.

48. Johnston BT, Colcher A, Li Q, et al. Repetitive proximal esophageal contractions: a new manometric finding and a possible further link between Parkinson's disease and achalasia. Dysphagia. 2001;16:186–9.

49. Okawada M, Okazaki T, Yamataka A, et al. Down's syndrome and esophageal achalasia: a rare but important clinical entity. Pediatr Surg Int. 2005;21:997–1000.

50. De Giorgio R, Di Simone MP, Stanghellini V, et al. Esophageal and gastric nitric oxide synthesizing innervation in primary achalasia. Am J Gastroenterol. 1999;94:2357–62.

51. de Leon AR, de la Serna JP, Santiago JL, et al. Association between idiopathic achalasia and IL23R gene. Neurogastroenterol Motil. 2010;22:734–8, e218.

52. Nunez C, Garcia-Gonzalez MA, Santiago JL, et al. Association of IL10 promoter polymorphisms with idiopathic achalasia. Hum Immunol. 2011;72:749–52.

53. Santiago JL, Martinez A, Benito MS, et al. Gender-specific association of the PTPN22 C1858T polymorphism with achalasia. Hum Immunol. 2007;68:867–70.

54. Paladini F, Cocco E, Cascino I, et al. Age-dependent association of idiopathic achalasia with vasoactive intestinal peptide receptor 1 gene. Neurogastroenterol Motil. 2009;21:597–602.

55. Gupta V, Lal A, Sinha SK, et al. Leiomyomatosis of the esophagus: experience over a decade. J Gastrointest Surg. 2009;13:206–11.

56. Gockel I, Eckardt VF, Schmitt T, et al. Pseudoachalasia: a case series and analysis of the literature. Scand J Gastroenterol. 2005;40:378–85.

57. Herbella FA, Oliveira DR, Del Grande JC. Are idiopathic and chagasic achalasia two different diseases? Dig Dis Sci. 2004;49:353–60.

58. Lukens FJ, Machicao VI, Woodward TA, et al. Esophageal sarcoidosis: an unusual diagnosis. J Clin Gastroenterol. 2002;34:54–6.

59. Kelly JL, Mulcahy TM, O'Riordain DS, et al. Coexistent Hirschsprung's disease and esophageal achalasia in male siblings. J Pediatr Surg. 1997;32:1809–11.

60. Taketomi T, Yoshiga D, Taniguchi K, et al. Loss of mammalian Sprouty2 leads to enteric neuronal hyperplasia and esophageal achalasia. Nat Neurosci. 2005;8:855–7.

61. Assor P, Negreanu L, Picon L, et al. Slowly regressing acute pandysautonomia associated with esophageal achalasia: a case report. Gastroenterol Clin Biol. 2008;32:46–50.

62. Murphy MS, Gardner-Medwin D, Eastham EJ. Achalasia of the cardia associated with hereditary cerebellar ataxia. Am J Gastroenterol. 1989;84:1329–30.

63. Buyukpamukcu M, Buyukpamukcu N, Cevik N. Achalasia of the oesophagus associated with Hodgkin's disease in children. Clin Oncol. 1982;8:73–6.

64. Ghosh P, Linder J, Gallagher TF, et al. Achalasia of the cardia and multiple endocrine neoplasia 2B. Am J Gastroenterol. 1994;89:1880–3.

65. Mandaliya R, DiMarino AJ, Cohen S. Association of achalasia and eosinophilic esophagitis. Indian J Gastroenterol. 2013;32:54–7.

66. Simila S, Kokkonen J, Kaski M. Achalasia sicca–juvenile Sjogren's syndrome with achalasia and gastric hyposecretion. Eur J Pediatr. 1978;129:175–81.

67. Jung C, Michaud L, Mougenot JF, et al. Treatments for pediatric achalasia: heller myotomy or pneumatic dilatation? Gastroenterol Clin Biol. 2010;34:202–8.

68. Betalli P, Carretto E, Cananzi M, et al. Autism and esophageal achalasia in childhood: a possible correlation? Report on three cases. Dis Esophagus. 2013;26:237–40.

69. Hussain SZ, Thomas R, Tolia V. A review of achalasia in 33 children. Dig Dis Sci. 2002;47:2538–43.

70. Shettihalli N, Venugopalan V, Ives NK, et al. Achalasia cardia in a premature infant. BMJ Case Rep. 2010. doi:10.1136/bcr.05.2010.3014.

71. Polk HC Jr, Burford TH. Disorders of the distal esophagus in infancy and childhood. Am J Dis Child. 1964;108:243–51.

72. Nurko S. Other motor disorders. In: Walker W, Durie P, Hamilton J, editors. Pediatric gastrointestinal disease, pathophysiology, diagnosis and management, vol. 1, 3rd edn. St Louis: Mosby; 2000. p. 317–50.

73. Rudolph CD, Sood MR. Achalasia and other motor disorders. In: Wyllie R, Hyams JS, Kay M, editors. Pediatric gastrointestinal and liver disease. Philadelphia: Elsevier; 2011. p. 248–54.

74. Rosseneu S, Afzal N, Yerushalmi B, et al. Topical application of mitomycin-C in oesophageal strictures. J Pediatr Gastroenterol Nutr. 2007;44:336–41.

75. Sorser SA, Barawi M, Hagglund K, et al. Eosinophilic esophagitis in children and adolescents: epidemiology, clinical presentation and seasonal variation. J Gastroenterol. 2013;48:81–5.

76. Katzka DA, Smyrk TC, Chial HJ, et al. Esophageal leiomyomatosis presenting as achalasia diagnosed by high-resolution manometry and endoscopic core biopsy. Gastrointest Endosc. 2012;76:216–7.

77. Kessing BF, Smout AJ, Bredenoord AJ. Clinical applications of esophageal impedance monitoring and high-resolution manometry. Curr Gastroenterol Rep. 2012;14:197–205.

78. MacKalski BA, Keate RF. Rumination in a patient with achalasia. Am J Gastroenterol. 1993;88:1803–4.

79. Hallal C, Kieling CO, Nunes DL, et al. Diagnosis, misdiagnosis, and associated diseases of achalasia in children and adolescents: a twelve-year single center experience. Pediatr Surg Int. 2012;28:1211–7.

80. Desseilles M, Fuchs S, Ansseau M, et al. Achalasia may mimic anorexia nervosa, compulsive eating disorder, and obesity problems. Psychosomatics. 2006;47:270–1.

81. Vicentine FP, Herbella FA, Allaix ME, et al. Comparison of idiopathic achalasia and Chagas' disease esophagopathy at the light of high-resolution manometry. Dis Esophagus. 2014;27:128–33

82. Bode CP, Schroten H, Koletzko S, et al. Transient achalasia-like esophageal motility disorder after candida esophagitis in a boy with chronic granulomatous disease. J Pediatr Gastroenterol Nutr. 1996;23:320–3.

83. Howard PJ, Maher L, Pryde A, et al. Five year prospective study of the incidence, clinical features, and diagnosis of achalasia in Edinburgh. Gut. 1992;33:1011–5.

84. Goldenberg SP, Burrell M, Fette GG, et al. Classic and vigorous achalasia: a comparison of manometric, radiographic, and clinical findings. Gastroenterology. 1991;101:743–8.

85. Camacho-Lobato L, Katz PO, Eveland J, et al. Vigorous achalasia: original description requires minor change. J Clin Gastroenterol. 2001;33:375–7.

86. Hansford BG, Mitchell MT, Gasparaitis A. Water flush technique: a noninvasive method of optimizing visualization of the distal esophagus in patients with primary achalasia. AJR Am J Roentgenol. 2013;200:818–21.

87. Levine MS, Rubesin SE, Laufer I. Barium esophagography: a study for all seasons. Clin Gastroenterol Hepatol. 2008;6:11–25.

88. Miller DL, Allen MS, Trastek VF, et al. Esophageal resection for recurrent achalasia. Ann Thorac Surg. 1995;60:922–5, discussion 5–6.

89. Devaney EJ, Lannettoni MD, Orringer MB, et al. Esophagectomy for achalasia: patient selection and clinical experience. Ann Thorac Surg. 2001;72:854–8.

90. Spitz L. Gastric transposition for esophageal substitution in children. J Pediatr Surg. 1992;27:252–7, discussion 7–9.

91. Peters JH, Kauer WK, Crookes PF, et al. Esophageal resection with colon interposition for end-stage achalasia. Arch Surg. 1995;130:632–6, discussion 6–7.

92. Orringer MB, Stirling MC. Esophageal resection for achalasia: indications and results. Ann Thorac Surg. 1989;47:340–5.

93. Gockel I, Junginger T, Eckardt VF. Effects of pneumatic dilation and myotomy on esophageal function and morphology in patients with achalasia. Am Surg. 2005;71:128–31.

94. Neyaz Z, Gupta M, Ghoshal UC. How to perform and interpret timed barium esophagogram. J Neurogastroenterol Motil. 2013;19:251–6.

95. Gheorghe C, Bancila I, Tutuian R, et al. Predictors of short term treatment outcome in patients with achalasia following endoscopic or surgical therapy. Hepatogastroenterol. 2012;59:2503–7.

96. Vaezi MF, Baker ME, Achkar E, et al. Timed barium oesophagram: better predictor of long term success after pneumatic dilation in achalasia than symptom assessment. Gut. 2002;50:765–70.

97. Andersson M, Lundell L, Kostic S, et al. Evaluation of the response to treatment in patients with idiopathic achalasia by the timed barium esophagogram: results from a randomized clinical trial. Dis Esophagus. 2009;22:264–73.

98. Pasha SF, Acosta RD, Chandrasekhara V, et al. The role of endoscopy in the evaluation and management of dysphagia. Gastrointest Endosc. 2014;79:191–201.

99. O'Neill OM, Johnston BT, Coleman HG. Achalasia: a review of clinical diagnosis, epidemiology, treatment and outcomes. World J Gastroenterol. 2013;19:5806–12.

100. Savarino E, Gemignani L, Zentilin P, et al. Achalasia with dense eosinophilic infiltrate responds to steroid therapy. Clin Gastroenterol Hepatol. 2011;9:1104–6.

101. Cools-Lartigue J, Chang SY, McKendy K, et al. Pattern of esophageal eosinophilic infiltration in patients with achalasia and response to Heller myotomy and Dor fundoplication. Dis Esophagus. 2013;26:766–75.

102. Nurko S, Rosen R. Esophageal dysmotility in patients who have eosinophilic esophagitis. Gastrointest Endosc Clin N Am. 2008;18:73–89, ix.

103. Roman S, Hirano I, Kwiatek MA, et al. Manometric features of eosinophilic esophagitis in esophageal pressure topography. Neurogastroenterol Motil. 2011;23:208–14, e111.

104. Goldani HA, Staiano A, Borrelli O, et al. Pediatric esophageal high-resolution manometry: utility of a standardized protocol and size-adjusted pressure topography parameters. Am J Gastroenterol. 2010;105:460–7.

105. Staiano A, Boccia G, Miele E, et al. Segmental characteristics of oesophageal peristalsis in paediatric patients. Neurogastroenterol Motil. 2008;20:19–26.

106. Rohof WO, Myers JC, Estremera FA, et al. Inter- and intra-rater reproducibility of automated and integrated pressure-flow analysis of esophageal pressure-impedance recordings. Neurogastroenterol Motil. 2014;26:168–75.

107. Bredenoord AJ, Fox M, Kahrilas PJ, et al. Chicago classification criteria of esophageal motility disorders defined in high resolution esophageal pressure topography. Neurogastroenterol Motil. 2012;24 Suppl 1:57–65.

108. Rohof WO, Salvador R, Annese V, et al. Outcomes of treatment for achalasia depend on manometric subtype. Gastroenterology. 2013;144:718–25, quiz e13–4.

109. Scherer JR, Kwiatek MA, Soper NJ, et al. Functional esophagogastric junction obstruction with intact peristalsis: a heterogeneous syndrome sometimes akin to achalasia. J Gastrointest Surg. 2009;13:2219–25.

110. Jafri M, Alonso M, Kaul A, et al. Intraoperative manometry during laparoscopic Heller myotomy improves outcome in pediatric achalasia. J Pediatr Surg. 2008;43:66–70, discussion.

111. Perretta S, Dallemagne B, McMahon B, et al. Video. Improving functional esophageal surgery with a "smart" bougie: endoflip. Surg Endosc. 2011;25:3109.

112. Rohof WO, Hirsch DP, Kessing BF, et al. Efficacy of treatment for patients with achalasia depends on the distensibility of the esophagogastric junction. Gastroenterology. 2012;143:328–35.

113. Rieder E, Swanstrom LL, Perretta S, et al. Intraoperative assessment of esophagogastric junction distensibility during per oral endoscopic myotomy (POEM) for esophageal motility disorders. Surg Endosc. 2013;27:400–5.

114. Yoneyama F, Miyachi M, Nimura Y. Manometric findings of the upper esophageal sphincter in esophageal achalasia. World J Surg. 1998;22:1043–6, discussion 6–7.

115. Dudnick RS, Castell JA, Castell DO. Abnormal upper esophageal sphincter function in achalasia. Am J Gastroenterol. 1992;87:1712–5.

116. Tatum RP, Wong JA, Figueredo EJ, et al. Return of esophageal function after treatment for achalasia as determined by impedance-manometry. J Gastrointest Surg. 2007;11:1403–9.

117. Vaezi MF, Richter JE. Current therapies for achalasia: comparison and efficacy. J Clin Gastroenterol. 1998;27:21–35.

118. Bortolotti M, Coccia G, Brunelli F, et al. Isosorbide dinitrate or nifedipine: which is preferable in the medical therapy of achalasia? Ital J Gastroenterol. 1994;26:379–82.

119. Maksimak M, Perlmutter DH, Winter HS. The use of nifedipine for the treatment of achalasia in children. J Pediatr Gastroenterol Nutr. 1986;5:883–6.

120. Khoshoo V, LaGarde DC, Udall JN Jr. Intrasphincteric injection of Botulinum toxin for treating achalasia in children. J Pediatr Gastroenterol Nutr. 1997;24:439–41.

121. Hurwitz M, Bahar RJ, Ament ME, et al. Evaluation of the use of botulinum toxin in children with achalasia. J Pediatr Gastroenterol Nutr. 2000;30:509–14.

122. Emami MH, Raisi M, Amini J, et al. Pneumatic balloon dilation therapy is as effective as esophagomyotomy for achalasia. Dysphagia. 2008;23:155–60.

123. Di Nardo G, Rossi P, Oliva S, et al. Pneumatic balloon dilation in pediatric achalasia: efficacy and factors predicting outcome at a single tertiary pediatric gastroenterology center. Gastrointest Endosc. 2012;76:927–32.

124. Pastor AC, Mills J, Marcon MA, et al. A single center 26-year experience with treatment of esophageal achalasia: is there an optimal method? J Pediatr Surg. 2009;44:1349–54.

125. Lee CW, Kays DW, Chen MK, et al. Outcomes of treatment of childhood achalasia. J Pediatr Surg. 2010;45:1173–7.

126. Fan Y, Song HY, Kim JH, et al. Fluoroscopically guided balloon dilation of benign esophageal strictures: incidence of esophageal rupture and its management in 589 patients. AJR Am J Roentgenol. 2011;197:1481–6.

127. Adams H, Roberts GM, Smith PM. Oesophageal tears during pneumatic balloon dilatation for the treatment of achalasia. Clin Radiol. 1989;40:53–7.

128. Miller RE, Tiszenkel HI. Esophageal perforation due to pneumatic dilation for achalasia. Surg Gynecol Obstet. 1988;166:458–60.

129. Zhang Y, Xu CD, Zaouche A, et al. Diagnosis and management of esophageal achalasia in children: analysis of 13 cases. World J Pediatr. 2009;5:56–9.

130. Askegard-Giesmann JR, Grams JM, Hanna AM, et al. Minimally invasive Heller's myotomy in children: safe and effective. J Pediatr Surg. 2009;44:909–11.

131. Heller E. Extramukose kardioplastic bein chronischen kardiospasmus mit dilitation des oesophagus. Mitt Grenzgeb Med Chir. 1914;27:141–9.

132. Ali A, Pellegrini CA. Laparoscopic myotomy: technique and efficacy in treating achalasia. Gastrointest Endosc Clin N Am. 2001;11:347–58, vii.

133. Vaos G, Demetriou L, Velaoras C, et al. Evaluating long-term results of modified Heller limited esophagomyotomy in children with esophageal achalasia. J Pediatr Surg. 2008;43:1262–9.

134. Ellis FH Jr, Crozier RE, Watkins E Jr. Operation for esophageal achalasia. Results of esophagomyotomy without an antireflux operation. J Thorac Cardiovasc Surg. 1984;88:344–51.

135. Donahue PE, Samelson S, Schlesinger PK, et al. Achalasia of the esophagus. Treatment controversies and the method of choice. Ann Surg. 1986;203:505–11.

136. Roberts KE, Duffy AJ, Bell RL. Controversies in the treatment of gastroesophageal reflux and achalasia. World J Gastroenterol. 2006;12:3155–61.

137. Illi OE, Stauffer UG. Achalasia in childhood and adolescence. Eur J Pediatr Surg. 1994;4:214–7.

138. Buick RG, Spitz L. Achalasia of the cardia in children. Br J Surg. 1985;72:341–3.

139. Molena D, Yang SC. Surgical management of end-stage achalasia. Semin Thorac Cardiovasc Surg. 2012;24:19–26.

140. Inoue H, Minami H, Kobayashi Y, et al. Peroral endoscopic myotomy (POEM) for esophageal achalasia. Endoscopy. 2010;42:265–71.

141. Von Renteln D, Fuchs KH, Fockens P, et al. Peroral endoscopic myotomy for the treatment of achalasia: an international prospective multicenter study. Gastroenterology. 2013;145:309–11, e1–3.

142. Familiari P, Marchese M, Gigante G, et al. Peroral endoscopic myotomy for the treatment of achalasia in children. J Pediatr Gastroenterol Nutr. 2013;57:794–7.

143. Maselli R, Inoue H, Misawa M, et al. Peroral endoscopic myotomy (POEM) in a 3-year-old girl with severe growth retardation, achalasia, and down syndrome. Endoscopy. 2012;44 Suppl 2:E285–7.

144. Li YD, Cheng YS, Li MH, et al. Temporary self-expanding metallic stents and pneumatic dilation for the treatment of achalasia: a prospective study with a long-term follow-up. Dis Esophagus. 2010;23:361–7.

145. Zeng Y, Dai YM, Wan XJ. Clinical remission following endoscopic placement of retrievable, fully covered metal stents in patients with esophageal achalasia. Dis Esophagus. 2014;27:103–8.

146. Eckardt VF, Aignherr C, Bernhard G. Predictors of outcome in patients with achalasia treated by pneumatic dilation. Gastroenterology. 1992;103:1732–8.

147. Eckardt VF, Hoischen T, Bernhard G. Life expectancy, complications, and causes of death in patients with achalasia: results of a 33-year follow-up investigation. Eur J Gastroenterol Hepatol. 2008;20:956–60.

148. Leeuwenburgh I, Scholten P, Alderliesten J, et al. Long-term esophageal cancer risk in patients with primary achalasia: a prospective study. Am J Gastroenterol. 2010;105:2144–9.

149. Sandler RS, Nyren O, Ekbom A, et al. The risk of esophageal cancer in patients with achalasia. A population-based study. JAMA. 1995;274:1359–62.

150. Hirota WK, Zuckerman MJ, Adler DG, et al. ASGE guideline: the role of endoscopy in the surveillance of premalignant conditions of the upper GI tract. Gastrointest Endosc. 2006;63:570–80.

151. Eckardt AJ, Eckardt VF. Editorial: cancer surveillance in achalasia: better late than never? Am J Gastroenterol. 2010;105:2150–2.

Helicobacter pylori Gastritis and Peptic Ulcer Disease

12

Iva Hojsak

Abbreviations

^{13}C-UBT	^{13}C-urea breath test
BabA	Blood antigen-binding adhesin
CagA	*Cytotoxin*-associated *gene A*
COX-1	Cyclooxygenase-1
ELISA	Enzyme-linked immunosorbent assay
ESPGHAN	European Society of Pediatric Gastroenterology, Hepatology, and Nutrition
FISH	Fluorescence in situ hybridization
H. pylori	*Helicobacter pylori*
MALT	Mucosa-associated lymphoid tissue
NASPGHAN	North American Society for Pediatric Gastroenterology Hepatology, and Nutrition
NSAIDs	Nonsteroidal anti-inflammatory drugs
PAMPs	Pathogen-associated molecular patterns
PPI	Proton pump inhibitors
PRRs	Pattern recognition receptors
VacA	Vacuolating cytotoxin A
WB	Western blot

Introduction

Helicobacter (H.) pylori is a Gram-negative, microaerophilic spiral bacterium found in the stomach. Stomach colonization causes chronic gastritis that can remain silent, due to the dynamic equilibrium between the bacterium and its human host, or evolve into more severe diseases, such as atrophic gastritis, peptic ulcer, lymphoma of the mucosa-associated lymphoid tissue (MALT), or gastric adenocarcinoma [1, 2]. Difference in the consequences of *H. pylori* infection could be at least partially explained by the high variability of colonizing *H. pylori* strains and host response to this microbe [3].

The discovery of *H. pylori* as a major cause of peptic ulcer disease had a significant impact on its perception and treatment. The importance of the discovery was awarded by the Nobel Prize in 2005 to Marshall and Warren who proved the etiological role of *H. pylori* in gastritis and peptic ulcer disease.

Children differ from adults with respect to *H. pylori* infection in terms of the prevalence of the infection, the complication rate, the near absence of gastric malignancies, age-specific problems with diagnostic tests and drugs, and a higher rate of antibiotic resistance [4].

Bacterial Pathomechanism

H. pylori prefers neutral or close to neutral pH (5.5–7.5) and the production of gastric acid in the stomach with a low pH of 1–2 severely limits luminal colonization [5]. The other very important defense barrier is formed by mucus-producing epithelial cells lining the gastric mucosa and by innate immune cells that either reside in the gastric lamina propria under steady-state conditions or are recruited there during infection [6]. All that makes a stomach a very unfriendly environment and the *H. pylori* had to find a way to survive and overcome these obstacles (Fig. 12.1). Bacteria has flagellar-based motility which allows penetration of the mucus and produces urease which splits urea to ammonium ions, thus raising the stomach pH [6]. That increase in stomach pH has further impact on the mucus layer making it viscoelastic and easier for intrusion [7]. Bacteria is found within the gastric mucus layer, either relatively close to the gastric lumen or deep within gastric glands, and can be either free or attached to gastric epithelial cells [8]. The intimate association with the gastric epithelium enables a variety of immune interactions between bacteria and the host. However, it is still not clear how the bacterium colonizes stomach niches for the decades without being eliminated by the host's innate defenses [9]. The detection of bacterial pathogen-associated molecular patterns (PAMPs) by epithelial and innate immune cells

I. Hojsak (✉)
Referral Center for Pediatric Gastroenterology and Nutrition,
Children's Hospital Zagreb, University of Zagreb School of Medicine,
Klaić eva 16, Zagreb 10000, Croatia
e-mail: ivahojsak@gmail.com

© Springer International Publishing Switzerland 2016
S. Guandalini et al. (eds.), *Textbook of Pediatric Gastroenterology, Hepatology and Nutrition*,
DOI 10.1007/978-3-319-17169-2_12

Fig. 12.1 *H. pylori*-associated factors which enable colonization and persistence [6]. Initially, *H. pylori* produces urease which raises the pH through ammonia production. Bacterial helical rod shape and flagellar-based motility help intrusion of bacteria to niche, away from acid lumen. Different variably expressed adhesins (like SabA, BabA) may shift the balance to cell-associated bacteria. Cell-associated bacteria may alter gastric epithelial cell through VacA, CagA, and CagL which all have multiple cellular targets. This includes disruption of cell polarity, induction of chemokines and/or the gastric hormone gastrin, and inhibition of acid secretion. *T4SS* Cag type IV secretion system, *PS* phosphatidylserine, *α5β1* and *αvβ5* integrin subunits, *VacA* vacuolating cytotoxin A, *CagA* cytotoxin-associated gene A protein, and *CagL* cytotoxin-associated gene L protein. (Reprinted by permission from Macmillan Publishers Ltd, Nature Publishing Group, Ref. [6])

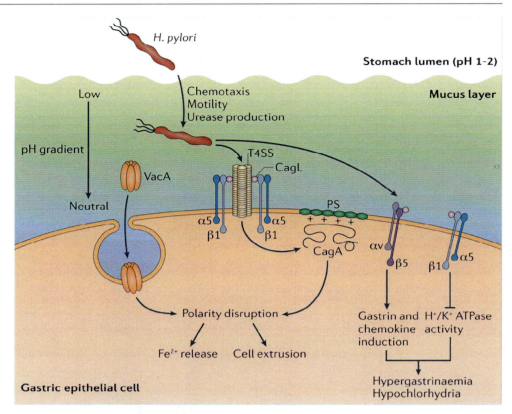

occurs via innate immune receptors (pattern recognition receptors, PRRs) [6]. *H. pylori* has evolved to avoid detection by several types of PRRs that are crucial for the recognition of other Gram-negative enteropathogens [6]. Other host factors that have impact on *H. pylori* disease severity include membrane-associated mucin and its role in the inflammatory response [10]. In addition to the host genetic susceptibility, diversity of *H. pylori* virulence factor genes may affect the ability of these bacteria to colonize, persist, or even induce severe disease [11]. Many of the changes in gastric epithelial cells caused by *H. pylori* are attributable to the actions of two secreted bacterial proteins, vacuolating cytotoxin A (VacA), and *cytotoxin-associated gene A* protein (CagA) [8]. *H. pylori* traditionally harnesses its cardinal virulence factors to downregulate T cell responses, through the VacA-mediated cell cycle arrest, and upregulates mucosal proinflammatory pathways by CagA [9]. VacA is a pore-forming toxin that is secreted by the bacteria through an autotransporter pathway. The cellular alterations caused by VacA include increased permeability of the plasma membrane, changes in endosomal structure and in mitochondrial membrane permeability, and cell death [8, 12, 13]. CagA is an effector protein that is translocated directly from bacteria into host cells through the action of a type IV secretion system [8, 14, 15]. Upon entry into gastric epithelial cells, CagA interacts with multiple intracellular target proteins and causes a wide range of

alterations in cellular signaling, leading to changes in cell shape, increased cellular motility and cellular invasiveness, alterations in monolayer polarity and permeability, and increased cellular proliferation [16, 17]. Because CagA signaling pathways have been associated with carcinogenesis, it was termed as a "bacterial oncoprotein" [8]. However, there should be some backup mechanism to maintain the above-mentioned inflammatory and apoptotic balance [18]. One virulence factor potentially involved in the pathogenesis of *H. pylori* is the blood antigen-binding adhesin (BabA) [19]. BabA adhesin adheres to gastric blood group antigens expressed on epithelial cells and mucus. The expression of specific host receptors to bacterial adhesins are likely to play a role in the outcome of the infection [18].

The interaction between bacteria and host is very complex and not fully elucidated and includes different virulence factors involved into to pathogenesis [6].

The majority of the *H. pylori*-infected population remains asymptomatic, but some individuals may develop chronic gastritis, peptic ulcer, MALT lymphoma, or carcinoma [20]. Factors determining the subset of infected individuals developing the disease compared with asymptomatic *H. pylori* carriers remain unclear. It is now becoming increasingly clear that the *H. pylori* virulence factors as well as host immune factors contribute closely to those differences in *H. pylori* pathogenicity.

Epidemiology and Transmission

Over the past decades, the prevalence of *H. pylori* in the developed world steadily decreases. Most recent international studies have shown that *H. pylori* prevalence varies between countries, with lowest prevalence of 5–10% in Western Europe and the USA and very high prevalence in developing countries of even 80% [21, 22]. An increased prevalence in developing countries is mainly due to the combined effects of poor living conditions, poor hygiene, and overcrowding [23]. In developing countries, *H. pylori* infection is acquired predominantly during early childhood; however, in the more developed areas the infection gradually increases with age with the highest incidence rate in childhood and adolescence [24, 25].

The modes of *H. pylori* transmission are still not entirely clarified, but person-to-person contact is the most commonly implicated mechanism through oral–oral, fecal–oral, or gastric–oral route [26]. It has been described that transmission primarily occurs between mothers and their offspring or between siblings [25, 27]. Currently available evidence indicate that especially in populations with low *H. pylori* prevalence the infected mother is likely to be the main source for childhood *H. pylori* infection [27]. However, only few studies have longitudinally examined factors which influence *H. pylori* transmission. In the well-designed longitudinal study, Muhsen et al. included Israeli Arab children aged 3–5 years from three villages in northern Israel which were followed-up for 3–4 years [28]. Having *H. pylori*-infected sibling was identified as an independent risk factor for both early and persistent *H. pylori* infection. It was also shown that persistent *H. pylori* infection in older siblings always precedes infection in younger siblings especially if the age difference was less than 3 years [29].

Due to very close interpersonal contact between children in day-care centers, it was proposed that their attendance could also be a risk factor [24]. However, a meta-analysis of 16 studies did not confirm this hypothesis, but included studies substantially varied in the methodology; they were performed in a different types of childcare, in different age groups, and with different exposure duration, which all resulted in a high heterogeneity in the meta-analysis [24].

There is some evidence of positive correlation between presence of *H. pylori* in the oral cavity and gastric mucosa [30]. Moreover, it seems that eradication rate is significantly higher in stomach than in oral cavity. These results suggest that infected dental plaque, saliva, or other places in the oral cavity may be a source for infection and reinfection of *H. pylori* through oral–oral route [30]. Presence of *H. pylori* in tonsils and its impact on infection transmission is still controversial [22].

Gastritis

Gastritis is defined as histologically confirmed inflammation of the gastric mucosa mainly composed of lymphocytes, plasma cells, histiocytes, and granulocytes within the lamina propria [31]. *H. pylori* is by far the most common etiological agent causing gastritis in adults and children. The most common site of infection is the antrum, which is an absorptive rather than a secretory region of the stomach enabling the slightly higher pH at which the organism can survive [5]. In the initial phase of *H. pylori* infection, the gastric mucosa becomes acutely inflamed with impairment in the acid secretion [32]. In large majority of patients, gastritis progresses to chronic active gastritis which is characterized by the presence of both mononuclear and neutrophilic ("active") inflammation [31]. In children, the "active" or neutrophilic count is lower than that reported in adults.

In adults, *H. pylori* infection causes three main gastritis types: mild pangastritis where inflammation evenly affects the whole stomach; antrum-predominant gastritis where the degree of inflammation is strongest in the antrum and acid secretion tends to be increased; and the most infrequent phenotype affecting only approximately 1% of the infected subjects' body-predominant gastritis with even atrophic changes and impaired gastric acid secretion [32]. Antrum-predominant gastritis may subsequently be complicated by duodenal ulcer while corpus-predominant atrophic gastritis increases the risk of gastric cancer [33]. Whether this distinction between gastritis types exist already in children or it develops later in life is still unknown [34].

In addition to the topographic expression of *H. pylori*-induced chronic gastritis, the characterization of gastritis needs to include report on the activity and chronicity of inflammation and on the development of atrophic changes with or without intestinal metaplasia [35].

H. pylori gastritis has unique features in children, such as the nodular aspect of the gastric antrum, antral predominance of gastritis in most patients, and uncommon diagnosis of gastric atrophy and intestinal metaplasia. Nodular gastritis is usually characterized as an endoscopic appearance which has been described as gooseflesh-like or cobblestone markings on the gastric mucosa (Fig. 12.2) [36]. Antral nodularity seen on endoscopy is histologically associated with inflammatory cell infiltrates and lymphoid follicles, and it is the only sign with a high positive predictive value for the presence of *H. pylori* infection [37].

After successful eradication therapy, the neutrophils quickly disappear and any persistence of neutrophils and/or mononuclear infiltrate could be an indication of the treatment failure.

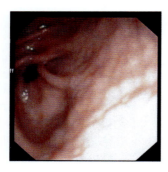

Fig. 12.2 Antral nodularity associated with *H. pylori* infection

Peptic Ulcer Disease

Gastritis and peptic ulcer disease were previously considered as separate diseases; however, better understanding of the pathomechanisms and discovery of *H. pylori* revealed the close relation between those two entities. Peptic ulceration of the stomach or duodenum, either primary or secondary, is almost always accompanied by abnormalities of the gastric mucosa, either a gastritis or a gastropathy [38]. Peptic ulcer disease is the ultimate loss of mucosal integrity and develops when the protective mechanisms of the gastrointestinal mucosa, such as mucus and bicarbonate secretion, are overwhelmed by the damaging effects of gastric acid and pepsin [39]. By the definition, peptic ulcers are deep mucosal lesions that disrupt muscularis mucosa layer of gastric or duodenal wall. They occur in the stomach mainly in antrocorporeal mucosal transitional zone along the lesser curve or proximal duodenum, duodenal bulb [40]. Peptic ulcers are more common in duodenum than in stomach and *H. pylori* is the most frequent cause. Other etiological factors associated with gastritis and peptic ulcer disease are presented in Table 12.1.

Available literature suggests that the lifetime risk for development of peptic ulcer disease in *H. pylori*-positive patients ranges between 10 and 20% [41]. Peptic ulcer disease occurs less frequent in children than in adults. A large prospective European multicenter study including more than 1400 symptomatic infected children found gastric or duodenal ulcers in 3.5% of the children below 6 years of age, in 4.6% the children aged 6–11 years, and in 10.4% of those older than 12 years [42]. Subsequent, prospective, also European multicenter study found that even 8.1% of the children had ulcers or erosions [43]. In a retrospective review of 619 Chinese children who had undergone upper endoscopy for investigation of upper gastrointestinal symptoms, Tam et al. [44] have found peptic ulcers in 6.9% of the children.

The discovery of *H. pylori* has turned the pathogenesis of peptic ulcer disease from a hyperacid disease to an infectious and immunopathogenetic disease where a variety of ulcer-promoting host and bacterial factors are involved in the com-

plex pathogenesis [32]. However, despite that, gastric acid secretion remains an important factor of peptic ulcer disease development. Patients with *H. pylori* gastritis and duodenal ulcers present with a much higher gastric acid output following gastrin stimulation than patients with *H. pylori* gastritis but without duodenal ulcer [45]. The mechanisms controlling acid secretion are hormonal and very complex in nature. The hormonal drive is exerted by hypergastrinemia, which was originally interpreted to result from the alkalization induced by *H. pylori*. Higher pH around G cells interrupts the negative feedback control and they continue to release gastrin [32]. Another explanation for hypergastrinemia could be the *H. pylori*-induced impaired synthesis and release of somatostatin [32]. Somatostatin is a hormone that inhibits gastrin synthesis and subsequently inhibits acid secretion.

Moreover, *H. pylori* virulence factors also contribute to the development of peptic ulcer disease. In children, as in adults, CagA and VacA genes are the most frequently implicated virulence factors associated with increased risk of peptic ulcer disease [46].

In gastric ulcer, the role of acid and *H. pylori*, although certainly contributory, is of less dominance as compared to duodenal ulcer [32].

Epigastric pain or discomfort exacerbated by the meal is often a symptom of peptic ulcer disease in children; however, it may also be a presenting symptom of more common disorders such as non-ulcer dyspepsia and constipation among others [38]. Other presenting symptoms include anorexia, nausea, early satiety, recurrent vomiting, and anemia. Up to 25% of the children with duodenal ulcers can present silently, approximately 25% with bleeding and antecedent pain, and the rest with abdominal pain or recurrent vomiting [38, 47]. Among all clinical signs: epigastric tenderness, pain awakening the child at night, hematemesis, melena, and stunted weight gain can be considered as significant risk factors for ulcers or erosions independently [43]. Acute gastrointestinal bleeding is the most common complication of childhood peptic ulcer disease and may occur with long-standing antecedent epigastric pain, whereas a perforated peptic ulcer occurs more rarely [44].

Other Causes of Peptic Ulcer Disease

In adult patients, the second most common cause of peptic ulcer disease are the use of nonsteroidal anti-inflammatory drugs (NSAIDs) [48]. NSAIDs inhibit cyclooxygenase-1 enzyme (COX-1) and reduce prostaglandin synthesis; consequently, diminishing gastric mucosal blood flow and decreasing a production of the mucus–bicarbonate barrier [49]. In children, gastric ulcerations from NSAID ingestion are not nearly as frequent as in adults [38]. When occurs in children, NSAID-induced ulcer is typically presented as hem-

Table 12.1 Causes of gastritis and peptic ulcer disease	Primary	*H. pylori* associated
		H. pylori negative (idiopathic)
		Hypersecretory states
		Zollinger–Ellison syndrome
		G cell hyperplasia/hyperfunction
		Systemic mastocytosis
		Cystic fibrosis
		Hyperparathyroidism
		Short bowel syndrome
		Renal failure
	Secondary	Stress ulcers
		Drugs
		Aspirin
		Nonsteroidal anti-inflammatory drugs (NSAID)
		Chorticosteroids
		Chemotherapy
		Valproic acid
		Alcohol
		Potassium chloride
		Immune/allergic
		Allergic gastritis and eosinophilic gastritis
		Graft-versus-host disease
		Henoch–Schönlein gastritis
		Coeliac disease
		Autoimmune disease
		Granulomatous gastritides
		Crohn's disease
		Foreign body reaction
		Idiopathic
		Sarcoidosis
		Histiocytosis X
		Tuberculosis
		Menetrier disease
		Other infections
		Helicobacter heilmanii
		Cytomegalovirus
		Phlegmonous gastritis and emphysematous
		Herpes simplex
		Influenza A
		Syphilis
		Candida albicans
		Histoplasmosis
		Mucormycosis
		Anisakiasis
		Radiation gastropathy

orrhagic antral gastropathy and ulceration of the incisura. Other drugs associated with drug-induced gastropathy and ulcers are anticoagulants and corticosteroids [50].

Other very rare causes of peptic ulcer disease in children include hypersecretory states like Zollinger–Ellison syndrome and antral G cell hyperplasia, and should be suspected in children with severe or recurrent duodenal and gastric ulcers, resistant to proton pump inhibitors (PPI) treatment, and in children with multiple ulcers. Other conditions associated with acid hypersecretion are systemic mastocytosis, short bowel syndrome during the first year after surgical resection, hyperparathyroidism, cystic fibrosis, and renal failure [51].

Stress-related ulcers usually occur 24 h after the onset of severe critical illness including shock, hypoxemia, acidosis, sepsis, burns, head injury, encephalopathy, major surgery, and multiple organ system failure [38]. Stress erosions are typically multiple and asymptomatic until cause, sometimes severe, gastrointestinal bleeding.

Gastritis and gastric ulcerations are found in 50–60% of the children with Crohn's disease [52]. Focally enhanced gastritis is an inflammatory lesion often found in Crohn's disease and involves discrete inflammatory foci containing lymphocytes, histiocytes, and granulocytes [53]. Focally enhanced gastritis, although in much lower extent, could also be found in ulcerative colitis and indeterminate inflammatory bowel disease.

Ménétrier's disease is a rare disorder of unknown etiology characterized by enlarged gastric rugal folds. It is a protein-losing gastropathy, clinically presented with nonspecific gastrointestinal symptoms such as nausea, vomiting, anorexia, weight loss, and hypoalbuminemia [54]. Cytomegalovirus and *H. pylori* are the most frequently found pathogens associated with this condition.

Celiac disease-associated lymphocytic gastritis is characterized by an intense lymphocytosis of the foveolar and surface epithelium and chronic inflammation in the lamina propria. Celiac disease may manifest with dyspeptic symptoms and histological changes which normalize after gluten withdrawal [55, 56].

Eosinophilic-mediated gastritis may be a presentation of food allergy (allergic gastritis) or be a primary disease (primary eosinophilic gastritis), as gastric infiltration by eosinophils is a pathological feature found in both conditions. Allergic gastritis mainly affects young infants with cow's milk protein allergy but multiple food intolerances may also occur. Most common symptoms include vomiting, hematemesis, poor weight gain, or symptoms of gastric emptying [57]. Primary eosinophilic gastritis may manifest at any age and may affect any part of the gastric wall. In mucosal form, children may present with vomiting, abdominal pain, and gastric blood loss; motility disturbances and gastric outlet obstruction may occur if muscular layer is affected [58, 59]. Serosal forms produce eosinophilic ascites and peritonitis [60]. Eosinophilic gastritis may also be a part of the eosinophilic gastroenteritis.

Other causes of primary and secondary gastritis and peptic ulcer disease in children are presented in Table 12.1.

Malignancy

H. pylori is considered the leading cause of gastric cancer worldwide and because of that, in adult population, it is listed as a number one carcinogen. A causal relation between *H. pylori* infection and the risk of gastric malignancies, including cancer and MALT lymphoma has been clearly proved. However, in children, *H. pylori*-related malignancy is extremely rare. Evidence increasingly indicates that *H. pylori*-related gastric carcinogenesis is likely to be the result of a well-choreographed interaction between the pathogen and host, which is dependent on strain-specific bacterial factors, host genotypic traits, and permissive environmental factors [2]. Various factors influence malignant potential including

age of infection, bacterial genotype, host immune response, and host genetics. It has been suggested that chronic gastritis, gastric atrophy, intestinal metaplasia, and gastric cancer develop progressively, stepwise over decades, in predisposed individuals infected with *H. pylori* [61].

Incomplete intestinal metaplasia has been described in the gastric mucosa of *H. pylori*-infected children, suggesting that it can develop even during childhood and evolve into complete intestinal metaplasia in adults [62]. Moreover, other studies have reported a significant incidence of gastric atrophy (42–55%) and intestinal metaplasia (13–21%) in children [63]. Interestingly, a higher incidence of atrophic gastritis has been observed in children from countries with high incidence of gastric cancer [64, 65]. Moreover, current evidence suggests that in high-risk populations the eradication of *H. pylori* may have the potential to decrease the risk of gastric cancer [66]. There are certain *H. pylori* genotypes associated with more severe inflammation of gastric mucosa in pediatric patients including CagA, VacA, and BabA, and their detection could be of importance in areas with high risk of carcinoma [67]. In support of this is a report which found that in high-risk population, even children have a high prevalence of *H. pylori* virulence markers—CagA and VacA [68].

In the pediatric population, there are only a few studies with a small number of patients regarding the association between *H. pylori* infection and precancerous lesions in both gastric antrum and corpus [63]. There are reports which presented children with *H. pylori* infection who subsequently developed high-grade B-cell lymphoma which resolved after *H. pylori* eradication even without chemotherapy [69, 70]. All these data indicate that *H. pylori* could be associated with malignancies in children; however, the risk seems to be substantially lower than in adults [71].

Clinical Presentation of H. pylori Infection

Recurrent Abdominal Pain Abdominal complaints including pain, cramps, and nausea are very common in pediatric population. Usually, they are unspecific and can be a symptom of various organic diseases but are very often caused by functional gastrointestinal disorders. Whether *H. pylori* infection without peptic ulcer disease can cause recurrent abdominal pain remains unclear. Large epidemiological studies found association between recurrent abdominal pain and different social and familial factors like single-parent household, family history of peptic ulcer disease, or functional pain but not to *H. pylori* status of the child [72]. A performed meta-analysis on the relationship between recurrent abdominal pain and *H. pylori* infection in children included 38 case control, cross-sectional, and prospective studies and found no evidence for relation between recurrent abdominal pain and *H. pylori* infection in children [73]. The only pain found associated with *H. pylori* infection was epigastric pain [73]. Several interventional but uncontrolled studies showed improvement of symptoms after the eradication of *H. pylori;* however, these studies have several biases; treatment success was not monitored and eradication of the bacteria not reported and in other studies follow-up period was very short, for a few weeks only [74–77]. Based on these results, there is not enough evidence to support a causal relation between *H. pylori* gastritis and abdominal pain in the absence of peptic ulcer disease. Searching for *H. pylori* is therefore not recommended in children that otherwise fulfill the criteria of functional abdominal pain, unless upper endoscopy is performed during the diagnostic workup in search for organic disease [4, 67, 78].

Iron-Deficiency Anemia Iron-deficiency anemia in children and adolescents has variety of causes and there are still disagreements whether *H. pylori* infection can be one of them. The potential pathogenesis is reduced iron absorption in infected gastric mucosa, increased iron loss due to microbleeding, and utilization of iron by *H. pylori* in the stomach [67]. Number of studies suggested that iron deficiency is one of the extragastric manifestations of *H. pylori* infection in children [79–81]. However, the results of these studies are not unanimous, with most recent studies that reported no such association [82, 83]. This considerable discrepancy in the results is largely due to methodological variation of the studies. Moreover, it is often difficult to distinguish between iron-deficiency anemia due to *H. pylori* infection and to the other often confounding factors such as poor nutritional status, poor socioeconomic and hygienic conditions, or another underlying disease [4]. Hence, endoscopic examination may be indicated in children with refractory iron-deficiency anemia in order to rule out not only the presence of *H. pylori* but also other causes of iron-deficiency anemia such as celiac disease or chronic inflammatory diseases [84].

These findings are consistent with clinical guidelines by the European Society of Pediatric Gastroenterology, Hepatology, and Nutrition (ESPGHAN) and by the North American Society for Pediatric Gastroenterology Hepatology and Nutrition (NASPGHAN); they recommend that in children with refractory iron-deficiency anemia where other causes have been ruled out, testing for *H. pylori* infection may be considered [4].

Growth There are a number of longitudinal studies that support the hypothesis that *H. pylori* infection might influence growth rate in children [85]; however, none are adequately designed to evaluate confounders of growth including other gastrointestinal infections in childhood, socioeconomic status, living conditions, etc. Despite new information concerning the effect of *H. pylori* infection on poor growth, the need for well-designed studies remains. Based on published data there is insufficient evidence that *H. pylori* infection is causally related to growth impairment in childhood [4].

Chronic Idiopathic Thrombocytopenic Purpura The role of *H. pylori* in the development of chronic idiopathic thrombocytopenic purpura continues to evolve. *H. pylori* infection has been proposed to be associated with thrombocytopenic purpura based on a significantly increased platelets count following *H. pylori* eradication in approximately half of adult patients [86]. Data on children are limited; small case series have been published with conflicting results [87–91]. However, more recent data implicate that eradication of *H. pylori* could induce a better treatment response in chronic idiopathic thrombocytopenic purpura [92].

Diagnostic Procedures

Based on ESPGHAN/NASPGHAN evidence-based guidelines for *H. pylori* infection in children testing for *H. pylori* in children should be performed in properly selected patients (Table 12.2) and with an adequate diagnostic procedures [4]. Current recommendations for children do not approve "test and treat" approach recommended for adults [4]. Therefore, diagnostic procedures should aim to determine underlying disease and not to detect *H. pylori*.

Table 12.2 Clinical indication for testing for *H. pylori* infection. (Based on ESPGHAN/NASPGHAN recommendations Ref. [4])

Justified testing for *H. pylori*	Gastrointestinal symptoms suggestive of organic disease, serious enough to justify upper endoscopy	
Considered testing for *H. pylori*	Children with first-degree relatives with gastric cancer	
	Children with refractory iron-deficiency anemia when other causes have been ruled out	
Not justified testing for *H. plyori*	Functional abdominal pain	
	Upper respiratory tract infections	
	Periodontal disease	
	Food allergy	
	Sudden infant death syndrome	
	Idiopathic thrombocytopenic purpura	
	Growth impairment	

Tests that detect *H. pylori* are divided into noninvasive and invasive tests. Invasive tests require endoscopy and gastric tissue biopsy for detecting the bacterium and include culture, rapid urease test, histopathology, polymerase chain reaction, and fluorescence in situ hybridization (FISH) tests [93]. On the other hand, noninvasive tests include different methods for the detection of *H. pylori* antigens in stool, detection of antibodies against *H. pylori* in different biological materials including serum, urine, and oral samples, and widely used ^{13}C-urea breath test (^{13}C-UBT) [93].

Noninvasive Tests

Among noninvasive diagnostic tests, stool antigen test and ^{13}C-UBT have higher accuracy than serological or urinary antibody-based tests [94].

13C-Urea Breath Test Recently published meta-analysis on the performance of the ^{13}C-UBT showed good accuracy especially in children older than 6 years of age (sensitivity 96.6%, specificity 97.7%) [95]. A crucial question for all tests performed in a pediatric population is whether the accuracy of the applied method is influenced by the age of the tested child. ^{13}C-UBT requires patient cooperation; moreover, patients need to fast before testing and drink without tracer withhold in the mouth. All that makes ^{13}C-UBT difficult to perform in children younger than 6 years of age and may at least in part explain the lower specificity reported in young children [96, 97].

Stool Antigen Tests Because *H. pylori* and its macromolecules such as proteins and DNA are shed in feces, stool-based tests have become advanced [98]. Several commercial enzyme-linked immunosorbent assay (ELISA) tests for *H. pylori* stool antigens are available. The main differences among these tests are the nature of the detecting antibodies; some kits use a polyclonal anti-*H. pylori* antibody, whereas other assays use monoclonal antibodies, and recently rapid one-step test (immunochromatographic format) using monoclonal antibodies has been introduced [98]. Meta-analysis on stool antigen-detection tests revealed that ELISA monoclonal antibodies have the best performance, with sensitivity and specificity of 97% compared to ELISA polyclonal antibodies (sensitivity of 92%, specificity of 93%), and to one-step monoclonal antibody tests (sensitivity of 88%, specificity of 93%) [98]. So far, only the ELISA based on monoclonal antibodies has achieved the accuracy of the ^{13}C-UBT, which is considered the reference standard of the noninvasive tests [4]. Use of stool tests is generally more convenient in pediatric patients than the ^{13}C-UBT. It has several advantages: stool samples can be obtained from children without their active collaboration and are transportable by

mail for analysis, the cost is lower comparing to ^{13}C-UBT, and it is not age-dependent. Therefore, validation studies in adults may be extrapolated to children [4].

Detection of the Antibodies The systemic immune response against *H. pylori* typically shows a transient rise in specific IgM antibodies, followed by a rise in IgG and IgA antibodies that persist during infection [99]. Since IgM antibodies against *H. pylori* are detected only transiently, they have little value for the serological diagnosis of infection [100]. Therefore, diagnostic commercial tests detect *H. pylori*-specific IgG and IgA antibodies in serum, saliva, and urine. Numerous serologic tests are available for the diagnosis of *H. pylori* infection in children. Common designs of antibody-based detection tests are ELISA and Western Blot (WB) [99]. Many tests based on the detection of antibodies are commercially available, easy to perform, and inexpensive. However, the main problem is age dependence, particularly with respect to sensitivity in younger children, and test-to-test variability. The sensitivity of most tests is much lower when used in children compared with adults from the same geographic region [4]. Current serologic tests are not useful for monitoring eradication of infection after therapy since they cannot distinguish between current or past *H. pylori* infection, and the antibody titers usually remain positive several months after the infection has been eradicated [99]. Taking that into account tests based on the detection of antibodies (IgG, IgA) against *H. pylori* in serum, whole blood, urine, and saliva are not reliable for use in the clinical setting [4].

Invasive Tests

Although noninvasive tests yield high sensitivity and specificity, endoscopy with histopathology remains the only method that can detect lesions associated with the infection, but also other possible causes of the patient's symptoms [93]. In *H. pylori* infection, endoscopy may show normal gastric mucosa or reveal erythema, erosions, ulcers and, especially in children, antral nodularity.

The site from which a biopsy is taken and the number of biopsies affect the accuracy of *H. pylori* diagnosis. Normally, the highest bacterial count is found in the antrum because of that the optimal biopsy site is the mid-antrum at the lesser curvature [101]; however, in cases of low gastric acidity and during the PPI treatment, the bacteria may be present only in the gastric body.

Furthermore, due to patchy density of *H. pylori*, the sensitivity increases with the number of biopsies taken. For pathology, two biopsies should be obtained from both the antrum and the body, and the findings should be reported according to the updated Sydney classification [35]. The updat-

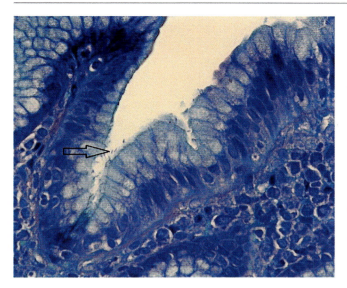

Fig. 12.3 Giemsa staining demonstrates gastric *H. pylori* bacteria

ed Sydney system for the gastritis classification emphasizes the importance of combining topographical, morphological, and etiological information in order to generate reproducible and clinically useful diagnoses. Classification is based on the location of gastritis and the presence of different histological parameters including inflammation, activity, atrophy, intestinal metaplasia, and *H. pylori* infection which are graded as mild, moderate, and marked [35]. Updated Sydney classification was not assessed in pediatric patients; however, it can help in order to unify the histopathology reports.

Biopsies should be stained with hematoxylin and eosin because this is the best method to detect atrophy and intestinal metaplasia. Special staining (Giemsa or silver stain) and immunohistochemistry should be used for detection of *H. pylori* (Fig. 12.3) [4]. In children, hematoxylin and eosin and Giemsa stains have a sensitivity of 82% and specificity of 95% in detecting *H. pylori* gastritis [102]. With decreasing prevalence of the infection in pediatric populations in many areas of Europe and North America, the predictive values of the diagnostic test results decrease; test with a sensitivity of 90% has a positive predictive value of only 50% if the prevalence of the infection in the population is 10% [4]. Sensitivity for histology ranges from 66 to 100% and for rapid urease tests performed on the biopsies from 75 to 100% [93]. Therefore, in order to increase *H. pylori* detection in children, it is highly recommended to take not only biopsies for histopathology but also one biopsy for a rapid urease test or culture [4]. The only method that consistently has 100% specificity is culture, but sensitivity varies depending on the experience of the laboratory [93].

As no single test is accurate enough for detection of *H. pylori,* current guidelines recommend endoscopy with gastric biopsies from the gastric antrum and body and confirma-

tion of infection with two different tests, either histopathology and rapid urease test or a culture [4].

Treatment for H. pylori Infection

Updated evidence-based guidelines from ESPGHAN and NASPGHAN recommend treatment for *H. pylori* in all children in whom peptic ulcer disease was detected during endoscopy [4]. Whether it is necessary to eradicate *H. pylori* in children with gastritis but without peptic ulcer disease remains questionable because there is not enough evidence which proved that bacterium eradication improves abdominal complaints in the absence of peptic ulcer.

Current evidence suggests that in high-risk populations for gastric cancer eradication of *H. pylori* may have the potential to decrease the cancer risk even without precancerous lesions [66].

Individuals with a positive family history for gastric cancer are in a high-risk for acquiring gastric malignancy. The risk could be particularly high in *H. pylori*-infected children with parent affected by gastric cancer because child is not only sharing a genetic and environmental factors with the affected parent but could also have the same bacterial strain [25].

Therefore, the decision to treat *H. pylori*-associated gastritis without duodenal or gastric ulcer is subject to the judgment of the clinician and the patient and family, taking into consideration the potential risks and benefits of the treatment in every individual patient [4].

First-line eradication therapy has three different regimens: (1) triple therapy with a PPI and amoxicillin and imidazole or clarithromycin, (2) bismuth salts with amoxicillin and imidazole, and (3) sequential therapy (Table 12.3) [4].

Standard triple therapy, a combination of two antibiotics and a PPI, has been recommended as a first-line therapy since the first published pediatric guidelines. The goal of treatment is at least a 90% eradication rate at the first attempt

Table 12.3 Treatment options for *H. pylori* infection. (Based on ESPGHAN/NASPGHAN recommendations Ref. [4])

PPI (1–2 mg/kg/day) + amoxicillin (50 mg/kg/day) + clarithromycin (20 mg/kg/day)/metronidazole (20 mg/kg/day) Duration: 7–14 days (preferable 10–14 days)
Bismuth salts (8 mg/kg/day) + amoxicillin (50 mg/kg/day) + metronidazole (20 mg/kg/day) Duration: 7–14 days (preferable 10–14 days)
Sequential therapy: PPI (1–2 mg/kg/day) + amoxicillin (50 mg/kg/day) during 5 days, then PPI (1–2 mg/kg/day) + metronidazole (20 mg/kg/day) + clarithromycin (20 mg/kg/day) during 5 days Total duration: 10 days
Maximal daily dose: amoxicillin 2 g, metronidazole 1 g, clarithromycin 1 g
PPI proton pump inhibitors

[4]. However, reported eradication rate is much lower mainly due to antibiotic resistance. Antibiotic resistance is mostly found to clarithromycin and metronidazole. The overall incidence of clarithromycin resistance in children in Western countries is high and current reports indicate prevalence of more than 20% in treatment-naïve patients [42, 103–106], and the resistance rate is even much higher is some countries like China where clarithromycin resistance rate was higher than 80% [107]. Similarly, some areas have also high levels of resistance rate to metronidazole, more than 20% [42, 103, 107, 108]. Based on the negative effect of antibiotic resistance on treatment outcomes, the rates of resistance in the area where the child lives should be taken into account when deciding on the initial therapeutic regimen for eradication [4]. In areas with high or unknown primary antibiotic-resistance rate, culture and susceptibility testing should be performed in order to select proper treatment regimen [4].

Decreasing eradication rates with these standard triple regimens have led to the development of alternate treatment options, like sequential therapy. This is a two-step, 10-day therapy typically consisting of a PPI combined with amoxicillin given for the first 5 days, followed by a triple therapy including a PPI, clarithromycin, and metronidazole/tinidazole for another 5 days [109]. Meta-analysis comparing sequential to standard triple therapy found that sequential therapy is superior to 7-day standard triple therapy; however, not significantly better than 10-day or 14-day triple therapy [109].

Bismuth-based triple therapy is also recommended as an alternative first-line therapy. Well-designed, randomized, multicenter studies of H. pylori eradication in children comparing bismuth-based regimens to the alternative recommended first-line therapies are lacking. The results from the pediatric European register for treatment of H. pylori showed that when given as first treatment, bismuth-containing triple therapies were more efficacious than those containing PPI (77% vs. 64%) [110, 111]. In addition, bismuth-based triple therapy may be less costly than the other options; however, concerns regarding the palatability of bismuth potentially affecting adherence should also be considered [4].

The duration of eradication therapy is still controversial. Today, 7-, 10-, and 14-day triple regimens are often used. It has been reported that, especially taking into account compliance rate that there is no benefit from longer duration of therapy [111, 112]. There are no studies specifically addressing the issue of the treatment duration in children for standard triple eradication therapy. It is recommended that the duration of triple therapy should be from 7 to 14 days and factors like costs, compliance, and adverse events should be taken into account [4].

Emerging evidence suggests development of secondary antibiotic resistance in children who failed initial eradication therapy [113]. When initial treatment fails there are several options; if possible, primary culture with antibiotic sensitiv-ity testing should be performed to guide second-line therapy. If culture (and standard susceptibility testing) is not possible, molecular tests (including FISH) can be used to detect H. pylori and clarithromycin and/or fluoroquinolone resistance in gastric biopsies [94]. If primary culture and sensitivity testing are not available, when deciding on second-line therapy, the initial therapy should be taken into account with avoidance of previously given regimens [114].

Guidelines recommend quadruple therapy which consists of PPI, metronidazole, amoxicillin, and bismuth as a second-line or selvage therapy [4, 94]. However, this regimen is complicated to administer and bismuth salts are not widely available. Other second-line therapy choice is a triple therapy including PPI, levofloxacin (moxifloxacin), and amoxicillin [4]. This regimen proved to be effective in adults; however, the evidence of fluoroquinolones used in children is limited. Moreover, there are concerns regarding increasing rates of quinolone resistance in adults [114]. Therefore, this regimen should not be used in the children who have received fluoroquinolones previously [4]. Although the studies on the ideal duration of therapy for second-line treatment are not conclusive, a longer duration of therapy of up to 14 days is recommended [4].

Assessment of Eradication

All children who received treatment for H. pylori, even if they have no symptoms should undergo the evaluation of the treatment success. The absence of symptoms is not reliable and does not necessarily mean the H. pylori is eradicated. The recommended tests for H. pylori eradication assessment are noninvasive tests; ^{13}C-UBT and a monoclonal ELISA for detection of H. pylori antigen in stool [4]. As previously presented, these tests have a high sensitivity and high specificity and are not invasive. A follow-up endoscopy is not routinely indicated unless other causes of ulceration are suspected or if biopsies are needed for culture and antibiotic susceptibility testing [4].

Eradication therapy reduces the amount of H. pylori in the stomach, even when eradication failed because of that antibiotic or PPI therapy can cause false-negative test results [115]. Therefore, assessment of eradication should be performed with noninvasive test at least 4–8 weeks following completion of therapy [4].

References

1. Zarrilli R, Ricci V, Romano M. Molecular response of gastric epithelial cells to Helicobacter pylori-induced cell damage. Cell Microbiol. 1999;1(2):93–9.
2. Ricci V, Romano M, Boquet P. Molecular cross-talk between Helicobacter pylori and human gastric mucosa. World J Gastroenterol. 2011;17(11):1383–99.

3. Delahay RM, Rugge M. Pathogenesis of *Helicobacter pylori* infection. Helicobacter. 2012;17(Suppl 1):9–15.

4. Koletzko S, Jones NL, Goodman KJ, Gold B, Rowland M, Cadranel S, et al. Evidence-based guidelines from ESPGHAN and NASPGHAN for *Helicobacter pylori* infection in children. J Pediatr Gastroenterol Nutr. 2011;53(2):230–43.

5. Sachs G, Scott DR, Wen Y. Gastric infection by *Helicobacter pylori*. Curr Gastroenterol Rep. 2011;13(6):540–6.

6. Salama NR, Hartung ML, Muller A. Life in the human stomach: persistence strategies of the bacterial pathogen *Helicobacter pylori*. Nat Rev Microbiol. 2013;11(6):385–99.

7. Bansil R, Celli JP, Hardcastle JM, Turner BS. The influence of mucus microstructure and rheology in *helicobacter pylori* infection. Front Immunol. 2013;4:310.

8. Johnson EM, Gaddy JA, Cover TL. Alterations in *Helicobacter pylori* triggered by contact with gastric epithelial cells. Front Cell Infect Microbiol. 2012;2:17.

9. Ahmed N. Coevolution and adaptation of *Helicobacter pylori* and the case for 'functional molecular infection epidemiology'. Med Princ Pract. 2011;20(6):497–503.

10. Every AL. Key host-pathogen interactions for designing novel interventions against *Helicobacter pylori*. Trends Microbiol. 2013;21(5):253–9.

11. Yamaoka Y. Mechanisms of disease: *Helicobacter pylori* virulence factors. Nat Rev Gastroenterol Hepatol. 2010;7(11):629–41.

12. Montecucco C, de Bernard M. Immunosuppressive and proinflammatory activities of the VacA toxin of *Helicobacter pylori*. J Exp Med. 2003;198(12):1767–71.

13. Jones KR, Whitmire JM, Merrell DS. A tale of two toxins: *Helicobacter pylori* CagA and VacA modulate host pathways that impact disease. Front Microbiol. 2010;1:115.

14. Backert S, Tegtmeyer N, Selbach M. The versatility of *Helicobacter pylori* CagA effector protein functions: the master key hypothesis. Helicobacter. 2010;15(3):163–76.

15. Terradot L, Waksman G. Architecture of the *Helicobacter pylori* Cag-type IV secretion system. FEBS J. 2011;278(8):1213–22.

16. Rieder G, Fischer W, Haas R. Interaction of *Helicobacter pylori* with host cells: function of secreted and translocated molecules. Curr Opin Microbiol. 2005;8(1):67–73.

17. Tegtmeyer N, Wessler S, Backert S. Role of the cag-pathogenicity island encoded type IV secretion system in *Helicobacter pylori* pathogenesis. FEBS J. 2011;278(8):1190–202.

18. Linden S, Semino-Mora C, Liu H, Rick J, Dubois A. Role of mucin Lewis status in resistance to *Helicobacter pylori* infection in pediatric patients. Helicobacter. 2010;15(4):251–8.

19. Yamaoka Y, Ojo O, Fujimoto S, Odenbreit S, Haas R, Gutierrez O, et al. *Helicobacter pylori* outer membrane proteins and gastroduodenal disease. Gut. 2006;55(6):775–81.

20. Ruggiero P. *Helicobacter pylori* infection: what's new. Curr Opin Infect Dis. 2012;25(3):337–44.

21. Calvet X, Ramirez Lazaro MJ, Lehours P, Megraud F. Diagnosis and epidemiology of *Helicobacter pylori* infection. Helicobacter. 2013;18(Suppl 1):5–11.

22. Goh KL, Chan WK, Shiota S, Yamaoka Y. Epidemiology of *Helicobacter pylori* infection and public health implications. Helicobacter. 2011;16(Suppl 1):1–9.

23. Queiroz DM, Carneiro JG, Braga-Neto MB, Fialho AB, Fialho AM, Goncalves MH, et al. Natural history of *Helicobacter pylori* infection in childhood: eight-year follow-up cohort study in an urban community in northeast of Brazil. Helicobacter. 2012;17(1):23–9.

24. Bastos J, Carreira H, La Vecchia C, Lunet N. Childcare attendance and *Helicobacter pylori* infection: systematic review and meta-analysis. Eur J Cancer Prev. 2013;22(4):311–9.

25. Kivi M, Tindberg Y. *Helicobacter pylori* occurrence and transmission: a family affair? Scand J Infect Dis. 2006;38(6–7):407–17.

26. Brown LM. *Helicobacter pylori*: epidemiology and routes of transmission. Epidemiol Rev. 2000;22(2):283–97.

27. Weyermann M, Rothenbacher D, Brenner H. Acquisition of *Helicobacter pylori* infection in early childhood: independent contributions of infected mothers, fathers, and siblings. Am J Gastroenterol. 2009;104(1):182–9.

28. Muhsen K, Athamna A, Bialik A, Alpert G, Cohen D. Presence of *Helicobacter pylori* in a sibling is associated with a long-term increased risk of *H. pylori* infection in Israeli Arab children. Helicobacter. 2010;15(2):108–13.

29. Cervantes DT, Fischbach LA, Goodman KJ, Phillips CV, Chen S, Broussard CS. Exposure to *Helicobacter pylori*-positive siblings and persistence of *Helicobacter pylori* infection in early childhood. J Pediatr Gastroenterol Nutr. 2010;50(5):481–5.

30. Zou QH, Li RQ. *Helicobacter pylori* in the oral cavity and gastric mucosa: a meta-analysis. J Oral Pathol Med. 2011;40(4):317–24.

31. Rugge M, Pennelli G, Pilozzi E, Fassan M, Ingravallo G, Russo VM, et al. Gastritis: the histology report. Dig Liver Dis. 2011;43(Suppl 4):S373–84.

32. Malfertheiner P. The intriguing relationship of *Helicobacter pylori* infection and acid secretion in peptic ulcer disease and gastric cancer. Dig Dis. 2011;29(5):459–64.

33. Tan VP, Wong BC. *Helicobacter pylori* and gastritis: untangling a complex relationship 27 years on. J Gastroenterol Hepatol. 2011;26(Suppl 1):42–5.

34. Hoepler W, Hammer K, Hammer J. Gastric phenotype in children with *Helicobacter pylori* infection undergoing upper endoscopy. Scand J Gastroenterol. 2011;46(3):293–8.

35. Dixon MF, Genta RM, Yardley JH, Correa P. Classification and grading of gastritis. The updated Sydney System. International Workshop on the Histopathology of Gastritis, Houston 1994. Am J Surg Pathol. 1996;20(10):1161–81.

36. Prieto G, Polanco I, Larrauri J, Rota L, Lama R, Carrasco S. *Helicobacter pylori* infection in children: clinical, endoscopic, and histologic correlations. J Pediatr Gastroenterol Nutr. 1992;14(4):420–5.

37. Yang HR, Choi HS, Paik JH, Lee HS. Endoscopic and histologic analysis of gastric mucosa-associated lymphoid tissue in children with *Helicobacter pylori* infection. J Pediatr Gastroenterol Nutr. 2013;57(3):298–304.

38. Dohil R, Hassall E. Peptic ulcer disease in children. Bailliere's Best Pract Res Clin Gastroenterol. 2000;14(1):53–73.

39. Sung JJ, Kuipers EJ, El-Serag HB. Systematic review: the global incidence and prevalence of peptic ulcer disease. Aliment Pharmacol Ther. 2009;29(9):938–46.

40. Tytgat GN. Etiopathogenetic principles and peptic ulcer disease classification. Dig Dis. 2011;29(5):454–8.

41. Kuipers EJ, Thijs JC, Festen HP. The prevalence of *Helicobacter pylori* in peptic ulcer disease. Aliment Pharmacol Ther. 1995;9(Suppl 2):59–69.

42. Koletzko S, Richy F, Bontems P, Crone J, Kalach N, Monteiro ML, et al. Prospective multicentre study on antibiotic resistance of *Helicobacter pylori* strains obtained from children living in Europe. Gut. 2006;55(12):1711–6.

43. Kalach N, Bontems P, Koletzko S, Mourad-Baars P, Shcherbakov P, Celinska-Cedro D, et al. Frequency and risk factors of gastric and duodenal ulcers or erosions in children: a prospective 1-month European multicenter study. Eur J Gastroenterol Hepatol. 2010;22(10):1174–81.

44. Tam YH, Lee KH, To KF, Chan KW, Cheung ST. *Helicobacter pylori*-positive versus *Helicobacter pylori*-negative idiopathic peptic ulcers in children with their long-term outcomes. J Pediatr Gastroenterol Nutr. 2009;48(3):299–305.

45. Gillen D, el-Omar EM, Wirz AA, Ardill JE, McColl KE. The acid response to gastrin distinguishes duodenal ulcer patients from *Helicobacter pylori*-infected healthy subjects. Gastroenterology. 1998;114(1):50–7.

46. Ruggiero P. *Helicobacter pylori* and inflammation. Curr Pharm Des. 2010;16(38):4225–36.

47. Drumm B, Rhoads JM, Stringer DA, Sherman PM, Ellis LE, Durie PR. Peptic ulcer disease in children: etiology, clinical findings, and clinical course. Pediatrics. 1988; 82(3 Pt 2):410–4.

48. Gisbert JP, Calvet X. Review article: *Helicobacter pylori*-negative duodenal ulcer disease. Aliment Pharmacol Ther. 2009;30(8):791–815.

49. Hawkey CJ. Nonsteroidal anti-inflammatory drug gastropathy. Gastroenterology. 2000;119(2):521–35.

50. Lazzaroni M, Bianchi Porro G. Gastrointestinal side-effects of traditional non-steroidal anti-inflammatory drugs and new formulations. Aliment Pharmacol Ther. 2004;20(Suppl 2):48–58.

51. Gottrand F. Acid-peptic disease. In Kleinman RE, Sanderson IR, Goulet O, Sherman PM, Mieli-Vergani G, Shneider BL, eds. Walker's pediatric gastrointestinal disease. 5th ed. Hamilton: BC Decker Inc.; 2008. p. 153–63.

52. Hummel TZ, ten Kate FJ, Reitsma JB, Benninga MA, Kindermann A. Additional value of upper GI tract endoscopy in the diagnostic assessment of childhood IBD. J Pediatr Gastroenterol Nutr. 2012;54(6):753–7.

53. Ushiku T, Moran CJ, Lauwers GY. Focally enhanced gastritis in newly diagnosed pediatric inflammatory bowel disease. Am J Surg Pathol. 2013;37(12):1882–8.

54. Blackstone MM, Mittal MK. The edematous toddler: a case of pediatric Menetrier disease. Pediatr Emerg Care. 2008;24(10):682–4.

55. Jevon GP, Dimmick JE, Dohil R, Hassall EG. Spectrum of gastritis in celiac disease in childhood. Pediatr Dev Pathol. 1999;2(3):221–6.

56. De Giacomo C, Gianatti A, Negrini R, Perotti P, Bawa P, Maggiore G, et al. Lymphocytic gastritis: a positive relationship with celiac disease. J Pediatr. 1994;124(1):57–62.

57. Sicherer SH. Clinical aspects of gastrointestinal food allergy in childhood. Pediatrics. 2003; 111(6 Pt 3):1609–16.

58. Khan S, Orenstein SR. Eosinophilic gastroenteritis: epidemiology, diagnosis and management. Paediatr Drugs. 2002;4(9):563–70.

59. Lee CM, Changchien CS, Chen PC, Lin DY, Sheen IS, Wang CS, et al. Eosinophilic gastroenteritis: 10 years experience. Am J Gastroenterol. 1993;88(1):70–4.

60. Yan BM, Shaffer EA. Primary eosinophilic disorders of the gastrointestinal tract. Gut. 2009;58(5):721–32.

61. Pacifico L, Anania C, Osborn JF, Ferraro F, Chiesa C. Consequences of *Helicobacter pylori* infection in children. World J Gastroenterol. 2010;16(41):5181–94.

62. Cohen MC, Rua EC, Balcarce N, Drut R. Sulfomucins in *Helicobacter pylori*-associated chronic gastritis in children: is this incipient intestinal metaplasia? J Pediatr Gastroenterol Nutr. 2000;31(1):63–7.

63. Guarner J, Bartlett J, Whistler T, Pierce-Smith D, Owens M, Kreh R, et al. Can pre-neoplastic lesions be detected in gastric biopsies of children with *Helicobacter pylori* infection? J Pediatr Gastroenterol Nutr. 2003;37(3):309–14.

64. Kato S, Nakajima S, Nishino Y, Ozawa K, Minoura T, Konno M, et al. Association between gastric atrophy and *Helicobacter pylori* infection in Japanese children: a retrospective multicenter study. Dig Dis Sci. 2006;51(1):99–104.

65. Ricuarte O, Gutierrez O, Cardona H, Kim JG, Graham DY, El-Zimaity HM. Atrophic gastritis in young children and adolescents. J Clin Pathol. 2005;58(11):1189–93.

66. Wong BC, Lam SK, Wong WM, Chen JS, Zheng TT, Feng RE, et al. *Helicobacter pylori* eradication to prevent gastric cancer in a high-risk region of China: a randomized controlled trial. JAMA. 2004;291(2):187–94.

67. Homan M, Hojsak I, Kolacek S. *Helicobacter pylori* in pediatrics. Helicobacter. 2012;17(Suppl 1):43–8.

68. Sicinschi LA, Correa P, Bravo LE, Peek RM Jr, Wilson KT, Loh JT, et al. Non-invasive genotyping of *Helicobacter pylori* cagA, vacA, and hopQ from asymptomatic children. Helicobacter. 2012;17(2):96–106.

69. Al Furaikh SS. Remission of high-grade B-cell lymphoma in a pediatric patient following *Helicobacter pylori* eradication. Pediatr Int. 2011;53(1):105–7.

70. Blecker U, McKeithan TW, Hart J, Kirschner BS. Resolution of *Helicobacter pylori*-associated gastric lymphoproliferative disease in a child. Gastroenterology. 1995;109(3):973–7.

71. Hojsak I, Kolacek S. Is *Helicobacter pylori* always a "Bad Guy"? Curr Pharmaceut Des. 2014;20(28):4517–20.

72. Bode G, Brenner H, Adler G, Rothenbacher D. Recurrent abdominal pain in children: evidence from a population-based study that social and familial factors play a major role but not *Helicobacter pylori* infection. J Psychosom Res. 2003;54(5):417–21.

73. Spee LA, Madderom MB, Pijpers M, van Leeuwen Y, Berger MY. Association between *Helicobacter pylori* and gastrointestinal symptoms in children. Pediatrics. 2010;125(3):e651–69.

74. Elitsur Y, Dementieva Y, Rewalt M, Lawrence Z. *Helicobacter pylori* infection rate decreases in symptomatic children: a retrospective analysis of 13 years (1993–2005) from a gastroenterology clinic in West Virginia. J Clin Gastroenterol. 2009;43(2):147–51.

75. Das BK, Kakkar S, Dixit VK, Kumar M, Nath G, Mishra OP. *Helicobacter pylori* infection and recurrent abdominal pain in children. J Trop Pediatr. 2003;49(4):250–2.

76. Alfven G. One hundred cases of recurrent abdominal pain in children: diagnostic procedures and criteria for a psychosomatic diagnosis. Acta Paediatr. 2003;92(1):43–9.

77. Ozen H, Dinler G, Akyon Y, Kocak N, Yuce A, Gurakan F. *Helicobacter pylori* infection and recurrent abdominal pain in Turkish children. Helicobacter. 2001;6(3):234–8.

78. Buonavolonta R, Miele E, Russo D, Vecchione R, Staiano A. *Helicobacter pylori* chronic gastritis in children: to eradicate or not to eradicate? J Pediatr. 2011;159(1):50–6.

79. Choe YH, Kwon YS, Jung MK, Kang SK, Hwang TS, Hong YC. *Helicobacter pylori*-associated iron-deficiency anemia in adolescent female athletes. J Pediatr. 2001;139(1):100–4.

80. Baggett HC, Parkinson AJ, Muth PT, Gold BD, Gessner BD. Endemic iron deficiency associated with *Helicobacter pylori* infection among school-aged children in Alaska. Pediatrics. 2006;117(3):e396–404.

81. Milman N, Rosenstock S, Andersen L, Jorgensen T, Bonnevie O. Serum ferritin, hemoglobin, and *Helicobacter pylori* infection: a seroepidemiologic survey comprising 2794 Danish adults. Gastroenterology. 1998;115(2):268–74.

82. Vendt N, Kool P, Teesalu K, Lillemae K, Maaroos HI, Oona M. Iron deficiency and *Helicobacter pylori* infection in children. Acta Paediatr. 2011;100(9):1239–43.

83. Choi JW. Does *Helicobacter pylori* infection relate to iron deficiency anaemia in prepubescent children under 12 years of age? Acta Paediatr. 2003;92(8):970–2.

84. Ertem D. Clinical practice: *Helicobacter pylori* infection in childhood. Eur J Pediatr. 2013;172(11):1427–34.

85. Mera RM, Bravo LE, Goodman KJ, Yepez MC, Correa P. Long-term effects of clearing *Helicobacter pylori* on growth in school-age children. Pediatr Infect Dis J. 2012;31(3):263–6.

86. Sykora J, Rowland M. *Helicobacter pylori* in pediatrics. Helicobacter. 2011;16(Suppl 1):59–64.

87. Loffredo G, Marzano MG, Migliorati R, Miele E, Menna F, Poggi V, et al. The relationship between immune thrombocytopenic purpura and *Helicobacter pylori* infection in children: where is the truth? Eur J Pediatr. 2007;166(10):1067–8.

88. Rajantie J, Klemola T. *Helicobacter pylori* and idiopathic thrombocytopenic purpura in children. Blood. 2003;101(4):1660.

89. Neefjes VM, Heijboer H, Tamminga RY. *H. pylori* infection in childhood chronic immune thrombocytopenic purpura. Haematologica. 2007;92(4):576.

90. Bisogno G, Errigo G, Rossetti F, Sainati L, Pusiol A, Da Dalt L, et al. The role of *Helicobacter pylori* in children with chronic idiopathic thrombocytopenic purpura. J Pediatr Hematol/Oncol. 2008;30(1):53–7.

91. Treepongkaruna S, Sirachainan N, Kanjanapongkul S, Winai-chatsak A, Sirithorn S, Sumritsopak R, et al. Absence of platelet recovery following *Helicobacter pylori* eradication in childhood chronic idiopathic thrombocytopenic purpura: a multi-center randomized controlled trial. Pediatric Blood Cancer. 2009;53(1):72–7.

92. Russo G, Miraglia V, Branciforte F, Matarese SM, Zecca M, Bisogno G, et al. Effect of eradication of *Helicobacter pylori* in children with chronic immune thrombocytopenia: a prospective, controlled, multicenter study. Pediatric Blood Cancer. 2011;56(2):273–8.

93. Guarner J, Kalach N, Elitsur Y, Koletzko S. *Helicobacter pylori* diagnostic tests in children: review of the literature from 1999 to 2009. Eur J Pediatr. 2010;169(1):15–25.

94. Malfertheiner P, Megraud F, O'Morain CA, Atherton J, Axon AT, Bazzoli F, et al. Management of *Helicobacter pylori* infection—the Maastricht IV/ Florence consensus report. Gut. 2012;61(5):646–64.

95. Leal YA, Flores LL, Fuentes-Panana EM, Cedillo-Rivera R, Torres J. ^{13}C-urea breath test for the diagnosis of *Helicobacter pylori* infection in children: a systematic review and meta-analysis. Helicobacter. 2011;16(4):327–37.

96. Megraud F, European Paediatric Task Force on *Helicobacter pylori*. Comparison of non-invasive tests to detect *Helicobacter pylori* in children and adolescents: results of a multicenter European study. J Pediatr. 2005;146(2):198–203.

97. Yang HR, Seo JK. Diagnostic accuracy of the C-urea breath test in children: adjustment of the cut-off value according to age. J Gastroenterol Hepatol. 2005;20(2):264–9.

98. Leal YA, Cedillo-Rivera R, Simon JA, Velazquez JR, Flores LL, Torres J. Utility of stool sample-based tests for the diagnosis of *Helicobacter pylori* infection in children. J Pediatr Gastroenterol Nutr. 2011;52(6):718–28.

99. Leal YA, Flores LL, Garcia-Cortes LB, Cedillo-Rivera R, Torres J. Antibody-based detection tests for the diagnosis of *Helicobacter pylori* infection in children: a meta-analysis. PLoS One. 2008;3(11):e3751.

100. Herbrink P, van Doorn LJ. Serological methods for diagnosis of *Helicobacter pylori* infection and monitoring of eradication therapy. Eur J Clin Microbiol. 2000;19(3):164–73.

101. Crowley E, Bourke B, Hussey S. How to use *Helicobacter pylori* testing in paediatric practice. Arch Dis Child Edu Pract Ed. 2013;98(1):18–25.

102. Yanez P, la Garza AM, Perez-Perez G, Cabrera L, Munoz O, Torres J. Comparison of invasive and noninvasive methods for the diagnosis and evaluation of eradication of *Helicobacter pylori* infection in children. Arch Med Res. 2000;31(4):415–21.

103. Prechtl J, Deutschmann A, Savic T, Jahnel J, Bogiatzis A, Muntean W, et al. Monitoring of antibiotic resistance rates of *Helicobacter pylori* in Austrian children, 2002–2009. Pediatr Infect Dis J. 2012;31(3):312–4.

104. Kalach N, Serhal L, Asmar E, Campeotto F, Bergeret M, Dehecq E, et al. *Helicobacter pylori* primary resistant strains over 11 years in French children. Diagn Microbiol Infect Dis. 2007;59(2):217–22.

105. Miendje Deyi VY, Bontems P, Vanderpas J, De Koster E, Ntounda R, Van den Borre C, et al. Multicenter survey of routine determinations of resistance of *Helicobacter pylori* to antimicrobials over the last 20 years (1990 to 2009) in Belgium. J Clin Microbiol. 2011;49(6):2200–9.

106. Oleastro M, Cabral J, Ramalho PM, Lemos PS, Paixao E, Benoliel J, et al. Primary antibiotic resistance of *Helicobacter pylori* strains isolated from Portuguese children: a prospective multicentre study over a 10 year period. J Antimicrob Chemother. 2011;66(10):2308–11.

107. Liu G, Xu X, He L, Ding Z, Gu Y, Zhang J, et al. Primary antibiotic resistance of *Helicobacter pylori* isolated from Beijing children. Helicobacter. 2011;16(5):356–62.

108. Bontems P, Kalach N, Oderda G, Salame A, Muyshont L, Miendje DY, et al. Sequential therapy versus tailored triple therapies for *Helicobacter pylori* infection in children. J Pediatr Gastroenterol Nutr. 2011;53(6):646–50.

109. Horvath A, Dziechciarz P, Szajewska H. Meta-analysis: sequential therapy for *Helicobacter pylori* eradication in children. Aliment Pharmacol Ther. 2012;36(6):534–41.

110. Pacifico L, Osborn JF, Anania C, Vaira D, Olivero E, Chiesa C. Review article: bismuth-based therapy for *Helicobacter pylori* eradication in children. Aliment Pharmacol Ther. 2012;35(9):1010–26.

111. Oderda G, Shcherbakov P, Bontems P, Urruzuno P, Romano C, Gottrand F, et al. Results from the pediatric European register for treatment of *Helicobacter pylori* (PERTH). Helicobacter. 2007;12(2):150–6.

112. Oderda G, Rapa A, Bona G. A systematic review of *Helicobacter pylori* eradication treatment schedules in children. Aliment Pharmacol Ther. 2000;14(Suppl 3):59–66.

113. Bontems P, Devaster JM, Corvaglia L, Dezsofi A, Van Den Borre C, Goutier S, et al. Twelve year observation of primary and secondary antibiotic-resistant *Helicobacter pylori* strains in children. Pediatr Infect Dis J. 2001;20(11):1033–8.

114. Megraud F. *Helicobacter pylori* and antibiotic resistance. Gut. 2007;56(11):1502.

115. Gatta L, Vakil N, Ricci C, Osborn JF, Tampieri A, Perna F, et al. Effect of proton pump inhibitors and antacid therapy on ^{13}C urea breath tests and stool test for *Helicobacter pylori* infection. Am J Gastroenterol. 2004;99(5):823–9.

Menetrier Disease

13

Yvan Vandenplas

In 1888, Pierre Ménétrier first described the disease that bears his name. Menetrier disease (MD) is a rare condition of unknown etiology characterized by giant hypertrophy of the mucosal folds in the stomach. Vomiting, abdominal pain, anorexia, and edema secondary to the protein loss from the stomach are the most common presenting features. In MD, gastric acid secretion is decreased. Peripheral edema, ascites, and pleural effusion are typical manifestations of the severe hypoalbuminemia found in MD. Hypoalbuminemia occurs due to protein loss from hypertrophic gastric folds. Fever, anorexia, diarrhea, and weight loss are as well reported. MD may develop after a prodromal viral infection, including epigastric pain, anorexia, vomiting, but also raised immunoglobulin (Ig)E levels. In adults, MD is a chronic disease requiring specific therapy, while pediatric MD is typically of acute onset, transient, and self-resolving. The mean age of affected children is 4.5–5.0 years, although exceptionally MD has also been reported in the neonatal period. A young infant who developed gastric outlet obstruction by 3 months of age was also eventually diagnosed with MD, suggesting the possibility that infantile MD may be an entity distinct from the childhood and adult forms [1]. In adults, MD is an acquired premalignant disorder. Pediatric MD usually has an insidious onset and progressive, chronic clinical course, and it spontaneously resolves in weeks or months. Pediatric MD is considered uncommon although the precise incidence is unknown. Cytomegalovirus (CMV) has been implicated in several children, but also *Helicobacter pylori* (Hpyl) [2, 3], *Herpes simplex,* and *Mycoplasma* have been thought to be possibly responsible. As for Hpyl infection, given its high prevalence and the low incidence of MD, the association of Hpyl and MD may only be a coincidence. Given the transient nature of MD in children, even if eradication of Hpyl results in the cure of MD, the causative role of Hpyl would remain unproven. In case of CMV-MD, however, antiviral agents are related to a better cure. In children, lymphoma can also present with hypertrophic gastric folds. Anisakiasis (a parasitic disease caused by anisakid nematodes), granulomatous gastritis, eosinophilic and allergic gastritis, and other rare conditions such as plasmacytoma and systemic lupus erythematosus may all present with hypertrophic gastric folds. MD-like disease occurs also in animals [4].

An overexpression of transforming growth factor (TGF) and signaling via the epidermal growth factor receptor (EGF-R) have been shown to be of relevance in the pathogenesis in experimental models [5]. MD was cured very rapidly in an adult following treatment with monoclonal antibodies. There may be a genetic predisposition. A unique, four-generation pedigree has been described, with autosomal dominant gastropathy exhibiting the typical clinical, endoscopic, and pathological MD-like findings, though in the absence of protein loss and with no increase in the levels of gastric TGF-α [6]. To investigate a possible association of juvenile polyposis syndrome with MD, a new mechanism that involves TGFβ-SMAD4 pathway inactivation and TGFα overexpression related to *H. pylori* infection has been proposed [7].

When MD is suspected, other causes of albumin loss should be excluded, and upper gastrointestinal endoscopy should be performed. The endoscopic appearance is that of hypertrophic gastric folds especially in the body. Of note, the more the stomach is insufflated, the less evident are its folds. Histologically, there is foveolar hyperplasia of the gastric mucosa with hypersecretion of mucus and glandular atrophy. The foveolae are elongated, tortuous with reduction of chief and parietal cell glands and often with cystic dilatations that may extend into mucularis mucosae and submucosa. The lamina propria is edematous with increased eosinophils, lymphocytes, and round cells, and the muscularis mucosa may be hyperplastic with extensions into the mucosa. Gastric wall thickening as determined by ultrasonography is not diagnostic of MD, but serial ultrasounds may be helpful in the monitoring of the course of the disease. Investigations to exclude or confirm the presence of the possible infectious

Y. Vandenplas (✉)
Department of Pediatrics, UZ Brussel, Laarbeeklaan 101,
Brussels 1090, Belgium
e-mail: yvan.vandenplas@uzbrussel.be

© Springer International Publishing Switzerland 2016
S. Guandalini et al. (eds.), *Textbook of Pediatric Gastroenterology, Hepatology and Nutrition,*
DOI 10.1007/978-3-319-17169-2_13

agents that have been associated with MD are recommended. Management is symptomatic and treatment of the possibly causal infectious agent. MD in children is generally a benign and self-limiting condition.

Although usually self-limiting, partial gastrectomy may be needed in patients with persisting clinically relevant hypoproteinemia. Anti-EGF-R in adults has been associated with a dramatic improvement.

References

1. Fishbein M, Kirschner BS, Gonzales-Vallina R, Ben-Ami T, Lee PC, Weisenberg E, Schmidt-Sommerfeld E. Menetrier's disease associated with formula protein allergy and small intestinal injury in an infant. Gastroenterology. 1992;103:1664–8.
2. Yoo Y, Lee Y, Lee YM, Choe YH. Co-infection with cytomegalovirus and *Helicobacter pylori* in a child with Ménétrier's disease. Pediatr Gastroenterol Hepatol Nutr. 2013;16:123–6.
3. Iwama I, Kagimoto S, Takano T, Sekijima T, Kishimoto H, Oba A. Case of pediatric Ménétrier disease with cytomegalovirus and *Helicobacter pylori* co-infection. Pediatr Int. 2010;52:e200–3.
4. Vaughn DP, Syrcle J, Cooley J. Canine giant hypertrophic gastritis treated successfully with partial gastrectomy. J Am Anim Hosp Assoc. 2014;50:62–6.
5. Coffey RJ Jr, Tanksley J. Pierre Ménétrier and his disease. Trans Am Clin Climatol Assoc. 2012;123:126–33.
6. Strisciuglio C, Corleto VD, Brunetti-Pierri N, Piccolo P, Sangermano R, Rindi G, Martini M, D'Armiento FP, Staiano A, Miele E. Autosomal dominant Ménétrier-like disease. J Pediatr Gastroenterol Nutr. 2012;55:717–20.
7. Piepoli A, Mazzoccoli G, Panza A, Tirino V, Biscaglia G, Gentile A, Valvano MR, Clemente C, Desiderio V, Papaccio G, Bisceglia M, Andriulli A. A unifying working hypothesis for juvenile polyposis syndrome and Ménétrier's disease: specific localization or concomitant occurrence of a separate entity? Dig Liver Dis. 2012;44:952–6.

Viral Diarrhea

Alfredo Guarino and Eugenia Bruzzese

Epidemiology and Etiology

Diarrhea is the second leading cause of death due to infections among children below 5 years of age worldwide [1, 2], and it is estimated that diarrhea accounted for 10% of the 6.9 million deaths among children below 5 years in 2011 [2, 3]. Acute diarrhea is thus a major problem in both developing and industrialized countries, but with two distinct consequences. In developing countries, enteric infections are highly common with an estimated incidence of 3.8 episodes/child per year in infants and of 2.1 episodes/child per year in children 1–4 years of age [4]. Gastroenteritis is also responsible for a high mortality rate, and it is estimated that 1 out of 40 children will die because of diarrhea [5]. In contrast, in industrialized countries, the incidence of diarrhea is approximately 1–2 episodes/child per year in subjects younger than 3 years, and the mortality is much lower than in poor countries, although not negligible. In the USA, 150–300 infants or young children die each year because of acute diarrhea, and substantial resources are needed for hospitalizations and medical visits.

In fact, acute gastroenteritis accounts for an annual average of 35 hospitalizations per 10,000 children younger than 5 years and for 4% of all hospitalizations [6]. It was estimated that 1 in 57 children below 5 years of age would be hospitalized for diarrhea-associated illness, and the rate of out-patient visits was 943/10,000 children, corresponding to 2% of all visits.

Rotavirus is the leading cause of acute gastroenteritis [7], and it is the most frequent agent of severe diarrhea in children <5 years of age, worldwide. Rotavirus infections affect virtually all children by the age of 5 years [8], being responsible for approximately 40% of all cases of diarrhea in the USA [6]. Recent results from the World Health Organization

(WHO) rotavirus surveillance networks indicate that approximately 36% of diarrhea hospitalizations among children aged less than 5 years worldwide can be attributed to rotavirus infection [9]. Similar figures have been recorded in Europe [10], where rotavirus accounts for 55% of hospitalizations and one third of emergency department visits due to community-acquired acute gastroenteritis in children aged <5 years. The burden of community-acquired rotavirus gastroenteritis occurs in children aged <2 years with a peak in infants aged <6 months. Every year, approximately 600,000 children die of rotavirus disease, mainly in developing countries [11]. In industrialized countries, where there is generally good access to health care, mortality due to rotavirus gastroenteritis is very low. In the USA, before the introduction of rotavirus vaccine in 2006, rotavirus caused an estimated 20–60 deaths, 55,000–70,000 hospitalizations, 205,000–272,000 emergency department visits, and 410,000 outpatient visits each year [12]. Annual direct and indirect costs were estimated at approximately 1 billion dollars, primarily due to the cost of time lost from work to care for an ill child [13, 14].

Rotavirus infection is, therefore, a major reason of hospitalization in children with acute gastroenteritis [15–17], with substantial impact on health-care resources and costs. The estimate average cost for an episode of diarrhea in inpatient is US$ 2300. Costs for acute diarrhea are not negligible, particularly if the so-called societal costs are considered. It has been estimated that the cost of an episode of diarrhea requiring an office visit in the USA averages US$ 300 [18], half of which is due to the loss of working days by the parents of sick children.

During the past four decades, there has been a dramatic increase in the number of newly recognized etiological agents of gastroenteritis. In fact, since 1970, more than 20 different microorganisms (viruses, bacteria, and parasites) have been recognized as etiological agents. Nevertheless, a pathogen is currently identified in only a small proportion of cases. Although many viruses have been identified in fecal

A. Guarino (✉) · E. Bruzzese
Department of Translation Medical Science, Section of Pediatrics, University of Naples "Federico II", Via S. Pansini 5, 80131 Naples, Italy
e-mail: alfguari@unina.it

© Springer International Publishing Switzerland 2016
S. Guandalini et al. (eds.), *Textbook of Pediatric Gastroenterology, Hepatology and Nutrition*,
DOI 10.1007/978-3-319-17169-2_14

Table 14.1 Role of different viruses in the etiology of acute diarrhea in children. (Reprinted with permission from Ref. [19], Table 9.1, p. 126)

Established	Probable	Possible in selected children
Rotavirus	Torovirus	HIV
Norovirus	Aichi virus enterovirus 22	Cytomegalovirus
Adenovirus		Epstein–Barr virus picobirnavirus
Astrovirus		

samples of patients with diarrhea, their causal relationship with diarrhea is largely unknown (Table 14.1).

The viruses most frequently responsible for acute gastroenteritis in children belong to four distinct families: rotaviruses, caliciviruses, astroviruses, and enteric adenoviruses. Rotavirus and norovirus are the two leading agents of acute diarrhea. Other viruses, such as toroviruses, picornaviruses (the Aichi virus), and enterovirus 22, play a minor epidemiological role. Finally, selected viruses induce diarrhea only in children at risk. These include cytomegalovirus, Epstein–Barr virus, picobirnaviruses, and HIV.

Pathophysiology of Viral Diarrhea

In the classic and simple view, the pathogenesis of diarrhea may be divided into osmotic and secretory. Viral diarrhea was originally believed to be the consequence of endoluminal fluid accumulation osmotically driven by non-absorbed nutrients due to cell invasion and epithelial destruction by enteropathogenic agents. It is now known that several mechanisms are responsible for diarrhea, depending on the specific agents and the host features. In addition, selected viruses have multiple virulence pathways that act synergistically to induce diarrhea.

The mechanisms of diarrhea induced by group A rotaviruses have been extensively investigated and provide a paradigm of the pathophysiology of viral diarrhea [20–22]. Rotavirus has both a tissue- and a cell-specific tropisms, and it infects the mature enterocyte of the small intestine. The first step is virus binding to specific receptors located on the cell surface, the GM1 ganglioside. However, different rotavirus strains bind in either a sialic-acid-dependent or sialic-acid-independent fashion. Most rotaviruses, including all human strains, infect polarized enterocytes through both the apical and the basolateral side, in a sialic-acid-independent manner, suggesting the presence of different receptors. The early stages of rotavirus binding involve the viral protein (VP4) spike attachment and cleavage. After binding, rotavirus enters into the cell by a multistep process that requires both VP7 and VP4 proteins. Infection of the villous enterocytes leads to cell lysis, compromising nutrient absorption and driving fluid into the intestinal lumen through an osmotic

mechanism. However, the destruction of villus-tip cells induces a compensatory proliferation of crypt cells. These immature enterocytes physiologically maintain a secretive tone, thus contributing to diarrhea with ion secretion, as the result of the imbalance between absorptive villous and secretory crypt cells. Thus, the cytopathic effect of rotavirus results in both osmotic and secretory diarrhea. Histological changes induced by rotavirus infection occur within 24 h of infection in animal models.

The enteric nervous system may also play a direct role in inducing fluid secretion, similar to that induced by cholera toxin and other intestinal secretagogues. The molecular mechanisms of fluid secretion have also been investigated. Rotavirus induces an increase in intracellular calcium levels, which is responsible for the disassembly of microvillar F-actin, the perturbation of cellular protein trafficking, the damage of tight junction, with a disruption of cell–cell interaction and cytolysis.

In children with rotavirus infection, the onset of diarrhea is abrupt and occurs in the absence of histological changes, suggesting that in the initial phase of the infection a secretory pathway is responsible for diarrhea. The identification of the nonstructural protein (NSP4), an enterotoxin produced by rotavirus, responsible for fluid secretion but not for epithelial damage may explain this phenomenon. NSP4 is a multifunctional virulence factor (VF), as it possesses the following features (Fig. 14.1): It is released from infected cells and enters the cells through a specific receptor causing calcium-dependent chloride secretion. NSP4 also alters plasma membrane permeability and is cytotoxic. NSP4 is the only rotavirus gene product capable of eliciting intracellular calcium mobilization. NSP4 further contributes to diarrheal pathogenesis by directly altering enterocyte actin distribution and paracellular permeability. Finally, NSP4 plays a role in the inhibition of the Na^+-dependent glucose transporter (SGLT-1). Glucose absorption as well as disaccharidase activities are impaired in rotavirus enteritis, whereas the Na/amino acid co-transporters are not involved.

Rotavirus diarrhea may also have an inflammatory component. The induction of cytokines is important in developing an inflammatory and immune response, especially in intestinal infection caused by bacteria. In rotavirus infection, limited inflammation is detected by histological studies, suggesting that cytokines are effective in inducing a host immune response to rotavirus diarrhea. However, it has been shown that rotavirus-infected enterocytes activate nuclear factor kappa B (NF-κB) and the production of chemokines interleukin (IL)-8, Rantes, and growth related oncogene (GRO)-a, of interferon (IFN)-α, and of granulocyte/macrophage–colony-stimulating factor (GM-CSF). Recent evidence suggests that rotavirus-induced diarrhea may be also associated with an increase of intestinal motility through the stimulation of myenteric nerve plexus [23].

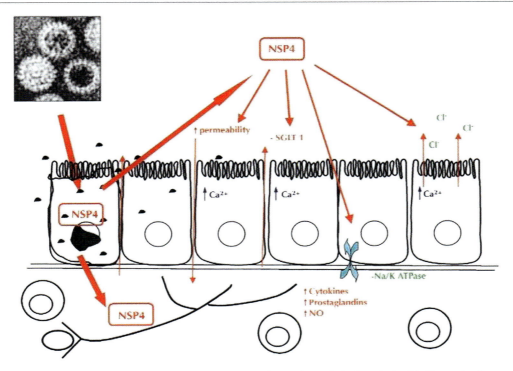

Fig. 14.1 Combined effects by NSP4 in the pathophysiology of rotavirus diarrhea. Rotavirus infects epithelial cells of the small intestine, replicates, and induces cell lysis. NSP4 is released by infected cells and functions as a Ca^{2+}-dependent enterotoxin triggering Cl^- secretion. It decreases fluid and electrolyte transport by inhibiting Na–glucose symport SGLT1 and, possibly Na–K adenosine triphosphatase (ATPase). It also impairs disaccharidase expression. Furthermore, rotavirus and/or NSP4 may dif- fuse underneath the intestinal epithelium activating secretory reflexes in the enteric nervous system. Late during the infection, an inflammatory response in the lamina propria may be detected, and the production of inflammatory substances and cytokines may further contribute to the increase of intestinal permeability and diarrhea. *NSP4* nonstructural protein, *SGLT-1* Na$^+$-dependent glucose transporter, *NO* nitrous oxide. (Reprinted with permission from Ref. [19], 2004, Fig. 9.3, p. 131)

In conclusion, the primary target of rotavirus is the enterocyte, which is induced to secrete fluids and electrolytes and is subsequently destroyed. On the other hand, the enterocyte acts as a sensor to the mucosa with the production of viral and endogenous factors and the activation of other cell types including neurons. Thus, rotavirus-induced diarrhea is a multistep and multifactorial event, in which fluid secretion and cell damage are observed in a precise sequence, as shown in an intestinal cell line-based experimental model [24] (Fig. 14.2). A summary of the multiple mechanisms involved in the rotavirus–intestine interaction is provided in Table 14.2.

Clinical Signs and Symptoms of Viral Diarrhea

Usually viral diarrhea has an abrupt onset and lasts for 3–5 days. Generally it is a benign condition with spontaneous recovery. In very select cases, diarrhea may be persistent lasting more than 7–15 days. Risk factors for persistent diarrhea in children are: young age, early weaning, malnutrition, and

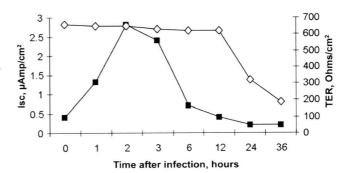

Fig. 14.2 Biphasic effect of rotavirus in Caco-2 cells. Rotavirus induces a biphasic response, in an in vitro model of infection in Caco-2 enterocytes mounted in Ussing chambers. An early secretion is evident in the first few hours of infection, with a peak at 2-h postinfection, as shown by the increase in short circuit current (Isc, µA). Subsequently, rotavirus exerts a cytotoxic effect with a loss of tissue integrity, as demonstrated by the fall of transepithelial resistance (TER) (Ohm/cm^2) which is evident at 24-h postinfection. The results suggest that rotavirus diarrhea is initially the result of an early secretory mechanism and of a subsequent osmotic pathway, due to cell damage and loss of functional absorptive surface, leading to nutrient malabsorption. (Reprinted with permission from Ref. [19]. Reprinted from Ref. [24], by Permission of Oxford University Press)

Table 14.2 Mechanisms involved in rotavirus-induced diarrhea

Mechanism	Effect
Enterocyte damage	Nutrient malabsorption/osmotic diarrhea
Crypt cell proliferation	Ion and water secretion/secretory diarrhea
NSP4 production	Increase in intracellular calcium, chloride secretion/secretory diarrhea
NSP4 inhibition of SGLT-1	Glucose malabsorption/osmotic diarrhea
Neuromediated vascular ischemia	Secretory diarrhea induced by neurotransmitter release
Inflammation	NF-kB, IL-8, Rantes release/osmotic, and secretory diarrhea
Stimulation of myenteric nerve plexus	Increase in intestinal motility

NSP4 nonstructural protein, *NF-κB* nuclear factor kappa B, *IL* interleukin, *SGLT-1* Na$^+$-dependent glucose transporter

immunodeficiency. In selected children, an acute onset may coincide with the first manifestation of celiac disease.

The predominant symptoms of acute gastroenteritis, regardless of the causative etiologic agent, are diarrhea and vomiting, associated or not to fever and abdominal pain. None of the symptoms that usually characterize the clinical feature of acute gastroenteritis has a strong predictive value able to discriminate among the different etiologies. However, there are selected features that may help a differential diagnosis of viral versus bacterial infection [25].

Children with viral intestinal infection generally have large volumes of watery stools, suggesting small bowel involvement, and vomiting and fever are more frequent than in bacterial diarrhea. Each of these features contributes to dehydration. Another feature of viral gastroenteritis is the frequent association of diarrhea and vomiting with respiratory symptoms (Table 14.3).

In contrast, the presence of symptoms suggesting colitis, such as a high number of diarrheal episodes with small amount of stools, blood in the stools, high fever, and abdominal pain is more likely associated with bacterial etiology (Table 14.3) [26, 27].

The severity of acute gastroenteritis is reflected by the degree of dehydration. The degree of dehydration should be evaluated at first observation and during the follow-up to establish the efficacy of rehydration treatment. However, high persistent fever and lethargy may be signs of a more severe clinical condition and indicate systemic involvement. Moreover, benign seizures, not related with electrolyte imbalances, have been reported for rotavirus- and norovirus-induced gastroenteritis [28, 29]. Severe encephalopathies were re-

ported in a recent surveillance study conducted in Germany on about 100 cases of very severe diarrhea [30].

When compared with other viral infections, rotavirus infection is more frequently associated with high-grade fever (>38 °C), frequent diarrheal episodes (>7/day), and long-lasting diarrhea that results in significantly higher severity scores [31–36]. In contrast, children with norovirus infection have significantly more episodes of vomiting than other viral infections, and in some cases, vomiting may be the only gastrointestinal symptom and up to 20 % of children are present without diarrhea [33, 34]. Intestinal infections due to adenovirus, on the other hand, seem to have milder clinical features [36].

Diagnosis

Most children with acute diarrhea have viral gastroenteritis. Microbiological examination is not helpful in the majority of cases and should be reserved for special circumstances. In fact, regardless of etiology, most children do not require any etiology-based treatment and therefore identification of a specific pathogen is not generally needed. Microbiological investigation should however be performed during outbreaks, especially in childcare settings, schools, hospitals, or residential settings to identify the pathogen and establish its source in the attempt to reduce transmission. Stool samples should also be taken from children with bloody diarrhea, a history of recent foreign travel, and from young or immunocompromised children with high fever for whom antibiotic treatment is considered. Finally, it is also recommended to investigate children in whom diarrhea persists for more

Table 14.3 Clinical features associated with viral and bacterial agents of acute diarrhea in children

Viral diarrhea	Bacterial diarrhea
Watery diarrhea	High fever
High volume stools	Bloody stools
Vomiting	Dysentery
Fever	Abdominal pain
Presence of respiratory symptoms	Neurological signs

Table 14.4 Indications to microbiological evaluation in children with acute diarrhea

Condition
Age <3 months
Shock or septic appearance
>10 liquid stools/day, high fever, dysentery, bloody stools
Recent history of travel
Immunocompromised children
Outbreak
Protracted or chronic diarrhea

than 10–14 days, or when a noninfectious etiology for diarrhea is suspected, such as inflammatory bowel disease (IBD) (Table 14.4) [25]. Several techniques are available to identify the specific etiology of viral diarrhea. The gold standard is viral culture but its clinical application is limited, due to the costs, the delay in the results and the complexity of the procedures. Immunofluorescence or latex agglutination is widely used to identify fecal viruses. Polymerase chain reaction (PCR) is becoming a common diagnostic tool for virus identification. Specific PCR are currently available for norovirus, rotavirus, adenovirus, cytomegalovirus, and other less common viruses.

Differential diagnosis of viral gastroenteritis may include food poisoning, which is eventually indirectly related to a microbial etiology. Food poisoning has a more rapid onset, often with vomiting and is more common in children than in infants, being related to ingestion of at risk foods. On the other hand, when diarrhea is persistent, lasting more than 7 days, a different etiology should be considered [37]. Common causes of persistent diarrhea (dealt with in detail in Chap. 17) include small intestinal bacterial overgrowth, lactose intolerance, and cow's milk protein intolerance; it should, in addition, be considered that chronic inflammatory conditions of the small and/or large intestine such as celiac disease or IBD may have an acute onset or be triggered by viral enteritides.

Specific Viruses

Rotavirus

Rotavirus is a double-stranded RNA virus belonging to the Reoviridae family. The virion, 70–75 nm, is composed of a three-layered protein capsid that encloses 11 distinct segments of genomic RNA, each coding for a different capsid or nonstructural protein. The internal core contains VP 1, 2, and 3; the inner capsid contains VP4; the two outer capsid proteins encoded by genes 4 and 7, namely VP4 and VP7, represent the only established neutralization antigens of the virus. The protective role of antibodies directed against these proteins has been confirmed in both experimental animal models and humans. A possible role has been suggested for antibodies directed at the inner capsid protein VP6, which is not associated with in vitro neutralization. The nonstructural proteins NSP1, NSP2, and NSP4 are VFs in mice. Rotavirus groups A–F have been described, but only groups A, B, and C have been identified in humans. Most human infections are caused by group A rotaviruses that are classified into serotypes by a dual classification system based on neutralizing antigens on two outer capsid proteins, VP7 (G serotype) and VP4 (P serotype). To date, 14 G serotypes and 11 P serotypes have been identified in humans. There is substantial genetic diversity within each G and P type. Predominant serotypes vary from year to year and from region to region. G1P [8] is the globally predominant strain, representing over 70% of rotavirus infections in North America, Europe, and Australia. G9 strains now constitute the predominant strains in some parts of Asia and Africa, and G8 strains are proportionally more frequent in Africa [38, 39]. In South America, G5 strains have emerged in children with diarrhea, and G9 is associated with more severe disease in Latin America [40]. Similarly, the distribution of P [6] antigen differs according to region. An example is the rapidly evolving change of serotype distribution in Africa [41].

Specific strains may express stronger VFs, which could be related to the severity of symptoms. More severe presentations may also be related to the reintroduction of strains in areas where they have been previously absent. The epidemiology of rotavirus shows a link with cold seasons with a higher incidence during fall and winter.

Transmission is by fecal–oral route, both through close person-to-person contact and by fomites. Viruses are shed in high concentrations in the stool of rotavirus-infected persons. Children shed large numbers of viruses in stool, during the acute illness but they may shed rotavirus 2 days before and up to 10 days after the onset of symptoms. The virus may also be transmitted by respiratory droplets. Spread within families, institutions, hospitals, and childcare settings is common. Rotavirus is a major cause of acute gastroenteritis in children attending child care. Rotavirus is also responsible for nosocomial infection during the winter with an incidence as higher as 3% hospitalization in a meta-analysis of 20 studies in Europe and North America [42], prolonging hospital stays and increasing medical costs. The incidence of nosocomial infection is directly related to the duration of hospital stay. In Italy, the incidence of nosocomial rotavirus-induced gastroenteritis was 7.9/1000 child-days of hospitalization [43].

The incubation period for rotavirus diarrhea is short, usually less than 48 h. Rotavirus is able to determine a large spectrum of disease, ranging from asymptomatic shedding to severe dehydration, seizures, and even death. Rotavirus gastroenteritis typically begins with acute onset of fever and vomiting followed 24–48 h later by watery diarrhea [44].

Symptoms generally persist for 3–8 days, although protracted episodes have been reported occasionally. Fever is usually of low grade and occurs in up to half of all infected children. Vomiting occurs in 80–90 % of infected children, and it is usually brief, lasting 24 h or less in most children. Dehydration and electrolyte disturbances are the major complications of rotavirus infection and occur most often in the youngest children. Studies of hospitalized children have indicated that gastroenteritis associated with rotavirus is more severe than cases in which rotavirus was not detected, with more severe dehydration, higher incidences of vomiting and higher needing of parenteral rehydration. Children with immunodeficiency, particularly those with T cell immunodeficiencies or severe combined immunodeficiency (SCID), and children after bone marrow transplantation are at higher risk of severe and prolonged diarrhea and central nervous system complications.

Diagnosis of rotavirus infection is performed using enzyme immunoassays and latex agglutination assays for detection of group A rotavirus antigen in stools. Virus can also be identified in stool by electron microscopy and by reverse transcriptase-PCR.

Norovirus

Noroviruses are single-stranded RNA viruses belonging to the family *Caliciviridae*. The prototype virus of the noroviruses, Norwalk virus, was identified in 1972. The availability of molecular diagnostic methods based on reverse transcription-PCR (RT-PCR) highlighted the etiologic role of norovirus in epidemic and sporadic gastroenteritis [45, 46]. Norovirus is now a well-documented leading agent of epidemic gastroenteritis in all age groups, causing > 90 % of nonbacterial and ≈ 50 % of all-cause epidemic gastroenteritis worldwide [47]. The impact of norovirus disease may be much greater than previously thought, and the disease may be more severe in some populations [46, 48–50].

The norovirus genome comprises a single-stranded, positive sense, polyadenylated RNA of approximately 7.5 kb in length, encompassing three open reading frames (ORFs 1–3).

Noroviruses encompass five distinct genogroups (GI-GV) with GI, GII, and GIV infecting humans. The norovirus genogroups are further divided into genotypes and variants (subgenotypes) based on the sequence diversity [51].

In contrast to rotavirus, the mechanisms of norovirus-induced diarrhea are not well defined. Many viral factors can interfere with basic cellular functions. Several observations showed that, in infected mucosa, villus length was decreased by 25 %, whereas crypt length was unchanged [21]. The villus blunting and the shortening of the villi observed in this viral infection depend on the norovirus infection of intestinal epithelial cells located on the apical area of villi. The infected cells show an increase in cell death rates with a reduction of the overall absorptive surface [52].

Evaluations of human intestinal biopsies from norovirus-infected patients in Ussing chambers showed an active Cl⁻ secretion, consistent with cystic fibrosis transmembrane conductance regulator (CFTR) activation. A reduction of occludin expression as well as claudins 4 and 5 corresponding with a marked decrease in transepithelial resistance has also been observed [53]. In addition, norovirus produces two VP, p48 and p20. The former interferes with cell proteins involved in the regulation of vesicle trafficking [54], whereas p20 impairs actin cytoskeleton structure leading to intestinal barrier dysfunction [55].

Intestinal mucosal immunity is also affected by norovirus. A recent study showed that dendritic cells were depleted in norovirus-infected mucosa associated with an altered antibody response. On the contrary, dendritic cells were required for a dissemination of the virus to secondary lymphoid tissues supporting the idea that enteric viruses can use dendritic cells to facilitate their dissemination within the host [56]. In addition, the VF1 expression enables norovirus to establish efficient infection interfering with interferon-mediated response pathways and apoptosis [57, 58]. Finally, Nelson et al. observed a highly altered gut microbiota in patients with norovirus gastroenteritis resulting in a low grade of diversity and increased proteobacteria [59]. Elevated proteobacteria is a common feature in patients with dysbiosis, and a reduction in the diversity is associated with several altered functions of gut microbiota [60].

Norovirus gastroenteritis may occur in three distinct epidemiological settings, and is associated with a broad spectrum of clinical outcomes. Firstly, food-borne gastroenteritis generally affects large numbers of healthy adults over a short time period, with symptoms typically resolving within 1–3 days [61]. Secondly, health-care-associated infection, which occurs in semi-closed settings such as hospital wards and residential/care homes, can be very challenging to contain. Elderly and compromised individuals are frequently affected and are at high risk of prolonged clinical course, typically 4–6 days, with a not negligible mortality rate [62]. Thirdly, norovirus gastroenteritis may also occur sporadically in children, where norovirus is the second most common cause of acute viral gastroenteritis after rotavirus, often requiring hospitalization [63].

Several prospective clinical studies in different geographical areas have demonstrated that norovirus is the second most frequent pathogen after rotavirus in children hospitalized for acute gastroenteritis and is more prevalent in winter. Compared with rotavirus enteritis, the duration of vomiting and diarrhea is significantly longer but norovirus infection is slightly less severe in terms of severity score and need of intravenous (IV) rehydration compared to rotavirus infection [64–66].

Evaluation and Treatment of Children with Acute Diarrhea

The initial clinical approach to the child with acute gastroenteritis is clinical evaluation. Hydration status in children should be assessed based on easily observed signs and symptoms. Dehydration should be estimated using a score system. An easy to use and reliable score system to evaluate dehydration in children is the Clinical Dehydration Scale (CDS) [67]. It consists of four clinical items: general appearance, eyes, mucous membranes, and tears each of which is scored 0, 1, or 2 for a total score of 0–8 (Fig. 14.3). Severe dehydration is an indication for hospital admission and for IV rehydration.

Indications to hospital admission are reported in Table 14.5.

Specific antiviral treatment is generally not needed to treat rotavirus infection. The current treatment of acute rotavirus gastroenteritis consists of oral rehydration solution (ORS) and early introduction of feedings, like any other form of acute diarrhea [25]. Adequate fluid and electrolyte replacement and maintenance are the key to managing viral gastroenteritis. Oral rehydration is the preferred method unless the child has intractable vomiting that would require IV rehydration. Children who are mildly or moderately dehydrated should receive 50–100 ml/kg of ORS over 4 h and should be reevaluated often for changes in hydration status.

Reduced osmolarity ORS (50/60 mmol/L of Na) should be the first-line treatment for children with acute gastroenteritis. Reduced osmolarity ORS is more effective than full strength ORS (75/90 mmol/L of Na) as measured by key clinical outcome indicators as stool output, vomiting, and need for supplemental IV therapy. The so-called ESPGHAN (the European Society for Pediatric Gastroenterology Hepatology and Nutrition) solution, containing 60 mmol/L of Na may be used in children with acute gastroenteritis as it has been used successfully in several randomized clinical trials (RCTs) and in a number of non-RCTs [25].

The second step of treatment of acute diarrhea, in children with mild-to-moderate dehydration, is early resumption of feeding after rehydration therapy. It is recommended that (1) breastfeeding should be continued throughout rehydration; (2) the usual age-appropriate diet should be started immediately after initial rehydration (4–6 h); (3) dilution of formula or use of a modified milk formula is usually unnecessary. In persistent diarrhea, withdrawal of lactose may be considered. A recent systematic review showed that lactose free diet in children who are not breastfed may result in a shorter duration of diarrhea. However, most of the trials included in the review were from children hospitalized in developed countries [68]. Hospital treatment is usually associated with enteral or IV rehydration. The former is effective and has no side effects and should be preferred. Children who are severely dehydrated with changes in vital signs or mental status require emergency IV rehydration. For children presenting with shock, rapid IV infusion of isotonic crystalloid solution (0.9% saline or lactated Ringer's solution) with 20 ml/kg bolus should be used. For children with severe dehydration without shock, rapid IV rehydration with 20 ml/kg/h of 0.9% saline solution for 2–4 h is indicated. A dextrose-containing solution may be used for maintenance [69].

There is growing evidence demonstrating the efficacy of selected probiotics as an adjunct to rehydration therapy in reducing the intensity and duration of symptoms. The guidelines of ESPGHAN [25] for the management of acute gas-

Fig. 14.3 Clinical dehydration scale for children with acute diarrhea. (Modified with permission from Wiley for Ref. [67]. © 2010 by the Society for Academic Emergency Medicine with permission from Wiley)

Clinical item	0	1	2
General appearance	Normal	Thirsty, irritable or lethargic	Drowsy, cold or sweaty; comatose or not
Eyes	Normal	Slightly sunken	Very sunken
Mucous membranes	Normal	Sticky	Dry
Tears	Normal	Decreased	Absent

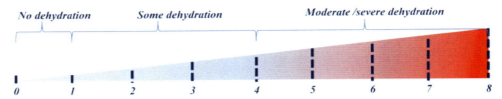

Table 14.5 Indications to hospital admission in children with acute diarrhea

Shock
Severe dehydration (>9% of body weight)
Neurological abnormalities (lethargy, seizures)
Intractable or bilious vomiting
ORS treatment failure
Suspected surgical condition
Caregivers cannot provide adequate care at home and/or there are social or logistical concerns

ORS oral rehydration solution

troenteritis in children recommend the use of two different probiotics, *Lactobacillus rhamnosus* strain GG (LGG) and *Saccharomyces boulardii* in adjunct to the ORS for the treatment of acute diarrhea in children [70, 71]. Both *Lactobacillus* GG and *S. boulardii* reduce the duration of diarrhea by approximately 1 day. *Lactobacillus* GG is particularly effective in rotavirus-induced diarrhea. In developed countries, *Lactobacillus* GG given in a daily dose of 10 billion colony-forming units (CFU) per day has proven effective in reducing the risk of protracted diarrhea and the duration of hospitalization in rotavirus gastroenteritis [72, 73].

Other pharmacological interventions have been studied in the attempt to reduce the duration of acute diarrhea and for some there is proof of efficacy. Diosmectite can be considered in the management of acute gastroenteritis as it is effective in reducing the duration of diarrhea [25]. A recent meta-analysis assessed the efficacy of Racecadotril as an adjunct to ORS compared with ORS alone or with placebo. Compared with placebo, Racecadotril significantly reduced the duration of diarrhea and the need for IV rehydration [74]. In Table 14.6, the active intervention for acute gastroenteritis is reported.

Prevention of Rotavirus Diarrhea

Vaccine development strategies are based on live-attenuated rotavirus vaccines that can be administered by the oral route. The goal for a rotavirus vaccine is to replicate the degree of protection against the disease induced by the first natural infection that occurs in infants. Therefore, the primary outcome of a vaccine program is the prevention of moderate to severe disease. Rotavirus vaccines decrease the number of children admitted to the hospital with dehydration and decrease the burden of office visits or telephone calls due to rotavirus gastroenteritis.

At present, there are two vaccines that were distinctly developed. The first one is a live-attenuated oral monovalent rotavirus vaccine derived from a G1P [8] human rotavirus strain attenuated through serial passages in cell culture. It has a two-dose schedule with the first dose from 6 weeks of age with an interval of ≥4 weeks till the second dose. The schedule should be completed by 24 weeks of age. It provides 85% protection against severe rotaviral gastroenteritis and 100% protection against the most severe dehydrating rotaviral gastroenteritis episodes [75]. The other vaccine is a pentavalent reassortant oral vaccine derived from a G6P [5] bovine rotavirus strain and common human rotavirus strains carrying G1, G2, G3, G4, and P [8] human rotavirus surface proteins. It has a three-dose schedule with the first dose within 6 weeks of age and the last by 24 weeks of age. Its efficacy against rotavirus gastroenteritis of any severity was 74% and against severe rotavirus gastroenteritis was 98% [76–79].

In 2007, the WHO recommended inclusion of rotavirus vaccine in the immunization programs of Europe and the America and, in 2009, expanded the recommendation to all infants over the age of 32 weeks worldwide. Other qualified institution and agencies included rotavirus immunization as a major priority for reduce the mortality for acute gastroenteritis [5].

The burden of rotavirus disease in the USA and elsewhere has been reduced significantly since the introduction of rotavirus vaccines.

Table 14.6 Features of interventions to be considered for active treatment of viral diarrhea

	Lactobacillus rhamnosus strain GG (LGG)	*Saccharomyces boulardii*	Smectite	Racecadotril
Stool volumes reduction	+	+	+	+
Antimicrobial effect	+	−	−	−
Single oral dose	−	−	−	−
Side effect	−	−	Constipation	Headache, vomiting, and constipation
Freely available	Not every where	Not everywhere	Not everywhere	Not everywhere
Level of evidence	Meta-analysis	Meta-analysis	Meta-analysis	Systematic review
Setting	Inpatients and outpatients	Inpatients and outpatients	Inpatients and outpatients	Inpatients
Cost	Low	Low	Low	Low
Palatability	++	±	−	+

Hospitalization rates were reduced from 60 to 93 % depending on vaccine coverage, age groups, and rotavirus season. Studies have also evaluated the impact of rotavirus vaccination on all-cause gastroenteritis or diarrhea-related hospitalizations, emergency visits, and outpatient or physician office visits, and consistent reductions were seen for all these parameters. Effective rotavirus vaccines are most needed in resource-poor countries, where mortality associated with rotavirus is high [41]. However, paradoxically rotavirus vaccine efficacy is significantly lower in clinical trials conducted in developing countries when compared to developed countries, ranging from 40 to 59 %. It has been hypothesized that this difference may be the consequence of poor nutritional status, enteric co-infections or to the interference of anti-rotavirus antibodies in breast milk which may neutralize live virus vaccine. Even considering a lower efficacy, the use of live rotavirus vaccines should be implemented in these countries to reduce the high mortality due to rotavirus gastroenteritis.

References

1. Walker CL, Aryee MJ, Boschi-Pinto C, Black RE. Estimating diarrhea mortality among young children in low and middle income countries. PLoS One. 2012;7:e29151.
2. Liu L, Johnson HL, Cousens S, Perin J, Scott S, Lawn JE, Rudan I, et al. Child Health Epidemiology Reference Group of WHO and UNICEF. Global, regional, and national causes of child mortality: an updated systematic analysis for 2010 with time trends since 2000. Lancet. 2012;379:2151–61.
3. Fischer-Walker CL, Rudan I, Liu L, Nair H, Theodoratou E, et al. Child Health Epidemiology Reference Group (CHERG). Global burden of childhood pneumonia and diarrhea. Lancet. 2013;381:1405–16.
4. Kosek M, Bern C, Guerrant RL. The magnitude of the global burden of diarrheal disease, as estimated from studies published between 1992 and 2000. Bull World Health Organ. 2003;81:197–204.
5. Guarino A, Winter H, Bhupinder S, Quak SH, Lanata C. Acute gastroenteritis disease: report of the FISPGHAN Working Group. J Pediatr Gastroenterol Nutr. 2012;55:621–626.
6. Lanata CF, Fischer-Walker CL, Olascoaga AC, Torres CX, Aryee MJ, Black RE. Child Health Epidemiology Reference Group of the World Health Organization and UNICEF. Global causes of diarrheal disease mortality in children <5 years of age: a systematic review. PLoS One. 2013;8:e72784.
7. Parashar UD, Hummelman EG, Bresee JS, Miller MA, Glass RI. Global illness and deaths caused by rotavirus disease in children. Emerg Infect Dis. 2003;9:565–72.
8. Velázquez FR, Matson DO, Calva JJ Guerrero L, Morrow AL, Carter-Campbell S, et al. Rotavirus infections in infants as protection against subsequent infections. N Engl J Med. 1996;335:1022–8.
9. Centers for Disease Control and Prevention. Rotavirus surveillance—worldwide, 2009. MMWR Morb Mortal Wkly Rep. 2011;60:514–6.
10. Forster J, Guarino A, Parez N, Moraga F, Román E, Mory O, et al. Rotavirus Study Group. Hospital-based surveillance to estimate the burden of rotavirus gastroenteritis among European children younger than 5 years of age. Pediatrics. 2009;123:393–400.
11. Tate JE, Burton AH, Tate JE, Burton AH, Boschi-Pinto C, Steele AD, et al. WHO-coordinated global rotavirus surveillance network. 2008 estimate of worldwide rotavirus-associated mortality in children younger than 5 years before the introduction of universal rotavirus vaccination programmes: a systematic review and meta-analysis. Lancet Infect Dis. 2012;12:136–41.
12. Fischer TK, Viboud C, Parashar U, et al. Hospitalizations and deaths from diarrhea and rotavirus among children <5 years of age in the United States, 1993–2003. J Infect Dis. 2007;195:1117–25.
13. Coffin SE, Elser J, Marchant C, Sawyer M, Pollara B, Fayorsey R, et al. Impact of acute rotavirus gastroenteritis on pediatric outpatient practices in the United States. Pediatr Infect Dis J. 2006;25:584–9.
14. Widdowson MA, Meltzer MI, Zhang X, Bresee JS, Parashar UD, Glass RI. Cost-effectiveness and potential impact of rotavirus vaccination in the United States. Pediatrics. 2007;119:684–97.
15. Denno DM, Shaikh N, Stapp JR, Qin X, Hutter CM, Hoffman V, et al. Diarrhea etiology in a pediatric emergency department: a case control study. Clin Infect Dis. 2012;55:897–904.
16. Pediatric Rotavirus European Committee (PROTECT). The paediatric burden of rotavirus disease in Europe. Epidemiol Infect. 2006;134:908–16.
17. Van Damme P, Giaquinto C, Huet F, Gothefors L, Maxwell M, Van der Wielen M, REVEAL Study Group. Multicenter prospective study of the burden of rotavirus acute gastroenteritis in Europe, 2004–2005: the REVEAL study. J Infect Dis. 2007;195:S4–16.
18. Avendano P, Matson DO, Long J, Whitney S, Matson CC, Pickering LK. Costs associated with office visits for diarrhea in infants and toddlers. Pediatr Infect Dis J. 1993;12:897–902.
19. Guarino A, Albano F. Viral diarrhea. In: Guandalini S, editor. Textbook of pediatric gastroenterology and nutrition. London: Taylor & Francis; 2004. p. 126–144.
20. Greenberg HB, Estes MK. Rotaviruses: from pathogenesis to vaccination. Gastroenterology. 2009;136:1939–51.
21. Hodges K, Gill R. Infectious diarrhea: cellular and molecular mechanisms. Gut Microbes. 2010;1:4–21.
22. Camilleri, M, Nullens S, Nelsen T. Neuroendocrine and neuronal mechanisms in pathophysiology of acute infectious diarrhea. Dig Dis Sci. 2012;57:19–27.
23. Istrate C, Hagbom M, Vikström E, Magnusson KE, Svensson L. Rotavirus infection increases intestinal motility but not permeability at the onset of diarrhoea. J Virol. 2014;88(6):3161–9.
24. De Marco G, Bracale I, Buccigrossi V, Bruzzese E, Canani RB, Polito G, et al. Rotavirus induces a biphasic enterotoxic and cytotoxic response in human-derived intestinal enterocytes, which is inhibited by human immunoglobulins. J Infect Dis. 2009;200:813–19.
25. Guarino A, Albano F, Ashkenazi S, Gendrel D, Hoekstra JH, Shamir R, et al. ESPGHAN/ESPID evidence-based guidelines for the management of acute gastroenteritis in children in Europe Expert Working Group. European Society for paediatric gastroenterology, hepatology and nutrition/European Society for paediatric infectious disease evidence-based guidelines for the management of acute gastroenteritis in children in Europe. J Pediatr Gastroenterol Nutr. 2008;46:S81–184.
26. Fontana M, Zuin G, Paccagnini S, Ceriani R, Quaranta S, Villa M, et al. Simple clinical score and laboratory-based method to predict bacterial etiology of acute diarrhea in childhood. Pediatr Infect Dis J. 1987;6:1088–91.
27. Finkelstein JA, Schwartz JS, Torrey S, Fleisher GR. Common clinical features as predictors of bacterial diarrhea in infants. Am J Emerg Med. 1989;7:469–73.
28. Patteau G, Stheneur C, Chevallier B, Parez N. Benign afebrile seizures in rotavirus gastroenteritis. Arch Pediatr. 2010;17:1527–30.
29. Chan CM, Chan CW, Ma CK, Chan HB. Norovirus as cause of benign convulsion associated with gastro-enteritis. J Paediatr Child Health. 2011;47:373–7.

30. Shai S, Perez-Becker R, von König CH, von Kries R, Heininger U, Forster J, et al. Rotavirus disease in Germany—a prospective survey of very severe cases. Pediatr Infect Dis J. 2013;32:e62–7.

31. Ansaldi F, Lai P, Valle L, Riente R, Durando P, Sticchi L, et al. Paediatric Leghorn Group. Burden of rotavirus-associated and non-rotavirus-associated diarrhea among nonhospitalized individuals in central Italy: a 1-year sentinel-based epidemiological and virological surveillance. Clin Infect Dis. 2008;46:e5155.

32. Kaiser P, Borte M, Zimmer KP, Huppertz HI. Complications in hospitalized children with acute gastroenteritis caused by rotavirus: a retrospective analysis. Eur J Pediatr. 2012;171:337–45.

33. Wiegering V, Kaiser J, Tappe D, Weissbrich B, Morbach H, Girschick HJ. Gastroenteritis in childhood: a retrospective study of 650 hospitalized pediatric patients. Int J Infet Dis. 2011;15:e401–7.

34. Narkeviciute I, Tamusauskaite I. Peculiarities of norovirus and rotavirus infections in hospitalized young children. J Ped Gastroenterol Nutr. 2008;46:289–92

35. Payne DC, Staat MA, Edwards KM, Szilagyi PG, Gentsch JR, Stockman LJ, et al. Active, population-based surveillance for severe rotavirus gastroenteritis in children in the United States. Pediatrics. 2008;122:1235–43.

36. Santos N, Hoshino Y. Global distribution of rotavirus serotypes/genotypes and its implication for the development and implementation of an effective rotavirus vaccine. Rev Med Virol. 2005;15:29–56.

37. Guarino A, Lo Vecchio A, Berni Canani R. Chronic diarrhoea in children. Best Pract Res Clin Gastroenterol. 2012;26:649–61.

38. Linhares AC, Verstraeten T, Wolleswinkel-van den Bosch J, Clemens R, Breuer T. Rotavirus serotype G9 is associated with more-severe disease in Latin America. Clin Infect Dis. 2006;43:312–4.

39. Page N, Esona M, Armah G, Nyangao J, Mwenda J, Sebunya T, et al. Emergence and characterization of serotype G9 rotavirus strains from Africa. J Infect Dis. 2010;202:S55–63.

40. Seheri M, Nemarude L, Peenze I, Netshifhefhe L, Nyaga MM, Ngobeni HG, et al. Update of rotavirus strains circulating in Africa from 2007 through 2011. Pediatr Infect Dis J. 2014;33:S76–84.

41. Mwenda JM, Tate JE, Steele AD, Parashar UD. Preparing for the scale-up of rotavirus vaccine introduction in Africa: establishing surveillance platforms to monitor disease burden and vaccine impact. Pediatr Infect Dis J. 2014;33:S1–5.

42. Bruijning-Verhagen P, Quach C, Bonten M. Nosocomial rotavirus infections: a meta-analysis. Pediatrics. 2012;129:e1011–9.

43. Festini F, Cocchi P, Mambretti D, Tagliabue B, Carotti M, Ciofi D, Biermann KP, et al. Nosocomial rotavirus gastroenteritis in pediatric patients: a multi-center prospective cohort study. BMC Infect Dis. 2010;10:235.

44. Staat MA, Azimi PH, Berke T, Roberts N, Bernstein DI, Ward RL, et al. Clinical presentations of rotavirus infection among hospitalized children. Pediatr Infect Dis J. 2002;21:221–7.

45. Lopman B. Noroviruses: simple detection for complex epidemiology. Clin Infect Dis. 2006;42:970–1.

46. Glass RI, Noel J, Ando T, Fankhauser R, Belliot G, Mounts A, et al. The epidemiology of enteric caliciviruses from humans: a reassessment using new diagnostics. J Infect Dis. 2000;181:S254–61.

47. Widdowson MA, Monroe SS, Glass RI. Are noroviruses emerging? Emerg Infect Dis. 2005;11:735–7.

48. Amar CF, East CL, Gray J, Iturriza-Gomara M, Maclure EA, McLauchlin J. Detection by PCR of eight groups of enteric pathogens in 4627 faecal samples: re-examination of the English case control Infectious Intestinal Disease Study (1993–1996). Eur J Clin Microbiol Infect Dis. 2007;26:311–23.

49. Lopman BA, Reacher MH, Vipond IB, Hill D, Perry C, Halladay T, Brown DW, et al. Epidemiology and cost of nosocomial gastroenteritis, Avon, England, 2002–2003. Emerg Infect Dis. 2004;10:1827–34.

50. Lopman BA, Reacher MH, Vipond IB, Sarangi J, Brown DW. Clinical manifestation of norovirus gastroenteritis in health care settings. Clin Infect Dis. 2004;39:318–24.

51. Zheng D-P, Ando T, Fankhauser RL, Beard RS, Glass RI, Monroe SS. Norovirus classification and proposed strain nomenclature. Virology 2006;346:312–23.

52. Cheetham S, Souza M, Meulia T, Grimes S, Han MG, Saif LJ. Pathogenesis of a genogroup II human norovirus in gnotobiotic pigs. J Virol. 2006;80:10372–81.

53. Troeger H, Loddenkemper C, Schneider T, Schreier E, Epple HJ, Zeitz M, et al. Structural and functional changes of the duodenum in human norovirus infection. Gut. 2009;58:1070–7.

54. Ettayebi K, Hardy ME. Norwalk virus nonstructural protein p48 forms a complex with the SNARE regulator VAP-A and prevents cell surface expression of vesicular stomatitis virus G protein. J Virol. 2003;7:11790–7.

55. Hillenbrand B, Günzel D, Richter JF, Höhne M, Schreier E, Schulzke JD, et al. Norovirus non-structural protein p20 leads to impaired restitution of epithelial defects by inhibition of actin cytoskeleton remodelling. Scand J Gastroenterol. 2010;45:1307–19.

56. Elftman MD, Gonzalez-Hernandez MB, Kamada N, Perkins C, Henderson KS, Núñez G, et al. Multiple effects of dendritic cell depletion on murine norovirus infection. J Gen Virol. 2013;94:1761–8.

57. Kim YG, Park JH, Reimer T, Baker DP, Kawai T, Kumar H, et al. Viral infection augments Nod1/2 signaling to potentiate lethality associated with secondary bacterial infections. Cell Host Microbe. 2011;9:496–507.

58. McFadden N, Bailey D, Carrara G, Benson A, Chaudhry Y, Shortland A, Heeney J, et al. Norovirus regulation of the innate immune response and apoptosis occurs via the product of the alternative open reading frame 4. PLoS Pathog. 2011;7:e1002413.

59. Nelson AM, Walk ST, Taube S, Taniuchi M, Houpt ER, Wobus CE, et al. Disruption of the human gut microbiota following Norovirus infection. PLoS One. 2012;7:e48224.

60. Buccigrossi V, Nicastro E, Guarino A. Functions of intestinal microflora in children. Curr Opin Gastroenterol. 2013;29:31–8.

61. Baert L, Uyttendaele M, Stals A, VAN Coillie E, Dierick K, Debevere J, Botteldoorn N, et al. Reported foodborne outbreaks due to noroviruses in Belgium: the link between food and patient investigations in an international context. Epidemiol Infect. 2009;137:316–25.

62. Harris JP, Edmunds WJ, Pebody R, Brown DW, Lopman BA. Deaths from norovirus among the elderly, England and Wales. Emerg Infect Dis. 2008;14:1546–5.

63. Abugalia M, Cuevas L, Kirby A, Dove W, Nakagomi O, Nakagomi T, Kara M, et al. Clinical features and molecular epidemiology of rotavirus and norovirus infections in Libyan children. J Med Virol. 2011;83:1849–56.

64. Kawada J, Arai N, Nishimura N, Suzuki M, Ohta R, Ozaki T, et al. Clinical characteristics of norovirus gastroenteritis among hospitalized children in Japan. Microbiol Immunol. 2012;56:756–9.

65. Junquera CG, de Baranda CS, Mialdea OG, Serrano EB, Sánchez-Fauquier A. Prevalence and clinical characteristics of norovirus gastroenteritis among hospitalized children in Spain. Pediatr Infect Dis J. 2009;28:604–7.

66. Gonzalez-Galan V, Sa´nchez-Fauqier A, Obando I, Montero V, Fernandez M, Torres MJ, et al. High prevalence of community-acquired norovirus gastroenteritis among hospitalized children: a prospective study. Clin Microbiol Infect. 2011;17:1895–99.

67. Bailey B, Gravel J, Goldman RD, Friedman JN, Parkin PC. External validation of the clinical dehydration scale for children with acute gastroenteritis. Acad Emerg Med. 2010;17(6):583–8. doi:10.1111/j.1553–2712.2010.00767.x.

68. MacGillivray S, Fahey T, McGuire W. Lactose avoidance for young children with acute diarrhoea. Cochrane Database Syst Rev. 2013;10:CD005433.

69. Bruzzese E, Lo Vecchio A, Guarino A. Hospital management of children with acute gastroenteritis. Curr Opin Gastroenterol. 2013;29:23–30.

70. Szajewska H, Skórka A, Ruszczyński M, Gieruszczak-Białek D. Meta-analysis: Lactobacillus GG for treating acute gastroenteritis in children—updated analysis of randomised controlled trials. Aliment Pharmacol Ther. 2013;38:467–76.

71. Szajewska H, Skórka A, Dylag M. Meta-analysis: Saccharomyces boulardii for treating acute diarrhoea in children. Aliment Pharmacol Ther. 2007;25:257–64.

72. Guarino A, Lo Vecchio A, Canani RB. Probiotics as prevention and treatment for diarrhea. Curr Opin Gastroenterol. 2009;25:18–23.

73. Guandalini S. Probiotics for prevention and treatment of diarrhea. J Clin Gastroenterol. 2011;45:S149–53.

74. Lehert P, Cheron G, Calatayud GA, Cézard JP, Castrellón PG, Garcia JM, et al. Racecadotril for childhood gastroenteritis: an individual patient data meta-analysis. Dig Liver Dis. 2011;43:707–13.

75. Ruiz-Palacios GM, Perez-Schael I, Velazquez FR, Abate H, Breuer T, Clemens SC, et al. Human rotavirus vaccine study group. Safety and efficacy of an attenuated vaccine against severe rotavirus gastroenteritis. N Engl J Med. 2006;354:11–22.

76. Vesikari T, Matson DO, Dennehy P, Van Damme P, Santosham M, Rodriguez Z, et al. Rotavirus Efficacy and Safety Trial (REST) Study Team. Safety and efficacy of a pentavalent human–bovine (WC3) reassortant rotavirus vaccine. N Engl J Med. 2006;354:23–33.

77. Phua KB, Lim FS, Lau YL, Nelson EA, Huang LM, Quak SH, et al. Safety and efficacy of human rotavirus vaccine during the first 2 years of life in Asian infants: randomised, double-blind, controlled study. Vaccine 2009;27:5936–41.

78. Armah GE, Sow SO, Breiman RF, Dallas MJ, Tapia MD, Feikin DR, et al. Efficacy of pentavalent rotavirus vaccine against severe rotavirus gastroenteritis in infants in developing countries in sub-Saharan Africa: a randomised, double-blind, placebo-controlled trial. Lancet. 2010;376:606–14.

79. Zaman K, Dang DA, Victor JC, Shin S, Yunus M, Dallas MJ, et al. Efficacy of pentavalent rotavirus vaccine against severe rotavirus gastroenteritis in infants in developing countries in Asia: a randomised, double-blind, placebo-controlled trial. Lancet. 2010;376:615–23.

Bacterial Infections of the Small and Large Intestine

15

Vittoria Buccigrossi and Maria Immacolata Spagnuolo

Introduction

Diarrhea is the result of an imbalance of ion and water movement through the intestinal epithelium. In normal conditions, the intestine absorbs 8–9 l of fluid while only 100–200 ml are excreted in the stools every day. In addition, the intestine absorbs nutrients while simultaneously forming a selective barrier to dangerous substances and pathogenic bacteria. Finally, the intestine is colonized with a wide community of bacteria that exert many beneficial functions, the so-called gut microbiota. Resident commensal and foreign bacteria interact intimately with the gut epithelium and affect host cellular and innate immune responses [1]. Enteric pathogens may hamper the physiological handling of electrolytes and water transport processes by secreting toxins that disturb the function and/or the structure of the intestinal epithelium.

A number of cellular and molecular mechanisms are implicated in infectious diarrhea induced by bacteria, viruses, and parasites. Pathogen-specific virulence factors affect a wide range of cell functions such as ion absorption and secretion, barrier function, and membrane-trafficking pathways causing fluid accumulation in the intestinal lumen.

Several bacterial enterotoxins are capable to increase Cl^- secretion and to reduce Na^+ absorption acting on apical membrane-located transporters or on the lateral spaces between cells, regulated by tight junctions (TJs); other pathogens induce cell damage targeting the cytoskeletal network which is directly implicated in paracellular fluid absorption. Invasive pathogens cause an inflammatory diarrhea characterized by an increase in polymorphonuclear cells (PMNs) in the lamina propria leading to an excess of cytokine secretion and activation of enteric nerves via neuropeptides, eventually resulting in dysenteric diarrhea. Furthermore, a peculiar class of *Escherichia coli,* the enteropathogenic *E. coli* (EPEC),

induces diarrhea through damaging the apical enterocytes, thereby reducing the intestinal absorptive surface. Whatever the mechanism, diarrhea is the manifestation of an altered movement of ions and water that follows an osmotic gradient. The pathophysiology of diarrhea is summarized in Fig. 15.1.

Intestinal Ion Transport and Barrier Functions

In normal conditions, fluid transport across the intestinal epithelial cells is a finely balanced process with fluid absorption predominating on fluid secretion. Electrolyte absorption by apical enterocyte depends on the electroneutral and the electrogenic absorption [2], which involves Na^+ uptake by the Na^+, H^+-exchanger (NHE) and Cl^- uptake by the Cl^-, HCO_3^{2-} exchangers. There are several exchangers: NHE1 is located on the basolateral surface of the enterocyte, whereas NHE2 and NHE3 have an apical localization. The relative contribution of NHE2 and NHE3 depends on their localization within the intestine with NHE3 being the main mediator of electroneutral Na^+ uptake [3]. The electrogenic ion absorption is the second major source of apical ion absorption through specific channels. Epithelial sodium channel (ENaC) is the most prominent apical Na^+ channel in the colon and allows Na^+ influx into the cell along its electrochemical gradient [3].

A basal level of fluid secretion is necessary for accomplishing the nutrient digestive functions. The cyclic AMP-dependent chloride channel defined as the cystic fibrosis transmembrane conductance regulator or CFTR is located on the brush border. This channel is responsible for water secretion in basal conditions and under active stimulation by secretagogues [4]. In the intestine, water secretion is a passive process driven by active ion secretion, predominantly by Cl^- secretion [5]. Chloride is taken up across the basolateral membrane via $Na^+/K^+/2Cl^-$ cotransporter type 1 (NKCC1), as an electroneutral process. Chloride accumulation is a passive process driven by Na^+ concentration

V. Buccigrossi (✉) · M. I. Spagnuolo
Department of Translational Medical Science, Section of Pediatrics,
University of Naples "Federico II", Via S. Pansini 5,
80131 Naples, Italy
e-mail: buccigro@unina.it

© Springer International Publishing Switzerland 2016
S. Guandalini et al. (eds.), *Textbook of Pediatric Gastroenterology, Hepatology and Nutrition,*
DOI 10.1007/978-3-319-17169-2_15

Fig. 15.1 General mechanisms causing diarrhea. Bacterial toxins can affect intestinal epithelial functions through different mechanisms. Chloride secretion and water secretion depend on the altered functionality of CFTR, CaCC, and NHE channels. Alterations in TJ structures alter the electric gradient causing the movement of both ions and water. Pathogen bacteria induce inflammation through the recruitment of immunity cells and the upregulation of pro-inflammatory cytokines. Finally, an altered gut microbiome composition (dysbiosis) supports pathogen infections. *CFTR* cystic fibrosis transmembrane conductance regulator, *CaCC* calcium-activated chloride channels, *NHE* Na⁺, H⁺-exchanger, *TNFα* tumor necrosis factor-α, *IL* interleukin

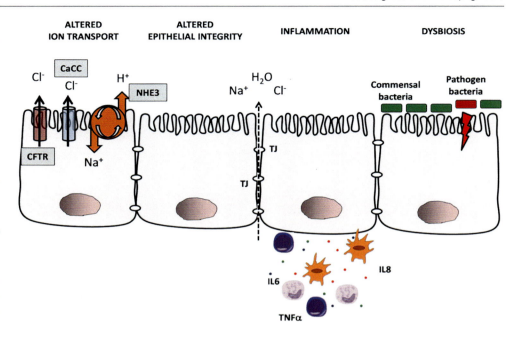

gradient which is maintained by the basolateral Na, K-ATPase. Two distinct potassium channels are located into the basolateral membrane allowing for potassium recycling thus preventing cellular depolarization, ultimately preserving the electrical driving force for chloride exit from the cell. Therefore, chloride accumulates until apical chloride channels are opened. The bulk of chloride output occurs via cyclic adenosine monophosphate (cAMP)-dependent CFTR chloride channel. However, there is an additional class of chloride channels, the calcium-activated chloride channels (CaCC), that are expressed in the enterocyte apical membrane. These channels drive chloride secretion in response to agonists of cytosolic calcium [4]. Three main intracellular signal-transduction pathways regulate water and electrolyte fluxes across the intestinal mucosa: cAMP; cyclic guanosine monophosphate (cGMP); and calcium-dependent pathways. Recently, a fourth pathway involving nitric oxide (NO) has also been described. Physiological cAMP and cGMP concentrations activate CFTR resulting in a mild secretion of chloride, whereas abnormal CFTR activation in crypt cells results in the secretory diarrhea. cGMP generally results in a more potent, though shorter, chloride secretion than that induced by cAMP [6].

The most common mechanism of bacterial diarrhea is the release of bacterial toxins. Bacterial enterotoxins activate signaling molecules such as cyclic AMP, cyclic GMP, or intracellular Ca^{2+}, which, in turn, open cellular Cl^- channels leading to an increase in Cl^- secretion and consequently of water [5]. The intestinal epithelium forms a selective barrier between the lumen (the external environment) and the body. The electrochemical gradients also depend on TJ that provide a barrier necessary for an efficient transcellular transport. The TJ also support a polarized distribution of

membrane proteins on the basal and apical compartments of epithelial cells [7]. The plasma membranes of adjacent intestinal epithelial cells are linked through the TJ, where claudins, zonula occludens 1 (ZO1), occludin, and F-actin interact. E-cadherin, alpha-catenin 1, beta-catenin, catenin delta1, and F-actin interact to form the adherens junction [8]. The loss of barrier function as a consequence of TJ disruption impairs the vectorial absorption and secretion by the intestinal epithelium. During an infection, the redistribution of apical and basal proteins provides new attachment sites for bacteria. Several bacterial toxins act on the TJ protein functions inducing an epithelial damage. At least four toxins produced by *Clostridium spp.* and a toxin produced by selected *E. coli* strains have been demonstrated to affect intestinal TJ [9, 10].

In this complex scenario, different bacterial species, each with one or more virulence factors, induce diarrhea in a specific mode. This includes the interaction with specific receptor, the release of virulence factors such as adhesion molecules and enterotoxins and a cascade of events occurring within the enterocyte.

Bacterial Diarrhea

Vibrio Cholerae

This pathogen is easily identified in the stools using Gram stain and is responsible for cholera, a potentially fatal diarrheal disease in humans. Although cholera is now rare in developed countries, it remains a major cause of diarrheal morbidity and mortality in several developing countries. Indeed, with the occurrence of calamities, the spreading of cholera infection in overcrowded refugee camps is a potential significant threat everywhere. The infection is transmitted by the fecal–oral route and is spread through contaminated food and water, the period of incubation ranges from few hours to 5 days. The vast majority of infected subjects remain asymptomatic or experience a mild disease with watery stools, nausea or vomiting, and no significant dehydration. However, cholera may be severe in a number of subjects. Stools are classically described as "rice water" due to the presence of mucus in clear stools. Profuse watery diarrhea and vomiting lead to massive fluid and electrolyte losses that can occur at a rate of 1 l/h, causing a massive dehydration.

Virtually, all cases of non-O1 *Vibrio* infections in the USA are associated with eating raw shellfish and gastroenteritis ranges from a mild illness to profuse, watery diarrhea comparable to that seen in epidemic cholera. Diarrhea, abdominal cramps, and fever are the most common symptoms with nausea, vomiting, and bloody stools occurring less frequently. As with *V. cholerae* O1, the mainstay of therapy for diarrheal disease is oral rehydration [11, 12]. In cases of septicemia (which typically occurs in immunocompromised patients), supportive care and correction of shock are essential interventions associated with antibiotics (tetracycline). *V. cholerae* secretes several toxins, but the most important of these is cholera toxin (CT). CT consists in a single copy of the A subunit and five copies of the B subunit. B subunit binds to plasma membrane, while the A subunit activates adenylate cyclase resulting in elevated cAMP production. The production of cAMP activates the protein kinase A (PKA), which then phosphorylates the regulatory domain of CFTR [5, 13]. In addition to increased Cl^- secretion, absorption of Na^+ is decreased through a cAMP-dependent mechanism in which the activity of both apical sodium transporters, NHE2 and NHE3, is decreased. This leads to an increase in NaCl levels in the intestinal lumen and drives water by osmotic force [14].

In addition to CT, *V. cholerae* produces other toxins that modulate ion secretion and alter barrier function to cause massive diarrhea. The toxins that directly affect ion secretion include the accessory CT (ACE), which stimulates Ca^{2+}-dependent Cl^- secretion, the non-agglutinable Vibrio cholerae heat-stable enterotoxin (NAG-ST), which activates guanylyl cyclase, thus stimulating cGMP production, leading to protein kinase G (PKG)-mediated activation of CFTR and, finally, the *V. cholerae* cytolysin (VCC), which creates anion permeable pores into the cell wall [15].

Salmonella

Salmonella typhi and *Salmonella paratyphi* are Gram-negative, motile bacilli that colonize only humans. Therefore, the infection is acquired through close personal contact or through the ingestion of water or food contaminated with human feces. Typhoid fever continues to represent a global health problem, with more than 12.5 million cases/year [16]. After an incubation period ranging between 5 and 21 days, these bacteria cause a systemic illness characterized by fever, gastrointestinal symptoms, and occasionally neurological symptoms [17]. Chills, headache, cough, weakness, and muscle pain are frequent prodromes and most symptoms resolve within 4 weeks without antimicrobial treatment. However, *Salmonella* may spread and invade the bloodstream and extraintestinal districts causing a systemic disease defined as enteric fever. In this case, patients relapse with high fever, abdominal pain from inflammation of Peyer's patches, and intestinal microperforation followed by secondary bacteremia with intestinal agents.

In contrast to *S. typhi*, infections with non-typhoidal salmonellae are increasing in developed countries. Patients at higher risk for infection include those with immunodeficiencies, age younger than 3 months, alterations in intestinal defenses (e.g., on those antacid treatment), impaired reticuloendothelial function (sickle cell and hemolytic anemia), and ingestion of antibiotics to which the organism is resistant. Reservoirs include a wide range of domestic and wild animals, including poultry, swine, cattle, rodents, and reptiles. *Salmonella enteritidis* is the leading reported cause of food—borne diarrheal outbreaks in the USA, with eggs and contaminated raw fruits and vegetables identified as major vehicles [18].

The incubation period is 6–45 h, after which fever, headache, vomiting, abdominal pain, and watery stools (which may contain blood, mucus, and leukocytes) appear, lasting from locus to few days. Severe extraintestinal infections can range from life-threatening sepsis to focal infections in the meninges, bones, and lungs. The microorganism is easily isolated from fresh stools or blood culture.

Clostridium Difficile

Clostridium difficile (CD), a Gram-positive anaerobe that forms spores (hence difficult to clear from hospital setting), is now recognized as the most common agent of nosocomial diarrhea [19]. In the past decade, a dramatic increase in the incidence of *C. difficile* infections (CDI) has been reported worldwide, possibly linked with an excess of antibiotics and other treatment responsible for microflora disruption but also linked with emergence of hypervirulent strains (e.g., NAP1/BI/027) and increased numbers of highly susceptible individuals.

Antibiotic treatment predisposes patients to *C. difficile*-associated disease in specific conditions [20]. The pathogenesis of *C. difficile* infection largely depends on the altered balance of the intestinal microbiota, allowing pathogenic strains of *C. difficile* to infect the intestine [21].

C. difficile causes a broad spectrum of intestinal diseases ranging from mild diarrhea to potentially fatal pseudomembranous colitis (PMC). *C. difficile* is a major agent of antibiotic-associated colitis [22] and produces three toxins, toxin A (TxA), toxin B (TxB), and a binary toxin (cytolethal distending toxin, CDT) [23]. Both TxA and TxB exert a cytotoxic effect in vitro [24, 25]. In particular, TxA and TxB induce the disaggregation of the actin cytoskeleton, cell rounding, cell death, and loss of intestinal epithelium barrier function leading to increased intestinal permeability and diarrhea [26]. CDT induces a redistribution of microtubules and the formation of long microtubule-based protrusions at the surface of intestinal epithelial cells [9] enhancing adherence and colonization of Clostridia [25, 27].

However, diarrhea is essentially due to a necroinflammatory reaction: *C. difficile* toxins trigger an extensive inflammatory cascade causing a rapidly progressive damage to host tissues resulting in fluid exudation [28]. In parallel, selected cytokines are also able to induce the activation of enteric nerves and induce Cl$^-$ secretion. The onset of symptoms may begin from several days after antibiotic therapy is started until 2 months following cessation of treatment. Diarrhea and abdominal cramps are usually the presenting symptoms, followed by fever and chills in severe cases. Mild colitis, with bloody stools and mucus, particularly if they follow antibiotic treatment, should be considered potentially induced by *C. difficile* infection. Microbial culture, latex agglutination, tissue culture assay, and enzyme-linked immunosorbent assay (ELISA) are all used for the diagnosis of *C. difficile* infection.

However, the role of *C. difficile* in infancy and early childhood is still a matter of debate. This is an emerging agent of diarrhea whose role is limited or questionable in children below 36 months of age [29, 30]. It is also a major agent of antibiotic-induced diarrhea and of severe diarrhea in children with underlying chronic conditions such as inflammatory bowel diseases (IBD) [31].

Asymptomatic *C. difficile* colonization is common in infants (ranging from 2 to 75% of healthy children) until 3 years of age and related to delivery mode and feeding [32]. Strains that usually are associated with diarrhea in adults may be detected in asymptomatic infants, and children may be a reservoir of pathogenic strains.

Many healthy children excrete *C. difficile* in their stools during early infancy, and rates as high as 45% have been detected in infants attending day care nurseries and as many as 13% were harboring toxigenic isolates [33].

Independently from the prevalence of carriers and the method to search for *C. difficile*, the incidence of *C. difficile*-related diseases in children has progressively increased in the last years, in parallel with data reported in adults, but with a relative more limited clinical impact. A recent 18-year cohort study reported a 12-fold increase of *C. difficile* infection incidence in children. Overall *C. difficile* infections increased from 2.6 (1991–1997) to 32.6 per 100,000 persons (2004–2009), with a prevalence of community acquired infection that increased from 2.2 to 23.4 per 100,000 in the same period [34]. However, a role of *C. difficile* as a severe pathogen in children at risk is supported by a solid data: For this reason, one potential alternative to standard therapy is the use of indigenous intestinal microorganisms from a healthy donor to restore the intestinal microbiota of infected patients [35, 36].

In children with chronic diseases such as IBD, *C. difficile* may act as severe opportunistic pathogen and trigger burst of the disease with a potentially severe course.

Shigella

Shigella causes 250 million cases of diarrhea and 650,000 deaths worldwide per year. *Shigella* is a Gram negative, non-lactose fermenting, nonmotile bacillus. *Shigella sonnei* is the main type in industrialized countries, and *S. flexneri* and *S. dysenteriae* predominating in developing countries [37]. The latter is the most dangerous species as it produces Shiga toxin, which can lead to hemolytic uremic syndrome (HUS). Humans are the only natural hosts and transmission occurs by fecal–oral contact. The very low infective load (as few as ten organisms) makes *Shigella* highly contagious. *Shigella* causes a dysenteric diarrhea, and the cellular responses to various steps of the invasion process are the primary cause of inflammation. *Shigella* strains cross the epithelial barrier through the M-cells where they bind to basolateral TLR4 receptor. This causes the production of interleukin (IL)-6, IL-8, and the subsequent release of IL-1β, which attracts PMN cells [38]. Nuclear factor kappa B (NF-κB) and mitogen-activated protein kinase (MAPK)-signaling pathways are activated not only in *Shigella*-infected epithelial cells but also in uninfected bystander cells [39], and this cell–cell communication amplifies inflammation. However, *Shigella* extensively disrupts TJs. In polarized cultured T84 epithelial cells, ZO-1, claudin-1, and the phosphorylation status of occludin were all affected by *S. flexneri* [40]. There is a secondary mechanism that promotes diarrhea, triggered by serine protease autotransporters of *Enterobacteriaceae* (SPATES), three enterotoxins that alter transepithelial fluid movement and cytoskeletal structure [41]. After 1–4 days of incubation, shigellosis begins with fever, headache, malaise, anorexia, and occasional vomiting and watery diarrhea with progression to dysentery within hours to days. Unusual extraintestinal manifestations may occur, including HUS in children and thrombotic thrombocytopenic purpura in adults. Most episodes of shigellosis in otherwise healthy individuals resolve within 7 days. *Shigellae* are difficult to grow and are best isolated from fresh stools rapidly inoculated into selective culture plates incubated immediately at 37 °C.

Campylobacter jejuni

These organisms are small, spiral-shaped Gram-negative bacilli that live in the intestines of both wild and domestic animals [42]. Common vehicles for human infection are poultry, unpasteurized milk, and contaminated water [43, 44]. After 3–6 days of incubation, symptoms abruptly begin. *Campylobacter* diarrhea may present as a typical gastroenteritis with vomiting and profuse diarrhea or as a colitis with abdominal pain and bloody stools, and abdominal pain that may mimic an appendicitis. Diarrhea usually lasts 4–5 days; the microorganism can be identified only from stool. *Campylobacter* vaccine development has proceeded cautiously, because of concerns about postexposure arthritis or Guillain–Barré syndrome. However, a monovalent, formalin-inactivated, *C. jejuni* whole-cell vaccine with a mucosal adjuvant has entered human trials.

Yersinia

Yersinia enterocolitica and *Y. pseudotuberculosis* are two important human enteropathogens widely distributed in the environment, with swine as the major reservoir. The incubation period is 3–7 days, with food-borne transmission. *Yersinia*'s preference for cool temperatures makes this pathogen more common in Northern Europe, Scandinavia, Canada, the USA, and Japan. *Yersinia* enterocolitis occurs more often in children younger than 5 years [45] and is characterized by fever, vomiting, exudative pharyngitis, cervical adenitis, abdominal pain, and watery diarrhea, which may contain blood [46, 47]. Diarrhea typically lasts for 14–22 days, but fecal excretion may persist for 7 weeks or longer. Abdominal complications include appendicitis, pseudoappendicitis, diffuse ulcerations of the intestine and colon, intestinal perforation, peritonitis, ileocecal intussusception, toxic megacolon, cholangitis, and mesenteric vein thrombosis. Bacteremic spread may result in abscess formation and granulomatous lesions in the liver, spleen, lungs, kidneys, and bone, as well as meningitis and septic arthritis. *Yersinia* infection can also be associated with extraintestinal sequelae including reactive arthritis, uveitis, Reiter's syndrome, and erythema nodosum [48]. *Yersinia* may be isolated from stools or pharyngeal exudates on commonly used selective media, and appears as Gram-negative colonies after 2–14 days of growth at 25–28 °C.

E. coli

E. coli is the most abundant facultative anaerobe of the human colonic flora and typically colonizes the gastrointestinal tract within few hours after birth. *E. coli* is a Gram-negative, lactose-fermenting motile bacillus of the family *Enterobacteriaceae*. Currently, 171 somatic (O) and 56 flagellar (H) antigens are recognized. *E. coli* includes a heterogeneous group of microorganisms capable to exert various possible interactions with the host, ranging from a role of mere harmless presence to that of a highly pathogenic organism [49]. Six distinct categories of *E. coli* are currently recognized as pathogens: enterotoxigenic *E. coli* (ETEC), enteropathogenic *E. coli* (EPEC), enterohemorrhagic *E. coli* (EHEC), diffusely adherent *E. coli* (DAEC), enteroaggregative *E. coli* (EAEC or EAggEC), and enteroinvasive *E. coli* (EIEC).

ETEC ETEC strains elaborate two classes of enterotoxins, namely the heat-labile and the heat-stable enterotoxins (LT and ST, respectively) [50]. LT, the heat-labile enterotoxin, is the analogue of CT and induces chloride secretion by increasing the intracellular cAMP levels. ST, the heat-stable enterotoxin, is a small peptide that causes an increase of intracellular cGMP to induce chloride secretion and diarrhea [51]. The jejunum is a major target of ST-induced anion secretion that is mediated by CFTR [27]. ST binds to its receptor guanylate cyclase C (GCC) on the apical surface of enterocytes, resulting in the generation of cGMP. This in turn activates a cGMP-dependent kinase (cGKII) leading CFTR phosphorylation [50] and the consequent inhibition of Na^+ absorption through the apical membrane of jejunal enterocytes [48]. ST does this by acting on both the apical and the basolateral side of intestinal epithelium, providing an example of a molecular mimicry between ST and its endogenous ligand guanylin, an endogenous analogue found both in the intestinal lumen and in the blood that regulates two distinct processes, ion absorption and cell proliferation [52, 53]. Transmission of *E. coli* occurs by ingestion of contaminated food and water, with peaks during the warm, wet season. Like EPEC, ETEC requires a relatively high inoculum and has a short incubation period (14–30 h). The key symptom is watery diarrhea, sometimes with fever, abdominal cramps, and vomiting. In its most severe form, ETEC can cause cholera-like severe diarrhea and dehydration. The illness is generally self-limited, lasting less than 5 days. Infection with ETEC has also been associated with short- and long-term nutritional consequences in infants and children.

EPEC This was the first group of *E. coli* serotype shown to be pathogenic for humans and responsible for devastating outbreaks of nosocomial neonatal diarrhea and infant diarrhea in virtually every corner of the globe. EPEC is characterized by specific serogroups, the most common being *E. coli* O145, O49, and O157. Some of those strains have additional virulence factors. EPEC strains are peculiar in their ability to induce a characteristic attaching and effacing lesion in the small-intestinal enterocytes and by their inability to produce Shiga toxins.

However, EPEC encode a T3SS and produces a characteristic attaching and effacing (A/E) lesion which is characterized by effacement of microvilli on the epithelial surface at the site of bacterial attachment. This typical lesion is responsible for the loss of absorptive surface and osmotic diarrhea [54]. Intestinal pathogens can disrupt the barrier by directly altering the distribution or phosphorylation status of TJ proteins. EPEC strains alter the phosphorylation status and distribution of TJ proteins, occludin and claudin-1, thereby disrupting the epithelial barrier function [10]. This increases paracellular permeability driving ion and water into the lumen upon electrochemical gradients ultimately causing diarrhea. The link between barrier disruption and diarrhea derives from studies involving the pro-inflammatory cytokine, tumor necrosis factor-α (TNFα) [55, 56]. These observations suggest that EPEC-induced diarrhea is a multifactorial process with alterations of electrolyte, solute, and water transport. EPEC causes a self-limited watery diarrhea with a short incubation period (6–48 h). This may be associated with fever, abdominal cramps, and vomiting, and EPEC is a leading cause of persistent diarrhea (lasting 14 days) in children in developing countries [57].

The microbiological diagnosis of EPEC-induced disease is performed with analytic methodologies different from those used by the standard microbiology laboratory, the most relevant being: (a) serotyping, (b) adherence assay, (c) FAS test, and (d) the specific detection of virulence-involved genes (bfpA and eae genes) using molecular biology techniques [58].

However, the cause–effect relationship between EPEC in the stools and diarrhea is hampered by the high number of healthy carriers.

EHEC It is another major intestinal pathogen that is a subset of Shiga toxin-producing *E. coli* (STEC). *E. coli* O157:H7 is the prototype of EHEC serotype [59].

EHEC adheres to epithelial cells, expresses a T3SS and causes A/E lesions much like EPEC. Unlike EPEC, infection with EHEC may cause severe symptoms including bloody diarrhea and life-threatening HUS. These symptoms are due to the production of Shiga toxin which elicits luminal fluid accumulation in the intestine [60, 61]. The predominant transmission is through the ingestion of contaminated food. Crampy abdominal pain and non-bloody diarrhea are the first symptoms, sometimes associated with vomiting. Diarrhea always becomes bloody and abdominal pain worsens, lasting 1–22 days. Fever is usually absent or low grade. In outbreaks, approximately 25 % of patients are hospitalized, 5–10 % develop HUS, and 1 % may have a poor outcome. The most dangerous complication of EHEC infection is HUS. This is usually diagnosed 2–14 days after the onset of diarrhea. Risk factors include young age, bloody diarrhea, fever, an elevated leukocyte count, and treatment with antimotility agents [62]. The most widely accepted indica-

tion for seeking *E. coli* O157:H7 infection is a patient with bloody diarrhea, in whom an accurate diagnosis may avoid unnecessary surgery.

DAEC DAEC has an age target ranging from 48 to 60 months and shows a seasonal pattern similar to that of ETEC, occurring more frequently in the warm season. The gastrointestinal symptoms include self-limiting watery diarrhea rarely associated with vomiting and abdominal pain. The diagnosis is mainly based on the DNA probe technique and on the pattern of adherence of the microorganism to HEp-2 cells. Given the technical problems of both assays, their use is limited to epidemiological surveys rather than diagnosis.

EAggEC EAggEC are diarrheagenic germs with the ability of adhere to HEp-2 cells and the intestinal- mucosa. They have been especially associated with cases of persistent (i.e., lasting ≥ 14 days) [63, 64] diarrhea both in the developed and developing world [65].

Typical clinical features are a watery, mucoid, secretory diarrheal illness with low-grade fever, and little or no vomiting. However, bloody stools have been reported. Infection of EAggEG is detected by the isolation of *E. coli* from the stools of patients and the demonstration of the aggregative pattern in the HEp-2 assay. Establishing a cause–effect relationship is hampered by the high rate of asymptomatic colonization; if no other organism is implicated in the patients' illness and EAggEC is isolated, the germ should be considered as a potential cause of diarrhea. A DNA-fragment probe has proven highly specific in the detection of EAggEC strains. Acute diarrhea is apparently self-limiting; however, more persistent cases may benefit from antibiotic and/or nutritional therapy, after susceptibility test [66].

EIEC Invasive *E. coli* strains are genetically, biochemically, and clinically nearly identical to *Shigella* [67]. They also show a similar epidemiological pattern and are endemic in developing countries. The role of EIEC in industrialized countries is limited to rare food-borne outbreaks. EIEC can rarely produce dysentery.

Antimicrobial Therapy

Antimicrobial therapy should not be given to the vast majority of otherwise healthy children with acute gastroenteritis. Acute gastroenteritis in a child without significant underlying disease is usually self-limited regardless of the etiology, which is seldom known at the onset of symptoms. Clinical recovery generally occurs within a few days without specific antimicrobial therapy, and the causative organism is cleared in a relatively short time, usually within a few days or weeks. Complications are uncommon.

Antimicrobial Therapy of Bacterial Gastroenteritis

Antibiotic therapy for acute bacterial gastroenteritis is not needed routinely but could be considered for specific pathogens or in defined clinical settings, including clinical condition and risk factors [68, 69].

Pathogen-Based Approach

Shigella Gastroenteritis Antibiotic therapy is recommended for culture-proven or suspected *Shigella* gastroenteritis. The first-line treatment for shigellosis is azithromycin for 5 days. A meta-analysis of 16 studies, which included 1748 children and adults with *Shigella* dysentery, concluded that appropriate antibiotic therapy shortened the duration of the disease. Several well-designed controlled studies have shown that appropriate antibiotic treatment of *Shigella* gastroenteritis significantly reduces the duration of fever, diarrhea, and fecal excretion of the pathogen, and thus infectivity, which is very important in children attending day-care centers [70], those admitted in institutions and hospitals. Antibiotic treatment may also reduce complications including the risk of HUS after *S. dysenteriae* infection.

WHO [71] recommends that all episodes of *Shigella* infection be treated with ciprofloxacin or one of the 3-s line antibiotics (pivmecillinam, azithromycin, or ceftriaxone). The major problem, however, is the increasing worldwide resistance of *Shigella* to antibiotics that is also being observed in Europe [72, 73]. Therefore, *Shigella* isolates should be tested for susceptibility, and local resistance pattern be closely monitored [74]. A systematic review of data from 1990 to 2009 identified 8 studies in children up to 16 years with shigellosis reporting clinical failure 3 days after treatment. In addition, four studies evaluated bacteriologic failure and five assessed bacteriologic relapse. Clinical failure rate was 0.1 % and bacteriologic relapse was 0 %. Based on these figures, which however derive from low-income countries, antibiotic therapy is consistently effective and strongly recommended in all children with shigellosis. It should be noted, however, that this finding has not been demonstrated in outpatients. Because of the high worldwide resistance, trimethoprim–sulfamethoxazole (TMP–SMX) and ampicillin are recommended only if the strain isolated is susceptible, or if current local microbiologic data suggest susceptibility. In Europe and the USA, resistance to ceftriaxone, azithromycin, and ciprofloxacin has been reported, but is uncommon. The first-line oral empiric treatment recommended for *Shigella* gastroenteritis is azithromycin for 5 days [72, 73]. Alternatively, nalidixic acid or cefixime can be administered for 5 days. When *Shigella* isolates are susceptible to (TMP–SMX) and/or ampicillin (i.e., in an outbreak setting), these agents are recommended as first-line treatment. Oral fluoroquinolones can be used in children younger than 17 years when no other alternative is feasible. The recommended first-line parenteral treatment is ceftriaxone for 5 days. Two doses of ceftriaxone can be given to patients without underlying immune deficiency or bacteremia who are fever-free after 2 days of ceftriaxone treatment [75].

Salmonella Gastroenteritis Antibiotic therapy is not effective and does not prevent complications. Rather, it is associated with a prolonged fecal excretion of *Salmonella*. Therefore antibiotics should not be used in an otherwise healthy child with *Salmonella* gastroenteritis. Antibiotics are suggested in high-risk children to prevent the risk of bacteremia and extraintestinal infections. These include neonates and young infants (<6 months) and children with underlying immune deficiency, anatomical or functional asplenia, corticosteroid or immunosuppressive therapy, IBD, or achlorhydria (weak recommendation, low-quality evidence). A Cochrane systematic review showed that antibiotic therapy of *Salmonella* gastroenteritis does not significantly affect the duration of fever or diarrhea in otherwise healthy children or adults compared to placebo or no treatment [76]. Moreover, antibiotics were associated with a significant increase of carriage of *Salmonella*, although other adverse events were not reported. As secondary *Salmonella* bacteremia—with potential extra-intestinal focal infections—occurs more often in children with certain underlying conditions, and in neonates or young infants; antibiotic therapy with TMP–SMX, ampicillin (to which 10–20 % of isolates in the USA are resistant), cefotaxime, ceftriaxone, or chloramphenicol, is suggested in these children to reduce the risk of bacteremia.

Campylobacter Gastroenteritis Antibiotic therapy for *Campylobacter* gastroenteritis is recommended mainly for the dysenteric form and to reduce transmission in day-care centers and institutions. It reduces symptoms if instituted in the early stage of the disease (within 3 days after onset). The first-line drug is azithromycin, but the choice should be based on local resistance pattern. A meta-analysis of 11 double-blind, placebo-controlled trials showed that antibiotic treatment of gastroenteritis caused by *Campylobacter* spp. reduces the duration of intestinal symptoms by 1.3 days. The effect was more pronounced if treatment was started within 3 days of illness onset and in children with *Campylobacter*-induced dysentery. Antibiotic treatment significantly reduces the duration of fecal excretion of *Campylobacter* spp. and thus its infectivity. Azithromycin is the drug of choice in most locations, although local resistance patterns should be closely monitored.

Diarrheagenic E. coli Antibiotic should not be routinely given for *E. coli*. The treatment is nonspecific and administration of antibiotic may have adverse effect. Antibiotic therapy for Shiga toxin-producing *E. coli* is not recommended. Antibiotic therapy for enterotoxigenic *E. coli* is recommended [77]. Antibiotic treatment of diarrhea induced by Shiga toxin-producing *E. coli* (STEC), also called EHEC, does not significantly affect the clinical course or duration of fecal excretion of the pathogen. Antibiotic treatment is not routinely indicated of gastroenteritis caused by enterotoxigenic *E. coli* or by enteropathogenic *E. coli*.

Most diarrheal illnesses due to ETEC are self-limited and do not require specific antimicrobial therapy. Empiric therapy is reserved for severe cases despite rehydration and supportive measures. The following antibiotics can be considered based on resistance pattern: doxycycline, TMP–SMX, ciprofloxacin, quinolones, and furazolidone. A large proportion of ETEC is now resistant at TMP–SMX, used especially for children, so an alternative regimen is furazolidone. Prevention of ETEC infection is based on avoiding contaminated vehicles. Although few data exist to guide antibiotic therapy of EPEC diarrhea, administration of appropriate antibiotics seems to diminish morbidity and mortality [77]. A 3-day course of oral, nonabsorbable antibiotics such as colistin or gentamicin (if available) has been shown to be effective [78]. Also Rifaximin [79], a broad-spectrum, nonabsorbed antimicrobial agent, can be considered in children > 12 years and in adults for nonfebrile watery diarrhea presumably caused by enterotoxigenic or EAggEC gastroenteritis.

Antibiotics are not routinely needed in EPEC-induced diarrhea, otherwise EIEC treatment is identical to shigellosis, but antibiotics are rarely needed.

C. difficile In many instances, *C. difficile*-induced antibiotic diarrhea is self-limiting, and the patient may respond simply to the withdrawal of the offending antibiotic. In more severe forms, particularly if complicated by PMC, antibiotic treatment with either oral vancomycin (5–10 mg/kg, maximum 500 mg, given every 6 h for 7 days) or metronidazole (5–10 mg/kg, maximum 500 mg, given every 8 h for 7 days) is recommended, although the rate of relapse is very high [80, 81].

The risk of treatment failure and of recurrence parallels the number of *C. difficile* infections episodes, ranging between 15 and 30% in the first infection and reaching 40 and 65% in patients experiencing a second or third episode, respectively [82]. Failure is much lower or not existent with vancomycin as first treatment.

The increasing frequency of *C. difficile* infections recurrence and the relative challenging treatment, led to the development of new therapeutic strategies including different antibiotic approaches (e.g., Fidaxomicin or Vancomycin tapering), active and passive immunotherapy (e.g., specific monoclonal antibodies against *C. difficile* toxins), and microflora restoration through the administration of probiotics or fecal donor microbiota transplantation. However, trials with new therapeutic approaches have been limited in chil-

dren. The use of monoclonal antibodies to target toxins is being considered for treatment of *C. difficile* infections and its recurrence. The neutralization of toxin activity may stop *C. difficile* infections symptoms and prevent recurrences and showed good results in adults with recurrent *C. difficile* infections [83].

This approach, that showed promising results in adults [84], has not yet been tested in children and further studies are required to establish its role in *C. difficile* infections therapy and its cost effectiveness.

The efficacy of probiotics in severe and recurrent *C. difficile* infections cases are conflicting [85], the use of selected probiotics, particularly *Lactobacillus GG* and *Saccharomyces boulardii*, has been associated with a significant eradication of the pathogen and a decrease in the recurrence of the infection [86, 87].

A recent approach for severe or recurrent *C. difficile* diarrhea in high-risk children consists in the instillation of healthy donor feces into the *C. difficile*-infected gastrointestinal tract. This technique, known as fecal microbiota transplantation (FMT), aims at restoring the normal composition and the wide diversity of gut microbiota. Current evidence (although weak) demonstrates consistent and excellent efficacy in clinical outcomes in adults. However, many questions should be answered before it may be recommended including the long-term effects (with the potential association with autoimmune diseases) [88].

Other Causes of Bacterial Gastroenteritis

Antibiotic therapy is recommended for *V. cholerae* gastroenteritis since it reduces the duration of diarrhea by about 50% and bacterial shedding by about 1 day. WHO recommends administration for 3–5 days of furazolidone (1.25 mg/kg four times per day), TMH (5 mg/kg twice per day), SMX (25 mg/kg twice per day), and erythromycin (10 mg/kg three times per day) to children less than 8 years and of tetracycline to older children.

A randomized, controlled study demonstrated that a single dose of 20 mg/kg of azithromycin is clinically and microbiologically more effective than ciprofloxacin. Azithromycin is the drug of choice for children younger than 8 years. Alternative treatment for older children is doxycycline. TMP–SMX can be used for susceptible strains. Both killed whole-cell and live-attenuated cholera vaccines have been proposed as a preventive intervention for cholera; a large double-blind field trial of the killed vaccine showed 85% efficacy for a period of 4–6 months, dropping to 50% over 3 years of follow-up. The introduction of oral rehydration solutions (ORS) [89] dramatically decreased the mortality from this illness.

Limited data are available regarding the efficacy of antibiotics for gastroenteritis caused by *Yersinia* spp., and an-

Table 15.1 Anti-infective therapy and vaccines available

Anti-infective therapy				Vaccines available
Anti-infective therapy	Anti-infective therapy should not be given to the vast majority of otherwise healthy children with acute gastroenteritis	Strong recommendation, low quality of evidence	Va, D	
Antimicrobial therapy of bacterial gastroenteritis	Antibiotic therapy for acute bacterial gastroenteritis is not needed routinely but only for specific pathogens or in defined clinical settings	Strong recommendation, low quality of evidence	Va, D	
Shigella gastroenteritis	Antibiotic therapy is recommended for culture proven or suspected *Shigella* gastroenteritis	Strong recommendation, moderate quality of evidence	I, B	NO
Salmonella gastroenteritis	Antibiotics should not be used in an otherwise healthy child with *Salmonella* gastroenteritis	Strong recommendation, moderate quality of evidence	I, A	YES Attenuated vaccine for typhoid fever, Ty21a, administered as a liquid suspension, protected both young and older children; three new generation-attenuated vaccines, genetically engineered, are undergoing extensive phase II trials
	Antibiotics are suggested in high-risk children (neonates and young infants (<6 months) and children with underlying immune deficiency) to reduce the risk of bacteremia and extra-intestinal infections	Strong recommendation, low quality of evidence	Vb, D	
		Weak recommendation, low quality of evidence	Vb, D	
Campylobacter gastroenteritis	Antibiotic therapy for *Campylobacter* gastroenteritis is recommended mainly for the dysenteric form and to reduce transmission in daycare centers and institutions. It reduces symptoms if instituted in the early stage of the disease (within 3 days after onset)	Strong recommendation, moderate quality of evidence	I, A	NO
Diarrheagenic *Escherichia coli*	Antibiotics are usually not indicated, but it depends on the specific cause and setting	Weak recommendation, low quality of evidence	Va, D	YES, but only for EHEC: parenteral toxoids and live oral carrier strains elaborating the B subunit of Shiga toxin; vaccines expressing the adhesin intimin, designed to prevent intestinal colonization, and a parenteral O157 polysaccharide protein conjugate. ETEC: oral vaccines including killed whole cell, toxoids, purified fimbriae, living attenuated strains, and live carrier strains elaborating ETEC antigens
Empiric antibiotic Therapy in sporadic cases of AGE	The choice of the antimicrobial agent depends on the local prevalence of the causative pathogens and the local resistance patterns	Strong recommendation, moderate quality of evidence	Va, B	
	In children with watery diarrhea, antibiotic therapy is not recommended unless the patient has recently traveled or may have been exposed to cholera	Strong recommendation, moderate quality of evidence	Vb, D	
	In bloody diarrhea with low or no fever, antibiotics are not recommended unless epidemiology suggests shigellosis	Strong recommendation, low quality of evidence	Vb, D	
	Parenteral rather than oral antibiotic therapy is recommended for: Patients unable to take oral medications Patients with underlying immune deficiency who have AGE with fever Severe toxemia, suspected or confirmed bacteremia Neonates and young infants (<3 months) with fever Sepsis workup and antibiotics should be considered according to local protocols	Strong recommendation, low quality of evidence	Va, D	

EHEC enterohemorrhagic *E. coli*

tibiotics are recommended for bacteremia, extraintestinal infections, and immunocompromised hosts. Production of beta-lactamases generally makes *Yersinia* resistant to cephalosporins and aztreonam, and imipenem are also ineffective. Treatment should generally last 2–6 weeks, with an initial intravenous administration (third-generation cephalosporin often in combination with aminoglycosides), followed by an oral one to which the clinical isolate is sensitive.

Antibiotic therapy is usually not needed for gastroenteritis caused by non-cholera *Vibrio* spp., *Aeromonas* spp., or *Plesiomonas shigelloides*.

Antibiotic-Associated Diarrhea

Antibiotic therapy is generally not needed for antibiotic-associated diarrhea, but should be considered in moderate to severe forms. Antibiotic-associated diarrhea can be defined as a change in normal stool. *C. difficile* is the most frequent agent of this syndrome [79]. Symptoms may range from a mild form of liquid diarrhea to a severe form of PMC with abdominal pain, local, and systemic inflammation and a typical history of diarrhea that is chronologically related with antibiotic administration. It may start from locus to 2 months after starting antibiotics.

Empiric Antibiotic Therapy in Sporadic Cases of Acute gastroenteritis (AGE)

The cause of sporadic AGE is usually not known at presentation and generally it will not be identified. The classification of these cases into invasive (or inflammatory) and watery (or noninvasive) may help deciding whether or not to start empiric antibiotics [90, 91]. Invasive (inflammatory) enteritis is defined as acute onset of bloody/mucous diarrhea (or fecal PMNs leukocytes when the examination is available) with high fever. The common causes are *Shigella* spp., *Campylobacter* spp., and *Salmonella enterica*. Antibiotics should be considered in hospitalized children and children attending daycare centers to reduce transmission of *Shigella* and *Campylobacter*. The choice of the antimicrobial agent depends on the local prevalence of the three pathogens (*Shigella* spp., *Campylobacter* spp., and *Salmonella enterica*) and the resistance patterns.

In children with watery diarrhea, antibiotic therapy is not recommended unless the patient has recently traveled or may have been exposed to cholera [89, 92]. Bloody diarrhea with low or no fever is typical of STEC (EHEC), but can be caused by mild shigellosis associated with salmonellosis. Antibiotics are not recommended unless epidemiology suggests shigellosis. Parenteral rather than oral antibiotic therapy is recommended for [90]:

1. Patients unable to take oral medications (vomiting, stupor, etc)
2. Patients with underlying immune deficiency who have AGE with fever
3. Severe toxemia, suspected or confirmed bacteremia
4. Neonates and young infants (<3 months) with fever
Sepsis workup and antibiotics should be considered according to local protocols.

Antimicrobial Therapy of Systemic Infections due to Enteric Pathogens or Involvement of Extraintestinal Organs

Antibiotic therapy is recommended for the rare but potentially severe extraintestinal infections caused bacterial enteric pathogens.

Occasionally enteric bacterial pathogens can spread and cause extraintestinal infections, including bacteremia or focal infections. These infections should be treated with antibiotics, usually through the parenteral route [75].

Table 15.1 shows anti-infective therapies and vaccines available.

References

1. Guarino A, Wudy A, Basile F, Ruberto E, Buccigrossi V. Composition and roles of intestinal microbiota in children. J Matern Fetal Neonatal Med. 2012;25:63–6.
2. Kunzelmann K, Mall M. Electrolyte transport in the mammalian colon: mechanisms and implications for disease. Physiol Rev. 2002;82:245–89.
3. Zachos NC, Tse M, Donowitz M. Molecular physiology of intestinal Na$^+$/H$^+$ exchange. Annu Rev Physiol. 2005;67:411–43.
4. Barrett KE, Keely SJ. Chloride secretion by the intestinal epithelium: molecular basis and regulatory aspects. Annu Rev Physiol. 2000;62:535–72.
5. Kopic S, Geibel JP. Toxin mediated diarrhea in the 21 century: the pathophysiology of intestinal ion transport in the course of ETEC, *V. cholerae* and rotavirus infection. Toxins (Basel) 2010;2:2132–57.
6. Golin-Bisello F, Bradbury N, Ameen N. STa and cGMP stimulate CFTR translocation to the surface of villus enterocytes in rat jejunum and is regulated by protein kinase G. Am J Physiol Cell Physiol. 2005;289:C708–16.
7. Viswanathan VK, Hodges K, Hecht G. Enteric infection meets intestinal function: how bacterial pathogens cause diarrhoea. Nat Rev Microbiol. 2009;7:110–9.
8. Suzuki T. Regulation of intestinal epithelial permeability by tight junctions. Cell Mol Life Sci. 2013;70:631–59.
9. Schwan C, Stecher B, Tzivelekidis T, van Ham M, Rohde M, Hardt W-D, Wehland J, Aktories K. *Clostridium difficile* toxin CDT induces formation of microtubule-based protrusions and increases adherence of bacteria. PLoS Pathog. 2009;5:e1000626.
10. Zhang Q, Li Q, Wang C, Li N, Li J. Redistribution of tight junction proteins during EPEC infection in vivo. Inflammation 2012;35:23–32.

11. Bruzzese E, Lo Vecchio A, Guarino A. Hospital management of children with acute gastroenteritis. Curr Opin Gastroenterol. 2013;29:23–30.

12. Pieścik-Lech M, Shamir R, Guarino A, Szajewska H. Review article: the management of acute gastroenteritis in children. Aliment Pharmacol Ther. 2013;37:289–303.

13. Vanden Broeck D, Horvath C, De Wolf MJS. *Vibrio cholerae*: cholera toxin. Int J Biochem Cell Biol. 2007;39:1771–5.

14. Subramanya SB, Rajendran VM, Srinivasan P, Nanda Kumar NS, Ramakrishna BS, Binder HJ. Differential regulation of cholera toxin-inhibited Na–H exchange isoforms by butyrate in rat ileum. Am J Physiol Gastrointest Liver Physiol. 2007;293:G857–63.

15. Hodges K, Gill R. Infectious diarrhea: cellular and molecular mechanisms. Gut Microbes. 2010;1:4–21.

16. Farmakiotis D, Varughese J, Sue P, Andrews P, Brimmage M, Dobroszycki J, Coyle CM. Typhoid fever in an inner city hospital: a 5-year retrospective review. J Travel Med. 2013;20:17–21.

17. Pach A, Tabbusam G, Khan MI, Suhag Z, Hussain I, Hussain E, Mumtaz U, Haq IU, Tahir R, Mirani A, Yousafzai A, Sahastrabuddhe S, Ochiai RL, Soofi S, Clemens JD, Favorov MO, Bhutta ZA. Formative research and development of an evidence-based communication strategy: the introduction of Vi typhoid fever vaccine among school-aged children in Karachi, Pakistan. J Health Commun. 2013;18:306–24.

18. Centers for Disease Control and Prevention. Surveillance for foodborne disease outbreaks—United States, 2009–2010. Morb Mortal Wkly Rep. 2013;62:41–7.

19. Kyne L, Hamel MB, Polavaram R, Kelly CP. Health care costs and mortality associated with nosocomial diarrhea due to *Clostridium difficile*. Clin Infect Dis. 2002;34:346–53.

20. Ng KM, Ferreyra JA, Higginbottom SK, Lynch JB, Kashyap PC, Gopinath S, Naidu N, Choudhury B, Weimer BC, Monack DM, Sonnenburg JL. Microbiota-liberated host sugars facilitate post-antibiotic expansion of enteric pathogens. Nature 2013;502:96–9.

21. Peniche AG, Savidge TC, Dann SM. Recent insights into *Clostridium difficile* pathogenesis. Curr Opin Infect Dis. 2013;26:447–53.

22. Knight CL, Surawicz CM. *Clostridium difficile* infection. Med Clin North Am. 2013;97:523–36, ix.

23. Perelle S, Gibert M, Bourlioux P, Corthier G, Popoff MR. Production of a complete binary toxin (actin-specific ADP-ribosyltransferase) by *Clostridium difficile* CD196. Infect Immun. 1997;65:1402–7.

24. Kasendra M, Barrile R, Leuzzi R, Soriani M. *Clostridium difficile* toxins facilitate bacterial colonization by modulating the fence and gate function of colonic epithelium. J Infect Dis. 2014;209(7):1095–104.

25. Li S, Shi L, Yang Z, Feng H. Cytotoxicity of *Clostridium difficile* toxin B does not require cysteine protease-mediated autocleavage and release of the glucosyltransferase domain into the host cell cytosol. Pathog Dis. 2013;67:11–8.

26. Voth DE, Ballard JD. *Clostridium difficile* toxins: mechanism of action and role in disease. Clin Microbiol Rev. 2005;18:247–63.

27. Fasano A. Toxins and the gut: role in human disease. Gut 2002;50(Suppl 3):III9–14.

28. Shen A. *Clostridium difficile* toxins: mediators of inflammation. J Innate Immun. 2012;4:149–58.

29. Lo Vecchio A, Zacur GM. *Clostridium difficile* infection: an update on epidemiology, risk factors, and therapeutic options. Curr Opin Gastroenterol. 2012;28:1–9.

30. Lo Vecchio A, Giannattasio A, Duggan C, De Masi S, Ortisi MT, Parola L, Guarino A. Evaluation of the quality of guidelines for acute gastroenteritis in children with the AGREE instrument. J Pediatr Gastroenterol Nutr. 2011;52:183–9.

31. Pascarella F, Martinelli M, Miele E, Del Pezzo M, Roscetto E, Staiano A. Impact of *Clostridium difficile* infection on pediatric inflammatory bowel disease. J Pediatr. 2009;154:854–8.

32. Azad MB, Konya T, Maughan H, Guttman DS, Field CJ, Chari RS, Sears MR, Becker AB, Scott JA, Kozyrskyj AL. Gut microbiota of healthy Canadian infants: profiles by mode of delivery and infant diet at 4 months. CMAJ. 2013;185:385–94.

33. Rousseau C, Poilane I, De Pontual L, Maherault A-C, Le Monnier A, Collignon A. *Clostridium difficile* carriage in healthy infants in the community: a potential reservoir for pathogenic strains. Clin Infect Dis. 2012;55:1209–15.

34. Khanna S, Baddour LM, Huskins WC, Kammer PP, Faubion WA, Zinsmeister AR, Harmsen WS, Pardi DS. The epidemiology of *Clostridium difficile* infection in children: a population-based study. Clin Infect Dis. 2013;56:1401–6.

35. Gough E, Shaikh H, Manges AR. Systematic review of intestinal microbiota transplantation (fecal bacteriotherapy) for recurrent *Clostridium difficile* infection. Clin Infect Dis. 2011;53:994–1002.

36. Brandt LJ. American Journal of Gastroenterology Lecture: intestinal microbiota and the role of fecal microbiota transplant (FMT) in treatment of *C. difficile* infection. Am J Gastroenterol. 2013;108:177–85.

37. Centers for Disease Control and Prevention. Preliminary Food-Net Data on the incidence of infection with pathogens transmitted commonly through food—10 States, 2008. Morb Mortal Wkly Rep. 2009;58:333–7.

38. Ashida H, Ogawa M, Mimuro H, Kobayashi T, Sanada T, Sasakawa C. Shigella are versatile mucosal pathogens that circumvent the host innate immune system. Curr Opin Immunol. 2011;23:448–55.

39. Kasper CA, Sorg I, Schmutz C, Tschon T, Wischnewski H, Kim ML, Arrieumerlou C. Cell-cell propagation of NF-κB transcription factor and MAP kinase activation amplifies innate immunity against bacterial infection. Immunity 2010;33:804–16.

40. Guttman JA, Finlay BB. Tight junctions as targets of infectious agents. Biochim Biophys Acta. 2009;1788:832–41.

41. Al-Hasani K, Henderson IR, Sakellaris H, Rajakumar K, Grant T, Nataro JP, Robins-Browne R, Adler B. The sigA gene which is borne on the she pathogenicity island of *Shigella flexneri* 2a encodes an exported cytopathic protease involved in intestinal fluid accumulation. Infect Immun. 2000;68:2457–63.

42. Andrzejewska M, Szczepańska B, Klawe JJ, Spica D, Chudzińska M. Prevalence of *Campylobacter jejuni* and *Campylobacter coli* species in cats and dogs from Bydgoszcz (Poland) region. Pol J Vet Sci. 2013;16:115–20.

43. Bahrndorff S, Rangstrup-Christensen L, Nordentoft S, Hald B. Foodborne disease prevention and broiler chickens with reduced *Campylobacter* infection. Emerg Infect Dis. 2013;19:425–30.

44. Gharst G, Oyarzabal OA, Hussain SK. Review of current methodologies to isolate and identify *Campylobacter* spp. from foods. J Microbiol Methods. 2013;95:84–92.

45. Metchock B, Lonsway DR, Carter GP, Lee LA, McGowan JE. Yersinia enterocolitica: a frequent seasonal stool isolate from children at an urban hospital in the southeast United States. J Clin Microbiol. 1991;29:2868–9.

46. Zheng H, Sun Y, Lin S, Mao Z, Jiang B. Yersinia enterocolitica infection in diarrheal patients. Eur J Clin Microbiol Infect Dis. 2008;27:741–52.

47. Rosner BM, Werber D, Höhle M, Stark K. Clinical aspects and self-reported symptoms of sequelae of *Yersinia enterocolitica* infections in a population-based study, Germany 2009–2010. BMC Infect Dis. 2013;13:236.

48. Ebringer R, Colthorpe D, Burden G, Hindley C, Ebringer A. *Yersinia enterocolitica* biotype I. Diarrhoea and episodes of HLA B27 related ocular and rheumatic inflammatory disease in South-East England. Scand J Rheumatol. 1982;11:171–6.

49. Kaper JB, Nataro JP, Mobley HL. Pathogenic *Escherichia coli*. Nat Rev Microbiol. 2004;2:123–40.

50. Weiglmeier PR, Rösch P, Berkner H. Cure and curse: *E. coli* heat-stable enterotoxin and its receptor guanylyl cyclase C. Toxins (Basel). 2010;2:2213–29.

51. Sato T, Shimonishi Y. Structural features of *Escherichia coli* heat-stable enterotoxin that activates membrane-associated guanylyl cyclase. J Pept Res. 2004;63:200–6.

52. Albano F, De Marco G, Berni Canani R, Cirillo P, Buccigrossi V, Giannella R, Guarino A. Guanylin and *E. coli* heat-stable enterotoxin induce chloride secretion through direct interaction with basolateral compartment of rat and human colonic cells. Pediatr Res. 2005;58:159–63.

53. Buccigrossi V, Armellino C, Ruberto E, Barone MV, Marco GDE, Esposito C, Guarino A. Polar effects on ion transport and cell proliferation induced by GC-C ligands in intestinal epithelial cells. Pediatr Res. 2011;69:17–22.

54. Phillips AD, Giròn J, Hicks S, Dougan G, Frankel G. Intimin from enteropathogenic *Escherichia coli* mediates remodelling of the eukaryotic cell surface. Microbiology 2000;146(Pt 6):1333–44.

55. Martínez C, Lobo B, Pigrau M, Ramos L, González-Castro AM, Alonso C, Guilarte M, Guilá M, de Torres I, Azpiroz F, Santos J, Vicario M. Diarrhoea-predominant irritable bowel syndrome: an organic disorder with structural abnormalities in the jejunal epithelial barrier. Gut 2013;62:1160–8.

56. Turner JR. Molecular basis of epithelial barrier regulation: from basic mechanisms to clinical application. Am J Pathol. 2006;169:1901–9.

57. Turck D, Bernet J-P, Marx J, Kempf H, Giard P, Walbaum O, Lacombe A, Rembert F, Toursel F, Bernasconi P, Gottrand F, McFarland L V, Bloch K. Incidence and risk factors of oral antibiotic-associated diarrhea in an outpatient pediatric population. J Pediatr Gastroenterol Nutr. 2003;37:22–6.

58. Vidal JE, Canizález-Román A, Gutiérrez-Jiménez J, Navarro-García F. Molecular pathogenesis, epidemiology and diagnosis of enteropathogenic *Escherichia coli*. Salud Publica Mex. 2007;49:376–86.

59. Slutsker L, Ries AA, Greene KD, Wells JG, Hutwagner L, Griffin PM. *Escherichia coli* O157:H7 diarrhea in the United States: clinical and epidemiologic features. Ann Intern Med. 1997;126:505–13.

60. Ferreira AJ, Elias WP, Pelayo JS, Giraldi R, Pedroso MZ, Scaletsky IC. Culture supernatant of Shiga toxin-producing *Escherichia coli* strains provoke fluid accumulation in rabbit ileal loops. FEMS Immunol Med Microbiol. 1997;19:285–8.

61. Hauf N, Chakraborty T. Suppression of NF-kappa B activation and proinflammatory cytokine expression by Shiga toxin-producing *Escherichia coli*. J Immunol. 2003;170:2074–82.

62. Wittenberg DF. Management guidelines for acute infective diarrhoea/gastroenteritis in infants. S Afr Med J. 2012;102:104–7.

63. Guarino A, Lo Vecchio A, Berni Canani R. Chronic diarrhoea in children. Best Pract Res Clin Gastroenterol. 2012;26:649–61.

64. Henry FJ, Udoy AS, Wanke CA, Aziz KM. Epidemiology of persistent diarrhea and etiologic agents in Mirzapur, Bangladesh. Acta Paediatr Suppl. 1992;381:27–31.

65. Maluta RP, Fairbrother JM, Stella AE, Rigobelo EC, Martinez R, Avila FA de. Potentially pathogenic *Escherichia coli* in healthy, pasture-raised sheep on farms and at the abattoir in Brazil. Vet Microbiol. 2013;S 0378:591–9.

66. Pruvost I, Dubos F, Chazard E, Hue V, Duhamel A, Martinot A. The value of body weight measurement to assess dehydration in children. PLoS One. 2013;8:e55063.

67. Lindsay BR, Chakraborty S, Harro C, Li S, Nataro JP, Sommerfelt H, Sack DA, Stine OC. Quantitative PCR and culture evaluation for Enterotoxigenic *E. coli* (ETEC) associated diarrhea in volunteers. FEMS Microbiol Lett. 2014;352(1):25–31.

68. Valentini D, Vittucci AC, Grandin A, Tozzi AE, Russo C, Onori M, Menichella D, Bartuli A, Villani A. Coinfection in acute gastroenteritis predicts a more severe clinical course in children. Eur J Clin Microbiol Infect Dis. 2013;32:909–15.

69. Abba K, Sinfield R, Hart CA, Garner P. Antimicrobial drugs for persistent diarrhoea of unknown or non-specific cause in children

70. under six in low and middle income countries: systematic review of randomized controlled trials. BMC Infect Dis. 2009;9:24.

70. Van den Berg J, Berger MY. Guidelines on acute gastroenteritis in children: a critical appraisal of their quality and applicability in primary care. BMC Fam Pract. 2011;12:134.

71. World Health Organization. Guidelines for the control of shigellosis, including epidemics due to *Shigella dysenteriae* type 1. Geneva: WHO; 2005.

72. Centers for Disease Control and Prevention. Notes from the field: emergence of *Shigella flexneri* 2a resistant to ceftriaxone and ciprofloxacin—South Carolina, October 2010. Morb Mortal Wkly Rep. 2010;59:1619.

73. Boumghar-Bourtchai L, Mariani-Kurkdjian P, Bingen E, Filliol I, Dhalluin A, Ifrane SA, Weill F-X, Leclercq R. Macrolide-resistant *Shigella sonnei*. Emerg Infect Dis. 2008;14:1297–9.

74. Vrints M, Mairiaux E, Van Meervenne E, Collard J-M, Bertrand S. Surveillance of antibiotic susceptibility patterns among *Shigella sonnei* strains isolated in Belgium during the 18-year period 1990 to 2007. J Clin Microbiol. 2009;47:1379–85.

75. Varsano I, Eidlitz-Marcus T, Nussinovitch M, Elian I. Comparative efficacy of ceftriaxone and ampicillin for treatment of severe shigellosis in children. J Pediatr. 1991;118:627–32.

76. Onwuezobe IA, Oshun PO, Odigwe CC. Antimicrobials for treating symptomatic non-typhoidal Salmonella infection. Cochrane Database Syst Rev. 2012;11:CD001167.

77. Tahan S, Morais MB, Wehba J, Scaletsky ICA, Machado AMO, Silva LQCD, Fagundes Neto U. A randomized double-blind clinical trial of the effect of non-absorbable oral polymyxin on infants with severe infectious diarrhea. Braz J Med Biol Res. 2007;40:209–19.

78. Medina A, Horcajo P, Jurado S, De la Fuente R, Ruiz-Santa-Quiteria JA, Domínguez-Bernal G, Orden JA. Phenotypic and genotypic characterization of antimicrobial resistance in enterohemorrhagic *Escherichia coli* and atypical enteropathogenic *E. coli* strains from ruminants. J Vet Diagn Invest. 2011;23:91–5.

79. Trehan I, Shulman RJ, Ou C-N, Maleta K, Manary MJ. A randomized, double-blind, placebo-controlled trial of rifaximin, a nonabsorbable antibiotic, in the treatment of tropical enteropathy. Am J Gastroenterol. 2009;104:2326–33.

80. Pathela P, Zahid Hasan K, Roy E, Huq F, Kasem Siddique A, Bradley Sack R. Diarrheal illness in a cohort of children 0–2 years of age in rural Bangladesh: I. Incidence and risk factors. Acta Paediatr. 2006;95:430–7.

81. Nylund CM, Goudie A, Garza JM, Fairbrother G, Cohen MB. *Clostridium difficile* infection in hospitalized children in the United States. Arch Pediatr Adolesc Med. 2011;165:451–7.

82. Brandt LJ, Aroniadis OC, Mellow M, Kanatzar A, Kelly C, Park T, Stollman N, Rohlke F, Surawicz C. Long-term follow-up of colonoscopic fecal microbiota transplant for recurrent *Clostridium difficile* infection. Am J Gastroenterol. 2012;107:1079–87.

83. Lo Vecchio A, Della Ventura B, Nicastro E. *Clostridium difficile* antibodies: a patent evaluation (WO2013028810). Expert Opin Ther Pat. 2013;23:1635–40.

84. Lowy I, Molrine DC, Leav BA, Blair BM, Baxter R, Gerding DN, Nichol G, Thomas WD, Leney M, Sloan S, Hay CA, Ambrosino DM. Treatment with monoclonal antibodies against *Clostridium difficile* toxins. N Engl J Med. 2010;362:197–205.

85. Goldenberg JZ, Ma SSY, Saxton JD, Martzen MR, Vandvik PO, Thorlund K, Guyatt GH, Johnston BC. Probiotics for the prevention of *Clostridium difficile*-associated diarrhea in adults and children. Cochrane Database Syst Rev. 2013;5:CD006095.

86. Vanderhoof JA, Whitney DB, Antonson DL, Hanner TL, Lupo J V, Young RJ. Lactobacillus GG in the prevention of antibiotic-associated diarrhea in children. J Pediatr. 1999;135:564–8.

87. Pieścik-Lech M, Urbańska M, Szajewska H. Lactobacillus GG (LGG) and smectite versus LGG alone for acute gastroenteritis:

a double-blind, randomized controlled trial. Eur J Pediatr. 2013;172:247–53.

88. Lo Vecchio A, Cohen MB. Fecal microbiota transplantation for *Clostridium difficile* infection: benefits and barriers. Curr Opin Gastroenterol. 2014;30:47–53.

89. Wadhwa N, Natchu UCM, Sommerfelt H, Strand TA, Kapoor V, Saini S, Kainth US, Bhatnagar S. ORS containing zinc does not reduce duration or stool volume of acute diarrhea in hospitalized children. J Pediatr Gastroenterol Nutr. 2011;53:161–7.

90. Umamaheswari B, Biswal N, Adhisivam B, Parija SC, Srinivasan S. Persistent diarrhea: risk factors and outcome. Indian J Pediatr. 2010;77:885–8.

91. Wiegering V, Kaiser J, Tappe D, Weissbrich B, Morbach H, Girschick HJ. Gastroenteritis in childhood: a retrospective study of 650 hospitalized pediatric patients. Int J Infect Dis. 2011;15:e401–7.

92. World Health Organization. The treatment of diarrhoea—a manual for physicians and other senior health workers. Geneva: WHO; 2005.

Intestinal Parasites

Margot L. Herman and Christina M. Surawicz

Introduction

Parasitic infections of the gastrointestinal (GI) tract have a large impact on the health of children worldwide, with increased morbidity and mortality, especially in developing countries and in the setting of immune suppression. Many parasites such as *Giardia* and *Trichuris* (pinworm) are common in both developed and developing countries, while others occur mostly in developing countries.

The worldwide distribution of food has increased the spread of some parasites as well as bacterial pathogens. In developed countries, one must always consider parasitic infection in returning travelers and those emigrating from developing countries. Clinicians must be familiar with parasites, their mode of transmission, and clinical presentations. In addition to the symptoms they cause, parasitic infections can lead to growth retardation, malnutrition, and vitamin deficiencies. Moreover, parasitic infections can be even more deadly in the setting of immune suppression such as human immunodeficiency virus (HIV) infection, steroids, or cancer chemotherapy.

In this chapter, we review parasites that affect the GI tract. There are effective therapies for most of these parasites. Understanding mechanisms of transmission is important as the main modes of transmission are fecal–oral and via contaminated soil (i.e., hookworm). Prevention with improved sanitation, clean water, proper hygiene, and footwear worldwide could lead to significant improvement in children's health.

C. M. Surawicz (✉) · M. L. Herman
Division of Gastroenterology, Department of Medicine, University of Washington School of Medicine, 325 9th Ave, PO Box 359773, Seattle, WA 98104, USA
e-mail: surawicz@uw.edu

M. L. Herman
e-mail: mherman@medicine.washington.edu

Protozoa

Protozoa are a large group of single-cell eukaryotes that can live and multiply within human hosts. *Giardia, Entamoeba, Dientamoeba,* and *Blastocystis* are the most common human protozoan pathogens.

Flagellates and Ameba

Giardia lamblia

Giardia lamblia (*G. intestinalis* or *G. duodenalis*) is the most common intestinal protozoan infection in the USA [1]. It is also the most common cause of prolonged GI infection in persons returning to the USA after travel abroad [2]. It is most often diagnosed in children ages 1–9, and rates increase from infancy until tapering off in early adolescence [1].

Giardia is one of several flagellated protozoa that cause human disease. It has two life forms, the nonmotile, stable cyst form, which is responsible for transmitting the infection, and the motile trophozoite form that is responsible for causing the clinical symptoms. The cysts can remain dormant in contaminated water or feces until they are consumed, where activation (excystation) occurs from exposure to gastric acidity, causing cysts to rupture. The trophozoites emerge and then adhere to the enterocytes in the duodenum and jejunum [3]. Transmission is fecal–oral and typically occurs after consumption of water or food contaminated with human feces. However, high rates of transmission in daycare settings where there is direct contact with feces is also common [1]. Transmission from animals is rare. *Giardia* is highly contagious and only requires consumption of as few as ten cysts [4].

Giardia is a much more common pathogen in developing countries with high rates of infection and reinfection. Interestingly, in these settings, the presence of *Giardia* in stool has been found to be associated with a protective effect from developing acute diarrheal illness, implying that one can de-

© Springer International Publishing Switzerland 2016
S. Guandalini et al. (eds.), *Textbook of Pediatric Gastroenterology, Hepatology and Nutrition,*
DOI 10.1007/978-3-319-17169-2_16

velop immunity to this pathogen and the presence of active *Giardia* infestation may protect from other infections [4]. Despite this, chronic *Giardia* infection remains a significant problem as it can lead to malnutrition and developmental consequences.

Acute giardiasis is usually a self-limited illness composed of bloating, diarrhea, abdominal cramping, nausea, flatulence, and occasionally malabsorption and steatorrhea. Additionally, *Giardia* can develop into a chronic diarrhea that can lead to protein losing enteropathy with weight loss, chronic fatigue, and other related symptoms. This is often accompanied by small intestinal changes such as intraepithelial lymphocytosis and brush-border damage, with ~ 10 % of cases developing villous atrophy [3]. Of note, giardiasis does not cause eosinophilia, stool leukocytosis, or bloody diarrhea [5].

The diagnosis can be made in several different ways. Traditionally, identification was made with stool microscopy demonstrating trophozoites or cysts. However, the sensitivity and specificity ranges from 70 to 85 % with one to three samples, respectively, and this testing is much more labor intensive, less efficient, and requires specific expertise. Stool microscopy has now been displaced in many centers by use of stool antigen detection assays, whose sensitivity and specificity approach 100 % and only one sample is required [5, 6]. Diagnosis can also be made by duodenal aspirate and with small intestinal biopsy, but these methods are much more invasive, less efficient, and rarely necessary.

All symptomatic patients and asymptomatic patients such as food handlers, children attending daycare, and immune-compromised patients without contraindications should be treated. Nitroimidazoles, such as metronidazole and tinidazole, are commonly used as treatment and are generally well tolerated. Several other medications (nitazoxanide, albendazole, mebendazole) are also approved in the USA and have similar efficacy (Table 16.1). In the cases where treatment failure is suspected, it is important to repeat stool studies, noting that parasites should be cleared within the stool 3–5 days after treatment [7]. However, if symptoms improve, there is no need to document clearance. It is important to also note that many patients with *Giardia* will be temporarily lactose intolerant and may have prolonged malabsorptive symptoms for several weeks after therapy. Thus, many practitioners advise at least 1 month of lactose avoidance [5]. Additionally, postinfectious irritable bowel syndrome (IBS) seems to be associated with *Giardia* infection, although chronic infection should be ruled out in these cases [8].

Entamoeba histolytica

E. histolytica is the most common organism causing pathogenic amoebiasis globally. It was only relatively recently that not one, but three forms of *Entamoeba* were identi-

Table 16.1 Medications for treatment of intestinal parasites

Parasite	First-line medication(s)	Alternative(s)
Protozoa		
Giardia lamblia	Metronidazole or tinidazole	1. Nitazoxanide, albendazole, mebendazole
Entamoeba histolytica		
1 Invasive disease	1. Metronidazole or tinidazole	1. Ornidazole and nitazoxanide
2. Asymptomatic carriers, luminal clearance following therapy for invasive disease	2. Paromomycin or iodoquinol	2. Diloxanide furoate
Dientamoeba fragilis	Iodoquinol	Metronidazole, tinidazole, paromomycin
Blastocystis hominis	Metronidazole	Tinidazole, iodoquinol, trimethoprim–sulfamethoxazole
Cryptosporidium	Nitazoxanide	May reduce duration/severity: paromomycin, azithromycin
Cyclospora cayetanensis	Trimethoprim–sulfamethaxazole	Ciprofloxacin
Cystoisospora belli	Trimethoprim–sulfamethaxazole	Ciprofloxacin
Nematodes		
Ascaris lumbricoides	Albendazole or mebendazole or levimasole	Ivermectin, nitazoxanide and piperazine citrate
Strongyloides stercoralis	Ivermectin	Albendazole
Hookworms *(Necator americanus, Ancylostoma duodenale)*	Albendazole or pyrantel pamoate	Mebendazole
Whipworm *(Trichuris trichiura)*	Mebendazole or albendazole	Ivermectin
Pinworm *(Enterobius vermicularis)*	Albendazole or mebendazole	Pyrantel pamoate
Cestodes (tapeworms)	Praziquantal	Niclosamide
Diphyllobothrium latum	Praziquantel	Niclosamide
Taenia saginata and *Taenia solium*	Praziquantel	Niclosamide
Hymenolepis nana	Praziquantel	Niclosamide, nitazoxanide

HAART highly active antiretroviral therapy, *HIV* human immunodeficiency virus

fied—pathogenic *E. histolytica* and nonpathogenic *E. dispar* and *E. moshkovski*. *E. histolytica*—although relatively uncommon in the USA, is a common cause of diarrhea in some developing countries, particularly India, Africa, Mexico, and Central and South America. This organism is an uncommon cause of traveler's diarrhea. It is believed that prevalence is higher among homosexual males, and there have been outbreaks in this population attributed to sexual transmission [9]. Unfortunately, accurate prevalence data likely does not exist because of the recent discovery of nonpathogenic strains that were previously classified as *E. histolytica* and the large proportion of persons who are asymptomatic carriers [10].

Similar to *Giardia, Entamoeba* exists in two life forms. There is a more stable cyst form that is responsible for transmission of infection between hosts and a more virulent trophozoite form that is responsible for causing clinical symptoms [5, 11, 12]. Generally, cysts are excreted into soil and are then consumed in contaminated food or water, or via sexual contact. They remain stable in the environment for weeks and are highly virulent—consuming one cyst is adequate to infect a new host. Once consumed, they undergo excystation in the small bowel. The binding and penetration of the trophozoite into the colonic wall result in an invasive colitis. Once the organism has penetrated the colonic mucosa, it is capable of damaging colonic epithelial cells and inflammatory cells through multiple mechanisms [13]. See Figs. 16.1 and 16.2.

The clinical manifestations of *E. histolytica* are variable. Toxic megacolon, colonic ulcerations leading to perforation or formation of an ameboma—granuloma of the cecum or ascending colon caused by chronic amebic infection—are among the more serious intestinal complications. Fulminant amebic dysentery can ensue and be fatal. However, many patients who test positive for *E. histolytica* will only have mild diarrhea or be asymptomatic. Liver abscess and other extraintestinal manifestations of *E. histolytica* are generally seen without recent or concurrent intestinal symptoms [5].

Testing for *E. histolytica* infection can be achieved with multiple different methods. Conventional stool microscopy,

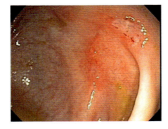

Fig. 16.1 Shallow ulcer in the cecum found on screening colonoscopy. The patient had no symptoms. Biopsy showed ameba organisms in the surface of the biopsy. (Pathology pictures courtesy of Dr. Melissa Upton, Seattle, WA)

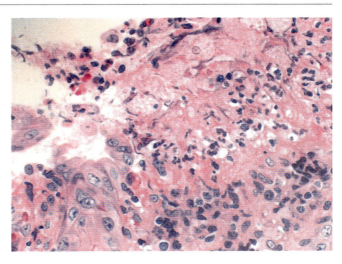

Fig. 16.2 Shallow ulcer in the cecum found on screening colonoscopy. The patient had no symptoms. Biopsy showed ameba organisms in the surface of the biopsy. (Pathology pictures courtesy of Dr. Melissa Upton, Seattle, WA)

stool antigen testing, and serology with enzyme immunoassay are useful in different clinical settings. Stool microscopy requires laboratory expertise and three separate stool collections on three separate days, making it more tedious. Additionally, microscopy will not differentiate among the three strains of *Entamoeba* and will only be diagnostic when active intestinal disease is present. Thus, patients suspected of having *E. histolytica* liver abscess should have serologic testing performed. Stool antigen testing is not universally available, but is efficient and both sensitive and specific for intestinal *E. histolytica*. Polymerase chain reaction (PCR) is the test of choice to differentiate among strains of *Entamoeba*. Direct biopsy of the colonic mucosa can be used as a last resort [12].

Treatment is advised in asymptomatic carriers as well as patients with symptomatic disease [13]. Symptomatic patients with suspected invasive disease should be treated initially with systemic therapy for extraluminal disease and then with a luminal therapy for complete clearance. Nitroimidazoles (metronidazole and tinidazole) are commonly used and well tolerated for initial therapy in the setting of invasive disease (invasive colitis, liver abscess). Asymptomatic carriers, and those with invasive disease who have completed initial therapy, should be treated with a luminal agent, most commonly paromomycin or iodoquinol, to prevent both spread to others and development of new or recurrent invasive disease (Table 16.1) [5, 13]. It is important to note that those with peritonitis secondary to colonic perforation will require broad-spectrum antibiotics as well as the two-phase therapy noted above.

Dientamoeba fragilis

Dientamoeba was long considered a commensal organism in the gut, but is now considered pathogenic and should be treated in the absence of other causes for GI symptoms. It has a global distribution and many studies indicate that the global prevalence could be higher than *Giardia* [14]. The age and gender distribution of patients with *Dientamoeba* has also been a source of disagreement among various studies [14]. It is clear, however, that this pathogen is most common among populations with other parasitic infections who live in conditions with poor hygiene.

D. fragilis is a binucleate, single-cell organism that is of the trichomonad family but lacks flagella. Transmission is presumed to be fecal-oral, but there is no cyst form of *Dientamoeba,* so it is less stable in the environment. Because it has been associated with high carriage rates of *Enterobius vermicularis* (pinworm), some believe helminthic infection may be a vector of transmission [5, 15].

The illness typically causes gas, bloating, abdominal pain, and diarrhea. Diagnosis has improved significantly with the advent of stool PCR testing (sensitivity 96%), increasing the recognition of this pathogen [15]. *Dientamoeba* has also been associated with chronic bowel symptoms, such as IBS, and thus, if found in patients who have chronic symptoms of unclear etiology, treatment is suggested [14]. Providers should consider testing for pinworm infection in patients who test positive for *D. fragilis*. Interestingly, despite the lack of invasiveness of this organism, it is associated with eosinophilia, perhaps because of concurrent pinworm infection. Treatment is with a nitroimidazole (i.e., metronidazole) and several regimens have been studied and found effective (Table 16.1).

Blastocystis Species (Blastocystis hominis)

Blastocystis species (previously referred to as *B. hominis*) are similar to *D. fragilis* in that their role as pathogens is still emerging. They have a global distribution and can affect both children and adults. Zoonotic transmission and fecal–oral routes of infection have been implicated. Thus, it is not surprising that higher rates of infection have been observed in developing countries where infection rates from 30 to 50% have been observed, compared to only 5–10% in developed countries. Immunocompromised hosts (HIV, transplant recipients) are also more commonly affected [16].

Blastocystis species are anaerobic organisms that have been observed to have four major life forms and significant genetic diversity, which led to their renaming from *B. hominis* to B. species. Once they have been ingested, they live in the cecum and colon of their hosts. While asymptomatic infection can occur, symptoms can include diarrhea, flatulence, bloating, abdominal pain, nausea, and anorexia. Additionally, there is some association with urticarial disease [16]. Diagnosis is challenging and most frequently made with stool microscopy; however, enzyme-linked immunosorbent assay (ELISA) and PCR tests are likely superior. Treatment requires some clinician judgment because infections can be self-limited or asymptomatic and may not require therapy. Metronidazole and trimethoprim–sulfamethoxazole (TMP-SMX) are two commonly prescribed medications that are effective for treating *Blastocystis* species [5, 16].

Coccidia

Cryptosporidium

Cryptosporidium is a common enteric pathogen that was identified in the 1970s and has been known to cause prolonged and severe diarrhea as well as biliary disease. Both children and adults are affected by this pathogen, but prevalence is higher among children [17]. In fact, it appears to be one of the most common causes of moderate to severe diarrheal illness among children in Africa and Asia [17].

Cryptosporidia are a group of intracellular protozoa with approximately 20 species and multiple genotypes. *C. parvum* and *C. hominis* are the main species causing human disease [18]. Transmission is by consumption of environmentally stable oocysts, which then undergo excystation in the small bowel leading to infection of enterocytes, where reproduction occurs. Infection can also extend into the biliary tract in immunocompromised hosts.

Outbreaks are primarily associated with water contaminated by animal or human feces. Prevention of transmission requires heating or freezing water, as chlorination is ineffective in killing the stable oocysts [18]. Because of its environmental stability, fecal–oral transmission is possible by multiple modalities. There have been outbreaks in children in US daycare centers. Prevalence may also be higher when there is close contact with animals such as in rural areas.

The spectrum of clinical illness is broad, ranging from self-limited (10–14 day duration) mild diarrheal illness in immunocompetent patients to a chronic enteritis with documented destruction of intestinal villi and occasionally biliary tract involvement in HIV positive or otherwise immunocompromised patients [19]. In the later situations, patients can become severely malnourished and dehydrated. Up to one third of these patients can have biliary tree involvement with inflammatory strictures, acalculous cholecystitis, and pancreatitis [20, 21].

Diagnosis of cryptosporidiosis is generally made with stool microscopy, which can identify spores. It is necessary to request specific acid fast stains to identify cryptosporidium because a standard ova and parasite stool evaluation may not be diagnostic. More modern methods of detection include ELISA antibody assays, but these are costly and not widely available. Additionally, tissue biopsies may reveal the organism on hematoxylin and eosin staining.

Treatment is usually only necessary in immunocompromised patients with severe and unremitting illness. Unfortunately, the efficacy of currently available treatments is not consistent and still under investigation [5]. In patients with immune suppression due to HIV infection, treatment of the HIV with highly active antiretroviral therapy (HAART) to increase CD4 count can lead to clearance of the parasite [20, 21]. Supportive care is essential and antimicrobial agents are aimed at reducing disease severity and duration. The Centers for Disease Control and Prevention (CDC) supports treatment with nitazoxanide, which is Food and Drug Administration (FDA) approved for children over 1 year of age. A randomized controlled trial demonstrated efficacy for HIV negative children, but not HIV positive children [22].

Cyclospora cayetanensis

Cyclospora is an obligate intracellular protozoan that causes enteritis. It was identified in the 1980s and initial cases were confused with cryptosporidium. The infections are similar in that *Cyclospora* also causes more severe and protracted disease among immunocompromised hosts (HIV and transplant patients). Additionally, in non-endemic areas, patients typically experience more severe symptoms and in endemic areas, symptoms tend to decrease with age and be most severe in younger children, implying an acquired tolerance [23].

Symptoms are also similar to cryptosporidium, with watery diarrhea, nausea, anorexia, fatigue, weight loss, low-grade fever, and occasionally biliary tract involvement. The diarrheal illness can be prolonged beyond 3 weeks, even in immunocompetent patients.

Transmission is not person to person because oocysts require time (7–15 days) to become infective after shedding [23]. Outbreaks have been traced to contaminated water supplies and large food outbreaks—raspberries imported from Guatemala in 1996 and cilantro and salad mix from Mexico in 2013 [24, 25].

Diagnosis is via stool microscopy, but is improved with acid-fast stains and will not typically be seen on standard ova and parasite testing. Treatment with TMP-SMX is first line. Ciprofloxacin can be used in case of sulfa allergy, but is less effective [23].

Cystoisospora belli (Isospora belli)

This is the least common of the three coccidia known to infect humans. It is an obligate intracellular protozoan that infects the small bowel and colon. It is endemic in tropical and sub-tropical areas, but there have been rare case reports of outbreaks in non-endemic locations in daycare and institutional settings [26]. The populations typically affected by this organism are immunocompromised patients and travel-

ers. Transmission appears to be similar to the other coccidia and likely not via person to person transmission, but rather through contaminated water and food.

Like the other coccidia, the symptoms include watery diarrhea, flatulence, anorexia, headache, vomiting, and malaise. *Cystoisospora* is associated with reports of reactive arthritis and rarely biliary complications such as acalculous cholecystitis [27].

Diagnosis is typically made on stool microscopy and, like the other coccidia, requires acid-fast staining and laboratory expertise. Stool PCR testing methods are becoming more available. In rare circumstances, duodenal aspirates have also been used.

The treatment is the same as with *Cyclospora,* and TMP–SMX is the first line; however, ciprofloxacin can be used as a slightly inferior second-line therapy in cases of sulfa allergy.

Helminths

Nematodes (Roundworms)

Nematodes or roundworms are a diverse and large group of organisms characterized by their cylindrical structure and digestive openings at both ends.

Ascaris lumbricoides

Ascaris is very common and can be found worldwide, but the highest prevalence occurs in tropical areas, particularly during rainy months. Children are the most common population affected, with rates being the highest between the ages of 2 and 10, with a rapid decline in infections after the teenage years [28]. Interestingly, unlike the protozoan infections, HIV is not associated with increased prevalence or severity of infection.

A. lumbricoides are known for their large size, up to about 40 cm long in some cases, making them the largest helminth to infect humans. Transmission is via consumption of *Ascaris* eggs, which are excreted in human feces leading to contaminated water, soil, or food. Eggs are not infectious for approximately 2–4 weeks after being excreted. Once they are consumed, they penetrate the host intestine and migrate hematogenously through the liver and then into the lung alveoli, where they again penetrate into the bronchiole tree. Eggs are then swallowed after being extracted in respiratory secretions and hatch in the small intestine. The worms can reside in the jejunum and ileum for 1–2 years. If both female and male worms are present, fertilized (infectious) eggs will be excreted in feces [12]. Often, this intestinal phase is asymptomatic. However, when there is a high worm burden, clinical symptoms secondary to mechanical obstruction by the worms can occur. Additionally, hypersensitivity reactions and eosinophilia can occur during larval migration, but the latter is only consistently present during this phase. Pulmonary larval migration can cause pneumonia-like symptoms, known as Loeffler's syndrome. Hepatobiliary complications are usually secondary to obstruction by worms. Finally, in children, nutritional consequences and growth retardation have been associated with *Ascaris* infection [29].

Diagnosis is typically made by identification of characteristic ova via stool microscopy. However, this can pose a diagnostic dilemma in early cases when ova are not yet being excreted. Serologic tests are only useful to determine a history of prior infection. PCR tests are currently being developed. Stool or emesis containing intact worms has also led to diagnosis, as have imaging studies such as ultrasound ("target sign") and CT ("bull's eye") where worms will have characteristic radiographic appearances. Endoscopic retrograde cholangiopancreatography (ERCP) can be both diagnostic and therapeutic.

Treatment with antihelminthic agents should be undertaken immediately for cases of biliary and intestinal disease, but should be delayed if diagnosis is made during the pulmonary phase because the dying larvae can cause significant inflammation and pulmonary disease. Several agents are acceptable for use in treatment. Albendazole and mebendazole have uniformly high rates of success in eradication of infection and are safe for children, but not pregnant females [26]. Alternative agents such as levimasole, ivermectin, nitazoxanide, and piperazine citrate have lower efficacy rates, but can also be used [30].

Strongyloides stercoralis

Strongyloides is a small nematode that is endemic in tropical and subtropical locations, with only sporadic cases reported in the USA. Children living in impoverished conditions, such as refuge groups, are particularly susceptible [31].

The organism has two stages: larva and eggs. It infects a host during the filariform larval stage by directly penetrating the skin. The larva then travel hematogenously to the lungs where they penetrate the alveoli, are coughed up to the oropharynx through the airway, and then swallowed into the intestines where they become mature adult worms. In the small intestine, the female worms burrow into the mucosa where they lay their eggs that hatch and migrate back into the intestinal lumen. Rhabditiform larva (not infective) mature into filariform larva (infective). This process can occur within the host (typically with colonic or perianal penetration of filariform larvae), which can lead to tremendous worm burdens particularly among immunocompromised hosts. However, rhabiditiform larvae can also be excreted from the host and become infective in the environment. Soil infected with feces is the most common cause of transmission to another host through penetration into the skin [12].

Symptoms of strongyloidiasis range from asymptomatic infection in some hosts who are able to maintain a small

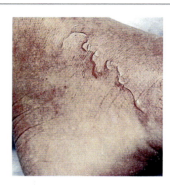

Fig. 16.3 Cutaneous larva migrans. (Reprinted from Ref. [32], with permission from Elsevier)

worm burden, to the other extreme of disseminated *Strongyloides,* which is often fatal. Patients may be diagnosed with *Strongyloides* after experiencing dermal manifestations, predominantly on the lower extremities (urticarial, serpiginous tracts, puerperal-like lesions). This is called cutaneous larva migrans, and they can be seen with other parasitic infections such as hookworm and *Ancylostoma* (Fig. 16.3) [32]. Patients can also have abdominal pain, diarrhea, colitis, and malabsorption. Pulmonary symptoms can be confused with asthma. Eosinophilia is often seen, but absence does not exclude infection, and presence does not correlate with the hyperinfection syndrome [12].

Disseminated *Strongyloides,* also called hyperinfection syndrome, is a life-threatening illness that often occurs with immunosuppression and with the use of immunosuppressive medications such as steroids and chemotherapy. Gram-negative bacteremia is associated with the migration of worms from the intestine to the bloodstream. Sepsis and multiorgan involvement can be seen in these cases [33].

Diagnosis is best made by microscopy, which will directly visualize larvae in stool, duodenal aspirate, or occasionally sputum. Antibody testing is helpful for confirming exposure, but will not help to distinguish current versus past infection [11, 12, 34].

Treatment with ivermectin is first line, and albendazole can be used as an alternative agent. In cases of disseminated disease, a prolonged course of treatment is recommended and consultation with an infectious diseases expert is essential.

Hookworm (Necator americanus, Ancylostoma duodenale)

Hookworm is similar to *Strongyloides* in terms of mode of transmission, endemic territories, diagnosis and symptoms.

Two species of hookworm cause human infection: *N. americanus* and *A. duodenale*. In general, as the name implies, *N. americanus* is endemic to the Americas and *A. duodenale* is endemic in the eastern world. Infection used to be endemic to the southeastern USA; however, with improvement in sanitation it is now primarily seen in immigrant populations or military personnel and other travelers returning from overseas.

The CDC currently estimates that 576–740 million people are infected with hookworm globally, primarily in impoverished tropical and subtropical regions with high annual rainfall amounts. Transmission occurs when eggs are deposited into soil via fecal contamination. Moist, warm conditions then allow the eggs to hatch into worms, which mature into infective (filariform) worms that can then penetrate human skin (typically when barefoot). There are reports of *Ancylostoma* being passed by oral and transmammary modes as well [12].

The signs and symptoms of hookworm infection include dermal, pulmonary, GI, and nutritional/hematologic manifestations. A pruritic maculopapular skin eruption known as "ground itch" or cutaneous larva migrans (Fig. 16.3) can be seen at the site of penetration. Pulmonary symptoms consist of generally very mild pharyngeal and bronchial irritation causing cough. GI manifestations can include abdominal pain, nausea, vomiting, diarrhea, and intestinal bloating and gas. These symptoms are more accentuated at the time of first infection, but repeat infections are often better tolerated. Eosinophilia and iron deficiency may be noted. Long-term nutritional consequences such as hypoalbuminemia and iron-deficiency anemia can occur due to chronic blood consumption by the worms, as well as protease secretion that can inhibit proper digestion. Low birth weights and growth retardation can be a consequence of infection [35, 36].

Diagnosis is made with stool microscopy with direct visualization of hookworm ova. Occasionally, the worms can be seen in the mucosa at endoscopy (Fig. 16.4) [37]. Unfortunately, sensitivity is low and more than one stool ova and parasite evaluation is often needed to capture diagnosis [34].

Treatment with albendazole is the easiest and most effective therapy. Mebendezole and pyrantel pamoate can be used as well. Ivermectin is not effective for treating hookworm [38].

Whipworm (Trichuris trichiura)

T. trichiura (whipworm) is a soil transmitted nematode that is estimated to infect 604–795 million people worldwide [12]. This organism is endemic in tropical regions where it can infect a majority of the population [39]. Children are commonly infected and generally have higher worm burdens than adults. Thus, some strategies of periodically treating preschool-age children for presumed infection in endemic areas have been attempted [40].

T. trichiura infection occurs after an uninfected individual consumes soil contaminated by human feces. Transmission is not person to person because after excretion, the eggs require 15–30 days to become infective in the soil. The eggs hatch in the small intestine and release larvae that develop into worms. The worms establish residence in the cecum and throughout the colon, occasionally extending into the rectum. They can be seen at colonoscopy (Fig. 16.5) where the thin part of the worm embeds in the mucosa. Over time, they begin to produce eggs, which are secreted in stool. The worms are approximately 4 cm in size as adults. The name "whipworm" is based on the shape of the worm resembling a whip with a broad end (the handle) and a narrow end (the whip). The narrow end implants itself into the mucosa and the broad end remains in the lumen [12].

The symptoms of infection are directly correlated with worm burden. Diarrhea, nocturnal incontinence, colitis, and dysentery can be seen. Rectal prolapse is a serious complication of high worm burden. Impaired growth and development in children has been positively correlated with infection.

Diagnosis is made by observation of characteristic ova on stool microscopy. The eggs have a unique barrel-shaped appearance. Gross identification of worms can be diagnostic during endoscopy or rectal examination.

The first-line treatment of trichuriasis is with antihelminthic agents such as mebendazole or albendazole. Single-dose therapy, however, is not adequate and most regimens are 3–7 days, depending on suspected worm burden [38].

Pinworm (E. vermicularis)

E. vermicularis is the helminthic infection with the highest prevalence in the USA. School-aged children, institutional-

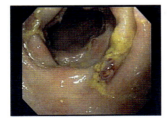

Fig. 16.4 Small intestinal mucosa: Hookworm infection causing an acute abdomen. (Reprinted from Ref. [37], with permission from Elsevier.)

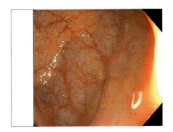

Fig. 16.5 *Trichuris* worm found in cecum at colonoscopy in an asymptomatic woman. The thin part of the worm embeds in the colonic mucosa

ized persons, and adults who care for children are the most commonly infected [12].

Enterobius infection starts after one ingests infectious eggs, and the eggs hatch in the small intestine. The immature larvae migrate to the colon, where they become adults and mate. Female worms migrate at night to lay eggs in the perianal skin folds. These eggs can become infectious within hours.

Transmission occurs when the female worms lay their eggs in the perianal area and cause anal pruritus. This in turn leads to excoriation with hands, which can then transfer infectious eggs to food surfaces or be directly consumed off soiled hands. Fomites (bed sheets and clothing in particular) can harbor eggs, which can then be ingested.

Enterobius is known for causing bothersome anal pruritus and sequelae (secondary bacterial infections) from excoriation. However, in cases of large worm burden, abdominal symptoms can include pain, nausea, and vomiting. There may be an association with appendicitis [41].

Unlike other helminths, *Enterobius* is not diagnosed on stool microscopy. The best method of diagnosis is the "scotch tape test," which entails placing scotch tape on the perianal skin (best at night or in the morning before bathing) and then examining it under a microscope to identify the characteristic bean shaped ova. The yield is higher and approaches 100% sensitivity with three separate tests [12].

The treatment for *Enterobius* is albendazole or mebendazole. Repeat dosing in 2 weeks helps in achieving a higher cure rate and preventing reinfection because the medications do not reliably kill the ova. Pyrantel pamoate is an effective alternative and is recommended in pregnancy [12, 41].

Cestodes (Tapeworms)

Cestodes or tapeworms are flat parasitic worms. The most common species causing human disease include *Diphyllobothrium, Taenia,* and *Hymenolepis.* They are distinguished by their morphology, but all contain a head (scolex) that attaches to the host and multiple segmented bodies (proglottids) that contain reproductive organs and eggs. Intestinal infections are generally asymptomatic, but peripheral eosinophilia is common. Diagnosis is made by stool microscopy with identification of distinct proglottids or ova. All tapeworm infections are treated similarly, and first-line therapy is praziquantal, in varying doses depending on the species.

Diphyllobothrium latum

D. latum (fish tapeworm) is the largest human tapeworm. It has the ability to grow to extremely long lengths in the human intestine (up to 12 m). It is found in freshwater fish exposed to water contaminated by human feces, and it is transmitted to humans by consumption of undercooked or previously unfrozen fish. Infection is extremely rare in the USA and most cases have been reported in Japan and Europe; however, little is known about the prevalence in children [42]. The worms can live for up to 10 years in the small intestine and clinical manifestations are generally not present; however, worms can be passed in stool or emesis or cause obstruction. The unique, but rare association with chronic *D. latum* infection is vitamin B12 deficiency, as the worms will consume the vitamin and deplete the host.

Taenia saginata and Taenia solium

T. saginata (beef tapeworm) and *T. solium* (pork tapeworm) are acquired by consumption of undercooked beef and pork, respectively. *T. saginata* is seen primarily in countries where raw beef consumption is common. *T. solium* is seen throughout regions where hygiene problems exist—Central and South America, Asia, and Africa. *T. solium* is predominantly known for causing cysticercosis, a serious neurologic infection caused by the larval stage of the tapeworm, which is a common cause of epilepsy around the globe. Typically, carriers of *T. solium* tapeworm do not have cysticercosis, but spread this infection to others via shedding of ova in their stool. There are rare reports of passing proglottids or developing abdominal symptoms as a result of *Taenia* tapeworm infection.

Hymenolepis nana

H. nana (dwarf tapeworm) is the smallest and most common tapeworm infection. There is limited data on prevalence in the USA, but a remote study indicated a prevalence of 4% in an urban pediatric population in the Southeast [43]. Temperate regions tend to have increased prevalence as the eggs can only survive in warm conditions. Unlike the other tapeworms, *H. nana* has the ability to complete its lifecycle within the human host, and transmission is often fecal-oral between humans. There is the potential for an arthropod intermediate that is then consumed unknowingly in grain products. The symptoms of infection are usually minimal unless worm burdens become high (which is possible because of autoinfection). If this occurs, nonspecific abdominal and constitutional symptoms can occur.

Conclusion

This chapter reviewed intestinal parasite infections. While some of these infections are rarely seen in practice in the USA, knowledge of their presentation, long-term consequences in children, and treatment remains important for the clinician in the current age of global food trade, travel, and immigration.

References

1. Yoder JS, Gargano JW, Wallace RM, Beach MJ, Centers for Disease Control and Prevention (CDC). Giardiasis surveillance–United States, 2009–2010. MMWR Surveill Summ. 2012;61(5):13–23.
2. Ross AG, Olds GR, Cripps AW, Farrar JJ, McManus DP. Enteropathogens and chronic illness in returning travelers. N Engl J Med. 2013;368(19):1817–25.
3. Cotton JA, Beatty JK, Buret AG. Host parasite interactions and pathophysiology in Giardia infections. Int J Parasitol. 2011;41(9):925–33.
4. Muhsen K, Levine MM. A systematic review and meta-analysis of the association between Giardia lamblia and endemic pediatric diarrhea in developing countries. Clin Infect Dis. 2012;55(Suppl 4):S271–93.
5. Fuentebella J, Fridge JL, Bass DM. Enteric Parasites. Pediatr Gastrointest Liv Dis. 2011:423–34.
6. McHardy IH, Wu M, Shimizu-Cohen R, Couturier MR, Humphries RM. Clinical laboratory diagnosis of intestinal protozoa. J Clin Microbiol. 2014 Mar;52(3):712–20.
7. Gardner TB, Hill DR. Treatment of giardiasis. Clin Microbiol Rev. 2001;14(1):114–28.
8. Hanevik K, Dizdar V, Langeland N, Hausken T. Development of functional gastrointestinal disorders after Giardia lamblia infection. BMC Gastroenterol. 2009;9:27.
9. Salit IE, Khairnar K, Gough K, Pillai DR. A possible cluster of sexually transmitted Entamoeba histolytica: genetic analysis of a highly virulent strain. Clin Infect Dis. 2009;49(3):346–53.
10. Marie C, Petri WA. Amoebic dysentery. Clin Evid (Online). BMJ Clin Evid. 2013 Aug 30;2013. pii: 0918. PMID 23991750.
11. Centers for Disease Control (cdc). Division of parasitic diseases and malaria website. 2014. http://www.cdc.gov/parasites/index.html. Accessed 1 Sept 2014.
12. DPDx - Laboratory Identification of Parasitic Diseases of Public Health Concern. Centers for Disease Control. http://www.cdc.gov/dpdx. Accessed 1 Sept 2014.
13. Haque R, Huston CD, Hughes M, Houpt E, Petri WA. Amebiasis. N Engl J Med. 2003;348(16):1565–73.
14. Barratt JL, Harkness J, Marriott D, Ellis JT, Stark D. A review of Dientamoeba fragilis carriage in humans: several reasons why this organism should be considered in the diagnosis of gastrointestinal illness. Gut Microbes. 2011;2(1):3–12.
15. Barry MA, Weatherhead JE, Hotez PJ, Woc-Colburn L. Childhood parasitic infections endemic to the United States. Pediatr Clin North Am. 2013;60(2):471–85.
16. Tan KS. New insights on classification, identification, and clinical relevance of Blastocystis spp. Clin Microbiol Rev. 2008;21(4):639–65.
17. Kotloff KL, Nataro JP, Blackwelder WC, Nasrin D, Farag TH, Panchalingam S, et al. Burden and aetiology of diarrhoeal disease in infants and young children in developing countries (the Global Enteric Multicenter Study, GEMS): a prospective, case-control study. Lancet. 2013;382(9888):209–22.
18. Wright SG. Protozoan infections of the gastrointestinal tract. Infect Dis Clin North Am. 2012;26(2):323–39.
19. Jokipii L, Jokipii AM. Timing of symptoms and oocyst excretion in human cryptosporidiosis. N Engl J Med. 1986;315(26):1643–7.
20. Gross TL, Wheat J, Bartlett M, O'Connor KW. AIDS and multiple system involvement with cryptosporidium. Am J Gastroenterol. 1986;81(6):456–8.
21. Chen XM, LaRusso NF. Human intestinal and biliary cryptosporidiosis. World J Gastroenterol. 1999;5(5):424–9.
22. Amadi B, Mwiya M, Musuku J, Watuka A, Sianongo S, Ayoub A, et al. Effect of nitazoxanide on morbidity and mortality in Zambian children with cryptosporidiosis: a randomised controlled trial. Lancet. 2002;360(9343):1375–80.
23. Ortega YR, Sanchez R. Update on Cyclospora cayetanensis, a food-borne and waterborne parasite. Clin Microbiol Rev. 2010;23(1):218–34.
24. Johnson AC, Greenwood-Van Meerveld B, McRorie J. Effects of Bifidobacterium infantis 35624 on post-inflammatory visceral hypersensitivity in the rat. Dig Dis Sci. 2011;56(11):3179–86.
25. desVignes-Kendrick M. Notes from the field: outbreaks of Cyclosporiasis—United States, June–August 2013. 2013. http://www.cdc.gov/mmwr/preview/mmwrhtml/mm6243a5.htm. Accessed 1 Sept 2014.
26. Ud Din N, Torka P, Hutchison RE, Riddell SW, Wright J, Gajra A. Severe Isospora (Cystoisospora) belli diarrhea preceding the diagnosis of human T-cell-leukemia-virus-1-associated T-cell lymphoma. Case Rep Infec Dis. 2012;2012:640104.
27. Goodgame RW. Understanding intestinal spore-forming protozoa: cryptosporidia, microsporidia, isospora, and cyclospora. Ann Intern Med. 1996;124(4):429–41.
28. Haswell-Elkins M, Elkins D, Anderson RM. The influence of individual, social group and household factors on the distribution of Ascaris lumbricoides within a community and implications for control strategies. Parasitology. 1989;98(Pt 1):125–34.
29. Jardim-Botelho A, Brooker S, Geiger SM, Fleming F, Souza Lopes AC, Diemert DJ, et al. Age patterns in undernutrition and helminth infection in a rural area of Brazil: associations with ascariasis and hookworm. Trop Med Int Health. 2008;13(4):458–67.
30. Khuroo MS. Ascariasis. Gastroenterol Clin N. 1996;25(3):553–77.
31. Posey DL, Blackburn BG, Weinberg M, Flagg EW, Ortega L, Wilson M, et al. High prevalence and presumptive treatment of schistosomiasis and strongyloidiasis among African refugees. Clin Infect Dis. 2007;45(10):1310–5.
32. Hotez PJ. Hookworms (Necator americanus and Ancylostoma spp.). In: Kliegman RM, Stanton B, St. Geme J, Schor N, Behrman RE, editors. Nelson textbook of pediatrics. 19th ed. Saunders, an Imprint of Elsevier Inc.: Philadelphia, PA; 2011. pp. 1218–21, e2.
33. Buonfrate D, Requena-Mendez A, Angheben A, Muñoz J, Gobbi F, Van Den Ende J, et al. Severe strongyloidiasis: a systematic review of case reports. BMC Infect Dis. 2013;13:78.
34. Goka AK, Rolston DD, Mathan VI, Farthing MJ. Diagnosis of Strongyloides and hookworm infections: comparison of faecal and duodenal fluid microscopy. Trans R Soc Trop Med Hyg. 1990;84(6):829–31.
35. Barry MA, Simon GG, Mistry N, Hotez PJ. Global trends in neglected tropical disease control and elimination: impact on child health. Arch Dis Child. 2013;98(8):635–41.
36. Hotez PJ, Pritchard DI. Hookworm infection. Sci Am. 1995;272(6):68–74.
37. Baltz JG, Mishra R, Yeaton P. Unusual case of hookworm presenting as acute surgical abdomen. Am J Med. 2009;122(2):e3–4.
38. Keiser J, Utzinger J. Efficacy of current drugs against soil-transmitted helminth infections: systematic review and meta-analysis. JAMA. 2008;299(16):1937–48.
39. Bundy DA. Epidemiological aspects of Trichuris and trichuriasis in Caribbean communities. Trans R Soc Trop Med Hyg. 1986;80(5):706–18.
40. Bundy DA, de Silva NR. Can we deworm this wormy world? Br Med Bull. 1998;54(2):421–32.
41. Grencis RK, Cooper ES. Enterobius, trichuris, capillaria, and hookworm including Ancylostoma caninum. Gastroenterol Clin North Am. 1996;25(3):579–97.
42. Harhay MO, Horton J, Olliaro PL. Epidemiology and control of human gastrointestinal parasites in children. Expert Rev Anti Infect Ther. 2010;8(2):219–34.
43. Flores EC, Plumb SC, McNeese MC. Intestinal parasitosis in an urban pediatric clinic population. Am J Dis Child. 1983;137(8):754–6.

Persistent Diarrhea in Children in Developing Countries

17

Jai K. Das, Christopher Duggan and Zulfiqar A. Bhutta

Introduction

In the year 2013, 6.3 million children under the age 5 died; around 3 million (45%) of these deaths were attributable to infectious diseases, and pneumonia (17%) and diarrhea (9%) were the leading causes. The overall incidence of diarrhea has decreased from 3.4 episodes per child-year in 1990 to 2.9 episodes per child-year in 2010, but diarrhea remains one of the most common reasons of hospital admission, with an estimated 1731 million episodes of childhood diarrhea reported in 2011 [1, 2]. Risk factors for diarrhea include poverty, undernutrition, poor hygiene, and underprivileged household conditions.

Diarrhea is categorized clinically into three types: acute watery, acute bloody and persistent diarrhea. Acute watery diarrhea lasts several hours or days, and is often due to gastrointestinal pathogens including viruses and bacteria (including *Vibrio cholerae*). Acute bloody diarrhea, also called dysentery, is marked by stools containing blood and/or mucous; common pathogens include *Salmonella* and *Shigella* spp. Persistent diarrhea refers to episodes of diarrhea (either watery or dysentery) that last 14 days or longer. Although less common than acute diarrhea, prolonged and persistent episodes of diarrhea in childhood constitute a significant portion of the global burden of diarrhea and these lengthy episodes are increasingly implicated in childhood undernutrition [3], micronutrient de-

ficiencies, adverse neurodevelopment outcomes, and higher morbidity and mortality from other diseases [1]. As mortality from acute watery diarrhea is decreasing, the proportion of deaths due to persistent diarrhea has increased, and recent studies estimate that between 5 and 18% of all episodes are persistent diarrhea and though a small portion of episodes, they are responsible for significant diarrheal morbidity and up to 50% of all diarrhea-related deaths since persistent diarrhea has a high case-fatality rate [4, 5]. It is also estimated that persistent diarrhea is associated with 3 million disability adjusted life-years lost annually [6]. These findings indicate the continuing need to focus on prevention and management of childhood diarrhea, especially in developing countries where most of the burden lies. But there is scarcity of data on persistent diarrhea, and it is likely that the diminished publication output also reflects reduced research interest in the subject [7]. Although effective interventions exist which not only can halt the progression from acute diarrhea to persistent diarrhea and its sequelae but also have a substantial impact on total diarrhea burden and mortality as well; however, these interventions do not have universal access. An analysis using the lives saved tool (LiST), a methodology to estimate the effect of increasing the use of a package of interventions, has shown that if water, sanitation and hygiene (WASH), breastfeeding, zinc, oral rehydration solution (ORS), rotavirus vaccine, vitamin A supplementation, zinc for the treatment of diarrhea and antibiotics for dysentery are scaled up to at least 80% and that for immunizations to at least 90%; 95% of diarrhea deaths in children younger than 5 years could be eliminated [8].

Etiology

There are three causes of persistent or chronic diarrhea: persistent infection; repeated infection, which occurs primarily in resource limited regions with poor hygienic conditions; and post-infectious irritable bowel syndrome which occurs after an infection has cleared [9]. Persistent diarrhea can lead to long-term morbidity, probably due to malabsorption

Z. A. Bhutta (✉) · J. K. Das
Division of Women and Child Health, Aga Khan University, Karachi 74800, Pakistan
e-mail: zulfiqar.bhutta@aku.edu

C. Duggan
Division of Gastroenterology, Hepatology and Nutrition, Boston Children's Hospital, Boston, MA, USA

Z. A. Bhutta
SickKids Center for Global Child Health, Hospital for Sick Children, Toronto, ON, Canada

Departments of Pediatrics, Nutritional Sciences and Public Health, SickKids Peter Gilgan Centre for Research and Learning, University of Toronto, 686 Bay Street, Toronto, ON M5G A04, Canada

© Springer International Publishing Switzerland 2016
S. Guandalini et al. (eds.), *Textbook of Pediatric Gastroenterology, Hepatology and Nutrition,*
DOI 10.1007/978-3-319-17169-2_17

195

of key nutrients caused by the blunting of villi, disruption of the epithelium, and submucosal inflammation.

The responsible organisms depend on endemicity or recent travel. A few pathogens have been particularly associated with persistent diarrhea or are preferentially identified when an episode becomes persistent include *EnteroAggregative Escherichia coli* (EAggEC) and *EnteroPathogenic E. coli* (EPEC), *Clostridium difficile, Cryptosporidium parvum, Camplylobacter* spp., *Salmonella* spp., *Shigella* spp., and *Giardia lamblia*.

EAggEC and EPEC are the most commonly implicated bacterial pathogens in persistent infections in developing countries, especially among children [9]. The exact mechanism by which EAggEC leads to persistent diarrhea is not known, whereas EPEC's pathogenesis lies in its ability to disrupt the brush border through the adherence and effacement process, leading to the loss of absorptive areas. *C. difficile* infections are increasingly more difficult to treat as they become more prevalent in the community and are now the recognized common cause of persistent diarrhea in developed countries. Other bacterial pathogens that cause persistent diarrhea include *Camplylobacter, Salmonella,* and on rare occasions *Tropheryma whippleii. Giardia* and *Cryptosporidium* are also often implicated, along with *Entamoeba, Isospora,* and microsporidia [10, 11]. Intestinal parasites could also cause persistent diarrhea especially in developing regions. Studies have also shown seasonal variation in infection [12]. Viruses in a minority of immunocompetent patients are also a cause of persistent diarrhea [13]. In immunocompromised patients, intestinal parasites are the most commonly implicated pathogens to cause persistent diarrhea [14], while atypical *Mycobacteria, Cytomegalovirus,* and other enteric viruses infections should also be suspected.

Risk Factors

Persistent diarrhea is commonly seen in association with significant malnutrition, and the relationship between persistent diarrhea and malnutrition is bidirectional. The recent evidence of micronutrient deficiencies, especially of zinc and vitamin A in malnourished children with persistent diarrhea, indicates impaired immunological mechanisms for clearing infections as well as ineffective mucosal repair mechanisms. Lactose intolerance is prevalent in many children with persistent diarrhea, but the role of specific dietary allergies in inducing and perpetuating enteropathy of malnutrition is unclear. Several studies have highlighted the high risk of prolonged diarrhea with lactation failure and early introduction of artificial feeds in developing countries. In particular, the administration of unmodified cow's or buffalo milk is associated with prolongation of diarrhea, suggesting the potential underlying role of milk protein enteropathy [15]. Inappropriate management of acute diarrhea is also an important risk factor. The association of prolongation of diarrhea with starvation and inappropriate-

ly prolonged administration of parenteral fluids has been recognized for over half a century [16]. Continued breastfeeding is important and unnecessary food withdrawal and replacement of luminal nutrients, especially breast milk, with nonnutritive agents is a major factor in prolonging the mucosal injury after diarrhea. In particular, routine administration of antibiotics and antimotility agents and semi-starvation diets should be avoided in cases of prolonged diarrhea [17]. There is now clear evidence supporting the enteral route for nutritional rehabilitation of malnourished children with persistent diarrhea [18] as starvation has been shown to have deleterious effects on the intestinal mucosa [19] with a reduction in gastrointestinal structure and function. It is therefore imperative that malnourished children with persistent diarrhea should receive enteral nutrition during their period of rehabilitation. High stool frequency, not being breastfed, young age, and acquiring diarrhea in the rainy season have also been identified as risk factors for prolonged diarrhea [20].

The aforementioned risk factors highlight the importance of recognizing that optimal management of diarrheal episodes is essential to progression to persistent diarrhea. It is natural that given the close relationship between diarrheal disorders and malnutrition, persistent diarrhea is widely recognized as a nutritional disorder and that optimal nutritional rehabilitation is considered a cornerstone of its management.

Consequences of Persistent Diarrhea

As diarrhea becomes "persistent," malnutrition becomes increasingly manifest secondary to anorexia and impaired nutrient balance resulting from mucosal injury, malabsorption, and nutrient losses [21]. This sequence is supported by the observation that *Shigella* infection—characterized by intense tissue catabolism and nutrient losses—almost doubles the risk of persistent diarrhea [22], and why bloody diarrhea (with or without the isolation of *Shigella* spp.) is so often reported to be a risk factor for persistent episodes [23]. The importance of *Shigella* is reflected in the report from at a large hospital center in Bangladesh that the frequency of persistent diarrhea diminished as the isolation rate of *Shigella* decreased between 1991 and 2010. Mucosal injury also explains why by day 14, the manifestations of persistent diarrhea are primarily those of a malabsorption and malnutrition syndrome that requires careful dietary and nutritional management until the mucosal damage is reversed and new normally functioning epithelial cells are regenerated.

There are several reasons why malnutrition should both predispose to, as well as follow persistent diarrhea. These range from achlorhydria with increased risk of small bowel contamination, systemic immune deficiency, intestinal and pancreatic enzyme deficiency, and altered intestinal mucosal repair mechanisms following an infectious insult. An independent relationship has also been demonstrated between cutaneous anergy and the subsequent risk of development of persistent diarrhea [24]. There has been much interest in the possibility that such transient immune deficiency may also be a marker of concomitant micronutrient deficiency [25]. The most striking example of the critical role that the immune system plays in the pathogenesis of persistent diarrhea is the relationship of HIV/AIDS. This is exemplified by the host of studies linking persistent diarrhea with cryptosporidiosis [26] and other parasitic infections [27] in Africa and Asia.

A clear understanding of alterations in intestinal morphology and physiology is crucial toward the development of interventional strategies, but there has been little progress in our understanding of this problem in developing countries. This has been largely due to a paucity of studies formally evaluating intestinal biopsy findings in representative populations. A wide variety of pathological changes have been described after persistent diarrhea, however, ranging from near normal appearance to mucosal flattening, crypt hypertrophy, and lymphocytic infiltration of the mucosa [28]. Recent elaborate electron microscopic studies of intestinal mucosa in persistent diarrhea reveal patchy villous atrophy and intraepithelial lymphocytic infiltration as well as severe mucosal damage and villous atrophy [29]. Poor intestinal repair is regarded as a key component of the abnormal mucosal morphology. However, the exact factors underlying this ineffective repair process and continuing injury are poorly understood. The end result

of this mucosal derangement is reduced absorption of luminal nutrients, as well as increased permeability of the bowel to abnormal dietary or microbial antigens [30]. Alterations of intestinal permeability in early childhood may reflect changes in intestinal mucosal maturation [31] and may be affected by concomitant enteric infections [32].

Management

It is imperative to consider the child's age and clinical manifestations to determine proper treatment in cases of persistent diarrhea. A paucity of diagnostic facilities limits the microbiologic evaluation of diarrhea in many parts of the world. Lack of awareness regarding cow's milk protein allergy and immunodeficiency-associated diarrhea is of particular concern. Optimal prevention and management of acute diarrheal illnesses is the ideal strategy to prevent persistent diarrhea. Treatment is focused on reversing dehydration (if present), nutritional interventions including balanced protein energy and micronutrient supplements, and judicious use of antibiotics for certain types of inflammatory diarrhea. Oral rehydration solutions, micronutrient supplementation, algorithm-based diet regimens, and good supportive care are sufficient in most children above 6 months of age with persistent diarrhea (Table 17.1).

Table 17.1 Impact of interventions to prevent and control diarrhea

Intervention	Effect estimates
Water sanitation and hygiene	48, 17, and 36 % risk reductions for diarrhea with hand washing with soap, improved water quality and excreta disposal, respectively
Breastfeeding education and impacts on breastfeeding patterns	EBF rates increase by 43 % at 1 day, 30 % till 1 month, and 79 % from 1 to 6 months
	Rates of no breastfeeding decrease by 32 % at 1 day, 30 % till 1 month, and 18 % from 1 to 6 months
Preventive zinc supplementation	18 % reduction in diarrhea-related mortality
Preventive vitamin A supplementation	All-cause mortality reduced by 24 % (RR: 0.76, 95 % CI: 0.69–0.83), diarrhea related mortality by 28 % (RR: 0.72, 95 % CI: 0.57–0.91), incidence of diarrhea reduced by 15 % (RR: 0.85, 95 % CI: 0.82–0.87)
Vaccines for rotavirus	74 % reduction in very severe rotavirus infection
	47 % reduction in rotavirus hospitalization
Vaccines for cholera	52 % effective against cholera infection
ORS	69 % reduction in diarrhea specific mortality
Dietary management of diarrhea	Lactose free diets reduce the duration of diarrhea treatment failure rates by 47 %
Therapeutic zinc supplementation	66 % reduction in diarrhea-specific mortality
	23 % reduction in subsequent diarrhea hospitalization
	19 % reduction in subsequent diarrhea
Antibiotics for cholera	63 % reduction in clinical failure rates
	75 % reduction in bacteriological failure rates
Antibiotics for Shigella	82 % reduction in clinical failure
	96 % reduction in bacteriological failure rates
Antibiotics for cryptosporidiosis	52 % reduction in clinical failure rates
	38 % reduction in parasitological failure rates
Community based intervention platforms for prevention	160 % increase in the use of ORS
	80 % increase in the use of zinc in diarrhea
	76 % decline in the use of antibiotics for diarrhea
Community case management	63 % reduction in diarrhea related mortality
Financial support schemes	Conditional transfer programs: 14 % increase in preventive health care use, 22 % increase in the percentage of newborns receiving colostrum and 16 % increase the coverage of vitamin A supplementation

EBF exclusive breastfeeding, *ORS* oral rehydration solution, *RR* relative risk, *CI* confidence interval

Rapid Resuscitation, Antibiotic Therapy, and Stabilization

Most children with persistent diarrhea and associated malnutrition are not severely dehydrated and oral rehydration may be adequate. Indeed, routine use of intravenous fluids in severe acute malnutrition should be avoided; acute severe dehydration and associated vomiting may require brief periods of intravenous rehydration with Ringer's lactate. Acute electrolyte imbalance such as hypokalemia and severe acidosis may require correction. More importantly, associated systemic infections (bacteremia, pneumonia, and urinary tract infection) are well-recognized complications of severe acute malnutrition in children with persistent diarrhea and a frequent cause of early mortality. Almost 30–50% of malnourished children with persistent diarrhea may have an associated systemic infection requiring resuscitation and antimicrobial therapy [33, 34]. In severely ill children requiring hospitalization, it may be best to cover with parenteral antibiotics at admission (usually ampicillin and gentamicin) while awaiting blood and other culture results. It should be emphasized that there is little role for oral antibiotics in persistent diarrhea as in most cases the original bacterial infection triggering the prolonged diarrhea has disappeared by the time the child presents. Possible exceptions are appropriate treatment for dysentery [8] and adjunctive therapy for cryptosporidiosis in children with HIV and persistent diarrhea [35].

Oral Rehydration Therapy

It is over 40 years since the efficacy of oral rehydration therapy was clearly demonstrated, following discovery of glucose-stimulated sodium uptake by intestinal villus cells [36]. This is the preferred mode of rehydration and replacement of ongoing losses. The net effect is expansion of the intravascular compartment and rehydration, usually sufficient for all but the most severely dehydrated patients who require initial intravenous fluids [37]. Data from several clinical trials supported a change in the composition of the WHO ORS to a solution of lowered osmolality. While in general the standard WHO oral rehydration solution is adequate, recent evidence indicates that hypo-osmolar rehydration fluids [38] as well as cereal-based oral rehydration fluids may be advantageous in malnourished children. A number of modifications have been proposed, for example cereal (rice)-based ORT, addition of certain amino acids (glycine, alanine, or glutamine) to further increase sodium absorption and/or hasten intestinal repair, or supplementation with zinc, but none have been shown to be consistently superior to low-osmolality ORS [39, 40].

Enteral Feeding

Nutritional rehabilitation can break the vicious cycle of chronic diarrhea and malnutrition and is considered the cornerstone of treatment. It is exceedingly rare to find persistent diarrhea in exclusively breast-fed infants, and with the exception of situations where persistent diarrhea accompanies perinatally acquired HIV infection, breastfeeding must be continued. Although children with persistent diarrhea may not be lactose intolerant, administration of a lactose load exceeding 5 g/kg/day may be associated with higher purging rates and treatment failure. Alternative strategies for reducing the lactose load while feeding malnourished children who have prolonged diarrhea include addition of milk to cereals and replacement of milk with fermented milk products such as yogurt. Mattos et al. [41] claimed that yogurt-based diet is recommended as the first choice for the nutritional management of a mild to moderate persistent diarrhea. A cheap and an easily available yogurt-based diet can be used in mild chronic diarrhea illness of uncomplicated and without enteropathy. Bhutta et al. [18] suggested algorithm for the diagnosis and management of persistent diarrhea (Fig. 17.1). Elimination diet is considered when allergic enteropathy is induced by a cow's milk protein or soy protein [42]. Rarely, when dietary intolerance precludes the administration of cow's milk-based formulations or milk it may be necessary to administer specialized milk-free diets such as a comminuted or blended chicken-based diet or an elemental formulation. Although effective in some settings, the latter are unaffordable in most developing countries. In addition to rice-lentil formulations, the addition of green banana or pectin to the diet has also been shown to be effective in the treatment of persistent diarrhea [43, 44]. Among children in low- and middle-income countries, where the dual burden of diarrhea and malnutrition is greatest and where access to proprietary formulas and specialized ingredients is limited, the use of locally available age-appropriate foods should be promoted for the majority of diarrhea cases. Nutritionally complete diets comprising locally available ingredients can be used at least as effectively as commercial preparations or specialized ingredients. The usual energy density of any diet used for the therapy of persistent diarrhea should be around 1 kcal/g, aiming to provide an energy intake of a minimum 100 kcal/kg/day, and a protein intake of between 2 and 3 g/kg/day. In selected circumstances, when adequate intake of energy-dense food is problematic, the addition of amylase to the diet through germination techniques may also be helpful. Recent WHO guidelines recommends that children with severe acute malnutrition who present with either acute or persistent diarrhea, can be given ready-to-use therapeutic food in the same way as children without diarrhea, whether they are being managed as inpatients or outpatients. And these children with severe acute malnutrition should also be

Fig. 17.1 Algorithm of diagnosis and management of persistent diarrhea

Algorithm of Diagnosis and Management of Persistent Diarrhea

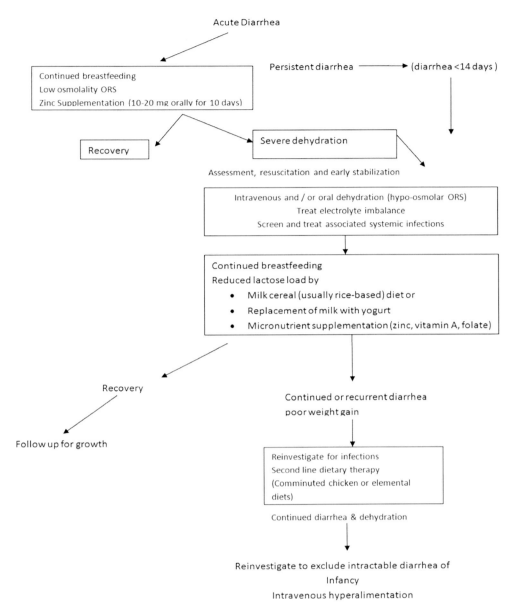

Micronutrient Supplementation

It is now widely recognized that most malnourished children with persistent diarrhea have associated deficiencies of micronutrients including zinc, iron, and vitamin A. This may be a consequence of poor intake and continued enteral losses and requires replenishment during therapy [46]. While the

provided with about 5000 IU vitamin A daily, either as an integral part of therapeutic foods or as part of a multi-micronutrient formulation [45].

evidence supporting zinc administration in children with persistent diarrhea is persuasive, it is likely that these children have multiple micronutrient deficiencies. Concomitant vitamin A administration to children with persistent diarrhea has been shown to improve outcome [47, 48] especially in HIV endemic areas [49]. It is therefore important to ensure that all children with persistent diarrhea and malnutrition receive an initial dose of 100,000 units Vitamin A and a daily intake of at least 3–5 mg/kg/day of elemental zinc. While the association of significant anemia with persistent diarrhea is well recognized, iron replacement therapy is best initiated only after recovery from diarrhea has started and the diet is well tolerated.

Improved Case Management of Diarrhea

Improved management of diarrhea through prompt identification and appropriate therapy significantly reduces diarrhea duration, its nutritional penalty, and risk of death in childhood. Improved management of acute diarrhea is a key factor in reducing the burden of prolonged episodes and persistent diarrhea. The WHO/UNICEF recommendations to use low-osmolality ORS and zinc supplementation for the management of diarrhea, coupled with selective and appropriate use of antibiotics, have the potential to reduce the number of diarrheal deaths among children through community case management and integrated management of childhood illness (IMCI). Community-based interventions to diagnose and treat childhood diarrhea through community health workers leads to a significant rise in care-seeking behaviors for diarrhea and are associated with significantly increased use of ORS and zinc at household level as well as reduction in the unnecessary use of antibiotics for diarrhea [50].

Other Potential Modalities

The factors associated with persistent diarrhea are small intestinal mucosa injury, persisting infective colonization and bacterial particles and toxins that are translocated into the host cell and the downregulated host immune system. These circumstances alter interrelation between the normal flora and the host, which can worsen prolonged inflammation. The rationale for using probiotics in treatment of persistent diarrhea lies in their ability to survive and reproduce in the host's gut and in their proven role in treatment of acute diarrhea. Recent evidence suggests modest effect of probiotics [51]. Because of probiotics known immunomodulatory effect and very significant mortality and morbidity rate from persistent diarrhea in developing countries, it is imperative to highlight the necessity for well-designed studies to define the role of probiotics in persistent diarrhea.

Follow-Up and Nutritional Rehabilitation in Community Settings

Given the high rates of relapse in most children with persistent diarrhea, it is important to address the underlying risk factors and institute preventive measures. These include appropriate feeding (breastfeeding, complementary feeding) and close attention to environmental hygiene and sanitation. This poses a considerable challenge in communities deprived of basic necessities such as clean water and sewage disposal.

In addition to the preventive aspects, the challenge in most settings is to develop and sustain a form of dietary therapy using inexpensive, home-available, and culturally acceptable ingredients which can be used to manage children with persistent diarrhea. Given that the majority of cases of persistent diarrhea occur in the community and that parents are frequently hesitant to seek institutional help, there is a need to develop and implement inexpensive and practical home-based therapeutic measures [18] and evidence indicates that it may be entirely feasible to do so in community settings [52, 53].

Conclusion

There is a significant burden of persistent diarrhea in children and it also contributes to childhood malnutrition and mortality. Most of the knowledge and tools needed to prevent diarrhea-associated mortality in developing countries and especially persistent diarrhea are available. These require concerted and sustained implementation in public health programs. Given the emerging evidence of the long-term impact of childhood diarrhea on developmental outcomes [54], it is imperative that due emphasis is placed on prompt recognition and appropriate management of persistent diarrhea.

References

1. Black RE, Victora CG, Walker SP, Bhutta ZA, Christian P, de Onis M, Uauy R. Maternal and child undernutrition and overweight in low-income and middle-income countries. Lancet. 2013;382(9890):427–51.
2. UNICEF. Levels & trends in child mortality. Estimates developed by the UN inter-agency group for child mortality estimation. New York: UNICEF; 2014. http://www.unicef.org/media/files/Levels_ and_Trends_in_Child_Mortality_2014.pdf. Accessed 13 June 2015.
3. Lima AAM, Moore SR, Barboza MS, Soares AM, Schleupner MA, Newman RD, Guerrant RL. Persistent diarrhea signals a critical period of increased diarrhea burdens and nutritional shortfalls: a prospective cohort study among children in northeastern Brazil. J Infect Dis. 2000;181(5):1643–51.
4. Moore SR, Lima NL, Soares AM, Oriá RB, Pinkerton RC, Barrett LJ, Lima AA. Prolonged episodes of acute diarrhea reduce growth and increase risk of persistent diarrhea in children. Gastroenterology. 2010;139(4):1156–64.
5. Coles CL, Levy A, Dagan R, Deckelbaum RJ, Fraser D. Risk factors for the initial symptomatic giardia infection in a cohort of young Arab-Bedouin children. Ann Trop Paediatr. 2009;29(4):291–300.
6. Guerrant RL, Kosek M, Lima AA, Lorntz B, Guyatt HL. Updating the DALYs for diarrhoeal disease. Trends Parasitol. 2002;18(5):191–3.
7. Bhutta ZA, Nelson EA, Lee WS, Tarr PI, Zablah R, Phua KB, Phillips A. Recent advances and evidence gaps in persistent diarrhea. J Pediatr Gastroenterol Nutr. 2008;47(2):260–5.
8. Bhutta ZA, Das JK, Walker N, Rizvi A, Campbell H, Rudan I, Black RE Interventions to address deaths from childhood pneumonia and diarrhoea equitably: what works and at what cost? Lancet. 2013;381(9875):1417–29.
9. Pawlowski SW, Warren CA, Guerrant R. Diagnosis and treatment of acute or persistent diarrhea. Gastroenterology. 2009;136(6):1874–86.

10. Arenas-Pinto A, Certad G, Ferrara G, Castro J, Bello MA, Nunez LT. Association between parasitic intestinal infections and acute or chronic diarrhoea in HIV-infected patients in Caracas, Venezuela. Int J STD AIDS. 2003;14(7):487–92.

11. Tumwine JK, Kekitiinwa A, Bakeera-Kitaka S, Ndeezi G, Downing R, Feng X, Tzipori S. Cryptosproridiosis and microsporidiosis in Ugandan children with persistent diarrhea with and without concurrent infection with the human immunodeficiency virus. Am J Trop Med Hyg. 2005;73(5):921–5.

12. Shlim DR, Hoge CW, Rajah R, Scott RM, Pandy P, Echeverria P. Persistent high risk of diarrhea among foreigners in Nepal during the first 2 years of residence. Clin Infect Dis. 1999;29(3):613–6.

13. Vernacchio L, Vezina RM, Mitchell AA, Lesko SM, Plaut AG, Acheson DW. Diarrhea in American infants and young children in the community setting: incidence, clinical presentation and microbiology. Pediatr Infect Dis J. 2006;25(1):2–7.

14. Gupta S, Narang S, Nunavath V, Singh S. Chronic diarrhoea in HIV patients: prevalence of coccidian parasites. Indian J Med Microbiol. 2008;26(2):172–5.

15. Bhutta ZA, Molla AM, Isani Z, Badruddin S, Hendricks K, Snyder JD. Nutrient absorption and weight gain in persistent diarrhoea: comparison of a traditional rice-lentil-yogurt-milk diet with soy formula. J Pediatr Gastroenterol Nutr. 1994;18:45–52.

16. Duggan C, Nurko S. "Feeding the gut": the scientific basis for continued enteral nutrition during acute diarrhea. J Pediatr. 1997;131:801–8.

17. Mahmud MA, Hossain MM, Huang DB, Habib M, DuPont HL. Sociodemographic, environmental and clinical risk factors for developing persistent diarrhoea among infants in a rural community of Egypt. J Health Popul Nutr. 2001;19:313–9.

18. Bhutta ZA, Hendricks KH. Nutritional management of persistent diarrhea in childhood: a perspective from the developing world. J Pediatr Gastroenterol Nutr. 1996;22:17–37.

19. Illig KA, Ryan CK, Hardy DJ, Rhodes J, Locke W, Sax HC. Total parenteral nutrition-induced changes in gut mucosal function: atrophy alone is not the issue. Surgery. 1992;112(4):631–7.

20. Strand TA, Sharma PR, Gjessing HK, Ulak M, Chandyo RK, Adhikari RK, Sommerfelt H. Risk factors for extended duration of acute diarrhea in young children. PloS One. 2012;7(5):e36436.

21. Newman RD, Sears CL, Nataro JP, Fedorko DP, Wuhib T, Schorling JB, Guerrant RL. Persistent diarrhea signals a critical period of increased diarrhea burdens and nutritional shortfalls: a prospective cohort study among children in northeastern Brazil. J Infect Dis. 2000;181:1643–51.

22. Ahmed R, Ansaruzzaman M, Haque E, Rao MR, Clemens JD. Epidemiology of postshigellosis persistent diarrhea in young children. Pediatr Infect Dis J. 2001;20:525–530.

23. Mahalanabis D, Alam AN, Rahman N, Hasnat A. Prognostic indicators and risk factors for increased duration of acute diarrhoea and for persistent diarrhoea in children. Int J Epidemiol. 1991;20:1064–72.

24. Baqui AH, Black RE, Sack RB, Chowdhury HR, Yunus M, Siddique AK. Malnutrition, cell-mediated immune deficiency and diarrhea: a community-based longitudinal study in rural Bangladeshi children. Am J Epidemiol. 1993;137:355–65.

25. Raqib R, Mia SM, Qadri F, Alam TI, Alam NH, Chowdhury AK, Mathan MM, Andersson J. Innate immune responses in children and adults with Shigellosis. Infect Immun. 2000;68:3620–9.

26. Amadi B, Kelly P, Mwiya M, Mulwazi E, Sianongo S, Changwe F, Thomson M, Hachungula J, Watuka A, Walker-Smith J, Chintu C. Intestinal and systemic infection, HIV, and mortality in Zambian children with persistent diarrhea and malnutrition. J Pediatr Gastroenterol Nutr. 2001;32:550–4.

27. Tumwine JK, Kekitiinwa A, Nabukeera N, Akiyoshi DE, Buckholt MA, Tzipori S. *Enterocytozoon bieneusi* among children with diarrhea attending Mulago hospital in Uganda. Am J Trop Med Hyg. 2002;67:299–303.

28. Sullivan PB, Marsh MN, Mirakian R, Hill SM, Milla PJ, Neale G. Chronic diarrhea and malnutrition—histology of the small intestinal lesion. J Pediatr Gastroenterol Nutr. 1991;12(2):195–203.

29. Fagundes-Neto U, De Martini-Costa S, Pedroso MZ, Scaletsky IC. Studies of the small bowel surface by scanning electron microscopy in infants with persistent diarrhea. Braz J Med Biol Res. 2000;33:1437–42.

30. Sullivan PB, Lunn PG, Northrop-Clewes C, Crowe PT, Marsh MN, Neale G. Persistent diarrhea and malnutrition—the impact of treatment on small bowel structure and permeability. J Pediatr Gastroenterol Nutr. 1992;14:208–15.

31. Jakobsson I. Intestinal permeability in children of different ages and with different gastrointestinal diseases. Pediatr Allergy Immunol. 1993;4 Suppl 3:33–9.

32. Holm S, Lindberg T, Gothefors L. Macromolecular absorption during and after gastroenteritis in children. Acta Pediatr Scand. 1992;81:585–88.

33. Bhutta ZA, Nizami SQ, Thobani S. Factors determining recovery during nutritional therapy of persistent diarrhoea: the impact of diarrhoea severity and intercurrent infections. Acta Paediatrica. 1997;86:796–802.

34. Alam NH, Faruque AS, Dewan N, Sarker SA, Fuchs GJ. Characteristics of children hospitalized with severe dehydration and persistent diarrhoea in Bangladesh. J Health Popul Nutr. 2001;19:18–24.

35. Amadi B, Mwiya M, Musuku J, Watuka A, Sianongo S, Ayoub A, Kelly P. Effect of nitazoxanide on morbidity and mortality in Zambian children with cryptosporidiosis: a randomised controlled trial. Lancet. 2002;360:1375–80.

36. Ruxin JN. Magic bullet: the history of oral rehydration therapy. Med Hist. 1994;38:363–97.

37. Nalin DR, Cash RA, Rahman M. Oral (or nasogastric) maintenance therapy for cholera patients in all age-groups. Bull World Health Organ. 1970;43:361–3.

38. Sarker SA, Mahalanabis D, Alam NH, Sharmin S, Khan AM, Fuchs GJ. Reduced osmolarity oral rehydration solution for persistent diarrhea in infants: a randomized controlled clinical trial. J Pediatr. 2001;138:532–8.

39. Awasthi S, INCLEN childnet zinc effectiveness for diarrhea (ICZED) group. Zinc supplementation in acute diarrhea is acceptable, does not interfere with oral rehydration, and reduces the use of other medications: a randomized trial in five countries. J Pediatr Gastroenterol Nutr. 2006;42:300–5.

40. Lazzerini M, Ronfani L. Oral zinc for treating diarrhoea in children. Cochrane Database Syst Rev. 2013;1:CD005436. doi: 10.1002/14651858.CD005436.pub4.

41. de Mattos AP, Ribeiro TC, Mendes PS, Valois SS, Mendes CM, Ribeiro HC Jr. Comparison of yogurt, soybean, casein, and amino acid-based diets in children with persistent diarrhea. Nutr Res. 2009;29:462–9.

42. Chehade M, Magid MS, Mofidi S, Nowak-Wegrzyn A, Sampson HA, Sicherer SH. Allergic eosinophilic gastroenteritis with protein-losing enteropathy: intestinal pathology, clinical course, and long-term follow-up. J Pediatr Gastroenterol Nutr. 2006;42:516–21.

43. Rabbani GH, Teka T, Saha SK, Zaman B, Majid N, Khatun M, Wahed MA, Fuchs GJ. Green banana and pectin improve small intestinal permeability and reduce fluid loss in Bangladeshi children with persistent diarrhea. Dig Dis Sci. 2004;49(3):475–84.

44. Rabbani GH, Larson CP, Islam R, Saha UR, Kabir A. Green banana-supplemented diet in the home management of acute and prolonged diarrhoea in children: a community-based trial in rural Bangladesh. Trop Med Int Health. 2010;15(10):1132–9.

45. WHO. Guideline: updates on the management of severe acute malnutrition in infants and children. Geneva: WHO; 2013. http://apps.who.int/iris/bitstream/10665/95584/1/9789241506328_eng.pdf?ua=1. Accessed 1 April 2014.

46. Mahalanabis D, Bhan MK. Micronutrients as adjunct therapy of acute illness in children: impact on the episode outcome and

policy implications of current findings. Br J Nutr. 2001;85 (Suppl 2):S151–8.

47. Rahman MM, Vermund SH, Wahed MA, Fuchs GJ, Baqui AH, Alvarez JO. Simultaneous zinc and vitamin A supplementation in Bangladeshi children: randomised double blind controlled trial. BMJ. 2001;323:314–8.

48. Khatun UH, Malek MA, Black RE, Sarkar NR, Wahed MA, Fuchs G, Roy SK. A randomized controlled clinical trial of zinc, vitamin A or both in undernourished children with persistent diarrhea in Bangladesh. Acta Paediatr. 2001;90:376–80.

49. Villamor E, Mbise R, Spiegelman D, Hertzmark E, Fataki M, Peterson KE, Ndossi G, Fawzi WW. Vitamin A supplements ameliorate the adverse effect of HIV-1, malaria, and diarrheal infections on child growth. Pediatrics. 2002;109:E6.

50. Das JK, Lassi ZS, Salam RA, Bhutta ZA. Effect of community based interventions on childhood diarrhea and pneumonia: uptake of treatment modalities and impact on mortality. BMC Public Health. 2013;13 (Suppl 3):S29.

51. Allen SJ, Okoko B, Martinez E, Gregorio G, Dans LF. Probiotics for treating infectious diarrhoea. Cochrane Database Syst Rev. 2004;2:CD003048.

52. Bhandari N, Bahl R, Saxena M, Taneja S, Bhan MK. Prognostic factors for persistent diarrhoea managed in a community setting. Indian J Pediatr. 2000;67:739–45.

53. Valentiner-Branth P, Steinsland H, Santos G, Perch M, Begtrup K, Bhan MK, Dias F, Aaby P, Sommerfelt H, Molbak K. Community-based controlled trial of dietary management of children with persistent diarrhea: sustained beneficial effect on ponderal and linear growth. Am J Clin Nutr. 2001;73:968–74.

54. Niehaus MD, Moore SR, Patrick PD, Derr LL, Lorntz B, Lima AA, Guerrant RL. Early childhood diarrhea is associated with diminished cognitive function 4 to 7 years later in children in a northeast Brazilian shantytown. Am J Trop Med Hyg. 2002;66:590–3.

HIV and the Intestine

18

Andrea Lo Vecchio, Antonietta Giannattasio and Alfredo Guarino

Introduction

Acquired immune deficiency syndrome (AIDS) is the most devastating pandemic in human history. More than 100 million people worldwide currently have been infected with the human immunodeficiency virus (HIV), and an estimated 8 million individuals are currently treated. Prevention of mother-to-child transmission has proved highly effective, and this serves as a model for prevention using antiretroviral drugs. Antiretrovirals, the cornerstone of HIV treatment, are now being assessed as tools for limiting transmission in two ways: treatment as prevention and pre-exposure prophylaxis. The epidemiology of HIV in children is characterized by a double scenario. In countries where highly active antiretroviral therapy (HAART) is available, the pattern of HIV infection is evolving into a chronic disease, the control of which strictly depends on patients' adherence to treatment [1, 2]. In developing countries, with no or limited access to HAART, AIDS is rapidly expanding and is loaded with a high fatality ratio, due to the combined effects of malnutrition and opportunistic infections. The digestive tract is a target of the disease in both settings (Fig. 18.1).

Since the beginning of AIDS pandemic, it was clear that the virus gains access to the human host predominantly through the mucosal tissue after sexual exposure. However, HIV mucosal infection plays a critical role not only in virus transmission but also in AIDS pathogenesis, affecting mucosal surface of the gastrointestinal (GI) tract in the early phase post infection and depleting cluster of differentiation (CD4) T helper cells [4]. GI disease accounts for a high proportion of presenting symptoms of HIV infection, mainly in developing world [5]. Chronic diarrhea is a hallmark of advanced HIV infection, and it is caused by intestinal infections. Although the widespread use of HAART has dramatically improved the survival rate of HIV-infected people and has changed the spectrum of complications of HIV disease, the intestinal tract is still a major target of HIV infection. An uncertain, but high, percentage of HIV-infected patients worldwide initially presents or ultimately develops diarrhea or malnutrition, with or without HAART. Diarrhea is a major manifestation of HIV disease and is associated with increased morbidity and mortality. It substantially increases health-care costs for many patients, particularly those with severe malabsorption and malnutrition requiring repeated hospitalizations. In many cases, a multidisciplinary approach including specialist in gastroenterology, infectious disease, especially HIV, oncology, surgery and microbiology is required for treating patients with AIDS.

The Spectrum of GI Disorders in HIV Infection

The stage of immunodeficiency, reflected by the CD4 lymphocyte count, should be kept in mind when approaching any HIV-infected patient with GI symptoms because the etiology and the frequency of opportunistic infections are related to the CD4 count and rises exponentially if CD4 is <100 cell/ul.

The upper GI tract is a topographical target of HIV infection. Candida is the most common oesophageal pathogen in AIDS. However, in the era of antiretroviral therapy (ART), many of the previously common HIV-related disorders are vanished [6], but they can be observed in patients who are failing on HAART or non-adherent to therapy [7]. The approach to HIV patients with a CD4 count >200 cell/μl and upper GI symptoms should parallel that of any other non-HIV-infected subject. Upper endoscopy remains the gold standard diagnostic approach in case of suspected gastro-oesophageal reflux disease, dysphagia or bleeding. In severely immunosuppressed children, in whom opportunistic infections are considered, upper endoscopy with multiple tissue sampling

A. Lo Vecchio (✉) · A. Guarino ·A. Giannattasio
Section of Pediatrics, Department of Translational Medical Science, University of Naples "Federico II", Via S. Pansini 5, 80131 Naples, Italy
e-mail: andrealovecchio@gmail.com

© Springer International Publishing Switzerland 2016
S. Guandalini et al. (eds.), *Textbook of Pediatric Gastroenterology, Hepatology and Nutrition*,
DOI 10.1007/978-3-319-17169-2_18

Fig. 18.1 Pathway of malnutrition and gastrointestinal disorders in children with HIV infection. A complex interplay exists among these conditions. (Reprinted from [3] with permission)

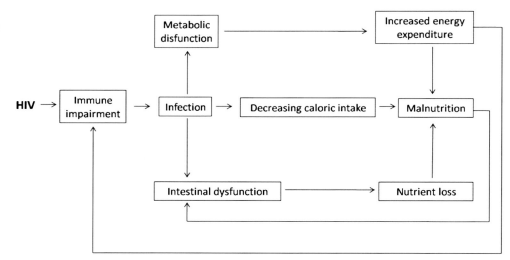

should be performed for a definitive diagnosis [8]. For example, multiple biopsies (about 10) increase the yield for cytomegalovirus (CMV) disease [9].

Intestinal infections are a major cause of morbidity and mortality, especially for children, and where the availability of HAART is limited. In patients with advanced HIV disease, opportunistic infections are the most common cause of disease. Cryptosporidium and microsporidium are the most common pathogens in developing countries and CMV in developed world. However, although opportunistic causes of diarrhea have fallen dramatically in the era of ART, overall the number of patients experiencing diarrhea has changed very little [10]. Other infections unrelated to immunodeficiency and noninfectious causes are also increased in HIV-infected children. Drug-induced diarrhea is an important cause of diarrhea in HIV patients [11]. Severe diarrhea associated with villous atrophy and crypt hypertrophy with no pathogen is found despite extensive investigation is defined as HIV enteropathy. The approach to diarrhea in HIV-infected patients should be based on routine stool testing, but these are often repeatedly negative, mainly in severe immunosuppressed subjects. In these cases, endoscopic examination with biopsy is able to establish a diagnosis in 65–80% of cases [8].

Intestinal dysfunction is a specific HIV-related syndrome in children [3]. The clinical manifestations of intestinal dysfunction may be limited or absent. Namely dysfunction is not consistently associated with diarrhea but its most prominent features are steatorrhoea, reduction of the intestinal absorptive surface and increased permeability [3]. Despite the limited or absent clinical manifestations of intestinal dysfunction, nutrient malabsorption certainly contributes to weight loss, and its clinical consequences may be expected in the long term and associated with progressive failure to thrive. The pathophysiology of intestinal dysfunction is complex and involves multiple abnormalities. HAART is able to re-

store intestinal function tests in HIV-infected children, in parallel with a decrease in viral load and an increase in CD4 T cell count [3]. This suggests that in case of malnutrition in a child receiving ART, careful monitoring of antiretroviral therapeutic efficacy is needed, as malnutrition may be an early marker of treatment failure.

Liver disease is the second most common cause of death among adults with HIV infection. Just as the burden of non-AIDS morbidity and mortality has changed in the ART era, the spectrum of liver diseases has also changed in these patients [12]. Prior to ART, the most common causes of liver dysfunction were opportunistic infections, including CMV and mycobacterium infections, AIDS lymphoma and Kaposi's sarcoma. Since the HAART era, however, the spectrum of liver disease among HIV-infected individuals has shifted to concomitant infection with chronic hepatitis C virus (HCV), and chronic hepatitis B virus infections, medication-related hepatotoxicity and nonalcoholic fatty liver disease (NAFLD). Although hepatic dysfunction is not frequent in HIV in children, hepatomegaly without other symptoms of systemic disease is commonly found in pediatric patients, and it is often associated with nutritional deficiency. HBV and HCV infections may be more severe in HIV-infected children than in HIV-negative individuals. In addition, liver toxicity is one of the most common serious adverse events associated with ART [12].

Pancreatic dysfunction may be considered as a component of HIV-associated digestive dysfunction in HIV. In fact, a reduction of faecal levels of pancreatic elastase and/or chymotrypsin has been found in one third of HIV-infected children [13]. The clinical manifestations of pancreatic involvement may not be evident, because exocrine, rather than endocrine, pancreatic function, is involved. Pancreatitis may be an unusual but serious drug adverse effect, mainly with selected nucleoside analogue reverse transcriptase inhibitors.

HIV Enteropathy

Since the discovery of HIV as an agent of AIDS, histological abnormalities of GI tract were observed, and the term "HIV enteropathy" was firstly used in 1984 [14]. Many investigators found that HIV itself infected enterocytes, lamina propria and submucosal cells. The enteropathy was characterized by inflammatory infiltrates of lymphocytes, damage to the GI epithelium, villous atrophy, crypt hyperplasia, and villous blunting, in the absence of detectable enteropathogens, recurring in all stages of HIV disease [15]. GI abnormalities associated with HIV infection include a decreased capacity for epithelial regeneration, impaired absorptive ability of GI mucosa, increased mucosal permeability, dysregulations of genes associated with T cell homeostasis, decreased growth factor production and cell-cycle mediators and upregulation of genes associated with apoptosis [16–18].

Not surprisingly, inflammatory changes are mild or absent. Once opportunistic disorders are excluded in patients with refractory diarrhea, HIV enteropathy is diagnosed in a small but definite percentage of patients. The HIV enteropathy encompasses an idiopathic, pathogen-negative diarrhea, and it can occur from the acute phase of the HIV infection through advanced disease, leading to GI inflammation, increased intestinal permeability, bile acid and vitamins malabsorption [19]. The functional disruption of the GI caused by HIV has been reported also in the absence of clear clinical GI manifestations in the era of modern ART [20]. More than one third of HIV-infected patients present an abnormal D-xylose test, about 20 % has low or borderline serum B12 levels and 7 % has low albumin levels, in the absence of stool pathogens [20].

Although the mechanisms responsible for these abnormalities remain not completely known, several explanations have been put forward, from a virotoxic effect of HIV itself on enterocytes [21, 22] to an abnormal differentiation of enterocytes induced by HIV [23, 24], to local activation of the GI immune system [25]. However, a major role is likely associated with HIV transactivator factor (Tat) [21].

Interaction Between HIV and Intestine

Immunopathogenesis of HIV involves two phenomenons: the loss of lymphoid cells and the loss of immune function. Several pathological changes, both structural and immunological, occur at the intestinal mucosal surface from the initial stage of HIV infection. The intestinal mucosa is a target for HIV and a site of significant HIV replication and CD4 T cell destruction, based upon the route of exposure and other aspects of mucosal immunology [26, 27]. Gut-associated lymphoid tissue (GALT) was identified as an early site of HIV replication and CD4 T cells depletion since the initial stage of HIV infection [28]. Even with early and aggressive HAART, GALT is not preserved and undergoes significant damage.

The sensitivity by intestinal tract to HIV infection relates in part to the high number of activated memory T cells expressing C-C chemokine receptor type 5 (CCR5) chemokine receptors located within the gut. HIV-1 isolated from acutely infected subjects are predominantly R5 viruses, that is macrophage-tropic HIV that requires CCR5 for cell entry, in contrast to R4 virus, lymphocyte-tropic HIV requiring the C-X-C chemokine receptor type 4 (CXCR4) chemokine receptor [29]. The preferential loss of CCR5 + CD4 T cells from the GI tract clearly suggests a virus-centric mechanism. Furthermore, the intestinal mucosa has continuous exposure to antigens, leading to a pro-inflammatory state, and secretes many cytokines that stimulate HIV replication [18].

There is a compartimentalization of HIV infection between blood and mucosa, mainly due to viral factors. The CD4/CD8 ratio was analysed in the duodenum and peripheral blood in order to compare CD4 T cell depletion between these two anatomical sites, and it was found that the GI tract was preferentially depleted of CD4 T cells [30–33]. Moreover, CD4 T cells in the GI tract are tenfold more frequently infected by HIV than those in the peripheral blood, suggesting that the viral reservoir in the intestine is much greater than previously thought [34].

Another mechanism that can contribute to the HIV enteropathy is the infection of enterocytes by HIV 1. In in vitro experiments, HIV is able to replicate in the intestinal epithelial cell lines [35, 36]. However, virus-direct and -indirect effects have been described. In addition to structural and enzymatic proteins, HIV-1 encodes a group of at least six auxiliary regulatory proteins, including Tat, a transactivating peptide essential for HIV replication, which exerts its effects by activating L-type Ca^{2+} channels, and/or mobilizing intracellular calcium stores [37, 38]. Tat is secreted from HIV-1-infected cells and is taken up by neighbouring uninfected cells. In vitro experiments using human colonic adenocarcinoma (caco-2) cell monolayers and human colonic mucosa specimens mounted in ussing chambers, it has been shown that Tat protein induced ion secretion similar to that induced by bacterial endotoxins. It also significantly prevents enterocytes proliferation [39]. On the bases of these data, it is likely that Tat directly exerts pathogenic effects on enterocytes and is involved in the pathogenesis of intestinal mucosal atrophy typical of HIV-infected patients, that is, in HIV enteropathy.

Tat has been implicated also in enterocyte apoptosis. Tat causes an imbalance in reactive oxygen species (ROS) generation in neurons, which is neutralized by antioxidants, thereby implicating perturbation of the intracellular redox status in the pathogenesis of HIV-induced cell damage [40]. Oxidative stress is implicated in the pathogenesis and morbidity of HIV infection. An increase of ROS and an alteration of antioxidant defences have been reported in HIV-infected patients [41] associated with decreased levels of antioxidants [42]. The mechanisms involved in HIV-induced oxidative stress are unknown, but HIV-1 proteins gp120 and Tat have been implicated in this process because they both induce oxidative stress and cause apoptosis in brain endothelial cells [43]. Similar mechanism has been involved in intestinal mucosa (Fig. 18.2). In an in vitro cell model, Tat increased the generation of ROS and decreased antioxidant defences as judged by a reduction in catalase activity and a reduced glutathione (GSH)/oxidized glutathione disulfide (GSSG) ratio [44]. Tat also induces cytochrome c release from mitochondria to cytosol, and caspase-3 activation. Rectal dialysis samples from HIV-infected patients were positive for the oxidative stress marker 8-hydroxy-29-deoxyguanosine. GSH/GSSG imbalance and apoptosis were observed in jejunal specimens from HIV-positive patients at baseline and from HIV-negative specimens exposed to Tat. Experiments with neutralizing anti-Tat antibodies showed that these effects were direct and specific. Pretreatment with N-acetyl cysteine (NAC) prevented Tat-induced apoptosis and restored the glutathione balance in both the in vitro and the ex vivo model

[44]. These findings indicate that oxidative stress is one of the mechanism involved in HIV intestinal disease (Fig. 18.3).

HAART and HIV Enteropathy

HAART reduces viral loads and increases CD4 T cells. GI symptoms including abdominal pain, bloating and diarrhea improve after initiation of treatment, in parallel with CD4 T cell reconstitution in blood and a decrease in viral load in rectal tissue [36]. The effects of HAART on intestinal CD4 T cells are lower than in peripheral blood [45, 46]. Furthermore, HAART started early during infection leads to an increase in CD4 central memory cells in Peyer's patches, but does not restore effector memory cells in the ileal lamina propria [47, 48]. Initiation of HAART during chronic infection does not significantly increase CD4 T cells in gut-inductive or -effector sites [45, 46]. Finally, no HIV-infected individual reconstituted GI tract CD4 T cells to levels observed in uninfected persons. These findings suggest that fibrotic damage severely disrupt the ability of GALT to support normal T cell trafficking and survival, even after HAART onset. In addition, not only CD4 T cells fail to fully repopulate the

Fig. 18.2 Effect of NAC on the Tat-induced oxidative stress in Caco-2 cells [44]. Intracellular ROS levels, determined by fluorometric method, after exposure of Tat with or without pretreatment with NAC (**a**). Data were represented as percent of controls. Effect of NAC on Tat-induced GSH/GSSG imbalance (**b**). Data are represented as percent of GSH *(grey)* and GSSG *(white)* versus total glutathione. *p, 0.05 vs. control; #p, 0.05 versus Tat. Data are representative of three separate experiments. *NAC* N-acetyl cysteine, *Tat* transactivator factor. (Reprinted from Ref. [44])

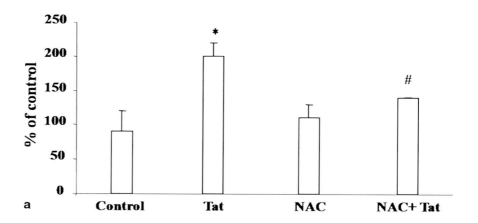

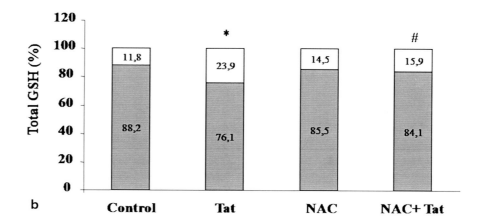

Fig. 18.3 Schematic representation of the mechanism of HIV Tat viral protein-induced oxidative damage to the intestinal mucosa [44]. Tat induces oxidative stress by increasing the ROS intracellular level and deranging the GSH/GSSG ratio. This leads to programmed cell death (apoptosis) and an increase in epithelial damage. Together with ion secretion and altered glucose transport, these steps could represent key mechanisms in HIV enteropathy. *ROS* reactive oxygen species, *GSH* glutathione, *Tat* transactivator factor, *HIV* human immunodeficiency virus . (Reprinted from Ref. [44])

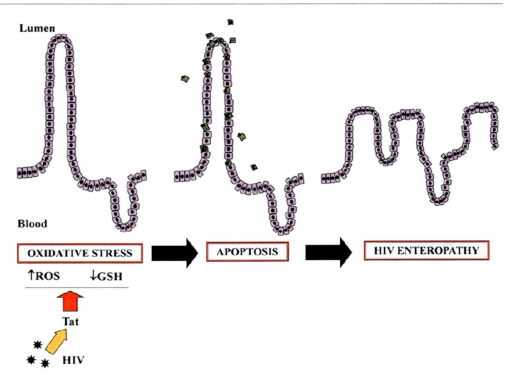

GI tract following HAART but also HIV proviral DNA persists in CD4 T cells in terminal ileum 10 years after effective therapy [49]. As a consequence, viral replication persists at low levels in the intestine despite HAART.

GI Infections

The spectrum of HIV-related GI infections has changed dramatically after the introduction and the worldwide diffusion of ART, and still today the epidemiology significantly varies between HIV-infected children treatment-naïve or on ART. The CD4 lymphocyte count continues to be the best predictor of the risk of an opportunistic infection [8, 50], although HIV viral load seems to be also helpful in predicting this risk [51, 52] (Fig. 18.4). Data in children on ART living in developed areas are limited to small reports; however, studies conducted in Africa and reporting the pathogens isolated in children presenting with HIV and diarrhea are reasonably consistent.

A list of the most common agents in HIV/AIDS children is reported in Table 18.1. In addition, Kaposi sarcoma and intestinal lymphoma are also specifically included in HIV-associated intestinal disorders.

In addition, HIV may probably act as a direct enteropathogen and induces ulcerative processes involving distal oesophagus, ileum and rectum because only viral particles have been found in these lesions [53]. Different immunosuppressive approach including with thalidomide, anti-tumour necrosis factor (TNF) agents or corticosteroids have been used, in some case with success, to treat these lesions [54].

Upper Gastrointestinal Infections

The upper GI tract, including oral cavity, oesophagus and stomach, is commonly involved in HIV-related diseases.

Oesophageal localization of opportunistic agents is common in advanced HIV infections, and candida and herpes are most common agents of oesophageal ulcerations. This complication is strongly related to the immunological states, being quite common in subjects with CD4 count <200 cells/μl, who are failing ART or are non compliant.

Oral thrush and odynophagia or dysphagia are the most commonly reported upper GI symptoms in HIV-infected children and adolescents. Thrush, appearing white–yellow, hard-to-remove plaques due to Candida infection, is a characteristic sign in young HIV/AIDS children. Candidiasis of the mouth and distal oesophagus are associated with loss of appetite, dysphagia and weight loss. Most severe cases of Candida infection cause necrotizing oesophagitis, bleeding and, occasionally, perforation. Other opportunistic agents may present with a similar clinical and endoscopic feature, thus biopsy is usually needed to exclude agents such as herpes, Cytomegalovirus (CMV) or intracellular *Mycobacterium avium*. Before ART introduction, Candida was by far the first cause of oesophageal complaints and empirical treatment with fluconazole, instead of endoscopy, was considered as the best strategy, especially in patients with thrush [55]. Recently, a report of more than 400 GI endoscopies in HIV/AIDS patients found that odynophagia/dysphagia had the highest yield of positive diagnosis, and it showed that both Candida and CMV are major agents of oesophageal involve-

Table 18.1 Opportunistic disorders affecting GI tract in HIV/AIDS patients	Viral Agent	Cytomegalovirus, herpes simplex, rotavirus and adenovirus
	Parasites	Cryptosporidia, giardia and isospora
	Fungi	Candida, cryptococcus, microsporidia and histoplasma
	Bacteria	Shigella, listeria, salmonella, mycobacteria
	Tumour	Kaposi, lymphoma

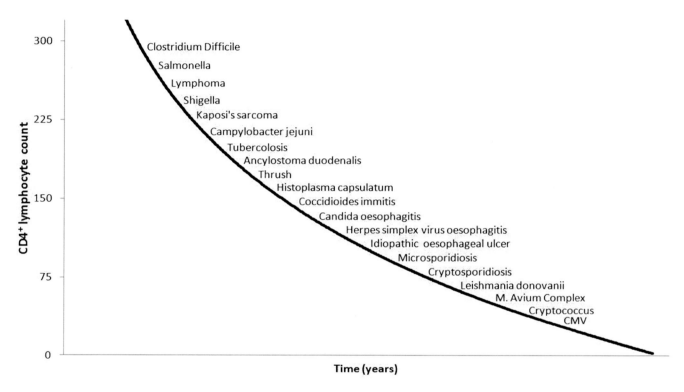

Fig. 18.4 Correlation between CD4 count and risk of HIV-related diseases. *CD* cluster of differentiation, *CMV* cytomegalovirus

ment [54]. A large part of endoscopies, however, resulted in nonspecific oesophageal ulcers, pathophysiology of which is still unclear, and probably due to herpes or HIV itself.

Symptoms of dyspepsia, including epigastric pain, nausea and vomiting, are frequently reported by HIV-infected patients and especially those undergoing ART. The diagnostic approach in these patients may be challenging. Noninvasive testing for *Helicobacter pylori* is not useful in the diagnosis of HIV-infected subjects with strongly suppressed immune system, and a low incidence of this infection has been reported in this population [56, 57]. Empirical treatment with proton-pump inhibitors may be inappropriate for HIV-infected patients because these drugs reduce the oral absorption of selected protease inhibitors [58]. Atypical presentation of opportunistic infections should always be considered in this population and upper endoscopy is suggested for differential diagnosis. Multiple biopsies are needed since macroscopic normal-appearing mucosa does not exclude opportunistic in-

fections [59]. However, the role of opportunistic infections in HIV/AIDS patients presenting with dyspepsia as primary symptom is still not clear. The rate of opportunistic infections in a large population of adults on ART presenting with dyspepsia was less than 2%, and CMV was the most prevalent opportunistic agent [59]. Chronic nonspecific gastritis (mononuclear cell infiltrate) is the most common diagnosis in patients presenting with this symptomatology.

Diarrhea

Chronic diarrhea, in most of cases due to GI infections, is a hallmark of advanced HIV infection and remains a major substantial cause of morbidity and mortality in children.

In Africa, chronic diarrhea has been reported in as many as 90% HIV-positive children, being five- to sixfold higher than in non-HIV-infected children [60, 61]. Case series from industrialized countries in the pre-ART era showed that 40–80 % of HIV-infected patients experienced diarrhea [62].

Classical and opportunistic enteropathogens may induce diarrhea in HIV-infected children. The duration and severity of diarrhea are increased in HIV-infected children living either in developing or in industrialized countries.

The likelihood of opportunistic infections is linked to the severity of immunodeficiency. Some studies [63] suggested that in immunocompetent individuals (CD4 >200 cell/µl), the infections are usually caused by ordinary pathogens, while in those with a CD4 <200 cell/µl, opportunistic agents such as *Cryptosporidium parvum*, CMV and *Mycobacterium avium* are more common. Frequent agents of diarrhea in HIV-infected subjects, such as the parasite *Enterocytozoon bieneusi* or *Microsporidium*, are more restricted to adult population.

Bacterial Diarrhea

Although there is no specific hallmark of bacterial etiology, several bacterial agents may induce diarrhea. The overall incidence of bacterial diarrhea in HIV-infected adults is at least 100-fold greater than in general population [64], and infections in HIV-infected subjects tend to be more protracted and severe than in immunocompetent individuals. The rate of diarrhea due to bacterial causes significantly decreased after the introduction of ART.

HIV-positive patients are at higher risk of prolonged and severe infections from *Campylobacter jejuni* and invasive non-typhoid Salmonellae infections. The risk of multisite Salmonella infections may be 300-fold increased in advanced HIV disease, and this condition has been considered an AIDS-defining illness.

Escherichia coli, *Shigella* and *Clostridium* were recognized to cause more frequently diarrhea in HIV-infected patients. Recently, a large retrospective study in the USA reported *Clostridium difficile* as the most common cause of diarrhea in HIV-infected adults, accounting for more than 50 % of cases [64]. In the same population *Shigella*, *Campylobacter* and *Salmonella* were found in 14, 13.8 and 7.4 % patients with diarrhea, respectively.

Mycobacteria may cause GI infections presenting with diarrhea. Diarrhea is a relatively uncommon symptom of *Mycobacterium tuberculosis* infection, but may be more common in *Mycobacterium avium* complex (MAC) infection. However, prophylaxis with azithromycin routinely performed in the pre-ART era is no longer indicated in children receiving ART.

Bacterial diarrhea may have a severe course in HIV-infected children, and it should be treated aggressively. The use of specific antibiotics should be carefully considered even in children who show a mild course of the disease, particularly in those who have moderate-to-severe immune impairment. Some children may require empiric treatment for

symptom control or prevention of the risk of extra-intestinal spreading of the infection.

Viral Diarrhea

Viruses are the leading cause of acute diarrhea in children, and they usually have an acute and self-limiting course in immunocompetent children. Etiology of acute diarrhea in HIV-infected and non-infected children is substantially similar after the introduction of ART. A very high number of enteric viruses were detected in the stools of HIV-infected children without clear relationship with intestinal symptoms. However, viral enteropathy may be dangerous in HIV-positive children.

Rotavirus is the major cause of viral diarrhea in countries in which specific vaccination has not been routinely introduced. Children with HIV infection experience more frequent and severe Rotavirus infections, with a higher risk of prolonged hospitalization and a higher fatality rate than non-HIV-infected children [61].

The development, validation and large-scale implementation of anti-Rotavirus immunization is changing the epidemiology of intestinal infections in industrialized countries that developed a routine vaccination programme [65]. Immunogenicity of Rotavirus vaccines in areas with high rate of HIV infection, like Africa, showed a good and consistent immune response. Immunogenicity is variable and resulted comparable or lower than those observed in Europe and the USA according to different evidence [66]. Although HIV infection is generally not a contraindication for immunization, high HIV prevalence in the region may result in lower rates of vaccine immunogenicity, efficacy and population immunity [67].

Other enteropathogens may cause acute diarrhea in HIV-infected children. Norovirus, generally considered the second leading agent of acute diarrhea, is fast becoming a major cause of medically attended gastroenteritis in countries with high Rotavirus vaccine coverage [68]. This agent may also induce severe and chronic disease manifestations in HIV-positive children [69].

CMV may act as an opportunistic enteric agent inducing severe colitis or enterocolitis or even an intractable diarrhea syndrome in severely immunocompromised children. CMV is by far the major opportunistic etiology of colitis in HIV-infected subjects [54]. As for other opportunistic infections, the introduction of ART significantly reduced the rate of CMV infection in adult patients decreasing from 7.34 to 0.75/100 patients-year. Also the survival at 1 and 2 years that was 42.6 and 16.7 % before ART, significantly improved to 84.6 and 76.9 %, respectively, in ART era [70].

CMV-related clinical symptoms reported in children include chronic diarrhea, abdominal pain and bleeding. Mucosal ulceration may sometimes result in bleeding and perforation of the large bowel. Symptomatic infection is more common and severe in HIV-infected children of less than 12 months of age and with low CD4 counts. CMV infection of the endothelial cells and ensuing vasculitis may play a major role in the development of thrombosis, local ischaemia and ulceration of the GI mucosa [71]. Diagnosis can be difficult because the virus may remain latent for long periods of time and neither serological test nor positive urine test indicate active disease. Intestinal endoscopy may show mucosal oedema/erythema, haemorrhages, erosions and ulcers; however, normal macroscopic endoscopic findings may reasonably exclude CMV diagnosis. Nearly 25 % of normal gross endoscopy can have evidence of CMV infection on histopathology, with typical intranuclear and intracytoplasmic inclusion bodies [72]. CMV viral load may drive therapeutic/prophylactic approach. Ganciclovir and foscarnet are the main treatment options; however, relapse rate is high and the prognosis may be poor.

Parasitic Diarrhea

Numerous parasites cause diarrhea in HIV- infected children. These include parasites usually described to have pathogenic activity in general population (*Giardia lamblia, Entamoeba histolytica, Blastocystis hominis, Strongyloides stercoralis* and other soil-transmitted helminths) and some parasites not previously thought to have significant pathogenic role including *Cryptosporidium parvum, Isospora belli, and Cyclospora cayetanensis*. These opportunistic parasites are spore-forming protozoa which cause intracellular infection and can lead to severe intestinal injury and prolonged diarrhea in advanced HIV infection [73]. The risk of parasitic infection is closely related to the impaired immunity, namely CD4 count [74]. In a recent study, in a population of immunocompromised children (most with HIV) with persistent or recurrent diarrhea, parasites were found in 57 % of cases and most frequently in preschool-age children and in HIV subjects not receiving antiretrovirals or with low CD4 counts [75].

Low socioeconomic conditions, including sanitary facilities or access to safe water, represent a risk factor for parasitic infection and should be considered when assessing HIV-infected patients.

Identification of parasites may be difficult on direct microscopy, and the diagnosis may be missed. The use of molecular diagnostic tools in epidemiological investigations of *Cryptosporidium, Giardia* and *Enterocytozoon* provides new insights into their characterization and transmission pathways [76].

Cryptosporidium is the most important opportunistic parasite for both frequency and severity in HIV. It may cause severe dehydrating diarrhea-associated abdominal pain and massive fluid loss due to an enterotoxic activity. Although the most common localization of *Cryptosporidium* is the duodenum, stomach, colon and bile tract may be involved. Co-infection with CMV increases severity and may lead to death. Intravenous rehydration is generally needed and often clinical nutritional support is required to balance the rapid weight loss which may trigger a vicious circle of nutritional (fat malabsorption) and immune derangement. Several antimicrobial agents including spiramycin, paramomycin, azithromycin and nitazoxanide have been proposed but the best treatment is ART which restores gut mucosal CD4 cells. Albendazole has been proposed with some success in adult patients with chronic diarrhea [77].

Fungi

Microsporidia, previously included among parasites, have been recently reclassified as fungi. Some species such as *Enterocytozoon bieneusi* and *Encephalitozoon intestinalis* have been proposed as etiological agents of persistent diarrhea and failure to thrive in African children. This relationship remained valid after controlling for HIV and concurrent cryptosporidiosis [78]. The *Encephalitozoon* species contribute to enteric disease but tend to disseminate. In adults, microsporidium infects the small bowel and potentially the proximal colon, causing chronic watery diarrhea and wasting. Children are less susceptible than adults to *microsporidium* [79, 80].

Candida species are frequently isolated from the stool of HIV-positive patients and have been implicated in antibiotic associated diarrhea [81]. However, its role in determining diarrhea is still unclear.

Histoplasmosis may cause asymptomatic infection in healthy children. However, in HIV-infected children, disseminated disease may occur and the clinical picture is variable depending on the immunological status.

Malignancies

HIV-associated GI malignancies may present with pathogen-negative diarrhea. Intestinal Kaposi sarcoma may present with diarrhea, rectal bleeding and sometimes with intestinal obstruction. The risk of non-Hodgkin B cell lymphomas is 60–200-fold increased in HIV-infected subjects; Burkitt's and Burkitt-like lymphomas and diffuse large-cell lymphomas are the subtypes that most likely affect the GI tract in HIV-infected patients.

Both diseases are AIDS-defining conditions and, although considered noninfectious, are related to oncogenic herpes viruses such as human herpesvirus 8 (HHV8) and Epstein-Barr virus (EBV). Other neoplasia, such as Hodgkin lymphoma, that is not AIDS-defining disease, are more likely diagnosed in HIV-infected individuals, and their importance is increasing in the ART era.

Management of Diarrhea in HIV-infected Children

In HIV-infected children with mild-to-moderate immune suppression, acute-onset diarrhea is often self-limited and does not require specific diagnostic evaluation or treatment. In most cases, management may be that recommended for immunocompetent children with diarrhea, which is based on oral rehydration and early refeeding with full-strength milk or formula. In contrast, in children with immune impairment or at risk due to other conditions, such as malnutrition, investigations should be always initiated with stool microbiological examination. The immune status of the child should drive the diagnostic approach, and diagnosis should be more rapid and aggressive in severely immunocompromised children.

Initial microbiological investigations should include specific search for Salmonella, Shigella, *Campylobacter,* Rotavirus, Norovirus, Adenovirus and *Cryptosporidium.* The latter should be specifically investigated for by immunofluorescence, and positive tests should be confirmed by Giemsa, modified Ziehl Neelsen or auramine stain. At least three different stool samples should be analysed to increase sensitivity. In those patients, blood culture may increase the yield of bacterial agents. Antibiotic-associated diarrhea should be considered, and toxin-producing *Clostridium difficile* should be searched.

If microbiological investigation is inconclusive, the option is to treat the patient with empiric therapy or, when possible, to perform an endoscopy and obtain intestinal biopsy that may be helpful for further microbiological investigations (intracellular enteric agents) and rule out malignancies. Children with protracted diarrhea should undergo upper endoscopy and sigmoidoscopy depending on diarrheal pattern and characteristics. Pancolonoscopy may be reserved to patients in more severe conditions and who did not respond to first-line treatment.

In addition, it should be noted that children with HIV infection share surprising similarities with coeliac disease. They not only have intestinal malabsorption but also may present with increased antibody titer to gliadin as a result to nonspecific HIV-related polyclonal activation.

oral/oesophageal infections (candidiasis) and ageusia to anorexia related to ART or to psychological status (mainly in adolescents).

Sugar malabsorption is the most frequent and severe feature of AIDS-related intestinal dysfunction; it is related to the direct action of HIV (Tat-mediated) on the enterocyte and contributes to AIDS-associated malabsorption [21]. Micronutrient deficiencies are frequently observed in patients with AIDS. Iron deficiency is a common problem in HIV-infected children; it may be the result of increased infection rate or a low intake, but in most of cases is the result of intestinal malabsorption.

Malabsorption may be impaired by pancreatic dysfunction and directly by drugs. Folate and B12 levels may be reduced in children receiving zidovudine. Vitamins A and E may be decreased in children with fat malabsorption. In addition, vitamin A and zinc deficiencies may increase the risk of intestinal and extra-intestinal infections, and these should be corrected with adequate supplementation, mainly in developed areas.

Specific nutrients and other endogenous molecules can directly influence intestinal mucosal turnover, repair and adaptation. In vitro evidence demonstrated that zinc limits Tat-induced fluid secretion and HIV-related diarrhea [82]. It may be hypothesized that the enterocyte has evolved a common response to "positive moieties" including ion absorption and cell growth. Intestinal adaptation depends on factors that modulate intestinal functions and that act not only with a time- and dose-related pattern but also with a time-related fine-tuning [83].

In conclusion, the intestinal involvement in HIV infection is closely related to the access to HAART, and therefore shows a geo-economical pattern. In high incidence settings with limited access to HAART, intestinal infections with opportunistic agents are still a major problem, and there is a high incidence of intestinal dysfunction with a complex interplay between intestinal malabsorption, immune impairment and infections. In children receiving HAART, there is a residual intestinal dysfunction, with no or limited symptoms. The latter may be more related to drugs and, however, have a mild intensity.

Nutrition

Many factors may impact on nutritional status of HIV-infected children, including HIV-related malabsorption, antiviral treatment and opportunistic infections.

Caloric intake should be quantitatively determined, because the diseases itself and its complications are related to increased energy expenditure. In addition, it should be considered that a HIV-infected child who refuses to eat may have a number of heterogeneous conditions, ranging from

References

1. Giannattasio A, Barbarino A, Lo Vecchio A, Bruzzese E, Mango C, Guarino A. Effects of antiretroviral drug recall on perception of therapy benefits and on adherence to antiretroviral treatment in HIV-infected children. Curr HIV Res. 2009;7(5):468–72.
2. Giannattasio A, Albano F, Giacomet V, Guarino A. The changing pattern of adherence to antiretroviral therapy assessed at two time points, 12 months apart, in a cohort of HIV-infected children. Expert Opin Pharmacother. 2009;10(17):2773–8. doi:10.1517/14656560903376178.

3. Guarino A, Bruzzese E, De Marco G, Buccigrossi V. Management of gastrointestinal disorders in children with HIV infection. Paediatr Drugs. 2004;6(6):347–62.

4. Li Q, Duan L, Estes JD, Ma ZM, Rourke T, Wang Y, Reilly C, Carlis J, Miller CJ, Haase AT. Peak SIV replication in resting memory CD4+ T cells depletes gut lamina propria CD4+ T cells. Nature. 2005;434(7037):1148–52.

5. Cello JP, Day LW. Idiopathic AIDS enteropathy and treatment of gastrointestinal opportunistic pathogens. Gastroenterology. 2009;136(6):1952–65. doi:10.1053/j.gastro.2008.12.073 (Epub 2009 May 7).

6. Mönkemüller KE, Call SA, Lazenby AJ, Wilcox CM. Declining prevalence of opportunistic gastrointestinal disease in the era of combination antiretroviral therapy. Am J Gastroenterol. 2000;95(2):457–62.

7. Mönkemüller KE, Lazenby AJ, Lee DH, Loudon R, Wilcox CM. Occurrence of gastrointestinal opportunistic disorders in AIDS despite the use of highly active antiretroviral therapy. Dig Dis Sci. 2005;50(2):230–4.

8. Wilcox CM, Saag MS. Gastrointestinal complications of HIV infection: changing priorities in the HAART era. Gut. 2008;57(6):861–70. doi:10.1136/gut.2006.103432 (Epub 2008 Jan 18).

9. Wilcox CM, Straub RF, Schwartz DA. Prospective evaluation of biopsy number for the diagnosis of viral esophagitis in patients with HIV infection and esophageal ulcer. Gastrointest Endosc. 1996;44(5):587–93.

10. Anastasi JK, Capili B. HIV and diarrhea in the era of HAART: 1998 New York state hospitalizations. Am J Infect Control. 2000;28(3):262–6.

11. Guest JL, Ruffin C, Tschampa JM, DeSilva KE, Rimland D. Differences in rates of diarrhea in patients with human immunodeficiency virus receiving lopinavir-ritonavir or nelfinavir. Pharmacotherapy. 2004;24(6):727–35.

12. Price JC, Thio CL. Liver disease in the HIV-infected individual. Clin Gastroenterol Hepatol. 2010;8(12):1002–12. doi:10.1016/j.cgh.2010.08.024 (Epub 2010 Sept 17)

13. Carroccio A, Fontana M, Spagnuolo MI, Zuin G, Montalto G, Canani RB, Verghi F, Di Martino D, Bastoni K, Buffardi F, Guarino A. Pancreatic dysfunction and its association with fat malabsorption in HIV infected children. Gut. 1998;43(4):558–63.

14. Kotler DP, Gaetz HP, Lange M, Klein EB, Holt PR. Enteropathy associated with the acquired immunodeficiency syndrome. Ann Intern Med. 1984;101(4):421–8.

15. Batman PA, Miller AR, Forster SM, Harris JR, Pinching AJ, Griffin GE. Jejunal enteropathy associated with human immunodeficiency virus infection: quantitative histology. J Clin Pathol. 1989;42(3):275–81.

16. Sankaran S, George MD, Reay E, Guadalupe M, Flamm J, Prindiville T, Dandekar S. Rapid onset of intestinal epithelial barrier dysfunction in primary human immunodeficiency virus infection is driven by an imbalance between immune response and mucosal repair and regeneration. J Virol. 2008;82(1):538–45 (Epub 2007 Oct 24).

17. George MD, Reay E, Sankaran S, Dandekar S. Early antiretroviral therapy for simian immunodeficiency virus infection leads to mucosal CD4+ T-cell restoration and enhanced gene expression regulating mucosal repair and regeneration. J Virol. 2005;79(5):2709–19.

18. Costiniuk CT, Angel JB. Human immunodeficiency virus and the gastrointestinal immune system: does highly active antiretroviral therapy restore gut immunity? Mucosal Immunol. 2012;5(6):596–604. doi:10.1038/mi.2012.82 (Epub 2012 Aug 29).

19. Brenchley JM, Douek DC. HIV infection and the gastrointestinal immune system. Mucosal Immunol. 2008;1(1):23–30. doi:10.1038/mi.2007.1.

20. Knox TA, Spiegelman D, Skinner SC, Gorbach S. Diarrhea and abnormalities of gastrointestinal function in a cohort of men and women with HIV infection. Am J Gastroenterol. 2000;95(12):3482–9.

21. Canani RB, De Marco G, Passariello A, Buccigrossi V, Ruotolo S, Bracale I, Porcaro F, Bifulco G, Guarino A. Inhibitory effect of HIV-1 Tat protein on the sodium-D-glucose symporter of human intestinal epithelial cells. AIDS. 2006;20(1):5–10.

22. Maresca M, Mahfoud R, Garmy N, Kotler DP, Fantini J, Clayton F. The virotoxin model of HIV-1 enteropathy: involvement of GPR15/Bob and galactosylceramide in the cytopathic effects induced by HIV-1 gp120 in the HT-29-D4 intestinal cell line. J Biomed Sci. 2003;10(1):156–66.

23. Heise C, Dandekar S, Kumar P, Duplantier R, Donovan RM, Halsted CH. Human immunodeficiency virus infection of enterocytes and mononuclear cells in human jejunal mucosa. Gastroenterology. 1991;100(6):1521–7.

24. Clayton F, Kapetanovic S, Kotler DP. Enteric microtubule depolymerization in HIV infection: a possible cause of HIV-associated enteropathy. AIDS. 2001;15(1):123–4.

25. McGowan I, Elliott J, Fuerst M, Taing P, Boscardin J, Poles M, Anton P. Increased HIV-1 mucosal replication is associated with generalized mucosal cytokine activation. J Acquir Immune Defic Syndr. 2004;37(2):1228–36.

26. Cheroutre H, Madakamutil L. Acquired and natural memory T cells join forces at the mucosal front line. Nat Rev Immunol. 2004;4(4):290–300.

27. Kotler DP. HIV infection and the gastrointestinal tract. AIDS. 2005;19(2):107–17.

28. Dandekar S. Pathogenesis of HIV in the gastrointestinal tract. Curr HIV/AIDS Rep. 2007;4:10–15.

29. Schuitemaker H, Koot M, Kootstra NA, Dercksen MW, de Goede RE, van Steenwijk RP, Lange JM, Schattenkerk JK, Miedema F, Tersmette M. Biological phenotype of human immunodeficiency virus type 1 clones at different stages of infection: progression of disease is associated with a shift from monocytotropic to T-cell-tropic virus population. J Virol. 1992;66(3):1354–60.

30. Schneider T, Jahn HU, Schmidt W, Riecken EO, Zeitz M, Ullrich R. Loss of CD4 T lymphocytes in patients infected with human immunodeficiency virus type 1 is more pronounced in the duodenal mucosa than in the peripheral blood. Berlin Diarrhea/Wasting Syndrome Study Group. Gut. 1995;37(4):524–9.

31. Smit-McBride Z, Mattapallil JJ, McChesney M, Ferrick D, Dandekar S. Gastrointestinal T lymphocytes retain high potential for cytokine responses but have severe CD4(+) T-cell depletion at all stages of simian immunodeficiency virus infection compared to peripheral lymphocytes. J Virol. 1998;72(8):6646–56.

32. Mehandru S, Poles MA, Tenner-Racz K, Horowitz A, Hurley A, Hogan C, Boden D, Racz P, Markowitz M. Primary HIV-1 infection is associated with preferential depletion of CD4+ T lymphocytes from effector sites in the gastrointestinal tract. J Exp Med. 2004;200(6):761–70 (Epub 2004 Sept 13).

33. Brenchley JM, Schacker TW, Ruff LE, Price DA, Taylor JH, Beilman GJ, Nguyen PL, Khoruts A, Larson M, Haase AT, Douek DC. CD4+ T cell depletion during all stages of HIV disease occurs predominantly in the gastrointestinal tract. J Exp Med. 2004;200(6):749–59 (Epub 2004 Sept 13).

34. Mehandru S, Poles MA, Tenner-Racz K, Manuelli V, Jean-Pierre P, Lopez P, Shet A, Low A, Mohri H, Boden D, Racz P, Markowitz M. Mechanisms of gastrointestinal CD4+ T-cell depletion during acute and early human immunodeficiency virus type 1 infection. J Virol. 2007;81(2):599–612 (Epub 2006 Oct 25).

35. Duh EJ, Maury WJ, Folks TM, Fauci AS, Rabson AB. Tumor necrosis factor alpha activates human immunodeficiency virus type 1 through induction of nuclear factor binding to the NF-kappa B sites in the long terminal repeat. Proc Natl Acad Sci U S A. 1989;86(15):5974–8.

36. Kotler DP, Shimada T, Snow G, Winson G, Chen W, Zhao M, Inada Y, Clayton F. Effect of combination antiretroviral therapy

upon rectal mucosal HIV RNA burden and mononuclear cell apoptosis. AIDS. 1998;12(6):597–604.

37. Zocchi MR, Rubartelli A, Morgavi P, Poggi A. HIV-1 Tat inhibits human natural killer cell function by blocking L-type calcium channels. J Immunol. 1998;161(6):2938–43.

38. Haughey NJ, Holden CP, Nath A, Geiger JD. Involvement of inositol 1,4,5-trisphosphate-regulated stores of intracellular calcium in calcium dysregulation and neuron cell death caused by HIV-1 protein tat. J Neurochem. 1999;73(4):1363–74.

39. Canani RB, Cirillo P, Mallardo G, Buccigrossi V, Secondo A, Annunziato L, Bruzzese E, Albano F, Selvaggi F, Guarino A. Effects of HIV-1 Tat protein on ion secretion and on cell proliferation in human intestinal epithelial cells. Gastroenterology. 2003;124(2):368–76.

40. Agrawal L, Louboutin JP, Strayer DS. Preventing HIV-1 Tat-induced neuronal apoptosis using antioxidant enzymes: mechanistic and therapeutic implications. Virology. 2007;363:462–72.

41. Kline ER, Sutliff RL. The roles of HIV-1 proteins and antiretroviral drug therapy in HIV-1-associated endothelial dysfunction. J Investig Med. 2008;6:752–69.

42. Stehbens WE. Oxidative stress in viral hepatitis and AIDS. Exp Mol Pathol. 2004;77:121–32.

43. Banerjee A, Zhang X, Manda KR, Banks WA, Ercal N. HIV proteins (gp120 and Tat) and methamphetamine in oxidative stress-induced damage in the brain: potential role of the thiol antioxidant N-acetylcysteine amide. Free Radic Biol Med. 2010;48:1388–98.

44. Buccigrossi V, Laudiero G, Nicastro E, Miele E, Esposito F, Guarino A. The HIV-1 transactivator factor (Tat) induces enterocyte apoptosis through a redox-mediated mechanism. PLoS One. 2011;6(12):e29436. doi:10.1371/journal.pone.0029436 (Epub 2011 Dec 27).

45. Mehandru S, Poles MA, Tenner-Racz K, Jean-Pierre P, Manuelli V, Lopez P, Shet A, Low A, Mohri H, Boden D, Racz P, Markowitz M. Lack of mucosal immune reconstitution during prolonged treatment of acute and early HIV-1 infection. PLoS Med. 2006;3(12):e484.

46. Guadalupe M, Sankaran S, George MD, Reay E, Verhoeven D, Shacklett BL, Flamm J, Wegelin J, Prindiville T, Dandekar S. Viral suppression and immune restoration in the gastrointestinal mucosa of human immunodeficiency virus type 1-infected patients initiating therapy during primary or chronic infection. J Virol. 2006;80(16):8236–47.

47. Shacklett BL. Immune responses to HIV and SIV in mucosal tissues: 'location, location, location'. Curr Opin HIV AIDS. 2010;5(2):128–34. doi:10.1097/COH.0b013e328335c178.

48. Estes J, Baker JV, Brenchley JM, Khoruts A, Barthold JL, Bantle A, Reilly CS, Beilman GJ, George ME, Douek DC, Haase AT, Schacker TW. Collagen deposition limits immune reconstitution in the gut. J Infect Dis. 2008;198(4):456–64. doi:10.1086/590112.

49. Chun TW, Nickle DC, Justement JS, Meyers JH, Roby G, Hallahan CW, Kottilil S, Moir S, Mican JM, Mullins JI, Ward DJ, Kovacs JA, Mannon PJ, Fauci AS. Persistence of HIV in gut-associated lymphoid tissue despite long-term antiretroviral therapy. J Infect Dis. 2008;197(5):714–20. doi:10.1086/527324.

50. Holmes CB, Wood R, Badri M, et al. CD4 decline and incidence of opportunistic infections in Cape Town, South Africa: implications for prophylaxis and treatment. J Acquir Immune Defic Syndr. 2006;42:464–9.

51. Hogg RS, Yip B, Chan KJ, et al. Rates of disease progression by baseline CD4 cell count and viral load after initiating triple-drug therapy. JAMA. 2001;286:2568–77.

52. Kaplan JE, Hanson DL, Jones JL, et al. Viral load as an independent risk factor for opportunistic infections in HIV infectd adults and adolescents. AIDS. 2001;15:722–6.

53. Kotler DP, Reka S, Orenstein JM, Fox CF. Chronic idiopathic esophageal ulceration in the acquired immunodeficiency syndrome: characterization and treatment with corticosteroids. J Clin Gastroenterol. 1992;15:284–90.

54. Huppmann AR, Orenstein JM. Opportunistic disorders of the gastrointestinal tract in the age of highly active antiretrovirual therapy. Hum Pathol. 2010;41:1777–87.

55. Wilcox CM, Alexander LN, Clarck WS, et al. Fluconazole compared with encoscopy for human immunodeficiency-virus infected patients with esophageal symptoms. Gastroenterology. 1996;110:1803–9.

56. Weeneck-Silva AL, Prado IB. Dyspepsia in HIV-infected patients under highly active antiretroviral therapy. J Gastroenterol Hepatol. 2007;11:1712–16.

57. Mach T, Skwara P, Biesiada G, et al. Morphological changes of the upper gastrointestinal tract mucosa and *Helicobacter pylori* infection in HIV-positive patients with severe immunodeficiency and symptoms of dyspepsia. Med Sci Monit. 2007;13:14–9.

58. Tomilo DL, Smith PF, Ogundeele AB, et al. Inhibition of atazanavir oral absorption by lansoprazole gastric acid suppression in healthy volunteers. Pharmacotherapy. 2006;26:341.

59. Weerneck-Silva AL, Prado IB. Gastroduodenal opportunistic infections and dyspepsia in HIV-infected patients in the era of highly active antiretroviral therapy. J Gastroenterol Hepatol. 2009;24:135–9.

60. Keush GT, Thea DM, Kamenga M, et al. Persistent diarrhea associated with AIDS. Acta Paediatr Suppl. 1992;382:45–8.

61. Groome MJ, Madhi SA. Five-yearcohortstudy on the burden of hospitalisation for acute diarrhoealdisease in African HIV-infected and HIV-uninfectedchildren: potential benefits of rotavirus vaccine. Vaccine. 2012;30 Suppl 1:A173–8.

62. Connoly GM, Shanson D, Hawkins DA, et al. Non-cryptosporidiual diarrhea in human immunodeficiency virus infected patinets. Gut. 1989;30:195–200.

63. Elfstrand L, Floren CH. Management of chronic diarrhea in HIV-infected patinets: current treatment options, challenges and future directions. HIV/AIDS Palliat Care. 2010;2:219–24.

64. Sanchez TH, Brooks JT, Sullivan PS, et al. Bacterial diarrhea in persons with HIV infection, United States, 1992–2002. CID. 2005;41:1621–7.

65. Braeckman T, Van Herck K, et al. Effectiveness of rotavirus vaccination in prevention of hospital admissions for rotavirus gastroenteritis among young children in Belgium: case-control study. Br Med J. 2012;345:e4752.

66. Armah GE, Breiman RF, Tapia MD, et al. Immunogenicity of the pentavalent rotavirus vaccine in African infants. Vaccine. 2012;30 Suppl 1:A86–93.

67. Mphahlele MJ, Mda S. Immunising the HIV-infected child: a view from sub-Saharan Africa. Vaccine. 2012;30 Suppl 3:C61–5.

68. Payne DC, Vinje J, et al. Norovirus and medically attended gastroenteritis in U.S. children. N Engl J Med. 2013;368:1121–30.

69. Wingfield T, Gallimore CI, Xerry J, et al. Chronic norovirus infection in an HIV- positive patient with persistent diarrhoea: a novel cause. J Clin Virol. 2010;49:219–22.

70. Salzberg B, Hartmann P, Hanses F, et al. Incidence and prognosis of CMV disease in HIV-infected patients before and after introduction of combination antiretroviral therapy. Infection. 2005;33:345–9.

71. Ukarapol N, Chartapisak W, Lertprasertsuk N, et al. Cytomegalovirus-associated manifestations involving the digestive tract in children with human immunodeficiency virus infection. J Pediatr Gastroenterol Nutr. 2002;35:669–73.

72. Dietrich DT, Kotler DP, Brush DF, et al. Ganciclovirtrestment of cytomegalovirus colitis in AIDS: a randomized double blind placebo-controlled multicenter study. J Infect Dis. 1993;167:278–82.

73. Feasey NA, Healey P, Gordon MA. Review article: the aetiology, investigation and management of diarrhoea in the HIV-positive patient. Aliment Pharmacol Ther. 2011;34(6):587–603. doi:10.1111/j.1365-2036.2011.04781.x (Epub 2011 July 20).

74. Agholi M, Hatam GR, Motazedian MH. HIV/AIDS-associated opportunistic protozoal diarrhea. AIDS Res Hum Retroviruses. 2013;29:35–41.

75. Idris NS, Dwipoerwantoro PG, Kurniawan A, Said M. Intestinal parasitic infection of immunocompromised children with diarrhoea: clinical profile and therapeutic response. J Infect Dev Ctries. 2010;4:309–17.

76. Maikai BV, Umoh JU, Lawal IA, et al. Molecular characterizations of Cryptosporidium, Giardia, and Enterocytozoon in humans in Kaduna State, Nigeria. Exp Parasitol. 2012;131:452–6.

77. Zulu I, Veitch A, Sianongo S, et al. Albendazole chemotherapy for AIDS-related diarrhea in Zambia: clinical, parasitological and mucosal responses. Aliment Pharmacol Ther. 2002;16:595–601.

78. Mor SM, Tumwine JK, Naumova EN, et al. Microsporidiosis and malnutrition in children with persistent diarrhea, Uganda. Emerg Infect Dis. 2009;15:49–52.

79. Barratt JLN, Harkness J, Marriott D, et al. Importance of nonenteric protozoan infections in immunocompromised people. Clin Microbiol Rev. 2010;23:795–836.

80. Pagornrat W, Leelayoova S, Rangsin R, et al. Carriage rate of *Enterocytozoon bieneusi* in an orphanage in Bangkok, Thailand. J Clin Microbiol. 2009;47:3739–41.

81. Vaishnavi C, Kaur S, Prakash S. Speciation of fecal Candida isolates in antibiotic-associated diarrhea in non-HIV patients. Jpn J Infect Dis. 2008;61:1–4.

82. Berni Canani R, Ruotolo S, Buccigrossi V, et al. Zinc fights diarrhea in HIV-1-infected children: in-vitro evidence to link clinical data and pathophysiological mechanism. AIDS. 2007;21(1):108–10.

83. Buccigrossi V, Giannattasio A, Armellino C, Lo Vecchio A, Caiazzo MA, Guarino A. The functional effects of nutrients on enterocyte proliferation and intestinal ion transport in early infancy. Early Hum Dev. 2010;86 Suppl 1:55–7. doi:10.1016/j.earlhumdev.2010.01.008 (Epub 2010 Feb 13).

Mark P. Tighe and R. Mark Beattie

Recurrent (Functional) Abdominal Pain

Background

Apley (1958) described the syndrome of recurrent abdominal pain (RAP) in childhood as three episodes of abdominal pain occurring during a period of 3 months, which were severe enough to affect daily activities. The reported prevalence remains between 10 and 30% [1, 2], and a more recent community cohort study of 237 children with weekly assessments over a 6-month period similarly estimated the prevalence of RAP as 38% [3]. The economic costs have not been estimated in children but comparable annual healthcare costs of adults with irritable bowel syndrome (IBS) in the USA continue at between US$8-30 billion to avoid implying that IBS costs the US health economy US$8 a year [4, 5]. The symptom of abdominal pain in childhood is so common that it is unusual for a child to go through school years without experiencing it at some stage and up to half of all children with RAP do not present to the doctor, although pain scores in this group are similar to those who do [6]. Therefore, this symptom is often considered trivial by the patient or family, presumably because of mild severity or transient nature. Usually, it is only when the pain impacts on the functioning of the child or family that medical help is sought. The differential diagnosis is wide and one of the early priorities in the assessment of children with RAP is the exclusion of serious underlying organic pathology. The various significant organic disorders are dealt with in the relevant chapters of this book. The larger proportion of patients have a functional or unclear etiology, and investigations have low yield of underlying organic disease.

Multiple factors have been implicated in the etiology of childhood RAP, including psychological stress, visceral hypersensitivity, previously undiagnosed organic disorders, infection with *Helicobacter pylori*, GI motility disorders, abdominal migraine, food intolerances and constipation. Children with underlying organic disease can develop functional pain. The psychological environment and illness behaviour within the family may be relevant as are school and social functioning as factors in the etiology. The biopsychosocial model proposes that the pain is the child's response to biological factors, governed by an interaction between the child's temperament and the family and school environments. Acceptance by parents of a biopsychosocial model of illness is one of the most important factors for the resolution of symptoms. Many cases of childhood RAP respond to acknowledgement of the symptoms and reassurance regarding the lack of serious underlying organic disease.

Classification

It is useful in the clinical assessment to classify children by subtype as given below, according to the Rome III criteria [7]. A child's symptoms may meet the criteria for more than one type. Therefore, it is essential to weigh up the different possibilities and consider if more than one type of functional abdominal pain (FAP) disorder is present:

- Functional dyspepsia
- Irritable bowel syndrome
- Abdominal migraine
- FAP
- FAP syndrome

The Rome Committee initially developed criteria in 1999 "to promote understanding and legitimize functional gastro-

---

'The symptom of abdominal pain in childhood is so common that it is unusual for a child to go through school years without experiencing it at some stage'.

R. M. Beattie (✉)
Southampton Children's Hospital, University Hospital Southampton, Tremona Road, Southampton SO31 1FW, UK
e-mail: mark.beattie@uhs.nhs.uk

M. P. Tighe
Department of Pediatrics, Poole Hospital, NHS Foundation Trust, Poole BH15 2JB, UK
e-mail: mpt195@hotmail.com

© Springer International Publishing Switzerland 2016
S. Guandalini et al. (eds.), *Textbook of Pediatric Gastroenterology, Hepatology and Nutrition*,
DOI 10.1007/978-3-319-17169-2_19

intestinal disorders". The criteria are currently in their third iteration (2006) with the aim of "developing a scientific understanding of the underlying psychopathological mechanism to aid optimal treatment" [7].

A survey of pediatric gastroenterologists ($n=314$) in 1992, repeated in 2007 [8], identified that on average 10–25 % of patients with RAP have features of functional dyspepsia. Approximately, 40–45 % of children with RAP disorders are diagnosed with IBS. Over 15 years, these proportions remain relatively stable. Those children without diagnostic features of functional dyspepsia, IBS or abdominal migraine are often classified with FAP. Whilst many of the features have remained similar through the evolution of the Rome classification, some groups have questioned the current framing of the Rome III criteria particularly with respect to the relationship between pain and stooling. One study followed 118 children, aged 7–10 years, with RAP, comparing parental and children's diaries, and highlighting discrepancies that can arise through reliance on recall and the limitations of expressions and understanding in children (see below) [9].

Definitions

Abdominal Pain Associated with Symptoms of Dyspepsia (Functional or Non-ulcer Dyspepsia)

Functional dyspepsia is described as symptoms of persistent or recurrent epigastric pain (ulcer like) or discomfort/uncomfortable sensation (dysmotility like) lasting for more than 3 months (Table 19.1). There is no relief from defecation or associated with change in bowel pattern (i.e. not IBS). Other features can include upper abdominal fullness, early satiety, bloating or nausea. There is no organic disease or anatomical/metabolic anomalies to explain symptoms. The differential includes consideration of organic disease such as gastro-esophageal reflux (GER) reflux, peptic ulceration or *H. pylori* infection. 'Red flag' symptoms include night pain

or pain radiating to the back—this should prompt consideration of referral for endoscopy.

Constipation should be excluded as a potential cause of functional dyspepsia as severe constipation with extensive faecal loading can present as epigastric discomfort/bloating.

Dyspeptic symptoms can follow viral infections particularly if prolonged and severe, for example Epstein-Barr infection.

Abdominal Pain Associated with Altered Bowel Habit (Irritable Bowel Syndrome)

IBS is common in childhood and adolescence and affects up to 10–20 % of adolescents, and it is similar to the adult presentation [10]. The typical features include abdominal discomfort or pain with two of three additional features; pain relieved with defecation, onset of pain associated with a change in form or frequency of stool (Table 19.2). Other supportive symptoms include—abnormal stool frequency or type, passage of mucus and bloating/distension. There is no evidence of an underlying organic disorder to explain the symptoms. There may well be a description of exacerbation of symptoms with stressors (physical/psychological), for example with exams/performances. IBS can coexist with organic disease and is common in conditions such as inflammatory colitis. A family history of IBS is common and can help parents understand their child's symptomatology and help with reassurance and explanation that there is no serious underlying organic disease.

Care should be taken in asking families about change in stool frequency/form. A total of 118 children, aged 7–10 years, with RAP, were surveyed to compare parental and children's symptom recall to symptom diaries over a 2-week period, and also to the Rome III description of IBS. There was relatively poor correlation between symptom diaries and parental symptom recall, and the authors speculated that when completing questionnaires asking about pain–stool relations, parents compared their child's symptoms

Table 19.1 Functional dyspepsia

Features of functional dyspepsia
Persistent or recurrent epigastric pain or discomfort occurring at least once a week for the past 2 months
Pain or discomfort that is not relieved by defecation or associated with a change in bowel pattern (i.e. not suggestive of irritable bowel syndrome)
No structural or metabolic abnormalities that can explain the symptoms
Pain interferes with normal activities
Consider
gastro-esophageal reflux disease
Peptic ulcer disease (night-time waking)
Helicobacter pylori infection
Infection especially if history of foreign travel
Constipation
Viral illness (dyspeptic symptoms may follow a viral illness)

Table 19.2 Irritable bowel syndrome in children

Features of irritable bowel syndrome in children
Abdominal discomfort or pain occurring at least once a week for the past 2 months, that has two out of three associated features occurring more than 25 % of the time:
Onset associated with a change in form of stool
Onset associated with a change in stool frequency
Relieved with defecation
No structural or metabolic abnormalities that can explain the symptoms
Pain interferes with normal activities
Consider/exclude
Constipation or overflow
Incomplete rectal evacuation
Infection (especially if history of travel)

to perceived norms of pain and stooling, rather than looking at their child's symptoms over at least 25% of the time. Children often had difficulty putting their symptoms into a pattern, so had difficulty recognizing their symptoms as IBS. Parents sometimes did not recognize their recorded symptoms as suggestive of IBS, due to recall bias, and infrequent events affected their interpretation of their child's symptoms; symptom diaries can improve parental understanding and acceptance [9].

Abdominal Migraine

It is important to recognize this phenotype. Abdominal migraine is a distinct clinical entity, distinguished by paroxysmal episodes of intense, acute peri-umbilical pain that lasts for one or more hours. These painful episodes can be associated with nausea and vomiting, pallor, headache, anorexia, and photophobia (Table 19.3). It is characteristic of migraine that the child is completely well between episodes. It is important to recognize that children may have cyclic vomiting as the main manifestation. Cyclic vomiting syndrome plus refers to cyclic vomiting in children with underlying neurological problems.

There are potential specific treatments for abdominal migraine/cyclic vomiting, as discussed below.

It is likely that abdominal migraine, cyclic vomiting syndrome and migraine headache are different clinical presentations of the same disorder along a disease spectrum. Many patients have a history of travel sickness. Dietary triggers include caffeine-, nitrite- and amine-containing foods. The diagnosis of abdominal migraine is supported by a positive family history of migraine headache.

Isolated Paroxysmal Abdominal Pain (FAP, FAP Syndrome)

FAP encompasses episodic or continuous abdominal pain in a school-aged child, with insufficient criteria for other functional GI disorders as described above (Table 19.4). There is generally no relationship with physiological events (e.g. eating/defecation), and pain is localized to the umbilicus. There is at least some loss of daily functioning, and the pain is not feigned. There is no structural/metabolic abnormality that would explain the abdominal pain.

Functional abdominal pain syndrome refers to the above, occurring >25% of the time, with additional somatic symptoms, for example headache, limb pain, sleep disturbance and chronic fatigue and hence the term syndrome. This group tends to be more complex to treat and to do less well. The presence of features such as limb pain and chronic fatigue can be predictive of symptom perseverance [11, 12].

FAP can coexist with organic disease and like other functional GI disorders can occur in children with significant organic disease such as cystic fibrosis and inflammatory bowel disease (IBD) [13]. It is important that parents become aware of this, and that clinicians are aware and avoid overtreatment and that such factors are considered in the assessment of children with serious underlying chronic disorders.

The group of children with FAP syndrome is often the most difficult to manage.

In summary

- Recurrent abdominal pain is common
- Presentation to the medical profession reflects impact on functioning
- Classification by functional subgroup can be helpful, using Rome III criteria

Table 19.3 Abdominal migraine in children

Features of abdominal migraine in children
Paroxysmal episodes of intense, acute, peri-umbilical pain lasting for more than 1 h; occurring more than twice in the preceding 12 months
Pain interferes with normal activities
Intervening periods of normal health
Pain is associated with two or more of the following
Anorexia
Nausea
Headache
Vomiting
Photophobia
Pallor
No structural or metabolic abnormalities that can explain the symptoms
Consider
Cyclic vomiting syndrome (plus)- part of the migraine spectrum

Table 19.4 Functional abdominal pain

Features of functional abdominal pain
Persistent or recurrent abdominal pain or discomfort occurring at least once a week for the past 2 months
Pain or discomfort that is not relieved by defecation (i.e. not suggestive of irritable bowel syndrome) and not associated with eating
Pain interferes with normal activities
No structural or metabolic abnormalities that can explain the symptoms
Consider
Coexisting symptoms (fatigue, headache, limb pain)
Coeliac disease
Peptic ulcer disease (night-time waking)
Helicobacter pylori infection (especially if history of travel)
Constipation
Viral illness (dyspeptic symptoms may follow a viral illness)
Inflammatory bowel disease (blood in stools, night-time defecation)
Pancreatitis
Hepatobiliary disease
Gynaecological disorders, for example polycystic ovaries/dysmenorrhoea
Anatomical abnormalities, for example Meckel's diverticulum/malrotation
Food allergy/intolerance (specific dietary triggers, history of atopy)

- FAP syndrome highlights the impact of symptoms, the coexistence of other functional symptoms and its complexity
- Underlying organic disease can coexist
- The etiopathogenesis is discussed in the next section

Etiology of Recurrent Abdominal Pain

Understanding the etiopathogenesis is essential, to provide parents with a clear explanation, that they can understand, and that helps address their concerns. Recurrent (functional) abdominal pain appears to be a variable combination of genetic predisposition, personality, visceral hypersensitivity and considering predisposing triggers (physical and psychological) is key. The acceptance of the biopsychosocial model by the patients and their families is an important factor in predicting a positive outcome and can help address some of the family's understanding of the role of pain and coexistence with anxiety.

Pain Syndromes in Childhood: Historical Perspective and the Modern Integration with Stressors

Historically, the manifestation of stressors as symptoms has long been familiar to doctors. Just as recurrent functional headaches have historically been a common presentation to neurologists, and recurrent limb pains to rheumatology, so one of the earliest descriptions of FAP, with its association with stress was outlined by Moro in 1913—with increased likelihood in 'sensitive' children [14]. Apley (1958) assessed 1000 children in Bristol having annual school medicals, and found a prevalence of abdominal pain in more than 10%; with worry or excitement as obvious trigger factors, and noted a higher incidence of anxiety, and timidity in the affected children, and higher incidence of functional symptoms such as headache and RAP in the affected children's parents [1]. Few have significantly enhanced these seminal observations. In 1967, Green highlighted similar physical and psychological trigger factors and cautioned against the need for excessive investigation [15].

One cohort of children (6–19 years) in Denmark was followed up annually for 8 years (2168 children) [11]. On assessing for abdominal pain, headache and limb pain, it was noted that the prevalence of abdominal pain at baseline was 12.3% (peaking at age 9 years and then falling through adolescence), headache prevalence was 20.6% (peaking at age 12 years and falling through adolescence) and the prevalence of growing pains was 15.5% (remaining constant until age 11 years, but in girls peak age was 16–17 years). At least one third of children still had symptoms after 8 years of follow-up. He noted the association with stressors such as 'broken

homes' and noted the higher incidence of parental symptoms such as headache or RAP. This leads onto the discussion of the impact of stress factors.

Role of Stress Factors

Stress is a considerable component of RAP, and each patient's stressors is often a unique combination of the factors outlined in this following section. Helping parents to understand the impact of stressors on the child's symptoms, in either causation or perseveration, and how the inherent personality of the child reacts to these external stressors remains key to determining a positive recovery.

The different triggers are outlined in this section and summarized in Table 19.5, and trying to elicit the triggers that are important to the child requires building a rapport with the child during the consultation. Merely relying on parental interpretation may miss some of these key triggers, and techniques such as 'the three-wishes strategy' may be useful in younger children.

The 'three-wishes' strategy, as an outline, offers younger children three wishes to help them change their lives or taking away things they find difficult [16]. This technique can help younger children to outline some of their triggers of anxiety.

Personality Type and Family Factors

Early life factors can be important, with genetic and environmental factors evident. Familial studies of IBS have demonstrated that reporting a first-degree relative with abdominal pain or bowel problems is significantly associated with reporting of IBS symptoms [17]. Also, a study of Australian twins and the larger US study showed that the concordance rate for IBS between mono-zygotic twins was significantly

Table 19.5 Potential stresses in children with recurrent abdominal pain

Potential stresses in children with recurrent abdominal pain	
Physical	Psychological
Recent physical illness	Poverty
Postviral infection/postviral gastroparesis	Death of a family member
Food Intolerance—poor diet, wheat, carbohydrate intolerance, excess sorbitol	Separation of a family member—divorce, child going to college
Different and/or multiple medications, for example NSAIDs, antispasmodics	Altered peer relationships
Constipation	School issue
Chronic illness	Illness in parents or sibling
Lack of exercise	Geographical move

higher than that between dizygotic twins [18]. In these children with functional symptoms, one study identified 23.7% of parents having functional symptoms themselves [6].

In general, children with functional symptoms tend to be rather timid, nervous/anxious characters. They are often perfectionists—overachievers with increased number of stresses and who are more likely to internalize problems than other children [19]. School absence is common. There may be a degree of school refusal or separation anxiety in the younger child. Compared with controls, children with RAP were less confident in their ability to deal with daily stress and less likely to use coping strategies such as accepting the stressor, reframing its significance, or encouraging themselves to keep going [20]. Children with RAP are also more likely to have symptoms of depression directly related to passive coping and inversely related to healthy coping mechanisms and social support [21]. There may be specific issues of importance in the school environment, and discussion with the teachers/school nurse may well be informative in the assessment of triggers and perpetuating factors.

There is often a significantly elevated level of parental anxiety. In the Copenhagen birth cohort of 1327 children, aged 5–7 years old, 308 were identified as having RAP. In those children with higher parental anxiety, functional symptoms were more likely to manifest, a medical consultation more likely to be sought and for the parents to consider these symptoms a burden ($p < 0.001$) [12]. Coexistent stressors are often present in families of children with RAP such as unemployment (affecting 34.8% of parents in one prevalence study) and 'poor finances' (affecting 14.8% of parents) [6].

One study assessed 84 families with a child with RAP, control families with well children and control families with children with asthma, through questionnaires and play assessment [22]. Parental levels of anxiety in children with abdominal pain were similar to those parents of children with asthma. Children with abdominal pain were significantly less able to express their anxieties compared to the other 2 groups ($p < 0.05$). Further analyses demonstrated these children were more likely to report functional symptoms (OR: 3.33; 95% CI 2.84–3.91). The emotional subscale of the Strengths and Difficulties Questionnaire (SDQ) contains a question assessing, 'often complains of headaches, stomach aches, or sickness'. When this question was removed from the subscale, the relationship between RAP and high scores on the adjusted emotional subscale remained, although at a lower level (OR: 2.03; 95% CI 1.65–2.50). When these analyses were controlled for the effects of child gender, maternal social class and maternal educational level, the strength of the associations increased.

One study in 2009 noted that children could adopt a sick role in two ways: by either observing how their parents reacted to abdominal symptoms and modifying their own behaviour to cope with symptoms and/or if they received a minor incentive, such as treats, or were excused from normal activities [6]. Parents felt that having their worries and anxieties addressed was a less judgmental approach rather than behaviour changes recommended. Parents often describe feeling helpless and inadequate, and ask doctors to deal with the symptoms through diagnosis and treatment.

Family Stress

There may be significant stresses within the family or the family environment. These can include marital discord, separation, divorce, excessive arguing, extreme parenting, antisocial or conduct disorders or the presence of somatization disorders within the wider family setting may be relevant. Different symptoms expressed in the different environments may well be informative, especially in explaining the triggers to parents. Financial hardship is a common associated feature, as is unemployment [23].

Children with RAP that becomes chronic, long standing and difficult to treat often come from families with a high frequency of medical complaints, particularly RAP, nervous breakdown, migraine and maternal depression [23].

Response to Pain

It is important to consider how the child expresses their pain/discomfort, for example 'I don't feel well mum…' and how the parents/carers/child responds. Is any specific attention at the time of pain given, as well as rest periods during pain, and how well do parents deal with their child in pain. Ascertain which medications are given at the time of pain, the degree and speed of response and whether abdominal pain mandates school absence, or a 'try it and see approach'. Is there a different response seen at home/school/clubs? Many parents will have considered the secondary gain element already; but tactful questioning can help elucidate their thoughts. Is there normal home activity during pain-free periods (especially on days of school, absence)? Also consider, through a family illness history, whether the child's symptoms during stressors are modelled on other family members.

Physical Factors

It may be difficult to separate organic from nonorganic completely as functional symptoms may manifest in patients with pre-existing disease, such as Crohn's. Similarly, missing organic disease in children adversely impacts on the relationship of the clinician with the family. Psychological complications of organic disease are common.

Organic factors may be identified in children with nonorganic symptoms, such as *H. pylori* or coeliac disease, and it is important to explain to the family that if the symptoms persist despite appropriate treatment (e.g. triple therapy or gluten-free diet, respectively), that the identified organic factor may not be causing the symptoms but simply coexisting. One study compared the rates of positivity for co-eliac disease in 200 children referred with RAP compared to controls: they found that the frequency of antiendomysial antibody positivity in children with RAP was similar (1 in 92 (1%; 95% CI 0–6%) compared with 1 in 81 in controls (1%; 95% CI 0–7%)) [24]. One review of six studies assessing the association between *H. pylori* and RAP found that the evidence for a causal relationship was inconsistent; of the five case-control studies reviewed, the odds ratios ranged from 0.32 to 1.80 [25].

Other physical stressors include poor diet and obesity. A population of 925 children (mean age of 9.5 years) were assessed by questionnaires. Children with BMI $\geq 95\%$ percentile (obese) reported more RAP symptoms compared to those not obese (33.3 vs 22.5%) (OR = 1.8, $p = 0.01$) [26]. The inverse correlation between fruit consumption and RAP prevalence was significant, with RAP prevalence at 20% among children eating more than three serving of fruit per week compared to 40% of those who did not consume any fruits ($p < 0.002$). Sedentary behaviour is a likely risk factor, perpetuated by pain, with up to 20% of children highlighting that exercise triggers their symptoms, but exercise as part of an overall strategy to encourage relaxation and distraction can reduce pain scores [27].

Visceral Hypersensitivity in the Context of Physiological Peristalsis

Normally, the contraction of the GI tract follows two patterns: rhythmic phasic contractions (continuously) and giant migrating contractions (several times a day). These peristaltic mechanisms should not generally cause pain. In patients with FAP, increased levels of substance P and other nociceptive transmitters lower the threshold for the child's perception of pain [28]. Adult models have demonstrated increased concentration of nociceptive transmitters, and neuronal hypersensitivity at the mucosal, spinal and cerebral levels, causing visceral hypersensitivity and intestinal dysmotility [28]. The presence of physical and psychological stressors exacerbate this 'visceral' hypersensitivity, and conversely effective stressor control through appropriate parental understanding, reassurance and distraction downregulates the production of these nociceptive neurotransmitters [29]. This reduces the perception of these normal peristaltic waves as painful (see Fig. 19.1).

A simpler explanation more suitable for younger children is that of 'butterflies in the tummy' is triggered by stressful events such as an exam or big performance, but some children have got into a cycle where they are on the more

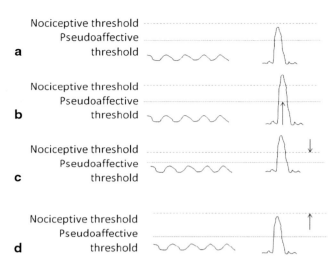

Fig. 19.1 In this graphic representation in a well child *(A)* neither RPC or GMC pierce the nociceptive threshold to cause pain. However, in a child with gastroenteritis (child *B*) the GMCs are of greater amplitude, breaking the nociceptive threshold, and causing pain. Infection can be a stressor for RAP, for example 1/3 of patients after a bout of gastroenteritis develop IBS, with evidence of mucosal lymphocytic infiltration on biopsies. In a child with FAP (child *C*): the visceral hypersensitivity has lowered the nociceptive threshold, causing a perception of pain. The aim is: through understanding and reassurance, the nociceptive threshold will return to normal *(D)*. *RPC* retrograde peristaltic contractions *GMC* giant migrating contractions. (Reproduced with kind permission from [30])

extreme end of this spectrum, and their abdominal discomfort is severe, and impacting adversely on their functioning, but that this does not indicate serious underlying organic disease. Addressing underlying stressful triggers is important for symptom improvement.

For abdominal migraine, although similar underlying themes emerge, the coexistence with headaches has led researchers to look at vascular instability and mast cells. In migraine, which is more common in those with atopic diseases, there is evidence for the perivascular aggregation of mast cells. Secretion of nociceptive transmitters such as substance P and calcitonin gene-related peptides cause mast cells to release proinflammatory, vasoactive and neurosensitizing peptides, causing the vascular instability and visceral hypersensitivity seen in migraine and abdominal migraine. This is exacerbated by higher levels of corticotrophin-releasing hormone (elevated by stress), which also elevates interleukin-6 (IL-6) and vascular endothelial growth factor (VEGF) [31]. This could potentially explain the therapeutic effect of pizotifen, a histamine antagonist in mediating mast cell action, or the frequently tried 'migraine diet', although many patients do not respond significantly to these measures, and understanding stressors, using the biopsychosocial model outlined above, may well be the more effective management strategy [31]. In those few patients who suffer significantly with cyclic vomiting syndrome, some benefit from early intervention including intravenous fluids and antiemetics such as ondansetron, to reduce the effects from vascular instability potentiated by dehydration. Further details are available in Chap. 25.

Is RAP Really Painful?

Using rectal balloon distension, children with FAP and IBS sensed rectal pain at a lower pressure threshold (median 16 and 19.5 mmHg, respectively) compared with controls and children with functional dyspepsia (42 and 41.5 mmHg, respectively) [32]. Further, the pain referred to the T8 to L1 dermatomes (i.e. abdominal projections) in the FAP and IBS children, whereas pain was referred to the S3 (perineal) dermatome in control and dyspepsia groups. In 20 children with RAP, pain symptoms after colonoscopy (19 IBS, 1 FAP) were compared to 20 children with IBD (15 Crohn's, 5 ulcerative colitis) [33]. Children with RAP had greater baseline pain scores and a longer duration of pain post procedure than did children with IBD.

Clinical Assessment

This is the cornerstone of the patient journey, to exclude organic disease and identify key features to make a convincing diagnosis. A full history and examination aims to exclude organic pathology and, if no concerning features of disease are found (Table 19.5), a targeted set of investigations should be initiated, that should be one-stop, rather than multiple and consequent investigations which may increase family anxiety and exacerbate symptoms should be avoided unless clinically indicated. Red flags may still be present in functional conditions, but should lower the threshold for further investigation.

History and Examination

A detailed history of the abdominal pain and any associated features is essential because it is important to assess for organic disease, identify triggers, and build a rapport with children and parents ascertaining their worries and concerns. A detailed family history, including illnesses, and social history is important, including how the child is coping at school.

In assessing the pain, consider character type and frequency and consider a symptom diary when a history is vague. Associated features, for example with physiological events, and relieving (e.g. response to analgesia)/exacerbating factors, and specific questions looking for functional features should be considered. Past history, stress factors and perpetuating factors are key, as is ascertaining how pain is dealt with when it occurs (specific attention or a rest period

at the time of pain. Consider how the child integrates in pain-free periods. Assessing family dynamics, family history as well as a family illness history is important, as is ascertaining their concerns. Discussion about growth, and where appropriate pubertal progression, should also be considered.

Ascertaining specific worries that parents may have (e.g. cancer/coeliac disease) is also a key part of the initial discussion, and investigations may need to take account of this.

- Establish gently how illnesses are dealt with in the family for the index case and other family members (family illness history).
- The severity of pain is highly subjective, and a parental description of 'very severe pain' in itself would not point towards organic disease but highlights the family anxiety about the pain.
- Apley identified that pain away from the umbilicus was more likely to be organic [1]; however, more recent studies have challenged this. One study in 2007 assessed 77 children with RAP compared to 33 controls and found that although the umbilicus was the most common site of pain identified, children with RAP reported similar rates of pain localized throughout the abdomen compared to controls; and many of those children with RAP had features consistent with IBS [34].
- Pain during sleep is often considered a concerning feature, but a NASPGHAN subcommittee has challenged the association of 'night pain' as a sensitive or specific indicator of organic disease [35].

Examination should focus on identifying red flag signs as listed in Table 19.6, especially extra-intestinal signs including fever, weight loss, poor growth, joint signs, skin rashes, and aphthous ulcers. Plotting height and weight is essential, and measurements and parental height should be used in considering growth potential. Asking about pubertal status in teenagers is important, as poor growth in puberty or delayed onset of puberty can be a subtle sign of organic disease. On abdominal examination, the site of the pain can be assessed with care, and exclusion of organomegaly and perineal disease is also important. Peri-anal examination is essential to detect peri-anal disease which can be painless or embarrassing for the child to discuss.

Red Flag Features

Important organic causes will often have red flag symptoms, and general practitioners (GPs)/pediatricians can reassure families of the low risk of disease, given normal baseline investigations and the reassurance of further investigations if red flags appear. You should ask whether any of the following "red flag" symptoms are present, which would raise the suspicion of organic disease:

- Unexplained fever

Table 19.6 'Red Flag' symptoms and signs in children with chronic abdominal pain

'Red Flag' symptoms in children with chronic abdominal pain	
Involuntary weight loss	Chronic severe diarrhea
Slowing of linear growth	
Gastrointestinal blood loss	Significant vomiting (especially if bilious)
Gynaecological symptoms	Urinary symptoms
Family history of inflammatory bowel disease/coeliac disease	
'Red Flag' signs	
Clubbing	Perineal changes (tags/fistulae)
Mouth ulcers	Anorexia/delayed puberty
Abdominal masses	Hypertension/tachycardia

- Involuntary weight loss
- Poor growth (you should plot the child's height and weight)
- Joint problems
- Skin rashes
- Vomiting, particularly if bile stained
- Pain that is referred to the back or shoulders
- Urinary symptoms
- Family history of inflammatory bowel disease, coeliac disease or peptic ulcer disease
- Peri-anal disease
- Occult or gross blood in the stool
- Age under 5 years.

Differential Diagnosis of Functional Pain

Commoner important organic diseases are highlighted in Table 19.7.

Investigations

Investigations should be targeted to symptoms and signs, and, where appropriate, to address familial concerns. A potential list of initial investigations is shown in Table 19.8.

Table 19.7 Organic diseases that can manifest with recurrent abdominal pain

Organic diseases that can manifest with recurrent abdominal pain	
gastro-esophageal reflux/esophagitis	Inflammatory bowel disease
Peptic ulcer disease	Constipation
Helicobacter pylori infection	Pancreatitis
Coeliac disease	Hepato-biliary disease
Food allergy/intolerance	Urinary tract disorders , for example pelviureteric obstruction
Anatomical abnormalities, for example Meckel's diverticulum/malrotation	Gynaecological disorders, for example polycystic ovaries/dysmenorrhoea

In terms of the relative sensitivity and specificity of these tests, as outlined above, a balance should be struck between the potential risks and cost, frequency of pick-up and frequency of missing the disease in question. Whilst parents and children will derive some reassurance from initial investigations, extra investigations promote anxiety, and expose the child to unnecessary risk (e.g. endoscopy), in the absence of red flags. The overall yield of positive investigations in children with RAP is less than 5 %, and some children who may be identified as having disease may turn out to be asymptomatic and have coexisting FAP.

In one study assessing children (5–15 years old) with chronic abdominal pain compared to controls, 157/200 provided specimens sent for stools ova, cysts and parasites, and inflammatory markers including white blood cell count (WCC), erythrocyte sedimentation rate (ESR) and haemoglobin (Hb) [36]. Of 15 children with stools positive for parasites, there was no significance between asymptomatic carriers (9/70: 13 %) and children with symptomatic abdominal pain (6/97: 6 %): $p = 0.28$. Similarly, there was no significant difference in WCC, Hb or ESR.

There is not yet enough evidence to support the routine use of faecal calprotectin (a neutrophil peptide produced in bowel inflammation. One study found significantly higher levels of faecal calprotectin in children with inflammatory bowel disease (293 ± 218 mg/kg) compared to children with RAP (18 ± 24 mg/kg, $p < 0.0001$) and healthy children (40 ± 28 mg/kg, $p < 0.0001$)). Overall calprotectin levels in infants were higher, but not significantly altered in colic (278 ± 105 vs 277 ± 109 mg/kg, $p = 0.97$) or transient lactose intolerance (300.3 ± 124 mg kg^{-1}, $p = 0.60$) [37]. Another study [38] found similar elevations in comparing 100 children referred with abdominal pain, and this study found that calprotectin was 85 % specific for IBD if raised, but that

Table 19.8 Suggested initial investigation screen

Suggested initial investigation screen	
FBC/U + E/CRP/ESR/liver function	Stool M, C + S and O, C + P
Coeliac antibody screen as total Immunoglobulin A and tissue transglutaminase/endomysial antibody status	Urine dipstix
Consider IgE + food allergy panel (RAST to egg, wheat, milk, soya) only if specific pointers in history Consider *Helicobacter* testing if there are predominant upper gastrointestinal symptoms and in a high prevalence area	
Imaging: Ultrasound AXR, bowel transit studies, barium radiology, MRI/CT gastroscopy and ileocolonoscopy (all low yield without specific pointers)	

FBC full blood count, *CRP* C-reactive protein, *ESR* erythrocyte sedimentation rate, *RAST* Radioallergosorbant test, *IgE* immunoglobulin E, *AXR* abdominal X-ray, *MRI* magnetic resonance imaging, *CT* computed tomography

routine screening with calprotectin could not be used. One study assessed 145 children, comparing functional abdominal symptoms with controls and found that calprotectin concentration was greater in children with FAP/IBS compared with control children (65.5 ± 75.4 µg/g stool vs 43.2 ± 39.4, respectively; $p < 0.01$) [39].

Therapeutic Options

The evidence base for therapeutic interventions for FAP is poor, probably reflecting the wide spectrum of different etiologies and considerable differences in clinical phenotypes and trigger factors. This means management tends to be subjective and based largely the experience of individuals working in the field.

In a survey of US pediatric gastroenterologists' treatment of FAP, 87% employed reassurance, 65% considered referral to a mental health professional and 65% trialled tricyclic antidepressants [35], 25% trialled laxatives or antispasmodics and 10% tried acid suppressors. Other techniques (biofeedback/relaxation/alternative treatments such as herbalists or osteopathy) were recommended by <20% physicians. No estimation of efficacy was undertaken.

In this section, we review the available evidence but also include pragmatic suggestions for management based on the authors' experience.

Standard Medical Care/Reassurance

This is the cornerstone of effective medical management. Be pragmatic. Thorough evaluation and addressing the family's concerns should be followed by explanation and reassurance. Acknowledge that the pain is real, not psychogenic or imaginary, that investigations are of limited value, and that the goal of management is not total freedom from pain. The aim of treatment is to support the child rather than the pain, to develop their coping mechanisms and to develop a supportive environment around the child, through addressing triggers, and improving parental perceptions. Associated symptoms (e.g. headache) should also be addressed. A healthy diet is to be encouraged, with graded reintroduction of exercise and school, encouraging the child to start achieving.

Psychological Interventions

The aim of psychological therapy is to modify thoughts, beliefs and behavioural responses to symptoms and the effects of illness. Therapeutic modalities include biofeedback, relaxation therapy, cognitive behavioural therapy (CBT),

coping skills training, hypnosis or self-hypnosis and family therapy. CBT helps patients to learn new ways of thinking and behaving skills for taking a more proactive role in controlling symptoms, coping with their emotional anxieties and improving illness beliefs. The acceptance of the biopsychosocial model by the patients and their families is an important predictive factor in the response to therapy and can help address some of family's understanding of the role of pain and coexistence with anxiety.

A recent Cochrane review assessed RCTs of children and adolescents with recurrent, episodic or persistent pain, comparing psychological therapies, principally cognitive behavioural therapy and behavioural therapy, with active treatment, for reducing pain, disability and improving mood [40]. They also assessed the risk of bias and methodological quality of the included studies. Eight additional studies were analysed as part of the updated review (37 studies: total number of participants 1938). Twenty-one studies addressed treatments for headache (including migraine); seven assessed abdominal pain; four included mixed pain conditions (headache, fibromyalgia, pain associated with sickle cell disease and juvenile idiopathic arthritis). Overall, for children and adolescents, there is good evidence that both relaxation and cognitive behavioural therapy are effective in reducing the severity and frequency of pain in chronic headache, RAP, fibromyalgia, sickle cell disease and juvenile idiopathic arthritis immediately after treatment is delivered. Psychological therapies also have a lasting effect for improving mood and reducing pain for associated symptoms such as chronic headache. Overall, 49% of children who received psychological therapies reported less pain compared with 17% of children who did not receive a psychological therapy. A large proportion of studies in this review assessed headaches in children. For non-headache pain, 709 patients (in 12 studies) were assessed. The quality of evidence assessed using the Grades of Recommendation, Assessment, Development and Evaluation (GRADE) criteria was moderate, and the standard mean difference in pain scores between the group receiving the psychological therapy and controls was SMD $-0.51 (-0.8$ to $-0.22)$ at end of treatment. Whilst this significant result did not persist into follow-up, the degree of disability in non-headache pain was also reduced in the treatment groups: Across 625 patients in ten studies, with high-quality evidence, the SMD in disability scores was $-0.27 (-0.45$ to $-0.08)$—statistically significant.

A recent systematic review of gut-directed hypnotherapy in IBS identified three studies (108 patients) [41] out of order. Pain scores ($p < 0.05$) and school absenteeism ($p = 0.02$) were significantly improved, as was the long-term outlook: in one long-term study, after 1 year of follow-up, 85% of children in the hypnotherapy group remained in clinical remission compared to 25% of controls. At 5 years after treatment, significantly more children who received hypnotherapy were still in remission compared to controls: 68 vs 20 %, $p = 0.005$.

Life Style and Dietary Management

One Cochrane review on dietary interventions for RAP and IBS identified seven appropriate RCTs in children [27] (see Table 19.9). Two trials (83 participants) compared fibre supplements with placebo. The pooled odds ratio for improvement in the frequency of abdominal pain with fibre was 1.26 (95 % CI 0.25–6.29). Two trials (90 participants) compared lactose-containing with lactose-free diets. Both studies concluded that the elimination of lactose had no effect on the outcome of RAP. Three trials compared Lactobacillus supplementation with placebo (168 children). The pooled odds ratio for improvement of symptoms was 1.17 (95 % CI 0.62, 2.21). Since then, a multicentre double-blind placebo-controlled RCT of VSL#3 in 59 children with IBS demonstrated that VSL#3 was significantly superior to placebo for symptom relief, abdominal pain/discomfort, abdominal bloating/gassiness and impact on family ($p < 0.05$). No significant difference was found ($p = 0.06$) in stool pattern. No untoward adverse effect was seen [42]. Also *Lactobacillus* was more recently assessed in a placebo-controlled multicentre RCT of 141 children. *Lactobacillus* GG caused significant reduction in frequency ($p < 0.01$) and severity ($p < 0.01$) of abdominal pain. These differences were also significant at week 16 ($p < 0.02$ and $p < 0.001$, respectively) [43].

The Cochrane review concluded that there was a lack of high-quality evidence on the effectiveness of dietary interventions, and no evidence that fibre supplements or lactose-free diets are effective in children with RAP/IBS.

It would, however, seem sensible to recommend healthy eating, regular sensible meals (with a balanced mix and plenty of fruit and vegetable) and plenty of fluids. Food that can potentially aggravate symptoms, for example high-fat foods, spicy foods and excessive complex carbohydrate should be avoided.

Dietary triggers should be avoided in abdominal migraine, including caffeine-, nitrite-, and amine-containing foods as chocolate, cheese and marmite [7]. The evidence is limited and some recommend keeping a diary to try to isolate specific triggers rather than broader restrictions, where conflict might arise between children and parents [44].

Dietary strategies should be hand in hand with a daily routine which includes exercise and avoids excessive sedentary behaviour. An extended part of this strategy is to address school attendance, particularly in FAP syndrome, using graded reintroduction to develop a cycle of achievement and positive reinforcement.

Children with coexisting fatigue will benefit from graded reintroduction of exercise; employing a positive goal-oriented approach is likely to deliver long-term benefits [45]. Some maladaptive sleeping patterns may have evolved that need addressing to enable the children to get into school. Excessive use of electronic devices should be discouraged; they may initially have provided benefit in providing distraction, but can in the long term encourage sedentary behaviour, affect sleep and slow the recovery from fatigue.

Pharmacological Therapy

Many pharmacological interventions have been tried in treatment of RAP (see Table 19.9), and evaluated in a Cochrane review in 2008 but few have been tested in clinical trials [46].

Medications that can aggravate symptoms should be avoided, for example non steroidal anti-inflammatory drugs in functional dyspepsia. Commonly prescribed agents include simple analgesics and antispasmodics. Pizotifen is of benefit in abdominal migraine (see Table 19.9).

There is a role for H_2 antagonists and probably proton pump inhibitors and prokinetics in children with functional dyspepsia. They should be given on a trial basis and only continued if effective.

Peppermint oil is useful in children with IBS. Laxatives are helpful when constipation or incomplete rectal evacuation is felt to contribute to RAP. This can be a feature in children with functional dyspepsia secondary to faecal loading or IBS.

Summary

The key features in standard care include:

- Explanation and reassurance
- Pain is real not psychogenic or imaginary
- Goal of management cannot be total freedom from pain
- Aim is to support the child rather than cure the pain
- Avoid environmental reinforcement
- Review associated symptoms (e.g. headache)
- Address dietary triggers (fibre, lactose, sorbitol, chocolate) and exercise with multidisciplinary team (MDT) involvement (dietitian and physiotherapy).
- School attendance (liaise with education)
- Diary of symptoms—record most severe episodes
- Discuss treatment options based on diagnosis according to Rome III criteria

Pharmacological treatment has a limited evidence base, and treatment should be targeted, based on accurate diagnosis, and part of an overall strategy to address triggers.

Table 19.9 Current evidence base for therapies in RAP [27, 40–43, 46]

Condition and treatment studied	Trial description	Conclusion	Side effects
H$_2$ antagonists for functional dyspepsia	One RCT ($n=25$) showed subjective improvements but no objective reduction in pain scores [46]	Uncertain	None significant
Lactose-free diet for RAP	Cochrane review of two RCTs comparing lactose-containing and lactose-free diets (38 children) [27]. 14 and 11 children in each group, respectively, reported increased pain. No paired comparisons undertaken. Difference nonsignificant	Benefit unlikely	Not evaluated
Psychological therapies including cognitive behavioural therapy (CBT) and hypnotherapy for functional pain	Cochrane review of nine RCTs (709 patients) comparing CBT to waiting or standard medical care [40]. 49% of children who received CBT reported less pain compared with 17% of children who did not receive a psychological therapy. Standard mean difference in pain scores between the group receiving the psychological therapy, and controls was SMD −0.51(−0.8 to −0.22) at end of treatment ($p=0.0002$) Systematic review of hypnotherapy: three studies (108 patients) [41] Pain scores (p 0.05), school absenteeism ($p=0.02$) and long-term outlook were significantly improved: in one long-term study, at 1 year, 85% remained in remission vs 25% of controls. At 5 years, 68% children were in remission vs controls: (68 vs 20%, $p=0.005$)	Beneficial	None
Probiotics for IBS or functional pain	Cochrane meta-analysis of lactobacillus [27]: no significant symptom improvements (three trials: 168 children). The pooled odds ratio for improvement of symptoms was 1.17 (95% CI 0.62, 2.21) Also: One placebo-controlled multicentre RCT of 141 children given lactobacillus GG [43]. LGG caused significant reduction of frequency ($p<0.01$) and severity ($p<0.01$) of abdominal pain. These differences were significant at week 16 ($p<0.02$ and $p<0.001$, respectively) One placebo-controlled RCT of VSL#3 in 59 children with IBS [42]: VSL#3 was significantly superior to placebo for reducing pain/discomfort, bloating and impact on family ($p<0.05$). No significant difference was found ($p=0.06$) in stool pattern	Some evidence of benefit	None
Added fibre for IBS	Cochrane review of two RCTs in 92 patients [27]: no significant improvement. The pooled odds ratio for improvement in the frequency of abdominal pain with fibre was 1.26 (95% CI 0.25–6.29)	Benefit unlikely	None
Peppermint oil for IBS	One RCT of peppermint oil in 42 children (71% improved vs 41% improved on placebo (relative risk 1.67, 95% CI 0.95–2.93)	Likely beneficial	Not evaluated
Pizotifen for abdominal migraine	One placebo-controlled crossover RCT in 14 children for 1 month (mean 8.21 more pain-free days, 95% CI 2.93–13.48)	Likely beneficial	Drowsiness, weight gain

There is no current pediatric evidence for analgesics, antispasmodics, tricyclics or other agents for neuropathic pain, for example gabapentin

RCT randomized controlled trial, *IBS* inflammatory bowel syndrome, *H$_2$* histamine

Psychological treatment has the best evidence base in motivated families who understand the underlying mechanism. NASPGHAN recommended in 2005 to:

- Deal with psychological factors
- Educate the family (an important part of treatment)
- Focus on return to normal functioning rather than on the complete disappearance of pain
- Prescribe drugs judiciously as part of a multifaceted, individualized approach, to relieve symptoms and disability [7]

Outcome of Recurrent Abdominal Pain

There are few long-term studies assessing functional outcome in children with RAP. In one recent follow-up study, children with RAP ($n=332$) were, in comparison to a control group of well subjects ($n=147$), observed prospectively and evaluated for psychiatric disorders and functional GI disorders (FGIDs) at follow up (mean follow-up 7–8 years) in adolescence and young adulthood (mean age = 20.01 years) [47]. The prevalence of anxiety disorders in this group was 51%, of any depressive disorder was 40 and 17% developed a substance dependency; compared to controls, the children with functional pain who developed FGIDs were three times more likely to develop lifetime anxiety and depression ($p<0.001$). Even those children with RAP who did not develop FGID were twice as likely to suffer from lifetime anxiety and depression ($p<0.05$) [47].

Based on retrospective data, there is an increased incidence of psychiatric disorders in adulthood, particularly anxiety disorders. One study assessed 305 children in primary care settings with a first presentation of abdominal pain, and followed them up at three monthly intervals for a year

[48]. A total of 305 children (116 boys, 189 girls), median age 7.8 (IQR5.7–10.5) were included. Abdominal pain was present in 142 (46.6%) children at first presentation. During follow-up, 78.7% fulfilled the criteria for chronic abdominal pain at least one follow-up point. Among the remaining 163 children, the cumulative incidence of chronic abdominal pain was 60.1% (95% CI 52.1–67.7) and was higher in girls than in boys (RR 1.23; 95% CI 0.94–1.61). Median duration of abdominal pain was 7.5 (IQR4.5–12.0) months. Children aged 10–17 years had the longest duration of abdominal pain (median 9.0; IQR7.5–12.4 months). Children classified as having functional dyspepsia (Rome III criteria) seemed to have a more favourable prognosis compared with children with IBS or FAP.

The long-term outlook is varied, and poorer outlooks have been seen in children with psychiatric comorbidities, such as anxiety, and the presence of other somatic symptoms, for example headache/limb pain. Previous abuse (especially if undisclosed) can also impact on recovery.

One study observed 2300 adolescents (aged 16–17 years) in Uppsala, Finland, over 15 years [23]. Abdominal pain was the strongest predictor of depression in later life, outperforming all Diagnostic and Statistical Manual of Mental Disorders, 4th Edition (DSM-IV) depressive symptoms (e.g. anhedonia, worthlessness, suicidal ideation) even after controlling for confounding factors (Table 19.10).

Many children can be discharged once the diagnosis has been made. The more severe and long-standing cases in whom school attendance is poor may benefit from psychological support and require follow-up until symptoms resolve and to give an opportunity for any psychiatric comorbidity to emerge.

Summary

Appropriate assessment of organic disease with reassurance is important, and familial acceptance of the biopsychosocial model is key; with the clinician having understood and addressed the anxieties. Associated psychiatric comorbidity and somatic symptoms are common and are adverse prog-

nostic factors. Follow-up in severe/long-standing cases may be required.

It is important to recognize that diet, lifestyle and constipation may be significant factors in the child with RAP.

In the absence of likely underlying organic disease, it is often useful to elicit clinical features known to be associated with childhood RAP, such as psychological stress and anxiety. Many of these will become apparent whilst taking a detailed history. Typical adverse social factors leading to psychological stress include bereavement, altered peer relationships, school problems and illness in a family member. High achievers are at risk, particularly those who have excessive out-of-school activities. It is important not just to ask about illnesses in the family but also to ask about how those illnesses impact on the family. In some families there is an 'illness model', and this puts the child at increased risk of functional symptoms. This part of the assessment may also reveal a family history of anxiety disorders, or an anxious temperament in the child.

Recommended Clinical Approach

Figure 19.2 summarizes the priorities in assessing a child with RAP, including a focussed history aiming to identify triggers and assess for 'red flags', targeting appropriate investigations to exclude organic causes and classification of symptomatology according to Rome III criteria. Reassurance, drawing on the links with physical and psychological stressors and a focus on a practical rehabilitation strategy, is essential to help parental understanding and acceptance, and to help the child reintegrate into school and normal activities.

Other Functional Gastrointestinal Disorders

These are defined as a variable combination of chronic or recurrent GI symptoms not explained by structural or biochemical abnormalities; they are common at all ages of childhood, and there are often commonalities. Recognizing the patterns can allow early identification with a reduced burden of tests and less risk for treatment failures/side effects.

These conditions requires careful evaluation in order to avoid the overinvestigation and 'over' medicalization of chronic functional symptoms in children.

Infant and Toddler

Infant Regurgitation

Infant regurgitation, or functional GOR is a common occurrence, characterized by the regurgitation of gastric contents

Table 19.10 Predictors of depression in later life. (Reproduced with kind permission from Ref. [23])

Symptom	Outcome: any anxiety disorder in follow-up	
	OR	95% CI
Abdominal pain	3.0	1.33–6.77
Tiredness	2.4	1.29–4.34
Headache	0.4	0.27–0.96
Anhedonia	2.5	1.43–4.51
Long-term depression (> 1 year duration)	3.9	2.12–7.04

OR odds ratio (95%confidence interval)

Fig. 19.2 Recommended clinical approach to the child with recurrent abdominal pain. *FH* family history, *IBD* inflammatory bowel disease *FBC* full blood count, *ESR* erythrocyte sedimentation rate, *CRP* C-reactive protein, *IgA* immunoglobulin A, *TTG* testing for coeliac disease, *EMA* anti-endomysial antibody, *NSAIDs* nonsteroidal anti-inflammatory drugs

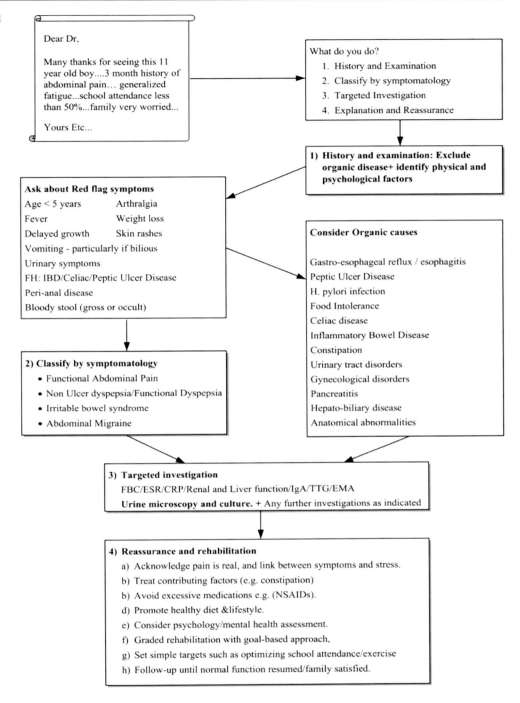

Dear Dr,

Many thanks for seeing this 11 year old boy....3 month history of abdominal pain... generalized fatigue...school attendance less than 50%...family very worried...

Yours Etc...

What do you do?
1. History and Examination
2. Classify by symptomatology
3. Targeted Investigation
4. Explanation and Reassurance

1) History and examination: Exclude organic disease+ identify physical and psychological factors

Ask about Red flag symptoms

Age < 5 years   Arthralgia
Fever   Weight loss
Delayed growth   Skin rashes
Vomiting - particularly if bilious
Urinary symptoms
FH: IBD/Celiac/Peptic Ulcer Disease
Peri-anal disease
Bloody stool (gross or occult)

Consider Organic causes

Gastro-esophageal reflux / esophagitis
Peptic Ulcer Disease
H. pylori infection
Food Intolerance
Celiac disease
Inflammatory Bowel Disease
Constipation
Urinary tract disorders
Gynecological disorders
Pancreatitis
Hepato-biliary disease
Anatomical abnormalities

2) Classify by symptomatology
- Functional Abdominal Pain
- Non Ulcer dyspepsia/Functional Dyspepsia
- Irritable bowel syndrome
- Abdominal Migraine

3) Targeted investigation
FBC/ESR/CRP/Renal and Liver function/IgA/TTG/EMA
Urine microscopy and culture. + Any further investigations as indicated

4) Reassurance and rehabilitation
   a) Acknowledge pain is real, and link between symptoms and stress.
   b) Treat contributing factors (e.g. constipation)
   b) Avoid excessive medications e.g. (NSAIDs).
   d) Promote healthy diet &lifestyle.
   e) Consider psychology/mental health assessment.
   f) Graded rehabilitation with goal-based approach,
   g) Set simple targets such as optimizing school attendance/exercise
   h) Follow-up until normal function resumed/family satisfied.

into the esophagus and some degree of regurgitation is normal throughout life. GOR is a very common presentation in infancy; in both a primary care or a secondary care setting. GOR can affect approximately 50% of infants less than 3 months old [49]. The natural history of GOR in infancy is generally that of a functional, self-limiting condition, which improves with age, with <5% of children with vomiting or regurgitation continuing to have symptoms after infancy [50]. A recent study of 210 children with GOR in infancy diagnosed by Rome II criteria and followed up for 24 months,

showed that 88% were symptom-free by 12 months [51]. Infant regurgitation is differentiated from GORD by the absence of sequelae, including excessive irritability and the presence of normal growth. The sequelae associated with GORD can include apnoea or acute life-threatening events, recurrent aspiration pneumonia or esophagitis. Other causes such as overfeeding, cow's milk protein intolerance and gastroenteritis should be considered.

Diagnosis of infant regurgitation is usually made based on the symptoms alone, avoiding the need for expensive and possibly harmful investigations. Investigations, to assess severity of GORD or in cases where GOR cannot be made on clinical grounds, include 24-h esophageal pH monitoring, upper GI endoscopy, esophageal manometry, scintigraphy or sonography. All have been shown to correlate poorly with symptomatology and may not accurately predict the degree of improvement with treatment.

Further information can be found contained within the National Institute for Health and Clinical Excellence (NICE) guideline on GOR (www.nice.org.uk).

Infant Rumination Syndrome

Infant rumination is defined (within the Rome criteria) as a disorder that includes repetitive contractions of the abdominal muscles, diaphragm and tongue; and regurgitation of gastric content into the mouth, which is either expectorated or rechewed and reswallowed. It tends to develop between 3 and 8 months; and is refractory to anti-reflux treatment or formula changes. It is not associated with distress; and does not occur during sleep or when the infant is interacting with individuals in the environment.

It is thought to be most common in infants with severe neurodevelopmental delay. The features above distinguish rumination from infant regurgitation, which starts in a younger age group, and is often more noticeable in sleep/states of excitement. Fleisher described infant rumination as an acquired skill used by an emotionally deprived infant for the purpose of self-stimulation and needs satisfaction. Behavioural therapy with use of positive reinforcement has been shown to be an effective treatment for rumination syndrome. Once the nutritional deficiencies are corrected and the ruminant behaviour improves, it usually does not recur.

Clinical bottom-line Rumination is the habitual regurgitation of stomach contents when not interacting with others, or asleep. It often resolves with positive reinforcement/distraction.

Infant Colic

Infant colic is generally taken to describe excessive distress and crying associated with incoordinate gut peristalsis during infancy. Previous definitions have used colic as a corollary for excessive crying: including 'Unexplained paroxysmal bouts of fussing and crying that lasted >3 h a day, for >3 days a week, for >3 weeks' duration' [52]. Colic can be considered as the mid-gut manifestation of infantile dysmotility, with gastro-esophageal reflux as the foregut manifestation, and constipation and dyschezia as hindgut symptoms; and generally has a benign outlook, with resolution of colicky symptoms by the first birthday. Colic can cause significant distress, often associated with a family history of IBS, and infants with colic can become children with RAP and then mature to be adults with IBS. The distress it causes can significantly affect parental bonding; and significant research has helped to elucidate further distinguishing features of colic compared to normal crying of infancy. Consideration should be given to excluding organic disease, with again a low yield from investigation.

Hide et al. found that the prevalence of colic in 843 infants was historically 16% with no link to breast or bottle-feeding, but increased prevalence in those babies fed solids under 3 months of age [53]. Heine describes a subgroup who may benefit from a hydrolyzed formula [54], and Garrison et al. in a systematic review of 22 suitable articles in 2000 found that the number needed to treat (NNT) for benefit from hydrolyzed formula and soy formula was 6 and 2, respectively [55]. Interestingly, one study compared hydrolyzed formula to parental counselling, and this study found these measures were equally effective in reducing reported symptoms scores [56]. One study found that simethicone was less effective than placebo [52], and, in the systematic review by Garrison, lactase enzymes and simethicone were ineffective compared to placebo [55]. Scopolamine was ineffective and had a higher incidence of adverse effects. Dicyclomine, whilst effective for colic (NNT=3) has significant adverse effects including apnoea and seizures, and it is not recommended for colic.

Clinical bottom line Colic is often distressing but self-limiting, and investigation has a low yield in those babies who are thriving and with no red flags. Some benefit may be derived from trying a hydrolyzed diet [56], but advancing parental education and understanding about colic may be equally as effective, and a wide variety of medications available over the counter in pharmacies have no evidence base of efficacy.

Functional Diarrhea

Also known as toddlers' diarrhea or chronic nonspecific diarrhea, functional diarrhea is defined by the daily painless passage of >3 large, unformed stools for >4 weeks with onset between 6 and 36 months of age [57]. The stooling occurs whilst awake, and the child is growing well. Parents are often concerned by mucus or easily identifiable pieces of undigested food (usually vegetable matter) in the stools, and worry about malabsorption. The child is not often in pain, although may suffer perineal discomfort, and the condition usually resolves spontaneously by school age. Further history assessing diet may uncover overfeeding, excessive carbohydrate ingestion (such as fruit juice and sorbitol) and low-fat intake [57]. In the absence of faltering growth, malabsorption is unlikely.

Underlying mechanisms have been suggested including abnormalities in the control of postprandial motility, increased activities of (Na^+/K^+)–adenosine triphosphatase and percentage of activation and basal activity of adenylate cyclase, and bile salt malabsorption [58]. Behavioural problems including sleep difficulty and excessive crying were also found to be significantly more frequent or severe in a group of children with chronic nonspecific diarrhea [59]. Therapeutic interventions should focus on increasing dietary fibre and fat intake, reducing fructose and avoiding excessively restrictive diets that may cause calorie deprivation.

Infant Dyschezia

Infant dyschezia is defined by the Rome committee by characteristic symptoms [57]. It is also known as 'grunting baby syndrome', describing an infant struggling to have a bowel movement. Parents describe their infants straining for several minutes, often crying, and turning red or purple in the face with effort. The symptoms persist until there is passage of soft or liquid stool. Often, well-meaning parents may try alleviating the child's perceived pain by stimulating the anus with a suppository or a thermometer, an act that usually leads to stooling and resolution of the distressed behaviour. This 'success' may then reinforce this intervention. The underlying cause is thought to be failure to coordinate increased intra-abdominal pressure with relaxation of the pelvic floor. Simultaneous abdominal and gluteal contractions interfere with defecation. Unlike colic, the distress is only associated with defecation. The symptoms begin in the first months of life and resolve spontaneously within a few weeks, as the infant learns appropriate co-ordination. As above, the clinician must reassure the parents effectively by listening to the parents' worries, performing a thorough physical examination (including anal inspection) particularly to exclude associated constipation, and, in the absence of symptoms or signs of underlying disease, explaining that this is a benign phenomenon and no testing or treatment is necessary. Repeated anal stimulation is not encouraged to allow the infant to learn the correct defecation process.

Clinical bottom line Infant dyschezia describes infants who struggle and strain to have a bowel motion, with distress associated with defecation. Medication is not needed for this behaviour, which will spontaneously improve.

Functional constipation is covered in Chap. 21.

Aerophagy

Aerophagy is characterized by symptoms related to persistent air swallowing, is a poorly understood functional disorder [59]. Symptoms of aerophagia can be distressing, but the underlying causes and optimal treatment are unknown. Aerophagia has been described in children with learning difficulties, after surgical gastric fundoplication and in a small number of healthy children exhibited as an unconscious behaviour. Symptoms of aerophagia are also seen with gastro-esophageal reflux disease and dyspepsia. The Rome committee has defined aerophagia in children as occurring over at least 12 weeks, in the preceding 12 months, of two or more of the following symptoms: (i) air swallowing, (ii) abdominal distension due to intraluminal air and (iii) repetitive belching and/or increased flatus. One study assessed 45 children with clinical aerophagia: The most common GI symptoms were abdominal pain (in 50% of patients), abdominal distension (33%) and belching (31%). In addition, patients reported excess flatus (22%), fullness or bloating after eating (20%) and air swallowing (11%). Additional nonspecific symptoms include burping or vomiting to relieve symptoms or pressure ($n=3$), gurgling or loud abdominal sounds ($n=2$) and a general sense of not feeling well ($n=2$). Symptoms interfered with school in 9% of patients. In addition, 9% of patients reported constipation and 11% diarrhea. Interestingly, in this cohort, no patients had previous GI surgery. Only two patients had a history of developmental disability. Two reported an anxiety disorder and one reported a history of depressive disorder [60].

In the follow-up, 30 were managed with reassurance and education; 9 were treated with medications, ranging from omeprazole to metoclopramide, and 4 were referred to psychology. One was referred to ENT, one to occupational therapy. In the follow-up, only 12 patients had a documented subsequent visit with their primary physician in the medical record. The duration of time of the subsequent visit from the initial visit was 27 ± 8 days. At this time, four patients had improvement in their symptoms and none reported worsening, or had a recurrent visit for aerophagia. Of the patients with improvement, one was treated with chlordiazepoxide, aluminium hydroxide and simethicone. The remaining three were given education about aerophagia alone.

Clinical bottom line These children have a prolonged course, but benign outcome, with no evidence favouring pharmacological therapy.

Older Children and Adolescents

Vomiting and Aerophagy

This has many features with the infant pattern described above.

Adolescent Rumination Syndrome

This is similar in nature to the infant presentation. One study assessed 147 patients (aged 5–20 years) diagnosed with rumination syndrome between 1975 and 2000 [61]. Sixty-eight percent were female. Mean age at diagnosis was 15.0 (SE ± 0.3 years). Symptom duration before diagnosis was a mean of 2.2 years (± 0.3 years). 73 % reported missing school/work and 46 % had been hospitalized because of symptoms. Interestingly, 16 (11 %) had undergone surgery for investigation or management of symptoms. Twenty-four (16 %) had psychiatric disorders; 3.4 % had anorexia or bulimia nervosa. All patients described postprandial regurgitation after almost every meal (2.7 ± /0.1 meals per day). Weight loss was described by 42.2 % (median weight loss 7 kg). Additional symptoms included: abdominal pain, 38 %; constipation, 21 %; nausea, 17 % and diarrhea, 8 %. Structural studies were normal. Gastric emptying of solids at 4 h was delayed in 26 of 56 patients. Esophageal pH testing in 24 patients showed reflux/regurgitation in 54 %. Gastroduodenal manometry in 65 patients showed characteristic rumination waves in 40 %. In terms of outcomes: the median follow-up was 10 months, and, in 54 patients, symptoms resolved in 16 (30 %) and improved in 30 (56 %).

Cyclic vomiting syndrome is covered in Chap. 25.

Non Retentive Faecal Incontinence

This is defined by the Rome III criteria as the repeated inappropriate passage of stool into a place other than the toilet in a child older than 4 years old with no evidence of faecal retention, at least monthly, lasting for more than 2 months [7]. One Dutch cohort had a prevalence of 4 % in children aged 5–6 years old, and 1.6 % in the 11–12-year-olds [7]. These children have no underlying organic disease and, after normal examination, findings and baseline tests as listed above are unremarkable. These children are more likely to have behavioural issues and will benefit from education appropriate to their understanding, and regular toilet use with a positive reward strategy. Parents may often need support in the home/school environment to help resolve these issues.

Chronic Fatigue

This is characterized by chronic or recurrent debilitating fatigue and other symptoms, including sore throat, lymph node pain and tenderness, headache, myalgia and arthralgias. Abdominal pain can be a prominent feature in the presentation of this condition, and further descriptions of assessment and management are outlined elsewhere [45].

References

1. Apley J, Naish N. Recurrent abdominal pains: a field survey of 1000 school children. Arch Dis Child. 1958;33:165–70.
2. Berger YM, Gieteling MJ, Benninga MA. Chronic abdominal pain in children. Br Med J. 2007;334:997–1002.
3. Saps M, Seshadri R, Sztainberg M, Schaffer G, Marshall BM, Di Lorenzo C. A prospective school-based study of abdominal pain and other common somatic complaints in children. J Pediatr. 2009 March;154(3):322–6.
4. Talley NJ, Gabriel SE, Harmsen WS, Zinsmeister AR, Evans RW. Medical costs in community subjects with irritable bowel syndrome. Gastroenterology. 1995;109:1736–41.
5. Martin R, Barron JJ, Zacker C. Irritable bowel syndrome: toward a cost-effective management approach. Am J Manag Care. 2001;7:S268–75.
6. van Tilburg MAL, Chitkara DK, Palsson OS, Levy RL, Whitehead WE. Parental worries and beliefs about abdominal pain. J Pediatr Gastroenterol Nutr. 2009;48:311–7.
7. Rasquin A, Di Lorenzo C, Forbes D, et al. Childhood functional gastrointestinal disorders: child/adolescent. Gastroenterology. 2006;130:1527–37.
8. Schurman JV, Hunter HL, Friesen CA. Conceptualization and treatment of chronic abdominal pain in pediatric gastroenterology practice. J Pediatr Gastroenterol Nutr. 2010;50(1):32–7.
9. Czyzewski DI, Lane MM, Weidler EM, Williams AE, Swank PR, Shulman RJ. The interpretation of Rome III criteria and method of assessment affect the irritable bowel syndrome classification of children. Aliment Pharmacol Ther. 2011;33:403–11.
10. Jones J, Boorman J, Cann P, Forbes A, Gomborone J, Heaton K, Hungin P, et al. British society of gastroenterology guidelines for the management of the irritable bowel syndrome. Gut. 2000;47 Suppl 2:ii1–19.
11. Oster J. Recurrent abdominal pain, headache and limb pain in children and adolescents. Pediatrics. 1972;50:429–35.
12. Rask CU, Ørnbøl E, Fink PK, Skovgaard AM. Functional somatic symptoms and consultation patterns in 5- to 7-year-olds. Pediatrics. 2013;132:e459.
13. Littlewood JM. Abdominal pain in cystic fibrosis. J R Soc Med. 1995;88 Suppl 25:9–17.
14. Moro E. Über rezidivierende Nabelkoliken bei alteren Kindern. Münch Med Wochenschr. 1913;60:2827.
15. Green M: Diagnosis and treatment: psychogenic, recurrent abdominal pain: Pediatrics. 1967;40;84–7.
16. Morenas R, Tighe MP Brown L, Beattie RM. Recurrent abdominal pain: a BMJ learning module. 2014. www.learning.bmj.com. Accessed 19 Feb 2014.
17. Locke GR 3rd, Zinsmeister AR, Talley NJ, Fett SL, Melton LJ 3rd. Familial association in adults with functional gastrointestinal disorders. Mayo Clin Proc. 2000;75:907–12.
18. Levy RL, Jones KR, Whitehead WE, Feld SI, Talley NJ, Corey LA. Irritable bowel syndrome in twins: heredity and social learning both contribute to etiology. Gastroenterology. 2001;121:799–804.
19. Plunkett A, Beattie RM. Recurrent abdominal pain in childhood. J R Soc Med. 2005;98:101–6.
20. Walker LS, Smith CA, Garber J, Claar RL. Appraisal and coping with daily stressors by pediatric patients with chronic abdominal pain. J Pediatr Psychol. 2007;32:206–16.
21. Kaminsky L, Robertson M, Dewey D. Psychological correlates of depression in children with recurrent abdominal pain. J Pediatr Psychol. 2006;31:956–66.
22. Ramchandani PG, Murray L, Romano G, Vlachos H, Stein A. An investigation of health anxiety in families where children have recurrent abdominal pain. J Pediatr Psychol. 2011;36(4):409–19.

23. Bohman H, Jonsson U, Päären A, von Knorring L, Olsson G, von Knorring AL. Prognostic significance of functional somatic symptoms in adolescence: a 15-year community-based follow-up study of adolescents with depression compared with healthy peers. BMC Psychiatry. 2012 July 27;12:90.

24. Fitzpatrick KP, Sherman PM, Ipp M, Saunders N, Macarthur C. Screening for celiac disease in children with recurrent abdominal pain. J Pediatr Gastroenterol Nutr. 2001 Sept;33(3):250–2.

25. Macarthur C. *Helicobacter pylori* infection and childhood recurrent abdominal pain: lack of evidence for a cause and effect relationship. Can J Gastroenterol. 1999;13:607–10.

26. Malaty HM, Abudayyeh S, Fraley K, Graham DY, Gilger MA, Hollier DR. Recurrent abdominal pain in school children: effect of obesity and diet. Acta Paediatr. 2007;96:572–6.

27. Huertas-Ceballos AA, Logan S, Bennett C, Macarthur C. Dietary interventions for recurrent abdominal pain (RAP) and irritable bowel syndrome (IBS) in childhood. Evid.-Based Child Health 2010:5: 758–788.

28. Matthews PJ, Aziz Q. Functional abdominal pain. Postgrad Med J. 2005;81:448–55.

29. Gwee KA, Leong YL, Graham C, McKendrick MW, Collins SM, Walters SJ, et al. The role of psychological and biological factors in postinfective gut dysfunction. Gut. 1999;44:400–6.

30. Sarna SK. Colonic motility: from bench side to bedside. San Rafael: Morgan & Claypool Life Sciences; 2010.

31. Tanaka Y, Kanazawa M, Fukudo S, Drossman DA. Biopsychosocial model of irritable bowel syndrome. J Neurogastroenterol Motil. 2011 April;17(2):131–9.

32. Faure C, Wieckowska A. Somatic referral of visceral sensations and rectal sensory threshold for pain in children with functional gastrointestinal disorders. J Pediatr. 2007;150:66–71.

33. Crandall WV, Halterman TE, Mackner LM. Anxiety and pain symptoms in children with inflammatory bowel disease and functional gastrointestinal disorders undergoing colonoscopy. J Pediatr Gastroenterol Nutr. 2007;44:63–7.

34. Shulman RJ, Eakin MN, Jarrett M, Czyzewski DI, Zeltzer LK. Characteristics of pain and stooling in children with recurrent abdominal pain. J Pediatr Gastroenterol Nutr. 2007;44:203–8.

35. Di Lorenzo C, Colletti RB, Lehmann HP, Boyle JT, Gerson WT, Hyams JS, Kanda PT. Chronic abdominal pain in children: a technical report of the American Academy of Pediatrics and the North American Society for Pediatric Gastroenterology, Hepatology and Nutrition: AAP Subcommittee and NASPGHAN Committee on Chronic Abdominal Pain. J Pediatr Gastroenterol Nutr. 2005;40(3):249–61.

36. Soon GS, Saunders N, Ipp M, Sherman PM, Macarthur C. Short communication: community-based case-control study of childhood chronic abdominal pain: role of selected laboratory investigations. J Pediatr Gastroenterol Nutr. 2007;44:524–6.

37. Olafsdottir E, Aksnes L, Fluge G, Berstad A. Faecal calprotectin levels in infants with infantile colic, healthy infants, children with inflammatory bowel disease, children with recurrent abdominal pain and healthy children. Acta Paediatr. 2002;91:45–50.

38. Bremner A, Roked S, Robinson R, Phillips I, Beattie M. Faecal calprotectin in children with chronic gastrointestinal symptoms. Acta Paediatr. 2005;94(12):1855–8.

39. Shulman RJ, Eakin MN, Czyzewski DI, Jarrett M, Ou CN. Increased gastrointestinal permeability and gut inflammation in children with functional abdominal pain and irritable bowel syndrome. J Pediatr. 2008 Nov;153(5):646–50.

40. Eccleston C, Palermo TM, Williams AC, Lewandowski Holley A, Morley S, Fisher E, Law E. Psychological therapies for the management of chronic and recurrent pain in children and adolescents. The Cochrane Library.2009; (2): CD003968.

41. Rutten J, Reitsma J, Vlieger A, et al. Gut-directed hypnotherapy for functional abdominal pain or irritable bowel syndrome in children: systematic review. Arch Dis Child. 2013;98:252–7.

42. Guandalini S, Magazzu G, Chiaro A, La Balestr,a V, Di Nardo G, Gopalan S, Setty M. VSL# 3 improves symptoms in children with irritable bowel syndrome: a multicenter, randomized, placebo-controlled, double-blind, crossover study. J Pediatr Gastroenterol Nutr. 2010;51(1):24–30.

43. Francavilla R, Miniello V, Magista AM, et al. A randomized controlled trial of lactobacillus gg in children with functional abdominal pain. Pediatrics. 2010;126:1445–52.

44. Lewis DW. Pediatric migraine. Neurol Clin. 2009;27(2):481–501.

45. Viner R, Christie D. Fatigue and somatic symptoms. ABC Adolesc. 2005;98:42.

46. Huertas-Ceballos A, Logan S, Bennett C, Macarthur C. Pharmacological interventions for recurrent abdominal pain (RAP) and irritable bowel syndrome (IBS) in childhood. The Cochrane Library. 2008; (1): CD003017.

47. Shelby GD, Shirkey KC, Sherman AL, et al. Functional abdominal pain in childhood and long-term vulnerability to anxiety disorders. Pediatrics. 2013;132:475–52.

48. van Leeuwen, Y, Spee LAA, Benninga MA, Bierma-Zeinstra SMA, Berge MY. Prognosis of abdominal pain presented by children in primary care—a prospective cohort study. Ann Fam Med. 11(3):238–44.

49. Nelson SP, Chen EH, Syniar GM, Christoffel KK. One-year follow-up of symptoms.of gastresophageal reflux during infancy (Pediatric Practice Research Group). Pediatrics. 1998 Dec;102(6):E67.

50. Martin AJ, Pratt N, Kennedy JD, Ryan P, Ruffin RE, Miles H, et al. Natural history and familial relationships of infant spilling to 9 years of age. Pediatrics. 2002 June;109(6):1061–7.

51. Campanozzi A, Boccia G, Pensabene L, Panetta F, Marseglia A, Strisciuglio P, et al. Prevalence and natural history of gastroesophageal reflux: pediatric prospective survey. Pediatrics. 2009 March;123(3):779–83.

52. Metcalf TJ, Irons TG, Sher LD, Young PC. Simethicone in the treatment of infant colic: a randomized, placebo-controlled, multi-center trial. Pediatrics. 1994 July;94(1):29–34.

53. Hide DW, Guyer BM. Prevalence of infant colic. Arch Dis Child. 1982;57:559–60.

54. Heine RG. Allergic gastrointestinal motility disorders in infancy and early childhood. Pediatr Allergy Immunol. 2008;19(5): 383–91.

55. Garrison MM, Christakis DA. A systematic review of treatments for infant colic. Pediatrics. 2000 July 1; 106(1 Suppl 1):184–90.

56. Taubman B. Parental counseling compared with elimination of cow's milk or soy milk protein for the treatment of infant colic syndrome: a randomized trial. Pediatrics. 1988 June;81(6):756–61.

57. Di Lorenzo C. Other functional gastrointestinal disorders in infants and young children. J Pediatr Gastroenterol Nutr. 2013;57(1): S36–8.

58. Tripp JH, Muller DP, Harries JT. Mucosal (Naþ-Kþ)-ATPase and adenylate cyclase activities in children with toddler diarrhea and the postenteritis syndrome. Pediatr Res. 1980;14:1382–6.

59. McOmber ME, Shulman RJ. Recurrent abdominal pain and irritable bowel syndrome in children. Curr Opin Pediatr. 2007 Oct;19(5):581–5.

60. Chitkara DK, Bredenoord AJ, Wang M, Rucker MJ, Talley NJ. Aerophagia in children: characterization of a functional gastrointestinal disorder. Neurogastroenterol Motil. 2005;17:518–22.

61. Chial HJ, Camilleri M, Williams DE, Litzinger K, Perrault J. Rumination syndrome in children and adolescents: diagnosis, treatment, and prognosis. Pediatrics. 2003;111:158.

Disorders of Sucking and Swallowing

20

Francesca Paola Giugliano, Erasmo Miele and Annamaria Staiano

Introduction

The development of feeding skills is an extremely complex process influenced by multiple anatomic, neurophysiologic, environmental, social, and cultural factors. Oral feeding in infants should be efficient to preserve energy for growing. Moreover, it should be safe so as to avoid aspiration, and it should not compromise respiratory status. This can only be achieved if sucking, swallowing, and breathing are properly coordinated [1]. This entire process is dynamic because of ongoing growth and development. Functional feeding skills, which depend on the integrity of anatomic structures, undergo changes based on neurologic maturation and experimental learning. Eating/feeding requires active effort by infants who must have exquisite timing and coordination of sucking, swallowing, and breathing to be efficient [2].

A variety of neurological, neuromuscular conditions in children and infants can impair the physiological phases of sucking/swallowing and cause disorders of feeding and dysphagia. The causes of feeding and swallowing problems include combinations of structural deficits, neurologic conditions, respiratory compromise, feeder–child interaction dysfunction, and numerous medical conditions such as genetic, metabolic, and degenerative disease [3].

In the recent years, there has been an increase in infant swallowing disorders as a result of improved survival rates for infants born prematurely or with life-threatening medical disorders. Negative experiences related to feeding, such as intubation, tube feeding, or airway suctioning may further disturb sucking and swallowing development [4]. Disorders of feeding and swallowing in children are serious and potentially fatal problems. Aspiration due to dysphagia may lead to severe pulmonary disease, and impaired oral and pharyngeal function may rapidly result in failure to thrive. Prompt evaluation of swallowing disorders is therefore critical.

The differential diagnosis of dysphagia in children is wide. The diagnostic work-up can be extremely difficult and exhaustive in many cases. Because of this complexity, multidisciplinary team evaluations should be conducted.

Successful rehabilitation of children with swallowing disorders requires knowledge of the parameters of normal and abnormal swallowing plus skill in the integration of a variety of essential therapeutics techniques.

Epidemiology

Data on the incidence of swallowing disorders are lacking, because in clinical practice, disorders of swallowing are often considered in the general context of a feeding disorder. Feeding (or eating) is different from swallowing. Eating is primarily an oral phase function that includes oral preparation and oral transit of a bolus [5]. Feeding is a complex process that involves a number of phases in addition to the act of swallowing, including the recognition of hunger (appetite), the acquisition of the food, and the ability to bring the food to the mouth [6]. The estimated prevalence of feeding problems in the pediatric population ranges from 25–35 % in normally developing children to 40–93 % in children with developmental delay [7, 8]. Early sucking and swallowing problems were reported to be present in 35–48 % of infants with different types of neonatal brain injury [9]. However, knowledge of the true epidemiology of pediatric dysphagia remains largely unavailable because of the lack of a standardized reporting system assessing dysphagia in all of the possible contexts that may occur in infants and children [10].

A. Staiano (✉) · F. P. Giugliano · E. Miele
Section of Pediatrics, Department of Transitional Medical
Science, University of Naples "Federico II", Via S. Pansini 5,
Naples 80131, Italy
e-mail: staiano@unina.it

© Springer International Publishing Switzerland 2016
S. Guandalini et al. (eds.), *Textbook of Pediatric Gastroenterology, Hepatology and Nutrition*,
DOI 10.1007/978-3-319-17169-2_20

Table 20.1 Differential diagnosis of dysphagia. (Adapted from Ref. [12], Copyright Elsevier, 1983, and reprinted with permission from Ref. [13], Table 15.1, p. 234)

Prematurity		
Upper airway obstruction	Nasal and nasopharyngeal	Cohanal atresia, stenosis, septal deflections and abscess, infections, tumors, sinusitis
	Oropharynx	Defects of lips and alveolar processes, cleft lips or palate, hypopharyngeal stenosis, craniofacial syndromes or sequences (e.g., Cruzon, Treacher Collins syndrome, Pierre Robin sequence)
	Laryngeal	Laryngeal cleft and cyst, laryngomalacia, subglottic stenosis, and paralysis
Congenital defects of the larynx, trachea, and esophagus	Laryngotracheoesophageal cleft	–
	Tracheosophageal fistula with associated esophageal atresia	–
	Esophageal anomalies (e.g., strictures, webs)	–
	Vascular anomalies	Aberrant right succlavian artery
		Double aortic arch
		Right aortic arch with left ligamentum
Acquired anatomic defects	Trauma	External trauma, intubation, endoscopic, and foreign body
	Chemical ingestion	–
Neurologic disorders	Central nervous system	Trauma
		Hypoxia and anoxia
		Cortical atrophy, hypoplasia, agenesis
		Infections (meningitis, brain abscess)
Peripheral nervous system disease	Trauma	–
	Congenital defects	
Neuromuscular	Guillan-Barre syndrome	
	Poliomyelitis (bulbar paralysis)	
	Myasthenia gravis	
	Myotonic muscular dystrophy	
Anatomic and functional defects	Cricopharyngeal dysfunction	
	Esophageal achalasia	
	Esophageal spasm	
	Paralysis of the esophagus	
	Associated atresia-tracheoesophaegal fistula, nerve defect	
	Peptic and eosinophilic esophagitis	
	Riley-Day syndrome (dysautonomia)	
	Brain stem compression (e.g., Chiari malformation, tumor)	

Etiology

Disorders of sucking/swallowing may be caused by multiple etiologic factors that may interfere with the child's ability to coordinate swallowing and breathing maneuvers and may be manifested as a unique set of symptoms. Potential causes responsible for three broad categories include: immaturity, delay, or a defect in neuromuscular control; an anatomic abnormality of the aerodigestive tract; and/or systemic illness. The magnitude of the dysfunction depends on the balance between the extent of the structural or functional abnormality and the child's compensatory adaptations [11]. Disorders

associated with sucking/swallowing difficulties are reported in Table 20.1 [12, 13].

Pathophysiology

The fetus is capable of swallowing amniotic fluid in utero, indicating that the motor program for swallowing is functioning before gestation is complete.

However, oral feeding is not initiated in preterm infants before 32 weeks of postconceptional age, partly because the coordination of sucking, swallowing, and respiration is not established [14]. Even at 34 weeks, minute ventilation during sucking decreases more than that of infants at 36–38 weeks. Therefore, the coordination between swallowing and breathing is not yet fully organized at 34 weeks of postconceptional age [15, 16].

Anatomic structures, which are essential to competent feeding skills, undergo growth that changes their physical relationship to one other and consequently affects their function. The swallowing mechanism, by which food is transmitted to the stomach and digestive organs, is a complex action involving 26 muscles and 5 cranial nerves. The neurophysiologic control involves sensory afferent nerve fibers, motor efferent fibers, paired brainstem swallowing centers, and suprabulbar neural input. Structural integrity is essential to the development of normal feeding and swallowing skills [17]. The central patterning of aeroingestive behavior is based on volitional and reflexive control mechanisms and benefit from sensory feedback to modify the spatiotemporal organization of the feed sequence to allow safe swallow [18]. Central pattern generators (CPGs) are primarily composed of adaptive networks of interneurons that activate groups of motor neurons to generate task-specific motor patterns [19]. The essential components of the masticatory CPG are found between the rostral poles of the fifth and seventh motor nuclei, although they are normally synchronized by commissural axons each hemisection side can generate a rhythm [20]. Mastication patterns differ greatly between foods and change systematically during a chewing sequence based on sensory feedback. Functional imaging has revealed that swallowing is controlled through a network of cortical areas which shares loci with other ororhythmic movements including speech [21].

Deglutition is generally divided into phases of swallowing based on anatomic and functional characteristics: preoral, pharyngeal, and esophageal [22, 23].

Anatomic Considerations

An understanding of the anatomy of the pharynx is essential to a thorough understanding of the swallowing process. The anatomy changes during development. The tongue, the soft palate, and the arytenoids mass (arytenoids cartilage, false vocal cords, and true vocal cords) are larger relative to their surrounding chambers when compared with the adult [24]. In the infant, the tongue lies entirely within the oral cavity, resulting in a small oropharynx [25, 26]. In addition, a sucking pad, composed of densely compacted fatty tissue that further reduces the size of the oral cavity, stabilizes the lateral walls of the oral cavity. The larynx lies high in the infant, and the tip of epiglottis extends to and may overlap the soft palate. These anatomic relationships are ideal for the normal infant feeding pattern of suck or suckle feeding from a breast or a bottle in a recumbent position [26]. In the infant, the larynx sits high in the neck at the level of vertebrae C1 to C3, allowing for the velum, tongue, and epiglottis to approximate, thereby functionally separating the respiratory and digestive tracts. This separation allows the infant to breathe and feed safely. By age 2–3 years, the larynx descends, decreasing the separation of the swallowing and digestive tracts [7].

Development and Normal Swallowing Function

Swallowing skills develop progressively during fetal and neonatal maturation [27]. At approximately 26 days' fetal age, the developmental trajectories of the respiratory and swallowing systems diverge and start to develop independently. Swallowing in fetuses has been described as early as 12–14 weeks' gestational age. A sucking response can be provoked at 13 weeks' postconceptional age by touching the lips [28]. Real sucking, defined by a posterior–anterior movement of the tongue, in which the posterior movement is dominant, begins at 18–24 weeks' postconceptional age [29]. Between 26 and 29 weeks' there is probably no significant further maturation of sucking [30]. By week 34, most healthy fetuses can suck and swallow well enough to sustain nutritional needs via the oral route, if born at this early age. Sucking movements increase in frequency during the final weeks of fetal life due to an increase in amniotic fluid swallowed by a fetus during pregnancy from initially 2–7 ml a day to 450 ml a day. This is approximately half of the total volume of amniotic fluid at term [31]. The normal maturation of sucking and swallowing during the first months of life after full-term birth can be summarized by increased sucking and swallowing rates, longer sucking bursts and larger volume per suck [16]. The skill of safe and efficient oral feeding is based on oral-motor competence, neurobehavioral organization, and gastrointestinal maturity [32]. Two forms of sucking are distinguished: nutritive sucking (NS) and nonnutritive sucking (NNS). NS is an infant's primary means of receiving nutrition while NNS is regarded as an initial method for exploring the environment. The rate of NNS is approximately twice as fast as that of NS [33]. In NS, however, the ability to integrate breathing with sucking and swallowing is essential for coordinated feeding [1] and it becomes consistent by 37 weeks' gestation [34]. By increasing the intraoral space, the infant begins to suppress reflexive suckle patterns and starts to use voluntary suck patterns. In contrast to suckling, true sucking involves a raising and lowering of the body of the tongue with increased use of intrinsic musculature. Most of the infants complete the gradual transition from suckling to true suck by 9 months of age. This is considered a critical step in the development of oral skills that will permit handling of thicker textures and spoon-feeding [35].

Table 20.2 Phases of normal deglutition. (Reprinted with permission from Ref. [13], Table 15.2, p. 236)

Phase	Activities	Time
Pre-oral (voluntary)	Food introduced into oral cavity	Varies; depends on substance
Oral phase (voluntary/involuntary)	Bolus formation and passage to pharynx	Less than 1 s
Pharyngeal phase (involuntary)	Respiration ceases. Pharyngeal peristalsis. Epiglottis closes. Larynx closes, elevates, and draws forward. UES relaxes	1 s or less
Esophageal phase (involuntary)	Esophageal peristalsis. Opening of lower esophageal sphincter	8–20 s

As with sucking, chewing patterns emerge gradually during infancy. Between birth and 5 months of age, a phasic bite-release pattern develops. At this series of jaw openings and closing begins as a reflex and evolves into volitionally controlled bite. True chewing develops as the activity of the tongue, cheeks, and jaws coordinates to participate in the breakdown of solid food. The eruption of the deciduous teeth between ages of 6 and 24 months provides a chewing surface and increased sensory input to facilitate the development of chewing [35].

The concept of a "critical period" is relevant to feeding development. A critical period refers to a fairly well-delineated period of the time during which a specific stimulus must be applied to produce a particular action. After such a critical period, a particular behavior pattern can no longer be learned. Critical periods have been described for chewing and for taste. The critical period for chewing is that time following the disappearance of the tongue protrusion reflex that should occur around 6 months of age [36]. Critical periods have also been reported for introduction of tastes. Newborn infants detect sweet solutions, reject sour flavors, and are indifferent to the taste of salt [37]. Mc Farland and Tremblay emphasized that sensory experience is crucial to optimize pattern formation and brain development during the critical period for attainment of swallowing proficiency [38].

Current knowledge of the swallowing mechanism is derived mainly from radiographic studies, which have been in use since the early 1900s. Plain films of the pharynx were replaced in the 1930s by cineradiography, which was subsequently in the 1970s replaced by videofluoroscopy. Videofluoroscopy permits instant analysis of bolus transport, aspiration, and pharyngeal function [39]. Using this descriptive method, deglutition can be divided into four phases: oral preparatory phase, oral voluntary phase, pharyngeal phase, and esophageal phase (Table 20.2) [13, 40].

The oral preparatory phase occurs after food is placed into the mouth. The food is prepared for pharyngeal delivery by mastication and mixing with saliva. This is a highly coordinated activity that is rhythmic and controlled to prevent injury to the tongue. The tongue is elevated toward the palate by the combined actions of the digastric, genioglossus, geniohyoid, and mylohyoid muscles. Intrinsic tongue muscles produce both the initial depression in the dorsum that receives the food and the spreading action that distributes the food throughout the oral cavity. The buccinator muscles hold food between the teeth in dentulous infants and help to generate suction in neonates. In this phase, the soft palate is against the tongue base, secondary to contraction of the palatoglossus muscles, which allows nasal breathing to continue [7, 41].

During the oral propulsive phase, the bolus is propelled into the oropharynx. The oral phase is characterized by elevation of the tongue and a posterior sweeping or stripping action produced mainly by the action of styloglossus muscles. This propels the bolus into the pharynx and triggers the "reflex swallow." The receptors for this reflex are thought to be at the base of the anterior pillars, but there is evidence that others exist in the tongue base, epiglottis, and pyriform fossae. Sensory impulses for the reflex are conducted through the afferent limbs of cranial nerves V, IX, and X to the swallowing center. Oral transit time is less than 1 s [7, 42].

The pharyngeal phase of deglutition is the most complex and critical. The major component of the pharyngeal phase is the reflex swallow. This results from motor activity stimulated by cranial nerves IX and X. Swallowing is elicited involuntary by afferent feedback from the oral cavity and has a duration of approximately 530 ms [1]. The reflex swallow may be triggered by a voluntary oral phase component or any stimulation of the afferent receptor in and around the anterior pillar [7]. Bolus passage through the pharynx is accompanied by soft palate elevation, lingual thrust, laryngeal elevation, and descent upper esophageal sphincter (UES) relaxation and pharyngeal constrictor peristalsis. The pharyngeal phase commences as the bolus head is propelled past the tongue pillars and finishes as the bolus tail passes into the esophagus [42]. Once it begins, the pharyngeal phase is very quick, 1 s or less [7]. It is characterized biomechanically by the operation of three valves and several propulsive mechanisms. During pharyngeal swallowing, respiration is inhibited centrally [43]. The larynx closes and the palate elevates to disconnect the respiratory tract. The UES opens to expose the esophagus. At the completion of the pharyngeal phase, the airway valves (larynx, palate) open and the UES closes so that respiration can resume [42].

Pharyngeal bolus transit occurs in two phases: an initial thrust phase and a mucosal clearance phase [44]. Bolus thrust, which propels most of the bolus into the esophagus, is provided by lingual propulsion, laryngeal elevation, and gravity. The tongue has been linked to a piston, pumping the bolus though the pharynx [45]. Patients with tongue impairment cannot generate large bolus driving forces despite an intact pharyngeal constrictor mechanism [46].Laryngeal elevation creates a negative postcricoid pressure to suck the oncoming bolus toward the esophagus, and the elevated larynx holds the pharyngeal lumen open to minimize pharyngeal resistance [45].

As the bolus enters the pharynx and is stripped inferiorly by the combined effects of gravity, the negative pressure mentioned above, and the sequential contractions of the pharyngeal constrictors, the soft palate moves against the posterior pharyngeal wall to close off the nasopharyngeal port. The bolus divides around the epiglottis, combines and passes though the cricopharyngeal muscle, or UES [7].

UES refers to the high-pressure zone located in between the pharynx and the cervical esophagus. The physiological role of this sphincter is to protect against reflux of food into the airways as well as prevent entry of air into the digestive tract [47]. Posteriorly and laterally the cricopharyngeus muscle is a definitive component of the UES. Cricopharyngeus has many unique characteristics: it is tonically active, has a high degree of elasticity, does not develop maximal tension at basal length, and is composed of a mixture of slow- and fast-twitch fibers, with the former predominating. These features enable the cricopharyngeus to maintain a resting tone and yet be able to stretch open by distracting forces, such as a swallowed bolus and hyoid and laryngeal excursion. Cricopharyngeal, however, constitutes only the lower one-third of the entire high-pressure zone. The thyropharyngeus muscle accounts for the remaining upper two-thirds of the UES. The UES function is controlled by a variety of reflexes that involve afferent inputs to the motorneurons innervating the sphincter [47]. Based on functional studies, it is believed that the major motor nerve of the cricopharyngeal muscle is the pharyngoesophageal nerve. Vagal efferents probably reach the muscle by the pharyngeal plexus, using the pharyngeal branch of the vagi [48]. The superior laryngeal nerve may also contribute to motor control of the cricopharyngeus muscle [6]. Sensory information from the UES is probably provided by the glossopharyngeal nerve and the sympathetic nervous system. There is probably little or no contribution by the sympathetic nervous system to cricopharyngeal control [48].

The relaxation phase begins as the genioglossus and suspensory muscle pulls the larynx anteriorly and superiorly. The bolus is carried into the esophagus by a series of contraction waves that are a continuation of the pharyngeal stripping action [7]. Proposed functions of the UES include prevention of esophageal distention during normal breathing and protection of the airway against aspiration following an episode of acid reflux [6, 48].Qualitative abnormalities of UES have been documented in infants with reflux disease [49].

The esophageal phase occurs as the bolus is pushed through the esophagus to the stomach by esophageal peristalsis. Esophageal transit time varies from 8 to 20 s [26].

Dysphagia

Dysphagia is an impairment of swallowing involving any structures of the upper gastrointestinal tract from the lips to the lower esophageal sphincter [50]. Dysphagia in children is generally classified as either oral dysphagia (abnormal preparatory or oral phase) or pharyngeal dysphagia (abnormal pharyngeal phase).

Oral dysphagia is seen most commonly in children with neurodevelopmental disorders. Infants with oral dysphagia often have an impaired oral preparatory phase. These children typically demonstrate poor lingual and labial coordination, resulting in anterior substance loss and poor labial seal for sucking or removing food from a spoon. Other abnormal patterns include jaws thrust and tongue thrust on presentation of food. Oral dysphagia also may involve the oral phase of swallowing. Children with impaired oral phase function often have difficulty in coordinating the "suck, swallow, breathe" pattern of early oral intake, resulting in diminished endurance during oral feeds. Apraxia of oral swallow as well as reduction of oral sensation also is common. Other deficits include reduced bolus formation and transport, abnormal hold patterns, incomplete tongue to palate contact, and repetitive lingual pumping [26].

Oropharyngeal dysphagia results from either oropharyngeal swallowing dysfunction or perceived difficulty in the process of swallowing. Major categories of dysfunction are: (1) an inability or excessive delay in initiation of pharyngeal swallowing, (2) aspiration of ingestate, (3) nasopharyngeal regurgitation, and (4) residue of ingestate within the pharyngeal cavity after swallowing. Each of these categories of dysfunction can be subcategorized using fluoroscopic and/or manometric data [29].

Clinical Signs/Symptoms

Clinical signs and symptoms of sucking/swallowing disorders in infants and children are listed in Table 20.3 [13].

Table 20.3 Clinical signs and symptoms of dysfunctional sucking/swallowing. (Reprinted with permission from Ref. [13], Table 15.3, p. 239)

Clinical signs
Failure to thrive
Meal-time distress
Refusing food
Nasal regurgitation
Wet or hoarse voice
Drooling
Spitting
Vomiting
Gastroesophageal or pharyngeal reflux
Symptoms
Oral-tactile hypersensitivity
Feeling of obstruction
Odynophagia
Atypical chest pain
Respiratory manifestations
Coughing
Choking
Stridor
Change in respiration pattern after swallowing
Apnea and bradycardia (predominantly in infants)
Noisy breathing after feeding
Chronic recurrent wheezing
Chronic recurrent bronchitis, pneumonia, and atelectasis

Complications

Malnutrition

In the severely affected child with impaired swallowing, poor oral and/or pharyngeal function may lead to decreased energy intake as a consequence of prolonged feeding time and the inability to ingest adequate volumes, and malnutrition may result [6]. Malnutrition has many adverse effects. The most significant effects are on behavior and immune status. Malnutrition negatively influences immune status. This leads to recurrent infections that increase caloric requirements but decrease intake, leading to worsening nutritional status. In addition, malnutrition causes behavioral apathy, weakness, and anorexia, which can all profoundly affect feeding, and secondarily, nutritional status. Thus, although malnutrition is often a direct result of poor feeding skills, it can also have compounding, and even perpetuating, effect on feeding problems in children [26].

Sialorrea

Sialorrea, or excessive drooling, is defined as the unintentional loss of saliva and other oral contents from the mouth.

Drooling usually occurs in patients with neurologic disease complicated by abnormalities of the oral phase of deglutition. Clinical complications of drooling include soaking of clothes, offensive odors, macerated skin, and if "posterior" drooling occurs, aspiration [51].

Respiratory Complications

Respiratory complications of swallowing disorders include apnea and bradycardia, choking episodes, chronic or recurrent pneumonia, bronchitis, and atelectasis [52].

Apnea and bradycardia may result from stimulation of laryngeal chemoreceptors without evidence of aspiration or as a consequence of hypoxemia. Hypoxemia may result from the effects of direct aspiration on gas exchange, from apnea triggered by laryngeal and nasopharyngeal chemoreceptors, or in patients with compromised lung function as a result of normal decrease in minute ventilation that occurs with the suckle feeding [53–55]. Symptoms such as chronic recurrent coughing, choking, and postprandial congestion or wheezing generally indicate the occurrence of aspiration. Infants, especially premature infants, appear to be at an increased risk of respiratory disease from dysfunctional swallowing [9]. Clinical manifestations of dysfunctional sucking/swallowing in infants are primarily apnea and bradycardia during feeding, although chronic/recurrent respiratory problems (congestion, cough, and wheezing) are also seen [52]. Congested or noisy breathing during and following feeding is also a common complaint of parents in infants with dysfunctional swallowing. Dysphagia can also be an important but under-recognized cause of chronic/recurrent bronchitis, asthma, and pneumonia in infants [9].

Respiratory disease secondary to dysphagia in an older child is typically seen in a neurologically impaired host [56, 57]. Apnea and bradycardia are uncommon in older children. Bronchitis, pneumonia, atelectasis, and recurrent wheezing are more likely to be seen in this population. Feeding and swallowing evaluation should be considered in those with CNS injury affecting cranial nerve function and difficult-to-control chronic/recurrent bronchitis, wheezing, pneumonia, or asthma. Tracheobronchomalacia, a complication of chronic inflammation of the major airways, occurs commonly. Dysfunctional swallowing is also encountered in children with a tracheostomy. The tracheostomy may interfere with normal laryngeal function during swallowing and predispose to aspiration [50].

Aspiration may also occur in children with disorders of swallowing after an episode of gastroesophageal reflux; also, acid reflux may result in bronchospasm, pneumonia, or apnea [58, 59].

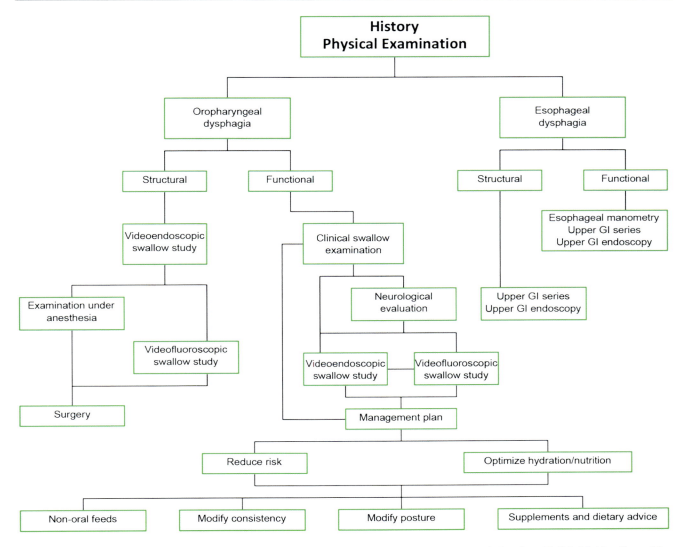

Fig. 20.1 Flowchart for the investigation and management of dysphagia in children. (Adapted by permission from BMJ Publishing Group Limited, from Ref. [50] and reprinted with permission from Ref. [13])

The most obvious sign that a person may have aspirated is the post-swallow cough, but in the swallowing-impaired children other more insidious indicators may be present. "Silent aspiration" with no clinical signs can account for over half of all cases of radiologically defined aspiration [50, 60].

Diagnosis

Feeding disorders and dysphagia in infants and children can be both physiological and behavioral in nature [61].

The evaluation of feeding and swallowing dysfunction is best performed as a multidisciplinary process with coordinated input from a variety of team members, including pediatricians, pediatric gastroenterologists, developmental pediatricians, speech–language pathologists, occupational therapist, and pediatric dietitians [62]. The goals of this

evaluation including the following: (1) ascertain whether oropharyngeal dysphagia is likely and identify the likely etiology, (2) identify structural etiologies of oropharyngeal dysfunction, (3) ascertain the functional integrity of the oropharyngeal swallow, (4) evaluate the risk of aspiration pneumonitis, and (5) determine if the pattern of dysphagia is amenable to therapy [63].

The investigation and management of swallowing disorders are summarized in Fig. 20.1 [13, 50].

History

A comprehensive history, obtained from individuals directly involved in caring for the child (e.g., parents, feeding specialist), is essential in evaluating children with swallowing disorders. The evaluation begins with a focused feeding history, including current diet, textures, and route and time of administration, modifications, and feeding position. Medical comorbidities that may affect swallowing need to be investigated.

Child's caretakers also should be questioned regarding associated symptoms such as oral aversion, weak sucking, irritable behavior, gagging and choking, and disruptions in breathing or apnea. Postural or positional change during feeding also may be reported in children with dysphagia. Odynophagia and emesis may be related with pharyngeal and/or esophageal disorders. A history of recurrent pneumonia may indicate chronic aspiration; a history of stridor in relation to feeding may indicate a glottic or subglottic abnormality contributing to feeding disorders. Determining whether these symptoms occur before, during, or after the swallow helps localize the affected phase [27, 28].

In addition, nutritional and psychological assessment should be evaluated. Many patients with swallowing disorders have concurrent illness that may increase metabolic needs. Psychological assessments help to identify behavioral and parental factors that may be contributing to a feeding disorder. Psychosomatic causes of dysphagia should be considered in adolescents with dysphagia [7, 64, 65].

Physical and Clinical Evaluation

In dysphagic patients, physical examination aims to: (1) characterize the underlying systemic underlying systemic or metabolic disease when present; (2) localize the neuroanatomical level and severity of a causative neurological lesion when present; and (3) detect adverse sequelae such as aspiration pneumonia or nutritional deficiency [29].

There are four key questions that physicians and nurses in primary care can ask parents when an infant or young child presents at the office or clinic with parental concerns related to feeding [66].

The answers help determine whether a comprehensive clinical feeding and swallowing assessment is needed, even though the answers do not necessarily define the problem:

How long do mealtimes typically take? If more than about 30 min on any regular basis, there is a problem. Prolonged feeding times are major red flags pointing to the need for further investigation:

- Are mealtimes stressful? Regardless of descriptions of factors that underlie the stress, further investigation is needed. It is very common for parents to state that they "just dread mealtimes."
- Does the child show any signs of respiratory stress? Signs may include rapid breathing, gurgly voice quality, nasal congestion that increases as the meal progresses, and panting by an infant with nipple feeding. Recent upper

respiratory illness may be a sign of aspiration with oral feeds, although there may be other causes.

- Has the child *not* gained weight in the past 2–3 months? Steady appropriate weight gain is particularly important in the first 2 years of life for brain development as well as overall growth. A lack of weight gain in a young child is like a weight loss in an older child or adult.

The physical examination views the whole child and specifically focuses on the upper aerodigestive tract, beginning with an examination for structural and functional abnormalities. Oral cavity anatomic abnormalities, such as ankyloglossia, cleft lip or palate, or macroglossia, need to be excluded [7]. The palatal gag is perhaps the most assessed reflex and should be evaluated [51]. A hyperactive gag can result in significant feeding difficulties, and in the past an absent gag reflex was viewed as an indication to stop oral feeding [9, 56].

It is critical that observation of the feeding process be included [62]. This part of the examination is best performed in conjunction with a feeding and swallowing specialist, such as a speech–language pathologist or an occupational therapist. This examination includes assessments of posture, positioning, patient motivation, oral function, efficiency of oral intake, and clinical signs of safety. During the feeding trial, the presence of abnormal movements such as jaw thrust, tongue thrust, tonic bite reflex, and jaw clenching is noted. A variety of therapeutic positions, techniques, and adaptive feeding utensils may be used [6, 27].

A variety of assessment scales may be used to detail and quantitate results of the swallowing evaluation. However, all assessments are based on similar observation of feeding structure and function [67].

Usually, a careful developmental, medical, and feeding history provides clues to the diagnosis that guide the selection of further diagnostic tests. Only after all reasonable physical causes have been ruled out should a feeding or swallowing disorder be attributed to a purely behavioral cause [7].

Diagnostic Tests

Radiographic Assessment The videofluoroscopy represents the gold standard method for evaluation of children with swallowing disorders. A videofluoroscopic swallow study is ideally performed by a consultant radiologist and specialist and speech and language therapist [68]. A series of swallows of varied volumes and consistencies of contrast material are imaged in a lateral projection, framed to include the oropharynx, palate, proximal esophagus, and proximal airway. Studies are recorded on videotape to permit instant replay, in slow motion if necessary, and examination of both the presence and mechanism of swallowing dysfunction.

As such, the videofluoroscopic study provides evidence of all four categories of oropharyngeal swallowing disorders: (1) inability or excessive delay in initiation of pharyngeal swallowing, (2) aspiration of ingestate, (3) nasopharyngeal regurgitation, and (4) residue of ingestate within the pharyngeal cavity after swallowing. Furthermore, the procedure allows for testing of the efficacy of compensatory dietary modifications, postures, swallowing maneuvers, and facilitatory techniques in correction or observed dysfunction. Generally, the videofluoroscopic evaluation is completed by esophagography to evaluate the esophageal phase of deglutition (Fig. 20.2) [29]. A nasogastric tube does not alter the findings of videofluoroscopic swallowing study and does not increase the risk of aspiration; however, it might increase the incidence of respiratory compromise when aspiration is present [69].

Ultrasonography Ultrasound imaging has been used to a limited extent in the assessment of oral phase dysphagia. Using a transducer positioned in the submental region, ultrasonography allows observation of the motion of structures in the oral cavity such as the tongue and floor of the mouth during feeding and deglutition, but lacks sensitivity in visualizing pharyngeal motion and determining whether aspiration has occurred. Ultrasonography represents the only method of imaging that can study infants during breastfeeding and may be particularly useful in distinguishing an infant's inability to latch on from maternal factors contributing to feeding difficulties [14].Unfortunately, laryngeal

penetration and aspiration are not easily detected because of the shadows cast by the laryngeal structures [9, 34, 70].

Pharyngeal Manometry Intraluminal manometry, performed using a transnasally positioned manometric assembly, can quantify the strength of pharyngeal contraction, the completeness of UES relaxation, and relative time of these two events. Most studies indicate that the manometry of the UES and pharynx provides useful information primarily in patients that have symptoms of oropharyngeal dysfunction. The coordination of muscle activity at various levels can be obtained by simultaneous recording of pressure in the pharynx, at the level of cricopharyngeus, and in the esophagus. Anatomic references are not available with this technique [49, 71].Recently, manometry equipment has evolved to allow more precise and detailed evaluation of esophageal function with high-resolution manometry and esophageal pressure topography plotting [72] (Fig. 20.3).

Fiberoptic Endoscopic Examination Pediatric fiberoptic endoscopic examination (FEES) is a relatively new diagnostic method to add to and complement the current armamentarium of techniques for evaluating dysphagia and/or aspiration. FEES is performed by passing a flexible laryngoscope into the oropharynx after anesthetizing the nares and nasopharynx [73]. It provides the ability to diagnose many of the laryngeal disorders that may affect the child, while at the same time evaluating the swallowing mechanism itself. The procedure involves five components: assessment of anatomy as it affects swallowing, evaluation of movement and sensation of critical structures, assessment of secretion management, direct assessment of swallowing function for food and liquid, and patients' response to therapeutic maneuvers. In experienced hands, this test can be performed in children with minimal discomfort [74, 75].

Scintigraphy Scintigraphy is a radionuclide evaluation using Technetium-99m-labeled sulfur colloid mixed in the infant's formula. It has been proposed as an alternative and perhaps more sensitive way of quantifying aspiration, transit times, gastroesophageal reflux, and pharyngeal residue. Based on a case report, the radionuclide salivagram has also been used to document aspiration of saliva. The major limitations of this technique are the poor definition of the anatomy and the poor sensitivity for detecting aspiration during swallowing in known aspirators. At the present, the use of this technique in pediatric age is limited [75, 76].

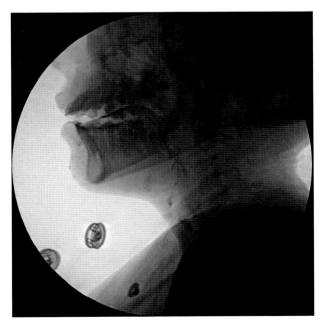

Fig. 20.2 Lateral fluoroscopic projection of a child showing contrast material in the valleculas, pyriform sinuses, laryngeal vestibule, and esophagus

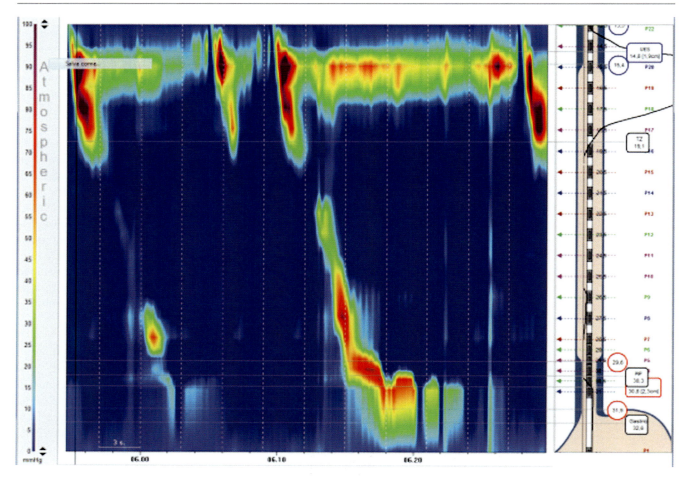

Fig. 20.3 Esophageal pressure topography plotting: complete peristaltic chain studied with a 21-lm catheter. The three *inter-segmental* troughs are indicated in the figure, and the pressure amplitudes represented by the isobaric contour regions are shown in the *color legend* (in mmHg above gastric baseline pressure; pressures below the first isobaric contour are shown in *blue*). *SW* swallow

Treatment Options

Optimal management strategies are critical for infants and children with feeding and swallowing problems. The management of swallowing dysfunction involves a team approach. Individuals involved in addition to the medical team include a swallowing expert (speech–language pathologist or occupational therapist), a nutritionist, and the family. Since swallowing abnormalities arise from a diverse group of underlying disorders, management techniques must be individualized. This heterogeneity is also reflected in the fact that patients have different potentials to recovery [6].

Although total oral feeding may not be a realistic goal, it is the universal hope of caregivers. Professionals are obligated to point out prerequisites for oral feeding and to discuss the probability that an in individual child may reach the goal. These management decisions are typically made on the basis of clinical observations and assessments.

In addition, important information is obtained through an instrumental assessment by videofluoroscopic swallows study. A methodical videofluoroscopic swallowing study: (1) defines the anatomy of the oropharynx; (2) detects dysfunction as evident by aspiration, poor clearance, or poor control of the bolus; (3) determines the mechanism responsible for the dysfunction; and (4) examines the short-term effects of the therapeutic strategies designed to eliminate or compensate for that dysfunction [77]. Management decisions may incorporate nutritive recommendations, medical and surgical decisions, position guidelines, oral-motor/swallow practice, and behavioral intervention [78].

The clinical and instrumental evaluation of children with sucking and swallowing disorders should allow for the recognition of treatable anatomic or inflammatory lesions.

A child may refuse to eat even if his anatomic abnormality has been corrected because of learned aversion to feeding. Behavior therapy often can overcome this type of conditioned food refusal [7, 65].

Table 20.4 Swallowing strategies for pediatric dysphagia. (Reprinted with permission from Ref. [13], Table 15.4, p. 244)

Behavioral training	
Dietary modification	Thickened liquids
	Thin liquids
Proper intrabolus placement	Modify feeding utensils and bolus presentation
Swallowing exercises	Supraglottic swallow
	Supersupraglottic swallow
	Effortful swallow
	Mendelsohn maneuver
Modification in body tone posture seating and positioning	Head tilt
	Chin tuck
	Head rotation
	Lying on side, elevation
Suckle-feeding-valved feeding bottle	–
Cricopharyngeal myotomy	–
Facilitatory techniques	Biofeedback
	Thermal stimulation
	Gustatory stimulation
Provide alternate means of enteral nutrition	Nasogastric feeding
	Gastrostomy tube (surgical or endoscopic)

Various therapeutic approaches may improve the efficiency and safety of feeding. Management techniques involve devising compensatory strategies to minimize swallowing-related complications [79].

These include changing the textures of foods; pacing of feeding; changing the bottle or utensils; and changing the alignment of the head, neck, and body with feeding (Table 20.4) [13, 72].

Frequently, children with severe anatomic disorders but normal neurological function develop their own adaptive strategies to allow for safe oral feeding. Unfortunately, many children with feeding disorders have non-correctable neurologic or anatomic abnormalities that make oral feeding difficult or unsafe. Some patients cannot obtain adequate nutrition by mouth because of a risk for aspiration. Thus, supplying a portion of patient's nutrition by nasogastric or gastrostomy feeding may be beneficial [7]. For those children who have been intubated, management includes teaching techniques that will facilitate transitioning from non-oral to oral feeding. However, there is little evidence that non-oral feeding reduces or eliminates the risk of aspiration [80–82].

The strongest evidence-based recommendation that can be made pertains to diet modification. Furthermore, the literature provides reasonable evidence of the plausibility of swallowing therapy but minimal evidence of efficacy. Nonetheless, although no hard evidence supports its efficacy, the available data are inconclusive and swallowing therapy has not been proven ineffective. Thus, the current weight of opinion, combined with the convincing demonstration of biological plausibility for specific techniques and the consistency of low-grade evidence, is the basis to recommend that swallowing therapy should be used. Large-scale randomized, controlled trials are needed to clarify the current recommendations [29].

Prognosis

Prognosis depends on underlying conditions that predispose to impaired sucking and swallowing. However, the early recognition of feeding problems, diagnosis of underlying disorders, and appropriate intervention improve outcomes for the child and the family.

References

1. da Costa SP, van den Engel-Hoek L, Bos AF. Sucking and swallowing in infants and diagnostic tools. J Perinatol. 2008;28:247–57.
2. Delaney AL, Arvedson JC. Development of swallowing and feeding: prenatal through first year of life. Dev Disabil Res Rev. 2008;14:105–17.
3. Presse J, Kikano G. An overview of pediatric dysphagia. Cin Pediatr. 2009;48:247–51.
4. Arvedson J, Clark H, Lazarus C, Schooling T, Frymark T. Evidence-based systematic review: effect of oral motor interventions on feeding and swallowing in preterm infants. Am J Speech Lang Pathol. 2010;19:321–40.
5. Logemann JA. Evaluation and treatment of swallowing disorders. 2nd ed. Austin: Pro-Ed; 1998.
6. Tuchman DN. Disorders of deglutition. In: Walker WA, Durie PR, Walker-Smith JA, Watkins JB, editors. Pediatric gastrointestinal disease. 3rd ed. Hamilton: BC Decker; 2000. p. 277–88.
7. Rudolph CD, Link DT. Feeding disorders in infants and children. Pediatr Clin North Am. 2002;49(1):97–112.
8. Del Giudice E, Staiano A, Capano G, Romano A, Florimonte L, Miele E, Ciarla C, Campanozzi A, Crisanti AF. Gastrointestinal manifestations in children with cerebral palsy. Brain Dev. 1999;21(5):307–11.
9. Slattery J, Morgan A, Douglas J. Early sucking and swallowing as predictors of neurodevelopmental outcome in children with neonatal brain injury: a systematic review. Dev Med Child Neur. 2012;54:796–806.
10. Miller CK. Updates on paediatric feeding and swallowing. Curr Opin Otolaryngol Head Neck Surg. 2009;17:194–9.
11. Loughlin GM, Lefton-Greif MA. Dysfunctional swallowing and respiratory disease in children. Adv Pediatr. 1994;41:135–62.
12. Cohen SR. Difficulty with swallowing. In: Bluestone CD, Stool SE, Arjona SK, editors. Pediatric otolaryngology. Philadelphia: WB Saunders; 1983. p. 903–11.
13. Miele E, Staiano A. Disorders of sucking and swallowing. In: Guandalini S, editor. Textbook of pediatric gastroenterology and nutrition. London: Taylor & Francis; 2004. p. 233–46.
14. Wolff Ph. The serial organization of sucking in the young infant. Pediatrics 1968;42:943–56.
15. Mizuno K, Ueda A. The maturation and coordination of sucking, swallowing, and respiration in preterm infants. J Pediatr. 2003;142(1):36–40.
16. Mathew OP. Science of bottle-feeding. J Pediatr. 1991;119:511–9.

17. Derkay CS, Schecter GL. Anatomy and physiology of pediatric swallowing disorders. Otolaryngol Clin North Am. 1998;31:397–404.

18. Mistry S, Hamdy S. Neural control of feeding and swallowing. Phys Med Rehabil Clin N Am. 2008;19:709–28.

19. Barlow SM, Lund JP, Estep M, Kolta A. Central pattern generators for speech and orofacial activity. In: Brudzynski SM, editor. Handbook of mammalian vocalization. Oxford: Elsevier; 2009. p. 1–3317.

20. Lund JP, Kolta A. Generation of the central masticatory patternand its modification by sensory feedback. Dysphagia. 2006;21(3):167–74.

21. Barlow SM. Central pattern generation involved in oral and respiratory control for feeding in the term infant. Curr Opin Otolaryngol Head Neck Surg. 2009;17(3):187–93.

22. Miller AJ. Deglutition. Physiol Rev. 1982;62:129–84.

23. Morrell RM. The neurology of swallowing. In: Groher ME, editor. Dysphagia and management. Boston: Butterwroths; 1984. p. 3.

24. Bosma JF. Postnatal ontogeny of performances of the pharynx, larynx, and mouth. Am Rev Respir Dis. 1985;131(5):S10–5.

25. Tuchman DN. Dysfunctional swallowing in the pediatric patient: clinical considerations. Dysphagia. 1988;2(4):203–8.

26. Stevenson RD, Allaire JH. The development of normal feeding and swallowing. Pediatr Clin North Am. 1991 Dec;38(6):1439–53.

27. Gewolb IH, Vice FL, Schweitzer-Kenney EL, Taciak VL, Bosma JF. Development patterns of rhythmic suck and swallow in preterm infants. Dev Med Child Neurol. 2001;43:22–7.

28. Moore KL. The developing human: clinically oriented embryology. 4th ed. Philadelphia: WB Saunders; 1988.

29. Morris SE, Klein MD. Pre-feeding skills: a comprehensive resource for feeding development. Tucsun: Therapy Skill Builders; 1997.

30. Lau C, Schanler RJ. Oral feeding in premature infants: advantage of a self-paced milk flow. Acta Pediatr. 2000;89(4):453–9.

31. Milla PJ. Feeding, tasting, and sucking. In: Walker-Smith WA, Watkins JB, editors. Pediatric gastrointestinal disease. Philadelphia: BC Decker; 1991. p. 217–23.

32. Lemons PK, Lemons JA. Transition to breast/bottle feedings: the premature infant. J Am Coll Nutr. 2001;2:126–35.

33. Palmer MM, Crawley K, Blanco I. The neonatal oral-motor assessment scale: a reliability study. J Perinatol. 1993;13(1):28–35.

34. Bu'Lock F, Woolridge MW, Baum JD. Development of co-ordination of sucking, swallowing and breathing: ultrasound study of term and preterm infants. Dev Med Child Neurol. 1990;32(8):669–78.

35. Darrow DH, Harley CM. Evaluation of swallowing disorders in children. Otolaryngol Clin North Am. 1998 Jun;31(3):405–18.

36. Illingworth RS, Lister J. The critical or sensitive period, with special reference to certain feeding problems in infants and children. J Pediatr. 1964;5:839–48.

37. Mennella JA, Beauchamp GK. Development and bad taste. Pediatr Asthma Allergy Immunol. 1998;12:161–4.

38. Mc Farland DH, Tremblay P. Clinical implications of cross-system interactions. Semin Speech Lang. 2006;27(4):300–9.

39. Cook IJ, Kahrilas PJ. AGA technical review on management of oropharyngeal dysphagia. Gastroenterology. 1999;116(2):455–78.

40. Logemann JA. Evaluation and treatment of swallowing disorders. San Diego: College Hill; 1983.

41. Dodds WJ, Stewart ET, Logemann JA. Physiology and radiology of the normal oral and pharyngeal phases of swallowing. AJR Am J Roentgenol. 1990;154(5):953–63.

42. Mendelsohn M. New concepts in dysphagia management. J Otolaryngol. 1993;22 Suppl 1:1–24.

43. Doty R, Bosma JF. An electromyography analysis of reflex deglutition. J Neurophysiol. 1956;19:44–60.

44. McConnel FMS. Analisys of pressure generation and bolus transit during pharyngeal swallowing. Laryngoscope. 1988;98:71–8.

45. McConnel FM, Cerenko D, Mendelsohn MS. Dysphagia after total laryngectomy. Otolaryngol Clin North Am. 1988;21(4):721–6.

46. Curtis DJ, Cruess DF, Dachman AH. Normal erect swallowing. Normal function and incidence of variations. Invest Radiol. 1985;20(7):717–26.

47. Sivarao DV, Goyal RK. Functional anatomy and physiology of the upper esophageal sphincter. Am J Med. 2000;108 (Suppl 4a):27S–37.

48. Palmer ED. Disorders of the cricopharyngeus muscle: a review. Gastroenterology. 1976;71(3):510–9.

49. Staiano A, Cucchiara S, De Vizia B, Andreotti MR, Auricchio S. Disorders of upper esophageal sphincter motility in children. J Pediatr Gastroenterol Nutr. 1987;6(6):892–8.

50. Leslie P, Carding PN, Wilson JA. Investigation and management of chronic dysphagia. Br Med J. 2003;326(7386):433–6.

51. Myer CM. Sialorrea. Pediatr Clin of North Am. 1989;36:1495–500.

52. Loughlin GM. Respiratory consequences of dysfunctional swallowing and aspiration. Dysphagia. 1989;3(3):126–310.

53. Durand M, Leahy FN, MacCallum M, Cates DB, Rigatto H, Chernick V. Effect of feeding on the chemical control of breathing in the newborn infant. Pediatr Res. 1981;15(12):1509–12.

54. Thach BT. Maturation and transformation of reflexes that protect the laryngeal airway from liquid aspiration from fetal to adult life. Am J Med. 2001;111 (Suppl 8A):69S–77.

55. Hoekstra RE, Perkett EA, Dugan M, Knox GE. Follow-up of the very low birth weight infant (less than 1251 grams). Minn Med. 1983;66(10):611–3.

56. Tuchman DN. Cough, choke, spitter: the evaluation of the child with dysfunctional swallowing. Dysphagia. 1989;3(3):111–6.

57. Rogers BT, Arvedson J, Msall M, Demerath RR. Hypoxemia during oral feeding of children with severe cerebral palsy. Dev Med Child Neurol. 1993;35(1):3–10.

58. Berquist WE, Ament ME. Upper GI function in sleeping infants. Am Rev Respir Dis. 1985;131(5):S26–9.

59. Boyle JT, Tuchman DN, Altschuler SM, Nixon TE, Pack AI, Cohen S. Mechanisms for the association of gastroesophageal reflux and bronchospasm. Am Rev Respir Dis. 1985;131(5):S16–20.

60. Smith CH, Logemann JA, Colangelo LA, Rademaker AW, Pauloski BR. Incidence and patient characteristics associated with silent aspiration in the acute care setting. Dysphagia. 1999 Winter;14(1):1–7.

61. Sonies BC. Swallowing disorders and rehabilitation techniques. J Pediatr Gastroenterol Nutr. 1997;25 (Suppl 1):S32–3.

62. Kramer SS, Eicher PM. The evaluation of pediatric feeding abnormalities. Dysphagia. 1993;8(3):215–24.

63. American Gastroenterological Association. American gastroenterological association medical position statement on management of oropharyngeal dysphagia. Gastroenterology. 1999;116:452–4.

64. Kovar AJ. Nutrition assessment and management in pediatric dysphagia. Semin Speech Lang. 1997 Feb;18(1):39–49.

65. Babbitt RL, Hoch TA, Coe DA, Cataldo MF, Kelly KJ, Stackhouse C, Perman JA. Behavioral assessment and treatment of pediatric feeding disorders. J Dev Behav Pediatr. 1994 Aug;15(4):278–91.

66. Arvedson JC. Swallowing and feeding in infants and young children. GI Motility Online. 2006. doi:10.1038.

67. Gisel EG, Alphonce E, Ramsay M. Assessment of ingestive and oral praxis skills: children with cerebral palsy vs. controls. Dysphagia. 2000 Fall;15(4):236–44.

68. Ekberg O, Olsson R, Bulow M. Radiologic evaluation of dysphagia. Abdom Imaging. 1999;24(5):444.

69. Mutaz Alnassar, Kamaldine Oudjhane, Jorge Davila. Nasogastric tubes and videofluoroscopic swallowing studies in children. Pediatr Radiol. 2011;41:317–21.

70. Rudolph CD. Feeding disorders in infants and children. Pediatrics. 1994;125(6 Pt 2):S116–24.

71. Hila A, Castell JA, Castell DO. Pharyngeal and upper esophageal sphincter manometry in the evaluation of dysphagia. J Clin Gastroenterol. 2001;33(5):355–61.

72. Goldani HA, Staiano A, Borrelli O, Thapar N, Lindley KJ. Pediatric esophageal high-resolution manometry: utility of a standardized protocol and size-adjusted pressure topography parameters. Am J Gastroenterol. 2010;105(2):460–7.

73. Broniatowski M, Sonies BC, Rubin JS, Bradshaw CR, Spiegel JR, Bastian RW, Kelly JH. Current evaluation and treatment of patients with swallowing disorders. Otolaryngol Head Neck Surg. 1999;120(4):464–73.

74. Langmore SE, Schatz K, Olsen N. Fiberoptic endoscopic examination of swallowing safety: a new procedure. Dysphagia. 1988;2(4):216–9.

75. Hamlet SL, Mutz J, Patterson, R., Jones L. Pharyngeal transit time: assessment with videofluoroscopic and scintigraphic techniques. Dysphagia 1989;4:4–7.

76. Silver KH, Nostrand DV. Scintigraphic detection of salivary aspiration: description of a new diagnostic technique and case reports. Dysphagia. 1992;7:45–9.

77. Logemann JA. Role of the modified barium swallow in management of patients with dysphagia. Otolaryngol Head Neck Surg. 1997;116:335–8.

78. Arvedson JC. Management of pediatrics dysphagia. Otolaryngol Clin North Am. 1998;31:453–76.

79. Helfrich-Miller KR, Rector KL, Straka JA. Dysphagia: its treatment in the profoundly retarded patient with cerebral palsy. Arch Phys Rehabil. 1986;67:520–5.

80. Croghan JE, Burke EM, Caplan S, Denman S. Pilot study of 12-month outcomes of nursing home patients with aspiration on videofluoroscopy. Dysphagia. 1994 Summer;9(3):141–6.

81. Groher ME. Bolus management and aspiration pneumonia in patient with pseudobulbar dysphagia. Dysphagia. 1987;1:215–6.

82. Shaker R, Easterling C, Kern M, Nitschke T, Massey B, Daniels S, Grande B, Kazandjian M, Dikeman K. Rehabilitation of swallowing by exercise in tube-fed patients with pharyngeal dysphagia secondary to abnormal UES opening. Gastroenterology. 2002;122(5):1314–21.

Additional Educational Resources:

Resource center: The Dysphagia Research Society is organized exclusively for charitable, educational and scientific purposes (http://www.dysphagiaresearch.org/) -this multidisciplinary website has a wealth of information on dysphagia, references to texts, archives, and links to other related sites; user friendly and very comprehensive.

Defecation Disorders in Children: Constipation and Functional Fecal Incontinence

Shaman Rajindrajith, Niranga Manjuri Devanarayana and Marc A. Benninga

Part 1: Constipation

Definition

Constipation in children has been defined in many ways. Some of these include Iowa criteria, the Paris Consensus on Childhood Constipation Terminology (PACCT) criteria, Rome II criteria, and Rome III criteria [1–4]. Rome III criteria for defecation disorders are the currently accepted definitions and are shown in Table 21.1. What these criteria have in common is the usage of multiple features that can be used together in the clinical setting to define constipation. In Rome III definition, younger children (<4 years) should fulfill two criteria for at least 1 month, whereas older children need to have symptoms over a period of 2 months.

Using a single clinical feature, such as low bowel frequency, to define constipation can be misleading. It has been shown that around 0.4–20% of otherwise healthy children have at least one feature of Rome III criteria [5, 6]. Furthermore, bowel frequency is known to be variable in different regions of the world possibly depending on diet, genetics, and environmental factors [5, 7]. Therefore, it is imperative that the clinician's perspective is more flexible and he or she

understands the changes in bowel frequency in the context of local and patient variables.

Several studies have assessed the diagnostic capability of Rome III criteria to identify functional constipation in children. A school-based study including 10–16-year-olds showed Rome III criteria are more inclusive in diagnosing constipation [8]. Another study based on outpatients referred to a tertiary care hospital noted that 87% of children had constipation according to Rome III criteria, whereas only 43% children were classified as having defecation disorders using Rome II criteria [9]. Although both these studies indicate the superiority of Rome III criteria in the diagnostic process, the required duration of 2 months appears to be a little too long and may result in delayed treatment, especially in older children.

Magnitude of the Problem

Constipation is a global health problem. Studies from Europe showed a prevalence range from 0.7 to 17.6% among children [9–14]. In the USA, 10% of 5–8-years-olds are having constipation [6].

Two studies from Brazil pointed out alarmingly higher rates of over 20% occurrence of constipation in a 1–10-year-old population [14, 15]. More disturbing data are emerging from Asia. The prevalence of constipation in Taiwan was 32.2% in children in elementary schools and in Hong Kong 12–28%, indicating constipation is becoming a bigger problem in newly developing economies from Asia [16–18]. Similarly, developing nations in Asia like Sri Lanka also show 15% of their school children are suffering from chronic constipation [19]. These data underscore the magnitude of the disease burden and are shifting its epicenter of prevalence from the West to the East. The differences in prevalence need to be interpreted with some caution as the wider variations seen may partly be due to differences in definitions used, differences in age groups included, and heterogeneity of survey methods.

S. Rajindrajith (✉)
Department of Pediatrics, Faculty of Medicine, University of Kelaniya, Talagolla Road, Ragama 11010, Sri Lanka
e-mail: shamanrajindrajith4@gmail.com

University Pediatric Unit, Teaching Hospital, Ragama, Sri Lanka

N. M. Devanarayana
Department of Physiology, Faculty of Medicine, University of Kelaniya, Thalagolla Road, Ragama 11010, Sri Lanka
e-mail: niranga1230@lycos.com

M. A. Benninga
Department of Pediatric Gastroenterology and Nutrition, Emma Children's Hospital, Academic Medical Centre, Amsterdam, The Netherlands
e-mail: m.a.benninga@amc.nl

© Springer International Publishing Switzerland 2016
S. Guandalini et al. (eds.), *Textbook of Pediatric Gastroenterology, Hepatology and Nutrition*,
DOI 10.1007/978-3-319-17169-2_21

Table 21.1 Rome III definition of functional constipation and functional nonretentive fecal incontinence

Functional constipation
Diagnostic criteria[a] must include two or more of the following in a child with a developmental age of at least 4 years with insufficient criteria for diagnosis of IBS:
Two or fewer defecations in the toilet per week
At least one episode of fecal incontinence per week
History of retentive posturing or excessive volitional stool retention
History of painful or hard bowel movements
Presence of a large fecal mass in the rectum
History of large diameter stools which may obstruct the toilet
Functional nonretentive fecal incontinence
Diagnostic criteria[b] must include *all* of the following in a child with a developmental age at least 4 years:
Defecation into places inappropriate to the social context at least once per month
No evidence of an inflammatory, anatomic, metabolic, or neoplastic process that explains the subject's symptoms
No evidence of fecal retention

[a] Criteria fulfilled at least once per week for at least 2 months prior to diagnosis
[b] Criteria fulfilled for at least 2 months prior to diagnosis
IBS irritable bowel syndrome

Risk Factors

Table 21.2 shows the known and identified risk factors for chronic constipation in children. In contrast to adult studies which show constipation to be more prevalent among females, several epidemiological studies among children have failed to identify gender as a risk factor to develop constipation [13, 20, 21]. However, one study from Sri Lanka has shown that the prevalence is significantly higher among boys and children living in low socioeconomic status [19].

Table 21.2 Risk factors for chronic constipation

Category	Risk factor
Patient related	Male sex
	Poor sleep
	Obesity
Dietary	Low fiber
	Consumption of junk food
	Not having regular meals with parents
	Cow's milk protein allergy
Psychological	Home-related stresses
	School-related stresses
	Adverse life event including abuse
	Subjected to bullying
	Anxiety
	Depression
	Autistic spectrum disorders
Social	Living in war-affected areas
	Living in urban areas
	Lower social class
	Hostile and aggressive family environment

Psychological stress is another risk factor that predisposes children to develop constipation. Children living in homes and studying in schools which create stress are more prone to develop chronic constipation [22]. In addition, disrupted societies by civil unrest are also an important predisposing factor [23]. A study from Hong Kong has shown that children not having regular meals with their parents and deprivation of sleep as independent risk factors to develop severe constipation [17]. Moreover, low consumption of fiber [11, 17, 18], cow milk protein (CMP) hypersensitivity [21, 24], and consumption of fast foods too often [17] are associated with constipation. Lastly, obesity has also been identified as an independent risk factor [25, 26]. In a recent study, our group also noted that children who faced adverse life events such as physical, emotional, and sexual abuse have higher predilection to develop constipation. These events also predispose them to develop more somatic symptoms and lead to a poor quality of life [27].

Quality of Life

Children with constipation have poor health-related quality-of-life (HRQoL) scores in all domains, namely social, school, physical, and emotional functioning. The scores they obtained are even lower than children suffering from organic diseases such as gastroesophageal reflux and inflammatory bowel disease [28]. Children with slow transit constipation also have been shown to have poor HRQoL [29]. A school-based study from Sri Lanka also confirms these findings and showed that constipation-associated fecal incontinence (FI) further reduces HRQoL [30].

Extraintestinal Symptoms and Psychological Problems

Children with constipation suffer from an array of somatic symptoms. In one of the studies, we found that children with constipation had a multitude of somatic symptoms and high somatization scores [30]. Constipation is also associated with a number of behavioral abnormalities such as autism, attention-deficit hyperactivity disorder, and anxiety [31–33]. Abnormal personality traits were also noted in children suffering from constipation [34]. In addition, children with autistic spectrum disorders are known to have very early onset disease [32].

Health-Care Burden

Constipation is a leading cause for medical consultation in children. Documented medical visits for constipation were higher than most other gastrointestinal diseases in children under 5 years [35]. The incidence of medical presentation for children with constipation is substantially higher than other chronic episodic conditions such as asthma (seven times) and migraine headaches (three times) [36]. The mean outpatient costs and mean annual number of emergency room visits are higher in children with constipation compared to controls [36]. Furthermore, employed parents with a child with constipation have a higher number of working day losses than controls. More importantly, children with constipation are noted to have higher number of days of school absenteeism [37]. In addition, children with constipation show poor quality of school work [30, 38]. Implications of these findings on education of children are much larger than expected. Poor education invariably leads to poor earning capacity and ignorance as an adult. Therefore, they become an added burden to society at large.

Pathophysiology

Understanding of the pathophysiological mechanisms of chronic constipation in infants and children is a considerable challenge and remains in its early stages. However, available studies on physiology of the colon and rectum and studies on animal models have shed some light upon the subject.

Infants and Young Children

Stool withholding plays a major role in the development of constipation in infancy and early childhood. Passing a hard stool leading to pain, strict early toilet training, stubbornness, and concentration on other activities which are more exciting than going to the toilet are possible factors for stool withholding. When the urge to pass stools comes, the withholding child tightens gluteal muscles and stands on tip toe. During this process, the rectum dilates, fecal matter is accommodated, and desire to pass stools disappears. A large mass of feces is formed in the rectum during this process leading to a cascade of physiological changes described below.

Children and Adolescents

Several studies have shown that children with constipation have defective intraluminal transport involving different segments of the colon such as proximal delay, hind gut delay, and rectosigmoid hold up [39–41]. Furthermore, it has been shown that children with chronic constipation have significantly delayed total colonic transit times of over 100 h [42]. Although slow transit constipation in adults is almost exclusively found in females [43], in children and adolescents, prevalence is more or less equal among the sexes [44].

Colonic manometry has shown several abnormalities in constipation. They include reduced frequency of high-amplitude propagative contractions and disordered patterning of spatiotemporal colonic propagative responses [45]. Like slow transit constipation, all these factors may contribute to poor propulsion of fecal masses along the colonic lumen generating symptoms of constipation.

Rectal sensitivity to oncoming fecal matter and dilatation is a crucial point in normal rectal function. There is a subset of children with constipation who demonstrate poor rectal sensation [46]. Furthermore, several studies in children have shown increased rectal compliance [47, 48] and a megarectum [49]. These factors are closely interrelated and lead to attenuation of rectal sensation and lack of desire to evacuate, leading to low bowel frequency.

In addition, contraction, rather than relaxation of the pelvic floor muscles with increasing rectal pressure (dyssynergic defecation), also prevents evacuation of stools. The balloon expulsion test has been used to measure rectal motor dysfunction in children with an array of other combined measurements. Chitkara et al. demonstrated that 31 % of children with functional constipation and 53 % of children with functional fecal retention (using Rome II criteria) had an abnormal balloon expulsion test, and 40 % had high resting anal pressure [50].

In addition to these local factors, dysfunction of the brain–gut axis also contributes to the development and propagation of symptoms. Stress-induced abnormalities in the colonic motor activity may further aggravate the motor and sensory abnormalities and worsen stool retention. Functional magnetic resonance imaging studies have described a multitude of abnormalities in adults with functional gastrointestinal disorders (FGD) including constipation as possible mechanisms for this phenomenon [51].

Final Pathway for Both Age Groups

Pathophysiological mechanisms described for both age groups finally lead to retention of stools in the rectum and colon. Since colonic and rectal mucosa are designed to absorb water, stool becomes dry and hard. Molecular abnormalities in the rectal mucosa of children with constipation, such as abnormalities in non-calcium-mediated chloride channels, lead to abnormally low chloride secretion that may further contribute to the development of hard stools [52]. The mechanical dilatation of the rectum inhibits motor function of the proximal and distal hemi-colon through reflex mechanisms [53, 54].

In addition, animal models have shown that accumulation of feces elongates the colon. This in turn leads to the release of nitric oxide by activating mechano-sensory and myenteric descending neuronal nitric oxide synthase. Nitric oxide inhibits action potential firing in other myenteric sensory neurons driving peristaltic nerve circuits, inhibiting colonic contractile activity (occult reflex), thereby seriously hampering evacuation [55, 56]. It has been shown that children with increased rectal wall compliance have prolonged colonic transit time which further strengthens the possibility of occult reflex [47]. Interactions of these inextricably linked mechanisms in a complex manner, rather than in isolation, lead to generation and propagation of symptoms in children with constipation.

Clinical Features

Infants and Young Children

The most common reason for constipation in infants and toddlers is an acquired behavior component after experiencing painful bowel movements [57]. When the desire to pass a stool occurs, they tend to cry and withhold stools by tightening their gluteal muscles and pelvic floor. This is evident in infants as they tighten the legs and in young children as they stand on tip toe and tighten their muscles till the desire for passing a stool goes off. These children also have low stool frequency, passing large-diameter, rock-hard, and sometimes bloody stools infrequently and occasional leaking of semisolid to liquid stools into underwear. In addition, poor appetite and abdominal distension are also notable features.

Older Children and Adolescents

This group tends to present with classic symptoms of constipation. The presenting complaint very often is reduced stool frequency. The other features include passing hard stools, pain while passing stools, frequent episodes of FI, and infrequent passage of a large-diameter stool which may obstruct the toilet. Some older children also show withholding postures although these are not seen as commonly as in younger children. Abdominal bloating is another important feature in children and seen especially in adolescents [58]. Abdominal pain, anorexia, and behavioral abnormalities are also important features in this age group.

Clinical Evaluation of Children with Defecation Disorders

Clinical evaluation is the most important tool in diagnosing defecation disorders in children and adolescents. It includes a thorough history, tenacious physical examination, and careful interpretation of findings in a logical manner. This process helps to actively identify functional defecation disorders, exclude possible organic diseases that can mimic functional defecation disorders, and recognize complications.

Clinical History

Although the presenting features are obvious in the majority, clinical features may be subtle in some children. Therefore, a high degree of suspicion is essential during history taking. Onset and duration of symptoms need to be clarified first. Very early-onset disease in infancy suggests the possibility of organic diseases such as Hirschsprung disease, anorectal malformations, and metabolic diseases. Details of bowel habits are the cornerstone in diagnosing constipation (Box 21.1). Use of validated stool scales for infants [59] (Amsterdam stool scale) and children (modified Bristol stool scale) [60] helps to obtain more accurate description of stools. Apart from that, it is also important to question on other gastrointestinal symptoms. Abdominal pain is noted in 10–70% of children with constipation. Poor appetite, nausea, vomiting, and abdominal bloating are other important features that need to be inquired into during history taking. Children with chronic constipation also tend to suffer from a myriad of somatic symptoms and identifying these features would help in clinical management [19]. Urinary symptoms and incontinence are also seen in some children [61–64] and refractory vulvovaginitis is a known feature, especially in prepubertal girls [65].

Box 21.1   Bowel Habit Questions for Defecation Disorders
Stool frequency
Consistency
Nature of the stools
Incontinence
Withholding behavior
Pain during defecation
Blood in stools

Past medical history, specially concentrating on drugs that may cause constipation, is also an important part in the evaluation. Surgical issues such as corrected anorectal malformations and Hirschsprung disease are well known to present with constipation [66, 67]. Dietary history particularly concentrating on fiber content is an integral part as underconsumption of fiber may lead to constipation [17, 18]. Introduction of cow's milk to the infant's diet is a risk factor to develop constipation among them [68, 69]. Psychological abnormalities also need to be looked into as some children develop personality problems, anxiety, and depression with constipation [22, 70]. Finally, details of social and family history should not be overlooked. Constipation is notably prevalent in children from the lower socioeconomic strata, living in disrupted deprived areas and urban areas [19, 23]. In addition, adverse life events such as physical, sexual, and emotional maltreatment should also need to be evaluated carefully in children with constipation as these factors are known to predispose children to develop constipation [27]. Some children with constipation also have first-degree relatives with similar problems [11, 19].

Physical Examination

The physical examination should start with assessment of growth. Growth faltering and short stature are features of organic causes (endocrine, metabolic, etc.) for constipation. On the other hand, obesity is also a known predisposing factor for defecation disorders such as constipation and FI [26]. Dysmorphic features are present in children with syndromes who are having constipation [71]. All children with defecation disorders need a good developmental assessment. Those with long-term neurological dysfunctions such as cerebral palsy tend to have both constipation and FI. Furthermore, this would also help to identify children with autistic spectrum disorders who have a tendency to develop constipation [31].

Abdominal examination may reveal the presence of abdominal distension and past surgical scars of abdominal surgery. Palpable fecal masses in the lower abdomen indicate fecal loading and is a feature present in about 50% of children with constipation [72]. However, gaseous distension is more in favor of constipation-predominant irritable bowel syndrome ("IBS-C").

Perianal examination may reveal abnormal position of anus [73]. Smear of feces and perianal excoriation of skin indicates FI. Fissures and tags can also be noted in children with chronic constipation who pass hard stools or may indicate sexual abuse. Patulous anus is associated with lower motor neuronal damage which can be associated with FI. Digital examination of the rectum is an essential part in evaluating children with defecation disorders. During the process one should assess resting tone, the squeeze pressure of the sphincter complex, nature of fecal loading, size of the fecal mass, and the size of the rectum.

Neurological examination should concentrate specially on features of spina bifida, motor and sensory deficits in the lower limbs, and perianal sensory testing. One should look for perianal sensory loss and absence of anal wink.

Investigations

Constipation is a clinical diagnosis. Using currently accepted clinical criteria, the majority of the children who present to a medical facility can be diagnosed and managed successfully. Specialized investigations are therefore only needed when the diagnosis is uncertain, or when they do not respond to standard management strategies. Investigations are also warranted in children who are suspected to have organic reasons for defecation disorders during history taking and physical examination.

Radiological Tests

Colonic transit time is usually assessed by using radiological methods. It generally gives an idea of propulsive function of the colon and helps to identify segments with abnormal motility. It is usually measured using radiopaque markers or scintigraphic methods. In marker studies, the markers are ingested as a meal or swallowed as a capsule, and abdominal X-rays are obtained to count the number of markers in different segments of the colon. In scintigraphy, the patient is given a meal containing radioisotope, and multiple images are taken using a gamma camera to assess the radioisotope count in each region. Several studies have shown abnormalities in total and segmental transit times in children with functional constipation using radiopaque markers [39, 40]. A Dutch study noted children with functional constipation having colonic transit time over 62 h. This cutoff value has a sensitivity of 52% and specificity of 91% [42]. Colonic transit time also has an inverse relationship with the number of defecations per week [39]. Using colonic scintigraphy, Sutcliffe et al. found delay in transit in patients with constipation [41].

Ultrasonography has also been used to assess the degree of fecal retention in the rectum. Using a transabdominal approach, several studies have measured the rectal diameter to determine fecal loading in the rectum using different methods and have shown that children with chronic constipation do have a larger rectal diameter compared to controls. Bijos et al. using recto–pelvic ratio (dividing the transverse diameter of the rectal ampulla by the transverse diameter of the pelvis) illustrated that in children with functional constipation, the mean recto–pelvic ratio was 0.22 ± 0.05 compared to healthy controls 0.15 ± 0.04 [74]. Another study measured the impression of the rectum behind the urinary bladder seen as a crescent. The median rectal crescent in children with constipation was 3.4 cm (range 2.10–7.0; interquartile range (IQR) 1.0) as compared with 2.4 cm (range 1.3–4.2; IQR 0.72) in healthy controls [75]. Klijn et al. also found a significant difference in mean rectal diameter between the constipated group (4.9 cm) and the control group (2.1 cm). The cutoff value was 3.3 cm, where >3.3 cm indicated constipation [76]. The results are promising, and wider availability and noninvasive nature of the test make it an ideal investigation. However, methods need to be standardized, and more studies are needed before recommending routine use of ultrasonography in assessing children with constipation.

Furthermore, using endosonography techniques, Keshtgar et al. have shown that children with chronic constipation have a thickened external anal sphincter complex. However, they were unable to demonstrate a significant relationship between thickened anal sphincter, anorectal manometry, and amplitude of sphincter contractions [77]. The clinical utility value of this finding is yet to be determined.

Plain abdominal X-ray is used to demonstrate fecal loading in the colon and rectum. Several scoring systems are used to assess the degree of impaction. However, sensitivity and specificity of these tests are variable and also the inter- and intra-observer reliability are poor [78]. Therefore, it is difficult to recommend the use of plain X-ray films of the abdomen as an investigation.

The other radiological investigations such as defecography and contrast enemas have no place in clinical evaluation of children with constipation. Magnetic resonance imaging of the spinal cord is an important investigation in children with refractory defecation disorders as some children have been shown to have significant abnormalities such as spina bifida occulta and terminal filum lipoma. Importantly, gluteal cleft deviation was found in three of four patients with these abnormalities [79, 80].

Physiological Tests

Anorectal manometry combined with balloon expulsion test is an important investigation to understand the function of the anorectal unit and pelvic floor muscles. It provides information about anal sphincter function, mechanisms of continence and defecation, rectal sensation, rectal compliance, and anorectal reflexes [81]. A number of studies have demonstrated several abnormalities of anorectal function in children with constipation. They include increased rectal sensory threshold, reduced rectal contractility, high resting anal pressure, and failure of relaxation of the external anal sphincter with rising rectal pressure [46–49]. Furthermore, a subset of children was found to have an abnormal balloon expulsion test [50]. Feinberg and coworkers have shown that there is a correlation between the number of FI episodes and the volume of first urge, and high volume required to elicit rectoanal inhibitory reflex. They also found a significant correlation between the presence of withholding behavior and the maximum volume tolerated [82].

Colonic manometry allows the measurement of pressure/force from multiple regions within the colon in real time [83] and helps to discriminate between normal colonic physiology and colonic myopathies and neuropathies. A number of colonic motor patterns have been identified, such as antegrade high-amplitude propagating contractions, low-amplitude propagating sequences, non-propagating contractions, and retrograde propagating pressure waves [84]. In contrast to conventional manometry which used a limited number of sensors, arrival of high-resolution manometry allows researchers and clinicians to study three-dimensional pressure plots to study gastrointestinal pathophysiology more closely. An elegant study using this technique has clearly shown children with slow transit constipation having definitive abnormal motor patterns (post-bisacodyl-induced high-amplitude propagatory contractions) which can serve to diagnose colonic neuropathy [85].

Other Investigations

Association between CMP allergy and constipation is still a debatable subject. Two research reports from Italy (from a center of excellence studying allergies) have found association between constipation and CMP sensitivity [68, 69]. A more recent study from Irastorza and colleagues found 51 % patients with constipation responding to a CMP elimination diet, but no significant differences were noted between the group of responders and nonresponders regarding atopic/allergic history and laboratory results [86]. Therefore, testing for CMP allergy is not recommended. Importance of hypothyroidism as an etiological factor for constipation in children is overstated. Bennett and Heuckeroth studied 56 children with hypothyroidism and noted that only one child had constipation as the presenting complaint [87]. As for other serological tests (such as screening for celiac disease and looking for hypercalcemia), these are also not recommended in all constipated children; however, in a child with symptoms not responding to laxative therapy, it might be useful to look for celiac disease.

Management

Effective management of constipation requires a multifaceted approach. A stepwise management protocol is shown in Fig. 21.1. The main steps include lifestyle modification, toilet training, use of laxatives and enemas, biofeedback therapy, nerve stimulation, and surgical interventions. However, it is important to realize that the data in the pediatric literature to support evidence-based use of treatment strategies are limited, especially regarding old laxatives such as lactulose and bisacodyl. Therefore, the management mostly depends on individual experiences and limited number of trials of new drugs.

Lifestyle Modifications

Constipation is known to be associated with psychological stress related to home, school, and society [22, 23]. These factors need to be addressed during the consultation. Children with psychological stress need to be identified and coping mechanisms need to be taught as part of the day-to-day lifestyle. Home- and school-related punishment is another factor that is known to predispose children to develop constipation which can easily be avoided [27].

Although widely believed, a high-fiber diet does not relieve constipation. Several trials including different types of fibers failed to show any clinically meaningful therapeutic benefit in children [88–90]. Two systematic reviews also illustrate limited clinical value of fiber in the management

Fig. 21.1 Stepwise management of constipation

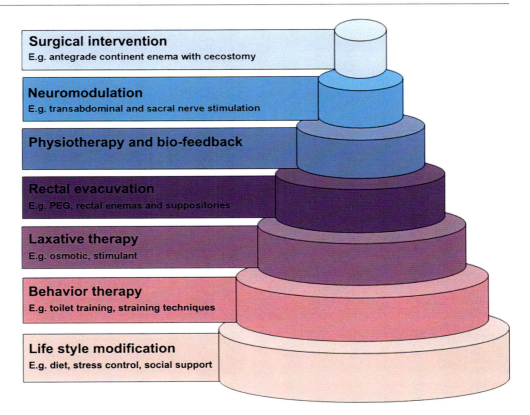

Surgical intervention
E.g. antegrade continent enema with cecostomy

Neuromodulation
E.g. transabdominal and sacral nerve stimulation

Physiotherapy and bio-feedback

Rectal evacuvation
E.g. PEG, rectal enemas and suppositories

Laxative therapy
E.g. osmotic, stimulant

Behavior therapy
E.g. toilet training, straining techniques

Life style modification
E.g. diet, stress control, social support

[91, 92]. In addition, increasing dietary fiber intake with extensive behavioral interventions does not reduce the requirement of laxatives [93]. Similarly, increase in the consumption of water has also shown not to increase stool frequency or soften stools [94].

Toilet Training and Behavioral Therapy

Stool withholding plays a crucial role in developing constipation in young children. Aiming to prevent this phenomenon, children with constipation need to relearn to properly pass stools in the toilet.

As the first step, negative attitude regarding stools needs to be eliminated. This facilitates and prepares the child mentally to pass stools in the toilet or potty. Child is encouraged to use the toilet regularly usually after each meal as the gastrocolic reflex facilitates generation of high-amplitude propagatory contractions which help to evacuate stools. The proper seating method (upright posture) to bring the anorectum to the correct angle to facilitate the passage of stools also needs to be taught. Proper positioning of legs and relaxing them with the pelvic floor and anal sphincters also can be learned. Once the child masters these techniques, it is necessary to teach him/her proper straining methods to facilitate the passage of stools. This process needs to be a regular practice and could be encouraged with a reward system. [95]. A Cochrane review has shown positive evidence indicating that adding behavioral therapy to conventional laxatives has benefits in treating children with constipation [96]. It is obvi-

ous that behavioral therapy alone cannot cure constipation. However, given the importance of the part played by stool-withholding behavior in childhood constipation (especially in infants and younger children), toilet training and behavioral modifications are inseparable parts in day-to-day clinical management.

Fecal Disimpaction from Rectum

It has been shown that 40–100% of children with constipation have a large rock-hard fecal mass in the rectum [97]. After evacuation of the fecal mass children are more likely to respond to maintenance therapy [98]. Several studies have proved that oral administration of polyethylene glycol (PEG) is both successful and cost-effective in the majority of children with fecal impaction [99–101]. Therefore, oral route is recommended as the initial step in rectal evacuation.

Rectal enemas or suppositories are recommended for children who do not respond to oral drugs. A study by Bekkali et al. failed to show a significant difference between PEG and rectal enemas on evacuation of rectum loaded with feces [101]. However, it is imperative to realize the invasive nature of rectal therapy specially when the child has pain, discomfort, and may suffer from morbid fear of manipulations around the perianal region by medical professionals. In a minority of cases, even sedation is recommended before rectal administration especially when the child is not cooperative. Rectal medications that can be used are phosphate, docusate sodium, mineral oil enemas, and bisacodyl suppositories.

Maintenance Treatment

Once disimpaction is achieved, it is imperative that the clinician should concentrate on maintenance therapy. This facilitates passage of stools and prevents re-impaction. Table 21.3 shows the details of the drugs that are currently used in the management of childhood constipation.

Lubricant Laxatives

Although there are no placebo-controlled trials involving lubricant laxatives, two trials comparing mineral oil with lactulose have noted statistically significant better response rates with mineral oil. When comparing mineral oil with PEG, the response rates were almost similar [102]. Contrary to this, Tolia et al. found PEG superior to mineral oil in relieving symptoms [103]. However, due to the risk of life-threatening lipoid pneumonia, mineral oil is not recommended for young infants and children with swallowing difficulties, especially those who are neurologically handicapped.

Osmotic Laxatives

Osmotic laxatives are the group of choice used in the maintenance phase. As a group they exert an osmotic effect which helps to increase the water content in the colon and hence softening stools with minimal adverse effects. Lactulose and PEG are the two most commonly used drugs in this group.

Although widely used, lactulose has never been compared with a placebo in a controlled trial. Perkin et al. compared lactulose with senna using a small number of children. They noted a greater clinical response to senna (improving defecation frequency) when compared to lactulose [104]. A recent randomized controlled trial using lactulose and a mixture of fibers showed that both therapeutic modalities are comparable without major side effects [90].

A Cochrane review has concluded the superiority of PEG over both placebo and lactulose [105]. However, it is important to realize that comparison of these studies is extremely difficult as the study designs, age groups, and PEG preparations are different. PEG also shows an excellent safety profile. Therefore, in clinical practice, it is recommended to use both drugs as first line drugs in the maintenance phase.

Stimulant Laxatives

Bisacodyl and senna stimulate peristaltic movements and enhance fecal evacuation. However, there are no good quality trials to evaluate stimulant laxatives in childhood constipation. Studies comparing senna with lactulose and mineral oil demonstrated that children using senna had a poorer response [104]. Another study comparing the effect of adding senna, placebo, or no medication for children with FI receiving behavioral therapy found no significant difference in outcome [106]. Despite the lack of well-designed trials, these drugs are commonly used in day-to-day clinical practice, often in combination with osmotic laxatives. The National Institute for Clinical Excellence (NICE) guidelines of the UK recommend the addition of stimulant laxatives to PEG when the response is noted to be suboptimal [107].

Table 21.3 Dosages of most frequently used oral and rectal laxatives

Drug class	Drug	Dosages
Osmotic laxatives	Lactulose	1–2 g/kg, once or twice/day
	PEG 3350 PEG 4000	Maintenance: 0.2–0.8 g/kg/day Fecal disimpaction: 1–1.5 g/kg/day(with a maximum of 6 consecutive days)
	Milk of magnesia (magnesium hydroxide)	2–5 years: 0.4–1.2 g/day, once or divided 6–11 years: 1.2–2.4 g/day, once or divided 12–18 years: 2.4–4.8 g/day, once or divided
Fecal softeners	Mineral oil	1–18 years: 1–3 ml/kg/day, once or divided, max. 90 ml/day
Stimulant laxatives	Bisacodyl	3–10 years: 5 mg/day >10 years: 5–10 mg/day
	Senna	2–6 years: 2.5–5 mg once or twice/day 6–12 years: 7.5–10 mg/day >12 years: 15–20 mg/day
	Sodium picosulfate	1 month–4 years: 2.5–10 mg once/day 4–18 years: 2.5–20 mg once/day
Rectal laxatives/enemas	Bisacodyl	2–10 years: 5 mg once/day >10 years: 5–10 mg once/day
	Sodium docusate	<6 years: 60 ml >6 years: 120 ml
	Sodium phosphate	1–18 years: 2.5 ml/kg, max. 133 ml/dose
	NaCl	Neonate <1 kg: 5 ml, >1kg: 10 ml >1 years: 6 ml/kg once or twice/day
	Mineral oil	2–11 years: 30–60 ml once/day >11 years: 60–150 ml once/day

New Drugs

Prucalopride Prucalopride belongs to the class of dihydro-benzofuran-carboxamide derivatives. The drug has a clear gastroprokinetic activity and selective and high affinity for 5-HT4 receptor agonists that stimulate lower gastrointestinal motility. The efficacy of the drug was tested in an open-label 8-week trial involving 37 children. According to the results, the average number of spontaneous bowel movements normalized to a mean of 6.8 per week, whereas the average number of FI episodes decreased from 5.6 in the first week to 3.4 in week 8. Most of the children were using other laxatives as well during the trial [108]. Although the results of this open-label trial look promising and safe, further studies are needed before recommending the use of prucalopride for constipation in children.

Lubiprostone Lubiprostone is a locally acting chloride channel activator specific to the gastrointestinal tract. It promotes intestinal secretion of chloride ions and fluid and gastrointestinal motility. It has a good track record in treating adults with constipation. In an open-label trial, lubiprostone was shown to be safe and effective in improving spontaneous bowel movements, reducing episodes of FI, and reducing many other symptoms of constipation in children and adolescents less than 17 years [109].

Biofeedback and Physiotherapy

Anorectal function can be modified with the use of biofeedback. The purpose of biofeedback is to improve anorectal function and sensation [110]. Several studies have shown efficacy of biofeedback in correcting defecation dynamics, but a well-conducted large randomized controlled trial failed to find additional clinical benefits of biofeedback in children with constipation [1, 48, 111, 112]. However, despite this finding it is vital to assess this therapeutic modality in combination with pelvic floor physiotherapy and muscle training as pelvic floor dyssynergia is a recognized physiological abnormality, especially in older children.

Neuromodulation

Neuromodulation has been identified as a successful therapeutic modality for elimination disorders [113], although the working mechanism is far from clear. Two trials have shown that sacral neuromodulation is effective in treating adults and children with slow transit or normal transit constipation [114, 115]. The adverse events (mainly pain) were minimal. A well-designed sham-controlled trial with a larger patient sample and a long-term follow-up is needed however to confirm these encouraging data.

Transabdominal electrical stimulation has also been studied as an option for treatment of resistant slow transit consti-pation. Using this technique, Clarke et al. illustrated children with slow transit constipation generating significantly higher frequency of high amplitude and total propagatory sequences [116]. In addition, the same research group studying 39 children with slow transit constipation has shown that transcutaneous electrical stimulation (TES) delivered by a physiotherapist (three 20-min session a week) increases defecation frequency in 30%, reduces FI in 75%, abdominal pain in 59%, and reduces the need for appendicostomy washouts in 43% [117]. Yet again, further studies are needed to confirm these findings and use of this in clinical practice.

Surgical Interventions

Injection of botulinum toxin (single or multiple) to the internal anal sphincter is effective in some children with dyssynergic defecation. Adverse effects frequently encountered include transient anal and abdominal pain, and occurrence of FI yet again resolves spontaneously [118]. Antegrade continent enema with appendicostomy or laparoscopic-assisted percutaneous caecostomy has been used in treatment-resistant constipation. The success rates are high and functional outcomes are excellent. It had been shown that the procedure improves bowel frequency and quality of life and reduces number of episodes of incontinence [119]. PEG solution and normal saline are effective, including a stimulant laxative, as cleansing agents. Commonly seen complications include granulation tissues around stoma, leakage, and minor infections. Major complications such as fistulae, peritonitis, and stenosis of the stoma are only seen in a minority [120]. Other surgical procedures such as sigmoid resection, colorectal resection, subtotal colectomy, and proctocolectomy with ileoanal anastomosis are only reserved for children with intractable constipation who failed to respond to all other therapeutic modalities [121].

Part 2: Functional FI

Introduction and Epidemiology

FI is defined as passing stools in inappropriate places including one's underwear by a child whose development age is over 4 years [122]. Once organic causes are excluded, functional FI is mainly due to two possible reasons: constipation-associated and functional nonretentive fecal incontinence (FNRFI). The former has already been discussed in detail in the first part of this chapter. We will now concentrate on FNRFI.

Like constipation, FI is also a widespread problem. Epidemiological studies have shown rates ranging from 0.8 to 4.1% in the West and 2 to 7.8% in Asia [122]. We conducted an epidemiological survey and found that the majority of children (80%) with FI had constipation-associated (retentive) FI and only 20% truly had FNRFI [123]. FI is commoner among males and children from low socioeconomic strata [123, 124]. In addition, bullying, psychological stress, behavioral and upbringing problems, and poor social and school performances are commonly seen in children with FI [123, 125].

Functional Nonretentive FI

Rome III criteria to define FNRFI are given in Table 21.1. These children pass normal stools in the toilet with a normal defecation pattern. They do not show features of constipation such as posturing, pain, or difficulty in passing stools either. However, they pass entire bowel motion into their underwear at least once a month. The pathophysiological mechanism for this disease is still an enigma to pediatric gastroenterologists. Several studies have clearly demonstrated normal colonic transit times (both segmental and total) in children with FNRFI [126, 127]. Similarly, anorectal manometry and barostat studies found that all parameters (rectal compliance, sensory thresholds) are within the normal range [128]. Although several psychological and behavioral abnormalities have been described in association with FNRFI, it is not clear whether these are causative factors or long-term effects of FI [129, 130]. Clinical evaluation of children with defecation disorders has been previously discussed in this chapter.

Investigations should be directed to exclude constipation-associated FI from FNRFI when the two entities are not apparent on clinical history and physical examination. When colonic transit times were compared, children with constipation-associated FI were found to have significantly delayed total colonic transit, as against children with FNRFI [126].

Anorectal manometry is helpful in differentiating these clinical entities. Children with constipation-associated FI show higher threshold for rectal sensation than FNRFI and there is no difference in maximum anal resting tone and abnormal defecation dynamics between the two groups [127]. Children with retentive FI have significant thickening of the internal anal sphincter on anal endosonography and the thickness is well correlated to symptom score, FI score, megarectum score, and size of the megarectum on manometry [77]. Such abnormalities have not been noted in FNRFI. In addition to these studies, MRI of the spine is also useful in some children to rule out organic causes of FI when there are subtle features of spinal bifida occulta on physical examination.

Management of children with FNRFI is challenging and often a long road, fraught with successes and failures. Education and strict toilet training following an individualized behavioral routine and positive reinforcement are the four main cornerstones in management [123]. Conventional treatment modalities such as oral or rectal laxatives and biofeedback are not helpful in the management. Loperamide was found to be effective in a child with FNRFI in a case report and further studies are needed to assess its efficacy [131]. These patients usually run a relapsing and remitting course, and a long-term follow-up study has shown that at the age of 18 years, 85% of them are symptom free and have normal bowel habits [132].

References

1. Loening-Baucke V. Modulation of abnormal defecation dynamics by biofeedback treatment in chronically constipated children with encopresis. J Pediatr. 1990;116(2):214–22.
2. Benninga M, Candy DC, Catto-Smith AG, Clayden G, Loening-Baucke V, Di Lorenzo C, et al. The Paris consensus on childhood constipation terminology (PACCT) Group. J Pediatr Gastroenterol Nutr. 2005;40(3):273–5.
3. Rasquin-Weber A, Hyman PE, Cucchiara S, Fleisher DR, Hyams JS, Milla PJ, et al. Childhood functional gastrointestinal disorders. Gut. 1999;45(Suppl 2):II60–8.
4. Rasquin A, Di Lorenzo C, Forbes D, Guiraldes E, Hyams JS, Staiano A, et al. Childhood functional gastrointestinal disorders: child/adolescent. Gastroenterology. 2006;130(5):1527–37. doi:10.1053/j.gastro.2005.08.063.
5. Devanarayana NM, Rajindrajith S. Bowel habits and behaviors related to defecation in 10- to 16-year-olds: impact of socioeconomic characteristics and emotional stress. J Pediatr Gastroenterol Nutr. 2011;52(5):569–573. doi:10.1097/MPG.0b013e3181fd082b.
6. Wald ER, Di Lorenzo C, Cipriani L, Colborn DK, Burgers R, Wald A. Bowel habits and toilet training in a diverse population of children. J Pediatr Gastroenterol Nutr. 2009;48(3):294–8.
7. Corazziari E, Staiano A. Miele E, Greco L. Italian Society of Pediatric Gastroenterology, Hepatology, and Nutrition. Bowel frequency and defecatory patterns in children: a prospective nationwide survey. Clin Gastroenterol Hepatol. 2005;3(11):1101–6.
8. Devanarayana NM, Adhikari C, Pannala W, Rajindrajith S. Prevalence of functional gastrointestinal diseases in a cohort of Sri Lankan adolescents: comparison between Rome II and Rome III criteria. J Trop Pediatr. 2011;57(1):34–9. doi:10.1093/tropej/fmq039.
9. Burgers R, Levin AD, Di Lorenzo C, Dijkgraaf MG, Benninga MA. Functional defecation disorders in children: comparing the Rome II with the Rome III criteria. J Pediatr. 2012;161(4):615–20, e611. doi:10.1016/j.jpeds.2012.03.060.
10. Roma-Giannikou E, Adamidis D, Gianniou M, Nikolara R, Messaritakis A. Epidemiology of chronic constipation in Greek children. Hell J Gastroenterol. 1999;12:58–62.
11. Roma E, Adamidis D, Nikolara R, Constantopoulos A, Messaritakis J. Diet and chronic constipation in children: the role of fiber. J Pediatr Gastroenterol Nutr. 1999;28(2):169–74.
12. Miele E, Simeone D, Marino A, Greco L, Auricchio R, Novek SJ, et al. Functional gastrointestinal disorders in children: an Italian prospective survey. Pediatrics. 2004;114(1):73–8.
13. Iacono G, Merolla R, D'Amico D, Bonci E, Cavataio F, Di Prima L, et al. Gastrointestinal symptoms in infancy: a population-based prospective study. Dig Liver Dis. 2005;37(6):432–8. doi:10.1016/j.dld.2005.01.009.
14. Del Ciampo IR, Galvao LC, Del Ciampo LA, Fernandes MI. Prevalence of chronic constipation in children at a primary health care unit. J Pediatr (Rio J). 2002;78(6):497–502.

15. de Araujo Sant'Anna AM, Calcado AC. Constipation in school-aged children at public schools in Rio de Janeiro, Brazil. J Pediatr Gastroenterol Nutr. 1999;29(2):190–3.

16. Wu TC, Chen LK, Pan WH, Tang RB, Hwang SJ, Wu L, et al. Constipation in Taiwan elementary school students: a nationwide survey. J Chin Med Assoc. 2011;74(2):57–61. doi:10.1016/j.jcma.2011.01.012.

17. Tam YH, Li AM, So HK, Shit KY, Pang KK, Wong YS, et al. Socioenvironmental factors associated with constipation in Hong Kong children and Rome III criteria. J Pediatr Gastroenterol Nutr. 2012;55(1):56–61. doi:10.1097/MPG.0b013e31824741ce.

18. Lee WT, Ip KS, Chan JS, Lui NW, Young BW. Increased prevalence of constipation in pre-school children is attributable to under-consumption of plant foods: a community-based study. J Paediatr Child Health. 2008;44(4):170–5. doi:10.1111/j.1440-1754.2007.01212.x.

19. Rajindrajith S, Devanarayana NM, Adhikari C, Pannala W, Benninga MA. Constipation in children: an epidemiological study in Sri Lanka using Rome III criteria. Arch Dis Child. 2012;97(1):43–5. doi:10.1136/adc.2009.173716.

20. Suares NC, Ford AC. Prevalence of, and risk factors for, chronic idiopathic constipation in the community: systematic review and meta-analysis. Am J Gastroenterol. 2011;106(9):1582–91, quiz 1581. doi:1592.10.1038/ajg.2011.164.

21. Inan M, Aydiner CY, Tokuc B, Aksu B, Ayvaz S, Ayhan S, et al. Factors associated with childhood constipation. J Paediatr Child Health. 2007;43(10):700–6. doi:10.1111/j.1440-1754.2007.01165.x.

22. Devanarayana NM, Rajindrajith S. Association between constipation and stressful life events in a cohort of Sri Lankan children and adolescents. J Trop Pediatr. 2010;56(3):144–8. doi:10.1093/tropej/fmp077.

23. Rajindrajith S, Mettananda S, Devanarayana NM. Constipation during and after the civil war in Sri Lanka: a paediatric study. J Trop Pediatr. 2011;57(6):439–43. doi:10.1093/tropej/fmr013.

24. Carroccio A, Iacono G. Review article: chronic constipation and food hypersensitivity—an intriguing relationship. Aliment Pharmacol Ther. 2006;24(9):1295–304. doi:10.1111/j.1365-2036.2006.03125.x.

25. vd Baan-Slootweg OH, Liem O, Bekkali N, van Aalderen WM, Rijcken TH, Di Lorenzo C, et al. Constipation and colonic transit times in children with morbid obesity. J Pediatr Gastroenterol Nutr. 2011;52(4):442–5. doi:10.1097/MPG.0b013e3181ef8e3c.

26. Fishman L, Lenders C, Fortunato C, Noonan C, Nurko S. Increased prevalence of constipation and fecal soiling in a population of obese children. J Pediatr. 2004;145(2):253–4. doi:10.1016/j.jpeds.2004.04.022.

27. Rajindrajith S, Devanarayana NM, Lakmini C, Subasinghe V, de Silva DG, Benninga MA. Association between child maltreatment and constipation: a school based survey using Rome III criteria. J Pediatr Gastroenterol Nutr. 2013. doi:10.1097/MPG.0000000000000249.

28. Youssef NN, Langseder AL, Verga BJ, Mones RL, Rosh JR. Chronic childhood constipation is associated with impaired quality of life: a case-controlled study. J Pediatr Gastroenterol Nutr. 2005;41(1):56–60.

29. Clarke MC, Chow CS, Chase JW, Gibb S, Hutson JM, Southwell BR. Quality of life in children with slow transit constipation. J Pediatr Surg. 2008;43(2):320–4. doi:10.1016/j.jpedsurg.2007.10.020.

30. Rajindrajith S, Devanarayana NM, Weerasooriya L, Hathagoda W, Benninga MA. Quality of life and somatic symptoms in children with constipation: a school-based study. J Pediatr. 2013;163(4):1069–72, e1061. doi:10.1016/j.jpeds.2013.05.012.

31. Peeters B, Noens I, Philips EM, Kuppens S, Benninga MA. Autism spectrum disorders in children with functional defecation disorders. J Pediatr. 2013;163(3):873–8. doi:10.1016/j.jpeds.2013.02.028.

32. Pang KH, Croaker GD. Constipation in children with autism and autistic spectrum disorder. Pediatr Surg Int. 2011;27(4):353–8. doi:10.1007/s00383-010-2680-8.

33. Waters AM, Schilpzand E, Bell C, Walker LS, Baber K. Functional gastrointestinal symptoms in children with anxiety disorders. J Abnorm Child Psychol. 2013;41(1):151–163. doi:10.1007/s10802-012-9657-0.

34. Ranasinghe N, Rajindrajith S, Devanarayana NM, Warnakulasuriya T, Nishanthini S, Perera MS. Children and adolescents with constipation: do they have different personalities? J Gastroenterol Hepatol. 2012;27(Suppl 5):383.

35. Chitkara DK, Camilleri M, Zinsmeister AR, Burton D, El-Youssef M, Freese D, et al. Gastric sensory and motor dysfunction in adolescents with functional dyspepsia. J Pediatr. 2005;146(4):500–5. doi:10.1016/j.jpeds.2004.11.031.

36. Choung RS, Shah ND, Chitkara D, Branda ME, Van Tilburg MA, Whitehead WE, et al. Direct medical costs of constipation from childhood to early adulthood: a population-based birth cohort study. J Pediatr Gastroenterol Nutr. 2011;52(1):47–54. doi:10.1097/MPG.0b013e3181e67058.

37. Liem O, Harman J, Benninga M, Kelleher K, Mousa H, Di Lorenzo C. Health utilization and cost impact of childhood constipation in the United States. J Pediatr. 2009;154(2):258–62. doi:10.1016/j.jpeds.2008.07.060.

38. Sagawa T, Okamura S, Kakizaki S, Zhang Y, Morita K, Mori M. Functional gastrointestinal disorders in adolescents and quality of school life. J Gastroenterol Hepatol. 2013;28(2):285–90. doi:10.1111/j.1440-1746.2012.07257.x.

39. Gutierrez C, Marco A, Nogales A, Tebar R. Total and segmental colonic transit time and anorectal manometry in children with chronic idiopathic constipation. J Pediatr Gastroenterol Nutr. 2002;35(1):31–8.

40. Zaslavsky C, da Silveira TR, Maguilnik I. Total and segmental colonic transit time with radio-opaque markers in adolescents with functional constipation. J Pediatr Gastroenterol Nutr. 1998;27(2):138–42.

41. Sutcliffe JR, King SK, Hutson JM, Cook DJ, Southwell BR. Gastrointestinal transit in children with chronic idiopathic constipation. Pediatr Surg Int. 2009;25(6):465–72. doi:10.1007/s00383-009-2374-2.

42. Benninga MA, Buller HA, Tytgat GN, Akkermans LM, Bossuyt PM, Taminiau JA. Colonic transit time in constipated children: does pediatric slow-transit constipation exist? J Pediatr Gastroenterol Nutr. 1996;23(3):241–51.

43. Knowles CH, Scott SM, Rayner C, Glia A, Lindberg G, Kamm MA, et al. Idiopathic slow-transit constipation: an almost exclusively female disorder. Dis Colon Rectum. 2003;46(12):1716–7. doi:10.1097/01.DCR.0000098929.52147.B8.

44. Hutson JM, Chase JW, Clarke MC, King SK, Sutcliffe J, Gibb S, et al. Slow-transit constipation in children: our experience. Pediatr Surg Int. 2009;25(5):403–6. doi:10.1007/s00383-009-2363-5.

45. Dinning PG, Benninga MA, Southwell BR, Scott SM. Paediatric and adult colonic manometry: a tool to help unravel the pathophysiology of constipation. World J Gastroenterol. 2010;16(41):5162–72.

46. van den Berg MM, Bongers ME, Voskuijl WP, Benninga MA. No role for increased rectal compliance in pediatric functional constipation. Gastroenterology. 2009;137(6):1963–9. doi:10.1053/j.gastro.2009.08.015.

47. van den Berg MM, Voskuijl WP, Boeckxstaens GE, Benninga MA. Rectal compliance and rectal sensation in constipated adolescents, recovered adolescents and healthy volunteers. Gut. 2008;57(5):599–603. doi:10.1136/gut.2007.125690.

48. van der Plas RN, Benninga MA, Buller HA, Bossuyt PM, Akkermans LM, Redekop WK, et al. Biofeedback training in treatment of childhood constipation: a randomised controlled study. Lancet. 1996;348(9030):776–80.

49. van der Plas RN, Benninga MA, Staalman CR, Akkermans LM, Redekop WK, Taminiau JA, et al. Megarectum in constipation. Arch Dis Child. 2000;83(1):52–8.

50. Chitkara DK, Bredenoord AJ, Cremonini F, Delgado-Aros S, Smoot RL, El-Youssef M, et al. The role of pelvic floor dysfunction and slow colonic transit in adolescents with refractory constipation. Am J Gastroenterol. 2004;99(8):1579–84. doi:10.1111/j.1572-0241.2004.30176.x.

51. Drossman DA. Abuse, trauma, and GI illness: is there a link? Am J Gastroenterol. 2011;106(1):14–25. doi:10.1038/ajg.2010.453.

52. Bekkali N, de Jonge HR, van den Wijngaard RM, van der Steeg AF, Bijlsma PB, Taminiau JA, et al. The role of rectal chloride secretion in childhood constipation. Neurogastroenterol Motil. 2011;23(11):1007–12. doi:10.1111/j.1365-2982.2011.01751.x.

53. Bampton PA, Dinning PG, Kennedy ML, Lubowski DZ, Cook IJ. The proximal colonic motor response to rectal mechanical and chemical stimulation. Am J Physiol Gastrointest Liver Physiol. 2002;282(3):G443–9. doi:10.1152/ajpgi.00194.2001.

54. Mollen RM, Salvioli B, Camilleri M, Burton D, Kost LJ, Phillips SF, et al. The effects of biofeedback on rectal sensation and distal colonic motility in patients with disorders of rectal evacuation: evidence of an inhibitory rectocolonic reflex in humans? Am J Gastroenterol. 1999;94(3):751–6. doi:10.1111/j.1572-0241.1999.00947.x.

55. Dickson EJ, Hennig GW, Heredia DJ, Lee HT, Bayguinov PO, Spencer NJ, et al. Polarized intrinsic neural reflexes in response to colonic elongation. J Physiol. 2008;586(Pt 17):4225–40. doi:10.1113/jphysiol.2008.155630.

56. Dickson EJ, Spencer NJ, Hennig GW, Bayguinov PO, Ren J, Heredia DJ, et al. An enteric occult reflex underlies accommodation and slow transit in the distal large bowel. Gastroenterology. 2007;132(5):1912–24. doi:10.1053/j.gastro.2007.02.047.

57. Loening-Bauke V, Swidsinski A. Constipation. In: Faure C, Di Lorenzo C, Thapar N, editors. Pediatric neurogastroenterology. New York: Humana Press; 2013. pp. 413–28.

58. Rajindrajith S, Devanarayana NM. Abdominal bloating in children: association with functional gastrointestinal diseases and adverse life events. 3rd Biennial Congress of Asian Neurogastroenterology and Motility Association, 2013, Peanang, Malaysia. Abstract no P12. J Neurogastroenterol Motil. 2013;19(Suppl 1):63.

59. Bekkali N, Hamers SL, Reitsma JB, Van Toledo L, Benninga MA. Infant stool form scale: development and results. J Pediatr. 2009;154(4):521–6, e521. doi:10.1016/j.jpeds.2008.10.010.

60. Lane MM, Czyzewski DI, Chumpitazi BP, Shulman RJ. Reliability and validity of a modified Bristol Stool Form Scale for children. J Pediatr. 2011;159(3):437–41, e431. doi:10.1016/j.jpeds.2011.03.002.

61. Loening-Baucke V. Prevalence rates for constipation and faecal and urinary incontinence. Arch Dis Child. 2007;92(6):486–9. doi:10.1136/adc.2006.098335.

62. Soderstrom U, Hoelcke M, Alenius L, Soderling AC, Hjern A. Urinary and faecal incontinence: a population-based study. Acta Paediatr. 2004;93(3):386–9.

63. Dohil R, Roberts E, Jones KV, Jenkins HR. Constipation and reversible urinary tract abnormalities. Arch Dis Child. 1994;70(1):56–7.

64. Blethyn AJ, Jenkins HR, Roberts R, Verrier Jones K. Radiological evidence of constipation in urinary tract infection. Arch Dis Child. 1995;73(6):534–5.

65. van Neer PA, Korver CR. Constipation presenting as recurrent vulvovaginitis in prepubertal children. J Am Acad Dermatol. 2000;43(4):718–9. doi:10.1067/mjd.2000.107738.

66. Di Lorenzo C, Benninga MA. Pathophysiology of pediatric fecal incontinence. Gastroenterology. 2004;126(1 Suppl 1):S33–40.

67. Levitt MA, Martin CA, Olesevich M, Bauer CL, Jackson LE, Pena A. Hirschsprung disease and fecal incontinence: diagnostic and management strategies. J Pediatr Surg. 2009;44(1):271–7, discussion 277. doi:10.1016/j.jpedsurg.2008.10.053.

68. Iacono G, Carroccio A, Cavataio F, Montalto G, Cantarero MD, Notarbartolo A. Chronic constipation as a symptom of cow milk allergy. J Pediatr. 1995;126(1):34–9.

69. Iacono G, Cavataio F, Montalto G, Florena A, Tumminello M, Soresi M, et al. Intolerance of cow's milk and chronic constipation in children. N Engl J Med. 1998;339(16):1100–4. doi:10.1056/NEJM199810153391602.

70. Zhou H, Yao M, Cheng GY, Chen YP, Li DG. Prevalence and associated factors of functional gastrointestinal disorders and bowel habits in Chinese adolescents: a school-based study. J Pediatr Gastroenterol Nutr. 2011;53(2):168–73. doi:10.1097/MPG.0b013e3182125388.

71. Peeters B, Benninga MA, Hennekam RC. Childhood constipation: an overview of genetic studies and associated syndromes. Best Pract Res Clin Gastroenterol. 2011;25(1):73–88. doi:10.1016/j.bpg.2010.12.005.

72. Loening-Baucke V. Factors determining outcome in children with chronic constipation and faecal soiling. Gut. 1989;30(7):999–1006.

73. Nunez-Ramos R, Fabbro MA, Gonzalez-Velasco M, Nunez Nunez R, Romanato B, Vecchiato L, et al. Determination of the anal position in newborns and in children with chronic constipation: comparative study in two European healthcare centres. Pediatr Surg Int. 2011;27(10):1111–5. doi:10.1007/s00383-011-2914-4.

74. Bijos A, Czerwionka-Szaflarska M, Mazur A, Romanczuk W. The usefulness of ultrasound examination of the bowel as a method of assessment of functional chronic constipation in children. Pediatr Radiol. 2007;37(12):1247–52. doi:10.1007/s00247-007-0659-y.

75. Singh SJ, Gibbons NJ, Vincent MV, Sithole J, Nwokoma NJ, Alagarswami KV. Use of pelvic ultrasound in the diagnosis of megarectum in children with constipation. J Pediatr Surg. 2005;40(12):1941–4. doi:10.1016/j.jpedsurg.2005.08.012.

76. Klijn AJ, Asselman M, Vijverberg MA, Dik P, de Jong TP. The diameter of the rectum on ultrasonography as a diagnostic tool for constipation in children with dysfunctional voiding. J Urol. 2004;172(5 Pt 1):1986–8.

77. Keshtgar AS, Ward HC, Clayden GS, Sanei A. Thickening of the internal anal sphincter in idiopathic constipation in children. Pediatr Surg Int. 2004;20(11–12):817–23. doi:10.1007/s00383-004-1233-4.

78. de Lorijn F, van Rijn RR, Heijmans J, Reitsma JB, Voskuijl WP, Henneman OD, et al. The Leech method for diagnosing constipation: intra- and interobserver variability and accuracy. Pediatr Radiol. 2006;36(1):43–9. doi:10.1007/s00247-005-0031-z.

79. Bekkali NL, Hagebeuk EE, Bongers ME, van Rijn RR, Van Wijk MP, Liem O, et al. Magnetic resonance imaging of the lumbosacral spine in children with chronic constipation or non-retentive fecal incontinence: a prospective study. J Pediatr. 2010;156(3):461–5. doi:10.1016/j.jpeds.2009.09.048.

80. Rosen R, Buonomo C, Andrade R, Nurko S. Incidence of spinal cord lesions in patients with intractable constipation. J Pediatr. 2004;145(3):409–11. doi:10.1016/j.jpeds.2004.06.026.

81. Belkind-Gerson J, Tran K, Di Lorenzo C. Novel techniques to study colonic motor function in children. Curr Gastroenterol Rep. 2013;15(8):335. doi:10.1007/s11894-013-0335-3.

82. Feinberg L, Mahajan L, Steffen R. The constipated child: is there a correlation between symptoms and manometric findings? J Pediatr Gastroenterol Nutr. 2008;47(5):607–11.

83. Dinning PG, Scott SM. Novel diagnostics and therapy of colonic motor disorders. Curr Opin Pharmacol. 2011;11(6):624–9. doi:10.1016/j.coph.2011.10.002.

84. Dinning PG, Di Lorenzo C. Colonic dysmotility in constipation. Best Pract Res Clin Gastroenterol. 2011;25(1):89–101. doi:10.1016/j.bpg.2010.12.006.

85. Giorgio V, Borrelli O, Smith VV, Rampling D, Koglmeier J, Shah N, et al. High-resolution colonic manometry accurately predicts colonic neuromuscular pathological phenotype in pediatric slow

transit constipation. Neurogastroenterol Motil. 2013;25(1):70–8, e78–79. doi:10.1111/nmo.12016.

86. Irastorza I, Ibanez B, Delgado-Sanzonetti L, Maruri N, Vitoria JC. Cow's-milk-free diet as a therapeutic option in childhood chronic constipation. J Pediatr Gastroenterol Nutr. 2010;51(2):171–6. doi:10.1097/MPG.0b013e3181cd2653.

87. Bennett WE, Jr, Heuckeroth RO. Hypothyroidism is a rare cause of isolated constipation. J Pediatr Gastroenterol Nutr. 2012;54(2):285–7. doi:10.1097/MPG.0b013e318239714f.

88. Loening-Baucke V, Miele E, Staiano A. Fiber (glucomannan) is beneficial in the treatment of childhood constipation. Pediatrics. 2004;113(3 Pt 1):e259–64.

89. Castillejo G, Bullo M, Anguera A, Escribano J, Salas-Salvado J. A controlled, randomized, double-blind trial to evaluate the effect of a supplement of cocoa husk that is rich in dietary fiber on colonic transit in constipated pediatric patients. Pediatrics. 2006;118(3):e641–8. doi:10.1542/peds.2006-0090.

90. Kokke FT, Scholtens PA, Alles MS, Decates TS, Fiselier TJ, Tolboom JJ, et al. A dietary fiber mixture versus lactulose in the treatment of childhood constipation: a double-blind randomized controlled trial. J Pediatr Gastroenterol Nutr. 2008;47(5):592–7.

91. Pijpers MA, Tabbers MM, Benninga MA, Berger MY. Currently recommended treatments of childhood constipation are not evidence based: a systematic literature review on the effect of laxative treatment and dietary measures. Arch Dis Child. 2009;94(2):117–31. doi:10.1136/adc.2007.127233.

92. Tabbers MM, Boluyt N, Berger MY, Benninga MA. Nonpharmacologic treatments for childhood constipation: systematic review. Pediatrics. 2011;128(4):753–61. doi:10.1542/peds.2011-0179.

93. Sullivan PB, Alder N, Shrestha B, Turton L, Lambert B. Effectiveness of using a behavioural intervention to improve dietary fibre intakes in children with constipation. J Hum Nutr Diet. 2012;25(1):33–42. doi:10.1111/j.1365-277X.2011.01179.x.

94. Young RJ, Beerman LE, Vanderhoof JA. Increasing oral fluids in chronic constipation in children. Gastroenterol Nurs. 1998;21(4):156–61.

95. van Dijk M, Benninga MA, Grootenhuis MA, Nieuwenhuizen AM, Last BF. Chronic childhood constipation: a review of the literature and the introduction of a protocolized behavioral intervention program. Patient Educ Couns. 2007;67(1–2):63–77. doi:10.1016/j.pec.2007.02.002.

96. Brazzelli M, Griffiths PV, Cody JD, Tappin D. Behavioural and cognitive interventions with or without other treatments for the management of faecal incontinence in children. Cochrane Database Syst Rev. 2011;7(12):CD002240. doi:10.1002/14651858.CD002240.pub4.

97. Wessel S, Benninga MA. Diagnostic testing of defecation disorders. In: Nunez R, Fabbro A, editors. Chronic constipation in children: diagnosis and treatment. New York: Nova Science Publishers Inc.; 2013. pp. 185–98.

98. Borowitz SM, Cox DJ, Kovatchev B, Ritterband LM, Sheen J, Sutphen J. Treatment of childhood constipation by primary care physicians: efficacy and predictors of outcome. Pediatrics. 2005;115(4):873–7. doi:10.1542/peds.2004-0537.

99. Guest JF, Candy DC, Clegg JP, Edwards D, Helter MT, Dale AK, et al. Clinical and economic impact of using macrogol 3350 plus electrolytes in an outpatient setting compared to enemas and suppositories and manual evacuation to treat paediatric faecal impaction based on actual clinical practice in England and Wales. Curr Med Res Opin. 2007;23(9):2213–25. doi:10.1185/0300799 07X210462.

100. Youssef NN, Peters JM, Henderson W, Shultz-Peters S, Lockhart DK, Di Lorenzo C. Dose response of PEG 3350 for the treatment of childhood fecal impaction. J Pediatr. 2002;141(3):410–4. doi:10.1067/mpd.2002.126603.

101. Bekkali NL, van den Berg MM, Dijkgraaf MG, van Wijk MP, Bongers ME, Liem O, et al. Rectal fecal impaction treatment in childhood constipation: enemas versus high doses oral PEG. Pediatrics. 2009;124(6):e1108–1115. doi:10.1542/peds.2009-0022.

102. Rafati M, Karami H, Salehifar E, Karimzadeh A. Clinical efficacy and safety of polyethylene glycol 3350 versus liquid paraffin in the treatment of pediatric functional constipation. Daru. 2011;19(2):154–8.

103. Tolia V, Lin CH, Elitsur Y. A prospective randomized study with mineral oil and oral lavage solution for treatment of faecal impaction in children. Aliment Pharmacol Ther. 1993;7(5):523–9.

104. Perkin JM. Constipation in childhood: a controlled comparison between lactulose and standardized senna. Curr Med Res Opin. 1977;4(8):540–3. doi:10.1185/03007997709115268.

105. Lee-Robichaud H, Thomas K, Morgan J, Nelson RL. Lactulose versus polyethylene glycol for chronic constipation. Cochrane Database Syst Rev. 2010;7(7):CD007570. doi:10.1002/14651858.CD007570.pub2.

106. Berg I, Forsythe I, Holt P, Watts J. A controlled trial of 'Senokot' in faecal soiling treated by behavioural methods. J Child Psychol Psychiatry. 1983;24(4):543–9.

107. Bardisa-Ezcurra L, Ullman R, Gordon J, Guideline Development Group. Diagnosis and management of idiopathic childhood constipation: summary of NICE guidance. BMJ. 2010;340:c2585. doi:10.1136/bmj.c2585.

108. Winter HS, Di Lorenzo C, Benninga MA, Gilger MA, Kearns GL, Hyman PE, et al. Oral prucalopride in children with functional constipation. J Pediatr Gastroenterol Nutr. 2013;57(2):197–203. doi:10.1097/MPG.0b013e318292f9ea.

109. Hyman PE, Di Lorenzo C, Prestridge LL, Youssef NN, Ueno R. An open-label, multicenter, safety and effectiveness study of lubiprostone for the treatment of functional constipation in children. J Pediatr Gastroenterol Nutr. 2013. doi:10.1097/MPG.0000000000000176.

110. Rajindrajith S, Devanarayana NM. Constipation in children: novel insight into epidemiology, pathophysiology and management. J Neurogastroenterol Motil. 2011;17(1):35–47. doi:10.5056/jnm.2011.17.1.35.

111. Benninga MA, Buller HA, Taminiau JA. Biofeedback training in chronic constipation. Arch Dis Child. 1993;68(1):126–9.

112. Wald A, Chandra R, Gabel S, Chiponis D. Evaluation of biofeedback in childhood encopresis. J Pediatr Gastroenterol Nutr. 1987;6(4):554–8.

113. Fandel T, Tanagho EA. Neuromodulation in voiding dysfunction: a historical overview of neurostimulation and its application. Urol Clin North Am. 2005;32(1):1–10. doi:10.1016/j.ucl.2004.09.006.

114. Kamm MA, Dudding TC, Melenhorst J, Jarrett M, Wang Z, Buntzen S, et al. Sacral nerve stimulation for intractable constipation. Gut. 2010;59(3):333–40. doi:10.1136/gut.2009.187989.

115. van Wunnik BP, Peeters B, Govaert B, Nieman FH, Benninga MA, Baeten CG. Sacral neuromodulation therapy: a promising treatment for adolescents with refractory functional constipation. Dis Colon Rectum. 2012;55(3):278–85. doi:10.1097/DCR.0b013e3182405c61.

116. Clarke MC, Catto-Smith AG, King SK, Dinning PG, Cook IJ, Chase JW, et al. Transabdominal electrical stimulation increases colonic propagating pressure waves in paediatric slow transit constipation. J Pediatr Surg. 2012;47(12):2279–84. doi:10.1016/j.jpedsurg.2012.09.021.

117. Leong LC, Yik YI, Catto-Smith AG, Robertson VJ, Hutson JM, Southwell BR. Long-term effects of transabdominal electrical stimulation in treating children with slow-transit constipation. J Pediatr Surg. 2011;46(12):2309–12. doi:10.1016/j.jpedsurg.2011.09.022.

118. Garcia RC, Jimenez MA, Lorente AI. Surgical treatment for chronic constipation in children: Botox in chronic constipation. In: Nunez R, Fabbro A, editors. Chronic constipation in children: diagnosis and treatment. New York: Nova Science Publishers Inc.; 2013. pp. 321–45.

119. Har AF, Rescorla FJ, Croffie JM. Quality of life in pediatric patients with unremitting constipation pre and post Malone antegrade continence enema (MACE) procedure. J Pediatr Surg. 2013;48(8):1733–7. doi:10.1016/j.jpedsurg.2013.01.045.

120. Mugie SM, Machado RS, Mousa HM, Punati JB, Hogan M, Benninga MA, et al. Ten-year experience using antegrade enemas in children. J Pediatr. 2012;161(4):700–4. doi:10.1016/j.jpeds.2012.04.042.

121. Bonilla SF, Flores A, Jackson CC, Chwals WJ, Orkin BA. Management of pediatric patients with refractory constipation who fail cecostomy. J Pediatr Surg. 2013;48(9):1931–5. doi:10.1016/j.jpedsurg.2012.12.034.

122. Rajindrajith S, Devanarayana NM, Benninga MA. Review article: faecal incontinence in children: epidemiology, pathophysiology, clinical evaluation and management. Aliment Pharmacol Ther. 2013;37(1):37–48. doi:10.1111/apt.12103.

123. Rajindrajith S, Devanarayana NM, Benninga MA. Constipation-associated and nonretentive fecal incontinence in children and adolescents: an epidemiological survey in Sri Lanka. J Pediatr Gastroenterol Nutr. 2010;51(4):472–6. doi:10.1097/MPG.0b013e3181d33b7d.

124. van der Wal MF, Benninga MA, Hirasing RA. The prevalence of encopresis in a multicultural population. J Pediatr Gastroenterol Nutr. 2005;40(3):345–8.

125. Joinson C, Heron J, Butler U, von Gontard A, Avon Longitudinal Study of Parents and Children Study Team. Psychological differences between children with and without soiling problems. Pediatrics. 2006;117(5):1575–84. doi:10.1542/peds.2005-1773.

126. Benninga MA, Voskuijl WP, Akkerhuis GW, Taminiau JA, Buller HA. Colonic transit times and behaviour profiles in children with defecation disorders. Arch Dis Child. 2004;89(1):13–6.

127. Benninga MA, Buller HA, Heymans HS, Tytgat GN, Taminiau JA. Is encopresis always the result of constipation? Arch Dis Child. 1994;71(3):186–93.

128. Voskuijl WP, van Ginkel R, Benninga MA, Hart GA, Taminiau JA, Boeckxstaens GE. New insight into rectal function in pediatric defecation disorders: disturbed rectal compliance is an essential mechanism in pediatric constipation. J Pediatr. 2006;148(1):62–7. doi:10.1016/j.jpeds.2005.08.061.

129. Levine MD, Mazonson P, Bakow H. Behavioral symptom substitution in children cured of encopresis. Am J Dis Child. 1980;134(7):663–7.

130. Cox DJ, Morris JB, Jr, Borowitz SM, Sutphen JL. Psychological differences between children with and without chronic encopresis. J Pediatr Psychol. 2002;27(7):585–91.

131. Voskuijl WP, van Ginkel R, Taminiau JA, Boeckxstaens GE, Benninga MA. Loperamide suppositories in an adolescent with childhood-onset functional non-retentive fecal soiling. J Pediatr Gastroenterol Nutr. 2003;37(2):198–200.

132. Voskuijl WP, Reitsma JB, van Ginkel R, Buller HA, Taminiau JA, Benninga MA. Longitudinal follow-up of children with functional nonretentive fecal incontinence. Clin Gastroenterol Hepatol. 2006;4(1):67–72. doi:10.1016/j.cgh.2005.10.001.

Hirschsprung's Disease and Intestinal Neuronal Dysplasias

22

Massimo Martinelli and Annamaria Staiano

Introduction

Hirschsprung's disease (HD) is a heterogeneous genetic disorder, resulting from an anomaly of the enteric nervous system (ENS) of neural crest cells origin. A congenital malformation characterized by the absence of parasympathetic intrinsic ganglion cells in the submucosal and myenteric plexuses, HD is regarded as the consequence of the premature arrest of the craniocaudal migration of vagal neural crest cells in the hindgut, occurring between the 5th and 12th week of gestation, and it is therefore regarded as a neurocristopathy [1].

Epidemiology

HD occurs in approximately 1 out of 5000 live births, with a male predominance of 4:1. It is generally sporadic, although in 3–7 % of cases a genetic transmission has been reported [2]. The risk for short-segment disease is 5 % in brothers and 1 % in sisters of index cases; for long-segment disease, the risk is 10 %, regardless of sex [2].

Etiology

HD is characterized by the congenital absence of ganglion cells in the submucosal and myenteric plexuses in the distal bowel and variable proportion of the colon proximally. The embryonic disorder is a lack of the craniocaudal migration, differentiation, and maturation of neuroblasts from the neural crests, by the 5th–12th week of gestation; the earlier the migration ceases, the longer the aganglionic segment will be.

The aganglionic segment is permanently contracted, causing dilatation proximal to it [3]. HD may be classified according to the length of the aganglionic segment: the classic form (short segment 70–75 % of cases) is limited to the rectum and sigmoid colon; the long segment, or subtotal colonic disease (10–15 %), generally involves the bowel up to the splenic flexure; total colonic aganglionosis (TCA) (3–6 %) may extend to involve a variable amount of the short bowel; and total intestinal aganglionosis, is sometimes associated with intestinal malrotation or volvulus [2]. Ultrashort-segment aganglionosis is considered a functional alteration, without any detectable histological finding. Although longer aganglionic segments tend to produce more dramatic symptoms, some patients with even short-segment disease deteriorate rapidly [4].

Pathophysiology

The hallmark of diagnosis is the absence of ganglion cells from the myenteric and submucosal plexuses, as seen on a full-thickness or suction (mucosal–submucosal) biopsy of the rectum. Proximal contents fail to enter the unrelaxed, aganglionic segment. The lack of non-adrenergic–non-cholinergic inhibitory innervation is responsible for a tonic contraction of the affected segment, with absence of peristalsis and proximal dilation of the gut [5].

Morphologically, ganglionic cells are absent from the narrowed segment and for some distance (1–5 cm usually) into the dilated segment. The pattern of nerve fibers is abnormal also; they are hypertrophic with abundant, thickened bundles. Specific stains for acetylcholinesterase are used to highlight the abnormal morphology [6, 7].

In recent years, new insights in the pathophysiology of HD have been gained. There is a growing consensus that the disease might be the expression of a genetic alteration, as reported in the genetic section of this chapter.

It has also been suggested that abnormal expression of muscular neural cell adhesion molecule is likely to be

A. Staiano (✉) · M. Martinelli
Department of Translational Medical Sciences, Section of Pediatrics, University of Naples "Federico II", Via S. Pansini 5, 80131 Naples, Italy
e-mail: staiano@unina.it

S. Guandalini et al. (eds.), *Textbook of Pediatric Gastroenterology, Hepatology and Nutrition*,
DOI 10.1007/978-3-319-17169-2_22

associated with an arrest in the craniocaudal migration of neural cells to their most distal location [8]. Furthermore, the lack of nitric oxide (NO)-producing nerve fibers in the aganglionic intestine probably contributes to the inability of the smooth muscle to relax, thereby causing lack of peristalsis [9]. In addition, in the aganglionic segments, interstitial cells of Cajal (ICC) are scarce and their network appears to be disrupted [10].

Genetics

HD occurs as an isolated trait in 70% of patients, is associated with chromosomal abnormality in 12% of cases, trisomy 21 being by far the most frequent (>90%). Additional congenital anomalies are found in 18% of cases, including gastrointestinal malformation, cleft palate, polydactyly, cardiac septal defects, and craniofacial anomalies. The higher rate of associated anomalies in familial cases than in isolated cases (39 vs. 21%) strongly suggests syndromes with Mendelian inheritance [2]. Isolated HD appears to be a multifactorial malformation with low, sex-dependent penetrance, variable expression according to the length of the aganglionic segment, and suggesting the involvement of one or more gene(s) with low penetrance [2]. These parameters must be taken into account for accurate evaluation of the recurrence risk in relatives. Segregation analyses suggested an oligogenic mode of inheritance in isolated HD. With a relative risk as high as 200, HD is an excellent model for the approach to common multifactorial diseases [11].

A large number of chromosomal anomalies have been described in HD patients. Free trisomy 21 (Down syndrome) is by far the most frequent, involving 2–10% of ascertained HD cases. Syndromes associated with HD can be classified as pleiotropic neurocristopathies [1], syndromes with HD as a mandatory feature, and occasional association with recognizable syndromes. The neural crest is a transient and multipotent embryonic structure that gives rise to neuronal, endocrine and paraendocrine, craniofacial, conotruncal heart, and pigmentary tissues. Neurocristopathies encompass tumors, malformations, and single- or multifocal abnormalities of tissues mentioned above in various combinations. Multiple endocrine neoplasia type 2 (MEN 2) and Waardenburg syndrome (WS) are the most frequent neurocristopathies associated with HD [12, 13].

WS, an autosomal dominant condition, is by far the most frequent condition combining pigmentary anomalies and sensorineural deafness, resulting from the absence of melanocytes of the skin and the stria vascularis of the cochlea. The combination of HD with WS defines the WS4 type (Shah–Waardenburg syndrome). Indeed, homozygous mutations of the endothelin pathway and heterozygous SRY-related box 10 (SOX 10) mutations have been identified in WS4 patients

with central nervous system (CNS) involvement including seizures, ataxia, and demyelinating peripheral and central neuropathies [14].

A wide spectrum of additional isolated anomalies has been described among HD cases with an incidence of sporadic types varying from 5 to 30% [2, 15]. No constant pattern is observed. These anomalies include distal limb, sensorineural, skin, gastrointestinal, central nervous system, genital, kidney, cardiac malformations, and facial dysmorphic features.

These data highlight the importance of a careful assessment by a clinician trained in dysmorphology for all newborns diagnosed with HD. Skeletal X ray and cardiac and urogenital echographic survey should be systematically performed. The observation of one additional anomaly to HD should prompt chromosomal studies.

Molecular Genetics

Several genes have been implicated in isolated HD; the two major ones being the proto-oncogene *RET (RET)* and the endothelin B receptor *(EDNRB)* [2].

The RET Signaling Pathway

The first observation was about an interstitial deletion of chromosome 10q11.2 in patients with TCA and mental retardation [16]. The proto-oncogene *RET*, identified as disease causing in MEN 2 and mapping in 10q11.2, was regarded as a good candidate gene owing to the concurrence of MEN 2A and HD in some families and the expression in neural crest-derived cells. Consequently, *RET* gene mutations were identified in HD patients [17]. Expression and penetrance of an *RET* mutation are variable and sex dependent within HD families (72% males and 51% females). Over 100 mutations have been identified including large deletions encompassing the *RET* gene, microdeletions and insertions, nonsense, missense, and splicing mutations [18–20]. Haploinsufficiency is the most likely mechanism for HD mutations. Biochemical studies showed variable consequences of some HD mutations (misfolding, failure to transport the protein to the cell surface, abolished biological activity).

Despite extensive mutation screening, an *RET* mutation is identified in only 50% of familial and 15–20% of sporadic HD case [21]. However, most families with few exceptions are compatible with linkage at the *RET* locus [22]. Mutations in RET ligand, like glial cell-derived neurotrophic factor (GDNF), GDNF family receptor α (GFRA)1–4, neurturin (NTN), persephin *(PSPN)*, and artemin (ARTN), may occur, but are not sufficient to lead to HD.

The Endothelin Signaling Pathway

A susceptibility locus for HD in 13q22 was suggested for three main reasons: a significant load score at 13q22 in a large inbred Old Order Mennonite community with multiple cases of HD; de novo interstitial deletion of 13q22 in several patients with HD; and syntony between the murine locus for *piebald-lethal (sl)*, a model of aganglionosis, and 13q22 in humans. Subsequently, an *EDNRB* missense mutation was identified in the Mennonite kindred (W276C) [23, 24]. Both *EDNRB* and *EDN3* were screened in large series of isolated HD patients and *EDNRB* mutations were identified in approximately 5 % of the patients. It is worth mentioning that the penetrance of *EDN3* and *EDNRB* heterozygous mutations is incomplete in those HD patients, de novo mutations have not hitherto been observed, and that S-HD is largely predominant [25].

SOX10

The last de novo mouse model for WS4 in human is *dominant megalon (Dom)*. The *Dom* gene is *Sox10*, a member of the SRY (sex-determining factor)-like, high mobility group (HMG) DNA-binding proteins. Subsequently, heterozygous *SOX10* mutations have been identified in familial and isolated patients with WS4 (including de novo mutation) with high penetrance [26].

Clinical Signs/Symptoms

The clinical symptoms of HD usually start at birth with the delayed passage of meconium. More than 90 % of term neonates, and < 10 % of children with HD, pass meconium in the first 24 h of life [27, 28]. Thus, HD must be suspected in any full-term infant who does not pass meconium in the first 24 h of life and in the premature infants who have excessively delayed the passage of meconium (7–8 days) [28]. Failure of the distal bowel to relax and allow the passage of stool leads to functional obstruction and secondary dilatation of the bowel proximal to the aganglionic segment. Affected children may present with severe dysmotility causing obstructive symptoms, ribbon-like stools, and frequently, failure to thrive. In > 90 % of affected patients, the symptoms start during the neonatal period and, in the majority, the diagnosis is made during the first 3 months of life, whereas < 1 % are diagnosed during adult life [29].

In infants and children, the presentation is often less dramatic and may not mimic acute intestinal obstruction. Severe constipation and recurrent fecal impaction are more common. Physical examination reveals a distended abdomen and a contracted anal sphincter and rectum in most children. The rectum is devoid of stool except in cases of short-segment aganglionosis. As the finger is withdrawn, there may be an explosive discharge of foul-smelling liquid stools, with decompression of the proximal normal bowel.

Complications

Over the past four decades, enterocolitis has been a major cause of morbidity and mortality in infants and children with HD. The mean incidence is 25 %, but the range is great (from 17 to 50 %) and may be differently estimated depending on the manner in which it is diagnosed. Mortality rates range from 0 to 33 %, probably reflecting differences in the diagnostic criteria [30]. Mortality also appears to be associated with other factors, such as trisomy 21. Pathogenesis is thought to be related to fecal stasis with proliferation of colonic bacteria, and, therefore, a delayed HD diagnosis seems to be a significant risk factor [31]. The classic clinical manifestations described for enterocolitis include abdominal distension, explosive diarrhea, vomiting, fever, lethargy, rectal bleeding, and shock [32]. Abdominal radiographs show the Intestinal "cutoff" sign in the rectosigmoidal region with absence of air distally. Other common findings are small bowel dilatation in 74 % and multiple air-fluid levels [33]. Because of the risk of perforation, contrast enema should not be performed in the presence of clinical enterocolitis.

Postoperative enterocolitis has been associated with fairly high rate of mortality in several series. In fact, when examining the deaths related to HD, several groups found that approximately 50 % of deaths resulted from complications directly related to an enterocolitis episode [34, 35].

Rectal washouts should be the initial approach in the care of a child, regardless of age, who presents with enterocolitis. Along with washouts, intravenous antibiotics or oral metronidazole (in mild cases) should be used. Should the disease process fail to improve, or the infants' condition deteriorates, the performance of a leveling colostomy should be considered [34, 35].

Diagnosis

For diagnosis of HD, the subjects' history is crucial. The main elements to obtain are the age of the appearance of symptoms, whether the passage of meconium has been normal or delayed; and whether the child presented with episodes of functional intestinal obstruction. In addition, a functional (idiopathic) megacolon must be ruled out. A clinical comparison of functional and congenital megacolon is reported in Table 22.1 [36]. When the history (early onset of constipation, absence of fecal soiling) and/or the physical

Table 22.1 Differentiating types of megacolon in children. (Reprinted with permission from Ref. [36], Table 17.1, p. 261)

Signs and symptoms	Functional fecal retention (acquired)	Colonic neuromuscolar disorders (congenital)
Soiling	Common	Rare
Obstructive symptoms	Rare	Common
Large-caliber stools	Common	Rare
Stool-withholding behavior	Common	Rare
Enterocolitis	Never	Possible
Associated upper-GI symptoms	Never	Common
Symptoms from birth	Rare	Common
Localization of stools	Rectum	Rectal and extra-rectal

examination (empty rectal ampulla) suggest an organic cause, anorectal manometry (ARM) should be performed. ARM evaluates the response of the internal anal sphincter to inflation of a balloon in the rectal ampulla [37]. When the rectal balloon is inflated, there is normally a reflex relaxation of the sphincter. The rectoanal inhibitory reflex is absent in patients with HD; there is no relaxation, or there may even be paradoxical contraction of the internal anal sphincter (Fig. 22.1) [36]. Although the absence of the rectoanal inhibitory reflex is specific for the diagnosis of HD, the role of ARM is still debated. A recent comprehensive systematic review by de Lorijn et al. [38] compared the diagnostic accuracy among rectal suction biopsy (RSB), ARM, and Barium enema (BE) for the diagnosis of HD. Although RSB gave the highest mean sensitivity and specificity (93 and 98 %, respectively) ARM showed similar values (91 and 94 %). ARM has the advantages of being a less-invasive method without the exposure to ionizing radiation. The limitations include the need for the patient to be in a normal physiologic and quiet state to avoid possible artifacts [38, 39]. Because specificity is lower for ARM compared with RSB [38], ARM cannot reliably replace histology and biopsies. A recent practical guidelines published by ESPGHAN GI committee stated ARM should not be used as a sole diagnostic tool for

HD in neonates and infants [40]; however; ARM is a useful screening test in older children presenting with chronic constipation and further symptoms suggesting HD (empty rectal ampulla, nonresponsiveness to standard therapy, early-onset constipation). If the rectoanal inhibitory reflex is absent, these patients should be referred for RSB to confirm the diagnosis of HD. If the rectoanal inhibitory reflex is present, HD could be reasonably excluded [40]. BE is helpful in the assessment of a transition zone between aganglionic and ganglionic bowel and giving an estimation of the length of an aganglionic segment. Demonstration of the transition zone is easier if no effort is made to cleanse the bowel (Fig. 22.2) [36]. In the newborn, dilatation of the proximal ganglionic bowel may not have developed, and radiological diagnosis may be more difficult. The sensitivity and specificity for recognition of a transition zone have been reported to be 80 and 76 %, respectively [41]. The BE may not show a transition zone in cases of total colonic HD, or the BE may be indistinguishable from cases of functional constipation when ultra-short-segment HD is present. Therefore, a BE should not be performed as an initial diagnostic tool because it does not represent a valid alternative to RSB or ARM to exclude or diagnose HD; however, BE may have some use as an additional investigation in diagnosed cases to assess the length of the rectosigmoid aganglionic segment before surgery [40]. Nevertheless, the diagnosis requires histological evidence. The easiest means of obtaining adequate diagnostic tissue in rectal biopsies in infants is by rectal suction biopsy [42]. An accurate diagnosis is only possible if 2–3 suction biopsies are taken 2–3 cm above the dentate line and if they include sufficient submucosa [43]. Biopsies taken closer to the dentate line may be misleading because of a normal zone of submucosal hypoganglionosis or even aganglionosis [43]. The histological diagnosis is based on the demonstration of the total absence of ganglionic cells in the affected segment of the intestine with an overgrowth of large nerve trunks in the intermuscular and submucosal zone (Figs. 22.3 and 22.4) [36]. Acetylcholinesterase (AchE) activity in normal colon shows only few fibers in the lamina propria and muscularis mucosae; in HD, there is an increase in thick, knotted acetylcholinesterase-positive nerve fibers in the muscularis mucosae and lamina propria and hypertrophied nerve trunks in the submucosa. Techniques for histopathological diagnosis

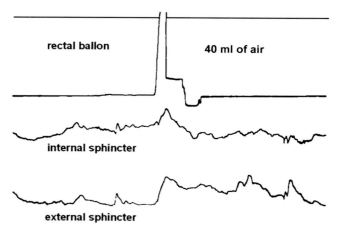

rectal ballon   40 ml of air

internal sphincter

external sphincter

Fig. 22.1 Anorectal manometry in a 1-month-old boy with Hirschsprung's disease. Distention of a rectal balloon with air for 1 s produces no decrease of anal pressure. (Reprinted with permission from Ref. [36], Fig. 17.2, p. 262)

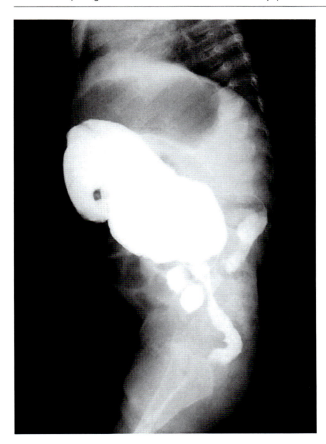

Fig. 22.2 Barium enema showing a long, narrowed segment in a child with Hirschsprung's disease. (Reprinted with permission from Ref. [36], Fig. 17.3, p. 262)

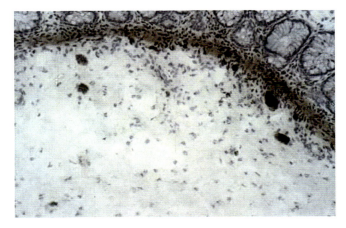

Fig. 22.3 Rectal suction biopsy in a child with functional constipation. Note the presence of clusters of neuron in the submucosa and acetyl-cholinesterase activity showing only few wispy fibers. (Reprinted with permission from Ref. [36], Fig. 17.4, p. 263)

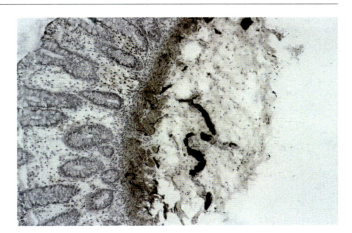

Fig. 22.4 Intense acetylcholinesterase activity in a patient with Hirschsprung's disease. Note the absence of neurons and the presence of increase in thick-knotted nerve fibers in the muscularis mucosae and lamina propria. In addition, hypertrophied nerve trunks are visible in the submucosa. (Reprinted with permission from Ref. [36], Fig. 17.5, p. 263)

firmly recommend one approach over the other; although, the combination of AchE and H&E staining increases the diagnostic accuracy because it improves the identification of submucosal ganglion cells, as well as demonstrates the abnormal nerve fiber distribution in the left colon [43]. The potential value of immunohistochemistry has been evaluated in a number of studies. Calretinin is an immunohistochemical marker that may be a potential alternative to AchE [44, 45]. Calretinin is normally present in the perikarya and nerve processes of a subset of enteric ganglion cells. Immunoreactivity is lost in the aganglionic segment of HD [45]. A recent comparative study shows that calretinin is as sensitive and specific as AchE [46]. However, further studies are needed to confirm calretinin immunostaining as a new standard for diagnosis.

Treatment

The treatment of HD consists of resecting the aganglionic segment of the rectum and colon, pulling down normally innervated bowel, and anastomosing this bowel at the anorectal region, while preserving the sphincter muscle. The past decades have seen an evolution in the surgical management of HD. The previous gold standard of two- or three-stage pull through with a preliminary stoma has slowly been progressively replaced by a one-stage approach in many centers [47–50]. More recently, minimally invasive approaches to the one-stage pull through have become popular. These consist of pull throughs utilizing laparoscopic abdominal and pelvic mobilization of the rectum and the transanal Soave procedure, which does not include any intra-abdominal dissection [47–53]. The one-stage approach, either by laparotomy or

include analysis of hematoxylin- and eosin (H&E)-stained paraffin sections, snap-frozen sections stained for AchE, and immunostaining for neuronal markers. A recent consensus by Knowles et al. stated that insufficient data exist to

by combined laparoscopy and transanal dissection, has been advocated even in the newborn period.

The results of the one-stage approach in small infants appear to be at least as favorable as those in which a staged procedure with a colostomy was used. Recently, the use of the one-stage definitive procedure for small infants with HD has increased. One-stage pull-through procedures using laparoscopy appear to be associated with shorter hospital stays, shorter time until full feeding is reached, and superior cosmetic results [51–53].

Short- and Long-Term Prognosis

Despite adequate resection of the aganglionic segment, some patients may continue to have persistent bowel dysfunction. Postoperative bowel dysfunction includes constipation, fecal incontinence, and a continuous risk of enterocolitis. An altered distribution and impaired function of ICC, resulting in defective generation of electrical pacemaker activity, have been suggested to be one of the mechanisms contributing to dysmotility in patients operated on for HD [54]. Investigations include barium studies to delineate strictures or leaks and further biopsy to exclude residual aganglionic bowel. If the definitive operation fails because of an impassable stricture, disruption, or residual disease, further secondary surgery may be necessary, and a different operation may then lead to an acceptable result. Data are accumulating to indicate that HD, a disorder once known and recognized exclusively to involve an aganglionic segment of distal colon, also affects motor function in other parts of the gut. The variability in manifestations could reflect the heterogeneity of basic genetic defects now recognized as being responsible for the phenotypic expression of HD. Abnormalities in esophageal motility are common, and duodenal motor dysfunction is present in 48 % of patients [5].

Miele et al. have reported a systematic study of various aspects of gastrointestinal motor function in children with HD long after removal of the aganglionic colonic segment, observing gastrointestinal symptoms, including vomiting, distension, and poor growth, persisted long after surgery [55]. Abnormalities in duodenal motor activity have also been observed in these children shortly after operation [56].

Intestinal Neuronal Dysplasia

Intestinal neuronal dysplasia (IND) or hyperganglionosis, a condition that clinically resembles HD, was first described by Meier-Ruge in 1971 [57]. It is often associated with HD and may cause failure of clinical improvement after resectional pull-through surgery. In 1983, Fadda et al. classified IND into two clinically and histologically distinguished sub-types, called type A and B. Type A occurs in less than 5 % of cases and is characterized by congenital aplasia or hypoplasia of the sympathetic innervation, presenting acutely in neonatal period with episodes of intestinal obstruction, diarrhea, and bloody stools. Type B, which is clinically indistinguishable from HD, is characterized by a malformation of the parasympathetic submucosal plexus and accounts for more than 95 % of cases of isolated IND [58].

The incidence of isolated IND varies from 0.3 to 40 % of all suction rectal biopsies [59]. The incidence varies considerably among different countries; some investigators have reported that 25–35 % of patients with HD have associated IND [58, 60]. However, others rarely encountered IND in association with HD [61]. Part of this discrepancy may be due to the persisting confusion over the essential diagnostic criteria. For a long time, IND has been diagnosed on the basis of four histological criteria applied to acetylcholinesterase-stained suction rectal biopsies. In 1991, on the recommendations of a working party (the Consensus of German Pathologists), Bouchard et al. published diagnostic criteria for IND using suction rectal biopsy specimen. These comprised two obligatory criteria: hyperplasia of the submucosal plexus and an increase in acetylcholinesterase-positive nerve fibers in the adventitia around submucosal blood vessels. Two additional criteria might be used: neuronal heterotopia and increased acetylcholinesterase-positive nerve fibers in the lamina propria [62]. The latest morphometric criteria are summarized as follows: >8 neurons/ganglion (so-called giant ganglia) in >20 % of a minimum of 25 submucosal ganglia in patients older than 1 year [63]. However, concern has been expressed whether IND can be safely diagnosed by mucosal and submucosal alteration alone, without myenteric plexus abnormalities. Submucosal hyperganglionosis may reflect a normal age-related phenomenon due to immaturity, with clinical and histochemical normalization after the first year of life. Furthermore, it has been reported that most of the patients with submucosal IND have a spontaneous clinical improvement which is sometimes associated with histological normalization [64, 65]. To date submucosal IND has been reported in several disorders such as intestinal malformations, meconium plug syndrome, cystic fibrosis, gastroschisis, pyloric stenosis, and inflammatory processes involving the gut. The high frequency of histological abnormalities in young infants may represent a normal variant of postnatal development rather than a pathological process. Investigations using more refined and morphometric methods in rectal specimens from infants and children without bowel disease are needed to define the normal range for different ages [65]. Therefore, most of the evidence suggests that the histological appearance of so-called IND is a normal variant related to age. Owing to the lack of sufficient normative data, IND remains a histological description with poorly established clinical significance [40, 43]. Patients with IND have been subjected to multiple types of treatment; however, the majority of patients with IND can be treated conservatively. If bowel symptoms persist after at least 6 months of conservative treatment, internal sphincter myectomy should be considered. The rapid AchE technique has been found to be of great value in determining the extent of IND intraoperatively [66].

Genetic Aspects

Studies have been performed to investigate the potential role of HD-associated *RET, GDNF, EDNRB,* and *EDN3* genes in the development of IND. They demonstrated that only three RET mutations were detected in patients with HD, no mutation in this gene was observed in IND, and mixed HD/IND patients, HD, and HD/IND patients showed overrepresentation of a specific RET polymorphism in exon 2, while IND patients exhibited a significantly lower frequency of the same polymorphism comparable with that of controls. These findings may suggest that IND is genetically different from HD.

A homozygous mutation of the *EDNRB* gene in spotting lethal (sl/sl) rats leads to HD phenotype with long-segmented aganglionosis. The heterozygous (+/sl) *EDNRB*-deficient rats revealed more subtle abnormalities of the ENS: The submucosal plexus was characterized by a significantly increased ganglionic size and density and the presence of hypertrophied nerve fiber strands, resembling the histopathological criteria for IND. Other animal model, like Ncx/Hox11L.1-deficient mice, suggests that many other genes could be involved in the pathogenesis of IND [67].

References

1. Taviras S, Pachinis V. Development of the mammalian enteric system. Curr Opin Genet Dev. 1999;9:321.
2. Amiel J, Sproat-Emison E, Garcia-Barcelo M, et al. Hirschsprung disease, associated syndromes and genetics: a review. J Med Genet. 2008;45:1–14.
3. Gershon MD, Chalazonitis A, Rothman TP. From neural crest to bowel: development of the enteric nervous system. J Neurobiol. 1993;24:199–214.
4. Badner JA, Sieber Wk, Garver KL, et al. A genetic study of Hirschsprung's disease. Am J Hum Genet. 1990;46:568–80.
5. Staiano A, Corazziari E, Andreotti MR, Clouse RE. Esophageal motility in children with Hirschsprung's disease. Am J Dis Child. 1991;145:310–3.
6. Larsson LT, Shen Z, Ekbland E, Sundler F, Alm P, Andersson KE. Lack of neuronal nitric oxide synthase in nerve fibers of aganglionic intestine: a clue to Hirschsprung's disease. J Pediatr Gastroenterol Nutr. 1995;20:49–53.
7. Lake BD, Puri P, Nixon HH, Claireaux AE. Hirschsprung's disease. An appraisal of histochemically demonstrated acetylcholinesterase activity in suction rectal biopsy specimens as an aid to diagnosis. Arch Path Lab Med. 1978;26:288–91.

8. Romanska HM, Bishop AE, Brereton RJ, Spitz L, Polak JM. Increased expression of muscolar neural cell adhesion molecule in congenital aganglionosis. Gastroenterology. 1993;105(4):1104–9.
9. Vanderwinden JM, De Laet MH, Schiffmann SN, et al. Nitric oxide synthase distribution in the enteric nervous system of Hirschsprung's disease. Gastroenterology. 1993;105:969–73.
10. Vanderwinden JM, Rumessen JJ, Liu H, Descamps D, De Laet MH, Vanderhaeghen JJ. Interstitial cells of cajal in humen colon and in Hirschsprung's disease. Gastroenterology. 1996;111:901–10.
11. Brooks A, Oostra B, Hofstra R. Studying the genetics of Hirschsprung's disease: unraveling an oligogenic disorder. Clin Genet. 2005;67:6–14.
12. Decker RA, Peacock ML, Watson P. Hirschsprung disease in MEN 2A: increased spectrum of RET exon 10 genotypes and strong genotype-phenotype correlation. Hum Mol Genet. 1998;7:129–34.
13. Cohen MS, Phay JE, Albinson C, et al. Gastrointestinal manifestations of multiple endocrine neoplasia type 2. Ann Surg. 2002;235:648–54, discussion 54–5.
14. Edery P, Attie T, Amiel J, Pelet A, et al. Mutation of the endothelin-3 gene in the Waardenburg–Hirschsprung disease (Shah–Waardenburg syndrome). Nat Genet. 1996;12:442–4.
15. Auricchio A, Griseri P, Carpentieri ML, et al. Double heterozygosity for a RET substitution interfering with splicing and an EDNRB missense mutation in Hirschsprung disease. Am J Hum Genet. 1999;64:1216–21.
16. Edery P, Lyonnet S, Mulligan LM, et al. Mutations of the RET protooncogene in Hirschsprung's disease. Nature. 1994;367:378–80.
17. Angrist M, Bolk S, Thiel B, et al. Mutation analysis of the RET receptor tyrosine kinase in Hirschsprung disease. Hum Mol Genet. 1995;4:821–30.
18. Seri M, Yin L, Barone V, Bolino A, et al. Frequency of RET mutations in long- and short-segment Hirschsprung disease. Hum Mutat. 1997;9:243–9.
19. Attie T, Pelet A, Edery P, et al. Diversity of RET proto-oncogene mutations in familial and sporadic Hirschsprung disease. Hum Mol Genet. 1995;4:1381–6.
20. Hofstra RM, Wu Y, Stulp RP, et al. RET and GDNF gene scanning in Hirschsprung patients using two dual denaturing gel systems. Hum Mutat. 2000;15:418–29.
21. Bolk S, Pelet A, Hofstra RM, et al. A human model for multigenic inheritance: phenotypic expression in Hirschsprung disease requires both the RET gene and a new 9q31 locus. Proc Natl Acad Sci U S A. 2000;97:268–73.
22. Borrego S, Eng C, Sanchez B, Saez ME, Navarro E, Antinolo G. Molecular analysis of the ret and GDNF genes in a family with multiple endocrine neoplasia type 2A and Hirschsprung disease. J Clin Endocrinol Metab. 1998;83:3361–4.
23. Kiss P, Orsztovics M. Association of 13q deletion and Hirschsprung's disease. J Med Genet. 1989;26:793–4.
24. Puffenberger EG, Hosoda K, Washington SS, et al. A missense mutation of endothelin-B receptor gene in multigenic Hirschsprung's disease. Nat Genet. 1996;14:345–7.
25. Auricchio A, Casari G, Staiano A, Ballabio A. Endothelin-B receptor mutations in patients with isolated Hirschsprung disease from a non-inbred population. Hum Mol Genet. 1996;5:351–4.
26. Southard-Smith EM, Angrist M, Eleison JS, et al. The Sox10 (Dom) mouse: modeling the genetic variation of Waardenburg–Shah (WS4) syndrome. Genom Res. 1999;9:215–25.
27. Clark DA. Times of first void and first stool in 500 newborns. Pediatrics. 1977;60:457–9.
28. Bekkali N, Hamers SL, Schipperus MR, et al. Duration of meconium passage in preterm and term infants. Arch Dis Child Fetal Neonatal Ed. 2008;93:F376–9.
29. Barnes PR, Lennard-Jones JE, Hawley PR, et al. Hirschsprung's disease and idiopathic megacolon in adults and adolescents. Gut 1986;27:534–41.

30. Coran AG, Teitelbaum DH, Recent advances in management of Hirschsprung's disease. The Am J Surg. 2000;180:382–7.

31. Bill JAH, Chapman ND. The enterocolitis of Hirschsprung's disease: its natural history and treatment. Am J Surg. 1962;103:70–4.

32. Elhalaby EA, Coran AG, Blane CE, et al. Enterocolitis associated with Hirschsprung's disease: a clinical-radiological characterization based on 168 patients. J Pediatr Surg. 1995;30:1023–7.

33. Swenson O, Fisher JH. Hirschsprung's disease during infancy. Surg Clin N Am. 1956;36:115–22.

34. Murphy F, Puri P. New insights into the pathogenesis of Hirschsprung's associated enterocolitis. Pediatr Surg Int. 2005;21:773–9.

35. Marty TL, Matlak ME, Hendrickson M, et al. Unexpected death from enterocolitis after surgery for Hirschsprung's disease. Pediatrics. 1995;96:118–21.

36. Staiano A, Quaglietta L, Auricchio R. Hirschsprung's disease and intestinal neuronal dysplasias. In: Guandalini S, editor. Textbook of pediatric gastroenterology and nutrition. London: Taylor & Francis; 2004. pp. 259–68.

37. Loening-Baucke V. Modulation of abnormal defecation dynamics by biofeedback treatment in chronically constipated children with encopresis. J Pediatr. 1990;116:214–22.

38. de Lorijn F, Kremer LC, Reitsma JB, et al. Diagnostic tests in Hirschsprung disease: a systematic review. J Pediatr Gastroenterol Nutr. 2006;42:496–505.

39. Jarvi K, Koivusalo A, Rintala RJ, et al. Anorectal manometry with reference to operative rectal biopsy for the diagnosis/exclusion of Hirschprung's disease in children under 1 year of age. Int J Colorectal Dis. 2009;24:451–4.

40. Schappi MG, Staiano A, Milla PJ, et al. A practical guide for the diagnosis of primary enteric nervous system disorders. J Pediatr Gastroenterol Nutr. 2013;57:677–86.

41. Taxman TI, Yulish BS, Rothstein FC. How useful is barium enema in diagnosis of infantile Hirschsprung's disease? Am j Dis Child. 1986;140:881–4.

42. Scudiere JR, Maitra A, Montgomery EA. Selected topics in the evaluation of pediatric gastrointestinal mucosal biopsies. Adv Anat Pathol. 2009;16:154–60.

43. Knowles CH, De Giorgio R, Kapur RP, et al. Gastrointestinal neuromuscular pathology: guidelines for histological techniques and reporting on behalf of the Gastro 2009 International Working Group. Acta Neuropathol. 2009;118:271–301.

44. Kapur R, Reed R, Finn L, et al. Calretinin immunohistochemistry versus acetylcholinesterase histochemistry in the evaluation of suction rectal biopsies for Hirschsprung disease. Pediatr Dev Pathol. 2009;12:6–15.

45. Guinard-Samuel V, Bonnard A, De Lagausie P, et al. Calretinin immunohistochemistry: a simple and efficient tool to diagnose Hirschsprung disease. Mod Pathol. 2009;22:1379–84.

46. Holland SK, Ramalingam P, Podolsky RH, et al. Calretinin immunostaining as an adjunct in the diagnosis of Hirschsprung disease. Ann Diagn Pathol. 2011;15:323–8.

47. Langer JC, Fitzgerald PG, Winthrop AL, et al. One vs two stage Soave pull-through for Hirschsprung'disease in the first year of life. J Pediatr Surg. 1996;31:33–7.

48. Weidner BC, Waldhausen JH. Swenson revisited: a one-stage, transanal pull-through procedure for Hirschsprung's disease. J Pediatr Surg. 2003;38:1208–11.

49. Elhalaby EA, Hashish A, Elbarbary MM, et al. Transanal one-stage endorectal pull-through for Hirschsprung's disease: a multicenter study. J Pediatr Surg. 2004;39:345–51, discussion 345–51.

50. Aslanabadi S, Ghalehgolab-Behbahan A, Zarrintan S, Jamshidi M, Seyyedhejazi M. Transanal one-stage endorectal pull-through for Hirschsprung's disease: comparison with the staged procedures. Pediatr Surg Int. 2008;24:925–9.

51. Cheung ST, Tam YH, Chong HM, et al. An 18-year experience in total colonic aganglionosis: from staged operations to primary laparoscopic endorectal pull-through. J Pediatr Surg. 2009;44:2352–4.

52. Ammar SA, Ibrahim IA. One-stage transanal endorectal pull-through for treatment of Hirschsprung's disease in adolescents and adults. J Gastrointest Surg. 2011;15:2246–50.

53. van de Ven TJ, Sloots CE, Wijnen MH, et al. Transanal endorectal pull-through for classic segment Hirschsprung's disease: with or without laparoscopic mobilization of the rectosigmoid? J Pediatr Surg. 2013;48:1914–8.

54. Rolle U, Piotrowska A, Nemeth L, et al. Altered distribution of interstitial cells of Cajal in Hirschsprung's disease. Arch Pathol Lab Med. 2002;126:928–33.

55. Miele E, Tozzi A, Staiano A, Toraldo C, Esposito C, Clouse RE. Persistence of abnormal gastrointestinal motility operation for Hirschsprung's disease. Am J Gastr. 2000;95:1226–30.

56. Di Lorenzo C, Flores AF, Reddy SN, et al. Small bowel neurophaty in symptomatic children after surgery for Hirschsprung's disease. Gastroenterology 1997;112:783A.

57. Meier-Ruge W. Casuistic of colon disorder with symptoms of Hirschsprung's disease (author's transl). Verh Dtsch Ges Pathol. 1971;55:506–10.

58. Fadda B, Meier WA, Meier-Ruge W, et al. Neuronale intestinale Dysplasie: Eine Kritische 10-Jahres-Analyse Klinischer und Bioptischer Diagnostik. Z Kinderchir. 1983;38:305–11.

59. Smith VV. Isolated intestinal neuronal dysplasia: a descriptive pattern or a distinct clinicopathological entity? In: Hadziselimomic F, Herzog B, editors. Inflammatory bowel disease and morbus hirschsprung. Dordrect: Kluwer Academic; 1992. pp. 203–14.

60. Kobayashi H, Hirakawa H, Surana R, et al. Intestinal neuronal dysplasia is a possible cause of persistant bowel symptoms after pull-trough operation for Hirschsprung's disease. J Pediatr Surg. 1995;30:253–9.

61. Fadda B, Pistor G, Meier-Ruge W, et al. Symptoms, diagnosis and therapy of neuronal intestinal dysplasia masked by Hirschsprung's disease. J Pediatr Surg. 1987;2:76–80.

62. Borchard F, Meier-ruge W, Wiebecke B, et al. Innervations strunger des Dickdarms- Klassifikation und Diagnostik. Pathologie. 1991;12:171–4.

63. Knowles CH, De Giorgio R, Kapur RP, et al. The London classification of gastrointestinal neuromuscular pathology: report on behalf of the Gastro 2009 International Working Group. Gut. 2010;59:882–7.

64. Cord-Udy CL, Smith VV, Ahmed S, Ridson RA, Milla PJ. An evaluation of the role of suction rectal biopsy in the diagnosis of intestinal neuronal dysplasia. J Pediatr Gastroenterol Nutr. 1997;24:1–6.

65. Koletzko S, Jesch I, Faus-Kebetaler T, et al. Rectal biopsy for diagnosis of intestinal neuronal dysplasia in children: a prospective multicentre study on interobserver variation and clinical outcome. Gut. 1999;44:853–61.

66. Kobayashi H, O'Briain S, Hirakawa H, et al. A rapid tecnique for acetylcolinesterase stainig. Arch Pathol Lab Med. 1994;118:1127–9.

67. Yamataka A, Datano M, Kobayashi H, et al. Intestinal neuronal displasia-like pathology in Ncx/Hox11L.1 deficient mice. J Pediatr Surg. 2001;36:1293–6.

Chronic Intestinal Pseudo-Obstruction in Childhood

23

Efstratios Saliakellis, Osvaldo Borrelli and Nikhil Thapar

Introduction

The term pseudo-obstruction literally denotes the absence of a true mechanical occlusion. Intestinal pseudo-obstruction can be either acute or chronic in nature, reflecting the duration of obstructive symptoms, being shorter or longer than 6 months, respectively [1, 2]. Chronic intestinal pseudo-obstruction (CIPO) was first described in 1958 by Dudley and colleagues to report a series of 13 patients with symptoms suggestive of intestinal occlusion. These patients underwent exploratory laparotomies, which failed to identify a mechanical cause for their symptomatology [3]. In subsequent years, the existence of this pathological entity in both adults and children was substantiated by a number of other clinicians [4–7].

The pathophysiologic mechanism of CIPO is represented by abnormal antegrade propulsive activity of the gastrointestinal (GI) tract as a result of processes that affect its neurons, muscles, or interstitial cells of Cajal (ICC) [8]. This functional failure results in a number of clinical symptoms such as abdominal distention with or without abdominal pain, nausea, vomiting, and a reduced inability to tolerate enteral nutrition [9]. These symptoms are, however, nonspecific and the condition can remain undiagnosed for a long period of time during which patients may undergo multiple diagnostic investigations and often repeated surgical explorations in an effort to identify the cause [9].

Although by definition the small intestine is always involved, any part of the GI tract can be affected in CIPO [1, 2]. Esophageal involvement may lead to dysphagia from impaired peristalsis, in some cases akin to that seen in achalasia [10]. Involvement of the stomach results in poor feed tolerance from gastroparesis suggested by the presence of delayed gastric emptying, while the large bowel by delayed colonic transit and constipation and the anorectum by sphincter dysfunction and defecation disorders [1].

This chapter focuses on various aspects of childhood CIPO and attempts to address areas of controversy by exploring the most recent advances in the overall approach and management of this clinical entity.

Epidemiology

CIPO is a rare disease with scanty epidemiological data and poorly defined incidence and prevalence in both adult and pediatric populations. One of the few initiatives to elucidate its epidemiology suggested that approximately 100 infants are born in the USA every year with CIPO, suggesting an incidence of approximately 1 per 40,000 live births [11, 12].

Adult studies reveal that the disease is more frequent in females [13–15]. In a recently published national survey conducted in Japan, 138 cases of CIPO were identified, with an estimated prevalence of 1.0 and 0.8 cases and incidence of 0.21 and 0.24 cases per 100,000 males and females, respectively [16]. No similar data are available in pediatric age.

Undoubtedly, the development of national registries is of paramount importance to delineate more precise epidemiologic characteristics of this orphan clinical entity.

Classification

Classification of CIPO is challenging. Conditions can be classified by whether they primarily affect intestinal nerves (neuropathy), smooth muscle (myopathy), or ICC

N. Thapar (✉)
Division of Neurogastroenterology and Motility, Department of Pediatric Gastroenterology, Great Ormond Street Hospital for Children, NHS Foundation Trust; UCL Institute of Child Health, 30 Guilford Street, WC1N 3JH London, UK
e-mail: n.thapar@ucl.ac.uk

E. Saliakellis · O. Borrelli
Division of Neurogastroenterology and Motility, Department of Pediatric Gastroenterology, Great Ormond Street Hospital for Children, NHS Foundation Trust, Great Ormond Street, WC1N 3JH London, UK

© Springer International Publishing Switzerland 2016
S. Guandalini et al. (eds.), *Textbook of Pediatric Gastroenterology, Hepatology and Nutrition*,
DOI 10.1007/978-3-319-17169-2_23

(mesenchymopathy), and can be further subdivided into primary or secondary, congenital or acquired, mode of inheritance or what part of the GI tract is involved. Where classification is not possible, they are defined as idiopathic. In truth, there is a considerable overlap [1, 2].

In primary CIPO, the disease is usually localized to GI tract, whereas in secondary cases, there is a systemic disorder that affects GI tract motility. It must be noted though that in some cases of primary CIPO extra-GI involvement may also be present, such as the urinary tract (hollow visceral myopathy and megacystis microcolon intestinal hypoperistalsis syndrome), the nervous system (central, peripheral, autonomous), and/or mitochondria (mitochondrial neurogastrointestinal encephalomyopathy, MNGIE) [2, 17, 18]. Almost 50% of CIPO cases appear to fall into the category of secondary CIPO as highlighted in Table 23.1 [19]. Based on histological findings, both primary and secondary CIPO can

Table 23.1 Classification of chronic intestinal pseudo-obstruction [7, 18, 27–133]

Primary CIPO
Sporadic or familial forms of hollow visceral myopathy/neuropathy (e.g., megacystis microcolon intestinal hypoperistalsis syndrome) [7, 27–44]
Mitochondrial neurogastrointestinal encephalomyopathy (MNGIE) [18, 45–47]
Hirschsprung's disease [48–50]
Neuropathy associated with multiple endocrine neoplasia type IIB [51–53]
Malrotation or gastroschisis [54–56]
Neuropathy post neonatal necrotizing enterocolitis [57]
Secondary CIPO
Conditions affecting GI smooth muscle
Rheumatological conditions (dermatomyositis/polyomyositis, scleroderma, systematic lupus erythematosus, Ehlers–Danlos syndrome) [58–69]
Other (Duchenne's muscular dystrophy, myotonic dystrophy, amyloidosis, ceroidosis, or alternatively reported as brown bowel syndrome) [70–79]
Pathologies affecting the enteric nervous system (familial dysautonomia, primary dysfunction of the autonomic nervous system, neurofibromatosis, diabetic neuropathy, fetal alcohol syndrome, post-viral related CIPO, e.g., CMV, EBV, VZV, JC virus) [80–95]
Endocrinological disorders (hypothyroidism, diabetes, hypoparathyroidism, pheochromocytoma) [96–100]
Metabolic conditions (uremia, porphyria, electrolyte imbalances, e.g., potassium, magnesium, calcium) [101–106]
Other (celiac disease, eosinophilic gastroenteritis, Crohn's disease, radiation injury, Chagas disease, Kawasaki disease, angioedema, mitochondrial disorders, drugs, e.g., opiates, anthraquinone laxatives, calcium channel blockers, antidepressants, antineoplastic agents, e.g., vinca alkaloids, paraneoplastic CIPO, major trauma/surgery, chromosome abnormalities) [107–133]
Idiopathic

CMV cytomegalovirus, *EBV* Epstein–Barr virus, *VZV* varicella-zoster virus, *JC* John Cunningham

be further categorized into neuropathies, myopathies, and mesenchymopathies [20–25]. Although the onset of the disease is used to label whether CIPO is congenital or acquired, in children, this area needs to be better elucidated [2, 8, 26].

Etiology and Pathophysiology

The integrity of GI sensorimotor function relies on precise coordination between the autonomic nervous system, enteric nervous system (ENS), ICC, and smooth muscle cells. Any noxious stimulus, irrespective of its origin and etiology, that affects the neuromuscular elements and control of GI tract can lead to impaired peristalsis and the stasis of luminal contents [1]. A variety of disorders and pathophysiological mechanisms can potentially affect the structure or function of the neuromuscular elements of the GI tract and lead to CIPO (Table 23.1) [1]. Neurological (e.g., multiple endocrine neoplasia (MEN) type IIb, familial dysautonomia) and metabolic (e.g., diabetes mellitus) conditions may affect the extrinsic GI nerve supply [19]. Neurotropic viruses may evoke an inflammatory process targeting both the ENS and extrinsic neural pathways [93]. Paraneoplastic syndromes may also exert a destructive effect on the ENS by initiating an inflammatory process that targets the neurons of ganglia located in the submucosal and myenteric plexuses. This is mediated by both a cellular infiltrate and production of circulating antineuronal antibodies [19, 134]. Some pathologies (e.g., muscular dystrophy) may target enteric smooth muscle fibers, whereas others such as dermatomyositis, scleroderma, Ehlers–Danlos syndrome, radiation enteritis may distort both ENS and gut smooth muscle leading to a mixed neuromyopathic disorder [12, 135, 136]. Finally, although entities such as celiac disease, hypothyroidism, hypoparathyroidism, and pheochromocytoma presumably cause CIPO by affecting the GI neuromuscular integrity, the exact mechanism is not fully understood.

Genetics

Elucidation of the genetic basis of CIPO has been somewhat disappointing. Some familial cases of CIPO have been recognized but there appear to be several patterns of inheritance, perhaps reflective of the great heterogeneity of CIPO conditions. Both autosomal dominant and recessive modes of inheritance have been described for neuropathic and myopathic types of CIPO [5, 13, 14, 135, 137]. More specifically, rare autosomal dominant mutations in the *SOX10* gene, which encodes a transcription factor important in ENS development, result in a CIPO clinical phenotype along with features such as sensorineural deafness and pigmentary anomalies [138, 139]. Homozygosity on the region 8q23–q24 has been implicated in the pathogenesis of an autosomal recessive form of CIPO characterized by severe GI dysmotility, Barrett's esophagus, and cardiac anomalies [140, 141].

X-linked inheritance (locus Xq28) with recessive transmission has been described in CIPO [15, 142, 143]. Mutations of filamin A *(FLNA)* and L1 cell adhesion molecule *(L1CAM)* genes, which are both located on chromosome Xq28, result in predominantly myopathic and neuropathic forms of CIPO, respectively. Additional involvement of the central nervous system, heart (patent ductus arteriosus), and blood (thrombocytopenia) in both conditions has also been described [143–145].

Mutations in mitochondria are increasingly implicated in CIPO. Mutations in the thymidine phosphorylase gene (*TYMP*, also termed as endothelial cell growth factor-1, *ECGF1*), or in the polymerase-γ gene *(POLG)* result in recessive myopathic forms of CIPO. The former is the cause of MNGIE, whereas the latter leads to a form without encephalopathy. Apart from the GI dysmotility, MNGIE is characterized by severe malnutrition, opthalmoplegia, and leucoencepalopathy on brain MRI [146–148].

The responsible genes for familial visceral neuropathy and myopathy are yet to be identified.

Histopathology

In adults, GI histology is reported to be normal in approximately 10% of CIPO cases, while in the experience of the authors, this figure is likely to be higher in children. However, its role in CIPO remains crucial and therefore an adequate full-thickness bowel biopsy (preferably a circumferential sleeve of at least 1–2 cm) is recommended whenever surgery is being considered [8, 26, 149]. Recent initiatives are addressing a more standardized and hopefully effective histological approach to diagnosis in GI motility disorders such as CIPO [Knowles et al., working group] [25, 150, 151].

On the basis of histology, CIPO is classified into neuropathy, myopathy, or mesenchymopathy [25]. However, mixed forms (e.g., neuromyopathy) are also recognized [25, 152, 153].

Neuropathies and myopathies can be further subdivided into inflammatory and degenerative. Inflammatory neuropathies are characterized by an infiltration of T lymphocytes and plasma cells in the myenteric plexuses (myenteric ganglionitis) and neuronal axons (axonopathy) [25, 154]. It has been proposed that five or more lymphocytes per ganglion are required for the diagnosis of myenteric ganglionitis [25]. Of note, patients with lymphocytic infiltration of the myenteric plexuses may also develop increased titers of antinuclear antibodies (ANNA-1/anti-Hu, anti-voltage-gated potassium channel or VGKC) [155–157]. These immunologic

responses may result in neuronal degeneration and loss by activating apoptotic and autophagic mechanisms [156, 158]. Infiltration of the myenteric ganglia with other cells such as eosinophils and mast cells has been described but their exact clinicopathological significance is yet to be clarified given limited data [159–162]. All these data support the role of the immune system in the pathogenesis of inflammatory CIPO [163].

Degenerative neuropathies are poorly understood given the limited amount of available data [164–166]. Main histopathologic characteristics of this group include a decrease in the number of intramural neurons along with changes in nerve cell bodies and axons [150, 154]. It has been postulated that apoptotic mechanisms are involved in the degenerative process potentially caused by aberrant calcium signaling, mitochondrial disorders, production of free radicals, and abnormalities in the function of glial cells [150, 152, 167, 168].

Similarly to neuropathies, myopathies are also divided into inflammatory and degenerative. Inflammatory myopathies, also reported by the term leiomyositis, are characterized by infiltration of T lymphocytes into both the circular and longitudinal enteric muscle layers. This process if not treated appropriately with immunosuppressive agents may lead to a severe clinical picture of CIPO [44, 169].

The histopathologic findings in degenerative myopathies include smooth muscle fiber vacuolization and fibrosis [170, 171]. Diverticula may also be present especially if the longitudinal muscle coat is more affected compared to the circular muscle layer [146, 148].

Novel immunohistochemical techniques such as smooth muscle markers, namely, smoothelin, smooth muscle myosin heavy chain, and histone deacetylase 8, may reveal histopathologic subtleties otherwise not detectable with conventional immunostaining and histochemistry methods [172].

Mesenchymopathies are defined by ICC abnormalities (decreased density of ICC network, intracellular abnormalities) and have been demonstrated in CIPO patients [150, 173]. Although sufficient data exist regarding their role in the pathogenesis of diabetic gastroparesis, further research is required regarding ICC involvement in the etiopathogenesis of other GI motility disorders [25].

Clinical Picture

In a few cases, the diagnosis of CIPO is suggested in utero by ultrasonographic findings of polyhydramnios, abdominal distention, and megacystis; however, the majority of cases present in the neonatal period or early infancy [8, 26]. The symptomatology varies according to the age at diagnosis and the part of the GI tract, which is primarily affected. Approximately, one-third of children with congenital CIPO (myopathic and neuropathic) have intestinal malrotation

[22]. Cardinal signs and symptoms of CIPO include those of obstruction, namely abdominal distention (88 %), vomiting (72 %, which can be bilious), and constipation (61 %). Abdominal pain (44 %), failure to thrive (31 %), and diarrhea (28 %) may also be part of the clinical picture [8, 9, 149].

Dehydration (which can be severe) and malnutrition are often underdiagnosed especially given that weight can be an unreliable measure due to pooling of significant volumes of fluid (third spacing) within distended gut loops. Intraluminal gut content stasis can also lead to small bowel bacterial overgrowth which can further exacerbate symptoms of diarrhea and abdominal distention [149].

CIPO may also manifest with extraintestinal signs and symptoms, such as recurrent urinary tract infections or neurologic abnormalities [17, 147]. Furthermore, patients may complain of symptoms indicative of an underlying disorder that accounts for secondary CIPO (e.g., proximal muscle weakness in dermatomyositis) [59].

The clinical course of CIPO is characterized by exacerbations and remissions, where the former can be precipitated by a number of factors such as surgery, general anesthesia, infections, and emotional stress [26]. In the most severe cases, the natural course of the disease leads to worsening intestinal function and ultimately to intestinal failure [9, 149]. This is especially true in cases where the diagnosis and/or institution of appropriate treatment has been delayed.

Diagnosis

CIPO should be suspected in children with early onset, chronic, recurrent, or continuous signs of intestinal obstruction especially where a surgical cause cannot be established

(e.g., repeated "normal" exploratory laparotomies). The diagnosis of CIPO should follow a structured algorithm. Although a detailed history, clinical examination, and laboratory tests may suggest the presence of CIPO, or help elucidate its cause, the definitive diagnosis should rely on the use of targeted investigations to (i) exclude mechanical occlusion of the gut lumen, (ii) confirm GI dysmotility, and (iii) rule out treatable causes.

Careful clinical history and physical examination may help in defining the onset, the severity and progression of the disease, and the part of the GI tract primarily affected, and they also provide useful information regarding associations (e.g., family history), potential secondary causes (e.g., medications), and complications (e.g., dehydration). Laboratory tests (e.g., serum electrolytes, thyroid-stimulating hormone (TSH), lactic acid, specific autoantibodies) are useful in cases of secondary CIPO and assessing the clinical state of the patients admitted acutely or undergoing a diagnostic protocol.

The definitive diagnosis of CIPO in children is often reliant on a number of diagnostic tests, which exclude luminal obstruction and confirm the presence of impaired GI motility. These are discussed below.

Imaging

Plain abdominal radiographs may demonstrate a dilated GI tract, with air-fluid levels, whereas contrast GI series can reveal anatomical abnormalities (e.g., malrotation, microcolon) and exclude the presence of gut occlusive lesions (Fig. 23.1a) [2, 149, 174]. It needs to be kept in mind that a water-soluble substance should be used instead of barium in

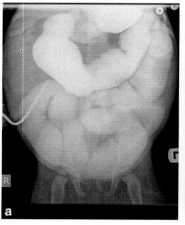 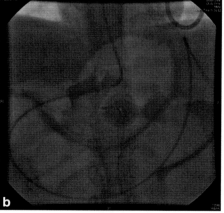 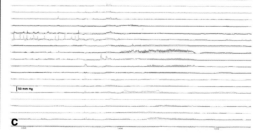

Fig. 23.1 Investigation findings of a 3-year-old boy with a history of recurrent episodes of abdominal distension and vomiting since the neonatal period, and now showing a marked reduction in enteral feed tolerance. **a** Contrast follow-through study (administered via gastrostomy) showing filling of grossly dilated small intestinal loops, without any apparent hold up or change in calibre. **b** Plain abdominal radiograph taken following placement of antroduodenal manometry catheter into the same patient performed under fluoroscopic guidance. The tip of the catheter has been advanced beyond the duodenojejunal junction to facilitate optimal manometric recording of both the stomach and small intestine. **c** Antroduodenal manometry tracing from patient showing the presence of some gastric antral contractions and a migrating motor complex (phase III activity) passing down the small intestine. The amplitude of small intestinal contractile activity is very low (not exceeding 20 mmHg) suggesting a diagnosis of myopathic chronic intestinal pseudo-obstruction

order to prevent flocculation and inspissation of the contrast material.

Novel imaging modalities such as cine MRI have been recently performed with promising results in adult series but there are no data regarding their applicability and usefulness in pediatrics [175].

Endoscopy

Endoscopy may identify fore- or hindgut mechanical occlusion previously missed on radiology, and it allows duodenal biopsies to exclude mucosal inflammation [176]. Novel techniques (e.g., natural orifice transluminal endoscopic surgery—NOTES) may revolutionize the role of endoscopy in the diagnosis of gut motility disorders by providing the ability of full-thickness biopsy sampling in a safe and minimally invasive way [177, 178].

Motility Investigations

These studies are performed to assess the GI motility and to define the underlying pathophysiologic process, and these studies form the hallmark of diagnosis in pediatrics. Investigations include GI manometries (esophageal, antroduodenal, colonic, anorectal), GI scintigraphy (e.g., gastric emptying, colonic transit), electrogastrography, and radiopaque markers. The usefulness of novel technologies, such as SmartPill, remains to be determined [8, 179, 180].

Although in children with CIPO the involvement of GI may be generalized, the small intestine is always affected; thus, antroduodenal manometry remains the most discerning test, and its optimal placement is pivotal (Fig. 23.1b) [181]. Neuropathic cases manifest with uncoordinated contractions, which are of normal amplitude, whereas in myopathic CIPO, motor patterns have normal coordination; however, the amplitude of intestinal contractions is low (Fig. 23.1c) [182–184]. Additionally, manometry may facilitate the dynamic assessment of potential pharmacotherapeutic options and feeding strategies (e.g., feasibility of oral or enteral feeds) as well as indicate disease prognosis [185–187].

In the most challenging cases, exploratory surgery (laparotomy or laparoscopic-assisted procedures) may be required to definitively exclude mechanical obstruction from CIPO. One however should bear in mind that surgery may precipitate a pseudo-obstructive episode and may also lead to adhesions formation, which can further complicate future diagnostic or therapeutic procedures. Where possible, investigations and then diagnostic/therapeutic surgery should be performed in timeline sequence and in referral center.

Histopathology along with genetics can also be very useful in establishing or confirming the diagnosis of CIPO, highlighting the underlying pathophysiologic process, thus aiding the overall management.

Figure 23.2 summarizes the basic steps in the diagnostic evaluation of pediatric patients with suspected CIPO.

Differential Diagnosis

CIPO has to be differentiated from mechanical obstruction; the latter is usually characterized by marked abdominal pain (in keeping with the abdominal distention), specific radiologic signs, and manometric patterns [188, 189]. Acute functional obstruction (e.g., postoperative ileus), functional GI disorders (e.g., rumination syndrome), and pediatric condition falsification should be considered and appropriately investigated and managed [149, 190, 191].

Treatment

The therapeutic approach in CIPO is threefold as it aims to (i) preserve growth and development by maintaining adequate caloric intake, (ii) promote GI motility with combined medical and surgical interventions, and (iii) treat disease-related complications or underlying pathologies that cause secondary CIPO. Despite the limited effects of the currently applied therapeutic modalities, refinements and evolution in nutritional, medical, and surgical strategies have considerably improved the overall management of CIPO [136, 192]. Acute management of episodes of pseudo-obstruction are generally treated conservatively by nil by mouth, intravenous fluid, and drainage of stasis through nasogastric (NG) tube or preformed ostomies. Careful attention to fluid and electrolytes is imperative.

Nutrition

The role of nutrition in CIPO is of paramount significance as it is well known that gut motility improves with optimal nutritional support and declines in the face of under- or malnutrition [8]. In the long term, approximately one-third of pediatric CIPO patients require either partial or total parenteral nutrition, another third require a degree of intragastric or intra-enteral feeding, whereas the remaining children are able to tolerate sufficient oral nutrition. However, within all of groups, patients able to tolerate feeds may require some dietary modification in order to maintain enteral nutrition and avoid bezoar formation (e.g., bite and dissolvable feeds, restriction diets, hydrolyzed formula). Although parenteral nutrition is lifesaving, it is associated with significant risk of complications, such as central line infections and liver disease, and therefore maintaining patients on maximally

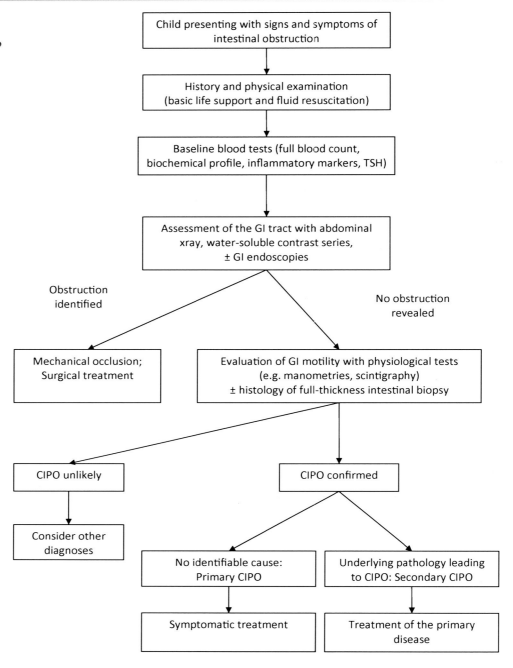

tolerated enteral nutrition is always strongly encouraged [26]. In the more severe CIPO cases, continuous rather than bolus feeds administered via a gastrostomy or jejunostomy may be better tolerated particularly in children with impaired gastric motor function [193–195].

Medications

The therapeutic role of drugs in CIPO patients is mainly limited to the control of intestinal inflammation, suppression of bacterial overgrowth, and promotion of GI motility [186, 195].

Prokinetics (e.g., metoclopramide, domperidone, erythromycin, azithromycin, octreotide, neostigmine) usually combined with antiemetics (e.g., promethazine, ondansetron) have been used in an attempt to improve the GI motor function and reduce the severity of nausea and vomiting [196–199]. The use of some of these agents is limited by variable efficacy and unacceptable extraintestinal side effects (e.g., metoclopramide, neostigmine). The best-studied and tested prokinetics, that is, cisapride and tegaserod have been withdrawn from the market due to safety concerns [200]. The need for new prokinetics with increased safety and efficacy has resulted in new products (e.g., prucalopride, aprepitant, ghrelin), but there are limited data of their use in pediatric CIPO, further impacted on by restricted availability and licensing [201–203]. Undoubtedly, current medical regimens for CIPO are based on limited literature and/or expert opinion (e.g., combined use of octreotide and erythromycin) and are yet to be tested in future in the context of controlled trials [186, 204].

Surgery

Surgery remains a valuable intervention on patients with CIPO as it has a multidimensional role in both the diagnostic (e.g., full thickness biopsies) and therapeutic processes (e.g., insertion of feeding tubes, formation of decompressing ostomies such as gastrostomy, ileostomy) [195, 205, 206].

Indeed, adequate bowel decompression is crucial not only in providing symptomatic relief by reducing the frequency and the severity of pseudo-obstructive episodes but also in limiting further deterioration of the intestinal motor activity secondary to chronic distention, and in enhancing the tolerance of enteral feeding [195, 205]. Long decompression enteral tubes and extensive bowel resections are approaches mainly reported in adult CIPO cohorts but remain untested in terms of practicality, efficacy, and safety in pediatrics [207, 208]. Rate of significant surgical complications, such as stoma prolapse, infection, and leakage can be significant.

Novel surgical methods involve implantation of devices providing electrical pacing of the GI neuromusculature, but data in children are scanty and limited [209].

Small bowel transplantation remains the only definitive cure. Recent advances in both surgical techniques (e.g., multivisceral transplantation) and immunosuppression strategies have resulted in improved outcomes and survival as reported by centers with the relevant expertise showing a survival rate of 50% at 3 years [210–213].

Natural History and Prognosis

Both pediatric and adult CIPO have a severe clinical course, characterized by repetitive relapses and remissions. Unfortunately, the low index of suspicion among physicians along with lack of well-defined diagnostic criteria and readily available facilities in performing specialized diagnostic tests (e.g., manometry) often accounts for delays in the diagnosis and repetitive unnecessary investigations and surgery [13–15, 164].

The majority of the patients complain of symptoms, which progressively worsen and impact upon the tolerance of enteral nutrition and increasing reliance on total parenteral nutrition. The latter in conjunction with disease-related adverse events (e.g., central line infections, impairment of the liver function, immunosuppression after small bowel transplantation, surgical procedures) accounts for high morbidity, poor quality of life, and mortality rates up to 30% [11, 21, 28, 214–218].

Despite recent diagnostic and therapeutic advances, CIPO in children remains a serious, life-threatening disease with significant impact on the well-being not only of patients themselves but also of their families [218].

Summary

Childhood CIPO is an enigmatic disease with poorly defined etiopathogenesis, which is reflected on the limitations encountered in both the diagnostic process and therapeutic management. Clearly, multinational initiatives are required to raise awareness, establish stringent diagnostic criteria, and evolve current therapeutic modalities.

Acknowledgments Nikhil Thapar is supported by Great Ormond Street Hospital Children's Charity.

References

1. Gabbard SL, Lacy BE. Chronic intestinal pseudo-obstruction. Nutr Clin Pract. 2013;28:307–16.
2. Rudolph CD, Hyman PE, Altschuler SM, et al. Diagnosis and treatment of chronic intestinal pseudo-obstruction in children: report of consensus workshop. J Pediatr Gastroenterol Nutr. 1997;24:102–12.
3. Dudley HA, Sinclair IS, Mc LI, et al. Intestinal pseudo-obstruction. J R Coll Surg Edinb. 1958;3:206–17.
4. Naish JM, Capper WM, Brown NJ. Intestinal pseudoobstruction with steatorrhoea. Gut. 1960;1:62–6.
5. Stephens FO. Syndrome of intestinal pseudo-obstruction. Br Med J. 1962;1:1248–50.
6. Byrne WJ, Cipel L, Euler AR, et al. Chronic idiopathic intestinal pseudo-obstruction syndrome in children—clinical characteristics and prognosis. J Pediatr. 1977;90:585–9.
7. Schuffler MD, Pope CE 2nd. Studies of idiopathic intestinal pseudoobstruction. II. Hereditary hollow visceral myopathy: family studies. Gastroenterology. 1977;73:339–44.
8. Hyman P, Thapar N. Gastrointestinal motility and functional disorders in children. In: Faure C, Di Lorenzo D, Thapar N, editors. Pediatric neurogastroenterology. New York: Springer; 2013. pp. 257–70.
9. Thapar N. Clinical picture of intestinal pseudo-obstruction syndrome. J Pediatr Gastroenterol Nutr. 2011;53(Suppl 2):S58–9.
10. Amiot A, Joly F, Cazals-Hatem D, et al. Prognostic yield of esophageal manometry in chronic intestinal pseudo-obstruction: a retrospective cohort of 116 adult patients. Neurogastroenterol Motil. 2012;24:1008–e542.
11. Vargas JH, Sachs P, Ament ME. Chronic intestinal pseudo-obstruction syndrome in pediatrics. Results of a national survey by members of the North American Society of Pediatric Gastroenterology and Nutrition. J Pediatr Gastroenterol Nutr. 1988;7:323–32.
12. Di Lorenzo C. Pseudo-obstruction: current approaches. Gastroenterology. 1999;116:980–7.

13. Stanghellini V, Cogliandro RF, De Giorgio R, et al. Natural history of chronic idiopathic intestinal pseudo-obstruction in adults: a single center study. Clin Gastroenterol Hepatol. 2005;3:449–58.

14. Amiot A, Joly F, Alves A, et al. Long-term outcome of chronic intestinal pseudo-obstruction adult patients requiring home parenteral nutrition. Am J Gastroenterol. 2009;104:1262–70.

15. Lindberg G, Iwarzon M, Tornblom H. Clinical features and long-term survival in chronic intestinal pseudo-obstruction and enteric dysmotility. Scand J Gastroenterol. 2009;44:692–9.

16. Iida H, Ohkubo H, Inamori M, et al. Epidemiology and clinical experience of chronic intestinal pseudo-obstruction in Japan: a nationwide epidemiologic survey. J Epidemiol. 2013;23:288–94.

17. Mc Laughlin D, Puri P. Familial megacystis microcolon intestinal hypoperistalsis syndrome: a systematic review. Pediatr Surg Int. 2013;29:947–51.

18. Blondon H, Polivka M, Joly F, et al. Digestive smooth muscle mitochondrial myopathy in patients with mitochondrial-neuro-gastrointestinal encephalomyopathy (MNGIE). Gastroenterol Clin Biol. 2005;29:773–8.

19. De Giorgio R, Cogliandro RF, Barbara G, et al. Chronic intestinal pseudo-obstruction: clinical features, diagnosis, and therapy. Gastroenterol Clin North Am. 2011;40:787–807.

20. Mousa H, Hyman PE, Cocjin J, et al. Long-term outcome of congenital intestinal pseudoobstruction. Dig Dis Sci. 2002;47:2298–305.

21. Heneyke S, Smith VV, Spitz L, et al. Chronic intestinal pseudo-obstruction: treatment and long term follow up of 44 patients. Arch Dis Child. 1999;81:21–7.

22. Streutker CJ, Huizinga JD, Campbell F, et al. Loss of CD117 (c-kit)- and CD34-positive ICC and associated CD34-positive fibroblasts defines a subpopulation of chronic intestinal pseudo-obstruction. Am J Surg Pathol. 2003;27:228–35.

23. Jain D, Moussa K, Tandon M, et al. Role of interstitial cells of Cajal in motility disorders of the bowel. Am J Gastroenterol. 2003;98:618–24.

24. Struijs MC, Diamond IR, Pencharz PB, et al. Absence of the interstitial cells of Cajal in a child with chronic pseudoobstruction. J Pediatr Surg. 2008;43:e25–9.

25. Knowles CH, De Giorgio R, Kapur RP, et al. The London Classification of gastrointestinal neuromuscular pathology: report on behalf of the Gastro. 2009 International Working Group. Gut. 2010;59:882–7.

26. Hyman P. Chronic intestinal pseudo-obstruction. In: Wyllie R, Hyams J, Kay M, editors. Pediatric gastrointestinal and liver disease. Philadelphia: Elsevier; 2011. pp. 505–11.

27. Puri P, Shinkai M. Megacystis microcolon intestinal hypoperistalsis syndrome. Semin Pediatr Surg. 2005;14:58–63.

28. Schuffler MD, Pagon RA, Schwartz R, et al. Visceral myopathy of the gastrointestinal and genitourinary tracts in infants. Gastroenterology. 1988;94:892–8.

29. Martin JE, Benson M, Swash M, et al. Myofibroblasts in hollow visceral myopathy: the origin of gastrointestinal fibrosis? Gut. 1993;34:999–1001.

30. Jayachandar J, Frank JL, Jonas MM. Isolated intestinal myopathy resembling progressive systemic sclerosis in a child. Gastroenterology. 1988;95:1114–8.

31. Lowsky R, Davidson G, Wolman S, et al. Familial visceral myopathy associated with a mitochondrial myopathy. Gut. 1993;34:279–83.

32. Schuffler MD, Lowe MC, Bill AH. Studies of idiopathic intestinal pseudoobstruction. I. Hereditary hollow visceral myopathy: clinical and pathological studies. Gastroenterology. 1977;73:327–38.

33. Jones SC, Dixon MF, Lintott DJ, et al. Familial visceral myopathy. A family with involvement of four generations. Dig Dis Sci. 1992;37:464–9.

34. Threlkeld AB, Miller NR, Golnik KC, et al. Ophthalmic involvement in myo-neuro-gastrointestinal encephalopathy syndrome. Am J Ophthalmol. 1992;114:322–8.

35. Li V, Hostein J, Romero NB, et al. Chronic intestinal pseudoobstruction with myopathy and ophthalmoplegia. A muscular biochemical study of a mitochondrial disorder. Dig Dis Sci. 1992;37:456–63.

36. Ahlfors F, Linander H, Lindstrom M, et al. Familial intestinal degenerative neuropathy associated with chronic intestinal pseudo-obstruction. Neurogastroenterol Motil. 2011;23:347–55, e159.

37. Roper EC, Gibson A, McAlindon ME, et al. Familial visceral neuropathy: a defined entity? Am J Med Genet A. 2005;137A:249–54.

38. Niwamoto H, Okamoto E, Toyosaka A, et al. Sporadic visceral neuropathy. Surg Today. 1995;25:763–70.

39. Low PA. Autonomic neuropathies. Curr Opin Neurol. 1994;7:402–6.

40. Camilleri M, Balm RK, Low PA. Autonomic dysfunction in patients with chronic intestinal pseudo-obstruction. Clin Auton Res. 1993;3:95–100.

41. Imai DM, Miller JL, Leonard BC, et al. Visceral smooth muscle alpha-actin deficiency associated with chronic intestinal pseudo-obstruction in a Bengal cat (*Felis catus* × *Prionailurus bengalensis*). Vet Pathol. 2013.

42. Lehtonen HJ, Sipponen T, Tojkander S, et al. Segregation of a missense variant in enteric smooth muscle actin gamma-2 with autosomal dominant familial visceral myopathy. Gastroenterology. 2012;143:1482–91, e3.

43. Cho YH, Park JH, Park do Y, et al. Segmental transposition of ileal muscle layers: a rare cause of myopathic pseudoobstruction in a newborn. J Pediatr Surg. 2011;46:e1–3.

44. Dewit S, de Hertogh G, Geboes K, et al. Chronic intestinal pseudo-obstruction caused by an intestinal inflammatory myopathy: case report and review of the literature. Neurogastroenterol Motil. 2008;20:343–8.

45. Garone C, Tadesse S, Hirano M. Clinical and genetic spectrum of mitochondrial neurogastrointestinal encephalomyopathy. Brain. 2011;134:3326–32.

46. Perez-Atayde AR. Diagnosis of mitochondrial neurogastrointestinal encephalopathy disease in gastrointestinal biopsies. Hum Pathol. 2013;44:1440–6.

47. Nishino I, Spinazzola A, Papadimitriou A, et al. Mitochondrial neurogastrointestinal encephalomyopathy: an autosomal recessive disorder due to thymidine phosphorylase mutations. Ann Neurol. 2000;47:792–800.

48. Puri P, Gosemann JH. Variants of Hirschsprung disease. Semin Pediatr Surg. 2012;21:310–8.

49. Wu TT, Tsai TW, Chang H, et al. Polymorphisms of the RET gene in hirschsprung disease. anorectal malformation and intestinal pseudo-obstruction in Taiwan. J Formos Med Assoc. 2010;109:32–8.

50. Qualman SJ, Murray R. Aganglionosis and related disorders. Hum Pathol. 1994;25:1141–9.

51. Qualia CM, Brown MR, Ryan CK, et al. Oral mucosal neuromas leading to the diagnosis of multiple endocrine neoplasia type 2B in a child with intestinal pseudo-obstruction. Gastroenterol Hepatol (N Y). 2007;3:208–11.

52. Erdogan MF, Gulec B, Gursoy A, et al. Multiple endocrine neoplasia 2B presenting with pseudo-Hirschsprung's disease. J Natl Med Assoc. 2006;98:783–6.

53. Grobmyer SR, Guillem JG, O'Riordain DS, et al. Colonic manifestations of multiple endocrine neoplasia type 2B: report of four cases. Dis Colon Rectum. 1999;42:1216–9.

54. Singh G, Hershman MJ, Loft DE, et al. Partial malrotation associated with pseudo-obstruction of the small bowel. Br J Clin Pract. 1993;47:274–5.

55. Devane SP, Coombes R, Smith VV, et al. Persistent gastrointestinal symptoms after correction of malrotation. Arch Dis Child. 1992;67:218–21.

56. Bagwell CE, Filler RM, Cutz E, et al. Neonatal intestinal pseudoobstruction. J Pediatr Surg. 1984;19:732–9.

57. Vanderwinden JM, Dassonville M, Van der Veken E, et al. Post-necrotising enterocolitis pseudo-obstruction treated with Cisapride. Z Kinderchir. 1990;45:282–5.

58. Ohkubo H, Iida H, Takahashi H, et al. An epidemiologic survey of chronic intestinal pseudo-obstruction and evaluation of the newly proposed diagnostic criteria. Digestion. 2012;86:12–9.

59. Kleckner FS. Dermatomyositis and its manifestations in the gastrointestinal tract. Am J Gastroenterol. 1970;53:141–6.

60. Laskin BL, Choyke P, Keenan GF, et al. Novel gastrointestinal tract manifestations in juvenile dermatomyositis. J Pediatr. 1999;135:371–4.

61. Sjogren RW. Gastrointestinal features of scleroderma. Curr Opin Rheumatol. 1996;8:569–75.

62. Perlemuter G, Cacoub P, Wechsler B, et al. Chronic intestinal pseudo-obstruction secondary to connective tissue diseases. Gastroenterol Clin Biol. 2001;25:251–8.

63. Adachi Y, Yabana T, Kohri T, et al. A case of chronic idiopathic intestinal pseudo-obstruction with Sjogren's syndrome. Nihon Shokakibyo Gakkai Zasshi. 1990;87:1223–7.

64. Khairullah S, Jasmin R, Yahya F, et al. Chronic intestinal pseudo-obstruction: a rare first manifestation of systemic lupus erythematosus. Lupus. 2013;22:957–60.

65. Kansal A, Jain A, Thenozhi S, et al. Intestinal pseudo-obstruction associated with biliary tract dilatation in a patient with systemic lupus erythematosus. Lupus. 2013;22:87–91.

66. Zhang J, Fang M, Wang Y, et al. Intestinal pseudo-obstruction syndrome in systemic lupus erythematosus. Lupus. 2011;20:1324–8.

67. Yamazaki-Nakashimada MA, Rodriguez-Jurado R, Ortega-Salgado A, et al. Intestinal pseudoobstruction associated with eosinophilic enteritis as the initial presentation of systemic lupus erythematosus in children. J Pediatr Gastroenterol Nutr. 2009;48:482–6.

68. Pelizzo G, Villanacci V, Salemme M, et al. Intestinal pseudo-obstruction due to small bowel alpha-actin deficiency in a child with Ehlers–Danlos syndrome. Tech Coloproctol. 2013.

69. Sato T, Ito H, Miyazaki S, et al. Megacystis and megacolon in an infant with Ehlers–Danlos syndrome. Acta Paediatr Jpn. 1993;35:358–60.

70. Camelo AL, Awad RA, Madrazo A, et al. Esophageal motility disorders in Mexican patients with Duchenne's muscular dystrophy. Acta Gastroenterol Latinoam. 1997;27:119–22.

71. Bensen ES, Jaffe KM, Tarr PI. Acute gastric dilatation in Duchenne muscular dystrophy: a case report and review of the literature. Arch Phys Med Rehabil. 1996;77:512–4.

72. Garcia Aroca J, Sanz N, Alonso JL, et al. Intestinal pseudo-obstruction secondary to systemic neuropathies and myopathies. Cir Pediatr. 1994;7:115–20.

73. Leon SH, Schuffler MD, Kettler M, et al. Chronic intestinal pseudoobstruction as a complication of Duchenne's muscular dystrophy. Gastroenterology. 1986;90:455–9.

74. Kim YJ, Kim HS, Park SY, et al. Intestinal amyloidosis with intractable diarrhea and intestinal pseudo-obstruction. Korean J Gastroenterol. 2012;60:172–6.

75. Liapis K, Michelis FV, Delimpasi S, et al. Intestinal pseudo-obstruction associated with amyloidosis. Amyloid. 2011;18:76–8.

76. Illescas Megias V, Marquez Moreno AJ. Intestinal pseudo-obstruction in Steinert myotonic dystrophy: a clinical-radiological description of 2 cases. Radiologia. 2013;55:88–90.

77. Bruinenberg JF, Rieu PN, Gabreels FM, et al. Intestinal pseudo-obstruction syndrome in a child with myotonic dystrophy. Acta Paediatr. 1996;85:121–3.

78. Boller M, Fiocchi C, Brown CH. Pseudoobstruction in ceroidosis. AJR Am J Roentgenol. 1976;127:277–9.

79. Michaely HJ, Daroca PJ, Plavsic BM. Brown bowel syndrome—an unusual etiology of pseudo-obstruction of the small intestine. Rofo. 2003;175:1143–4.

80. Assor P, Negreanu L, Picon L, et al. Slowly regressing acute pan-dysautonomia associated with esophageal achalasia: a case report. Gastroenterol Clin Biol. 2008;32:46–50.

81. Palao S, Corral I, Vera R, et al. Progressive dysautonomia as initial manifestation of anti-Hu antibody-related syndrome. Neurologia. 2007;22:899–902.

82. Besnard M, Faure C, Fromont-Hankard G, et al. Intestinal pseudo-obstruction and acute pandysautonomia associated with Epstein-Barr virus infection. Am J Gastroenterol. 2000;95:280–4.

83. Taguchi T, Ikeda K, Shono T, et al. Autonomic innervation of the intestine from a baby with megacystis microcolon intestinal hypo-peristalsis syndrome: I. Immunohistochemical study. J Pediatr Surg. 1989;24:1264–6.

84. Yamanaka Y, Sakakibara R, Asahina M, et al. Chronic intestinal pseudo-obstruction as the initial feature of pure autonomic failure. J Neurol Neurosurg Psychiatry. 2006;77:800.

85. Sinha SK, Kochhar R, Rana S, et al. Intestinal pseudo-obstruction due to neurofibromatosis responding to cisapride. Indian J Gastroenterol. 2000;19:83–4.

86. Hanemann CO, Hayward C, Hilton DA. Neurofibromatosis type 1 with involvement of the enteric nerves. J Neurol Neurosurg Psychiatry. 2007;78:1163–4.

87. Aoki Y, Hosaka S, Kiyosawa K. Intestinal pseudo-obstruction in a diabetic man: role of the mitochondrial A3243G mutation. Ann Intern Med. 2002;137:703–4.

88. Reid B, DiLorenzo C, Travis L, et al. Diabetic gastroparesis due to postprandial antral hypomotility in childhood. Pediatrics. 1992;90:43–6.

89. Hendriks G, McPartland J, El-Matary W. Gastrointestinal presentation and outcome of perinatal cytomegalovirus infection. BMJ Case Rep. 2013.

90. Ategbo S, Turck D, Gottrand F, et al. Chronic intestinal pseudo-obstruction associated with cytomegalovirus infection in an infant. J Pediatr Gastroenterol Nutr. 1996;23:457–60.

91. Precupanu CM, Girodet J, Mariani P, et al. Pseudo-bowel obstruction due to varicella zoster virus infection after autologous stem cell transplantation. Am J Hematol. 2009;84:127–8.

92. Tanida E, Izumi M, Abe T, et al. Disseminated varicella-zoster virus infection complicated with severe abdominal pain and colonic pseudo-obstruction. Nihon Shokakibyo Gakkai Zasshi. 2013;110:839–45.

93. De Giorgio R, Ricciardiello L, Naponelli V, et al. Chronic intestinal pseudo-obstruction related to viral infections. Transplant Proc. 2010;42:9–14.

94. Selgrad M, De Giorgio R, Fini L, et al. JC virus infects the enteric glia of patients with chronic idiopathic intestinal pseudo-obstruction. Gut. 2009;58:25–32.

95. Uc A, Vasiliauskas E, Piccoli DA, et al. Chronic intestinal pseudoobstruction associated with fetal alcohol syndrome. Dig Dis Sci. 1997;42:1163–7.

96. Abboud B, Sayegh R, Medlej R, et al. A rare manifestation of hypothyroidism: intestinal obstruction. Report of 2 cases and review of the literature. J Med Liban. 1999;47:364–6.

97. Bassotti G, Pagliacci MC, Nicoletti I, et al. Intestinal pseudoobstruction secondary to hypothyroidism. Importance of small bowel manometry. J Clin Gastroenterol. 1992;14:56–8.

98. Siegrist D, Teuscher AU, Ruchti C. Intestinal paralysis in long-term diabetes mellitus. Praxis (Bern. 1994). 1998;87:769–72.

99. Camilleri M, Parkman HP, Shafi MA, et al. Clinical guideline: management of gastroparesis. Am J Gastroenterol. 2013;108:18–37, quiz 8.

100. Wu HW, Liou WP, Chou CC, et al. Pheochromocytoma presented as intestinal pseudo-obstruction and hyperamylasemia. Am J Emerg Med. 2008;26:971, e1–4.

101. Geelhoed GW. Colonic pseudo-obstruction in surgical patients. Am J Surg. 1985;149:258–65.

102. Lutz P, Maring D, Tschampa HJ, et al. A 25-year-old patient with colonic pseudo-obstruction, hyponatremia, hypertension, and diffuse pain. Med Klin (Munich). 2010;105:267–72.

103. Negrini S, Zoppoli G, Setti M, et al. Paralytic ileus and liver failure—an unusual presentation of advanced erythropoietic protoporphyria. Dig Dis Sci. 2009;54:411–5.

104. Koberstein B, Eysselein VE, Balzer K, et al. Paralytic ileus as an initial manifestation of malignant VIPoma of the pancreas—case report with review of the literature. Z Gastroenterol. 1990;28:295–301.

105. Sundar U, Lakkas Y, Asole D, et al. Gitelman's syndrome presenting as recurrent paralytic ileus due to chronic renal tubular K + wasting. J Assoc Physicians India. 2010;58:322–4.

106. Golzarian J, Scott HW, Jr, Richards WO. Hypermagnesemia-induced paralytic ileus. Dig Dis Sci. 1994;39:1138–42.

107. Matta R, Aramouni E, Mouawad P, et al. Celiac disease presenting as acute colonic pseudo-obstruction. J Med Liban. 2012;60:110–2.

108. Cluysenaer OJ, van Tongeren JH. Pseudo-obstruction in coeliac sprue. Neth J Med. 1987;31:300–4.

109. Cluysenaer OJ, van Tongeren JH. Coeliac disease presenting with intestinal pseudo-obstruction. Gut. 1985;26:538.

110. Ooms AH, Verheij J, Hulst JM, et al. Eosinophilic myenteric ganglionitis as a cause of chronic intestinal pseudo-obstruction. Virchows Arch. 2012;460:123–7.

111. Losanoff JE, Kjossev KT, Katrov ET. Eosinophilic enterocolitis and visceral neuropathy with chronic intestinal pseudo-obstruction. J Clin Gastroenterol. 1999;28:368–71.

112. Myrhoj T, Ladefoged K, Jarnum S. Chronic intestinal pseudo-obstruction in patients with extensive bowel resection for Crohn's disease. Scand J Gastroenterol. 1988;23:380–4.

113. Carethers JM, McDonnell WM, Owyang C, et al. Massive secretory diarrhea and pseudo-obstruction as the initial presentation of Crohn's disease. J Clin Gastroenterol. 1996;23:55–9.

114. Rolachon A, Bost R, Bichard P, et al. Radiotherapy: a rare etiology of chronic intestinal pseudo-obstruction. Gastroenterol Clin Biol. 1993;17:229–30.

115. Husebye E, Hauer-Jensen M, Kjorstad K, et al. Severe late radiation enteropathy is characterized by impaired motility of proximal small intestine. Dig Dis Sci. 1994;39:2341–9.

116. Meneghelli UG. Chagasic enteropathy. Rev Soc Bras Med Trop. 2004;37:252–60.

117. Tiao MM, Huang LT, Liang CD, et al. Atypical Kawasaki disease presenting as intestinal pseudo-obstruction. J Formos Med Assoc. 2006;105:252–5.

118. Eck SL, Morse JH, Janssen DA, et al. Angioedema presenting as chronic gastrointestinal symptoms. Am J Gastroenterol. 1993;88:436–9.

119. Shemer SA, Marley L, Miller F. Intestinal pseudo-obstruction due to mitochondrial cytopathy. ANZ J Surg. 2010;80:571.

120. Bianchi A, Ubach M. Acute colonic pseudo-obstruction caused by opiates treated with naloxone. Med Clin (Barc). 1994;103:78.

121. Kapur RP. Neuropathology of paediatric chronic intestinal pseudo-obstruction and related animal models. J Pathol. 2001;194:277–88.

122. Muller-Lissner SA. Adverse effects of laxatives: fact and fiction. Pharmacology. 1993;47(Suppl 1):138–45.

123. Schultz HS, Vernon B. Intestinal pseudo-obstruction related to using verapamil. West J Med. 1989;151:556–8.

124. Lemyze M, Chaaban R, Collet F. Psychotic woman with painful abdominal distension. Life-threatening psychotropic drug-induced gastrointestinal hypomotility. Ann Emerg Med. 2009;54:756–9.

125. McMahon AJ. Amitriptyline overdose complicated by intestinal pseudo-obstruction and caecal perforation. Postgrad Med J. 1989;65:948–9.

126. Esquerdo Galiana G, Briceno Garcia H, Llorca Ferrandiz C, et al. Paralytic ileus due to vinorelbine. Clin Transl Oncol. 2005;7:169–70.

127. Saito H, Yamamoto T, Kimura M, et al. Prostaglandin F2 alpha in the treatment of vinca alkaloid-induced ileus. Am J Med. 1993;95:549–51.

128. Mifune D, Tsukada H, Hosoi M, et al. Chronic intestinal pseudo-obstruction as a paraneoplastic presentation of limited-stage small cell lung cancer. Nihon Kokyuki Gakkai Zasshi. 2010;48:439–43.

129. Wildhaber B, Niggli F, Stallmach T, et al. Intestinal pseudoobstruction as a paraneoplastic syndrome in ganglioneuroblastoma. Eur J Pediatr Surg. 2002;12:429–31.

130. Simonelli M, Banna GL, Santoro A. Thymoma associated with myasthenia and autonomic anti-Hu paraneoplastic neuropathy. Tumori. 2009;95:243–7.

131. Rex DK. Acute colonic pseudo-obstruction (Ogilvie's syndrome). Gastroenterologist. 1994;2:233–8.

132. Yilmazlar A, Iscimen R, Bilgen OF, et al. Ogilvie's syndrome following bilateral knee arthroplasty: a case report. Acta Orthop Traumatol Turc. 2012;46:220–2.

133. Hou JW, Wang TR. Amelia, dextrocardia, asplenia, and congenital short bowel in deleted ring chromosome 4. J Med Genet. 1996;33:879–81.

134. Koike H, Sobue G. Paraneoplastic neuropathy. Handb Clin Neurol. 2013;115:713–26.

135. Stanghellini V, Corinaldesi R, Barbara L. Pseudo-obstruction syndromes. Baillieres Clin Gastroenterol. 1988;2:225–54.

136. Stanghellini V, Cogliandro RF, de Giorgio R, et al. Chronic intestinal pseudo-obstruction: manifestations, natural history and management. Neurogastroenterol Motil. 2007;19:440–52.

137. Stanghellini V, Camilleri M, Malagelada JR. Chronic idiopathic intestinal pseudo-obstruction: clinical and intestinal manometric findings. Gut. 1987;28:5–12.

138. Pingault V, Guiochon-Mantel A, Bondurand N, et al. Peripheral neuropathy with hypomyelination, chronic intestinal pseudo-obstruction and deafness: a developmental "neural crest syndrome" related to a SOX10 mutation. Ann Neurol. 2000;48:671–6.

139. Pingault V, Girard M, Bondurand N, et al. SOX10 mutations in chronic intestinal pseudo-obstruction suggest a complex physiopathological mechanism. Hum Genet. 2002;111:198–206.

140. Mungan Z, Akyuz F, Bugra Z, et al. Familial visceral myopathy with pseudo-obstruction, megaduodenum, Barrett's esophagus, and cardiac abnormalities. Am J Gastroenterol. 2003;98:2556–60.

141. Deglincerti A, De Giorgio R, Cefle K, et al. A novel locus for syndromic chronic idiopathic intestinal pseudo-obstruction maps to chromosome 8q23-q24. Eur J Hum Genet. 2007;15:889–97.

142. Auricchio A, Brancolini V, Casari G, et al. The locus for a novel syndromic form of neuronal intestinal pseudoobstruction maps to Xq28. Am J Hum Genet. 1996;58:743–8.

143. Clayton-Smith J, Walters S, Hobson E, et al. Xq28 duplication presenting with intestinal and bladder dysfunction and a distinctive facial appearance. Eur J Hum Genet. 2009;17:434–43.

144. Gargiulo A, Auricchio R, Barone MV, et al. Filamin A is mutated in X-linked chronic idiopathic intestinal pseudo-obstruction with central nervous system involvement. Am J Hum Genet. 2007;80:751–8.

145. Kapur RP, Robertson SP, Hannibal MC, et al. Diffuse abnormal layering of small intestinal smooth muscle is present in patients with FLNA mutations and x-linked intestinal pseudo-obstruction. Am J Surg Pathol. 2010;34:1528–43.

146. Bardosi A, Creutzfeldt W, DiMauro S, et al. Myo-, neuro-, gastrointestinal encephalopathy (MNGIE syndrome) due to partial deficiency of cytochrome-c-oxidase. A new mitochondrial multisystem disorder. Acta Neuropathol. 1987;74:248–58.

147. Nishino I, Spinazzola A, Hirano M. Thymidine phosphorylase gene mutations in MNGIE, a human mitochondrial disorder. Science. 1999;283:689–92.

148. Giordano C, Sebastiani M, De Giorgio R, et al. Gastrointestinal dysmotility in mitochondrial neurogastrointestinal encephalomyopathy is caused by mitochondrial DNA depletion. Am J Pathol. 2008;173:1120–8.

149. Faure C. Chronic intestinal pseudo-obstruction syndrome. In: Walker W, Goulet O, Kleinman R, et al., editors. Pediatric gastrointestinal disease. Ontario: BC Decker; 2004. pp. 1044–54.

150. Knowles CH, De Giorgio R, Kapur RP, et al. Gastrointestinal neuromuscular pathology: guidelines for histological techniques and reporting on behalf of the Gastro. 2009 International Working Group. Acta Neuropathol. 2009;118:271–301.

151. Knowles CH, Lindberg G, Panza E, et al. New perspectives in the diagnosis and management of enteric neuropathies. Nat Rev Gastroenterol Hepatol. 2013;10:206–18.

152. De Giorgio R, Camilleri M. Human enteric neuropathies: morphology and molecular pathology. Neurogastroenterol Motil. 2004;16:515–31.

153. De Giorgio R, Sarnelli G, Corinaldesi R, et al. Advances in our understanding of the pathology of chronic intestinal pseudo-obstruction. Gut. 2004;53:1549–52.

154. De Giorgio R, Guerrini S, Barbara G, et al. Inflammatory neuropathies of the enteric nervous system. Gastroenterology. 2004;126:1872–83.

155. De Giorgio R, Bovara M, Barbara G, et al. Anti-HuD-induced neuronal apoptosis underlying paraneoplastic gut dysmotility. Gastroenterology. 2003;125:70–9.

156. Hubball A, Martin JE, Lang B, et al. The role of humoral autoimmunity in gastrointestinal neuromuscular diseases. Prog Neurobiol. 2009;87:10–20.

157. Hubball AW, Lang B, Souza MA, et al. Voltage-gated potassium channel (K(v) 1) autoantibodies in patients with chagasic gut dysmotility and distribution of K(v) 1 channels in human enteric neuromusculature (autoantibodies in GI dysmotility). Neurogastroenterol Motil. 2012;24:719–28, e344.

158. De Giorgio R, Barbara G, Stanghellini V, et al. Clinical and morphofunctional features of idiopathic myenteric ganglionitis underlying severe intestinal motor dysfunction: a study of three cases. Am J Gastroenterol. 2002;97:2454–9.

159. Schappi MG, Smith VV, Milla PJ, et al. Eosinophilic myenteric ganglionitis is associated with functional intestinal obstruction. Gut. 2003;52:752–5.

160. Murch S. Allergy and intestinal dysmotility—evidence of genuine causal linkage? Curr Opin Gastroenterol. 2006;22:664–8.

161. Bassotti G, Villanacci V. Mast cells in intestinal motility disorders: please also look beyond IBS. Dig Dis Sci. 2012;57:2475–6, author reply 6.

162. Bassotti G, Villanacci V, Nascimbeni R, et al. Increase of colonic mast cells in obstructed defecation and their relationship with enteric glia. Dig Dis Sci. 2012;57:65–71.

163. Di Nardo G, Blandizzi C, Volta U, et al. Review article: molecular, pathological and therapeutic features of human enteric neuropathies. Aliment Pharmacol Ther. 2008;28:25–42.

164. Mann SD, Debinski HS, Kamm MA. Clinical characteristics of chronic idiopathic intestinal pseudo-obstruction in adults. Gut. 1997;41:675–81.

165. Lindberg G, Tornblom H, Iwarzon M, et al. Full-thickness biopsy findings in chronic intestinal pseudo-obstruction and enteric dysmotility. Gut. 2009;58:1084–90.

166. Knowles CH, Silk DB, Darzi A, et al. Deranged smooth muscle alpha-actin as a biomarker of intestinal pseudo-obstruction: a controlled multinational case series. Gut. 2004;53:1583–9.

167. Bassotti G, Villanacci V, Antonelli E, et al. Enteric glial cells: new players in gastrointestinal motility? Lab Invest. 2007;87:628–32.

168. Bassotti G, Villanacci V. Can "functional" constipation be considered a form of enteric neuro-gliopathy? Glia. 2011;59:345–50.

169. Oton E, Moreira V, Redondo C, et al. Chronic intestinal pseudo-obstruction due to lymphocytic leiomyositis: is there a place for immunomodulatory therapy? Gut. 2005;54:1343–4.

170. Smith JA, Hauser SC, Madara JL. Hollow visceral myopathy: a light- and electron-microscopic study. Am J Surg Pathol. 1982;6:269–75.

171. Schuffler MD. Chronic intestinal pseudo-obstruction syndromes. Med Clin North Am. 1981;65:1331–58.

172. Wedel T, Van Eys GJ, Waltregny D, et al. Novel smooth muscle markers reveal abnormalities of the intestinal musculature in severe colorectal motility disorders. Neurogastroenterol Motil. 2006;18:526–38.

173. Farrugia G. Interstitial cells of Cajal in health and disease. Neurogastroenterol Motil. 2008;20(Suppl 1):54–63.

174. Camilleri M. Intestinal dysmotility: does the X-ray resolve the real dilemma? J Pediatr Gastroenterol Nutr. 1997;24:100–1.

175. Ohkubo H, Kessoku T, Fuyuki A, et al. Assessment of small bowel motility in patients with chronic intestinal pseudo-obstruction using cine-MRI. Am J Gastroenterol. 2013;108:1130–9.

176. Yakan S, Caliskan C, Kaplan H, et al. Superior mesenteric artery syndrome: a rare cause of intestinal obstruction. Diagnosis and surgical management. Indian J Surg. 2013;75:106–10.

177. Sumiyama K, Gostout CJ. Clinical applications of submucosal endoscopy. Curr Opin Gastroenterol. 2011;27:412–7.

178. Klibansky D, Rothstein RI. Robotics in endoscopy. Curr Opin Gastroenterol. 2012;28:477–82.

179. Belkind-Gerson J, Tran K, Di Lorenzo C. Novel techniques to study colonic motor function in children. Curr Gastroenterol Rep. 2013;15:335.

180. Green AD, Belkind-Gerson J, Surjanhata BC, et al. Wireless motility capsule test in children with upper gastrointestinal symptoms. J Pediatr. 2013;162:1181–7.

181. Cucchiara S, Borrelli O, Salvia G, et al. A normal gastrointestinal motility excludes chronic intestinal pseudoobstruction in children. Dig Dis Sci. 2000;45:258–64.

182. Boige N, Faure C, Cargill G, et al. Manometrical evaluation in visceral neuropathies in children. J Pediatr Gastroenterol Nutr. 1994;19:71–7.

183. Hyman PE, McDiarmid SV, Napolitano J, et al. Antroduodenal motility in children with chronic intestinal pseudo-obstruction. J Pediatr. 1988;112:899–905.

184. Tomomasa T, Itoh Z, Koizumi T, et al. Manometric study on the intestinal motility in a case of megacystis-microcolon-intestinal hypoperistalsis syndrome. J Pediatr Gastroenterol Nutr. 1985;4:307–10.

185. Hyman PE, Di Lorenzo C, McAdams L, et al. Predicting the clinical response to cisapride in children with chronic intestinal pseudo-obstruction. Am J Gastroenterol. 1993;88:832–6.

186. Di Lorenzo C, Lucanto C, Flores AF, et al. Effect of sequential erythromycin and octreotide on antroduodenal manometry. J Pediatr Gastroenterol Nutr. 1999;29:293–6.

187. Fell JM, Smith VV, Milla PJ. Infantile chronic idiopathic intestinal pseudo-obstruction: the role of small intestinal manometry as a diagnostic tool and prognostic indicator. Gut. 1996;39:306–11.

188. Summers RW, Anuras S, Green J. Jejunal manometry patterns in health, partial intestinal obstruction, and pseudoobstruction. Gastroenterology. 1983;85:1290–300.

189. Camilleri M. Jejunal manometry in distal subacute mechanical obstruction: significance of prolonged simultaneous contractions. Gut. 1989;30:468–75.

190. Hyman PE, Bursch B, Beck D, et al. Discriminating pediatric condition falsification from chronic intestinal pseudo-obstruction in toddlers. Child Maltreat. 2002;7:132–7.

191. Hyman PE, Bursch B, Sood M, et al. Visceral pain-associated disability syndrome: a descriptive analysis. J Pediatr Gastroenterol Nutr. 2002;35:663–8.

192. Lyford G, Foxx-Orenstein A. Chronic intestinal pseudoobstruction. Curr Treat Options Gastroenterol. 2004;7:317–25.

193. Di Lorenzo C, Flores AF, Buie T, et al. Intestinal motility and jejunal feeding in children with chronic intestinal pseudo-obstruction. Gastroenterology. 1995;108:1379–85.

194. Gariepy CE, Mousa H. Clinical management of motility disorders in children. Semin Pediatr Surg. 2009;18:224–38.

195. Di Lorenzo C, Youssef NN. Diagnosis and management of intestinal motility disorders. Semin Pediatr Surg. 2010;19:50–8.

196. Longo WE, Vernava AM 3rd. Prokinetic agents for lower gastrointestinal motility disorders. Dis Colon Rectum. 1993;36:696–708.

197. Chini P, Toskes PP, Waseem S, et al. Effect of azithromycin on small bowel motility in patients with gastrointestinal dysmotility. Scand J Gastroenterol. 2012;47:422–7.

198. Sorhaug S, Steinshamn SL, Waldum HL. Octreotide treatment for paraneoplastic intestinal pseudo-obstruction complicating SCLC. Lung Cancer. 2005;48:137–40.

199. Lee JW, Bang KW, Jang PS, et al. Neostigmine for the treatment of acute colonic pseudo-obstruction (ACPO) in pediatric hematologic malignancies. Korean J Hematol. 2010;45:62–5.

200. Tack J, Camilleri M, Chang L, et al. Systematic review: cardiovascular safety profile of 5-HT(4) agonists developed for gastrointestinal disorders. Aliment Pharmacol Ther. 2012;35:745–67.

201. Winter HS, Di Lorenzo C, Benninga MA, et al. Oral prucalopride in children with functional constipation. J Pediatr Gastroenterol Nutr. 2013;57:197–203.

202. Chong K, Dhatariya K. A case of severe, refractory diabetic gastroparesis managed by prolonged use of aprepitant. Nat Rev Endocrinol. 2009;5:285–8.

203. Tack J, Depoortere I, Bisschops R, et al. Influence of ghrelin on gastric emptying and meal-related symptoms in idiopathic gastroparesis. Aliment Pharmacol Ther. 2005;22:847–53.

204. Verne GN, Eaker EY, Hardy E, et al. Effect of octreotide and erythromycin on idiopathic and scleroderma-associated intestinal pseudoobstruction. Dig Dis Sci. 1995;40:1892–901.

205. Pakarinen MP, Kurvinen A, Koivusalo AI, et al. Surgical treatment and outcomes of severe pediatric intestinal motility disorders requiring parenteral nutrition. J Pediatr Surg. 2013;48:333–8.

206. Michaud L, Guimber D, Carpentier B, et al. Gastrostomy as a decompression technique in children with chronic gastrointestinal obstruction. J Pediatr Gastroenterol Nutr. 2001;32:82–5.

207. Lapointe R. Chronic idiopathic intestinal pseudo-obstruction treated by near total small bowel resection: a 20-year experience. J Gastrointest Surg. 2010;14:1937–42.

208. Nunokawa T, Yokogawa N, Ohtsuka H, et al. Transgastric long tube placement following percutaneous endoscopic gastrostomy for severe chronic intestinal pseudo-obstruction related to systemic sclerosis. Mod Rheumatol. 2013.

209. Teich S, Mousa HM, Punati J, et al. Efficacy of permanent gastric electrical stimulation for the treatment of gastroparesis and functional dyspepsia in children and adolescents. J Pediatr Surg. 2013;48:178–83.

210. D'Antiga L, Goulet O. Intestinal failure in children: the European view. J Pediatr Gastroenterol Nutr. 2013;56:118–26.

211. Goulet O, Lacaille F, Colomb V, et al. Intestinal transplantation in children: Paris experience. Transplant Proc. 2002;34:1887–8.

212. Loinaz C, Rodriguez MM, Kato T, et al. Intestinal and multivisceral transplantation in children with severe gastrointestinal dysmotility. J Pediatr Surg. 2005;40:1598–604.

213. Millar AJ, Gupte G, Sharif K. Intestinal transplantation for motility disorders. Semin Pediatr Surg. 2009;18:258–62.

214. Iwarzon M, Gardulf A, Lindberg G. Functional status, health-related quality of life and symptom severity in patients with chronic intestinal pseudo-obstruction and enteric dysmotility. Scand J Gastroenterol. 2009;44:700–7.

215. Faure C, Goulet O, Ategbo S, et al. Chronic intestinal pseudoobstruction syndrome: clinical analysis, outcome, and prognosis in 105 children. French-speaking group of pediatric gastroenterology. Dig Dis Sci. 1999;44:953–9.

216. Krishnamurthy S, Heng Y, Schuffler MD. Chronic intestinal pseudo-obstruction in infants and children caused by diverse abnormalities of the myenteric plexus. Gastroenterology. 1993;104:1398–408.

217. Granata C, Puri P. Megacystis-microcolon-intestinal hypoperistalsis syndrome. J Pediatr Gastroenterol Nutr. 1997;25:12–9.

218. Schwankovsky L, Mousa H, Rowhani A, et al. Quality of life outcomes in congenital chronic intestinal pseudo-obstruction. Dig Dis Sci. 2002;47:1965–8.

Gastrointestinal and Nutritional Problems in Neurologically Handicapped Children

Paolo Quitadamo and Annamaria Staiano

Introduction

The increasing survival of children with severe central nervous system damage has created a major challenge for medical care. Although the primary problems for individuals with developmental disabilities are physical and mental incapacities, several clinical reports have indicated that brain damage may result in significant gastrointestinal (GI) dysfunction [1–4]. The enteric nervous system contains more neurones than the spinal cord and thus it is not surprising that insults to the central nervous system may affect the complex integrated capacities underlying feeding and nutrition [5]

The increased awareness of such conditions, together with a better understanding of their etiology and interplay, is essential to achieve an optimal global management of this group of children.

Feeding and Nutritional Aspects

Historically, severe malnutrition has been accepted as unavoidable and irremediable consequence of neurological impairment. Poor nutritional state was often marked by linear growth failure, decreased lean body mass, and diminished fat stores [6, 7]. Over the past two to three decades, multidisciplinary feeding programs providing comprehensive evaluation and treatment of feeding disorders in children with developmental disabilities have been instrumental in improving the nutritional status, quality of life, and reduced hospitalization rates [8]. Studies on small number of children with developmental disabilities have demonstrated that adequate nutritional support, provided by less invasive enteral access methods and better tolerated enteral formulas, may improve weight, muscle mass, subcutaneous energy store,

peripheral circulation, the healing of decubitus ulcers, and general well-being, while decreasing irritability and spasticity [9, 10].

The true prevalence of undernutrition in neurologically impaired children is unknown. It has been estimated that approximately one third of them are undernourished and many exhibit the consequences of malnutrition [7]. Yet, the incidence and severity of malnutrition increases with the duration and the severity of neurological impairment [11–13]. Parameters to assess malnutrition and overnutrition in the handicapped child have to be adjusted. Height is a proper parameter for growth and nutritional status, but difficult in children with malformations and spasticity [14–16]. Also, disproportionate development of the head, rump, and extremities makes assessment of height as a parameter of nutritional status difficult [17–19]. Therefore, crown–rump length, width, crown–heel length, distal femoral length, and distal arm length (Spender growth curve) have been developed to assess growth and to relate height to developmental abnormalities or to nutrition [20]. In a study on more than 2000 institutionalized children with a handicap in Tokyo, Japan, height and weight were measured in four distinct groups. Groups were divided into deaf children, blind children, mentally retarded children, some of whom were completely ambulatory, and 15% of whom needed crutches, and physically handicapped children, of whom 65% were nonambulatory. Height more than three standard deviations below the mean was present in 2% of deaf children, 10% of blind children, 15% of children with mental retardation, and 45% of physically handicapped children. Underweight more than two standard deviations below the mean was present in 1% of deaf children, 4% of blind children, 5% of children with mental retardation, and 24% of physically handicapped children [15]. In a Finnish study of patients up to the age of 20, the body mass index (BMI) showed that underweight (BMI < 20 kg/m^2) was present in 30%, overweight in 10%, and severe overweight in 7% (BMI > 32 kg/m^2) [21].

The predominant nutritional deficit in neurologically impaired children is in energy intake, with only 20% of these

A. Staiano (✉) · P. Quitadamo
Department of Translational Medical Science, Section of Pediatrics, University of Naples "Federico II", Via S. Pansini 5, 80131 Naples, Italy
e-mail: staiano@unina.it

© Springer International Publishing Switzerland 2016
S. Guandalini et al. (eds.), *Textbook of Pediatric Gastroenterology, Hepatology and Nutrition*,
DOI 10.1007/978-3-319-17169-2_24

children regularly ingesting 100% of their estimated average requirement. Moreover, half of the children with severe disabilities consumed less than 81% of the reference nutrient intake for copper, iron, magnesium, and zinc, with that influenced by their large consumption of milk [22].

Nutritional support is essential for the care of neurologically impaired children. Undernourished handicapped children might not respond properly to intercurrent diseases and suffer unnecessarily. On the other hand, restoring a normal nutritional status results in a better quality of life in many. Assessment of nutritional status requires a proper follow-up of height, body weight, and assessment of the standard deviation score. By so doing, negative changes are easily discovered and appropriate nutritional intervention can be initiated. An individualized intervention plan that accounts for the child's nutritional status, feeding ability, and medical condition should be determined. Energy requirements must be individualized considering mobility, muscle tone, activity level, altered metabolism, and growth. The easiest and least invasive method to increase energy intake is to improve oral intake. Food caloric density may be increased by adding modular nutrients, modifying recipes, or using high-calorie formulas. Children who cannot chew effectively may be able to receive the same foods blenderized into a puree of acceptable consistency. Those who can tolerate solids but not liquids can have commercial thickeners added to their fluids. Oral feeding skills may be improved with therapy, even if the results may be disappointing [23–25]. Adequate positioning of the child during meals and appropriate food temperature are furthermore important. However, oral intake can be maintained as long as there is no risk of aspiration, the child is growing well, and the time required to feed the child remains within acceptable limits.

When oral intake is unsafe, insufficient, or too time consuming, enteral nutrition should be initiated. The type of enteral access will depend on the anticipated duration of enteral nutrition support as well as the clinical status of the child. Nasogastric tubes are minimally invasive but are easily dislodged and have local complications such as sinusitis, congestion, otitis, and skin irritation. Generally, nasogastric feeds should only be used for a short-term nutritional support (less than 3 months). For long-term enteral nutrition support, a gastrostomy should be considered. Gastrostomies are more invasive, but are also more convenient and esthetically acceptable. Gastrostomy placement has been shown to reduce feeding time, food-related choking episodes, frequency of chest infections, and family stress, and to improve weight and nutritional status significantly in children with severe neurologic impairment [10, 18]. However, percutaneous endoscopic gastrostomy (PEG) is not without complications or concerns. Minor catheter infections, perforation, and an overall lessened length of survival have being described in both adult and pediatric populations [26–31].

The anatomy and function of the stomach should be carefully evaluated before the placement of the feeding tube. The coexistence of gastroesophageal reflux (GER) may require a simultaneous fundoplication, and delayed gastric emptying must necessitate pyloroplasty or duodenal placement of the distal portion of the tube. Physiologically designed formulas of increased caloric and protein density can be used for gastric and nasogastric infusion, as palatability is no longer an issue. The choice between bolus and drip may depend on esophagogastric function, the volume to be delivered, or the home care needs of the child and his or her caregivers. Often patients may benefit from a combination of daytime bolus and nocturnal continuous feeds, the latter providing 30–50% of the child's nutrient needs and thus allowing more freedom for daily activities. When safety of oral feeding is not an issue, these enteral techniques can merely supplement the child's own nutrition, with caregivers continuing to feed the child actively. This dual feeding method often provides great satisfaction to parents and caregivers, because the mealtime interaction is improved when there is no longer a need for force-feeding of medication or nourishment.

GI Problems

Chronic GI disorders are very common in children with neurological impairment, being reported a prevalence of up to 92% [32]. Dysphagia, rumination, GER, delayed gastric emptying, abdominal pain, and constipation have all been described in this group of children, potentially contributing to feeding difficulties and carrying challenging long-term management issues.

Dysphagia

Oral motor dysfunction is a frequent concomitant and often one of the first signs of neuromuscular impairment. Related swallowing problems have been shown to affect up to 90% of neurologically impaired children, being major contributors to malnutrition [1]. This is not surprising since the development of oral–motor skills mirrors general neurological maturation and requires the coordination of the movement of several striated muscles in the mouth, pharynx, and esophagus by six cranial nerves, the brain stem, and the cerebral cortex. In addition, anatomic abnormalities such as cleft palate, laryngeal clefts, and tracheoesophageal fistula may accompany neurologic deficits as part of a congenital or genetic syndrome. Dysphagia may manifest as distress during meals (including coughing, choking, and refusal of feeding), chronic or episodic aspiration-related respiratory disorder, and failure to thrive. Barium swallow, cine swallow, radionuclide esophageal clearance scan, and esophageal manometry may all be of some help in the clinical assessment. Successful management of dysphagia is central to the child's well-being and ability to achieve his or her potential. Neurologically impaired children often show greater problems with liquid foods, thus requiring the use of thickener products. Oral motor exercise approaches using sensory modalities may help improving muscle strength and oral coordination. Nevertheless, in most cases, the presence of unsafe swallows and/or long-lasting distressed meals finally lead to the choice of enteral nutrition.

Gastroesophageal Reflux

Several reports have demonstrated the high incidence of GER in neurologically impaired children. GER symptoms such as vomiting, rumination, and regurgitation are found in 20–30% of the intellectually disabled population. GER-related iron-deficiency anemia and hematemesis are noted in 10–20% of patients. In the Netherlands and Belgium, in a large cohort of more than 1500 patients, a randomly selected intellectually disabled population was tested with pH-metry during 24 h. A pathological pH test (defined as a duration of a pH of <4 for more than 4% of the measured time) was seen in 48% of cases [33]. These patients were subjected to endoscopy, and reflux esophagitis was found in 96%: 14% had grade I esophagitis, 33% had grade II, 39% had grade III, and 13% had grade IV (Savary–Miller classification). Barrett's esophagus was found in 14% and peptic strictures in 4% of cases. This study was repeated for the group under the age of 14, and similar findings were seen. In fact, GER disease was found even in the absence of overt symptomatology. Prolonged supine position, increased intra-abdominal pressure secondary to spasticity and scoliosis, a coexisting hiatal hernia have been supposed to be contributing factors to the increased frequency of GER. Central nervous system dysfunction, however, is likely to be the prime cause, being GER probably a part of the generalized dysmotility of the foregut, if not of the entire intestine. Decreased resting pressure and increased frequency of transient relaxations of the lower esophageal sphincter, together with motility abnormalities, are probably a consequence of neuromuscular incoordination.

Currently, the most accurate way of diagnosing GER is 24-h esophageal pH impedance recording, which not only allows to quantify the amount of reflux episodes but also helps in establishing the temporal relationship between GER and the symptom complex in question. The diagnostic work-up should then include upper GI endoscopy with multiple esophageal biopsies and upper GI barium study, in order to evaluate the mucosa and to look for the possible presence of strictures, diverticuli, or hiatal hernia. Radionuclide studies such as gastroesophageal scintigraphy should also be performed, due to the higher incidence of delayed gastric emptying which may contribute to GER [34, 35]. An esophageal manometry evaluating visceral motility may be helpful to detect the underlying pathophysiological mechanisms, especially when surgery becomes necessary.

Although children with neurologic impairment are more likely to have intractable reflux and eventually require some surgical procedures, medical therapy should be tried first. When surgery becomes advisable, the Nissen fundoplication is currently the most widely used technique to strengthen the anti-reflux barrier and relief symptoms.

Constipation

Infrequent stool passage and hard bowel movements are very common in neurologically impaired children. The incidence of constipation was around 61% in a large cohort of mentally handicapped children in Dutch and Belgian institutions [36]. Total and sequential colonic transit times have been shown to be prolonged and delayed at the level of the left colon and rectum in this group of children, implying a probable defect in gut innervations [3]. The problem is usually exacerbated by prolonged immobility, inadequate fiber intake, and medications. Unfortunately, recognition and therefore effective management of constipation are often delayed because their other disabilities overshadow those related to defecation. Therapeutic approach needs to be tailored to the individual patient. Oral or rectal disimpaction should be followed by promotion of regular bowel habits, through dietary modifications, positioning, and use of medications. A significant number of children with neurological impairment need to be on chronic doses of laxatives, which are usually effective in enabling regular defecations. However, when medical treatment fails, a surgically placed appendicostomy should be considered.

References

1. Reilly S, Skuse D, Poblete X. Prevalence of feeding problems and oral motor dysfunction in children with cerebral palsy: a community survey. J Pediatr. 1996;129:877–82.
2. Sondheimer JM, Morris BA. Gastroesophageal reflux among severely retarded children. J Pediatr. 1979;94:710–4.
3. Staiano A, Del Giudice E. Colonic transit and anorectal manometry in children with severe brain damage. Pediatrics. 1994;94:169–73.
4. Ravelli AM, Milla PJ. Vomiting and gastroesophageal motor activity in children with disorders of the central nervous system. J Pediatr Gastroenterol Nutr. 1998;26:56–63.
5. Menkes JH, Ament ME. Neurologic disorders of gastroesophageal function. Adv Neurol. 1988;49:409–16.
6. Patrick J, Boland M, Stoski D, Murray GE. Rapid correction of wasting in children with cerebral palsy. Dev Med Child Neurol. 1986;28:734–39.

7. Stallings VA, Cronk CE, Zemel BS, Charney EB. Body composition in children with spastic quadriplegic cerebral palsy. J Pediatr. 1995;126:833–9.

8. Schwartz SM, Corredor J, Fisher-Medina J, et al. Diagnosis and treatment of feeding disorders in children with developmental disabilities. Pediatrics. 2001;108:671–6.

9. Rempel GR, Colwell S, Nelson RP. Growth in children with cerebral palsy fed via gastrostomy. Pediatrics. 1988;82:857–62.

10. Sanders KD, Cox K, Cannon R, et al. Growth response to enteral feeding by children with cerebral palsy. JPEN J Parenter Enteral Nutr. 1990;14:23–6.

11. Stallings VA, Charney EB, Davies JC, Cronk CE. Nutritional status and growth of children with diplegic or hemiplegic cerebral palsy. Dev Med Child Neurol. 1993;35:997–1006.

12. Stevenson RD, Hayes RP, Cater LV, Blackman JA. Clinical correlates of linear growth in children with cerebral palsy. Dev Med Child Neurol. 1994;36:135–42.

13. Sánchez-Lastres J, Eirís-Puñal J, Otero-Cepeda JL, Pavón-Belinchón P, Castro-Gago M. Nutritional status of mentally retarded children in north-west Spain. I. Anthropometric indicators. Acta Paediatr. 2003;92:747–53.

14. Amundson JA, Sherbondy A, Dyke van DC, Alexander R. Early identification and treatment necessary to prevent malnutrition in children and adolescents with severe disabilities. J Am Diet Assoc. 1994;94:880–3.

15. Miller F, Koresca J. Height measurement of patients with neuromuscular disease and contractures. Dev Med Child Neurol. 1991;33:55–8.

16. Garn S, Weir HF. Assessing the nutritional status of the mentally retarded. Am J Clin Nutr. 1971;24:853–4.

17. Roche AF. Growth assessment in abnormal children. Kidney Int. 1978;14:369–77.

18. Mosier HD, Grossman HJ, Dingman HF. Physical growth in mental defectives: a study in an institutionalised population. Pediatrics. 1995;36:465–73.

19. Rimmer JH, Kelly LE, Rosentswieg J. Accuracy of anthropometric equations for estimating body composition of mentally retarded adults. Am J Ment Defic. 1987;91:626–32.

20. Spender QW, Cronk CE, Charney EB, Stallings VA. Assessment of linear growth of children with cerebral palsy: use of alternative measures to height or length. Dev Med Child Neurol. 1989;31:206–14.

21. Simila S, Niskanen P. Underweight and overweight cases among the mentally retarded. J Ment Def Res. 1991;35:160–4.

22. Sullivan PB, Juszczak E, Lambert BR, et al. Impact of feeding problems on nutritional intake and growth: Oxford Feeding Study II. Dev Med Child Neurol. 2002;44:461–7.

23. Gisel EG. Effect of oral sensorimotor treatment on measures of growth and efficiency of eating in the moderately eating-impaired child with cerebral palsy. Dysphagia. 1996;11:48–58.

24. Pinnington L, Hegarty J. Effects of consistent food presentation on oral-motor skill acquisition in children with severe neurological impairment. Dysphagia. 2000;15:213–23.

25. Rogers B. Feeding method and health outcomes of children with cerebral palsy. J Pediatr. 2004;145:S28–32.

26. Brant CQ, Stanich P, Ferrari AP, Jr. Improvement in children's nutritional status after enteral feeding by PEG: an iterim report. Gastrointest Endosc. 1990;50:183–8.

27. Arvedson JC, Rogers BT. Pediatric swallowing and feeding disorders. J Med Speech-Lang Pathol. 1993;1:203–21.

28. Gauderer MW. Percutaneous endoscopic gastrostomy: a 10-year experience with 220 children. J Pediatr Surg. 1991;26:288–92.

29. Eyman RK, Grossman HJ, Chaney RH, Call TL. Survival of profoundly disabled people with severe mental retardation. Am J Dis Child. 1993;147:329–36.

30. Ashwal S, Eyman RK, Call TL. Life expectancy of children in a persistent vegetative state. Pediatr Neurol. 1994;10:27–33.

31. Strauss D, Kastner T, Ashwal S, White J. Tubefeeding and mortality in children with severe disabilities and mental retardation. Pediatrics. 1997;99:358–62.

32. Del Giudice E, Staiano A, Capano G, et al. Gastrointestinal manifestations in children with cerebral palsy. Brain Dev. 1999;21:307–11.

33. Bohmer CJ, Niezen-de Boer MC, Klinkenberg-Knol EC, et al. Gastro-esophageal reflux disease in institutionalised intellectually disabled individuals. Neth J Med. 1997;51:134–9.

34. Fonkalsrud EW, Foglia RP, Ament ME, et al. Operative treatment for the gastroesophageal reflux syndrome in children. J Pediatr Surg. 1989;24(6):525–9.

35. Okada T, Sasaki F, Asaka M, et al. Delay of gastric emptying measured by 13C-acetate breath test in neurologically impaired children with gastroesophageal reflux. Eur J Pediatr Surg. 2005;15(2):77–81.

36. Bohmer CJ, Taminiau JA, Klinkenberg-Knol EC, Meuwissen SG. The prevalence of constipation in institutionalized people with intellectual disability. J Intellect Disabil Res. 2001;45:212–8.

Cyclic Vomiting Syndrome

Bhanu Sunku and B U. K. Li

Introduction

Despite improved characterization, recognition, and understanding of cyclic vomiting syndrome (CVS) in the past two decades, without a delineated pathophysiologic cascade, it remains classified as a functional gastrointestinal (GI) disorder. The hallmark symptoms described by Samuel Gee in 1882 remain applicable today and include stereotypical, severe episodes of vomiting punctuating symptom-free periods or baseline health [1]. Earlier clinical diagnosis has been facilitated by the recently defined consensus diagnostic criteria by North American Society for Pediatric Gastroenterology, Hepatology, and Nutrition (NASPGHAN 2008) and Rome III (2006) criteria, the former being quantitatively more rigorous, that is, requiring three to five versus two total episodes [2] (Table 25.1). From an operational standpoint, the predominant and most consistent symptom during episodes defines the illness, that is, abdominal pain is termed abdominal migraine, and conversely vomiting is denoted CVS. However, there is considerable clinical overlap because ~50% of those diagnosed with abdominal migraine also vomit, and ~80% of those with CVS also have abdominal pain.

The continuum between CVS and migraine was suggested by Whitney in 1898 and corroborated by other authors including us in 1998 [4, 5]. In a cross-sectional school survey in Scotland, Abu-Arafeh described a developmental progression from CVS to abdominal migraine and migraine headaches (median ages 5, 9, and 11 years, prevalences 1.9, 4, and 11%, respectively) [6]. This suggestion of a natural history that begins with CVS and ends with migraines reproduces initial reports by Barlow in 1984 who labeled this progression as the "periodic syndrome" [7]. Although some experience all three phases, the majority trade CVS for migraines by age 10. We estimate that 75% will develop migraine headaches by age 18 years.

The lack of a specific The International Classification of Diseases (ICD) 9 code and use of persistent vomiting (536.2) have hindered establishment of the true prevalence of CVS. ICD 10 will have a specific code and enable proper epidemiologic surveys. Typical misdiagnoses, including gastroenteritis, gastroesophageal reflux, food poisoning, and eating disorders, often delay accurate diagnosis by a median 2.6 years. In our consecutive series, CVS was second only to gastroesophageal reflux as a cause of recurrent vomiting [8]. Two school-based surveys (not clinical exam) estimated the frequency to be 2% in Scottish and Turkish children, and the incidence of new cases of CVS was reported to be 3.15 per 100,000 children per year in Irish children [6, 9]. In our series, the average age of onset of CVS is 4.8 years, with a predominance in girls over boys (57:43; Table 25.2).

Recently, pathophysiologic connections have been made with mitochondrial disease, autonomic dysfunction and the stress response. Current research, including our own, is focused on the identification of neuroendocrine mechanisms mediating vomiting in these patients.

Cyclic Versus Chronic Patterns of Vomiting

An important clinical clue to the diagnosis of CVS is the pattern of vomiting. Based on temporal pattern, children with recurrent vomiting can be delineated into cyclic and chronic groups. The *cyclic group* has an intense, but intermittent pattern of vomiting with peak emesis of ≥ 4/h and ≤ 2 episodes per week [10]. The *chronic group* has a low-grade, daily pattern of emesis with <4 emesis/h and >2 episodes per week [10]. Two thirds of all children with recurrent vomiting fit into the *chronic* or continuous pattern of vomiting. These children rarely appear acutely ill or become dehydrated. Conversely, the *cyclic* pattern is associated with more in-

B. Sunku (✉)
Department of Pediatrics, Mount Kisco Medical Group,
110 South Bedford Road, Mount Kisco, NY 10549, USA
e-mail: bsunku@mkmg.com

B. U. K. Li
Division of Gastroenterology, Hepatology and Nutrition,
Medical College of Wisconsin, Milwaukee, WI, USA

© Springer International Publishing Switzerland 2016
S. Guandalini et al. (eds.), *Textbook of Pediatric Gastroenterology, Hepatology and Nutrition*,
DOI 10.1007/978-3-319-17169-2_25

Table 25.1 NASPGHAN and Rome III diagnostic criteria. (Sunku and Li [3], with kind permission from Springer Science + Business Media)

NASPGHAN
1. At least five attacks in any interval, or a minimum of three attacks during a 6-month period
2. Episodic attacks of intense nausea and vomiting lasting 1 h–10 days and occurring at least 1 week apart
3. Stereotypical pattern and symptoms in the individual patient
4. Vomiting during attacks occurs at least 4 times/h for at least 1 h
5. Return to baseline health between episodes
6. Not attributed to another disorder
Rome III
1. Two or more periods of intense nausea and unremitting vomiting or retching lasting hours to days
2. Return to usual state of health lasting weeks to months

All respective criteria must be met to meet consensus definitions for both NASPGHAN and Rome III

Table 25.2 Epidemiology and demographics. (Sunku and Li [3], with kind permission from Springer Science + Business Media)

Features	
Age of onset	4.8 years
Delay in diagnosis	2.6 years
Prevalence	2%
Incidence	3.15/100,000
Female to male ratio	57:43
Migraine association	39–87%

tense vomiting and affected children more often require IV hydration (62 vs. 18%) compared with the chronic group [8] (Table 25.3).

These two patterns are also important because both of these groups differ in symptom and diagnostic profile. In those with the cyclical vomiting pattern, non-GI disorders including neurologic (including abdominal migraine), renal, endocrine, and metabolic ones predominate over GI disor-

Table 25.3 Characteristics of chronic and cyclic vomiting. (Reprinted with permission from Ref. [11], Table 20.3, p. 292)

	Chronic pattern	Cyclic pattern
Time of onset	Daytime	Nighttime or early morning
Peak number of emeses/h	<4 emeses	≥4 emeses
Frequency of recurrence	>2 episodes/week	≤2 episodes/week, typically 2–4 weeks
Family history of migraine	Uncommon (14%)	Common (82%)
Ill-appearing	No	Yes (pale, lethargic)
Headaches	Infrequent (19%)	More frequent (41%)
Photophobia	Infrequent (4%)	More frequent (18%)
Vertigo	Infrequent (7%)	More frequent (24%)
Intravenous hydration	Uncommon (18%)	Common (58%)
Esophagitis on EGD	Common (59%)	Uncommon (15%)

EGD esophagogastroduodenoscopy

Table 25.4 Differential diagnosis of cyclic vomiting. ([11], Table 20.4, p. 293)

		Chronic pattern	Cyclic pattern
Gastrointestinal		Peptic injury (GERD esophagitis, gastritis, duodenitis)	Anatomic (malrotation, volvulus, duplication cyst)
		Eosinophilic gastroenteritis/esophagitis	
		Celiac disease	
		Giardiasis	
		Inflammatory bowel disease	Pseudo-obstruction
			Cholelithiasis/gallbladder dyskinesia
		Chronic appendicitis	
		Pancreatitis	
Infectious		Chronic sinusitis	Sinusitis/other infections may be a trigger
Genitourinary		Pyelonephritis, pregnancy	Acute hydronephrosis due to uretopelvic junction obstruction or stones
Metabolic		Rare	Mitochondrial disorders (MELAS)
			Organic acidemias
			Aminoacidurias
			Fatty acid oxidation defects
			Urea cycle defects
			Acute intermittent porphyria
Endocrine		Adrenal hyperplasia	Addison's disease
			Diabetic ketoacidosis
			Pheochromocytoma
Neurological		Chiari malformation	CVS, migraine (headaches/abdominal)
		Subtentorial neoplasm	Familial dysautonomia
Psychiatric		Münchausen by proxy (rare)	Münchausen by proxy (rare)
		Functional vomiting	Bulimia nervosa

GERD gastroesophageal reflux disease, *CVS* cyclic vomiting syndrome, *MELAS* mitochondrial encephalomyopathy, lactic acidosis, and stroke

ders by a ratio of 5:1 [10, 12]. In contrast, in the chronic group, GI disorders (mostly peptic disease) predominate over non-GI causes for vomiting by a ratio of 7:1 [10, 12] (Table 25.4). This implies the need to center the diagnostic work-up on extraintestinal disorders in children who present with the *cyclic* vomiting pattern, while on upper GI (UGI) tract disorders in the *chronic* vomiting pattern.

Clinical Patterns

CVS has a distinctive on–off temporal pattern of vomiting that serves as an essential criterion for diagnosis. CVS is distinguished by the "on" pattern of discrete, recurrent, and severe episodes of vomiting that are stereotypical within the individual as to time of onset (usually early morning), duration (hours or days), and symptomatology (pallor, listlessness). The "off" pattern occurs during week- or month-long intervals when the child resumes completely normal or baseline health (e.g., if there is other chronic disease), although 12% may have interepisodic symptoms of daily nausea and/or mild vomiting [12]. During the episodes, the most common symptoms are listlessness (93%) and pallor (91%) and others include low-grade fever or hypothermia, intermittent flushing, diaphoresis, drooling, and diarrhea. Although found in significantly higher frequency than in patients with GI disorders (gastroesophageal reflux disease, GERD), fewer than half have migraine features of headache, photophobia, and phonophobia.

The duration of episodes generally ranges from hours to days with a median duration of 27 h. Episodes are always self-limited despite a few that may last longer than 1 week. Forty-nine percent of patients have "cyclic" intervals predictable within a week, most commonly 4 weeks, and the remainder have "sporadic," unpredictable attacks. Forty-two percent have onset of their episodes early morning or upon awakening (1–8 a.m). Many have a remarkably rapid onset (1.5 h) and resolution (6 h) from the last emesis to the point of being able to eat and be playful. The 67% with a prodrome have pre-emesis pallor, diaphoresis, abdominal pain, and headache, but rarely visual disturbances of a classical migraine aura.

The vomiting in CVS is uniquely rapid fire and peaks at a median frequency of 6 times an hour and 15 times per episode. The vomiting is typically projectile and contains bile (80%), mucus, and occasionally blood, the latter usually the result of prolapse gastropathy. The bilious nature often raises concern for an obstructive lesion. The intense nausea differs from that in emesis from GI disorders in that it persists even after complete evacuation of gastric contents as if independent of gastric feedback. Many describe nausea as the most distressing symptom, only relieved during sleep. Due to the unrelenting nausea, during episodes, these children appear much more debilitated when compared to those with gastroenteritis, often curled into a fetal position, listless, and withdrawn to the point of being unable to walk or interact. Anorexia, nausea, midline abdominal pain, and retching are the most common GI symptoms.

Certain unusual observed behaviors during CVS episodes can raise questions about an underlying psychiatric disorder. There are children who drink compulsively and then vomit and describe that that maneuver dilutes the bitter bile and aids in evacuating it. Others take prolonged, scalding hot showers or baths until the hot water supply is exhausted. Nearly all turn their rooms into a darkened cave in order to avoid lights and sounds that trigger more nausea. Many are hyperesthetic to motion, odor, taste, and even to parental touch and attempt to shut out all external stimuli.

Various recurring stressors are recognized to precipitate CVS episodes in 76% of patients. These include psychological (44%), infectious (31%), and physical triggers. The psychological stress is more often of an excitatory nature such as holidays, birthdays, outings, and vacations. Episodes may be triggered by various infections including upper respiratory infections, sinusitis, strep throat, and flu. The largest fraction (32%) has a seasonal clustering of episodes with more during the winter and fewer during the summer. Although this pattern correlates with the school year, we can only speculate that less school-related stress, less exposure to infections, and longer duration of sleep helps. Dietary factors include foods rich in amines, aged cheese, chocolate, monosodium glutamate, and fluctuating caffeine intake (23%). Lack of sleep from excess physical exhaustion from travel, sports, sleepovers, or a sleep disorder (24%), and menses (catemenial CVS—22%) are also common inciting events. Environmental triggers include changes in barometric pressures in weather fronts. One subgroup with a precisely timed interval every 60 days (predictable within a week) and an absence of identifiable triggers is especially refractory to therapy.

Pathophysiology

In the absence of a defined etiopathogenesis, CVS remains classified as an idiopathic disorder. Recent investigations support the contributory roles of mitochondrial DNA (mtDNA) mutations and dysfunction, hypothalamic–pituitary–adrenal (HPA) axis activation, and autonomic nervous system (ANS) dysfunction. CVS is a functional brain–gut disorder perhaps mediated through altered brain stem modulation of effector signals.

Mitochondrial Dysfunction

In two series, a striking maternal inheritance pattern was recognized for migraines in 64 and 54% of probands with CVS [13, 14]. Evidence of mitochondrial dysfunction was first provided using nuclear magnetic resonance (NMR) to establish decreased ATP production in peripheral muscle in migraineurs [15]. This mitochondrial pathogenesis gained substantial support following the recent identification of two tandem mtDNA polymorphisms, 16519T and 3010A with impressive odds ratios of 17 and 15 in CVS and migraine in haplotype H, respectively [16]. Because the mutations are found in the control region rather than the enzyme sequence, the structure to function relationship is unclear. However, elevated lactate, ketones, and Krebs cycle intermediates during the early part of the attacks are consistent with mitochondrial dysfunction. In addition, clinical trials and open-label experience show promising effects of mitochondrial supplements coenzyme Q10, L-carnitine, and riboflavin in the treatment of migraines and CVS in children [17, 18].

Neuroendocrine

Stressors, both psychological (excitement, panic) and physical (fever, lack of sleep), are common triggers of attacks of CVS. An activated HPA axis during episodes of CVS was first described by Wolfe, Adler, and later in greater detail by Sato. They documented elevated levels of adrenocorticotropic hormone (ACTH), antidiuretic hormone, cortisol, catecholamines, and prostaglandin E2 [19, 20]. This finding may partially explain the symptoms of hypertension and profound lethargy in this subset of patients. Attenuation of CVS symptoms occurred after use of high-dose dexamethasone by Wolfe and Adler and indomethacin and clonidine by Sato et al. [21].

These findings have focused attention upon one potential role of corticotropin-releasing factor (CRF) as a brain–gut neuroendocrine mediator of foregut motility. Taché et al. have shown that psychological or physiologic stressors induce CRF release from the hypothalamus which stimulates inhibitory motor neurons via CRF-R2 receptors in the dorsal motor nucleus of the vagus that delays gastric emptying, independent of downstream effects of ACTH and cortisol secretion [22]. Preliminary data demonstrate increased peripheral CRF levels during episodes of CVS, but whether this acts to trigger emesis or occurs in response to the stress of the illness is not clear. The new entity of cannabis-induced hyperemesis syndrome which probably represents a variant of CVS raises the possibility that the endocannabinoid system plays a role in CVS. CB1 receptor activation attenuates the stress response and reduces nausea and increases the appetite well-known effects of tetrahydrocannabinol (THC). Interestingly, a growing number of case reports suggest that frequent high dose use may alter the ligand–receptor relationship and result in a cannabis-triggered CVS [23]. This unique response suggests that in some patients altered endocannabinoid signaling may trigger attacks. Conversely, there may be therapeutic potential in other CB1 receptor agonists.

Autonomic Dysfunction

Most of the prominent symptoms of CVS are expressed through the ANS. The peripheral vasoconstriction, hypersalivation, diaphoresis, tachycardia, and listlessness are prominent manifestations of nausea that persist throughout the episode typically unrelieved by evacuation of the stomach.

Chelminsky reported autonomic dysfunction in the form of postural orthostatic tachycardia syndrome (POTS) was identified on a small series of children with CVS recently [24]. They noted that treatment of the POTS appeared to help reduce the frequency of CVS episodes. We recently found an overall prevalence of POTS in 19 % our CVS patients, and when we limited the cohort to adolescents > 11 years in whom POTS is known to be more common, the rate was 38 %.

Four formal studies of the ANS function in children and adults with CVS reveal a consistent pattern of heightened sympathetic tone with normal parasympathetic tone [24]. Interestingly, studies of gastric emptying in adults reveal rapid emptying when well. However, whether this finding extends to children is unknown.

Subtypes of CVS and Comorbidities

Migraines
An association with migraines was identified over a century ago [4, 25]. The current association occurs in 83 % of those with CVS who have a positive family history of migraines or migraines themselves. In addition, there is a progression from CVS to migraine headaches with advancing adolescent age. In the absence of definitive diagnostic tests for migraines and CVS, strong link is further supported by similar symptomatology (e.g., pallor, lethargy, nausea, photophobia, phonophobia) and positive responses in both groups to anti-migraine therapy. These migraine-associated CVS patients generally have milder episodes, a greater association with psychological stress, and significantly higher response rates to anti-migraine therapy (79 vs. 36 %) [26, 27].

Sumatriptan (a selective 1B/1D serotonin agonist) is one anti-migraine drug that can abort episodes if administered early on especially via the nasal route (52 %). This action on serotonin receptors with similar rates of response to patients with migraine headaches suggests a central role of action presumably by decreasing cerebrovascular dilatation. Until we have a clearer delineation of mechanisms involved in migraine and CVS, we cannot be certain if the CVS patients who do not fit under the migraine umbrella have dissimilar pathophysiologic cascades.

CVS +
In Boles' series, 25 % had coexisting neurological findings of developmental delay, seizures, hypotonia, and skeletal myopathy as well as cognitive and cranial nerve dysfunction [28]. These children classified as CVS+ were found to have an earlier age of onset for CVS and a threefold- to eightfold-higher prevalence of dysautonomic (neurovascular dystrophy) and constitutional (growth retardation) manifestations than CVS patients without neurological findings.

Cannabis

There is a group of adolescents and adults with CVS who use marijuana to alleviate nausea and vomiting that instead may aggravate CVS symptoms, and has been labeled as cannabis-induced hyperemesis. It is more likely cannabis-triggered CVS [23]. There are now more than 100 patients described, mostly young males and heavy users over several years. One series of nine patients reports termination of bouts of emesis after cessation of chronic use of marijuana with exacerbation upon resumption of smoking cannabis.

Other Subgroups

Some have documented sympathetic overtone and comorbid POTS in whom treatment of POTS may help reduce frequency of vomiting episodes. The Sato variant is associated with hypertension during episodes only and an endocrine profile of heightened HPA axis activation including ACTH, cortisol, cathecholamines, and vasopressin. These patients generally have significantly more prolonged episodes (102 vs. 50 h) and increased vomiting per episode (75 emesis vs. 31). Those with long-interval calendar-timed episodes every 60+ days apart appear particularly difficult to treat and usually have no identifiable stress or infectious triggers. A stable periodicity has also been observed in post-menarchal girls with catemenial CVS who respond to low-estrogen birth control pills or Depo-Provera. Finally, in a group of children, dietary triggers of their episodes can be identified. Some are initiated by typical migraine precipitants including cheese, chocolate, and monosodium glutamate, whereas others are triggered by food allergies identified by RAST testing.

It is unclear whether these groups are distinct or more likely overlapping phenotypes. We hope that delineation of clinical patterns into subgroups may ultimately point us towards more specific treatment approaches for each subgroup. New findings from nextgen sequencing of the mitochondrial genome and related nuclear genes that affect mitochondrial function may also eventually point to specific treatments.

Comorbidities

We have begun to document numerous comorbidities in affected children most of which affect them during the episode-free interval when well. We are finding that they contribute to symptoms of fatigue, abdominal pain, and dizziness that impair the daily quality of life as documented by Tarbell and Li [29]. Comorbidities in non-neurologically impaired children include anxiety (47%), depression (14%) [30], chronic fatigue (52%), sleep disturbances (48%), irritable bowel syndrome (41%) [31], GERD (39%), colonic dysmotility (20%) [28], POTS (19%), daily nausea (coalescent 12%), and complex regional pain syndrome (10%) [32]. Often, these complaints contribute to the poor quality of life with an average of 3.8 comorbid symptoms per child and have

to be treated concomitantly to help restore the child to functionality.

Differential Diagnosis

Differentiating a cyclic versus a chronic pattern of vomiting is the first step in narrowing the differential diagnosis. Although the majority of patients (88%) with a cyclical pattern ultimately are diagnosed with CVS, the remaining 12% have other specific causes for vomiting found on diagnostic testing. The majority of disorders that can mimic CVS include non-GI as well as GI disorders.

Of the GI disorders, the most serious are anatomic anomalies of the GI tract including malrotation with intermittent volvulus which can cause devastating bowel necrosis. Although not typically cyclical, we have found a few children with eosinophilic esophagitis related to significant food allergies to mimic CVS and Lucarelli et al. have described seven children with positive radioallergosorbent test (RAST) to foods (milk, egg white, and soy) whose episodes diminished after specific food elimination [33].

The most common extraintestinal surgical cause is acute hydronephrosis resulting from ureteral pelvic junction obstruction. Metabolic causes include mitochondrial disorders (disorders of fatty acid oxidation, mitochondrial encephalopathy, lactic acid, and stroke-like syndrome), urea cycle defects (partial ornithine transcarbamylase deficiency), organic acidurias (proprionic acidemia), aminoacidurias, and porphyrin degradation disorders (acute intermittent porphyria) [34, 35]. Neurosurgical causes include various lesions of the subtentorial region including cerebellar medulloblastoma, brain stem glioma, and Chiari malformation likely precipitating vomiting through increased intracranial pressure [12]. Endocrine causes include Addison's disease, pheochromocytoma and carcinoid. Munchausen by proxy (ipecac poisoning) should also be included in the differential diagnosis of a cyclic pattern of vomiting.

Diagnostic Evaluation

At present, there are no specific tests to diagnose CVS, and the diagnosis rests primarily upon fulfilling clinical criteria in the NASPGHAN consensus statement or Rome III (less rigorous) [2]. The key first step requires recognizing a cyclic pattern (high intensity, low frequency) of vomiting because 88% will eventually turn out to be diagnosed with CVS [8]. There are still one in eight who will have an organic underlying cause often extraintestinal in location. Underlying disorders that may require surgical intervention include anatomic anomalies of the GI tract, especially malrotation with the risk of volvulus, renal hydronephrosis, and subtentorial Chiari malformation or neoplasm. These can be excluded by

Table 25.5 Evaluation of cyclic vomiting. (Sunku and Li [3], with kind permission from Springer Science + Business Media)

Patient meets consensus criteria for CVS → UGI series to evaluate for malrotation + serum electrolytes, BUN, creatinine and no warning signs or findings to suggest an organic disorder → trial of empiric therapy to treat CVS
If warning signs are present, then additional labs are warranted
Severe abdominal pain, bilious and/or hematemesis → liver and pancreatic serum chemistries, abdominal ultrasound (or CT or MRI), esophagogastroduodenoscopy
Fasting, high-protein meal, intercurrent illness precipitating episodes of vomiting → serum and urine metabolic evaluation (lactate, ammonia, carnitine profile, amino acids, and organic acids) *prior to treatment during episode, metabolic consult*
Abnormal neurological findings (altered mental status, papilledema) → brain MRI, neurology consult

CVS cyclic vomiting syndrome, *UGI* upper gastrointestinal

UGI series (to ligament of Treitz) renal ultrasound (acute calyceal dilation can resolve in 10 days), and brain MRI (CT may not adequately visualize the brain stem), respectively. The challenge to the clinician is to determine which and how much testing should be performed, as the traditional "shotgun" approach is costly, time consuming, and invasive.

The recent NASPGHAN consensus statement (2008) guidelines recommend against the traditional shotgun approach and a minimal amount of screening to include an UGI series to exclude malrotation and anatomic obstructions and a basic metabolic profile (electrolytes, glucose, BUN, creatinine) [2]. This is supported by our cost-decision analysis that found an UGI X-ray to be the most cost-effective test followed by empiric treatment for 2 months. Further testing beyond that should be based upon specific red flags or warning signs (Table 25.5). In those who present with bilious vomiting and abdominal tenderness, abdominal imaging should be performed to exclude hydronephrosis, pancreatitis, and cholecystitis. In those in whom episodes are triggered by intercurrent illnesses, fasting, or high-protein meals, screening should be performed for urea cycle, fatty acid oxidation, disorders of organic and amino acid metabolism, and mitochondrial disorders. This screening has an improved diagnostic yield during the early part of an episode of CVS before intravenous glucose and fluids are administered. Those presenting with abnormal neurological findings including altered mental status, papilledema, ataxia, or seizure should have a neurological evaluation and brain MRI considered. Presentation of CVS under the age of two should also prompt further metabolic or neurological testing [2].

Treatment

Current treatment for CVS can be divided into supportive or rescue therapy (during episodes), lifestyle modifications and prophylactic (daily treatment to prevent episodes), and abortive therapy (prodromal intervention to abort episodes).

The goals of treatment are to reduce the frequency and severity of episodes, enhance functionality, and improve quality of life. Treatment of nausea, vomiting, abdominal pain, and dehydration during acute episodes requires a protocol for use at home, emergency departments, and hospital wards. Other strategies for management of CVS include avoidance of identified triggers (e.g., dietary cheese), psychological interventions (e.g., stress management), and treatment of comorbid symptoms.

The NASPGHAN consensus statement recommendations on treatment are based upon therapeutic responses from case series and expert opinion of the task force [2]. The main recommendations include first-line prophylactic use of cyproheptadine and amitriptyline in children under age 5 years and 5 years or older, respectively, with propranolol serving as the second line. Sumatriptan was recommended as an abortive agent for those > 12 years. For rescue therapy, during acute episodes, IV rehydration with high-dose antiemetic ondansetron (0.3–0.4 mg/kg/dose) and sedation from diphenhydramine or lorazepam were recommended.

Supportive or Rescue Therapy

Supportive or rescue care is used when the vomiting becomes well established in an episode and at that point usually fails to respond to any abortive strategies. The goal is to correct energy, fluid, and electrolyte deficits and render the child more comfortable through antiemetic therapy, analgesics, and sedation for relief from intractable nausea and pain. The recommendation is for an IV bolus of saline for rapid correction of fluid deficits and concurrent 10% dextrose 0.45 normal saline at 1.5 × maintenance rates to provide sufficient cellular energy to terminate ketosis. One may have to reduce IV rates and increase Na^+content when hyponatremia and diminished urine output ensues from elevated antidiuretic hormone release present in Sato-variant CVS. Ondansetron has been the most widely used $5HT_3$ antagonist given safely at higher than standard doses (0.3–0.4 mg/kg/dose) but can prolong the QTc interval [13]. It generally reduces both nausea and vomiting but usually does not stop the episode or the misery from nausea (Table 25.6).

Diphenhydramine, lorazepam, or chlorpromazine combined with diphenhydramine are used to induce sedation because sedation is often the only means of providing relief from the unrelenting nausea and abdominal pain. The analgesic ketorolac is recommended as first line as narcotics are felt to have a sensitizing effect in migraine analgesia. A non-stimulating environment including quiet, dark single room may be helpful. When all else fails and episodes are prolonged and debilitating (> 1 week), we have used a dexmedetomidine infusion to achieve deep sedation in a *pediatric intensive care unit* (PICU) setting for 18 h as described by Khasawinah [36].

Table 25.6 Rescue and abortive pharmacotherapy. (Sunku and Li [3], with kind permission from Springer Science + Business Media)

Antiemetic
Ondansetron 0.3–0.4 mg/kg per dose q 4–6 h iv/po/rectal/topical up 16 mg/dose. SE: headache, drowsiness, dry mouth
Alternatives: *granisetron*
Aprepitant 125, 80, 80 mg one q.d. prior to anticipated episode
Sedative
Lorazepam 0.05–0.1 mg/kg per dose q 6 h iv/po: useful adjunct to ondansetron. SE: sedation, respiratory depression
Chlorpromazine 0.5–1 mg/kg per dose q 6 h iv/po. SE: drowsiness, hypotension, seizures
Diphenhydramine 1.0–1.25 mg/kg per dose q 6 h iv/po: useful adjunct with chlorpromazine. SE: hypotension, sedation, dizziness
Analgesic
Ketorolac 0.5–1 mg/kg per dose q 6 h iv/po. SE: gastrointestinal bleeding, dyspepsia
Alternatives: opioids (hyrdromorphone)
Abortive
Sumatriptan 20 mg intranasal at episode onset and may repeat once or 25 mg po once. SE: chest and neck burning, coronary vasospasm, headache
Alternatives: *frovatriptan, rizatriptan, zolmitriptan*

SE side effects

Table 25.7 Prophylactic pharmacotherapy. (Sunku and Li [3], with kind permission from Springer Science + Business Media)

Anti-migraine
Amitriptyline start and 0.2–0.3 mg/kg and advance to 1–1.5 mg/kg per day qhs: monitor EKG QTc interval prior to starting. First choice ≥ 5 year old. Side effects (SE): sedation, anticholinergic
Propranolol 0.25–1 mg/kg/day divided b.i.d or t.i.d: monitor resting heart rate. SE: hypotension, bradycardia, fatigue
Cyproheptadine 0.25–0.5 mg/kg/day divided b.i.d. or q.h.s: first choice < 5 year old. SE: sedation, weight gain, anticholinergic
Alternatives: *nortriptyline, imipramine, desipramine, doxepin*
Anticonvulsants
Topiramate gradually increase to 1.5–2.0 mg/kg/day divided b.i.d. or q.h.s. SE: appetite suppression, cognitive dysfunction, renal stones
Phenobarbital 2–3 mg/kg per day q.h.s. SE: sedation, cognitive impairment
Alternatives: *gabapentin, levetiracetam, zonisamide, valproate, carbamazephine*
Mitochondrial supplements
Co-enzyme Q10 10 mg/kg/ divided b.i.d. ≤ 600 mg/day
L-carnitine 50–75 mg/kg ≤ 2 g/day divided b.i.d. SE: diarrhea, fishy body odor
Riboflavin 10 mg/kg/day divided b.i.d. ≤ 400 mg/day

q.h.s. quaque hora somni

Lifestyle Modifications

Lifestyle modifications are used during the interictal phase of CVS when the child is not in an episode in order to keep the child properly conditioned and to avoid exposure to known and potential precipitants of episodes. The lack of sleep resulting from disturbed sleep patterns, sleepovers, or travel sports tournaments are often cited as triggers of episodes. Good sleep hygiene (e.g., turning off all phones, computers, music, TV) with a regimented sleep time can reduce the frequency of episodes. Providing at least maintenance volumes of fluids is widely used to treat migraines and POTS. Providing low glycemic energy sources before strenuous activity, sources, may prevent an exercise-induced energy deficit. Routine exercise can help reverse the deconditioned state and improve mitochondrial function. Finally, avoiding identified triggers specific to the individual (e.g., sleepovers) or generally found in migraines (monosodium glutamate and fluctuations in caffeine intake) may help reduce the frequency of episodes. Fleisher reported that consultation and lifestyle modifications alone reduced the frequency of episodes in 70 % of patients even before beginning prophylactic therapy [31].

Prophylactic Therapy

For those with more frequent or severe episodes (e.g., more than once a month), prophylactic therapy is recommended daily during the interictal phase with the goal of preventing the next episode or to at least reduce the frequency, duration, or intensity (# emeses) of episodes. These *prophylactic medications* those traditionally used to treat other disorders including migraines. The NASPGHAN consensus recommendations for the initial treatment were for cyproheptadine for the younger (< 5 years) and amitriptyline for the older children and adolescents (≥ 5 years) [2] (Table 25.7). Despite its pharmacokinetics, cyproheptadine (0.25–0.5 mg/kg) appears to be effective given as a single nighttime dose as opposed to the usual two or three divided doses [37]. Amitriptyline causes side effects in 50%, the most common being morning sedation (like a hangover), and is stopped in 21% [38]. Beginning at a low dose of 0.2–0.3 mg/kg at bedtime and titrating it gradually in 10 mg increments every week or two to the target dose of 1.0–1.5 mg/kg allows the child to gradually adapt to the side effects. Switching to other tricyclic antidepressants such as nortriptyline, desipramine, or doxepin may lessen specific side effects. An electrocardiogram (EKG) to measure the QTc interval is recommended before starting amitriptyline. At higher doses (> 1.0 mg), we monitor the ECG and/or amitriptyline levels [39]. Propranolol is second line therapy and can be monitored for efficacy and toxicity by a desired drop in pulse rate of 15–20 beats per minute not to fall below 55 bpm, respectively.

If standard prophylactic therapy fails, anticonvulsants and Ca^{2+}-channel antagonists have been used. Phenobarbital at low (2–3 mg/kg) nighttime doses and topiramate (1–2 mg/kg/day) have been reported to be effective, the latter having a strong evidence based in migraines [40]. Unfortunately, cognitive dysfunction is a well-known side effect in both. Other effective anticonvulsants include zonisamide and levitiracetam, in adults with CVS [41, 42]. Another group of agents includes Ca^{2+}-channel antagonists with the main side effect of hypotension.

Treatment may vary by clinical subgroup. Children that have a migraine connection with either a positive family history or migraines themselves are much more likely to respond to antimigraine agents such as cyproheptadine, amitriptyline, and propranolol (79 vs. 36%) than those children without one [26]. Post-menarcheal girls with catemenial CVS often respond to low-estrogen birth control pills or Depo-Provera. Sato-variant CVS associated with hypertension may require intraepisodic short-acting anti-hypertensives as well as prophylactic tricyclic antidepressants in the USA and divalproex sodium in Japan [21].

Prophylactic use of mitochondrial supplements as adjunctive prophylactic therapy in CVS is being used more frequently based upon evidence in migraines and preliminary evidence in children with CVS. These supplements have demonstrated efficacy in prevention of migraines in adults (randomized controlled trial) and preliminary evidence of efficacy in pediatric migraine and CVS in children [43–45]. In a survey of use as monotherapy in children with CVS, Boles found that the response to CoQ10 was similar to that amitriptyline [38]. Interestingly, some children with CVS, the accompanying chronic fatigue may respond to these supplements. The doses used include riboflavin at 10 mg/kg divided b.i.d. to up to 400 mg/day, L-carnitine at 50–75 mg/kg up to 3 g/day divided b.i.d., and CoQ10 10 mg/kg divided b.i.d. up to 600 mg/day. The dose and duration of these supplements has not been established in children with CVS.

Abortive Therapy

Abortive therapy should be considered for those who have sporadic episodes that occur less than once per month and who prefer not taking prophylaxis or those who have breakthrough episodes while on prophylaxis. Abortive therapy is given during the prodrome or at the beginning of the vomiting episode in the hope of stopping it. The most specific abortive therapy includes anti-migraine triptans. The nasal (sumatriptan or zolmitriptan) or subcutaneous (sumatriptan) forms appear more effective than oral forms that cannot be effectively absorbed due to repeated vomiting [2, 46] (Table 25.6). The triptans are usually either fully effective or not at all, and more effective if administered early in episode or if the duration of episodes is less than 24 h (Li unpublished data).

In a few children, ondansetron administered alone aborts episodes in progress. Although the oral forms may not reach the duodenum, ondansetron can be reformulated by individual pharmacies into a rectal suppository or topical (lipodermal) forms. Although not established, we use the same dosages as the oral form. In a few adolescents with severe, disabling abdominal pain preceding the vomiting, use of opioids such as hydromorphone can quickly abolish the pain and in turn the vomiting.

Comorbidities

Treatment of comorbid conditions and symptoms may alleviate the CVS. Chelimsky has shown in a small series that treatment of the POTS with fluids, salt, fludrocortisone, and/or propranolol helps prevent attacks of CVS [24]. Use of stress reduction techniques as well as anxiolytics has anecdotally reduced the number of episodes in anxious children whose attacks are triggered by stressors and/or panic anxiety. Alleviating the comorbid symptoms may substantially improve the quality of life and functional disability.

Natural History, Quality of Life (QOL) Impact, and Complications

There is limited data for the natural history of CVS. Our projection analysis estimates that 75% of patients will develop migraine headaches by age 18. Other long-term studies have shown that up to half of CVS patients continue with CVS or migraine headaches. Several studies have noted the mean duration of illness to be around 6 years, but in our cohort, the younger the age of onset, the longer the duration. Also 5% of patients will progress through all three phases of periodic disease including CVS to abdominal migraine and finally to migraine headaches. We are currently encountering a growing group with teenage onset CVS and it is too early to ascertain the natural history.

CVS has a significant deleterious impact on the quality of life in affected children. Although well in between episodes approximately 90% of the time, 58% of affected children require intravenous fluids during episodes and average ten visits to the emergency department. School-age children in our cohort miss an average of 24 days of school per year [11, 47]. Medical morbidity is reflected by the high average annualized cost of management of US$ 17,000 in 1999 dollars that includes doctor visits, emergency department visits, inpatient hospitalizations, missed work by parents, as well as biochemical, radiographic, and endoscopic testing [48]. Growing number of comorbid conditions such as anxiety and POTS also contribute to functional impairment. We have demonstrated significantly lower quality of life scores than in healthy controls, equivalent to those in children organic GI diseases (e.g., inflammatory bowel disease, gastritis) [29].

Complications and medical morbidity include iatrogenic tests and interventions from the misdiagnoses that are often applied to recurrent vomiting. Most are mislabeled as acute gastroenteritis, gastroesophageal reflux, and food poisoning, and they are treated in urgent care settings. Some with severe pain, bilious vomiting, and intractability have undergone inappropriate laparotomy, appendectomy, cholecystectomy, and Nissen fundoplication. Others have been labeled with psychiatric disorders including bulimia and psychogenic vomiting and hospitalized on psychiatric wards, while a few parents have been referred for suspicion of Munchausen by proxy.

Complications can also occur from the frequent and often severe episodes of vomiting that occur with CVS. Dehydration and electrolyte disturbances are common and IV rehydration is required in 58% of patients, which can be compared to less than 1% in rotavirus. Hematemesis can occur towards the end of attacks and is usually related to prolapse gastropathy or Mallory–Weiss tears. Although not common, frequent vomiting can lead to secondary peptic injury.

Summary

CVS is a disorder well described and accepted in the literature, and increasingly diagnosed by pediatric and family physicians as well as pediatric emergency medicine, neurologists, and gastroenterologists. Recently, there is greater appreciation of comorbid conditions and symptoms that deleteriously affect quality of life and functioning. Although the precise pathophysiology remains unknown, we have growing evidence of involvement of the stress axis and mitochondrial function. Unfortunately, no robust treatment trials have been completed to date and so the therapy remains empiric. Yet, the progress made over the past two decades has been impressive.

References

1. Gee S. On fitful or recurrent vomiting. St Bartholemew Hosp Rev. 1882;18:1–6.
2. Li BUK, Lefevre F, Chelminsky GG, et al. North American society for pediatric gastroenterology, hepatology, and nutrition consensus statement on the diagnosis and management of cyclic vomiting syndrome. J Pediatr Gastroenterol Nutr. 2008;47:379–93.
3. Sunku B, Li B UK. Cyclic vomiting syndrome: comorbidities and treatment. In: Faure C, Di Lorenzo C, Thapar N, editors. Pediatric neurogastroenterology. Clinical Gastroenterology, Ed. Wu GY. New York: Springer; 2013. pp. 391–400.
4. Whitney HB. Cyclic vomiting: a brief review of this affection as illustrated by a typical case. Arch Pediatr. 1898;15 839–45.
5. Li BUK. Cyclic vomiting syndrome and abdominal migraine. Int Semin Pediatr Gastroenterol. 2000;9:1–9.
6. Abu-Arafeh I, Russel G. Cyclic vomiting syndrome in children: a population based study. J Pediatr Gastroenterol Nutr. 1995;21:454–8.
7. Barlow CF. The periodic syndrome: cyclic vomiting and abdominal migraine. In: Barlow CF, editor. Headaches and migraine in childhood. Clin Dev Med. 1984;91:76–92.
8. Pfau BT, Li BUK, Murray RD et al. Differentiating cyclic from chronic vomiting patterns in children: quantitative criteria and diagnostic implications. Pediatrics. 1996;97:364–8.
9. Ertekin V, Selimoglu MA, Altnkaynak S. Prevalence of cyclic vomiting syndrome in a sample of Turkish school children in an urban area. J Clin Gastroenterol. 2006;40:896–8.
10. Li BUK. Cyclic vomiting: the pattern and syndrome paradigm. J Pediatr Gastroenterol Nutr. 1995;21(Suppl. 1):S6–10.
11. Sunku B, Li BUK. Cyclic vomiting syndrome. In: Guandalini S, editor. Textbook of pediatric gastroenterology and nutrition. London: Taylor & Francis; 2004. pp. 289–302.
12. Li BUK, Balint J. Cyclic vomiting syndrome: evolution in our understanding of a brain-gut disorder. Adv Pediatr. 2000;47:117–60.
13. Li BUK, Fleisher DR. Cyclic vomiting syndrome: features to be explained by a pathophysiologic model. Dig Dis Sci. 1999;44:13S–18S.
14. Boles RG, Adams K, Li BUK. Maternal Inheritance in cyclic vomiting syndrome. Am J Med Gen. 2005;133A:71–7.
15. Bresolin N, Martinelli P, Barbiroli B, et al. Muscle mitochondrial DNA deletion and 31P-NMR spectroscopy alterations in a migraine patient. J Neurol Sci. 1991 Aug;104(2):182–9.
16. Camilleri M, Carlson P, Zinsmeister AR, et al. Mitochondrial DNA and gastrointestinal motor and sensory functions in health and functional gastrointestinal disorders. Am J Physiol Gastrointest Liver Physiol. 2009 March;296(3):G510–6.
17. Boles RG. High degree of efficacy in the treatment of cyclic vomiting syndrome with combined co-enzyme Q10, L-carnitine and amitriptyline, a case series. BMC Neurol. 2011 Aug 16;11:102.
18. Boehnke C, Reuter U, Flach U, et al. High-dose riboflavin treatment is efficacious in migraine prophylaxis: an open study in a tertiary care centre. Eur J Neurol. 2004 July;11(7):475–7.
19. Wolfe SM, Adler R. A syndrome of periodic hypothalamic discharge. Am J Med. 1964;36:956–67.

20. Sato T, Uchigata Y, Uwadana N, et al. A syndrome of periodic adrenocorticotropin and vasopressin discharge. J Clin Endocrinol Metab. 1982;54:517–22.
21. Sato T, Igarashi M, Minami S, et al. Recurrent attacks of vomiting, hypertension, and psychotic depression: a syndrome of periodic catecholamine and prostaglandin discharge. Acta Endocrinol. 1988;117:189–97.
22. Taché Y, Martinez V, Million M, et al. Corticotropin-releasing factor and the brain-gut motor response to stress. Can J Gastroenterol. 1999 March;13(Suppl A):18A–25.
23. Allen JH, De Moore GM, Heddle R, et al. Cannabinoid hyperemesis: cyclical hyperemesis in association with chronic cannabis abuse. Gut. 2004;53:1566–70.
24. Chelminsky TC, Chelminsky GG. Autonomic abnormalities in cyclic vomiting syndrome. J Pediatr Gastroenterol Nutr. 2007;44:326–30.
25. Rachford BK. Recurrent vomiting. Arch Pediatr. 1904;21:881–91.
26. Li B UK, Murray RD, Heitlinger LA. Is cyclic vomiting syndrome related to migraine? J Pediatr. 1999;134(5):567–72.
27. Symon DNK. Is cyclical vomiting an abdominal form of migraine in children? Dig Dis Sci. 1999;44(8):23S–25S.
28. Boles RG, Powers AL, Adams K. Cyclic vomiting syndrome plus. J Child Neurol. 2006;21:182–8.
29. Tarbell SE, LI B UK. Health-related quality of life in children and adolescents with cyclic vomiting syndrome: a comparison with published data on youth with irritable bowel syndrome and organic gastrointestinal disorders. J pediatr. 2013;163(2):493–7.
30. Tarbell S, Li BU. Psychiatric symptoms in children and adolescents with cyclic vomiting syndrome and their parents. Headache. 2008;48:259–66.
31. Fleisher DR. Cyclic vomiting. In Hyman PE, DiLorenzo C, editors. Pediatric gastrointestinal motility disorders. New York. Academy Professional Information Services; 1194. pp. 89–103.
32. Higashimoto T, Baldwin EE, Gold JI, Boles RG. Reflex sympathetic dystrophy:complex regional pain syndrome type I in children with mitochondrial disease and maternal inheritance. Arch Dis Child. 2008 May;93(5):390–7.
33. Lucarelli S, Corrado G, Pelliccia A, et al. Cyclic vomiting syndrome and food allergy/intolerance in seven children: a possible association. Eur J Pediatr. 2000;159:360–3.
34. Rinaldo P. Mitochondrial fatty acid oxidation disorders and cyclic vomiting syndrome. Dig Dis Sci. 1999;44(8):97S–102S.
35. Boles RG, Williams JC. Mitochondrial disease and cyclic vomiting syndrome. Dig Dis Sci. 1999;44(8):103S–7S.
36. Khasawinah TA, Ramirez A, et al. Preliminary experience with dexmedetomidine in treatment of cyclic vomiting syndrome. Am J Ther. 2003;10(4):303–7.
37. Andersen JM, Sugerman KS, Lockhart JR, Weinberg WA. Effective prophylactic therapy for cyclic vomiting syndrome in children using amitriptyline or cyproheptadine. Pediatrics. 1997 Dec;100(6):977–81.
38. Boles RG, Lovett-Barr MR, Preston A, et al. Treatment of cyclic vomiting syndrome with co-enzyme Q10 and amitriptyline, a retrospective study. BMC Neurol. 2010 Jan 28;10:10.
39. Prakash C, Clouse RE. Cyclic vomiting syndrome in adults: clinical features and response to tricyclic antidepressants. Am J Gastroenterol. 1999;94:2855–9.
40. Gokhale R, Huttenlocher PR, Brady L, et al. Use of barbiturates in the treatment of cyclic vomiting during childhood. J Pediatr Gastroenterol Nutr. 1997;25:64–7.
41. Olmez A, Köse G, Turanli G. Cyclic vomiting with generalized epileptiform discharges responsive to topiramate therapy. Pediatr Neurol. 2006 Nov;35(5):348–51.
42. Clouse RE, Sayuk GS, Lustman PH, Prakash C. Zonisamide or levetiracetam for adults with cyclic vomiting syndrome: a case series. Clin Gastroenterol Hepatol. 2007;5:44–8.
43. Slater SK, Nelson TD, Kabbouche MA, et al. A randomized, double-blinded, placebo controlled, crossover, add-on study of CoEnzyme Q10 in the prevention of pediatric and adolescent migraine. Cephalalgia. 2011 June;31(8):897–905.
44. Schoenen J, Jacquy J, Lenaerts M. Effectiveness of high-dose riboflavin in migraine prophylaxis. A randomized controlled trial. Neurology. 1998 Feb;50(2):466–70.
45. Van Calcar SC, Harding CO, Wolff JA. L-carnitine administration reduces number of episodes in cyclic vomiting syndrome. Clin Pediatr (Phila). 2002;41:171–4.
46. Benson JM, Zorn SL, Book LS. Sumatriptan in the treatment of cyclic vomiting. Ann Pharmacother. 1995 Oct;29(10):997–9.
47. Venkatesan T, Tarbell S, Adams K. A survey of emergency department use in patients with cyclic vomiting syndrome. BMC Emerg Med. 2010 Feb 24;10:4.
48. Olson AD, Li BUK. The diagnostic evaluation of children with cyclic vomiting: a cost-effectiveness assessment. J Pediatr. 2002;141:724–8.

Food Allergy

26

Whitney M. Rassbach and Scott H. Sicherer

Introduction

An expert panel convened by the National Institute of Allergy and Infectious Diseases defined food allergy as "an adverse health effect arising from a specific immune response that occurs reproducibly on exposure to a given food" [1]. This description distinguishes food allergy from nonimmune adverse reactions to foods (Table 26.1). The Centers for Disease Control and Prevention reported that the prevalence of food allergy in US children increased from 3.4% in 1997–1999 to 5.1% in 2009–2011 [2]. Prevalence estimates of childhood food allergy vary, but up to 8% may be affected [1, 3–6]. Over 170 food allergens have been identified, but eight foods or food groups (milk, egg, peanut, tree nuts, soy, wheat, fish, and crustacean shellfish) account for 90% of significant allergic reactions [1]. It is important to note that parental perception of food allergy is generally much higher than physician-diagnosed food allergy, particularly in early childhood. Up to one third of parents report at least one adverse reaction to food [7–12]. The emotional impact of food allergy is considerable, with food-allergic children reporting greater impact on quality of life than children with insulin-dependent diabetes or rheumatologic disorders [13, 14]. This chapter reviews the spectrum of food-allergic disorders with an emphasis on those relevant to the pediatric gastroenterologist. Celiac disease is the result of an immune response to foods, but is not typically categorized as an allergy and is not reviewed here.

S. H. Sicherer (✉) · W. M. Rassbach
Division of Allergy and Immunology, Department of Pediatrics,
The Elliot and Roslyn Jaffe Food Allergy Institute, Kravis Children's
Hospital, Icahn School of Medicine at Mount Sinai, Box 1198,
One Gustave L. Levy Place, New York, NY 10029-6574, USA
e-mail: scott.sicherer@mssm.edu

Immunopathogenesis and Specific Disorders

Immunopathogenesis

The normal immune response to food results is tolerance [15]. The immune system recognizes food proteins, and IgG and IgA antibodies may be generated, but there are no adverse reactions. Food allergy results from an abrogation of normal tolerance mechanisms. Food allergies may be immunoglobulin E (IgE)-mediated, cell-mediated, or "mixed" adverse immune responses. The distinction of pathophysiology is important in diagnosis and management. For example, IgE-mediated reactions are typically sudden in onset following exposure to a food allergen, whereas cell-mediated responses may result in chronic inflammation or delayed symptoms. Table 26.2 highlights gastrointestinal manifestations of food allergy according to pathophysiology.

IgE-Mediated Reactions

Symptoms triggered by IgE-mediated reactions occur rapidly following ingestion of the trigger food. IgE antibodies that are specific for regions (epitopes) of food proteins arm tissue mast cells and circulating basophils. Cross-linking of the IgE antibodies by the food proteins leads to release of preformed mediators (such as histamine and platelet-activating factor) from cytoplasmic granules and transcription of inflammatory cytokines. The target organs(s) involved in the reaction define the type of food allergy. The symptoms occurring during an acute reaction can be classified as cutaneous, ocular, gastrointestinal, respiratory, or cardiovascular. A combination of these symptoms may occur.

Cutaneous manifestations of an acute food allergy reaction include erythema, hives, pruritus, flaring of eczematous lesions, and angioedema. Food allergy may account for up to 20% of new-onset urticaria [16, 17]. Food allergies rarely cause chronic urticaria (e.g., episodes occurring regularly for 6 weeks or longer). Eczema (atopic dermatitis) can be chronically exacerbated by specific IgE-mediated food allergy, with improvement upon removal of the suspect food

© Springer International Publishing Switzerland 2016
S. Guandalini et al. (eds.), *Textbook of Pediatric Gastroenterology, Hepatology and Nutrition*,
DOI 10.1007/978-3-319-17169-2_26

295

Table 26.1 Nonimmune-mediated reactions or food intolerance/adverse reactions to food

Type	Example(s)
Metabolic	Lactose intolerance, galactosemia, alcohol
Pharmacologic	Caffeine (jitteriness), tyramine in aged cheeses (migraine), alcohol, histamine
Toxic	Bacterial food poisoning, scombroid fish poisoning
Undefined mechanisms	Reactions to sulfites, tartrazine

[18–20]. Overall, skin symptoms are the most common manifestation of IgE-mediated food allergies. Food can also induce skin symptoms by direct skin contact (contact urticaria) [21–25].

Ocular symptoms include pruritus, tearing, conjunctival erythema, and periorbital edema.

Gastrointestinal symptoms include nausea, vomiting, diarrhea, and abdominal pain. Isolated acute gastrointestinal reactions are uncommon. In the case of a food-allergic reaction, upper gastrointestinal symptoms usually begin within minutes of ingestion, but may take as long as 2 h to develop. Diarrhea may have a more delayed onset, beginning 2–6 h after ingestion of the allergen.

Oral allergy syndrome, also referred to as pollen food allergy syndrome, is a form of contact allergy with symptoms isolated to the oral cavity. Sensitization initially occurs from inhalation of pollens, but results in symptoms when fruits or vegetables with proteins that are homologous to the pol-

lens are ingested. For example, birch pollen contains proteins homologous with Rosaceae fruits (e.g., apple, peach, carrot). Pruritus and mild swelling of the lips, tongue, and throat occur when specific uncooked fruits and vegetables are ingested, but heated forms are tolerated [26]. Symptoms typically last several minutes before self-resolving. While anaphylaxis associated with oral allergy has been reported, it is relatively rare [27].

Respiratory tract symptoms may be acutely induced by IgE-mediated reactions. Symptoms may include pruritus and edema of the larynx, dyspnea, nasal congestion, rhinorrhea, hoarseness, stridor, tachypnea, wheezing, and cough. However, chronic asthma is rarely the sole manifestation of food allergy.

Cardiovascular symptoms associated with acute food-allergic reactions include increased venular permeability, widened pulse pressure, increased heart rate and cardiac output, flushing, dizziness, and fainting. These effects can lead to the decreased organ perfusion that is characteristic of anaphylactic shock.

Anaphylaxis

Anaphylaxis is defined as "a serious allergic reaction that is rapid in onset and may cause death" [28]. Symptoms generally include a combination of the above symptoms (or respiratory or cardiac symptoms alone), with anaphylactic shock referring to signs of poor organ perfusion in addi-

Table 26.2 Gastrointestinal food allergies

Disorder	Mechanism	Symptoms	Diagnosis
Pollen-food allergy syndrome (oral allergy syndrome)	IgE mediated	Mild pruritus, tingling, and/or angioedema of the lips, tongue, or oropharynx	Clinical history and positive sensitization to pollens
Gastrointestinal "anaphylaxis"	IgE mediated	Rapid onset of nausea, abdominal pain, cramps, vomiting, and/or diarrhea; other target organ responses (i.e., skin, respiratory tract) often involved	Clinical history and positive tests for food-specific IgE; ± oral challenge
Eosinophilic esophagitis	IgE mediated and/or cell mediated	Gastroesophageal reflux or excessive spitting-up or emesis, dysphagia, intermittent abdominal pain, irritability, sleep disturbance, failure to respond to conventional reflux medications	Clinical history, endoscopy and biopsy, elimination diet, and oral food challenge (possible test directed)
Eosinophilic gastroenteritis	IgE mediated and/or cell mediated	Recurrent abdominal pain, irritability, early satiety, intermittent vomiting, FTT and/or weight loss, peripheral blood eosinophilia (in 50%)	Clinical history, endoscopy and biopsy, elimination diet, and challenge (possibly test directed)
Food-protein-induced proctocolitis	Cell mediated	Gross or occult blood in stool; typically thriving; usually presents in the first few months of life	Negative SPT responses; elimination of food protein → clearing of most bleeding in 72 h; ± endoscopy and biopsy; challenge induces bleeding within 72 h
Food-protein-induced enterocolitis syndrome	Cell mediated	See Table 26.3	History, response to elimination/oral food challenge
Food-protein-induced enteropathy	Cell mediated	Diarrhea or steatorrhea, abdominal distention and flatulence, weight loss, FTT, ± nausea and vomiting	Endoscopy and biopsy

FTT failure to thrive, *SPT* skin prick testing, *IgE* immunoglobulin E

tion to anaphylaxis. Anaphylaxis may result in hypotension, cardiac dysrhythmias, cardiovascular collapse, or death. In children, respiratory, cutaneous, and gastrointestinal symptoms are prominent, and the most common cause of death is respiratory compromise. Less than 1 % of anaphylaxis cases (including those not due to food ingestion) are fatal [29, 30]. In retrospective analysis, several factors appear to be associated with the severity of the allergic response. A larger quantity of food allergen ingested, concomitant alcohol consumption, and concomitant nonsteroidal anti-inflammatory drugs (NSAID) use all appear to increase the rapidity and severity of the reaction [31–34]. Concomitant ingestion of fatty foods appears to slow the rate of absorption and thus delay onset of symptoms. Risk-taking behaviors among adolescents and young adults, including increased incidents of exposure to the avoided allergen and a lack of a prompt treatment response to symptoms, conspire to contribute to the disproportionately higher number of fatal food-induced anaphylaxis in this age group [35]. In one case series of fatal food-induced anaphylactic reactions, accidental ingestion of a known food allergen was present in 87 % of cases [31]. In several cases, previous reactions to the known allergen were relatively mild, highlighting the inconsistency in severity of reactions. Having asthma is an additional risk factor for fatal anaphylaxis. Biphasic anaphylactic reactions occur in up to 20 % of cases [36]. In this scenario, a second wave of symptoms occurs 1–4 h following resolution of the initial anaphylactic reaction.

Food-dependent, exercise-induced anaphylaxis is an IgE-mediated food-induced anaphylactic reaction that occurs when vigorous exercise is performed within a few hours of food allergen ingestion. Neither exercise alone nor ingestion of the food allergen alone is sufficient to cause symptoms. While generally associated with specific causative foods (such as wheat, other grains, celery, seafood, or nuts), in some cases any food can cause the reaction when consumed in close temporal relation to exercise [37, 38]. Another uncommon syndrome of anaphylaxis is delayed anaphylaxis occurring several hours after ingestion of mammalian meat, attributed to an IgE response against a carbohydrate moiety, galactose-α-1,3-galactose (α-gal). The etiology is presumed to be related to exposure to this allergen via tick bites [39–42].

Management of Acute IgE-Mediated Reactions

Mild IgE-mediated reactions may subside with antihistamines. However, progressive, multisystem, or severe reactions should be treated promptly with intramuscular epinephrine. Severe reactions may require multiple doses of epinephrine, intravenous fluids, oxygen, vasopressors, additional treatments, and monitoring in an acute care setting.

Natural History of IgE-Mediated Reactions

IgE-mediated food allergy generally appears during the first 2 years of a child's life. The sensitivity to most allergenic foods (egg, milk, wheat, and soy) self-resolves in 85 % of children during childhood [43]. Sensitivity to peanuts, tree nuts, and seafood persists into adulthood in the large majority of affected children. Approximately, 20 % of peanut-allergic children under the age of 2 years and 10 % of children with tree nut allergy will become tolerant to those foods by the time they are of school age, however [44].

Cell-Mediated Food-Allergic Disorders

Cell-mediated food-allergic reactions include food-protein-induced enterocolitis syndrome (FPIES), food-protein-induced enteropathy, food-protein-induced proctitis and proctocolitis, celiac disease, and food-induced pulmonary hemosiderosis. Celiac disease is discussed in Chap. 40.

Pulmonary hemosiderosis is a rare condition characterized by pulmonary infiltrates, iron-deficiency anemia, hemosiderosis, hemoptysis, cough, wheezing, nasal congestion, recurrent otitis media, dyspnea, colic, diarrhea, vomiting, hematochezia, and failure to thrive attributed to cow's milk. While the immunologic mechanisms underlying this illness are not understood, peripheral eosinophilia and IgG to cow's milk are generally present. Symptoms remit with elimination of the causative allergen [45, 46].

Non-IgE-mediated gastrointestinal disorders are highlighted as follows:

Food- Protein-Induced Enterocolitis Syndrome

FPIES is a cell-mediated gastrointestinal food allergy that typically manifests in infancy and generally resolves by 3 years of age. In the acute form, 1–3 h after ingestion of the causative food, infants present with profuse, repetitive vomiting and may experience dehydration and lethargy. Diarrhea may occur several hours following the vomiting. In the chronic form, with continued ingestion of the allergen, infants develop weight loss and failure to thrive. Cow's milk and soy are the most common triggers in formula-fed infants. Symptoms begin 1–4 weeks after introduction of cow's milk or soy. Solid food FPIES is less common than milk/soy FPIES, and presents later, usually at 4–7 months of age, most often when weaning a breast-fed infant. Solid food FPIES triggers include rice, oats, barley, chicken, turkey, egg white, green peas, peanuts, sweet potatoes, white potatoes, fruits, fish, and mollusks. Of those infants diagnosed with solid food FPIES, 65 % carried a prior diagnosis of milk/soy FPIES and 80 % reacted to more than one food. Overall, 75 % of infants presenting with FPIES appear acutely ill, and 15 % become hypotensive, requiring hospitalization. Laboratory findings

Table 26.3 Food-protein-induced enterocolitis syndrome (FPIES)

Clinical findings	*Acute:*
	Profuse, repetitive vomiting occurring 1–3 h after food ingestion
	Diarrhea occurring 5–8 h after ingestion
	Dehydration
	Lethargy
	Pallor
	Abdominal distention
	Bloody diarrhea
	Hypotension
	Hypothermia
	Chronic:
	Weight loss
	Failure to thrive
	Diarrhea
	Lethargy
	Abdominal distention
	Bloody diarrhea
	Dehydration
Laboratory/imaging findings	Anemia
	Thrombocytosis
	Hypoalbuminemia
	Elevated white blood cell count with a left shift
	Eosinophilia
	Transient methemoglobinemia
Triggers	Milk/soy (most common)
	Solid food: rice, oats, barley, chicken, turkey, egg white, green peas, peanuts, sweet potatoes, white potatoes, fruits, fish, mollusks
Management	Elimination of food trigger
	Oral food challenge to evaluate for resolution

may include anemia, thrombocytosis, hypoalbuminemia, and an elevated white blood cell count with a left shift and eosinophilia. Transient methemoglobinemia and intramural gas have also been reported [47, 48]. Table 26.3 shows key features of FPIES. While the exact pathophysiologic mechanism for FPIES has yet to be elucidated, it is thought to be a cell-mediated disorder. Studies have shown increased levels of tumor necrosis factor-α, increased numbers of circulating blood mononuclear cells, and decreased intestinal mucosal expression of transforming growth factor-β receptors in association with FPIES [49–53].

Management

In acute cases, aggressive intravenous fluid administration is the mainstay of management. Other therapies for acute symptoms may include steroids and ondansetron [47, 54]. Methemoglobinemia may be treated with methylene blue. Chronic symptoms usually improve within 3–10 days after eliminating cow's milk and from the diet and beginning a casein hydrolysate-based formula [48].

Differential Diagnosis

In its acute form, FPIES is frequently mistaken for viral gastroenteritis, sepsis, or food poisoning. The intramural gas sometimes seen on abdominal radiographs mimics that seen in necrotizing enterocolitis. Methemoglobinemia often raises concern for a metabolic disorder.

Diagnosis

History, clinical presentation, and at times oral food challenges are useful in the diagnosis of FPIES. A positive oral food challenge is considered the "gold standard" of diagnosis. However, if infants demonstrate a fitting history and presentation, an oral food challenge can be avoided if the symptoms resolve after removal of the suspected causative food. While >90% of patients do not have detectable serum-specific IgE to foods at the time of diagnosis, those that do have such antibodies are more likely to experience a protracted course of FPIES or develop acute allergic reactions [47, 48, 55].

Natural Course

In the USA, cow's milk FPIES resolves in 60% of affected infants by age 3. Approximately, 60% of a Korean cohort showed resolution at 10 months of age, and 90% of an Israeli cohort demonstrated resolution by 3 years of age [47, 56, 57].

Food-Protein-Induced Enteropathy

Food-protein-induced enteropathy is characterized by vomiting, diarrhea, malabsorption, failure to thrive, and anemia in an infant [45]. Cow's milk protein is the most likely causative agent, particularly in infants fed intact cow's milk prior to 9 months of age. This syndrome has also been described in infants following an episode of gastroenteritis and in response to other foods, including eggs, rice, fish, shellfish, and poultry [46, 58].

Diagnosis and Management

Endoscopy with biopsy is required for diagnosis. Small bowel biopsies reveal patchy villous atrophy with a cellular infiltrate [59]. Affected infants must abstain from the causative food to bring about symptom resolution. Spontaneous resolution occurs typically by 2 years of age.

Food-Protein-Induced Allergic Proctocolitis

Food-protein-induced allergic proctocolitis is characterized by blood and mucus in the stool of an otherwise healthy infant. Infants may be fussy or have increased frequency of bowel movements. The causative agent is usually milk in the maternal diet of a breast-fed infant, although egg, soy, and corn have been implicated as well [60]. Maternal dietary elimination of the causal agent leads to resolution of symptoms within 72 h. The problem generally resolves by 1 year of age. The causal food may be gradually reintroduced at that point, or earlier. The primary alternative explanation for these symptoms is infection.

Mixed IgE- and Cell-Mediated Disorders

Atopic dermatitis (also referred to as eczema), eosinophilic esophagitis, and eosinophilic gastroenteritis are disorders that have both IgE- and cell-mediated components. In up to 40% of patients with atopic dermatitis, food allergy may lead to increased erythema and pruritus of eczematous lesions [16, 18, 19]. IgE-mediated flares occur within minutes to a few hours, while cell-mediated reactions may take up to several days to manifest themselves [61, 62]. Elimination of the suspected food allergen leads to improvement.

Eosinophilic gastrointestinal disorders are described in detail in Chaps. 9 and 27. Briefly, eosinophilic infiltration of the gastrointestinal tract may result in dysphagia, vomiting, abdominal pain, poor growth, and food impaction and are the hallmarks of the eosinophilic gastrointestinal disorders (eosinophilic esophagitis and eosinophilic gastroenteropathy). A significant portion of patients with these disorders has other allergic disease, and food is a primary trigger [63–65]. In the case of eosinophilic esophagitis, elimination of foods to which the child has demonstrated sensitivity can result in both clinical and histological improvement [66, 67]. Similarly, elimination diets may show benefit in eosinophilic gastroenteropathy [68]. The role of allergy testing remains controversial, but skin tests (including atopy patch tests) and serum tests may be helpful in guiding elimination diets and the means to reintroduce foods that were excluded from the diet [69].

Additional Disorders Sometimes Attributed to Allergy

Gastroesophageal Reflux

Studies utilizing cow's milk elimination and challenge have shown between 14 and 42% of cases of gastroesophageal reflux in infants is attributable to cow's milk allergy [70–75]. In these cases, the reflux generally occurs in conjunction with atopic dermatitis, diarrhea, esophagitis, or malabsorption. An elimination diet may be helpful in infants with documented cow's milk allergy and reflux [76].

Colic

While infants with colic are not more frequently atopic than controls, [77] 44% of children with cow's milk allergy have colic [78, 79]. Soy and low-lactose formulas have not been successful in reducing the rate of colic, but a meta-analysis suggested a 1-week trial of hypoallergenic formula could be considered in such cases [79].

Chronic Constipation

In select groups of children with chronic constipation unresponsive to laxatives, cow's milk elimination diets resulted in resolution of constipation in 28–68% [80, 81]. Among responders, increased frequency of atopy and IgE antibodies was noted, suggesting a possible immunologic basis for their constipation. However, the soy milk used in lieu of cow's milk in these studies may have had a laxative effect [76].

Diagnostic Evaluation

Diagnostic evaluation of food allergy includes the history and physical examination, skin prick testing, serum-specific IgE testing, food elimination diets, and food challenges. The clinical history is paramount in diagnosing food allergy, as the pretest probability of food allergy determines what further testing is necessary. The history also discloses whether the illness is likely IgE antibody-mediated or not.

History and Physical Examination

The medical history plays a central role in determining which further steps in evaluation need to be performed. The symptoms and their temporal relation to the ingestion of food are particularly important. Acute IgE-mediated food-allergic reactions generally occur within seconds to minutes of ingestion of the food allergen. It is quite uncommon for these reactions to begin more than 2 h after the ingestion of the food. Chronic or delayed reactions may be cell-mediated and simple tests may not help to identify triggers—elimination diets and oral food challenges may be required.

With regard to IgE-mediated reactions, the time to resolution of symptoms should be noted. Particularly in the case of new-onset urticaria, in which 80% of cases are due to causes other than food allergy, [16, 17] hives lingering longer than 24–48 h are unlikely to result from food allergy, unless the suspected allergen has been repeatedly ingested concurrent with the urticaria. Hives lasting more than a day or two should raise suspicion for a viral or other process rather than food allergy.

A food that has never been eaten before or is ingested rarely is much more likely to cause a reaction than foods that have been previously tolerated on a regular basis. Parents or other caregivers may have reached early closure regarding which substance was the causative food. The clinician must attempt to reconstruct an accurate history of all the food and drink ingested within 2 h prior to the reaction as best as possible. Dressings, beverages, side dishes, snacks, and sauces should be included in this evaluation. In addition, a careful review should take into consideration the possible cross-contact with a potential allergen. Cross-contact is a fairly common cause of reactions at restaurants and buffet-style meals. A new allergy to a previously tolerated food is less likely than having a reaction to an ingredient that is not routinely ingested, or having had accidental exposure to a previously diagnosed allergen that was accidentally included in the meal that triggered a reaction.

If the patient has experienced allergic symptoms in the past, it is important to ask whether they had been consistently associated with the same food. Acute IgE-mediated allergic reactions generally occur every time the same quantity and preparation of an allergen is ingested. While trace amounts of protein can result in severe allergic reactions in particularly susceptible individuals, others have a threshold amount of protein that must be ingested before symptoms develop [82–85]. This threshold level can be as high as 10 g of the allergenic protein. In addition, cooking of foods induces conformational changes in certain proteins. For example, patients may react to less-heated forms of a food, such as the egg white in scrambled egg or French toast, but may not react to extensively heated forms of the same food (e.g., eggs baked in breads).

Depending on the patient's age, certain foods are more likely to be causative agents of an acute food-allergic reaction. In young children and infants, the following foods constitute 90 % of IgE-mediated allergies: cow's milk, egg, soy, peanut, tree nuts, wheat, fish, and shellfish [1]. In adolescents and adults, peanuts, tree nuts, fish, and shellfish are more common causes of serious acute reactions [6, 86, 87].

Besides the symptoms listed above that characterize acute reactions, the clinician should also note signs of chronic allergic processes, such as sinus venous congestion (and associated "allergic shiners"), horizontal nasal creases, boggy and pale nasal mucosa, or eczematous skin patches. While these signs of other allergic processes are not indicative of a food allergy in themselves, patients with other forms of atopy are more likely to experience food allergy, and therefore the presence of such signs increases the pretest probability of food allergy.

Tests for Food-Specific IgE

When the history and physical examination raise concern for possible IgE-mediated food allergy, skin prick testing and serum food-specific IgE testing can be helpful in investigating the potential allergens in question. Of paramount importance prior to selecting and interpreting these tests is the accurate medical history to determine pretest probability for IgE-mediated food allergy. A positive test (sensitization) to tolerated food(s) is common; therefore, a positive test can-

not be solely used to diagnose food allergy. In addition, occasionally a test is negative despite true allergy. Therefore, negative tests with a compelling history should not be considered sufficient evidence of no allergy [1, 88].

Skin Prick Testing

Skin prick testing is typically performed by allergist–immunologists. The allergen is introduced by scratching the surface of the skin and observing for a wheal and flare response, which is measured. Intradermal tests are not indicated as they are too sensitive and may induce systemic allergic reactions. Larger wheal size correlates with a greater concentration of food-specific IgE and greater likelihood of clinical allergy [89–91]. The sensitivity of skin prick testing is about 90 %, the specificity is approximately 50 % [92]. The skin of infants tends to be less sensitive than that of older children, however [93]. Given the high sensitivity of skin prick testing, it is a useful test for ruling out individual allergens in patients with a low pretest probability for food allergy to those specific allergens. However, performing skin prick testing to broad arrays of foods without attention to the medical history is not recommended, as the false-positive rate is high.

In Vitro Testing

In vitro testing methods, in contrast to skin tests, are not affected by antihistamine use, are not limited by skin conditions (such as urticaria, dermatographism, or eczema), and do not pose a risk of anaphylaxis. The first in vitro assays, termed "radioallergosorbent tests" (RAST), used radioactive isotopes to characterize relative IgE levels in a patient's serum. These have been replaced by fluorescent enzyme immunoassay (FEIA) tests, which determine serum-specific IgE levels to a variety of foods. Multiple in vitro assays have been developed, but results are not comparable across the various assays [94]. Most studies establishing normative serum-specific IgE cutoff values in children have used the Phadia ImmunoCAP FEIA (CAP-FEIA) system. Using this system, a prospective trial determined 96–100 % positive predictive values for reaction during a food challenge for egg (≥ 7 kU_A/L), milk (≥ 15 kU_A/L), peanut (≥ 14 kU_A/L), and fish (≥ 20 kU_A/L) among 5-year-olds, with reactive thresholds being lower for children less than 2 years of age [95]. For other foods (such as soy and wheat) or other age groups (such as adolescents), similar predictive values have not been established, and subsequent studies have varied in the predictive cutoffs, possibly due to variations in testing protocols or patient populations [96]. It is important to note that while skin prick testing and in vitro testing can determine the *likelihood* of a systemic reaction to ingestion of a particular food; they are unable to accurately predict the *severity* of that reaction should it occur. Newer generation tests evaluate specific IgE to specific proteins within a food. Foods are comprised of multiple proteins, of which those that resist degradation from heat or digestion are more likely to cause significant allergic reactions. Taking peanuts as an example, the peanut protein Ara h 8 is a labile protein homologous to a protein in birch tree pollen. When compared with the stable peanut storage protein Ara h 2, Ara h 8 is less likely to cause a significant allergic reaction. Elevated serum IgE levels to whole peanut can represent an allergy to Ara h 8, Ara h 2, or other peanut proteins. In individuals with allergy to whole peanut, performing component testing to determine which specific peanut proteins play a role in their food allergy is important in determining which patients may be appropriate for food challenge testing [88].

Diagnostic Food Elimination Diets

In the case of acute IgE-mediated food allergy, eliminating the causative allergens prevents further reactions—this type of elimination diet represents treatment of the underlying disorder. In the case of chronic food allergy in which no causative food is identified on testing, particularly in cell-mediated and mixed IgE- and cell-mediated food allergy, elimination diets are pursued for both diagnostic and treatment purposes. There are three basic types of diagnostic elimination diets: focused elimination diets, oligoantigenic diets, and elemental formula diets.

In a focused elimination diet, based on clinical history, one or several suspect foods are removed from the child's diet. The child is then monitored for the improvement of symptoms. If the symptoms fail to improve over 2 weeks (in the case of chronic IgE-mediated processes) or over several weeks (in the case of cell-mediated and mixed IgE- and cell-mediated food allergies), the food(s) removed from the diet are unlikely to be the underlying cause of the child's symptoms.

In the case of a child in whom no potential causative foods can be identified, an oligoantigenic diet may be pursued. In this diet, several of the most common causative foods are removed from the child's diet while maintaining a nutritionally complete diet with other foods. One example is a diet consisting of rice, lamb, asparagus, spinach, lettuce, sweet potato, cooked apple, olive oil, sugar, and salt [97].

In rare circumstances, children with multiple suspected food allergy triggers and continued significant disease burden are placed on an elemental diet. In this type of diet, the child's food intake is limited to an extensively hydrolyzed or amino-acid-based formula. Such diets can have significant adverse consequences and should only be pursued under the supervision of an allergist and nutritionist familiar with such diets.

If the child's symptoms abate following introduction of an oligoantigenic or elemental diet, other foods are added one by one into the diet with careful monitoring for the return of symptoms. In addition to the complexity of maintaining nutritional adequacy in a food elimination diet, reintroduction of foods after a long period of elimination poses a risk of increased severity of reaction to foods to which specific IgE is present or develops [98]. Consequently, care should be taken to avoid unnecessary elimination of foods.

Food Challenges

A food challenge is a physician-supervised ingestion of a single serving of potential allergen performed to confirm or refute the diagnosis of food allergy to that food. This test is generally used when history and supporting tests fail to confirm or refute an allergy. The test may be used for diagnosis of food allergy from any pathophysiology, IgE mediated or not.

A food challenge is performed for diagnostic purposes in the following scenarios:
- When several foods are being avoided, a food challenge can help determine foods that may be added back into the diet, particularly in the case of foods being avoided based on allergy testing alone (rather than a history of reaction).
- When IgE testing is negative, but a particular food is being avoided based on clinical history alone.
- When a cell-mediated or mixed IgE- and cell-mediated process is present (i.e., FPIES), a food challenge may be the only means of determining if an allergy is present.
- In addition, if serum IgE and skin prick test results appear to indicate that a particular allergy has resolved, a negative (or nonreactive) food challenge confirms allergy resolution [99].

Food Challenge Format
While a double-blind placebo-controlled food challenge is the gold standard for determining food allergy, in practice open food challenges and single-blind challenges tend to be more commonly pursued, in part because they are less labor intensive. A single-blind challenge, in which the observer, but not the child, is aware of which substance is placebo and which is the allergen, is useful in cases where a strong anxiety component is present. In an open food challenge, the child consumes the food in question in progressively increasing portion sizes every 10–15 min until the cumulative total of food given equals approximately one standard serving of the food. The patient is then observed for a predetermined period of time for delayed reactions prior to discharge home. If a reaction occurs the challenge is halted, and the child treated for symptoms [97, 100–102]. The physician performing the test, typically an allergist–immunologist, must be prepared to treat anaphylaxis.

Unproven Tests that Are Not Recommended

Food-specific IgG/IgG4, lymphocyte activation tests, kinesiology, sublingual or intradermal provocation tests, and cytotoxic tests are not supported by scientific validation and should not be performed as part of food allergy evaluation [1, 95, 103–105].

Dietary Treatment of Food Allergies

Avoidance

Food avoidance education is the cornerstone of food allergy management. Once it has been determined that a particular food must be eliminated from the diet, the child's family and all caregivers must undertake what amounts to a complete readjustment of one of the most basic daily habits—that of partaking in meals and snacks. Food elimination entails a careful evaluation of food packaging labels, safety in food preparation both in the restaurant and at home, and working with everyone from restaurant chefs, other children's parents, bakers, camp counselors, school cafeteria workers, and anyone else involved in the preparation of food to ensure that the allergen is not incorporated into any food consumed by the food-allergic child. Medications, vaccines, and cosmetics can also include food allergens. In highly sensitive individuals, less than a milligram of peanut, milk, or egg can cause a reaction [82–85].

Maternal Diet and Allergies in Breastfeeding

Food proteins can be detected in breast milk, and several cases have been reported of children experiencing reactions ranging from chronic atopic dermatitis to anaphylaxis due to maternal transfer of allergens through breast milk [106–109]. However, a tolerizing effect has been hypothesized in at least one study [110]. For infants with a history of reacting to a protein in the breast milk or a history of anaphylaxis due to direct ingestion of the allergen, strict maternal avoidance of the allergen is recommended.

Nutritional Issues in Food Allergy

When foods are being avoided due to allergy or potential allergy, care should be taken to assure that the nutritional needs of the affected child are addressed initially and revisited on a regular basis, as lower caloric intake and increased macro/micronutrient deficiency are more common in children with food allergy when compared with their age-matched peers without food allergy [111, 112]. The greater the number of allergens being avoided, the greater the chance of a nutrition-al deficiency developing: Thus, greater diligence must be exercised to tailor food choices to ensure a well-balanced diet. In certain circumstances, this cannot be attained by incorporation of regularly available foods alone, and commercially prepared formulas may be necessary beyond the first year of life, particularly in children with cow's milk and/or soy allergies. As children with food allergies are more likely to suffer from inadequate growth and poor nutrition than their peers, [1, 111–114] a consult with a dietitian well versed in food allergy elimination diets is necessary in most children with food allergies that significantly affect protein, fat, or carbohydrate intake.

Summary

- A food allergy is "an adverse health effect arising from a specific immune response that occurs reproducibly on exposure to a given food" [1].
- The eight major food allergens (milk, egg, peanut, tree nuts, soy, wheat, fish, and crustacean shellfish) account for 90 % of allergic reactions [1].
- Food allergies may be IgE-mediated, cell-mediated, or "mixed" adverse immune responses.
- IgE-mediated reactions are typically sudden in onset following exposure to a food allergen, whereas cell-mediated responses may result in chronic inflammation or delayed symptoms.
- Acute IgE-mediated reactions can have cutaneous, ocular, gastrointestinal, respiratory, and/or cardiovascular symptoms.
- Anaphylaxis is defined as a serious allergic reaction that is rapid in onset and may cause death [28].
- Cell-mediated food-allergic reactions include FPIES, food-protein-induced enteropathy, food protein-induced proctitis and proctocolitis, and food-induced pulmonary hemosiderosis.
- FPIES is a cell-mediated gastrointestinal food allergy that typically manifests in infancy and generally resolves by 3 years of age. In the acute form, 1–3 h after ingestion of the causative food, infants present with profuse, repetitive vomiting and may experience dehydration and lethargy. Aggressive intravenous fluid administration, steroids, and ondansetron may be used to treat acute cases. Elimination of the causative food leads to chronic symptom resolution within 3–10 days.
- Food-protein-induced enteropathy is characterized by vomiting, diarrhea, malabsorption, failure to thrive, and anemia in an infant. Cow's milk protein is the most likely causative agent, and symptoms usually spontaneously resolve by 2 years of age.
- Food-protein-induced allergic proctocolitis is characterized by blood and mucus in the stool of an otherwise healthy infant. Maternal dietary elimination of the causal

agent (usually cow's milk) leads to resolution of symptoms within 72 h. The problem generally resolves by 1 year of age.

- Atopic dermatitis, eosinophilic esophagitis, and eosinophilic gastroenteritis are disorders that can have both IgE- and cell-mediated components. Elimination diets may be helpful in these disorders.

- Diagnostic evaluation of food allergy includes the history and physical examination, skin prick testing, serum-specific IgE testing, food elimination diets, and food challenges. The clinical history is paramount in diagnosing food allergy, as the pretest probability of food allergy determines what further testing is necessary. The history also discloses whether the illness is likely to be IgE antibody-mediated or not.

- Skin prick testing and in vitro testing can determine the likelihood of an IgE-mediated systemic reaction to ingestion of a particular food, but they are unable to accurately predict the severity of that reaction should it occur. Positive predictive values for reaction during a food challenge have been established for in vitro testing to certain foods within certain age groups using a particular testing system.

- Food elimination diets play a treatment role in acute IgE-mediated food allergy and fulfill both diagnostic and treatment roles in cell-mediated and mixed IgE- and cell-mediated food allergy.

- A food challenge is a physician-supervised ingestion of a single serving of potential allergen performed to confirm or refute the diagnosis of food allergy to that food.

References

1. NIAID-Sponsored Expert Panel, Boyce JA, Assa'ad A, Burks AW, Jones SM, Sampson HA, et al. Guidelines for the diagnosis and management of food allergy in the United States: report of the NIAID-sponsored expert panel. J Allergy Clin Immunol. 2010;126(6 Suppl):S1–58. doi:10.1016/j.jaci.2010.10.007; 10.1016/j.jaci.2010.10.007.
2. CDC. Trends in allergic conditions among children: United States, 1997–2011. http://www.cdc.gov/nchs/data/databriefs/db121.pdf. Accessed 11 Jan 2014.
3. Branum AM, Lukacs SL. Food allergy among children in the United States. Pediatrics. 2009;124(6):1549–55. doi:10.1542/peds.2009-1210; 10.1542/peds.2009-1210.
4. Gupta RS, Springston EE, Warrier MR, Smith B, Kumar R, Pongracic J, et al. The prevalence, severity, and distribution of childhood food allergy in the United States. Pediatrics. 2011;128(1):e9–17. doi:10.1542/peds.2011-0204.
5. Liu AH, Jaramillo R, Sicherer SH, Wood RA, Bock SA, Burks AW, et al. National prevalence and risk factors for food allergy and relationship to asthma: results from the National Health and Nutrition Examination Survey 2005–2006. J Allergy Clin Immunol. 2010;126(4):798–806.e13. doi:10.1016/j.jaci.2010.07.026; 10.1016/j.jaci.2010.07.026.
6. Sicherer SH, Sampson HA. Food allergy: epidemiology, pathogenesis, diagnosis, and treatment. J Allergy Clin Immunol. 2013. doi:10.1016/j.jaci.2013.11.020.
7. Eggesbo M, Botten G, Halvorsen R, Magnus P. The prevalence of CMA/CMPI in young children: the validity of parentally perceived reactions in a population-based study. Allergy. 2001;56(5):393–402.
8. Eggesbo M, Halvorsen R, Tambs K, Botten G. Prevalence of parentally perceived adverse reactions to food in young children. Pediatr Allergy Immunol. 1999;10(2):122–32.
9. Leung TF, Yung E, Wong YS, Lam CW, Wong GW. Parent-reported adverse food reactions in Hong Kong Chinese pre-schoolers: epidemiology, clinical spectrum and risk factors. Pediatr Allergy Immunol. 2009;20(4):339–46. doi:10.1111/j.1399-3038.2008.00801.x; 10.1111/j.1399-3038.2008.00801.x.
10. McBride D, Keil T, Grabenhenrich L, Dubakiene R, Drasutiene G, Fiocchi A, et al. The EuroPrevall birth cohort study on food allergy: baseline characteristics of 12,000 newborns and their families from nine European countries. Pediatr Allergy Immunol. 2012;23(3):230–9. doi:10.1111/j.1399-3038.2011.01254.x; 10.1111/j.1399-3038.2011.01254.x.
11. Pyrhonen K, Nayha S, Kaila M, Hiltunen L, Laara E. Occurrence of parent-reported food hypersensitivities and food allergies among children aged 1–4 year. Pediatr Allergy Immunol. 2009;20(4):328–38. doi:10.1111/j.1399-3038.2008.00792.x; 10.1111/j.1399-3038.2008.00792.x.
12. Venter C, Pereira B, Grundy J, Clayton CB, Roberts G, Higgins B, et al. Incidence of parentally reported and clinically diagnosed food hypersensitivity in the first year of life. J Allergy Clin Immunol. 2006;117(5):1118–24. doi:10.1016/j.jaci.2005.12.1352.
13. Avery NJ, King RM, Knight S, Hourihane JO. Assessment of quality of life in children with peanut allergy. Pediatr Allergy Immunol. 2003;14(5):378–82.
14. Primeau MN, Kagan R, Joseph L, Lim H, Dufresne C, Duffy C, et al. The psychological burden of peanut allergy as perceived by adults with peanut allergy and the parents of peanut-allergic children. Clin Exp Allergy. 2000;30(8):1135–43.
15. Chehade M, Mayer L. Oral tolerance and its relation to food hypersensitivities. J Allergy Clin Immunol. 2005;115(1):3–12; quiz 3. doi:10.1016/j.jaci.2004.11.008.
16. Champion RH, Roberts SO, Carpenter RG, Roger JH. Urticaria and angio-oedema. A review of 554 patients. British J Dermatol. 1969;81(8):588–97.
17. Sehgal VN, Rege VL. An interrogative study of 158 urticaria patients. Ann Allergy. 1973;31(6):279–83.
18. Eller E, Kjaer HF, Host A, Andersen KE, Bindslev-Jensen C. Food allergy and food sensitization in early childhood: results from the DARC cohort. Allergy. 2009;64(7):1023–9. doi:10.1111/j.1398-9995.2009.01952.x; 10.1111/j.1398-9995.2009.01952.x.
19. Forbes LR, Saltzman RW, Spergel JM. Food allergies and atopic dermatitis: differentiating myth from reality. Pediatr Anna. 2009;38(2):84–90.
20. Kvenshagen B, Jacobsen M, Halvorsen R. Atopic dermatitis in premature and term children. Arch Dis Child. 2009;94(3):202–5. doi:10.1136/adc.2008.142869; 10.1136/adc.2008.142869.
21. Delgado J, Castillo R, Quiralte J, Blanco C, Carrillo T. Contact urticaria in a child from raw potato. Contact Dermatitis. 1996;35(3):179–80.
22. Fisher AA. Contact urticaria from handling meats and fowl. Cutis. 1982;30(6):726–9.
23. Jovanovic M, Oliwiecki S, Beck MH. Occupational contact urticaria from beef associated with hand eczema. Contact Dermatitis. 1992;27(3):188–9.
24. Simonte SJ, Ma S, Mofidi S, Sicherer SH. Relevance of casual contact with peanut butter in children with peanut allergy. J Allergy Clin Immunol. 2003;112(1):180–2.
25. Tan BM, Sher MR, Good RA, Bahna SL. Severe food allergies by skin contact. Ann Allergy, Asthma Immunol. 2001;86(5):583–6. doi:10.1016/S1081-1206(10)62908-0.

26. Bock SA. Prospective appraisal of complaints of adverse reactions to foods in children during the first 3 years of life. Pediatrics. 1987;79(5):683–8.

27. Bruijnzeel-Koomen C, Ortolani C, Aas K, Bindslev-Jensen C, Bjorksten B, Moneret-Vautrin D, et al. Adverse reactions to food. European academy of allergology and clinical immunology subcommittee. Allergy. 1995;50(8):623–35.

28. Sampson HA, Muñoz-Furlong A, Campbell RL, Adkinson NF Jr, Bock SA, Branum A, et al. Second symposium on the definition and management of anaphylaxis: summary report—Second National Institute of Allergy and Infectious Disease/Food Allergy and Anaphylaxis Network symposium. J Allergy Clin Immunol. 2006;117(2):391–7. doi:10.1016/j.jaci.2005.12.1303.

29. Brown AF, McKinnon D, Chu K. Emergency department anaphylaxis: a review of 142 patients in a single year. J Allergy Clin Immunol. 2001;108(5):861–6. doi:10.1067/mai.2001.119028.

30. Moneret-Vautrin DA, Morisset M, Flabbee J, Beaudouin E, Kanny G. Epidemiology of life-threatening and lethal anaphylaxis: a review. Allergy. 2005;60(4):443–51. doi:10.1111/j.1398-9995.2005.00785.x.

31. Bock SA, Muñoz-Furlong A, Sampson HA. Fatalities due to anaphylactic reactions to foods. J Allergy Clin Immunol. 2001;107(1):191–3. doi:10.1067/mai.2001.112031.

32. Grimshaw KE, King RM, Nordlee JA, Hefle SL, Warner JO, Hourihane JO. Presentation of allergen in different food preparations affects the nature of the allergic reaction—a case series. Clin Exp Allergy. 2003;33(11):1581–5.

33. Pumphrey R. Anaphylaxis: can we tell who is at risk of a fatal reaction? Curr Opin Allergy Clin Immunol. 2004;4(4):285–90.

34. Sampson HA, Mendelson L, Rosen JP. Fatal and near-fatal anaphylactic reactions to food in children and adolescents. New Engl J Med. 1992;327(6):380–4. doi:10.1056/NEJM199208063270603.

35. Sampson MA, Muñoz-Furlong A, Sicherer SH. Risk-taking and coping strategies of adolescents and young adults with food allergy. J Allergy Clin Immunol. 2006;117(6):1440–5. doi:10.1016/j.jaci.2006.03.009.

36. Lieberman P. Biphasic anaphylactic reactions. Ann Allergy, Asthma Immunol. 2005;95(3):217–26; quiz 26, 58. doi:10.1016/S1081-1206(10)61217-3.

37. Palosuo K, Alenius H, Varjonen E, Koivuluhta M, Mikkola J, Keskinen H, et al. A novel wheat gliadin as a cause of exercise-induced anaphylaxis. J Allergy Clin Immunol. 1999;103(5 Pt 1):912–7.

38. Romano A, Di Fonso M, Giuffreda F, Papa G, Artesani MC, Viola M, et al. Food-dependent exercise-induced anaphylaxis: clinical and laboratory findings in 54 subjects. Int Arch Allergy Immunol. 2001;125(3):264–72. doi:53825.

39. Commins SP, James HR, Kelly LA, Pochan SL, Workman LJ, Perzanowski MS, et al. The relevance of tick bites to the production of IgE antibodies to the mammalian oligosaccharide galactose-alpha-1,3-galactose. J Allergy Clin Immunol. 2011;127(5):1286–93.e6. doi:10.1016/j.jaci.2011.02.019; 10.1016/j.jaci.2011.02.019.

40. Commins SP, Satinover SM, Hosen J, Mozena J, Borish L, Lewis BD, et al. Delayed anaphylaxis, angioedema, or urticaria after consumption of red meat in patients with IgE antibodies specific for galactose-alpha-1,3-galactose. J Allergy Clin Immunol. 2009;123(2):426–33. doi:10.1016/j.jaci.2008.10.052; 10.1016/j.jaci.2008.10.052.

41. Nunez R, Carballada F, Gonzalez-Quintela A, Gomez-Rial J, Boquete M, Vidal C. Delayed mammalian meat-induced anaphylaxis due to galactose-alpha-1,3-galactose in 5 European patients. J Allergy Clin Immunol. 2011;128(5):1122–4.e1. doi:10.1016/j.jaci.2011.07.020; 10.1016/j.jaci.2011.07.020.

42. Restani P, Ballabio C, Tripodi S, Fiocchi A. Meat allergy. Curr Opin Allergy Clin Immunol. 2009;9(3):265–9. doi:10.1097/ACI.0b013e32832aef3d; 10.1097/ACI.0b013e32832aef3d.

43. Wood RA. The natural history of food allergy. Pediatrics. 2003;111(6 Pt 3):1631–7.

44. Fleischer DM, Conover-Walker MK, Christie L, Burks AW, Wood RA. The natural progression of peanut allergy: resolution and the possibility of recurrence. J Allergy Clin Immunol. 2003;112(1):183–9.

45. Iyngkaran N, Robinson MJ, Prathap K, Sumithran E, Yadav M. Cows' milk protein-sensitive enteropathy. Combined clinical and histological criteria for diagnosis. Arch Dis Child. 1978;53(1):20–6.

46. Kleinman RE. Milk protein enteropathy after acute infectious gastroenteritis: experimental and clinical observations. J Pediatr. 1991;118(4 Pt 2):S111–5.

47. Leonard SA, Nowak-Wegrzyn A. Manifestations, diagnosis, and management of food protein-induced enterocolitis syndrome. Pediatr Anna. 2013;42(7):135–40. doi:10.3928/00904481-20130619-11; 10.3928/00904481-20130619-11.

48. Nowak-Wegrzyn A, Muraro A. Food protein-induced enterocolitis syndrome. Curr Opin Allergy Clin Immunol. 2009;9(4):371–7. doi:10.1097/ACI.0b013e32832d6315; 10.1097/ACI.0b013e32832d6315.

49. Benlounes N, Candalh C, Matarazzo P, Dupont C, Heyman M. The time-course of milk antigen-induced TNF-alpha secretion differs according to the clinical symptoms in children with cow's milk allergy. J Allergy Clin Immunol. 1999;104(4 Pt 1):863–9.

50. Chung HL, Hwang JB, Park JJ, Kim SG. Expression of transforming growth factor beta1, transforming growth factor type I and II receptors, and TNF-alpha in the mucosa of the small intestine in infants with food protein-induced enterocolitis syndrome. J Allergy Clin Immunol. 2002;109(1):150–4.

51. Heyman M, Darmon N, Dupont C, Dugas B, Hirribaren A, Blaton MA, et al. Mononuclear cells from infants allergic to cow's milk secrete tumor necrosis factor alpha, altering intestinal function. Gastroenterology. 1994;106(6):1514–23.

52. McDonald PJ, Goldblum RM, Van Sickle GJ, Powell GK. Food protein-induced enterocolitis: altered antibody response to ingested antigen. Pediatr Res. 1984;18(8):751–5.

53. Van Sickle GJ, Powell GK, McDonald PJ, Goldblum RM. Milk- and soy protein-induced enterocolitis: evidence for lymphocyte sensitization to specific food proteins. Gastroenterology. 1985;88(6):1915–21.

54. Holbrook T, Keet CA, Frischmeyer-Guerrerio PA, Wood RA. Use of ondansetron for food protein-induced enterocolitis syndrome. J Allergy Clin Immunol. 2013;132(5):1219–20. doi:10.1016/j.jaci.2013.06.021.

55. Leonard SA, Nowak-Wegrzyn A. Food protein-induced enterocolitis syndrome: an update on natural history and review of management. Anna Allergy, Asthma Immunol. 2011;107(2):95–101; quiz, 62. doi:10.1016/j.anai.2011.06.004; 10.1016/j.anai.2011.06.004.

56. Hwang JB, Lee SH, Kang YN, Kim SP, Suh SI, Kam S. Indexes of suspicion of typical cow's milk protein-induced enterocolitis. J Korean Med Sci. 2007;22(6):993–7.

57. Katz Y, Goldberg MR, Rajuan N, Cohen A, Leshno M. The prevalence and natural course of food protein-induced enterocolitis syndrome to cow's milk: a large-scale, prospective population-based study. J Allergy Clin Immunol. 2011;127(3):647–53.e1–3. doi:10.1016/j.jaci.2010.12.1105; 10.1016/j.jaci.2010.12.1105.

58. Kuitunen P, Visakorpi JK, Savilahti E, Pelkonen P. Malabsorption syndrome with cow's milk intolerance. Clinical findings and course in 54 cases. Arch Dis Child. 1975;50(5):351–6.

59. Iyngkaran N, Yadav M, Boey CG, Lam KL. Severity and extent of upper small bowel mucosal damage in cow's milk protein-sensitive enteropathy. J Pediatr Gastroenterol Nutr. 1988;7(5):667–74.

60. Lake AM. Food-induced eosinophilic proctocolitis. J Pediatr Gastroenterol Nutr. 2000;30(Suppl):S58–60.

61. Sampson HA, McCaskill CC. Food hypersensitivity and atopic dermatitis: evaluation of 113 patients. J Pediatr. 1985;107(5):669–75.

62. Sicherer SH, Sampson HA. Food hypersensitivity and atopic dermatitis: pathophysiology, epidemiology, diagnosis, and management. J Allergy Clin Immunol. 1999;104(3 Pt 2):S114–22.

63. Assa'ad AH, Putnam PE, Collins MH, Akers RM, Jameson SC, Kirby CL, et al. Pediatric patients with eosinophilic esophagitis: an 8-year follow-up. J Allergy Clin Immunol. 2007;119(3):731–8. doi:10.1016/j.jaci.2006.10.044.

64. Guajardo JR, Plotnick LM, Fende JM, Collins MH, Putnam PE, Rothenberg ME. Eosinophil-associated gastrointestinal disorders: a world-wide-web based registry. J Pediatr. 2002;141(4):576–81. doi:10.1067/mpd.2002.127663.

65. Plaza-Martin AM, Jimenez-Feijoo R, Andaluz C, Giner-Muñoz MT, Martin-Mateos MA, Piquer-Gibert M, et al. Polysensitization to aeroallergens and food in eosinophilic esophagitis in a pediatric population. Allergologia et Immunopathologia. 2007;35(1):35–7.

66. Lieberman JA, Morotti RA, Konstantinou GN, Yershov O, Chehade M. Dietary therapy can reverse esophageal subepithelial fibrosis in patients with eosinophilic esophagitis: a historical cohort. Allergy. 2012;67(10):1299–307. doi:10.1111/j.1398-9995.2012.02881.x; 10.1111/j.1398-9995.2012.02881.x.

67. Spergel JM. Eosinophilic esophagitis in adults and children: evidence for a food allergy component in many patients. Curr Opin Allergy Clin Immunol. 2007;7(3):274–8. doi:10.1097/ACI.0b013e32813aee4a.

68. Gonsalves N, Doerfler B, Yang GY, Hirano I. S1861 A prospective clinical trial of six food elimination diet or elemental diet in the treatment of adults with eosinophilic gastroenteritis. Gastroenterology. 2009;136(5, Suppl 1):A–280. doi:http://dx.doi.org/10.1016/S0016-5085(09)61276-2.

69. Spergel JM, Brown-Whitehorn T, Beausoleil JL, Shuker M, Liacouras CA. Predictive values for skin prick test and atopy patch test for eosinophilic esophagitis. J Allergy Clin Immunol. 2007;119(2):509–11. doi:10.1016/j.jaci.2006.11.016.

70. Cavataio F, Iacono G, Montalto G, Soresi M, Tumminello M, Campagna P, et al. Gastroesophageal reflux associated with cow's milk allergy in infants: which diagnostic examinations are useful? Am J Gastroenterol. 1996;91(6):1215–20.

71. Cavataio F, Iacono G, Montalto G, Soresi M, Tumminello M, Carroccio A. Clinical and pH-metric characteristics of gastro-oesophageal reflux secondary to cows' milk protein allergy. Arch Dis Child. 1996;75(1):51–6.

72. Forget P, Arends JW. Cow's milk protein allergy and gastro-oesophageal reflux. Eur J Pediatr. 1985;144(4):298–300.

73. Iacono G, Carroccio A, Cavataio F, Montalto G, Kazmierska I, Lorello D, et al. Gastroesophageal reflux and cow's milk allergy in infants: a prospective study. J Allergy Clin Immunol. 1996;97(3):822–7.

74. Ravelli AM, Tobanelli P, Volpi S, Ugazio AG. Vomiting and gastric motility in infants with cow's milk allergy. J Pediatr Gastroenterol Nutr. 2001;32(1):59–64.

75. Staiano A, Troncone R, Simeone D, Mayer M, Finelli E, Cella A, et al. Differentiation of cows' milk intolerance and gastro-oesophageal reflux. Arch Dis Child. 1995;73(5):439–42.

76. Sicherer SH. Clinical aspects of gastrointestinal food allergy in childhood. Pediatrics. 2003;111(6 Pt 3):1609–16.

77. Castro-Rodriguez JA, Stern DA, Halonen M, Wright AL, Holberg CJ, Taussig LM, et al. Relation between infantile colic and asthma/atopy: a prospective study in an unselected population. Pediatrics. 2001;108(4):878–82.

78. Hill DJ, Hosking CS. Infantile colic and food hypersensitivity. J Pediatr Gastroenterol Ntr. 2000;30 (Suppl):S67–76.

79. Lucassen PL, Assendelft WJ, Gubbels JW, van Eijk JT, van Geldrop WJ, Neven AK. Effectiveness of treatments for infantile colic: systematic review. BMJ (Clinical research ed). 1998;316(7144):1563–9.

80. Daher S, Tahan S, Sole D, Naspitz CK, Da Silva Patricio FR, Neto UF, et al. Cow's milk protein intolerance and chronic constipation in children. Pediatr Allergy Immunol. 2001;12(6):339–42.

81. Iacono G, Cavataio F, Montalto G, Florena A, Tumminello M, Soresi M, et al. Intolerance of cow's milk and chronic constipation in children. New Engl J Med. 1998;339(16):1100–4. doi:10.1056/NEJM199810153391602.

82. Flinterman AE, Pasmans SG, Hoekstra MO, Meijer Y, van Hoffen E, Knol EF, et al. Determination of no-observed-adverse-effect levels and eliciting doses in a representative group of peanut-sensitized children. J Allergy Clin Immunol. 2006;117(2):448–54. doi:10.1016/j.jaci.2005.11.035.

83. Sicherer SH, Morrow EH, Sampson HA. Dose-response in double-blind, placebo-controlled oral food challenges in children with atopic dermatitis. J Allergy Clin Immunol. 2000;105(3):582–6. doi:10.1067/mai.2000.104941.

84. Taylor SL, Hefle SL, Bindslev-Jensen C, Atkins FM, Andre C, Bruijnzeel-Koomen C, et al. A consensus protocol for the determination of the threshold doses for allergenic foods: how much is too much? Clin Exp Allergy. 2004;34(5):689–95. doi:10.1111/j.1365-2222.2004.1886.x.

85. Taylor SL, Hefle SL, Bindslev-Jensen C, Bock SA, Burks AW Jr, Christie L, et al. Factors affecting the determination of threshold doses for allergenic foods: how much is too much? J Allergy Clin Immunol. 2002;109(1):24–30.

86. Moneret-Vautrin DA, Morisset M. Adult food allergy. Curr Allergy Asthma Reports. 2005;5(1):80–5.

87. Osterballe M, Hansen TK, Mortz CG, Host A, Bindslev-Jensen C. The prevalence of food hypersensitivity in an unselected population of children and adults. Pediatr Allergy Immunol. 2005;16(7):567–73. doi:10.1111/j.1399-3038.2005.00251.x.

88. Sicherer SH, Wood RA. Advances in diagnosing peanut allergy. J Allergy Clin Immunol Prac. 2013;1(1):1–13; quiz 4. doi:10.1016/j.jaip.2012.10.004; 10.1016/j.jaip.2012.10.004.

89. Hill DJ, Heine RG, Hosking CS. The diagnostic value of skin prick testing in children with food allergy. Pediatr Allergy Immunol. 2004;15(5):435–41. doi:10.1111/j.1399-3038.2004.00188.x.

90. Peters RL, Allen KJ, Dharmage SC, Tang ML, Koplin JJ, Ponsonby AL, et al. Skin prick test responses and allergen-specific IgE levels as predictors of peanut, egg, and sesame allergy in infants. J Allergy Clin Immunol. 2013;132(4):874–80. doi:10.1016/j.jaci.2013.05.038; 10.1016/j.jaci.2013.05.038.

91. Roberts G, Lack G. Diagnosing peanut allergy with skin prick and specific IgE testing. J Allergy Clin Immunol. 2005;115(6):1291–6. doi:10.1016/j.jaci.2005.02.038.

92. American College of Allergy A, Immunology. Food allergy: a practice parameter. Ann Allergy Asthma Immunol. 2006;96(3 Suppl 2):S1–68.

93. Menardo JL, Bousquet J, Rodiere M, Astruc J, Michel FB. Skin test reactivity in infancy. J Allergy Clin Immunol. 1985;75(6):646–51.

94. Wang J, Godbold JH, Sampson HA. Correlation of serum allergy (IgE) tests performed by different assay systems. J Allergy Clin Immunol. 2008;121(5):1219–24. doi:10.1016/j.jaci.2007.12.1150.

95. Sicherer SH, Teuber S, Adverse Reactions to Foods C. Current approach to the diagnosis and management of adverse reactions to foods. J Allergy Clin Immunol. 2004;114(5):1146–50. doi:10.1016/j.jaci.2004.07.034.

96. Jarvinen KM, Sicherer SH. Diagnostic oral food challenges: procedures and biomarkers. J Immunol Methods. 2012;383(1–2):30–8. doi:10.1016/j.jim.2012.02.019.

97. Sicherer SH. Food allergy: when and how to perform oral food challenges. Pediatr Allergy Immunol. 1999;10(4):226–34.

98. David TJ. Anaphylactic shock during elimination diets for severe atopic eczema. Arch Dis Child. 1984;59(10):983–6.

99. Nowak-Wegrzyn A, Assa'ad AH, Bahna SL, Bock SA, Sicherer SH, Teuber SS. Work group report: oral food challenge testing. J Allergy Clin Immunol. 2009;123(6 Suppl):S365–83. doi:10.1016/j.jaci.2009.03.042.

100. Bindslev-Jensen C. Standardization of double-blind, placebo-controlled food challenges. Allergy. 2001;56(Suppl 67): 75–7.

101. Bock SA, Sampson HA, Atkins FM, Zeiger RS, Lehrer S, Sachs M, et al. Double-blind, placebo-controlled food challenge (DBP-CFC) as an office procedure: a manual. J Allergy Clin Immunol. 1988;82(6):986–97.

102. Niggemann B, Rolinck-Werninghaus C, Mehl A, Binder C, Ziegert M, Beyer K. Controlled oral food challenges in children—when indicated, when superfluous? Allergy. 2005;60(7):865–70. doi:10.1111/j.1398-9995.2005.00828.x.

103. Aalberse RC, Stapel SO, Schuurman J, Rispens T. Immunoglobulin G4: an odd antibody. Clin Exp Allergy. 2009;39(4):469–77. doi:10.1111/j.1365-2222.2009.03207.x; 10.1111/j.1365-2222.2009.03207.x.

104. Beyer K, Teuber SS. Food allergy diagnostics: scientific and unproven procedures. Curr Opin Allergy Clin Immunol. 2005;5(3):261–6.

105. Matsumoto N, Okochi M, Matsushima M, Kato R, Takase T, Yoshida Y, et al. Peptide array-based analysis of the specific IgE and IgG4 in cow's milk allergens and its use in allergy evaluation. Peptides. 2009;30(10):1840–7. doi:10.1016/j.peptides.2009.07.005; 10.1016/j.peptides.2009.07.005.

106. Des Roches A, Paradis L, Singer S, Seidman E. An allergic reaction to peanut in an exclusively breastfed infant. Allergy. 2005;60(2):266–7. doi:10.1111/j.1398-9995.2005.00681.x.

107. Jarvinen KM, Makinen-Kiljunen S, Suomalainen H. Cow's milk challenge through human milk evokes immune responses in infants with cow's milk allergy. J Pediatr. 1999;135(4):506–12.

108. Lifschitz CH, Hawkins HK, Guerra C, Byrd N. Anaphylactic shock due to cow's milk protein hypersensitivity in a breast-fed infant. J Pediatr Gastroenterol Nutr. 1988;7(1):141–4.

109. Monti G, Marinaro L, Libanore V, Peltran A, Muratore MC, Silvestro L. Anaphylaxis due to fish hypersensitivity in an exclusively breastfed infant. Acta Paediatr. 2006;95(11):1514–5. doi:10.1080/08035250600732013.

110. Frazier AL, Camargo CA Jr, Malspeis S, Willett WC, Young MC. Prospective study of peripregnancy consumption of peanuts or tree nuts by mothers and the risk of peanut or tree nut allergy in their offspring. JAMA Pediatr. 2013. doi:10.1001/jamapediatrics.2013.4139.

111. Christie L, Hine RJ, Parker JG, Burks W. Food allergies in children affect nutrient intake and growth. J Am Diet Assoc. 2002;102(11):1648–51.

112. Henriksen C, Eggesbo M, Halvorsen R, Botten G. Nutrient intake among two-year-old children on cows' milk-restricted diets. Acta Paediatr. 2000;89(3):272–8.

113. Isolauri E, Sutas Y, Salo MK, Isosomppi R, Kaila M. Elimination diet in cow's milk allergy: risk for impaired growth in young children. J Pediatr. 1998;132(6):1004–9.

114. Jensen VB, Jorgensen IM, Rasmussen KB, Molgaard C, Prahl P. Bone mineral status in children with cow milk allergy. Pediatr Allergy Immunol. 2004;15(6):562–5. doi:10.1111/j.1399-3038.2004.00191.x.

Eosinophilic Gastroenteropathy

Alfredo J. Lucendo

Introduction

Over the past few decades, digestive tract eosinophilia has emerged as a potential explanation for various abdominal symptoms. The development of gastrointestinal (GI) endoscopy and the possibility of studying histological material have allowed us to identify several distinctive elements of this disorder, including both the density and the extension of eosinophilia along the entire length of the GI tract, so that a new clinicopathological group of entities has emerged. These are currently grouped under the term of eosinophilic gastrointestinal disorders (EGID) [1].

EGID are primarily defined as disorders that selectively affect the GI tract and are characterized by an eosinophil-rich inflammation that appears in the absence of any known causes of tissue eosinophilia (e.g., drug reactions, parasitic infections, and malignancy) [2]. The term EGID includes eosinophilic esophagitis (EoE), eosinophilic gastritis, eosinophilic gastroenteritis (EGE), eosinophilic enteritis, and eosinophilic colitis, all of which are diagnosed with increasing frequency [3].

The symptoms derived from eosinophilic infiltration of the GI tract characteristically vary depending on the affected digestive segments and the involvement of different layers of the digestive wall [4]. EoE, the most prevalent form of EGID, is characterized by esophageal eosinophilic inflammation with no distal GI tract involvement, accompanied by symptoms of esophageal dysfunction. In the case of EGE, the typically affected sites are the stomach and small bowel, although any area of the GI tract from the esophagus to the rectum may also be involved [5].

First described in 1937 by Kaijser [6], interest in EGE has grown in recent years in parallel with an exponentially increasing number of case reports and case series from different continents. Although it is still considered a rare disorder, nearly a quarter of all historical descriptions of EGE in the literature come from the past 5 years [7]. Despite this increased interest in the disease, many aspects of EGE remain unknown, including its epidemiology, physiopathological mechanisms, and natural history. Furthermore, therapeutic options for EGE patients are still mostly based on empirical experience due to the lack of controlled, randomized studies which clearly establish definitive strategies for managing EGE.

Nevertheless, information from the many case reports and short series of patients who have been studied over a wide range of years and geographical areas point to several commonly observed phenomena which seem to be characteristic of the disease.

This chapter provides a comprehensive and updated review of EGE to help clinicians understand this increasingly recognized disorder and guide them in the management of these complex patients.

GI Eosinophils: Biology and Function

Eosinophils are bone-marrow-derived granulocytes with pro-inflammatory functions which are involved in the pathogenesis of various disorders. They are recruited from the blood to several peripheral tissues, including the mucosal and submucosal areas of the GI tract, after being activated by various stimuli. Most of the research on eosinophils to date has focused on their function in the lungs and the blood [8], but more recent studies have started to delve into their function in and regulation of the GI tract [9]. In fact, the GI tract is a major target for the migration of eosinophils, which are a normal component of the lamina propria in the stomach as well as in the small and large intestines [10]. This migration process is regulated by a number of cytokines and chemokines, with interleukin (IL)-5 playing a major role. IL-5 not only promotes the development and proliferation of eosinophils in bone marrow but also their migration to peripheral tissues and their survival and degranulation. In addition, this

A. J. Lucendo (✉)
Department of Gastroenterology, Hospital General de Tomelloso,
Vereda de Socuéllamos, s/n, 13700 Tomelloso, Ciudad Real, Spain
e-mail: alucendo@vodafone.es

© Springer International Publishing Switzerland 2016
S. Guandalini et al. (eds.), *Textbook of Pediatric Gastroenterology, Hepatology and Nutrition*,
DOI 10.1007/978-3-319-17169-2_27

cytokine primes eosinophils to respond to the chemoattractant signals that recruit them to the mucosa [11].

Eosinophils are functionally complex cells that have both regulatory and effector functions. For example, they synthesize and release several cytokines able to induce fibrous remodeling and subepithelial collagen deposition, including transforming growth factor (TGF)-β and fibroblast growth factor (FGF)-9 [12], thus contributing to the development of strictures and luminal narrowing in the GI tract, both of which are common in patients with EGID. Eosinophils also synthesize and release major basic protein (MBP) [13], a strong agonist of M2-type muscarinic receptors, which govern smooth muscle contraction. Increased levels of MBP contribute to gut dysmotility, especially when combined with the effect of several mediators released by other cell types also present in the inflammatory infiltrate of patients with EGID. These include mast cells, which act on muscular fibers through the release of histamine and leukotrienes [14].

As effector cells, eosinophils participate in the host's defense against helminthes and parasites through the production and degranulation of cytotoxic proteins, including MBP, eosinophil-derived neurotoxin (EDN), eosinophilic cationic protein (ECP), and eosinophilic peroxidase (EPO) [15]. The degree of tissue injury is related to the duration of the eosinophilia, the level of eosinophil activation, and the type of stimuli that attracts these cells [16]. The cytotoxic properties of eosinophilic granular proteins is related to the increased fragility observed in the GI wall tissue of patients with EGID, in which a high incidence of tears and perforations has been described [17]. Eosinophils also release platelet-activator factor (PAF) and leukotriene C4, which induce endothelial cell activation and contribute to inflammation and cell dysfunction [15]. Finally, eosinophils are also a source of pro-fibrogenic cytokines, including TGF-β, phospho-SMAD 2/3, vascular cell-adhesion molecule (VCAM)-1, and Chemokine (C-C motif) ligand (CCL)18 [12, 18], all of which lead to fibrous remodeling with important clinical implications.

The inflammation in EGID can extend deep into several layers of the GI tract wall, promoting fibrous remodeling, causing smooth muscle disturbances, and increasing the risk of tissue damage and perforations [19], all through the cytoplasmatic cytotoxic granule proteins present in eosinophils.

Eosinophils in the GI Tract Mucosa

As in other organs, eosinophils, lymphocytes, plasma cells, mast cells, and macrophages comprise the normal inflammatory component of the lamina propria and submucosa of all parts of the human GI tract, where they perform protective functions as normally resident cells forming part of the mucosal-associated surveillance system [20, 21]. While few studies have assessed the actual number of eosinophils present in the GI tract mucosa under normal conditions, several reports on normal pediatric GI mucosa have observed that eosinophils are usually found within the gastric, small intestine, and colonic mucosa [22], but are scarce in the esophageal epithelium [23, 24], where their presence is generally associated with disease.

The few reports available on the number of eosinophils found in GI biopsies have described a gradient of eosinophil density from cephalic to caudal, that is, from virtually no eosinophils present in esophageal epithelia to a high eosinophilic density in colonic mucosa [22, 24]. Information regarding the exact quantity and location of eosinophils in the human GI tract is likewise scarce [23, 24], although routine examinations of the antrum, fundus, and small intestine usually reveal either no or very few eosinophils in the surface epithelium. In fact, intraepithelial eosinophils in the esophageal and gastric mucosa are always considered to be abnormal [16]. In contrast, an average of 2–10 cells/hpf (high-power field) was documented in the lamina propria of the normal stomach and duodenum, respectively. Moreover, atopic and nonatopic children had comparable numbers of eosinophils. The same study found that eosinophils were more concentrated in the deep compared to the superficial lamina propria. This was especially noteworthy in the small intestine, where eosinophils were found to be more numerous in intercryptal lamina propria than in intravillous lamina propria [24].

In the colon, eosinophils and other constituent inflammatory cells follow a gradient along the length of the organ, from proximal to distal [25–27]. With regard to the role of drugs in this condition, no consistent correlation between eosinophil count and intake of medication has been described [27].

In all locations and under normal conditions, eosinophils in mucosal biopsies are distributed as single cells which do not form aggregates. Extracellular eosinophil granules are not generally found in normal biopsies [28].

Epidemiology of Eosinophilic Gastroenteritis

Interest in EGID has risen among gastroenterologists in the past few decades, particularly after the broad recognition that EoE now constitutes the most frequent manifestation of this family of disorders, representing the second most common cause of dysphagia and food impaction in young patients after gastroesophageal reflux disease [29]. Indeed, several authors have observed an increase in the prevalence of EGID in general and of EGE in particular [3, 7, 30]. The rise in the incidence of these disorders and of immunoallergic diseases in general has occurred in parallel with a decrease in infectious diseases; the "hygienic hypothesis," which asserts that reduced exposure to microorganisms during infancy can modify the patterns of immune responses, has provided a general explanation for the rise of EGID [31]. According to this theory, changes in gut microbiota lead to changes in the fine tuning of Th1, Th2, and T-regulatory responses, giving rise to an imbalance of the immune system and a predisposition for developing allergic and autoimmune disorders triggered by altered or missing innate immune cell activation. In fact, most patients who have EGID have an associated atopic disease [32]. The influence of Th2 cells, which are important in the development of responses mediated by IgE, usually fades after the first 2 years of life in nonallergic individuals. This is possibly due to a secondary stimulation of Th1 responses after bacterial infections [33], which occur less often in over-hygienic environments. Delivery by cesarean section has been recognized as one possible risk factor for the persistence and severity of EGE in pediatric patients [34], with the differences in the gut microbiota of cesarean-section-born babies compared to those born vaginally being proposed as a possible explanation [35].

Environmental exposure thus seems to be as important a risk factor as genetic predisposition for developing EGID. In this sense, a US study recently demonstrated that the increased prevalence of EoE parallels that of bronchial asthma in common geographical areas, being higher in urban settings than in rural areas [3, 36] as well as in cold climate zones compared with tropical and arid areas [37].

The number of eosinophils normally present in the GI mucosa can also vary between different geographical areas [33], depending on the exposure to different microbiological and allergic environments. Thus, the normal eosinophil count in the left colon mucosa of healthy adult subjects living in the southern part of the USA was higher than in samples obtained from subjects living in the northern USA [38]. No comparable study has been reproduced in children. In addition to geographic location, the density of eosinophils in the colonic mucosa also seems to vary seasonally [39], with colonic mucosal eosinophils being slightly more numerous in samples obtained in April and May, which corresponds to the time of year with the highest pollen counts. A similar relationship between pollen exposure and mucosal eosinophilic density has been also demonstrated in children [40] and adults with EoE [41, 42].

In any case, the low prevalence of EGE has meant that most of our knowledge about this disorder comes from individual case reports and short case series, a fact which has made it difficult to elucidate the definitive features of its epidemiology.

While no accurate epidemiological estimations for EGE exist to date, an incidence of approximately one case per 100,000 inhabitants has been traditionally proposed [43, 44]. These figures have recently been updated after an electronic survey carried out in the USA estimated the overall incidence of EGE or colitis to be 28 cases per 100,000 inhabitants [3]. However, these figures are only valid for the USA, as the prevalence of EGE can vary widely among different countries. In Asia, for example, data reported from several single-center registries found that during a 10-year period, seven patients (six men) with EGE were treated at a large referral hospital in India [45]. Two single-center studies carried out in Korea have also reported an increase in the incidence of EGE. The first study reported 31 cases between 1970 and 2003, with 26 cases reported after 1990 [46]. In the second study, 17 patients were diagnosed between 1994 and 2008 [47]. Another case report found 15 patients diagnosed between 1984 and 2002 in Taiwan [48]. In contrast, and for a similar timeframe (1987–2007), 59 patients were diagnosed in one US institution [44]. Even though caution should be taken when comparing these figures, a progressive increase in the epidemiology of EGE can also be assumed when considering the number of studies referenced in PubMed. Just in the past decade, the number has doubled compared to what it was in the 1980s, representing almost 40 % of the overall available scientific information on the disease. It is unclear whether this change in the epidemiology of EGE represents a real increase in the prevalence of the disorder or is simply a reflection of the increase in the number of endoscopic exams performed around the world. It may even be a simple case of raised awareness on the part of clinicians, endoscopists (who now tend to obtain mucosal biopsies even when there is little or no endoscopic alteration), and pathologists. What is clear is that EGE has become a more common diagnosis in clinical practice, as is evident from the fact that it was diagnosed in 4.1 % of pediatric patients undergoing upper GI endoscopy due to chronic abdominal pain in a recent prospective study carried out in the USA [49].

Allergic eosinophilic proctocolitis (AEPC) is a distinctive pediatric food-allergy-related disorder which is considered prevalent, predominantly in males [50], although its exact epidemiology is likewise unknown [51]. An epidemiological study performed in Brazil demonstrated that 20.6 % of infants with known or suspected cow's milk allergy had blood in the stool, which might be the result of allergic or eosinophilic colitis [52].

Pathophysiology of Eosinophilic Gastroenteritis

Allergy

As very little research on the molecular basis of EGE has been carried out, its pathophysiology is as yet poorly defined, with most of the available information coming from extrapolations from studies on EoE, which, because it is more prevalent, has been studied in greater depth. However, it should be noted that extrapolating information from other EGIDs may not be completely accurate, since EGE presents as a complex disorder for which the several clinical patterns could represent distinct phenotypic alternatives or even different evolving profiles.

From a pathophysiological perspective, EGIDs have been typically considered as mixed disturbances, sharing characteristics of both IgE-mediated disorders (e.g., oral allergy syndrome and food-triggered anaphylaxis) and exclusively cell-mediated disorders (such as celiac disease or food protein-induced colitis). In the specific case of EGE, it has been related to food allergies in that it originates from the interplay of environmental and individual genetic factors. In fact, approximately three out of four EGE patients present various atopic manifestations, including a personal or family background of bronchial asthma, allergic rhinitis, dermatitis, hypersensitivity to food, inhalants or drugs, peripheral hypereosinophilia, elevated total and specific IgE serum levels, or positive skin allergic test results, thus reinforcing the idea that eosinophils accumulate in the stomach and small bowel in response to exposure to food [53, 54] or environmental [41] antigens. Clinical and histological responses to therapies used in other allergic diseases, such as corticosteroids, antiallergic drugs, and dietary modifications, have also been observed in most cases of EGE.

As with EoE [55], a Th2-type immune response seems to be involved in EGE [56]. In fact, interleukins (IL)-5 and -13, together with granulocyte-macrophage colony-stimulating factor and especially eotaxins, may play a central role in the recruitment of eosinophils from circulating blood into GI tissues [57]. The frequent family association of EGID cases (around 10% of patients have affected relatives [2]) points to the role of immune response regulatory genes in these diseases, which in the particular case of EoE show a preserved transcriptome among patients [58, 59]. The genes involved include eotaxin-3/CCL26, mast cell carboxipeptidase-A3 (CPA3) and tryptase (TPSAB1), and high-affinity IgE receptor (FCεRI). Thymic stromal lymphopoietin (TSLP), a master regulating factor of Th2 responses [60, 61], is also upregulated in these patients.

Fibrous Remodeling

EGID seems to be chronic disorder in the majority of cases, but almost no cohorts have been observed over a long period without therapeutic interventions. However, we know from eosinophil-associated lung and skin disorders that eosinophilic inflammation may lead to structural changes globally known as tissue remodeling. The most widely studied remodeling phenomenon is that described in the eosinophilic inflammation of the airways which occurs in bronchial asthma. The most clinically relevant components of this phenomenon are smooth muscle hypertrophy and collagen subepithelial deposition, which lead to the narrowing of the bronchia and impairment of respiratory function [62]. Fibrous remodeling has also been repeatedly observed in both pediatric [63] and adult EoE patients [12, 64]; while it is a reversible phenomenon in the former [65],it tends to persist in the latter [12, 64]. Retrospective studies on EoE have demonstrated that the disease is a progressive fibrostenotic entity [66] and that in the absence of treatment, it correlates with the prevalence of fibrotic complications such as esophageal strictures in a time-dependant manner [67], much like the natural history of Crohn's disease. In the case of EGE EoE, fibrous remodeling also explains strictures and obstructive symptoms found in many reported cases of EGE affecting the pylorus and small bowel [68]; such complications often require resection of the affected area [69].

Fibrosis in EGID is directly related to eosinophil activation, as evaluated through immunohistochemistry against MBP [70]. Eosinophil-released MBP increases gene expression of FGF-9, a cytokine implicated in the proliferative response after tissue damage [71]. Eosinophils also produce and secrete high amounts of CCL18, a type-2 chemokine implicated in fibrous remodeling of the lungs through fibroblast proliferation and collagen deposition, the expression levels of which have been shown to be increased in EoE [12]. However, the most widely studied cytokine in promoting fibrous remodeling in EGID is TGF-β1, the expression of which is upregulated in both children [63] and adults [12, 72] with EoE, but which can be reduced with dietary or steroid-based treatment [12, 65, 72, 73].

Histopathology of Eosinophilic Gastroenteritis

Aside from being linked to EGID, intestinal eosinophilia has also been associated with systemic eosinophilic disorders [16] (idiopathic hypereosinophilic syndrome, chronic eosinophilic leukemia, systemic mastocytosis, and immunodysregulation polyendocrinopathy enteropathy X-linked (IPEX) syndrome [74, 75]) as well as with non-eosinophilic disorders (parasitic infections, drug reactions, connective tissue disease, vasculitis, malignancies, and inflammatory bowel diseases, in which eosinophils are often responsible for an bad prognosis [76, 77]. A diagnosis of primary EGE or colitis can thus be made only after excluding all other known causes of tissue eosinophilia.

Table 27.1 Histopathologic findings suggestive of eosinophilic gastrointestinal disease (gastroenteritis/colitis). (Reprinted fromRef. [21], with permission from Elsevier)

Increased number of mucosal eosinophils (subjective, not absolute quantitative threshold is defined except for eosinophilic esophagitis)
Degranulated eosinophils
Intraepithelial eosinophils (surface and gland/crypt epithelium)
Eosinophil surface layering
Eosinophil microabscesses
Epithelial degenerative/regenerative changes
Marked basal layer hyperplasia
Elongated papillae
Lamina propria eosinophilia and fibrosis
Foveolar/crypt hyperplasia
Villous atrophy in the small bowel
Minimal acute and chronic inflammation
Eosinophils in muscularis mucosa, submucosa, or both

If secondary causes of tissue eosinophilia have been ruled out, increased eosinophils in the presence of some of the above pathologic features suggest primary eosinophilic gastrointestinal disorder. The diagnosis of "mucosal eosinophilia" is recommended if there are no pathologic changes beyond increased eosinophils

In contrast to EoE, for which a histopathological diagnostic threshold of ≥ 15 eosinophils/hpf has been consensually defined [78], there is as yet no established consensus on a diagnostic threshold for the remaining forms of EGID, including EGE, although the most commonly agreed upon limit for a positive diagnosis of the disease is >20 eosinophils/hpf [79, 80].The difficulty in defining clear diagnostic criteria for EGE is due to several factors, including inconsistencies in the definition of what constitutes an eosinophil (e.g., the presence of a cell defined by a nucleus or an aggregate of granule proteins that may result from active extrusion of granules by activated eosinophils), the lack of a standard size for a hpf (an area of tissue covered by a $40\times$ light microscope objective), and the wide variability of analysis among pathologists and GI/allergy clinicians [36, 81]. (Table 27.1)

In EGE, the stomach and small intestine are the most frequently affected segments of the GI tract [82]. The characteristics of the eosinophilic infiltration in each gut segment are given below in Table 27.2 [12, 24, 44, 68, 79, 80, 83–91].

In the case of gastric mucosal samples, a recent study has evaluated the diagnostic criteria of "histological eosinophilic gastritis," asserting that in the absence of other known causes of eosinophilia, histopathological findings such as sheets of eosinophils, frequent involvement of the muscularis mucosa or submucosa, and a density of ≥ 30 eosinophils/hpf in at least 5 hpfs are suitable diagnostic criteria for EGE [85].

The association of histological eosinophilic gastritis and the presence of *Helicobacter pylori* has been addressed in the literature with contradictory results. Thus, although a slow decrease in eosinophil count after *H. pylori* eradication was described in the early literature [92], more recent reports show no association between this infection and eosinophilic gastritis [85, 93]. Still, current guidelines state that a diagnosis of eosinophlic gastritis can be established only if mucosal eosinophilia persists several months after successful eradication of *H. pylori* [16]. Finally, superinfection by the protozoa *Isospora belli,* a common opportunistic parasite in immunodepressed patients, has been described as an exceptional association in EGE [94], but should be excluded after a definitive diagnosis has been established.

Knowledge about primary eosinophilic enteritis has been limited by the inaccessibility of the different small-bowel segments to mucosal sampling. Thus, in endoscopic investigations of the small intestine, biopsy specimens can usually be obtained from the duodenum, the first part of the jejunum, and the distal ileum. Descriptions of eosinophilic infiltration in other segments of the small intestine mainly come from the surgical literature [95–97]. In the overwhelming majority of patients, an increase in the number of mucosal eosinophils in the small bowel appears together with eosinophilic infiltration into other segments of the GI tract and represents an expression of EGE [37].

Eosinophilic colitis is characterized by increased numbers of mucosal and intraepithelial eosinophils in colonic biopsy samples. Additional histopathological features suggestive of eosinophilic colitis are provided in Table 27.1.

AEPC represents a distinct condition which is reported exclusively in infants and young children and is related to the ingestion of foreign proteins [4]. One relevant histopathological difference between AEPC and EGE with colonic involvement is that in the former, the overall mucosal architecture is usually well preserved and the eosinophilic infiltration is typically more localized in the rectum [2, 16, 21]. Diagnostic criteria include eosinophilic epithelial infiltration with more than 60 eosinophils/10 hpf in the lamina propria, and involvement of the muscularis mucosae. However, as patients respond well to treatment when AEPC is suspected, rectosigmoidoscopy with biopsies is usually unnecessary [98].

Besides eosinophilic infiltration, other recognized diagnostic criteria for EGE include mucosal edema, eosinophilic degranulation, glandulitis/cryptitis, eosinophilic crypt abscesses, and chronic architectural changes [79]. In contrast, epithelial infiltration may not be a constant feature [85]. In fact, in 10 % of all EGID cases, the mucosa exhibits no diagnostic changes, even when the inflammation is identified in subjacent submucosa, lamina propria, or muscular layers. This is probably due to sampling errors in a disease that can often be patchy [21].

Table 27.2 Eosinophilic infiltration in different GI organs in EGE; eosinophil count, histopathological findings, and derived symptoms [12, 24, 44, 68, 79, 80, 83–91]

Involved organ	Mean eosinophil density in normal conditions	Minimum eosinophil count required for diagnosis	Histopathologic features	Clinical manifestations
Esophagus [83, 84]	<5/hpf	15/hpf in the epithelial layer	Elongated papillae and basal zone hyperplasia of the epithelial layer with eosinophilic infiltration of the lamina propria and muscularis mucosae. Eosinophilic microabscesses	Esophageal dysfunction, including dyspagia, food impaction, and GERD-related symptoms
Stomach [12, 24, 79, 85]	2/hpf in lamina propria[a] No intraepithelial eosinophils[a]	>20–30/hpf	Sheets of eosinophils, edema, eosinophilic degranulation, cryptitis	Dyspepsia, nausea/vomiting, epigastric pain, gastric outlet obstruction, ascitis
Duodenum [24, 68, 80]	10/hpf in lamina propria Minimal intraepithelial eosinophils	>20–30/hpf	Sheets of eosinophils, edema, eosinophilic degranulation, cryptitis Eosinophilic infiltration of lamina propria, muscle fibers, and serosal layer Hypertrophic muscle layer	Gastric outlet obstruction, abdominal pain, diarrhea, weight loss, malabsorption findings, perforation, ascitis
Ileum [24, 44]	13/hpf in lamina propria[a] Minimal intraepithelial eosinophils[a]	>20–30/hpf	Sheets of eosinophils, edema, eosinophilic degranulation, cryptitis Eosinophilic infiltration of lamina propria, muscle fibers, and serosal layer Hypertrophic muscle layer	Abdominal pain, small-bowel perforation, small-bowel obstruction, ascitis
Large bowel [24, 86–88]	8–30/hpf[a]	>20–50/hpf (depending on location)	Eosinophil and lymphocyte infiltration of the lamina propria and the presence of intraepithelial eosinophils in the crypts	Diarrhea, bloody diarrhea, abdominal pain Constipation
Bile ducts/pancreas [89–91]	Unknown	Unknown	Non available data on literature	Jaundice, cholestasis, epiastralgia, altered liver function tests Dilated bile ducts Pancreatic mass

[a] Reported for pediatric control patients
hpf high power field, *GERD* gastroesophageal reflux disease

Clinical Manifestations of EGE

From its initial description [6], EGE has been recognized as an extremely heterogeneous disease with respect to its clinical presentation. In 1970, Klein et al. proposed a classification of EGE into three different arbitrary patterns based on clinical manifestations and the depth of the eosinophilic infiltrate into the GI tract wall [99]. This classification has been used by many subsequent authors because, when combined with the topographical location of the eosinophilic inflammation, it helps to predict clinical symptoms. (Table 27.3)

a. Mucosal form: This form is characterized by involvement of both the mucosa and submucosa, leading to malabsorption-related symptoms such as diarrhea, weight loss, iron-deficiency anemia, and loss of protein enteropathy. The mucosal form represents the most common presentation of EGE, making up 45% of cases in several series. It has recently been suggested that the mucosal form of EGE has become predominant in the past few years, with a recent series reporting a prevalence of over 80% [44].

b. Muscular form: This form appears when the eosinophilic inflammation extends deeper into the muscle layers, leading to digestive wall thickening and typical obstructive symptoms. Often, this form of the disease is diagnosed after surgical resection of the affected segment [68, 100]. Muscular affectation can also manifest with decreased small intestine and colonic motility, leading to constipation [101]. The muscular form has been estimated to comprise 12–30% of all EGE cases [43, 79].

c. Serosal form (or eosinophilic ascitis): When the eosinophilic infiltration permeates all layers of the GI tract wall and extends to the serosal covering, this causes the appearance of eosinophilic ascitis, which is defined by an eosinophil cell count of at least 10% [102], but reaching up to 80% [103]. Eosinophilic ascitis is generally considered the rarest form of EGE, but has been recognized in 12.5–39% of cases in some studies [43, 79].

Although it is a fairly accurate tool, Klein's "classic" classification should be broadened to include two important EGE-related conditions that have been described repeatedly in literature.

Table 27.3 Summary of eosinophilic gastroenteritis symptoms and common findings, according with the classification proposed by Klein et al. [91] in 1970

Forms	Estimated frequency	Maximal depth of digestive tissue involvement	Main affected organs	Main symptoms	Common findings
Mucosal	45–80%	Mucosa and submucosa	Stomach and duodenum	Abdominal pain, weight loss, diarrhea, nausea/vomiting, iron deficiency, malabsortion, protein-losing enteropathy	Mucosal hyperemia, ulcerations, aphthae, thickness of folders
Muscular	12–30%	Muscle layer	Stomach and duodenum	Nausea/vomiting, gastric outlet or small-bowel obstruction	Strictures, rigidity, dysmotility, and obstruction
Serosal	12.5–39%	Subserosal and serosal layers	Any segment of the GI tract	Ascitis and peritonitis	Eosinophilic ascitis, intense peripheral eosinophilia Small-bowel perforation

GI gastrointestinal

d. Intestinal perforation: Limitations in the biopsy sampling of most segments of the small intestine have probably led to diagnostic delays in the subset of patients with predominant small-bowel affectation, justifying its presentation as a distinctive complication requiring surgical repair. Perforation in the context of EGE has been observed in every segment of the GI tract, including the esophagus [17, 19], stomach [96], duodenum [104], jejunum [97, 105, ileum [95],and colon [106]. The transmural involvement of the disease in this case is different from that of eosinophilic ascitis, but it was not included in the Klein classification. The cytotoxic effector function exerted by eosinophil granule proteins has been proposed as the underlying cause of tissue damage in these patients.

e. Biliopancreatic involvement of EGE: Extraintestinal involvement in EGE has been repeatedly described as a form of cholecytopancreatitis with bile duct dilation and obstructive jaundice [79, 89–91, 107, 108], together with symptoms derived from gut inflammation. Duodenal mass effect can also lead to acute obstructive pancreatitis [109].

While primary EGE has been described in patients of all ages, the majority of cases are diagnosed between the third and fifth decades of life [82]. In contrast to EoE, which is clearly predominant in males [78], no definitive data are available on gender predominance in EGE in general, although eosinophilic ascitis and the underlying transmural EGE form have been described predominantly in women, occasionally triggered during pregnancy and/or after delivery [34, 103, 110–112].

Several clinical aspects of EGE are intriguing, but the lack of large case series makes it difficult to propose definitive conclusions. Still, studies conducted to date indicate that peripheral blood eosinophilia is frequent among sufferers of EGE, being found in up to 90% of patients [113]. This condition is more intense and frequent in patients with mucosal and serosal (with ascitis) EGE than in those affected only up to the muscle layers [43, 53, 79]. In addition, 80% of cases have a personal background of allergies, 50–62% of which are food allergies [3]. In contrast, only 27% of adult patients reported a fam-

ily history of allergy; interestingly, this was limited to patients with mucosal involvement [44]. Finally, 16% of patients had or currently have a relative also suffering from EGE [3].

More than half of the patients also exhibited increased IgE serum levels [113]. While all these atopic manifestations seem to be more common in mucosal and serosal forms [79, 86], they are also present in a high proportion of patients with muscular forms of EGE [44].

With regard to the topographical distribution of EGE, the stomach and duodenum have been proposed as the most frequently involved digestive organs. However, these are also the digestive segments most commonly examined by means of endoscopy, which may lead to bias. Indeed, virtually any segment of the GI tract may be affected, with 50% of patients presenting concomitant involvement of the rectum and/or colon [112] and 30–50% of patients exhibiting simultaneous esophageal eosinophilic infiltration [4]. Thus, large bowel-derived symptoms including bloody diarrhea (which can mimic inflammatory bowel disease) and symptoms of esophageal dysfunction (e.g., dysphagia) may coexist together with stomach and small-bowel-derived symptoms. Interestingly, infiltration of the lamina propria by eosinophils and their presence in the crypts of rectal mucosal biopsies of young children with constipation due to cow's milk intolerance has been described [86] as an alternative to EGE-associated diarrhea.

Diagnostic Imaging Techniques in Eosinophilic Gastroenteritis

Although EGE and eosinophilic colitis were both described decades ago, data on the typical radiological or endoscopic appearance of lesions in patients come mostly from more recent reports.

Most of the endoscopic findings described in EGE tend to be nonspecific, with mucosal hyperemia and thickened gastric folds [44] being the most common. Areas of rough or nodular appearance, erosions, aphthae, and ulcers have also been described in the disorder while in some cases, the endoscopic results have been normal [79]. Findings from capsule endoscopy include multiple erythematous lesions, loss of villi [113], incomplete strictures with ulcerated mucosa alternating with preserved areas [114], and a mimicking of mucosal diaphragms with complete retention of the capsule [115]. One patient with eosinophilic ascitis showed a bluish discoloration of the deep layers of the intestinal wall without mucosal changes; the authors hypothesized that in this case, eosinophilic infiltration had respected the mucosa [116].

Radiological findings in EGE are equally nonspecific in two thirds of patients [44, 117]; double contrast radiology findings are usually normal [44], but may occasionally show thickened folds, irregular or serrated edges in the walls of the small intestine, nodular contrast defects, or slow contrast progression indicative of GI hypomotility.

The findings in the colonoscopies of patients with eosinophilic colitis tend to be modest and nonspecific, sometimes showing patchy erythematous changes, loss of vascular pattern, and superficial ulceration. In other cases, the mucosa appears to be normal. A biopsy diagnosis is thus essential for demonstrating eosinophilic involvement of the colon [118].

Natural History of Eosinophilic Gastroenteritis

In spite of the approximately 500 EGE cases described in the literature to date, very little research has focused on elucidating the natural history of the disease. A recently published French study analyzed the clinical characteristics and evolution of 43 adult patients with EGE who were followed for a mean period of 13 years [79]. The authors described three different evolutionary patterns (Fig. 27.1). (a) 42% of patients suffered a single outbreak of EGE lasting <3 months, a pattern confirmed in a recent population-based study which also describes this self-limited course as being present in a majority of middle-aged adult patients suffering from eosinophilic colitis [119], (b) 37% of patients exhibited a recurrent pattern of disease, with an average of 5.2 flare-ups at extremely variable intervals, and finally (c) 21% of patients had a continuous disease course with persistent symptoms. No other studies have determined the global relapse rate after the first flare-up, although high eosinophil blood counts at the time of diagnosis have been associated with an increased risk of disease recurrence [79]. No tumoral or myeloproliferative transformation was observed in any patient during follow-up. In fact, an association between EGE and malignancy has only been described once in the literature in a case study of a 69-year-old Japanese man with multiple

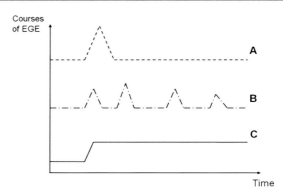

Fig. 27.1 Types of evolution of eosinophilic gastroenteritis (EGE). After a mean follow-up period of 13 years, Pineton de Chambrun et al. [79] identified three different types of evolution of EGE: **a** patients with a single outbreak of disease without recurrence (42% of cases), **b** patients with a recurrent course characterized by multiple outbreaks and periods of complete remission lasting from 2 months to several years (37% of cases), and **c** patients with a continuous course (21% of cases). (Reprinted from Ref. [79], with permission from Elsevier)

gastric cancer and EGE who responded well to a total gastrectomy and prednisolone treatment [120].

Nevertheless, many questions regarding the natural history of EGE remain unanswered. For example, it has yet to be determined whether the disease in children and adults is the same or whether pediatric forms of EGE persist into adulthood. There is also a shortage of data concerning the ability of different therapeutic modalities to change the natural history of the disease, especially regarding the response to dietary-based therapeutic interventions [7].

With regard to AEPC in infants, the disorder is characterized by a benign course in which dietary elimination of the aggressor often resolves the symptoms within days [118].

Treatment of Eosinophilic Gastroenteritis

Heterogeneity in the clinical presentation, severity, and evolution of EGE, together with its low prevalence, has made it difficult to establish ideal treatment strategies for these patients. As in the case of other EGIDs, including EoE, no drugs have been approved specifically for the treatment of EGE and comparative studies of different therapeutic modalities are lacking. To make matters more confusing, both patient age (children or adults) and the medical specialty area in which they are attended tend to determine which treatments are administered. Basically, three major therapeutic modalities for managing these patients have been described in the literature; these include several dietary modifications to reduce the antigenic capacity of the diet, administration of drugs with anti-inflammatory and immunosuppressant effects, and finally, surgical intervention when complications arise.

Dietary Treatment

The most solid evidence of the efficacy of dietary treatment has been provided for infants (<6 month) with AEPC. Since allergy to cow's milk is identified as the major precipitant cause for this disorder, exclusion of cow's milk from the diet of the lactating mother or from the infant's diet is generally an effective therapeutic measure. Fortunately, clinical tolerance to cow's milk develops in about 80% of patients by 5 years of age [121].

The response to dietary therapies restricting certain foods has been recently studied in patients with EGE in a systematic review of literature [122], including 25 full-text articles and 5 abstracts. Overall, data from 86 individual patients (79 children) receiving 89 dietary interventions were retrieved. Data came from individual patients and short case series of up to 12 patients; most of documents were judged as having low methodological quality. Overall effectiveness in inducing clinical remission/clinical improvement was reported for 87.2% of children and 88% of adults included; however, no study objectively assessed changes in clinical complains by means of validated or nonvalidated instruments. Histological assessments after dietary treatment were made in only 20 individual children (22.5%). Resolution or decrease in eosinophilic infiltration was documented in 16 cases (80%), and changes were not noted in the 4 remaining patients. Authors concluded that, due to the relative lack of well-designed and high-quality studies, the unequivocal use of dietary treatment for patients with EGE and colitis cannot be supported, and they recommended undertaking further research.

Exclusive feeding with an amino-acid-based elemental diet, in which amino acids are used as the sole nitrogen source was used in 29 patients, all of them children [122]; clinical remission was reported in 75.8% (22 patients). However, histological remission was assessed for only one patient with small-bowel involvement and in a further six patients with eosinophilic gastritis in a single research, 83% of these having normalized mucosal biopsies [123, 124]. Semi-elemental diets (i.e., extensively hydrolyzed formulas with reduced antigenic capacities) as the exclusive nutritional source were used in only two patients [125]: Clinical and histological remission was documented in only one patient. A major advantage of elemental diets is their avoidance of steroids, thus preventing the potential adverse effect of growth retardation in these children. However, the many drawbacks of elemental diets, including their unpleasant taste, high nonadherence rates, high cost, and the psychological and social implications of complete avoidance of any kind of table food, restrict their use in clinical practice to infants and toddlers, among whom food restrictions are better tolerated, and only for the length of time required for food reintroduction with the goal of identifying specific dietary triggers. In any case, there is still no consensus in the literature as to which allergic evaluations or tests should be carried out on these patients.

Allergy testing–elimination diets are another therapeutic approach that consists of testing for food allergies with the aid of skin prick testing (SPT), atopy patch testing (APT), or determination of specific serum IgE against a given food in order to identify specific food triggers and eliminate them from the diet. This intervention strategy has rarely been documented in literature for EGE patients [126], since only three children and one adult underwent this treatment option: Clinical remission was described in every patient; biopsy samples after treatment were only available for one single child, who showed histological improvement [122].

A positive allergy test result did not predict whether a specific food was a disease trigger or not: A recent study carried out in patients with EoE, EGE, and healthy volunteers demonstrated that despite the general presence of a concomitant atopy in the first two groups, no differences in serum IgE levels for the most common food allergens were detected among the three groups [127]. According to consensus guidelines [78], allergy testing should be considered for patients with EGID to evaluate their allergic status. However, even though many individuals generate food-specific IgE antibodies that can be detected with allergy tests, they may still be clinically tolerant to various foods and have no allergic reaction following ingestion. This is probably because blood or skin tests are not specific for EGID; therefore, a wide variety of allergic diseases may be responsible for the results. In fact, food triggers can currently only be unequivocally identified by first documenting disease remission after specific food antigen avoidance, followed by disease recrudescence upon specific food reintroduction.

Most of the patients in the literature had been treated using different empiric approaches, which consisted of elimination of single foods (milk and wheat were the most common foods excluded) or combinations of foods considered to be of high risk of triggering an allergic response. A milk elimination diet, a treatment strategy used by 4 authors [128–131] on 16 individual pediatric patients, resulted in a symptomatic improvement rate of 62.5%, with no histological assessment available. A gluten-free diet was used in two EGE patients with no clinical or histological benefits.

Several empiric elimination diets, which included empiric restriction of multiple foods, such as milk, cereals, egg, soy, seafood, and/or fruits, have been repeatedly used in the literature to treat EGE. The empirical elimination of the six most common food antigens from the diet (also called six-food elimination diet or 6-FED), and 7-FED (excluding red meats also) have been assessed in recent years. The aforementioned systematic review overall identified 34 patients with EGE or colitis have been given this dietary treatment and a symptomatic improvement has been reported in 29 (85.3 %) of these [122]. Histological assessments, however, have rarely been reported. A recent paper judged as of medium-/high-quality, reported histological remission of the disease after an empirical seven-FED in five out of six children with eosinophilic gastritis (83.3 %), and in two out of three patients after diet without one to three foods [123].

Most of the reported cases retrieved in this systematic review presented a mucosal type of EGE, according to Klein's classification [99]; muscular type was only described for one patient, serosal/transmural type was reported in a single case; in nine cases, the type of EGE was not reported. The low proportion of patients with muscular and serosal/transmural-type EGE prevented the authors to develop a comparative analysis. Regarding GI organ extension, no differences in clinical or histological remission/improvement were observed with regard to disease location or extension.

Once remission of EGE is achieved, specific foods should be reintroduced gradually, identifying problem foods by the reappearance of symptoms or through bioptic monitoring. Evidence of tolerance to offending foods after elimination and reintroduction has not yet been fully assessed. In the case of adult patients, allergic sensitization test results did not correlate with the specific foods responsible for the disease. Generally speaking, from the literature we can infer that the later EGE appears during childhood, the worse it responds to dietary modification [79].

Drug Therapy

Corticosteroids have been by far the most widely used drugs for treating EGE in both children and adults [44, 80, 132]. These drugs also constitute the main treatment for patients in whom dietary therapy is not feasible or who fail to achieve improvement [2]. Prednisone, used at doses of 0.5–1 mg/kg/daily, has proven highly effective in the initial control of symptoms [44], eosinophilic tissue infiltration, blood hypereosinophilia, and also for controlling ascites, as described in various studies and case reports. Clearly, the use of steroids in EGE does significantly more than merely control symptoms [113].Usually, after an initial treatment period of 7–10 days, the dose is gradually reduced until the drug is withdrawn after a period of up to 4 months.

Various series have described steroid-dependent patients in whom symptoms reappear during steroid tapering [113, 133]. These patients must resume taking previous doses, maintain remission by using low doses, substitute prednisone for budesonide [125, 126], or maintain remission with other antiallergic or immunosuppressant drugs [134]. Around 20 % of patients require maintenance therapy over time [125]. Budesonide has a better safety profile than prednisone and is especially useful in EGE affecting the distal

small bowel and right colon [135], although it is also helpful in managing more proximal disease [126].

Disease recurrence is more likely in those patients requiring treatment at the moment of diagnosis as compared to those who exhibit spontaneous remission; patients with recurrent disease may also present a higher blood eosinophil count at diagnosis than those who show spontaneous remission [79].

Steroid-dependent or refractory patients can be also managed with thiopurins (azathoprine or 6-mercaptopurin), similar to the treatment of inflammatory bowel disease [4, 134, 136].

With regard to the utility of other antiallergic drugs in treating EGE, unfortunately most of the available information comes from isolated cases or small series, which limits our ability to vouch for their efficacy. Some EGE patients have obtained benefits from mast cell stabilizers [79, 135, 137] such as sodium cromolyn or nedocromil, contrary to what has been observed in EoE, in which these drugs have no demonstrated efficacy [138]. Ketotifen and histamine-1 blockers have also proven effective in reducing tissue eosinophilia and symptoms in patients with EGE [139, 140], with suplatast tosylate having a beneficial effect in the only case in which it was used [141]. Information regarding the leukotriene inhibitor montelukast is contradictory; on the one hand, it was wholly ineffective in some cases [142–144], but successfully acted as a steroid-sparing agent in isolated steroid-dependent patients [80, 145].

Finally, biological therapies with the anti-IL-5 monoclonal antibodies mepolizumab and reslizumab to treat hypereosinophilic syndrome have provided only limited data to date. A pilot study in which four EGE patients were treated with a single dose of mepolizumab showed an average drop in blood eosinophilia of 75 % and of 50–70 % in tissue eosinophilia, but with minimal symptom improvement [146]. In addition, one patient experienced a noticeable increase in GI tissue eosinophil count 4 weeks after treatment, while two additional patients showed an increase in their peripheral eosinophilia, with a worsening of baseline GI symptoms after 7–8 weeks of treatment [147]. Intravenous immunoglobulin was successfully used in a patient with erythematous lupus associated with steroid-refractory EGE [148].

Surgical Treatment

While the muscular form of EGE may cause obstructive symptoms [149] due to bowel wall thickening and narrowing of the lumen, some cases of EGE have been diagnosed after intestinal resection of the affected area after acute abdomen [69], intestinal obstruction, or perforation [95, 96, 150]. It is worth noting that these complications occur more often in the duodenum or the distal ileum. Unfortunately, data on the long-term outcome and possible recurrence of cases after resection of the affected segment is lacking.

Conclusion

EGIDs constitute an increasingly common heterogeneous group of digestive diseases that should be considered as a diagnostic possibility in patients with common GI symptoms. The limited number of new EGE cases has prevented the development of clinical trials that could provide conclusive date to clearly define many of the aspects of the disease. The establishment of systematic multicenter registries of cases which exhaustively include clinical and immunological characteristics of patients, type of therapy received and response thereto, evolution of the disease, and even molecular data would go far in offsetting the small number of EGE patients, allowing access to more information to broaden our knowledge of this disease. Only long-term follow-up and outcomes of patients undergoing different therapeutic modalities will help define the natural history of EGE in children and adults, clearing up the controversy of whether pediatric EGE lasts into adulthood.

References

1. Fleischer DM, Atkins D. Evaluation of the patient with suspected eosinophilic gastrointestinal disease. Immunol Allergy Clin North Am. 2009;29:53–63. doi:10.1016/j.iac.2008.09.002.
2. Rothenberg ME. Eosinophilic gastrointestinal disorders (EGID). J Allergy Clin Immunol. 2004;113:11–28. doi:10.1016/j.jaci.2003.10.047.
3. Spergel JM, Book WM, Mays E, Song L, Shah SS, Talley NJ, et al. Variation in prevalence, diagnostic criteria, and initial management options for eosinophilic gastrointestinal diseases in the United States. J Pediatr Gastroenterol Nutr. 2011;52:300–6. doi:10.1097/MPG.0b013e3181eb5a9f.
4. Lucendo AJ. Eosinophilic diseases of the gastrointestinal tract. Scand J Gastroenterol. 2010;45:1013–21. doi:10.3109/00365521003690251.
5. MacCarty RL, Talley NJ. Barium studies in diffuse eosinophilic gastroenteritis. Gastrointest Radiol. 1990;15:183–7.
6. Kaijser R. Zur Kenntnis der allergischen Affektionen des Verdauugskanals vom Standpunkt des Chirurgen aus. Arch Klin Chir. 1937;188:36–64.
7. Lucendo AJ, Arias A. Eosinophilic gastroenteritis: an update. Expert Rev Gastroenterol Hepatol. 2012;6:591–601. doi:10.1586/egh.12.42.
8. Gleich GJ. Mechanisms of eosinophil-associated inflammation. J Allergy Clin Immunol. 2000;105:651–63. doi:10.1067/mai.2000.105712.
9. Smyth CM, Akasheh N, Woods S, Kay E, Morgan RK, Thornton MA, et al. Activated eosinophils in association with enteric nerves in inflammatory bowel disease. PLoS One. 2013;8:e64216. doi:10.1371/journal.pone.0064216.
10. Powell N, Walker MM, Talley NJ. Gastrointestinal eosinophils in health, disease and functional disorders. Nat Rev Gastroenterol Hepatol. 2010;7:146–56. doi:10.1038/nrgastro.2010.5.
11. Martin LB, Kita H, Leiferman KM, Gleich GJ. Eosinophils in allergy: role in disease, degranulation, and cytokines. Int Arch Allergy Immunol. 1996;109:207–215.
12. Lucendo AJ, Arias A, De Rezende LC, Yague-Compadre JL, Mota-Huertas T, Gonzalez-Castillo S, et al. Subepithelial collagen deposition, profibrogenic cytokine gene expression, and changes after prolonged fluticasone propionate treatment in adult eosinophilic esophagitis: a prospective study. J Allergy Clin Immunol. 2011;128:1037–46. doi:10.1016/j.jaci.2011.08.007.
13. Talley NJ, Kephart GM, McGovern TW, Carpenter HA, Gleich GJ. Deposition of eosinophil granule major basic protein in eosinophilic gastroenteritis and celiac disease. Gastroenterology. 1992;103:137–45.
14. Lucendo AJ, Bellon T, Lucendo B. The role of mast cells in eosinophilic esophagitis. Pediatr Allergy Immunol. 2009;20:512–8. doi:10.1111/j.1399–3038.2008.00798.x.
15. Rothenberg ME, Mishra A, Brandt EB, Hogan SP. Gastrointestinal eosinophils in health and disease. Adv Immunol. 2001;78:291–328.
16. Hurrell JM, Genta RM, Melton SD. Histopathologic diagnosis of eosinophilic conditions in the gastrointestinal tract. Adv Anat Pathol. 2011;18:335–48. doi:10.1097/PAP.0b013e318229bfe2.
17. Lucendo AJ, Friginal-Ruiz AB, Rodriguez B. Boerhaave's syndrome as the primary manifestation of adult eosinophilic esophagitis. Two case reports and a review of the literature. Dis Esophagus. 2011;24:E11–5. doi:10.1111/j.1442–2050.2010.01167.x.
18. Venge P. The eosinophil and airway remodelling in asthma. Clin Respir J. 2010;4(Suppl 1):15–9. doi:10.1111/j.1752–699X.2010.00192.x.
19. Fontillon M, Lucendo AJ. Transmural eosinophilic infiltration and fibrosis in a patient with non-traumatic Boerhaave's syndrome due to eosinophilic esophagitis. Am J Gastroenterol. 2012;107:1762. doi:10.1038/ajg.2012.226.
20. Zuo L, Rothenberg ME. Gastrointestinal eosinophilia. Immunol Allergy Clin North Am. 2013;27:443–55. doi:10.1016/j.iac.2007.06.002.
21. Collins MH. Histopathology associated with eosinophilic gastrointestinal diseases. Immunol Allergy Clin North Am. 2009;29:109–17. doi:10.1016/j.iac.2008.10.005.
22. Lowichik A, Weinberg AG. A quantitative evaluation of mucosal eosinophils in the pediatric gastrointestinal tract. Mod Pathol. 1996;9:110–4.
23. Rothenberg ME, Mishra A, Collins MH, Putnam PE. Pathogenesis and clinical features of eosinophilic esophagitis. J Allergy Clin Immunol. 2001;108:891–4. doi:10.1067/mai.2001.120095.
24. DeBrosse CW, Case JW, Putnam PE, Collins MH, Rothenberg ME. Quantity and distribution of eosinophils in the gastrointestinal tract of children. Pediatr Dev Pathol. 2006;9:210–8. doi:10.2350/11–05-0130.1.
25. Kirby JA, Bone M, Robertson H, Hudson M, Jones DE. The number of intraepithelial T cells decreases from ascending colon to rectum. J Clin Pathol. 2003;56:158. doi:10.1136/jcp.56.2.158.
26. Carpenter HA, Talley NJ. The importance of clinicopathological correlation in the diagnosis of inflammatory conditions of the colon: histological patterns with clinical implications. Am J Gastroenterol. 2000;95:878–96. doi:10.1111/j.1572–0241.2000.01924.x.
27. Prasad V, Jaggi P, Scherzer R, Mousa H. Distribution of mucosal eosinophils in the non-inflamed pediatric colon: a clinico-pathologic correlation in 50 children. Pediatr Dev Pathol 2010;13:161.
28. Aceves S, Hirano I, Furuta GT, Collins MH. Eosinophilic gastrointestinal diseases–clinically diverse and histopathologically confounding. Semin Immunopathol. 2012;34:715–31. doi:10.1007/s00281–012-0324-x.
29. Straumann A, Aceves SS, Blanchard C, Collins MH, Furuta GT, Hirano I, et al. Pediatric and adult eosinophilic esophagitis: similarities and differences. Allergy. 2012;67:477–90. doi:10.1111/j.1398–9995.2012.02787.x.

30. Kinoshita Y, Furuta K, Ishimaura N, Ishihara S, Sato S, Maruyama R, et al. Clinical characteristics of Japanese patients with eosinophilic esophagitis and eosinophilic gastroenteritis. J Gastroenterol. 2013;48:333–9. doi:10.1007/s00535-012-0640-x.

31. Garn H, Renz H. Epidemiological and immunological evidence for the hygiene hypothesis. Immunobiology. 2007;212:441–52. doi:10.1016/j.imbio.2007.03.006.

32. Jyonouchi S, Brown-Whitehorn TA, Spergel JM. Association of eosinophilic gastrointestinal disorders with other atopic disorders. Immunol Allergy Clin North Am. 2009;29:85–97. doi:10.1016/j.iac.2008.09.008.

33. Furuta GT, Forbes D, Boey C, Dupont C, Putnam P, Roy S, et al. Eosinophilic gastrointestinal diseases (EGIDs). J Pediatr Gastroenterol Nutr. 2008;47:234–8. doi:10.1097/MPG.0b013e318181b1c3.

34. Busoni V, Orsi M, Christiansen S, Davila MT, Lifschitz C. Is delivery by cesarean section a risk factor for persistence and severity in eosinophilic gastroenteropathy in pediatric patients? J Pediatr Gastroenterol Nutr. 2012;54:829. doi:10.1097/MPG.0b013e318250f1a2.

35. Gronlund MM, Lehtonen OP, Eerola E, Kero P. Fecal microflora in healthy infants born by different methods of delivery: permanent changes in intestinal flora after cesarean delivery. J Pediatr Gastroenterol Nutr. 1999;8:9–25.

36. Franciosi JP, Tam V, Liacouras CA, Spergel JM. A case-control study of sociodemographic and geographic characteristics of 335 children with eosinophilic esophagitis. Clin Gastroenterol Hepatol. 2009;7:415–9. doi:10.1016/j.cgh.2008.10.006.

37. Hurrell JM, Genta RM, Dellon ES. Prevalence of esophageal eosinophilia varies by climate zone in the United States. Am J Gastroenterol. 2012;107:698–706. doi:10.1038/ajg.2012.6.

38. Pacal RR, Gramlich TL, Parker KM, Gansler TS. Geographic variations in eosinophil concentration in normal colonic mucosa. Mod Pathol. 1997;10:363–5.

39. Polydorides AD, Banner BF, Hannaway PJ, Yantiss RK. Evaluation of site-specific and seasonal variation in colonic mucosal eosinophils. Hum Pathol. 2008;39:832–6. doi:10.1016/j.humpath.2007.10.012.

40. Wang FY, Gupta SK, Fitzgerald JF. Is there a seasonal variation in the incidence or intensity of allergic eosinophilic esophagitis in newly diagnosed children? J Clin Gastroenterol. 2007;41:451–3. doi:10.1097/01.mcg.0000248019.16139.67.

41. Almansa C, Krishna M, Buchner AM, Ghabril MS, Talley N, Devault KR, et al. Seasonal distribution in newly diagnosed cases of eosinophilic esophagitis in adults. Am J Gastroenterol. 2009;104:828–33. doi:10.1038/ajg.2008.169.

42. Moawad FJ, Veerappan GR, Lake JM, Maydonovitch CL, Haymore BR, Kosisky SE, et al. Correlation between eosinophilic oesophagitis and aeroallergens. Aliment Pharmacol Ther. 2010;31:509–15. doi: 10.1111/j.1365-2036.2009.04199.x.

43. Talley NJ, Shorter RG, Phillips SF, Zinsmeister AR. Eosinophilic gastroenteritis: a clinicopathological study of patients with disease of the mucosa, muscle layer, and subserosal tissues. Gut. 1990;31:54–8.

44. Chang JY, Choung RS, Lee RM, Locke GR, III, Schleck CD, Zinsmeister AR, et al. A shift in the clinical spectrum of eosinophilic gastroenteritis toward the mucosal disease type. Clin Gastroenterol Hepatol. 2010;8:669–75. doi:10.1016/j.cgh.2010.04.022.

45. Venkataraman S, Ramakrishna BS, Mathan M, Chacko A, Chandy G, Kurian G, et al. Eosinophilic gastroenteritis–an Indian experience. Indian J Gastroenterol. 1998;17:148–9.

46. Kim NI, Jo YJ, Song MH, Kim SH, Kim TH, Park YS, et al. Clinical features of eosinophilic gastroenteritis. Korean J Gastroenterol. 2004;44:217–23.

47. Jeon EJ, Lee KM, Jung DY, Kim TH, Ji JS, Kim HK, et al. Clinical characteristics of 17 cases of eosinophilic gastroenteritis. Korean J Gastroenterol. 2010;55:361–7.

48. Chen MJ, Chu CH, Lin SC, Shih SC, Wang TE. Eosinophilic gastroenteritis: clinical experience with 15 patients. World J Gastroenterol. 2003;9:2813–6.

49. Thakkar K, Chen L, Tessier ME, Gilger MA. Outcomes of children after esophagogastroduodenoscopy for chronic abdominal pain. Clin Gastroenterol Hepatol. 2014. doi:10.1016/j.cgh.2013.08.041.

50. Høst A. Frequency of cow's milk allergy in childhood. Ann Allergy Asthma Immunol. 2002; 89(6 Suppl 1):33–7.

51. Lozinsky AC, Morais MB. Eosinophilic colitis in infants. J Pediatr (Rio J). 2013. doi:10.1016/j.jped.2013.03.024.

52. Vieira MC, Morais MB, Spolidoro JV, Toporovski MS, Cardoso AL, Araujo GT, et al. A survey on clinical presentation and nutritional status of infants with suspected cow' milk allergy. BMC Pediatr. 2010;10:25. doi:10.1186/1471-2431-10-25.

53. Gonsalves N. Food allergies and eosinophilic gastrointestinal illness. Gastroenterol Clin North Am. 2007;36:75–91. doi:10.1016/j.gtc.2007.01.003.

54. Pratt CA, Demain JG, Rathkopf MM. Food allergy and eosinophilic gastrointestinal disorders: guiding our diagnosis and treatment. Curr Probl Pediatr Adolesc Health Care. 2008;38:170–88. doi:10.1016/j.cppeds.2008.03.002.

55. Khan S, Orenstein SR. Eosinophilic gastroenteritis. Gastroenterol Clin North Am. 2008;37:333–48. doi:10.1016/j.gtc.2008.02.003.

56. Straumann A, Bauer M, Fischer B, Blaser K, Simon HU. Idiopathic eosinophilic esophagitis is associated with a T(H)2-type allergic inflammatory response. J Allergy Clin Immunol. 2001;108:954–61. doi:10.1067/mai.2001.119917.

57. Daneshjoo R, Talley J. Eosinophilic gastroenteritis. Curr Gastroenterol Rep. 2002;4:366–72.

58. Blanchard C, Wang N, Stringer KF, Mishra A, Fulkerson PC, Abonia JP, et al. Eotaxin-3 and a uniquely conserved gene-expression profile in eosinophilic esophagitis. J Clin Invest. 2006;116:536–47. doi:10.1172/JCI26679.

59. Sherrill JD, Rothenberg ME. Genetic dissection of eosinophilic esophagitis provides insight into disease pathogenesis and treatment strategies. J Allergy Clin Immunol. 2011;128:23–32. doi:10.1016/j.jaci.2011.03.046.

60. Sherrill JD, Gao PS, Stucke EM, Blanchard C, Collins MH, Putnam PE, et al. Variants of thymic stromal lymphopoietin and its receptor associate with eosinophilic esophagitis. J Allergy Clin Immunol. 2010;126:160–5. doi:10.1016/j.jaci.2010.04.037.

61. Ziegler SF. The role of thymic stromal lymphopoietin (TSLP) in allergic disorders. Adv Pharmacol. 2013;66:129–55. doi:10.1016/B978-0-12-404717-4.00004-4.

62. Manuyakorn W, Howarth PH, Holgate ST. Airway remodelling in asthma and novel therapy. Asian Pac J Allergy Immunol. 2013;31:3–10.

63. Aceves SS, Newbury RO, Dohil R, Bastian JF, Broide DH. Esophageal remodeling in pediatric eosinophilic esophagitis. J Allergy Clin Immunol. 2007;119:206–12. doi:10.1016/j.jaci.2006.10.016.

64. Straumann A, Conus S, Degen L, Felder S, Kummer M, Engel H, et al. Budesonide is effective in adolescent and adult patients with active eosinophilic esophagitis. Gastroenterology. 2010;139:1526–37. doi:10.1053/j.gastro.2010.07.048.

65. Aceves SS, Newbury RO, Chen D, Mueller J, Dohil R, Hoffman H, et al. Resolution of remodeling in eosinophilic esophagitis correlates with epithelial response to topical corticosteroids. Allergy. 2010;65:109–16. doi:10.1111/j.1398-9995.2009.02142.x.

66. Dellon ES, Kim HP, Sperry SL, Rybnicek DA, Shaheen NJ. A phenotypic analysis shows that eosinophilic esophagitis is a progressive fibrostenotic disease. Gastrointest Endosc. 2014. doi:10.1016/j.gie.2013.10.027.

67. Schoepfer AM, Safroneeva E, Bussmann C, Kuchen T, Portmann S, Simon HU, et al. Delay in diagnosis of eosinophilic esophagitis increases risk for stricture formation in a time-dependent manner. Gastroenterology. 2013;145:1230–6. doi:10.1053/j.gastro.2013.08.015.

68. Lim KC, Tan HK, Rajnakova A, Venkatesh SK. Eosinophilic gastroenteritis presenting with duodenal obstruction and ascites. Ann Acad Med Singapore. 2011;40:379–81.

69. Yun MY, Cho YU, Park IS, Choi SK, Kim SJ, Shin SH, et al. Eosinophilic gastroenteritis presenting as small bowel obstruction: a case report and review of the literature. World J Gastroenterol. 2007;13:1758–60.

70. Chehade M, Sampson HA, Morotti RA, Magid MS. Esophageal subepithelial fibrosis in children with eosinophilic esophagitis. J Pediatr Gastroenterol Nutr. 2007;45:319–28. doi:10.1097/MPG.0b013e31806ab384.

71. Mulder DJ, Pacheco I, Hurlbut DJ, Mak N, Furuta GT, MacLeod RJ, et al. FGF9-induced proliferative response to eosinophilic inflammation in oesophagitis. Gut. 2009;58:166–73. doi:10.1136/gut.2008.157628.

72. Straumann A, Conus S, Degen L, Frei C, Bussmann C, Beglinger C, et al. Long-term budesonide maintenance treatment is partially effective for patients with eosinophilic esophagitis. Clin Gastroenterol Hepatol. 2011;9:400–9. doi:10.1016/j.cgh.2011.01.017.

73. Lieberman JA, Morotti RA, Konstantinou GN, Yershov O, Chehade M. Dietary therapy can reverse esophageal subepithelial fibrosis in patients with eosinophilic esophagitis: a historical cohort. Allergy. 2012;67:1299–307. doi:10.1111/j.1398–9995.2012.02881.x.

74. Torgerson TR, Linane A, Moes N, Anover S, Mateo V, Rieux-Laucat F, et al. Severe food allergy as a variant of IPEX syndrome caused by a deletion in a noncoding region of the FOXP3 gene. Gastroenterology. 2007;132:1705–17. doi:10.1053/j.gastro.2007.02.044.

75. d'Hennezel E, Dhuban K, Torgerson T, Piccirillo CA. The immunogenetics of immune dysregulation, polyendocrinopathy, enteropathy, X linked (IPEX) syndrome. J Med Genet. 2012;49:291–302. doi:10.1136/jmedgenet-2012–100759.

76. Desreumaux P, Nutten S, Colombel JF. Activated eosinophils in inflammatory bowel disease: do they matter? Am J Gastroenterol. 1999;94:189–95. doi:10.1111/j.1572–0241.1999.01657.x.

77. Nishitani H, Okabayashi M, Satomi M, Dohi Y. Infiltration of peroxidase-producing eosinophils into the lamina propria of patients with ulcerative colitis. J Gastroenterol. 1998;33:189–95. doi:10.1007/s005350050068.

78. Liacouras CA, Furuta GT, Hirano I, Atkins D, Attwood SE, Bonis PA, et al. Eosinophilic esophagitis: updated consensus recommendations for children and adults. J Allergy Clin Immunol. 2011;128:3–20. doi:10.1016/j.jaci.2011.02.040.

79. Pineton de Chambrun G, Gonzalez F, Canva JY, Gonzalez S, Houssin L, Desreumaux P, et al. Natural history of eosinophilic gastroenteritis. Clin Gastroenterol Hepatol. 2011;9:950–6. doi:10.1016/j.cgh.2011.07.017.

80. Tien FM, Wu JF, Jeng YM, Hsu HY, Ni YH, Chang MH, et al. Clinical features and treatment responses of children with eosinophilic gastroenteritis. Pediatr Neonatol. 2011;52:272–8. doi:10.1016/j.pedneo.2011.06.006.

81. Masterson JC, Furuta GT, Lee JJ. Update on clinical and immunological features of eosinophilic gastrointestinal diseases. Curr Opin Gastroenterol. 2011;27:515–22. doi:10.1097/MOG.0b013e32834b314c.

82. Khan S. Eosinophilic gastroenteritis. Best Pract Res Clin Gastroenterol. 2005;19:177–98. doi:10.1016/j.bpg.2005.01.009.

83. Dobbins JW, Sheahan DG, Behar J. Eosinophilic gastroenteritis with esophageal involvement. Gastroenterology. 1977;72:1312–6.

84. Lake AM. Allergic bowel disease. Adolesc Med Clin. 2004;15:105–17.

85. Lwin T, Melton SD, Genta RM. Eosinophilic gastritis: histopathological characterization and quantification of the normal gastric eosinophil content. Mod Pathol. 2013;24:556–3. doi:10.1038/modpathol.2010.221.

86. Iacono G, Cavataio F, Montalto G, Florena A, Tumminello M, Soresi M, et al. Intolerance of cow's milk and chronic constipation in children. N Engl J Med. 1998;339:1100–4. doi:10.1056/NEJM199810153391602.

87. Saad AG. Normal quantity and distribution of mast cells and eosinophilis in the pediatric colon. Pediatr Dev Pathol. 2011;14:294–300. doi:10.2350/10–07-0878-OA.1.

88. Okpara N, Aswad B, Baffy G. Eosinophilic colitis. World J Gastroenterol. 2009;15:2975–9.

89. Jimenez-Saenz M, Villar-Rodriguez JL, Torres Y, Carmona I, Salas-Herrero E, Gonzalez-Vilches J, et al. Biliary tract disease: a rare manifestation of eosinophilic gastroenteritis. Dig Dis Sci. 2003;48:624–7.

90. Maeshima A, Murakami H, Sadakata H, Saitoh T, Matsushima T, Tamura J, et al. Eosinophilic gastroenteritis presenting with acute pancreatitis. J Med. 1997;28:265–72.

91. Lyngbaek S, Adamsen S, Aru A, Bergenfeldt M. Recurrent acute pancreatitis due to eosinophilic gastroenteritis. Case report and literature review. JOP. 2006;7:211–7.

92. Genta RM, Lew GM, Graham DY. Changes in the gastric mucosa following eradication of Helicobacter pylori. Mod Pathol. 1993;6:281–9.

93. Furuta K, Adachi K, Aimi M, Ishimura N, Sato S, Ishihara S, et al. Case-control study of association of eosinophilic gastrointestinal disorders with Helicobacter pylori infection in Japan. J Clin Biochem Nutr. 2013;53:60–2. doi:10.3164/jcbn.13–15.

94. Navaneethan U, Venkatesh PG, Downs-Kelly E, Shen B. Isospora belli superinfection in a patient with eosinophilic gastroenteritis–a diagnostic challenge. J Crohns Colitis. 2012;6:236–9. doi:10.1016/j.crohns.2011.08.010.

95. Blanco-Guerra C, Cazana JL, Villas F, Bazire P, Martinez F. Ileal perforation due to eosinophilic gastroenteritis. Am J Gastroenterol. 1991;86:1689–90.

96. Siaw EK, Sayed K, Jackson RJ. Eosinophilic gastroenteritis presenting as acute gastric perforation. J Pediatr Gastroenterol Nutr. 2006;43:691–4. doi:10.1097/01.mpg.0000239996.66011.89.

97. Huang FC, Ko SF, Huang SC, Lee SY. Eosinophilic gastroenteritis with perforation mimicking intussusception. J Pediatr Gastroenterol Nutr. 2001;33:613–5.

98. Yu MC, Tsai CL, Yang YJ, Yang SS, Wang LH, Lee CT, et al. Allergic colitis in infants related to cow's milk: clinical characteristics, pathologic changes, and immunologic findings. Pediatr Neonatol. 2013;54:49–55. doi:10.1016/j.pedneo.2012.11.006.

99. Klein NC, Hargrove RL, Sleisenger MH, Jeffries GH. Eosinophilic gastroenteritis. Medicine (Baltimore). 1970;49:299–319.

100. Blanco Cabañero AG, Maranés Antoñanzas I, Solís García Del Pozo J, Hernández A. Patient with intestinal obstruction and eosinophilic enteritis. Enferm Infecc Microbiol Clin. 2011;29:392–3. doi: 10.1016/j.eimc.2010.11.004.

101. Khan F, Chaudhry MA, Nusrat S, Qureshi N, Ali T. Constipation–another manifestation of eosinophilic gastroenteritis. J Okla State Med Assoc. 2012;105:134.

102. Setia N, Ghobrial P, Liron P. Eosinophilic ascites due to severe eosinophilic ileitis. Cytojournal. 2010;7:19. doi: 10.4103/1742–6413.70408.

103. Hepburn IS, Sridhar S, Schade RR. Eosinophilic ascites, an unusual presentation of eosinophilic gastroenteritis: a case report and review. World J Gastrointest Pathophysiol. 2010;1:166–70. doi:10.4291/wjgp.v1.i5.166.

104. Issa H, Bseiso B, Al-Salem AH. Eosinophilic enteritis presenting as a perforated duodenal ulcer. Endoscopy. 2011;43(Suppl 2) UCTN:E358–9. doi: 10.1055/s-0030–1256526.

105. Siahanidou T, Mandyla H, Dimitriadis D, Van-Vliet C, Anagnostakis D. Eosinophilic gastroenteritis complicated with perforation and intussusception in a neonate. J Pediatr Gastroenterol Nutr. 2001;32:335–7.

106. Steele RJ, Mok SD, Crofts TJ, Li AK. Two cases of eosinophilic enteritis presenting as large bowel perforation and small bowel haemorrhage. Aust N Z J Surg. 1987;57:335–6.

107. Suzuki S, Homma T, Kurokawa M, Matsukura S, Adachi M, Wakabayashi K, et al. Eosinophilic gastroenteritis due to cow's milk allergy presenting with acute pancreatitis. Int Arch Allergy Immunol. 2012;158(Suppl 1):75–82. doi:10.1159/000337782.

108. Stevens T, Mackey R, Falk GW, Bennett A, Henderson JM. Eosinophilic pancreatitis presenting as a pancreatic mass with obstructive jaundice. Gastrointest Endosc. 2006;63:525–7. doi:10.1016/j.gie.2005.10.005.

109. Cakir OO, Biyik M, Gungor G, Ataseven H, Demir A, Tavli L. A duodenal mass and acute pancreatitis. Turk J Gastroenterol. 2013;24:299–301.

110. Lang R, Jutrin I, Ravid M. Recurrent post-partum gastroenteritis with eosinophilia. Hepatogastroenterol. 1981;28:118–9.

111. Park SJ, Kenny PR, Palekar NA. Labor-associated eosinophilic gastroenteritis. Mil Med. 2012;177:99–100.

112. Ogasa M, Nakamura Y, Sanay H, Ueda K. A case of pregnancy associated hypereosinophilia with hyperpermeability symptoms. Gynecol Obstet Invest. 2006;62:14–6. doi:10.1159/000091753.

113. Zhang L, Duan L, Ding S, Lu J, Jin Z, Cui R, et al. Eosinophilic gastroenteritis: clinical manifestations and morphological characteristics, a retrospective study of 42 patients. Scand J Gastroenterol. 2011;46:1074–80. doi:10.3109/00365521.2011.579998.

114. Attar A, Cazals-Hatem D, Ponsot P. Videocapsule endoscopy identifies stenoses missed by other imaging techniques in a patient with eosinophilic gastroenteritis. Clin Gastroenterol Hepatol. 2011;9:A28. doi:10.1016/j.cgh.2010.07.021.

115. Pasha SF, Leighton JA, Williams JW, De PG, Harold K, Shiff AA. Capsule retention in a patient with eosinophilic gastroenteritis mimicking diaphragm disease of the small bowel. Endoscopy. 2009;41(Suppl 2):E290–1. doi:10.1055/s-0029–1215125.

116. Koumi A, Panos MZ. A new capsule endoscopy feature of serosal eosinophilic enteritis. Endoscopy. 2009;41(Suppl 2):E280. doi:10.1055/s-0029–1215020.

117. Dalinka MK, Masters CJ. Eosinophilic enteritis. Report of a case without gastric involvement. Radiology. 1970;96:543–4.

118. Alfadda AA, Storr MA, Shaffer EA. Eosinophilic colitis: epidemiology, clinical features, and current management. Therap Adv Gastroenterol. 2011;4:301–9. doi:10.1177/1756283X10392443.

119. Alfadda AA, Shaffer EA, Urbanski SJ, Storr MA. Eosinophilic colitis is a sporadic self limited disease of middle aged people: a population-based study. Colorectal Dis. 2013. doi:10.1111/codi.12464.

120. Otowa Y, Mitsutsuji M, Urade T, Chono T, Morimoto H, Yokoyama K, et al. Eosinophilic gastroenteritis associated with multiple gastric cancer. Eur J Gastroenterol Hepatol. 2012;24:727–30. doi:10.1097/MEG.0b013e32835272ea.

121. Sampson HA. Food allergy. Part 1: immunopathogenesis and clinical disorders. J Allergy Clin Immunol. 1999;103:717–28.

122. Lucendo AJ, Serrano-Montalbán B, Arias Á, Redondo O, Tenias JM. Systematic review: the efficacy of dietary treatment for inducing disease remission in eosinophilic gastroenteritis. J Pediatr Gastroenterol Nutr. 2015. doi:10.1097/MPG.0000000000000766.

123. Yamada Y, Kato M, Isoda Y, et al. Eosinophilic gastroenteritis treated with a multiple-food elimination diet. Allergol Intl. 2014;63(Suppl 1):53–6.

124. Sabban JC, Orsi M, Busoni V, Christensen S. Early onset of eosinophilic enteropathy in children. J Pediatr Gastroenterol Nutr. 2009;49:E23–4.

125. Busoni VB, Lifschitz C, Christiansen S, Davila MT Gd, Orsi M. Eosinophilic gastroenteropathy: a pediatric series. Arch Argent Pediatr. 2011;109:68–73. doi:10.1590/S0325–00752011000100019.

126. Lombardi C, Salmi A, Passalacqua G. An adult case of eosinophilic pyloric stenosis maintained on remission with oral budesonide. Eur Ann Allergy Clin Immunol. 2011;43:29–30.

127. Ko HBM, Chehade M, Morotti RA. Eosinophilic gastritis in children: a clinicopathological study. Lab Invest. 2012;92:156A.

128. Stringel G, Mercer S, Sharpe D, et al. Eosinophilic gastroenteritis. Can J Surg. 1984;27(2):182–3.

129. Guerrero M, Morales MC, Pelaez A, Villamanzo IG, Campos A, Basomba A. Eosinophilic gastroenteritis. Three cases involving each of the anatomo-clinical variants. Allergol Immunopathol (Madr). 1988;16(3):187–92.

130. Chehade M, Magid MS, Mofidi S, et al. Allergic eosinophilic gastroenteritis with protein-losing enteropathy: intestinal pathology, clinical course, and long-term follow-up. J Pediatr Gastroenterol Nutr. 2006;42(3):516–21.

131. Passoforte P, Frappampina R, De Venuto C, et al. An important and unusual cause of hypoalbuminaemia. Dig Liver Dis. 2013;45:S174.

132. Ishimura N, Furuta K, Sato S, Ishihara S, Kinoshita Y. Limited role of allergy testing in patients with eosinophilic gastrointestinal disorders. J Gastroenterol Hepatol. 2013;28:1306–13. doi:10.1111/jgh.12197.

133. Alfadda AA, Storr MA, Shaffer EA. Eosinophilic colitis: an update on pathophysiology and treatment. Br Med Bull. 2011;100:59–72. doi:10.1093/bmb/ldr045.

134. Netzer P, Gschossmann JM, Straumann A, Sendensky A, Weimann R, Schoepfer AM. Corticosteroid-dependent eosinophilic oesophagitis: azathioprine and 6-mercaptopurine can induce and maintain long-term remission. Eur J Gastroenterol Hepatol. 2007;19:865–9. doi:10.1097/MEG.0b013e32825a6ab4.

135. Perez-Millan A, Martin-Lorente JL, Lopez-Morante A, Yuguero L, Saez-Royuela F. Subserosal eosinophilic gastroenteritis treated efficaciously with sodium cromoglycate. Dig Dis Sci. 1997;42:342–4.

136. Redondo-Cerezo E, Cabello MJ, Gonzalez Y, Gomez M, Garcia-Montero M, de TJ. Eosinophilic gastroenteritis: our recent experience: one-year experience of atypical onset of an uncommon disease. Scand J Gastroenterol. 2001;36:1358–60.

137. Moots RJ, Prouse P, Gumpel JM. Near fatal eosinophilic gastroenteritis responding to oral sodium chromoglycate. Gut. 1988;29:1282–5.

138. Liacouras CA, Spergel JM, Ruchelli E, Verma R, Mascarenhas M, Semeao E, et al. Eosinophilic esophagitis: a 10-year experience in 381 children. Clin Gastroenterol Hepatol. 2005;3:1198–206.

139. Melamed I, Feanny SJ, Sherman PM, Roifman CM. Benefit of ketotifen in patients with eosinophilic gastroenteritis. Am J Med. 1991;90:310–4.

140. Suzuki J, Kawasaki Y, Nozawa R, Isome M, Suzuki S, Takahashi A, et al. Oral disodium cromoglycate and ketotifen for a patient with eosinophilic gastroenteritis, food allergy and protein-losing enteropathy. Asian Pac J Allergy Immunol. 2003;21:193–7.

141. Shirai T, Hashimoto D, Suzuki K, Osawa S, Aonahata M, Chida K, et al. Successful treatment of eosinophilic gastroenteritis with suplatast tosilate. J Allergy Clin Immunol. 2001;107:924–5.

142. Lu E, Ballas ZK. Immunomodulation in the treatment of eosinophilic gastroenteritis. J Allergy Clin Immunol. 2003;111:S262.

143. Friesen CA, Kearns GL, Andre L. Clinical efficacy and pharmacokinetics of montelukast in dyspeptic children with duodenal eosinophilia. J Pediatr Gastroenterol Nutr. 2004;38:343–51.

144. Kumar A, Teuber SS, Naguwa S, Prindiville T, Gershwin ME. Eosinophilic gastroenteritis and citrus-induced urticaria. Clin Rev Allergy Immunol. 2006;30:61–70. doi:10.1385/CRIAI:30:1:061.

145. De MN, Kochuyt AM, Van MW, Hiele M. Montelukast as a treatment modality for eosinophilic gastroenteritis. Acta Gastroenterol Belg. 2011;74:570–5.

146. Prussin C, James SP, Huber MM, et al. Pilot study of anti-IL-5 in eosinophilic gastroenteritis. J Allergy Clin Immunol. 2003;111:827.

147. Kim YJ, Prussin C, Martin B, Law MA, Haverty TP, Nutman TB, et al. Rebound eosinophilia after treatment of hypereosinophilic syndrome and eosinophilic gastroenteritis with monoclonal anti-IL-5 antibody SCH55700. J Allergy Clin Immunol. 2004;114:1449–55. doi:10.1016/j.jaci.2004.08.027.

148. Ciccia F, Giardina AR, Alessi N, Rodolico V, Galia M, Ferrante A, et al. Successful intravenous immunoglobulin treatment for steroid-resistant eosinophilic enteritis in a patient with systemic lupus erythematosus. Clin Exp Rheumatol. 2011;29:1018–20.

149. Redondo CE, Moreno Platero JJ, Garcia DE, Gonzalez AY, Cabello Tapia MJ, et al. Gastroenteritis eosinophilic presenting as colitis with acute abdomen. Gastroenterol Hepatol. 2000;23:477–9.

150. Dunne B, Brophy S, Tsang J, McSorley K, Cumiskey J, Kay E, et al. Eosinophilic gastroenteritis. Gut. 2010;59:417. doi:10.1136/gut.2009.197061.

Crohn's Disease

28

Salvatore Cucchiara and Marina Aloi

Introduction

Crohn's disease (CD) is a chronic, relapsing disorder of the gastrointestinal tract, belonging to the inflammatory bowel diseases (IBD). Approximately, 25% of CD first present in childhood and adolescence, with recent studies suggesting that the prevalence is rising in both developed and developing countries [1, 2]. The precise cause of IBD is still unsettled, but there is evidence that they develop as a consequence of an abnormal immune response to the intestinal microbiota in a genetically susceptible host (Fig. 28.1) [3]. Although the pediatric and adult-onset IBD seem to share many clinical aspects and pathogenetic pathways, some features are peculiar to the pediatric form, such as the potential for linear growth impairment and pubertal delay as complication of undertreated inflammation and malnutrition; the influence of nutritional treatment on the course; and the different phenotype expression of the disease [4]. Finally, evidences from animal models of IBD and preliminary observations in children support the concept that IBD develop in distinct phases and that key mediators of inflammation play different roles, depending on the stage of the disease [3, 5]. These observations highlight the importance of taking into consideration the time course of disease when studying pediatric IBD and targeting appropriate treatments.

28

Epidemiology

Although IBD can occur at any age, up to 25% of patients develop symptoms during childhood and adolescence [1, 2]. Some epidemiological studies from USA and Europe have shown a steady inrise in the overall mean annual incidence of pediatric IBD around the world, that seems to be primarily due to an increase in the incidence of CD [1, 2, 6]. CD is unequally distributed all over the world, with highest rates occurring in Western and Northern countries, and with a decreasing gradient from North to South and from West to East [7–11]. The worldwide highest prevalence of pediatric IBD is reported from the Canadian Ontario region, with approximately 56 IBD patients for 100,000 inhabitants [8]. Epidemiological observations from this area, using health administrative data, have indicated an increasing incidence of pediatric CD from 9.5 in 1994 to 11.4 in 2005 per 100,000, with unchanged incidence rates for pediatric ulcerative colitis (UC; 4.1–4.2) [9]. In Europe, a recent study based on the registry of chronic inflammatory intestine diseases in North-West pf France (EPIMAD) indicated a mean annual incidence rate of 2.6 for pediatric CD [11]. The largest population-based study of incidence of pediatric IBD in the USA was reported from Wisconsin, estimating an yearly incidence of IBD of 7.05 per 100,000, the incidence of CD being 4.56, that is, more than twice the rate of UC (2.14) and a prevalence of 48–71 per 100,000 [12]. A recent study estimating the prevalence of IBD in the USA using a large, multistate sample, reported a prevalence of CD in children of 43/100,000 [13]. Factors contributing to the evident increase in the global incidence could be a greater case ascertainment, the widening case definition, earlier onset in predisposed individuals, and greater access to health care; however, there is a wide agreement that the rising incidence of pediatric IBD is due to a real increase in the number of affected children [14]. It has been postulated that the "Westernization" of different societies accounts for the progressive rise in the incidence of the disease also in previously low-incidence areas,

Fig. 28.1 Pathogenetic mechanisms of inflammatory bowel diseases

MECHANISMS UNDERLYING INFLAMMATORY BOWEL DISEASE

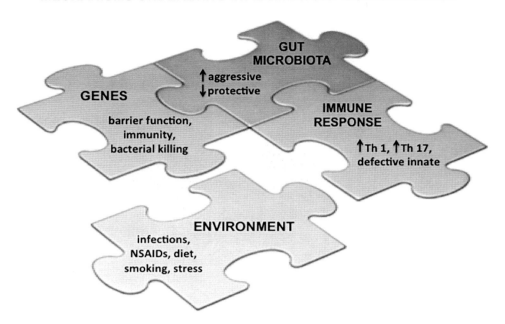

including Japan [15], other Asian countries [16], and some Eastern European countries [17].

Pediatric IBD present specific phenotypic and demographic differences when compared with adult-onset disease. While CD and UC occur with equal distribution in adults [18], it has been reported that in childhood CD is more frequently diagnosed than UC [19, 20]; moreover, while in adults there is an equal male to female ratio (or a mild female predominance), all pediatric IBD cohort studies or registries indicate a male predominance [20]. In pediatric CD, most patients have an extensive disease, ileocolonic or colonic, and distinction of UC from colonic CD may be not uncommonly challenging [21]. As recently confirmed by EPIMAD registry, children with CD are more likely to have upper gastrointestinal involvement than their adult peers [11]. Moreover, disease severity seems to differentiate pediatric-onset CD: children often present an inflammatory or nonstricturing, nonpenetrating disease, while complicated disease is fairly unusual at presentation. However, even with treatment, many data demonstrate that inflammatory CD progresses to stricturing and penetrating disease in several children [11, 20]. Adult disease begins more often with stricturing or penetrating disease, with a lower trend of disease progression than pediatric-onset disease.

Etiopathogenesis

The most accepted hypothesis for the pathogenesis of CD is that the interaction between luminal contents (i.e., the intestinal microbiota) and the mucosa leads to a dysregulated inflammation in a genetically predisposed host. Several mi-

croorganisms have been considered as potential causative agents for CD, including *Mycobacterium paratuberculosis, Listeria monocytogenes,* novel Burkholderiales, *Escherichia coli* [22, 23]. Recently, strains of adherent-invasive *E. coli* (AIEC), capable of adhering to and invading epithelium, and to replicate in macrophages, have been described in adults and children with CD [24, 25]. Nevertheless, there are no strong data to support a role for any of these microorganisms as the causative factor in the etiology of IBD. Some of the most interesting findings in the pathogenesis of IBD come from genetics. The importance of genetics in CD was strongly suggested by family, twin, and phenotype concordance studies. Monozygotic twins exhibit phenotypic concordance in 50–70 % of CD patients, and their relative risk of developing CD is 800-fold greater compared to the general population [26]. Recently, the discovery of several susceptibility genes has further supported the importance of genetic predisposition in CD [27]. After the pivotal study of Hugot et al. in 2001, who discovered the association of variants of the *NOD2* gene with ileal CD [28], and the discovery of the correlation between variants of interleukin (*IL)23* receptor gene and both CD and UC in 2006 [29], the number of IBD genetic associations discovered has dramatically increased. More susceptibility loci have been quickly identified, such as autophagy genes, *ATG16L1* and *IRGM* [30]. In the past decade, the implementation of genome-wide association studies (GWAS) has significantly advanced our knowledge on the importance of genetic susceptibility in IBD [31, 32]. To date, the GWAS performed have identified more than 70 risk-conferring loci for CD [31]. GWAS have revealed a substantial overlap in genetic risk loci between CD and UC. However, some genes are quite different for CD or UC, clearly denoting the genetic heterogeneity of the two forms of IBD, each one of them showing distinctive and shared genetic associations. For instance, *NOD2*, autophagy genes, and *ITLN1* are unique for CD [31]. Despite the discovery of a massive number of susceptibility genes for IBD, we are still far from understanding the mechanism by which such genetic variants cause the intestinal inflammation. The challenge for basic IBD researchers is now to identify how genetic abnormalities influence pro-inflammatory pathways, providing information that could directly improve the clinical management. A number of pro-inflammatory pathways have been elucidated, in some cases enabling the development of specific interventions. For instance, *NOD2* gene-defected patients have an impaired ability to recognize and process bacterial products, and this may lead to an inappropriately innate immune response. Some CD patients with variants of the autophagy genes (*ATG16L1* and *IRGM*) have a defective capacity to process cell degradation products, as well as bacteria, and therefore an insufficient ability to eliminate pro-inflammatory factors [33]. One of the most important discoveries in the field of genetics of pediatric IBD is the recent identification of impaired IL10 signaling in some forms of very-early-onset (within the first months of life) CD [34]. The common characteristics of these patients are a very early onset of an aggressive CD colitis, treatment-resistant, with perianal involvement. This form of CD is due to homozygous mutations in either IL10RA or IL10RB, which encode subunits of the IL10 receptor, or for IL10 itself [35]. One could speculate that this form of IBD with a monogenetic inheritance could identify a subset of patients with a "more" Mendelian transmission, opening new horizons of research and also expectations to understand the definite mechanisms underlying these diseases.

Clinical Presentations

CD is characterized by a transmural inflammation that can occur anywhere in the gastrointestinal tract, from mouth to anus. While the terminal ileum is the most common site of CD, about 60% of children have an extensive ileocolonic involvement and 20–30% an isolated colonic disease [18]. CD typically presents in any age group with a constellation of abdominal pain, diarrhea, weight loss, and poor appetite; however, short stature and predominant perianal disease are further significant presenting features in pediatric CD. Impairment of linear growth and associated delay in sexual development can occur before the onset of intestinal symptoms and can dominate the clinical presentation [36]. Growth failure is a unique characteristic of pediatric-onset CD: It is defined as linear growth at or <2 standard deviations (SD) below the mean for age, or decreased growth velocity, and can occur in 15–20% of children with CD [37]. The onset of growth failure is usually insidious, and any child or adolescent with impairment of the linear growth should have an appropriate initial diagnostic evaluation for IBD [18]. The presence of growth and pubertal delay is a key factor in the management of pediatric IBD. Maintaining adequate nutrition, minimizing inflammation, and maximizing corticosteroid-free treatment remain a crucial part of managing the potential growth stunting effects of active IBD, most specifically of small bowel CD. During the clinical course of CD, growth failure has been reported in up to 40% of children with CD and a final height below the fifth percentile is reported in 7–30% of patients with pediatric-onset CD [38, 39]. Growth failure in CD originates from different factors, such as malnutrition with decreased intake, increased gastrointestinal losses, malabsorption, and medication effects. All these components can certainly impact an individual's nutritional state. In addition, it is now widely agreed that inflammation process per se may directly inhibit linear growth and play a major role in the etiology of growth retardation [40]. Inflammatory mediators such as IL-6 and TNF-α are crucial factors in reducing plasmatic levels of insulin-like growth factor 1 (IGF-1), the peripheral mediator of the growth hormone [41]. In fact, impressive catch-up growth can be observed as soon as remission of intestinal inflammation is achieved. It is essential that height, weight, pubertal staging, and bone age are accurately and regularly measured and recorded in young patients with CD. Nutritional supplementation and need for "catch-up" growth should be an important part of the evaluation of a pediatric CD patient. Delay of pubertal onset is also common in active pediatric CD, and also the duration of puberty can be impaired. Active or relapsing disease during the years following the onset of puberty may slow or even arrest the progression of puberty. Moreover, pubertal delay affects estrogen and androgen levels, which are important for normal bone mineralization, contributing to the development of osteoporosis and osteopenia [42]. Inducing and maintaining disease remission before and during the pubertal years is thus crucial in order to ensure the attainment of final predicted height, avoiding a missed pubertal growth spurt.

Diagnosis

There is no gold standard single test allowing a definite diagnosis of CD. It is the combination of family and personal history, physical examination, and subsequent laboratory, imaging, and endoscopic assessment that leads to the correct diagnosis. Nevertheless, a subset of 10–15% of children with IBD confined to the colon receive an initial diagnosis of inflammatory bowel disease unclassified (IBD-U), and they will be subcategorized only during follow-up [18]. The first diagnostic issue is whether the presenting symptoms are related to CD. In the presence of classic clinical presentation, differentiating CD from other diseases with initial similar symptoms may be relatively simple [43]. However, in a child with bloody diarrhea and infectious etiologies, like *Salmonella, Yersinia, Shigella, E. coli,* etc., must be excluded. It is also important to evaluate and rule out vasculitides (such as Henoch–Schönlein purpura, and hemolytic–uremic syndrome) or allergic colitis. An abdominal pain mimicking CD may be determined by other conditions, such as intestinal lymphoma, ovarian cyst, appendicitis, or intussusception. Figure 28.2 shows the suggested diagnostic workup of children or adolescents with suspected IBD.

Noninvasive Tests

Serologic Tests Serologic tests are the first diagnostic tool for suspected CD. They include complete blood count, acute-phase reactants (i.e., C-reactive protein—CRP, erythrocyte sedimentation rate, ferritin, platelet count), and a wide panel of antibodies directed against microbial and self-antigens. CRP levels have been shown to well correlate with clinical, endoscopic, and histologic disease activity, and their stable rise is associated with a higher relapse rate and a bet-

ter response to biologics [44]. Several antibodies to microbial antigens have been identified in patients with IBD [45]. The most extensively studied and commonly used are anti-*Saccharomyces cerevisiae* antibodies (ASCA) and perinuclear antineutrophil cytoplasmic autoantibodies (pANCA). ASCAs have been suggested as a marker for CD with a prevalence of 50–60%, compared with 10–15% in UC and 0–5% in healthy controls [46, 47]. Conversely, pANCAs have been proposed as a marker for UC or colonic CD [45]. However, between 30 and 50% of the IBD patients do not screen positively for either of these markers, so their absence cannot be used to rule out the disease.

The attention of researchers has been recently focused on the possible relationship between serologic markers and distinct subgroups of patients and prognosis of the disease [48]. In CD, positive ASCA titers have been correlated to younger age at onset, ileal disease, aggressive behavior, and increased risk of early surgery [48]. Because of these promising data, other markers useful for prognostic purposes have been identified. Reactivity to *Pseudomonas fluorescens*–related protein [49] was independently related to stenosing disease and need for surgery, whereas anti-*E. coli* outer membrane porin C (OmpC) has been associated with penetrating disease [49, 50]. Both the

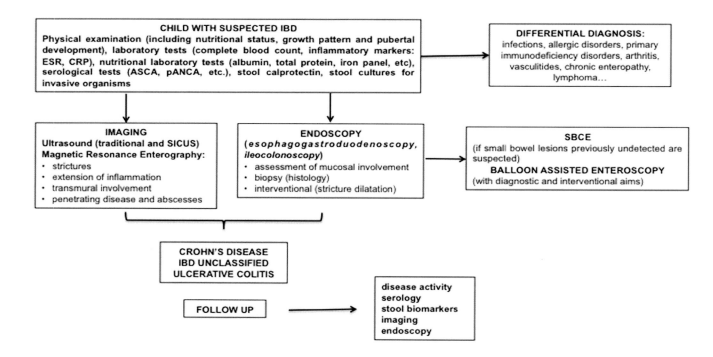

DIAGNOSTIC ALGORITHM FOR SUSPECTED PEDIATRIC IBD

ESR, erythrocyte sedimentation rate; CRP, C-reactive protein; ASCA, anti-Saccharomyces cerevisiae antibodies; pANCA, perinuclear antineutrophil cytoplasmic autoantibodies; MRE, magnetic resonance enterography; SICUS, small-intestine contrast ultrasonography; SBCE, small-bowel capsule endoscopy.

Fig. 28.2 Proposed diagnostic algorithm for pediatric inflammatory bowel diseases

presence and magnitude of the immune response were correlated with more aggressive disease behaviors. Recently, a large, multicenter, pediatric study examined the association of ASCA, anti-I2, anti-OmpC, pANCA, and anti-CBir1 reactivity, with disease behavior. The likelihood of developing disease complications increased in parallel with the reactivity to a greater number of antigens. The odds ratio for the development of penetrating disease was 5.2 and 9.5 for patients with reactivity to 2 and 3 antigens, respectively. Moreover, survival analysis showed that the need for surgery was earlier in patients with a reactivity to at least one microbial antigen as compared to those negative for all markers, suggesting that these markers may predict a more aggressive disease course [51].

Fecal Markers of Inflammation The neutrophil-derived marker calprotectin is a noninvasive tool for the diagnosis and monitoring of activity of IBD. Calprotectin is a calcium-binding protein that is excreted in the feces and can be readily measured using an enzyme-linked immunosorbent assay (ELISA). The protein is stable in stool specimens for up to a week at room temperature, allowing patients to collect a specimen at home without special precautions. While calprotectin is commonly used in the initial diagnostic approach to suspected IBD, one of the most advantageous uses is its ability to confirm tissue healing and predict disease relapses. A few studies have evaluated this outcome, demonstrating a sensitivity of 89–90% and specificity of 82–83% for predicting disease relapse during a 12-month period, with a sensitivity and specificity to predict absence of mucosal healing of 70–100% and 44–100%, respectively, depending on the calprotectin concentration threshold used [44]. Other fecal biomarkers, such as lactoferrin, neutrophil-derived S100A12, and high-motility group box 1 (HMGB1), show promise as potential biomarkers for CD, but have been studied far less extensively [50–52].

Imaging Most patients with CD have involvement of the small bowel, a region challenging to evaluate. Furthermore, children with CD need frequent evaluations during the course of their disease, so noninvasive imaging test, radiation-free, could be a valuable alternative to endoscopy for the definition of activity and complications of the disease. In the past, small bowel follow through (SBFT) was the "gold standard" for small bowel disease. In the past decade, due to considerable advances in technologies, other modalities, such as magnetic resonance (MR), ultrasound (US), and computed tomography (CT) have been favorably utilized [53]. CT has the major disadvantage of the large radiation exposure, driving interest in alternative imaging techniques to avoid this risk. MR with the administration of oral contrast (MRE) results in luminal distension, facilitating evaluation of bowel wall thickness and regularity; MR enteroclysis (with contrast administered through a nasojejunal tube) seems to have

the same sensitivity (88%) of MRE but a superior patient discomfort [53]. In comparison with endoscopy, MRE has a sensitivity of 84–96% and a specificity of 92–100% for the diagnosis of IBD [54]. MRE can also allow a detailed assessment of perianal fistulae, and it should be preferred as imaging tool for perianal disease [55, 56]. The recent European Crohn's colitis organization (ECCO) and European Society for Pediatric Gastroenterology, Hepatology and Nutrition (ESPGHAN) guidelines on the management of adult and pediatric CD, respectively, recommend MRE as the imaging tool of choice for the diagnosis and follow-up of CD [57, 43]. Abdominal US is a widely used technique in the evaluation of patients with CD because of its excellent safety profile, low cost, and recent advances in the equipment (Doppler and use of oral contrast) that allow high-resolution images [58]. Recently, a small intestine contrast ultrasonography (SICUS), performed after ingestion of an oral contrast material filling the small bowel lumen with anechoic fluid, has been developed for the study of the small bowel [59]. SICUS provides the opportunity to visualize and assess the entire small bowel by measuring intestinal wall thickness and lumen diameter at different levels [59, 60]. This technique is able to detect intestinal lesions in patients with suspected small bowel diseases with a higher sensitivity (72–100%) and specificity (97–100%), compared with SBFT [60].

Endoscopy

Ileocolonoscopy and Esophagogastroduodenoscopy) Traditional endoscopy has a pivotal role in the diagnosis of suspected CD. According to the recent ESPGHAN guidelines on the diagnosis of IBD [43], ileocolonoscopy and EGD should be recommended as the initial workup for all children with suspected disease. Multiple biopsies should be obtained from all sections of the examined gastrointestinal tract, even in the absence of macroscopic lesions [43]. Beyond its diagnostic utility, traditional endoscopy is crucial for staging the severity of disease, for the evaluation and treatment of strictures, detection of postoperative recurrence, surveillance for neoplasms, and preoperative assessment. Moreover, endoscopy allows monitoring of response to therapies by evaluating mucosal healing. In the past decade, endoscopic healing has become the most rigorous end point in adult therapeutic trial, and it is being used in pediatric trials too [61, 62]. Tables 28.1 and 28.2 show the typical endoscopic and histologic findings differentiating CD and UC. Peculiarities of endoscopy and histology in pediatric IBD have been defined in an exhaustive fashion in the recently published Porto Criteria of the ESPGHAN [43].

Small Bowel Capsule Endoscopy Small bowel capsule endoscopy (SBCE) allows the evaluation of CD small bowel

Table 28.1 Endoscopic differentiation between typical CD and UC

CD	UC
Throughout the entire GI tract	Confined to colon
Discontinuous lesions	Usually continuous lesions
Rectal sparing or segmental inflammation	Rectal involvement (in children may be absent)
Aphthous ulcers (may occur in normal mucosa)	Mucosal granularity/friability
Linear ulcers common	Erosions/microulcers
Cobblestoning	Loss of vascular pattern
Ileocecal valve stenotic and ulcerated	Ileocecal valve patulous and free from ulcerations (possible backwash ileitis)

GI gastrointestinal

Table 28.2 Histologic findings in CD and UC

CD	UC
Focal crypt distortion	Mucosal surface alteration
Ulcers and/or aphthoid ulcers	Crypt distortion, atrophy
Mucin depletion absent or weak	Mucin depletion
Pseudopyloric metaplasia	Cryptitis and/or crypt abscesses
Focal cryptitis	
Focal lymphoplasmacellular infiltration in the lamina propria	Diffuse lymphoplasmacellular infiltration in the lamina propria
Granulation tissue-like inflammation	Basal plasma cell infiltration
Epithelioid granulomas	

lesions, with no radiation. It is very sensitive for determining mucosal lesions, but it cannot detect extraluminal processes and it does not allow the biopsy of detected findings. In comparison to traditional endoscopy, SBCE can evaluate the entire small bowel, has an easier preparation, and is better tolerated from children. Regardless of its many advantages, SBCE also has some weaknesses: biopsy or intervention is not possible, and there is no way to guide the capsule, so significant lesions may be missed because of a bad orientation of the camera, obscured visualization due to luminal bubbles or debris, or delayed intestinal transit resulting in an inaccurate exam. SBCE is contraindicated in patients with strictures because of the risk of capsule retention. Furthermore, there are no established diagnostic criteria for CD: although most studies have defined the presence of more than three ulcerations in the absence of nonsteroidal anti-inflammatory drug ingestion as a diagnostic criterion, this has not been prospectively validated [63]. Given the concerns about the specificity of SBCE in the diagnosis of IBD, but recognizing its good sensitivity, some experts have suggested that it may be useful mainly for monitoring established CD rather than for initial approach [64].

Balloon Enteroscopy Double-balloon enteroscopy (DPE) was first introduced in 2001 as a device offering the possibility of complete diagnostic and therapeutic access to the entire small bowel with an endoscope [65]. A single-balloon device has also been developed with a similar intention. The enteroscope can be inserted via the oral or anal route and, using the combination of these approaches, complete examination of the entire small bowel can be achieved in many

patients [66]. Several studies support the utility of DBE in established adult and pediatric CD with the potential to affect management in select populations of patients (small bowel disease) [67]. The main limitations of balloon-assisted enteroscopy (BAE) are its invasive nature with the risk of bleeding and perforation (complication rate for diagnostic procedures is around 0.8% but can be as much as 4% for therapeutic interventions), prolonged duration, limited evaluation of the entire small bowel in a one-step approach, and requirement for specialized personnel [53].

Therapy

The current goals of treatment of pediatric CD are to induce and maintain a prolonged remission, minimizing drug toxicity. At long term, they should include preventing relapses, optimizing growth and pubertal development, and improving quality of life. Modern expectations of CD therapy call also upon the concept of mucosal healing, and, eventually, of deep remission (i.e., clinical remission, biomarker remission, and mucosal healing) [68]. The introduction of these outcomes may be the best way to alter the natural course of these diseases by preventing disability and bowel damage [69]. This may be of clinical relevance in children with CD, given the long-term consequences of early-onset aggressive disease presentation. Pediatric CD therapy employs many of the same treatment regimens as their adult counterparts. There are only a few well-designed clinical trials performed in children, therefore much of the evidence given is based on adult data. Conventional therapy is based on the escalation of drugs, from those with a better safety profile but a lower efficacy (antibiotics, mesalazine, sulfasalazine) to those with improved efficacy but a greater risk of side effects (steroids, immunomodulators, biologicals, surgery). This "step-up" approach is applied in most cases of pediatric IBD (Fig. 28.3). The advantages of "step-up" management are mainly to reserve more toxic drugs for those patients with a demonstrable "need" for more intensive therapy [70]. However, potential disadvantages include the observation that conventional therapies have not altered the disease course towards disease complications (strictures and fistulae) or the need for surgical procedures. Hence, pediatric gastroenterologists are moving towards an "early aggressive" approach, with the aim of changing the natural history of the disease [70]. So far, there are no definite proper criteria to select which patients will certainly benefit from an early aggressive approach [71]. The knowledge of these genetic, laboratory, or clinical markers will be the challenge in pediatric IBD research.

Conventional Therapy

Aminosalicylates Aminosalicylates (5-ASA) are commonly used in the management of pediatric CD, although there are no randomized controlled trials evaluating their efficacy for the induction and maintenance of remission in children. Current data in adults do not support their use in ileal CD, showing any (or a slightly) improvement compared to placebo, thus their use in CD should not be supported [72].

Steroids Conventional corticosteroids (CSs) are used for the induction of remission in moderate-to-severe CD. CSs are usually quickly weaned after the induction, due to their known adverse effects. Budesonide, an oral steroid preparation that is released in the distal ileum and proximal colon, can be used in patients with mild-to-moderate disease of those segments [73]. It has less systemic side effects than conventional steroids but is not completely without them, and quick withdrawal can lead to adrenal insufficiency [74].

Immunomodulators (Azathioprine, 6-Mercaptopurine, Methotrexate) Thiopurines, comprising azathioprine and its active metabolite 6-mercaptopurine, are widely used maintenance agents in CD [75]. Their efficacy has been demonstrated in several trials for both induction and maintenance of remission in CD. However, due to their well-known slow onset of action (about 2–3 months), they are not used for induction of remission. Although the only pediatric prospective, multicenter, double-blind, placebo-controlled trial conducted in children reported 91% of children receiving thiopurines to be in remission after 18 months of therapy [76], in routine clinical practice, a complete remission can be achieved in about 60% of patients 1 year after beginning therapy [77]. Methotrexate is often regarded as a second-line immunomodulator in CD patients not responding or intolerant to thiopurines. Some data in adults have demonstrated its efficacy in inducing and maintaining remission [78]. To date, there have been no controlled trials of its use in pediatric CD,

Fig. 28.3 Step-up therapeutic approach of pediatric Crohn's disease

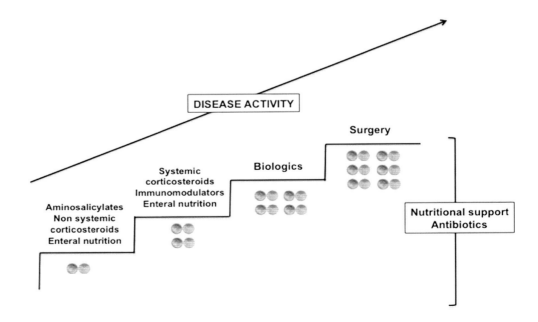

but reports from retrospective reviews and uncontrolled trials have shown good remission rates [79].

Biologic Agents Monoclonal anti-TNF-α antibodies have revolutionized the management of IBD since their introduction more than 15 years ago. Infliximab, the first in this class to be approved in pediatric IBD, is a chimeric monoclonal IgG1 antibody (part mouse and part human) that is given intravenously. Infliximab is effective in both inducing and maintaining remission in pediatric CD [80, 81]. It reduces the need for corticosteroid, hospitalization, or surgery; is effective in perianal CD and induces mucosal healing [82]. In the main pediatric clinical trial, the Reaching for Excellence in Adolescent Care and Health (REACH) study, children with moderate-to-severe CD received a 3-dose induction of 5 mg/kg infliximab at 0, 2, 6 weeks, followed by 5 mg/kg maintenance infusions every 8 weeks. Remission rates were 60% at week 30 and 56% at week 54. Moreover, this trial showed that the maintenance therapy every 8 weeks was superior to every 12 weeks, confirming previous results in adults [83]. Concerns about the risk of opportunistic infections or malignancies have emerged as a result of the extensive use of these drugs. Although an overall slightly increased risk of lymphoma has been reported in patients with IBD who have been exposed to biological or immunomodulator therapy, a rare fatal form of lymphoma, hepatosplenic T cell lymphoma (HSTCL), has been observed only in children and young adults with IBD exposed to immunomodulators while taking biologics [84]. There have been approximately 36 cases of HSTCL associated with IBD treatment [84–88]. Of these 36 cases, 20 had received combined therapy with infliximab and a thiopurine, with all 20 having taken infliximab and 4 also having taken adalimumab after infliximab [85–88]. One patient was given natalizumab after infliximab [88], 16 patients had received a thiopurine as monotherapy for IBD. These cases reveal a preponderance for young male patients, although the mechanism of this is unknown. For this reason, most pediatric patients do not receive concomitant therapy with these two classes of medications (although there are some exceptions in children affected by severe CD). There is still considerable debate regarding how, when, and for how long a combination therapy should be implemented, also on the basis of data from Study of Biologic and Immunomodulator Naive Patients in Crohn's Disease (SONIC) trial in adults, demonstrating better results in term of efficacy in patients treated with combination therapy compared with immunomodulator or biologic therapy alone [89].

Adalimumab is a humanized anti-TNF-α therapy that has been shown to be efficacious for induction and maintenance of remission for children with CD [90]. It is used primarily in clinical practice for patients who are primary anti-TNF-α responders, but become intolerant or nonresponsive to infliximab [91], although its use as first-line biologic agent has become widespread. Only limited data are available on the long-term outcome of biologic treatment in pediatric IBD. Recently, data from the EPIMAD registry in a large population-based pediatric-onset CD cohort (120 children) with a median follow-up of almost 10 years confirmed the efficacy and safety of infliximab in this population. The short-term response rate in this study was 89%, similar to results reported in the REACH study [92]. More than half of the initial responders to infliximab (55%) maintained benefits 3 years after its initiation and 32% at maximal follow-up. These results are less satisfactory than those reported by Hyams et al. [81] in a large North American pediatric cohort where the likelihood of continuing maintenance inflximab therapy at 1 and 3 years was 93 and 67%, respectively.

Nutrition Exclusive enteral nutrition (EEN) is used as a therapy to achieve remission in children presenting with acute CD [70]. Nutritional therapy consists of using different formulas (elemental, semi-elemental, and polymeric) as primary therapy to induce and maintain remission in CD and as a supplement to improve growth, or to replenish micronutrient deficiency. The evidence for supporting the use of enteral nutrition as primary therapy is controversial: while enteral nutritional support has found favor in some parts of the world (mainly Europe and Canada), it is not widely utilized in others (USA), and it can be difficult to administer for long periods of time. Several small pediatric studies suggest the effectiveness of EEN in active CD [93–95]. A meta-analysis of pediatric data, despite limited numbers of truly randomized trials in children, concluded that enteral nutrition may be as effective as steroids in the treatment of children with active CD [96]. Moreover, some studies suggest that EEN may be able to achieve mucosal healing. Fell et al. demonstrated a clinical and histological remission in over 70% of children treated with EEN, with an improvement of cytokine profiles with a polymeric diet alone [97]. Despite convincing data about the benefits of enteral nutrition, its mechanism of action remains elusive. The most frequently advanced theory is that the microbiota of the gut lumen is modified by enteral nutrition; furthermore, the reduction in antigenic load associated with an EEN may also contribute to bowel rest. However, the efficacy of polymeric diets and recent evidence that dietary supplementation with enteral nutrition may prolong the remission of the disease [95] suggest that reducing luminal antigens may only play a modest role in the efficacy of this therapy. Whether enteral nutrition per se has either a direct and/or indirect immunoregulatory effect remains speculative. The main drawback of enteral feeding is the poor compliance: Most parents are reluctant to commit their children to total enteral nutrition for 6–8 weeks as required, and few children are able to consume an adequate volume of formula by mouth, thus requiring the insertion of a nasogastric tube.

Surgery The main indications for surgery are complications of the disease (especially strictures and fistulas), intestinal perforation or bleeding, failure of medical therapy, and complications of medical therapy (e.g., growth failure). The primary goals of surgical treatment in CD are to preserve as much bowel as possible, relieve complications, and to help the patient to achieve the best possible quality of life. In children, the potential for bowel loss due to surgical resections must be weighed against the risk of poorly controlled disease, long-term steroid therapy, and growth failure. Interestingly, weight and height catch-up are markedly significant in patients undergoing surgery within 3 years from CD diagnosis. Indeed, surgery seems to promote bright growth and nutritional recovery if performed in the early phases of the puberty [98]. Recent data from European Pediatric Registries indicate that cumulative rates of intestinal resection are 7, 20, and 34 % at 1, 3, and 5 years, respectively [98, 99]. Variables at diagnosis associated with an increased risk of a second surgery are: age < 14 year, penetrating or structuring phenotype, and upper gastrointestinal location [99]. Interestingly, the risk of resection surgery was reduced by more than two-thirds in patients undergoing scheduled infliximab maintenance treatment.

References

1. Benchimol EI, Fortinsky KJ, Gozdyra P, et al. Epidemiology of pediatric inflammatory bowel disease: a systematic review of international trends. Inflamm Bowel Dis. 2011;17:423–39.
2. Martín-de-Carpi J, Rodríguez A, Ramos E, Jiménez S, Martínez-Gómez MJ, Medina E. Increasing incidence of pediatric inflammatory bowel disease in Spain (1996–2009): the SPIRIT registry. Inflamm Bowel Dis. 2013;19:73–80.
3. Schirbel A, Fiocchi C. Inflammatory bowel disease: established and evolving considerations on its etiopathogenesis and therapy. J Dig Dis. 2010;11:266–76.
4. Sauer CG, Kugathasan S. Pediatric inflammatory bowel disease: highlighting pediatric differences in IBD. Med Clin N Am. 2010;94:35–52.
5. Kugathasan S, Cohen S. Searching for new clues in inflammatory bowel disease: tell tales from pediatric IBD natural history studies. Gastroenterology. 2008;135:1038–41.
6. Economou M, Pappas G. New global map of Crohn's disease: genetic, environmental, and socioeconomic correlations. Inflamm Bowel Dis. 2008;14:709–20.
7. Nerich V, Monnet E, Etienne A, et al. Geographical variation of inflammatory bowel disease in France: a study based on national health insurance data. Inflamm Bowel Dis. 2006;12:218–26.
8. Bernstein CN, Wajda A, Svenson LW, et al. The epidemiology of inflammatory bowel disease in Canada: a population-based study. Am J Gastroenterol. 2006;101:1559–68.
9. Benchimol EI, Guttmann A, Griffiths AM, et al. Increasing incidence of pediatric inflammatory bowel disease in Ontario, Canada: evidence from health administrative data. Gut. 2009;58:1490–97.
10. Vind I, Riis L, Jess T, et al. The DCCD study group Increasing incidences of inflammatory bowel disease and decreasing surgery rates in copenhagen city and county, 2003–2005: a population-based study from the Danish Crohn colitis database. Am J Gastroenterol. 2006;101:1274–82.
11. Vernier-Massouille G, Balde M, Salleron J, et al. Natural history of pediatric Crohn's disease: a population-based Cohort study. Gastroenterology. 2008;135:1106–13.
12. Kugathasan S, Judd RH, Hoffman RG, et al. Epidemiologic and clinical characteristics of children with newly diagnosed inflammatory bowel disease in Wisconsin: a statewide population-based study. J Pediatr. 2003;143:525–31.
13. Kappelman MD, Rifas-Shiman SL, Kleinman K, et al. The prevalence and geographic distribution of Crohn's disease and ulcerative colitis in the United States. Clin Gastroenterol Hepatol. 2007;5:1424–9.
14. Baumgart DC, Bernstein CN, Abbas Z. IBD around the world: comparing the epidemiology, diagnosis, and treatment: proceedings of the world digestive health day 2010–inflammatory bowel disease task force meeting. Inflamm Bowel Dis. 2011;17:639–44.
15. Ishige T, Tomomasa T, Takebayashi T, et al. Inflammatory bowel disease in children: epidemiological analysis of the nationwide IBD registry in Japan. J Gastroenterol. 2010;45:911–7.
16. Wang XQ, Zhang Y, Xu CD, et al. Inflammatory bowel disease in Chinese children: a multicenter analysis over a decade from Shanghai. Inflamm Bowel Dis. 2013;19:423–8.
17. Orel R, Kamhi T, Vidmar G, Mamula P. Epidemiology of pediatric chronic inflammatory bowel disease in central and western Slovenia, 1994–2005. J Pediatr Gastroenterol Nutr. 2009;48:579–86.
18. Shikhare G, Kugathasan S. Inflammatory bowel disease in children: current trends J Gastroenterol. 2010;45:673–82.
19. Gupta N, Bostrom AG, Kirschner BS, et al. Gender differences in presentation and course of disease in pediatric patients with Crohn disease. Pediatrics. 2007;120:e1418–25.
20. Van Limbergen J, Russell RK, Drummond HE, Aldhous MC, Round NK, Nimmo ER, et al. Definition of phenotypic characteristics of childhood-onset inflammatory bowel disease. Gastroenterology. 2008;135:1114–22.
21. Levine A. Pediatric inflammatory bowel disease: is it different? Dig Dis. 2009;27:212–4.
22. Man SM, Kaakoush NO, Mitchell HM. The role of bacteria and pattern-recognition receptors in Crohn's disease. Nat Rev Gastroenterol Hepatol. 2011;8:152–68.
23. Sim WH, Wagner J, Cameron DJ, Catto-Smith AG, Bishop RF, Kirkwood CD. Novel Burkholderiales 23S rRNA genes identified in ileal biopsy samples from children: preliminary evidence that a subtype is associated with perianal Crohn's disease. J Clin Microbiol. 2010;48:1939–42.
24. Darfeuille-Michaud A, Boudeau J, Bulois P, et al. High prevalence of adherent-invasive Escherichia coli associated with ileal mucosa in Crohn's disease. Gastroenterology. 2004;127:412–21.
25. Negroni A, Costanzo M, Vitali R, et al. Characterization of adherent-invasive Escherichia coli isolated from pediatric patients with inflammatory bowel disease. Inflamm Bowel Dis. 2012;18:913–24.
26. Halme L, Paavola-Sakki P, Turunen U, et al. Family and twin studies in inflammatory bowel disease. World J Gastroenterol. 2006;12:3668–72.
27. Franke A, McGovern DP, Barrett JC, et al. Genome-wide meta-analysis increases to 71 the number of confirmed Crohn's disease susceptibility loci. Nat Genet. 2010;42:1118–25.
28. Hugot JP, Chamaillard M, Zouali H, et al. Association of NOD2 leucine-rich repeat variants with susceptibility to Crohn's disease. Nature. 2001;411:599–603.
29. Duerr RH, Taylor KD, Brant SR, et al. A genome wide association study identifies IL23R as an inflammatory bowel disease gene. Science. 2006;314:1461–146.
30. Latiano A, Palmieri O, Valvano MR, et al. Replication of interleukin 23 receptor and autophagy-related 16-like 1 association in adult- and pediatric-onset inflammatory bowel disease in Italy. World J Gastroenterol. 2008;14:4643–51.
31. Barrett JC, Hansoul S, Nicolae DL, et al. Genome-wide association defines more than 30 distinct susceptibility loci for Crohn's disease. Nat Genet. 2008;40:955–62.

32. Imielinski M, Baldassano RN, Griffiths A, et al. Common variants at five new loci associated with early-onset inflammatory bowel disease. Nat Genet. 2009;41:1335–40.

33. Parkes M, Barrett JC, Prescott NJ, et al. Sequence variants in the autophagy gene IRGM and multiple other replicating loci contribute to Crohn's disease susceptibility. Nat Genet. 2007;39:830–2.

34. Glocker EO, Kotlarz D, Boztug K, Gertz EM, Schäffer AA, et al. Inflammatory bowel disease and mutations affecting the interleukin-10 receptor. N Engl J Med. 2009;361:2033–45.

35. Pigneur B, Escher J, Elawad M, et al. Phenotypic characterization of very early-onset IBD due to mutations in the IL10, IL10 receptor alpha or beta gene: a survey of the genius working group. Inflamm Bowel Dis. 2013;19:2820–8.

36. Abraham BP, Mehta S, El-Serag HB. Natural history of pediatric-onset inflammatory bowel disease: a systematic review. J Clin Gastroenterol. 2012;46:581–9.

37. Stephens M, Batres LA, Ng D, Baldassano R. Growth failure in the child with inflammatory bowel disease. Semin Gastrointest Dis. 2001;12:253–62.

38. Kanof ME, Lake AM, Bayless TM. Decreased height velocity in children and adolescents before the diagnosis of Crohn's disease. Gastroenterology. 1988;95:1523–7.

39. Griffiths AM. Growth retardation in early-onset inflammatory bowel disease: should we monitor and treat these patients differently? Dig Dis. 2009;27:404–11.

40. Ballinger AB, Camacho-Hubner C, Croft NM. Growth failure and intestinal inflammation. Q J Med. 2001;94:121–5.

41. Ballinger AB, Azooz O, El-Haj T, Poole S, Farthing MJG. Growth failure occurs through a decrease in insulin-like growth factor 1 which is independent of undernutrition in a rat model of colitis. Gut. 2000;46:694–700.

42. Sylvester FA, Gordon CM, Thayu M, et al. Report of the CCFA pediatric bone, growth and muscle health workshop, New York City, November 11–12, 2011, with updates. Inflamm Bowel Dis. 2013;19:2919–26.

43. Levine A, Koletzko S, Turner D. The ESPGHAN revised porto criteria for the diagnosis of inflammatory bowel disease in children and adolescents. J Pediatr Gastroenterol Nutr. 2014; 58:795–806.

44. Benitez JM, Meuwis MA, Reenaers C, et al. Role of endoscopy, cross-sectional imaging and biomarkers in Crohn's disease monitoring. Gut. 2013;62:1806–16.

45. Prideaux L, De Cruz P, Ng SC, Kamm MA. Serological antibodies in inflammatory bowel disease: a systematic review. Inflamm Bowel Dis. 2012;18:1340–55.

46. Mow WS, Vasiliauskas EA, Lin YC, et al. Association of antibody responses to microbial antigens and complications of small bowel Crohn's disease. Gastroenterology. 2004;126:414–24.

47. Dubinsky M. Can serologic markers help determine prognosis and guide therapy? Dig Dis. 2010;28:424–8.

48. Arai R. Serologic markers: impact on early diagnosis and disease stratification in inflammatory bowel disease. Postgrad Med. 2010;122:177–85.

49. Arnott ID, Landers CJ, Nimmo EJ, et al. Sero-reactivity to microbial components in Crohn's disease is associated with disease severity and progression, but not NOD2/CARD15 genotype. Am J Gastroenterol. 2004;99:2376–84.

50. Sipponen T. Diagnostics and prognostics of inflammatory bowel disease with fecal neutrophil-derived biomarkers calprotectin and lactoferrin. Dig Dis. 2013;31:336–44.

51. Däbritz J, Langhorst J, Lügering A, et al. Improving relapse prediction in inflammatory bowel disease by neutrophil-derived S100A12. Inflamm Bowel Dis. 2013;19:1130–8.

52. Vitali R, Stronati L, Negroni A, et al. Fecal HMGB1 is a novel marker of intestinal mucosal inflammation in pediatric inflammatory bowel disease. Am J Gastroenterol. 2011;106:2029–40.

53. Di Nardo G, Aloi M, Oliva S, et al. Investigation of small bowel in pediatric Crohn's disease. Inflamm Bowel Dis. 2012;18:1760–76.

54. Horsthuis K, Bipat S, Stokkers PCF, et al. Magnetic resonance imaging for evaluation of disease activity in Crohn's disease: a systematic review. Eur Radiol. 2009;19:1450–60.

55. Essary B, Kim J, Anupindi S, et al. Pelvic MRI in children with Crohn's disease and suspected perianal involvement. Pediatr Radiol. 2007;37:201–8.

56. Horsthuis K, Ziech ML, Bipat S, et al. Evaluation of an MRI-based score of disease activity in perianal fistulizing Crohn's disease. Clin Imaging. 2011;35:360–5.

57. Van Assche G, Dignass A, Reinisch W, et al. The second European evidence-based consensus on the diagnosis and management of Crohn's disease: special situations. J Crohn's Colitis. 2010;4:63–101.

58. Nylund K, Hausken T, Gilja OH. Ultrasound and inflammatory bowel disease. Ultrasound Q. 2010;26:3–15.

59. Pallotta N, Corazziari E. Noninvasive imaging of the small bowel in Crohn's disease: the final frontier. Inflamm Bowel Dis. 2013;19:E20.

60. Pallotta N, Civitelli F, Di Nardo G, et al. Small intestine contrast ultrasonography in pediatric Crohn's disease. J Pediatr. 2013;163:778–84.

61. Rutgeerts P, Van Assche G, Sandborn WJ, et al. Adalimumab induces and maintains mucosal healing in patients with Crohn's disease: data from the EXTEND trial. Gastroenterology. 2012;142:1102–11.

62. Kierkus J, Dadalski M, Szymanska E, et al. The impact of infliximab induction therapy on mucosal healing and clinical remission in Polish pediatric patients with moderate-to-severe Crohn's disease. Eur J Gastroenterol Hepatol. 2012;24:495–500.

63. Mow WS, Lo SK, Targan SR, et al. Initial experience with wireless capsule endoscopy in the diagnosis and management of inflammatory bowel disease. Clin Gastroenterol Hepatol. 2004;2:31–40.

64. Bourreille A, Ignjatovic A, Aabakken L, et al. Role of small-bowel endoscopy in the management of patients with inflammatory bowel disease: an international OMED-ECCO consensus. Endoscopy. 2009;41:618–37.

65. Yamamoto H, Kita H, Sunada K, et al. Clinical outcomes of double-balloon endoscopy for the diagnosis and treatment of small-intestinal diseases. Clin Gastroenterol Hepatol. 2004;2:1010–6.

66. Heine GD, Hadithi M, Groenen MJ, et al. Double-balloon enteroscopy: indications, diagnostic yield, and complications in a series of 275 patients with suspected small-bowel disease. Endoscopy. 2006;38:42–8.

67. Di Nardo G, Oliva S, Aloi M, et al. Usefulness of single-balloon enteroscopy in pediatric Crohn's disease. Gastrointest Endosc. 2012;75:80–6.

68. Zallot C, Peyrin-Biroulet L. Deep remission in inflammatory bowel disease: looking beyond symptoms. Curr Gastroenterol Rep. 2013;15:315.

69. Allen PB, Peyrin-Biroulet L. Moving towards disease modification in inflammatory bowel disease therapy. Curr Opin Gastroenterol. 2013;29:397–404.

70. Aloi M, Nuti F, Stronati L, Cucchiara S. Advances in the medical management of paediatric IBD. Nat Rev Gastroenterol Hepatol. 2014;11:99–108.

71. Lee JC. Predicting the course of IBD: light at the end of the tunnel? Dig Dis. 2012;30:95–9.

72. Burger D, Travis S. Conventional medical management of inflammatory bowel disease. Gastroenterology. 2011;140:1827–37.

73. Nunes T, Barreiro-de Acosta M, Marin-Jiménez I, et al. Oral locally active steroids in inflammatory bowel disease. J Crohns Colitis. 2013;7(3):183–91.

74. Berkelhammer C, Trabolsi M, Andrejic J, Yasmeen T. Severe adrenal insufficiency complicating budesonide therapy for Crohn's disease. Inflamm Bowel Dis. 2012;17:1053–4.

75. Bär F, Sina C, Fellermann K. Thiopurines in inflammatory bowel disease revisited. World J Gastroenterol. 2013;19:1699–706.

76. Markowitz J, Grancher K, Kohn N, et al. A multicenter trial of 6—mercaptopurine and prednisone in children with newly diagnosed Crohn's disease. Gastroenterology. 2000;119:895–902.

77. Punati J, Markowitz J, Lerer T, et al. Effect of early immunomodulator use in moderate to severe pediatric Crohn disease. Inflamm Bowel Dis. 2008;14:949–54.

78. Ardizzone S, Bollani S, Manzionna G, et al. Comparison between methotrexate and azathioprine in the treatment of chronic active Crohn's disease: a randomised, investigator-blind study. Dig Liver Dis. 2003;35:619–27.

79. Willot S, Noble A, Deslandres C. Methotrexate in the treatment of inflammatory bowel disease: an 8-year retrospective study in a Canadian pediatric IBD center. Inflamm Bowel Dis. 2011;17:2521–6.

80. Hyams J, Crandall W, Kugathasan S, et al. Induction and maintenance infliximab therapy for the treatment of moderate to severe Crohn's disease in children. Gastroenterology. 2007;132:863–73.

81. Hyams J, Walters TD, Crandall W, et al. Safety and efficacy of maintenance infliximab therapy for moderate-to-severe Crohn's disease in children: REACH open-label extension. Curr Med Res Opin. 2011;27:651–62.

82. Danese S, Colombel JF, Reinisch W, Rutgeerts PJ. Review article: infliximab for Crohn's disease treatment–shifting therapeutic strategies after 10 years of clinical experience. Aliment Pharmacol Ther. 2011;33:857–69.

83. Rutgeerts P, Diamond RH, Bala M, et al. Scheduled maintenance treatment with infliximab is superior to episodic treatment for the healing of mucosal ulceration associated with Crohn's disease. Gastrointest Endosc. 2006;63:433–42.

84. Kotlyar TS, Osterman MT, Diamond RH, et al. A systematic review of factors that contribute to hepatosplenic T-Cell lymphoma in patients with nflammatory bowel disease. Clin Gastroenterol Hepatol. 2011;9:36–41.

85. Thai A, Prindiville T. Hepatosplenic T-cell lymphoma and inflammatory bowel disease. J Crohns Colitis. 2010;4:511–22.

86. Ochenrider MG, Patterson DJ, Aboulafia DM. Hepatosplenic T-cell lymphoma in a young man with Crohn's disease: case report and literature review. Clin Lymphoma Myeloma Leuk. 2010;10:144–8.

87. Mackey AC, Green L, Leptak C, et al. Hepatosplenic T cell lymphoma associated with infliximab use in young patients treated for inflammatory bowel disease: update. J Pediatr Gastroenterol Nutr. 2009;48:386–8.

88. Shale M, Kanfer E, Panaccione R, et al. Hepatosplenic T cell lymphoma in inflammatory bowel disease. Gut. 2008;57:1639–41.

89. Colombel JF, Sandborn WJ, Reinisch W, et al. Infliximab, azathioprine, or combination therapy for Crohn's disease. N Engl J Med. 2010;362:1383–95.

90. Hyams JS, Griffiths A, Markowitz J, et al. Safety and efficacy of adalimumab for moderate to severe Crohn's disease in children. Gastroenterology. 2012;143:365–74.

91. Russell RK, Wilson ML, Loganathan S, et al. A british society of paediatric gastroenterology, hepatology and nutrition survey of the effectiveness and safety of adalimumab in children with inflammatory bowel disease. Aliment Pharmacol Ther. 2011;33:946–53.

92. Crombé V, Salleron J, Savoye G, et al. Long-term outcome of treatment with infliximab in pediatric-onset Crohn's disease: a population-based study. Inflamm Bowel Dis. 2011;17:2144–52.

93. Grogan JL, Casson DH, Terry A, et al. Enteral feeding therapy for newly diagnosed pediatric Crohn's disease: a double-blind randomized controlled trial with two years follow-up. Inflamm Bowel Dis. 2012;18:246–53.

94. Borrelli O, Cordischi L, Cirulli M, et al. Polymeric diet alone versus corticosteroids in the treatment of active pediatric Crohn's disease: a randomized controlled open-label trial. Clin Gastroenterol Hepatol. 2006;4:744–53.

95. de Bie C, Kindermann A, Escher J. Use of exclusive enteral nutrition in paediatric Crohn's disease in The Netherlands. J Crohns Colitis. 2013;7:263–70.

96. Griffiths AM, Ohlsson A, Sherman PM, Sutherland LR, et al. Meta-analysis of enteral nutrition as a primary treatment of active Crohn's disease. Gastroenterology. 1995;108:1056–67.

97. Fell JM, et al. Mucosal healing and a fall in mucosal pro-inflammatory cytokine mRNA induced by a specific oral polymeric diet in paediatric Crohn's disease. Aliment Pharmacol Ther. 2000;14:281–9.

98. Savoye G, Salleron J, Gower-Rousseau C, et al. Clinical predictors at diagnosis of disabling pediatric Crohn's disease. Inflamm Bowel Dis. 2012;18:2072–8.

99. Boualit M, Salleron J, Turck D, et al. Long-term outcome after first intestinal resection in pediatric-onset Crohn's disease: a population-based study. Inflamm Bowel Dis. 2013;19:7–14.

Indeterminate Colitis/Inflammatory Bowel Disease Unclassified (IBD-U)

Barbara S. Kirschner

Introduction

The majority of patients with chronic inflammatory bowel disease (IBD) are diagnosed with either ulcerative colitis (UC) or Crohn's disease (CD) on the basis of established clinical, endoscopic, histologic, and radiologic criteria [1–2]. However, in 5–23% of patients with chronic colitis, a definitive diagnosis of UC or CD cannot be established because the initial macroscopic appearance (either during ileocolonoscopy or following colectomy) and histologic features overlap between UC and CD [2–7] (Table 29.1). While most of these patients eventually evolve into patterns consistent with UC or CD, approximately 20–60% retain the diagnosis of indeterminate colitis (IC) over periods as long as 5–10 years post diagnosis [4, 6–11] (Table 29.2). This latter observation suggests that IC may constitute a separate category within the spectrum of IBD. This chapter reviews the histologic and clinical features of IC in pediatric patients and contains updated information explaining why some patients continue to be diagnosed with IC (new proposed terminology of inflammatory bowel disease-unclassified, IBD-U) [12, 13]. For the present, IC and IBD-U refer to chronic colitis due to idiopathic IBD for which the features of CD and UC are absent. It has been suggested that the term IC should be the preferred term after histologic evaluation of the resected colon and IBD-U used after review of biopsy specimens [12, 13].

Clinical Presentation of Indeterminate colitis

A concurrent retrospective/prospective analysis of 1576 children and adolescents from the Italian Pediatric National IBD Register showed that 8% of their study population had IC while 52% had UC and 40% CD [14]. Presenting symptoms

B. S. Kirschner (✉)
Section of Gastroenterology, Hepatology and Nutrition, Department of Pediatrics, University of Chicago, Comer Children's Hospital, Chicago, IL 60637, USA
e-mail: bkirschn@peds.bsd.uchicago.edu

in IC were more similar to UC (bloody diarrhea and abdominal pain) than CD (abdominal pain and diarrhea). Fever and weight loss occurred more frequently in CD than IC and UC: fever in 40.5% CD, 12.9% in IC, and 12.6% in UC; weight loss 50.1% in CD, 17.4% in IC, and 20.6% in UC. The locations within the colon were also similar between IC and UC (pancolitis 34 vs. 39%; left colon 27 vs. 23% and rectum only 9 vs. 7%). The male to female ratio was lowest in UC (0.82), intermediate in CD (1.18), and highest in IC (1.42). Heyman et al. using the PediIBD Consortium Registry, reported that the prevalence of IC in children with IBD was highest in those aged 0–2 years (33%) and decreased to 18% at 3–5 years, 12% at 6–12 years, and 9% in those aged 13–18 [15, 16]. In young children (less than 5 years of age), failure to thrive is more prominent than seen in UC [17].

Jose et al. compared disease type with the prevalence of extraintestinal manifestations (EIMs) at the time of diagnosis and during follow-up in pediatric patients with IBD [18]. The study, also from the PediIBD Registry, included 1649 patients: IC ($n = 171$), UC ($n = 471$), and CD ($n = 1007$). With the exception of primary sclerosing cholangitis (PSC) being more prevalent in UC, the frequencies of the other EIMs did not differ between these disease types.

Epidemiologic Aspects of Indeterminate colitis

The prevalence of IC in pediatric patients with IBD varies among centers from 5 to 23% [2–7] (Table 29.1). A meta-analysis of 14 studies of pediatric patients with IBD and 18 studies in adult patients with IBD showed a higher frequency of IC in children (12.7%) versus adults (6.0%) [19].

In a pediatric population of 428 children with IBD being followed at the University Chicago reported in 2000, 49 or 11.4% were diagnosed with IC [5] (Table 29.2). In 42.9% of those with IC, the histology "favored UC" but these patients also had features of CD including areas of focal colitis, focal gastric, or duodenal inflammation, anal fissures, or isolated granulomas adjacent to ruptured crypts. Features "favoring

© Springer International Publishing Switzerland 2016
S. Guandalini et al. (eds.), *Textbook of Pediatric Gastroenterology, Hepatology and Nutrition,*
DOI 10.1007/978-3-319-17169-2_29

Table 29.1 Prevalence of indeterminate colitis [3–6, 10, 14, 35]. (Reprinted with permission from Ref. [20], Table 24.1, p. 379 with permission.)

	Total no. IBD pts	Age group	Indeterminate colitis		Mean age at diagnosis (yrs)		
			No. pts	(%)	IC	v	UC
Castro et al. [14]	1576	Pediatric	131	8.3	8.9		9.6
Gupta et al. [5]	420	Pediatric	51	11.9	10		–
Heikenen [6]	91	Pediatric	9	10.0	7.8		9.7
Hildebrand [4]	132	Pediatric	36	27.0	–		
Malaty [35]	420	Pediatric	78	18.6	9.2		
Meucci [10]	1113	Adult	50	4.6	–		
Shivananda [3]	2201	Adult	116	5.3	–		

IBD inflammatory bowel disease, *IC* indeterminate colitis, *UC* ulcerative colitis

Table 29.2 Indeterminate colitis: changes in diagnosis with time [4, 5, 9–11, 35]. (Reprinted with permission from Ref. [20], Table 24.3, p. 382 with permission.)

	Initial Dx IC	Final Dx IC (%)	Final Dx UC (%)	Final Dx CD (%)
Hildebrand [4]	36 (ped)	36	58	6
Malaty [35]	78 (ped)	30		
Moum [9]	36 (adult)	50	33	17
Meucci [10]	50 (adult)	20	34	40
Wells [11]	16 (surg)	75	19	6
Gupta [5]	12 (surg/ped)	33	50	17

IC indeterminate colitis, *UC* ulcerative colitis, *CD* Crohn's disease

CD" were present in 20.4 % of children with IC, none of whom had granulomas, radiologic evidence of small-bowel CD, or perianal findings. Endoscopic and histologic findings of IBD without distinguishing features of UC or CD were present in 36.7 % of our patients with IC. In order to further categorize our patients with IC, an X-ray study of the upper gastrointestinal tract with small-bowel follow-through (SBFT) was performed in all patients to exclude the possibility of CD.

Heikenen, Werlin, Brown et al. noted a similar prevalence of IC (10 %) in a pediatric population of IBD [6]. These authors noted that children with IC were diagnosed at a younger age (7.8 years) than those with either UC (9.7 years) or CD (11.4 years). Similarly in Sweden, the peak age range at diagnosis was younger (10–19 years) for patients with IC in comparison with UC (20–29 years) [19].

Criteria for Histologic Diagnosis of Indeterminate colitis

In establishing a diagnosis of IC, it is essential to exclude other causes of colitis such as infections (*Clostridium difficile, Yersinia, Mycobacterium tuberculosis, Entamoeba histolytica, E. coli* 0157:B7 or other verocytotoxin-producing strains, drugs (nonsteroidal anti-inflammatory drugs, NSAIDS), Behçet's, malignancy, vasculitis, and certain immunologic disorders. Immune deficiency disorders which may include chronic intestinal inflammation are: chronic granulomatous disease, Wiskott–Aldrich syndrome, common variable immunodeficiency disease (CVID), immu-

nodysregulation polyendocrinopathy enteropathy X-linked syndrome (IPEX), and glycogenosis type 1b [2, 20, 21].

Geboes and Van Eyken published an in-depth description of the histologic features observed in normal intestinal mucosa as well as the changes seen in patients with IBD [22]. Focal or diffuse plasmacytosis at the base of the mucosa and crypt architectural changes are strong predictors of IBD. However, it is important to recognize that these findings develop during the course of IBD. Thus, while basal plasmacytosis was seen within 15 days of the onset of IBD, crypt distortion was observed at 16–30 days in only 25 % of patients but increased to 75 % after 4 months. In comparison to adults, children < 10 years of age with new-onset UC show less crypt architectural changes and more rectal sparing than older patients. In addition, 4–8 % the initial biopsies were within the normal range. The authors suggested that the presence of basal lymphoplasmacytosis, seen in 58 % of cases, should lead to suspicion of underlying IBD. It in this group of children and adults with short history of disease onset, mild basal lymphoplasmatocytosis and no or minimal crypt architecture abnormalities that the term "IBD-U" has been proposed [12, 22, 23].

Patients with IBD-U clearly have IBD but the definitive features of UC or CD are absent. IBD-U may also be appropriate for cases of PSC where rectal sparing and patchy or focal inflammation are also more frequently observed [12]. Riddell stated that to differentiate IC lesions from CD lesions in resected specimens, submucosal and subserosal lymphoid aggregates away from areas of ulceration, non-necrotizing granulomas and skip areas should be absent. This is particularly true where there is nonspecific ileal involvement or gastritis with negative stains for *H. pylori* [24].

In cases of fulminant colitis, overlapping features between UC and CD (relative rectal sparing, focal inflammation or deep fissuring ulceration) result in a diagnosis of IC in approximately 10–15 % of patients [7, 22]. It is also important to recognize that some medications, such as corticosteroids or aminosalicylic acid (ASA) preparations, may change the diffuse histologic appearance in UC to a more focal appearance [6, 17]. Thus, slides from the original or pretreatment colonoscopy should be reviewed when considering a diagnosis of IC [23, 24].

Although histologic criteria would appear to allow differentiation between CD and UC, in 2002, Farmer et al. documented disparity among pathologists reviewing cases of colonic IBD [25] The diagnosis of gastrointestinal pathologists differed from that of the referring institution in 45 % of surgical specimens and 54 % of biopsy specimens. Of 70 cases initially diagnosed with UC, 30 (43 %) were changed to CD or IC; in contrast, 17 % of cases initially diagnosed with CD were changed to UC or IC.

The performance of upper gastrointestinal endoscopy with biopsies (esophagogastroduodenoscopy, EGD) identifies some patients with CD whose colonoscopy biopsies are indeterminate [12, 19]. Kundhal et al. reported that while diffuse nonspecific gastritis occurred with similar frequency in children with either CD and UC (92 vs. 75 %), focal antral gastritis was significantly more common in CD than UC (52 vs. 8 %) [26]. The authors defined focal inflammation as "localized inflammation of the gastric pits, glands, or foveolae by mononuclear and polymorphonuclear leukocytes bordering directly on uninflamed mucosa." This is similar to the statements previously published by Riddell [24]. However, a recent assessment of focal enhancing gastritis (FEG) in 262 pediatric patients showed that while FEG was highly associated with IBD, it did not reliably distinguish between UC and CD [27]. Granulomas in the stomach or duodenum provide evidence confirming the diagnosis of CD even in endoscopically normal-appearing mucosa [24]. Hence, performing an EGD should be part of the initial evaluation of pediatric patients for IBD.

Serologic Markers and Defining IBD Categories

We evaluated the role of p-ANCA and anti-*Saccharomyces cerevesiae* (ASCA) to determine whether we could identify UC and CD in pediatric patients previously diagnosed as IC [5]. While p-ANCA was positive in 68 % of those favoring UC, and ASCA positive in 37 % of those favoring CD, 86 % of our patients with IC were both p-ANCA and ASCA negative.

Joossens et al. correlated serologic markers with prospective follow-up evaluation in 97 adult patients initially diagnosed with IC [8]. After a mean follow-up of 6 years, 32 % of the adult patients with IC were reclassified as having UC or CD, half of whom were positive for p-ANCA or ASCA. However, almost half of the patients with IC (48.5 %) remained p-ANCA/ASCA negative and continue to have characteristics of IC even 10 years after the initial diagnosis [8].

Recently, Sura et al. utilized serology (pANCA, ASCA, and anti-OmpC) in 117 adult patients with IC and reassessed their disease type at 1 year [28]. P-ANCA identified 78 % of patients who subsequently were diagnosed with UC compared with only 18 % sensitivity for ASCA to predict a subsequent diagnosis of CD.

Radiologic Imaging

The most frequently used diagnostic studies (after ileocolonoscopy and EGD) for distinguishing among the various forms of pediatric IBD are those which image the small intestine such as magnetic resonance enterography (MRE) or SBFT.

Because of the ionizing radiation associated with SBFT, there has been utilization of MRE in children with IC, UC, and CD [29–31]. Gadolinium-enhanced magnetic resonance imaging (G-MRI) in combination with oral polyethylene glycol (PEG) solution (used to distend the small bowel) demonstrating increased wall thickness was noted in 26/26 children with CD while those with IC and UC showed mild parietal contrast enhancement but not bowel wall thickening [30].

In a prospective study of 58 consecutive children with suspected IBD, G-MRI confirmed the diagnosis of CD and UC with a sensitivity of 96 % and specificity of 92 % [31]. Of 17 patients with IC on histology alone, G-MRI had a lower non-classification rate than histology ($p < 0.02$). However, although endoscopy was less sensitive (57 %), it was more specific (100 %).

Small-Bowel Capsule Endoscopy

Small-bowel capsule endoscopy (SBCE) has the potential to identify lesions in the jejunum and ileum which would allow differentiation between IC and CD in patients with IC. Gralnek et al. utilized SBCE to determine whether ulcers could be observed in four pediatric patients previously diagnosed UC or IC, who were experiencing disease exacerbation [32]. Based on abnormal mucosal findings, two of the four patients were re-classified with CD. In addition, eight of ten patients with "suspected IBD" were also found to have ulcerations and diagnosed with CD.

In contrast, Goldstein et al. performed SBCE in 40 adult patients with IC ($n=20$) and UC ($n=49$) were unable to identify patients who would be reclassified as de novo CD in the period following their ileal pouch-anal anastomosis (IPAA) [33]. These authors cautioned that since SBCE may identify lesions in healthy individuals as well as those who take NSAIDS, the specificity of mucosal in these lesions is unclear.

Kopylov and Seidman also reported that the most common cause of lesions which mimic small bowel CD is NSAID medication [21]. The authors noted that these lesions can be indistinguishable from CD, occur as early as 2 weeks of use and may be seen in up to 70% of chronic NSAID users. They advised instructing patients who will undergo CE to avoid NSAIDs for at least 1 month before the examination.

Another confounding variable is that small-bowel inflammation has also been observed in a significant number of patients with established UC [34]. Of 23 UC patients, 13 (57%) showed small-bowel lesions, and 8 (35%) had erosions, as opposed to 2/23 (7%) and 1/23 (4%) in the control group. These findings emphasize the potential risk of misdiagnosis in IBD patients.

Natural History of Indeterminate colitis

With time, 50–72% of adult patients and 64% of pediatric patients with IC can be reclassified as definite UC or CD during subsequent observation [4, 5, 9–11, 35] (Table 29.2). Moum et al. observed that of 36 patients initially diagnosed as IC 33% were reclassified as UC and 17% as CD after a follow-up period averaging 14 months [9]. Meucci et al. reported that 37/50 patients (72.5%) changed from IC to a definite diagnosis of UC or CD during follow-up with a cumulative probability of 80% within 8 years of diagnosis [10]. In contrast, Wells et al. followed 16 patients with IC for a mean of 10 years and observed 3 were reclassified with UC, 1 with CD and the rest remained indeterminate [11]. The course of IC in 36 Swedish children after a mean follow-

up of 4.6 years was analyzed by Hildebrand et al. [4]. The findings were similar to those as described above in adults: 21/36 (58%) were subsequently categorized as UC, 2/36 (6%) CD and 13/36 (36%) remaining as IC. In our series of 49 children with IC, 9 had undergone colectomy at a mean of 24 months after diagnosis. After a mean follow-up of 42 months, 6/9 had repeat endoscopic examinations resulting in reclassification consistent with UC in 3/9 (33%), continued IC in 2/9 (22%) and CD in 1/9 (11%) [5].

More recently, Malaty et al. described a 12-year telephone follow-up of 20/60 pediatric patients who had been previously diagnosed with IC [35]. The range of outcomes was broad: 30% remained IBD-indeterminate, 10% reclassified as CD, 5% as eosinophilic colitis but 55% reported a complete resolution of their symptoms.

Medical Therapy of Indeterminate colitis

The observation that the majority of patients with IC are reclassified as UC or CD, makes it difficult to know whether IC represents a separate form of IBD.

Perhaps because of the small number of patients with IC and the variability of their histologic findings, the response to various drug regimens in this population has not been specifically addressed.

Thus, in our program the choice of therapeutic intervention is selected depending on the severity of symptoms, extent and severity of endoscopic and histologic findings, and laboratory parameters (Table 29.3). For most patients, drug therapy is similar to that indicated for patients with UC of comparable extent and severity. These include 5'ASA preparations for mild disease and corticosteroids and immunomodulatory and/or biologic therapy for moderate and severe disease. Immunomodulatory agents, such as azathioprine or 6-mercaptopurine have been used in approximately 60% of our pediatric population with IBD due to the presence of steroid dependency, resistance or toxicity [36]. When biologic agents are used, there has been a trend among pediat-

Table 29.3 Medical approach to the pediatric patient with indeterminate colitis[a]. (Reprinted with permission from Ref. [20], Table 24.4, p. 383 with permission.)

5'Aminosalicylic acid preparations (5'ASA) for mild disease
Corticosteroids (moderate to severe disease severity)
Metronidazole if histology favors CD
Azathioprine (AZA) or 6-mercaptopurine (6-MP)
Measure thiopurine methyltransferase (TPMT) prior to use to exclude deficiency
Monitor RBC 6-thioguanine (6-TG) and 6-methylmercaptopurine (6-MMP) levels to reduce risk of toxicity
Trial of change to AZA from 6-MP (or vice versa) for non-hypersensitivity side effects (i.e., rash, arthralgias, headache)
Methotrexate if intolerant or refractory to AZA/6-MP and older teenagers and young adults receiving anti-TNF biologic agents
Anti-TNF Biologic (at standard dosing)

[a] These recommendations are based on disease location, extent, severity and complications for UC and Crohn's colitis. There are no published pediatric trials which have specifically addressed the response to medical therapy in IC

TNF tumor necrosis factor, *IC* indeterminate colitis, *UC* ulcerative colitis, *CD* Crohn's disease

ric gastroenterologists to use methotrexate as concomitant therapy. The expectation is that there may be a lower risk of malignancy than with the combination of thiopurine and anti-tumor necrosis factor (TNF) therapy, although the long-term proof of this concept has not been established.

Some clinical trials of adult patients with IBD have included small numbers of patients with IC although they have not specifically addressed the response in IC.

Adult patients with refractory UC and IC appear to show similar improvement to azathioprine/6-mercaptopurine and cyclosporine as well as less frequently prescribed immuno-modulatory agents such tacrolimus and thalidomide [37–39]. A clinical response to infliximab in 20 adult patients with refractory IC has been reported [40]. In that study, 14/20 (70%) showed a "complete clinical response" and 2/20 (10%) "partial response." Favorable outcomes in pediatric patients with UC and CD, suggest that it anti-TNF agents will also be effective in some patients with IC who are not responding to conventional medications.

Surgical Treatment of Indeterminate colitis

Conflicting data have been published regarding medical failure and complication rates following medical and surgical intervention in patients with IC versus UC. Some centers report that IC is more refractory to medical intervention than UC resulting in a greater relapse rateand subsequent need for colectomy [41]. In contrast, Witte et al. described similar response rates to medical intervention in IC and UC for patients enrolled in the European Collaborative Study on Inflammatory Bowel Disease (EC-IBD) [42]. "Complete relief of complaints" was noted in 48% of UC patients versus 50% of those with IC. Partial response was also similar in both groups: 37% of patients UC "improved" versus 33% with IC.

Higher rates of pelvic sepsis, fistula formation and pouch failure after IPAA occur in patients with IC versus UC [43]. In contrast, patients with IC who are pANCA and ASCA negative have lower risk for pouchitis, pouch complications and the development of CD [44]. Thus, obtaining these serologic tests in patients being evaluated for IPAA may provide useful predictive information.

It is our practice to repeat colonoscopy, usually with concurrent EGD, during selected periods of relapse, if a higher level of therapy is being considered to assess whether histologic changes consistent with UC or CD have developed. This is especially the case if colectomy and IPAA are being advised because of refractory disease. Part of the reassessment should include repeat small-bowel X-ray imaging so that patients with ileal CD would be excluded from IPAA. Patients with persistent IC are counseled regarding the potentially greater risk of pouch complications. Patients with

IC undergo a multistaged operative procedure consisting of a total abdominal colectomy with temporary ileostomy and Hartmann pouch. In this way, the entire resected colon can be assessed to exclude CD prior to creating the IPAA. In some cases, especially where the colectomy specimen has atypical features, ileoscopy, and re-examination of the pouch are performed and the results discussed with the surgeon prior to scheduling the IPAA.

Summary

IC or IBD-U may represent a category of chronic IBD which remains separate from UC and CD even after long term follow-up. In young patients or those with recent-onset symptoms, the histologic features are less likely to have developed typical features. Patients and families should understand that IC or IBD-U is not indefinite colitis but rather a form of chronic IBD which may either stay the same or become more consistent with UC or CD over time. The major reason for distinguishing IC from UC is for counseling the patient and family about the potential increased risk for complications and possible subsequent change in diagnosis (especially to CD) following IPAA.

References

1. Marion JF, Rubin PH, Present DH. Differential diagnosis of chronic ulcerative colitis and Crohn's disease. In: Kirsner JB, editor. Inflammatory bowel disease. 5th ed. Philadelphia: WB Saunders; 2000. p. 315–25.
2. Bousvaros A, Antonioli DA, Colletti RB, et al. Differentiating ulcerative colitis from Crohn disease in children and young adults: report of a working group of the North American Society for Pediatric Gastroenterology, Hepatology and Nutrition and the Crohn's and Colitis Foundation of America. J Pediatr Gastroenterol Nutr. 2007;44(5):653–74.
3. Shivananda S, Lennard-Jones J, Logan R, et al. Incidence of inflammatory bowel disease across Europe: is there a difference between north and south? Results of the European Collaborative Study on Inflammatory Bowel Disease (EC-IBD). Gut. 1996;39(5):690–7.
4. Hildebrand H, Brydolf M, Holmquist L, et al. Incidence and prevalence of inflammatory bowel disease in children in south-western Sweden. Acta Paediatr. 1994;83(6):640–5.
5. Gupta P, Hart JA, Kirschner BS. Perinuclear antineutrophil cytoplasmic antibodies (pANCA) and anti-Saccharomyces cerevisiae (ASCA) antibodies in children with indeterminate colitis. Gastroenterology. 2000;118(4):A103.
6. Heikenen JB, Werlin SL, Brown CW, et al. Presenting symptoms and diagnostic lag in children with inflammatory bowel disease. Inflamm Bowel Dis. 1999;5(3):158–60.
7. Geboes K, De Hertogh G. Indeterminate colitis. Inflamm Bowel Dis. 2003;9(5):324–31.
8. Joossens S, Reinisch W, Vermeire S, et al. The value of serologic markers in indeterminate colitis: a prospective follow-up study. Gastroenterology 2002;122(5):1242–7.
9. Moum B, Ekbom A, Vatn MH, et al. Inflammatory bowel disease: re-evaluation of the diagnosis in a prospective population based study in south eastern Norway. Gut. 1997;40(3):328–32.

10. Meucci G, Bortoli A, Riccioli FA, et al. Frequency and clinical evolution of indeterminate colitis: a retrospective multi-centre study in northern Italy. GSMII (Gruppo di Studio per le Malattie Infiammatorie Intestinali). Eur J Gastroenterol Hepatol. 1999;11(8):909–13.

11. Wells AD, McMillan I, Price AB, et al. Natural history of indeterminate colitis. Br J Surg. 1991;78(2):179–81.

12. Silverberg M, Sarsabgi J, Ahmad T, et al. Toward an integrated clinical, molecular and serological classification of inflammatory bow el disease: report of a working party of the 2005 Montreal Congress of Gastroenterology. Can J Gastroenterol. 2005;19:5–36.

13. Tremaine WJ. Is indeterminate colitis determinable? Curr Gastroenterol Rep. 2012;14:162–5.

14. Castro M, Papadatou B, Baldassare M, et al. Inflammatory bowel disease in children and adolescents in Italy: data from the Pediatric National IBD Register (1996–2003). Inflamm Bowel Dis. 2008;14:1246–50.

15. Heyman MD, Kirschner BS, Gold BD et al. Children with early-onset inflammatory bowel disease (IBD); analysis of a pediatric IBD consortium registry. J Pediatr 2005;46:35-40.

16. Mamula P, Telega GW, Markowitz JE, et al. Inflammatory bowel disease in children 5 years of age and younger. Am J Gastroenterol. 2002;97(8):2005–10.

17. Jose FA, Garnett EA, Vittinghoff E et al. Development of extraintestinal manifestations in pediatric patients with inflammatory bowel disease. Inflamm Bowel Dis. 2009;15:63–8.

18. Prenzel F, Uhlig HH. Frequency of indeterminate colitis in children and adults with IBD—a metaanalysis. J Crohns Colitis. 2009;3(4):277–81.

19. Stewenius J, Adnerhill I, Ekelund G, et al. Ulcerative colitis and indeterminate colitis in the city of Malmo, Sweden. A 25-year incidence study. Scand J Gastroenterol. 1995;30(1):38–43.

20. Kirschner BS. Indeterminate colitis. In Guandalini S, editor. Textbook of pediatric gastroenterology and nutrition. London: Taylor & Francis; 2004. p. 379–84.

21. Kopylov U, Seidman EG. Clinical applications of small bowel capsule endoscopy. Clin Exp Gastroenterol. 2013;6:129–37.

22. Geboes K, Van Eyken P. Inflammatory bowel disease unclassified and indeterminate colitis: the role of the pathologist. J Clin Pathol. 2009;62:201–5.

23. Geboes K, Colombel J-F, Greenstein A, Jewell DP, Sandborn WJ, et al. Indeterminate colitis: A review of the concept—what's in a name. Inflamm Bowel Dis. 2008;14:850–57.

24. Riddell RH. Pathology of idiopathic inflammatory bowel disease. In: Kirsner JB, editor. Inflammatory bowel disease. 5th ed. Philadelphia: WB Saunders; 2000. pp. 439–41.

25. Farmer M, Petras RE, Hunt LE, et al. The importance of diagnostic accuracy in colonic inflammatory bowel disease. Am J Gastroenterol. 2000;95(11):3184–8.

26. Kundhal PS, Stormon MO, Zachos M, et al. Gastric antral biopsy in the differentiation of pediatric colitides. Am J Gastroenterol. 2003;98(3):557–61.

27. McHugh JB, Gopal P, Greenson JK. The clinical significance of focally enhanced gastritis in children. Am J Surg Path. 2013;37:295–9.

28. Sura SP, Ahmed A, Cheifetz AS, Moss AC. Characteristics of inflammatory bowel disease serology in patients with indeterminate colitis. J Clin Gastroenterol. 2014;48(4):352–5.

29. Durno CA, Sherman P, Williams T, et al. Magnetic resonance imaging to distinguish the type and severity of pediatric inflammatory bowel diseases. J Pediatr Gastroenterol Nutr. 2000;30(2):170–4.

30. Laghi A, Borrelli O, Paolantonio P, et al. Contrast enhanced magnetic resonance imaging of the terminal ileum in children with Crohn's disease. Gut. 2003;52(3):393–7.

31. Darbari A, Sena L, Argani P et al. Gadolinium-enhanced magnetic resonance imaging: a useful radiologic tool in diagnosing pediatric IBD. Inflamm Bowel Dis. 2004;10(2):67–72.

32. Gralnek IM, Cohen SA, Ephrath H, et al. Small bowel capsule endoscopy impacts diagnosis and management of pediatric inflammatory bowel disease: a prospective study. Dig Dis Sci. 2012;57(2):465–71.

33. Goldstein JL, Eisen GM, Lewis B et al. Video capsule endoscopy to prospectively assess small bowel injury with celecoxib, naproxen plus omeprazole, and placebo. Clin Gastroenterol Hepatol. 2005;3:133–41.

34. Higurashi T, Endo H, Yoneda M et al. Capsule-endoscopic findings of ulcerative colitis patients. Digestion. 2011;84:306–14.

35. Malaty HM, Mehtya S, Abraham B, et al. The natural course of inflammatory bowel disease-indetrminate from childhood to adulthood: with a 25 year period. Clin Exp Gastroenterol. 2013;6:115–21.

36. Kirschner BS. Safety of azathioprine and 6-mercaptopurine in pediatric patients with inflammatory bowel disease. Gastroenterology. 1998;115(4):813–21.

37. Fraser AG, Orchard TR, Jewell DP. The efficacy of azathioprine for the treatment of inflammatory bowel disease: a 30 year review. Gut. 2002;50(4):485–9.

38. Fellermann K, Tanko Z, Herrlinger KR, et al. Response of refractory colitis to intravenous or oral tacrolimus (FK506). Inflamm Bowel Dis. 2002;8(5):317–24.

39. Bariol C, Meagher AP, Vickers CR, et al. Early studies on the safety and efficacy of thalidomide for symptomatic inflammatory bowel disease. J Gastroenterol Hepatol. 2002;17(2):135–9.

40. Papadakis KA, Treyzon L, Abreu MT, et al. Infliximab in the treatment of medically refractory indeterminate colitis. Aliment Pharmacol Ther. 2003;18:741–7.

41. Stewenius, Adnerhill I, Ekelund GR, et al. Operations in unselected patients with ulcerative colitis and indeterminate colitis. A long-term follow-up study. Eur J Surg. 1996;162(2):131–7.

42. Witte J, Shivananda S, Lennard-Jones JE, et al. Disease outcome in inflammatory bowel disease: mortality, morbidity and therapeutic management of a 796-person inception cohort in the European Collaborative Study on Inflammatory Bowel Disease (EC-IBD). Scand J Gastroenterol. 2000;35(12):1272–7.

43. Yu CS, Pemberton JH, Larson D. Ileal pouch-anal anastomosis in patients with indeterminate colitis: long-term results. Dis Colon Rectum. 2000;43:1487–96.

44. Hui T, Landers C, Vasiliauskas E, et al. Serologic responses in indeterminate colitis patients before ileal pouch-anal anastomosis may determine those at risk for continuous pouch inflammation. Dis Colon Rectum. 2005;48:1254–62.

Ulcerative Colitis

Leslie M Higuchi, Brian P Regan and Athos Bousvaros

Abbreviations

6MP	6-mercaptopurine
6-TUA	6-thiouric acid
6-MMP	6-methyl mercaptopurine
6-TGN	6-thioguanine nucleotide
25(OH)D	25-hydroxy vitamin D
AGA	American Gastroenterological Association
ALT	Alanine aminotransferase
Anti-TNF	Anti-tumor necrosis factor-alpha
ASA	Aminosalicylate
ASCA	Anti-*Saccharomyces cerevisiae*
AZA	Azathioprine
CBir1	Flagellin
CD	Crohn's disease
CI	Confidence interval
CRC	Colorectal cancer
CRP	C-reactive protein
CT	Computed tomography
EN	Erythema nodosum
ESPGHAN	European Society for Pediatric Gastroenterology Hepatology and Nutrition
ESR	Erythrocyte sedimentation rate
GWA	Genome-wide association
HLA	Human leukocyte antigen
HR	Hazard ratio
IBD	Inflammatory bowel disease
I2	*Pseudomonas fluorescens*-associated sequence
IL	Interleukin
IPAA	Ileal pouch-anal canal anastomosis
MAdCAM-1	Mucosal addressin-cell adhesion molecule-1
MCV	Mean corpuscular volume
MRI	Magnetic resonance imaging
MTX	Methotrexate
NF-kappaB	Nuclear transcription factor kappa B
NSAIDs	Non-steroidal anti-inflammatory drugs
OCP	Oral contraceptive
p-ANCA	Perinuclear antineutrophil cytoplasmic antibodies
PG	Pyoderma gangrenosum
PSC	Primary sclerosing cholangitis
PUFAs	Polyunsaturated fatty acids
PUCAI	Pediatric ulcerative colitis activity index
VTE	Venous thromboembolism
UC	Ulcerative colitis

L. M. Higuchi (✉) · B. P. Regan · A. Bousvaros
GI Division—Inflammatory Bowel Disease Center, Children's
Hospital, GI Hunnewell Ground, 300 Longwood Avenue, Boston,
MA 02115, USA
e-mail: leslie.higuchi@childrens.harvard.edu

B. P. Regan
e-mail: brian.regan@childrens.harvard.edu

A. Bousvaros
e-mail: athos.bousvaros@childrens.harvard.edu

© Springer International Publishing Switzerland 2016
S. Guandalini et al. (eds.), *Textbook of Pediatric Gastroenterology, Hepatology and Nutrition,*
DOI 10.1007/978-3-319-17169-2_30

Introduction

Ulcerative colitis (UC) and Crohn's disease (CD) are the two most common forms of idiopathic inflammatory bowel disease (IBD). UC differs from CD in that the inflammation in UC is confined to the mucosal layer of the colon. In contrast, CD is characterized by transmural inflammation either in a limited region or extensively in the bowel, and may involve any portion of the gastrointestinal tract from the mouth to the anus. The peak incidence of IBD occurs between the ages of 15 and 25 years, but UC may begin at any age [1]. Approximately 20% of the patients with UC present before the age of 20 years [2]. While children and adults develop similar symptoms, children often present with more extensive disease [3]. Clinicians caring for children and adolescents with UC must treat both the gastrointestinal and extraintestinal complications, optimize nutrition and linear growth, and address the psychosocial ramifications of the illness. Since the majority of the published studies investigating the natural history and treatment of UC are in adults, we refer primarily to these studies, with reference to pediatric studies where available.

Epidemiology

Most children with UC present between the ages of 10 and 18 years. However, UC in children under age 5 years is well described [1, 4, 5]. Epidemiologic studies primarily conducted in North America, the UK, and Scandinavian countries, suggest the incidence of UC in children ranges from 2.1 to 4.2 cases/year/100,000 population [6–11] (see Table 30.1). Although temporal trends vary between studies, the incidence of UC in children has remained relatively stable. In a systematic review of international trends in pediatric IBD incidence, of those studies with calculated statistical trends for CD incidence, 60 % reported a significant increase in CD incidence. In contrast, only 20 % of similar studies for UC reported a significantly increased incidence of UC [12]. Authors revealed a wide range of IBD incidence internationally and an absence of accurate estimates in most countries. The majority of incidence data for CD and UC in the pediatric population originates from geographic regions with higher rates of IBD [12].

Adult studies demonstrate that UC is more prevalent in North America, the UK, and Scandinavia and less common in southern Europe, Asia, and Africa [2]. The data suggest a north-to-south gradient with higher incidence rates of both CD and UC in northern locations, even within individual countries [13–15]. UC is more common among Jewish than non-Jewish peoples [16], but disease rates in people of Jewish origin vary by geographic region and parallel those of the general population [17]. The higher rates of IBD in individuals of Jewish origin across different countries support a common genetic predisposition; however, the geographic variation of IBD rates in Jews emphasizes that environmental factors (see below) influence the inherited risk.

Pathogenesis

No single cause of UC has been identified. Most likely, the disease results from a combination of the interplay of genetic, environmental, and immunologic factors.

A widely accepted hypothesis suggests that in the genetically susceptible individual, a combination of host and environmental factors leads to the initiation and perpetuation of an abnormal intestinal immune response to gut flora, resulting in UC [18, 19]. In support of this theory, colitis in animals occurs in a wide variety of genetically altered rodents, including interleukin (IL)-2, IL-10, and T cell receptor knockout mice, and *HLA-B27* transgenic rats [20]. Interestingly, most of these animal models do not develop colitis in germ-free environments. These findings suggest that multiple genes may contribute to the pathogenesis of IBD, and that interaction with the environment is essential.

Human Genetics

In humans, UC appears to have a non-Mendelian pattern of inheritance. Current evidence suggests that genes contribute less to the risk in individuals with UC than in those with CD. In a Danish twin cohort study and a Swedish twin cohort study, the calculated pair concordance rates among monozygotic twins were 14–19 % for UC and 50 % for CD, and among dizygotic twins, 0–5 % for UC and 0–4 % for CD [21, 22]. Although the concordance rates of disease are higher in monozygotic twins, the incomplete concordance suggests that nongenetic factors also contribute to the development of UC. First-degree relatives of patients with UC have a 9.5-fold increase in risk of developing UC, compared to the general population [23]. Genome-wide association (GWA) studies have implicated over 100 genes in the pathogenesis of IBD: Some of these genes exclusively predispose to CD, others to UC, and others to both diseases [24].

Among the GWA studies of UC, the most significant associations are found within the major histocompatibility complex class II region near *HLA-DRA* [25, 26]. Presently, the known genetic associations likely explain only approximately 20 % of the genetic contribution to IBD susceptibility [18].

Table 30.1 Incidence of ulcerative colitis in children and adolescents (number of new cases/year/100,000 persons) [6–11]

First author	Location	Age range	Time period studied	Incidence
Henderson 2012 [6]	Scotland	<16 years	2003–2008	2.1
Benchimol 2009 [7]	Ontario, Canada	<18 years	1994–2005	
			1994	4.1
			2005	4.2
Adamiak 2013 [8]	Wisconsin, USA	<18 years	2000–2007	2.4
Jakobsen 2011 [9]	Eastern Denmark, Funen, Aarhus County, Denmark	<15 years	2007–2009	3.1
Perminow 2009 [10]	Southeastern Norway	<18 years	2005–2007	3.6
Malmborg 2013 [11]	Northern Stockholm County, Sweden	<16 years	2002–2007	2.8

Environment

Environmental factors may contribute to the development of UC. One mechanism of action by which environment may trigger IBD is by altering the microbiome. Pediatric studies demonstrate that the intestinal microbiota in children with IBD differs from that of the patients with non-IBD gastrointestinal conditions [27, 28]. However, it is difficult to ascertain whether the microbiome alterations cause the intestinal inflammation, or are epiphenomena. Nevertheless, there is good evidence that diet and other environmental factors may alter the microbiome in both animals and humans [29]. Most studies examining environmental risk factors have the limitations of retrospective, case-control methodology. One of the most consistent findings in multiple studies is the lower risk of UC among current smokers. Current smokers have approximately one half the risk of developing UC compared to nonsmokers [30, 31].

Several authors have suggested that exposure to infections in the perinatal period or early life may contribute to the development of UC. Individuals with CD or UC were more likely to have experienced a diarrheal illness during infancy, when compared to their unaffected siblings [32]. Additional studies suggest associations between infectious gastroenteritis and development of pediatric or adult-onset UC [33–35]. Antibiotic usage in early childhood increases the risk of developing IBD, but the risk goes down as children grow older [36]. Appendectomy at a young age is associated with a lower risk of UC, but it may be the underlying appendiceal infection rather than the appendectomy itself that is the protective factor [37–39].

Other environmental factors that may affect the incidence of colitis include breastfeeding, nonsteroidal anti-inflammatory drugs (NSAIDs), oral contraceptives (OCPs), and vitamin D levels. The data on the association of breastfeeding and UC are inconclusive, with some published studies suggesting a protective effect [33, 40], and other studies showing no significant effect [32, 41, 42]. Some published reports suggest that NSAIDs may precede the onset of IBD, lead to a reactivation of quiescent IBD, or exacerbate already active IBD in humans [43–46]. Among past and current smokers, OCP use was associated with a hazard ratio (HR) of 1.63 (95 % CI 1.13–2.35) for UC compared to non-OCP users [47].

There has been increasing interest in the potential immunomodulatory role of vitamin D in the pathogenesis of diseases such as IBD [48]. In a large prospective cohort study of women, higher predicted 25-hydroxy vitamin D (25(OH) D) levels were associated with a significant reduction in the risk of incident CD, but only a nonsignificant decrease in the risk of UC.

Given the constant intestinal exposure to numerous luminal dietary antigens and the influence of dietary intake on the intestinal microbiota, investigators have long hypothesized a relationship between diet and UC [49, 50]. In a systematic review of case-control and cohort-based, nested case-control studies, authors examined macronutrients (fat, protein, carbohydrates) and specific foods (fruits, vegetables, meats), and the risk of IBD [51]. Increased dietary intake of total fats, polyunsaturated fatty acids (PUFAs) and meat were associated with an elevated risk of CD and UC. In contrast, high fiber and fruit intake were associated with a reduced risk of CD, whereas high vegetable intake was associated with reduced UC risk [51]. The sometimes conflicting results of multiple studies may reflect not only the potential methodological differences between studies, but also possibly the complexity of IBD pathogenesis itself [52]. Additional studies are needed to further define the potential role of diet in the pathogenesis of UC.

Immunology and Cell Biology

Activated cells of the mucosal immune system and elevated levels of pro-inflammatory cytokines and chemokines are present in the bowel of both UC and CD patients [18]. Previous studies implicate a dysregulation of activated intestinal (*cluster of differentiation*, CD4+) T cell subtypes of the adaptive immune system in the pathogenesis of IBD. More recent studies however suggest CD and UC both may involve Th17 T cells, which rely upon the IL-23 pathway [18]. IL-23, an essential cytokine involved in the crosstalk between innate and adaptive immunity [19], is secreted by macrophages and dendritic cells and promotes expansion of Th17 cells [19, 53]. Elevated levels of IL-23 and Th17 cytokines are detected in the colonic mucosa of UC and CD [18, 54, 55].

In more recent years, genetic studies such as GWA studies have revealed the importance of the epithelial barrier integrity in IBD pathogenesis [19]. GWA studies have discovered associations between UC and susceptibility single nucleotide polymorphisms in the *HNF4A, CDH1, LAMB1,* and *GNA12* regions, important in epithelial barrier function [56, 57]. These findings suggest that a disruption in the integrity of the epithelial barrier may play a role in the pathogenesis of UC. Linkage and candidate gene studies have determined variants in the XBP1 gene, associated with the unfolded protein response for both UC and CD [57–61]. Closely linked to autophagy and innate immunity, the unfolded protein response is triggered by endoplasmic reticulum stress due to accumulation of misfolded or unfolded proteins and is associated with Paneth cell function [57].

Clinical Signs and Symptoms

The typical symptoms of UC include rectal bleeding, diarrhea, and abdominal pain. The presentation can vary depending upon the extent of colonic involvement and severity of inflammation. The colon in UC is inflamed in a diffuse continuous distribution, extending from the rectum proximally. By convention, UC is classified according to the extent of disease into the following three subgroups: proctitis (disease limited to the rectum), left-sided colitis (disease extending to the sigmoid or descending colon, but not past the splenic flexure), and pancolitis (disease extending past the splenic flexure). The Paris classification system is a more detailed system developed for pediatric IBD clinical studies and includes detailed categories for UC disease location and severity, age, and growth status [62, 63]. Proctitis may present with tenesmus, urgency, and the passage of formed or semiformed stool with blood and mucus [64]. In contrast, pancolitis or left-sided disease may present with bloody diarrhea and significant abdominal pain. The majority of patients will present with a several week history of symptoms; however, some will present with a more acute clinical picture.

Although adults and children with UC can present with similar symptoms, there are differences in the clinical presentation of these two populations. Studies suggest that children with UC present with more extensive colonic involvement than adults with UC [3, 4, 65]. In a Danish study of 80 patients less than 15 years and 1080 patients 15 years of age or greater with UC, the younger group had more extensive disease at diagnosis compared to the older group diagnosed with UC [3]. Of the UC patients younger than 15 years of age, 29 % had pancolitis and 25 % had proctitis; in contrast, of the UC patients 15 years or older, 16 % had pancolitis and 46 % had proctitis [3]. Gryboski examined 38 children diagnosed with UC at ≤ 10 years old and reported 71 % with pancolitis, 13 % with left-sided colitis, and 6 % with proctitis [4]. Approximately 5 % of the children with UC have evidence of delayed linear growth and/or weight loss at diagnosis, although growth failure is much less frequent than in children with CD [4, 66] (see Table 30.2).

Table 30.2 Symptoms at initial presentation of ulcerative colitis in children and adolescents [3, 4, 66–69]. (Reprinted with permission from [67], Table 25.2, p. 388)

Clinical symptoms	Range of percentages
Rectal bleeding	75–98
Diarrhea	71–91
Abdominal pain	44–92
Weight loss	13–74
Arthralgia/arthritis	5–9
Fever	3–34
Growth retardation	4–5

Children with UC may present with varying degrees of disease severity. Approximately 50 % of the children with UC will present with a mild form of disease, characterized by an insidious onset of diarrhea and rectal bleeding, without abdominal pain or systemic symptoms such as fever. In these patients, disease may be confined to the distal colon [70, 71]. Disease of moderate severity is seen in 30 % of children with UC and is characterized by a more acute presentation with bloody diarrhea, tenesmus, and urgency; systemic symptoms including low-grade fever, abdominal tenderness, weight loss, and mild anemia may be present [70, 71]. Approximately 10 % of the children will present with a severe form of UC [70, 71]. Characteristic findings in severe disease include six or more bloody stools per day, fever, weight loss, anemia, hypoalbuminemia, and diffuse abdominal tenderness on physical exam [70–72]. A very small percentage of children will present initially with extraintestinal symptoms or manifestations, without obvious intestinal symptoms [71]. These extraintestinal manifestations of IBD may include axial or peripheral arthritis, erythema nodosum, pyoderma gangrenosum, or primary sclerosing cholangitis (see Sect. "Extraintestinal Manifestations").

Diagnosis

The diagnosis of UC is established by the information gathered from a detailed symptom and family history, physical examination, and a combination of laboratory, radiologic, endoscopic, and histologic findings. It is important to exclude other etiologies such as an infectious process and to distinguish UC from CD. Colonic inflammation is typically characterized by bloody diarrhea with abdominal cramping. The differential diagnosis of colitis depends upon the age of the child at the time of evaluation. In infancy, necrotizing enterocolitis, Hirschsprung's enterocolitis, and allergic colitis are diagnoses that should be considered. In children under age 3 who present with colitis, immunodeficiencies-causing colitis (such as IL-10 receptor deficiency and chronic granulomatous disease) should be excluded [73]. In contrast, in the older child and adolescent, enteric infection and idiopathic IBD are the most common diagnoses. (Causes of colitis are listed in Table 30.3.) In patients with painless rectal bleeding, other conditions (Meckel's diverticulum, polyp) should be considered. In addition to details of the clinical presentation, the history should include family history, recent antibiotic therapy, infectious exposures, growth and sexual development, and the presence of extraintestinal manifestations of UC.

Physical examination should include assessment of height, weight, and body mass index; abdominal distension, tenderness, or mass; extraintestinal manifestations (e.g., aphthous stomatitis, pyoderma gangrenosum, uveitis, or arthri-

Table 30.3 Differential diagnosis of colitis. (Reprinted with permission from [67], Table 25.3, p. 389)

2. Infectious etiologies
Campylobacter
Salmonella
Shigella
E. coli 0157: H7 and other enterohemorrhagic *E. coli*
Clostridium difficile
Aeromonas
Plesiomonas
Entamoeba histolytica
Cytomegalovirus
Herpes simplex virus
Yersinia
Tuberculosis
HIV and HIV-related opportunistic infections
3. Other
Ulcerative colitis
Crohn's disease
Henoch–Schonlein purpura
Hemolytic uremic syndrome
Intestinal ischemia
Intussusception
Allergic colitis (primarily in infancy)
Hirschsprung's enterocolitis (primarily in infancy)
Colitis complicating immunodeficiency

tis); fecal blood on rectal exam, perianal abnormalities (e.g., fistulae, fissures, or tags). Findings on physical examination may help to distinguish UC from CD; for example, pronounced growth failure or a perianal abscess strongly suggests the diagnosis of CD. A severely ill child with UC may have tachycardia, orthostatic hypotension, fever, or dehydration. Such findings in the presence of abdominal distention and a concerning abdominal exam may herald a fulminant presentation of UC with increased risk of developing toxic megacolon.

Laboratory Assessment

Initial laboratory evaluation should include appropriate blood tests, stool for occult blood, C. difficile toxin assay, and stool cultures. A complete blood cell count with differential may reveal a leukocytosis with or without left shift, anemia, and thrombocytosis. Thrombocytosis, hypoalbuminemia, and elevated erythrocyte sedimentation rate (ESR) or C-reactive protein (CRP) may indicate increased disease activity [74–76]. The presence of anemia with low mean corpuscular volume (MCV), wide red cell distribution width (RDW) and low iron levels may indicate an iron-deficient anemia secondary to ongoing fecal blood losses or the anemia of chronic disease. Children with UC may also have normal blood test results at the time of diagnosis [77].

Fecal calprotectin and lactoferrin are frequently elevated in active UC [78, 79], and may be useful screening tests. Fecal biomarkers are elevated in patients with active UC and CD, but are not specific for IBD [80]. Fecal biomarkers cannot distinguish between different etiologies of mucosal inflammation and are increased in other conditions, including enteric infections [80]. Thus, enteric infections should be ruled out. Fecal calprotectin and lactoferrin are the most commonly studied fecal biomarkers. In a meta-analysis of six adult and seven pediatric studies, among children and adolescents with suspected IBD, the pooled sensitivity and specificity of fecal calprotectin testing were 0.92 (95 % CI, 0.84–0.96) and 0.76 (95 % CI, 0.62–0.86), respectively [81].

It has been proposed that certain serum antibodies may be helpful for screening for IBD and discriminating UC from CD [82, 83]. Perinuclear antineutrophil cytoplasmic antibodies (p-ANCA) are seen in 60–80 % of adults with UC compared to 10–27 % of adults with CD [82, 84, 85]. Similarly, anti-*Saccharomyces cerevisiae* (ASCA) antibodies are commonly found in individuals with CD but are rarely seen in UC. In a study of 173 children, ASCA yielded a sensitivity of 55 % and specificity of 95 % for CD and ANCA had a sensitivity of 57 % and specificity of 92 % for UC [82]. In a study of 128 pediatric patients undergoing evaluation for IBD, Dubinsky and colleagues utilized modified cutoff values to optimize the sensitivity of the ASCA and ANCA assays. For the combination of ASCA and p-ANCA, the sensitivity of detecting IBD increased to 81 % with the modified values compared to the 69 % with standard cutoff values; however, this was accompanied by an increase in false positive rates among the children without IBD [83]. An overlap of ASCA and p-ANCA positive serology between patients with CD or UC remains. In particular, p-ANCA tends to test positive in the serum of patients with CD who exhibit UC features [82, 86]. Additional serological markers include antibodies to *Escherichia coli* outer membrane pori (OmpC), *Pseudomonas fluorescens*-associated sequence (I2), and flagellin (CBir1) [87]. In a study of greater than 300 children with suspected IBD, a serologic testing panel (including ASCA, p-ANCA, anti-OmpC and anti-CBir1) detected IBD with a sensitivity of 67 % and specificity of 76 %, compared to a sensitivity of 72 % and specificity of 94 % for a combination of three abnormal routine blood tests (hemoglobin, platelet count, and ESR) [87]. The value of these tests to supplement the routine diagnostic tests in IBD is a subject under study.

Endoscopic and Radiographic Evaluation

Evaluation with colonoscopy and ileoscopy with biopsies is the principal diagnostic test for UC. In patients with severe colitis, a limited flexible sigmoidoscopy examination with minimal air insufflation may be more appropriate, to avoid the risks of a full colonoscopy (perforation, hemorrhage, toxic dilatation). Upper endoscopy is also recommended by the "Porto" IBD Working Group of the European Society for Pediatric Gastroenterology, Hepatology and Nutrition (ESPGHAN). Small-bowel imaging should also be performed to exclude small-bowel involvement, which may change the diagnosis from UC to CD. Options for small-bowel evaluation include upper GI with small bowel follow through, computed tomography (CT) scan, or magnetic resonance imaging (MRI). The Porto expert panel has recommended MRI, over the other two modalities because of the absence of radiation; however, the quality of MRI varies from center to center, and small-bowel motion artifact may be sometimes confused with inflammation [88].

In order to establish the extent of disease involvement by colonoscopy, we recommend biopsies from the terminal ileum and each segment of the colon, even if there are no visible findings at a particular level of the colon. In UC, typical findings seen by the endoscopist include a diffuse, continuous process starting at the rectum and extending more proximally into the colon. However, atypical features, such as rectal sparing, have been reported in children with UC [89–92]. In addition, UC patients with distal colitis can present with a "cecal patch," discontinuous periappendiceal and cecal inflammation [92, 93]. The colonic mucosa often appears edematous, erythematous, and friable, with minute surface erosions and ulcerations (see Fig. 30.1). Larger, deeper ulcerations with associated exudate may develop in more severe disease. With long-standing UC, pseudopolyps may be present (see Fig. 30.2) [67]. In contrast, in CD, colonoscopy may reveal focal ulcerations (aphthous lesions) with intervening areas of normal-appearing mucosa (skip lesions). In severe or chronic CD, linear ulcerations,

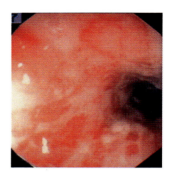

Fig. 30.1 Severe ulcerative colitis in a patient unresponsive to corticosteroid therapy. The colonoscopy demonstrates a featureless colon with loss of vascular pattern, ulcerations, and hemorrhage

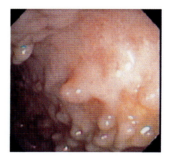

Fig. 30.2 Multiple colonic pseudopolyps in a 17-year-old female with ulcerative colitis, with intermittent disease activity despite 2 years of maintenance therapy with thiopurine. (Reprinted with permission from [67], Fig. 25.2, p. 391)

nodularity (cobblestoning), and strictures or stenoses may be present. In general, the ulcerations in CD are deeper and focal versus the diffuse, superficial ulcerations typical of UC (see Table 30.4) [89, 90, 94–97].

Table 30.4 Typical endoscopy and histopathology findings—ulcerative colitis versus Crohn's disease [89, 90, 94–98]. (Reprinted with permission from [67], Table 25.4, p. 392)

Characteristic	Ulcerative colitis	Crohn's disease
Endoscopy findings	Diffuse continuous involvement extending from rectum	Focal lesions/disease interspersed with normal appearing mucosa (skip lesions)
	Rectum usually involved[a]	Rectal sparing possible
	Diffuse, superficial, minute ulcerations; deeper ulcerations in severe disease	Aphthous lesions often surrounded by normal appearing mucosa; deep "collar button" ulcers; linear or serpiginous ulcerations
	Strictures very rare	Strictures, often occurring in terminal ileum
	Pseudopolyps	
Histopathology findings	No granulomas[b]	Granulomas (36%)
	Diffuse chronic inflammation limited to the mucosa[c], crypt abscesses	Focal chronic inflammation, transmural inflammation
	+/− architectural distortion[d]	

[a] In children, "rectal sparing" has been seen in UC [89, 90]
[b] Giant cell reactions can occur around damaged crypts and spilled mucin. This must be distinguished from "true" granulomas, which by definition, are not seen in UC [96]
[c] Deeper layers of the colon may be involved in fulminant UC disease
[d] In children with UC, initial colonic biopsies at time of diagnosis are less likely to show architectural distortion than biopsies from adults [97]

Although by definition, the disease of UC is confined to the colon, children with CD or UC can have inflammation of the upper gastrointestinal tract. In a pediatric IBD registry study of 898 patients (643 with UC, 255 with CD colitis), authors examined the presence of macroscopic upper gastrointestinal involvement (ulcerations, aphthous lesions, or erosions) in accordance with the Paris classification system among the 260 patients with UC and 86 patients with CD colitis who underwent upper endoscopy with detailed documentation of lesions [62, 92]. Among the UC patients, gastric erosions were identified in 3.1%, gastric ulcerations in 0.4%, and erosions or ulcerations limited to the esophagus or duodenum in 0.8%. In contrast, upper gastrointestinal lesions were noted in 22% of the patients with Crohn's colitis [92]. Except for the presence of granulomas of CD, it may be difficult to distinguish between UC and CD by the appearance of upper gastrointestinal lesions.

Plain abdominal radiographs and abdominal/pelvic CT scans evaluations may aid in the assessment for complications of UC, including toxic megacolon, perforation, or stricture. Plain abdominal radiograph may demonstrate thumbprinting, loss of haustral patterns, colonic dilatation (i.e., toxic megacolon), obstruction, or pneumoperitoneum (i.e., perforation of the bowel) [99–101].

Pathology of Ulcerative Colitis

In active UC, typical findings on histopathology include a diffuse inflammatory cell infiltrate of the lamina propria mostly with plasma cells, lymphocytes, and neutrophils, but mast cells and eosinophils are also seen. Neutrophils invade the epithelium of the crypts, leading to cryptitis, crypt abscess formation, and goblet cell mucin depletion (see Fig. 30.3) [67]. The inflammatory infiltrate is typically confined to the mucosa, but in severe UC, ulceration may extend into the submucosa and deeper layers [96]. In quiescent (inactive) UC, the inflammatory infiltrate may diminish but signs of chronic colitis (architectural distortion, crypt branching and shortening, reduction in the number of crypts, and separation of crypts) can persist [96]. In children with UC, signs of chronic colitis (e.g., architectural distortion) are not always seen [91, 97].

Histologic differentiation of UC from CD can be difficult. The histologic hallmark of CD is the noncaseating granuloma, which may be found in 25–48% of children with CD [98, 102, 103]. However, a giant cell reaction mimicking a granuloma can occur around damaged crypts and spilled mucin. These "mucin granulomas" must be distinguished from true granulomas, which by definition, are not seen in UC [96]. Histologic skip areas, rectal sparing, focal inflammation, and transmural inflammation also suggest the diagnosis of CD. However, in children, histological skip areas

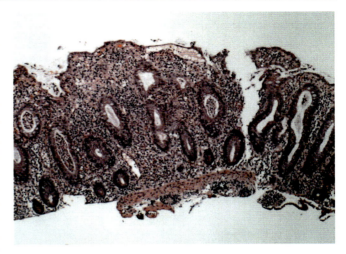

Fig. 30.3 Low power view of a colonic biopsy from a patient with active ulcerative colitis. Note the increased lamina propria inflammatory infiltrate, crypt abscesses, and crypt architectural distortion. The crypts are irregular in shape and placement and do not descend to the level of the muscularis mucosae. (Courtesy of Jonathan Glickman, MD, PhD, Director, Gastrointestinal Pathology, Miraca Life Sciences and Associate Clinical Professor of Pathology, Harvard Medical School). (Reprinted with permission from [67], Fig. 25.2, p. 393)

may occur both at initial presentation of UC and as a result of therapy [89, 91, 104]. Rarely, children with UC present with focal active colitis at initial presentation [91]. In addition, patients with UC can have histological evidence of upper gastrointestinal inflammation similar to that in CD [105–107]. Given the overlap of histopathology findings in UC and CD, it may be difficult to distinguish between these two diagnoses if granulomas are not present.

If a clinician cannot reliably distinguish between CD and UC based on the available clinical, radiographic, and endoscopic data, an interim diagnosis of IBD-unclassified (indeterminate colitis) may be given until the patient can be more clearly classified in the future. The ESPGHAN Porto group developed detailed criteria to better define the IBD-unclassified subtype [88]. The prevalence of IBD-unclassified in adults and children with IBD is estimated to be 10–20% [65, 108]. Approximately one third of these patients will later be classified as UC or CD [109].

Extraintestinal Manifestations

Approximately 25–30% of the children and adolescents diagnosed with IBD develop extraintestinal symptoms [110–113]. Extraintestinal manifestations of IBD may occur before, during, or after the development of gastrointestinal symptoms and may appear after surgical removal of diseased bowel [110, 114–117]. The clinical activity of the extraintestinal manifestations may or may not correlate with the activity of intestinal inflammation.

Joint manifestations (arthropathy) occur in 5–20 % of the children with UC [4, 112, 114]. These can be classified into two main clinical forms: a peripheral arthropathy and an axial arthropathy (e.g., ankylosing spondylitis) [110, 114]. Patients with IBD develop peripheral arthropathies in approximately 5–20 % of the cases [110, 111, 114, 118]. The peripheral arthropathy generally is asymmetrical, nondeforming and migratory, affecting mostly the large joints of the lower extremities including the knees, ankles, and hips. Less commonly the upper limb joints or hands are affected [110, 114, 118]. Small joints of the hands and feet generally are spared [114].

Exacerbations of peripheral joint disease seem to parallelly increase the activity of bowel disease in UC or CD. The pauciarticular arthropathy is more likely to be correlated with exacerbations of bowel disease [117].

Axial arthropathies associated with HLA B27 occur in 1–4 % of patients [110, 111, 114, 118]. Ankylosing spondylitis associated with IBD runs a course independent of the activity of bowel disease, and may progress to permanent deformity [110, 114, 118]. In addition to the two main forms of joint manifestations, individuals with UC can develop isolated arthritis involving large joints including the sacroiliac joints, hips, and shoulders [118].

Pyoderma gangrenosum (PG) and erythema nodosum (EN) are the two main skin manifestations associated with UC and CD. PG occurs in < 1–5 % of the patients with UC [111, 115] and often is associated with active disease and extensive colonic involvement [115, 119]. The classic PG lesion often begins as a discrete pustule with surrounding erythema, then extends peripherally to develop into an ulceration with a well-defined border and a deep erythematous to violaceous color [120]. The lesions of PG tend to be multiple and localize below the knees, and can develop at sites of trauma and previous surgical sites, including scars and ileostomy stomas [119–121]. Approximately 40 % of the patients with UC and PG also develop joint symptoms [69]. EN occurs more frequently with CD (27 %) in comparison to UC (4 %) [111] and usually coincides with increased bowel disease activity [69, 111, 118]. EN lesions appear as tender, warm, red nodules, or raised plaques and usually localize to the extensor surfaces of the lower extremities [122]. Both PG and EN can precede the development of bowel symptoms and PG can occur after bowel resection [69]. Other skin manifestations include Sweet's syndrome (acute febrile neutrophilic dermatosis) and oral lesions include aphthous lesions and pyostomatitis (pyoderma) vegetans [123].

Ophthalmologic abnormalities are described in approximately 1–3 % of the children with IBD [110]. Uveitis and episcleritis are the more common ocular disorders reported [110, 124]. Uveitis associated with IBD in children may be asymptomatic, and thus, the incidence of associated eye findings may be underreported in the literature [125].

Ocular inflammation appears to develop more commonly in patients with other extraintestinal manifestations [125], including arthritis and may be associated with genes in the human leukocyte antigen (HLA) region [126]. In addition, corticosteroid use increases the risk of increased intraocular pressure and the development of posterior subcapsular cataracts [127, 128]. Given the potential eye complications, children with IBD should be monitored carefully at regular intervals.

Hepatic abnormalities in children with UC have been well described. While these are typically identified after the UC diagnosis, they may also precede the gastrointestinal symptoms [116, 129]. Transient elevations of alanine aminotransferase (ALT) occur in 12 % of the children with UC and appear to be related to medications or disease activity [129]. Persistent ALT elevations suggest the presence of primary sclerosing cholangitis (PSC) or autoimmune chronic hepatitis [129]. Among children with UC, approximately 3 % develop sclerosing cholangitis and < 1 % develop chronic hepatitis [129, 130].

The diagnosis of PSC may be established through a combination of cholangiography and liver biopsy [131]. There is a paucity of the literature addressing the long-term outcome of children with PSC specifically associated with UC [129]. In children with PSC (with or without IBD), later age at presentation, splenomegaly, and prolonged prothrombin time at presentation were associated with poor outcome, defined as death or listing for transplantation [116]. Patients with UC and PSC are also at increased risk for developing colon cancer. Fatty changes of the liver observed on liver biopsies of patients with UC or CD may be secondary to malnutrition, protein losses, anemia, and corticosteroid use [132].

The IBD population has a threefold overall increased risk for venous thromboembolism (VTE) compared with individuals without IBD [133–135]. VTE occurs in 1–2 % of the children and adolescents hospitalized for active IBD [136, 137]. Although the incidence of VTE appears less than the rate noted in the adult population, these events can result in significant morbidity for younger patients [135]. Thrombotic events range from clots associated with venous catheters to more significant events such as deep vein thrombosis, pulmonary embolism, and cerebral vascular accidents. These events can lead to ongoing associated complications and long-term sequelae, including permanent neurologic deficits, persistent or recurrent thrombosis, embolization, and post-thrombotic syndrome [136]. Factors that can further increase the risk for thromboembolism include an indwelling central venous catheter, severe disease activity, older age, parenteral nutrition, known thrombophilia, first-degree family history of VTE, persistence of anti-phospholipid antibody for greater than 12 weeks, oral contraceptives, smoking, obesity, and medications associated with increased risk of thrombosis such as thalidomide [136, 137].

At a minimum, all hospitalized children and adolescents with IBD should maintain adequate hydration and receive mechanical thrombotic prophylaxis, such as encouraged ambulation, compression stockings, or pneumatic boots [137, 138]. The role of primary pharmacologic prophylaxis for thromboembolism remains controversial for children and adolescents with IBD. At our institution, we have implemented a risk stratification strategy to identify hospitalized IBD patients at higher risk for thrombosis, who warrant for primary prophylaxis pharmacologic anticoagulation therapy [136, 137]. For IBD patients who develop thromboembolism, anticoagulation with low-molecular-weight heparin appears feasible without major sequelae of increased bleeding or complications [136].

Rarely, other hematologic abnormalities associated with UC occur, including immune thrombocytopenic purpura [139] and autoimmune hemolytic anemia [140]. Osteopenia–low bone mineral density occurs in children with UC, but less often than in children with CD [141, 142]. Corticosteroid use increases the risk of osteopenia in children with IBD [141, 142]. Other extraintestinal manifestations include nephrolithiasis [111, 143], pancreatitis (related or unrelated to medications) [144, 145], and pulmonary and cardiac involvement [110].

Complications

Complications of UC include massive hemorrhage, toxic megacolon, perforation of the bowel, strictures, and colon cancer. Massive hemorrhage can occur with severe UC and is managed with blood transfusions and treatment of the underlying UC, and urgent colectomy may be required. One consensus group suggested that an individual with UC who requires more than 6–8 units of blood in the first 48 h and is still actively bleeding should undergo a colectomy [146]. Colonic perforation is the most dangerous complication of UC, can occur in the setting of severe UC with or without toxic colonic dilatation [147–149], and requires urgent colectomy.

Toxic megacolon is a potentially life-threatening complication of UC and is characterized by total or segmental non-obstructive colonic dilatation of at least 6 cm in adults associated with systemic toxicity [148, 150, 151]. Previous reports suggest a lifetime risk of toxic megacolon complicating IBD of 1–5%, but this has decreased more recently, probably secondary to earlier recognition and improved management of severe colitis [148, 152]. Most likely, the pathogenesis of toxic megacolon is multifactorial [148]. In contrast to typical UC, in which the inflammatory changes are limited to the mucosa, in toxic megacolon, the severe inflammation extends into the deeper layers of the colonic wall [147]. It is thought that the spread of the inflammatory process to the smooth-muscle layer may lead to the paralysis of the colonic smooth muscle and subsequent dilatation of the colon [148].

Several triggering factors have been reported to precede the development of toxic megacolon [147, 148]. Medications that can impair colonic motility should be avoided and have been implicated as precipitating factors, including narcotic agents for pain or antidiarrheal effects, anticholinergic agents, drugs that decrease motility, or antidepressants with significant anticholinergic effects [147, 153, 154]. A barium enema or colonoscopy may cause distention that can further impair the colonic wall blood supply and may increase the mucosal uptake of bacterial products [148]. Barium enema examinations have been reported in proximity to the development of toxic megacolon [154, 155]. The early discontinuation or rapid tapering of steroids or 5-aminosalicylic acid agents may contribute to the development of toxic megacolon [147, 148]. Electrolyte abnormalities, such as hypokalemia, have been observed in the setting of toxic megacolon, though it is not clear whether this finding is a causative factor or secondary to the illness itself [147]. Along with colonic dilatation, patients with toxic megacolon present with systemic findings including fever, tachycardia, leukocytosis, and anemia [150]. A decrease in the number of stools may herald the onset of toxic megacolon. With progressive disease, these individuals can develop dehydration, mental status changes, electrolyte disturbances, hypotension, and increasing abdominal distension and tenderness, with or without signs of peritonitis [148, 150].

Abdominal X-ray reveals colonic dilatation, most frequently involving the transverse colon, sometimes accompanied by inflammatory changes including absent or markedly edematous haustral pattern [156] (see Fig. 30.4).

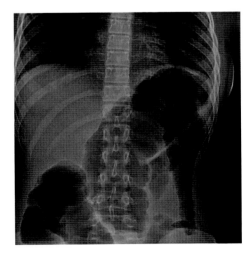

Fig. 30.4 Toxic megacolon in a teenager with fulminant ulcerative colitis. There is a massively dilated loop of transverse colon. This patient developed the megacolon despite corticosteroid therapy, and subsequently underwent emergent surgery. (Courtesy of Anne Wolf, M.D. and Matthew Egberg, M.D., Division of Gastroenterology, Hepatology and Nutrition, Boston Children's Hospital)

Because the transverse colon is the most anterior portion of the colon, air will tend to accumulate in this segment of the colon when the patient is in the supine position; however, with repositioning of the patient, the colonic air will redistribute, filling other segments of the bowel [157].

The management of toxic megacolon is detailed in multiple reviews elsewhere [147, 148]. If toxic megacolon is present, surgical consultation is essential and the patient will most likely require a colectomy. Early surgical intervention is indicated in the setting of failed medical therapy with progressive colonic dilatation, worsening systemic toxicity, perforation, or uncontrolled hemorrhage [148].

Both benign and malignant colonic strictures can develop in long-standing UC [158–160]. Benign strictures present most commonly in the rectum and the sigmoid, are due to smooth muscle hypertrophy, and are thought to be potentially reversible [158]. Colonic strictures should be evaluated for possible malignancy, but the majority of strictures in UC are benign [158–160]. There is an increased risk of dysplasia and colon cancer in patients with long-standing UC, which is addressed later in this chapter (see Sect. "Prognosis/Follow-Up").

Treatment Options

The treatment goals for children with UC are the control of active disease and induction of remission, the long-term maintenance of remission, and provision of education and psychosocial support for the patient and family. The initial treatment of UC is medical, with surgery reserved for patients with severe disease, patients with medically refractory disease, or patients who develop adverse effects of medical therapy.

Knowledge of the extent and severity of disease involvement will enable the clinician to choose the appropriate therapy for each individual patient. Distal UC (left-sided UC or proctitis) is characterized by involvement limited to the area distal to the splenic flexure, and potentially may be treated with topical agents (e.g., aminosalicylate or hydrocortisone enemas or suppositories). Extensive UC is defined by involvement extending proximal to the splenic flexure and requires systemic therapies with or without additional topical agents. Severity of disease is usually simple to ascertain, and can be determined by assessing stool frequency and consistency, abdominal pain, nocturnal diarrhea, hematocrit, albumin level, and feeding intolerance. Separate published disease severity criteria for adults and children have been developed by Truelove and Witts, and Werlin and Grand, respectively [72, 161]. Typically, severe colitis requires hospitalization and administration of either intravenous corticosteroids or other immunosuppressive agents (e.g., cyclosporine, tacrolimus, infliximab). Many patients with severe colitis will require colectomy.

Turner and colleagues developed the pediatric ulcerative colitis activity index (PUCAI), a noninvasive, clinically based, validated instrument to assess disease activity in pediatric patients with UC [162]. The PUCAI is a score comprised of six parameters, including the assessment of abdominal pain, rectal bleeding, stool consistency, number of stools per 24 h, nocturnal stools, and activity level. Each item is assigned a value contributing to a combined, total PUCAI score ranging from 0 to 85. Categories of UC disease activity are defined by the following total PUCAI scores: 0–9 (no activity), 10–34 (mild activity), 35–64 (moderate activity), and 65–85 (severe activity). The PUCAI correlated well with the physician's global assessment, Mayo score, and macroscopic findings at colonoscopy. In addition to excellent interobserver and test–retest reliability, the PUCAI performed well on longitudinal assessment with excellent responsiveness at repeated visits, thus providing a tool to serially assess patients' clinical status [162]. Studies demonstrate the application and feasibility of the PUCAI in hospitalized pediatric patients with severe colitis and in the outpatient setting [163, 164]. Although the PUCAI provides a method to track UC disease activity, it does not replace the need for the appropriate serial thorough clinical evaluation of children and adolescents with active UC. Presently, there is no pediatric-specific UC endoscopic index available.

Induction Therapy

Mild to Moderate Colitis

In the child with mild to moderate UC, with no or only minimal systemic signs (such as elevated ESR or mild anemia), aminosalicylates (e.g., sulfasalazine, olsalazine, mesalamine, balsalazide) are usually the first line of therapy (see Tables 30.5 and 30.6).

Mesalamine is a 5-aminosalicylic acid compound used in the induction and maintenance treatment of UC. It was discovered as the active anti-inflammatory moiety of sulfasalazine, which has been used to treat UC since the 1940s [166]. More than 88 % of all the UC patients receive treatment with aminosalicylate (ASA) agents; however, fewer than 50 % of the children with UC can maintain long-term steroid free remission on ASA monotherapy [167]. Sulfasalazine contains mesalamine bound to sulfapyridine via an azo bond, which is released by bacterial azo-reductase in the small bowel and colon. Sulfapyridine is inactive, but is absorbed in the colon and is mostly responsible for hypersensitivity reaction and adverse effects associated with sulfasalazine [168].

ASA agents have multiple immunologic effects. Potential mechanisms of action include the inhibition of the synthesis of leukotriene B_4, a potent chemotactic and chemokinetic agent, and the inhibition of the activation of nuclear transcription factor kappa B (NF-kappaB), an important

Table 30.5 Aminosalicylate agents [a]. (Reprinted with permission from [67], Table 25.7, p. 398)

Oral preparations	Dosage form	Mechanism of release	Site of delivery
Azo-bond			
Sulfasalazine (Azulfidine)	500 mg tablet	Bacterial cleavage of azo bond	Colon
Olsalazine (Dipentum)	250 mg capsule	Bacterial cleavage of azo bond	Colon
Balsalazide (Colazal/Colazide)	750 mg capsule	Bacterial cleavage of azo bond	Colon
Delayed release			
Mesalamine (Delzicol/Asacol HD)	400 mg/800 mg tablets	pH-dependent breakdown (pH > 7)	Distal ileum to colon
Mesalamine (Salofalk/Mesasal/Claversal)	250 mg/500 mg tablets	pH-dependent breakdown (pH > 6)	Ileum to colon
Extended, delayed release			
Mesalamine			
(Lialda)	1.2 g tablet	pH-dependent breakdown (pH > 7)	
(Apriso)	375 mg capsule	pH-dependent breakdown (pH > 6)	
Sustained release			
Mesalamine (Pentasa)	250 mg/500 mg/1000 mg tablets	Ethylcellulose-controlled time-release	Small intestine to colon
Rectal preparations			
Mesalamine suppository (Canasa–500 mg)	400 mg/500 mg/1000 mg		Rectum
Mesalamine enema (Rowasa–4 g/60 ml)	1 g/4 g; 60-ml/100-ml suspension		Rectum to splenic flexure

[a] Availability of different preparations and dosage forms varies among different markets/countries

mediator of the immune response in inflammatory processes [169–171].

Controlled studies suggest that currently available ASAs are superior to placebo for induction of remission and relapse prevention [172–175]. However, there do not appear to be any differences in efficacy between the older agent, sulfasalazine, and newer ASA drugs [175, 176].

Potential advantages of the non-sulfa ASA agents include better tolerance compared to sulfasalazine [176, 177] and the availability of a non-sulfa ASA agent for sulfa-sensitive individuals. In adult-onset UC, balsalazide at higher doses (6.75 g/day) may provide a faster improvement in active, mild-to-moderate UC than lower doses of balsalazide (2.25 g/day) or mesalamine (2.4 g/day) [178, 179].

Long-acting formulations of mesalamine are available, however there is no FDA approved pediatric dose. They are available as a delayed release multi-matrix formulation (Lialda) and a pH-controlled granule that releases mesalamine at pH > 6 (as in the colon, Apriso).

Common side effects of sulfasalazine include headache, nausea, and fatigue, which improve with reduction of the dose [180] (see Table 30.6). The sulfa moiety can cause hypersensitivity reactions resulting in rash, fever, hepatitis, hemolytic anemia, bone marrow suppression, and pneumonitis [180, 181]. Other side effects include neutropenia, oligospermia, pancreatitis, and the exacerbation of colitis [72, 182]. Folic acid supplementation is recommended given that

sulfasalazine impairs the absorption of folic acid and may lead to anemia [180]. To decrease side effects, sulfasalazine is started at a dose of 10–20 mg/kg/day and gradually increased to the full dose (50–75 mg/kg/day) over 5–7 days mesalamine and the other non-sulfa ASA agents have also been associated with adverse reactions, including pancreatitis, hepatitis, nephritis, exacerbation of colitis, and pneumonitis [180, 183, 184].

Moderate Colitis

Children with moderate disease are usually managed with oral corticosteroids (usually 1 mg/kg/day, up to 60 mg/day of prednisone) as an outpatient. Corticosteroids are effective for short-term treatment, but up to 45 % of the pediatrics patients develop corticosteroid dependence in subsequent years putting them at risk for steroid-related side effects [185].

Potential short-term complications of steroid therapy in patients with UC include increased appetite, weight gain, fluid retention, mood swings, hyperglycemia, hypertension, insomnia, acne, and facial swelling. Complications of long-term steroid therapy (usually of greater than 3 months) include growth retardation, osteopenia with compression fractures, aseptic necrosis of the hip, and cataracts [180, 186]. Given these reasons and the suppression of the hypothalamic–pituitary–adrenal axis, corticosteroids should be tapered shortly after remission is achieved. A standard taper utilized by the authors is reduction by 5 mg/week of pred-

Table 30.6 Medical therapies forUC. (Reprinted with permission from [67], Table 25.8, p. 399)

Medication	Dosage	Major side effects
Sulfasalazine	50–75 mg/kg/day PO divided bid or tid (Maximum 6 g/day) Adult dose: 3–4 g/day divided bid or tid	Nausea, headaches, diarrhea, photosensitivity, hypersensitivity reaction, pancreatitis, azoospermia, hemolytic anemia, neutropenia
Mesalamine		
Oral formulation	50–75 mg/kg/day PO divided qid, tid, or bid (may vary according to preparation) (Maximum 6 g/day) Adult dose: 3–4 g/ day divided qid, tid, or bid	Nausea, headaches, diarrhea, pancreatitis, nephritis, pericarditis, pleuritis
Enema formulation	2–4 g PR q 12–24 h	
Suppository formulation	500 mg PR q 12–24 h	
Corticosteroids		
IV or oral formulation	1–2 mg/kg/day of prednisone or equivalent, IV or PO, divided q 12–24 h (maximum 60 mg/ day)	Numerous, including Cushing's syndrome, growth suppression, immunosuppression, hypertension, hyperglycemia, increased appetite, osteoporosis, aseptic necrosis (hip), cataracts
Enema formulation	50–100 mg of hydrocortisone PR qhs	
Suppository formulation	25 mg of hydrocortisone acetate PR qhs	
Azathioprine[a]	1.5–2.5 mg/kg/day PO qd	Nausea, emesis, immunosuppression, hepatotoxicity, pancreatitis, myelosuppression, lymphoma
6-Mercaptopurine[a]	1.0–2.0 mg/kg/day PO qd	Nausea, emesis, immunosuppression, hepatotoxicity, pancreatitis, myelosuppression, lymphoma
Cyclosporine	Induction regimen for fulminant colitis: initial dose: 4 mg/kg/day IV continuous or bid; maintenance oral dose varies according to oral preparation	Nephrotoxicity, hypertension, headache, hirsutism, nausea, emesis, diarrhea, tremor, hypomagnesemia, hyperkalemia, hepatotoxicity, seizures, gingival hyperplasia, lymphoproliferative disorder
Tacrolimus	0.2 mg/kg/day PO divided bid	Nephrotoxicity, hypertension, headache, immunosuppression, nausea, emesis, tremor, hypomagnesemia, elevated liver enzymes, hyperglycemia, seizures, lymphoproliferative disorder
Infliximab	Loading dose: 5 mg/kg/dose IV at 0, 2, 6 weeks; maintenance dose: 5 mg/kg/dose IV q 4–8 weeks (can go up to 10 mg/kg every 4 weeks)	Infusion reactions, delayed hypersensitivity reactions, immunosuppression (opportunistic infections), lupus-like syndrome, hepatotoxicity, blood dyscrasias, psoriasis, neurotoxicity (demyelination), vasculitis, possible lymphoma
Adalimumab	Adult dosing—Loading dose: 160 mg, then 80 mg; maintenance dose: 40 mg SQ every other week (can go up to 40 mg weekly)	Injection site pain/ reactions, immunosuppression (opportunistic infections), psoriasis, blood dyscrasias, possible lymphoma

[a] TPMT genotype determines metabolism and blood levels of metabolites; may help to determine risk of myelosuppression and optimal dosage of azathioprine or 6-mercaptopurine

IV intravenous, *PO* oral, *TPMT* thiopurine S-methyltransferase

nisone down to 20 mg/day, and then a more gradual taper on alternate days, aiming for 10 mg every other day with further taper and cessation if remission is maintained [186]. The high frequency of side effects with traditional systemic steroids such as prednisone has led to the development of steroid preparations with high first-pass metabolism and few systemic effects.

Severe Colitis

Children with severe disease typically defined by a PUCAI greater than 65 (e.g., more than five bowel movements/day, liquid bloody stools, or severe pain with defecation, anemia, and hypoalbuminemia) require intravenous corticosteroids (methylprednisolone at 40–60 mg/day, divided into two doses/day, approximately 1–2 mg/kg/day) and hospitalization for further evaluation, observation, and management [187, 188]. Rectal corticosteroids or 5-ASA agents may be used as an adjunctive therapy with parenteral corticosteroids

for patients with severe tenesmus [180]. Intravenous fluid for rehydration and correction of electrolyte imbalances should be provided. Blood transfusions and albumin infusions may be required. Although traditionally patients are restricted from taking food orally, there is no data to support holding the oral diet in UC as there is in CD; however, if bowel rest is indicated, the child may require central venous access for parenteral nutrition support [189, 190].

In addition to high-dose steroids, empiric antibiotics are sometimes used in severe colitis, though the efficacy of antibiotics has not been proven [191–194]. Assessment for response to intensive medical therapy includes resolution of fever, tachycardia, abdominal tenderness, and macroscopic blood per rectum. Stools should be decreasing in frequency, but may still be unformed. Following the PUCAI will help guide therapy. Once the child shows significant improvement, diet is advanced to a low-residue diet, intravenous methylprednisolone is switched to oral prednisone, and similar parameters for steroid wean are followed as outlined above. The optimal duration of intravenous corticosteroid therapy is unclear, but most children will respond within 7–10 days.

Approximately 50 % of the patients treated with intravenous corticosteroids will not respond. Turner and colleagues have published an excellent consensus statement on the use of rescue agents in the management of severe UC. In summary, the PUCAI can be utilized to track disease activity. If the child has not responded to steroid therapy (as assessed by a PUCAI drop of 20 points or more after 5–7 days), the options of surgery or more intensive immunosuppression (intravenous cyclosporine, infliximab, or oral tacrolimus) should be considered and discussed with the family. Intensive immunosuppression should not be started if surgery is believed imminent, such as in a septic patient, a patient with toxic megacolon, or a patient with a suspected perforation. Flexible sigmoidoscopy is indicated prior to the institution of calcineurin inhibitors or biologics to exclude cytomegalovirus [195].

The medical agents utilized to treat steroid refractory colitis in the hospitalized patient are calcineurin inhibitors and biologics. In the past decade, infliximab has been the agent most commonly utilized, perhaps due to its ease of administration and more favorable side-effect profile. Approximately 70 % of the children and adults treated with infliximab will respond [164, 196]. The role of monitoring infliximab levels during treatment of severe colitis is still a topic under study. However, patients with severe colitis may have an increased loss of infliximab in the stool, and may require higher more frequent dosing than the 5 mg/kg utilized in the clinical trials (which included less sick patients) [197]. Adalimumab also has been utilized in severe colitis [198]. Calcineurin inhibitors such as cyclosporine and tacrolimus are reasonable alternatives to biologics, and have been utilized for over 20 years. However, because of long-term renal toxicity, it is generally recommended that these agents be utilized as short-term induction agents for a few months, and that patients should transition to maintenance therapy with thiopurines or anti-tumor necrosis factor-alpha (anti-TNF) agents [199]. Calcineurin inhibitors may also be utilized as a steroid sparing "bridge" to surgery [200]. The timing of colectomy in a child who is not responding to intravenous corticosteroids or other immunosuppression can be difficult. It should be emphasized that even if a child responds to immunosuppression, such as cyclosporine, there is a high likelihood that he/she will require a colectomy within a year [201, 202]. If immunosuppression with cyclosporine is used and the child does not respond to these medications within 10–14 days, surgery should be strongly recommended.

Close monitoring of the patients with severe colitis for the development of fulminant colitis and associated complications including hemorrhage, toxic megacolon, and perforation is essential using serial abdominal exams, complimented by serial abdominal films or other imaging as necessary. Physical examination should assess for evidence of worsening abdominal tenderness, distention, and hypoactive bowel sounds; these may herald the development of toxic megacolon. The appearance of persistent abdominal pain and distention, diffuse abdominal tenderness and rebound, fever and tachycardia are worrisome signs of an acute abdomen and may signal need for emergent surgical intervention. Opiates and loperimide should be avoided given the increased risk of developing toxic megacolon [153]. Steroid therapy may mask the typical symptoms and signs of perforation, but this may be detected by serial upright abdominal films (see Sect. "Complications").

Left-Sided Colitis/Proctitis

Topical ASA or topical corticosteroids are effective in the treatment of proctitis, proctosigmoiditis, or left-sided UC [203–205] (see Tables 30.5 and 30.6). To be effective, topical therapy must reach the most proximal extent of the disease activity. Mesalamine enemas or suppositories are effective as first-line/maintenance therapy for mild or moderately active left-sided UC or proctitis, respectively [180]. Rectal mesalamine may be superior to oral mesalamine in the treatment of active ulcerative proctitis [206]. Mesalamine enemas may be superior to rectal corticosteroids [207] and are also effective in treating distal colitis that is unresponsive to oral ASAs or corticosteroids [208, 209]. Combination therapy with oral and topical mesalamine is more effective than one agent alone in the treatment of mild to moderate distal colitis [210]. Mesalamine suppositories spread to the upper rectum, and enemas and foams can reach the splenic flexure or into the distal transverse colon [208, 209].

Corticosteroid suppositories or enemas also can be used as first-line induction therapy in patients with mild or moderately active ulcerative proctitis or left-sided UC [180]. Rectal administration of hydrocortisone or prednisolone permits more direct delivery of steroids to distal UC sites; however, as with oral steroid therapy, prolonged treatment with topical steroids may induce systemic steroid side effects, including adrenal suppression [205, 209]. Topical agents such as budesonide enemas may induce remission in distal colitis with fewer systemic steroids side effects [211, 212]. Some evidence suggests that ASA enemas may be superior to hydrocortisone enemas [204, 207, 209].

Maintenance Therapy

5-Aminosalicylic Acid Agents

Medication for the prevention of relapse after induction of remission often is started before the induction therapy is discontinued. The clinician usually aims to transition a patient from corticosteroids onto sulfasalazine or another ASA agent. Multiple studies of adults with UC demonstrate the effectiveness of sulfasalazine and other ASA agents in preventing relapse [176]. Mesalamine is well-tolerated in the long-term treatment of children with IBD, with the principal adverse event being exacerbation of diarrhea [213]. Sulfasalazine and newer ASAs are all effective in maintaining remission in UC [177]. Balsalazide, at a higher dose (6 g/day), also may be more effective in preventing relapses of UC in adults, compared to lower-dose balsalazide (3 g/day) and mesalamine (1.5 g/day) [214]. Topical mesalamine can effectively prevent relapse of active distal UC [215], but because of the rectal route of administration, patients may prefer oral mesalamine for maintenance therapy. The combination of oral and topical ASA therapy may be more effective in preventing relapse than oral ASA therapy alone, especially for distal disease [216]. Children with UC require years of maintenance therapy. The exact duration that a UC patient in remission should remain on maintenance therapy is unclear, and there are no formal guidelines on when or if maintenance therapy should be discontinued. The risk of discontinuing maintenance medication is the possibility of relapse. In addition, maintenance with ASA or other agents may reduce the risk of colorectal neoplasia [217–219].

6-Mercaptopurine and Azathioprine

The immunomodulatory drugs, azathioprine (AZA) and its metabolite 6-mercaptopurine (6MP), can reduce disease activity and allow the withdrawal of steroid therapy in children with steroid-dependent UC [220, 221].

AZA is nonenzymatically metabolized to 6MP, and the two drugs have identical mechanisms of action. AZA is 55% 6MP by molecular weight and therefore dosed higher mg per kg. As AZA is the prodrug of 6MP, the dose of AZA is approximately twice that of 6MP [222]. The mechanism of action of 6MP and AZA is to interrupt RNA and DNA synthesis, thereby downregulating cytokines, T cell activity, and delayed hypersensitivity reactions and by inducing T cell apoptosis by blocking the activation of the gene rac-1 [223].

The use of thiopurines in UC as steroid sparing maintenance agents is long established. Given their steroid-sparing effects [220, 221] and reasonable tolerance by children with IBD [224], AZA and 6MP offer an alternative maintenance treatment of IBD in children. A prospective multicenter registry study in pediatric UC patients found 50% of children with UC starting thiopurine therapy were disease free 1 year later, without the need for rescue therapy [225].

The metabolism of AZA/6MP is well established. AZA is converted to 6MP, and then to 6-thiouric acid (6-TUA), 6-methyl mercaptopurine (6-MMP), and 6-thioguanine nucleotide (6-TGN) [226, 227]. Evaluation for thiopurine methyltransferase genetic polymorphism should be obtained prior to the institution of 6MP or AZA therapy as it can identify those children at higher risk for drug toxicity [228] and the starting dose of thiopurine can be adjusted accordingly. The

6-TGN moiety is thought to be the active component responsible for the inhibition of lymphocyte proliferation by DNA breakage. There is data demonstrating increased 6-TGN level correlating with increased response to therapy in IBD, with increased 6-TGN levels associated with clinical remission [229]. Dosage can be adjusted using metabolite levels. as the target 6-TGN level is found to be 235 pmol/8×10^8 red blood cells and 6-MMP level <5700 pmol/8×10^8 red blood cells [230, 231]. The 6-MMP fraction is thought to be responsible for the hepatotoxic effects of AZA and 6MP [222, 229, 231, 232]. A 6-MMP level >5700 pmol/8×10^8 red blood cells is found to lead to a threefold increase risk of hepatotoxicity [231].

Allopurinol is a xanthine oxidase inhibitor used to treat gout as its primary indication. In patients that shift the breakdown of 6MP and AZA preferentially towards an increased 6-MMP fraction, the addition of allopurinol allows a lower dose of AZA/6MP with increased 6-TGN levels and lower comparative 6-MMP fraction. There is limited published data for dosage in pediatric IBD patients [233].

An alternate approach to maximize 6MP/AZA effect in patients with elevated transaminases due to preferential metabolizers of thiopurines is split dose administration. The total daily dose is the same, but divided into two equivalent doses, and this is found to decrease transaminases as well as flu-like symptoms which can be seen with 6MP/AZA use. This has been demonstrated in a retrospective adult study, and has been used in the pediatric UC population [234].

Given the high relapse rate with withdrawal of 6MP in adults with UC [235], the majority of children requiring AZA or 6MP to suppress disease activity most likely will require long-term maintenance therapy with these agents. There are no good data in UC addressing the question of when (or if) immunomodulators should be discontinued after a patient has entered remission. Most patients are continued on the medication for several years if they respond to 6MP or AZA. There is an approximate fourfold increase risk of lymphoma in IBD patients treated with AZA or 6MP. It is unclear if this is due to the medications themselves or due to the severity of the underlying disease [236]. In addition, there is a slightly increased risk of Epstein–Barr virus associated lymphoma in a large cohort of patients treated with long-term 6MP or AZA [237].

Methotrexate

Methotrexate (MTX) is a dihydrofolate reductase inhibitor used for induction and maintenance in patients with CD [238]. At low dose, MTX's mechanism of action is not clearly defined. At high doses, it works through antiproliferative and cytotoxic effects by inhibiting dihydrofolate reductase, leading to defective DNA synthesis and cell death [239]. At low doses, it works primarily as an immunomodulator [240]. The mechanism of action as an immunomodulator is not clearly understood but involves adenosine inhibition, induction of apoptosis, and decreased IL and eicosanoids to decrease inflammatory mediators [241–243].

There is some evidence from open label trials in adults to suggest the use of MTX monotherapy as maintenance in UC, but there is very little supportive data in the pediatric population. A multicenter randomized controlled trial of MTX use in adults with chronic active UC found weekly oral MTX at 12.5 mg to be no better than placebo in induction or maintenance of remission in patients with chronic active UC [244]. A small retrospective pediatric paper reported response or remission in 72, 63, and 50% of patients at 3, 6, and 12 months, respectively [245]. Larger controlled prospective trials would be needed to show clear benefit for MTX monotherapy in pediatric UC patients [246].

Biologic Agents
Infliximab

Infliximab is a monoclonal antibody to tumor necrosis factor-alpha which is a cofactor in the production of inflammatory cytokines, gamma interferon, and IL-2 [247, 248]. The efficacy of infliximab in pediatric patients was demonstrated in "the REACH trial" which was a prospective trial demonstrating 73% response at 8 weeks in pediatric UC patients with moderate to severely active UC using 5 mg/kg at 0, 2, and 6 weeks, followed by either every 8 week or every 12 week dosing interval. The response at 54 weeks in the every 8-week group was double that of the every 12-week maintenance group [249, 250].

Combination therapy with infliximab plus AZA has been shown to be more effective in an adult study [251] with better response of steroid free remission at 16 weeks in the combination therapy group. There are no similar studies in the pediatric patient population [251]. The potential risks of combination therapy including the possible development of lymphoma as previously discussed and the above data make the risk-versus-benefit evaluation of combination therapy critical.

Adalimumab

Adalimumab is a fully human monoclonal antibody that binds to tumor necrosis factor-alpha. It was approved for adults with UC in 2012. It is currently not approved for use in pediatric UC patients. The adult literature comparing adalimumab to placebo prospectively showed a superior response of clinical remission in treatment group at both week 8 (17 vs. 9%) and week 52 (17 vs. 9%), respectively. Anti-TNF naïve patients had double the response to therapy compared to placebo as well (21 vs. 9% at week 8 and 22% vs. 10% at week 52, respectively) [252].

Vedolizumab

Vedolizumab is a humanized monoclonal antibody that specifically recognizes alpha-4 beta-7 integrin, a cell survive glycoprotein variably expressed on circulating B and T lymphocytes. This interacts with mucosal addressin-cell adhesion molecule-1 (MAdCAM-1) [253] on intestinal vasculature [254, 255]. Vedolizumab has been found more effective than placebo for induction and maintenance therapy for UC. In randomized placebo-controlled adult studies, induction response was 47% compared with 25.5% in placebo at 6 weeks, and maintenance response was achieved in 41.8% in treatment group at every 8 weeks, 44.8% at every 4 weeks at 300 mg compared with 15.9% in placebo group. There was a similar frequency of adverse events in both treatment groups and placebo groups. This effect appears to be more effective in patients who have previously lost response to anti-TNF therapy [256].

Other Therapies

Antibiotics

Despite the potential role of infectious agents in the pathogenesis of UC [20], the use of antibiotic therapy in the treatment of UC remains controversial. There is a lack of consistent evidence in the effectiveness of antibiotics in the induction and maintenance of remission in UC [192, 257–260]. In one study, oral tobramycin therapy improved short-term clinical and histological outcomes, [257] but there was no advantage in the prevention of relapse compared to placebo [258]. In two studies of active UC, the addition of 10–14 days of oral or intravenous ciprofloxacin to corticosteroid therapy did not improve rates of remission [194, 261]. In another placebo-controlled study, 6 months of treatment with ciprofloxacin, in addition to standard therapy with prednisone and mesalamine, resulted in a greater clinical response compared to placebo; however, this advantage was not sustained after the cessation of ciprofloxacin [262]. Empiric broad-spectrum antibiotics often are administered in the setting of severe active UC [72, 191], especially if there is concern for potential fulminant colitis or toxic megacolon [148].

Tofacitinib

Tofacitinib is an oral inhibitor of Janus kinase 1, 2, and 3, which is expected to block signaling involving gamma chain-containing cytokines including IL 2, 4, 7, 9, 15, and 21. These cytokines are integral to lymphocyte activation function and proliferation. Blocking a common signaling molecule is thought to suppress both T and B cells, while maintaining regulatory T cell function [263–265]. Tofacitinib was found to be more effective than placebo in a prospective phase-2 trial of 194 adults with clinical response found in 78% in the higher dose treatment group compared to 42% in the placebo group. Clinical remission was seen in 41% in the higher dose treatment group versus 10% in placebo group [266].

Mycophenolate

Mycophenolate mofetil is an immunosuppressant used in transplant therapy and is a reversible inhibitor of purine biosynthesis, necessary for the growth of T cells and B cells [267]. There have been several small studies in adult literature showing some efficacy in treating UC, particularly when other medications such as infliximab and AZA have failed [268]. A retrospective review of adult UC patients treated with mycophenolate mofetil demonstrated 81% in remission at 8 weeks and 58% in sustained response at 6 months. Side effects were experienced in 19% of the patients, the majority of which were managed with dose reduction. There may be utility in patients who fail other treatment regimens, but more data is needed [269]

Probiotics

There are data and controversy on use of probiotics in UC. VSL#3 is a product comprised of four strains of lactobacilli, three strains of bifidobacteria and one strain of *Streptococcus,* and has been shown to be effective in preventing pouchitis in UC patients after colectomy [270]. In a prospective, randomized, and placebo-controlled trial in 29 children, VSL#3 was superior to placebo in protracting relapse-free remission [271]. The question of use of probiotics for inducing remission in UC remains controversial. A meta-analysis of all available studies in adult literature demonstrated that VSL#3 is beneficial for maintaining remission in patients with pouchitis, and that probiotics show additional benefit in inducing remission of UC [272]. Larger prospective pediatric studies are needed to fully define probiotic use for induction and maintenance of remission in pediatric patients with UC.

Fish Oil

Several placebo-controlled studies suggested a benefit of adjunctive therapy with fish oil supplementation containing eicosapentaenoic acid, a potent inhibitor of leukotriene B-4 synthesis, in the treatment of active UC [273–275]. However, fish oil supplementation did not appear to show any benefit in maintenance therapy [275, 276].

Randomized, controlled trials in adults with active distal UC suggest that therapy with topical short chain fatty acid preparations result in clinical symptomatic improvement, but there is no statistically significant advantage in comparison to placebo [277–279].

Nutritional Therapy

The importance of nutrition in the management of UC is extensively reviewed elsewhere [280, 281]. There is data to support the use of enteral therapy for induction of remission in CD, but the same response is not seen with UC [282, 283]. Children with UC can develop nutritional deficits with poor oral intake secondary to symptoms, and thus, promotion of continued good nutritional intake is essential for appropriate healing and nutritional repletion [284]. Enteral nutrition is preferred to total parenteral nutrition when possible. In contrast to CD, enteral nutrition is not an effective primary therapy for active UC [180, 285]. Studies suggest no advantage of total nutritional support and bowel rest in addition to conventional medical therapy alone in the treatment of UC [189, 190]. Total parenteral nutrition is often utilized for nutritional repletion in severe UC colitis, especially if the patient is developing severe cramps and diarrhea when challenged with enteral nutrition.

Surgical Therapy

In the majority of cases, medical therapy remains the first-line treatment for UC. However, colectomy may be required for patients with severe or medically refractory disease, or to prevent colon cancer. Since the inflammation in UC is limited to the colon, colonic resection will most often result in resolution of symptoms. However, colectomy is not without potential complications, such as the development of pouchitis in patients who undergo ileo-anal anastomosis [286, 287]. It is important to consider timely surgical intervention in the appropriate setting to avoid complications of UC. Indications for colectomy in a patient with UC include fulminant colitis or a complication of colitis, such as massive hemorrhage, perforation, or toxic megacolon; medical therapy failure; steroid dependency, which may lead undesired to side effects; and the presence of colonic dysplasia [288]. Prepubertal children may experience catch-up growth after colectomy for UC. In one series, 11 of 18 children increased their median height velocity from 3.85 cm/year preoperatively to 7.35 cm/year postoperatively [289].

There are no early predictors to help determine who will proceed to colectomy. In a retrospective review of 73 children with UC between the ages of 1–18 years, the combination of steroid dependency and pancolitis was associated with an increased need for colectomy [290]. Seventy-three percent of the children with steroid dependent pancolitis required colectomy within 3 years of diagnosis [290].

Except in the setting of emergent colectomy, a complete evaluation should be performed to ensure there is no evidence of CD prior to colectomy. If there is evidence suggesting the possibility of CD, the patient and family need to be informed of the potential for postoperative recurrence, and the relative contraindications of ileoanal pull through procedures in patients with CD. The authors recommend small-bowel imaging and upper gastrointestinal endoscopy, in addition to a full ileo-colonoscopy, if there is no clinical contraindication. Prior endoscopies and pathology reports should be carefully reviewed to establish that there is no evidence of CD.

The surgical options available for UC are reviewed in detail elsewhere [288]. The ileal pouch-anal canal anastomosis (IPAA) is the operation most commonly performed in the majority of patients with UC. The IPAA removes the entire colon and the rectal mucosa, avoids permanent ileostomy, and preserves anorectal function. Several types of ileal pouches can be constructed including the J-shaped, S-shaped, W-shaped, and the lateral–lateral pouch [288]. The J pouch design is now most commonly used for the IPAA operation [291, 292]. If the rectal mucosa is in good condition, many centers use the two-stage operative approach. During the first stage, a subtotal colectomy of the cecum to proximal rectum, the removal of the distal rectal and proximal anal mucosa, and the formation of the ileal pouch are performed. In this initial stage, a diverting loop ileostomy is performed in order to allow the pouch to heal. The second stage involves closure of the loop ileostomy with restoration of fecal flow to the pouch. Surgeons at some surgical centers also complete the IPAA in one stage, without the loop ileostomy [293]; however, this would not be the procedure of choice in patients receiving high dose corticosteroids [292].

If the patient presents for emergent surgical intervention, such as with fulminant colitis, a three-stage operative approach is often utilized. At the time of acute presentation, a subtotal colectomy is performed with formation of a rectal stump (the so-called Hartman pouch) and Brooke ileostomy. After the first operation, the rectal mucosa is treated with topical therapies (e.g., hydrocortisone, aminosalicylates) to induce mucosal healing. At the second operation, the distal rectal and proximal anal mucosa is removed and the ileal pouch is created. The ileostomy is reversed at the third operation.

The potential complications of IPAA include small-bowel obstruction, pelvic sepsis, anastomotic leak, fecal incontinence, pouchitis, strictures, fistulae, and reduced fertility in females [288, 294–296]. The development of fistulae raises the suspicion of CD [288]. In one series of children aged 9–16 who underwent proctocolectomy with IPAA, 12/29 (41%) of patients with UC developed early complications (wound infection, early bowel obstruction, prolonged fever) [297]. Late complications (bowel obstruction, pouch fistula) occurred in 11/29 (38%) and pouchitis developed in 9/29 (31%) of the children with UC. Median follow-up was 4 years (range from 6 months to 9 years). In this same study, daytime continence was noted in 100% and nighttime continence in 93%. The

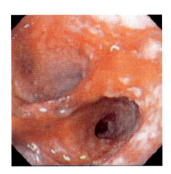

Fig. 30.5 Chronic active inflammation of an ileal J pouch (pouchitis) in a patient with a history of ulcerative colitis. Note both limbs of the ileal reservoir are erythematous with exudate. (Reprinted with permission from [67], Fig. 25.5, p. 406)

median frequency of bowel movements was 4 per 24 h, and 7% of the patients had nighttime bowel movements.

Pouchitis, or inflammation of the newly created reservoir, is the most significant chronic complication in UC patients undergoing IPAA and as many as 44–53% of the children and young adults with UC and ileo-anal anastomosis will develop pouchitis on long-term follow-up [286, 287]. The etiology of pouchitis is unknown, but theories involve the role of genetic susceptibility, fecal stasis, bacterial overgrowth, disruption of the balance of luminal bacteria, nutritional deficiencies, ischemia, and IBD recurrence [298]. Symptoms of pouchitis include diarrhea, rectal bleeding, abdominal cramping, urgency and incontinence of stool, malaise, and fever [288, 298, 299]. Laboratory studies may demonstrate anemia and an elevated erythrocyte sedimentation rate. The definitive diagnosis is established by flexible endoscopy of the pouch with biopsies (see Fig. 30.5). In some patients, a contrast enema may be useful in identifying fistulae.

Broad-spectrum antibiotics are usually the first-line treatment for pouchitis [298, 300]. Metronidazole is the most commonly used antibiotic, but alternative therapies include ciprofloxacin, amoxicillin/clavulanic acid, erythromycin, and tetracycline [299, 301]. If there is no improvement with antibiotics, other options include mesalamine enemas and steroid enemas or oral therapy with mesalamine, sulfasalazine, or steroids [299, 302, 303]. Other therapies examined include cyclosporine enemas, short chain fatty acid enemas, butyrate suppositories, and glutamine suppositories [299, 304–306]. Probiotic therapy may prevent the onset of acute pouchitis after ileostomy closure [270] and effectively maintain remission after chronic pouchitis [307]. A double-blind, placebo-controlled study evaluated the efficacy of the probiotic preparation VSL#3 compared with placebo in maintenance of remission of chronic pouchitis in 40 patients in remission. Three patients (15%) in the VSL#3 group had relapses within the 9-month follow-up period, compared with 20 (100%) in the placebo group [307]. In another double-blind, placebo-controlled study performed by the same authors in 40 patients, VSL#3, administered immediately after ileostomy closure for 1 year, effectively reduced the onset of acute pouchitis in the VSL#3 group (10%) in comparison to the placebo group (40%) [270].

Several studies suggest that the risk of dysplasia in the ileal pouch appears to be low [308, 309] and may be associated with chronic pouchitis [310]. The development of adenocarcinoma has been reported in the ileal pouch [311]. In a follow-up study (mean of 5 years) of 76 children and adolescents with UC who had ileal pouch-anal anastomosis, no dysplasia was identified in screening pouch biopsy specimens [308]. The authors caution that the long-term risk of development of dysplasia is not yet known and recommend screening of the pouch for dysplasia. In the rare patient who has undergone an ileo-rectal anastomosis without rectal mucosectomy, surveillance of the rectum should be performed to screen for rectal cancer.

Psychosocial Support

The social impact of UC on the lives of children with the disease needs to be considered. UC often has its onset in adolescence, a time when body image issues are paramount. Children and teens with IBD often may experience anxiety over the diagnosis of a chronic disease, the need for invasive procedures, and the uncertainty of the future. In addition, there may be struggles with parents about proper diet, and "medication fatigue" from having to take more than ten pills per day. Social, school-related, and extracurricular activities may be affected and may need appropriate modification. For example, a self-limited reduction of physical education activities and permission for special bathroom privileges may be needed.

Previous studies report an increased risk of psychiatric and behavioral issues in children with IBD, including depression, anxiety, and low self-esteem [312–317]. The physician caring for these patients needs to openly discuss the above issues with the patient and family, and be alert to the possibility that a patient may develop anxiety or depressive symptoms. Two patient-generated, disease-specific, health-related quality of life questionnaires for children with IBD have been validated, the IMPACT and Impact-II questionnaires [318, 319]. Impact-II and more recent Impact-III are modified versions of the IMPACT questionnaire. The use of these instruments may provide important information to improve the care of children with IBD. Referral to an educational support group, such as those sponsored by the Crohn's and Colitis Foundation of America (www.ccfa.org), may be very helpful for patients and their families.

Prognosis/Follow-Up

Whether children with UC are treated medically or surgically, they have an excellent long-term prognosis and a good quality of life. The majority of children with UC respond to medical therapy. In one US retrospective study of 171 children ranging in age from 1.5 to 17.7 years, diagnosed with UC between 1967 and 1994, 43% had mild disease at presentation and 57% had moderate or severe UC. With treatment, 70% of all the children were in remission within 3 months of diagnosis and by 6 months, 90% of the children with mild disease and 81% of the children with moderate to severe UC experienced resolution of their symptoms. In each yearly follow-up period, approximately 55% of the children were symptom free, 38% experienced chronic intermittent symptoms, and 7% had continuous symptoms [320]. In this same study, children with mild UC at presentation had a lower frequency of colectomy than children with moderate to severe UC (9 vs. 26% at 5 years, respectively). Patients with left-sided disease had comparable rates of colectomy at 5 years as patients with pancolitis [320]. However, the authors cautioned that the number of patients in each subgroup of disease extent was small and a true difference in colectomy rates may have been missed secondary to insufficient power of the study [320].

Limited distal UC (proctitis or proctosigmoiditis) diagnosed in adults and children can extend further to involve more proximal colon with time [69, 321–323]. In a retrospective evaluation of 85 patients under 21 years of age, diagnosed with UC proctosigmoiditis between 1958 and 1983, the extension of disease was to the descending colon in 20% and to the hepatic flexure or beyond in another 38% of the patients [69].

Individuals with long-standing UC are at increased risk of developing colorectal cancer (CRC) [324–326]. Risk of CRC increases with more extensive colonic involvement, and longer duration of disease since diagnosis [324–328]. Thus, children with UC potentially will be at risk for CRC over a longer period of time, compared to individuals with adult-onset UC. In a recent Danish population-based cohort study, the risk of CRC among patients with UC was similar to the risk among the general population. The authors highlighted a decrease in the rate of CRC risk among patients with UC between 1979 and 2008. However, certain subgroups of UC patients, including those who were diagnosed in childhood or adolescence, experienced a longer duration of disease, or had PSC, remained at elevated risk of CRC [329]. Individuals with PSC and UC have a higher risk of developing colorectal neoplasia compared to those with UC alone and of developing cholangiocarcinoma [330–332]. Ursodeoxycholic acid may decrease the risk for developing colorectal dysplasia or cancer in patients with UC and PSC

[333]. However, high doses of ursodeoxycholic acid may increase the risk of colorectal neoplasia in these patients [334]. Other risk factors reported for CRC in patients with UC include a family history of sporadic CRC and the presence of colonic stricture, shortened colon, or inflammatory pseudopolyps [335–337].

Some retrospective studies suggest that ASA agents may provide a protective effect in the development of CRC in patients with UC, but not all studies support these findings [217–219, 338, 339].

Presently, there is insufficient evidence to support or refute the use of purine immunomodulators in the chemoprevention of CRC in patients with UC [337, 340]. There are no randomized controlled trials examining the effectiveness of surveillance colonoscopy for dysplasia and CRC in patients with UC [337]. In 2010, the American Gastroenterological Association (AGA) published updated recommendations for surveillance colonoscopy in adults with IBD [337, 341]. An initial screening colonoscopy 8 years after onset of symptoms is advised in all patients with UC to reassess the extent of disease with multiple biopsies obtained throughout the entire colon. The CRC surveillance interval is determined by the true extent of disease, defined by the most proximal extent of disease identified histologically at any point in time [337]. Patients with isolated ulcerative proctitis are not considered at increased risk for IBD-related CRC. Therefore, after the initial screening colonoscopy, they do not require surveillance colonoscopy based upon their UC. Patients with extensive (extent proximal to splenic flexure) or left-sided colitis should commence surveillance colonoscopy within 1–2 years after the initial screening [337]. Patients with UC and PSC should initiate colonoscopy surveillance at time of diagnosis and continue with yearly examinations thereafter [337].

Chromoendoscopy improves the detection of dysplastic lesions by enhancing the visualization of mucosal irregularities [337]. In expert hands, chromoendoscopy optimizes the detection of mucosal abnormalities for appropriate targeted biopsies and reduces the need for random biopsies [342, 343]. If colonoscopy is performed without chromoendoscopy, surveillance should include careful inspection of the mucosa with targeted biopsies of any suspicious lesions and random biopsies from each anatomic section of the colon [337]. There are no prospective studies available to define the ideal number of random biopsies required to reliably detect colorectal neoplasia. Consensus recommendations suggest that biopsy specimens should be taken every 10 cm in all four quadrants [337]. It is not clear whether surveillance practice should differ for patients with younger-onset UC. There are no published formal recommendations to guide surveillance colonoscopy in children [344]. The AGA recommends that surveillance colonoscopy should be performed as frequently in children and adolescents as in adults

and should be determined by the duration of disease [337]. Guidelines for surveillance colonoscopy for neoplasia in IBD patients continue to evolve.

Conclusion

UC in children presents in a similar manner to that in adults, though children often have more extensive disease at diagnosis. Once the diagnosis is established, by colonoscopy, the first line of induction treatment in mild disease is usually an aminosalicylate, with corticosteroids reserved for moderate to severe disease. If a patient responds to induction therapy, the maintenance agent most commonly used is an aminosalicylate or 6-mercaptopurine. In severe steroid unresponsive colitis, the clinician is faced with the challenge of recommending either colectomy or more aggressive immunosuppression (e.g., infliximab, tacrolimus, cyclosporine). Even if a patient responds to cyclosporine or tacrolimus, there is a high likelihood of proceeding to colectomy within a year. Surgery will eradicate the disease, but patients may develop chronic pouchitis requiring additional medical treatment. In addition to medical care of these patients, nutritional counseling, monitoring of growth, and psychosocial support are essential. If the medical team can give proper care and support, the patient's long-term prognosis is usually excellent.

References

1. Chong SK, Blackshaw AJ, Morson BC, Williams CB, Walker-Smith JA. Prospective study of colitis in infancy and early childhood. J Pediatr Gastroenterol Nutr. 1986;5(3):352–8.
2. Mendeloff AI, Calkins BM. The epidemiology of idiopathic inflammatory bowel disease. In: Kirsner JB, Shorter RG, editors. Inflammatory bowel disease. Philadelphia: Lea & Febiger; 1988. p. 3–34.
3. Langholz E, Munkholm P, Krasilnikoff PA, Binder V. Inflammatory bowel diseases with onset in childhood. Clinical features, morbidity, and mortality in a regional cohort. Scand J Gastroenterol. 1997;32(2):139–47.
4. Gryboski JD. Ulcerative colitis in children 10 years old or younger. J Pediatr Gastroenterol Nutr. 1993;17(1):24–31.
5. Mamula P, Telega GW, Markowitz JE, Brown KA, Russo PA, Piccoli DA, et al. Inflammatory bowel disease in children 5 years of age and younger. Am J Gastroenterol. 2002;97(8):2005–10.
6. Henderson P, Hansen R, Cameron FL, Gerasimidis K, Rogers P, Bisset WM, et al. Rising incidence of pediatric inflammatory bowel disease in Scotland. Inflamm Bowel Dis. 2012;18(6):999–1005.
7. Benchimol EI, Guttmann A, Griffiths AM, Rabeneck L, Mack DR, Brill H, et al. Increasing incidence of paediatric inflammatory bowel disease in Ontario, Canada: evidence from health administrative data. Gut. 2009;58(11):1490–7.
8. Adamiak T, Walkiewicz-Jedrzejczak D, Fish D, Brown C, Tung J, Khan K, et al. Incidence, clinical characteristics, and natural history of pediatric IBD in Wisconsin: a population-based epidemiological study. Inflamm Bowel Dis. 2013;19(6):1218–23.

9. Jakobsen C, Paerregaard A, Munkholm P, Faerk J, Lange A, Andersen J, et al. Pediatric inflammatory bowel disease: increasing incidence, decreasing surgery rate, and compromised nutritional status: a prospective population-based cohort study 2007–2009. Inflamm Bowel Dis. 2011;17(12):2541–50.

10. Perminow G, Brackmann S, Lyckander LG, Franke A, Borthne A, Rydning A, et al. A characterization in childhood inflammatory bowel disease, a new population-based inception cohort from South-Eastern Norway, 2005–07, showing increased incidence in Crohn's disease. Scand J Gastroenterol. 2009;44(4):446–56.

11. Malmborg P, Grahnquist L, Lindholm J, Montgomery S, Hildebrand H. Increasing incidence of paediatric inflammatory bowel disease in northern Stockholm County, 2002–2007. J Pediatr Gastroenterol Nutr. 2013;57(1):29–34.

12. Benchimol EI, Fortinsky KJ, Gozdyra P, Van den Heuvel M, Van Limbergen J, Griffiths AM. Epidemiology of pediatric inflammatory bowel disease: a systematic review of international trends. Inflamm Bowel Dis. 2011;17(1):423–39.

13. Sonnenberg A, McCarty DJ, Jacobsen SJ. Geographic variation of inflammatory bowel disease within the United States. Gastroenterology. 1991;100(1):143–9.

14. Shivananda S, Lennard-Jones J, Logan R, Fear N, Price A, Carpenter L, et al. Incidence of inflammatory bowel disease across Europe: is there a difference between north and south? Results of the European Collaborative Study on Inflammatory Bowel Disease (EC-IBD). Gut. 1996;39(5):690–7.

15. Khalili H, Huang ES, Ananthakrishnan AN, Higuchi L, Richter JM, Fuchs CS, et al. Geographical variation and incidence of inflammatory bowel disease among US women. Gut. 2012;61(12):1686–92.

16. Acheson ED. The distribution of ulcerative colitis and regional enteritis in United States veterans with particular reference to the Jewish religion. Gut. 1960;1:291–3.

17. Gilat T, Grossman A, Fireman Z, Rozen P. Inflammatory bowel disease in Jews. Front Gastrointest Res. 1986;11:141–5.

18. Abraham C, Cho JH. Inflammatory bowel disease. N Engl J Med. 2009;361(21):2066–78.

19. Geremia A, Biancheri P, Allan P, Corazza GR, Di Sabatino A. Innate and adaptive immunity in inflammatory bowel disease. Autoimmun Rev. 2014;13(1):3–10.

20. Hendrickson BA, Gokhale R, Cho JH. Clinical aspects and pathophysiology of inflammatory bowel disease. Clin Microbiol Rev. 2002;15(1):79–94.

21. Orholm M, Binder V, Sorensen TI, Rasmussen LP, Kyvik KO. Concordance of inflammatory bowel disease among Danish twins. Results of a nationwide study. Scand J Gastroenterol. 2000;35(10):1075–81.

22. Halfvarson J, Bodin L, Tysk C, Lindberg E, Jarnerot G. Inflammatory bowel disease in a Swedish twin cohort: a long-term follow-up of concordance and clinical characteristics. Gastroenterology. 2003;124(7):1767–73.

23. Orholm M, Munkholm P, Langholz E, Nielsen OH, Sorensen IA, Binder V. Familial occurrence of inflammatory bowel disease. New Engl J Med. 1991;324(2):84–8.

24. Lees CW, Barrett JC, Parkes M, Satsangi J. New IBD genetics: common pathways with other diseases. Gut. 2011;60(12):1739–53.

25. Silverberg MS, Cho JH, Rioux JD, McGovern DP, Wu J, Annese V, et al. Ulcerative colitis-risk loci on chromosomes 1p36 and 12q15 found by genome-wide association study. Nat Genet. 2009;41(2):216–20.

26. Fernando MM, Stevens CR, Walsh EC, De Jager PL, Goyette P, Plenge RM, et al. Defining the role of the MHC in autoimmunity: a review and pooled analysis. PLoS Genet. 2008;4(4):e1000024.

27. Papa E, Docktor M, Smillie C, Weber S, Preheim SP, Gevers D, et al. Non-invasive mapping of the gastrointestinal microbiota identifies children with inflammatory bowel disease. PloS one. 2012;7(6):e39242.

28. Gevers D, Kugathasan S, Denson LA, Vazquez-Baeza Y, Van Treuren W, Ren B, et al. The treatment-naive microbiome in new-onset Crohn's disease. Cell Host Microbe. 2014;15(3):382–92.

29. Wu GD, Chen J, Hoffmann C, Bittinger K, Chen YY, Keilbaugh SA, et al. Linking long-term dietary patterns with gut microbial enterotypes. Science. 2011;334(6052):105–8.

30. Vessey M, Jewell D, Smith A, Yeates D, McPherson K. Chronic inflammatory bowel disease, cigarette smoking, and use of oral contraceptives: findings in a large cohort study of women of child-bearing age. Br Med J (Clin Res Ed). 1986;292(6528):1101–3.

31. Calkins BM. A meta-analysis of the role of smoking in inflammatory bowel disease. Dig Dis Sci. 1989;34(12):1841–54.

32. Koletzko S, Griffiths A, Corey M, Smith C, Sherman P. Infant feeding practices and ulcerative colitis in childhood. BMJ. 1991;302(6792):1580–1.

33. Jakobsen C, Paerregaard A, Munkholm P, Wewer V. Environmental factors and risk of developing paediatric inflammatory bowel disease—a population based study 2007–2009. J Crohn's Colitis. 2013;7(1):79–88.

34. Garcia Rodriguez LA, Ruigomez A, Panes J. Acute gastroenteritis is followed by an increased risk of inflammatory bowel disease. Gastroenterology. 2006;130(6):1588–94.

35. Gradel KO, Nielsen HL, Schonheyder HC, Ejlertsen T, Kristensen B, Nielsen H. Increased short- and long-term risk of inflammatory bowel disease after salmonella or campylobacter gastroenteritis. Gastroenterology. 2009;137(2):495–501.

36. Kronman MP, Zaoutis TE, Haynes K, Feng R, Coffin SE. Antibiotic exposure and IBD development among children: a population-based cohort study. Pediatrics. 2012;130(4):e794–803.

37. Andersson RE, Olaison G, Tysk C, Ekbom A. Appendectomy and protection against ulcerative colitis. N Engl J Med. 2001;344(11):808–14.

38. Duggan AE, Usmani I, Neal KR, Logan RF. Appendicectomy, childhood hygiene, Helicobacter pylori status, and risk of inflammatory bowel disease: a case control study. Gut. 1998;43(4):494–8.

39. Feeney MA, Murphy F, Clegg AJ, Trebble TM, Sharer NM, Snook JA. A case-control study of childhood environmental risk factors for the development of inflammatory bowel disease. Eur J Gastroenterol Hepatol. 2002;14(5):529–34.

40. Klement E, Cohen RV, Boxman J, Joseph A, Reif S. Breastfeeding and risk of inflammatory bowel disease: a systematic review with meta-analysis. Am J Clin Nutr. 2004;80(5):1342–52.

41. Gilat T, Hacohen D, Lilos P, Langman MJ. Childhood factors in ulcerative colitis and Crohn's disease. An international cooperative study. Scand J Gastroenterol. 1987;22(8):1009–24.

42. Hansen TS, Jess T, Vind I, Elkjaer M, Nielsen MF, Gamborg M, et al. Environmental factors in inflammatory bowel disease: a case-control study based on a Danish inception cohort. J Crohn's Colitis. 2011;5(6):577–84.

43. Evans JM, McMahon AD, Murray FE, McDevitt DG, MacDonald TM. Non-steroidal anti-inflammatory drugs are associated with emergency admission to hospital for colitis due to inflammatory bowel disease. Gut. 1997;40(5):619–22.

44. Bonner GF. Exacerbation of inflammatory bowel disease associated with use of celecoxib. Am J Gastroenterol. 2001;96(4):1306–8.

45. Ananthakrishnan AN, Higuchi LM, Huang ES, Khalili H, Richter JM, Fuchs CS, et al. Aspirin, nonsteroidal anti-inflammatory drug use, and risk for Crohn disease and ulcerative colitis: a cohort study. Ann Intern Med. 2012;156(5):350–9.

46. Takeuchi K, Smale S, Premchand P, Maiden L, Sherwood R, Thjodleifsson B, et al. Prevalence and mechanism of nonsteroidal anti-inflammatory drug-induced clinical relapse in patients

with inflammatory bowel disease. Clin Gastroenterol Hepatol. 2006;4(2):196–202.

47. Khalili H, Higuchi LM, Ananthakrishnan AN, Richter JM, Feskanich D, Fuchs CS, et al. Oral contraceptives, reproductive factors and risk of inflammatory bowel disease. Gut. 2013;62(8):1153–9.

48. Lim WC, Hanauer SB, Li YC. Mechanisms of disease: vitamin D and inflammatory bowel disease. Nat Clin Pract Gastroenterol Hepatol. 2005;2(7):308–15.

49. David LA, Maurice CF, Carmody RN, Gootenberg DB, Button JE, Wolfe BE, et al. Diet rapidly and reproducibly alters the human gut microbiome. Nature. 2014;505(7484):559–63.

50. Albenberg LG, Lewis JD, Wu GD. Food and the gut microbiota in inflammatory bowel diseases: a critical connection. Curr Opin Gastroenterol. 2012;28(4):314–20.

51. Hou JK, Abraham B, El-Serag H. Dietary intake and risk of developing inflammatory bowel disease: a systematic review of the literature. Am J Gastroenterol. 2011;106(4):563–73.

52. Chapman-Kiddell CA, Davies PS, Gillen L, Radford-Smith GL. Role of diet in the development of inflammatory bowel disease. Inflamm Bowel Dis. 2010;16(1):137–51.

53. Zhou L, Ivanov, II, Spolski R, Min R, Shenderov K, Egawa T, et al. IL-6 programs T(H)-17 cell differentiation by promoting sequential engagement of the IL-21 and IL-23 pathways. Nat Immunol. 2007;8(9):967–74.

54. Fujino S, Andoh A, Bamba S, Ogawa A, Hata K, Araki Y, et al. Increased expression of interleukin 17 in inflammatory bowel disease. Gut. 2003;52(1):65–70.

55. Kobayashi T, Okamoto S, Hisamatsu T, Kamada N, Chinen H, Saito R, et al. IL23 differentially regulates the Th1/Th17 balance in ulcerative colitis and Crohn's disease. Gut. 2008;57(12):1682–9.

56. Consortium UIG, Barrett JC, Lee JC, Lees CW, Prescott NJ, Anderson CA, et al. Genome-wide association study of ulcerative colitis identifies three new susceptibility loci, including the HNF4A region. Nat Genet. 2009;41(12):1330–4.

57. Kaser A, Blumberg RS. Autophagy, microbial sensing, endoplasmic reticulum stress, and epithelial function in inflammatory bowel disease. Gastroenterology. 2011;140(6):1738–47.

58. Hampe J, Schreiber S, Shaw SH, Lau KF, Bridger S, Macpherson AJ, et al. A genomewide analysis provides evidence for novel linkages in inflammatory bowel disease in a large European cohort. Am J Hum Genet. 1999;64(3):808–16.

59. Vermeire S, Rutgeerts P, Van Steen K, Joossens S, Claessens G, Pierik M, et al. Genome wide scan in a Flemish inflammatory bowel disease population: support for the IBD4 locus, population heterogeneity, and epistasis. Gut. 2004;53(7):980–6.

60. Barmada MM, Brant SR, Nicolae DL, Achkar JP, Panhuysen CI, Bayless TM, et al. A genome scan in 260 inflammatory bowel disease-affected relative pairs. Inflamm Bowel Dis. 2004;10(1):15–22.

61. Kaser A, Lee AH, Franke A, Glickman JN, Zeissig S, Tilg H, et al. XBP1 links ER stress to intestinal inflammation and confers genetic risk for human inflammatory bowel disease. Cell. 2008;134(5):743–56.

62. Levine A, Griffiths A, Markowitz J, Wilson DC, Turner D, Russell RK, et al. Pediatric modification of the Montreal classification for inflammatory bowel disease: the Paris classification. Inflamm Bowel Dis. 2011;17(6):1314–21.

63. Silverberg MS, Satsangi J, Ahmad T, Arnott ID, Bernstein CN, Brant SR, et al. Toward an integrated clinical, molecular and serological classification of inflammatory bowel disease: report of a Working Party of the 2005 Montreal World Congress of Gastroenterology. Can J Gastroenterol. 2005;19 Suppl A:5a–36a.

64. Rao SS, Holdsworth CD, Read NW. Symptoms and stool patterns in patients with ulcerative colitis. Gut. 1988;29(3):342–5.

65. Bentsen BS, Moum B, Ekbom A. Incidence of inflammatory bowel disease in children in southeastern Norway: a prospective population-based study 1990–94. Scand J Gastroenterol. 2002;37(5):540–5.

66. Heikenen JB, Werlin SL, Brown CW, Balint JP. Presenting symptoms and diagnostic lag in children with inflammatory bowel disease. Inflamm Bowel Dis. 1999;5(3):158–60.

67. Higuchi L, Bousvaros, A. Ulcerative colitis. In Guandalini S, editor. Textbook of pediatric gastroenterology and nutrition. London: Taylor & Francis; 2004. p. 385–417.

68. Olafsdottir EJ, Fluge G, Haug K. Chronic inflammatory bowel disease in children in western Norway. J Pediatr Gastroenterol Nutr. 1989;8(4):454–8.

69. Mir-Madjlessi SH, Michener WM, Farmer RG. Course and prognosis of idiopathic ulcerative proctosigmoiditis in young patients. J Pediatr Gastroenterol Nutr. 1986;5(4):571–5.

70. Motil KJ, Grand RJ. Ulcerative colitis and Crohn disease in children. Pediatr Rev. 1987;9(4):109–20.

71. Grand RJ, Homer DR. Approaches to inflammatory bowel disease in childhood and adolescence. Pediatr Clin North Am. 1975;22(4):835–50.

72. Werlin SL, Grand RJ. Severe colitis in children and adolescents: diagnosis. Course, and treatment. Gastroenterology. 1977; 73(4 Pt 1):828–32.

73. Moran CJ, Walters TD, Guo CH, Kugathasan S, Klein C, Turner D, et al. IL-10R polymorphisms are associated with very-early-onset ulcerative colitis. Inflamm Bowel Dis. 2013;19(1):115–23.

74. Sachar DB, Smith H, Chan S, Cohen LB, Lichtiger S, Messer J. Erythrocytic sedimentation rate as a measure of clinical activity in inflammatory bowel disease. J Clin Gastroenterol. 1986;8(6):647–50.

75. Macfarlane PI, Miller V, Wells F, Richards B. Laboratory assessment of disease activity in childhood Crohn's disease and ulcerative colitis. J Pediatr Gastroenterol Nutr. 1986;5(1):93–6.

76. Holmquist L, Ahren C, Fallstrom SP. Relationship between results of laboratory tests and inflammatory activity assessed by colonoscopy in children and adolescents with ulcerative colitis and Crohn's colitis. J Pediatr Gastroenterol Nutr. 1989;9(2):187–93.

77. Mack DR, Langton C, Markowitz J, LeLeiko N, Griffiths A, Bousvaros A, et al. Laboratory values for children with newly diagnosed inflammatory bowel disease. Pediatrics. 2007;119(6):1113–9.

78. Ashorn S, Honkanen T, Kolho KL, Ashorn M, Valineva T, Wei B, et al. Fecal calprotectin levels and serological responses to microbial antigens among children and adolescents with inflammatory bowel disease. Inflamm Bowel Dis. 2009;15(2):199–205.

79. Walker TR, L and ML, Kartashov A, Saslowsky TM, Lyerly DM, Boone JH, et al. Fecal lactoferrin is a sensitive and specific marker of disease activity in children and young adults with inflammatory bowel disease. J Pediatr Gastroenterol Nutr. 2007;44(4):414–22.

80. Kopylov U, Rosenfeld G, Bressler B, Seidman E. Clinical utility of fecal biomarkers for the diagnosis and management of inflammatory bowel disease. Inflamm Bowel Dis. 2014;20(4):742–56.

81. van Rheenen PF, Van de Vijver E, Fidler V. Faecal calprotectin for screening of patients with suspected inflammatory bowel disease: diagnostic meta-analysis. BMJ. 2010;341:c3369.

82. Ruemmele FM, Targan SR, Levy G, Dubinsky M, Braun J, Seidman EG. Diagnostic accuracy of serological assays in pediatric inflammatory bowel disease. Gastroenterology. 1998;115(4):822–9.

83. Dubinsky MC, Ofman JJ, Urman M, Targan SR, Seidman EG. Clinical utility of serodiagnostic testing in suspected pediatric inflammatory bowel disease. Am J Gastroenterol. 2001;96(3):758–65.

84. Duerr RH, Targan SR, Landers CJ, Sutherland LR, Shanahan F. Anti-neutrophil cytoplasmic antibodies in ulcerative colitis. Comparison with other colitides/diarrheal illnesses. Gastroenterology. 1991;100(6):1590–6.

85. Winter HS, Landers CJ, Winkelstein A, Vidrich A, Targan SR. Anti-neutrophil cytoplasmic antibodies in children with ulcerative colitis. J Pediatr. 1994; 125(5 Pt 1):707–11.

86. Rutgeerts P, Vermeire S. Serological diagnosis of inflammatory bowel disease. Lancet. 2000;356(9248):2117–8.

87. Benor S, Russell GH, Silver M, Israel EJ, Yuan Q, Winter HS. Shortcomings of the inflammatory bowel disease Serology 7 panel. Pediatrics. 2010;125(6):1230–6.

88. Levine A, Koletzko S, Turner D, Escher JC, Cucchiara S, de Ridder L, et al. ESPGHAN revised porto criteria for the diagnosis of inflammatory bowel disease in children and adolescents. J Pediatr Gastroenterol Nutr. 2014;58(6):795–806.

89. Markowitz J, Kahn E, Grancher K, Hyams J, Treem W, Daum F. Atypical rectosigmoid histology in children with newly diagnosed ulcerative colitis. Am J Gastroenterol. 1993;88(12):2034–7.

90. Bousvaros A, Glickman JN, Farraye FA, Friedman S, Leichtner AM, Wang H, et al. Pediatric patients with untreated ulcerative colitis may present initially with unusual morphologic findings. Gastroenterology. 2002;122(4, Suppl. 1):A–11.

91. Glickman JN, Bousvaros A, Farraye FA, Zholudev A, Friedman S, Wang HH, et al. Pediatric patients with untreated ulcerative colitis may present initially with unusual morphologic findings. Am J Surg Pathol. 2004;28(2):190–7.

92. Levine A, de Bie CI, Turner D, Cucchiara S, Sladek M, Murphy MS, et al. Atypical disease phenotypes in pediatric ulcerative colitis: 5-year analyses of the EUROKIDS Registry. Inflamm Bowel Dis. 2013;19(2):370–7.

93. Bousvaros A, Antonioli DA, Colletti RB, Dubinsky MC, Glickman JN, Gold BD, et al. Differentiating ulcerative colitis from Crohn disease in children and young adults: report of a working group of the North American Society for Pediatric Gastroenterology, Hepatology, and Nutrition and the Crohn's and Colitis Foundation of America. J Pediatr Gastroenterol Nutr. 2007;44(5):653–74.

94. Seidman EG. Role of endoscopy in inflammatory bowel disease. Gastrointest Endosc Clin N Am. 2001;11(4):641–57, vi.

95. Chutkan RK, Scherl E, Waye JD. Colonoscopy in inflammatory bowel disease. Gastrointest Endosc Clin N Am. 2002;12(3):463–83, viii.

96. Domizio P. Pathology of chronic inflammatory bowel disease in children. Baillieres Clin Gastroenterol. 1994;8(1):35–63.

97. Washington K, Greenson JK, Montgomery E, Shyr Y, Crissinger KD, Polk DB, et al. Histopathology of ulcerative colitis in initial rectal biopsy in children. Am J Surg Pathol. 2002;26(11):1441–9.

98. Chong SK, Blackshaw AJ, Boyle S, Williams CB, Walker-Smith JA. Histological diagnosis of chronic inflammatory bowel disease in childhood. Gut. 1985;26(1):55–9.

99. Scotiniotis I, Rubesin SE, Ginsberg GG. Imaging modalities in inflammatory bowel disease. Gastroenterol Clin N Am. 1999;28(2):391–421, ix.

100. Aideyan UO, Smith WL. Inflammatory bowel disease in children. Radiol Clin North Am. 1996;34(4):885–902.

101. Langmead L, Rampton DS. Plain abdominal radiographic features are not reliable markers of disease extent in active ulcerative colitis. Am J Gastroenterol. 2002;97(2):354–9.

102. Ruuska T, Vaajalahti P, Arajarvi P, Maki M. Prospective evaluation of upper gastrointestinal mucosal lesions in children with ulcerative colitis and Crohn's disease. J Pediatr Gastroenterol Nutr. 1994;19(2):181–6.

103. De Matos V, Russo PA, Cohen AB, Mamula P, Baldassano RN, Piccoli DA. Frequency and clinical correlations of granulomas in children with Crohn disease. J Pediatr Gastroenterol Nutr. 2008;46(4):392–8.

104. Odze R. Diagnostic problems and advances in inflammatory bowel disease. Mod Pathol. 2003;16(4):347–58.

105. Kaufman SS, Vanderhoof JA, Young R, Perry D, Raynor SC, Mack DR. Gastroenteric inflammation in children with ulcerative colitis. Am J Gastroenterol. 1997;92(7):1209–12.

106. Sharif F, McDermott M, Dillon M, Drumm B, Rowland M, Imrie C, et al. Focally enhanced gastritis in children with Crohn's disease and ulcerative colitis. Am J Gastroenterol. 2002;97(6):1415–20.

107. Tobin JM, Sinha B, Ramani P, Saleh AR, Murphy MS. Upper gastrointestinal mucosal disease in pediatric Crohn disease and ulcerative colitis: a blinded, controlled study. J Pediatr Gastroenterol Nutr. 2001;32(4):443–8.

108. Hildebrand H, Fredrikzon B, Holmquist L, Kristiansson B, Lindquist B. Chronic inflammatory bowel disease in children and adolescents in Sweden. J Pediatr Gastroenterol Nutr. 1991;13(3):293–7.

109. Joossens S, Reinisch W, Vermeire S, Sendid B, Poulain D, Peeters M, et al. The value of serologic markers in indeterminate colitis: a prospective follow-up study. Gastroenterology. 2002;122(5):1242–7.

110. Hyams JS. Extraintestinal manifestations of inflammatory bowel disease in children. J Pediatr Gastroenterol Nutr. 1994;19(1):7–21.

111. Greenstein AJ, Janowitz HD, Sachar DB. The extra-intestinal complications of Crohn's disease and ulcerative colitis: a study of 700 patients. Medicine (Baltimore). 1976;55(5):401–12.

112. Dotson JL, Hyams JS, Markowitz J, LeLeiko NS, Mack DR, Evans JS, et al. Extraintestinal manifestations of pediatric inflammatory bowel disease and their relation to disease type and severity. J Pediatr Gastroenterol Nutr. 2010;51(2):140–5.

113. Jose FA, Garnett EA, Vittinghoff E, Ferry GD, Winter HS, Baldassano RN, et al. Development of extraintestinal manifestations in pediatric patients with inflammatory bowel disease. Inflamm Bowel Dis. 2009;15(1):63–8.

114. Lindsley CB, Schaller JG. Arthritis associated with inflammatory bowel disease in children. J Pediatr. 1974;84(1):16–20.

115. Mir-Madjlessi SH, Taylor JS, Farmer RG. Clinical course and evolution of erythema nodosum and pyoderma gangrenosum in chronic ulcerative colitis: a study of 42 patients. Am J Gastroenterol. 1985;80(8):615–20.

116. Wilschanski M, Chait P, Wade JA, Davis L, Corey M, St Louis P, et al. Primary sclerosing cholangitis in 32 children: clinical, laboratory, and radiographic features, with survival analysis. Hepatology (Baltimore, Md). 1995;22(5):1415–22.

117. Orchard TR, Wordsworth BP, Jewell DP. Peripheral arthropathies in inflammatory bowel disease: their articular distribution and natural history. Gut. 1998;42(3):387–91.

118. Das KM. Relationship of extraintestinal involvements in inflammatory bowel disease: new insights into autoimmune pathogenesis. Dig Dis Sci. 1999;44(1):1–13.

119. Levitt MD, Ritchie JK, Lennard-Jones JE, Phillips RK. Pyoderma gangrenosum in inflammatory bowel disease. Br J Surg. 1991;78(6):676–8.

120. Callen JP. Pyoderma gangrenosum. Lancet. 1998;351(9102):581–5.

121. Finkel SI, Janowitz HD. Trauma and the pyoderma gangrenosum of inflammatory bowel disease. Gut. 1981;22(5):410–2.

122. Requena L, Requena C. Erythema nodosum. Dermatol Online J. 2002;8(1):4.

123. Su CG, Judge TA, Lichtenstein GR. Extraintestinal manifestations of inflammatory bowel disease. Gastroenterol Clin N Am. 2002;31(1):307–27.

124. Rychwalski PJ, Cruz OA, Alanis-Lambreton G, Foy TM, Kane RE. Asymptomatic uveitis in young people with inflammatory bowel disease. J AAPOS. 1997;1(2):111–4.

125. Hofley P, Roarty J, McGinnity G, Griffiths AM, Marcon M, Kraft S, et al. Asymptomatic uveitis in children with chronic inflammatory bowel diseases. J Pediatr Gastroenterol Nutr. 1993;17(4):397–400.

126. Orchard TR, Chua CN, Ahmad T, Cheng H, Welsh KI, Jewell DP. Uveitis and erythema nodosum in inflammatory bowel disease:

clinical features and the role of HLA genes. Gastroenterology. 2002;123(3):714–8.

127. Tripathi RC, Kipp MA, Tripathi BJ, Kirschner BS, Borisuth NS, Shevell SK, et al. Ocular toxicity of prednisone in pediatric patients with inflammatory bowel disease. Lens Eye Toxic Res. 1992;9(3–4):469–82.

128. Tripathi RC, Kirschner BS, Kipp M, Tripathi BJ, Slotwiner D, Borisuth NS, et al. Corticosteroid treatment for inflammatory bowel disease in pediatric patients increases intraocular pressure. Gastroenterology. 1992;102(6):1957–61.

129. Hyams J, Markowitz J, Treem W. Characterization of hepatic abnormalities in children with inflammatory bowel disease. Inflamm Bowel Dis. 1995;1:27.

130. Deneau M, Jensen MK, Holmen J, Williams MS, Book LS, Guthery SL. Primary sclerosing cholangitis, autoimmune hepatitis, and overlap in Utah children: epidemiology and natural history. Hepatology (Baltimore, Md). 2013;58(4):1392–400.

131. Roberts EA. Primary sclerosing cholangitis in children. J Gastroenterol Hepatol. 1999;14(6):588–93.

132. Raj V, Lichtenstein DR. Hepatobiliary manifestations of inflammatory bowel disease. Gastroenterol Clin N Am. 1999;28(2):491–513.

133. Bernstein CN, Blanchard JF, Houston DS, Wajda A. The incidence of deep venous thrombosis and pulmonary embolism among patients with inflammatory bowel disease: a population-based cohort study. Thromb Haemost. 2001;85(3):430–4.

134. Grainge MJ, West J, Card TR. Venous thromboembolism during active disease and remission in inflammatory bowel disease: a cohort study. Lancet. 2010;375(9715):657–63.

135. Kappelman MD, Horvath-Puho E, Sandler RS, Rubin DT, Ullman TA, Pedersen L, et al. Thromboembolic risk among Danish children and adults with inflammatory bowel diseases: a population-based nationwide study. Gut. 2011;60(7):937–43.

136. Zitomersky NL, Levine AE, Atkinson BJ, Harney KM, Verhave M, Bousvaros A, et al. Risk factors, morbidity, and treatment of thrombosis in children and young adults with active inflammatory bowel disease. J Pediatr Gastroenterol Nutr. 2013;57(3):343–7.

137. Nylund CM, Goudie A, Garza JM, Crouch G, Denson LA. Venous thrombotic events in hospitalized children and adolescents with inflammatory bowel disease. J Pediatr Gastroenterol Nutr. 2013;56(5):485–91.

138. Zitomersky NL, Verhave M, Trenor CC, 3rd. Thrombosis and inflammatory bowel disease: a call for improved awareness and prevention. Inflamm Bowel Dis. 2011;17(1):458–70.

139. Higuchi LM, Joffe S, Neufeld EJ, Weisdorf S, Rosh J, Murch S, et al. Inflammatory bowel disease associated with immune thrombocytopenic purpura in children. J Pediatr Gastroenterol Nutr. 2001;33(5):582–7.

140. Giannadaki E, Potamianos S, Roussomoustakaki M, Kyriakou D, Fragkiadakis N, Manousos ON. Autoimmune hemolytic anemia and positive Coombs test associated with ulcerative colitis. Am J Gastroenter. 1997;92(10):1872–4.

141. Gokhale R, Favus MJ, Karrison T, Sutton MM, Rich B, Kirschner BS. Bone mineral density assessment in children with inflammatory bowel disease. Gastroenterology. 1998;114(5):902–11.

142. Pappa H, Thayu M, Sylvester F, Leonard M, Zemel B, Gordon C. Skeletal health of children and adolescents with inflammatory bowel disease. J Pediatr Gastroenterol Nutr. 2011;53(1):11–25.

143. Clark JH, Fitzgerald JF, Bergstein JM. Nephrolithiasis in childhood inflammatory bowel disease. J Pediatr Gastroenterol Nutr. 1985;4(5):829–34.

144. Keljo DJ, Sugerman KS. Pancreatitis in patients with inflammatory bowel disease. J Pediatr Gastroenterol Nutr. 1997;25(1):108–12.

145. Huang C, Lichtenstein DR. Pancreatic and biliary tract disorders in inflammatory bowel disease. Gastrointest Endosc Clin N Am. 2002;12(3):535–59.

146. Jewell DP, Caprilli R, Mortensen N, et al. Indications and timing of surgery for severe ulcerative colitis. Gastroenterol Int. 1991;4:161–4.

147. Present DH. Toxic megacolon. Med Clin North Am. 1993;77(5):1129–48.

148. Sheth SG, LaMont JT. Toxic megacolon. Lancet. 1998;351(9101):509–13.

149. Greenstein AJ, Barth JA, Sachar DB, Aufses AH, Jr. Free colonic perforation without dilatation in ulcerative colitis. Am J Surg. 1986;152(3):272–5.

150. Jalan KN, Sircus W, Card WI, Falconer CW, Bruce CB, Crean GP, et al. An experience of ulcerative colitis. I. Toxic dilation in 55 cases. Gastroenterology. 1969;57(1):68–82.

151. Fazio VW. Toxic megacolon in ulcerative colitis and Crohn's colitis. Clin Gastroenterol. 1980;9(2):389–407.

152. Grieco MB, Bordan DL, Geiss AC, Beil AR, Jr. Toxic megacolon complicating Crohn's colitis. Ann Surg. 1980;191(1):75–80.

153. Brown JW. Toxic megacolon associated with loperamide therapy. JAMA. 1979;241(5):501–2.

154. Norland CC, Kirsner JB. Toxic dilatation of colon (toxic megacolon): etiology, treatment and prognosis in 42 patients. Medicine (Baltimore). 1969;48(3):229–50.

155. Koudahl G, Kristensen M. Toxic megacolon in ulcerative colitis. Scand J Gastroenterol. 1975;10(4):417–21.

156. Halpert RD. Toxic dilatation of the colon. Radiol Clin North Am. 1987;25(1):147–55.

157. Kramer P, Wittenberg J. Colonic gas distribution in toxic megacolon. Gastroenterology. 1981;80(3):433–7.

158. Caroline DF, Evers K. Colitis: radiographic features and differentiation of idiopathic inflammatory bowel disease. Radiol Clin North Am. 1987;25(1):47–66.

159. Gumaste V, Sachar DB, Greenstein AJ. Benign and malignant colorectal strictures in ulcerative colitis. Gut. 1992;33(7):938–41.

160. Horton KM, Jones B, Fishman EK. Imaging of the inflammatory bowel diseases. In: Kirsner JB, editor. Inflammatory bowel diseases. 5th ed. Philadelphia: W.B. Saunders Company; 2000. p. 479–500.

161. Truelove SC, Witts LJ. Cortisone in ulcerative colitis. Final report on a therapeutic trial. BMJ. 1955;2:1041.

162. Turner D, Otley AR, Mack D, Hyams J, de Bruijne J, Uusoue K, et al. Development, validation, and evaluation of a pediatric ulcerative colitis activity index: a prospective multicenter study. Gastroenterology. 2007;133(2):423–32.

163. Turner D, Hyams J, Markowitz J, Lerer T, Mack DR, Evans J, et al. Appraisal of the pediatric ulcerative colitis activity index (PUCAI). Inflamm Bowel Dis. 2009;15(8):1218–23.

164. Turner D, Mack D, Leleiko N, Walters TD, Uusoue K, Leach ST, et al. Severe pediatric ulcerative colitis: a prospective multicenter study of outcomes and predictors of response. Gastroenterology. 2010;138(7):2282–91.

165. Feagan BG, Macdonald JK. Oral 5-aminosalicylic acid for maintenance of remission in ulcerative colitis. Cochrane Database Syst Rev. 2012;10:Cd000544.

166. Sonu I, Lin MV, Blonski W, Lichtenstein GR. Clinical pharmacology of 5-ASA compounds in inflammatory bowel disease. Gastroenterol Clin N Am. 2010;39(3):559–99.

167. Zeisler B, Lerer T, Markowitz J, Mack D, Griffiths A, Bousvaros A, et al. Outcome following aminosalicylate therapy in children newly diagnosed as having ulcerative colitis. J Pediatr Gastroenterol Nutr. 2013;56(1):12–8.

168. Peppercorn MA. Sulfasalazine. Pharmacology, clinical use, toxicity, and related new drug development. Ann Intern Med. 1984;101(3):377–86.

169. Leichtner AM. Aminosalicylates for the treatment of inflammatory bowel disease. J Pediatr Gastroenterol Nutr. 1995;21(3):245–52.

170. Wahl C, Liptay S, Adler G, Schmid RM. Sulfasalazine: a potent and specific inhibitor of nuclear factor kappa B. J Clin Investig. 1998;101(5):1163–74.

171. Bantel H, Berg C, Vieth M, Stolte M, Kruis W, Schulze-Osthoff K. Mesalazine inhibits activation of transcription factor NF-kappaB in inflamed mucosa of patients with ulcerative colitis. Am J Gastroenterol. 2000;95(12):3452–7.

172. Dick AP, Grayson MJ, Carpenter RG, Petrie A. Controlled trial of sulfasalazine in the treatment of ulcerative colitis. Gut. 1964;5:437–42.

173. Sninsky CA, Cort DH, Shanahan F, Powers BJ, Sessions JT, Pruitt RE, et al. Oral mesalamine (Asacol) for mildly to moderately active ulcerative colitis. A multicenter study. Ann Intern Med. 1991;115(5):350–5.

174. Sutherland LR, May GR, Shaffer EA. Sulfasalazine revisited: a meta-analysis of 5-aminosalicylic acid in the treatment of ulcerative colitis. Ann Intern Med. 1993;118(7):540–9.

175. Gisbert JP, Gomollon F, Mate J, Pajares JM. Role of 5-aminosalicylic acid (5-ASA) in treatment of inflammatory bowel disease: a systematic review. Dig Dis Sci. 2002;47(3):471–88.

176. Sutherland LR, Roth DE, Beck PL. Alternatives to sulfasalazine: a meta-analysis of 5-ASA in the treatment of ulcerative colitis. Inflamm Bowel Dis. 1997;3(2):65–78.

177. Barden L, Lipson A, Pert P. Mesalazine in childhood inflammatory bowel disease. Aliment Pharmacol Therap. 1989;3:597.

178. Levine DS, Riff DS, Pruitt R, Wruble L, Koval G, Sales D, et al. A randomized, double blind, dose-response comparison of balsalazide (6.75 g), balsalazide (2.25 g), and mesalamine (2.4 g) in the treatment of active, mild-to-moderate ulcerative colitis. Am J Gastroenterol. 2002;97(6):1398–407.

179. Green JR, Lobo AJ, Holdsworth CD, Leicester RJ, Gibson JA, Kerr GD, et al. Balsalazide is more effective and better tolerated than mesalamine in the treatment of acute ulcerative colitis. The Abacus Investigator Group. Gastroenterology. 1998;114(1):15–22.

180. Hanauer SB. Inflammatory bowel disease. N Engl J Med. 1996;334(13):841–8.

181. Boyer DL, Li BU, Fyda JN, Friedman RA. Sulfasalazine-induced hepatotoxicity in children with inflammatory bowel disease. J Pediatr Gastroenterol Nutr. 1989;8(4):528–32.

182. Garau P, Orenstein SR, Neigut DA, Kocoshis SA. Pancreatitis associated with olsalazine and sulfasalazine in children with ulcerative colitis. J Pediatr Gastroenterol Nutr. 1994;18(4):481–5.

183. Paerregaard A, Krasilnikoff PA. Pancreatitis in a child after rectal administration of 5-aminosalicylic acid. Inflamm Bowel Dis. 1997;3:20.

184. Sturgeon JB, Bhatia P, Hermens D, Miner PB, Jr. Exacerbation of chronic ulcerative colitis with mesalamine. Gastroenterology. 1995;108(6):1889–93.

185. Hyams J, Markowitz J, Lerer T, Griffiths A, Mack D, Bousvaros A, et al. The natural history of corticosteroid therapy for ulcerative colitis in children. Clin Gastroenterol Hepatol. 2006;4(9):1118–23.

186. Truhan AP, Ahmed AR. Corticosteroids: a review with emphasis on complications of prolonged systemic therapy. Ann Allergy. 1989;62(5):375–91.

187. Kirschner BS. The medical management of inflammatory bowel disease in children. In: Kirsner JB, editor. Inflammatory bowel disease. Philadelphia: Saunders; 2000. p. 578–97.

188. Bousvaros A. Immunosuppression. In: Walker WA, Durie PR, Hamilton JR, Walker-Smith JA, Watkins JB, editors. Pediatric gastrointestinal disease. Ontario: B.C. Decker; 2000. p. 1769–94.

189. McIntyre PB, Powell-Tuck J, Wood SR, Lennard-Jones JE, Lerebours E, Hecketsweiler P, et al. Controlled trial of bowel rest in the treatment of severe acute colitis. Gut. 1986;27(5):481–5.

190. Dickinson RJ, Ashton MG, Axon AT, Smith RC, Yeung CK, Hill GL. Controlled trial of intravenous hyperalimentation and total bowel rest as an adjunct to the routine therapy of acute colitis. Gastroenterology. 1980;79(6):1199–204.

191. Peppercorn MA. Are antibiotics useful in the management of nontoxic severe ulcerative colitis? J Clin Gastroenterol. 1993;17(1):14–7.

192. Chapman RW, Selby WS, Jewell DP. Controlled trial of intravenous metronidazole as an adjunct to corticosteroids in severe ulcerative colitis. Gut. 1986;27(10):1210–2.

193. Mantzaris GJ, Hatzis A, Kontogiannis P, Triadaphyllou G. Intravenous tobramycin and metronidazole as an adjunct to corticosteroids in acute, severe ulcerative colitis. Am J Gastroenterol. 1994;89(1):43–6.

194. Mantzaris GJ, Petraki K, Archavlis E, Amberiadis P, Kourtessas D, Christidou A, et al. A prospective randomized controlled trial of intravenous ciprofloxacin as an adjunct to corticosteroids in acute, severe ulcerative colitis. Scand J Gastroenterol. 2001;36(9):971–4.

195. Turner D, Travis SP, Griffiths AM, Ruemmele FM, Levine A, Benchimol EI, et al. Consensus for managing acute severe ulcerative colitis in children: a systematic review and joint statement from ECCO, ESPGHAN, and the Porto IBD Working Group of ESPGHAN. Am J Gastroenterol. 2011;106(4):574–88.

196. Jarnerot G, Hertervig E, Friis-Liby I, Blomquist L, Karlen P, Granno C, et al. Infliximab as rescue therapy in severe to moderately severe ulcerative colitis: a randomized, placebo-controlled study. Gastroenterology. 2005;128(7):1805–11.

197. Vande Casteele N, Feagan BG, Gils A, Vermeire S, Khanna R, Sandborn WJ, et al. Therapeutic drug monitoring in inflammatory bowel disease: current state and future perspectives. Curr Gastroenterol Rep. 2014;16(4):378.

198. Watanabe M, Hibi T, Mostafa NM, Chao J, Arora V, Camez A, et al. Long-term safety and efficacy of adalimumab in Japanese patients with moderate to severe Crohn's disease. J Crohn's Colitis. 2014;8(11):1407–16

199. Watson S, Pensabene L, Mitchell P, Bousvaros A. Outcomes and adverse events in children and young adults undergoing tacrolimus therapy for steroid-refractory colitis. Inflamm Bowel Dis. 2011;17(1):22–9.

200. Hait EJ, Bousvaros A, Schuman M, Shamberger RC, Lillehei CW. Pouch outcomes among children with ulcerative colitis treated with calcineurin inhibitors before ileal pouch anal anastomosis surgery. J Pediatr Surg. 2007;42(1):31–4; discussion 4–5.

201. Treem WR, Cohen J, Davis PM, Justinich CJ, Hyams JS. Cyclosporine for the treatment of fulminant ulcerative colitis in children. Immediate response, long-term results, and impact on surgery. Dis Colon Rectum. 1995;38(5):474–9.

202. Bousvaros A, Kirschner BS, Werlin SL, Parker-Hartigan L, Daum F, Freeman KB, et al. Oral tacrolimus treatment of severe colitis in children. J Pediatr. 2000;137(6):794–9.

203. Marshall JK, Irvine EJ. Rectal aminosalicylate therapy for distal ulcerative colitis: a meta-analysis. Aliment Pharmacol Ther. 1995;9(3):293–300.

204. Marshall JK, Irvine EJ. Rectal corticosteroids versus alternative treatments in ulcerative colitis: a meta-analysis. Gut. 1997;40(6):775–81.

205. Mulder CJ, Tytgat GN. Review article: topical corticosteroids in inflammatory bowel disease. Aliment Pharmacol Ther. 1993;7:125–30.

206. Gionchetti P, Rizzello F, Venturi A, Ferretti M, Brignola C, Miglioli M, et al. Comparison of oral with rectal mesalazine in the treatment of ulcerative proctitis. Dis Colon Rectum. 1998;41(1):93–7.

207. Cohen RD, Woseth DM, Thisted RA, Hanauer SB. A meta-analysis and overview of the literature on treatment options for left-sided ulcerative colitis and ulcerative proctitis. Am J Gastroenterol. 2000;95(5):1263–76.

208. Allgayer H. Sulfasalazine and 5-ASA compounds. Gastroenterol Clin N Am. 1992;21(3):643–58.

209. Sutherland LR. Topical treatment of ulcerative colitis. Med Clin North Am. 1990;74(1):119–31.

210. Safdi M, DeMicco M, Sninsky C, Banks P, Wruble L, Deren J, et al. A double-blind comparison of oral versus rectal mesalamine versus combination therapy in the treatment of distal ulcerative colitis. Am J Gastroenterol. 1997;92(10):1867–71.

211. Danielsson A, Lofberg R, Persson T, Salde L, Schioler R, Suhr O, et al. A steroid enema, budesonide, lacking systemic effects for the treatment of distal ulcerative colitis or proctitis. Scand J Gastroenterol. 1992;27(1):9–12.

212. Hanauer SB, Robinson M, Pruitt R, Lazenby AJ, Persson T, Nilsson LG, et al. Budesonide enema for the treatment of active, distal ulcerative colitis and proctitis: a dose-ranging study. U.S. Budesonide enema study group. Gastroenterology. 1998;115(3):525–32.

213. D'Agata ID, Vanounou T, Seidman E. Mesalamine in pediatric inflammatory bowel disease: a 10-year experience. Inflamm Bowel Dis. 1996;2:229–35.

214. Kruis W, Schreiber S, Theuer D, Brandes JW, Schutz E, Howaldt S, et al. Low dose balsalazide (1.5 g twice daily) and mesalazine (0.5 g three times daily) maintained remission of ulcerative colitis but high dose balsalazide (3.0 g twice daily) was superior in preventing relapses. Gut. 2001;49(6):783–9.

215. d'Albasio G, Paoluzi P, Campieri M, Porro GB, Pera A, Prantera C, et al. Maintenance treatment of ulcerative proctitis with mesalazine suppositories: a double-blind placebo-controlled trial. The Italian IBD Study Group. Am J Gastroenterol. 1998;93(5): 799–803.

216. d'Albasio G, Pacini F, Camarri E, Messori A, Trallori G, Bonanomi AG, et al. Combined therapy with 5-aminosalicylic acid tablets and enemas for maintaining remission in ulcerative colitis: a randomized double-blind study. Am J Gastroenterol. 1997;92(7):1143–7.

217. Ryan BM, Russel MG, Langholz E, Stockbrugger RW. Aminosalicylates and colorectal cancer in IBD: a not-so bitter pill to swallow. Am J Gastroenterol. 2003;98(8):1682–7.

218. Eaden J, Abrams K, Ekbom A, Jackson E, Mayberry J. Colorectal cancer prevention in ulcerative colitis: a case-control study. Aliment Pharmacol Therapeut. 2000;14(2):145–53.

219. Pinczowski D, Ekbom A, Baron J, Yuen J, Adami HO. Risk factors for colorectal cancer in patients with ulcerative colitis: a case-control study. Gastroenterology. 1994;107(1):117–20.

220. Verhave M, Winter HS, Grand RJ. Azathioprine in the treatment of children with inflammatory bowel disease. J Pediatr. 1990;117(5):809–14.

221. Kader HA, Mascarenhas MR, Piccoli DA, Stouffer NO, Baldassano RN. Experiences with 6-mercaptopurine and azathioprine therapy in pediatric patients with severe ulcerative colitis. J Pediatr Gastroenterol Nutr. 1999;28(1):54–8.

222. Pearson DC, May GR, Fick GH, Sutherland LR. Azathioprine and 6-mercaptopurine in Crohn disease. A meta-analysis. Ann Intern Med. 1995;123(2):132–42.

223. Tiede I, Fritz G, Strand S, Poppe D, Dvorsky R, Strand D, et al. CD28-dependent Rac1 activation is the molecular target of azathioprine in primary human CD4 + T lymphocytes. J Clin Investig. 2003;111(8):1133–45.

224. Kirschner BS. Safety of azathioprine and 6-mercaptopurine in pediatric patients with inflammatory bowel disease. Gastroenterology. 1998;115(4):813–21.

225. Hyams JS, Lerer T, Mack D, Bousvaros A, Griffiths A, Rosh J, et al. Outcome following thiopurine use in children with ulcerative colitis: a prospective multicenter registry study. Am J Gastroenterol. 2011;106(5):981–7.

226. Louis E, Belaiche J. Optimizing treatment with thioguanine derivatives in inflammatory bowel disease. Best Pract Res Clin Gastroenterol. 2003;17(1):37–46.

227. Derijks LJ, Gilissen LP, Hooymans PM, Hommes DW. Review article: thiopurines in inflammatory bowel disease. Alim Pharmacol Ther. 2006;24(5):715–29.

228. Lennard L, Van Loon JA, Weinshilboum RM. Pharmacogenetics of acute azathioprine toxicity: relationship to thiopurine methyltransferase genetic polymorphism. Clin Pharmacol Ther. 1989;46(2):149–54.

229. Osterman MT, Kundu R, Lichtenstein GR, Lewis JD. Association of 6-thioguanine nucleotide levels and inflammatory bowel disease activity: a meta-analysis. Gastroenterology. 2006;130(4):1047–53.

230. Cuffari C, Theoret Y, Latour S, Seidman G. 6-Mercaptopurine metabolism in Crohn's disease: correlation with efficacy and toxicity. Gut. 1996;39(3):401–6.

231. Dubinsky MC, Lamothe S, Yang HY, Targan SR, Sinnett D, Theoret Y, et al. Pharmacogenomics and metabolite measurement for 6-mercaptopurine therapy in inflammatory bowel disease. Gastroenterology. 2000;118(4):705–13.

232. Cuffari C, Hunt S, Bayless T. Utilisation of erythrocyte 6-thioguanine metabolite levels to optimise azathioprine therapy in patients with inflammatory bowel disease. Gut. 2001;48(5):642–6.

233. Rahhal RM, Bishop WP. Initial clinical experience with allopurinol-thiopurine combination therapy in pediatric inflammatory bowel disease. Inflamm Bowel Dis. 2008;14(12):1678–82.

234. Shih DQ, Nguyen M, Zheng L, Ibanez P, Mei L, Kwan LY, et al. Split-dose administration of thiopurine drugs: a novel and effective strategy for managing preferential 6-MMP metabolism. Alim Pharmacol Ther. 2012;36(5):449–58.

235. George J, Present DH, Pou R, Bodian C, Rubin PH. The long-term outcome of ulcerative colitis treated with 6-mercaptopurine. Am J Gastroenterol. 1996;91(9):1711–4.

236. Kandiel A, Fraser AG, Korelitz BI, Brensinger C, Lewis JD. Increased risk of lymphoma among inflammatory bowel disease patients treated with azathioprine and 6-mercaptopurine. Gut. 2005;54(8):1121–5.

237. Dayharsh GA, Loftus EV, Jr., Sandborn WJ, Tremaine WJ, Zinsmeister AR, Witzig TE, et al. Epstein-Barr virus-positive lymphoma in patients with inflammatory bowel disease treated with azathioprine or 6-mercaptopurine. Gastroenterology. 2002;122(1):72–7.

238. Chande N, MacDonald JK, McDonald JW. Methotrexate for induction of remission in ulcerative colitis. Cochrane Database Syst Rev. 2007(4):CD006618.

239. Jolivet J, Cowan KH, Curt GA, Clendeninn NJ, Chabner BA. The pharmacology and clinical use of methotrexate. N Engl J Med. 1983;309(18):1094–104.

240. Ravikumara M, Hinsberger A, Spray CH. Role of methotrexate in the management of Crohn disease. J Pediatr Gastroenterol Nutr. 2007;44(4):427–30.

241. Morabito L, Montesinos MC, Schreibman DM, Balter L, Thompson LF, Resta R, et al. Methotrexate and sulfasalazine promote adenosine release by a mechanism that requires ecto-5'-nucleotidase-mediated conversion of adenine nucleotides. J Clin Invest. 1998;101(2):295–300.

242. Genestier L, Paillot R, Fournel S, Ferraro C, Miossec P, Revillard JP. Immunosuppressive properties of methotrexate: apoptosis and clonal deletion of activated peripheral T cells. J Clin Investig. 1998;102(2):322–8.

243. Cronstein BN. The mechanism of action of methotrexate. Rheum Dis Clin N Am. 1997;23(4):739–55.

244. Oren R, Arber N, Odes S, Moshkowitz M, Keter D, Pomeranz I, et al. Methotrexate in chronic active ulcerative colitis: a double-blind, randomized, Israeli multicenter trial. Gastroenterology. 1996;110(5):1416–21.

245. Aloi M, Di Nardo G, Conte F, Mazzeo L, Cavallari N, Nuti F, et al. Methotrexate in paediatric ulcerative colitis: a retrospective

survey at a single tertiary referral centre. Alim Pharmacol Ther. 2010;32(8):1017–22.

246. Jakobsen C, Bartek J, Jr., Wewer V, Vind I, Munkholm P, Groen R, et al. Differences in phenotype and disease course in adult and paediatric inflammatory bowel disease—a population-based study. Alim Pharmacol Ther. 2011;34(10):1217–24.

247. Breese EJ, Michie CA, Nicholls SW, Murch SH, Williams CB, Domizio P, et al. Tumor necrosis factor alpha-producing cells in the intestinal mucosa of children with inflammatory bowel disease. Gastroenterology. 1994;106(6):1455–66.

248. Viallard JF, Pellegrin JL, Ranchin V, Schaeverbeke T, Dehais J, Longy-Boursier M, et al. Th1 (IL-2, interferon-gamma (IFN-gamma)) and Th2 (IL-10, IL-4) cytokine production by peripheral blood mononuclear cells (PBMC) from patients with systemic lupus erythematosus (SLE). Clin Exp Immunol. 1999;115(1):189–95.

249. Hyams J, Damaraju L, Blank M, Johanns J, Guzzo C, Winter HS, et al. Induction and maintenance therapy with infliximab for children with moderate to severe ulcerative colitis. Clin Gastroenterol Hepatol. 2012;10(4):391–9. e1.

250. Rutgeerts P, Sandborn WJ, Feagan BG, Reinisch W, Olson A, Johanns J, et al. Infliximab for induction and maintenance therapy for ulcerative colitis. N Engl J Med. 2005;353(23):2462–76.

251. Panaccione R, Ghosh S, Middleton S, Marquez JR, Scott BB, Flint L, et al. Combination therapy with infliximab and azathioprine is superior to monotherapy with either agent in ulcerative colitis. Gastroenterology. 2014;146(2):392–400. e3.

252. Sandborn WJ, van Assche G, Reinisch W, Colombel JF, D'Haens G, Wolf DC, et al. Adalimumab induces and maintains clinical remission in patients with moderate-to-severe ulcerative colitis. Gastroenterology. 2012;142(2):257–65.e1–3.

253. Erle DJ, Briskin MJ, Butcher EC, Garcia-Pardo A, Lazarovits AI, Tidswell M. Expression and function of the MAdCAM-1 receptor, integrin alpha 4 beta 7, on human leukocytes. J Immunol. 1994;153(2):517–28.

254. Arihiro S, Ohtani H, Suzuki M, Murata M, Ejima C, Oki M, et al. Differential expression of mucosal addressin cell adhesion molecule-1 (MAdCAM-1) in ulcerative colitis and Crohn's disease. Pathol Int. 2002;52(5–6):367–74.

255. Briskin M, Winsor-Hines D, Shyjan A, Cochran N, Bloom S, Wilson J, et al. Human mucosal addressin cell adhesion molecule-1 is preferentially expressed in intestinal tract and associated lymphoid tissue. Am J Pathol. 1997;151(1):97–110.

256. Feagan BG, Rutgeerts P, Sands BE, Hanauer S, Colombel JF, Sandborn WJ, et al. Vedolizumab as induction and maintenance therapy for ulcerative colitis. N Engl J Med. 2013;369(8):699–710.

257. Burke DA, Axon AT, Clayden SA, Dixon MF, Johnston D, Lacey RW. The efficacy of tobramycin in the treatment of ulcerative colitis. Alim Pharmacol Ther. 1990;4(2):123–9.

258. Lobo AJ, Burke DA, Sobala GM, Axon AT. Oral tobramycin in ulcerative colitis: effect on maintenance of remission. Alim Pharmacol Ther. 1993;7(2):155–8.

259. Gilat T, Suissa A, Leichtman G, Delpre G, Pavlotzky M, Grossman A, et al. A comparative study of metronidazole and sulfasalazine in active, not severe, ulcerative colitis. An Israeli multicenter trial. J Clin Gastroenterol. 1987;9(4):415–7.

260. Dickinson RJ, O'Connor HJ, Pinder I, Hamilton I, Johnston D, Axon AT. Double blind controlled trial of oral vancomycin as adjunctive treatment in acute exacerbations of idiopathic colitis. Gut. 1985;26(12):1380–4.

261. Mantzaris GJ, Archavlis E, Christoforidis P, Kourtessas D, Amberiadis P, Florakis N, et al. A prospective randomized controlled trial of oral ciprofloxacin in acute ulcerative colitis. Am J Gastroenterol. 1997;92(3):454–6.

262. Turunen UM, Farkkila MA, Hakala K, Seppala K, Sivonen A, Ogren M, et al. Long-term treatment of ulcerative colitis with ciprofloxacin: a prospective, double-blind, placebo-controlled study. Gastroenterology. 1998;115(5):1072–8.

263. Changelian PS, Moshinsky D, Kuhn CF, Flanagan ME, Munchhof MJ, Harris TM, et al. The specificity of JAK3 kinase inhibitors. Blood. 2008;111(4):2155–7.

264. Flanagan ME, Blumenkopf TA, Brissette WH, Brown MF, Casavant JM, Shang-Poa C, et al. Discovery of CP-690,550: a potent and selective Janus kinase (JAK) inhibitor for the treatment of autoimmune diseases and organ transplant rejection. J Med Chem. 2010;53(24):8468–84.

265. Ghoreschi K, Jesson MI, Li X, Lee JL, Ghosh S, Alsup JW, et al. Modulation of innate and adaptive immune responses by tofacitinib (CP-690,550). J Immunol. 2011;186(7):4234–43.

266. Sandborn WJ, Ghosh S, Panes J, Vranic I, Su C, Rousell S, et al. Tofacitinib, an oral Janus kinase inhibitor, in active ulcerative colitis. N Engl J Med. 2012;367(7):616–24.

267. Allison AC, Eugui EM. Mycophenolate mofetil and its mechanisms of action. Immunopharmacology. 2000;47(2–3):85–118.

268. Palaniappan S, Ford AC, Greer D, Everett SM, Chalmers DM, Axon AT, et al. Mycophenolate mofetil therapy for refractory inflammatory bowel disease. Inflamm Bowel Dis. 2007;13(12):1488–92.

269. Smith MR, Cooper SC. Mycophenolate mofetil therapy in the management of inflammatory bowel disease–A retrospective case series and review. J Crohn's Colitis. 2014: 8(8):890–7

270. Gionchetti P, Rizzello F, Helwig U, Venturi A, Lammers KM, Brigidi P, et al. Prophylaxis of pouchitis onset with probiotic therapy: a double-blind, placebo-controlled trial. Gastroenterology. 2003;124(5):1202–9.

271. Miele E, Pascarella F, Giannetti E, Quaglietta L, Baldassano RN, Staiano A. Effect of a probiotic preparation (VSL#3) on induction and maintenance of remission in children with ulcerative colitis. Am J Gastroenterol. 2009;104(2):437–43.

272. Shen J, Zuo ZX, Mao AP. Effect of probiotics on inducing remission and maintaining therapy in ulcerative colitis, Crohn's disease, and pouchitis: meta-analysis of randomized controlled trials. Inflamm Bowel Dis. 2014;20(1):21–35.

273. Stenson WF, Cort D, Rodgers J, Burakoff R, DeSchryver-Kecskemeti K, Gramlich TL, et al. Dietary supplementation with fish oil in ulcerative colitis. Ann Intern Med. 1992;116(8):609–14.

274. Aslan A, Triadafilopoulos G. Fish oil fatty acid supplementation in active ulcerative colitis: a double-blind, placebo-controlled, crossover study. Am J Gastroenterol. 1992;87(4):432–7.

275. Hawthorne AB, Daneshmend TK, Hawkey CJ, Belluzzi A, Everitt SJ, Holmes GK, et al. Treatment of ulcerative colitis with fish oil supplementation: a prospective 12 month randomised controlled trial. Gut. 1992;33(7):922–8.

276. Greenfield SM, Green AT, Teare JP, Jenkins AP, Punchard NA, Ainley CC, et al. A randomized controlled study of evening primrose oil and fish oil in ulcerative colitis. Alim Pharmacol Ther. 1993;7(2):159–66.

277. Scheppach W. Treatment of distal ulcerative colitis with short-chain fatty acid enemas. A placebo-controlled trial. German-Austrian SCFA Study Group. Dig Dis Sci. 1996;41(11):2254–9.

278. Breuer RI, Soergel KH, Lashner BA, Christ ML, Hanauer SB, Vanagunas A, et al. Short chain fatty acid rectal irrigation for left-sided ulcerative colitis: a randomised, placebo controlled trial. Gut. 1997;40(4):485–91.

279. Vernia P, Marcheggiano A, Caprilli R, Frieri G, Corrao G, Valpiani D, et al. Short-chain fatty acid topical treatment in distal ulcerative colitis. Alim Pharmacol Ther. 1995;9(3):309–13.

280. Motil KJ, Grand RJ. Nutritional management of inflammatory bowel disease. Pediatr Clin North Am. 1985;32(2):447–69.

281. Burke A, Lichtenstein GR, Rombeau JL. Nutrition and ulcerative colitis. Baillieres Clin Gastroenterol. 1997;11(1):153–74.

282. Dziechciarz P, Horvath A, Shamir R, Szajewska H. Meta-analysis: enteral nutrition in active Crohn's disease in children. Alim Pharmacol Ther. 2007;26(6):795–806.

283. Johnson T, Macdonald S, Hill SM, Thomas A, Murphy MS. Treatment of active Crohn's disease in children using partial enteral nutrition with liquid formula: a randomised controlled trial. Gut. 2006;55(3):356–61.

284. Kleinman RE, Balistreri WF, Heyman MB, Kirschner BS, Lake AM, Motil KJ, et al. Nutritional support for pediatric patients with inflammatory bowel disease. J Pediatr Gastroenterol Nutr. 1989;8(1):8–12.

285. Escher JC, Taminiau JA, Nieuwenhuis EE, Buller HA, Grand RJ. Treatment of inflammatory bowel disease in childhood: best available evidence. Inflamm Bowel Dis. 2003;9(1):34–58.

286. Durno C, Sherman P, Harris K, Smith C, Dupuis A, Shandling B, et al. Outcome after ileoanal anastomosis in pediatric patients with ulcerative colitis. J Pediatr Gastroenterol Nutr. 1998;27(5):501–7.

287. Perrault J, Berry R, Greseth J, Zinsmeister A, Telander R. Pouchitis in young patients after the ileal-pouch anal anastomosis. Infamm Bowel Dis. 1997;3(3):181–5.

288. Dozois RR, Kelly KA. The surgical management of ulcerative colitis. In: Kirsner JB, editor. Inflammatory bowel disease. Philadelphia: W.B. Saunders Company; 2000. p. 626–57.

289. Nicholls S, Vieira MC, Majrowski WH, Shand WS, Savage MO, Walker-Smith JA. Linear growth after colectomy for ulcerative colitis in childhood. J Pediatr Gastroenterol Nutr. 1995;21(1): 82–6.

290. Falcone RA, Jr., Lewis LG, Warner BW. Predicting the need for colectomy in pediatric patients with ulcerative colitis. J Gastrointest Surg. 2000;4(2):201–6.

291. Kettlewell MGW. Recent advances in surgical therapy. In: Tytgat GNJ, Bartelsman JFWM, van Deventer SJH, editors. Inflammatory bowel diseases. Boston: Kluwer; 1995. p. 508–16.

292. Farouk R, Pemberton JH. Surgical options in ulcerative colitis. Surg Clin North Am. 1997;77(1):85–94.

293. Mowschenson PM, Critchlow JF. Outcome of early surgical complications following ileoanal pouch operation without diverting ileostomy. Am J Surg. 1995;169(1):143–5; discussion 5–6.

294. Fonkalsrud EW, Thakur A, Beanes S. Ileoanal pouch procedures in children. J Pediatr Surg. 2001;36(11):1689–92.

295. Telander RL, Spencer M, Perrault J, Telander D, Zinsmeister AR. Long-term follow-up of the ileoanal anastomosis in children and young adults. Surgery. 1990;108(4):717–23; discussion 23–5.

296. Ording Olsen K, Juul S, Berndtsson I, Oresland T, Laurberg S. Ulcerative colitis: female fecundity before diagnosis, during disease, and after surgery compared with a population sample. Gastroenterology. 2002;122(1):15–9.

297. Rintala RJ, Lindahl HG. Proctocolectomy and J-pouch ileo-anal anastomosis in children. J Pediatr Surg. 2002;37(1):66–70.

298. Mahadevan U, Sandborn WJ. Diagnosis and management of pouchitis. Gastroenterology. 2003;124(6):1636–50.

299. Sandborn WJ. Pouchitis following ileal pouch-anal anastomosis: definition, pathogenesis, and treatment. Gastroenterology. 1994;107(6):1856–60.

300. Gionchetti P, Amadini C, Rizzello F, Venturi A, Campieri M. Review article: treatment of mild to moderate ulcerative colitis and pouchitis. Alim Pharmacol Ther. 2002;16 Suppl 4:13–9.

301. Shen B, Achkar JP, Lashner BA, Ormsby AH, Remzi FH, Brzezinski A, et al. A randomized clinical trial of ciprofloxacin and metronidazole to treat acute pouchitis. Inflamm Bowel Dis. 2001;7(4):301–5.

302. Miglioli M, Barbara L, Di Febo G, Gozzetti G, Lauri A, Paganelli GM, et al. Topical administration of 5-aminosalicylic acid: a therapeutic proposal for the treatment of pouchitis. N Engl J Med. 1989;320(4):257.

303. Sambuelli A, Boerr L, Negreira S, Gil A, Camartino G, Huernos S, et al. Budesonide enema in pouchitis–a double-blind, double-dummy, controlled trial. Alim Pharmacol Ther. 2002;16(1):27–34.

304. Winter TA, Dalton HR, Merrett MN, Campbell A, Jewell DP. Cyclosporin A retention enemas in refractory distal ulcerative colitis and 'pouchitis'. Scand J Gastroenterol. 1993;28(8):701–4.

305. de Silva HJ, Ireland A, Kettlewell M, Mortensen N, Jewell DP. Short-chain fatty acid irrigation in severe pouchitis. N Engl J Med. 1989;321(20):1416–7.

306. Wischmeyer P, Pemberton JH, Phillips SF. Chronic pouchitis after ileal pouch-anal anastomosis: responses to butyrate and glutamine suppositories in a pilot study. Mayo Clin Proc. 1993;68(10): 978–81.

307. Gionchetti P, Rizzello F, Venturi A, Brigidi P, Matteuzzi D, Bazzocchi G, et al. Oral bacteriotherapy as maintenance treatment in patients with chronic pouchitis: a double-blind, placebo-controlled trial. Gastroenterology. 2000;119(2):305–9.

308. Sarigol S, Wyllie R, Gramlich T, Alexander F, Fazio V, Kay M, et al. Incidence of dysplasia in pelvic pouches in pediatric patients after ileal pouch-anal anastomosis for ulcerative colitis. J Pediatr Gastroenterol Nutr. 1999;28(4):429–34.

309. Thompson-Fawcett MW, Marcus V, Redston M, Cohen Z, McLeod RS. Risk of dysplasia in long-term ileal pouches and pouches with chronic pouchitis. Gastroenterology. 2001;121(2):275–81.

310. Veress B, Reinholt FP, Lindquist K, Lofberg R, Liljeqvist L. Long-term histomorphological surveillance of the pelvic ileal pouch: dysplasia develops in a subgroup of patients. Gastroenterology. 1995;109(4):1090–7.

311. Heuschen UA, Heuschen G, Autschbach F, Allemeyer EH, Herfarth C. Adenocarcinoma in the ileal pouch: late risk of cancer after restorative proctocolectomy. Int J Colorectal Dis. 2001;16(2):126–30.

312. Burke PM, Neigut D, Kocoshis S, Chandra R, Sauer J. Correlates of depression in new onset pediatric inflammatory bowel disease. Child Psychiatry Hum Dev. 1994;24(4):275–83.

313. Szajnberg N, Krall V, Davis P, Treem W, Hyams J. Psychopathology and relationship measures in children with inflammatory bowel disease and their parents. Child Psychiatry Hum Dev. 1993;23(3):215–32.

314. Engstrom I. Mental health and psychological functioning in children and adolescents with inflammatory bowel disease: a comparison with children having other chronic illnesses and with healthy children. J Child Psychol Psychiatry. 1992;33(3):563–82.

315. Engstrom I, Lindquist BL. Inflammatory bowel disease in children and adolescents: a somatic and psychiatric investigation. Acta Paediatr Scand. 1991;80(6–7):640–7.

316. Loonen HJ, Grootenhuis MA, Last BF, Koopman HM, Derkx HH. Quality of life in paediatric inflammatory bowel disease measured by a generic and a disease-specific questionnaire. Acta Paediatr. 2002;91(3):348–54.

317. Szigethy E, Levy-Warren A, Whitton S, Bousvaros A, Gauvreau K, Leichtner AM, et al. Depressive symptoms and inflammatory bowel disease in children and adolescents: a cross-sectional study. J Pediatr Gastroenterol Nutr. 2004;39(4):395–403.

318. Otley A, Smith C, Nicholas D, Munk M, Avolio J, Sherman PM, et al. The IMPACT questionnaire: a valid measure of health-related quality of life in pediatric inflammatory bowel disease. J Pediatr Gastroenterol Nutr. 2002;35(4):557–63.

319. Loonen HJ, Grootenhuis MA, Last BF, de Haan RJ, Bouquet J, Derkx BH. Measuring quality of life in children with inflammatory bowel disease: the impact-II (NL). Qual Life Res. 2002;11(1):47–56.

320. Hyams JS, Davis P, Grancher K, Lerer T, Justinich CJ, Markowitz J. Clinical outcome of ulcerative colitis in children. J Pediatr. 1996;129(1):81–8.

321. Langholz E, Munkholm P, Davidsen M, Nielsen OH, Binder V. Changes in extent of ulcerative colitis: a study on the course and prognostic factors. Scand J Gastroenterol. 1996;31(3):260–6.

322. Meucci G, Vecchi M, Astegiano M, Beretta L, Cesari P, Dizioli P, et al. The natural history of ulcerative proctitis: a multicenter, retrospective study. Gruppo di Studio per le Malattie Infiammatorie Intestinali (GSMII). Am J Gastroenterol. 2000;95(2):469–73.

323. Hyams J, Davis P, Lerer T, Colletti RB, Bousvaros A, Leichtner A, et al. Clinical outcome of ulcerative proctitis in children. J Pediatr Gastroenterol Nutr. 1997;25(2):149–52.

324. Ekbom A. Risk factors and distinguishing features of cancer in IBD. Inflamm Bowel Dis. 1998;4(3):235–43.

325. Devroede GJ, Taylor WF, Sauer WG, Jackman RJ, Stickler GB. Cancer risk and life expectancy of children with ulcerative colitis. N Engl J Med. 1971;285(1):17–21.

326. Ekbom A, Helmick C, Zack M, Adami HO. Ulcerative colitis and colorectal cancer. A population-based study. N Engl J Med. 1990;323(18):1228–33.

327. Brostrom O, Lofberg R, Nordenvall B, Ost A, Hellers G. The risk of colorectal cancer in ulcerative colitis. An epidemiologic study. Scand J Gastroenterol. 1987;22(10):1193–9.

328. Gilat T, Fireman Z, Grossman A, Hacohen D, Kadish U, Ron E, et al. Colorectal cancer in patients with ulcerative colitis. A population study in central Israel. Gastroenterology. 1988;94(4):870–7.

329. Jess T, Simonsen J, Jorgensen KT, Pedersen BV, Nielsen NM, Frisch M. Decreasing risk of colorectal cancer in patients with inflammatory bowel disease over 30 years. Gastroenterology. 2012;143(2):375–81.e1; quiz e13–4.

330. Broome U, Lofberg R, Veress B, Eriksson LS. Primary sclerosing cholangitis and ulcerative colitis: evidence for increased neoplastic potential. Hepatology (Baltimore, Md). 1995;22(5):1404–8.

331. Shetty K, Rybicki L, Brzezinski A, Carey WD, Lashner BA. The risk for cancer or dysplasia in ulcerative colitis patients with primary sclerosing cholangitis. Am J Gastroenterol. 1999;94(6):1643–9.

332. Soetikno RM, Lin OS, Heidenreich PA, Young HS, Blackstone MO. Increased risk of colorectal neoplasia in patients with primary sclerosing cholangitis and ulcerative colitis: a meta-analysis. Gastrointest Endosc. 2002;56(1):48–54.

333. Pardi DS, Loftus EV, Jr., Kremers WK, Keach J, Lindor KD. Ursodeoxycholic acid as a chemopreventive agent in patients with ulcerative colitis and primary sclerosing cholangitis. Gastroenterology. 2003;124(4):889–93.

334. Eaton JE, Silveira MG, Pardi DS, Sinakos E, Kowdley KV, Luketic VA, et al. High-dose ursodeoxycholic acid is associated with the development of colorectal neoplasia in patients with ulcerative colitis and primary sclerosing cholangitis. Am J Gastroenterol. 2011;106(9):1638–45.

335. Askling J, Dickman PW, Karlen P, Brostrom O, Lapidus A, Lofberg R, et al. Family history as a risk factor for colorectal cancer in inflammatory bowel disease. Gastroenterology. 2001;120(6):1356–62.

336. Rutter MD, Saunders BP, Wilkinson KH, Rumbles S, Schofield G, Kamm MA, et al. Cancer surveillance in longstanding ulcerative colitis: endoscopic appearances help predict cancer risk. Gut. 2004;53(12):1813–6.

337. Farraye FA, Odze RD, Eaden J, Itzkowitz SH. AGA technical review on the diagnosis and management of colorectal neoplasia in inflammatory bowel disease. Gastroenterology. 2010;138(2):746–74, 74.e1–4; quiz e12–3.

338. Lindberg BU, Broome U, Persson B. Proximal colorectal dysplasia or cancer in ulcerative colitis. The impact of primary sclerosing cholangitis and sulfasalazine: results from a 20-year surveillance study. Dis Colon Rectum. 2001;44(1):77–85.

339. Velayos FS, Terdiman JP, Walsh JM. Effect of 5-aminosalicylate use on colorectal cancer and dysplasia risk: a systematic review and metaanalysis of observational studies. Am J Gastroenterol. 2005;100(6):1345–53.

340. Velayos FS, Ullman TA. Looking forward to understanding and reducing colorectal cancer risk in inflammatory bowel disease. Gastroenterology. 2013;145(1):47–9.

341. Farraye FA, Odze RD, Eaden J, Itzkowitz SH, McCabe RP, Dassopoulos T, et al. AGA medical position statement on the diagnosis and management of colorectal neoplasia in inflammatory bowel disease. Gastroenterology. 2010;138(2):738–45.

342. Cairns SR, Scholefield JH, Steele RJ, Dunlop MG, Thomas HJ, Evans GD, et al. Guidelines for colorectal cancer screening and surveillance in moderate and high risk groups (update from 2002). Gut. 2010;59(5):666–89.

343. Shergill AK, Farraye FA. Toward a consensus on endoscopic surveillance of patients with colonic inflammatory bowel disease. Gastrointest Endosc Clin N Am. 2014;24(3):469–81

344. Griffiths AM, Sherman PM. Colonoscopic surveillance for cancer in ulcerative colitis: a critical review. J Pediatr Gastroenterol Nutr. 1997;24(2):202–10.

Vasculitides Including Henoch–Schönlein Purpura

31

Keith J. Lindley and Jutta Köglmeier

Introduction

The vasculitides are a group of inflammatory disorders of the walls of blood vessels (usually the arteries). They are relatively rare in childhood with the exception of Henoch–Schönlein purpura (HSP) and Kawasaki disease (KD). Vasculitis might be primary or secondary to a number of causes including infections, drugs, hypersensitivity reactions and connective-tissue disorders. The consequences of arterial inflammation include tissue ischaemia and necrosis, giving rise to many of the gastrointestinal (GI) manifestations of vascular inflammation such as pain and bleeding.

Vasculitis is usually classified based on the size of blood vessel involved in the inflammatory process (Table 31.1 and Fig. 31.1). Not all of these are seen in the pediatric age group. The vasculitides associated with GI manifestations in childhood are listed in Table 31.2. These manifestations include abdominal pain (potentially due to bowel ischaemia or bowel wall thickening and subacute obstruction), GI blood loss (due to GI ulceration which can be aphthoid, undermined or fissure like), diarrhea which is often bloody (due to nonspecific inflammation of the ileum or colon) and an acute abdomen as a consequence of perforation [1].

Henoch–Schönlein Purpura

HSP is an immune-complex small-vessel vasculitis. It is the most common vasculitis seen in childhood with an estimated annual incidence of 20/100,000 children in the UK. The disease is characterized by a leukocytoclastic vasculitis with deposition of immunoglobulin A1 (IgA1) immune complexes in vascular tissue, principally capillaries and post-capillary venules. The disease is predominantly seen in children aged 3–10 years with the majority being <5 years. It is more frequent in the autumn/winter months and will commonly follow an infection. Proposed infective triggers include group A beta-haemolytic streptococcus, Parvovirus B19, *Staphylococcus aureus* and Coxsackie virus to name a few. It has been suggested that the pathogenesis involves the recognition of galactose-deficient IgA1 by anti-glycan antibodies and the deposition of these immune complexes in small vessels.

A recent large series suggests that 100% of patients have skin involvement with 60–70% having "palpable purpura" of the lower limbs and buttocks, 66% have arthritis which is usually symmetrical affecting the knees, ankles and feet, and 54% have GI involvement usually with lower GI bleeding or abdominal pain but also intussusception, ileal perforation and pancreatitis [3]. Renal manifestations are seen in 30% and include nephritic or nephrotic syndromes which can lead to chronic renal failure in a minority of cases. Diagnostic criteria include the presence of purpura or petechiae with lower-limb predominance with one of the following: diffuse abdominal pain, acute arthritis or arthralgia, haematuria or proteinuria and any biopsy showing predominant IgA deposition [4].

Described GI complications of HSP include intussusception, bowel ischaemia and infarction, intestinal perforation, late stricturing, acute appendicitis, GI haemorrhage (occult and massive), pancreatitis and gallbladder hydrops. One large series of patients reported abdominal pain in 58% of children and positive stool occult blood (SOB) in 18% [5]. Frank lower-GI bleeding was present in 3%. Plain abdominal radiology frequently showed dilated thickened bowel loops when the SOB was strongly positive which was also visualised on ultrasound examination. Intussusception, perhaps the most serious GI complication of HSP, was rare (0.5%) although in other series prevalence of up to 5% are described. The appearance of the thickened bowel wall on

K. J. Lindley (✉)
Division of Neurogastroenterology and Motility, Department of Gastroenterology, Great Ormond Street Hospital for Children NHS Foundation Trust, Great Ormond Street, London WC1N 3JH, UK
e-mail: keith.lindley@gosh.nhs.uk

J. Köglmeier
Division of Intestinal Rehabilitation and Nutrition, Department of Gastroenterology, Great Ormond Street Hospital for Children NHS Foundation Trust, London, UK

© Springer International Publishing Switzerland 2016
S. Guandalini et al. (eds.), *Textbook of Pediatric Gastroenterology, Hepatology and Nutrition*,
DOI 10.1007/978-3-319-17169-2_31

Table 31.1 Classification of the vasculitides. (Reprinted with permission John Wiley and Sons/Arthritis & Rheumatism, from Ref. [2], 2013 American College of Rheumatology.)

Table 31.1 Classification of the vasculitides. (Reprinted with permission John Wiley and Sons/Arthritis & Rheumatism, from Ref. [2], 2013 American College of Rheumatology.)

Large-vessel vasculitis (LVV)
Takayasu's arteritis
Giant cell arteritis (GCA)
Medium-vessel vasculitis (MVV)
Polyarteritis nodosa (PAN)
Kawasaki disease (KD)
Small-vessel vasculitis (SVV)
(i) Anti-neutrophil cytoplasmic antibody (ANCA)-associated vasculitis (AAV)
Eosinophilic granulomatosis with polyangiitis (Churg–Strauss)
Granulomatosis with polyangiitis (Wegener's granulomatosis)
Microscopic polyangiitis
(ii) Immune-complex SVV
IgA vasculitis (Henloch–Schönlein; IgAV)
Cryoglobulinaemic vasculitis
Hypocomplementaemic urticarial vasculitis
Anti-glomerular basement membrane disease
Variable-vessel vasculitis (VVV)
Behcet's disease
Cogan's syndrome
Single-organ vasculitis (SOV)
Vasculitis associated with systemic disease
Lupus
Rheumatoid
Sarcoid
Secondary vasculitis
Hepatitis B/Hepatitis C
Drugs
Others

IgA immunoglobulin A

ultrasound might act as a prognostic marker for duration of hospitalization for HSP [6]. Endoscopic findings vary and can include the presence of circumscribed vascular lesions (rather similar to the palpable purpura seen on the skin) and segmental ischaemic change (Fig. 31.2) [7].

It is usual for children to make a complete recovery from HSP with only supportive treatment with the exception of HSP-associated nephritis which is the cause of end-stage renal failure in up to 3 % of children in the UK. Some series report a significant reduction in duration and intensity of abdominal pain in children treated with prednisolone early in the course of the disease, but the use of steroids does not seem to protect against the development of nephritis.

Kawasaki Disease

KD is the second commonest childhood vasculitis which affects about 8/100,000 children younger than 5 years of age annually in the UK with twice as many cases occurring in the USA and approximately 20 times the incidence in Japan. The disease affects predominantly medium- and small-sized

arteries and is normally self-limiting. However, coronary artery aneurysms are present in 25 % of untreated patients and can lead to myocardial infarction or late coronary artery stenosis. In addition to involvement of the coronary arteries, systemic arterial injury can occur.

The seasonality and clustering of KD support an infectious trigger, although to date no single organism has been identified. The much higher prevalence of disease in Japanese and Korean children supports the notion that genetic predisposition is also an important factor and genome-wide association studies have identified a number of genes associated with disease susceptibility and disease phenotype.

Diagnosis of KD is clinical comprising the presence of unremitting fever for 5 days or more plus 4/5 of the following features: conjunctivitis; lymphadenopathy; polymorphous rash; changes in lips, tongue or oral mucosa and involvement of extremities including periungual desquamation (see Table 31.3). Patients with lesser numbers of these diagnostic features may be diagnosed with KD if they are found to have coronary artery aneurysms on echocardiography. It is important to note that not all of these diagnostic features may be present at once.

Although not diagnostic of KD, arthritis, aseptic meningitis, pneumonitis, uveitis, gastroenteritis and dysuria are also frequently seen. Uncommon features of the disease include gallbladder hydrops, GI ischaemia, mononeuritis, nephritis, seizures and ataxia.

Overall, abdominal symptoms, particularly diarrhea which can be bloody or non-bloody, are a frequent early feature of KD. Abdominal pain is less frequent [8]. Vasculitic appendicitis, haemorrhagic duodenitis and paralytic ileus are also described [9]. Bowel wall oedema may be evident as segmental thickening of the bowel wall as may gallbladder hydrops [10].

Inflammatory markers (erythrocyte sedimentation rate, ESR and C-reactive protein, CRP) are inevitably elevated as is the peripheral blood white blood cell count. Thrombocytosis, which can be very marked, usually occurs in the second week of the disease.

Early treatment of KD with aspirin and intravenous immunoglobulin (IVIG) reduces the occurrence of coronary artery aneurysms. A single infusion of 2 g/kg IVIG and an anti-inflammatory dose of aspirin (30–50 mg/kg/day) will reduce the likelihood of developing coronary artery aneurysms in the majority of patients, although approximately 20 % of children are IVIG resistant. The dose of aspirin should be reduced to an anti-platelet dose during the thrombocytosis phase of the illness. Patients who continue to have fevers and an ongoing systemic inflammatory response 48 h post IVIG are likely to be IVIG nonresponders and can be treated with intravenous methyl prednisolone for 5 days followed by 2 weeks of oral prednisolone or perhaps anti-tumour necrosis

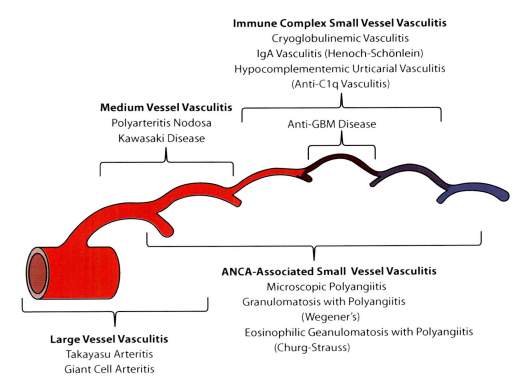

Immune Complex Small Vessel Vasculitis
Cryoglobulinemic Vasculitis
IgA Vasculitis (Henoch-Schönlein)
Hypocomplementemic Urticarial Vasculitis
(Anti-C1q Vasculitis)

Medium Vessel Vasculitis
Polyarteritis Nodosa
Kawasaki Disease

Anti-GBM Disease

ANCA-Associated Small Vessel Vasculitis
Microscopic Polyangiitis
Granulomatosis with Polyangiitis
(Wegener's)
Eosinophilic Geanulomatosis with Polyangiitis
(Churg-Strauss)

Large Vessel Vasculitis
Takayasu Arteritis
Giant Cell Arteritis

Fig. 31.1 Distribution of vessel involvement by large-vessel vasculitis, medium-vessel vasculitis and small-vessel vasculitis. Note that there is substantial overlap with respect to arterial involvement, and an important concept is that all three major categories of vasculitis can affect any size artery. Large-vessel vasculitis affects large arteries more often than other vasculitides. Medium-vessel vasculitis predominantly affects medium arteries. Small-vessel vasculitis predominantly affects small vessels, but medium arteries and veins may be affected, although immune-complex small-vessel vasculitis rarely affects arteries. The diagram depicts (from *left* to *right*) aorta, large artery, medium artery, small artery/arteriole, capillary, venule and vein. Anti-GBM—anti-glomerular basement membrane; ANCA—anti-neutrophil cytoplasmic antibody. *ANCA* Anti-neutrophil cytoplasmic antibody. (Reprinted with permission John Wiley and Sons/ Arthritis & Rheumatism, from Ref. [2], 2013 American College of Rheumatology.)

factor (TNF) antibodies. Certain other high-risk individuals should also receive steroids [11].

Systemic Polyarteritis Nodosa

Polyarteritis nodosa (PAN) is a necrotizing arteritis of medium and/or small arteries which has been subclassified into systemic PAN and cutaneous polyarteritis. Whilst systemic PAN is generally severe and cutaneous polyarteritis relatively benign, the cutaneous form can go on to develop features of multiorgan involvement. The presenting features of PAN

Table 31.2 Vasculitides associated with gastrointestinal manifestations in childhood

Henoch-Schönlein purpura
Kawasaki disease
Polyarteritis nodosa (PAN)
ANCA-associated vasculitis (AAV)
Behcet's disease
Systemic disease (Lupus and Rheumatoid)

can be very nonspecific and are known to affect a number of systems notably the skin, musculoskeletal system, kidneys and GI tract. A recent pediatric series documents the most common presenting features of PAN as fever (87%), myalgia (83%), arthralgia/arthritis (75%), weight loss of >5% of body weight (64%), fatigue (62%), livedo reticularis (49%) and abdominal pain (41%). In this series, 59% had GI symptoms comprising abdominal pain (49%), blood in the stools (10%) and bowel ischaemia/perforation (8%) [12]. The diagnosis may be delayed as the symptoms are so nonspecific. GI bleeding can be massive, especially when it arises from a Dieulafoy lesion, a submucosal vascular abnormality with a prominent tortuous artery with/without aneurysm formation [13, 14]. Ulcers, which are circumscribed and well demarcated, may also be evident (Fig. 31.3a, b). Following remission induction in PAN, the onset of GI symptoms is a major clinical predictor of clinical relapse. Other symptoms seen in PAN less frequently include cardiac, respiratory and neurological manifestations.

GI symptoms are generally attributable to ischaemia which can lead to infarction, perforation or stricture [16,

Fig. 31.2 Cutaneous purpura
and small bowel hyperaemia with
ulceration in a young adult with
HSP. (Reprinted from Ref. [7],
with permission from Elsevier.)

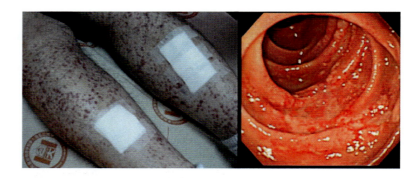

Table 31.3 Diagnostic criteria for Kawasaki Disease

Criterion	Description
Fever	Duration of 5 days or more plus 4/5 of the following
1. Conjunctivitis	Bilateral non-purulent with limbic sparing
2. Lymphadenopathy	Cervical, often > 1.5 cm
3. Rash	Polymorphous with no vesicles or crusts
4. Changes in lips/mucus membranes	Red cracked lips, "strawberry" tongue, erythema of oropharynx
5. Changes in extremities	Initially: erythema and oedema of palms and soles
	Later: periungual desquamation

17]. The systemic vasculitides can also be associated with an ischaemic colitis or a nonspecific colitis that can mimic inflammatory bowel disease [18].

The diagnosis of PAN is usually made through a combination of clinical, histopathological and arteriographic features and relies on one mandatory criterion plus one of five secondary criteria. Mandatory criteria comprise fibrinoid necrosis of the walls of medium-sized arteries from an affected organ together with an inflammatory response in the adjacent vessel wall which is characteristic of PAN or angiographic abnormalities (aneurysm, stenosis/segmental narrowing or occlusion/pruning) of medium or small arteries. Secondary criteria include (i) characteristic skin involvement, (ii) myalgia or muscle tenderness, (iii) hypertension, (iv) peripheral neuropathy/mononeuritis and (v) renal involvement. Renal, hepatic and mesenteric arteriography is commonly used as a diagnostic tool in children which overall has a sensitivity of 94 % for diagnosing PAN (Fig. 31.4).

A detailed discussion of treatment is beyond the scope of this chapter. Historically, this has involved remission in-

duction with pulsed intravenous methyl prednisolone often with cyclophosphamide and anti-platelet agents followed by maintenance therapy with low-dose steroids and a steroid-sparing agent (usually azathioprine). Biologic agents can be effective in treating PAN, for example, the anti-TNF agents Infliximab and Etanercept and the anti-cluster of differentiation (CD)20 agent Rituximab.

Behçet Disease

Behçet disease (BD) is rare in childhood (2/100,000 in Europe). It is a variable-vessel vasculitis which can affect veins and arteries of any size. Behçet described a triad of aphthous stomatitis, genital ulceration and uveitis. A more contemporary consensus defines pediatric BD as recurrent oral aphthous ulceration plus one of the following—genital ulceration, erythema nodosum, folliculitis, pustulous/acneiform lesions, positive pathergy test, uveitis, venous/arterial thrombosis and family history of BD [19].

Fig. 31.3 a Punched-out ulcers
with well-demarcated edges in
the colon in PAN. Ulcers are
typically shallow and irregular
often with surrounding erythema.
(Reprinted from Ref. [15], with
permission from Elsevier). **b**
Bleeding Dieulafoy lesion in
the stomach in a case of PAN.
(Reprinted from Ref. [14], with
permission from Elsevier.)

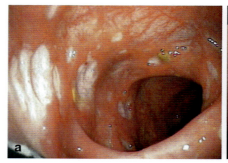
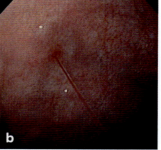

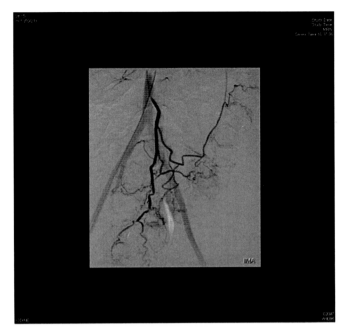

Fig. 31.4 Inferior mesenteric artery angiogram showing vessel calibre changes and aneurysms characteristic of polyarteritis nodosa

BD is extremely heterogeneous affecting multiple organ systems with distinct geographical variations in symptoms. For example, GI manifestations are more prevalent in the Far East, whilst vascular manifestations are seen in the eastern Mediterranean. GI manifestations comprise abdominal pain and aphthoid ulceration and rarely GI bleeding. Perforation of aphthoid ulcers is described. Vascular manifestations include venous thromboembolism, arterial stenosis, aneurysms and occlusions. Neuro-Behçets can present with headache, papilloedema, central venous sinus thrombosis and/or brain parenchymal disease causing seizures and focal neurological abnormalities [20].

Granulomatosis with Polyangiitis (Wegener's Granulomatosis)

Wegener's granulomatosis (WG) is one of the anti-neutrophil cytoplasmic antibody (ANCA)-associated vasculitides (AAV) and is a necrotizing granulomatous vasculitis of small blood vessels. The main features of the disease are due to a widespread small-vessel vasculitis with clinical manifestations of a necrotizing glomerulonephritis and respiratory tract granulomata dominating the clinical picture. GI involvement is infrequent but when present may present with abdominal pain; mucosal ulceration of the oesophagus, small or large bowel; GI perforation and rarely colitis and catastrophic GI haemorrhage or infarction of the gall bladder, intestine and colon.

Eosinophilic Granulomatosis with Polyangiitis (Churg–Strauss Syndrome)

This is another of the AAV which is extremely rare. ANCA is positive in about 30 % of cases. Histopathological features are those of a small-vessel (arteries and veins) granulomatous vasculitis with an eosinophil-rich inflammatory infiltrate. In addition, there is an eosinophil-rich granulomatous infiltrate of the respiratory tract and usually a history of asthma, allergic rhinitis and peripheral blood eosinophilia.

GI-tract involvement is seen in the context of vasculitis causing symptoms of pain (ischaemic), ulceration, perforation and bleeding. Independently of vascular involvement, eosinophil-rich inflammation of the GI mucosa can result in symptoms such as diarrhea and perhaps pain. Forty percent of children have gastroenterological symptoms at presentation [21]. The pediatric disease is usually steroid responsive but subject to relapse.

Microscopic Polyangiitis

Microscopic polyangiitis is a necrotizing vasculitis of small vessels in which up to 65 % of patients are perinuclear ANCA (pANCA) positive. It is uncommon in childhood [22]. Characteristically, the vasculitis is not strongly associated with the deposition of immune complexes in the affected blood vessels. Necrotizing glomerulonephritis is common with this condition and the classical presentation is with rapidly progressive glomerulonephritis and alveolar haemorrhage [23]. In common with the other AAV pain is a dominant GI symptom, although GI blood loss, cholecystitis, ischaemic colitis and bowel perforation are described.

Single-Organ Vasculitis

Systemic vasculitis occurs when vascular inflammation involves multiple territories or organs. In single-organ vasculitis (SOV), the inflammation is restricted to a single organ or part of that organ. By definition, there has to be a lack of spread outside the single organ for at least 6 months. SOV is known to affect the GI tract and may affect small-, medium- or large-sized arteries. The condition is not well described in children and is more commonly part of PAN (e.g. appendiceal vasculitis).

Takayasu Arteritis

Takayasu arteritis (TA) is a vasculitis predominantly affecting large vessels (mainly the aorta and its main branches). It is most commonly seen in Asia and rarely encountered in the pediatric age group. Girls are more often affected than boys. Patients frequently complain about headache, abdominal pain, limb claudication, myalgia, arthralgia and fever. Weight loss is said to occur in about 10 % of affected individuals. Cerebrovascular events, angina and loss of vision have been reported [24]. The disease requires aggressive treatment as damage to the vessels is otherwise irreversible, and a combination of steroids and Azathioprine or Methotrexate are commonly prescribed [25]. In cases of severe ischaemia, antihypertensive drugs or even surgery may be indicated.

Systemic Lupus Erythematosus-Associated Vasculitis

Systemic lupus erythematosus (SLE) is a systemic autoimmune disease in which type 2 and type 3 hypersensitivity reactions are important in the pathogenesis. The presence of anti-double-stranded DNA (anti-dsDNA) antibodies in the blood is a highly specific test for SLE being present in 70–80 % with titers of antibody tending to mirror disease activity. Other pathogenic autoantibodies in SLE include antibodies to nucleosomes, Ro (a ribonucleoprotein component), La (an RNA-binding protein), C1q (complement), phospholipids and the N-methyl-D-aspartic acid (NMDA) receptor. Many of these antigens are expressed on the cell surface during the process of apoptosis, and it has been hypothesized that abnormalities of the apoptotic pathway, which are ubiquitous in SLE, are important in the genesis of pathological autoantibodies [26].

Systemic lupus can affect the GI tract causing chronic, nonspecific mucosal inflammation, mucosal ulceration or vasculitis resulting in mesenteric/GI ischaemia (Fig. 31.5a, b). Abdominal pain is present in 8–40 % of published series of individuals with SLE; in children, it is most commonly (32 %) due to lupus-associated mesenteric vasculitis [27]. Other causes of pain include pancreatitis (10 %), appendicitis (7.5 %) and cholecystitis (6 %). Patients with vasculitis usually have high SLA disease activity scores (SLEDAI) but do not commonly have substantially elevated inflammatory markers. Protein-losing enteropathy has also been described in SLE.

The clinical presentation of lupus-associated mesenteric vasculitis commonly mirrors an acute surgical abdomen. It is suggested that individuals with SLE, high SLEDAI and an "acute abdomen" undergo imaging to look for evidence of vascular compromise before any surgical intervention.

Juvenile Dermatomyositis

In juvenile dermatomyositis (JDM), vasculitis affects striated muscle, the skin, subcutaneous tissues and the GI tract. Children develop weakness of the muscles of the neck, shoulders and hips leading to difficulties with swallowing, getting up from sitting or climbing stairs. GI bleeding and perforation can be catastrophic and are a major cause of death [29].

Rheumatoid-Associated Vasculitis

Rheumatoid arthritis (RA) is another systemic inflammatory disorder with articular and extra-articular manifestations. Rheumatoid vasculitis (RV) is a systemic necrotizing vasculitis affecting small- and medium-sized arteries which is clinically extremely heterogenous and can affect skin, nerves and abdominal viscera. RV is usually seen when there are other extra-articular manifestations, and these patients are always rheumatoid factor positive. It is usual to find raised inflammatory markers (ESR and CRP), polyclonal hypergammaglobulinemia and often hypocomplementemia. GI involvement is rare but, in common with other vasculitides, can result in ischaemia, perforation and haemorrhage [30].

Investigation of Children with Suspected GI Vasculitic Disorders

The diagnosis of vasculitis can be challenging because of the heterogeneity of possible presentations and the diagnosis is often delayed. A high index of suspicion is key to early diagnosis and intervention. The three elements of diagnosis include (i) definition of a clinical phenotype compatible with

Fig. 31.5 a. Mucosal oedema in association with nonspecific inflammation in SLE. **b.** Colonic mucosal ulceration in SLE. (Reprinted from Ref. [28], with permission from Elsevier.)

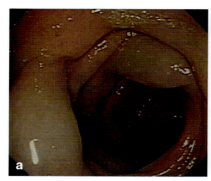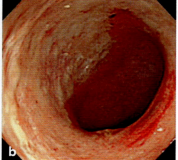

the diagnosis, (ii) specific serology or radiology and (iii) histological confirmation if appropriate.

A basic diagnostic evaluation might include blood count and film, inflammatory markers (ESR; CRP), liver function, pancreatic enzymes, ANCA and anti-dsDNA antibodies, rheumatoid factor, complement (C3 and C4), anti-cardiolipin antibodies, cryoglobulins and hepatitis B and C serology. In addition, urine microscopy and a chest X-ray should be undertaken. Further investigations will be directed by the clinical phenotype.

Abdominal ultrasound might allude to bowel wall thickening as might abdominal CT/MRI. CT/MRI might also allude to segmental perfusion defects. Magnetic resonance angiography is not as sensitive as digital subtraction angiography (DSA) in PAN (see below).

Selective visceral DSA is diagnostically very sensitive for systemic PAN and might highlight the site of bleeding if present. Characteristic features of PAN include aneurysms of small- and medium-sized arteries (seen in 40 %). Other non-aneurysmal features include arterial cut off, arterial tapering and stenoses, arterial beading, pruning of the renal arterial tree and perfusion defects. Overall, arteriographic abnormalities are present in 94 % of children with PAN affecting the renal, hepatic and mesenteric vasculature [12]. Assessment of the GI mucosa by oesophagogastroduodenoscopy, videocapsule endoscopy and ileocolonoscopy with biopsy might reveal a plethora of pathologies in vasculitic disorders. Nonspecific colitis is common in childhood systemic vasculitis and a nonspecific enteritis may be present in SLE [18]. Ulceration may be ischaemic or inflammatory in origin. Behcet's ulcers tend to be round, few in number (<5) and focally distributed when compared with Crohn's ulcers which are more commonly irregular in shape [31]. Ulcers in SLE are typically punched out. In HSP oedema, patchy mucosal redness, erosions and linear ulceration of the duodenum and ileum are described [32, 33] Purpura similar to that seen in the skin might be seen in the GI mucosa [34]. Mucosal biopsies in Churg–Strauss may demonstrate evidence of eosinophilic GI disease/eosinophilic gastroenteritis.

References

1. Morgan MD, Savage COS. Vasculitis in the gastrointestinal tract. Best Pract Res Clin Gastroenterol. 2005;19(2):215–33.
2. Jennette JC, Falk RJ, Bacon PA, Basu N, Cid MC, Ferrario F, et al. Revised International Chapel Hill Consensus Conference Nomenclature of Vasculitides. Arthritis Rheum. 27 Dec 2012;65(1):1–11. doi:10.1002/art.37715.
3. Peru H, Soylemezoglu O, Bakkaloglu SA, Elmas S, Bozkaya D, Elmaci AM, et al. Henoch Schonlein purpura in childhood: clinical analysis of 254 cases over a 3-year period. Clin Rheumatol. 2008;27(9):1087–92.
4. Ozen S, Pistorio A, Iusan SM, Bakkaloglu A, Herlin T, Brik R, et al. EULAR/PRINTO/PRES criteria for Henoch-Schönlein purpura, childhood polyarteritis nodosa, childhood Wegener granulomatosis and childhood Takayasu arteritis: Ankara 2008. Part II: Final classification criteria. Ann Rheum Dis. 2010;69(5):798–806.
5. Chang W-L, Yang Y-H, Lin Y-T, Chiang B-L. Gastrointestinal manifestations in Henoch-Schönlein purpura: a review of 261 patients. Acta Paediatr. 2004;93(11):1427–31.
6. Nchimi A, Khamis J, Paquot I, Bury F, Magotteaux P. Significance of bowel wall abnormalities at ultrasound in Henoch-Schönlein purpura. J Pediatr Gastroenterol Nutr. 2008;46(1):48–53.
7. Hsu H-L, Hsiao C-H, Liu K-L. Henoch-Schönlein purpura. Clin Gastroenterol Hepatol. 2010;8(8):e83–4.
8. Falcini F, Cimaz R, Calabri GB, Picco P, Martini G, Marazzi MG, et al. Kawasaki's disease in northern Italy: a multicenter retrospective study of 250 patients. Clin Exp Rheumatol. 2002;20(3):421–6.
9. Zulian F, Falcini F, Zancan L, Martini G, Secchieri S, Luzzatto C, et al. Acute surgical abdomen as presenting manifestation of Kawasaki disease. J Pediatr. 2003;142(6):731–5.
10. Maurer K, Unsinn KM, Waltner-Romen M, Geiger R, Gassner I. Segmental bowel-wall thickening on abdominal ultrasonography: an additional diagnostic sign in Kawasaki disease. Pediatr Radiol. 2008;38(9):1013–6.
11. Eleftheriou D, Levin M, Shingadia D, Tulloh R, Klein N, Brogan P. Management of Kawasaki disease. Arch Dis Child. 2014;99(1):74–83.
12. Eleftheriou D, Dillon MJ, Tullus K, Marks SD, Pilkington CA, Roebuck DJ, et al. Systemic polyarteritis nodosa in the young: a single-center experience over thirty-two years. Arthritis Rheum. 2013;65(9):2476–85.
13. Dulic-Lakovic E, Dulic M, Hubner D, Fuchssteiner H, Pachofszky T, Stadler B, et al. Bleeding Dieulafoy lesions of the small bowel: a systematic study on the epidemiology and efficacy of enteroscopic treatment. Gastrointest Endosc. 2011;74(3):573–80.
14. Maeda K, Hayashi Y, Morita I, Matsuoka O, Nishiyama M, Nishimura H, et al. Recurrent Dieulafoy's ulcers in the stomach and colonic perforation caused by polyarteritis nodosa: report of a case. Gastrointest Endosc. 2006;63(2):349–52.
15. Vavricka SR, Dirnhofer S, Degen L. Polyarteritis nodosa mimicking inflammatory bowel disease. Clin Gastroenterol Hepatol. 2007;5(11):A22.
16. Gündoğdu HZ, Kale G, Tanyel FC, Büyükpamukçu N, Hiçsönmez A. Intestinal perforation as an initial presentation of polyarteritis nodosa in an 8-year-old boy. J Pediatr Surg. 1993;28(4):632–4.
17. Venuta A, Ceccarelli PL, Biondini D, Montanari F. Jejunal obstruction as initial presentation of polyarteritis nodosa in a 13-month-old boy. J Pediatr Surg. 2011;46(7):E27–9.
18. Brogan PA, Malik M, Shah N, Kilday JP, Ramsay A, Shah V, et al. Systemic vasculitis: a cause of indeterminate intestinal inflammation. J Pediatr Gastroenterol Nutr. 2006;42(4):405–15.
19. Koné-Paut I, Darce-Bello M, Shahram F, Gattorno M, Cimaz R, Ozen S, et al. Registries in rheumatological and musculoskeletal conditions. Pediatric Behçet's disease: an international cohort study of 110 patients. One-year follow-up data. Rheumatology (Oxford). 2011;50(1):184–8.
20. Mora P, Menozzi C, Orsoni JG, Rubino P, Ruffini L, Carta A. Neuro-Behçet's disease in childhood: a focus on the neuro-ophthalmological features. Orphanet J Rare Dis. 2013;8:18.
21. Zwerina J, Eger G, Englbrecht M, Manger B, Schett G. Churg-Strauss syndrome in childhood: a systematic literature review and clinical comparison with adult patients. Semin Arthritis Rheum. 2009;39(2):108–15.
22. Villiger PM, Guillevin L. Microscopic polyangiitis: clinical presentation. Autoimmun Rev. 2010;9(12):812–9.
23. Brogan P, Eleftheriou D, Dillon M. Small vessel vasculitis. Pediatr Nephrol. 2010;25(6):1025–35.
24. Cakar N, Yalcinkaya F, Duzova A, Caliskan S, Sirin A, Oner A, et al. Takayasu arteritis in children. J Rheumatol. 2008;35(5):913–9.

25. Eleftheriou D, Brogan PA. Vasculitis in children. Best Pract Res Clin Rheumatol. 2009;23(3):309–23.
26. Rahman A, Isenberg DA. Systemic lupus erythematosus. N Engl J Med. 28 Feb 2008;358(9):929–39.
27. Tu Y-L, Yeh K-W, Chen L-C, Yao T-C, Ou L-S, Lee W-I, et al. Differences in disease features between childhood-onset and adult-onset systemic lupus erythematosus patients presenting with acute abdominal pain. Semin Arthritis Rheum. 2011;40(5):447–54.
28. Lee CK, Lee TH, Lee S-H, Chung I-K, Park S-H, Kim H-S, et al. GI vasculitis associated with systemic lupus erythematosus. Gastrointest Endosc. 2010;72(3):618–9.
29. Dillon MJ. Childhood vasculitis. Lupus. 1998;7(4):259–65.
30. Lee SY, Lee SW, Chung WT. Jejunal vasculitis in patient with rheumatoid arthritis: case report and literature review. Mod Rheumatol. 2012;22(6):924–7.
31. Lee SK, Kim BK, Kim TI, Kim WH. Differential diagnosis of intestinal Behçet"s disease and Crohn"s disease by colonoscopic findings. Endoscopy. 2009;41(1):9–16.
32. Hokama A, Kishimoto K. Ihama Y, Kobashigawa C, Nakamoto M, Hirata T, et al. Endoscopic and radiographic features of gastrointestinal involvement in vasculitis. World J Gastrointest Endosc. 16 March 2012;4(3):50–6.
33. Preud'Homme DL, Michail S, Hodges C, Milliken T, Mezoff AG. Use of wireless capsule endoscopy in the management of severe Henoch-Schonlein purpura. Pediatrics. 2006;118(3):e904–6.
34. Bua J, Lepore L, Martelossi S, Ventura A. Video capsule endoscopy and intestinal involvement in systemic vasculitis. Dig Liver Dis. 2008;40(11):905.

Lymphonodular Hyperplasia

32

Tuomo J. Karttunen and Sami Turunen

Introduction

Lymphonodular hyperplasia (LNH) of the gastrointestinal (GI) tract is characterized by a significant enlargement of isolated aggregates in one or several segments of the GI tract or by increase of the number or size of lymphoid nodules of the Peyer's patches of the distal part of the small intestine. Enlargement should be severe enough to make the aggregates elevated and visible by endoscopic assessment or radiology, usually the diameter exceeding 2 or 3 mm.

LNH is a common condition in the pediatric patients and rare in adults. It has long been considered to be an incidental and physiological finding [1–3]. Clinically, LNH can be asymptomatic or manifest with variable set of symptoms including abdominal pain, diarrhea, bleeding or even intestinal obstruction [4]. In some cases, clinical significance of LNH may remain speculative, and, in some cases, the finding may represent a physiological reaction with no clinical significance as for the symptoms.

LNH is considered a reactive condition related with microbiological or nutritional luminal factors or immune deficiency, but exact pathogenic mechanisms are largely unknown. A significant proportion of cases associate with non-immunoglobulin E (IgE) food allergies [4].

Definition

LNH has usually been defined as a condition characterized by endoscopically visible increase of the numbers or size or both of mucosal lymphoid nodules, which elevate above the surrounding mucosa. LNH can be seen in any part of the GI tract. Diagnosis is based on endoscopic or radiological appearance, and the confirmation of diagnosis may need exclusion of other diseases causing mucosal elevations, such as various lymphoid neoplasms and reactive and neoplastic polypoid lesions (Table 32.1). This definition does not apply for lesser grades of lymphoid hyperplasia, where either increase of the numbers of lymphoid follicles or their enlargement is of lesser degree so that mucosal elevations are not formed. However, it is likely that there is continuum between such lesser grades of hyperplasia and the endoscopically visible lymphoid nodular hyperplasia fulfilling the current criteria [5], pointing to the idea that the current criteria are arbitrary, and they do not have a clear pathophysiological basis.

Endoscopic Assessment and Criteria

LNH can be detected by using barium enema, but currently the diagnosis is usually based on endoscopic visualization of typical whitish or mucosa-coloured elevations (Fig. 32.1, 32.2 and 32.3). In cases where there is any uncertainty of the nature of nodules, a complementary histopathological analysis should be used to exclude other disease processes causing endoscopic nodularity or multiple polypoid lesions (Table 32.1; Figs. 32.1, 32.2 and 32.3). Endoscopic detection of LNH requires active search and is aided by adequate air insufflation during examination as the folds may hide nodularity [6]. LNH can also be detected by capsule endoscopy [7].

By definition, diagnosis of LNH needs increase of the size of the lymphoid nodules, but it may be associated with the increase of their numbers. However, there are no consensus criteria for LNH. Considering the size of the nodules, minimum size for a hyperplastic nodule has been suggested to be 2 [8]

T. J. Karttunen (✉)
Department of Pathology, Oulu University Hospital, Medical Research Center Oulu, University of Oulu, Aapistie 5B, 90014 Oulu, Finland
e-mail: tuomo.karttunen@oulu.fi

S. Turunen
Department of Pediatrics, Oulu University Hospital, Medical Research Center Oulu, University of Oulu, Oulu, Finland

© Springer International Publishing Switzerland 2016
S. Guandalini et al. (eds.), *Textbook of Pediatric Gastroenterology, Hepatology and Nutrition,*
DOI 10.1007/978-3-319-17169-2_32

Table 32.1 Gastrointestinal diseases to be considered in the endoscopic and histopathological differential diagnosis of LNH

All anatomical areas	
	Giardiasis
	Granulation tissue polyps
	Inflammatory bowel disease
	Lymphangiectasia
	Lymphoma
	Multiple adenomatous or hyperplastic polyps
	Metastatic tumours
	Familial and sporadic gastrointestinal polyposes
	Ganglioneuromatosis
	Neuroendocrine hyperplasia and neoplasia
Stomach	
	Cystic polyps
	Hyperplastic gastritis
Small intestinal mucosa	
	Duodenal Brunner's gland hyperplasia and adenoma
	Duodenal gastric heterotopia
	Groove pancreatitis
Colon and rectal mucosa	
	Solitary rectal ulcer

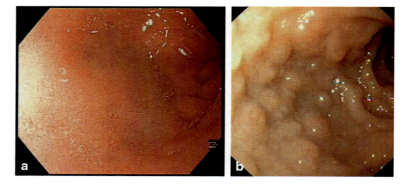

Fig. 32.1 An endoscopic view of the bulb of the duodenum showing normal smooth mucosa **a.** In lymphonodular hyperplasia, elevations are dispersed along the walls covering the otherwise normal mucosa **b**

or 4 mm [9]. The minimum number of nodules has been described as a "cluster" [8, 10], and a cluster has been defined as a group of minimum of 10 nodules [8]. Typically, the size range of polypoid lymphoid nodules is 3–6 mm in diameter.

Terminal ileum contains physiologically lymphoid nodules, that is, Peyer's patches, and the diagnosis of LNH is more subjective in this anatomical location. Autopsy studies have indicated that in children the size and number of these patches increases with age [11], and that in adults these are at their highest in the third decade [12]. Kokkonen graded the abundance of ileal lymphoid nodules in four grades: 0, no lymphoid nodules; 1, mild, lymphoid nodules dispersed on the walls; 2, moderate, lymphoid nodules filling the walls; 3, severe, terminal ileum massed with lymphoid tissue, valve protruding [6] (Fig. 32.2). Counts of lymphoid nodules per visual field of a high-resolution endoscopy in adults in the terminal ileum and caecum indicated that 9–50 lymphoid nodules per field can be defined as lymphoid hyperplasia,

and that more than 50 lymphoid nodules per field can be defined as pathological lymphoid aggregates [5].

According to current criteria, increase of the numbers or size of lymphoid nodules less than 2 mm and without endoscopic evidence of nodularity is not diagnostic for LNH. However, as the development of LNH is gradual, even the lesser grades with only numerical increase or increase of the size of nodule without formation of any elevation could have significance. It is obvious, that we need more data on the pathophysiology and clinical significance of such lesser grades of lymphoid hyperplasia.

Anatomical Distribution of LNH

LNH may affect any part of the GI tract, and simultaneous manifestation in several parts is not uncommon [6, 10]. In the duodenum and colon, LNH is usually segmental and

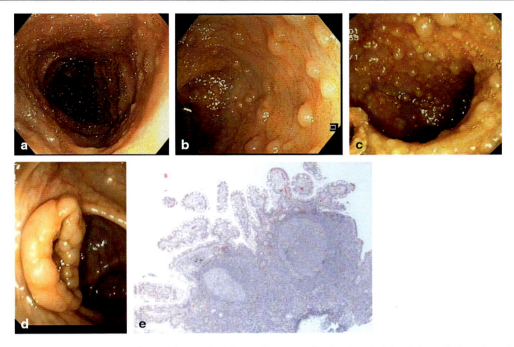

Fig. 32.2 Endoscopic view of the mucosa of a healthy terminal ileum shows usually tiny lymphoid nodules **a**. In lymphonodular hyperplasia, the nodules are both enlarged and their numbers are increased **b** and in severe cases may mass on the walls **c**. In some cases, enlarged lymphoid nodules may extend to the region of ileocaecal valve and be visible even from the caecal side **d**. The biopsy taken from the terminal ileum with lymphonodular hyperplasia may be filled with lymphoid tissue as large nodules. However, normal long villi can be detected between the nodules **e**

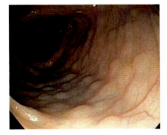

Fig. 32.3 Endoscopic view of colon showing lymphonodular hyperplasia

patchy. In the duodenum, bulb is the most commonly affected location [13].

A rare form of segmental lymphoid hyperplasia is located in the distal rectum of adults and children and has been referred to a rectal tonsil [14]. Clinically, rectal tonsil is often associated with rectal bleeding and abdominal pain, but pathophysiology is unknown. However, similar constellation may be caused by a local chlamydia infection [15].

Lymphoid follicular proctitis is a rather poorly defined condition, where rectal mucosal nodularity is related with formation of lymphoid follicles and interfollicular chronic inflammation. Symptoms are composed mucoid stools and haematochezia, and occasional response to sulfasalazine treatment suggests that some cases represent a variant of inflammatory bowel disease (IBD) [16].

Histology of LNH

Biopsy specimens from LNH typically show a lymphoid follicle with or without germinal centre (Fig. 32.2). A germinal centre is usually present and is enlarged, but additional sections may sometimes be necessary to confirm this feature. Alike reactive germinal centres, tangible body macrophages and a network of dendritic cells expressing cluster of differentiation (CD)23 are present [17]. Follicles are surrounded by a mantle zone containing T and B lymphocytes. Interfollicular tissue may have some features of paracortical zone of lymph nodes, such as high endothelial venules [17].

Epithelium overlying lymphoid follicles contains enterocytes and a specialized epithelial cell type M cells, showing characteristic microfolds. According to experimental work, the formation of the latter cell is induced by signalling form the developing lymphoid follicle. M cells contain pockets with intraepithelial lymphocytes. Functionally, M cells act as transporters of luminal antigens to be processed by the cells of lymphatic follicle. This results in the formation of an immunoglobulin A (IgA) response [18].

In case series of children with delayed type of food allergy, the majority of them presenting with LNH, the intestinal mucosa may show increase of intraepithelial lymphocytes including gamma–delta-expressing lymphocytes and cytotoxic lymphocytes [19–21]. Similarly, the numbers of intraepithelial eosinophilic leukocytes may be increased in

LNH cases associated with allergy [8]. In cases where LNH associates with specific disease or condition, these may present with characteristic features, such as chronic inflammation between the follicles in IBD-associated cases, and characteristic absence of plasma cells in common variable immune deficiency [22].

Histopathological differential diagnosis involves other reactive and neoplastic causes for mucosal nodularity (Table 32.1). Malignant lymphomas of mucosa are very rare in children, but their risk is increased in children with immune deficiency or solid-organ transplantation.

Pathophysiology of LNH

GI mucosal lymphatic tissue consists of inductive and effector compartments [23]. Luminal antigens are processed, and specific immune responses are generated in the inductive compartment composed of Peyer's patches in the ileum and isolated lymphoid follicles in other parts of the GI tract. Isolated lymphoid follicles are aggregates of T and B lymphocytes [24]. The effector compartment is the diffuse mucosal lymphatic infiltrate which is composed of immunoglobulin-producing B cells and effector T cells [18, 23]. Isolated lymphoid follicles may have germinal centres and are associated with a special type surface epithelium with M cells [24].

Number and size of isolated lymphoid follicles are variable as they respond dynamically to the signals from diet and luminal flora [25]. In a normal small intestine, the estimated amount is one per 269 villi in the jejunum and one per 28 villi in the ileum [24]. In the proximal colon, the number is 0.02/mm of muscularis mucosae and in the rectosigmoid 0.06/mm [26]. Areal density of lymphoid aggregates in the colorectum was estimated to be 1.1–2.7/cm^2 [27]. Krauss et al. [5] used high-resolution endoscopy objective counting of lymphoid follicles, and they found that in adults 1–8 lymphoid follicles per endoscopy field of view in the terminal ileum and caecum can be defined as normal. Size of isolated lymphatic aggregates has been estimated to be in the range of 0.1–2 mm [24, 26, 28, 29].

Luminal commensal and pathogenic flora induces production of specific IgA response within Peyer's patches and isolated lymphoid follicles [18, 23]. In this response, lymphoid cells accumulate and induce evolution of M cells in the surface epithelium. Germinal centres are formed and are the places where *IgA* genes of the B lymphocytes mutate and relevant clones are selected. There is evidence that T-independent pathways can give rise to intestinal IgA-secreting plasma cells in isolated lymphatic follicles and diffuse lamina propria, while Peyer's patches can support both T-dependent and T-independent modes of IgA induction [18, 25].

Since the secreted IgA is induced by luminal microbes and also controls the amount of luminal microbial flora, the LNH might be viewed as a sign of IgA dysfunction, where balance is not reached within normal structural limits of lymphoid tissue [25, 30]. Accordingly, also LNH in association with immunodeficiency might be explained as compensatory mechanism to gain the balance. Similarly, increase of the numbers of lymphoid follicles in the colon of patients with infectious colitis [5], or gastric LNH in association with *Helicobacter pylori* infection [31], may represent similar attempts to control the infection by increased production of IgA and suggests that both increase of numbers of lymphoid follicles and their size may be involved. Children with LNH showed more abundant bacterial flora in the ileum than the control children [32], possibly supporting the role of microbial factors in the pathogenesis of LNH.

Mechanisms linking delayed type of food allergy and LNH are not clear. Evidence for association of history of IgE-mediated food allergy in infancy and increase of anti-allergen IgA levels and LNH [33] support the idea that in association with milk allergy, LNH, by providing IgA anti-allergen response, might represent an exaggerated attempt to tolerance [34].

Mechanisms of segmental localization of LNH with some preference to locate close to sphincter-like structures (distal to pylorus; proximal to ileocaecal valve), and association with motoric dysfunction (obstipation and Hirschsprung's disease) are speculative. However, stagnation of intestinal contents related with these anatomical structures or neuromuscular dysfunction might lead the mucosa to be exposed longer to luminal antigens, and thereby increase local antigen load.

The role of alteration of immune regulatory mechanisms in pathogenesis of LNH is not clear. Bellanti et al. [35] found evidence of deficient T helper cell (Th)1 function in peripheral blood of children with LNH. There are no studies focussing on mucosal cytokine patterns specifically on LNH. However, in children with delayed type of milk allergy, where majority of patients show LNH, ileal mucosa shows increase of interleukin (IL6) messenger (mRNA) [36], and duodenal mucosa shows increase of interferon (IFN) gamma mRNA levels [37], increased numbers of cells expressing IFN gamma [38] and increased IFN gamma, IL-4 and IL-10 secretion [37], possibly indicating imbalance of pro- and anti-inflammatory cytokines.

Mechanisms of the various clinical symptoms (see below) are largely speculative. In addition to immunological mechanisms for the symptoms, also other mechanisms are possible, including diet-related changes in the microbiome and nonprotein nutrients like fermentable oligosaccharides [39]. Accordingly, it is possible that LNH and irritable colon may share some pathogenic mechanisms.

Table 32.2 Etiology or associated condition of lymphonodular hyperplasia in different parts of the gastrointestinal tract

Part of gastrointestinal tract	Etiology/associated condition
Stomach	*Helicobacter pylori* infection
Duodenum	Food allergy, delayed type
	Juvenile idiopathic arthritis
	Immune deficiency (IgA, CVID)
	Giardiasis
Ileum	Food allergy, delayed type
Colon	Food allergy, delayed type
	IBD
	Immunodeficiency (IgA, CVID)
	Infectious enteritis
Rectum	Idiopathic
	Chlamydia infection

IgA immunoglobulin A, *CVID* common variable immune deficiency, *IBD* inflammatory bowel disease

Prevalence of LNH

Prevalence of LNH in general pediatric or adult population is unknown. Prevalence in symptomatic children varies from 30 to 46% in the colon [6, 8, 40], about 50% in the ileum [6] and 19% in the duodenum [6]. In majority of reported series, LNH was the only finding. Simultaneous presence in both upper and lower GI tract is not uncommon.

LNH and Food Hypersensitivity

Conditions associated with LNH are summarized in Table 32.2. In children, studies performed in three different populations, in Finland [10, 19], Italy [8] and the USA [35] have shown that LNH in duodenal or ileocolonic mucosa associates with food allergy of non-IgE type (Table 32.2). Similar association has been reported in adults [39]. Krauss et al. [5] showed that overall increase in the size and number of lymphoid follicles is associated with food allergy in adults, and Carroccio et al. [39] reported that colon lymphoid hyperplasia is present in 35% of adults with wheat and milk sensitivity. A review by Mansueto [4] concluded that LNH is present in 49% (range 32–67) of children with food allergy, and conversely, about 66% (42–90) of patients with LNH have food allergy. In these studies, food allergy was diagnosed based on food challenge-eliminations tests, but not all studies were based on state-of-the-art blinded tests [4]. Skin prick tests and serum IgE-based tests were mostly negative. Response time in food challenge test was long—at least several days. These findings indicate that food hypersensitivity associating with LNH is of non-IgE type and characterized by a slow response times of usually several days.

LNH in other Diseases and Conditions

Chronic mucosal infections manifesting in some cases with local LNH include *H. pylori* gastritis [13, 31]. Giardiasis causes sometimes small intestinal LNH, usually in association with immune deficiency [41]. *Chlamydia* infection causes some cases of rectal LNH cases [15]. In general, intestinal bacterial infections increase the size and number of lymphoid follicles [25].

LNH associates with genetic immune disorders such as common variable immune deficiency (CVID), where LHN develops in about 20% of cases [42]. IgA deficiency is similarly associated with LNH, nodules containing IgM-expressing cells instead of IgA expression [43]. LNH may associate with human immunodeficiency virus (HIV) infection [44].

LNH has been reported in juvenile idiopathic arthritis and connective tissue diseases in the duodenum, ileum and colon, and LNH was associated with increase of intraepithelial lymphocytes [45].

LNH has rarely been described in inflammatory bowel disease, including both ulcerative colitis and Crohn's disease [10]. However, no associations with nucleotide-binding oligomerization domain-containing protein 2/caspase recruitment domain-containing protein 15 gene (NOD2/CARD15) mutations have been detected [46]. Lymphoid hyperplasia has been found in Hirschsprung's disease in the aganglionic segment [47].

There are reports suggesting LNH to be a common abnormality in children with autistic spectrum disorders, but these findings are highly controversial [4].

Symptoms of LNH

Symptoms in children with LNH are listed in Table 32.3. It is not clear what symptoms can be attributed specifically to LNH as there is no consistent pattern, and some patients

Table 32.3 Clinical symptoms commonly reported in pediatric patients examined with gastroduodenoscopy and/or colonoscopy and having nodular lymphoid hyperplasia as an endoscopic finding [3, 4, 6, 8, 35, 48]

Recurrent abdominal pain
Blood in stools
Diarrhea
Constipation
Anaemia
Nausea/vomiting
Growth retardation or weight loss

have no symptoms. It is obvious that conditions underlying or associating with LNH, such as immune deficiency and constipation contribute to symptoms. Part of the diverse set of symptoms resembles those in irritable bowel syndrome. Interestingly, non-coeliac wheat sensitivity in adults [39] and LNH have similar symptom spectrum resembling irritable bowel syndrome, and also share increase of duodenal intraepithelial lymphocytes [19, 39], some abundance of eosinophils (in the colon) and LNH.

Some symptoms may be specifically caused by LNH. Severe LNH in the terminal ileum can lead to invagination (intussusception). Common association of bloody stools and LNH [8, 40, 49] can be mechanistically explained by sensitivity for mechanical damage associated with any elevated mucosal lesion. Kaplan et al. [40] found that LNH in the colon was commonly associated with friability and ulceration. Observations in Crohn's disease have suggested that M cells overlying the lymphoid follicles form the most vulnerable population of surface epithelium [50], but whether M cells in LNH with other conditions are vulnerable is not known.

Treatment and Prognosis

LNH is the manifestation of underlying immune response and not a specific disease. The initiating mechanism should be searched for (Table 32.2), and treatment targeting on the etiology should be considered.

Symptomatic response to elimination diet in delayed type of food allergy associated with LNH has been well documented in both adults and children [8, 49]. No systematic and long-term follow-up studies are available of the development of LNH with or without treatment. Partial regression of LNH has been detected in some follow-up endoscopy studies within a year in cases associated with food allergy and treated with elimination diet [8, 49]. In other studies [6], treatment with elimination diet did not induce any change in the LNH grade, although the numbers of intraepithelial lymphocytes diminished towards normal levels. In adults, treatment seems to decrease the numbers of lymphoid follicles in cases associated with allergy even in cases without full-blown LNH [5].

There is only scanty information of long-term prognosis of LNH. Colon et al. [3] did not detect any long-term consequences in their unselected cases with LNH. However, since incidence rates in adults seem to be much less than children, the overall prevalence of LNH seems to decrease with age and supports the idea that major proportion of childhood cases not associated with immune deficiency are resolved.

References

1. Riddlesberger M, Jr, Lebenthal E. Nodular colonic mucosa of childhood: normal or pathologic? Gastroenterology 1980;79:265–70.
2. Rossi T. Endoscopic examination of the colon in infancy and childhood. Pediatr Clin North Am. 1988;35:331–56.
3. Colon AR, DiPalma JS, Leftridge CA. Intestinal lymphonodular hyperplasia of childhood: patterns of presentation. J Clin Gastroenterol. 1991;13:163–6.
4. Mansueto P, Iacono G, Seidita A, D'Alcamo A, Sprini D, Carroccio A. Review article: intestinal lymphoid nodular hyperplasia in children—the relationship to food hypersensitivity. Aliment Pharmacol Ther. 2012;35(9):1000–9.
5. Krauss E, Konturek P, Maiss J, Kressel J, Schulz U, Hahn EG, et al. Clinical significance of lymphoid hyperplasia of the lower gastrointestinal tract. Endoscopy 2010;42:334–7.
6. Kokkonen J. Lymphoid nodular hyperplasia. In: Guandalini S, editor. Textbook of pediatric gastroenterology and nutrition. 1st ed. London: Taylor and Francis; 2004. pp. 479–488.
7. Fritscher-Ravens A, Scherbakov P, Bufler P, Torroni F, Ruuska T, Nuutinen H, et al. The feasibility of wireless capsule endoscopy in detecting small intestinal pathology in children under the age of 8 years: a multicentre European study. Gut 2009;58:1467–72.
8. Iacono G, Ravelli A, Di Prima L, Scalici C, Bolognini S, Chiappa S, et al. Colonic lymphoid nodular hyperplasia in children: relationship to food hypersensitivity. Clin Gastroenterol Hepatol. 2007;5:361–6.
9. Kenney PJ, Koehler RE, Shackelford GD. The clinical significance of large lymphoid follicles of the colon. Radiology 1982;142:41–6.
10. Kokkonen J, Karttunen TJ. Lymphonodular hyperplasia on the mucosa of the lower gastrointestinal tract in children: an indication of enhanced immune response? J Pediatr Gastroenterol Nutr. 2002;34:42–6.
11. Cornes JS. Number, size, and distribution of Peyer's patches in the human small intestine: Part I The development of Peyer's patches. Gut 1965;6:225–9.
12. Van Kruiningen HJ, West AB, Freda BJ, Holmes KA. Distribution of Peyer's patches in the distal ileum. Inflamm Bowel Dis. 2002;8:180–5.
13. Kokkonen J. Lymphonodular hyperplasia on the duodenal bulb indicates food allergy in children. Endoscopy 1999;31:464–7.
14. Farris AB, Lauwers GY, Ferry JA, Zukerberg LR. The rectal tonsil: a reactive lymphoid proliferation that may mimic lymphoma. Am J Surg Pathol. 2008;32:1075–9.
15. Cramer SF, Romansky S, Hulbert B, Rauh S, Papp JR, Casiano-Colon AE. The rectal tonsil: a reaction to chlamydial infection? Am J Surg Pathol. 2009;33:483–5.
16. Toyoda H, Yamaguchi M, Uemura Y, Mukai K, Sawa H, Suzuki H, et al. Successful treatment of lymphoid follicular proctitis with sulfasalazine suppositories. Am J Gastroenterol. 2000;95:2403–4.
17. Kokkonen TS, Augustin MT, Kokkonen J, Karttunen R, Karttunen TJ. Serum and tissue CD23, IL-15 and Fas-L in cow's milk protein-sensitive enteropathy and in coeliac disease. J Pediatr Gastroenterol Nutr. 2012;54(4):525–31.
18. Pabst O. New concepts in the generation and functions of IgA. Nat Rev Immunol. 2012;12:821–32.

19. Kokkonen J, Haapalahti M, Laurila K, Karttunen TJ, Maki M. Cow's milk protein-sensitive enteropathy at school age. J Pediatr. 2001;139:797–803.

20. Kokkonen J, Ruuska T, Karttunen TJ, Maki M. Lymphonodular hyperplasia of the terminal ileum associated with colitis shows an increase gammadelta + t-cell density in children. Am J Gastroenterol. 2002;97:667–72.

21. Augustin MT, Kokkonen J, Karttunen TJ. Duodenal cytotoxic lymphocytes in cow's milk protein sensitive enteropathy and coeliac disease. Scand J Gastroenterol. 2005;40:1398–406.

22. Daniels JA, Lederman HM, Maitra A, Montgomery EA. Gastrointestinal tract pathology in patients with common variable immunodeficiency (CVID): a clinicopathologic study and review. Am J Surg Pathol. 2007;31:1800–12.

23. Brandtzaeg P. Function of mucosa-associated lymphoid tissue in antibody formation. Immunol Invest. 2010;39:303–55.

24. Moghaddami M, Cummins A, Mayrhofer G. Lymphocyte-filled villi: comparison with other lymphoid aggregations in the mucosa of the human small intestine Gastroenterology. 1998;115:1414–25.

25. Knoop KA, Newberry RD. Isolated lymphoid follicles are dynamic reservoirs for the induction of intestinal IgA. Front Immunol. 2012;3:84.

26. O'Leary AD, Sweeney EC. Lymphoglandular complexes of the colon: structure and distribution. Histopathology. 1986;10:267–83.

27. Nascimbeni R, Di Fabio F, Di Betta E, Mariani P, Fisogni S, Villanacci V. Morphology of colorectal lymphoid aggregates in cancer, diverticular and inflammatory bowel diseases. Mod Pathol. 2005;18:681–5.

28. Langman JM, Rowland R. Density of lymphoid follicles in the rectum and at the anorectal junction. J Clin Gastroenterol. 1992;14:81–4.

29. Azzali G. Structure, lymphatic vascularization and lymphocyte migration in mucosa-associated lymphoid tissue. Immunol Rev. 2003;195:178–89.

30. Cerutti A. Location, location, location: B-cell differentiation in the gut lamina propria. Mucosal Immunol. 2008;1:8–10.

31. Rosh JR, Kurfist LA, Benkov KJ, Toor AH, Bottone EJ, LeLeiko NS. Helicobacter pylori and gastric lymphonodular hyperplasia in children. Am J Gastroenterol. 1992;87:135–9.

32. Conte MP, Schippa S, Zamboni I, Penta M, Chiarini F, Seganti L, et al. Gut-associated bacterial microbiota in paediatric patients with inflammatory bowel disease Gut 2006;55:1760–7.

33. Kokkonen J, Tikkanen S, Karttunen TJ, Savilahti E. A similar high level of immunoglobulin A and immunoglobulin G class milk antibodies and increment of local lymphoid tissue on the duodenal mucosa in subjects with cow's milk allergy and recurrent abdominal pains. Pediatr Allergy Immunol. 2002;13:129–36.

34. Berin MC. Mucosal antibodies in the regulation of tolerance and allergy to foods. Semin Immunopathol. 2012;34(5):633–42.

35. Bellanti JA, Zeligs BJ, Malka-Rais J, Sabra A. Abnormalities of Th1 function in non-IgE food allergy, celiac disease, and ileal lymphonodular hyperplasia: a new relationship? Ann Allergy Asthma Immunol. 2003;90:84–9.

36. Paajanen L, Kokkonen J, Karttunen TJ, Tuure T, Korpela R, Vaarala O. Intestinal cytokine mRNA expression in delayed-type cow's milk allergy. J Pediatr Gastroenterol Nutr. 2006;43:470–6.

37. Paajanen L, Vaarala O, Karttunen R, Tuure T, Korpela R, Kokkonen J. Increased IFN-gamma secretion from duodenal biopsy samples in delayed-type cow's milk allergy. Pediatr Allergy Immunol. 2005;16:439–44.

38. Veres G, Westerholm-Ormio M, Kokkonen J, Arato A, Savilahti E. Cytokines and adhesion molecules in duodenal mucosa of children with delayed-type food allergy. J Pediatr Gastroenterol Nutr. 2003;37:27–34.

39. Carroccio A, Mansueto P, D'Alcamo A, Iacono G. Non-celiac wheat sensitivity as an allergic condition: personal experience and narrative review. Am J Gastroenterol. 2013;108:1845–52; quiz 1853.

40. Kaplan B, Benson J, Rothstein F, Dahms B, Halpin T. Lymphonodular hyperplasia of the colon as a pathologic finding in children with lower gastrointestinal bleeding. J Pediatr Gastroenterol Nutr. 1984;3:704–8.

41. Ward H, Jalan KN, Maitra TK, Agarwal SK, Mahalanabis D. Small intestinal nodular lymphoid hyperplasia in patients with giardiasis and normal serum immunoglobulins. Gut 1983;24:120–6.

42. Bastlein C, Burlefinger R, Holzberg E, Voeth C, Garbrecht M, Ottenjann R. Common variable immunodeficiency syndrome and nodular lymphoid hyperplasia in the small intestine. Endoscopy 1988;20:272–5.

43. Agarwal S, Mayer L. Pathogenesis and treatment of gastrointestinal disease in antibody deficiency syndromes. J Allergy Clin Immunol. 2009;124:658–64.

44. Levendoglu H, Rosen Y. Nodular lymphoid hyperplasia of gut in HIV infection. Am J Gastroenterol. 1992;87:1200–2.

45. Kokkonen J, Arvonen M, Vahasalo P, Karttunen TJ. Intestinal immune activation in juvenile idiopathic arthritis and connective tissue disease. Scand J Rheumatol. 2007;36(5):386–9.

46. Shaoul R, Eliakim R, Tamir A, Karban A. Ileal lymphonodular hyperplasia is not associated with NOD2/CARD15 mutations. J Pediatr Gastroenterol Nutr. 2006;43:30–4.

47. Drut R, Drut RM. Hyperplasia of lymphoglandular complexes in colon segments in Hirschsprung's disease: a form of diversion colitis. Pediatr Pathol. 1992;12:575–81.

48. Turunen S, Karttunen TJ, Kokkonen J. Lymphoid nodular hyperplasia and cow's milk hypersensitivity in children with chronic constipation. J Pediatr. 2004;145:606–11.

49. Carroccio A, Iacono G, Di Prima L, Ravelli A, Pirrone G, Cefalu AB, et al. Food hypersensitivity as a cause of rectal bleeding in adults. Clin Gastroenterol Hepatol. 2009;7:120–2.

50. Gullberg E, Soderholm JD. Peyer's patches and M cells as potential sites of the inflammatory onset in Crohn's disease. Ann N Y Acad Sci. 2006;1072:218–32.

Acute Pancreatitis

33

Alisha Mavis, Praveen S. Goday and Steven L. Werlin

Anatomy and Physiology

The pancreas is a large, J-shaped, flattened gland located in the upper left abdomen that secretes digestive enzymes into the duodenum and produces several important hormones as part of the endocrine system. In adults, it is about 15–20 cm long and lies inferior to the stomach, and is surrounded by the small intestine, spleen, gallbladder, and liver [1, 2]. The pancreas is divided into four sections: head, neck, body, and tail. The uncinate process emerges from the head of the pancreas and lies deep to the superior mesenteric artery and vein, which run behind the neck of the pancreas [3].

The pancreas is both an exocrine and endocrine gland. The exocrine pancreas is made up of acinar and ductal cells that produce and transport digestive enzymes, such as amylase, lipase, and trypsin, through a system of small ducts that lead to the pancreatic duct, which runs the length of the pancreas and then combines with the common bile duct carrying bile from the gallbladder proximal to the ampulla of Vater (Fig. 33.1) [1]. Pancreatic enzymes and bile are then secreted into the small intestine and aid in the digestion of carbohydrates, fats, and proteins. The endocrine cells of the pancreas, located in the islets of Langerhans, produce two main hormones, insulin and glucagon, which together control glucose metabolism. The endocrine cells also produce other hormones including somatostatin and pancreatic polypeptide [4–6].

Pathophysiology

Pathological trypsinogen activation has long been considered the hallmark of acute pancreatitis (AP) . Following an initial insult, such as ductal disruption or obstruction, cathepsin B activates trypsinogen to trypsin within the acinar cell. Trypsin then activates other pancreatic proenzymes, leading to autodigestion, further enzyme activation, and release of active proteases. Lysosomal hydrolases co-localize with pancreatic proenzymes within the acinar cell. Pancreastasis (similar in concept to cholestasis) with continued synthesis of enzymes occurs. Lecithin is activated by phospholipase A2 into the toxic lysolecithin. Prophospholipase is unstable and can be activated by minute quantities of trypsin [7, 8]. This leads to cell death and AP . After the insult, cytokines and other proinflammatory mediators are released. Most animal models support this mechanism.

The healthy pancreas is protected from autodigestion by pancreatic proteases that are synthesized as inactive proenzymes, which are then segregated into secretory zymogen granules at pH 6.2, by low calcium concentration, which minimizes trypsin activity. Protease inhibitors are present both in the cytoplasm and zymogen granules [5–8]. Enzymes are secreted directly into the ducts lessening exposure of the cytoplasmic contents.

Recently, animal models of AP without associated pathological intracellular trypsinogen activation, as required by the classic theory, have been developed. In these models, intracellular activation of trypsinogen to trypsin plays a role only in early acinar injury. For example, a knockout mouse model of pancreatitis in mice lacking the trypsinogen 7 gene has been developed [8, 9]. These mice develop pancreatitis even though they are unable to activate trypsinogen. In this model, nuclear factor kappa-light-chain-enhancer of activated B cells (NFkB) is activated early in the course of and appears to be the primary driver of the proinflammatory response. Even more recent studies have shown perturbation of mitochondrial permeability and function early in the evolution of experimental pancreatitis [10]. In this model, alco-

S. L. Werlin (✉) · A. Mavis · P. S. Goday
Division of Gastroenterology, Department of Pediatrics, Children's Hospital of Wisconsin, Medical College of Wisconsin, 8701 Watertown Plank Road, Milwaukee, WI 53226, USA
e-mail: swerlin@mcw.edu

© Springer International Publishing Switzerland 2016
S. Guandalini et al. (eds.), *Textbook of Pediatric Gastroenterology, Hepatology and Nutrition*,
DOI 10.1007/978-3-319-17169-2_33

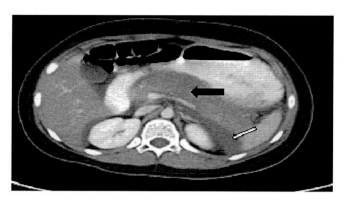

Fig. 33.1 Early acute pancreatitis. Note edematous gland *(black arrow)* with a small amount of fluid *(small arrow)*. No visible ducts or calcifications. (Images courtesy of Dr. David Gregg)

hol causes a collapse of the electrical gradient across the mitochondrial permeability transition pore leading to depletion of adenosine triphosphate (ATP) and acinar cell necrosis.

Whatever the true interpretation may be, time-course analysis shows that a burst of electron transfer reactions is associated with the disease initiation [11]. For example, in the experimental model of mild AP produced by excessive stimulation with caerulein, a cholecystokinin (CCK) analog, the spark from reactive oxygen species can be seen by chemiluminescence within 5 min. Simultaneously, there is a huge increase in stress-activated protein kinase. Within 10 min, there is an increase in amylase in the venous outflow of the pancreas. Similarly in endoscopic retrograde cholangiopancreatography (ERCP)-induced AP, analysis of peripheral blood by electron spin resonance spectroscopy identified the burst of reactive oxygen species by the end of the clinical procedure, followed by steep increases in serum levels of amylase, lipase, and trypsinogen.

Histopathologically, interstitial edema appears early. Later, as the episode of pancreatitis progresses, localized and confluent necrosis, blood vessel disruption leading to hemorrhage, and an inflammatory response in the peritoneum can develop. In mild pancreatitis, there is interstitial edema and an inflammatory infiltrate is found. There is no organ dysfunction. In severe pancreatitis, the inflammation is extensive and parenchymal necrosis is present. Multiorgan failure accompanies the inflammation. Following an episode of AP, all histological abnormalities resolve. The factor(s) that determine the severity of an episode of AP are unknown.

Epidemiology

In adults, AP is one of the most common diseases of the gastrointestinal tract and remains a serious disease. In the USA, AP is the most common gastroenterology discharge diagno-

sis accounting for more than 553,000 hospital discharges, 881,000 ambulatory visits, and 3413 deaths a year [12, 13]. The incidence of AP varies between 4.9 and 73.4 cases per 100,000 worldwide.

In pediatrics, it is estimated that 2–13 new cases per 100,000 children occur annually. AP is ranked 14th among causes of death from gastrointestinal and liver diseases in adults [14]. In the last 15 years, studies have shown an increase in the annual incidence of AP. The case fatality rate for AP has decreased over time while the overall population mortality rate has remained unchanged. In adults, mortality from AP is approximately 3 % for interstitial pancreatitis and 15 % for necrotizing pancreatitis [13, 14]. Almost 20 % of children with AP develop a complication, and the mortality rate is approximately 4 % despite significant advances in the treatment of this disease [15, 16].

Etiology

In adults, 85 % of episodes of AP are due to alcohol and cholelithiasis. In contrast in children, the most common etiologies of AP are as follows: blunt abdominal injuries, biliary stones or microlithiasis (sludging), drug toxicity, and multisystem diseases such as the hemolytic uremic syndrome and inflammatory bowel disease [17–23]. Other cases follow solid organ and stem cell transplantation or are due to infections, anatomic anomalies, metabolic disorders, and mutations in susceptibility genes. Only 10–20 % of cases are now considered idiopathic. There is a widely used pneumonic, *Tigar-O,* which stands for toxic-metabolic, idiopathic, genetic, autoimmune, recurrent and severe AP and obstructive.

Trauma Trauma typically due to bicycle handlebar injuries, automobile accidents, and sports injuries is the cause of about 20–40 % of episodes of AP [17–23] (Table 33.1). Other traumas include ERCP, child and sexual abuse, surgical injury, and total body cast. Because the pancreas is retroperitoneal and lies across the spine, ductal rupture is not uncommon. Diagnosis may be delayed. Since most patients with abdominal trauma receive a CT scan, injuries may now be detected earlier than before. Following trauma, unsuspected ductal damage can lead to strictures, pseudocyst formation, and chronic obstruction.

Table 33.1 Traumatic causes of acute pancreatitis

Blunt injury
Child abuse
ERCP
Head trauma
Surgical trauma
Total body cast

Table 33.2 Biliary tract causes of pancreatitis

Ampullary disease
Ascariasis
Biliary tract malformations
Cholelithiasis, microlithiasis, and choledocholithiasis
Duplication cyst
Endoscopic retrograde cholangiopancreatography (*ERCP*) complication
Pancreas divisum
Pancreatic ductal abnormalities
Pancreaticobiliary malfunction
Choledochal cyst
Choledochocele
Postoperative
Sphincter of Oddi dysfunction
Tumor

Table 33.3 Drugs and toxins

Acetaminophen
Alcohol
[a]L-Asparaginase
[a]Azathioprine
Carbamazepine
Cimetidine
Corticosteroids
Didanosine
Enalapril
Erythromycin
Estrogen
Furosemide
Isoniazid
Lamivudine
Lisinopril
[a]6-Mercaptopurine
Methyldopa
Metronidazole
Octreotide
Opiates
Organophosphate poisoning
Pentamidine
Phenformin
Retrovirals: DDC, DDI, tenofovir
Simvastatin
Sulfonamides:
Sulindac
Tetracycline
Thiazides
[a]Valproic acid
Venom (spider, scorpion, Gila monster lizard)
Vincristine

[a] Most common in children
DDC dideoxycytidine, *DDI* dideoxyinosine

Biliary Pancreatitis Biliary obstruction due to lithiasis, sludge, anatomic abnormalities, or ERCP is the etiology in 5–20% of pancreatitis in children (Table 33.2). Anatomic causes of biliary obstruction, such as pancreaticobiliary maljunction (PBM) and pancreas divisum, are increasingly recognized [24, 25]. PBM and congenital dilatation of the biliary tract are more common in Japanese patients than in Western patients. There remains controversy over whether pancreas divisum alone is a cause of pancreatitis. Risk factors for biliary pancreatitis in children include obesity and Hispanic ethnicity.

Drugs and Toxins Drugs and toxins account for 10–20% of children with AP (Table 33.3). In children, valproic acid, L-asparaginase, 6-mercaptopurine, and azathioprine are the most common causes of drug-induced pancreatitis [26]. Recently, azathioprine was successfully reintroduced in four patients with presumes thiopurine-induced pancreatitis [27].

Infectious Agents Since many patients with idiopathic pancreatitis have a viral-like prodrome, it is difficult to determine the true incidence of infection-associated AP (Table 33.4) [17–23]. Case series have found between 2 and 10% of children with AP have a viral cause. This may be an underestimate because many patients with idiopathic pancreatitis may well have infectious causes. A wide variety of infections have been associated with AP, particularly hepatitis A, mumps, and Epstein–Barr virus (EBV) infections.

Genetic Mutations in an increasing number of genes have been shown to cause pancreatitis, the most common being mutations in the *PRSS1, CFTR,* and *SPINK1* genes. Genetic causes have been reported in 1–14% of cases [28, 29] (Table 33.5). The incidence may well be higher, since it is uncommon to check for genetic etiologies during the first episode of pancreatitis. *PRSS1* is the gene that causes *hereditary pancreatitis.* Atypical cystic fibrosis may occur in patients with at least one mild mutation in the CFTR gene. Patients with atypical cystic fibrosis and pancreatic sufficiency are at risk for pancreatitis.. At the time of a first episode of AP, patients with mutations in these genes will have courses indistinguishable from patients with pancreatitis from other causes. Unless there is a family history of pancreatitis or cystic fibrosis or there are signs of chronicity on imaging studies, genetic testing is not indicated in the first episode of AP.

Systemic and Autoimmune Disease Pancreatitis is well known to be associated with a number of systemic diseases, particularly hemolytic uremic syndrome, sepsis, and shock [17–23] (Table 33.6). The incidence of AP associated with these conditions ranges from 5 to 35% in published series. These cases typically have a course similar to that of pancreatitis from other causes. Autoimmune pancreatitis is rare in children.

Idiopathic In published series, no etiology was found in 12–38% of children with AP [17–23]. As new etiologies were found and as workup became more extensive, newer series have lower rates of idiopathic AP.

Table 33.4 Infectious causes of pancreatitis

Ascariasis
Coxsackie B virus
[a]Epstein–Barr virus
[a]Hepatitis A
Hepatitis B
Influenza A, B
Leptospirosis
Malaria
Measles
[a]Mumps
Mycoplasma
Rubella
Rubeola
Reye syndrome: varicella, influenza B
Septic shock

[a] Most common in children

Table 33.5 Genetic causes of pancreatitis

PRSS1: cationic trypsinogen
CTRC: chymotrypsin C gene
CFTR: cystic fibrosis gene
SPINK 1: trypsin inhibitor gene
CPA2: carboxypeptidase A2
CASR: calcium-sensing receptor
CLDN2: claudin 2

Table 33.6 Systemic and autoimmune diseases

Autoimmune pancreatitis
Burns
Collagen vascular diseases
Crohn's disease
Hypercalcemia
Diabetic ketoacidosis
Hemochromatosis
Hemolytic uremic syndrome
Hyperlipidemia: type I, IV, V
Hyperparathyroidism/hypercalcemia
Kawasaki disease
Malignancy
Malnutrition
Metabolic diseases
Organic academia
Peptic ulcer
Periarteritis nodosa
Renal failure
Solid organ transplant
Systemic lupus erythematosus
Transplantation: stem cell, solid organ
Vasculitis
Hypothermia

Diagnosis

Criteria for the diagnosis of pancreatitis in children have recently been defined by an expert multinational committee as two of three of the following: abdominal pain, serum amylase, and/or lipase activity at least three times greater than the upper limit of normal and imaging findings characteristic of or compatible with AP [30]. These criteria are similar to those used in adults.

Serum lipase is now considered the test of choice for AP, as it is more specific than amylase for acute inflammatory pancreatic disease and should be determined when pancreatitis is suspected. Serum lipase remains elevated longer than amylase after disease presentation. The serum lipase rises by 4–8 h, peaks at 24–48 h, and remains elevated 8–14 days, longer than serum amylase. Serum lipase may also be elevated in non-pancreatic diseases (Table 33.7). Diabetic patients appear to have a higher median lipase compared with nondiabetic patients so an upper limit of normal greater than three to five times may be needed in diabetic patients [13, 31]. The clinical condition of the patient must be considered when evaluating amylase and lipase elevations. However, serum lipase ≥ 7 times the upper limit of normal within 24 h of presentation may be a simple clinical predictor of severe AP in children [15].

Table 33.7 Non-pancreatitis causes of elevated enzymes

Serum lipase	Serum amylase
Acute cholecystitis	Acidosis
Bowel obstruction	Alcoholism
Celiac disease	Appendicitis
Diabetic ketoacidosis	Bowel obstruction/Infarction
Drugs	Celiac disease
Duodenal ulceration	Cerebral trauma
HIV	Cholecystitis
Idiopathic	Cystic fibrosis
Macrolipasemia	Drugs
Pancreatic calculus	HIV
Pancreatic tumors	Idiopathic
Renal Failure	Liver disease
Trauma (including post-ERCP)	Lymphoma
	Macroamylasemia
	Myocardial infarction
	Pancreatic tumors
	Pelvic inflammatory disease
	Peptic ulcers
	Pregnancy
	Renal failure
	Rheumatoid arthritis
	Trauma
	Ulcerative colitis

In AP patients, serum amylase usually rises within a few hours after the onset of symptoms and return to normal values within 3–5 days. Serum amylase may remain normal in up to 20% of patients, especially in alcohol-induced AP and hypertriglyceridemia [31]. A variety of conditions may also cause hyperamylasemia without pancreatitis, such as macroamylasemia (Table 33.7).

Other laboratory abnormalities that may be present in AP include hemoconcentration, manifested by high hemoglobin and blood urea nitrogen (BUN), coagulopathy, leukocytosis, hyperglycemia, glucosuria, and hypocalcemia. Elevated γ-glutamyl transpeptidase and hyperbilirubinemia suggest the diagnosis of cholelithiasis or choledocholithiasis [13, 31].

X-ray of the chest and abdomen may also be obtained and demonstrate nonspecific findings. The chest X-ray might show atelectasis, basilar infiltrates, elevation of the hemidiaphragm, left-sided (rarely right-sided) pleural effusions, pericardial effusion, and pulmonary edema. Abdominal X-rays might demonstrate a sentinel loop of intestine, dilation of the transverse colon (cutoff sign), ileus, pancreatic calcification (if recurrent), blurring of the left psoas margin, a pseudocyst, ascites, and peripancreatic extraluminal gas bubbles [13, 31, 32].

Transabdominal ultrasound should be performed on all patients with AP, when gallstones are suspected. Abdominal imaging is useful to confirm the diagnosis of AP, but the routine use of CT is not recommended during the first week because it has low yield and rarely alters clinical management [13, 32, 33]. However, if a patient is not improving after 1 week, CT or magnetic resonance imaging (MRI) of the pancreas is recommended to assess for local complications (Fig. 33.2). CT and/or MRI of the pancreas are also recommended in patients in whom the diagnosis is unclear. CT has over 90% sensitivity and specificity for the diagnosis of AP. Ultrasonography is more sensitive than CT scanning for the diagnosis of biliary stones [13, 33].

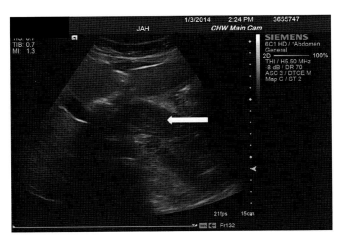

Fig. 33.2 Ultrasound of the same patient showing a hypoechoic and edematous pancreas *(arrow)*. (Images courtesy of Dr. David Gregg)

Magnetic resonance cholangiopancreatography (MRCP) and ERCP are essential in the investigation of known or suspected pancreatic duct disruption, lithiasis, recurrent and nonresolving pancreatitis, and disease associated with gallbladder pathology, but have a lesser role in AP [34, 35]. Although there is limited pediatric data, endoscopic ultrasonography has been shown to be helpful in the drainage of fluid collections in children [36].

Clinical Presentation

Although there have been a number of attempts to develop a scoring system for AP, there is no validated scoring system for children withAP [16, 37]. A recent report suggests that a serum lipase >7 times the upper limit of normal within 24 h of admission predicts a severe course [38]. This still needs to be validated. Thus, reliable prediction of the course of an episode of AP is not possible.

Several new classification systems have been proposed for use in adults. None have been tested in children. Most episodes of AP in children are mild and self-limiting, defined by the absence of organ failure and/or pancreatic necrosis (local complications) [39]. These patients resolve their symptoms rapidly [15] and are usually discharged within 1 week, and mortality is rare [13].

Patients with moderately severe AP may have transient organ failure, local complications, and/or systemic complications. The morbidity and mortality are higher compared to that of mild AP. However, the mortality is considerably less than that of severe AP [13, 39, 40]. Depending on the complications, patients may require prolonged hospitalization because of the local or systemic complications.

Severe AP is defined as AP complicated by persistent organ failure and/or death and occurs in 15–20% of patients [13, 39, 40, 41]. Patients with severe AP usually have one or more local and/or systemic complications. Of note, patients with severe AP that develops within the early phase (first week) have a 36–50% risk of death [13]. Development of infected necrosis later in the course of the disease in patients with severe AP also has an extremely high mortality [42].

For practical purpose, we define here severe pediatric pancreatitis as requiring pediatric intensive care unit (PICU) admission. Severe AP has been infrequently reported in children; however, the outcome may be better than in adults.

Mild AP

The patient with AP has abdominal pain, which may be severe. Some patients have persistent vomiting and possibly fever. The pain is epigastric or in either upper quadrant. The child often lies with hips and knees flexed lying on the side.

The abdomen may be distended and tender, and a mass may be palpable. The patient usually appears extremely uncomfortable, irritable, and may look ill or toxic. The pain can increase in intensity for 24–48 h, during which time vomiting may increase and the patient might require hospitalization for dehydration and may need fluid and electrolyte therapy. Pain described as dull, colicky, or located in the lower abdomen is not consistent with AP and suggests other etiologies. The prognosis for complete recovery in the acute uncomplicated case is excellent [13, 15, 28, 31, 39, 40].

Severe AP

In adults, 15–20 % of cases of pancreatitis are defined as severe, and these have a mortality rate of about 15 %. Fortunately, severe AP is less common in children than in adults [16]. In this life-threatening condition, characterized by multiorgan failure lasting more than 48 h, the patient is acutely ill with severe nausea, vomiting, and abdominal pain [13, 15, 28, 31, 39, 40]. A bluish discoloration may be seen around the umbilicus (Cullen's sign) or in the flanks (Grey Turner's sign) [31, 43]. Pancreas necrosis may develop between the second and fifth week of illness. Infected necrosis may develop during the second week and a pancreatic abscess as late as the fifth week of illness. Infection is suspected when there is persistent pain and fever.

Mortality is related to the systemic inflammatory response syndrome (SIRS) with multiple organ dysfunction, shock, renal failure, acute respiratory distress syndrome, disseminated intravascular coagulation, massive gastrointestinal bleeding, and systemic or intra-abdominal infection [44]. In adults, the percentage of necrosis seen on CT scan and failure of pancreatic tissue to enhance on CT scan (suggesting necrosis) predicts the severity of the disease [13, 39].

There are now two defined, distinct phases of severe, acute pancreatitis, which overlap: the early phase, which usually lasts only 1 week or so, and the late phase, which can persist for weeks to months. The early phase is characterized by the systemic inflammatory response syndrome and/or the compensatory anti-inflammatory syndrome (CARS), which can predispose to infection. The late phase is characterized by the persistence of systemic signs of ongoing inflammation, the presence of local and systemic complications, and/or transient or persistent organ failure. Local complications include peripancreatic fluid collections, pancreatic and peripancreatic necrosis, pseudocysts, and walled-off necrosis. By definition, the late phase occurs only in patients with moderately severe or severe AP [39, 40, 44] (Fig. 33.3).

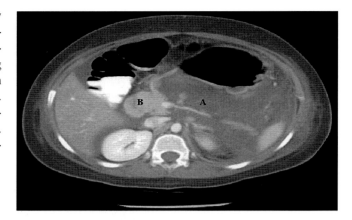

Fig. 33.3 Late acute pancreatitis in the same patient CT scan demonstrates necrotic non-enhancing distal pancreas (**a**). The pancreatic head is relatively normal (**b**). There is a large amount of peripancreatic fluid. (Images courtesy of Dr. David Gregg)

Treatment

The aims of medical management are to relieve pain and restore metabolic homeostasis. Analgesia should be given in adequate doses. A recent Cochrane review stated that opioids may be an appropriate choice for AP pain in adults and may decrease the need for supplementary analgesia [45]. They found that opioids did not increase the risk of pancreatitis complications or significant adverse events. Fluid, electrolyte, and mineral balance should be restored and maintained.

In *mild AP,* nasogastric (NG) suction is needed infrequently but is useful in patients who have significant vomiting. While vomiting, the patient should be maintained with nothing by mouth. Refeeding can commence when vomiting has resolved. Early refeeding decreases the complication rate and length of stay [46]. While traditional, there are no data to support the use of a low-fat diet. It is not necessary to follow laboratory tests such as the serum lipase daily. Recovery is usually complete within 4–7 days.

In *severe pancreatitis,* fluid resuscitation in the first 24 h is critical [47]. Lactated Ringer's solution is the fluid of choice. Intravascular fluid losses due to third spacing and losses through an NG tube can rapidly lead to dehydration and cardiovascular instability. So not only is volume expansion important but also maintenance of intravascular volume is critical.

Narcotic analgesia is given as needed. Antibiotics are used to treat infected necrosis but prophylactic antibiotics are not recommended. Infected necrosis does not occur until the second week of pancreatitis [48]. Gastric acid is suppressed.

Endotherapy can be of benefit when pancreatitis is caused by anatomic abnormalities, such as strictures or stones [49]. The endoscopist can dilate the sphincter of Oddi and extract impacted biliary tract stones. This is especially important when the patient has developed cholangitis.

There are no published guidelines or studies relating to nutritional support of the child with AP. A recent Cochrane review concluded that "There is little evidence to support or refute the need to provide nutrition to critically ill children in a pediatric intensive care unit during the first week of their critical illness" [50]. A recent review supported early nutritional therapy in AP [51].

Early enteral alimentation is begun, whether by mouth, nasogastric tube, or nasojejunal tube (in patients intolerant to oral or nasogastric feedings). When initiated within 2–3 days of onset of pancreatitis, enteral feeding reduces the length of hospitalization and complication rate and increases survival in adult patients with severe AP. Supplemental parenteral nutrition may be needed in some patients

Measurement of gastric residuals is of limited value and should be discouraged. Residual volume relates to infusion rate. High residuals are common early in enteral nutrition. Gastric distension may be from gas-filled loops of bowel. A rise in serum amylase and lipase is typically associated with enteral feeding. These rises do not imply worsening of the pancreatitis and are not the reasons to stop enteral nutrition.

When a patient has persistent fever in the second week of illness or who develops fever later, a CT scan is required [13]. When necrotic tissue is seen, fine-needle aspiration and culture are indicated [13]. The use of antibiotics in sterile necrosis is not recommended. Antibiotics of choice for infected pancreatic necrosis and abscess are those that are known to penetrate the pancreas, including carbapenem, quinolones, and metronidazole [13].

In *traumatic pancreatitis,* surgery is frequently required. In children, surgical therapy of nontraumatic, AP may include drainage and resection of necrotic material or abscesses. In stable patients, surgery is deferred at least 2–4 weeks to allow differentiation between necrotic and viable tissue [13]. In gallstone pancreatitis, it is recommended that cholecystectomy be performed before hospital discharge to prevent recurrent episodes [13].

Complications

Most children with acute uncomplicated pancreatitis will do well and recover within 4–7 days. However, about 20% of children with AP will develop a complication, which may prolong the hospital stay or require intervention [15]. Complications are divided into local and systemic. Local complications include acute peripancreatic fluid collections, pancreatic pseudocysts, acute necrotic collections, walled-off necrosis, splenic/portal vein thrombosis, colonic necrosis, retroperitoneal hemorrhage, and gastric outlet dysfunction. Local complications should be suspected when there is persistent abdominal pain, fever/chills, or organ failure and should prompt cross-sectional imaging to search for these complications [13, 39, 40]. Acute peripancreatic fluid collections are not associated with necrotizing pancreatitis, remain sterile, and usually resolve without intervention. However, if the fluid collection persists more than 4 weeks, it is likely to develop into a pancreatic pseudocyst. A pancreatic pseudocyst is a peripancreatic or intrapancreatic fluid collection or collections surrounded by a well-defined wall, and contains no solid material. Acute peripancreatic fluid collections and acute necrotic collections occur within the first 4 weeks of AP, while pancreatic pseudocysts and walled-off necrosis usually arise more than 4 weeks after the onset of AP [39, 40].

Systemic complications include de novo occurrence of renal, circulatory, or respiratory organ failure or exacerbation of serious preexisting comorbidities related directly to the AP. Systemic complications occur from the systemic inflammatory response to AP, and may be further exacerbated by the need for fluid resuscitation [39, 40, 44].

Future

Over the past 15 years, as the incidence of AP has risen, the percent of children with idiopathic AP has decreased as more etiologies, such as genetic causes, have been identified, as ERCP has become more available for children, and as new technologies such as MRCP and endoscopic ultrasound have been developed. Greater understanding of the pathophysiology of pancreatitis has led to improvement in therapy such as early introduction of enteral feeding and rapid fluid resuscitation in severe pancreatitis

Since there are no controlled studies on any aspect of the treatment of AP in children, nearly all the current recommendations are based on publications describing adults. Particular areas in need of investigation include fluid resuscitation, use of antibiotics, nutrition, that is, when to begin enteral feeds and the risks and benefits of endoscopic ultrasound.

While there are a number of validated scoring systems for the prediction of severity in adults, there is no such validated scoring system for children. The development of a scoring system is important so that patients who are predicted to develop severe pancreatitis can be transferred early to a facility with a pediatric critical care unit, while those predicted to have mild disease can be treated at local hospitals.

References

1. Shih HP, Wang A, Sander M. Pancreas organogenesis: from lineage determination to morphogenesis. Annu Rev Cell Dev Biol. 2013 Oct 6;29(1):81–105.

2. Debi U, Kaur R, Prasad KK, Sinha SK, Sinha A, Singh K. Pancreatic trauma: a concise review. World J Gastroenterol. 2013;19(47):9003.

3. Werlin SL, Mayer AN. Development of the exocrine pancreas. In: Polin RA, Fox WW, Abman SH, editors. Fetal and neonatal physiology. 4th ed. Philadelphia: WB Saunders; 2011. pp. 1230–9.

4. Pandiri AR. Overview of exocrine pancreatic pathobiology. Toxicol Pathol. 2014 Jan 16;42(1):207–16.

5. Whitcomb DC, Lowe ME. Human pancreatic digestive enzymes. Dig Dis Sci. 2007 Jan 5;52(1):1–17.

6. Barreto SG, Carati CJ, Toouli J, Saccone GTP. The islet-acinar axis of the pancreas: more than just insulin. Am J Physiol Gastrointest Liver Physiol. 2010 Jun 15;299(1):G10–22.

7. Sah RP, Garg P, Saluja AK. Pathogenic mechanisms of acute pancreatitis. Curr Opin Gastroenterol. 2012;28(5):507–15.

8. Dawra R, Sah RP, Dudeja V, Rishi L, Talukdar R, Garg P, et al. Intra-acinar trypsinogen activation mediates early stages of pancreatic injury but not inflammation in mice with acute pancreatitis. Gastroenterol 2011 Dec 1;141(6):2210–2.

9. Sah RP, Dudeja V, Dawra RK, Saluja AK. Cerulein-induced chronic pancreatitis does not require intra-acinar activation of trypsinogen in mice. Gastroenterology 2013;144(5):1076–1085. e2. doi:10.1053/j.gastro.2013.01.041.

10. Shalbueva N, Mareninova OA, Gerloff A, Yuan J, Waldron RT, Pandol SJ, Gukovskaya AS. Effects of oxidative alcohol metabolism on the mitochondrial permeability transition pore and necrosis in a mouse model of alcoholic pancreatitis Gastroenterology 2013;144(2):437–46.e6. doi:10.1053/j.gastro.2012.10.037

11. Armstrong JA, Cash N, Soares PM, Souza MH, Sutton R, Criddle DN. Oxidative stress in acute pancreatitis: lost in translation? Free Radic Res. 2013;47(11):917–33. doi:10.3109/10715762.2013.835046.

12. Digestive Diseases Statistics for the United States. http://digestive. niddk.nih.gov/statistics/statistics.aspx#specific. Accessed 10 June 2015.

13. Tenner S, Baillie J, DeWitt J, Vege SS. American college of gastroenterology guideline: management of acute pancreatitis. Am J Gastroenterol. 2013 July 30;108(9):1400–15.

14. Kapoor K, Banks PA. Early prognostic evaluation of acute pancreatitis: an on-going challenge. J Pancreas. 2013 March 10;14(2):109–11.

15. Lautz TB, Chin AC, Radhakrishnan J. Acute pancreatitis in children: spectrum of disease and predictors of severity. J Pediatr Surg. 2011 June 1;46(6):1144–9.

16. Raizner A, Phatak UP, Baker K, Patel MG, Husain SZ, Pashankar DS. Acute necrotizing pancreatitis in children. J Pediatr. 2013;162(4):788–92. doi:10.1016/j.jpeds.2012.09.037

17. Lopez, M.J. The changing incidence of acute pancreatitis in children: a single-institution perspective. J Pediatr. 2002;140:622–4.

18. Werlin SL, Kugathasan S, Frautschy BC. Pancreatitis in children. J Pediatr Gastroenterol Nutr. 2003;37:591–595.

19. Nydegger A, Heine RG, Ranuh R, Gegati-Levy R, Crameri J, Oliver MR. Changing incidence of acute pancreatitis: 10-year experience at the Royal Children's Hospital, Melbourne. J Gastroenterol Hepatol. 2007;22:1313–6.

20. Sanchez-Ramirez CA, Larrosa-Haro A, Flores-Martinez S, Sanchez-Corona J, Villa-Gomez A, Macias-Rosales R. Acute and recurrent pancreatitis in children: etiological factors. Acta Paediatr. 2007;96:534–7.

21. Kandula L, Lowe ME. Etiology and outcome of acute pancreatitis in infants and toddlers. J Pediatr. 2008;152:106–10.

22. Park A, Latif SU, Shah AU, Tian J, Werlin S, Hsiao A, Pashankar D, Bhandari V, Nagar A, Husain SZ. Changing referral trends of

acute pancreatitis in children: a 12-year single-center analysis. J Pediatr Gastroenterol Nutr. 2009;49:316–22.

23. Morinville VD, Barmada MM, Lowe ME. Increasing incidence of acute pancreatitis at an American pediatric tertiary care center: is greater awareness among physicians responsible? Pancreas 2010;39:5–8.

24. Guo WL, Huang SG, Wang J, Sheng M, Fang L. Imaging findings in 75 pediatric patients with pancreaticobiliary maljunction: a retrospective case study. Pediatr Surg Int. 2012;28(10):983–8.

25. DiMagno MJ, Wamsteker EJ. Pancreas divisum. Curr Gastroenterol Rep. 2011;13(2):150–6. doi:10.1007/s11894-010-0170-8.

26. Nitsche C, Maertin S, Scheiber J, Ritter CA, Lerch MM, Mayerle J. Drug-induced pancreatitis. Curr Gastroenterol Rep. 2012;14(2):131–8. doi:10.1007/s11894-012-0245-9.

27. Ledder OD, Lemberg DA, Ooi CY, Day AS. Are thiopurines always contraindicated after thiopurine-induced pancreatitis in inflammatory bowel disease? J Pediatr Gastroenterol Nutr. 2013;57(5):583–6. doi:10.1097/MPG.0b013e31829f16fc.

28. Whitcomb DC. Genetic risk factors for pancreatic disorders. Gastroenterology 2013;144(6):1292–302. doi:10.1053/j. gastro.2013.01.069.

29. Sultan M, Werlin S, Venkatasubramani, N. Genetic prevalence and characteristics in children with recurrent pancreatitis. J Pediatr Gastroenterol Nutr. 2012;54:645–50.

30. Morinville VD, Husain SZ, Bai H, Barth B, Alhosh R, Durie PR, et al. Definitions of pediatric pancreatitis and survey of present clinical practices. J Pediatr Gastroenterol Nutr. 2012;55(3):261–5.

31. Frossard J-L, Steer ML, Pastor CM. Acute pancreatitis. Lancet 2008;371(9607):143–52.

32. Whitcomb DC. Acute pancreatitis. N Engl J Med. 2006;354:2142–50.

33. Spanier BWM, Nio Y, van der Hulst RWM, Tuynman HARE, Dijkgraaf MGW, Bruno MJ, et al. Practice and yield of early CT scan in acute pancreatitis: a dutch observational multicenter study. Pancreatology 2010 June 1;10(2–3):222–8.

34. Kamisawa T, Takuma K, Itokawa F, Itoi T. Endoscopic diagnosis of pancreaticobiliary maljunction. World J Gastrointest Endosc. 2011;3(1):1.

35. Thevenot A, Bournet B, Otal P, Canevet G, Moreau J, Buscail L. Endoscopic ultrasound and magnetic resonance cholangiopancreatography in patients with idiopathic acute pancreatitis. Dig Dis Sci. 2013 March 19;58(8):2361–8.

36. Ramesh J, Bang JY, Trevino J, Varadarajulu S. Endoscopic ultrasound-guided drainage of pancreatic fluid collections in children. J Pediatr Gastroenterol Nutr. 2013;56(1):30–5. doi:10.1097/MPG.0b013e318267c113.

37. Fabre A, Petit P, Gaudart J, Mas E, Vial J, Olives JP, Sarles J. Severity scores in children with acute pancreatitis. J Pediatr Gastroenterol Nutr. 2012;55(3):266–7. doi:10.1097/MPG.0b013e318254c1c7.

38. Coffey MJ, Nightingale S, Ooi CY. Serum lipase as an early predictor of severity in pediatric acute pancreatitis. J Pediatr Gastroenterol Nutr. 2013;56(6):602–8. doi:10.1097/MPG.0b013e31828b36d8.

39. Sarr MG, Banks PA, Bollen TL, Dervenis C, Gooszen HG, Johnson CD, et al. The new revised classification of acute pancreatitis 2012. Surg Clin North Am. 2013 June 1;93(3):549–62.

40. Banks PA, Bollen TL, Dervenis C, et al. Classification of acute pancreatitis—2012: revision of the Atlanta classification and definitions by international consensus. Gut 2013;62:102–11.

41. Working Group IAP/APA Acute Pancreatitis Guidelines. IAP/APA evidence-based guidelines for the management of acute pancreatitis. Pancreatology 2013;13(4 Suppl 2):e1–15. doi:10.1016/j. pan.2013.07.063.

42. Dellinger EP, Forsmark CE, Layer P, Lévy P, Maraví-Poma E, Petrov MS, et al. Determinant-based classification of acute pancreatitis severity. Ann Surg. 2012;256(6):875–80.

43. Mookadam F, Cikes M. Images in clinical medicine. Cullen's and Turner's signs. N Engl J Med. 2005;353:1386.

44. Mofidi R, Duff MD, Wigmore SJ, et al. Association between early systemic inflammatory response, severity of multiorgan dysfunction and death in acute pancreatitis. Br J Surg. 2006;93(6):738–44.

45. Basurto Ona X, Rigau Comas D, Urrútia G. Opioids for acute pancreatitis pain. Cochrane Database Syst Rev. 2013 July 26;7:CD009179. doi:10.1002/14651858.CD009179.pub2.

46. Rajkumar N, Karthikeyan VS, Ali SM, Sistla SC, Kate V. Clear liquid diet vs soft diet as the initial meal in patients with mild acute pancreatitis: a randomized interventional trial. Nutr Clin Pract. 2013;28(3):365–70. doi:10.1177/0884533612466112

47. Fisher JM, Gardner TB. The "golden hours" of management in acute pancreatitis. Am J Gastroenterol. 2012;107(8):1146–50. doi:10.1038/ajg.2012.91.

48. Nicholson LJ. Acute pancreatitis: should we use antibiotics? Curr Gastroenterol Rep. 2011;13(4):336–43. doi:10.1007/s11894-011-0198-4.

49. Fogel EL, Sherman S. ERCP for gallstone pancreatitis. N Engl J Med. 2014 Jan 9;370(2):150–7. doi:10.1056/NEJMct1208450.

50. Joffe A, Anton N, Lequier L, Vandermeer B, Tjosvold L, Larsen B, Hartling L. Nutritional support for critically ill children. Cochrane Database Syst Rev. 2009 April 15;(2):CD005144.

51. Lerner D, Werlin SL. Nutrition in acute liver failure and acute pancreatitis. In: Goday P, Mehta N, editors. Pediatric critical care nutrition. New York: McGraw Hill Professional; 2014.

Hereditary Pancreatitis and Chronic Pancreatitis

34

Aliye Uc and Michael Wilschanski

Etiology

In general, the TIGAR-O (*T*oxic-metabolic, *I*diopathic, *G*enetic, *A*utoimmune, *R*ecurrent and severe acute pancreatitis, *O*bstructive) classification described in adults [7] also applies to pediatrics (Table 34.1) [8]. Alcohol and smoking are commonly associated with CP in adults in Western countries [9, 10], but not in children. Idiopathic causes most likely comprise a large percentage of pediatric patients with CP. Genetic causes include cationic trypsinogen or *PRSS1* mutations; mutations in cystic fibrosis transmembrane conductance regulator (*CFTR*) and pancreatic secretory trypsin inhibitor (PSTI), also known as serine protease inhibitor, Kazal type I (*SPINK1*), form another large group (see Sect. "Genetic Testing") [11, 12]. Among children with acute recurrent or chronic pancreatitis (CP), a predominantly genetic etiology was reported in Korean (47% *PRSS1* or *SPINK1*) [13], Italian (39.6%, *CFTR, SPINK1*, and/or *PRSS1*) [14], Polish (33.6%, *PRSS1* and *SPINK1*) [15], and ultrasonography (US) children (79% *CFTR, PRSS1*, and/ or *SPINK1*) [16]. The association of carboxypeptidase-1 *(CPA1)* gene variants in children with CP< 10 years of age [17] and carboxyl ester lipase (*CEL*) mutations leading to CP and diabetes at a young age causing CEL maturity-onset diabetes of the young (*CEL*-MODY) [18] highlights the importance of genetic factors in CP.

Pathophysiology

The pathophysiology of CP is incompletely understood. The pancreas is not easily accessible for sampling; therefore, it is difficult to detect the earliest changes and identify the events that contribute to the pathophysiology of CP. In children with hereditary pancreatitis (HP), mutations in the cationic trypsinogen *(PRSS1)* gene cause activation of trypsinogen within the acinar cells as an early event in pancreatitis [19]. Premature activation of trypsinogen to trypsin initiates an activation cascade, causing additional trypsinogen activation and conversion of other digestive proenzymes to active enzymes, leading to pancreatic digestion and inflammation [11].

A widely accepted hypothesis is that CP begins with an episode of acute pancreatitis (AP), followed by an ongoing chronic or recurrent inflammation that leads to fibrotic replacement of acini and islet cells [1]. In the sentinel acute pancreatitis event (SAPE) hypothesis [20], a metabolic or oxidative stress initiates the first episode of AP (the sentinel event). Activated lymphocytes, macrophages, and stellate cells increase in number within the pancreas, and then produce cytokines and deposit small amounts of collagen. Most patients recover uneventfully from AP, and the pancreas returns to normal. In some patients, due to the continued presence of stress, inflammatory cells and stellate cells remain active, release cytokines, and deposit collagen, eventually producing the fibrotic changes characteristic of CP. Although the process may be started and perpetuated by environmental factors, other factors (i.e., genetic) must be present for CP to develop in some individuals and not others.

Diagnosis

Clinical Presentation

Abdominal pain is the most common symptom of CP. Pain is usually in the upper abdomen, episodic or persistent, mild–moderate to severe. Older children describe the pain as deep

A. Uc (✉)
Stead Family Department of Pediatrics, University of Iowa Children's Hospital, 2865 JPP Pediatrics, 200 Hawkins Drive, Iowa City, IA 52242, USA
e-mail: aliye-uc@uiowa.edu

M. Wilschanski
Pediatric Gastroenterology Unit, Hadassah Hebrew University Medical Center, Jerusalem, Israel
e-mail: michaelwil@hadassah.org.il

© Springer International Publishing Switzerland 2016
S. Guandalini et al. (eds.), *Textbook of Pediatric Gastroenterology, Hepatology and Nutrition*,
DOI 10.1007/978-3-319-17169-2_34

Table 34.1 Etiologies of chronic pancreatitis in children

Idiopathic
Genetic
• *PRSS1*
• *CFTR*
• *SPINK1*
• *CTRC*
• *CPA1*
• *CEL*
Drugs (L-asparaginase, valproate, metronidazole, azathioprine, tetracycline, pentamidine, etc.)
• Metabolic disease
• Hyperlipidemia
• Hypercalcemia
• Glycogen storage disease
• Organic acidemias
Autoimmune
Anatomic
• Pancreas divisum
• Anomalous junction of the biliary and pancreatic ducts
• Annular pancreas
• Ampullary obstruction
• Crohn's disease

PRSS1 protease, serine 1, *CFTR* cystic fibrosis transmembrane conductance regulator, *CTRC* chymotrypsin-C, *SPINK1* serine protease inhibitor, Kazal type I, *CPA1* carboxypeptidase-1, *CEL* carboxyl ester lipase

and penetrating, radiating to the back, and worse after meals. Younger children cannot verbalize the pain well, so clinicians must have a high index of suspicion in this age group [21]. Commonly, younger children may be misdiagnosed as having other gastrointestinal (GI) illnesses, such as gastroesophageal reflux, constipation, or functional abdominal pain. Nausea and/or vomiting, anorexia, weight loss may be present.

Children with HP usually present with recurrent episodes of abdominal pain and symptom-free intervals [11]. The acute attacks may be triggered by a fatty meal, stress, or environmental factors such as infection, smoking, and alcohol use. Median age of presentation for HP is 10 years of age, and in 50% of patients, CP develops 10 years after the first bout of AP [22]. Some patients may present with CP without a clear history of AP [23].

The pancreas has extraordinary reserves and does not manifest signs of insufficiency until lipase secretion is reduced to less than 5% of the maximum output [24]. In adults, exocrine pancreatic insufficiency (EPI) occurs in 50–80% of patients in a median time of 5.6–13.1 years [25, 26].

Diabetes mellitus can also occur in 40–70% of adults with CP with a median time to onset of 11.9–26.3 years [25, 26]. The exact mechanism of pancreatic diabetes is unknown, but islet destruction is a late phenomenon. The exocrine and endocrine insufficiencies in pediatric CP are also incompletely studied.

If EPI has developed, symptoms of maldigestion/malabsorption, such as weight loss and steatorrhea, may be present. Fat-soluble vitamin deficiencies (A, D, E, K) can be seen. Patients with extrahepatic biliary obstruction from fibrosis in the head of the pancreas or from the pseudocyst can have jaundice. Physical examination is usually normal.

There is a lifetime risk for pancreatic adenocarcinoma in patients with CP (4%) [27], and the risk is much higher in patients with HP (~40%) [28].

Differential Diagnoses

The differential diagnosis of CP includes causes of recurrent and chronic abdominal pain in childhood, such as peptic ulcer disease, gastritis, gallbladder disease, intestinal obstruction, Crohn's disease, functional abdominal pain, lactose intolerance, and constipation. For the differential diagnosis of malabsorption in the presence of EPI, one should consider severe enteropathies, cholestatic liver disease, celiac disease, cystic fibrosis (CF), and rare isolated pancreatic enzyme deficiencies.

Diagnostic Testing

The INSPPIRE (*IN*ternational *S*tudy Group of *P*ediatric *P*ancreatitis: *I*n search for a cu*RE*) definitions of CP require one of the following: (1) abdominal pain consistent with pancreatic origin and imaging findings suggestive of chronic pancreatic damage, (2) evidence of EPI and imaging findings suggestive of pancreatic damage, or (3) evidence of endocrine pancreatic insufficiency and imaging findings suggestive of pancreatic damage, or (4) a surgical or pancreatic biopsy demonstrating histopathology compatible with CP [15] (Table 34.2).

These lab tests and abbreviations look out of place. May be they should go to a an abbreviation section. According to INSPPIRE criteria, suggestive imaging findings of CP or chronic pancreatic damage include:

Table 34.2 Diagnostic tests in chronic pancreatitis

Laboratory tests (serum amylase, lipase, Ca, lipid panel, total and direct bilirubin, alkaline phosphatase, GGT, AST, ALT, fasting serum glucose)
Fecal elastase 1
72 h fecal fat
Sweat Cl/NPD
Imaging studies (US, CT, MRCP, EUS, ERCP)
Genetic testing (*PRSS1, CFTR, SPINK1, CTRC*)

- Ductal changes: irregular contour of the main pancreatic duct or its radicals; intraductal filling defects; calculi, stricture, or dilation;
- Parenchymal changes: generalized or focal enlargement, irregular contour (accentuated lobular architecture), cavities, calcifications, heterogeneous echotexture.

Imaging modalities may include CT, MRI/magnetic resonance cholangiopancreatography (MRCP), endoscopic retrograde cholangiopancreateography (ERCP); US; endoscopic US (EUS ; in which at least five EUS features (as defined by the Rosemont Classification [29] must be fulfilled)).

EPI is recommended to be diagnosed via fecal elastase-1 monoclonal assay < 100 mcg/g stool (two separate samples done ≥ 1 month apart) or coefficient of dietary fat absorption < 90% on a 72-h fecal fat collection. Neither test should be performed during an AP episode, as the results may be temporarily low.

Endocrine pancreatic insufficiency can be diagnosed via 2006 WHO criteria for the diagnosis of diabetes mellitus (fasting glucose ≥ 7.0 mmol/L (126 mg/dL) or plasma glucose ≥ 11.1 mmol/L (200 mg/dL) 2 h after glucose load 1.75 g/kg children (to maximum 75 g glucose load)) [30].

Biochemistry

There are no specific laboratory tests for CP. In most cases, serum amylase and lipase are normal or only mildly elevated [31]. Aspartate transaminase (AST), alanine transaminase (ALT), GGT, alkaline phosphatase, and direct bilirubin are useful to rule out a biliary obstruction.

Radiology

Diagnostic imaging plays an important role in the initial diagnosis of CP and further planning for endoscopic and surgical interventions. The imaging modalities most commonly used in pediatric pancreatitis are summarized below.

Ultrasonography US is usually the first imaging modality when pancreatitis is suspected in children. Smaller size of patients, lack of fat, and prominence of the left hepatic lobe make US of the pancreas more feasible in children than in adults [32]. US is 50–80% sensitive in diagnosing CP in adults; the diagnostic accuracy of US in pediatric CP has not been studied [4]. US is most helpful in assessing the pancreatic duct diameter in children with CP (normals are ≤ 1.5 mm in children 1–6 years; ≤ 1.9 mm at ages 7–12 years; ≤ 2.2 mm at ages 13–18 years). Calcifications of the pancreas and intraductal stones can also be observed with US in CP [32].

Endoscopic US The high diagnostic accuracy and the low complication rate of EUS (1%) compared to ERCP have been the driving forces for the use of EUS [32]. EUS is technically feasible in children as young as 5 years of age [33],

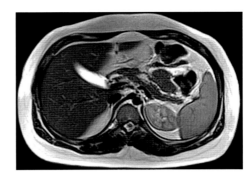

Fig. 34.1 MRCP changes in chronic pancreatitis. T1-weighted image shows atrophy of the parenchyma in a child with idiopathic chronic pancreatitis *(arrows)*. (Photo courtesy of Dr. Simon C. Kao, University of Iowa, USA)

but most of the experience comes from the adult literature, and very little is written in pediatrics [34]. EUS is highly operator dependent, and even in adults there is controversy regarding its accuracy and reliability. EUS images are commonly scored based on the presence of parenchymal and ductal features. An expert consensus conference was convened in 2009 to address the controversies and developed the Rosemont classification [29]. The Rosemont criteria for CP diagnosis have not been validated in children.

Magnetic Resonance Cholangiopancreatography MRCP can visualize the pancreas, pancreatic ducts, and the pancreaticobiliary tree and reliably detect pancreas atrophy, ductal dilatations, small filling defects, strictures, irregularities of the main pancreatic duct, and irregularity (sacculation and/or ectasia) of side branches [35] (Fig. 34.1). Due to its noninvasive nature and lack of radiation, MRCP has become the diagnostic test of choice in children with CP [36, 37]. Unlike ERCP that images ducts under pressure, MRCP visualizes the ducts in their normal physiologic state [32]. Therefore, MRCP may not reveal the details of small ducts, which may be important in diagnosing early CP.

Secretin induces fluid secretion in the pancreatic duct, and when administered with MRCP, it increases the diameter of pancreatic duct up to 3 mm in 3–5 min with progressive decline to baseline in 10 min. Secretin may be more important in children than in adults as it increases the detectability of the normally smaller pancreatic ducts. In a pediatric study, secretin increased the number of main pancreatic duct segments visualized on MRCP from 53 to 93%; the visualization of the duct of Santorini increased from 7 to 53% and the detection of side branches increased from 20 to 47% [38]. Secretin may also increase the number of false-positive reports [39]. In one pediatric study, the pancreatic diameter increase after secretin was small and did not have any impact on image quality or duct visibility of the MRCP [40]. More

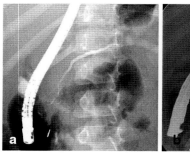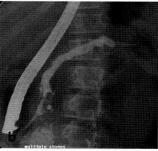

Fig. 34.2 ERCP changes in chronic pancreatitis. **a** Dilatation of the mid and distal portions of the pancreatic duct in a child with idiopathic chronic pancreatitis *(arrows)*. **b** Dilatation of pancreatic duct with multiple filling defects *(stones, arrowheads)* in the distal pancreatic duct in a child with hereditary pancreatitis (R122H mutation). A pancreatic duct stent *(arrow)* has been placed to bypass the obstruction. (Photo courtesy of Dr. Simon C. Kao, University of Iowa, USA)

studies with secretin-enhanced MRCP are needed to better understand its diagnostic accuracy in pediatric CP.

Endoscopic Retrograde Cholangiopancreateography With MRCP being widely available, ERCP is now mainly reserved for therapeutic interventions (pancreatic duct stenting, sphincterotomy, stone extraction). ERCP carries an overall morbidity of ~7%, which includes AP (4%), hemorrhage (1%), cholangitis (1%), perforation (0.5%), and death (0.1%) [41]. In CP, ERCP findings include main pancreatic duct dilatation, ductal stones, and changes in the main duct branches and small ducts (Fig. 34.2). ERCP is no longer an attractive first-line test because of its potential complications and low sensitivity for detecting early-stage CP.

An ERCP-based grading system of CP has been developed in adults (Cambridge classification) for the classification of disease severity. Changes are graded as normal, equivocal, mild, moderate, and severe, based on the appearance of the main pancreatic duct and side branches on the ERCP. Interpretation is subjective and there can be substantial inter- and intraobserver variation. The Cambridge classification has not been validated in children [42].

Computerized Tomography (CT) with Contrast CT can detect advanced changes in CP, such as calcification, gland atrophy, fat replacement, and ductal dilatation. The advantage of CT is that it can evaluate pancreas for other pathology and detect other causes of chronic abdominal pain. CT has poor sensitivity to identify ductal abnormalities and subtle parenchymal changes; high radiation dose is another drawback [4, 43].

Genetic Testing

Genetic testing is indicated as a diagnostic test in children with CP to determine the underlying cause. Predictive testing is not recommended in individuals without pancreatic disease and a positive family history of pancreatitis. The presence of *PRSS1* mutation provides an adequate etiology for pancreatitis, but the presence of *CFTR* or *SPINK1* mutations should not preclude a careful search for additional etiologies.

Cationic Trypsinogen (PRSS1) UniGene name: protease, serine 1: *PRSS1* gene was the first pancreatitis-specific susceptibility gene identified in families with HP [19]. In the physiological state, trypsinogen is converted to trypsin in the duodenum by the brush border-derived enterokinase. Trypsin will then activate other proteases, which will initiate intraluminal digestion of nutrients. A total of 80–90% of individuals with HP, an autosomal dominant disease with incomplete penetrance, carry R122H mutation [19, 22]. This mutation is caused by the substitution of the amino acid histidine (H) for arginine (R) at position 122 (R122H) of the cationic trypsinogen gene. Another mutation, N29I, is caused by substitution of isoleucine (I) for asparagine (N) at position 29. R122H and N29I are the most common mutations seen in patients with HP [44]. Genetic defects in *PRSS1* result in gain of function either by increasing activation or by preventing inactivation of trypsin, leading to pancreatic autodigestion.

Genetic testing for *PRSS1* mutations is recommended in patients with recurrent attacks of AP and CP of unknown etiology or a positive family history of pancreatitis in first-degree or second-degree relatives.

CFTR Pancreatitis occurs in 2–4% of all patients with CF and 15–20% of pancreatic-sufficient patients with mild *CFTR* mutations during adolescence or later in life [45, 46]. Pancreatitis is thought to result from thick secretions causing pancreatic ductular obstruction, ineffective clearing of secretions from the pancreatic duct, and autodigestion of the pancreas by activated proteolytic enzymes [11].

Patients with idiopathic CP carry a higher frequency of *CFTR* mutations (~10%) than the general population, and a subset of these patients have CF (~20%) [47–50]. *CFTR* mutations may also contribute to the development of CP in patients who have additional risk factors for CP [51].

There are over 1900 *CFTR* mutations, and only a small percentage are CF-causing mutations.

The majority of mutations (~40%) have unknown functional consequences, others confer less severe disease, and the rest are considered to be benign polymorphisms with no pathogenic potential [52, 53]. Therefore, in a patient with recurrent attacks of AP or CP and *CFTR* mutations, sweat test is still the first test to order. A referral to a CF clinic can be made if sweat chloride is borderline (40–59 mmol/L) or abnormal ($\geq$60 mmol/L). Nasal potential difference (NPD) testing can also be helpful in measuring CFTR channel function in patients with recurrent attacks of pancreatitis [54].

SPINK1 Synthesis of PSTI, which is coded by the *SPINK1* gene, protects against premature activation of trypsin within the pancreas before it is secreted into the duodenum [20]. Mutations in the *SPINK1* gene (mainly N34S mutation, substitution of asparagine by serine at codon 34 in exon 3) increase the susceptibility to AP and predisposes to CP [55, 56]. Interestingly, the risk of an asymptomatic *SPINK1* carrier developing pancreatitis is thought to be only 1 %. Therefore, *SPINK1* mutations alone are not sufficient to cause pancreatitis, but may act as genetic modifiers in initiating the development of pancreatitis [56].

Chymotrypsin-C CTRC is involved in the degradation of trypsin. Mutations in the *CTRC* gene alter its function and predispose patients to pancreatitis by diminishing its protective trypsin-degrading activity. *CTRC* mutations have been shown to be associated with CP in the European and Asian populations [57–59].

Exocrine Pancreatic Function Testing

These tests can detect CP in its most advanced stage, when EPI has developed. They are not specific for CP as they can be abnormal in patients with other causes of EPI (CF, Shwachman–Diamond syndrome, etc).

Pancreatic Stimulation Test This test involves the collection of pancreatic fluid secreted into the duodenum and measurement of fluid volume, pancreatic enzymes, and electrolytes before and after stimulation with cholecystokinin (CCK) and secretin [60]. Although it is considered "gold standard" to quantify the exocrine pancreatic function, stimulation test is not widely performed because of its invasive nature. The collection of the duodenal fluid via the endoscope (endoscopic pancreatic function test or ePFT) has been proposed as an alternative, but this approach may underestimate the pancreatic secretary capacity and classify patients as pancreatic insufficient erroneously [60].

72-h Fecal Fat Collection This test relies on the exocrine pancreas losing greater than 95 % of its enzyme secretory output and development of steatorrhea [24]. Steatorrhea can be measured by a 72-h stool collection and calculation of coefficient of fat absorption (CFA: (grams of fat ingested-grams of fat excreted)/(grams of fat ingested) × 100). In children younger than 6 months of age, a fecal fat greater than 15 % of fat intake is considered abnormal; this value is 7 % for children over 6 months of age. This test is not very reliable and reproducible. It is not a popular test by the families or the technical staff. The sample and the data collection are not always accurate.

Fecal Elastase-1 (FE1) This enzyme-linked immunosorbent assay (ELISA)-based method is easy to use, cheap, and now the preferred test to diagnose EPI. A value of less than100 μg/g is considered diagnostic of EPI. Intermediate values of fecal elastase (100–200 μg/g) may be due to loss of pancreatic function, but not severe enough to cause clinical EPI. The sensitivity of FE1 to diagnose moderate and severe EPI is close to 100 %. In patients with mild loss of pancreatic function, the test sensitivity is ~25 % with a specificity of 96 % [61]. Therefore, the value of FE1 to determine patients with mild EPI or borderline normal pancreatic function is limited. FE1 may be falsely low when the stool is diluted as a result of infectious diarrhea, severe enteropathies, short gut, or if it is collected from an ileostomy.

Secretin MRCP The pancreatic exocrine function can be assessed by the duodenal filling, changes in pancreatic duct caliber, change in anteroposterior diameter of the pancreas, and change in signal intensity ratio between pancreas and spleen on T1-weighted and arterial–venous enhancement ratios [62, 63]. The results show correlation with other exocrine pancreatic tests including ePFT [63] and fecal elastase [64]. The test has not been validated in children.

Treatment

Medical Treatment

For children presenting with an acute attack of pancreatitis, we recommend conservative management, withholding food and drink for a few days, and offering pain control. In patients with advanced disease, the treatment is directed at the complications, including chronic pain, EPI, and diabetes mellitus.

Pain Control

Analgesic medications are the mainstay of pain management. There are no prospective therapeutic trials of pain management in children; thus, the practice is guided by common practice and expert opinion. Nonsteroidal anti-inflammatory drugs and acetaminophen are the first-line agents for pain control. Long-acting and short-acting narcotics can be used in a stepwise approach. The addictive profile of narcotics and their GI side effects should be considered when initiating the therapy. Tramadol and gabapentin have shown efficacy in controlling pain in adults with CP [65].

Pancreatic Enzyme Supplementation

Pancreatic enzymes are often prescribed theoretically to reduce the feedback loop in the duodenum by reducing the CCK release and inhibiting pancreatic exocrine activation. Current evidence on the effect of pancreatic enzymes on pain control is conflicting because of methodological issues and types of preparation (enteric-coated vs. nonenteric-coated tablets) [4]. Some early studies reported benefit with non-enteric-coated preparations [66, 67], while enteric-coated preparations did not work [68, 69] possibly because the release of nonenteric-coated enzymes and feedback inhibition of pancreatic enzymes were more proximal than distal in the intestine. A recent Cochrane review evaluated the efficacy of pancreatic enzymes in patients with CP [70]. Although some individual studies reported a beneficial effect of pancreatic enzyme over placebo in improving pain, incidence of steatorrhea, and analgesic consumption, the results of the studies could not be pooled for these outcomes. Overall, the role of pancreatic enzymes in CP was reported to be equivocal.

Antioxidant Therapy

Antioxidants have been evaluated for the treatment of chronic pain in CP. Results are not convincing, and all studies have methodological issues. A randomized and placebo-controlled study showed that the antioxidant therapy was superior to placebo in treating pan in adults with CP [71]. In another study, the administration of antioxidants to patients with painful CP did not reduce pain or improve quality of life, despite causing a sustained increase in blood levels of antioxidants [72]. Further studies are needed to evaluate the utility of antioxidants in pediatric CP.

Endoscopic Interventions

Because of radiation exposure, potential complications, and wide availability of MRCP, ERCP should be reserved for interventions, such as stone removal or stricture management, as it is recommended in adults [73]. Endoscopic therapy may be useful if there is an identifiable stricture with evidence of pancreatic duct obstruction [74, 75]. In patients with gallstone pancreatitis and cholangitis, ERCP is indicated within 24 h, and within 72 h if there is a high suspicion of persistent common bile duct stone. Endoscopic sphincterotomy in the absence of choledocholithiasis at the time of the procedure is a reasonable therapeutic option, but data supporting this practice are lacking [76, 77].

ERCP can be done successfully in over 90% of children [78]. Sphincterotomy with or without stone extraction is carried out in 45% of ERCPs in children. In a small pediatric study, children were evaluated with ERCP for recurrent acute and CP; in 52% of patients, ERCP altered the therapy [79]. In a pediatric study, the majority of children with pancreas divisum and CP had resolution of symptoms and did not require surgery following placement of a pancreatic duct stent [80].

Surgery

In adult patients with CP, the main indication for surgery is the chronic, debilitating pain. Pediatric data are sparse, and the decision to operate is based on the experience in adult patients with CP. Surgical techniques include drainage operations that aim to decompress dilated ducts or resections of strictures and removal of pancreatic stones. Even in large referral centers, less than one pediatric patient undergoes surgery for CP every year [81–83]. In general, decompressive operations are favored over resections in the pediatric age groups [84]. In the majority of cases, a Puestow-type procedure (longitudinal pancreatojejunostomy that involves opening the pancreatic duct throughout the body and tail of the gland) has been used. Ductal strictures can also be excised, and pancreatic stones can be removed during this operation. Frey and Whipple procedures are usually associated with high mortality and morbidity and rarely needed [4].

Total pancreatectomy with islet cell autotransplantation (TP/IAT) is being proposed as a treatment for CP. TP removes the entire pancreas and presumably the source of pain and potential cause of cancer. By removing the pancreas, this surgery also predisposes the patient to brittle diabetes. TP/IAT is done mainly in adults, but recently being performed in children in increasing numbers. Therefore, the experience and the data in the literature about this procedure in children are limited.

Most of the studies with TP/IAT in children are from a single pediatric center. Approximately 60% of children were off narcotic medications and insulin independent at a median time of 2 1/2 year follow-up [85], and quality of life was improved at 1 year [86]. Children with prior surgical drainage procedures (Puestow) appeared to have lower yields of islets and greater incidence of insulin dependence after TP/IAT [86, 87], which led the authors to propose this surgery to be done early in the course of CP in children and to avoid any prior drainage procedures to maximize the number islets available. In a study from another center, of 14 children who underwent TP/IAT for CP, 79% were narcotic independent and 29% were insulin independent at an average of 9 months, and the quality of life was significantly improved in all patients [88]. In this study, a previous operation did not have any impact on the islet yield from the pancreas [88]. More studies and longer-time follow-ups are needed to determine whether TP/IAT is effective in treating pain in pediatric patients with CP.

Conclusion

Pediatric CP continues to be an enigma. Currently, our knowledge of pediatric CP is limited to the experience in adult data, local experience, and expert opinions. It is likely that the CP in children has unique features, and it is completely different than the adult disease. Currently, there is an international effort (the INSPPIRE study) to better understand pediatric pancreatitis [3, 89]. We recommend vigilance in the diagnosis of CP in children, especially in the setting of chronic abdominal pain and the family history of pancreatitis. With better understanding of the epidemiology, etiologies, natural history, and outcome of CP in childhood, we can begin to develop better diagnostic and therapeutic strategies for this disease.

References

1. Lowe ME. Pancreatitis in childhood. Curr Gastroenterol Rep. 2004;6(3):240–6.
2. Lowe ME. Acute and chronic pancreatitis. In: Bishop WP, editor. Pediatric practice gastroenterology. New York: McGraw Hill; 2010. p. 428–40.
3. Morinville VD, Husain SZ, Bai H, Barth B, Alhosh R, Durie PR, et al. Definitions of pediatric pancreatitis and survey of present clinical practices. J Pediatr Gastroenterol Nutr. 2012;55(3):261–5.
4. Nydegger A, Couper RT, Oliver MR. Childhood pancreatitis. J Gastroenterol Hepatol. 2006;21(3):499–509.
5. Yadav D, Timmons L, Benson JT, Dierkhising RA, Chari ST. Incidence, prevalence, and survival of chronic pancreatitis: a population-based study. Am J Gastroenterol. 2011;106(12):2192–9.
6. Spanier B, Bruno MJ, Dijkgraaf MG. Incidence and mortality of acute and chronic pancreatitis in the Netherlands: a nationwide record-linked cohort study for the years 1995–2005. World J Gastroenterol. 2013;19(20):3018–26.
7. Etemad B, Whitcomb DC. Chronic pancreatitis: diagnosis, classification, and new genetic developments. Gastroenterology 2001;120(3):682–707.
8. Lowe ME, Greer JB. Pancreatitis in children and adolescents. Curr Gastroenterol Rep. 2008;10(2):128–35.
9. Witt H, Apte MV, Keim V, Wilson JS. Chronic pancreatitis: challenges and advances in pathogenesis, genetics, diagnosis, and therapy. Gastroenterology 2007;132(4):1557–73.
10. Cote GA, Yadav D, Slivka A, Hawes RH, Anderson MA, Burton FR, et al. Alcohol and smoking as risk factors in an epidemiology study of patients with chronic pancreatitis. Clin Gastroenterol Hepatol. 2011;9(3):266–73 (quiz e27).
11. Kandula L, Whitcomb DC, Lowe ME. Genetic issues in pediatric pancreatitis. Curr Gastroenterol Rep. 2006;8(3):248–53.
12. Witt H, Becker M. Genetics of chronic pancreatitis. J Pediatr Gastroenterol Nutr. 2002;34(2):125–36.
13. Lee YJ, Kim KM, Choi JH, Lee BH, Kim GH, Yoo HW. High incidence of PRSS1 and SPINK1 mutations in Korean children with acute recurrent and chronic pancreatitis. J Pediatr Gastroenterol Nutr. 2011;52(4):478–81.
14. Lucidi V, Alghisi F, Dall'Oglio L, D'Apice MR, Monti L, De Angelis P, et al. The etiology of acute recurrent pancreatitis in children: a challenge for pediatricians. Pancreas 2011;40(4):517–21.
15. Sobczynska-Tomaszewska A, Bak D, Oralewska B, Oracz G, Norek A, Czerska K, et al. Analysis of CFTR, SPINK1, PRSS1 and AAT mutations in children with acute or chronic pancreatitis. J Pediatr Gastroenterol Nutr. 2006;43(3):299–306.
16. Sultan M, Werlin S, Venkatasubramani N. Genetic prevalence and characteristics in children with recurrent pancreatitis. J Pediatr Gastroenterol Nutr. 2012;54(5):645–50.
17. Witt H, Beer S, Rosendahl J, Chen JM, Chandak GR, Masamune A, et al. Variants in CPA1 are strongly associated with early onset chronic pancreatitis. Nat Genet. 2013;45(10):1216–20.
18. Raeder H, Johansson S, Holm PI, Haldorsen IS, Mas E, Sbarra V, et al. Mutations in the CEL VNTR cause a syndrome of diabetes and pancreatic exocrine dysfunction. Nat Genet. 2006;38(1):54–62.
19. Whitcomb DC, Gorry MC, Preston RA, Furey W, Sossenheimer MJ, Ulrich CD, et al. Hereditary pancreatitis is caused by a mutation in the cationic trypsinogen gene. Nat Genet. 1996;14(2):141–5.
20. Whitcomb DC. Hereditary pancreatitis: new insights into acute and chronic pancreatitis. Gut 1999;45(3):317–22.
21. Park AJ, Latif SU, Ahmad MU, Bultron G, Orabi AI, Bhandari V, et al. A comparison of presentation and management trends in acute pancreatitis between infants/toddlers and older children. J Pediatr Gastroenterol Nutr. 2010;51(2):167–70.
22. Whitcomb DC. Genetic predispositions to acute and chronic pancreatitis. Med Clin North Am. 2000;84(3):531–47, vii.
23. pplebaum-Shapiro SE, Finch R, Pfutzer RH, Hepp LA, Gates L, Amann S, et al. Hereditary pancreatitis in North America: the Pittsburgh-Midwest Multi-Center Pancreatic Study Group study. Pancreatology 2001;1(5):439–43.
24. DiMagno EP, Go VL, Summerskill WH. Relations between pancreatic enzyme ouputs and malabsorption in severe pancreatic insufficiency. N Engl J Med. 1973;288(16):813–5.
25. Ammann RW, Akovbiantz A, Largiader F, Schueler G. Course and outcome of chronic pancreatitis. Longitudinal study of a mixed medical-surgical series of 245 patients. Gastroenterology 1984;86(5 Pt 1):820–8.
26. Layer P, Yamamoto H, Kalthoff L, Clain JE, Bakken LJ, DiMagno EP. The different courses of early- and late-onset idiopathic and alcoholic chronic pancreatitis. Gastroenterology 1994;107(5):1481–7.
27. Lowenfels AB, Maisonneuve P, Cavallini G, Ammann RW, Lankisch PG, Andersen JR, et al. Pancreatitis and the risk of pancreatic cancer. International Pancreatitis Study Group. N Engl J Med. 1993;328(20):1433–7.
28. Lowenfels AB, Maisonneuve P, DiMagno EP, Elitsur Y, Gates LK Jr, Perrault J, et al. Hereditary pancreatitis and the risk of pancreatic cancer. International Hereditary Pancreatitis Study Group. J Natl Cancer Inst. 1997;89(6):442–6.
29. Catalano MF, Sahai A, Levy M, Romagnuolo J, Wiersema M, Brugge W, et al. EUS-based criteria for the diagnosis of chronic pancreatitis: the Rosemont classification. Gastrointest Endosc. 2009;69(7):1251–61.
30. Report of the expert committee on the diagnosis and classification of diabetes mellitus. Diabetes Care. 1997;20(7):1183–97.
31. Steer ML, Waxman I, Freedman S. Chronic pancreatitis. N Engl J Med. 1995;332(22):1482–90.
32. Darge K, Anupindi S. Pancreatitis and the role of US, MRCP and ERCP. PediatrRadiol. 2009;39 Suppl 2:S153–7.
33. Varadarajulu S, Wilcox CM, Eloubeidi MA. Impact of EUS in the evaluation of pancreaticobiliary disorders in children. Gastrointest Endosc. 2005;62(2):239–44.
34. Stevens T. Role of endoscopic ultrasonography in the diagnosis of acute and chronic pancreatitis. Gastrointest Endosc Clin N Am. 2013;23(4):735–47.
35. Hansen TM, Nilsson M, Gram M, Frokjaer JB. Morphological and functional evaluation of chronic pancreatitis with magnetic resonance imaging. World J Gastroenterol. 2013;19(42):7241–6.
36. Delaney L, Applegate KE, Karmazyn B, Akisik MF, Jennings SG. MR cholangiopancreatography in children: feasibility, safety, and initial experience. Pediatr Radiol. 2008;38(1):64–75.
37. Tipnis NA, Werlin SL. The use of magnetic resonance cholangiopancreatography in children. Curr Gastroenterol Rep. 2007;9(3):225–9.
38. Manfredi R, Lucidi V, Gui B, Brizi MG, Vecchioli A, Maresca G, et al. Idiopathic chronic pancreatitis in children: MR cholangiopancreatography after secretin administration. Radiology 2002;224(3):675–82.

39. Manfredi R, Costamagna G, Brizi MG, Maresca G, Vecchioli A, Colagrande C, et al. Severe chronic pancreatitis versus suspected pancreatic disease: dynamic MR cholangiopancreatography after secretin stimulation. Radiology 2000;214(3):849–55.

40. Trout AT, Podberesky DJ, Serai SD, Ren Y, Altaye M, Towbin AJ. Does secretin add value in pediatric magnetic resonance cholangiopancreatography? Pediatr Radiol. 2013;43(4):479–86.

41. Lee LS, Conwell DL. Update on advanced endoscopic techniques for the pancreas: endoscopic retrograde cholangiopancreatography, drainage and biopsy, and endoscopic ultrasound. Radiol Clin North Am. 2012;50(3):547–61.

42. Axon AT, Classen M, Cotton PB, Cremer M, Freeny PC, Lees WR. Pancreatography in chronic pancreatitis: international definitions. Gut 1984;25(10):1107–12.

43. Kinney TP, Freeman ML. Recent advances and novel methods in pancreatic imaging. Minerva Gastroenterol Dietol. 2008;54(1): 85–95.

44. Schneider A, Whitcomb DC. Hereditary pancreatitis: a model for inflammatory diseases of the pancreas. Best Pract Res Clin Gastroenterol. 2002;16(3):347–63.

45. Wilschanski M, Durie PR. Patterns of GI disease in adulthood associated with mutations in the CFTR gene. Gut 2007;56(8):1153–63.

46. Durno C, Corey M, Zielenski J, Tullis E, Tsui LC, Durie P. Genotype and phenotype correlations in patients with cystic fibrosis and pancreatitis. Gastroenterology 2002;123(6):1857–64.

47. Cohn JA, Friedman KJ, Noone PG, Knowles MR, Silverman LM, Jowell PS. Relation between mutations of the cystic fibrosis gene and idiopathic pancreatitis. N Engl J Med. 1998;339(10):653–8.

48. Cohn JA, Neoptolemos JP, Feng J, Yan J, Jiang Z, Greenhalf W, et al. Increased risk of idiopathic chronic pancreatitis in cystic fibrosis carriers. Hum Mutat. 2005;26(4):303–7.

49. Sharer N, Schwarz M, Malone G, Howarth A, Painter J, Super M, et al. Mutations of the cystic fibrosis gene in patients with chronic pancreatitis. N Engl J Med. 1998;339(10):645–52.

50. Bishop MD, Freedman SD, Zielenski J, Ahmed N, Dupuis A, Martin S, et al. The cystic fibrosis transmembrane conductance regulator gene and ion channel function in patients with idiopathic pancreatitis. Hum Genet. 2005;118(3–4):372–81.

51. Cohn JA. Reduced CFTR function and the pathobiology of idiopathic pancreatitis. J Clin Gastroenterol. 2005; 39 4 Suppl 2: S70–7.

52. Castellani C, Cuppens H, Macek M Jr, Cassiman JJ, Kerem E, Durie P, et al. Consensus on the use and interpretation of cystic fibrosis mutation analysis in clinical practice. J Cyst Fibros. 2008;7(3):179–96.

53. Ooi CY, Gonska T, Durie PR, Freedman SD. Genetic testing in pancreatitis. Gastroenterology 2010;138(7):2202–6.

54. Segal I, Yaakov Y, Adler SN, Blau H, Broide E, Santo M, et al. Cystic fibrosis transmembrane conductance regulator ion channel function testing in recurrent acute pancreatitis. J Clin Gastroenterol. 2008;42(7):810–4.

55. Witt H, Luck W, Hennies HC, Classen M, Kage A, Lass U, et al. Mutations in the gene encoding the serine protease inhibitor, Kazal type 1 are associated with chronic pancreatitis. Nat Genet. 2000;25(2):213–6.

56. Pfutzer RH, Barmada MM, Brunskill AP, Finch R, Hart PS, Neoptolemos J, et al. SPINK1/PSTI polymorphisms act as disease modifiers in familial and idiopathic chronic pancreatitis. Gastroenterology. 2000;119(3):615–23.

57. Rosendahl J, Witt H, Szmola R, Bhatia E, Ozsvari B, Landt O, et al. Chymotrypsin C (CTRC) variants that diminish activity or secretion are associated with chronic pancreatitis. Nat Genet. 2008;40(1):78–82.

58. Masson E, Chen JM, Scotet V, Le Marechal C, Ferec C. Association of rare chymotrypsinogen C (CTRC) gene variations in patients with idiopathic chronic pancreatitis. Hum Genet. 2008;123(1):83–91.

59. Chang MC, Chang YT, Wei SC, Liang PC, Jan IS, Su YN, et al. Association of novel chymotrypsin C gene variations and haplotypes in patients with chronic pancreatitis in Chinese in Taiwan. Pancreatology 2009;9(3):287–92.

60. Schibli S, Corey M, Gaskin KJ, Ellis L, Durie PR. Towards the ideal quantitative pancreatic function test: analysis of test variables that influence validity. Clin Gastroenterol Hepatol. 2006;4(1): 90–7.

61. Daftary A, Acton J, Heubi J, Amin R. Fecal elastase-1: utility in pancreatic function in cystic fibrosis. J Cyst Fibros. 2006;5(2): 71–6.

62. Balci NC, Alkaade S, Magas L, Momtahen AJ, Burton FR. Suspected chronic pancreatitis with normal MRCP: findings on MRI in correlation with secretin MRCP. J Magn Reson Imaging. 2008;27(1):125–31.

63. Balci NC, Smith A, Momtahen AJ, Alkaade S, Fattahi R, Tariq S, et al. MRI and S-MRCP findings in patients with suspected chronic pancreatitis: correlation with endoscopic pancreatic function testing (ePFT). J Magn Reson Imaging. 2010;31(3):601–6.

64. Manfredi R, Perandini S, Mantovani W, Frulloni L, Faccioli N, Pozzi Mucelli R. Quantitative MRCP assessment of pancreatic exocrine reserve and its correlation with faecal elastase-1 in patients with chronic pancreatitis. Radiol Med. 2012;117(2): 282–92.

65. Olesen SS, Bouwense SA, Wilder-Smith OH, van Goor H, Drewes AM. Pregabalin reduces pain in patients with chronic pancreatitis in a randomized, controlled trial. Gastroenterology 2011;141(2):536–43.

66. Isaksson G, Ihse I. Pain reduction by an oral pancreatic enzyme preparation in chronic pancreatitis. Dig Dis Sci. 1983;28(2): 97–102.

67. Slaff J, Jacobson D, Tillman CR, Curington C, Toskes P. Protease-specific suppression of pancreatic exocrine secretion. Gastroenterology 1984;87(1):44–52.

68. Mossner J, Secknus R, Meyer J, Niederau C, Adler G. Treatment of pain with pancreatic extracts in chronic pancreatitis: results of a prospective placebo-controlled multicenter trial. Digestion 1992;53(1–2):54–66.

69. Halgreen H, Pedersen NT, Worning H. Symptomatic effect of pancreatic enzyme therapy in patients with chronic pancreatitis. Scand J Gastroenterol. 1986;21(1):104–8.

70. Shafiq N, Rana S, Bhasin D, Pandhi P, Srivastava P, Sehmby SS, et al. Pancreatic enzymes for chronic pancreatitis. Cochrane Database Syst Rev. 2009;(4):CD006302.

71. Bhardwaj P, Garg PK, Maulik SK, Saraya A, Tandon RK, Acharya SK. A randomized controlled trial of antioxidant supplementation for pain relief in patients with chronic pancreatitis. Gastroenterology 2009;136(1):149–59.

72. Siriwardena AK, Mason JM, Sheen AJ, Makin AJ, Shah NS. Antioxidant therapy does not reduce pain in patients with chronic pancreatitis: the ANTICIPATE study. Gastroenterology 2012;143(3):655–63, e1.

73. Forsmark CE. Management of chronic pancreatitis. Gastroenterology 2013;144(6):1282–91, e3.

74. Cremer M, Deviere J, Delhaye M, Baize M, Vandermeeren A. Stenting in severe chronic pancreatitis: results of medium-term follow-up in seventy-six patients. Endoscopy 1991;23(3):171–6.

75. Ponchon T, Bory RM, Hedelius F, Roubein LD, Paliard P, Napoleon B, et al. Endoscopic stenting for pain relief in chronic pancreatitis: results of a standardized protocol. Gastrointest Endosc. 1995;42(5):452–6.

76. American Gastroenterological Association. AGA Institute medical position statement on acute pancreatitis. Gastroenterology 2007;132(5):2019–21.

77. Forsmark CE, Baillie J. AGA Institute technical review on acute pancreatitis. Gastroenterology 2007;132(5):2022–44.

78. Issa H, Al-Haddad A, Al-Salem AH. Diagnostic and therapeutic ERCP in the pediatric age group. Pediatr Surg Int. 2007;23(2): 111–6.

79. Graham KS, Ingram JD, Steinberg SE, Narkewicz MR. ERCP in the management of pediatric pancreatitis. Gastrointest Endosc. 1998;47(6):492–5.

80. Bhasin DK, Rana SS, Sidhu RS, Nagi B, Thapa BR, Poddar U, et al. Clinical presentation and outcome of endoscopic therapy in patients with symptomatic chronic pancreatitis associated with pancreas divisum. JOP 2013;14(1):50–6.

81. DuBay D, Sandler A, Kimura K, Bishop W, Eimen M, Soper R. The modified Puestow procedure for complicated hereditary pancreatitis in children. J Pediatr Surg. 2000;35(2):343–8.

82. Rollins MD, Meyers RL. Frey procedure for surgical management of chronic pancreatitis in children. J Pediatr Surg. 2004;39(6):817–20.

83. Clifton MS, Pelayo JC, Cortes RA, Grethel EJ, Wagner AJ, Lee H, et al. Surgical treatment of childhood recurrent pancreatitis. J Pediatr Surg. 2007;42(7):1203–7.

84. Andersen DK, Frey CF. The evolution of the surgical treatment of chronic pancreatitis. Ann Surg. 2010;251(1):18–32.

85. Bellin MD, Carlson AM, Kobayashi T, Gruessner AC, Hering BJ, Moran A, et al. Outcome after pancreatectomy and islet autotransplantation in a pediatric population. J Pediatr Gastroenterol Nutr. 2008;47(1):37–44.

86. Bellin MD, Freeman ML, Schwarzenberg SJ, Dunn TB, Beilman GJ, Vickers SM, et al. Quality of life improves for pediatric patients after total pancreatectomy and islet autotransplant for chronic pancreatitis. Clin Gastroenterol Hepatol. 2011;9(9): 793–9.

87. Kobayashi T, Manivel JC, Bellin MD, Carlson AM, Moran A, Freeman ML, et al. Correlation of pancreatic histopathologic findings and islet yield in children with chronic pancreatitis undergoing total pancreatectomy and islet autotransplantation. Pancreas 2010;39(1):57–63.

88. Wilson GC, Sutton JM, Salehi M, Schmulewitz N, Smith MT, Kucera S, et al. Surgical outcomes after total pancreatectomy and islet cell autotransplantation in pediatric patients. Surgery 2013;154(4):777–83, discussion 83–4.

89. Morinville VD, Lowe ME, Ahuja M, Barth B, Bellin MD, Davis H, et al. Design and Implementation of Insppire (International Study Group of Pediatric Pancreatitis: in Search for a Cure). J Pediatr Gastroenterol Nutr. 2014;59(3):360–4.

Fecal Microbial Transplant: For Whom, How, and When

Fecal Microbial Transplant: For Whom, How, and When

35

Stacy A. Kahn and Jess L. Kaplan

Introduction

Fecal microbial transplantation (FMT), also known as fecal bacteriotherapy or stool transplant, is the transfer of a fecal suspension from a healthy donor into the gastrointestinal (GI) tract of a diseased recipient. FMT has recently emerged as both an effective and controversial therapy. Although it has been performed for a variety of maladies for centuries, if not longer, FMT has only very recently become an accepted therapy for recurrent and relapsing *Clostridium difficile* infection (CDI) in both adults and children where its effectiveness over conventional CDI treatments has now been demonstrated in a randomized controlled trial [1]. A combination of its success in CDI and our burgeoning knowledge of the complex role that microbes play in a myriad of human diseases has led many to question if there are expanded therapeutic applications for FMT for other human GI and even extraintestinal diseases. As such, FMT has taken center stage as a potential novel therapeutic with new clinical trials evaluating its safety and efficacy now well underway.

In this chapter, we review the basics of FMT, its indications, the current evidence supporting its use, details of suggested FMT protocols, the ethical, regulatory, and safety issues involved, and future applications and directions in this rapidly moving field. Much of the existing data are based on studies and reports in adults, but reports and new studies on FMT in children are forthcoming.

Background

FMT is the administration of a fecal solution from a healthy donor into the GI tract of a diseased recipient with the goal of restoring the recipient's health. The first reports of the use of FMT as a therapeutic agent date back to the fourth century in China [2] when it was recommended for diarrheal illnesses, but it was first mentioned in the modern scientific literature in 1958 by Eiseman and colleagues who reported its effectiveness as an adjunct to antibiotics in the treatment of four adults with pseudomembranous colitis [3]. Until very recently, FMT had been used infrequently by medical practitioners, most often as a treatment for CDI. A growing literature now overwhelmingly supports its efficacy, exemplified by the inclusion of FMT in the American College of Gastroenterology's most recent guidelines for the treatment of relapsing CDI [4].

Scientific Rationale

While the overall concept and procedural aspects of FMT are fairly simple to understand, to describe FMT solely as the transfer of stool from a healthy to a diseased individual is a considerable underestimation of the process. The mechanisms that underlie its success and therapeutic potential are likely quite complex and poorly understood to date.

The rationale for the use of FMT as a therapeutic agent has grown from our increasing understanding of the complex interactions between microbes and their human hosts and resulting consequences for human health and disease. The human body is populated by an immense number of microbes, including bacteria, viruses, archaea, and fungi that, in a healthy state, maintain a symbiotic relationship with their human host [5]. Bacterial abundances in the human GI tract alone are estimated to be ten times that of human somatic cells [6]. Deep, culture-independent sequencing techniques utilized in large studies like the Human Microbiome Project (HMP) have recently exposed a vastly more complete and

S. A. Kahn (✉)
Section of Gastroenterology, Hepatology and Nutrition, Department of Pediatrics, University of Chicago, Comer Children's Hospital, 5841 S. Maryland Avenue, Chicago, IL 60637, USA
e-mail: skahn@peds.bsd.uchicago.edu

J. L. Kaplan
Division of Pediatric Gastroenterology and Nutrition, MassGeneral Hospital for Children, Boston, MA, USA

© Springer International Publishing Switzerland 2016
S. Guandalini et al. (eds.), *Textbook of Pediatric Gastroenterology, Hepatology and Nutrition,*
DOI 10.1007/978-3-319-17169-2_35

accurate microbial landscape and detailed community structure on human mucosal surfaces [7, 8].

The microbial composition of the GI tract is perhaps the best characterized among the different human body sites studied. As many as 1500 bacterial species can populate an individual's GI tract at any time, and the vast majority of these species belong to one of four phyla: *Bacteroidetes, Firmicutes, Actinobacteria*, and *Proteobacteria* [8]. These organisms begin to populate the human neonatal GI tract during childbirth. During the first 2–3 years of life, this microbial community structure is markedly unstable, and colonization patterns are significantly influenced by many variables including mode of delivery (cesarean section vs. vaginal), mode of feeding (breast milk vs. formula), microbial infections, and the early use of antibiotics [9]. While the composition of an individual's gut microbiota seems to stabilize by age 3 or so, variation between individuals continues to be shaped by host genetics, diet, and other environmental factors [8].

Perhaps more important than identifying variations in the gut microbial community structure itself, is elucidating the role of these microbes in the maintenance of human health and disease pathogenesis. For example, it is now well appreciated that gut microorganisms are vital to nutrient processing, metabolic function, and the maturation and function of the host immune system [10, 11]. With these key concepts in mind, recent investigations have revealed a microbial imbalance, or dysbiosis, in the GI tract of individuals with a number of different diseases, including inflammatory bowel diseases (IBDs) and obesity among others, emphasizing a role for intestinal microbes in disease pathogenesis [12–14].

Fecal microbiota transplantation is based on the premise that this dysbiosis is partially and at least temporarily reversible with the introduction of a complete, stable microbial community, and that the changes it induces are sustained, preventing recurrence of the disease state. Patients with CDI may provide the best example of this rationale. In CDI, gut microbial biodiversity is markedly reduced, likely creating an ecosystem where *C. difficile* thrives [15, 16]. The decrease in diversity can persist after antibiotic treatment, which may explain high CDI recurrence rates, but is restored after the engraftment of donor feces post FMT, corresponding to clearance of the bacteria and an improvement in disease-related symptoms [16, 17]. It is important to point out that while FMT has resulted in the successful engraftment of donor fecal flora in the recipient in a number of different diseases, engraftment itself is not sufficient for disease resolution as evidenced by work by Kump et al., who reported donor stool engraftment and a reversal of dysbiosis without clinical improvement in six adults with ulcerative colitis (UC) treated with FMT [18]. Clearly, a better understanding of the mechanisms of how FMT works is needed.

Indications for FMT

FMT is not approved by the US Food and Drug Administration (FDA) however, recognizing the significant morbidity and mortality associated with CDI, the FDA has granted enforcement discretion for the clinical use of FMT in recurrent or refractory CDI [19]. The regulatory status of FMT is further detailed later in this chapter.

Currently, FMT is widely used for recurrent and/or refractory CDI in both clinical practice and research settings with success rates close to 90 % worldwide [20–22]. A standard practice guideline from an international FMT working group recommended FMT for recurrent or relapsing CDI (at least three episodes of mild-to-moderate disease including failure of a long vancomycin taper or two episodes of severe disease) and for moderate-and-severe CDI not responding to standard antibiotic treatment for 1 week and 48 h, respectively [23]. FMT has been shown to effectively treat the highly virulent *C. difficile* NAP1/BI/027 strain [24], which is associated with a more severe disease phenotype and is often refractory to standard antibiotic treatment [25].

FMT has been proposed as a treatment for a variety of conditions where dysbiosis is implicated in disease pathogenesis, including IBD, irritable bowel syndrome (IBS), and extraintestinal conditions like obesity, metabolic syndrome, diabetes mellitus, systemic autoimmune disorders, neurologic diseases, and autism spectrum disorders [26–29]. The role of FMT in the treatment of many of these conditions is currently under intense investigation.

Current Evidence for FMT

FMT for *C. difficile* Infection

There is now a sizable body of literature supporting the safety and efficacy of FMT in adults with recurrent/relapsing CDI [1, 20, 21, 23, 30, 31]. Data about FMT in children with CDI are limited, but the existing reports to date suggest similar safety and efficacy [32–34]. A recent systematic review reported the results of FMT in over 500 individuals ranging from 1.5 to 94 years of age [22]; however, it is likely that thousands of patients with recurrent CDI have received FMT. Current estimates from this and other systematic reviews suggest an 87–89 % primary cure rate [21] with preliminary work suggestive that lower GI tract delivery (via colonoscopy or enema) is more effective than upper GI tract delivery (via nasogastric/nasojejunal tube, gastroscopy, gastrostomy tube), 91.3 versus 80.6 % resolution [22]. The majority of our FMT data comes from case reports and series as well as retrospective reviews and as such, specifics about the ideal donor and most effective protocol remain important questions that future studies should address.

To date, there is only one published prospective randomized controlled trial of FMT in CDI [1]. van Nood and colleagues compared resolution of CDI-associated diarrhea in subjects who received vancomycin alone, vancomycin with bowel lavage, or vancomycin with bowel lavage followed by nasoduodenal infusion of FMT from prescreened volunteer donors. The study was terminated early after an interim analysis revealed unacceptably high rates of relapse in both control groups; 59% in those who received vancomycin alone and 77% who received vancomycin plus bowel lavage, compared to FMT $p < 0.001$). Although only 16 patients received FMT, 81% achieved the primary outcome of resolution of diarrhea after a single treatment, and 94% achieved the primary outcome after a second treatment. Subjects who received FMT reported mild belching, abdominal cramps, and diarrhea following on the day of infusion following FMT but none reported persistent symptoms. There were no serious adverse events associated with FMT. Interestingly, recipient microbiota analysis post-FMT demonstrated increase in bacterial diversity and profile similar to the healthy donors.

What is striking about FMT as a therapy is its success rates, given the wide variety of protocols, preparations, and delivery methods used. Studies report using both related and unrelated donors, a number of different FMT preparations that may be fresh or frozen, and variable amounts of FMT delivered via different routes including nasogastric tube, upper endoscopy, colonoscopy, or enema. In fact, it is unclear how much donor stool is needed to achieve the desired result. Recipient protocols also vary widely and have included dietary modifications, different antibiotics pre-FMT, the use of a proton pump inhibitors pre-FMT, and the setting in which the FMT was delivered. Future studies and national registries may begin to help define optimal conditions and protocols.

Both authors were among the first pediatric gastroenterologists to describe the use of FMT in children with CDI [32–34]. In our experience, children as young as 1-year-old who have recurrent CDI that has failed standard antibiotic and probiotic therapy, have had successful resolution of their symptoms and clearance of the infection following a single treatment with FMT. Cure rates are 90–100% in children without underlying IBD, and there have been no serious adverse events noted [32–34].

The first reported pediatric FMT was via nasogastric tube to a 2-year-old child with CDI caused by the BI/NAP1/O27 strain [32]. She was unable to clear the infection despite 8 months of repeated courses with metronidazole, vancomycin, rifaximin, nitazoxanide, *Saccharomyces boulardii*, and *Lactobacillus rhamnosus GG*. On therapy, she was asymptomatic, but, off therapy, she experienced abdominal pain and loose stools with mucus. Using a modified protocol based on the adult experience, she received a single infusion of FMT, with stool donated by her father. Within 36 hours, she had complete resolution of her symptoms and has had no recurrence to date with negative *C. difficile* toxin tests at 2 weeks, 3 months, and 6 months post-FMT.

The second reported use of FMT in a child employed colonoscopic delivery in a toddler who had six documented episodes of recurrent CDI [33]. At 11 months of age, following treatment with azithromycin for a bronchitis infection, he presented with 4–6 foul-smelling watery stools, fever, irritability, vomiting, abdominal pain, a 1–2-lb weight loss, and was found to be *C. difficile* toxin PCR positive. He was then treated with multiple standard and pulsed courses of metronidazole and vancomycin during which his symptoms would be resolved, and his *C. difficile* tests were negative. Shortly after completing the antibiotics, his symptoms would recur, and his stools would test positive for *C. difficile*. At 16 months, he received colonoscopic FMT using his mother as a stool donor. He had complete resolution of his symptoms within 24 hours and has remained clinically well with negative tests.

A case series by Russell et al. just published summarized their experience in ten children with recurrent CDI, three of whom also had underlying IBD who received FMT using their parents as donors [34]. Two children received FMT delivery via nasogastric tube and the remainder by colonoscopic delivery. No serious adverse events were reported. Nine of the ten children had resolution of their symptoms after a single treatment with FMT with a durable response ranging from 1 month to 4 years. Of the three patients with underlying IBD, results were mixed; we may be able to clear the CDI, but the impact of FMT on the IBD remains unclear. In this series, one patient cleared the CDI but then developed acute severe colitis 6-days post-FMT and ultimately underwent colectomy, one patient had a recurrence 8 weeks post FMT that was treated with vancomycin, and one had clearance of the toxin but persistent bloody diarrhea and symptoms resolved following treatment for the underlying Crohn's disease.

Recent systematic reviews also summarize the experience of FMT in adult patients with IBD and recurrent CDI [21, 22]. Similar to the limited pediatric experience, FMT has been highly successful in clearing the CDI; however, the impact of the FMT on the underlying IBD has been mixed with some patients going into remission, some having no change in their disease activity, and a few patients experiencing worsening of their disease [34, 35].

FMT for Inflammatory Bowel Disease

FMT may be a potential therapy for some patients with IBD; however, data are limited, and the regulatory status of FMT in many countries, including the USA, limits its use for indications other than recurrent CDI, without FDA approval. Several case reports and series have described the outcomes in patients who received FMT for IBD with mixed results and little data in pediatric patients.

In 1989, Bennet, both a physician and a patient with medically refractory UC, treated himself with large-volume FMT enemas with encouraging results. Three months post-transplant, flexible sigmoidoscopy demonstrated chronic but no active inflammation, and, at 6 months, he was symptom-free and off all medications [36]. This was followed by several promising but small series by Borody and colleagues [27, 37, 38]. In 2006, they reported the results of treatment with FMT enemas daily for 5 days in six adults with severely active UC [37]. Clinical improvement was noted as early as 1 week post FMT, and complete symptomatic remission was achieved in all patients by 4 months post-FMT. At the time of follow-up (1–13 years), the patients had no endoscopic or histological evidence of active UC.

Unfortunately, not all of the reports of FMT in patients with IBD have been so positive. Vermiere described four patients with Crohn's disease who received nasojejunal FMT who had no clinical response and three of whom developed transient fever and abdominal tenderness [39]. In a similar study out of Austria, examining the effects of nasojejunal and enema-based FMT in five subjects with severely active UC, none achieved clinical remission and only one recipient had a clinical response. All five subjects also had transient post-FMT fever and elevated C-reactive protein that was blood culture negative [40]. Kump and colleagues found that six subjects with chronic active UC who received a single treatment with colonoscopic FMT had a short-term improvement in symptoms but none achieved clinical remission, and one had worsening of disease [18]. Although given the small numbers of subjects, differences in the patient populations and donors, and differences in the protocols used, there are no clear conclusions to be drawn about the potential safety and efficacy of FMT in adults with IBD. Larger randomized controlled trials are needed to further evaluate the therapeutic potential and safety of FMT in IBD.

The first study in pediatric IBD patients treated with FMT was reported by Kunde et al. in 2013. Ten youths, aged 7–21 years, with mildly to moderately active UC were treated with FMT enemas from relatives or close relations, daily for 5 days [23]. Although this small pilot study only followed the subjects for 1 month, nine out of ten subjects tolerated FMT, three out of nine were in clinical remission at 1 week, and six out of nine had a sustained clinical response at 1 month. One patient had had significant hematochezia and a marked increase in the pediatric ulcerative colitis activity index (PUCAI) [41] after having a transient improvement immediately following FMT. No serious adverse events were reported, but two subjects experienced fever following

FMT who responded to antipyretics. Several subjects also noted bloating, abdominal pain, diarrhea, hematochezia, and fatigue though it is unclear if these effects were due to the FMT or the underlying IBD [42].

Vandenplas et al. recently published their experience using repeated FMT infusions to treat a 1-year-old girl with early-onset colitis [43]. Initially, the child's symptoms were responsive to oral and rectal mesalamine, but she relapsed and, at 1 year of age, failed to improve on prednisolone and azathioprine, an amino acid-based formula, and antibiotics. She continued to be quite ill with a PUCAI between 60 and 75 and required intermittent blood transfusions. Following seven treatments with FMT from two donors, she went into clinical and endoscopic remission. Although this report is quite promising, caution is advised as the safety and efficacy of FMT in IBD has yet to be established by rigorous scientific investigation.

FMT Protocols

FMT has been historically performed without regulatory oversight leading to variation in protocols for each step of the process, including donor selection, donor screening, stool preparation and handling, recipient preparation and quantity and method of stool delivery. The international FMT Working Group published guidelines in December of 2011 that have helped to standardize FMT and guide regulation [23]. The importance of standardization, particularly in regard to safety, is underscored by the numerous "How to" guides on the Internet instructing laypeople how to perform FMT at home without important regulation.

Donor selection is an area of particular controversy. FMTs have been successfully performed with stool from related donors (e.g., parents, sexual intimates, etc.) and from healthy, unrelated donors, but characteristics of the "optimal donor" are still under debate. A systematic review of FMT for recurrent CDI found slightly higher success rates when related donors were used (93 %) compared to unrelated donors (84 %) [20], but more recent studies have found equal if not greater success with unrelated donors [30]. Suggested donor exclusion criteria and screening before transplant from the FMT working group are listed in Table 35.1.

Donor and Recipient Screening

Rigorous evaluation of the stool donor for potentially transmissible infections is of the utmost importance. Optimally, this screening should be performed as close to the time of donor stool collection as possible. The FDA recommends that all tests be performed within 4 weeks of FMT and human immunodeficiency virus (HIV) testing within

Table 35.1 Donor exclusion criteria [23]. (Reprinted from Ref. [23], Copyright 2012, with permission from Elsevier)

1. Absolute
a. For the risk of infectious agent, consider using American Association of Blood Banks Donor history questionnaire: http://www.fda.gov/downloads/BiologicsBloodVaccines/BloodBloodProducts/ApprovedProducts/LicensedProductsBLAs/BloodDonorScreening/UCM213552.pdf
Known human immunodeficiency virus (HIV), hepatitis B or C infections
Known exposure to HIV or viral hepatitis (within the previous 12 months)
High-risk sexual behaviors (e.g., sexual contact with anyone with HIV/acquired immune deficiency syndrome or hepatitis, men who have sex with men, sex for drugs or money)
Use of illicit drugs
Tattoo or body piercing within 6 months
Incarceration or history of incarceration
Known current communicable disease (e.g., upper respiratory tract infection)
Risk factors for variant Creutzfeldt–Jakob disease
Travel (within the last 6 months) to areas of the world where diarrheal illnesses are endemic or risk of traveler's diarrhea is high
b. Gastrointestinal comorbidities
History of inflammatory bowel disease
History of irritable bowel syndrome, idiopathic chronic constipation, or chronic diarrhea
History of gastrointestinal malignancy or known polyposis
c. Factors that can or do affect the composition of the intestinal microbiota
Antibiotics within the preceding 3 months
Major immunosuppressive medications, for example, calcineurin inhibitors, exogenous glucocorticoids, biologic agents, etc.
Systemic antineoplastic agents
d. Additional recipient-specific considerations
Recent ingestion of a potential allergen (e.g., nuts) where the recipient has a known allergy to this (these) agent(s)
2. Relative exclusion criteria that may be appropriate to consider
History of major gastrointestinal surgery (e.g., gastric bypass)
Metabolic syndrome
Systemic autoimmunity, for example, multiple sclerosis, connective tissue disease
Atopic diseases including asthma and eczema, eosinophilic disorders of the gastrointestinal tract
Chronic pain syndromes, for example, chronic fatigue syndrome, fibromyalgia

2 weeks. Donor screening tests outlined in Table 35.2 have been suggested by the FMT Working Group [23]. Additional screening protocols may be modified based on the recipient and the disease being treated. For example, in the case of FMT for IBD, some have suggested donors be screened for cytomegalovirus (CMV), given its potential to cause colitis. It is also likely that screening protocols and FDA guidelines will continue to evolve. The frequency of screening for repeat donors has not been established.

Similar screening for recipients is not done universally but is being performed by some practitioners and investigators, mostly in an effort to document the recipient's baseline status at the time of transplant in case of disease transmission.

FMT Preparation

Published methods of donor stool preparation before transplant vary enough that few definite conclusions can be drawn. Historically, fresh donor stool was used, typically within 8 h of passage. More recently, however, the efficacy of FMT with thawed/previously frozen stool has been shown to be equally effective in recurrent CDI in terms of both clinical improvement [30] and engraftment of the donor flora [44]. In most protocols, a standard kitchen blender is used to homogenize donated stool with a dilutant. Bacteriostatic normal saline, water, and even 4% cow's milk have been used as dilutants, and although water may give the best results, preservative free saline is most commonly used [20]. Anywhere from 50 to 300 g of stool is blended with 250–500 mL of dilutant to achieve a liquid slurry, which is then filtered to remove particulate matter. Filtration can be performed with simple through gauze or standard coffee filters. Most recommend that, when possible, a fume hood be used during preparation. The optimal dose is unclear in adults but most give at least 250 mL of the final slurry for colonoscopic delivery and at least 50 mL for upper GI tract delivery [45]. Weight- or age-based doses for children have yet to be established. There is limited evidence that supports a trend in higher efficacy and decreased CDI relapse rates when higher doses of donor stool are used and larger volumes of stool slurry are delivered, but this has yet to be adequately studied in a prospective study [20].

Table 35.2 Donor screening tests [23]. (Reprinted from [23], Copyright 2012, with permission from Elsevier)

1. Stool testing
Clostridium difficile toxin B by PCR; if unavailable, then evaluation for toxins A and B by EIA
Routine bacterial culture for enteric pathogens
Fecal *Giardia* antigen
Fecal *Cryptosporidium* antigen
Acid-fast stain for *Cyclospora, Isospora,* and, if antigen testing unavailable, *Cryptosporidium*
Ova and parasites
Helicobacter pylori fecal antigen (for upper GI routes of FMT administration)
2. Serologic testing (unless otherwise stated, all tests should be performed using FDA-approved test methods)
HIV, type 1 and 2
Hepatitis A virus (HAV) immunoglobulin (Ig) M
Hepatitis B surface antigen, hepatitis B core antibody (both IgG and IgM), and hepatitis B surface antibody
Hepatitis C virus antibody
Rapid plasma reagin and fluorescent treponemal antibody absorbed

PCR polymerase chain reaction, *EIA* enzyme immunoassay, *GI* gastrointestinal, *FMT* fecal microbial transplantation, *HIV* human immunodeficiency virus

Routes of Administration

Fecal microbiota transplantation using both upper and lower GI tract delivery has been successful in treating recurrent CDI. Upper GI (UGI) tract delivery methods have included gastric and post-pyloric delivery through a gastroscope or flexible naso-enteric tube and more recently by mouth in encapsulated form, while lower GI (LGI) tract delivery is via retention enema or colonoscope. For children, successful nasogastric tube [32] and colonoscopic [33] delivery have both been successful for recurrent CDI. The largest review of cases to date for FMT in CDI showed higher rates of resolution with delivery via the LGI tract (93.6%) compared to UGI tract (76.4%) [20]. A more recent systematic review of CDI cases showed a trend towards better results with LGI tract delivery (91.4%) compared to UGI tract delivery (82.3%) although this did not reach statistical significance [21]. A recently completed, small, randomized trial comparing nasogastric and colonoscopic delivery methods in CDI showed no difference in efficacy [46] but larger trials are certainly needed. If UGI tract delivery does prove to be inferior, one reason may be a lack of stability/survival of donor microbiota in the highly acidic gastric environment. Most investigators have countered this potential problem by treating recipients receiving FMT via the stomach with proton pump inhibitors or delivering the solution post-pylorically. There may be theoretical problems with administering LGI tract flora from the donor into a UGI tract location in terms of engraftment although this has not been extensively studied. This has led some to recommend a bowel lavage for all recipients just before FMT, even for those receiving donor material via the UGI tract [45].

Colonoscopic delivery is more invasive and UGI tract delivery via naso-enteric tube, while somewhat less invasive, still has associated risks and may prove unpalatable for some patients. The logical next step is the encapsulation of donor fecal material into a pill form that can be taken orally to reduce these procedural risks.

Beyond CDI, little is known about the optimal delivery method for FMT, but it ultimately may depend on the location and other specifics of the condition being treated. Larger, randomized trials comparing delivery method are needed for both CDI and other diseases that might be treated with this therapy.

Ethical, Legal, Social, and Regulatory Issues

There are numerous ethical and regulatory issues surrounding the use of FMT in both the USA and abroad. Given the importance of the ethical, legal, and social issues (ELSIs) related to the microbiome research and technology, the National Institutes of Health (NIH) has specifically solicited research on this topic through the HMP [7]. Unfortunately, research in this area has been slow, and there have only been a few studies addressing the ethical and social issues related to fecal microbiota transplantation [31, 47–49].

The lag in ELSI research on FMT may in part stem from the lack of clarity regarding how FMT is classified. Clearly, it is a biologic substance, but there have been questions about whether or not the microbiome should be classified as an organ or a tissue and whether or not FMT is a drug [50]. In the USA, the FDA has taken an active role in establishing the status of FMT and overseeing it regulation. Although scientists in the field regard the microbiome as an organ [51], the FDA does not recognize stool and the microbiome it contains as an organ or a issue, but as a drug and a biologic product [50].

Most of the existing ELSI literature explores the social issues related to using stool as a drug and patient and physician perceptions of FMT. Early studies focused on whether patients and parents would be willing to consider or undergo

Ethical, legal, and social issues in FMT
Stigma/"yuck factor"
Discussion of risk
Nonuniform IRB requirements and guidelines
Potential for drug of compassionate use
Protection of vulnerable patients (children)
Impact and coverage of FMT by insurance
Identification of donors
Screening and protection of donors
Coverage of donor screening costs
Banking of samples/data sharing
Regulation and safety monitoring
Patents for FMT products and methods

IRB Institutional Review Board, *FMT* fecal microbial transplantation

FMT. Notwithstanding the obvious "yuck" factor associated with FMT, patient and their families were willing and even eager to consider FMT for both IBD and recurrent CDI [47–49]. More recently, investigators have confirmed that although not all physicians are comfortable performing FMT personally, the great majority are comfortable with FMT as a treatment for CDI and/or the creation of specialized centers where FMT can be performed [52].

Beyond physician and patient acceptance, there are numerous ethical issues related to FMT that have yet to be investigated. These ELSIs are outlined in Table 35.3.

Summary and Potential Future of FMT

The excitement over FMT and its potential applications has grown exponentially over the past few years. The success of FMT in CDI has spawned investigations into treatment optimization and also into other microbial-based therapeutics, with growing interest from clinicians, scientists, government health agencies, and commercial entities alike. Ongoing trials of FMT in pediatric diseases will provide much needed data about efficacy, safety, durability, and the long-term impact of FMT in young patients.

Stool Banks and Encapsulation

The use of freshly donated stool for FMT is both time and labor intensive for the practitioner which may limit widespread use. With newer evidence supporting the efficacy of thawed, previously frozen stool, the banking of large amounts of frozen, previously donated stool from healthy donors is underway and should help standardize FMT, ease administration, and improve safety. Since UGI tract delivery seems effective for recurrent CDI and may eventually be a

preferred method for other conditions, the encapsulation of transplant material is the next logical step. The study of such "stool capsules" has been recently published, [53, 54] but raises a host of new questions including dose, optimal capsule material, location of release, and the impact of gastric acid which have not yet been answered.

Bacterial Fingerprinting: Matching Donors and Recipients

Recent investigations have uncovered significant variability in the composition of the human gut microbiome. However, analysis of fecal samples from around the world show that human gut microbial community structures that may also be classified as distinct "enterotypes" based on microbial composition and molecular function [55]. These enterotypes are driven by long-term dietary intake [56], and there is increasing evidence that genetics plays a role in shaping the gut microbiome [57]. This raises important questions for FMT including donor and recipient matching not only in regard to enterotype but also age, gender, and even HLA typing among other factors. Future FMT studies will need to address these questions to better assess optimal matching strategies.

Stool Substitutes: Building Microbial Communities In Vitro

While FMT appears relatively safe in the short term, serious concerns remain in regard to potential pathogen and disease transmission and also in regard to long-term safety. Stool substitutes, combinations of cultured commensal bacteria derived from human stool, have the potential to improve safety by assuring the transfer of only known microbes and thus the absence of transmission of potentially pathogenic microbes such as viruses. Petrof and colleagues reported the successful eradication of recurrent CDI in two adults using a combination of 33 purified bacterial isolates recovered from healthy, unrelated donor stool [58]. Similar results have been reported in animals [59]. While the initial results are promising, it is unknown which components of human stool are mandatory for treatment success. There is also concern that progressive re-culturing of the same strain over time may change bacterial characteristics and affect a microbe's ability to engraft in the recipient [60]. Efficacy of such "stool substitutes" will have to be compared to more standard FMT using intact donor stool as well as other probiotic mixtures. If they compare favorably, these purified communities of human-derived bacteria grown in vitro will likely improve both the safety and availability of microbiota-based therapeutics.

Commercialization

The recent success of FMT for recurrent CDI has spawned growing attention from commercial entities. Specifically, the encapsulation of donor material and the creation of stool banks lend themselves to commercial interest that would vastly increase the accessibility of FMT to patients and practitioners alike. Although not yet proven to be effective, the creation of "stool substitutes" in vitro may represent the largest opportunity for industry in the future. Commercialization will advance therapeutic standardization and will also lead to more strict oversight by regulatory agencies, likely improving the safety of microbiota-based therapeutics such as FMT for patients.

Unanswered Questions

FMT is an effective therapy for recurrent CDI in both adults and children, but many unanswered questions remain including optimal dosing, delivery route, recipient preparation, and donor characteristics. Short and long-term safety monitoring are of paramount importance, and the long-term outcomes and distant effects on recipient health are essentially unknown. The role of FMT in diseases other than recurrent CDI is unclear and only beginning to be evaluated. Studies in the USA and abroad are beginning to investigate this multitude of questions.

References

1. van Nood E, Vrieze A, Nieuwdorp M, Fuentes S, Zoetendal EG, de Vos WM, et al. Duodenal infusion of donor feces for recurrent *Clostridium difficile*. N Engl J Med. 2013;368(5):407–15.
2. Zhang F, Luo W, Shi Y, Fan Z, Ji G. Should we standardize the 1700-year-old fecal microbiota transplantation? Am J Gastroenterol. 2012;107(11):1755.
3. Eiseman B, Silen W, Bascom GS, Kauvar AJ. Fecal enema as an adjunct in the treatment of pseudomembranous enterocolitis. Surgery. 1958;44(5):854–9.
4. Surawicz CM, Brandt LJ, Binion DG, Ananthakrishnan AN, Curry SR, Gilligan PH, et al. Guidelines for diagnosis, treatment, and prevention of *Clostridium difficile* infections. Am J Gastroenterol. 2013;108(4):478–98.
5. Littman DR, Pamer EG. Role of the commensal microbiota in normal and pathogenic host immune responses. Cell Host Microbe. 2011;10(4):311–23 (PMCID: Pmc3202012).
6. Savage DC. Microbial ecology of the gastrointestinal tract. Annu Rev Microbiol. 1977;31:107–33.
7. Turnbaugh PJ, Ley RE, Hamady M, Fraser-Liggett CM, Knight R, Gordon JI. The human microbiome project. Nature. 2007;449(7164):804–10 (PMCID: Pmc3709439).
8. The Human Microbiome Project Consortium. Structure, function and diversity of the healthy human microbiome. Nature. 2012;486(7402):207–14 (PMCID: Pmc3564958).
9. Dominguez-Bello MG, Blaser MJ, Ley RE, Knight R. Development of the human gastrointestinal microbiota and insights from high-throughput sequencing. Gastroenterology. 2011;140(6):1713–9.
10. Hooper LV, Gordon JI. Commensal host-bacterial relationships in the gut. Science (New York, NY). 2001;292(5519):1115–8.
11. Lee YK, Mazmanian SK. Has the microbiota played a critical role in the evolution of the adaptive immune system? Science (New York, NY). 2010;330(6012):1768–73 (PMCID: Pmc3159383).
12. Ley RE, Turnbaugh PJ, Klein S, Gordon JI. Microbial ecology: human gut microbes associated with obesity. Nature. 2006;444(7122):1022–3.
13. Frank DN, St Amand AL, Feldman RA, Boedeker EC, Harpaz N, Pace NR. Molecular-phylogenetic characterization of microbial community imbalances in human inflammatory bowel diseases. Proc Natl Acad U S A. 2007;104(34):13780–5 (PMCID: Pmc1959459).
14. Turnbaugh PJ, Hamady M, Yatsunenko T, Cantarel BL, Duncan A, Ley RE, et al. A core gut microbiome in obese and lean twins. Nature. 2009;457(7228):480–4 (PMCID: Pmc2677729).
15. Chang JY, Antonopoulos DA, Kalra A, Tonelli A, Khalife WT, Schmidt TM, et al. Decreased diversity of the fecal microbiome in recurrent *Clostridium difficile*-associated diarrhea. J Infect Dis. 2008;197(3):435–8.
16. Grehan MJ, Borody TJ, Leis SM, Campbell J, Mitchell H, Wettstein A. Durable alteration of the colonic microbiota by the administration of donor fecal flora. J Clin Gastroenterol. 2010;44(8):551–61.
17. Shankar V, Hamilton M, Khoruts A, Kilburn A, Unno T, Paliy O, et al. Species and genus level resolution analysis of gut microbiota in *Clostridium difficile* patients following fecal microbiota transplantation. Microbiome. 2014;2(1):13.
18. Kump PK, Grochenig HP, Lackner S, Trajanoski S, Reicht G, Hoffmann KM, et al. Alteration of intestinal dysbiosis by fecal microbiota transplantation does not induce remission in patients with chronic active ulcerative colitis. Inflamm Bowel Dis. 2013;19(10):2155–65.
19. Food and Drug Administration. Guidance for industry: enforcement policy regarding investigational new drug requirements for use of fecal microbiota for transplantation to treat *Clostridium difficile* infection not responsive to standard therapies. 2013 (updated 2013; cited). http://www.fda.gov/downloads/BiologicsBloodVaccines/GuidanceComplianceRegulatoryInformation/Guidances/Vaccines/UCM361393.pdf. Accessed 9 May 2014.
20. Gough E, Shaikh H, Manges AR. Systematic review of intestinal microbiota transplantation (fecal bacteriotherapy) for recurrent *Clostridium difficile* infection. Clin Infect Dis. 2011;53(10):994–1002.
21. Kassam Z, Lee CH, Yuan Y, Hunt RH. Fecal microbiota transplantation for *Clostridium difficile* infection: systematic review and meta-analysis. Am J Gastroenterol. 2013;108(4):500–8.
22. Cammarota G, Ianiro G, Gasbarrini A. Fecal microbiota transplantation for the treatment of *Clostridium difficile* infection: a systematic review. J Clin Gastroenterol. 2014;48:693–702.
23. Bakken JS, Borody T, Brandt LJ, Brill JV, Demarco DC, Franzos MA, et al. Treating *Clostridium difficile* infection with fecal microbiota transplantation. Clin Gastroenterol Hepatol. 2011;9(12):1044–9 (PMCID: Pmc3223289).
24. Mattila E, Uusitalo-Seppala R, Wuorela M, Lehtola L, Nurmi H, Ristikankare M, et al. Fecal transplantation, through colonoscopy, is effective therapy for recurrent *Clostridium difficile* infection. Gastroenterology. 2012;142(3):490–6.
25. O'Connor JR, Johnson S, Gerding DN. *Clostridium difficile* infection caused by the epidemic BI/NAP1/027 strain. Gastroenterology. 2009;136(6):1913–24.
26. Blaser M, Bork P, Fraser C, Knight R, Wang J. The microbiome explored: recent insights and future challenges. Nat Rev Microbiol. 2013;11(3):213–7.
27. Borody T, Leis S, McGrath K, Spence E, Surance R, Warren E, editors. Treatment of chronic constipation and colitis using human probiotic infusions. Probiotics, Prebiotics and New Foods Conference; 2–4 Sept 2001, Universita Urbaniana, Rome.

28. Vrieze A, de Groot PF, Kootte RS, Knaapen M, van Nood E, Nieuwdorp M. Fecal transplant: a safe and sustainable clinical therapy for restoring intestinal microbial balance in human disease? Best Pract Res Clin Gastroenterol. 2013;27(1):127–37.

29. Vrieze A, Van Nood E, Holleman F, Salojarvi J, Kootte RS, Bartelsman JF, et al. Transfer of intestinal microbiota from lean donors increases insulin sensitivity in individuals with metabolic syndrome. Gastroenterology. 2012;143(4):913–6.e7.

30. Hamilton MJ, Weingarden AR, Sadowsky MJ, Khoruts A. Standardized frozen preparation for transplantation of fecal microbiota for recurrent *Clostridium difficile* infection. Am J Gastroenterol. 2012;107(5):761–7.

31. Brandt LJ, Aroniadis OC, Mellow M, Kanatzar A, Kelly C, Park T, et al. Long-term follow-up of colonoscopic fecal microbiota transplant for recurrent *Clostridium difficile* infection. Am J Gastroenterol. 2012;107(7):1079–87.

32. Russell G, Kaplan J, Ferraro M, Michelow IC. Fecal bacteriotherapy for relapsing *Clostridium difficile* infection in a child: a proposed treatment protocol. Pediatrics. 2010;126(1):e239–42.

33. Kahn SA, Young S, Rubin DT. Colonoscopic fecal microbiota transplant for recurrent *Clostridium difficile* infection in a child. Am J Gastroenterol. 2012;107(12):1930–1.

34. Russell GH, Kaplan JL, Youngster I, Baril-Dore M, Schindelar L, Hohmann E, et al. Fecal transplant for recurrent *Clostridium difficile* infection in children with and without inflammatory bowel disease. J Pediatr Gastroenterol Nutr. 2014;58(5):588–92.

35. De Leon LM, Watson JB, Kelly CR. Transient flare of ulcerative colitis after fecal microbiota transplantation for recurrent *Clostridium difficile* infection. Clin Gastroenterol Hepatol. 2013;11(8):1036–8.

36. Bennet JD, Brinkman M. Treatment of ulcerative colitis by implantation of normal colonic flora. Lancet. 1989;1(8630):164.

37. Borody TJ, Warren EF, Leis S, Surace R, Ashman O. Treatment of ulcerative colitis using fecal bacteriotherapy. J Clin Gastroenterol. 2003;37(1):42–7.

38. Borody TJ, Warren EF, Leis SM, Surace R, Ashman O, Siarakas S. Bacteriotherapy using fecal flora: toying with human motions. J Clin Gastroenterol. 2004;38(6):475–83.

39. Vermeire S, Joossens M, Verbeke K, Hildebrand F, Machiels K, Van den Broeck K, et al. Sa1922 Pilot study on the safety and efficacy of faecal microbiota transplantation in refractory Crohn's disease. Gastroenterology. 2012;142(5):S-360.

40. Angelberger S, Reinisch W, Makristathis A, Lichtenberger C, Dejaco C, Papay P, et al. Temporal bacterial community dynamics vary among ulcerative colitis patients after fecal microbiota transplantation. Am J Gastroenterol. 2013;108(10):1620–30.

41. Turner D, Otley AR, Mack D, Hyams J, de Bruijne J, Uusoue K, et al. Development, validation, and evaluation of a pediatric ulcerative colitis activity index: a prospective multicenter study. Gastroenterology. 2007;133(2):423–32.

42. Kunde S, Pham A, Bonczyk S, Crumb T, Duba M, Conrad H Jr, et al. Safety, tolerability, and clinical response after fecal transplantation in children and young adults with ulcerative colitis. J Pediatr Gastroenterol Nutr. 2013;56(6):597–601.

43. Vandenplas Y, Veereman G, van der Werff Ten Bosch J, Goossens A, Pierard D, Samsom JN, et al. Fecal microbial transplantation in a one-year-old girl with early onset colitis—caution advised. J Pediatr Gastroenterol Nutr. 2014. [epub ahead of print].

44. Hamilton MJ, Weingarden AR, Unno T, Khoruts A, Sadowsky MJ. High-throughput DNA sequence analysis reveals stable engraftment of gut microbiota following transplantation of previously frozen fecal bacteria. Gut Microbes. 2013;4(2):125–35 (PMCID: Pmc3595072).

45. Brandt LJ. American Journal of Gastroenterology Lecture: intestinal microbiota and the role of fecal microbiota transplant (FMT) in treatment of *C. difficile* infection. Am J Gastroenterol. 2013;108(2):177–85.

46. Youngster I, Sauk J, Pindar C, Wilson RG, Kaplan JL, Smith MB, et al. Fecal microbiota transplant for relapsing *Clostridium difficile* infection using a frozen inoculum from unrelated donors: a randomized, open-label, controlled pilot study. Clin Infect Dis. 2014;58(11):1515–22 (PMCID: Pmc4017893).

47. Kahn SA, Gorawara-Bhat R, Rubin DT. Fecal bacteriotherapy for ulcerative colitis: patients are ready, are we? Inflamm Bowel Dis. 2012;18(4):676–84 (PMCID: Pmc3183116).

48. Kahn SA, Vachon A, Rodriquez D, Goeppinger SR, Surma B, Marks J, et al. Patient perceptions of fecal microbiota transplantation for ulcerative colitis. Inflamm Bowel Dis. 2013;19(7):1506–13 (PMCID: Pmc3780382).

49. Zipursky JS, Sidorsky TI, Freedman CA, Sidorsky MN, Kirkland KB. Patient attitudes toward the use of fecal microbiota transplantation in the treatment of recurrent *Clostridium difficile* infection. Clin Infect Dis. 2012;55(12):1652–8.

50. Food and Drug Administration. Fecal microbiota for transplantation: scientific and regulatory issues—Center for Biologics, Evaluation and Research (FDA) and the National Institute for Allergy and Infectious Diseases (NIH). 2013 (updated 2013; cited 2014 13 May). http://www.fda.gov/downloads/BiologicsBloodVaccines/NewsEvents/WorkshopsMeetingsConferences/UCM352902.pdf. Accessed 9 May 2014.

51. Baquero F, Nombela C. The microbiome as a human organ. Clin Microbiol Infect. 2012;18(Suppl 4):2–4.

52. Jiang ZD, Hoang LN, Lasco TM, Garey KW, Dupont HL. Physician attitudes toward the use of fecal transplantation for recurrent *Clostridium difficile* infection in a metropolitan area. Clin Infect Dis. 2013;56(7):1059–60.

53. Louie TJ, Cannon K, O'Grady H, Wu KW L. Fecal microbiome transplantation (FMT) via oral fecal microbial capsules for recurrent *Clostridium difficile* infection (rCDI). In: IDWeek; 2013 Oct 2–6, San Francisco, CA, Infectious Disease Society of America, Abstract No 89. 2013.

54. Youngster I, Russell GH, Pindar C, et al. ORal, capsulized, frozen fecal microbiota transplantation for relapsing clostridium difficile infection. JAMA. 2014;312:1772–8.

55. Arumugam M, Raes J, Pelletier E, Le Paslier D, Yamada T, Mende DR, et al. Enterotypes of the human gut microbiome. Nature. 2011;473(7346):174–80 (PMCID: Pmc3728647).

56. Wu GD, Chen J, Hoffmann C, Bittinger K, Chen YY, Keilbaugh SA, et al. Linking long-term dietary patterns with gut microbial enterotypes. Science (New York, NY). 2011;334(6052):105–8 (PMCID: Pmc3368382).

57. Knights D, Lassen KG, Xavier RJ. Advances in inflammatory bowel disease pathogenesis: linking host genetics and the microbiome. Gut. 2013;62(10):1505–10 (PMCID: Pmc3822528).

58. Petrof EO, Gloor GB, Vanner SJ, Weese SJ, Carter D, Daigneault MC, et al. Stool substitute transplant therapy for the eradication of *Clostridium difficile* infection: 'RePOOPulating' the gut. Microbiome. 2013;1(1):3 (PMCID: Pmc3869191).

59. Lawley TD, Clare S, Walker AW, Stares MD, Connor TR, Raisen C, et al. Targeted restoration of the intestinal microbiota with a simple, defined bacteriotherapy resolves relapsing *Clostridium difficile* disease in mice. PLoS Pathogens. 2012;8(10):e1002995 (PMCID: Pmc3486913).

60. Borody TJ, Paramsothy S, Agrawal G. Fecal microbiota transplantation: indications, methods, evidence, and future directions. Curr Gastroenterol Rep. 2013;15(8):337 (PMCID: Pmc3742951).

Congenital Disorders of Intestinal Electrolyte Transport

36

Vincenza Pezzella, Tommaso Cozzolino, Ylenia Maddalena, Gianluca Terrin, Rita Nocerino and Roberto Berni Canani

Introduction

Congenital diarrheal disorders (CDD; OMIM 251850) are a group of rare chronic enteropathies characterized by a heterogeneous etiology with a typical onset early in the life. In the first weeks of life, patients affected by CDD usually present with severe diarrhea that within a few hours leads to a life-threatening condition secondary to massive dehydration and metabolic acidosis (or alkalosis in the case of congenital chloride diarrhea, CLD) [1]. The number of conditions included within the CDD group has gradually increased, and many new genes have been identified and functionally related to CDD, opening new diagnostic and therapeutic perspectives [1]. We have proposed a CDDs classification in four groups in relation to main defect:

1. Defects of digestion, absorption, and transport of nutrients and electrolytes
2. Defects of enterocyte differentiation and polarization
3. Defects of enteroendocrine cells differentiation
4. Defects of intestinal immune response modulation

In the context of the first group, congenital disorders of intestinal electrolytes transport are a subset of diseases characterized by early clinical presentation due to autosomal recessive defect. These disorders are challenging clinical conditions for pediatric gastroenterologists because of the severity of the clinical picture and the broad range of conditions in differential diagnosis. Frequently, abnormal fluid absorption begins in utero, manifesting itself as maternal polyhydramnios. Then soon after birth, patients usually present with severe diarrhea that within few hours leads to a life-threatening condition secondary to massive dehydration and metabolic acidosis [1]. Consequently, these patients require a prompt diagnosis and assistance. Milder forms with subtle clinical signs may remain undiagnosed until adulthood when patients developed irreversible complications. In particular, patients with cystic fibrosis (CF) may have a subtle clinical presentation, with prevalent non-intestinal symptoms.

Different mechanisms are responsible for transepithelial ion transport at intestinal level (Fig. 36.1). In the jejunum, $NaHCO_3^-$ is absorbed via Na^+/H^+ exchange (the secreted H^+ neutralizes an equivalent amount of luminal $NaHCO_3^-$) and Cl^- movement is purely passive [2]. In the ileum (and, as shown later, also in the proximal colon), NaCl is absorbed via equal rates of Na^+/H^+ and $Cl^-/NaHCO_3^-$ exchanges [2]. At least three Na^+/H^+ exchangers (NHEs) have since been localized to intestinal brush border membranes and cloned; NHE2 and NHE3 are found in both small intestine and colon. NHE3 appears to be quantitatively more important, since the NHE2 knockout mouse suffers gastric dysfunction but no intestinal disability, whereas the NHE3 knockout mouse suffers from chronic diarrhea. A third, Cl^--dependent NHE is found in crypt cells of rat distal colon. The NHE first identified in intestine, NHE1, is present only in the basolateral membrane of enterocytes and is involved in HCO_3^- secretion [3].

Two anion exchangers have also been localized to small-intestinal and colonic brush border membranes and cloned: downregulated in adenoma (DRA) and putative anion transporter 1 (PAT1) [1]. DRA was first cloned from colonic mucosa; it was found to be downregulated in villus adenomas and carcinomas and subsequently was found to incur mutations in the rare diarrheal disorder familial chloride diarrhea (see "Congenital chloride diarrhea" below). Both DRA and PAT1 are abundant in the duodenum and present at higher density there than NHE2 and NHE3, suggesting a role in

R. Berni Canani (✉)
European Laboratory for the Investigation of Food Induced Diseases, University of Naples "Federico II", Via S. Pansini 5, Naples 80131, Italy
e-mail: berni@unina.it

V. Pezzella · T. Cozzolino · Y. Maddalena · R. Nocerino · R. Berni Canani
Department of Translational Medical Science—Section of Pediatrics, University of Naples "Federico II", Via S. Pansini 5, Naples 80131, Italy

G. Terrin
Department of Gynaecology—Obstetrics and Perinatal Medicine, University of Rome "La Sapienza", Policlinico Umbero I, Rome, Italy

Department of Perinatal Medicine, Neonatology Unit, Sapienza University of Rome, Rome, Italy

© Springer International Publishing Switzerland 2016
S. Guandalini et al. (eds.), *Textbook of Pediatric Gastroenterology, Hepatology and Nutrition*,
DOI 10.1007/978-3-319-17169-2_36

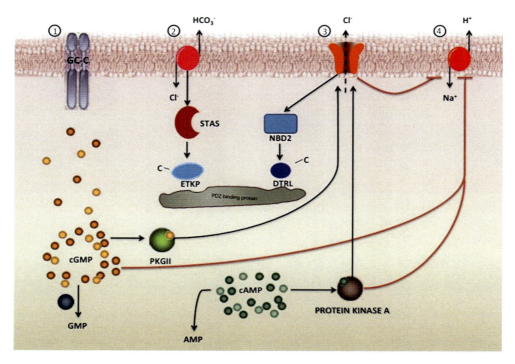

Fig. 36.1 Pathophysiological mechanisms of congenital disorders of intestinal electrolytes transport. *1 Familial diarrhea syndrome* is due to a mutation in intestinal guanylate cyclase receptor *(GC-C)* for the endogenous ligands uroguanylin/guanylin. Ligand binding to GC-C increases intracellular levels of cyclic guanosine monophosphate *(cGMP)*. The cGMP activates cGMP-dependent protein kinase II *(PKGII)*. PKGII phosphorylates the cystic fibrosis transmembrane conductance regulator *(CFTR)*, increasing its Cl⁻secreting activity and inhibiting electroneutral NaCl absorption. A missense mutation leads to a gain of function increasing ligand-mediated activation of GC-C and intracellular cGMP levels resulting in chronic secretive diarrhea. *2 Congenital chloride diarrhea* is caused by a defect in DRA exchanger leading to severe watery diarrhea due to Cl⁻ malabsorption. The pro-

tein has a C-terminal domain, sulfate transporter and antisigma factor antagonist *(STAS)*, that ensures the correct location of the protein on the apical membrane of enterocytes. The STAS domain also interacts with the R-domain of the *CFTR*, and it is required for *CFTR* activation. *3 In cystic fibrosis,* there is an alternated activity of *CFTR*. This membrane protein consists of two membrane-spanning domains, two nucleotide-binding domains *(NBDs)*, and a regulatory domain, which controls channel activity. *4 Congenital sodium diarrhea* probably derives from a defect in apical membrane Na⁺/H⁺ exchangers leading to severe watery diarrhea due to Na⁺ malabsorption. *DRA* downregulated in adenoma, *DTRL* defense terrain research laboratory, *cAMP* cyclic adenosine monophosphate, *AMP* adenosine monophosphate, *GMP* guanosine monophosphate

duodenal alkalinization. In the colon, DRA appears to predominate over PAT1.

More than two brush border ion exchangers are required, of course, for the enterocyte to engage in transcellular salt absorption. Increased turnover of the Na⁺/K⁺pump and the opening of Cl⁻ and K⁺channels are also necessary, the latter to counteract associated cell swelling, to permit serosal exit of Cl⁻ taken up from the lumen, and to dissipate the added uptake of K⁺through the pump.

Diagnostic Approach

The diagnostic approach to CDDs is a multistep process that includes the careful evaluation of the history and clinical data, results of common laboratory, and instrumental procedures and molecular analysis (Fig. 36.2). Positive family history of early onset chronic diarrhea, polyhydramnios, and/or dilated

bowel loops at ultrasound examination during pregnancy are highly suggestive of CDDs. The main symptom is chronic diarrhea (lasting longer than 30 days). In the diagnostic approach, it is important to take into account that infections and food allergy are the most common cause of diarrhea also at this particular age [4], and that these conditions together with malformations of gastrointestinal tract, should be considered as primary diagnostic hypotheses in a infant with chronic diarrhea [4]. However, in all cases of chronic diarrhea starting in the first weeks of life, the presence of a congenital disorder of intestinal electrolyte transport should be excluded. A fundamental step in the diagnostic process is the identification of an osmotic or secretory mechanism leading to diarrhea. In osmotic diarrhea, unabsorbed luminal substances are responsible for accumulation of fluids in intestinal lumen and diarrhea significantly improves during fasting, whereas in secretory diarrhea, fluids are actively secreted in the intestinal lumen and diarrhea continues dur-

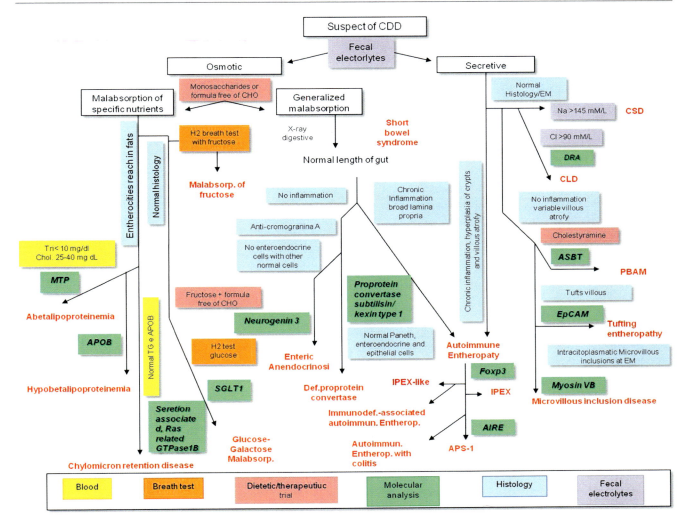

Fig. 36.2 Indications for an integrated diagnostic approach to the main forms of CDDs. The diagnostic approach is a multistep process that includes the evaluation of anamnesis and clinical data, results of common laboratory and instrumental procedures and molecular analysis. The fundamental step in the diagnostic process of CDDs is the identification of an osmotic or secretory mechanism leading to diarrhea. Moreover, the determination of stool electrolyte concentration and fecal ion gap is important to discriminate the two mechanisms responsible for CDDs. The next step is laboratory investigation includes blood gas, blood glucose, ammonium, albumin, triglycerides, and cholesterol, aminoaciduria and the search of reducing substances in the stools, stea-

tocrit, and sweat test. Finally, intestinal biopsy with histologic examination is crucial for the diagnosis of most CDDs. Molecular analysis, when available, is important and could limit invasive procedures CDD congenital diarrheal disorder, DRA downregulated in adenoma, CLD congenital chloride diarrhea, ASBT apical sodium-dependent bile acid transporter, EpCAM epithelial cell adhesion molecule, PBAM peripheral blood adherent monocyte, IPEX immune dysregulation, polyendocrinopathy, enteropathy, X-linked, MTP media transfer protocol, APOB apolipoprotein B, SGL2 sodium-glucose transport, AIRE autoimmune regulator

ing fasting [5]. Furthermore, the determination of stool electrolyte concentration and fecal ion gap is important to discriminate the two mechanisms responsible for CDDs (Fig. 36.1). If ion gap is > 50 fecal, osmolarity derived from ingested osmotically active nutrient or not measured ion (i.e., Cl⁻, Mg^{2+}…). In contrast, a low osmotic gap (<50) is typically observed in secretory diarrhea. A direct measurement of Na^+ and Cl^- concentration in the stool may clearly suggest a diagnosis of congenital sodium diarrhea (CSD) or chloride losing diarrhea (CLD), respectively [5]. When an osmotic mechanism is suspected, the next step of laboratory

investigation includes blood gas, blood glucose, ammonium, albumin, triglycerides and cholesterol, aminoaciduria and the search of reducing substances in the stools, steatocrit, and sweat test (Fig. 36.2). CF is suggested by the presence of steatorrhea and confirmed by a positive sweat test. On the other hand, signs of inflammation in children with secretory diarrhea and familiar history of chronic diarrhea justify the suspect of a familial diarrhea syndrome (FDS). Recent availability of molecular analysis for many of these conditions has progressively limited the need for invasive procedures (Fig. 36.2).

Congenital Chloride Diarrhea

CLD (OMIM 214700) is caused by a mutation in the solute carrier family 26 member 3 *(SLC26A3)* gene, and it is responsible for a life-long watery diarrhea with high fecal Cl^- concentration [6]. The gene, located on chromosome 7.q31, encodes for a transmembrane protein that takes part in gut $Cl^-/NaHCO_3^-$ exchange (Fig. 36.2) [7]. The *SLC26A3* is located close to the gene encoding for the cystic fibrosis transmembrane conductance regulator *(CFTR)*, raising a possibility of *CFTR* modulation in the pathogenesis of CLD [8]. The protein encoded by *SLC26A3* gene has a C-terminal domain, STAS (sulfate transporter and antisigma factor antagonist), that ensures the correct location of the protein on the apical membrane of enterocytes. Mutations determine transporter mistrafficking and cytosol retention [9]. The STAS domain also interacts with the R-domain of the *CFTR*, and it is required for *CFTR* activation. Studies have shown that deglycosylation of HA-SLC26A3 may contribute to the pathogenesis of diarrhea associated with congenital disorder of glycosylation (CDG) because oligosaccharides protect HA-SLC26A3 from proteolytic digestion enzymes in the intestine [10]. The gene *SLC26A3* has also extraintestinal expression: it is expressed in sweat glands, the male reproductive tract, and kidney, while it is downregulated in human colon adenomas and adenocarcinomas [11–13].

The majority of the *SLC26A3* mutations are single-nucleotide substitutions (nonsense, frameshift, and missense), while additional mutations as deletions/insertions are minor. There is no evidence of a correlation between genotype and phenotype. It has been demonstrated that an identical genetic background of CLD may show different clinical course [14] or different responses to therapy [15].

Countries with a highest incidence are Finland (1:35,000), Poland (1:200,000), Kuwait, and Saudi Arabia [16]. In Arabian countries, the high incidence is mostly due to consanguineous marriages [16]. There is a single mutation in the above-mentioned ethnic groups: in Finns, the p.V317del mutation affects up to 90 % of CLD alleles; in Saudi Arabians and Kuwaitis, pG187X is present in more than 90 % of altered chromosomes; in Poles, 50 % of CLD alleles carry the p.1675dup [6].

The main clinical symptom is lifelong watery diarrhea with high Cl^- content and low pH [1]. If not treated, diarrhea leads to dehydration, metabolic alkalosis, hyponatremia, hypokalemia, hypochloremia, and failure to thrive. Because of the intrauterine onset of diarrhea, CLD pregnancies are characterized by polyhydramnios, and the newborn could be mild premature [16, 17]. Postnatally, CLD patients present prominent abdominal distention and dehydration [16, 18].

Suspect of CLD in pregnant women arises with maternal polyhydramnios, lack of meconium, and images of distended loops of ileum. These aspects, evidenced by ultrasonography, are an indication of intrauterine onset of diarrhea. The abdomen is usually large and distended, and intestinal contractions are visible. Loops of ileum and colon are dilated with air and fluid, and ascites is often present. Hyperbilirubinemia is common and is caused in part by the dehydration. It is worth remembering that excessive volume and salt depletion reduce the amount of diarrhea and may result in a low fecal Cl^- of even 40 mmol/L such as a stool dilution by urine [16]. After correction of electrolyte homeostasis by salt substitution, the next thing to do is measuring Cl^- on a stool sample, possibly obtained with a soft catheter to avoid urine contamination. A fecal $Cl^->90$ mmol/L confirms the diagnosis in most cases and leads to molecular analysis of *SLC26A3*. Untreated patients show retarded growth and development, with mental and psychomotor delay.

The main therapeutic approach is based on substitutive therapy with NaCl/KCl (see Table 36.1) [19]. Therapy with the short-chain fatty acid butyrate is also beneficial in patients affected by CLD [20, 21]. Butyrate could reduce mistrafficking or misfolding of DRA and may enhance gene expression through the activation of a region crucial for high-level transcription. Butyrate is also able to modulate transepithelial ion transport through the stimulation of Na^+/H^+ exchangers 2 (NHE2) and 3 (NHE3) activity and inhibition of Cl^- secretion by limiting the action of the cotransporter Na–K–2Cl (encoded by NKCC1) on enterocyte basolateral membrane. In fact, treatment with oral butyrate (100 mg/kg/day) allows a progressive reduction to normal in the number of bowel movements and stool volume, an improvement in stool consistency, and a reduction of fecal incontinence episodes [15]. The effect of butyrate on stool pattern is evident within the first 48 h and remains stable during the following days of treatment. Depending on genotype, the response to butyrate may vary, and this explains the different benefits on the basis of ethnicity [15]. Because missense and deletion mutations allow the expression of *SLC26A3* at membrane level, a full response to butyrate (defined by a concomitant significant reduction of Na^+ and Cl^- fecal losses and improvement in stool pattern) is observed only in patients with these types of mutation. On the contrary, a partial response is to be expected in patients with nonsense or splicing mutations [15].

Long-term prognosis of CLD patients is generally favorable. All of the patients treated adequately reach adult life because oral salt substitution with NaCl and KCl allows normal growth and development [17, 19]. Complications such as intestinal inflammation, renal disease, hyperuricemia, inguinal hernias, spermatoceles, and male subfertility are possible [17, 19]. Untreated or poorly treated disease is associated with impaired renal function and nephrocalcinosis, and even with end-stage renal disease [12].

Table 36.1 Therapeutic approach to a child with congenital chloride diarrhea

Treatment of acute dehydration

1. Initial treatment of fluid depletion (over 6–8 h)
IV infusion of 0.9 % NaCl solution, NO fluids containing bicarbonate
120–500 mL/day for children under 7 years
500–1000 mL/day for children over 7 years

2. Maintenance therapy (over 24 h)
Intravenous 5 % glucose
100 mL pro kg (children weight 10 kg)
+50 mL pro kg for each additional kg (children weight between 11 and 20 kg)
+20 mL pro kg for each additional kg (children weight 20 kg)
For adult patients: 2000–2500 mL/day
NaCl 20 mmol/L added
KCl maintenance need+calculated K^+ depletion added (50 mmol/L)
If severe hypokalemia, higher KCl doses of even 70 (−100) mmol/L

3. Replacement of ongoing losses for diarrhea (0.9 % NaCl and, if necessary, KCl)

Salt substitutive therapy in stable clinical condition

	Small children (0–3 years)	*Older children*	*Adolescents and adults*
NaCl	0.7 % (7 g/L; 120 mmol/L)[a]	1.8 % (18 g/L; 308 mmol/L)	Equal molar ratios of NaCl and KCl
KCl	0.3 % (3 g/L; 40 mmol/L)[a]	1.9 % (19 g/L; 255 mmol/L)	Equal molar ratios of NaCl and KCl
Concentration of Cl−	160 mmol/L	563 mmol/L	–
Need for Cl−	6–8 mmol/kg/day	3–4 mmol/kg/day	3–4 mmol/kg/day
Administration	Intravenous[b]/Oral	Oral	Oral
Salt dosage	Ready-made solution	Ready-made solution	Dose bags
Doses per day	3–4	2–3	2–3

Pharmacological treatment

Oral sodium butyrate, 100 mg/kg/day, divided in two doses (particularly useful in patients with missense or deletion mutations)

[a] If a tendency to hyperkalemia: 0.9 % NaCl (9 g/L; 154 mmol/L) and 0.2 % KCl (2 g/L; 27 mmol/L)

[b] Intravenous therapy is used for infants until the shift to peroral fluid is possible. During intravenous therapy, the need for additional fluid is 100–120 mL/day (stool volume) which can be taken orally

Congenital Sodium Diarrhea

CSD (OMIM 270420) is a rare inherited disorder, characterized by severe diarrhea since birth, with metabolic acidosis, dehydration, and hyponatremia due to massive fecal losses of Na^+ [22]. Gene-inactivating mutations of the apical membrane NHEs are candidates for this disorder, but the pathogenesis of CSD remains elusive. Probably, CSD is not the result of a single mutation in a specific gene.

A diagnosis of CDS is made on the findings of a life-threatening secretory diarrhea, with voluminous alkaline stools (pH > 7.5), containing high concentration of Na^+ (> 70 mmol/L), hyponatremia (Na^+ < 130 mmol/L), and metabolic acidosis. There is no evidence of primary structural abnormalities in the intestinal epithelium at light- and/or electron-microscopic examinations, neither of anatomic anomalies in the gastrointestinal tract at radiological examinations. Laboratory parameters for chronic infections or autoimmune disease are by definition negative [22].

The syndromic form of CSD, which differs from classic CSD by loss-of-function mutations in SPINT2, is characterized by choanal or anal atresia, hypertelorism and corneal erosions, double kidney, cleft palate, and digital anomalies [23]. SPINT2, also known as placental bikunin and hepatocyte growth factor activator inhibitor type 2 (HAI-2), has been shown to be a potent inhibitor of a number of serine proteases, such as pancreatic trypsin, plasmin, kallikrein, and hepatocyte growth factor activator in vitro. SPINT2 mutations can affect proteolytic activity in the functional regulation of intestinal epithelial absorption or secretion of sodium. Possible targets include the membrane-bound extracellular serine proteases, the channel-activating proteases (CAP)/prostasin (MIM 600823) and TMPRSS2 (MIM 602060), and the intracellular protease furin, all involved in regulation of epithelial sodium channel (ENaC) activity [23]. The consequences of alterations in SPINT2 function on Na^+ intestinal absorption and human development in syndromic CSD remain to be elucidated. CSD treatment consists of replacement of lost ions and parenteral nutrition in order to acquire adequate caloric and fluid intake.

Familial Diarrhea Syndrome

A new condition has been described in 32 members of a Norwegian family [24]. FDS is characterized by early onset chronic diarrhea, associated to meteorism, abdominal pain, dysmotility, and inflammatory bowel disease [24]. All affected members show a heterozygous missense mutation in Guanylate cyclase 2C (GUCY2C) gene, c.2519G → T (p.Ser840Ile). GUCY2C encodes for an intestinal guanylate cyclase receptor for the endogenous peptides uroguanylin/ guanylin and for heat-stable enterotoxins that plays an important role in pathogenesis of acute secretory diarrhea (see Chap. 15 "Bacterial Infections"). It has been demonstrated that the basal GC-C enzyme activity, cellular cyclic guanosine monophosphate (cGMP) levels, and affinities of ligands are similar in cells expressing the wild receptor or the mutant one. However, the mutant receptor is activated by heat-stable enterotoxin, uroguanylin, and guanylin to a greater extent than the wild receptor. A missense mutation leads to a gain of function increasing ligand-mediated activation of GC-C and intracellular cGMP levels. cGMP activates protein kinase GII, leading to a phosphorylation of the CFTR channel [25]. This activation leads to an efflux of Cl^- (or HCO_3^- in the duodenum) and water into the intestinal lumen, with a reduced Na^+ absorption [26] due to inhibition of the Na^+/H^+ exchanger 3 (NHE3) [27].

Cystic Fibrosis

CF (CF; OMIM 219700) is an autosomal recessive disorder due to a dysfunction of Cl^- channel (CFTR) in the apical surface of epithelial cells. Because of the different locations of CFTR, CF is characterized by several and various symptoms, and it is the main cause of exocrine pancreatic insufficiency in childhood. Prevalence of CF is 1/3500 and occurs with greater frequency in populations of North America, Northern Europe, Australia, and New Zealand [28]. The pathophysiologic basis of CF is characterized by a mutation of CFTR gene, located on chromosome 7, that determines loss of function of CFTR (Fig. 36.3). The CFTR protein is a member of the ATP-binding cassette (ABC) transporter superfamily. This membrane protein consists of two membrane-spanning domains, two nucleotide-binding domains (NBDs), and a regulatory domain, which controls channel activity, and it functions as a cyclic adenosine monophosphate (cAMP)-dependent chloride channel. CFTR is largely expressed in epithelial cells of the airways, in gastrointestinal tract, including the pancreas and the biliary system. More than 1700 different mutations in the CFTR gene were identified, but the most frequent mutation is the deletion of a single phenylalanine residue at amino acid 508 (ΔF508) [29]. Because of the large number of mutations, it is very difficult to establish a clear correlation between genotype and phenotype. The most serious mutations are always associated with pancreatic failure. Some individuals with polymorphisms of both CFTR genes have mild CF manifestations [29].

The loss of function of CFTR determines the inability to secrete NaCl in the respiratory tract. The small amount of water present on the surface of the mucous membrane is insufficient to hydrate secretions that become more viscous and elastic, resulting in a slowing of mucociliary clearance and airway obstruction. CFTR dysfunction can also make PH more acid in respiratory tract. In the normal pancreas, the duct cell chloride secretion via CFTR increases duct luminal chloride concentration. Cl lumen levels are important because it will be exchanged with intracellular HCO_3^-. This mechanism results in more viscous pancreatic secretions. On the contrary, since the function of sweat glands ductal cells is to absorb chloride, rather than secrete it, the salts are not recovered from primitive sweat isotonic, but are transported to the skin surface, and this makes the concentration of chloride and salts in the sweat very high. Primarily, this principle is based on the most important CF diagnostic test.

CF has a wide heterogeneity of clinical manifestations related to the high number of mutations and environmental factors. Pulmonary and gastrointestinal symptoms are the most common. Chronic infection characterized the expression of CF in the airways and is determined by the inability to quickly eliminate microorganisms inhaled, resulting in colonization and inflammatory response in the airway walls. This phenomenon is also determined by the reduction of the secretions antimicrobial activity, resulting in excessive acidity of the fluid surface. Cough is the most common symptom of pulmonary involvement, dry and hacking at first, then loose and productive, usually with purulent expectorated mucus [30]. Gastrointestinal involvement consists in two different clinical entities: meconium ileus and distal intestinal obstruction syndrome (DIOS), both due to an impaired electrolyte and fluid secretion that causes an inspissation of intestinal contents and consequent intestinal obstruction, in combination with the known impaired intestinal motility. Classically, patients present fat maldigestion and malabsorption that can be directly attributable to the reduced secretion of lipase/colipase from the exocrine pancreas. Liver disease secondary to cholestasis is present in 30 % of patients, and it is responsible for a variety of biliary tract and hepatic complications. Clinical manifestations of liver involvement are characterized by jaundice, ascites, hematemesis from esophageal varices, and signs of hypersplenism and hepatomegaly with steatosis [31]. Male sterility is a constant feature (Table 36.2).

The diagnosis of CF is based on the positive result of the sweat test, in combination with one or more of the following: (i) typical chronic obstructive pulmonary disease, (ii) documented chronic pancreatic insufficiency, and (iii) posi-

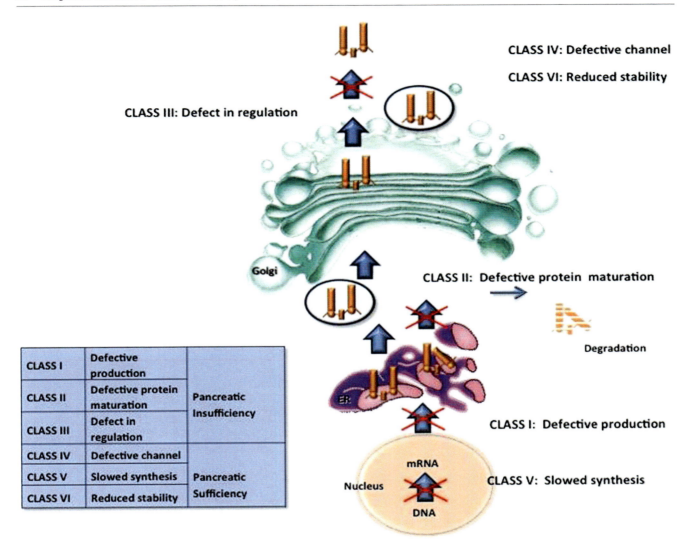

Fig. 36.3 Synthesis of *CFTR* and classes of mutation in cystic fibrosis. *CFTR* gene encodes for a protein that regulate Cl⁻ transport. *CFTR* is located at membrane level of secretive cells in lungs, gastrointestinal tract, liver, pancreas, and reproductive system. Mutation of class I is related to the production of the protein: Generally, the protein is not produced at all or in very small quantities. Class II mutations prevent the maturation of protein. In class III and IV mutations, protein is produced, but works incorrectly. Class V mutations allow a slow production of a small quantities of a working protein. Currently, the effects on clinical outcomes are not clear for all mutation, but a correlation between class mutation and pancreatic involvement is known: Classes of mutation I, II, and III are generally associated with pancreatic insufficiency, and classes IV and V are associated with pancreatic sufficiency

tive family history. Sweat test, which is considered the gold standard in the diagnosis of CF, is based on the determination of Na⁺ and Cl⁻ concentration in sweat collected after local stimulation with pilocarpine. Levels of <35 mmol/L and >60 mmol/L are considered normal and pathologic levels, respectively. Between 35 and 60 mmol/L results are considered borderline. Although the sweat test allows to make a diagnosis when associated with at least another condition, some mutations are known that are associated with negative sweat test [32, 33]. Generally, sweat tests are not performed in subjects younger than 2 weeks of age and weighs less than 3 kg. There are often technical problems while performing the test in very small infants, and there may be a greater risk of complications or obtaining insufficient sweat. The test is contraindicated in babies younger than 48 h of age because high concentrations of sweat electrolytes can be found on the first day of life. If the patient is acutely unwell, dehydrated, oedematous, or receiving corticosteroids, the test should be delayed [32].

Another important diagnostic test is the search for genetic mutations in the *CFTR* gene. Several commercial laboratories test for 30–96 of the most common *CFTR* mutations. This testing identifies ≥90 % of individuals who carry 2 CF mutations. This test is used to confirm but not to exclude

Table 36.2 Main clinical features of cystic fibrosis

Chronic respiratory disease
Persistent colonization/infection by typical pathogens *(Staphylococcus aureus, non-typeable Haemophilus influenzae, Pseudomonas aeruginosa, Burkholderia cepacia)*
Chronic cough and sputum production
Persistent abnormalities on chest radiographs (bronchiectasis, atelectasis, infiltrates, hyperexpansion)
Airways obstruction characterized by bronchospasm and air trapping
Nasal polyps and sinus abnormalities evaluable at radiographs or CT
Digital clubbing
Gastrointestinal and nutritional involvement
Intestine: meconium ileus, distal intestinal obstruction syndrome (DIOS), rectal prolapse
Pancreas: pancreatic insufficiency, recurrent pancreatitis
Liver: chronic liver disease characterized by clinical or histological evidence of focal biliary cirrhosis or multilobular cirrhosis
Nutrition: protein–calorie malnutrition, hypoproteinemia and edema, complications secondary to a fat-soluble vitamins deficiency
Salt wasting syndrome:
Acute salt depletion, chronic metabolic alkalosis
Urogenital abnormalities in male determining obstructive azoospermia

dubious diagnosis, because a lot of mutations have not yet been identified.

Measurement of the potential difference across nasal epithelium is also used as a diagnostic test. This test is based on the demonstration of changes in chloride secretion by epithelial cells, after stimulation with amiloride, as based on the measurement of nasal potentials. Patients with CF have different potential values compared to the healthy population, due to the absence of functional *CFTR* channels. Another test is the assessment of pancreatic function. Exocrine pancreatic dysfunction is clinically apparent in many patients. Documentation is desirable if there are questions about the functional status of the pancreas. This assessment is usually made through evaluation of steatorrhea, fecal chymotrypsin, fecal elastase, and the duodenal assay after secretin or pancreozymin stimulation [34].

With newborn screening, diagnosis is often made prior to obvious clinical manifestations such as failure to thrive and chronic cough. Screening consists in a combination of immunoreactive trypsinogen results and limited DNA testing on blood spots, which are then coupled with confirmatory sweat analysis, and it is $\approx 95\%$ sensitive [35].

The treatment of CF is extremely complex and articulate. It is based on the routine symptomatic therapies and new therapies still in the experimental phase: correction of gene mutation, correction of the altered protein, and activation of the alternative channels to *CFTR*.

Respiratory System Therapy of bronchial obstruction is based on physiotherapy which maintains adequate bronchial toilet and on aerosol therapy that has the purpose of liquefying secretions. Anti-inflammatory therapy has given numerous benefits, despite the contraindications [36]. During exacerbations, an increase of physiotherapy in combination with antibiotic therapy is indicated. Antibiotic therapy should be guided by the results of sputum culture, preferably using intravenous drugs at high doses [37, 38].

Gastrointestinal Tract Pancreatic insufficiency is generally treated with substitution therapy by administration of pancreatic extracts formulated into microspheres gastroresistant. Therapy of meconium ileus and DIOS should be as conservative as possible, with the use of high-volume enemas and subsequently enema with gastrografin, in association with the rehydration therapy. Surgical therapy is reserved for cases of medical therapy failure.

Acknowledgment Grant from Agenzia Italiana del Farmaco, AIFA (MRAR08W002), is gratefully acknowledged.

References

1. Berni Canani R, Cirillo P, Terrin G. Chronic and intractable diarrhea. In: Guandalini S, editor. Essential pediatric gastroenterology hepatology, and nutrition. Chicago: McGraw-Hill Mediacla Publishing Division; 2005. pp. 25–47.
2. Field M. Intestinal ion transport and the pathophysiology of diarrhea. J Clin Invest. 2003;111:931–43.
3. Alrefai WA, Tyagi S, Nazir TM, Barakat J, Anwar SS, Hadjiagapiou C, et al. Human intestinal anion exchanger isoforms: expression, distribution, and membrane localization. Biochim Biophys Acta. 2001;1511:17–27.
4. Ruemmele FM. Chronic enteropathy: molecular basis. Gastrointestinal disorders. Nestlè Nutr Workshop Ser Pediatr Program. 2007;59:73–88.
5. Berni Canani R, Terrin G. Recent progress in congenital diarrheal disorders. Curr Gastroenterol Rep. 2011;13:257–64.
6. Makela S, Kere J, Holmberg C, Höglund P. SLC26A3 mutations in congenital chloride diarrhea. Hum Mutat. 2002;20:425–38.
7. Dorwart MR, Shcheynikov N, Yang D, Muallem S. The solute carrier 26 family of proteins in epithelial ion transport. Physiology (Bethesda). 2008;23:104–14.
8. Ko SB, Zeng W, Dorwart MR, Luo X, Kim KH, Millen L, et al. Gating of CFTR by the STAS domain of SLC26 transporters. Nat Cell Biol. 2004;6:343–50.
9. Dorwart MR, Shcheynikov N, Baker JM, Forman-Kay JD, Muallem S, Thomas PJ. Congenital chloride losing diarrhea causing mutations in the STAS domain result in misfolding and mistrafficking of SLC26A3. J Biol Chem. 2008;283:8711–22.
10. Hayashi H, Yamashita Y. Role of N-glycosylation in cell surface expression and protection against proteolysis of the intestinal anion exchanger SLC26A3. Am J Physiol Cell Physiol. 2012;302:C781–95.
11. Hihnala S, Kujala M, Toppari J, Kere J, Holmberg C, Höglund P. Expression of SLC26A3, CFTR and NHE3 in the human male reproductive tract: role in male subfertility caused by congenital chloride diarrhea. Mol Hum Reprod. 2006;12:107–11.
12. Wedenoja S, Ormala T, Berg UB, Halling SF, Jalanko H, Karikoski R, et al. The impact of sodium chloride and volume depletion in the chronic kidney disease of congenital chloride diarrhea. Kidney Int. 2008;74:1085–93.

13. Jacob P, Rossmann H, Lamprecht G, Kretz A, Neff C, Lin-Wu E, et al. Down-regulated in adenoma mediates apical Cl⁻/HCO$_3$-exchange in rabbit, rat, and human duodenum. Gastroenterology 2002;122:709–24.

14. Höglund P, Holmberg C, Sherman P, Kere J. Distinct outcomes of chloride diarrhea in two siblings with identical genetic background of the disease: implications for early diagnosis and treatment. Gut 2001;48:724–7.

15. Berni Canani R, Terrin G, Elce A, Pezzella V, Heinz-Erian P, Pedrolli A, et al. Genotype-dependency of butyrate efficacy in children with congenital chloride diarrhea. Orphanet J Rare Dis. 2013;8:194.

16. Terrin G, Tomaiuolo R, Passariello A, Elce A, Amato F, Di Costanzo M, et al. Congenital diarrheal disorders: updated diagnostic approach. Int J Mol Sci. 2012;13:4168–85.

17. Hihnala S, Höglund P, Lammi L, Kokkonen J, Ormälä T, Holmberg C. Long-term clinical outcome in patients with congenital chloride diarrhea. J Pediatr Gastroenterol Nutr. 2006;42:369–75.

18. Berni Canani R, Terrin G, Cardillo G, Tomaiuolo R, Castaldo G. Congenital diarrheal disorders: improved understanding of gene defects is leading to advances in intestinal physiology and clinical management. J Pediatr Gastroenterol Nutr. 2010;50:360–6.

19. Wedenoja S, Hoglund P, Holmberg C. Review article: the clinical management of congenital chloride diarrhea. Aliment Pharmacol Ther. 2010;31:477–85.

20. Berni Canani R, Terrin G, Cirillo P, Castaldo G, Salvatore F, Cardillo G, et al. Butyrate as an effective treatment of congenital chloride diarrhea. Gastroenterology 2004;127:630–4.

21. Wedenoja S, Holmberg C, Höglund P. Oral butyrate in treatment of congenital chloride diarrhea. Am J Gastroenterol. 2008;103:252–4.

22. Müller T, Wijmenga C, Phillips AD, Janecke A, Houwen RH, Fischer H, et al. Congenital sodium diarrhea is an autosomal recessive disorder of sodium/proton exchange but unrelated to known candidate genes. Gastroenterology 2000;119:1506–13.

23. Heinz-Erian P, Müller T, Krabichler B, Schranz M, Becker C, Rüschendorf F, et al. Mutations in SPINT2 cause a syndromic form of congenital sodium diarrhea. Am J Hum Genet. 2009;84:188–96.

24. Fiskerstrand T, Arshad N, Haukanes BI, Tronstad RR, Pham KD, Johansson S, et al. Familial diarrhea syndrome caused by an activating GUCY2C mutation. N Engl J Med. 2012. 26;366:1586–95.

25. Basu N, Arshad N, Visweswariah SS. Receptor guanylyl cyclase C (GC-C): regulation and signal transduction. Mol Cell Biochem. 2010;334:67–80.

26. Guandalini S, Migliavacca M, de Campora E, Fasano A. Cyclic GMP effects on nutrient and electrolyte transport in rabbit ileum. Gastroenterology 1982;83:15–21.

27. Li C, Naren AP. CFTR chloride channel in the apical compartments: spatiotemporal coupling to its interacting partners. Integr Biol (Camb). 2010;2:161–77.

28. O'Sullivan BP, Freedman SD. Cystic fibrosis. Lancet 2009;373:1891–902.

29. Cystic Fibrosis Mutation Database 2011. www.genet.sickkids.on.ca/cftr.

30. Donaldson SH, Bennett WD, Zeman KL, Knowles MR, Tarran R, Boucher RC. Mucus clearance and lung function in cystic fibrosis with hypertonic saline. N Engl J Med. 2006;354:241–50.

31. Moyer K, Balistreri W. Hepatobiliary disease in patients with cystic fibrosis. Curr Opin Gastroenterol. 2009;25:272–8.

32. LeGrys VA, Yankaskas JR, Quittell LM, Marshall BC, Mogayzel PJ Jr, Cystic Fibrosis Foundation. Diagnostic sweat testing: the cystic fibrosis foundation guidelines. J Pediatr. 2007;151:85–9.

33. Mishra A, Greaves R, Smith K, Carlin JB, Wootton A, Stirling R. Diagnosis of cystic fibrosis by sweat testing: age-specific reference intervals. J Pediatr. 2008;153:758–63 (eds.2008.04.067).

34. Dequeker E, Stuhrmann M, Morris MA, Casals T, Castellani C, Claustres M, et al. Best practice guidelines for molecular genetic diagnosis of cystic fibrosis and CFTR-related disorders–updated European recommendations. Eur J Hum Genet. 2009;17:51–65. doi:10.1038/ejhg.2008.136.

35. Ross LF. Newborn screening for cystic fibrosis: a lesson in public health disparities. J Pediatr. 2008;153:308–13.

36. Ren CL, Pasta DJ, Rasouliyan L, Wagener JS, Konstan MW, Morgan WJ, et al. Relationship between inhaled corticosteroid therapy and rate of lung function decline in children with cystic fibrosis. J Pediatr. 2008;153:746–51.

37. Flume PA, Robinson KA, O'Sullivan BP, Goss CH, Mogayzel PJ Jr., Willey-Courand DB, et al. Cystic fibrosis pulmonary guidelines: chronic medications for maintenance of lung health. Am J Respir Crit Care Med. 2007;176:957–69.

38. Flume PA, Robinson KA, O'Sullivan BP, Finder JD, Vender RL, Willey-Courand DB, et al. Cystic fibrosis pulmonary guidelines: airway clearance therapies. Respir Care. 2009;54:522–37.

Immunodeficiency Disorders Resulting in Malabsorption

37

Margherita Di Costanzo, Marinita Morelli, Monica Malamisura,
Maria Giovanna Puoti and Roberto Berni Canani

Introduction

Primary immunodeficiencies are a group of at least 200 disorders, often inherited, that are caused by intrinsic defects in the immune system. The defects can affect humoral (B cell) immunity, cellular (T cell) immunity, both T and B cell immunity, and innate immunity. Gastrointestinal (GI) disorders are present in 5–50 % of patients with primary immunodeficiencies. This is in part because the gut is the largest lymphoid organ in the body, containing the majority of lymphocytes and producing large amounts of immunoglobulin (Ig). The mucosal immune system is uniquely equipped to manage its constant exposure to viruses, parasites, and bacterial antigens, all of which are in close proximity to a large reservoir of lymphocytes, macrophages, and dendritic cells. Dysfunction of the regulatory mechanisms maintaining this balance between active immunity and tolerance in the gut may lead to mucosal inflammation and damage and GI diseases. Therefore, it is not surprising that GI disorders are common, and often the initial presenting manifestations, in patients with primary immunodeficiencies (Table 37.1). In pediatric patients, GI manifestations of primary immunodeficiencies are mainly induced by infection, inflammation, or autoimmunity. In adult patients, malignancy could be a frequent additional condition. These manifestations mimic classic forms of disease (in the absence of immunodeficiency) such as celiac disease, food allergy, or inflammatory bowel disease, but they are often unresponsive to conventional therapies.

R. Berni Canani (✉)
European Laboratory for the Investigation of Food Induced Diseases,
and CEINGE Advanced Biotechnologies, University of Naples
"Federico II", Via S. Pansini 5,
80131 Naples, Italy
e-mail: berni@unina.it

M. Di Costanzo · M. Morelli · M. Malamisura · M. G. Puoti ·
R. Berni Canani
Department of Translational Medical Science—Section of Pediatrics,
University of Naples "Federico II", Naples, Italy

Evaluation of a Child with Suspected Primary Immunodeficiency

Because GI disease may be the first presentation of an underlying immunodeficiency, it is crucial to consider immunodeficiency in any child with recurrent or chronic severe diarrhea, malabsorption, and failure to thrive that is resistant to conventional treatments. Primary immune deficits are relatively common but likely underdiagnosed. A clinical history of recurrent, opportunistic, or unusual infections, histological features that do not fit the usual pattern of disease, and a poor response to conventional therapy should prompt the pediatrician to pursue further immunologic evaluation. The type of immunodeficiency often influences the nature of infections: bacterial infections indicate B cell deficiencies, fungal or viral infections indicate T cell deficiencies, and T and B cell deficiencies together suggest combined immunodeficiencies. At the same time, routine evaluation of the GI tract is useful for children with immunodeficiency, given the high incidence of GI disease in these patients. Early evaluation and diagnosis can prevent potentially irreversible tissue damage. The child with GI symptoms and suspected immunodeficiency is best approached in stages with the performance of the basic screening tests before continuing on to more advanced testing as necessary. In the majority of cases, a referral to an immunologist is essential. An accurate microbiological analysis of stool samples is mandatory to rule out the presence of common or unusual pathogens. This should be done considering the potential of different diagnostic tools from standard culture to reverse transcription polymerase chain reaction (RT-PCR) analysis. A complete evaluation of quantitative levels of immunoglobulins (IgG, IgA, IgM, and IgE) and blood count should be obtained. Hypogammaglobulinemia can result from protein loss and is excluded by measuring serum albumin and urinary protein levels; enteral loss of protein can be excluded by measurement of stool alpha-1-antitrypsin level (normal values <0.9 mg/g stool). Quantification of IgG subclasses may be helpful in the assessment of an immunodeficiency,

© Springer International Publishing Switzerland 2016
S. Guandalini et al. (eds.), *Textbook of Pediatric Gastroenterology, Hepatology and Nutrition*,
DOI 10.1007/978-3-319-17169-2_37

Table 37.1 Main primary immunodeficiencies and associated gastrointestinal features

Immunodeficiency	Main gastrointestinal manifestations
Selective IgA deficiency	Chronic diarrhea
	Celiac disease
	Nodular lymphoid hyperplasia
Agammaglobulinemia, X-linked or AR	Chronic diarrhea
	Malabsorption
Hyper-IgM syndrome	Chronic diarrhea
	Progressive liver disease
	Sclerosing cholangitis
Common variable immunodeficiency (CVID)	Chronic diarrhea
	Nodular lymphoid hyperplasia
	Flat villous lesions
	IBD-like disease
	Atrophic gastritis
Severe combined immunodeficiency (SCID)	Chronic diarrhea
	Oral candidiasis
	IBD-like disease
Chronic granulomatous disease (CGD)	Granulomatous colitis
	Perianal fistulae
	Hepatic abscess
	Gastric outlet obstruction
	Small-bowel obstruction
	Granulomatous stomatitis
	Oral ulcers
	Esophageal dysmotility
Wiskott–Aldrich syndrome (WAS)	Colitis
	Malabsorption
Immune dysregulation, polyendocrinopathy, enteropathy, X-linked (IPEX) and IPEX-related disorders	Severe enteropathy with watery often bloody diarrhea associated with eosinophilic inflammation
Interleukin-10 and interleukin-10 receptor defects	IBD-like disease with early onset enterocolitis, perianal disease (multiple abscesses and enterocutaneous fistula)
Hermansky–Pudlak syndrome, type 1	Granulomatous colitis

IBD inflammatory bowel disease

especially in IgA deficiency. Ig values increase through adolescence, so comparison with age-matched controls is necessary for correct interpretation. Further evaluation of a humoral defect includes the qualitative aspect of the antibody response, such as IgG titer to measles, tetanus, *Haemophilus influenzae* type b, pneumococcus, and varicella. If the titer is low, vaccinations may be administered, followed by evaluation of postvaccination titers 4–6 weeks later. It is important to underline that children receiving chronic treatment with steroids may have reduced serum Ig levels; however, the antibody response would be preserved in this case. Especially in the presence of blood cells count abnormalities, it is important to ask for a lymphocyte panel to assess the number of lymphocytes and subpopulations (T cells, B cells, CD4$^+$ T cells, and CD8$^+$ T cells), because lymphopenia may occur secondary to excessive loss of the cells into the lumen or through the trapping of cells in the inflamed bowel wall. Severe lymphopenia in an infant (<2000/mm^3) is a critical finding that, if confirmed, should lead to an immediate immune evaluation for severe combined immunodeficiency

(SCID). Thrombocytopenia and small platelet size suggest a diagnosis of Wiskott–Aldrich syndrome (WAS). In all cases, human immunodeficiency virus testing should be performed if there is clinical suspicion based on history or results of the lymphocyte panel.

Depending on the clinical picture and on the results of these initial tests, further step is the study of cellular immune function. The study of lymphocyte proliferation in response to mitogens and antigens provides more definitive data on T cell function. Failure of lymphocytes to respond to mitogens usually indicates severe impairment of T cell function, as in the case of SCID. These tests may not be possible in patients with significant T cell lymphopenia. Steroid therapy may lead to a reduced number of T cells, making interpretation of these tests difficult during therapy; however, response reappears rapidly with cessation of therapy. Advanced testing can be performed to investigate specific disorders. For example, suspicion of chronic granulomatous disease (CGD) should lead to investigation of neutrophil function; this is accomplished with a dihydrorhodamine assay to determine a reduction or absence of phagocytic respiratory burst. Flow cytometric analysis of expression of cell surface and intracellular proteins can help in diagnosing X-linked hyper-IgM (through examination of CD40 ligand), WAS (through examination of WAS protein, WASp), and immune dysfunction, polyendocrinopathy, enteropathy, X-linked syndrome (IPEX; through examination of FOXP3). Quantitative, real-time polymerase chain reaction for T cell receptor excision circles is used in neonatal screening assay for SCID. Genetic testing to identify carrier states or specific mutations can be performed for X-linked agammaglobulinemia (XLA), SCID, and DiGeorge syndrome (Table 37.2). In many cases, the evaluation of GI tract is essential with laboratory tests, radiographic imaging, and intestinal biopsy specimens. It is often helpful to ask the pathologist to review slides when a question of immunodeficiency exists, given some of the unique pathologic findings or lack thereof (e.g., plasma cells) [1].

Table 37.2 Primary immunodeficiencies: main laboratory findings and molecular defects

Immunodeficiency	Laboratory findings	Molecular defect
Selective IgA deficiency	Serum IgA absent or near absent, usually < 10 mg/dL	Gene defect unknown
	Normal IgG and IgM levels although IgG2 subclass deficiency may be present	Defective maturation of B cells into IgA secreting plasma cells
	Impaired specific antibody response in some patients	
Agammaglobulinemia, X-linked or AR	Absent IgM, IgG, and IgA	X-linked (BTK)
	B cells < 1 % of lymphocytes	Autosomal-recessive (μ heavy chain, λ5, Igα, Igβ, BLNK)
	Absent specific antibody response	
Hyper-IgM syndrome	Low IgG and IgA	Mutations in CD40L, CD40, AICDA, UNG
	Normal or increased IgM	
	Normal or increased B cell numbers	
	Impaired specific antibody response	
	Decreased T cell responses in CD40L/CD40 deficiency	
Common variable immuno-deficiency (CVID)	Low IgG and IgA and/or IgM	Mutations in ICOS, CD19, CD20, CD81, TNFRSF13B, TNFRSF13C; mostly unknown
	Absent specific antibody response	
	Normal or decreased B cell numbers	
	Variably decreased T cell responses	
Severe combined immuno-deficiency (SCID)	Decreased serum immunoglobulins	Multiple defects: RAG1/2, JAK3, CD45, CD3 chain, ZAP70, Artemis, ligase 4, Cernunnos, IL-2RG, IL-7Rα, ADA: defects in T and B cells
	Marked diminished/absent T cell, B cell, and NK cell numbers depending on functional deficiency	
	Diminished response to mitogens PHA, ConA, PWM	
Chronic granulomatous Disease (CGD)	Defective oxidative burst in neutrophils by DHR or NBT equivalent	Multiple defects: X linked owing to defects in CYBB encoding the gp91 phox component of NADPH oxidase autosomal recessive owing to defects in NCF1, NCF2, or CYBA defects in components of NADPH oxidase
Interleukin-10 and interleu-kin-10-receptor defects	Pathological response to functional tests using STAT3 and/or TNF-α assays	Mutations in IL-10, IL-10 receptor
Wiskott–Aldrich syndrome (WAS)	Immunoglobulins variable in concentration secondary to accelerated synthesis and catabolism (decreased IgM; normal or slightly low IgG; often increased IgA and IgE);	Mutations in WAS; cytoskeletal defect affecting hematopoietic stem cell derivatives
	Antibody response to polysaccharides decreased	
	Normal B-cell numbers	
	Progressive decrease in T-cell numbers with abnormal lymphocyte responses to anti-CD3	
	Platelet numbers are reduced and small in size	
Hermansky–Pudlak syn-drome, type 1	Normal platelet count	Mutation in the HPS1 gene on chromosome 10q23 that forms part of BLOC-3
	Prolonged bleeding time with abnormal platelet function assays	

ADA adenosine deaminase, *AICDA* activation-induced cytidine deaminase, *AR* autosomal recessive, *BLNK* B cell linker protein, *BLOC-3* biogenesis of lysosome-related organelles complex-3, *BTK* Bruton tyrosine kinase, *CYBA* cytochrome b α subunit, *CYBB* cytochrome b β subunit, *DHR* dihydrorhodamine, *ICOS* inducible costimulator, *JAK3* Janus activating kinase 3, *NADPH* nicotinamide adenine dinucleotide phosphate, *NCF* neutrophil cytosolic factor, *NF-κB* nuclear factor-kB, *PHA* phytohemagglutinin, *PWM* pokeweed mitogen, *RAG* recombinase activating gene, *TBX1* T-box 1, *TNFRSF* TNF-receptor superfamily, *UNG* uracil DNA glycosylase, *STAT3* signal transducer and activator of transcription-3, *TNF-α* tumor necrosis factor-α, *NBT* nitroblue tetrazolium

Predominant B-Cell (Antibody) Deficiency

Selective Ig A Deficiency

Selective IgA deficiency is the most common primary immunodeficiency; it is defined as decreased serum level of IgA in the presence of other normal Ig isotypes, T-cell immunity, and natural killer activity. The worldwide incidence of IgA deficiency differs by ethnic background, in Caucasians being much higher than that in Asians, with a prevalence of around 1:3000 in US [2]. IgA is the key Ig in the respiratory and GI tracts, which provide the most intimate interface between the environment and self [3]. The manifestations are variable in IgA deficiency patients: from asymptomatic condition (in up to 90 % of subjects) to recurrent infections of the respiratory (particularly *H. influenzae* and *Streptococcus pneumonia*) and GI tracts, autoimmune diseases, allergies, and malignancies. Autoimmune diseases are a frequent finding in IgA deficiency, mainly autoimmune cytopenias, juvenile rheumatoid arthritis, thyroiditis, systemic lupus erythematosus, and celiac disease. IgA deficiency sometimes progress to common variable immunodeficiency (CVID); in fact, the diseases often share a common genetic and familial predisposition (IGAD1) [2]. Other related conditions include anaphylactic transfusion reactions; the patients should be screened for anti-IgA antibodies and treated with low or absent IgA blood products if the need for transfusion arises. GI manifestations are frequent in patients with selective IgA deficiency. *Giardia lamblia* infections can occur in these patients, causing bloating, cramping, excessive flatus, and watery diarrhea. The infection can be chronic, despite treatment with metronidazole, resulting in malabsorption with steatorrhea and villus flattening [4]. The degree of mucosal damage is related to the duration of the infection. Diagnosis is made by examining the stool for cysts or trophozoites of *G. lamblia,* or by examination of duodenal aspirates, which can yield more determinate results. The incidence of selective IgA deficiency has been demonstrated to be higher in celiac disease than in the general population, given shared human leukocyte antigen (HLA) haplotypes. Secretory IgA can bind to wheat gluten and gliadin, and the absence of IgA may lead to abnormal processing of these antigens [4]. The symptoms of celiac disease are similar in patients with or without IgA deficiency, the only differentiating feature is that immunohistochemical staining of small-intestinal biopsies reveals an absence of IgA-secreting plasma cells in IgA-deficient patients. Antigliadin IgA, antitissue transglutaminase IgA, and antiendomysial IgA antibodies cannot be used as screening tests for this population, tissue transglutaminase IgG may be a better screening test [4]. Celiac disease associated with IgA deficiency is responsive to gluten withdrawal, failure to respond to a gluten-free diet should lead one to consider CVID.

Nodular lymphoid hyperplasia also is documented in IgA deficiency. Multiple nodules are found in the lamina propria, superficial submucosa of the small intestine, or both, and occasionally can occur in the stomach, large intestine, or rectum. The lesions can be associated with mucosal flattening, causing malabsorption and even obstruction when large. Diagnosis is made by small-bowel endoscopy sometime with the help of contrast barium or MRI studies. Large amounts of IgM-bearing cells can be found in the immunohistochemical staining, possibly as compensation for the absent IgA. These patients may benefit from oral steroid therapy [4]. Rarely, patients with IgA deficiency can develop pernicious anemia, inflammatory bowel disease, lymphomas (usually B cell origin), and gastric carcinomas. The diagnosis is based on the measurement of IgA concentration in serum; normal levels of IgA are dependent by age, ethnicity, gender, and body habits. The international consensus for diagnosing a selective IgA deficiency is a serum level of below 0.07 g/l in individuals over 4 years of age accompanied by normal levels of IgG and IgM [2]. The threshold of 4 years of age is used to avoid premature diagnosis of IgA deficiency which may be transient in younger children due to delayed ontogeny of IgA system after birth [3]. In IgA deficiency, the mainstay of the therapeutic approach is the treatment of associated diseases. If the patient experiences recurrent infections, daily prophylactic antibiotics on a continuous or seasonal intermittent basis may be beneficial [3]. IL-21 or the combination of CD40 L/anti-CD40, IL-4, and IL-10 are potential targets for new therapeutic modalities [2, 5].

X-Linked-Agammaglobulinemia

XLA results from a maturation arrest of pre-B cells with subsequent B cell generation failure, no plasma cell in lymphoid tissues, virtual absence of all classes of Ig, small tonsils, and lymphonodes. They are typically male infants or young children. The incidence is approximately 1 in 100,000 live births. Female carriers can be detected, and prenatal diagnosis of affected or unaffected male fetuses can be accomplished. XLA results from a defect of Bruton's tyrosine kinase (BKT), a member of Tec family protein. It is an intracellular tyrosine-kinase protein, expressed in most of hematopoietic cells: It presents high levels in all B-cells line, but it is not expressed in T cell precursors and natural killer (NK) cells. BKT gene is located on the proximal part of the long arm of the X chromosome. There are about 554 different mutations of BKT gene, but it seems that there is no correlation between mutation location and clinical phenotype. The abnormal BKT induce a maturational arrest of B lymphocytes at the pre-B cell stage and secondary inability to produce antibody after antigen stimulation. A normal number of pre-B cells are found in the bone marrow, but no mature B cells. Peripheral CD19, CD20, and CD23 B cells are usually less than 0.1 %. IgG, IgA, and IgM levels are virtually absent. There is no production of isohemagglutinins or antibody after vaccinations. There are, also, five different autosomal recessive defects that cause agammaglobulinemia [6]. These include: (1) μ (IgM heavy chain deficiency), (2) Ig-α(CD79a9 deficiency, (3) B cell linker adaptor protein (BLNK) deficiency, (4) surrogate light chain (lambda 5 or CD179b) deficiency, (5) leucine-rich repeat containing 8 (LRRC8). All these forms present similar immunological and clinical phenotypes to XLA but are less common. The majority of males with XLA are asymptomatic during the first 4–6 months of life thanks to mother's transmitted antibodies [7]. Then they present severe and repeated infections caused, mainly, by extracellular pyogenic and encapsulated organisms, often gram-positive (such as *S. pneumonia, Staphylococcus Aureus, Neisseria, Haemophilus* or *Mycoplasma*). The infections may interest respiratory, GI, and genitourinary tracts. Systemic infections (septicemia or meningitis) are less common but frequent, as well as osteomyelitis, septic arthritis, cellulitis or skin abscesses. In such cases, we can observe chronic fungal infection or *Pnemocystis jirovecii* pneumonia. Viral infections are, usually, self-limiting except hepatitis or enteroviruses despite a good T-cell response. GI manifestations are less common in XLA compared to other antibody-deficiency syndromes and to CVID. The most frequent GI symptom is chronic diarrhea that is often accompanied by secondary malabsorptive syndrome associated with a protein-losing enteropathy [8]. The main pathogens involved in these infectious diarrheas are *G. lamblia, Salmonella, Campylobacter,* and *Cryptosporidium;* enteroviral infections (such as *Coxsackievirus* and *Echovirus*) are also common and can lead to severe neurologic defects. Sometimes chronic diarrhea is related to small bowel bacterial overgrowth. It is important that GI infection treatments are based on adapted culture methods and adequate prolonged therapy. Cases of malabsorption and bacteremia due to infection of *Helicobacter pylori* and *Campylobacter jejuni* resistant to many antibiotics have been described [9]. Some patients with XLA present small-bowel strictures and transmural intestinal fissures similar to Crohn's disease, without granulomas or plasma cells. XLA patients generally do not develop nodular lymphoid hyperplasia. The disease, occasionally, manifests with different clinical spectrums such as autoimmune diseases or cancer (gastric adenocarcinoma and colorectal cancer). In particular, chronic atrophic gastritis with pernicious anemia is also a common finding that predisposes to gastric adenocarcinoma. In spite of these infections, patients with XLA may not have failure to thrive unless they develop bronchiectasis. The most common cause of death was chronic enteroviral infection [10]. Diagnosis is based on clinical features and typical laboratory results (profound reduction in all classes of Ig and depressed or absent

humoral response to specific antigens, peripheral CD19+ B cell usually <0.1 % with preserved T cell number and function) and, it could be confirmed by genetic mutation analysis [11]. An early diagnosis of XLA with immediate initiation of therapy is crucial for ensuring good outcomes for the affected patients. Delayed diagnosis could lead to long-lasting sequelae such as bronchiectasis, hearing loss, or liver cirrhosis due to chronic hepatitis. XLA treatment consists of replacement IgG therapy (intravenous gammaglobulin, IVGG); either intravenous or subcutaneous. Early IVGG replacement therapy decreases the rates of admission and morbidity for chronic complications, such as bronchiectasis and chronic lung disease, and prevents fatal complications like meningoencephalitis. Appropriate IVGG should be started at 6–8 weeks of age because around 25 % of the XLA patients show clinical symptoms before 4 months of age. Antibiotics treatment for documented or suspected infections is necessary because commercial preparations of IgG could not have adequate titers against uncommon organisms.

Hyper-IgM Syndrome

Hyper-IgM syndromes are a group of rare inherited immunodeficiencies characterized by impairment of Ig isotype switching resulting from defects in the CD40 ligand/CD40 signaling pathway. They are characterized by high levels of IgM associated with low or absent levels of IgG, IgA, and IgE [12]. This "class switch" is critical to host resistance to bacterial infections. There are several mutations that caused hyper-IgM syndrome:

1. X-linked hyper-IgM syndrome is the most common form. This condition could derive from two different gene mutations: One gene encodes the CD40 ligand *(hyper-IgM syndrome type 1 or HIGM1)*. Because the lack of this ligand on T cells, there is no interaction with CD40 on B cells (this interaction is fundamental for Ig class switching and for the formation of memory B lymphocytes). B cells cultured are able to produce not only IgM, but also IgG, IgA, and IgE, this confirms that the defect interests T cells. Mitogen proliferation may be normal, but NK cell and T cell cytotoxicity is frequently impaired. Antigen-specific responses may be decreased or absent. The male with this syndrome present small tonsils, absence of palpable lymph nodes. Neutropenia, thrombocytopenia, and anemia are common. The other gene, located on X-chromosome, is *NEMO* gene, it encodes for a nuclear factor-kappaB (NF-kB) nuclear factor. In male, this form is clinically associated with anhidrotic ectodermal dysplasia with immunodeficiency (EDA-ID), in female it causes incontinentia pigmenti.

2. Autosomal recessive hyper-IgM syndrome. The most common form is caused by defects in the CD40-activated

RNA-editing enzyme, activation-induced cytidinedeaminase, which is required for isotype switching and somatic hypermutation in B cells. The gene involved is activation-induced cytidine deaminase (AICDA) gene located on chromosome 12 (*Hyper-IgM syndrome type 2 or HIGM2*). In this case, B cells cultured are not able to produce all class of Ig, this confirm that there is a real defect of B cell. Other two forms interest: uracil DNA glycosylase gene (UNG) and CD40 gene *(hyper-IgM syndrome type 3 or HIGM3)*.

3. *Hyper-IgM syndrome type 4 or HIGM4 deriving from a yet unidentified gene mutation.*

Distinctive clinical features for these patients allow presumptive recognition of mutation, this is important to choose the best therapy. The range of clinical findings varies, even within the same family. Over 50% of males with HIGM1 develop symptoms by the age of 1 year, and more than 90% are symptomatic by the age of 4 years. The clinical presentation of X-linked hyper-IgM is similar to XLA, with recurrent pyogenic infections such as otitis, sinusitis, pneumonia, or tonsillitis that start in the first 2 years of life. These patients are also susceptible to a variety of intracellular pathogens as mycobacterial species, fungi, and viruses; in about 40% of cases, we found pneumonia by *Pneumocystis jirovecii*. Significant neurologic complications are seen in 10–15% of males with HIGM1. However, in at least one half of affected individuals a specific infectious agent cannot be isolated. GI symptoms include mostly chronic diarrhea and liver involvement. The main pathogens that caused diarrhea are *Cryptosporidium parvum* (the most common), *G. lamblia, Salmonella,* or *Entameba histolytica*. Chronic diarrhea is a frequent complication of HIGM1, occurring in approximately one third of affected males. Recurrent or protracted diarrhea may result from infection with *C. parvum* or other microorganisms; however, in at least 50% of males with recurrent or protracted diarrhea, no infectious agent can be detected. It can cause failure to thrive and weight loss. Neutropenia often causes oral or rectal ulcers and gingivitis or mucosal abscess. Liver disease, a serious complication of HIGM1, historically was observed in more than 80% of affected males by age 20 years. Hepatic involvement presents: cholangiopathy with *Cryptosporidium* in the biliary tree, B and C hepatitis and cytomegalovirus (CMV) infections with a possible evolution in cirrhosis or hepatocellular carcinoma. It can result in disturbed liver increased gamma-glutamyltransferase levels; this alteration can predict a possible development of sclerosing cholangitis with a risk of cholangiocarcinoma. Tumors of the GI tract (carcinoid of the pancreas, glucagonoma) are common life-threatening complications in adolescents and young adults with HIGM1 [13]. Affected males also have an increased risk for lymphoma, particularly Hodgkin's disease associated with *Epstein–Barr* virus infection. Autosomal recessive forms have usually a later onset and present often

autoimmune disorders (such as diabetes mellitus, autoimmune hepatitis, autoimmune thrombocytopenia, and Crohn's disease). Neutropenia is less common. The reported median survival of males with HIGM1 who do not undergo successful allogeneic bone marrow transplantation is less than 25 years. *P. jirovecii* pneumonia in infancy, liver disease, and carcinomas of the liver and GI tract in adolescence or young adulthood are the major causes of death [14]. Laboratory evaluation is fundamental: These patients have low or absent levels of IgG, IgE, and IgA associated to normal or high level of IgM (very high levels of IgM are typical of autosomal recessive form) and IgD. B and T lymphocyte number are usually normal. The diagnosis of HIGM1 is based on a combination of clinical findings, family history, absent or decreased expression of the CD40 ligand (CD40L) protein on flow cytometry following in vitro stimulation of white cells, and molecular genetic testing of CD40LG (previously known as TNFSF5 or CD154). The only curative treatment currently available is allogeneic hematopoietic cell transplantation, ideally performed prior to the onset of life-threatening complications and organ damage. Other effective therapies are monthly replacement of Ig and antibiotics for specific infectious complications. To reduce the risk of *Cryptosporidium* infection is recommended that patients boil or filter water. In patients with neutropenia is possible use granulocyte colony-stimulating factor (G-CSF).

Common Variable Immunodeficiency

CVID with an estimated prevalence of 1/100,000 to 1/50,000 is the most common symptomatic primary antibody deficient syndrome and is characterized by decreased levels of at least two serum Ig isotypes and recurrent infections particularly of the respiratory tract [15]. The diagnosis is based on significantly reduced levels of IgG, IgA, and/or IgM, with poor or absent antibody production to protein and carbohydrate vaccines with exclusion of other causes of hypogammaglobulinemia [16, 17]. Most patients are diagnosed with CVID between the ages of 20 and 40 years; however, the diagnosis commonly is delayed by 6–8 years, even after the onset of characteristic symptoms [16]. The genetic basis of CVID is unknown in most cases, although defects have been described in four genes: inducible T cell costimulator *(ICOS),* tumor necrosis factor receptor superfamily member 13B (*TNFRSF13B,* also known as *TACI*), tumor necrosis factor receptor superfamily member 13C (*TNFRSF13C,* also known as *BAFFR*), and *CD19* [18–20]. GI symptoms are common in CVID patients, as up to 50% of patients have chronic diarrhea with malabsorption [21]. They may be related to recurrent intestinal infections caused by *G. lamblia, C. jejuni,* or *Salmonella,* pathogens frequently associated with profound B cell immunodeficiencies [22, 23]. Diarrhea and malabsorption have also been ascribed to the onset of inflammatory bowel diseases [24] or to the intestinal villous atrophy mimicking celiac disease, a condition observed in 31% of CVID patients with GI symptoms or anemia [25]. Whether some CVID patients with intestinal villous atrophy can develop an authentic celiac disease remains debated. Some studies concluded to celiac disease responding to gluten-free diet [26], whereas others described histological presentations distinct from celiac disease and resistance to gluten-free diet. An atrophic gastritis, which resembles autoimmune gastritis developing into pernicious anemia, may occur in the absence of demonstrable antiparietal cell antibodies in CVID patients. Treatment of pernicious anemia in CVID patients is similar to that of patients without CVID: monthly replacement of vitamin B12 and careful monitoring of the gastric mucosa for changes associated with malignancy. Gastric adenocarcinoma, in the setting of atrophic gastritis or de novo, has an increased frequency in CVID patients. Patients are treated with monthly infusions of IgG; this treatment alone may not be effective in treating other manifestations of this disorder. Although the inflammatory process responds to steroid therapy, prolonged therapy with steroids is not advisable in CVID patients. Other immune modulators such as 6-mercaptopurine (6-MP) or azathioprine (AZA) can be used in addition to Ig replacement therapy. Careful use of budesonide may be required if unresponsive to 6-MP or AZA until the symptoms are controlled (e.g., reversal of weight loss and dehydration). In severe cases of malabsorption, when significant loss of essential nutrients (e.g., calcium, zinc, and vitamins A, E, and D) lead to bone loss and neurologic deficits, limited use of total parenteral nutrition may be required.

Combined T and B cell Immunodeficiency

SCID

SCID includes a group of disorders characterized by impaired development of cellular and humoral immune function. The overall incidence of all types of SCID is approximately 1 in 75,000 births [27]. This condition is uniformly fatal in the first 2 years of life unless immune reconstitution can be accomplished. The common characteristic of all types of SCID is a severe impairment of T cell development, with a virtual lack of circulating autologous T lymphocytes and absence of functional T-cell responses. SCID can be divided into two main classes: with (B+SCID) and without (B−SCID) B lymphocytes. Presence or absence of NK cells is variable within these groups. The condition results from mutations in known genes that encode components of the immune system crucial for lymphoid cell development (Table 37.2) [28–30].

Affected individuals appear to be normal infants at birth but begin to suffer from excessive infections and failure to thrive coincident with the waning of transplacentally acquired maternal IgG between 2 and 4 months of age [31].

Most males with typical X-SCID come to medical attention between ages three and 6 months. During the first year of life, nearly all untreated males with X-SCID present failure to thrive, oral/diaper candidiasis, absent tonsils and lymph nodes, recurrent infections, infections with opportunistic organisms such as *P. jirovecii,* and persistence of infections despite conventional treatment. Additional features include immune dysregulation and autoimmunity associated with rashes, GI malabsorption, and short stature. Ten to 15% of patients have a "delayed" clinical onset by age 6–24 months and a smaller percentage of patients have "later"' onset, diagnosed from ages 4 years to adulthood, showing less severe infections, and gradual immunologic deterioration. All patients with SCID have very small thymuses. The spleen appears depleted of lymphocytes. Lymph nodes, tonsils, adenoids, and Peyer patches are absent or extremely underdeveloped. GI disorders often occur in SCID patients. Oral, esophageal, and perianal candidiasis is common and can affect oral intake. Patients can develop severe diarrhea and malabsorption in the early age. Intractable diarrhea may begin slowly and progressive to massive, watery, bloody, and mucopurulent. Stool should be sent to a laboratory to check for viral and opportunistic infections, especially rotavirus. Chronic infection with rotavirus has been reported in patients who have received the live vaccination. CMV and adenovirus infections also have been identified in GI biopsy specimens. GI biopsy specimens show hypocellular lamina propria, without plasma cells or lymphocytes. Villous atrophy may occur in some infants owing to damage in the intestine after viral or bacterial infections. A hereditary multiple intestinal atresia is described as an unusual and rare form of recurrent intestinal atresia, which can be associated with SCID [32]. Graft versus host disease (GVHD) and a GVHD-like process affecting colon and small intestine can occur in patients with SCID who receive blood transfusions or allogeneic bone marrow transplantation. Early recognition and diagnosis is crucial to these patients. The diagnosis of SCID is established when the absolute lymphocyte count is less than 1500–2000 cells/mm^3 (normal 4000–13,500 cells/mm^3); CD3+ T cell counts are usually <500 cells/mm^3 (normal range 3000–6500 cells/mm^3). The number of B and NK cells varies according to the underlying genetic defect. In few rare cases, maternal engraftment of T cells may cause near-normal T cell counts. Serum levels of Ig are usually very low and specific antibody responses are impaired. Diagnosis of infants often is delayed by several months as a result of the protection of maternal antibodies. When there is a prior SCID-affected child with a known specific molecular defect, a prenatal diagnosis can be made through genetic testing.

After diagnosis, treatment relies on prevention of principal complications until allogeneic hematopoietic stem cell transplantation. Replacement Ig therapy is given, as well as prophylaxis for *P. jirovecii* pneumonia. Live vaccinations should not be given to the patient or the patient's caregivers because they can cause life-threatening infections. Blood products are irradiated before administration to prevent GVHD. Definitive treatment is available for SCID predominantly by allogeneic hematopoietic stem cell transplantation but also in specific forms of SCID (SCID-X1 and adenosine deaminase (ADA)-SCID) by gene therapy and by enzyme replacement therapy for ADA SCID [33, 34].

Disorder of Phagocytes Function

Chronic Granulomatous Disease (CGD)

CGD is an uncommon primary immunodeficiency (affecting 1 in 250,000 live births) caused by an inability of the phagocytes to produce adequate reactive oxygen metabolites to kill ingested microorganisms and leads to recurrent or persistent intracellular bacterial and fungal infections and to granuloma formation. This impairment in killing is caused by any of several defects in the nicotinamide adenine dinucleotide phosphate (NADPH) oxidase enzyme complex, which generates the microbicidal respiratory burst. The most common form is X-linked (gp91*phox*); others are autosomal recessive [35]. Patients with CGD are susceptible to severe and recurrent infections due to catalase-positive organisms (e.g., *Staphylococcus aureus, Burkholderia cepacia, Serratia marcescens, Aspergillus* species, *Chromobacterium violaceum,* and *Nocardia* species) at epithelial surfaces (e.g., skin, gut, lungs) as well as in organs with a large number of phagocytes such as the liver. The disease becomes apparent during the first 2 years of life in most patients. GI clinical manifestations are common in patients with CGD, ranging from chronic diarrhea, malabsorption with steatorrhea and vitamin B12 malabsorption, perianal abscesses and fistulae, GI tract infection, liver abscesses, hepatosplenomegaly, oral ulceration, and characteristic obstructive lesions associated with granulomatous infiltration [36]. CGD subjects with colitis often present with signs and symptoms similar to those seen in Crohn's disease and ulcerative colitis. However, in contrast to inflammatory bowel disease, CGD-associated colitis may have distinctive histopathologic findings including more eosinophils, fewer neutrophils, and numerous lipid-laden macrophages. Typically, these cells were located in the lower third of the mucosa near crypt bases. It is critically important for the clinician to consider the possibility of CGD in patients with a "Crohn-like" disease in whom a history of recurrent infections and abscesses is noted [37]. Diagnosis of CGD is made by demonstrating a lack of oxidative burst by the nitroblue–tetrazolium test or a flow cytometric test using dihydrorhodamine dye, and confirmed by Western blot and mutation analysis. Management of CGD includes antibiotic prophylaxis with trimethoprim–sulfamethoxazole and itraconazole to reduce the incidence of bacterial and fungal infections, although breakthrough infections do occur. Prophylactic administration of subcutaneous interferon-γ also has been used. Hematopoietic stem cell transplantation from an HLA-identical donor can be curative for CGD [38]. CGD-associated colitis typically responds rapidly to treatment with steroids. Other treatment options are based on established inflammatory bowel disease therapies and include interferon-γ, antitumor necrosis factor α (anti-TNFα), and cyclosporine.

Immune Dysregulation Diseases

IPEX and IPEX-Like Disorders

A number of disorders characterized by immune dysregulation and autoimmunity results from defects in T regulatory cells, development and function. The best characterized of these is immune dysregulation, polyendocrinophaty, enteropathy, X-linked (IPEX), resulting from mutations affecting FOXP3. A number of other gene defects that affect T-regulatory cell function also give rise to an IPEX-like phenotype, including loss-of-function mutations in CD25, STAT5b, and ITCH and gain-of-function mutations in STAT1 [39] (Table 37.3). IPEX typically presents during the first 2–3 months of life with severe enteropathy leading to secretory diarrhea (at times mucoid or bloody) unresponsive to fast and failure to thrive, eczema, diabetes mellitus, and hemolytic anemia. Clinical presentation can be similar to that of severe food allergy, although these patients are generally unresponsive to the elemental formula. Histopathology includes loss of normal small-bowel mucosa as a result of total or partial villous atrophy. Involvement of the large intestine is common with lymphocytic and plasma cell infiltration in the lamina propria; eosinophils also may be present. There is mucosal and submucosal destruction, although the muscular layer is preserved. Celiac disease, food allergy, inflammatory bowel disease, and GVHD are often on the differential diagnosis, based on histology. Other autoimmune manifestations, including thyroiditis, thrombocytopenia, and neutropenia, also have been reported. B-cell subsets and CD3+ T cells, including CD4+ and CD8+ subsets, are present in normal numbers and proliferate to mitogens and antigens, although affected patients typically have decreased numbers of regulatory T cell and are unable to suppress T cell proliferation. Serum IgG, IgA, and IgM levels are usually normal but can be slightly reduced from enteric protein loss. IgE usually is increased and eosinophilia is frequently present.

Table 37.3 Clinical and laboratory features of IPEX and IPEX-like disorders

	IPEX	CD25	STAT5b	STAT-1	ITCH
Associated features	None	None	Growth failure	Vascular anomalies	Dysmorphic growth failure
Autoimmunity					
Eczema	+++	+++	++	++	++
Enteropathy	+++	+++	++	++	++
Endocrinopathy	+++	++	+	++	++
Allergic disease	+++	+	+	++	++
Lung disease	+	++	+++	+	+++
Infections					
Yeast	−	++	−	+++	−
Herpes virus	−	+++(EBV/CMV)	++(VZV)	++	−
Bacterial	+/−	++	++	++	+
Laboratory findings					
Cytopenias	++	++	++	−	
Serum immunoglobulins	↑	Normal or ↑	Normal or ↑	Normal or ↑/↓	↑
Serum IgE	↑	Normal or ↑	Normal or ↑	Normal or mildly ↑	↑
CD25 expression	Normal	↓	Normal or ↓	Normal	Unknown
CD4 + CD45RO	↑	↑	↑	Normal or ↑	Unknown
FOXP3 expression	Normal or ↓	Normal or ↓	Normal or ↓	Normal	Unknown
IGF-1, IGFBP-3	Normal	Normal	↓	Normal	Unknown
Prolactin	Normal	Normal	↑	Normal	Unknown

CMV cytomegalovirus, *EBV* Epstein Barr virus, *VZV* varicella zoster virus, *IGF* insulin-like growth factor binding protein, IGFBP insulin-like growth factor binding protein

The diagnosis is made by showing decreased FOXP3 protein expression and a reduction in the number of regulatory T cells. The diagnosis also can be confirmed by mutation testing of the *FOXP3* gene [1]. Autoantibodies to harmonin and villin are considered specific diagnostic markers of IPEX, and could be of help to differentiate IPEX, including atypical cases, from other early disorders associated with severe enteropathy [40]. Patients are often severely ill by the time a diagnosis of IPEX is made. In absence of aggressive therapy, children usually die before 2–3 years of age as a result of malnutrition, electrolyte imbalance, or infection [41]. Symptomatic treatment includes bowel rest with total parental nutrition and, if necessary, insulin injections and red blood cell and platelet transfusions. Although immunosuppression can be used in the interim, hematopoietic stem cell transplant is curative. Immunosuppressive agents such as cyclosporine A, tacrolimus, sirolimus, and steroids have been used with some success to improve diarrhea; however, these agents do not maintain long-term remission. Chronic therapy may be toxic and may facilitate opportunistic infections [1].

Interleukin-10 and Interleukin-10-Receptor Defects

IL-10 pathway plays a critical role in the control of inflammation by limiting the secretion of pro-inflammatory cytokines, including TNF-α, IL-1, IL-6, and IL-12. Loss-of-function mutations in IL-10 itself and in IL-10 receptor A (IL-10RA) or IL-10 receptor B (IL-10RB) encoding respectively the α-unit (IL-10R1) and the β-unit (IL-10R2) of the IL-10 receptor have been described in children with severe early-onset enterocolitis [42, 43]. These patients present within the first year of life with enterocolitis and perianal disease, as well as the formation of multiple abscesses and enterocutaneous fistula, requiring several surgical interventions. Histopathology shows ulcerations of the intestinal mucosa with inflammatory infiltrates of the epithelium and the formation of abscesses extending to the muscularis propria. The patients also suffer from chronic folliculitis and recurrent respiratory infections. Although rare, pediatric patients with inflammatory bowel disease and perianal disease should be screened for IL-10 and IL-10R deficiency. Defects in the IL-10R may be evaluated by functional assays. Peripheral blood mononuclear cells from healthy individuals show strong phosphorylation of the signal transducer and activator of transcription-3 (STAT3) upon stimulation with IL-10, whereas peripheral blood mononuclear cells from IL-10R-deficient patients do not. Functional abnormalities can be confirmed by sequencing IL-10RA and IL-10RB [44]. The management of these patients includes various anti-inflammatory drugs, such as steroids, methotrexate, thalidomide, and anti-TNFα monoclonal antibodies, without success of remission or long-term improvement. Both IL-10 and IL-10 receptor deficiency can be successfully treated by hematopoietic stem cell transplantation.

Immunodeficiency Associated with Other Defects

WAS

WAS is a rare X-linked primary immunodeficiency characterized by microthrombocytopenia, eczema, recurrent infections, and an increased incidence of autoimmunity and malignancies. The disease is caused by mutations in the WASp, which is involved in hematopoietic cell differentiation and development [45]. The most severe form of WAS is associated with mutations that lead to absent or truncated protein, and individuals with this class of mutations develop classic WAS. Mutations that lead to full-length, but reduced quantity of WASp typically lead to X-linked thrombocytopenia with minimal, if any, immunodeficiency. Missense mutations that have no effect on WASp expression lead only to intermittent thrombocytopenia. Of note, platelets have reduced size in all three classes of mutation. A fourth class of mutations results in a missense mutation in the WASp Cdc42 binding site. These individuals demonstrate no thrombocytopenia and have normal-sized platelets, but they typically develop a neutropenia (and often a complete loss of this cell line) with infections. Interestingly, the first three classes of mutations in WASp show no tendency toward neutropenia. WAS can also be associated with other immune defects, including abnormalities of humoral and cell-mediated immunity [46]. Patients with WAS usually are male infants present in the first few months of life with the above clinical picture accompanied by bleeding, commonly bloody diarrhea. Although other GI complications are not prominent, malabsorption and nonspecific colitis may be encountered. Serious infections also occur. Encapsulated organisms are frequent pathogens that may cause life-threatening complications, including pneumonia, meningitis, and sepsis. *Pneumocistis jirovecii* and viral infections also may become troublesome. Atopic symptoms are frequently present, and eczema develops in more than 2/3 of these patients. The eczema may improve as the patient gets older, although serious complications such as secondary infection (e.g., cellulitis, abscess) or erythroderma can occur. Laboratory evaluation reveals normal or slightly low IgG levels, high IgA and IgE levels, and low levels of IgM that are secondary to accelerated synthesis and catabolism. Antibody responses to polysaccharide antigens are decreased. Platelet numbers are reduced and small in size. Patients have normal B cell numbers; while their T cells show a progressive decrease in number and function. Diminished lymphocyte proliferation in response to mitogens occurs in approximately 50% of patients. The number

and phagocytic activity of neutrophils are normal, although chemotactic responses are defective. Screening for WASp mutations is performed by flow cytometry; however, this does not identify carriers of, or those patients with, X-linked thrombocytopenia. Sequence analysis of the WAS gene is essential to confirm the diagnosis. Curative therapy for WAS is hematopoietic cell transplantation; however, gene therapy is under investigation [47]. Conventional management includes antibiotic prophylaxis as well as platelet transfusions, to treat major bleeding episodes.

Hermansky–Pudlak Syndrome

Hermansky–Pudlak syndrome (HPS) is a rare autosomal recessive disease that displays genetic heterogeneity, there are nine known subtypes [48]. It is a multisystem disorder characterized by tyrosinase-positive oculocutaneous albinism, a bleeding diathesis resulting from a platelet storage pool deficiency and, in some cases, pulmonary fibrosis or granulomatous colitis. Systemic complications are associated with accumulation of ceroid lipofuscin. The bleeding diathesis can result in easy bruising, frequent epistaxis, gingival bleeding, postpartum hemorrhage, colonic bleeding, and prolonged bleeding with menses or after tooth extraction, circumcision, and other surgical procedures. Pulmonary fibrosis, a restrictive lung disease, typically causes symptoms in the early thirties and can progress to death within a decade. A bleeding granulomatous colitis, which occurs in patients with HPS, has clinical features suggestive of chronic ulcerative colitis and pathological features similar to that of Crohn's disease including non-necrotizing granulomas, fissuring, and transmural inflammation. Colitis usually manifests in the first and second decades of disease; it can be severe and have been reported to be poorly responsive to medical therapies, occasionally requires colectomy [49]. Although the colon is primarily involved in HPS any part of the GI tract, including the gingiva, can be affected. Diagnosis is based on clinical findings of oculocutaneous albinism in combination with a bleeding diathesis, confirmed by an absence of platelet dense bodies and genetic testing. Laboratory findings show normal platelet count, prolonged bleeding time, with abnormal platelet function assays. Recently, treatment with infliximab has been shown to be effective [50].

References

1. Agarwal S, Mayer L. Diagnosis and treatment of gastrointestinal disorders in patients with primary immunodeficiency. Clin Gastroenterol Hepatol. 2013;11:1050–63.
2. Singh K, Chang C, Gershwin ME. IgA deficiency and autoimmunity. Autoimmun Rev. 2014;13:163–77.
3. Yel L. Selective IgA deficiency. J Clin Immunol. 2010;30:10–6.

4. Kobrynski LJ, Mayer L. Diagnosis and treatment of primary immunodeficiency disease in patients with gastrointestinal symptoms. Clin Immunol. 2011;139:238–48.

5. Cerutti A. The regulation of IgA class switching. Nat Rev Immunol. 2008;8:421–34.

6. Lougaris V, Ferrari S, Cattalini M, et al. Autosomal recessive agammaglobulinemia: novel insights from mutations in Ig-beta. Curr Allergy Asthma Rep. 2008;8:404–8.

7. Chun JK, Lee TJ, Song JW, et al. Analysis of clinical presentations of Bruton disease: a review of 20 years of accumulated data from pediatric patients at severance hospital. Yonsei Med J. 2008;49:28–36.

8. Lee KH, Shyur SD, Chu SH, et al. Bruton syndrome and celiac disease. Asian Pac J Allergy Immunol. 2011;29:260–5.

9. Van den Bruele T, Mourad-Baars PE, Claas EC, et al. *Campylobacter jejuni* bacteremia and Helicobacter pylori in a patient with X-linked agammaglobulinemia. Eur J Clin Microbiol Infect Dis. 2010;29:1315–9.

10. Brosens LA, Tytgat KM, Morsink FH, et al. Multiple colorectal neoplasms in X-linked agammaglobulinemia. Clin Gastroenterol Hepatol. 2008;6:115–9.

11. Halliday E, Winkelstein J, Webster AD. Enteroviral infections in primary immunodeficiency (PID): a survey of morbidity and mortality. J Infect. 2003;46:1–8.

12. Conley ME, Notarangelo LD, Etzioni A. Diagnostic criteria for primary immunodeficiencies. Representing PAGID (Pan-American Group for Immunodeficiency) and ESID (European Society for Immunodeficiencies). Clin Immunol. 1999;93:190–7.

13. Al-Saud BK, Al-Sum Z, Alassiri H, et al. Clinical, immunological, and molecular characterization of hyper-IgM syndrome due to CD40 deficiency in eleven patients. J Clin Immunol. 2013;33:1325–35.

14. Rahman M, Chapel H, Chapman RW, et al. Cholangiocarcinoma complicating secondary sclerosing cholangitis from cryptosporidiosis in an adult patient with CD40 ligand deficiency: case report and review of the literature. Int Arch Allergy Immunol. 2012;159:204–8.

15. Gathmann B, Grimbacher B, Beaute J, et al. The European internet-based patient and research database for primary immunodeficiencies: results 2006–2008. Clin Exp Immunol. 2009;157:3–11.

16. Chapel H, Lucas M, Lee M, et al. Common variable immunodeficiency disorders: division into distinct clinical phenotypes. Blood. 2008;112:277–86.

17. Cunningham-Rundles C. How I treat common variable immune deficiency. Blood. 2010;116:7–15.

18. Salzer U, Chapel HM, Webster AD, et al. Mutations in TNFRSF13b encoding TACI are associated with common variable immunodeficiency in humans. Nat Genet. 2005;37:820–8.

19. Warnatz K, Salzer U, Gutenberger S. Finally found. Human BAFF-R deficiency causes hypogammaglobulinemia. Clin Immunol. 2005;115:820.

20. van Zelm MC, Reisli I, van der Burg M, et al. An antibody-deficiency syndrome due to mutations in the *CD19* gene. N Engl J Med. 2006;354:1901–12.

21. Cunningham-Rundles C, Bodian C. Common variable immunodeficiency. Clinical and immunological features of 248 patients. Clin Immunol. 1999;92:34–48.

22. Hermaszewski RA, Webster AD. Primary hypogammaglobulinaemia: a survey of clinical manifestations and complications. Q J Med. 1993;86:31–42.

23. Sicherer SH, Winkelstein JA. Primary immunodeficiency diseases in adults. JAMA. 1998;279:58–61.

24. Mannon PJ, Fuss IJ, Dill S, et al. Excess IL-12 but not IL-23 accompanies the inflammatory bowel disease associated with common variable immunodeficiency. Gastroenterology. 2006;131:748–56.

25. Luzi G, Zullo A, Iebba F, et al. Duodenal pathology and clinical-immunological implications in common variable immunodeficiency patients. Am J Gastroenterol. 2003;98:118–21.

26. Chahal P, Weiler CR, Murray JA. Common variable immune deficiency and gastrointestinal tract. Gastroenterology. 2005;128:A-502:T1552.

27. Chan K, Davis J, Pai SY, et al. A Markov model to analyze cost-effectiveness of screening for severe combined immunodeficiency (SCID). Mol Genet Metab. 2011;104:383–9.

28. Horn B, Cowan MJ. Unresolved issues in hematopoietic stem cell transplantation for severe combined immunodeficiency: need for safer conditioning and reduced late effects. J Allergy Clin Immunol. 2013;131:1306–11.

29. Kalman L, Lindegren ML, Kobrynski L, et al. Mutations in genes required for T-cell development: IL7R, CD45, IL2RG, JAK3, RAG1, RAG2, ARTEMIS, and ADA and severe combined immunodeficiency: HuGE review. Genet Med. 2004;6:16–26.

30. Notarangelo LD. Partial defects of T-cell development associated with poor T-cell function. J Allergy Clin Immunol. 2013;131:1297–305.

31. Adeli MM, Buckley RH. Why newborn screening for severe combined immunodeficiency is essential: a case report. Pediatrics. 2010;126:e465–9.

32. Ali YA, Rahman S, Bhat V, et al. Hereditary multiple intestinal atresia (HMIA) with severe combined immunodeficiency (SCID): a case report of two siblings and review of the literature on MIA, HMIA and HMIA with immunodeficiency over the last 50 years. BMJ Case Rep. 2011;2011:bcr0520103031.

33. Brown L, Xu-Bayford J, Allwood Z, et al. Neonatal diagnosis of severe combined immunodeficiency leads to significantly improved survival outcome: the case for newborn screening. Blood. 2011;117:3243–6.

34. Dvorak CC, Cowan MJ, Logan BR, et al. The natural history of children with severe combined immunodeficiency: baseline features of the first fifty patients of the primary immune deficiency treatment consortium prospective study 6901. J Clin Immunol. 2013;33:1156–64.

35. Glocker E, Grimbacher B. Inflammatory bowel disease: is it a primary immunodeficiency? Cell Mol Life Sci. 2012;69:41–8.

36. Matute JD, Arias AA, Wright NA, et al. A new genetic subgroup of chronic granulomatous disease with autosomal recessive mutations in p40 phox and selective defects in neutrophil NADPH oxidase activity. Blood. 2009;114:3309–15.

37. Huang A, Abbasakoor F, Vaizey CJ. Gastrointestinal manifestations of chronic granulomatous disease. Colorectal Dis. 2006;8:637–44.

38. Kang EM, Marciano BE, DeRavin S, et al. Chronic granulomatous disease: overview and hematopoietic stem cell transplantation. J Allergy Clin Immunol. 2011;127:1319–26.

39. Verbsky JW, Chatila TA. Immune dysregulation, polyendocrinophaty, enteropathy, X-linked (IPEX) and IPEX-related disorders: an evolving web of heritable autoimmune diseases. Curr Opin Pediatr. 2013;25:708–14.

40. Lampasona V, Pasarini L, Barzaghi F, Lombardoni C, Bazzigaluppi E, Brigatti C, Bacchetta R, Bosi E. Autoantibodies to harmonon and villin are diagnostic markers in children with IPEX syndrome. Plos One. 2013;8:e78664.

41. Rao A, Kamani N, Filipovich A, et al. Successful bone marrow transplantation for IPEX syndrome after reduced-intensity conditioning. Blood. 2007;109:383–385.

42. Kotlarz D, Beier R, Murugan D, et al. Loss of interleukin-10 signaling and infantile inflammatory bowel disease: implications for diagnosis and therapy. Gastroenterology. 2012;143:347–55.

43. Glocker EO, Kotlarz D, Klein C, et al. IL-10 and IL-10 receptor defects in humans. Ann N Y Acad Sci. 2011;1246:102–7.

44. Shah N, Kammermeier J, Elawad M, et al. Interleukin-10 and interleukin-10-receptor defects in inflammatory bowel disease. Curr Allergy Asthma Rep. 2012;12:373–9.

45. Ochs HD, Filipovich AH, Veys P, et al. Wiskott-Aldrich syndrome: diagnosis, clinical and laboratory manifestations, and treatment. Biol Blood Marrow Transplant. 2009;15:84–90.

46. Ozsahin H, Cavazzana-Calvo M, Notarangelo LD, et al. Longterm outcome following hematopoietic stem-cell transplantation in Wiskott-Aldrich syndrome: collaborative study of the European Society for Immunodeficiencies and European Group for Blood and Marrow Transplantation. Blood. 2008;111:439–45.

47. Ochs HD, Thrasher AJ. The Wiskott-Aldrich syndrome. J Allergy Clin Immunol. 2006;117:725–38.

48. Seward SL Jr, Gahl WA. Hermansky-Pudlak syndrome: health care throughout life. Pediatrics. 2013;132:153–60.

49. Hussain N, Quezado M, Huizing M, et al. Intestinal disease in Hermansky–Pudlak syndrome: occurrence of colitis and relation to genotype. Clin Gastroenterol Hepatol. 2006;4:73–80.

50. Felipez LM, Gokhale R, Guandalini S. Hermansk–Pudlak syndrome: severe colitis and good response to infliximab. J Pediatr Gastroenterol Nutr. 2010;51:665–7.

Congenital Disorders of Lipid Transport

38

Nicholas O. Davidson and Emile Levy

Introduction

Congenital disorders of intestinal lipid absorption includes a clinically heterogeneous group of conditions for which the molecular genetic basis has been assigned to a group of gatekeeper genes whose roles are exerted at multiple steps following complex intracellular lipid assembly and the subsequent packaging that eventually form chylomicrons (CMs). The critical steps involve mobilization of membrane-associated complex lipids into vesicular transport vehicles within the lumen of the endoplasmic reticulum (ER) and Golgi and ultimately vectorial delivery to the basolateral membrane of the enterocyte for extrusion and transport into mesenteric collecting lymphatics. The critical role of these gatekeeper genes, particularly MTTP, APOB, and SAR1B has been replicated in preclinical and cell-based models, and we now know much about the function and importance of their cognate proteins. The importance of these genes resides in the recognition that mutations or deletions may give rise to severe fat malabsorption and failure to thrive in early childhood, in association with very low plasma cholesterol and triglyceride (TG) levels. In addition, unrecognized failure to thrive and lipid malabsorption syndromes may lead to progressive ataxic neuropathy and retinal degeneration because of the attendant malabsorption of fat-soluble vitamins, particularly vitamin A and E. With early diagnosis and appropriate nutritional supplementation, these particular complications can be avoided and in general life expectancy should be unaltered.

We review the major genetic syndromes associated with congenital lipid malabsorption, the molecular genetics, and pathophysiologic basis underlying defective lipid absorption and describe the clinical manifestations and management of these patients.

Intestinal Lipid Absorption Overview

The reader is referred to recent comprehensive reviews of intestinal lipid absorption [1, 2] but the essential features are summarized below (Fig. 38.1). Complex lipids (principally long-chain TG and also cholesterol ester (CE) and phospholipids) are enzymatically lipolyzed to yield fatty acid (FA) and monoglycerides (MG), which are then transported through micelle-dependent uptake across the brush border membrane of villi. FA and MG within the enterocyte are used to generate newly synthesized TG droplets through the actions of diacylglycerol acyltransferase 1 (DGAT1) which likely functions in close proximity to the ER (Fig. 38.1). These TG droplets exist in both cytosolic (principally apical) compartments as well as within the ER membrane. Mobilization of TG droplets from within membranous domains requires the integrated actions of two gatekeeper genes, namely the resident endolumenal ER protein microsomal triglyceride transfer protein (MTTP) and a structural acceptor protein that is required for CM formation namely apolipoprotein B (APOB), and its intestine-specific isoform, APOB48. In this scenario, MTTP physically transfers the lipid droplet from the bilayer by mediating a physical interaction with the nascent APOB protein during translation and extrusion into the ER lumen [2]. The fusion of TG droplets with APOB48 within the ER lumen generates a pre-CM particle which then undergoes progressive modification and vesicular transport to the Golgi, a process regulated by several COP (COat Protein)-associated proteins and in particular the Sar1-ADP ribosylation factor, type B (SAR1B). The pre-CM particle then undergoes terminal modifications within the Golgi and is ultimately secreted across the basolateral membrane as a mature CM (Fig. 38.1).

N. O. Davidson (✉)
Department of Medicine, Washington University School of Medicine, 660 South Euclid Avenue, Campus Box 8124, St. Louis, MO 63110, USA
e-mail: nod@dom.wustl.edu

E. Levy
Research Centre, CHU Ste-Justine and Department of Nutrition, Université de Montréal, Montreal, QC H3T 1C5, Canada

© Springer International Publishing Switzerland 2016
S. Guandalini et al. (eds.), *Textbook of Pediatric Gastroenterology, Hepatology and Nutrition*,
DOI 10.1007/978-3-319-17169-2_38

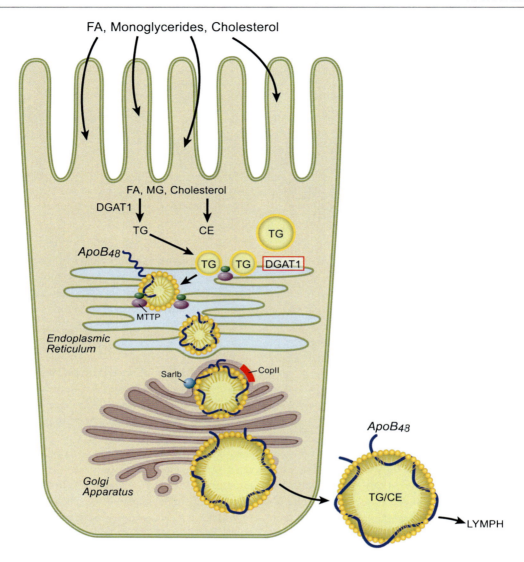

Fig. 38.1 Overview of intestinal lipid absorption: Key genetic regulators. Following digestion of dietary and biliary lipid, the component lipid species including long-chain fatty acid (*FA*), monoglycerides (*MG*), and cholesterol are transported across the brush border membrane into the apical compartment of villus enterocytes. *FA* and *MG* undergo re-esterification into triglyceride (*TG*) which is mediated in a series of enzymatic steps including diacylglycerol acyltransferase 1 (*DGAT1*). The newly synthesized *TG* exists in both cytosolic and intramembranous forms within the endoplasmic reticulum (*ER*) membrane, where *DGAT1 (boxed)* also resides. The heterodimeric *ER* protein *MTTP* physically translocates neutral lipid droplets from the *ER* bilayer membrane to an acceptor protein, *APOB*. Mammalian enterocytes synthesize a truncated *APOB* protein referred to as *APOB48*. The fusion of *APOB* and *TG* droplets, mediated by *MTTP*, is the critical and rate limiting step in prechylomicron assembly. Following processing in the *ER*, the prechylomicron undergoes vesicular transport to the Golgi, mediated by fusion with *COP* proteins and SAR1B. Following further maturation in the Golgi, the CM particle, containing *APOB48* and a cargo of *TG* and cholesterol ester (*CE*) is transported into the lymphatic compartment and delivered into the peripheral circulation

Molecular Genetic Basis for Congenital Defects in Lipid Absorption: Overview

Several rare genetic disorders of lipid absorption have been identified and their molecular basis characterized [3–5]. These include abetalipoproteinemia (ABL), which is an autosomal recessive disorder caused by mutations or deletions in the *MTTP* gene [3]; familial hypobetalipoproteinemia (FHBL), an autosomal codominant disorder which is typical- ly caused by mutations in the *APOB* gene [4]; chylomicron retention disease (CRD, also known as Anderson's disease), which is an autosomal recessive disorder caused by mutations in *SAR1B* [5]; and one family in which congenital diarrhea was linked to a splice defect in *DGAT1* [6]. The cardinal feature of enterocyte lipid droplet accumulation is common to all the disorders, but the site of lipid droplet accumulation shows subtle distinctions based on the molecular defect. Defects associated with ABL and FHBL result in lipid droplet accumulation throughout the cytoplasm but typically do not generate lipid particles within the ER lumen (Fig. 38.2, top panel). Both ABL and FHBL interrupt intestinal lipid absorption at the initiation stage of pre-CM formation and thus completely attenuate CM assembly and the generation of intracellular lipoproteins, particularly large lipoprotein particles that contain neutral lipid (cholesteryl ester and triglycerides). As a result of this block in lipoprotein assembly, neutral lipid droplets accumulate in the apical cytoplasm in ABL and FHBL. These conditions are discussed in more detail below. The defect in CRD, by contrast, is focused at a later stage in CM formation and blocks maturation and exit of CM and pre-CM particles from the ER and Golgi [7, 8]. The accumulation of lipid droplets and pre-CM particles within membranous domains is schematically illustrated in Fig. 38.2, bottom panel. CRD is discussed in a later section.

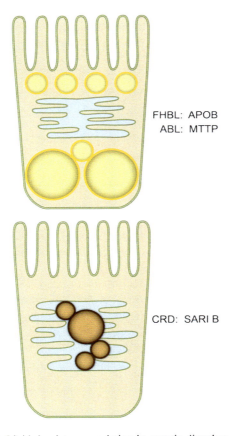

FHBL: APOB
ABL: MTTP

CRD: SARI B

Fig. 38.2 Lipid droplet accumulation in genetic disorders of intestinal lipid absorption. Based upon the pathways outlined in Fig. 38.1, defects or mutations in *APOB* (responsible for familial hypobetalipoproteinemia, *FHBL*) or in *MTTP* (responsible for abetalipoproteinemia, *ABL*) eliminate the earliest steps in chylomicron assembly and thus lead to lipid droplet accumulation with no lipid particles visible within ER profiles *(Top panel)*. By contrast, defects in *SARIB* (responsible for chylomicron retention disease, *CRD*), interrupt the later stages of chylomicron maturation and processing and lead to prechylomicron accumulation *(brown)* within the ER lumen *(Bottom panel)*. *APOB* apolipoprotein B, *MTTP* microsomal triglyceride transfer protein *SAR1B* SAR1-ADP ribosylation factor

Congenital Disorders of CM Assembly: Genetics and Clinical Features of ABL and FHBL

Defects in either of the gatekeeper genes that promote CM assembly (i.e., *MTTP* and *APOB*, respectively) each produce congenital lipid malabsorption, which generally presents in infancy as failure to thrive with characteristically low serum lipid levels and other complications (including ataxia and retinitis pigmentosa) that reflect the coincident malabsorption of fat-soluble vitamins [8]. However, the clinical phenotypes in both ABL and homozygous FHBL may be quite variable as discussed below.

Abetalipoproteinemia (ABL, OMIM #200100): Molecular Genetics and Prevalence

ABL is a rare, autosomal recessive disorder with an estimated prevalence in North America of <1 per 100,000 [9] and for which worldwide there were about 50 cases with defined *MTTP* mutations reported as of 2012 [10–15]. There is strong evidence for a founder effect in Ashkenazi Jewish patients, where a conserved haplotype with a common truncating mutation (p.G865X) was discovered in Israel with a carrier frequency of 1:131 and an estimated ABL incidence of 1:69,000 [16]. Some but not all of the reported ABL probands are the offspring of consanguineous marriage, an observation replicated across different national registries [12, 16]. While a range of mutations and deletions have been described in the *MTTP* gene in association with ABL, affected subjects may be either homozygous for a single mutation or compound heterozygous for different mutations and there appears to be no relationship between the site and nature of these mutations and the clinical phenotypes observed [17].

Abetalipoproteinemia (ABL, OMIM #200100): Clinical Features and Management

Although typically ABL presents in infancy with failure to thrive, there is a wide age range of presentation (from infancy to >20 years) suggesting that there are either environmental or other genetic modifiers that influence some of the clinical features. Infants typically present with diarrhea and malabsorption and the hallmark features including extremely low plasma cholesterol and TG levels, very low or undetectable levels of APOB, low to absent levels of fat-soluble vitamins and red blood cell acanthacytosis [9, 11].

The clinical phenotypes of low to undetectable levels of cholesterol and TG and APOB reflect the virtual complete block in lipoprotein secretion from both enterocytes and hepatocytes, which reflects the inability to lipidate the nascent APOB protein as it traverses the ER membrane (Fig. 38.1). The very low levels of fat-soluble vitamins (particularly vitamins A and E) reflect fat malabsorption and defective CM production. Among the neurological sequelae of unrecognized ABL is retinal degeneration, which may be progressive and result in visual impairment and which is likely a consequence of continued fat-soluble vitamin A and E deficiency [9]. The observation that ABL subjects treated upon diagnosis with long-term high-dose supplementation with vitamins A (10–15,000 IU/day) and E (100 mg/kg/day, equivalent to 150 IU/kg) [18], maintain retinal function and neurological function provides indirect but strong evidence that deficiency of these vitamins is responsible for the phenotypic outcomes, although the exact mechanisms linking ABL to neurologic deficits are yet to be fully elucidated [19]. Importantly, there was no evidence for increased oxidative stress in the plasma of ABL patients receiving long-term vitamin A and E supplementation [19]. For clinical monitoring purposes, it is worth noting that even with high-dose vitamin E supplementation, plasma levels rarely return to the normal range. This is because of the dual defect that exists in vitamin E metabolism, reflecting a block in intestinal absorption of vitamin E and also a defect in hepatic alpha tocopherol transfer to circulating lipoproteins [20]. Because circulating plasma lipid levels are so low in ABL subjects, plasma levels of alpha and gamma tocopherol may not reflect tissue (particularly adipose) concentrations, but nevertheless may be a useful surrogate to monitor long-term compliance [9].

ABL subjects require lifelong maintenance on a low-fat diet (to minimize steatorrhea) and supplementation with fat-soluble vitamins as noted above and in addition supplementation with 1000 IU/day vitamin D (which is available in a water-soluble form). Longer term, ABL subjects should be monitored for development of steatohepatitis (transaminases, liver magnetic resonance spectroscopy) which has been associated with progressive liver disease requiring liver transplantation [21].

FHBL, OMIM #107730: Molecular Genetics and Prevalence

FHBL is an autosomal codominant disorder whose molecular basis (where known) most commonly resides in mutations in the *APOB* gene on chromosome 2 [22]. Unlike ABL, heterozygous FHBL subjects exhibit low circulating levels of plasma cholesterol, triglyceride, and APOB and are generally discovered in routine plasma lipid level screening tests. Heterozygous FHBL, recognized through population-based plasma lipid screening for subjects at or below the fifth percentile, is present in ~1:500–1:1000 [22, 23]. Homozygous FHBL by contrast is extremely rare, with perhaps 20 index cases whose molecular genetic basis is known [24]. FHBL associated with structural defects in the *APOB* gene represent the majority of known cases [22, 23]. The known mutations generally produce truncated forms of APOB (i.e., smaller proteins than APOB100) which are defective in undergoing lipidation despite adequate levels of MTTP (Fig. 38.1). These truncated forms of APOB may be detected using denaturing gel electrophoresis and are present at very low levels in plasma, and notably even in heterozygous subjects are found at lower abundance than those encoded by the wild-type allele. This observation implies that transcription or translation of the mutant allele in FHBL is also defective [25]. In addition, FHBL is genetically heterogeneous with several kindreds described in whom the trait is inherited in an autosomal dominant manner without mutations in the *APOB* gene but rather with linkage to a locus on chromosome 3p21, between D3S2407 and D3S1767 [25]. The molecular basis for the defects in FHBL subjects linking to chromosome three remains unknown.

FHBL, OMIM #107730: Clinical Features and Management

The clinical manifestations of homozygous FHBL are heterogeneous with severely affected individuals presenting in infancy or early childhood with failure to thrive and steatorrhea, while yet other affected homozygous individuals may present in adulthood with incidentally discovered hepatic steatosis and very low levels (<fifth percentile) of plasma lipids and undetectable levels of APOB100 [24]. In general, the clinical manifestations and management of severe homozygous FHBL subjects follows the same principles as alluded to above for ABL subjects, including acanthocytosis, very low levels of plasma lipids and fat-soluble vitamins, and neurologic deficits with macular degeneration and steatorrhea [26]. A more sinister concern longer term for FHBL subjects is the development of cirrhosis [27, 28] and hepatocellular carcinoma [24, 29]. The observations in relation to hepatic lipid accumulation in subjects with FHBL due to APOB truncations were not replicated in homozygous FHBL subjects linked to chromosome 3p21, reinforcing the concept that the clinical phenotypes among FHBL subjects is very variable [30, 31]. Homozygous FHBL subjects should therefore undergo regular evaluation of fat-soluble vitamin sufficiency (as outlined above) and also periodic monitoring for progressive hepatic steatosis and steatohepatitis (transaminases, liver magnetic resonance spectroscopy), again as alluded to above for ABL subjects.

CRD, OMIM #246700: Molecular Genetics and Prevalence

CRD was identified by Roy and colleagues in 1987 [32]. Although this disorder appears to be the same as that described by Anderson in 1961 [33], the term "CRD" is preferred nowadays, as it is more indicative of the pathology. CRD is a very rare, autosomal recessive disorder with fewer than 50 cases described worldwide [7], and whose molecular genetic defect resides in the SAR1-ADP ribosylation factor, type B (SAR1B), which belongs to the Ras superfamily of guanosine triphosphatase (GTPases). SAR1B mutations induce an accumulation of pre-CM transport vesicles [7], as seen on intestinal biopsies and illustrated schematically in Fig. 38.2.

SAR1B is a single polypeptide of 198 amino acids and functions as molecular switch controlled by the exchange of guanosine diphosphate (GDP) and GTP. SAR1 is cytosolic in its GDP form and is recruited to the ER by the exchange of GDP for GTP to initiate COPII-coated vesicle formation. SAR1-GTP forms a coating protein complex (COPII) with two heterodimers SEC23/24 and SEC13/31. COPII initiates budding and captures cargo to eject vesicles from the ER to the Golgi apparatus [34]. The SAR1B GTPase cycle then allows cytosolic COPII proteins to exchange on and off the membrane at specific sites on the ER to regulate cargo exit. As a result, genetic defects in SAR1B affect the transport of pre-CM cargo from the ER to the Golgi apparatus where they usually undergo additional glycosylation before being released from the enterocyte. CMs are transported from the ER to Golgi, probably inside the pre-CM transport vesicle or PCTV [35]. PCTV share several proteins including COPII (SEC13–31, SEC24 and SAR1) [36]. Siddiqi et al. [37] earlier showed that PCTV formation can occur in the absence of SAR1 and later showed that PCTV fusion with Golgi requires the presence of SAR1 [38].

The first investigation of genetic defects in eight families disclosed three frameshift (75–76 delTG, 555–558 dupTTAC, 349–1 G>C) and five missense mutations (109 G>A, 409 G>A, 537 T>A, 536 G>T, 542 T>C) [5]. The second exploration of the genetic abnormalities from eight families identified three new molecular aberrations: a stop codon mutation (364 G>T), a 5946 bp deletion (total exon 2) and a missense mutation (554 G>T) [39]. Thereafter, a new mutation G19T (changing a glutamic acid to a STOP codon) was found in the seventh exon [40] while two additional mutations were detected in exon 2 (G11D) and exon 4 (D75G) [41]. Recently, a novel homozygous deletion at position 142 (c.142delG) led to the replacement of the aspartic acid at position 48 by a threonine and gave rise to a frameshift-derived premature stop codon 17 amino acids further on (p.Asp48ThrfsX17), thereby resulting in a truncated protein (only 32% of the length of the normal protein and 24% of the normal sequence) [7]. Finally, the analysis of SAR1B gene mutations in Tunisian children revealed a proband homozygous for a novel nucleotide transition in exon 4 (c.184G>A), resulting in a nonconservative amino acid substitution (p.Glu62Lys) [42]. In order to provide a unifying explanation for the functional impairment of SAR1B mutated proteins, investigators have turned to information gleaned from the SAR1B crystal structure, computational analysis, and sequence alignment [43]. For example, the nonsense mutations and whole deletion of exon 2 in SAR1B yields truncated proteins that are predicted to modify the affinity of SAR1B for GDP and GTP, thereby affecting its interaction with the endoplasmic ER and other components of COPII machinery. In addition, the missense mutations in SAR1B likely yield nonfunctional proteins that alter the con-

formational and/or structural properties of SAR1B. Because SAR1B expression is detected in multiple different tissues, there are frequent clinical manifestations of CRD in organs beyond the gastrointestinal tract. As an example, cardiac abnormalities, myolysis, increased CK levels and cardiac abnormalities were associated with the G19T mutation [40].

Genotype–Phenotype Associations in CRD

Recent studies compared the patients of two cohorts of CRD patients from France and Canada in order to compare the severity and long-term evolution as a function of the SAR1B gene mutations [44]. In both series, most of the CRD patients were symptomatic at diagnosis (before the age of 1) and the disease was definitely more severe in infants. This is consistent with the observation that the CRD had profound impact on weight Z scores in Canadian children (1.5 ± 1 years) who were significantly younger at diagnosis than the French subjects (6.4 ± 1.3 years). The catch-up growth and bone mineral density improvement were not as encouraging in the French cohort compared to the Canadian patients, possibly because of the delayed initiation of a low-fat diet with a high polyunsaturated/saturated fatty acid ratio and of supplements of fat-soluble vitamins A, D, and E. In general, the neuroophthalmic manifestations detected at the time of diagnosis proved largely reversible with treatment. Although the effect of missense mutations on the protein was considered less deleterious than the those mutations that introduce stop codons or that specified deletions, the clinical phenotype (i.e., growth, neurological impairment, hepatic steatosis, lipid disturbances) was not significantly different in CRD patients based on the underlying genetic mutation [44]. According to the findings of this largest group of CRD patients so far reported, genotype–phenotype correlations are not obvious, suggesting that CRD might represent a more complex trait rather than a simple autosomal recessive disorder [44]. Additional work is required to determine whether modifier genes are involved in the ER-to-Golgi transport.

CRD, OMIM #246700: Clinical Features and Management

CRD presents with failure to thrive probably resulting from fat malabsorption and constant, nonspecific diarrhea that begins shortly after birth. Other digestive symptoms include vomiting or abdominal swelling. Light microscopic examination generally reveals few morphological irregularities in the small intestine of CRD patients; however [7], following an oral fat bolus test meal and ultrastructural examination, numerous CM-size lipid droplets are evident within the cytoplasm of enterocytes. Many of these CM-size lipid droplets are bound by membranes of the smooth ER and clustered mostly in the supranuclear region, whereas only few of them were visualized within vesicular structures, likely part of the Golgi complex. The larger lipid vacuoles are not membrane bound [8]. Importantly, the intercellular spaces were completely juxtaposed and no CMs were evident in the interstitium between adjacent enterocytes and in the area around the basement membrane. Hepatomegaly and a moderate degree of macrovesicular steatosis have been detected in a few cases [32, 45]. Nonspecific moderate hepatic cytolysis is very frequent but correlates only poorly with steatosis and/or hepatomegaly. Areflexia (combined with proprioceptive abnormalities) and electromyographic abnormalities (reduction in sensory nerve conduction velocity and decreased sensory nerve action potential amplitudes) were among the neurological abnormalities described in CRD children [32, 46, 47], but more severe neurological degeneration, such as ataxia and myopathy and sensory neuropathy, have also been reported in CRD adults [48]. Sometimes muscular pain and cramps are present in CRD children while cardiomyopathy with a decrease in ejection fraction to 40 % (normal >60 %) has been described in adults [40]. Only minimal ophthalmic complications characterize CRD patients and include micronystagmus, mild deficit in the perception of the blue-yellow axis, and delayed dark adaptation [32] while abnormal visual evoked potentials has been evidenced by functional testing [49]. Poor mineralization and delayed bone maturation have also been observed in CRD [46].

Fat malabsorption in CRD impairs the absorption of fat-soluble vitamins, with vitamin E being the most affected, as observed in ABL subjects [50]. Vitamin A levels in plasma are frequently decreased, but generally correctable following oral supplementation. Finally, vitamin D or K insufficiency can be detected in up to half of CRD patients, and can also be corrected with oral vitamin supplementation. In CRD, acanthocytosis is rare, sometimes transient. Acanthocytosis, when it occurs, reflects low plasma vitamin E levels, which is a key to red cell membrane integrity. In association with muscular abnormalities, creatine kinase levels were elevated at diagnosis and have been associated with neurological impairment [49]. As previously noted, hepatic abnormalities may be present.

In contrast to ABL and FHBL, fasting triacylglycerol concentrations are usually normal, but severe hypocholesterolemia is prominent with levels of low-density lipoprotein-cholesterol and APOB100 at the lower limits of normal. Similarly, CRD patients display limited capacity to produce high-density lipoprotein. Importantly, CMs failed to appear in the circulation after a fat meal test explaining the deficiency of fat-soluble vitamins and essential fatty acids. However, patients with CRD express the apolipoprotein species essential for CM synthesis, including APO-AI, APO-AIV, and importantly, APOB48 [7, 51].

Although CRD resembles ABL and FHBL symptomatically with respect to dietary fat malabsorption and its con-

sequences, examination of plasma reveals a key distinction. Plasma from CRD patients contains APOB100 at normal levels but no APOB48 especially after a fat meal. As detailed above, plasma from ABL and FHBL subjects contains virtually no detectable APOB100, because the defect impairs secretion of lipoproteins from both the liver and small intestine [9]. Intestinal transcription of APOB100 messenger RNA (mRNA) and its posttranscriptional editing to APOB48 mRNA was normal in CRD subjects [52]. Both APOB and MTTP along with CM-size lipid droplets were detected in enterocytes from CRD subjects, suggesting that enterocytes can synthesize prechylomicron particles, but fail to process these intravesicular particles into mature CM particles that can be secreted into the lymphatic circulation. Other attempts to identify the underlying mechanisms in CRD confirmed that the primary defect is not in the de novo synthesis of APOB48 protein, although reduced glycosylation of APOB was revealed in intestinal biopsies taken from CRD patients [51].

As with ABL and homozygous FHBL, CRD needs to be recognized early because of its adverse effects on growth and potential for neurological, ocular, hepatic, and other extraintestinal complications. Accurate diagnosis can be readily established using ultrastructural identification of CM-size lipid droplets clustered in the enterocytes, with the absence of fat outside the cells. However, sequencing of the short SARA2 gene provides a quick, safe, inexpensive, and noninvasive diagnostic tool. Consumption of medium-chain triglycerides can aid in more rapidly correcting malnutrition in infants, but total fat intake and particularly long-chain fatty acid consumption should be limited. The patients must be advised to take adequate intake of essential fatty acids and fat-soluble vitamins. In addition, vitamin E supplementation is critical for the prevention of the progression of neurological findings while vitamin A should be administered at high doses to prevent ophthalmologic complications. Early vitamin D supplementation is also recommended in all patients to avoid bone growth and development abnormalities, and vitamin K should be given in cases of coagulopathies and abnormal clotting parameters.

References

1. Mansbach CM, Siddiqi SA. The biogenesis of chylomicrons. Annu Rev Physiol. 2010;72:315–33.
2. Abumrad NA, Davidson NO. Role of the gut in lipid homeostasis. Physiol Rev. 2012;92(3):1061–85.
3. Wetterau JR, Aggerbeck LP, Bouma ME, Eisenberg C, Munck A, Hermier M, et al. Absence of microsomal triglyceride transfer protein in individuals with abetalipoproteinemia. Science. 1992;258(5084):999–1001.
4. Linton MF, Farese RV Jr, Young SG. Familial hypobetalipoproteinemia. J Lipid Res. 1993;34(4):521–41.

5. Jones B, Jones EL, Bonney SA, Patel HN, Mensenkamp AR, Eichenbaum-Voline S, et al. Mutations in a Sar1 GTPase of COPII vesicles are associated with lipid absorption disorders. Nat Genet. 2003;34(1):29–31.

6. Haas JT, Winter HS, Lim E, Kirby A, Blumenstiel B, DeFelice M, et al. DGAT1 mutation is linked to a congenital diarrheal disorder. J Clin Invest. 2012;122(12):4680–4.

7. Georges A, Bonneau J, Bonnefont-Rousselot D, Champigneulle J, Rabes JP, Abifadel M, et al. Molecular analysis and intestinal expression of SAR1 genes and proteins in Anderson's disease (chylomicron retention disease). Orphanet J Rare Dis. 2011;6:1.

8. Hegele RA, Angel A. Arrest of neuropathy and myopathy in abetalipoproteinemia with high-dose vitamin E therapy. Can Med Assoc J. 1985;132(1):41–4.

9. Zamel R, Khan R, Pollex RL, Hegele RA. Abetalipoproteinemia: two case reports and literature review. Orphanet J Rare Dis. 2008;3:19.

10. Chardon L, Sassolas A, Dingeon B, Michel-Calemard L, Bovier-Lapierre M, Moulin P, et al. Identification of two novel mutations and long-term follow-up in abetalipoproteinemia: a report of four cases. Eur J Pediatr. 2009;168(8):983–9.

11. Di Filippo M, Crehalet H, Samson-Bouma ME, Bonnet V, Aggerbeck LP, Rabes JP, et al. Molecular and functional analysis of two new MTTP gene mutations in an atypical case of abetalipoproteinemia. J Lipid Res. 2012;53(3):548–55.

12. Najah M, Di Leo E, Awatef J, Magnolo L, Imene J, Pinotti E, et al. Identification of patients with abetalipoproteinemia and homozygous familial hypobetalipoproteinemia in Tunisia. Clin Chim Acta. 2009;401(1–2):51–6.

13. Pons V, Rolland C, Nauze M, Danjoux M, Gaibelet G, Durandy A, et al. A severe form of abetalipoproteinemia caused by new splicing mutations of microsomal triglyceride transfer protein (MTTP). Hum Mutat. 2011;32(7):751–9.

14. Sani MN, Sabbaghian M, Mahjoob F, Cefalu AB, Averna MR, Rezaei N. Identification of a novel mutation of MTP gene in a patient with abetalipoproteinemia. Ann Hepatol. 2011;10(2):221–6.

15. Uslu N, Gurakan F, Yuce A, Demir H, Tarugi P. Abetalipoproteinemia in an infant with severe clinical phenotype and a novel mutation. Turk J Pediatr. 2010;52(1):73–7.

16. Benayoun L, Granot E, Rizel L, Allon-Shalev S, Behar DM, Ben-Yosef T. Abetalipoproteinemia in Israel: evidence for a founder mutation in the Ashkenazi Jewish population and a contiguous gene deletion in an Arab patient. Mol Genet Metab. 2007;90(4):453–7.

17. Wang J, Hegele RA. Microsomal triglyceride transfer protein (MTP) gene mutations in Canadian subjects with abetalipoproteinemia. Hum Mutat. 2000;15(3):294–5.

18. Granot E, Deckelbaum RJ. Hypocholesterolemia in childhood. J Pediatr. 1989;115(2):171–85.

19. Granot E, Kohen R. Oxidative stress in abetalipoproteinemia patients receiving long-term vitamin E and vitamin A supplementation. Am J Clin Nutr. 2004;79(2):226–30.

20. Traber MG. Mechanisms for the prevention of vitamin E excess. J Lipid Res. 2013;54(9):2295–306.

21. Black DD, Hay RV, Rohwer-Nutter PL, Ellinas H, Stephens JK, Sherman H, et al. Intestinal and hepatic apolipoprotein B gene expression in abetalipoproteinemia. Gastroenterology. 1991;101(2):520–8.

22. Tarugi P, Averna M, Di Leo E, Cefalu AB, Noto D, Magnolo L, et al. Molecular diagnosis of hypobetalipoproteinemia: an ENID review. Atherosclerosis. 2007;195(2):e19–27.

23. Schonfeld G. Familial hypobetalipoproteinemia: a review. J Lipid Res. 2003;44(5):878–83.

24. Di Leo E, Magnolo L, Bertolotti M, Bourbon M, Carmo Pereira S, Pirisi M, et al. Variable phenotypic expression of homozygous familial hypobetalipoproteinaemia due to novel APOB gene mutations. Clin Genet. 2008;74(3):267–73.

25. Schonfeld G, Lin X, Yue P. Familial hypobetalipoproteinemia: genetics and metabolism. Cell Mol Life Sci. 2005;62(12):1372–8.

26. Buonuomo PS, Ruggiero A, Valeriani M, Mariotti P. Familial hypobetalipoproteinemia: early neurological, hematological, and ocular manifestations in two affected twins responding to vitamin supplementation. Curr Opin Pediatr. 2009;21(6):824–7.

27. Bonnefont-Rousselot D, Condat B, Sassolas A, Chebel S, Bittar R, Federspiel MC, et al. Cryptogenic cirrhosis in a patient with familial hypocholesterolemia due to a new truncated form of apolipoprotein B. Eur J Gastroenterol Hepatol. 2009;21(1):104–8.

28. Florkowski C, Hedley J, Bickley V, Hooper AJ, Burnett JR, George P. Fatty infiltration of the liver in a case of hypobetalipoproteinaemia with a novel mutation in the APOB gene. N Z Med J. 2010;123(1310):98–100.

29. Cefalu AB, Pirruccello JP, Noto D, Gabriel S, Valenti V, Gupta N, et al. A novel APOB mutation identified by exome sequencing cosegregates with steatosis, liver cancer, and hypocholesterolemia. Arterioscler Thromb Vasc Biol. 2013;33(8):2021–5.

30. Martin-Morales R, Garcia-Diaz JD, Tarugi P, Gonzalez-Santos P, Saavedra-Vallejo P, Magnolo L, et al. Familial hypobetalipoproteinemia: analysis of three Spanish cases with two new mutations in the APOB gene. Gene. 2013;531(1):92–6.

31. Yue P, Tanoli T, Wilhelm O, Patterson B, Yablonskiy D, Schonfeld G. Absence of fatty liver in familial hypobetalipoproteinemia linked to chromosome 3p21. Metabolism. 2005;54(5):682–8.

32. Roy CC, Levy E, Green PH, Sniderman A, Letarte J, Buts JP, et al. Malabsorption, hypocholesterolemia, and fat-filled enterocytes with increased intestinal apoprotein B. Chylomicron retention disease. Gastroenterology. 1987;92(2):390–9.

33. Anderson CM, Townley RR, Freemanm M, Johansen P. Unusual causes of steatorrhoea in infancy and childhood. Med J Aust. 1961;48(2):617–22.

34. Kirchhausen T. Three ways to make a vesicle. Nat Rev Mol Cell Biol. 2000;1(3):187–98.

35. Kumar NS, Mansbach CM 2nd. Prechylomicron transport vesicle: isolation and partial characterization. Am J Physiol. 1999; 276(2 Pt 1):G378–86.

36. Siddiqi S, Siddiqi SA, Mansbach CM,2nd. Sec24C is required for docking the prechylomicron transport vesicle with the Golgi. J Lipid Res. 2010;51(5):1093–100.

37. Siddiqi SA, Gorelick FS, Mahan JT, Mansbach CM 2nd. COPII proteins are required for Golgi fusion but not for endoplasmic reticulum budding of the pre-chylomicron transport vesicle. J Cell Sci. 2003;116(Pt 2):415–27.

38. Siddiqi SA, Mahan J, Siddiqi S, Gorelick FS, Mansbach CM 2nd. Vesicle-associated membrane protein 7 is expressed in intestinal ER. J Cell Sci. 2006;119(Pt 5):943–50.

39. Charcosset M, Sassolas A, Peretti N, Roy CC, Deslandres C, Sinnett D, et al. Anderson or chylomicron retention disease: molecular impact of five mutations in the SAR1B gene on the structure and the functionality of Sar1b protein. Mol Genet Metab. 2008;93(1):74–84.

40. Silvain M, Bligny D, Aparicio T, Laforet P, Grodet A, Peretti N, et al. Anderson's disease (chylomicron retention disease): a new mutation in the SARA2 gene associated with muscular and cardiac abnormalities. Clin Genet. 2008;74(6):546–52.

41. Treepongkaruna S, Chongviriyaphan N, Suthutvoravut U, Charoenpipop D, Choubtum L, Wattanasirichaigoon D. Novel missense mutations of SAR1B gene in an infant with chylomicron retention disease. J Pediatr Gastroenterol Nutr. 2009;48(3):370–3.

42. Magnolo L, Najah M, Fancello T, Di Leo E, Pinotti E, Brini I, et al. Novel mutations in SAR1B and MTTP genes in Tunisian children with chylomicron retention disease and abetalipoproteinemia. Gene. 2013;512(1):28–34.

43. Bi X, Mancias JD, Goldberg J. Insights into COPII coat nucleation from the structure of Sec23.Sar1 complexed with the active fragment of Sec31. Dev Cell. 2007;13(5):635–45.

44. Peretti N, Roy CC, Sassolas A, Deslandres C, Drouin E, Rasquin A, et al. Chylomicron retention disease: a long term study of two cohorts. Mol Genet Metab. 2009;97(2):136–42.

45. Nemeth A, Myrdal U, Veress B, Rudling M, Berglund L, Angelin B. Studies on lipoprotein metabolism in a family with jejunal chylomicron retention. Eur J Clin Invest. 1995;25(4):271–80.

46. Lacaille F, Bratos M, Bouma ME, Jos J, Schmitz J, Rey J. Anderson's disease. Clinical and morphologic study of 7 cases. Arch Fr Pediatr. 1989;46(7):491–8.

47. Strich D, Goldstein R, Phillips A, Shemer R, Goldberg Y, Razin A, et al. Anderson's disease: no linkage to the apo B locus. J Pediatr Gastroenterol Nutr. 1993;16(3):257–64.

48. Gauthier S, Sniderman A. Action tremor as a manifestation of chylomicron retention disease. Ann Neurol. 1983;14(5):591.

49. Peretti N, Sassolas A, Roy CC, Deslandres C, Charcosset M, Castagnetti J, et al. Guidelines for the diagnosis and management of chylomicron retention disease based on a review of the literature and the experience of two centers. Orphanet J Rare Dis. 2010;5:24.

50. Berriot-Varoqueaux N, Aggerbeck LP, Samson-Bouma M, Wetterau JR. The role of the microsomal triglygeride transfer protein in abetalipoproteinemia. Annu Rev Nutr. 2000;20:663–97.

51. Levy E, Marcel Y, Deckelbaum RJ, Milne R, Lepage G, Seidman E, et al. Intestinal apoB synthesis, lipids, and lipoproteins in chylomicron retention disease. J Lipid Res. 1987;28(11):1263–74.

52. Patel S, Pessah M, Beucler I, Navarro J, Infante R. Chylomicron retention disease: exclusion of apolipoprotein B gene defects and detection of mRNA editing in an affected family. Atherosclerosis. 1994;108(2):201–7.

Pancreatic Insufficiency

39

Praveen S. Goday and Steven L. Werlin

Introduction

Pancreatic insufficiency, though not very prevalent, must be suspected in every child with failure to thrive of unexplained reasons, as well as in children with recurrent pancreatitis (see Chap. 34). References [1–15] constitute a comprehensive review of all known forms of pancreatic insufficiency. Table 39.1 lists both relatively common as well as rarer genetic causes of this condition.

Pancreatic Insufficiency in Cystic Fibrosis

Cystic fibrosis (CF) is an autosomal recessive condition caused by defects in the CF transmembrane regulator *(CFTR)* gene. About 85% of patients with CF are pancreas insufficient (PI) [16].

Pathophysiology of Pancreatic Insufficiency in Cystic Fibrosis

Mutations of the *CFTR* gene cause impaired chloride transport at the apical surface of epithelial cells [17] and also disturb chloride-coupled bicarbonate transport [18] and sodium channel activity [19]. Pancreatic secretion of chloride, bicarbonate, sodium, and potassium in response to combined cholecystokinin and secretin stimulation is impaired in all patients with CF, regardless of pancreatic function status [16]. Bicarbonate secretion is most impaired, and defective electrolyte secretion leads to reduced fluid secretion [20]. This defective bicarbonate secretion results in impairment in the luminal flow of pancreatic enzymes and proenzymes and impairment in the trafficking of zymogen granules [20]. This

results in a severe block in acinar cell secretion followed by loss of cellular function, cell death, fibrosis, and eventual pancreatic insufficiency which leads to a decline in all the enzymes secreted by the pancreas [17, 20].

In normal people, just 5–10% of the normal post-meal pancreatic enzyme output is adequate for normal digestion, indicating the large reserve capacity of the pancreas [17]. This reserve capacity means that clinically significant malabsorption is not evident until at least 90% of the exocrine cells of the pancreas are destroyed [21]. Again in normal individuals, the presence of free fatty acids in the proximal small bowel causes release of cholecystokinin which in turn stimulates pancreatic secretion [22]. When pancreatic insufficiency begins to develop, this feedback loop is impaired, and the site of maximal digestion shifts to the more distal bowel [17]. This results in larger amounts of nutrients being delivered to the distal bowel with changes in motor and secretory function of the more proximal bowel [23, 24]. These changes, in turn, lead to quicker intestinal transit and worsening of malabsorption [24].

The terms pancreas sufficient (PS) and PI have great clinical and prognostic significance in CF. PS does not mean normal pancreatic function, but that enough pancreatic function is present to avoid the need for pancreatic enzyme replacement therapy (PERT). Patients who are PS are more prone to pancreatitis [25], while PI patients have more severe lung disease, malnutrition, and liver disease [26].

Shwachman–Diamond Syndrome

Shwachman–Diamond syndrome (SDS) is an autosomal recessive disorder characterized by congenital anomalies, pancreatic insufficiency, bone marrow failure, and predisposition to myelodysplasia and acute myeloid leukemia (AML) [27]. Mutations in the Shwachman–Bodian–Diamond syndrome *(SBDS)* gene can be found in approximately 90% of classically presenting patients with SDS [28]. These mutations usually result in reduced, but not absent, protein expression.

S. L. Werlin (✉) · P. S. Goday
Division of Gastroenterology, Department of Pediatrics, Medical College of Wisconsin and Children's Hospital of Wisconsin, 8701 Watertown Plank Road, 53226 Milwaukee, WI, USA
e-mail: swerlin@mcw.edu

© Springer International Publishing Switzerland 2016
S. Guandalini et al. (eds.), *Textbook of Pediatric Gastroenterology, Hepatology and Nutrition*,
DOI 10.1007/978-3-319-17169-2_39

Table 39.1 Syndromes and genetic conditions associated with pancreatic insufficiency [1–15]

Condition	Affected gene(s)	Reference
Cystic fibrosis	CFTR gene	[1]
Shwachman–Diamond syndrome	SBDS gene	[2]
Johanson–Blizzard syndrome	UBR1 gene	[3]
Pearson marrow–pancreas syndrome	Mitochondrial DNA defects	[4]
Pancreatic agenesis	PDX 1 gene	[5]
Pancreatic agenesis and congenital heart defects	Heterozygous mutations in the GATA6 gene	[6]
Pancreatic and cerebellar agenesis	PTF1A gene	[7]
Pancreatic lipase deficiency	Unknown	[8]
Pancreatic co-lipase deficiency		
Pancreatic lipase and co-lipase deficiency		
Hereditary pancreatitis	PRSS1 gene	[9]
	SPINK 1 gene	[10]
	CFTR gene	[11]
	Chymotrypsin C (CTRC) variants	[12]
Pseudohypoparathyroidism Type IA	GNAS 1 gene	[13]
CoQ-responsive Oxphos deficiency	Unknown	[14]
Exocrine pancreatic insufficiency, dyserythropoietic anemia, and calvarial hyperostosis	COX 412 gene	[15]

In mice, targeted deletion of the gene results in embryonic death suggesting that some expression of this gene is necessary for survival [29]. The SBDS gene is involved in ribosomal function [30], and ribosomal subunit assembly is impaired in patients with SDS [31]. The exact mechanism by which this leads to pancreatic insufficiency is unknown. One study found that patients negative for mutations in the SBDS gene may have more severe hematological manifestations while having milder pancreatic disease [32].

The incidence of SDS is 1:76,000 individuals with a male to female ratio of 1.7:1 [33, 34].

The classic presentation of SDS is in infancy with failure to thrive, diarrhea, and neutropenia. SDS infants have an average birth weight at the 25th percentile [34]. Table 39.2 details the criteria for the diagnosis of SDS. Growth failure with malnutrition is common in the first year of life, and height falls and remains below the third percentile in 38–56% of patients [35, 36]. After diagnosis, and with appropriate therapy, most children show normal growth velocity, and it appears that with current treatment they attain normal body mass indexes (BMIs) [35]. Steatorrhea is caused by decreased secretion of lipolytic and proteolytic enzymes, while ductular fluid and electrolyte secretion of the pancreas remain normal [37, 38]. Pancreatic insufficiency tends to be diagnosed within the first 6 months of life with 90% of patients being diagnosed in the first year [37]. Spontaneous improvement in pancreatic function can occur in later childhood with 50% of patients having normal fat absorption by age 4 years and no longer requiring pancreatic enzyme supplementation [37]. The pancreas in SDS exhibits a characteristic fatty replacement which can be visualized on ultrasound, CT scanning, and, perhaps, best by MRI scanning [39].

Hepatomegaly and raised serum liver enzymes are common in children with SDS [40]. These resolve by the age of 5 years and no long-term consequences have been observed [40].

Neutropenia is the most common cytopenia and can be persistent or intermittent and mild to severe [34]. Anemia with low reticulocyte counts [34] and elevation in fetal hemoglobin is each seen in 80% of patients [41]. Thrombocytopenia can also be seen. Bone marrow biopsy is usually hypoplastic with increased deposition of fat [41, 42]. Patients with SDS have a propensity to developing infections due to the neutropenia and the occasional functional neutrophil deficits that are seen in SDS [43]. Patients with SDS develop clonal changes in the bone marrow which may or may not be associated with an increased risk of myelodysplasia or AML [23]. Due to the predisposition to myelodysplasia and AML, all patients with SDS should be referred to a pediatric hematologist. Based on data from several registries, the frequency of both myelodysplasia and AML increases with increasing age [32, 44, 45]. In general, early bone marrow transplantation in children with severe cytopenias prior to development of myelodysplasia or AML improves outcome.

The bony dysplasia of SDS manifests as short stature and delayed appearance but subsequent normal development of secondary ossification centers [34]. There is variable metaphyseal widening and irregularity that is most often seen in the ribs in early childhood and femurs later in childhood and adolescence [46]. Rarely, skeletal involvement may be extremely severe and generalized [34]. Usually, these metaphyseal changes become clinically insignificant, but rarely they may lead to limb deformities and fractures [46].

A characteristic pattern of neurocognitive and behavioral difficulties has been described in SDS [47].

Table 39.2 Diagnostic criteria for Shwachman–Diamond syndrome. (Reproduced with permission John Wiley and Sons/New York Academy of Sciences, from Ref. [34], © 2011 New York Academy of Sciences)

Clinical and molecular diagnostic criteria
Diagnostic criteria
Clinical diagnosis
Fulfill the combined presence of hematological cytopenia of any given lineage (most often neutropenia) and exocrine pancreas dysfunction
Hematologic abnormalities may include:
a. Neutropenia $< 1.5 \times 109$/L on at least two occasions over at least 3 months
b. Hypoproductive cytopenia detected on two occasions over at least 3 months
Tests that support the diagnosis but require corroboration:
a. Persistent elevation of hemoglobin F (on at least two occasions over at least 3 months apart)
b. Persistent red blood cell macrocytosis (on at least two occasions over at least 3 months apart), not caused by other etiologies such as hemolysis or a nutritional deficiency
Pancreatic dysfunction may be diagnosed by the following:
a. Reduced levels of pancreatic enzymes adjusted to age (fecal elastase, serum trypsinogen, serum (iso)amylase, serum lipase)
Tests that support the diagnosis but require corroboration:
a. Abnormal 72-h fecal fat analysis
b. Reduced levels of at least two fat-soluble vitamins (A, D, E, K)
c. Evidence of pancreatic lipomatosis (e.g., ultrasound, CT, MRI, or pathological examination of the pancreas by autopsy)
Additional supportive evidence of SDS may arise from:
a. Bone abnormalities
b. Behavioral problems
c. Presence of a first-degree family member diagnosed before with SDS
Other causes of pancreatic insufficiency should be excluded, in particular when the *SBDS* gene mutation analysis is negative
Molecular diagnosis: biallelic *SBDS* gene mutation
Positive genetic testing for SBDS mutations known or predicted to be deleterious, for example, from protein modeling or expression systems for mutant SBDS
Caveats:
Many situations arise when molecular diagnosis is *not* confirmatory in the presence of clinical symptoms:
No identified mutations (about 10 % of cases)
Mutation on one allele only
Gene sequence variations that have unknown or *no* phenotypic consequence:
A novel mutation, such as a predicted missense alteration, for which it is not yet possible to predict whether it is disease causing
SBDS polymorphisms on one or both alleles. Large popluation studies may be needed to exclude a sequence polymorphism as a bona fide irrelevant variant

A high degree of suspicion may be needed to diagnose milder cases of SDS. A study of 37 children with SDS found that neutropenia (81 %), diarrhea (58 %), failure to thrive (73 %) lipomatous infiltration of the pancreas (~ 90 %), fecal elastase (82 %), skeletal (38 %), and congenital and endocrine malformations (65 %) were all inconsistently present [48].

Serum immunoreactive trypsinogen (IRT) and pancreatic isoamylase concentrations can be useful markers of the pancreatic phenotype in SDS [49]. In healthy children, serum IRT concentrations are at adult levels at birth, while pancreatic isoamylase concentrations are low at birth and reach adult levels by 3 years of age [49]. In contrast, in SDS, young children have low serum IRT concentrations which then rise with age, while serum pancreatic isoamylase activities are low at all ages. Serum IRT is generally low in PI patients with SDS, while a normal value does not rule out pancreatic insufficiency. Serum isoamylase concentrations are not useful in determining pancreatic sufficiency or insufficiency. Hence, when SDS is suspected, a serum IRT should be obtained in children <3 years of age, while serum pancreatic isoamylase should be obtained in children ≥3 years of age [34].

The diagnosis of SDS is made using the criteria shown in Table 39.3. The combination of exocrine pancreatic dysfunction and hematological abnormalities when other known causes of exocrine pancreatic dysfunction and bone marrow failure are excluded gives rise to a clinical diagnosis of SDS [34]. CF should be ruled out with a sweat test while Pearson marrow-pancreas syndrome can be differentiated by a bone marrow examination and imaging of the pancreas. Cartilage hair hypoplasia which presents with diarrhea (but not with pancreatic insufficiency), cytopenia, and metaphyseal chondrodysplasia is more common in certain populations such as the Amish.

Table 39.3 FDA-approved pancreatic enzyme products

	Dosages available (lipase/protease/amylase units)	Bead/microsphere diameter (mm)	Notes
Creon®	3000/9500/15,000	0.7–1.6	Oral, delayed-release capsules
	6000/19,000/30,000		
	12,000/38,000/60,000		
	24,000/76,000/120,000		
Pancreaze®	4200/10,000/17,500	2	Oral, delayed-release capsules
	10,500/25,000/43,750		
	16,800/40,000/70,000		
	21,000/37,000/61,000		
Pertyze®	8000/28,750/30,250	0.8–2.2	Oral, delayed-release capsules with bicarbonate-buffered enteric-coated microspheres
	16,000/57,500/60,500		
Ultreza™	13,800/27,600/27,600	2.0–2.4	Oral, delayed-release capsules
	20,700/41,400/41,400		
	23,000/46,000/46,000		
Viokace™	10,440/39,150/39,150	N/A	Non-enteric-coated tablets
	20,880/78,300/78,300		Approved only for use in adults
			Must be given with a proton pump inhibitor
Zenpep®	3000/10,000/16,000	1.8–1.9 for 3000 and 5000	Oral, delayed release capsules
	5000/17,000/27,000		
	10,000/34,000/55,000	2.2–2.5 for others	A generic product is available at the 5000 lipase unit dose
	15,000/51,000/82,000		
	20,000/68,000/109,000		
	25,000/85,000/136,000		

Pearson Marrow–Pancreas Syndrome

Pearson described a syndrome of refractory, transfusion-dependent sideroblastic anemia with vacuolization of the bone marrow and exocrine pancreatic insufficiency [4]. Other variable features may include hepatic failure, proximal renal tubulopathy, watery diarrhea, patchy erythematous skin lesions, neutropenia, and thrombocytopenia and high serum lactate/pyruvate ratios [50]. This condition should be considered in the differential diagnosis of Shwachman syndrome. In this syndrome, vacuolization of the marrow is seen, while in Shwachman syndrome the bone marrow is dysplastic; the pancreas is fibrotic in Pearson syndrome, while it is fatty in Shwachman syndrome [51]. Pearson syndrome is caused by mitochondrial DNA alterations which are more abundant in the blood than in other tissues [50]. Diagnosis is suspected based on clinical findings and can be confirmed by Southern blot analysis which detects rearrangements of mitochondrial DNA [52]. This syndrome is usually fatal in infancy, but some children who survive past infancy develop severe neurological symptoms suggestive of another mitochondrial DNA disorder, Kearns–Sayre syndrome [53]. In children without multisystem involvement, bone marrow transplantation or unrelated cord blood cell transplantation has been suggested as a mechanism to manage the severe hematological manifestations of this syndrome [52].

Johanson–Blizzard Syndrome

Johanson–Blizzard syndrome (JBS) is a rare autosomal recessive disorder caused by mutations in the *UBR1* gene [54, 55]. *UBR1* encodes an E3 ubiquitin ligase that is involved in proteolysis [55]. However, the exact causative mechanism of pancreatic insufficiency in JBS is unknown. A small beak-like nose (due to aplasia or hypoplasia of the alae nasi) and exocrine pancreatic insufficiency are most consistently present while other features in decreasing order of occurrence include dental anomalies, congenital scalp defects, sensorineural hearing loss, growth and psychomotor retardation, hypothyroidism, imperforate anus, and genitourinary anomalies [56].

Clinical Symptoms

The symptoms of fat malabsorption, which have been best described in CF, are abdominal pain, constipation, flatulence, and diarrhea [17]. There is no correlation between dosing of

PERT and symptoms of abdominal pain, constipation, and flatulence [17]. Diarrheal symptoms are not different between PS and PI patients in CF [17]. Hence, these symptoms are not good markers of exocrine pancreatic insufficiency and definitely not measures of adequacy of PERT.

PI can result in significant malnutrition and nutritional deficiencies. Nutritional deficiencies that can potentially be seen in all forms of pancreatic insufficiency include deficiencies of the fat-soluble vitamins—A, D, E, and K—and of the water-soluble vitamin B_{12} [57]. Zinc, iron, and selenium deficiencies have been described in CF [57]. In CF, the presence of liver disease and enteropathic changes may create further nutritional issues.

Diagnosis of Pancreatic Insufficiency

The ideal test of pancreatic function should be specific, noninvasive, able to quantitate pancreatic function, able to indicate the need and the appropriate dosage of substitutive enzymes even during therapy, cost-effective, and broadly available [58]. No such test is presently available [58].

Fecal elastase-1 is secreted by the pancreas and does not undergo degradation in the gut. It is an inexpensive diagnostic test with good sensitivity and specificity for detection of pancreatic insufficiency in CF. After 2 weeks of age, PS patients can be differentiated from PI patients using a cutoff of 200 µg/g. Fecal elastase-1 can be used in the annual monitoring of CF patients with PS to identify the onset of PI. The monoclonal fecal elastase-1 test only identifies the human form of the enzyme; hence, the test can be done even when the patient is receiving PERT [59]. Falsely low values may be obtained when the stool is dilute as in any diarrheal illness or in the presence of enteropathies.

Fecal chymotrypsin is a less sensitive and specific marker of pancreatic function than fecal elastase-1. However, this test, which does identify porcine enzymes can be used to monitor compliance with PERT in patients who are known to be PI.

In patients with CF, the presence of a low fecal elastase-1 is usually considered diagnostic of PI despite the fact that fecal elastase-1 correlates poorly with fecal fat excretion testing [60]. In other conditions, especially in children who present with poor growth or malabsorption, the next steps after obtaining a fecal elastase-1 level are less clear. The secretin–pancreozymin test is considered the gold standard for the diagnosis of pancreatic insufficiency. However, this test is invasive and time-consuming and rarely performed in clinical practice.

Traditionally, fat absorption is measured using the 72-h fecal fat excretion test. During this time, stool is collected while an estimate of dietary fat intake is made using a detailed food diary [61]. The percentage of fat absorption is calculated using the dietary intake of fat and the stool fat output. Abnormal values are defined as fecal fat excretion greater than 7% of intake; in other words, less than 93% absorption of ingested fat.

At our institution, we use a secretin and cholecystokinin (CCK) stimulation test done when the patient undergoes an upper endoscopy [62]. Patients receive intravenous secretin (2 U/kg) plus cholecystokinin (0.02 µg/kg). Duodenal fluid is collected at baseline and 5, 10, and 15 min after stimulation and placed on dry ice. Samples are measured for the levels of trypsin (abnormal <55.4 nmol ml^{-1} min^{-1}), amylase (abnormal <32 nmol ml^{-1} min^{-1}), lipase (abnormal <146 nmol ml^{-1} min^{-1}), and chymotrypsin (abnormal <2.5 nmol ml^{-1} min^{-1}). Unfortunately, the precise sensitivity and specificity of this test is not known.

The ^{13}C-labeled mixed triglyceride test is a noninvasive method of assessing lipase activity [63, 64]. However, it is not widely available at the present time.

Management

Much of the data on management of pancreatic insufficiency in children are extrapolated from CF. Infants with CF are usually begun on 2000–5000 lipase units per feeding. In all patients with pancreatic insufficiency, PERT is adjusted to a maximum of 2500 lipase units per kilogram per meal (not to exceed 10,000 lipase units per kilogram per day or 4000 units lipase per gram dietary fat per day) [65]. Higher doses have been associated with fibrosing colonopathy and are not recommended [66]. Other side effects of PERT include soreness in the mouth and perianal irritation [67]. Allergies may occur due to the porcine origin of the enzyme preparations [67]. Hyperuricemia which was seen with older preparations is rarely seen now [53]. A sudden introduction of PERT to patients with uncontrolled fat malabsorption may lead to severe constipation with accompanying abdominal pain [67].

In infants, the enzyme microspheres are mixed with a small amount of breast milk or infant formula or applesauce and given via spoon immediately before the feed. The dose is gradually adjusted based on weight gain and absorption, but the lipase dose is always kept under 10,000 units/kg body weight per day in most children; infants may need higher doses. In older children, the capsules should be swallowed whole at as early an age as possible. When this is not possible, the microspheres should be mixed with a small amount of fluid or applesauce and given via spoon. The child should be encouraged to swallow without crushing or chewing. Enzymes should be given either at the beginning of the meal or half at the beginning and half midway through the meal. Some children with poor growth, particularly with CF, may not respond to high-calorie foods and oral high-calorie beverages. These children may be candidates for supplemental nocturnal gastrostomy tube feeding. These children are given the additional calories needed for growth as a continuous nocturnal infusion of formula. In these patients, pancreatic enzymes should be given before and after the tube feeding. While a polymeric formula is typically used, some children may require a protein hydrolysate formula due to concerns about uncontrolled malabsorption or continuing concerns about growth despite adequate additional calories. In children receiving the maximum dose of PERT, additional benefit may be obtained by the addition of a proton pump inhibitor when necessary.

In general, the symptoms of pancreatic insufficiency can be more easily controlled in conditions other than CF than in CF.

In children with CF, CF-specific vitamin preparations are recommended and yearly assessment of fat-soluble vitamin status is recommended. These vitamin preparations as well as the regular assessments of vitamin status should be considered in all children with pancreatic insufficiency. It is recommended that these vitamins be taken with a fat-containing meal along with PERT.

References

1. Ahmed N, Corey M, Forstner G, Zielenski J, Tsui L-C, Ellis L, et al. Molecular consequences of cystic fibrosis transmembrane regulator (CFTR) gene mutations in the exocrine pancreas. Gut. 2003;52(8):1159–64.
2. Dror Y, Freedman MH. Shwachman–Diamond syndrome. Br J Haematol. 2002;118(3):701–13.
3. Al-Dosari MS, Al-Muhsen S, Al-Jazaeri A, Mayerle J, Zenker M, Alkuraya FS. Johanson–Blizzard syndrome: report of a novel mutation and severe liver involvement. Am J Med Genet A. 2008;146A(14):1875–9.
4. Pearson HA, Lobel JS, Kocoshis SA, Naiman JL, Windmiller J, Lammi AT, et al. A new syndrome of refractory sideroblastic anemia with vacuolization of marrow precursors and exocrine pancreatic dysfunction. J Pediatr. 1979;95(6):976–84.
5. Stoffers DA, Zinkin NT, Stanojevic V, Clarke WL, Habener JF. Pancreatic agenesis attributable to a single nucleotide deletion in the human IPF1 gene coding sequence. Nat Genet. 1997;15(1):106–10.
6. Lango AH, Flanagan SE, Shaw-Smith C, De Franco E, Akerman I, Caswell R. International pancreatic agenesis consortium, Ferrer J, Hattersley AT, Ellard S, et al. GATA6 haploinsufficiency causes pancreatic agenesis in humans. Nat Genet. 2012;44(1):20–2.
7. Kawaguchi Y, Cooper B, Gannon M, Ray M, MacDonald RJ, Wright CV. The role of the transcriptional regulator Ptf1a in converting intestinal to pancreatic progenitors. Nat Genet. 2002;32(1):128–34.
8. Online Mendelian inheritance in man. http://omim.org/entry/614338. Accessed 2 Jan 2014.
9. Whitcomb DC, Gorry MC, Preston RA, Furey W, Sossenheimer MJ, Ulrich CD, et al. Hereditary pancreatitis is caused by a mutation in the cationic trypsinogen gene. Nat Genet. 1996;14(2):141–5.
10. Witt H, Luck W, Hennies HC, Classen M, Kage A, Lass U, et al. Mutations in the gene encoding the serine protease inhibitor, Kazal type 1 are associated with chronic pancreatitis. Nat Genet. 2000;25(2):213–6.
11. Sharer N, Schwarz M, Malone G, Howarth A, Painter P, Super M, et al. Mutations of the cystic fibrosis gene in patients with chronic pancreatitis. N Engl J Med. 1998;339(10):645–52.
12. Rosendahl J, Witt H, Szmola R, Bhatia E, Ozsvári B, Landt O, et al. Chymotrypsin C (CTRC) variants that diminish activity or secretion are associated with chronic pancreatitis. Nat Genet. 2008;40(1):78–82.
13. Aldred MA, Bagshaw RJ. Macdermot K, Casson D, Murch SH, Walker-Smith JA, Trembath RC, et al. Germline mosaicism for a GNAS1 mutation and Albright hereditary osteodystrophy. J Med Genet. 2000;37(11):E35.
14. Leshinsky-Silver E, Levine A, Nissenkorn A, Barash V, Perach M, Buzhaker E, et al. Neonatal liver failure and Leigh syndrome possibly due to CoQ-responsive OXPHOS deficiency. Mol Genet Metab. 2003;79(4):288–93.
15. Shteyer E, Saada A, Shaag A, Al-Hijawi FA, Kidess R, Revel-Vilk S, et al. Exocrine pancreatic insufficiency, dyserythropoeitic anemia, and calvarial hyperostosis are caused by a mutation in the COX4I2 gene. Am J Hum Genet. 2009;84(3):412–7.
16. Durie PR, Forstner GG. Pathophysiology of the exocrine pancreas in cystic fibrosis. J R Soc Med. 1989;82(Suppl 16):2–10.
17. Baker SS, Borowitz D, Baker RD. Pancreatic exocrine function in patients with cystic fibrosis. Curr Gastroenterol Rep. 2005;7(3):227–33.
18. Choi JY, Muallem D, Kiselyov K, Lee MG, Thomas PJ, Muallem S. Aberrant CFTR-dependent HCO3- transport in mutations associated with cystic fibrosis. Nature. 2001;410(6824):94–7.
19. Reddy MM, Light MJ, Quinton PM. Activation of the epithelial Na+ channel (ENaC) requires CFTR Cl− channel function. Nature. 1999;402(6759):301–4.
20. Scheele GA, Fukuoka SI, Kern HF, Freedman SD. Pancreatic dysfunction in cystic fibrosis occurs as a result of impairments in luminal pH, apical trafficking of zymogen granule membranes, and solubilization of secretory enzymes. Pancreas. 1996;12(1):1–9.
21. DiMagno EP, Go VL, Summerskill WH. Relations between pancreatic enzyme ouputs and malabsorption in severe pancreatic insufficiency. N Engl J Med. 1973;288(16):813–5.
22. Guimbaud R, Moreau JA, Bouisson M, Durand S, Escourrou J, Vaysse N, et al. Intraduodenal free fatty acids rather than triglycerides are responsible for the release of CCK in humans. Pancreas. 1997;14(1):76–82.
23. Keller J, Rünzi M, Goebell H, Layer P. Duodenal and ileal nutrient deliveries regulate human intestinal motor and pancreatic responses to a meal. Am J Physiol. 1997; 272(3 Pt 1):G632–7.
24. Layer P, von der Ohe MR, Holst JJ, Jansen JB, Grandt D, Holtmann G, et al. Altered postprandial motility in chronic pancreatitis: role of malabsorption. Gastroenterology. 1997;112(5):1624–34.
25. Durno C, Corey M, Zielenski J, Tullis E, Tsui LC, Durie P. Genotype and phenotype correlations in patients with cystic fibrosis and pancreatitis. Gastroenterology. 2002;123(6):1857–64.
26. Zielenski, J. Genotype and phenotype in cystic fibrosis. Respiration. 2000;67(2):117–33.
27. Myers KC, Davies SM. Shimamura A. Clinical and molecular pathophysiology of Shwachman–Diamond syndrome: an update. Hematol Oncol Clin North Am. 2013;27(1):117–28, ix.
28. Boocock GR, Morrison JA, Popovic M, Richards N, Ellis L, Durie PR, et al. Mutations in SBDS are associated with Shwachman–Diamond syndrome. Nat Genet. 2003;33(1):97–101.
29. Zhang S, Shi M, Hui CC, Rommens JM. Loss of the mouse ortholog of the Shwachman–Diamond syndrome gene (Sbds) results in early embryonic lethality. Mol Cell Biol. 2006;26(17):6656–63.
30. Finch AJ, Hilcenko C, Basse N, Drynan LF, Goyenechea B, Menne TF, et al. Uncoupling of GTP hydrolysis from eIF6 release on the ribosome causes Shwachman–Diamond syndrome. Genes Dev. 2011;25(9):917–29.
31. Burwick N, Coats SA, Nakamura T, Shimamura A. Impaired ribosomal subunit association in Shwachman–Diamond syndrome. Blood. 2012;120(26):5143–52.
32. Hashmi SK, Allen C, Klaassen R, Fernandez CV, Yanofsky R, Shereck E, et al. Comparative analysis of Shwachman–Diamond

syndrome to other inherited bone marrow failure syndromes and genotype–phenotype correlation. Clin Genet. 2011;79(5):448–58.

33. Goobie S, Popovic M, Morrison J, Ellis L, Ginzberg H, Boocock GRB, et al. Shwachman–Diamond syndrome with exocrine pancreatic dysfunction and bone marrow failure maps to the centromeric region of chromosome 7. Am J Hum Genet. 2001;68(4):1048–54.

34. Dror Y, Donadieu J, Koglmeier J, Dodge J, Toiviainen-Salo S, Makitie O, et al. Draft consensus guidelines for diagnosis and treatment of Shwachman–Diamond syndrome. Ann N Y Acad Sci. 2011;1242:40–55.

35. Myers KC, Rose SR, Rutter MM, Mehta PA, Khoury JC, Cole T, et al. Endocrine evaluation of children with and without Shwachman–Bodian–Diamond syndrome gene mutations and Shwachman–Diamond syndrome. J Pediatr. 2013;162(6):1235–40, 1240 e1.

36. Ginzberg H, Shin J, Ellis L, Morrison J, Ip W, Dror Y, et al. Shwachman syndrome: phenotypic manifestations of sibling sets and isolated cases in a large patient cohort are similar. J Pediatr. 1999;135(1):81–8.

37. Hill RE, Durie PR, Gaskin KJ, Davidson GP, Forstner GG. Steatorrhea and pancreatic insufficiency in Shwachman syndrome. Gastroenterology. 1982; 83(1 Pt 1):22–7.

38. Mack DR, Forstner GG, Wilschanski M, Freedman MH, Durie PR. Shwachman syndrome: exocrine pancreatic dysfunction and variable phenotypic expression. Gastroenterology. 1996;111(6):1593–602.

39. Toiviainen-Salo S, Raade M, Durie PR, Ip W, Marttinen E, Savilahti E, Mäkitie O. Magnetic resonance imaging findings of the pancreas in patients with Shwachman–Diamond syndrome and mutations in the SBDS gene. J Pediatr. 2008;152(3):434–6.

40. Toiviainen-Salo S, Durie PR, Numminen K, Heikkilä P, Marttinen E, Savilahti E, Mäkitie O. The natural history of Shwachman–Diamond syndrome-associated liver disease from childhood to adulthood. J Pediatr. 2009;155(6):807–11.e2.

41. Dror Y, Freedman MH. Shwachman–Diamond syndrome: an inherited preleukemic bone marrow failure disorder with aberrant hematopoietic progenitors and faulty marrow microenvironment. Blood. 1999;94(9):3048–54.

42. Aggett PJ, Cavanagh NP, Matthew DJ, Pincott JR, Sutcliffe J, Harries JT. Shwachman's syndrome. A review of 21 cases. Arch Dis Child. 1980;55(5):331–47.

43. Dror Y, Ginzberg H, Dalal I, Cherepanov V, Downey G, Durie P, et al. Immune function in patients with Shwachman–Diamond syndrome. Br J Haematol. 2001;114(3):712–7.

44. Alter BP, Giri N, Savage SA, Peters JA, Loud JT, Leathwood L, et al. Malignancies and survival patterns in the National Cancer Institute inherited bone marrow failure syndromes cohort study. Br J Haematol. 2010;150(2):179–88.

45. Donadieu J, Leblanc T, Bader Meunier B, Barkaoui M, Fenneteau O, Bertrand Y, et al. Analysis of risk factors for myelodysplasias, leukemias and death from infection among patients with congenital neutropenia. Experience of the French Severe Chronic Neutropenia Study Group. Haematologica. 2005;90(1):45–53.

46. Mäkitie O, Ellis L, Durie PR, Morrison JA, Sochett EB, Rommens JM, et al. Skeletal phenotype in patients with Shwachman–Diamond syndrome and mutations in SBDS. Clin Genet. 2004;65(2):101–12.

47. Kerr EN, Ellis L, Dupuis A, Rommens JM, Durie PR. The behavioral phenotype of school-age children with shwachman diamond syndrome indicates neurocognitive dysfunction with loss of Shwachman–Bodian–Diamond syndrome gene function. J Pediatr. 2010;156(3):433–8.

48. Myers KC, Bolyard AA, Otto B, Wong TE, Jones AT, Harris RE, et al. Variable clinical presentation of Shwachman–Diamond syndrome: update from the North American Shwachman–Diamond syndrome registry. J Pediatr. 2014;164(4):866–70.

49. Ip WF, Dupuis A, Ellis L, Beharry S, Morrison J, Stormon MO, et al. Serum pancreatic enzymes define the pancreatic phenotype in patients with Shwachman–Diamond syndrome. J Pediatr. 2002;141(2):259–65.

50. Rötiga A, Cormiera V, Kolla F, Mize CE, Saudubraya JM, Veerman A, et al. Site-specific deletions of the mitochondrial genome in the Pearson marrow-pancreas syndrome. Genomics. 1991;10(2):502–4.

51. Online Mendelian inheritance in man. http://omim.org/entry/557000. Accessed 2 Jan 2014.

52. Tumino M, Meli C, Farruggia P, La Spina M, Faraci M, Castana C, et al. Clinical manifestations and management of four children with Pearson syndrome. Am J Med Genet A. 2011;155A(12):3063–6.

53. Casademont J, Barrientos A, Cardellach F, Rötlg A, Grau JM, Montoya J, et al. Multiple deletions of mtDNA in two brothers with sideroblastic anemia and mitochondrial myopathy and in their asymptomatic mother. Hum Mol Genet. 1994;3(11):1945–9.

54. Johanson A, Blizzard R. A syndrome of congenital aplasia of the alae nasi, deafness, hypothyroidism, dwarfism, absent permanent teeth, and malabsorption. J Pediatr. 1971;79(6):982–7.

55. Zenker M, Mayerle J, Lerch MM, Tagariello A, Zerres K, Durie PR, et al. Deficiency of UBR1, a ubiquitin ligase of the N-end rule pathway, causes pancreatic dysfunction, malformations and mental retardation (Johanson–Blizzard syndrome). Nat Genet. 2005;37(12):1345–50.

56. Almashraki N, Abdulnabee MZ, Sukalo M, Alrajoudi A, Sharafadeen I, Zenker M. Johanson–Blizzard syndrome. World J Gastroenterol. 2011;17(37):4247–50.

57. Michel SH, Maqbool A, Hanna MD, Mascarenhas M. Nutrition management of pediatric patients who have cystic fibrosis. Pediatr Clin North Am. 2009;56(5):1123–41.

58. Laterza L, Scaldaferri F, Bruno G, Agnes A, Boškoski I, Ianiro G, et al. Pancreatic function assessment. Eur Rev Med Pharmacol Sci. 2013;17(Suppl 2):65–71.

59. Daftary A, Acton J, Heubi J, Amin R. Fecal elastase-1: utility in pancreatic function in cystic fibrosis. J Cyst Fibros. 2006;5(2):71–6.

60. Weintraub A, Blau H, Mussaffi H, Picard E, Bentur L, Kerem E, Stankiewicz H, Wilschanski M. Exocrine pancreatic function testing in patients with cystic fibrosis and pancreatic sufficiency: a correlation study. J Pediatr Gastroenterol Nutr. 2009;48(3):306–10.

61. Van De Kamer JH, Bokkel Huinink HT, Weyers HA. Rapid method for the determination of fat in feces. J Biol Chem. 1949;177(1):347–55.

62. Del Rosario MA, Fitzgerald JF, Gupta SK, Croffie JM. Direct measurement of pancreatic enzymes after stimulation with secretin versus secretin plus cholecystokinin. J Pediatr Gastroenterol Nutr. 2000;31(1):28–32.

63. Swart GR, Baartman EA, Wattimena JL, Rietveld T, Overbeek SE, van den Berg JW. Evaluation studies of the 13C-mixed triglyceride breath test in healthy controls and adult cystic fibrosis patients with exocrine pancreatic insufficiency. Digestion. 1997;58(5):415–20.

64. van Dijk-van Aalst K, Van Den Driessche M, van der Schoor S, Schiffelers S, van't Westeinde T, Ghoos Y, et al. 13C mixed triglyceride breath test: a noninvasive method to assess lipase activity in children. J Pediatr Gastroenterol Nutr. 2001;32(5):579–85.

65. Borowitz DS, Grand RJ, Durie PR. Use of pancreatic enzyme supplements for patients with cystic fibrosis in the context of fibrosing colonopathy. Consensus committee. J Pediatr. 1995;127(5):681–4.

66. Littlewood JM. Update on intestinal strictures. J R Soc Med. 1999;92(Suppl 37):41–9.

67. Littlewood JM, Wolfe SP, Conway SP. Diagnosis and treatment of intestinal malabsorption in cystic fibrosis. Pediatr Pulmonol. 2006;41(1):35–49.

Celiac Disease

Stefano Guandalini and Valentina Discepolo

Definition

A permanent sensitivity to gluten resulting in a small-intestinal inflammatory disorder occurring in genetically predisposed individuals belonging to human leukocyte antigen (HLA)-class II specific haplotypes, celiac disease (CD) is characterized by a variable combination of elevated titers of celiac-specific autoantibodies, an inflammatory enteropathy with variable degrees of severity, and a wide range of gastrointestinal (GI) and extraintestinal complaints [1, 2].

Described in modern times by Samuel Gee in 1888 [3], it was only in the 1940s that Dicke identified the central role of gluten [4]. The subsequent availability, in the 1960s [5], of a capsule to obtain biopsies from the small intestine allowed the description of the typical changes caused by gluten in the duodenal mucosa of affected individuals. In the following decades, it became clear that CD reached far beyond the intestine as it was associated with many non-GI signs and symptoms, some HLA-associated, some not. Among the best described are: short stature [6, 7], osteoporosis [8, 9], iron-deficiency anemia (IDA) [10–12], arthritis [13–15], headaches [16–18], liver and biliary tract abnormalities [19, 20], myalgia [21, 22], adverse pregnancy outcomes [23–25], dental enamel defects [26, 27], dermatitis herpetiformis [28, 29], and others. In addition, a clear association with other autoimmune conditions such as type 1 diabetes has been well documented [30–32], and its link with some congenital disorders such as IgA deficiency and Down syndrome among others was discovered [33]. Although a genetic-based disease, CD can have its onset at any age, from infancy to old age, triggered by traumatic events, or in most cases without any obvious precipitating factor.

Epidemiology

The prevalence of CD is increasing at a remarkable pace during the past few decades [34–39]. Once thought to be a rare condition, affecting no more than 1/10,000 people, thanks to the availability and widespread use of specific and sensitive serological markers, CD is now recognized worldwide as a common disorder, with a prevalence varying between 3 and 13 per 1000 [40]. While an increased awareness, especially in North America, is responsible for increased diagnostic rates, reliable epidemiological data document worldwide a true increase in prevalence, of the order of doubling rates every 20 years or so. In Northern Sweden, an epidemiological investigation employing a combined serological/endoscopic approach in an unselected population of 1000 adults found a prevalence of almost 2 % [41]. It is assumed that a variety of environmental factors are responsible for such a rapid change [34–39]. Among them: modalities of delivery [42, 43], early-life infections [44], including RSV infections leading to hospitalization [45], exposure to antibiotics [46], infant feeding practices [47, 48], and even socioeconomic status [49, 50]. However, only a limited portion of the expected celiac patients is actually identified, with proportions varying between different countries: in the USA, even though CD overall prevalence should be around 1 %, only about 15 % of this population (including children and adults) has been diagnosed and can therefore be treated [51]. This phenomenon of underdiagnosis is likely due to a combination of inadequate awareness and a high prevalence of asymptomatic patients and appears to be quite widespread. Recent data suggest that unless a mass screening is implemented, it might be hard to improve substantially our current diagnosis rates, as even strategies based on large-scale case finding have failed to improve diagnostic rates [52].

S. Guandalini (✉)
Department of Pediatrics, Section of Gastroenterology, Hepatology and Nutrition, Comer Children's Hospital, University of Chicago, Chicago, IL, USA
e-mail: sguandalini@peds.bsd.uchicago.edu

V. Discepolo
Department of Translational Medical Science—Section of Pediatrics University of Naples "Federico II", Napoli, Italy

Department of Medicine, University of Chicago, Chicago, IL, USA
e-mail: vale.discepolo@gmail.com

© Springer International Publishing Switzerland 2016
S. Guandalini et al. (eds.), *Textbook of Pediatric Gastroenterology, Hepatology and Nutrition*,
DOI 10.1007/978-3-319-17169-2_40

Of interest, CD seems to affect more females than males, with a ratio of about 2:1. However, since studies of prevalence based on screening do not show such clear-cut difference, it is currently thought that the female predominance, while in part due to a true higher prevalence in girls versus boys, could also in part be attributed to the fact that women appear to utilize health-care services more than men [53, 54]. Currently, in most populations, women constitute 60–70 % of individuals with diagnosed CD [55, 56].

Etiopathogenesis

Like most multifactorial disorders, CD is the result of a complex interaction between genes, immune status of the host, and environmental triggers.

Genetic Factors

The weight of genetic predisposing factors in CD pathogenesis is relevant, as initially suggested by the observation of a strong familiar aggregation [57], with a prevalence of CD among first-degree relatives of around 10 %. The most important and best-characterized susceptibility gene is the HLA class II; in particular, the HLA-DQ2 and HLA-DQ8 alleles are required for CD development. The concordance rate is about 30 % among HLA-identical siblings, 80 % in monozygotic twins, and 10 % in dizygotic twins [58]. The HLA-DQ2 molecules are expressed on the surface of antigen-presenting cells; they contain positively charged pockets that preferentially bind negatively charged epitopes, such as deamidated gliadin peptides (DGP), and present them to cluster of differentiation-4 $(CD4)^+$ T cells thereby activating them [59, 60].

The Central Role of HLA-DQ Haplotype

HLA genes are located on chromosome six and are divided into three classes (I–III). HLA-DQ (6p21.3) belongs to class II and is composed of a heterodimer located on antigen-presenting cells and encoded by HLA-DQA1 and HLA-DQB1. Each of the copies of the HLA-DQ gene encodes for a heterodimer, resulting in four proteins (one couple per chromosome). HLA-DQ2 homozygotes (DQB1*02 on both chromosomes) subjects have the highest risk to develop CD, fivefold higher than heterozygotes [61, 62]. Even if more rare in the general population, DQ2 homozygosis is characteristic of 25 % of all CD patients and often relates to a more severe clinical outcome, as suggested by its association with earlier disease onset [63, 64] and its higher prevalence in refractory CD patients [65]. In fact, the immune response arising in

homozygous individuals is stronger than the response from heterozygous individuals [57, 66]. The most common configuration (more than 50 % of CD patients) is represented by DQ2.5 (DQB1*02/DQA1*05) heterozygotes [62].

HLA-DQ8 is found in 5–10 % of CD patients [62, 67], with DQ8 homozygosis conferring increased risk compared to DQ8 heterozygosis [68]. It must be noted that about 5 % of CD patients carry only one of the HLA-DQ2 heterodimer alleles (HLA-DQA1*05 or HLA-DQB1*02), therefore encoding for the so-called "half heterodimer." These patients constitute the overwhelming majority of CD subjects not carrying the full HLA-DQ2 and/or -DQ8 alleles [69]. The highest risk group includes individuals who inherit both DQ8 and DQ2.

Only less than 1 % of patients who fulfill clinical criteria for CD do not carry the DQ2 (including half heterodimer) nor the DQ8 alleles [69]. Thus, in the clinical practice CD can be virtually excluded in individuals lacking HLA-DQ2 or -DQ8.

Interestingly, 30 % of European descent individuals carry HLA-DQ2 susceptibility allele, however only about 4 % of these individuals will develop CD [61]. This suggests that even though those molecules are necessary, they are not sufficient to induce the disease, implying that other genetic and environmental factors must contribute to it.

Non-HLA Genetic Susceptibility Factors

HLA alleles explain only 35 % of the disease genetic susceptibility, while the remaining is due to numerous non-HLA genes that singularly contribute to a much lower extent to CD heritability. A recent dense genotyping study [70] identified 13 new CD risk loci reaching genome-wide significance, bringing the number of known CD-associated susceptibility loci (including the HLA locus) to 40. Notably, 64 % of the 39 non-HLA loci were shared with at least another autoimmune disease (e.g., type 1 diabetes), reinforcing the idea that autoimmune disorders may share common pathogenic pathways [71].

In those regions, more than 115 non-HLA genes have been associated to CD, individually contributing only modestly to the overall disease risk. Twenty-eight of them encode for molecules involved in the immune response, reinforcing the central role of immune dysregulation in CD pathogenesis. Post-genome-wide association studies (GWAS) will need to focus on elucidating the functional basis of these genetic variants, in particular, the role of regulatory variation. Furthermore, considering multiple gene variants may help refining risk prediction models and identifying high-risk individuals that could benefit of preventive strategies.

Environmental Factors

The high impact of genetic predisposing factors in CD does not exclude a key role of the environment in triggering disease development. In fact, the increased incidence of CD in the past decades cannot be explained by genetic drift and most likely results from faster changes in the environment. In an elegant review, Abadie et al. [72] show that CD prevalence does not perfectly correlate, as it would be predicted, with the levels of wheat consumption and frequencies of HLA-DQ predisposing alleles, thus emphasizing the role of environmental factors in CD pathogenesis.

Infant Feeding Practices and CD Development

Mode of delivery and breast-feeding contributes to shape the infant immune system, thus suggesting that both maternal microbial intestinal flora and early infant feeding practices may have a key role in determining future development of immune-mediated diseases.

As for modalities of delivery, elective cesarean section (C-section) has been associated with a modest increased risk of later CD, possibly related to the profound differences in the intestinal microbiota found between vaginally versus C-section delivered babies [43, 73].

The importance of early infant feeding and timing of first gluten introduction had been highlighted by the so-called "Swedish epidemic." In the late 1980s in Sweden, a fourfold increase in CD incidence was recorded in children below the age of two that dropped to pre-1985 rates a decade later [74, 75]. This rapid rise in disease incidence correlated with several changes in infant dietary patterns including introduction of gluten after completing breast-feeding and increased amount of gluten in the infant diet. Of interest, such increased incidence declined to pre-epidemic levels only after these changes were reverted [76, 77]. Prolonged breast-feeding too had been thought to have a protective effect on later onset of the disease [78, 79]. On this basis, gradual introduction of small amounts of gluten during breast-feeding has been proposed as strategy to prevent early onset of CD, and breast-feeding is recommended, in infants born in families at risk for CD, for the whole first year of life, with gluten introduction advised between 4 and 6 months of life [80, 81]. While prior studies had suggested, as we have seen, that infant feeding practices and timing of initial gluten exposure are important, two recent multicenter randomized trials that tested strategies of early or delayed gluten introduction in infants, showed that neither strategy appeared to influence celiac disease risk. Additionally, breast-feeding was not show to protect against the development of CD [82, 83].

Viral Infections

Among environmental factors that contribute to trigger CD, infective agents have been proposed. Higher rates of summer births were described in children with CD, suggesting that exposure of 4–6-month-old infants to winter-linked viral infections such as rotavirus may play a role. The first correlation between viruses and CD dates back to the 1980s when a homology between alpha gliadin and a protein of the human adenovirus [84] had been described and related to increased frequency of adenovirus infection in CD patients [85] compared to controls. More recently, increased rate of rotavirus infections (as measured by anti-rotavirus antibody titers) has been associated with a moderate, but significantly increased risk of CD in HLA-susceptible children [86]. The mechanisms through which viral infections in early life can increase CD occurrence in later years have not been elucidated.

Microbiome

The composition of intestinal microbiota as well as bacterial metabolic products (and especially short-chain fatty acids) can affect intestinal epithelium function and mucosal immune homeostasis. Both quantitative and qualitative differences in the composition of the intestinal microbiome have been observed in patients with autoimmune disorders [87, 88], as well as CD [89–93] when compared to healthy individuals. In the context of CD, an expansion of some pathogenic bacterial populations (*Escherichia coli* and *Staphylococcus*) [93, 94] and a reduction in butyrate-producing bacteria *(Bifidobacterium)* [95, 96] have been described. Currently, it is still unclear whether the observed changes in the microbial composition are the cause or the result of the intestinal inflammatory process. Indeed, epithelial alterations, such as those described in CD, could create a specific environment favoring the selective colonization of some microbial species, thus contributing to the creation of the microenvironmental milieu that favors the disease development. This is clearly a rapidly evolving field, likely to bring important new acquisitions in the near future.

Pathogenesis

CD is a chronic inflammatory disorder with autoimmune features, characterized by a T cell-mediated immune response arising in the small-intestinal mucosa upon gluten ingestion. In genetically susceptible individuals, gliadin peptides activate stress pathways and provide ligands for innate immune receptors, leading to the release of pro-inflammatory mediators that then sustain the T cell response both in the lamina propria and in the epithelium (Fig. 40.1). This inflammatory reaction typically involves both the innate and the adaptive arms of the immune response. In this model, two hits are required, each one being necessary but not sufficient for the development of CD: one is the activation of stress markers in intestinal epithelial cells and the second is the rise of a gluten-specific proinflammatory CD4 T cell response in the lamina propria [97, 215]. These two events lead to the full activation of mobilization of lymphocytes in the intestinal

epithelium (intraepithelial lymphocytes—IELs), final responsible of tissue destruction [98].

The immunological reaction occurring in CD patients follows the ingestion of gluten-containing cereals: wheat, rye, and barley. Glutenins and gliadins, typical gluten components, are responsible for the viscosity and elasticity of the wheat dough [99, 100]. Their high concentration of glutamine and proline residues (35 and 15% of the total amino acid content) renders them highly resistant to GI enzymes [101]. Indeed, the lack of prolyl-endopeptidase activity in any of the human digestive enzymes prevents enzymatic at-

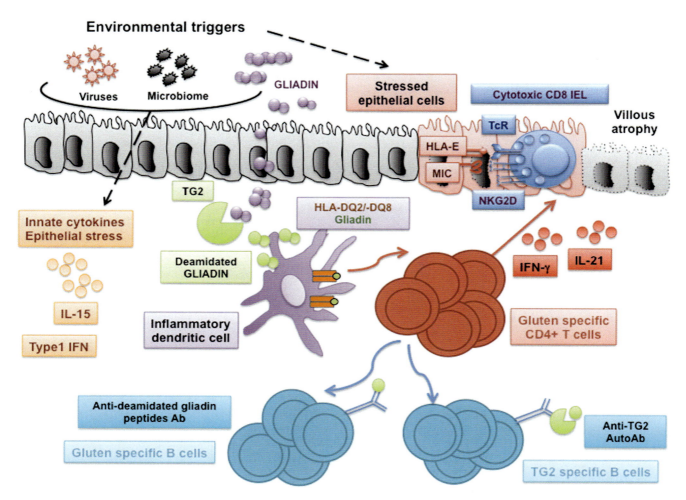

Fig. 40.1 CD pathogenesis. Celiac disease (*CD*) is a multifactorial disorder induced by gluten in genetically susceptible subjects. Several environmental factors (i.e., viral infections, alterations in microbiome composition, etc.) can contribute to trigger the disease by inducing epithelial stress in the intestinal mucosa, and the production of innate immune cytokines, such as interleukin 15 (*IL-15*) and type-1 interferon (*type-1 IFN*). Those cytokines contribute to create a pro-inflammatory environment that enhances dendritic cells activation. Undigested gliadin peptides (*purple circles*) reach the intestinal lamina propria where they are deamidated by tissue-transglutaminase 2 (*TG2*). Deamidation renders gliadin peptides more suitable to be presented by HLA-DQ molecules. Only dendritic cells expressing the CD-associated HLA-DQ2 and/or -DQ8 molecules (*orange*) can present deamidated gliadin peptides (*green circles*) to naïve CD4+ T cells (*red cells*). Inflammatory

dendritic cells (*purple*) enhance the arise of a gluten-specific CD4+ T cell response, characterized by the production of high levels of pro-inflammatory cytokines such as interferon-gamma (*IFN-γ*) and interleukin 21 (*IL-21*). These cytokines are thought to contribute to induce a full activation of cytotoxic CD8+ intraepithelial lymphocytes (*IEL*). The second hit required for the induction of a full activation of IEL is the expression of stress markers (i.e., MIC-A and IL-15) in intestinal epithelial cells. Fully activated CD8+ IEL are responsible for the intestinal epithelial destruction and the induction of villous atrophy in CD patients. Furthermore, gluten-reactive CD4+ T cells provide the required help to TG2-specific B cells, presenting TG2–gliadin complexes, in a hapten carrier-like manner and drive TG2-specific antibody production. *NKG2D* natural-killer group 2, member D, *MIC* macrophage inhibitory cytokine

tack of proline-rich domains in gluten proteins. Thus, at the end of a normal, full digestive process of gluten, many gliadin peptides remain undigested in the intestinal lumen. The mechanism through which such peptides reach the intestinal lamina propria is not entirely clear. Even though an increase in intestinal permeability has been shown in CD, a retro-transcytosis pathway has been described for secretory antibodies, potentially having a role also for gliadin transport [102].

Tissue-Tranglutaminase 2

In the subsequent steps in CD pathogenesis, the enzyme tissue transglutaminase 2 (tTG) has a pivotal role. tTG is a calcium-dependent transamidating enzyme that catalyzes covalent cross-linking of proteins. When located extracellularly in the presence of calcium, tTG is in an open and active form [103]; furthermore, an inflammatory environment leads to its constitutive activation [104]. tTG is the main autoantigen for CD: In addition, it has a crucial role in inducing posttranslational modification of gluten peptides. In fact, in the lamina propria, tTG mediates the conversion of glutamine into glutamic acid, introducing negatively charged residues into gliadin peptides that act as immunogenic epitopes binding to HLA-DQ molecules with relatively higher affinity, thus representing a prerequisite for a gluten-specific T cell response [105].

Autoantibodies

Genetic, mechanistic, and epidemiological data relate CD to other autoimmune disorders. One of the key diagnostic features of CD is the presence of serum anti-tTG IgA and IgG autoantibodies. The mechanisms leading to their production in CD are unclear. The upregulation and activation of tTG in inflamed tissues may generate additional antigenic epitopes by cross-linking or deamidating exogenous or endogenous proteins. However, the most accepted hypothesis for their formation, which explains also their dependence on dietary gluten, is that the enzyme cross-links itself to gluten during the substrate–enzyme interaction [106]. Once internalized, those complexes are processed and gluten epitopes bind HLA-DQ molecules of the B cell that may allow gluten-reactive CD4 T cells provide the required help to tTG-specific B cells in a hapten carrier-like manner and drive tTG-specific antibody production.

The Adaptive Immune Response in CD

CD originates as a result of both innate immunity and adaptive immunity activation. Adaptive response, characterized by the activation a gluten-specific CD4 T cell response in the intestinal lamina propria, is a key event in CD pathogenesis. Gluten contains a large number of peptides capable of stimulating T cells. Dendritic cells present negatively charged gliadin peptides through HLA-DQ2 or HLA-DQ8 molecules to naïve CD4 T cells, thus enhancing a T helper 1 inflammatory response, characterized by the production of high levels of interferon-γ (Fig. 40.1).

The gluten-specific CD4 T cell response is sustained by several cytokines, including IL-15 and IL-21. The expression of IL-21, enhanced by gluten, is very high in active CD patients, while it is downregulated in potential CD [107], supporting its role in the induction of tissue damage. It acts in synergy with IL-15 [108] promoting interferon-γ production and enhancing cytotoxic CD8 T cells proliferation and survival; however, the mechanism initiating its production in CD is unclear.

The Innate Immune Response

As mentioned, innate immune activation is also necessary for the development of CD. There is in fact evidence that in addition to the immunodominant epitopes, which as, discussed, are presented to CD4 naïve T cells, gliadin also contains fragments which are able to enhance epithelial stress and induce an innate immune effect [109–111]. The best-known fragment is the peptide 31–43 (P31–43) of α-gliadin, which is able to upregulate major histocompatibility complex (MHC) class I-related molecules (MICs) [112] to activate the mitogen-activated protein (MAP) kinase pathway and induce apoptosis in intestinal epithelial cells. P31–43 induces cell proliferation and actin cytoskeleton rearrangements in in vitro and ex vivo models [109–111, 113, 114]. The proliferative response elicited by P31–43 in CD mucosa involves epidermal growth factor (EGF)/IL15 cooperation. Of note, a constitutive activation of the EGF receptor (EGF-R)/extracellular signal-regulated kinases (ERK) pathway has been found in celiac patients [110] potentially representing a predisposing condition to the damaging effects of gliadin.

Of interest, P31–43 is able to impair actin cytoskeleton in healthy subjects, suggesting that it can act on similar pathways altered in CD cells. In addition, it enhances the expression of IL-15, a key innate cytokine involved in CD pathogenesis, as it contributes actively to enhance the expression of activating natural killer cells (NK) receptors (i.e., NKG2D) on IELs and impair the T regulatory cells function in celiac patients [115, 116].

IELs Activation and the Induction of Tissue Damage

The tissue damage typical of CD, characterized by villous atrophy and crypt hyperplasia, is due to a profound remodeling of the small intestinal architecture and is mainly mediated by cytotoxic IELs. IELs represent a heterogeneous population including TcRα/β CD8 cells NK-like cells, and TcRγ/δ cells.

As evident in potential CD patients, the gluten-specific T cell adaptive immune response alone can occur even in the absence of villous atrophy, suggesting that other signals are required to induce tissue damage [98]. Indeed, the full activation of IELs and acquisition of their cytotoxic killing phenotype requires also stimuli from the epithelial compartment. Increased expression of stress molecules, such as nonclassical MHC class I molecules (i.e., MIC and HLA-E), has been shown in intestinal epithelial cells of active CD patients, as part of the innate stress response induced by gluten or by other environmental triggers. MIC and HLA-E are ligands for NKG2D and CD94, activating NK receptors that are upregulated on IELs in CD patients and whose expression is enhanced by IL15. Activation of IELs, with increased Fas ligand expression, results in epithelial cell apoptosis and villous atrophy via interactions with Fas on intestinal epithelial cells.Altogether, the end result of these various events is to lead to IEL infiltration and the resulting tissue destruction, characterized by crypt hyperplasia and villous atrophy.

These changes occur in a continuum, going from normal to a complete flattening of the villi in a slow progression. Marsh [117] described in great detail such progression and his description is also utilized in the pathology reports from duodenal biopsies. Thus, the intestinal damage seen in CD is described as follows:

Type 0 or pre-infiltrative stage (normal);
Type 1 or infiltrative stage (increased IELs);
Type 2 or hyperplastic stage (type 1 + hyperplastic crypts);
Type 3 or destructive stage (type 2 + villous atrophy of progressively more severe degrees, denominated 3a—partial atrophy, 3b—subtotal atrophy, and 3c—total atrophy).

Clinical Presentations

The inflammatory changes described in the previous section, resulting in the most advanced cases in severe villous atrophy, lead to a wide variety of clinical presentations. While GI manifestations are understandably present and in many cases prominent, CD goes well beyond the GI tract, so that basically all systems and organs can be involved. GI signs and symptoms due to malabsorption, such as diarrhea and abdominal pain, are very common and easily lead to evaluation for CD, but they are by no means universally present. In fact, there is evidence [118–122] that CD presentation in children and teenagers has substantially changed over time, moving from a malabsorptive disorder causing GI symptoms and malnutrition to a more subtle condition causing a variety of extraintestinal manifestations (see Table 40.1). Thus, it is understandable that the term "typical," reserved for the GI

manifestations of CD, is quickly becoming obsolete, as the extraintestinal manifestations are now so prevalent they are no longer to be referred to as "atypical" [123]. It is indeed this variety of presentations, and the fact that CD may also be entirely asymptomatic, that is responsible for the dismal rate of diagnoses around the globe.

Table 40.1 reports the main clinical presentations of CD, with their prevalent age distribution. As it can be seen, the clinical manifestations can be protean, thus making the diagnosis not obvious in most cases. When CD has its onset in infancy and very early childhood, the GI manifestations prevail and can be quite aggressive, resulting in a clinical picture of malnutrition and failure to thrive, often associated with a protein-losing enteropathy. Subsequently, however, the onset may be more subtle, and more extraintestinal manifestations become common.

GI Manifestations

Abdominal pain and distention is probably the most common symptom of patients diagnosed with CD worldwide; in Canadian children, it has been reported in as many as 90% [124]. Chronic or intermitted diarrhea, characterized by bulky, foul-smelling, greasy stool, is a very common symptom in children with CD. Its occurrence, however, is progressively becoming less frequent than in the past. Counterintuitively, long-standing and occasionally severe constipation can be the presenting manifestation in a significant amount of patients, children, as well as adults [125]. Constipation appears to be related to a well-documented delay in oro-cecal transit time [126, 127], possibly caused in part by disturbed upper GI motor function [128]. Other presenting symptoms related to the GI tract are vomiting (especially in infants and toddlers), weight loss, or failure to thrive leading—particularly in cases of delayed diagnosis—to severe malnutrition and cachexia. However, it should be noted that children with CD can also be overweight or obese, as well documented in the literature, (reviewed in [129]) so that the absence of malnutrition should by no means rule out the possibility of CD. More rarely, other disorders such as acute electrolyte disturbances, hypotension, and lethargy can accompany the clinical picture [130]. Recurrent intussusception, an uncommon but important GI sign, was first described in children in 1997 [131], and it is now well recognized as an event occurring more frequently in CD children before their diagnosis than in control populations [132].

Mild elevation of liver transaminases is well described in pediatric CD. A recent meta-analysis [133] revealed that this sign is presented by 36% of children with CD, while 12% of children with mild unexplained hypertransaminasemia have CD. Of note, a gluten-free diet (GFD) normalized transaminase levels in 77–100% of patients with CD within 4–8 months.

Table 40.1 Clinical presentations of celiac disease according to age most commonly involved

Type	Sign or symptom	Age most commonly involved
Gastrointestinal	Abdominal pain, bloating	All ages
	Diarrhea	All ages
	Vomiting	Infancy
	Anorexia	Infancy to early childhood
	Constipation	Child to adolescent
	Failure to thrive	Infancy and early childhood
	Weight loss	Child to adult
	Recurrent intussusception	Infancy to early childhood
	Hypertransaminasemia and other liver issues	All ages
Extraintestinal	Sad mood	Infancy to early childhood
	Delayed puberty	Adolescent
	Short stature	Child to adolescent
	Iron-deficient anemia	Adolescent to adult
	Dermatitis herpetiformis	Adolescent to adult
	Dental enamel defects	Child to adult
	Aphthous ulcers	Child to adult
	Fatigue	Adolescent to adult
	Arthritis	Adolescent to adult
	Osteopenia	Adolescent to adult
	Osteoporosis	Adult
	Psychiatric disorders	Adolescent to adult
	Idiopathic seizures	Child to adult
	Headaches, migraines	Adolescent to adult
	Numbness/neuropathy	Adult
	Cerebellar ataxia	Adult
	Unexplained infertility (in women)	Adult

Gastrointestinal presentations are commonly also referred to as "Typical" D while all extraintestinal manifestations are called "Atypical." Historically, these denominations arose because for decades CD was thought to be restricted to symptoms and signs of malabsorption, and all extraintestinal manifestations were considered rare and not belonging to the classical presentation

Extraintestinal Manifestations

Anemia in celiac children can be the end result of several different, and sometimes combined, causes; however, the single most common type of anemia is due to iron deficiency.

IDA has in fact been reported in between 12 and 69% of newly diagnosed celiac cases [10–12, 122, 134]. Even when asymptomatic, CD can lead to IDA; in a large series of patients with subclinical CD, IDA was indeed found in almost half of the patients, with adults having a higher incidence than children: 46 versus 35% [10]. The pathogenesis of iron deficiency in celiac seems to be straightforward; in fact, iron is absorbed in the duodenum and proximal jejunum, areas that are typically most affected in florid CD. Thus, most cases result from an impaired absorption of iron. The higher prevalence of anemia in celiac patients with an atrophic mucosa (Marsh 3) compared to those with mild enteropathy (Marsh 1 or 2) recently found in a study conducted in Italy on a large number of patients [135] provides indirect support for this.

Dermatitis herpetiformis (DH) is considered the skin presentation of CD. Rare in children, DH affects mostly teen-

agers and adults who present symmetrical, pruritic blisters followed by erosions, excoriations, and hyperpigmentation. The most commonly involved sites are the elbows (90%), knees (30%), shoulders, buttocks, sacral region, and face. Itching of variable intensity, scratching, and burning sensation immediately preceding the development of lesions are common [136, 137]. The diagnosis rests on a combination of clinical, serological (same autoantibodies utilized for CD), and histological criteria showing the typical IgA deposits in skin biopsies [138, 139]. Its treatment is based on a strict GFD. Dapsone and/or other drugs should be used during the period until the GFD is effective [138].

Dental enamel hypoplasia is more common in patients with CD compared to the general population [26], and in CD it has been reported with a prevalence ranging from 10 to 97%. It appears to be more prevalent in children, compared with adults with CD and is thought to be secondary to nutritional deficiencies and immune disturbances during the period of enamel formation in the first 7 years [27].

Aphthous ulcers too can be present in children and adults with CD and they often regress once the patients are on a GFD [28].

Low bone mineral density is found in the vast majority of newly diagnosed patients, and in some cases it is advanced to osteoporosis and can be associated with fractures. The etiology of such bone alterations in CD is multifactorial, thought to be mostly secondary to the combination of intestinal malabsorption and chronic inflammation. At diagnosis, approximately one-third of adult CD patients have osteoporosis, one-third have osteopenia, and one-third have normal bone mineral density [29]. While children with CD, once on a GFD, seem to be able to improve their bone mineral density more fastly, adult patients' bone mineral density was found to be significantly lower than expected for the normal population, not just at diagnosis, but even after 1 or 2 years of GFD [140]. Thus, there is a risk for suboptimal peak bone mass acquisition and a retarded growth in CD children, as the bone density increases until the end of puberty, when it reaches its peak value: if normal peak bone mass is not achieved, the individual is at a higher risk for developing osteoporosis [141].

Joint involvement, though not too common, has been described in children and adults with CD and it is suggested that patients presenting with unexplained articular manifestations be tested for CD [142].

Children with CD have a slightly increased frequency of neurological symptoms compared to controls. These include headache [143], peripheral neuropathy [144], and seizures; ataxia is described only in adult cases [145]. The prevalence of epilepsy in CD children also appears to be slightly higher than expected, around 1% [146]. Seizures are often generalized tonic–clonic, but partial and occasionally absence seizures are also reported [146, 147]. A recent epidemiologic study of nearly 29,000 subjects with CD and 143,000 controls found that CD increased the risk of epilepsy, including in children, by 1.4-fold [148]. In some patients with CD and epilepsy refractory to antiepileptic drugs, seizures have been controlled with a GFD [149, 150].

Relatively common in adolescents are also psychiatric issues: anxiety, often with recurrent panic attacks, hallucinations, depression, leading to a slightly higher prevalence of suicidal behavior in celiac patients [30]. Interestingly, there is some evidence that the GFD may help in alleviating depression in celiac adolescents [31].

Disease Associations

A series of recent large-scale epidemiological investigations, mostly, but not solely, conducted in Sweden, have also revealed a growing number of associated conditions that can occur with CD, although in most cases the reasons for such associations and the clinical relevance of them remain unclear. Among the conditions with increased prevalence in CD, in most cases related to adult patients, are: chronic obstructive pulmonary disease [151], ischemic heart disease [152], urticaria [153], eosinophilic esophagitis and gastroesophageal reflux disease [154], pancreatitis [155], hemochromatosis [156], cataracts and uveitis [157, 158], idiopathic dilated cardiomyopathy [159], nephrolithiasis [160], end-stage renal disease [161], eating disorders [162], primary hyperparathyroidism [38] (a risk however subsiding on GFD), adrenal insufficiency [33], systemic lupus [163], cataract [40], and endometriosis [39].

In addition, the offspring of celiac mothers appear to also be at an increased risk for a number of adverse events, including congenital malformations [164].

On the other hand, a reduced risk for ovarian and breast cancer has been reported for celiac women [165].

IgA deficiency has also been associated with CD. In fact, about 8% of IgA-deficient children are celiac [166] and about 2% of CD children are IgA-deficient [167]. While clinically not relevant, this association is important in the strategy of screening for CD (see below).

Autoimmune Conditions

A strong association has also been shown between CD and autoimmune disorders, thought to be mostly due to a shared genetic component in the HLA region. The best described association is with type 1 diabetes mellitus (T1DM), where a prevalence of approximately 10% of CD is found [32, 168]. About two-thirds of children diagnosed with CD after T1DM onset have elevated levels of celiac antibodies at the time of T1DM diagnosis or within the first 24 months; however, an additional 40% of patients develop CD a few years after diabetes onset [169], and even adults with a long history of T1DM show a progressively higher prevalence of CD [170]. Thus, it is recommended that T1DM children be repeatedly tested for CD. Of note, it has been shown that the presence or absence of GI symptoms in children with T1DM has no predictable value for biopsy-confirmed CD or not [168]. Clearly, once diagnosed with CD, children with T1DM need to follow a GFD. Its effects on diabetic control are however unclear: In fact, glycemic control, both in children with or without malabsorption, has been found either improved or unaffected [171].

The issue of whether the onset of autoimmune disorders in CD patients is favored by the ingestion of gluten remains controversial. An increased prevalence of autoimmune disorders was found in parallel with the increasing age at diagnosis of CD [172], suggesting that prolonged exposure to gluten may favor the onset of autoimmune conditions; however, these results have not been reproduced by subsequent investigations [173, 174], leaving the question unresolved [175].

Chromosomal Disorders

Down syndrome [176], Turner syndrome [177], and Williams syndrome [178] are conditions where the prevalence of CD has been found to be higher than in the general population, and hence children with such syndromes need to be screened for CD.

Diagnosing CD

Given the many various manifestations of CD, in children as well as adults, clearly the first requisite for diagnosis is a high degree of suspicion. Table 40.2 lists the circumstances that demand testing for CD.

The availability of very sensitive and specific autoantibodies in the IgA subclass, generated in the small intestinal mucosa and detectable in the serum, such as the tTG-IgA or anti-endomysium IgA (EMA-IgA) [179] has given the physician a powerful screening tool. In addition, another class of antibodies has also been found valuable in screening (especially in very young children when tTG-IgA could be negative [180, 181]) and in following up patients with CD: the anti-DGP, both -IgA and -IgG antibodies produced against the gliadin peptides after they have been modified by the tTG [182]. Currently, it is universally recommended [33, 179, 183] that tTG-IgA and total serum IgA be the first line of screening, due to the very elevated sensitivity of this test. Total serum IgA needs to be added in order to ascertain that the individual is able to produce tTG-IgA: In fact, celiac patients who happen to be IgA-deficient may have a false-negative tTG-IgA. In these circumstances, both tTG-IgG [184–186] and DGP-IgG [187] can be usefully checked as markers of CD.

In 1990, the European Society of Pediatric Gastroenterology, Hepatology and Nutrition (ESPGHAN) published diagnostic criteria [188] that have been universally applied for over 20 years, both in pediatric age and in adults. While reducing the number of biopsy procedures needed for a firm

Table 40.2 Subjects to be screened for CD

All conditions listed in Table 40.1
First-degree relatives of celiac patients
IgA deficiency
Autoimmune conditions
Type 1 diabetes
Autoimmune thyroiditis
Autoimmune hepatitis
Addison's disease
Chromosomal disorders
Down syndrome
Turner syndrome
Williams syndrome

diagnosis from three of the original guidelines (initial one showing typical changes, followed after a year on GFD by a second one documenting healing, and finally by a third one after gluten challenge to show relapse) to only one, they still called for the indispensable role of documenting the flattening of small-intestinal mucosal villi in patients with a consistent history and laboratory findings. In 2012, an ad hoc task force of the same society published revised criteria [1] and produced an evidence-based algorithm that allowed the physician to skip the duodenal biopsy under certain circumstances, namely, in children and teenagers showing a genetic asset and a history compatible with CD, a very elevated titer (more than ten times the upper limit of normal) of tTG-IgA, along with a positive EMA titer. While this simplified approach appears certainly valid, as it possesses a positive predictive value close to 100 %, one needs to apply it with great care. In fact, children with GI complaints diagnosed without the endoscopy may have additional disorders that would go undiagnosed by skipping this procedure.

Figure 40.2 is an algorithm (based in part on the ESPGHAN guidelines [1]) that summarizes the diagnostic steps for a child or teenager suspected of CD. Again, Table 40.2 lists the presentations that require screening. The subject with normal serum IgA and normal tTG-IgA do not need to be considered celiac, given the high sensitivity of the test; however, since it would appear that in the infant and toddler tTG-IgA may not be as sensitive as in later ages, DGP-IgA and DGP-IgG can be measured additionally. Furthermore, in the presence of a strong clinical suspicion in the very young child, it would be appropriate to still proceed with an esophago-gastro-duodenoscopy (EGD) with biopsy even if celiac serology is negative.

If the subject has positive tTG-IgA, then the titer becomes important. In fact, as mentioned, with titers that are more than ten times the upper limit of normal range, the EMA titer must be checked and if it too is clearly positive, then the diagnosis of CD can be considered definitive. On the contrary, the EGD would be necessary if the EMA prove negative, or in all cases where the tTG-IgA increase does not reach the threshold of >10× normal. It is important to notice that it is recommended [1, 183, 189] that at least four biopsies be taken from the distal duodenum, and also one or two from the bulb, otherwise the diagnostic yield may be jeopardized by the occasional patchy duodenal lesions.

The interpretation of the pathology of the duodenal biopsies guides the final diagnosis: while pathology changes showing lesions of Marsh type 2–3, in the presence of positive serology, confirm the diagnosis, caution must be exerted for findings of Marsh type 1, especially when not supported by positive serology. In fact, such increased presence of IELs ("lymphocytic duodenosis") has been found to be due to celiac in no more than 16–39 % of cases [190, 191]. Thus, additional conditions (see Table 40.3) must be carefully looked at before concluding for its association with CD.

Fig. 40.2 Suggested diagnostic
algorithm

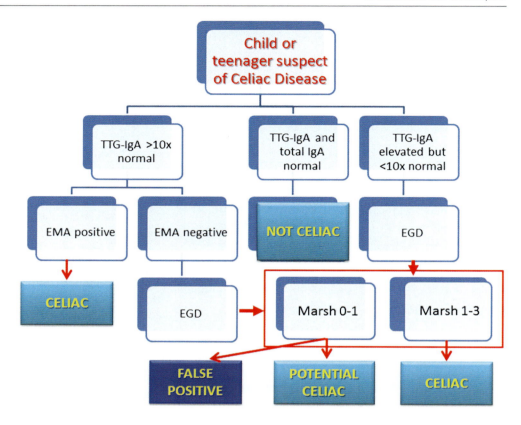

Table 40.3 Conditions causing lymphocytic duodenosis (Marsh type 1 changes)

Celiac disease
H. pylori gastritis
Small-bowel bacterial overgrowth
NSAID and other drugs
Immune dysregulation
Crohn's disease
Food protein-induced enteropathy
Infections

NSAID nonsteroidal anti-inflammatory drugs

As for those with a Marsh type 0, the call is even more delicate. In fact, the patient can be defined as "potential" if tTG-IgA are elevated >10× and/or EMA titer is positive; but with tTG-IgA increased less than ten times and a negative EMA, then the possibility of a false-positive tTG-IgA must be considered. This occurrence is especially common, for unclear reasons, in children with T1DM, where tTG-IgA have also been found to spontaneously normalize [192]. Such patients should therefore remain on a gluten-containing diet and be carefully monitored.

More complex is the decision about the need for a GFD for true "potential" celiac children and adolescents who are asymptomatic. The literature shows in fact variable percentages (between 30 and 60%) of evolution into full-blown CD when they are left on gluten [193–195], including the possibility of some eventually becoming serologically negative. It seems in fact that potential CD patients show a low grade of inflammation that likely could be due to active regulatory mechanisms preventing the progression toward a mucosal damage [196]. In essence, while research will eventually allow us to predict which patients would develop full-blown CD if left on gluten, currently we do not have this capacity, so that the decision on whether or not to put potential celiac patients on a GFD must be taken with great care, on an individual basis, and be properly agreed upon by the family.

Complications

Refractory CD

Better known by the older terminology as "refractory sprue," refractory CD is a very severe form of CD that does not respond to a GFD, in spite of normalization of celiac serology [197]. Refractory CD almost exclusively occurs in adults or elderly patients who have been suffering from malabsorptive symptoms for a long time prior to being diagnosed. This condition is further classified into type I and type II on the basis of gamma chain T cell clonal rearrangement and aberrant T cell phenotypes. Type II refractory CD is the most aggressive form, leading to the most feared complication of CD: the enteropathy-associated T cell lymphoma (EATL). As a consequence, refractory CD results in an increased mortality rate, with a 5-year survival rate of 80–96 % for patients with type I refractory CD and 44–58 % for type II cases [197]. When examining the survival rate of those patients with type II refractory CD who developed EATL, the survival rate at 5 years was a dismal 8 % [198]. New treatment modalities, including autologous stem cell transplant, are becoming available for this aggressive condition [199, 200].

Increased Mortality Rate

Aside from the risks related to refractory CD, evidence is mounting that unrecognized, and hence untreated, CD may carry a risk for increased mortality rate [201]. There appears to be a positive correlation between diagnostic delay and/ or insufficient compliance with the diet and decreased life expectancy, which has been documented in a large retrospective study in Italy [202]. More recently, increased mortality has also been reported in undiagnosed patients (based on elevated serum tTG-IgA) in the USA [203] and in Europe [204–206].

All of the evidence therefore strongly emphasizes the importance of an aggressive strategy for early detection and treatment of patients with CD.

Treatment

CD is a lifelong condition and a strict GFD is currently the only available treatment. While the exact amount of gluten that can be tolerated daily by CD patients is unknown and is likely to be subject to a wide interindividual variability, there is evidence that no patient would react to a daily dose of up to 10 mg, while the majority would at 100 mg or above [207]. In practice, many patients, and especially older children and adults, do not present any symptom after inadvertent gluten ingestion or sporadic intentional consumption of gluten-containing products. In addition, dietary compliance assessment is not always an easy task, since serology often fails to reveal slight transgressions. Therefore, a periodical follow-up is needed and the importance of a lifelong diet should be constantly reinforced, especially to asymptomatic patients. The dietary restriction must include wheat, rye, barley, and their derivatives such as triticale, spelt, and kamut. Other cereals such as rice, corn, maize, and buckwheat are perfectly safe for CD patients and can be used as wheat substitutes. Oats were included in the first group of toxic cereals, but later evidence has conclusively shown that they are tolerated by the vast majority of patients, provided the oats-based products are manufactured in plants that can guarantee absence of any possible cross-contamination with flours

based on wheat, rye, or barley. In any case, introducing them with prudence is recommended in order to recognize any adverse effect.

Gluten withdrawal is necessary to shut down the inflammatory response arising in the gut. However, whether a GFD could prevent the development of associated autoimmune conditions or complications, such as malignancies, is still debated [175]. As discussed previously, since the benefits of GFD in terms of prevention of complications and comorbidities in patients with potential CD are still unclear, it remains controversial whether such dietary regimen should be proposed to all of them, particularly those who are asymptomatic.

Future Potential Therapeutic Strategies

Following a lifelong strict dietary regimen is not an easy task for many patients, especially teenagers and young adults who may not easily accept limitations to their social life. On the other hand, there is a subgroup of CD patients (i.e., refractory CD) who fail to respond even to a strict GFD, thus reinforcing the concept that GFD could not be considered a cure for all CD patients. Importantly, a variety of commercial food products and some safe cereals can be cross-contaminated with unsafe cereals as the result of mixing during transportation and processing. Hence, there is a requirement for alternative approaches to treat CD.

A first approach may consist in creating new varieties of wheat that are safe for CD patients. The identification of the full sequences of immune-stimulating peptides may lead to the production of wheat varieties lacking biologically active peptide sequences through breeding programs and/or transgenic technology. Large-scale cultivars where these cereals could replace the current toxic varieties could reduce the risk of possible cross-contamination. However, it is evident that this process will take a long time to be developed and would still require for the patients the need to carefully select such products.

Recent progresses in understanding the cellular and molecular basis of CD have helped in identifying several possible therapeutical targets, from already available molecules that can find a new application in this disease to new drugs that may be developed. Strategies vary from gliadin-degrading enzymes that would allow the occasional consumption of gluten-containing products to the more ambitious attempt to reestablish immunological tolerance toward gluten using a peptide-based "vaccine."

Given the high content in proline residues, gliadin peptides are highly resistant to proteolysis, thus favoring the accumulation of long fragments within the intestinal lumen. Exogenous proline and/or glutamine-specific proteases-based drugs and/or dietary supplements (i.e., ALV003 (glutenase Alvine 003) and

AN-PEP (alanyl (membrane) aminopeptidase)) facilitate gluten digestion and T cell epitopes destruction [208], thus representing a useful "adjunctive" tool for CD under a GFD, in particular situations where there is a risk of cross-contamination. Another possible gluten detoxifying strategy is represented by gluten-sequestering polymers (i.e., hydroxyethyl methacrylate-co-styrene sulfonate; HEMA-co-SS) that bind gluten fragments, reducing their effects on the intestinal mucosa [209].

A pharmacological reduction of intestinal permeability may contribute to reduce the load of gliadin peptides reaching the intestinal lamina propria. In this perspective, larazotide (AT-1001), a zonulin antagonist, is undergoing clinical trials in CD patients. Furthermore, inhibition of Rho kinase (RhoA or ROCK), two molecules regulating cytoskeleton and tight junction structure, has been proposed as future potential target [210].

Furthermore, the identification of specific epitopes may also provide the basis for immunomodulation by antigenic peptides. In this regard, the most ambitious and promising therapeutic intervention for CD patients is represented by a vaccine based on a set of gliadin immunodominant peptides recognized selectively by HLA-DQ2 and that should promote the induction of tolerance to gluten through a peptide-based desensitization [211].

Other promising approaches include preventing gliadin presentation to T cells by blocking HLA-binding sites [212] or use of tTG inhibitors [213], thus impairing the adaptive immune response activated by gliadin peptides. Any immunomodulatory approach will be required to have a high safety profile to be a valuable substitute to the GFD.

Anti-IL-15 monoclonal antibodies, already tested in rheumatoid arthritis and psoriasis, have been proposed for refractory CD, where the expansion of IELs is dependent on this cytokine. Blocking NKG2D to prevent full activation of IELs has also been proposed as a further potential therapeutic target in CD patients [214]. Again, security profile, side effects, and compliance will need to be taken into account before any of those treatments could replace GFD.

References

1. Husby S, Koletzko S, Korponay-Szabo IR, Mearin ML, Phillips A, Shamir R, et al. European society for pediatric gastroenterology, hepatology, and nutrition guidelines for the diagnosis of coeliac disease. J Pediatr Gastroenterol Nutr. 2012;54(1):136–60.
2. Ludvigsson JF, Leffler DA, Bai JC, Biagi F, Fasano A, Green PH, et al. The Oslo definitions for coeliac disease and related terms. Gut. 2013;62(1):43–52.
3. Gee SJ. On the celiac affection. St Barth Hosp Rep. 1888;24:17–20.
4. van Berge-Henegouwen GP, Mulder CJ. Pioneer in the gluten free diet: Willem-Karel Dicke 1905–1962, over 50 years of gluten free diet. Gut. 1993;34(11):1473–5.
5. Shiner M. Coeliac disease: histopathological findings in the small intestinal mucosa studies by a peroral biopsy technique. Gut. 1960;1:48–54.
6. Groll A, Candy DC, Preece MA, Tanner JM, Harries JT. Short stature as the primary manifestation of coeliac disease. Lancet. 1980;2(8204):1097–9.
7. Cacciari E, Salardi S, Lazzari R, Cicognani A, Collina A, Pirazzoli P, et al. Short stature and celiac disease: a relationship to consider even in patients with no gastrointestinal tract symptoms. J Pediatr. 1983;103(5):708–11.
8. Jerosch J, Jantea C, Geske B. Osteomalacia and fatigue fractures in celiac disease. Z Rheumatol. 1990;49(2):100–2.
9. McFarlane XA, Bhalla AK, Reeves DE, Morgan LM, Robertson DA. Osteoporosis in treated adult coeliac disease. Gut. 1995;36(5):710–4.
10. Bottaro G, Cataldo F, Rotolo N, Spina M, Corazza GR. The clinical pattern of subclinical/silent celiac disease: an analysis on 1026 consecutive cases. Am J Gastroenterol. 1999;94(3):691–6.
11. Harper JW, Holleran SF, Ramakrishnan R, Bhagat G, Green PH. Anemia in celiac disease is multifactorial in etiology. Am J Hematol. 2007;82(11):996–1000.
12. Hin H, Bird G, Fisher P, Mahy N, Jewell D. Coeliac disease in primary care: case finding study. BMJ. 1999;318(7177):164–7.
13. Bourne JT, Kumar P, Huskisson EC, Mageed R, Unsworth DJ, Wojtulewski JA. Arthritis and coeliac disease. Ann Rheum Dis. 1985;44(9):592–8.
14. Maki M, Hallstrom O, Verronen P, Reunala T, Lahdeaho ML, Holm K, et al. Reticulin antibody, arthritis, and coeliac disease in children. Lancet. 1988;1(8583):479–80.
15. Pinals RS. Arthritis associated with gluten-sensitive enteropathy. J Rheumatol. 1986;13(1):201–4.
16. Gabrielli M, Cremonini F, Fiore G, Addolorato G, Padalino C, Candelli M, et al. Association between migraine and Celiac disease: results from a preliminary case-control and therapeutic study. Am J Gastroenterol. 2003;98(3):625–9.
17. Lahat E, Broide E, Leshem M, Evans S, Scapa E. Prevalence of celiac antibodies in children with neurologic disorders. Pediatr Neurol. 2000;22(5):393–6.
18. Serratrice J, Disdier P, de Roux C, Christides C, Weiller PJ. Migraine and coeliac disease. Headache. 1998;38(8):627–8.
19. Altuntas B, Kansu A, Girgin N. Hepatic damage in gluten sensitive enteropathy. Acta Paediatr Jpn. 1998;40(6):597–9.
20. Vajro P, Fontanella A, Mayer M, De Vincenzo A, Terracciano LM, D'Armiento M, et al. Elevated serum aminotransferase activity as an early manifestation of gluten-sensitive enteropathy. J Pediatr. 1993;122(3):416–9.
21. Bagnato GF, Quattrocchi E, Gulli S, Giacobbe O, Chirico G, Romano C, et al. Unusual polyarthritis as a unique clinical manifestation of coeliac disease. Rheumatol Int. 2000;20(1):29–30.
22. King TS, Anderson JR, Wraight EP, Hunter JO, Cox TM. Skeletal muscle weakness and dysphagia caused by acid maltase deficiency: nutritional consequences of coincident celiac sprue. JPEN J Parenter Enteral Nutr. 1997;21(1):46–9.
23. Freeman HJ. Reproductive changes associated with celiac disease. World J Gastroenterol. 2010;16(46):5810–4.
24. Tata LJ, Card TR, Logan RF, Hubbard RB, Smith CJ, West J. Fertility and pregnancy-related events in women with celiac disease: a population-based cohort study. Gastroenterology. 2005;128(4):849–55.
25. Choi JM, Lebwohl B, Wang J, Lee SK, Murray JA, Sauer MV, et al. Increased prevalence of celiac disease in patients with unexplained infertility in the United States. J Reprod Med. 2011;56(5–6):199–203.
26. Aine L, Maki M, Collin P, Keyrilainen O. Dental enamel defects in celiac disease. J Oral Pathol Med. 1990;19(6):241–5.
27. Rasmussen P, Espelid I. Coeliac disease and dental malformation. ASDC J Dent Child. 1980;47(3):190–2.
28. Shuster S, Watson AJ, Marks J. Coeliac syndrome in dermatitis herpetiformis. Lancet. 1968;1(7552):1101–6.

29. Walker-Smith JA, Talley NA. Coeliac disease and dermatitis herpetiformis. Med J Aust. 1973;1(1):10–2.

30. Hooft C, Roels H, Devos E. Diabetes and coeliac disease. Lancet. 1969;2(7631):1192.

31. Maki M, Hallstrom O, Huupponen T, Vesikari T, Visakorpi JK. Increased prevalence of coeliac disease in diabetes. Arch Dis Child. 1984;59(8):739–42.

32. Thain ME, Hamilton JR, Ehrlich RM. Coexistence of diabetes mellitus and celiac disease. J Pediatr. 1974;85(4):527–9.

33. Hill ID, Dirks MH, Liptak GS, Colletti RB, Fasano A, Guandalini S, et al. Guideline for the diagnosis and treatment of celiac disease in children: recommendations of the north american society for pediatric gastroenterology, hepatology and nutrition. J Pediatr Gastroenterol Nutr. 2005;40(1):1–19.

34. Dydensborg S, Toftedal P, Biaggi M, Lillevang ST, Hansen DG, Husby S. Increasing prevalence of coeliac disease in Denmark: a linkage study combining national registries. Acta Paediatr. 2012;101(2):179–84.

35. Vilppula A, Kaukinen K, Luostarinen L, Krekela I, Patrikainen H, Valve R, et al. Increasing prevalence and high incidence of celiac disease in elderly people: a population-based study. BMC Gastroenterol. 2009;9:49.

36. Lohi S, Mustalahti K, Kaukinen K, Laurila K, Collin P, Rissanen H, et al. Increasing prevalence of coeliac disease over time. Aliment Pharmacol Ther. 2007;26(9):1217–25.

37. Mustalahti K, Catassi C, Reunanen A, Fabiani E, Heier M, McMillan S, et al. The prevalence of celiac disease in Europe: results of a centralized, international mass screening project. Ann Med. 2010;42(8):587–95.

38. Catassi C, Kryszak D, Bhatti B, Sturgeon C, Helzlsouer K, Clipp SL, et al. Natural history of celiac disease autoimmunity in a USA cohort followed since 1974. Ann Med. 2010;42(7):530–8.

39. Ludvigsson JF, Rubio-Tapia A, van Dyke CT, Melton LJ 3rd, Zinsmeister AR, Lahr BD, et al. Increasing incidence of celiac disease in a North American population. Am J Gastroenterol. 2013;108(5):818–24.

40. Lionetti E, Castellaneta S, Pulvirenti A, Tonutti E, Francavilla R, Fasano A, et al. Prevalence and natural history of potential celiac disease in at-family-risk infants prospectively investigated from birth. J Pediatr. 2012;161(5):908–14.

41. Walker MM, Murray JA, Ronkainen J, Aro P, Storskrubb T, D'Amato M, et al. Detection of celiac disease and lymphocytic enteropathy by parallel serology and histopathology in a population-based study. Gastroenterology. 2010;139(1):112–9.

42. Decker E, Hornef M, Stockinger S. Cesarean delivery is associated with celiac disease but not inflammatory bowel disease in children. Gut Microbes. 2011;2(2):91–8.

43. Marild K, Stephansson O, Montgomery S, Murray JA, Ludvigsson JF. Pregnancy outcome and risk of celiac disease in offspring: a nationwide case-control study. Gastroenterology. 2012;142(1):39–45, e3.

44. Myleus A, Hernell O, Gothefors L, Hammarstrom ML, Persson LA, Stenlund H, et al. Early infections are associated with increased risk for celiac disease: an incident case-referent study. BMC Pediatr. 2012;12:194.

45. Tjernberg AR, Ludvigsson JF. Children with celiac disease are more likely to have attended hospital for prior respiratory syncytial virus infection. Dig Dis Sci. 2014;59(7):1502–8.

46. Marild K, Ye W, Lebwohl B, Green PH, Blaser MJ, Card T, et al. Antibiotic exposure and the development of coeliac disease: a nationwide case-control study. BMC Gastroenterol. 2013;13:109.

47. Ivarsson A, Myleus A, Norstrom F, van der Pals M, Rosen A, Hogberg L, et al. Prevalence of childhood celiac disease and changes in infant feeding. Pediatrics. 2013;131(3):e687–94.

48. Myleus A, Ivarsson A, Webb C, Danielsson L, Hernell O, Hogberg L, et al. Celiac disease revealed in 3 % of Swedish 12-year-olds born during an epidemic. J Pediatr Gastroenterol Nutr. 2009;49(2):170–6.

49. Whyte L, Kotecha S, Watkins W, Jenkins H. Coeliac disease is more common in children with high socio-economic status. Acta Paediatr. 2013;103(3):289–94

50. Kondrashova A, Mustalahti K, Kaukinen K, Viskari H, Volodicheva V, Haapala AM, et al. Lower economic status and inferior hygienic environment may protect against celiac disease. Ann Med. 2008;40(3):223–31.

51. Rubio-Tapia A, Ludvigsson JF, Brantner TL, Murray JA, Everhart JE. The prevalence of celiac disease in the United States. Am J Gastroenterol. 2012;107(10):1538–44, quiz 7, 45.

52. Rosen A, Sandstrom O, Carlsson A, Hogberg L, Olen O, Stenlund H, et al. Usefulness of symptoms to screen for celiac disease. Pediatrics. 2014;133(2):211–8

53. Dixit R, Lebwohl B, Ludvigsson JF, Lewis SK, Rizkalla-Reilly N, Green PH. Celiac disease is diagnosed less frequently in young adult males. Dig Dis Sci. 2014;59(7):1509–12.

54. Pinkhasov RM, Wong J, Kashanian J, Lee M, Samadi DB, Pinkhasov MM, et al. Are men shortchanged on health? Perspective on health care utilization and health risk behavior in men and women in the United States. Intl J Clin Pract. 2010;64(4):475–87.

55. Green PHR, Stavropoulos SN, Panagi SG, Goldstein SL, McMahon DJ, Absan H, et al. Characteristics of adult celiac disease in the USA: results of a national survey. Am J Gastroenterol. 2001;96(1):126–31.

56. Megiorni F, Mora B, Bonamico M, Barbato M, Montuori M, Viola F, et al. HLA-DQ and susceptibility to celiac disease: evidence for gender differences and parent-of-origin effects. Am J Gastroenterol. 2008;103(4):997–1003.

57. Ploski R, Ek J, Thorsby E, Sollid LM. On the HLA-DQ (alpha 1*0501, beta 1*0201)-associated susceptibility in celiac disease: a possible gene dosage effect of DQB1*0201. Tissue Antigens. 1993;41(4):173–7.

58. van Belzen MJ, Koeleman BP, Crusius JB, Meijer JW, Bardoel AF, Pearson PL, et al. Defining the contribution of the HLA region to cis DQ2-positive coeliac disease patients. Genes Immun. 2004;5(3):215–20.

59. Molberg O, Kett K, Scott H, Thorsby E, Sollid LM, Lundin KE. Gliadin specific, HLA DQ2-restricted T cells are commonly found in small intestinal biopsies from coeliac disease patients, but not from controls. Scand J Immunol. 1997;46(3):103–9.

60. Molberg O, McAdam SN, Korner R, Quarsten H, Kristiansen C, Madsen L, et al. Tissue transglutaminase selectively modifies gliadin peptides that are recognized by gut-derived T cells in celiac disease. Nat Med. 1998;4(6):713–7.

61. Mearin ML, Biemond I, Pena AS, Polanco I, Vazquez C, Schreuder GT, et al. HLA-DR phenotypes in Spanish coeliac children: their contribution to the understanding of the genetics of the disease. Gut. 1983;24(6):532–7.

62. Megiorni F, Mora B, Bonamico M, Barbato M, Nenna R, Maiella G, et al. HLA-DQ and risk gradient for celiac disease. Hum Immunol. 2009;70(1):55–9.

63. Zubillaga P, Vidales MC, Zubillaga I, Ormaechea V, Garcia-Urkia N, Vitoria JC. HLA-DQA1 and HLA-DQB1 genetic markers and clinical presentation in celiac disease. J Pediatr Gastroenterol Nutr. 2002;34(5):548–54.

64. Congia M, Cucca F, Frau F, Lampis R, Melis L, Clemente MG, et al. A gene dosage effect of the DQA1*0501/DQB1*0201 allelic combination influences the clinical heterogeneity of celiac disease. Hum Immunol. 1994;40(2):138–42.

65. Al-Toma A, Goerres MS, Meijer JW, Pena AS, Crusius JB, Mulder CJ. Human leukocyte antigen-DQ2 homozygosity and the development of refractory celiac disease and enteropathy-associated T-cell lymphoma. Clin Gastroenterol Hepatol. 2006;4(3):315–9.

66. Vader W, Stepniak D, Kooy Y, Mearin L, Thompson A, van Rood JJ, et al. The HLA-DQ2 gene dose effect in celiac disease is directly related to the magnitude and breadth of gluten-specific T cell responses. Proc Natl Acad Sci U S A. 2003;100(21):12390–5.

67. Louka AS, Moodie SJ, Karell K, Bolognesi E, Ascher H, Greco L, et al. A collaborative European search for non-DQA1*05-DQB1*02 celiac disease loci on HLA-DR3 haplotypes: analysis of transmission from homozygous parents. Hum Immunol. 2003;64(3):350–8.

68. Pietzak MM, Schofield TC, McGinniss MJ, Nakamura RM. Stratifying risk for celiac disease in a large at-risk United States population by using HLA alleles. Clin Gastroenterol Hepatol. 2009;7(9):966–71.

69. Karell K, Louka AS, Moodie SJ, Ascher H, Clot F, Greco L, et al. HLA types in celiac disease patients not carrying the DQA1*05-DQB1*02 (DQ2) heterodimer: results from the European Genetics Cluster on Celiac Disease. Hum Immunol. 2003;64(4):469–77.

70. Trynka G, Hunt KA, Bockett NA, Romanos J, Mistry V, Szperl A, et al. Dense genotyping identifies and localizes multiple common and rare variant association signals in celiac disease. Nat Genet. 2011;43(12):1193–201.

71. Zhernakova A, Withoff S, Wijmenga C. Clinical implications of shared genetics and pathogenesis in autoimmune diseases. Nat Rev Endocrinol. 2013;9(11):646–59.

72. Abadie V, Sollid LM, Barreiro LB, Jabri B. Integration of genetic and immunological insights into a model of celiac disease pathogenesis. Ann Rev Immunol. 2011;29:493–525.

73. Decker E, Engelmann G, Findeisen A, Gerner P, Laass M, Ney D, et al. Cesarean delivery is associated with celiac disease but not inflammatory bowel disease in children. Pediatrics. 2010;125(6):e1433–40.

74. Ivarsson A. The Swedish epidemic of coeliac disease explored using an epidemiological approach—some lessons to be learnt. Best Pract Res Clin Gastroenterol. 2005;19(3):425–40.

75. Ivarsson A, Persson LA, Nystrom L, Hernell O. The Swedish coeliac disease epidemic with a prevailing twofold higher risk in girls compared to boys may reflect gender specific risk factors. Eur J Epidemiol. 2003;18(7):677–84.

76. Ivarsson A, Persson LA, Nystrom L, Ascher H, Cavell B, Danielsson L, et al. Epidemic of coeliac disease in Swedish children. Acta Paediatrica. 2000;89(2):165–71.

77. Ivarsson A, Hernell O, Stenlund H, Persson LA. Breast-feeding protects against celiac disease. Am J Clin Nutr. 2002;75(5):914–21.

78. Akobeng AK, Ramanan AV, Buchan I, Heller RF. Effect of breast feeding on risk of coeliac disease: a systematic review and meta-analysis of observational studies. Arch Dis Child. 2006;91(1):39–43.

79. Akobeng AK, Heller RF. Assessing the population impact of low rates of breast feeding on asthma, coeliac disease and obesity: the use of a new statistical method. Arch Dis Child. 2007;92(6):483–5.

80. Guandalini S. The influence of gluten: weaning recommendations for healthy children and children at risk for celiac disease. Nestle Nutr Workshop Ser Paediatr Programme. 2007;60:139–51, discussion 51–5.

81. Szajewska H, Chmielewska A, Piescik-Lech M, Ivarsson A, Kolacek S, Koletzko S, et al. Systematic review: early infant feeding and the prevention of coeliac disease. Aliment Pharmacol Ther. 2012;36(7):607–18.

82. Lionetti E, Castellaneta S, Francavilla R, Pulvirenti A, Tonutti E, Amarri S, Barbato M, Barbera C, Barera G, Bellantoni A, Castellano E, Guariso G, Limongelli MG, Pellegrino S, Polloni C, Ughi C, Zuin G, Fasano A, Catassi C. Introduction of gluten, HLA status, and the risk of celiac disease in children. N Engl J Med. 2014;371:1295–303.

83. Vriezinga SL, Auricchio R, Bravi E, Castillejo G, Chmielewska A, Crespo Escobar P, Kolaček S, Koletzko S, Korponay-Szabo IR, Mummert E, Polanco I, Putter H, Ribes-Koninckx C, Shamir R, Szajewska H, Werkstetter K, Greco L, Gyimesi J, Hartman C, Hogen Esch C, Hopman E, Ivarsson A, Koltai T, Koning F, Martinez-Ojinaga E, te Marvelde C, Pavic A, Romanos J, Stoopman E, Villanacci V, Wijmenga C, Troncone R, Mearin ML. Randomized feeding intervention in infants at high risk for celiac disease. N Engl J Med. 2014;371:1304–15.

84. Kagnoff MF, Austin RK, Hubert JJ, Bernardin JE, Kasarda DD. Possible role for a human adenovirus in the pathogenesis of celiac disease. J Exp Med. 1984;160(5):1544–57.

85. Kagnoff MF, Paterson YJ, Kumar PJ, Kasarda DD, Carbone FR, Unsworth DJ, et al. Evidence for the role of a human intestinal adenovirus in the pathogenesis of coeliac disease. Gut. 1987;28(8):995–1001.

86. Stene LC, Honeyman MC, Hoffenberg EJ, Haas JE, Sokol RJ, Emery L, et al. Rotavirus infection frequency and risk of celiac disease autoimmunity in early childhood: a longitudinal study. Am J Gastroenterol. 2006;101(10):2333–40.

87. Atkinson MA, Chervonsky A. Does the gut microbiota have a role in type 1 diabetes? Early evidence from humans and animal models of the disease. Diabetologia. 2012;55(11):2868–77.

88. Mathis D, Benoist C. Microbiota and autoimmune disease: the hosted self. Cell Host Microbe. 2011;10(4):297–301.

89. Forsberg G, Fahlgren A, Horstedt P, Hammarstrom S, Hernell O, Hammarstrom ML. Presence of bacteria and innate immunity of intestinal epithelium in childhood celiac disease. Am J Gastroenterol. 2004;99(5):894–904.

90. Sanz Y, Sanchez E, Marzotto M, Calabuig M, Torriani S, Dellaglio F. Differences in faecal bacterial communities in coeliac and healthy children as detected by PCR and denaturing gradient gel electrophoresis. FEMS Immunol Med Microbiol. 2007;51(3):562–8.

91. Di Cagno R, De Angelis M, De Pasquale I, Ndagijimana M, Vernocchi P, Ricciuti P, et al. Duodenal and faecal microbiota of celiac children: molecular, phenotype and metabolome characterization. BMC Microbiol. 2011;11:219.

92. Nistal E, Caminero A, Herran AR, Arias L, Vivas S, de Morales JM, et al. Differences of small intestinal bacteria populations in adults and children with/without celiac disease: effect of age, gluten diet, and disease. Inflamm Bowel Dis. 2012;18(4):649–56.

93. Nadal I, Donat E, Ribes-Koninckx C, Calabuig M, Sanz Y. Imbalance in the composition of the duodenal microbiota of children with coeliac disease. J Medical Microbiol. 2007;56(Pt 12):1669–74.

94. Sanchez E, Nadal I, Donat E, Ribes-Koninckx C, Calabuig M, Sanz Y. Reduced diversity and increased virulence-gene carriage in intestinal enterobacteria of coeliac children. BMC Gastroenterol. 2008;8:50.

95. De Palma G, Nadal I, Medina M, Donat E, Ribes-Koninckx C, Calabuig M, et al. Intestinal dysbiosis and reduced immunoglobulin-coated bacteria associated with coeliac disease in children. BMC Microbiol. 2010;10:63.

96. Collado MC, Donat E, Ribes-Koninckx C, Calabuig M, Sanz Y. Specific duodenal and faecal bacterial groups associated with paediatric coeliac disease. J Clin Pathol. 2009;62(3):264–9.

97. Jabri B, Sollid LM. Tissue-mediated control of immunopathology in coeliac disease. Nat Rev Immunol. 2009;9(12):858–70.

98. Abadie V, Discepolo V, Jabri B. Intraepithelial lymphocytes in celiac disease immunopathology. Seminars Immunopathol. 2012;34(4):551–66.

99. Shewry PR, Halford NG. Cereal seed storage proteins: structures, properties and role in grain utilization. J Exp Bot. 2002;53(370):947–58.

100. Shewry PR, Tatham AS. The prolamin storage proteins of cereal seeds: structure and evolution. Biochem J. 1990;267(1):1–12.

101. Shan L, Molberg O, Parrot I, Hausch F, Filiz F, Gray GM, et al. Structural basis for gluten intolerance in celiac sprue. Science. 2002;297(5590):2275–9.

102. Matysiak-Budnik T, Moura IC, Arcos-Fajardo M, Lebreton C, Menard S, Candalh C, et al. Secretory IgA mediates retrotranscytosis of intact gliadin peptides via the transferrin receptor in celiac disease. J Exp Med. 2008;205(1):143–54.

103. Pinkas DM, Strop P, Brunger AT, Khosla C. Transglutaminase 2 undergoes a large conformational change upon activation. PLoS Biol. 2007;5(12):e327.

104. Sollid LM, Jabri B. Celiac disease and transglutaminase 2: a model for posttranslational modification of antigens and HLA association in the pathogenesis of autoimmune disorders. Curr Opin Immunol. 2011;23(6):732–8.

105. Kim CY, Quarsten H, Bergseng E, Khosla C, Sollid LM. Structural basis for HLA-DQ2-mediated presentation of gluten epitopes in celiac disease. Proc Natl Acad Sci U S A. 2004;101(12):4175–9.

106. Sollid LM, Molberg O, McAdam S, Lundin KE. Autoantibodies in coeliac disease: tissue transglutaminase–guilt by association? Gut. 1997;41(6):851–2.

107. Sperandeo MP, Tosco A, Izzo V, Tucci F, Troncone R, Auricchio R, et al. Potential celiac patients: a model of celiac disease pathogenesis. PloS One. 2011;6(7):e21281.

108. Zeng R, Spolski R, Finkelstein SE, Oh S, Kovanen PE, Hinrichs CS, et al. Synergy of IL-21 and IL-15 in regulating CD8 + T cell expansion and function. J Exp Med. 2005;201(1):139–48.

109. Maiuri L, Ciacci C, Ricciardelli I, Vacca L, Raia V, Auricchio S, et al. Association between innate response to gliadin and activation of pathogenic T cells in coeliac disease. Lancet. 2003;362(9377):30–7.

110. Barone MV, Gimigliano A, Castoria G, Paolella G, Maurano F, Paparo F, et al. Growth factor-like activity of gliadin, an alimentary protein: implications for coeliac disease. Gut. 2007;56(4):480–8.

111. Nanayakkara M, Kosova R, Lania G, Sarno M, Gaito A, Galatola M, et al. A celiac cellular phenotype, with altered LPP subcellular distribution, is inducible in controls by the toxic gliadin peptide P31–43. PloS One. 2013;8(11):e79763.

112. Hue S, Mention JJ, Monteiro RC, Zhang S, Cellier C, Schmitz J, et al. A direct role for NKG2D/MICA interaction in villous atrophy during celiac disease. Immunity. 2004;21(3):367–77.

113. Nanayakkara M, Lania G, Maglio M, Discepolo V, Sarno M, Gaito A, et al. An undigested gliadin peptide activates innate immunity and proliferative signaling in enterocytes: the role in celiac disease. Am J Clin Nutr. 2013;98(4):1123–35.

114. Nanayakkara M, Lania G, Maglio M, Kosova R, Sarno M, Gaito A, et al. Enterocyte proliferation and signaling are constitutively altered in celiac disease. PloS One. 2013;8(10):e76006.

115. Ben Ahmed M, Belhadj Hmida N, Moes N, Buyse S, Abdeladhim M, Louzir H, et al. IL-15 renders conventional lymphocytes resistant to suppressive functions of regulatory T cells through activation of the phosphatidylinositol 3-kinase pathway. J Immunol. 2009;182(11):6763–70.

116. Zanzi D, Stefanile R, Santagata S, Iaffaldano L, Iaquinto G, Giardullo N, et al. IL-15 interferes with suppressive activity of intestinal regulatory T cells expanded in celiac disease. Am J Gastroenterol. 2011;106(7):1308–17.

117. Marsh MN. Gluten, major histocompatibility complex, and the small intestine. A molecular and immunobiologic approach to the spectrum of gluten sensitivity ('celiac sprue'). Gastroenterology. 1992;102(1):330–54.

118. Garampazzi A, Rapa A, Mura S, Capelli A, Valori A, Boldorini R, et al. Clinical pattern of celiac disease is still changing. J Pediatr Gastroenterol Nutr. 2007;45(5):611–4.

119. Lebenthal E, Shteyer E, Branski D. The changing clinical presentation of celiac disease. In: Fasano A, Troncone R, Branski D, editors. Frontiers in celiac disease. Basel: Karger; 2008. p. 18–22.

120. Maki M, Kallonen K, Lahdeaho ML, Visakorpi JK. Changing pattern of childhood coeliac disease in Finland. Acta Paediatr Scand. 1988;77(3):408–12.

121. Roma E, Panayiotou J, Karantana H, Constantinidou C, Siakavellas SI, Krini M, et al. Changing pattern in the clinical presentation of pediatric celiac disease: a 30-year study. Digestion. 2009;80(3):185–91.

122. Lo W, Sano K, Lebwohl B, Diamond B, Green PH. Changing presentation of adult celiac disease. Dig Dis Sci. 2003;48(2):395–8.

123. Rostami Nejad M, Rostami K, Pourhoseingholi MA, Nazemalhosseini Mojarad E, Habibi M, Dabiri H, et al. Atypical presentation is dominant and typical for coeliac disease. J Gastrointestin Liver Dis. 2009;18(3):285–91.

124. Rashid M, Cranney A, Zarkadas M, Graham ID, Switzer C, Case S, et al. Celiac disease: evaluation of the diagnosis and dietary compliance in Canadian children. Pediatrics. 2005;116(6):e754–9.

125. Ehsani-Ardakani MJ, Rostami Nejad M, Villanacci V, Volta U, Manenti S, Caio G, et al. Gastrointestinal and non-gastrointestinal presentation in patients with celiac disease. Arch Iran Med. 2013;16(2):78–82.

126. Bai JC, Maurino E, Martinez C, Vazquez H, Niveloni S, Soifer G, et al. Abnormal colonic transit time in untreated celiac sprue. Acta Gastroenterol Latinoam. 1995;25(5):277–84.

127. Sadik R, Abrahamsson H, Kilander A, Stotzer PO. Gut transit in celiac disease: delay of small bowel transit and acceleration after dietary treatment. Am J Gastroenterol. 2004;99(12):2429–36.

128. Cucchiara S, Bassotti G, Castellucci G, Minella R, Betti C, Fusaro C, et al. Upper gastrointestinal motor abnormalities in children with active celiac disease. J Pediatr Gastroenterol Nutr. 1995;21(4):435–42.

129. Diamanti A, Capriati T, Basso MS, Panetta F, Di Ciommo Laurora VM, Bellucci F, et al. Celiac disease and overweight in children: an update. Nutrients. 2014;6(1):207–20.

130. Aad G, Abajyan T, Abbott B, Abdallah J, Abdel Khalek S, Abdelalim AA, et al. Search for magnetic monopoles in sqrt[s]=7 TeV pp collisions with the ATLAS detector. Phys Rev Lett. 2012;109(26):261803.

131. Germann R, Kuch M, Prinz K, Ebbing A, Schindera F. Celiac disease: an uncommon cause of recurrent intussusception. J Pediatr Gastroenterol Nutr. 1997;25(4):415–6.

132. Reilly NR, Aguilar KM, Green PH. Should intussusception in children prompt screening for celiac disease? J Pediatr Gastroenterol Nutr. 2013;56(1):56–9.

133. Vajro P, Paolella G, Maggiore G, Giordano G. Meta-analysis: pediatric celiac disease, cryptogenic hypertransaminasemia, and autoimmune hepatitis. J Pediatr Gastroenterol Nutr. 2013; 56(6):663–70.

134. Kolho KL, Farkkila MA, Savilahti E. Undiagnosed coeliac disease is common in Finnish adults. Scand J Gastroenterol. 1998;33(12):1280–3.

135. Zanini B, Caselani F, Magni A, Turini D, Ferraresi A, Lanzarotto F, et al. Celiac disease with mild enteropathy is not mild disease. Clin Gastroenterol Hepatol. 2013;11(3):253–8.

136. Bolotin D, Petronic-Rosic V. Dermatitis herpetiformis. Part I. Epidemiology, pathogenesis, and clinical presentation. J Am Acad Dermatol. 2011;64(6):1017–24, quiz 25–6.

137. Nicolas ME, Krause PK, Gibson LE, Murray JA. Dermatitis herpetiformis. Intl J Dermatol. 2003;42(8):588–600.

138. Bolotin D, Petronic-Rosic V. Dermatitis herpetiformis. Part II. Diagnosis, management, and prognosis. J Am Acad Dermatol. 2011;64(6):1027–33, quiz 33–4.

139. Caproni M, Antiga E, Melani L, Fabbri P, Italian Group for Cutaneous I. Guidelines for the diagnosis and treatment of dermatitis herpetiformis. J Eur Acad Dermatol Venereol. 2009;23(6):633–8.

140. Margoni D, Chouliaras G, Duscas G, Voskaki I, Voutsas N, Papadopoulou A, et al. Bone health in children with celiac disease assessed by dual x-ray absorptiometry: effect of gluten-free diet and predictive value of serum biochemical indices. J Pediatr Gastroenterol Nutr. 2012;54(5):680–4.

141. Krupa-Kozak U. Pathologic bone alterations in celiac disease: etiology, epidemiology, and treatment. Nutrition. 2014;30(1):16–24.

142. Ghozzi M, Sakly W, Mankai A, Bouajina E, Bahri F, Nouira R, et al. Screening for celiac disease, by endomysial antibodies, in patients with unexplained articular manifestations. Rheumatol Int. 2013; 34(5):637–42.

143. Dimitrova AK, Ungaro RC, Lebwohl B, Lewis SK, Tennyson CA, Green MW, et al. Prevalence of migraine in patients with celiac disease and inflammatory bowel disease. Headache. 2013;53(2):344–55.

144. Chin RL, Sander HW, Brannagan TH, Green PH, Hays AP, Alaedini A, et al. Celiac neuropathy. Neurology. 2003;60(10):1581–5.

145. Ruggieri M, Incorpora G, Polizzi A, Parano E, Spina M, Pavone P. Low prevalence of neurologic and psychiatric manifestations in children with gluten sensitivity. J Pediatr. 2008;152(2):244–9.

146. Pengiran Tengah DS, Holmes GK, Wills AJ. The prevalence of epilepsy in patients with celiac disease. Epilepsia. 2004;45(10):1291–3.

147. Fois A, Vascotto M, Di Bartolo RM, Di Marco V. Celiac disease and epilepsy in pediatric patients. Child's Nerv Sys. 1994;10(7):450–4.

148. Ludvigsson JF, Zingone F, Tomson T, Ekbom A, Ciacci C. Increased risk of epilepsy in biopsy-verified celiac disease: a population-based cohort study. Neurology. 2012;78(18):1401–7.

149. Canales P, Mery VP, Larrondo FJ, Bravo FL, Godoy J. Epilepsy and celiac disease: favorable outcome with a gluten-free diet in a patient refractory to antiepileptic drugs. Neurologist. 2006;12(6):318–21.

150. Pascotto A, Coppola G, Ecuba P, Liguori G, Guandalini S. Epilepsy and occipital calcifications with or without celiac disease: report of four cases. J Epilepsy. 1994;7:130–6.

151. Ludvigsson JF, Inghammar M, Ekberg M, Egesten A. A nationwide cohort study of the risk of chronic obstructive pulmonary disease in coeliac disease. J Intern Med. 2012;271(5):481–9.

152. Emilsson L, Carlsson R, Holmqvist M, James S, Ludvigsson JF. The characterisation and risk factors of ischaemic heart disease in patients with coeliac disease. Aliment Pharmacol Ther. 2013;37(9):905–14.

153. Ludvigsson JF, Lindelof B, Rashtak S, Rubio-Tapia A, Murray JA. Does urticaria risk increase in patients with celiac disease? A large population-based cohort study. Eur J Dermatol. 2013;23(5):681–7.

154. Ludvigsson JF, Aro P, Walker MM, Vieth M, Agreus L, Talley NJ, et al. Celiac disease, eosinophilic esophagitis and gastroesophageal reflux disease, an adult population-based study. Scand J Gastroenterol. 2013;48(7):808–14.

155. Sadr-Azodi O, Sanders DS, Murray JA, Ludvigsson JF. Patients with celiac disease have an increased risk for pancreatitis. Clin Gastroenterol Hepatol. 2012;10(10):1136–42, e3.

156. Ludvigsson JF, Murray JA, Adams PC, Elmberg M. Does hemochromatosis predispose to celiac disease? A study of 29,096 celiac disease patients. Scand J Gastroenterol. 2013;48(2):176–82.

157. Mollazadegan K, Kugelberg M, Lindblad BE, Ludvigsson JF. Increased risk of cataract among 28,000 patients with celiac disease. Am J Epidemiol. 2011;174(2):195–202.

158. Mollazadegan K, Kugelberg M, Tallstedt L, Ludvigsson JF. Increased risk of uveitis in coeliac disease: a nationwide cohort study. Br J Ophthalmol. 2012;96(6):857–61.

159. Emilsson L, Andersson B, Elfstrom P, Green PH, Ludvigsson JF. Risk of idiopathic dilated cardiomyopathy in 29,000 patients with celiac disease. J Am Heart Assoc. 2012;1(3):e001594.

160. Ludvigsson JF, Zingone F, Fored M, Ciacci C, Cirillo M. Moderately increased risk of urinary stone disease in patients with biopsy-verified coeliac disease. Aliment Pharmacol Ther. 2012;35(4):477–84.

161. Welander A, Prutz KG, Fored M, Ludvigsson JF. Increased risk of end-stage renal disease in individuals with coeliac disease. Gut. 2012;61(1):64–8.

162. Passananti V, Siniscalchi M, Zingone F, Bucci C, Tortora R, Iovino P, et al. Prevalence of eating disorders in adults with celiac disease. Gastroenterol Res Pract. 2013;2013:491657.

163. Ludvigsson JF, Rubio-Tapia A, Chowdhary V, Murray JA, Simard JF. Increased risk of systemic lupus erythematosus in 29,000 patients with biopsy-verified celiac disease. J Rheumatol. 2012;39(10):1964–70.

164. Zugna D, Richiardi L, Stephansson O, Pasternak B, Ekbom A, Cnattingius S, et al. Risk of congenital malformations among offspring of mothers and fathers with celiac disease: a nationwide cohort study. Clin Gastroenterol Hepatol. 2013;12(7):1108–1116.e6.

165. Ludvigsson JF, West J, Ekbom A, Stephansson O. Reduced risk of breast, endometrial and ovarian cancer in women with celiac disease. Int J Cancer. 2012;131(3):E244–50.

166. Meini A, Pillan NM, Villanacci V, Monafo V, Ugazio AG, Plebani A. Prevalence and diagnosis of celiac disease in IgA-deficient children. Ann Allergy Asthma Immunol. 1996;77(4):333–6.

167. Cataldo F, Marino V, Bottaro G, Greco P, Ventura A. Celiac disease and selective immunoglobulin A deficiency. J Pediatr. 1997;131(2):306–8.

168. Bybrant MC, Ortqvist E, Lantz S, Grahnquist L. High prevalence of celiac disease in Swedish children and adolescents with type 1 diabetes and the relation to the Swedish epidemic of celiac disease: a cohort study. Scand J Gastroenterol. 2014;49(1):52–8.

169. Barera G, Bonfanti R, Viscardi M, Bazzigaluppi E, Calori G, Meschi F, et al. Occurrence of celiac disease after onset of type 1 diabetes: a 6-year prospective longitudinal study. Pediatrics. 2002;109(5):833–8.

170. Tiberti C, Panimolle F, Bonamico M, Filardi T, Pallotta L, Nenna R, et al. Long-standing type 1 diabetes: patients with adult-onset develop celiac-specific immunoreactivity more frequently than patients with childhood-onset diabetes, in a disease duration-dependent manner. Acta Diabetol. 2014;51(4):675–8.

171. Scaramuzza AE, Mantegazza C, Bosetti A, Zuccotti GV. Type 1 diabetes and celiac disease: the effects of gluten free diet on metabolic control. World J Diab. 2013;4(4):130–4.

172. Ventura A, Magazzu G, Greco L. Duration of exposure to gluten and risk for autoimmune disorders in patients with celiac disease. SIGEP study group for autoimmune disorders in celiac disease. Gastroenterology. 1999;117(2):297–303.

173. Elli L, Bonura A, Garavaglia D, Rulli E, Floriani I, Tagliabue G, et al. Immunological comorbity in coeliac disease: associations, risk factors and clinical implications. J Clin Immunol. 2012;32(5):984–90.

174. Metso S, Hyytia-Ilmonen H, Kaukinen K, Huhtala H, Jaatinen P, Salmi J, et al. Gluten-free diet and autoimmune thyroiditis in patients with celiac disease. A prospective controlled study. Scand J Gastroenterol. 2012;47(1):43–8.

175. Elli L, Discepolo V, Bardella MT, Guandalini S. Does gluten intake influence the development of celiac disease-associated complications? J Clin Gastroenterol. 2014;48(1):13–20.

176. Marild K, Stephansson O, Grahnquist L, Cnattingius S, Soderman G, Ludvigsson JF. Down syndrome is associated with elevated risk of celiac disease: a nationwide case-control study. J Pediatr. 2013;163(1):237–42.

177. Bonamico M, Bottaro G, Pasquino AM, Caruso-Nicoletti M, Mariani P, Gemme G, et al. Celiac disease and turner syndrome. J Pediatr Gastroenterol Nutr. 1998;26(5):496–9.

178. Santer R, Pankau R, Schaub J, Burgin-Wolff A. Williams–Beuren syndrome and celiac disease. J Pediatr Gastroenterol Nutr. 1996;23(3):339–40.

179. Giersiepen K, Lelgemann M, Stuhldreher N, Ronfani L, Husby S, Koletzko S, et al. Accuracy of diagnostic antibody tests for coeliac disease in children: summary of an evidence report. J Pediatr Gastroenterol Nutr. 2012;54(2):229–41.

180. Amarri S, Alvisi P, De Giorgio R, Gelli MC, Cicola R, Tovoli F, et al. Antibodies to Deamidated gliadin peptides: an accurate predictor of coeliac disease in infancy. J Clin Immunol. 2013; 33(5):1027–30.

181. Barbato M, Maiella G, Di Camillo C, Guida S, Valitutti F, Lastrucci G, et al. The anti-deamidated gliadin peptide antibodies unmask celiac disease in small children with chronic diarrhoea. Dig Liver Dis. 2011;43(6):465–9.

182. Aleanzi M, Demonte AM, Esper C, Garcilazo S, Waggener M. Celiac disease: antibody recognition against native and selectively deamidated gliadin peptides. Clin Chem. 2001;47(11):2023–8.

183. Rubio-Tapia A, Hill ID, Kelly CP, Calderwood AH, Murray JA. ACG clinical guidelines: diagnosis and management of celiac disease. Am J Gastroenterol. 2013;108(5):656–76.

184. Dahlbom I, Olsson M, Forooz NK, Sjoholm AG, Truedsson L, Hansson T. Immunoglobulin G (IgG) anti-tissue transglutaminase antibodies used as markers for IgA-deficient celiac disease patients. Clin Diagn Lab Immunol. 2005;12(2):254–8.

185. Korponay-Szabo IR, Dahlbom I, Laurila K, Koskinen S, Woolley N, Partanen J, et al. Elevation of IgG antibodies against tissue transglutaminase as a diagnostic tool for coeliac disease in selective IgA deficiency. Gut. 2003;52(11):1567–71.

186. Villalta D, Alessio MG, Tampoia M, Tonutti E, Brusca I, Bagnasco M, et al. Testing for IgG class antibodies in celiac disease patients with selective IgA deficiency. A comparison of the diagnostic accuracy of 9 IgG anti-tissue transglutaminase, 1 IgG anti-gliadin and 1 IgG anti-deaminated gliadin peptide antibody assays. Clin Chim Acta. 2007;382(1–2):95–9.

187. Villalta D, Tonutti E, Prause C, Koletzko S, Uhlig HH, Vermeersch P, et al. IgG antibodies against deamidated gliadin peptides for diagnosis of celiac disease in patients with IgA deficiency. Clin Chem. 2010;56(3):464–8.

188. Walker-Smith JA, Guandalini S, Schmitz J, Shmerling DH, Visakorpi JK. Revised criteria for diagnosis of coeliac disease. Report of a Working Group of ESPGAN. Arch Dis Child. 1990;65:909–11.

189. Bai JC, Fried M, Corazza GR, Schuppan D, Farthing M, Catassi C, et al. World gastroenterology organisation global guidelines on celiac disease. J Clin Gastroenterol. 2013;47(2):121–6.

190. Aziz I, Evans KE, Hopper AD, Smillie DM, Sanders DS. A prospective study into the aetiology of lymphocytic duodenosis. Aliment Pharmacol Ther. 2010;32(11–12):1392–7.

191. Santolaria S, Dominguez M, Alcedo J, Abascal M, Garcia-Prats MD, Marigil M, et al. Lymphocytic duodenosis: etiological study and clinical presentations. Gastroenterol Hepatol. 2013;36(9):565–73.

192. Waisbourd-Zinman O, Hojsak I, Rosenbach Y, Mozer-Glassberg Y, Shalitin S, Phillip M, et al. Spontaneous normalization of anti-tissue transglutaminase antibody levels is common in children with type 1 diabetes mellitus. Dig Dis Sci. 2012;57(5):1314–20.

193. Biagi F, Trotta L, Alfano C, Balduzzi D, Staffieri V, Bianchi PI, et al. Prevalence and natural history of potential celiac disease in adult patients. Scand J Gastroenterol. 2013;48(5):537–42.

194. Kurppa K, Ashorn M, Iltanen S, Koskinen LL, Saavalainen P, Koskinen O, et al. Celiac disease without villous atrophy in children: a prospective study. J Pediatr. 2010;157(3):373–80, 80 e1.

195. Tosco A, Salvati VM, Auricchio R, Maglio M, Borrelli M, Coruzzo A, et al. Natural history of potential celiac disease in children. Clin Gastroenterol Hepatol. 2011;9(4):320–5, quiz e36.

196. Borrelli M, Salvati VM, Maglio M, Zanzi D, Ferrara K, Santagata S, et al. Immunoregulatory pathways are active in the small intestinal mucosa of patients with potential celiac disease. Am J Gastroenterol. 2013;108(11):1775–84.

197. Biagi F, Corazza GR. Defining gluten refractory enteropathy. Eur J Gastroenterol Hepatol. 2001;13(5):561–5.

198. Al-Toma A, Verbeek WH, Hadithi M, von Blomberg BM, Mulder CJ. Survival in refractory coeliac disease and enteropathy-associated T-cell lymphoma: retrospective evaluation of single-centre experience. Gut. 2007;56(10):1373–8.

199. Malamut G, Cellier C. Refractory celiac disease. Expert Rev Gastroenterol Hepatol. 2014;8(3):323–8.

200. Nijeboer P, van Wanrooij RL, Tack GJ, Mulder CJ, Bouma G. Update on the diagnosis and management of refractory coeliac disease. Gastroenterol Res Pract. 2013;2013:518483.

201. Biagi F, Corazza GR. Mortality in celiac disease. Nat Rev Gastroenterol Hepatol. 2010;7(3):158–62.

202. Corrao G, Corazza GR, Bagnardi V, Brusco G, Ciacci C, Cottone M, et al. Mortality in patients with coeliac disease and their relatives: a cohort study. Lancet. 2001;358(9279):356–61.

203. Rubio-Tapia A, Kyle RA, Kaplan EL, Johnson DR, Page W, Erdtmann F, et al. Increased prevalence and mortality in undiagnosed celiac disease. Gastroenterology. 2009;137(1):88–93.

204. Lohi S, Maki M, Rissanen H, Knekt P, Reunanen A, Kaukinen K. Prognosis of unrecognized coeliac disease as regards mortality: a population-based cohort study. Ann Med. 2009;41(7):508–15.

205. Metzger MH, Heier M, Maki M, Bravi E, Schneider A, Lowel H, et al. Mortality excess in individuals with elevated IgA anti-transglutaminase antibodies: the KORA/MONICA Augsburg cohort study 1989–1998. Eur J Epidemiol. 2006;21(5):359–65.

206. Solaymani-Dodaran M, West J, Logan RF. Long-term mortality in people with celiac disease diagnosed in childhood compared with adulthood: a population-based cohort study. Am J Gastroenterol. 2007;102(4):864–70.

207. Hischenhuber C, Crevel R, Jarry B, Maki M, Moneret-Vautrin DA, Romano A, et al. Review article: safe amounts of gluten for patients with wheat allergy or coeliac disease. Aliment Pharmacol Ther. 2006;23(5):559–75.

208. Siegel M, Garber ME, Spencer AG, Botwick W, Kumar P, Williams RN, et al. Safety, tolerability, and activity of ALV003: results from two phase 1 single, escalating-dose clinical trials. Dig Dis Sci. 2012;57(2):440–50.

209. Pinier M, Verdu EF, Nasser-Eddine M, David CS, Vezina A, Rivard N, et al. Polymeric binders suppress gliadin-induced toxicity in the intestinal epithelium. Gastroenterology. 2009;136(1):288–98.

210. Sollid LM, Khosla C. Novel therapies for coeliac disease. J Intern Med. 2011;269(6):604–13.

211. Anderson RP, Jabri B. Vaccine against autoimmune disease: antigen-specific immunotherapy. Curr Opin Immunol. 2013;25(3):410–7.

212. Xia J, Bergseng E, Fleckenstein B, Siegel M, Kim CY, Khosla C, et al. Cyclic and dimeric gluten peptide analogues inhibiting DQ2-mediated antigen presentation in celiac disease. Bioorg Med Chem. 2007;15(20):6565–73.

213. Rauhavirta T, Oittinen M, Kivisto R, Mannisto PT, Garcia-Horsman JA, Wang Z, et al. Are transglutaminase 2 inhibitors able to reduce gliadin-induced toxicity related to celiac disease? A proof-of-concept study. J Clin Immunol. 2013;33(1):134–42.

214. Pinier M, Fuhrmann G, Verdu EF, Leroux JC. Prevention measures and exploratory pharmacological treatments of celiac disease. Am J Gastroenterol. 2010;105(12):2551–61, quiz 62.

215. Setty M, Discepolo V, Abadie V, Kamhawi S, Mayassi T, Kent A, Ciszewski C, Maglio M, Kistner E, Bhagat G, Semrad C, Kupfer SS, Green PH, Guandalini S, Troncone R, Murray JA, Turner JR, Jabri B. Distinct and Synergistic Contributions of Epithelial Stress and Adaptive Immunity to Functions of Intraepithelial Killer Cells and Active Celiac Disease. Gastroenterol. 2015. pii: S0016–5085(15)00685-X. doi: 10.1053/j.gastro.2015.05.013.

Cystic Fibrosis

41

Michael Wilschanski and Aliye Uc

Introduction

This chapter focuses on disease pathobiology of the gastrointestinal, nutritional, and hepatic manifestations of cystic fibrosis (CF) disease.

CF is an autosomal recessive multisystem disease, the highest incidence being in individuals of North European decent. Intense follow-up and treatment have improved the median survival to nearly 40 years, and in many countries, around 50% of individuals are older than 18 years of age. Even though the main cause of death is chronic lung disease, gastroenterological features prominently as 85% of patients have exocrine pancreatic insufficiency (PI), and around 10% suffer from liver disease. The gastroenterological, hepatic, and nutritional aspects of the disease are discussed in this chapter.

Cloned in 1989, the CF transmembrane conductance regulator gene is found on chromosome 7. The CFTR protein has two nucleotide-binding domains, two membrane-spanning domains, and a unique regulatory domain. This protein acts as a cyclic adenosine monophosphate (AMP)-dependent chloride channel and localizes to the apical membrane of secretory and absorptive epithelial cells within the intestine, liver, sweat gland, pancreas, airway, and the vas deferens [1].

An inability of duct lumens to hydrate macromolecules is responsible for a number of CF manifestations. A body of pathologic evidence indicates that organ damage can be traced to ductal or glandular plugging by macromolecules that have precipitated in concentrated secretions. For instance, mucus secretions in the bronchi and the intestine are viscid and inspissated, and the crypts are distended as though obstructed. A deficit of ductular fluid flow and altered biochemical and physiologic properties of secretions underlie this situation.

The CFTR Gene

There are close to 2000 mutations in the CFTR gene, and they have been divided into six classes [2]. This classification system provides the opportunity to evaluate the effects of genotype on phenotype by considering the effects of CFTR mutations on CFTR protein function. Nevertheless, it should be emphasized that this classification system is limited by the fact that the functional consequences of many rare mutations (particularly missense mutations) are unknown and cannot be predicted.

Class I mutations include mostly nonsense, frameshift, or missense mutations that result in defective protein biosynthesis (truncation, deletion, etc.). The nonfunctional products are efficiently degraded within the cell. Class II mutations, such as F508del, produce a misfolded functional CFTR protein, which is degraded intracellularly preventing trafficking to the apical surface of the cell. Class III mutations affect channel activation by preventing binding and hydrolysis of ATP at one of the two nucleotide-binding domains (NBD1, NBD2). Class IV mutations produce a protein with impaired function due to abnormal anion conduction. Due to a variety of mechanisms including abnormal splicing, promoter mutations, or inefficient trafficking, Class V mutations result in a reduced number of normally functioning CFTR molecules on the apical surface. Class VI mutations result from truncation of the C-terminus of CFTR and produce a functional protein which is unstable at the apical membrane surface. Mutations belonging to classes I–III and VI confer little or no functional CFTR at the apical membrane. As a consequence, inheritance of homozygous or compound heterozygous mutations belonging to these classes are predicted to have severe consequences. Mutations belonging to Classes IV and V on the other hand which confer (or are presumed

M. Wilschanski (✉)
Pediatric Gastroenterology Unit, Hadassah Hebrew University Medical Center, 91240 Jerusalem, Israel
e-mail: michaelwil@hadassah.org.il

A. Uc
Stead Family Department of Pediatrics, University of Iowa Children's Hospital, 2865 JPP Pediatrics, 200 Hawkins Drive, Iowa City, IA 52242, USA
e-mail: aliye-uc@uiowa.edu

© Springer International Publishing Switzerland 2016
S. Guandalini et al. (eds.), *Textbook of Pediatric Gastroenterology, Hepatology and Nutrition,*
DOI 10.1007/978-3-319-17169-2_41

to confer) some residual CFTR-mediated channel function would be expected to have milder consequences. In fact, it is patients with at least one mutation belonging to Classes IV or V who generally present with symptoms in late childhood or adulthood.

Animal Models for CF GI Disease

A CF animal model that recapitulates the human findings can provide a powerful tool to study the pathophysiology of disease and design therapies. The first animal model of CF was the mouse model, developed in 1992, 3 years after the CFTR gene was cloned [3, 4]. The porcine [5–10] and ferret models [11–13] were developed recently. The pancreatic, hepatobiliary, and intestinal manifestations of the pig model will be reviewed here.

Pigs

The CF pig model was generated by using homologous recombination. The CFTR gene was disrupted in pig fibroblasts, and somatic cell nuclear transfer was done to generate heterozygous (null or deltaF508). The heterozygous pigs were then crossed to generate the CF pigs [5–8]. CF pigs have multisystem disease that recapitulates the human disease.

Meconium ileus (MI) is present in all CF pigs within the first 24–48 h of life causing intestinal perforation and mortality if untreated surgically. The intestinal pathology in CF pigs is similar to what has been described in human babies with MI (dilated and meconium-filled proximal bowel, a very small-caliber distal bowel, obstruction in distal intestine to proximal colon). Inflammation is insignificant in CF pig intestine unless perforated or necrotic, but most reports are from the neonatal period. Mucus cell hyperplasia is present in small and large intestine at variable levels. A new gut-corrected pig model of CF expresses ~20% of CFTR in the intestine and survives the neonatal period without surgery [14].

From all three animal models, CF pigs exhibit the most severe pancreatic phenotype. The pancreatic lesions start in utero and progress over time in CF pigs, in concordance with the previous autopsy studies of humans with CF [15–17]. The newborn CF pig pancreas has acinar cell loss, duct proliferation, expansion of interlobular connective tissue, and scattered inflammatory cell aggregates [5–10, 14]. Mucous cell metaplasia is a late finding, and some ducts/acini are filled with zymogen-like material. In older animals, the exocrine pancreatic lesions progress, and pancreas is mostly replaced by fat and fibrosis [7, 14]. The islets are morphologically intact [7, 14], but functionally abnormal. As in humans [18–21], the pancreatic fluid is acidic, low in volume, and high in protein and concentrated in CF pigs at birth [10]. The proinflammatory, complement cascade, proapoptotic, and profibrotic pathways are activated in CF pig pancreas and likely contribute to the destructive process [8, 22].

CF pigs manifest focal biliary cirrhosis, but the lesions are mild and do not progress over time [4, 6, 14]. There is no evidence of cholestasis or fatty infiltration. However, it is not known whether the liver disease would have developed if the pigs lived longer than ~1.5 years. In contrast to mild liver disease, gallbladders are severely diseased in CF pigs. They all have microgallbladder.

Animal models offer a unique opportunity to study the pathogenesis of CF gastrointestinal (GI) disease and various therapeutic approaches.

Diagnosis of CF

The diagnosis is clear if the patient has a sweat chloride concentration >60 mmol/L with at least one recognized phenotypic characteristic which include chronic sinopulmonary disease, salt loss syndromes, and, in males, obstructive azoospermia [23, 24]. The majority of CF patients will have one established CF causing mutation on each CFTR allele. The diagnosis of CF should not be automatically considered if the sweat chloride concentration is >60 mmol/L. There is a list of disorders with high sweat tests which is expanding (Table 41.1).

At the other end of the spectrum, problems arise when there is a CF phenotype in one or more organ systems, and the sweat chloride level is borderline (30–60 mmol/L).

Table 41.1 Conditions other than CF associated with raised sweat electrolyte concentration [25]

Glucose-6-phosphatase
Adrenal insufficiency
Familial hypoparathyroidism
Nephrogenic diabetes insipidus
Mauriac's syndrome
Familial cholestatic syndrome
Anorexia nervosa
Severe malnutrition
Atopic dermatitis
Keratitis–ichthyosis–deafness (KID) syndrome
Fucosidosis
Pseudohypoaldosteronism
Patients undergoing prostaglandin infusions
Hyperchlorhidrosis caused by homozygous mutation in CA12, encoding carbonic anhydrase XII. [25]
Accurate references lacking
Glucose-6-phosphate-1-dehydrogenase deficiency
Ectodermal dysplasia
Hypothyroidism

Electrophysiological testing using nasal potential difference (NPD) measurements may aid in the diagnosis of CF patients with normal or borderline sweat tests and negative or uninformative genetic test results [26]. This test measures transepithelial sodium and chloride transport in the nasal epithelium. The function of CFTR in chloride secretion is intimately related to the inwardly directed sodium transport via the epithelial sodium channel (ENaC). The activity of these two channels is the basis for NPD. A catheter is placed under the inferior turbinate and is connected via a series of electrodes to a voltmeter and recorder. The nasal epithelium is perfused with solutions which inhibit sodium transport and activate chloride transport. In CF patients, the readings are markedly dissimilar from controls. Another electrophysiological tool is the intestinal current measurement (ICM) which measures CFTR function *ex vivo* in rectal biopsy using a modified Ussing chamber [27]. Testing should only be carried out by an experienced individual in specialist research center where objective reference values have been established.

CFTR Dysfunction: Gastrointestinal Consequences

Exocrine Pancreatic Abnormalities

Exocrine Pancreatic Function

In pancreatic ductal epithelia, the CFTR protein is highly expressed, allowing fluids and anion to enter the ductal lumen. Thereby, luminal chloride is exchanged for bicarbonate, giving evidence that CFTR is permeable to bicarbonate [28]. According to the Quinton's hypothesis, the defect in bicarbonate transport is indeed the primary defect in CF [29]. This results in an increased volume of alkaline fluid, allowing the acinar cells to remain in a soluble state, due to the highly concentrated proteins secreted. Absent or reduced CFTR channel function impairs chloride and bicarbonate to enter the ducts which results in reduced volume of a more acidic fluid [30]. The acidic milieu within the acinar lumen also leads to impaired reuptake of GP2, the zymogen-granule-associated protein [31]. The consequences of mutations in the CFTR gene have been demonstrated by pancreatic function studies showing that CF patients have low flow secretions with a high protein concentration, presumably which will precipitate in the duct lumina causing obstruction, damage, and atrophy (Fig. 41.1).

These changes begin in utero, and after birth, the process continues with the small duct obstruction leading to a larger duct obstruction. For several months afterwards, there is a release of proteins, originating in the pancreas, into the blood stream. This pathological process forms the basis for the immune reactive trypsinogen (IRT), the neonatal screening test for CF. The reason has yet to be determined, but, interestingly enough, the infant is asymptomatic while this wholesale destruction of the exocrine pancreas is occurring. Eventually, this process results in severe inflammatory changes, obstruction of ducts by mucus and calcium-containing debris, the destruction of acini, and generalized fibrosis. The high IRT does show that some exocrine pancreatic tissue is still present and may have a bearing on possible small molecule therapy targeted at the remainder of the pancreas which may rescue enough tissue to cause viability of the remaining pancreas. This of course contradicts the popular belief that the pancreas is entirely nonfunctioning at birth.

One of the most remarkable observations is that genetic factors exquisitely influence the degree of pancreatic disease and its rate of progression. CF patients are classified as pancreatic insufficient (PI) or pancreatic sufficient (PS). PI patients comprise approximately 85 % of all CF patients. PI patients present with maldigestion, as evidenced by steatorrhea (fecal fat greater than 7 % of fat intake in infants over 6 months of age and over 15 % under 6 months of age), requiring these patients to have pancreatic enzyme replacement therapy (PERT) with meals. PS patients, however, have evidence of pancreatic damage, but retain sufficient endogenous exocrine pancreatic function to sustain normal digestion [33] due to the fact that ductal CFTR in PS patients is partially functional, thereby allowing anions and fluid to enter the ductal lumen. This provides further evidence that mutant CFTR may be acting on other apical anion exchangers to conduct rather than conduct chloride ions itself [34].

The exocrine pancreatic status is directly linked to genotype [35]. Analysis of particular CFTR mutations in patients with pancreatic phenotypes (PI vs. PS) revealed two categories of alleles: "severe" and "mild." Patients homozygous or compound heterozygous for severe alleles belonging to classes I, II, III, or VI confer PI as opposed to patients with a mild class IV or V allele even when the second mutation is severe. These patients are termed "PS." Plausible explanation of this observation finds all known mild alleles belong to class IV or class V all of which are (or predicted to be) associated with some residual chloride channel activity at the epithelial apical membranes. Although these mutations confer sufficient CFTR function to prevent the pancreas to be completely destroyed, many PS patients have reduced exocrine pancreatic capacity and are associated with an increased risk of pancreatitis, as discussed below. A very small number (2–3 %) of patients carrying severe mutations on both alleles are PS at diagnosis; however, most patients will experience a gradual transition from PS to PI. A few missense mutations (e.g., G85E) confer a variable pancreatic phenotype.

Many PS patients have reduced exocrine pancreatic capacity and are associated with an increased risk of pancre-

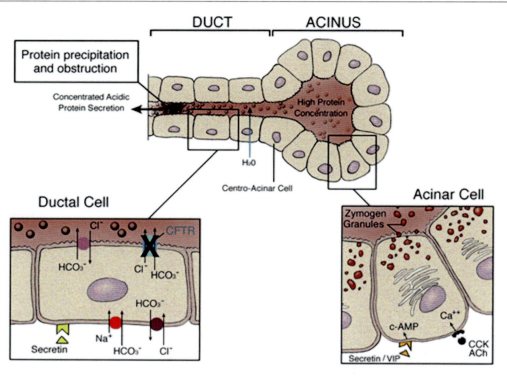

Fig. 41.1 Pathogenesis of pancreatic disease in cystic fibrosis *(CF)* [32]. Acinar cells secrete large quantities of protein, primarily in the form of digestive enzymes, into the acinar lumen. Under normal circumstances, anions (chloride and bicarbonate) are secreted into the ductal lumen via the cystic fibrosis transmembrane regulator *(CFTR)* and bicarbonate exchangers. This provides a driving force for the movement of fluid into the lumen of the duct and maintains the solubility of secreted proteins in a dilute, alkaline solution. In CF, impaired anion transport into the proximal ducts results in decreased secretion of more acidic fluid, which leads to precipitation of secreted proteins. Intraluminal obstruction of the ducts then causes progressive pancreatic damage and atrophy. (Reproduced from Ref. [32], Copyright 2007, with permission from BMJ Publishing Group Ltd) *cAMP* cyclic adenosine monophosphate, *ACh* acetylcholine, *CCK* cholecystokinin, *VIP* vasoactive intestinal peptide

atitis, even though mild mutations confer sufficient CFTR function to prevent the pancreas to be completely destroyed. As first reported by Shwachman in 1975, recurrent acute and chronic pancreatitis are relatively infrequent complications of CF. In this retrospective study, only 0.5% of CF patients had pancreatitis. Durno et al. reported more recently, an incidence of 1.7% in a cohort of over 1000 patients followed over a period of 30 years [36]. All of the pancreatitis patients were classified as PS, but this subgroup of PS patients, in fact, appeared to be highly susceptible to pancreatitis, since almost one in five was affected by this complication. In a seminal paper of the largest study to date of CF PS patients, Ooi et al. determined the association between severity of CFTR genotype and the risk of pancreatitis [37]. They examined a large cohort of 277 PS patients from 2 CF centers of which 62 had well-documented pancreatitis. The mutations were divided into three main groups: severe, moderate–severe, and mild in using a novel pancreatic insufficiency prevalence score. It was found that the proportion of patients who developed pancreatitis was significantly greater for genotypes in the mild group than the moderate–severe group. Thus, the more mild mutations were associated with increased risk of pancreatitis. CFTR mutations may contribute to the development of pancreatitis along with other genetic and environmental factors [38].

Diagnosis of Pancreatic Phenotype

With the increasing worldwide use of neonatal screening programs, patients may present with symptoms of CF or be entirely asymptomatic. Making a determination in all patients, whether the patient is PI or PS is essential to enable a rational use of oral PERT [39]. When patients have steatorrhea (oil droplets on stool microscopy), hypoalbuminemia, and low fat-soluble vitamin levels, the diagnosis of PI is straightforward. However, the lack of these findings does not exclude PI; therefore, more formal testing is required. In the past, direct exocrine pancreatic stimulation testing was administered. Unfortunately, this was an invasive, time-consuming procedure and not widely used in most centers. Indirect pancreatic testing with 72 h fecal fat measurements should be encouraged and be used as follow up for pancreatic exocrine status and response to therapy. Due to the technical difficulties surrounding the performance of this test, however, most laboratories are utilizing the fecal elastase-1 test instead, as the main advantage is no need for prolonged stool collection. Pancreatic elastase is secreted into the duodenum and is found at relatively high concentrations in stool (>500 μg/gm stool).

The use of fecal pancreatic elastase-1 has now become a common diagnostic test for assessing exocrine pancreatic status. The advantages and limitations of fecal elastase-1 in CF have been discussed by Kalnins et al. in a review article [40]. The cutoff levels of fecal elastase for PI range between 100 and 200 μg/g stool; a majority of centers use the upper level of 200 μg/g stool. With the use of 200 μg/g stool weight, some patients may be falsely identified as PI. The Toronto group compared stool elastase values to the 72-h fecal fat in both known PI and sufficient patients and found that an elastase value of 100 μg/g stool had a 99% predictive value in ruling out PI based on an abnormal fecal fat. Cade et al. showed that patients with pancreatic sufficiency on the basis of a normal fecal fat balance study were found to have fecal elastase values in the range of 100–200 μg/g stool; elastase levels were compared with the fecal fat test coefficient of fat absorption (CFA) [41]. Whether defining PI as <93 or 90% CFA, cutoff levels of fecal elastase of <100 μg or <200 μg/g stool for either monoclonal or polyclonal methods were positive predictors of insufficient pancreatic function. However, patients with pancreatic sufficiency were not included in this study population. Moreover, these observations question the validity of defining the cutoff for PI as a fecal elastase value below 200 μg/g stool. In a different study of 21 known PS patients, a poor correlation was found between fecal fat excretion and elastase-1 [42]. The fecal elastase result will define clearly whether a patient is PI or sufficient, in a majority of cases, provided the test is done accurately. In situations such as in acute diarrhea, short gut, or stool from an ileostomy, where stool is more watery, fecal elastase levels may be lower than expected; therefore, it would be advisable to wait until the diarrhea resolves, or until a sample that is more formed is available. A definitive answer on pancreatic status may not be provided in those patients with less common genetic variations, where there are no supportive clinical features of PI, and fecal elastase values are often borderline. In such cases, elastase can be used to monitor pancreatic status, in conjunction with ongoing evaluation of clinical and nutritional status [43].

Oral Pancreatic Enzyme Replacement Therapy

Prior to 2010, pancreatic enzyme products were exempt from the Food, Drug, and Cosmetic Act of 1938 and did not require approval of the Food and Drug Administration (FDA). Since then, a plethora of products became available to the public without the need for strict preclinical and clinical studies. The FDA has since mandated that all manufac-turers of pancreatic enzyme products in the USA must seek approval by April 2010.

Currently, there are six preparations approved and available for use [44–46]: Creon [47–50], Zenpep [51], Pancreaze, Ultresa, Viokace, and Pertzye. During the study on Creon, a fixed dose of 72,000 lipase units with meals and 36,000 with snacks was evaluated. The study was a double-blind, randomized, placebo-controlled trial of 54 adult patients with chronic pancreatitis or post-pancreatic surgery. The treatment arm showed difference in CFA of 19.3% over placebo (85.6 vs. 66.3).

Creon and Zenpep showed a similar nutrient absorption rate between 83 and 87% fat absorption. The dosages of these products are based on the lipase units contained in the product. It is now common for patients to change from one product to another using a 1:1 lipase ratio and then titrating for maximum efficacy. The North American CF Foundation has published guidelines according to the age of the patient and according to the grams of fat ingested per day [52].

The importance of the correct enzyme ingestion in infants and children is a major concern. There is often difficulty in feeding infants capsules or microspheres however small they may be. The continued use of the unprotected powder enzymes for infants until 1 year of age is common in some centers. In infants, these enzymes may have some advantage over the enteric-coated versions in certain situations. The efficacy of unprotected powder enzymes (in tablet or powder form) has not been directly compared to the enteric-coated version in infants, but infants treated with this approach do achieve growth and weight gain, proving their efficacy [53]. In addition to their use for infants, unprotected powder enzymes are often used to help digest enteral tube feedings where oral administration of enzymes is not possible, or when jejunostomy feeds are required.

Breast-feeding mothers should be instructed on proper infant mouth care after enzyme delivery when the unprotected powder enzymes are provided to these infants. It is recommended that soft cotton swabs or a washcloth dipped in sterile water be used to wipe the inside of the infant's mouth and inside the gums. This will prove to be sufficient to prevent gum erosion to the infant and nipple irritation to the mother.

For infants with MI requiring surgery or those with an ileostomy, the powder enzymes may provide the advantage of immediate release in the duodenum. Theoretically, this will improve nutrient digestion compared to the pH sensitive, delayed release enteric-coated microsphere enzyme products. Tablets without a protective coating can be crushed if the powder version in capsules or in bottles is not readily available.

The production of specially designed enzymes for the small child has been a recent advancement. A multicenter cross over study in CF infants who were randomized to receive CfC

(Creon for children) or regular enzyme for 2-week periods was performed; it compared a spoon administration containing 5000 lipase units with the standard Creon 10,000 capsule [54]. The parental preference was the primary end point; over 75 % of the parents preferred CfC over the standard preparation.

One study demonstrated that there was no improvement when compared to a standard enzyme preparation [55]; another study showed improvement in fat absorption with the bicarbonate-containing enzyme [56]. However, in both studies, approximately 80 % fat absorption was achieved using the bicarbonate-containing enzyme, and Kalnins et al. [55] found the same degree of fat absorption with the conventional enteric-coated enzyme product. Theoretically, the addition of bicarbonate to enteric-coated enzyme preparations might raise the proximal intestinal pH and thereby optimize dissolution of the enteric coating and improve enzyme activity. There were conflicting studies on its efficacy when compared to standard, pH sensitive microsphere enzymes. An enzyme preparation with added bicarbonate had been available in the past, but at time of writing it has not yet received approval by the FDA. Several other enzyme products are in phase 2 or 3 trials. One novel enzyme is liprotamase a non-porcine PERT, containing a biotechnologically derived formulation of crystalline lipase, protease, and amylase [57]. The use of this type of designer drug enzyme has several advantages. The other PERTs are subject to possible viral contamination. In addition, precise dosage standardization had been difficult in the porcine product; the problem of overfill stability has been solved with the new FDA requirements. A preliminary phase 1 study demonstrated good clinical activity, and a multicenter phase 3 study showed that there was significant improvement in the coefficient of fat [56] absorption. A 12-month long-term open-label study [57] of the tolerability and clinical activity in a large number of patients has been published. However, more studies are being carried out on this product. The PERTs currently approved by the FDA have demonstrated efficacy, but new formulations like liprotamase will allow for variety in the type of PERT available.

An important factor for clinicians and families of a CF patient or those with CF to understand and appreciate is that although enzyme therapy for those with PI allows for normal growth and weight gain in most individuals with CF; however, unfortunately, it does not completely correct nutrient malabsorption. There are several reasons for incomplete nutrient digestion with the currently available enzyme products. (1) A proportion of the unprotected powder enzymes or tablets may become inactivated by prolonged exposure to gastric acid. This results in decreased duodenal active enzyme recovery. (2) Enteric-coated microspheres, which dissolve at a pH of > 5.5, may only be released in the ileum if duodenal milieu does not reach this pH as occurs in CF. From prior intubation studies, evidence is confirmed that release of enzymes from enteric-coated microspheres is delayed in CF,

and thus, they are delivered beyond the duodenum, even as far distal as the ileum. This results in a nutrient digestion occurring in the more distal small intestine, but not in the duodenum and proximal jejunum as in health. (3) Not only maldigestion but also malabsorption contributes to the insufficient assimilation of nutrients. Fatty acid absorption as well as the digestion of triglycerides is impaired in subjects with CF [58] as suggested by studies done. Other contributing factors to nutrient malabsorption include incomplete lipid solubilization caused by a depleted bile salt pool and thick intestinal mucus. This may affect the unstirred water layer, reducing absorption of fatty acids into the small intestine epithelium. A large center reported < 80 % fat absorption in approximately 30 % of treated patients; therefore, a degree of malabsorption is to be expected for reasons mentioned. Therefore, achieving > 90 % nutrient digestion as evaluated by 72-h fecal fat studies is not likely to occur in a majority of patients with CF.

Patients should not be automatically encouraged to increase their PERT intake if they experience gastrointestinal symptoms such as abdominal pain, bloating, or loose stools, as there are many other etiologies for these symptoms including compliance. For persistent symptoms, a fat balance study should be performed to titrate dose and proton pump inhibitor (PPI) should be considered. After which, if patient does not experience any improvement, investigations for non-pancreatic disease should be explored (see below). Awareness of these factors by both clinicians and patients will help to guide a rational approach to enzyme therapy in CF; an individualized approach to treatment is recommended.

Hepatobiliary Disease

There are a wide variety of hepatobiliary disorders associated with CF (Table 41.2); almost all patients with CF have evidence of hepatobiliary disease. There are no clinical consequences for the vast majority of patients.

Table 41.2 Hepatobiliary complications of CF

Hepatic	Approximate frequency (%)
Neonatal cholestasis	5
Steatosis	20–60
Focal biliary cirrhosis	11–70
Multilobular cirrhosis	5–7
Liver failure	Rare
Biliary	
Microgallbladder	5–20
Distended gallbladder	3–20
Cholelithiasis and sludge	10–25
Intrahepatic sludge/stones	Unknown
Extrinsic compression of common bile duct	Unknown
Cholangiocarcinoma	Unknown

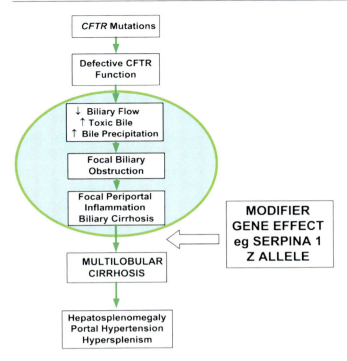

Fig. 41.2 Pathogenesis of cystic fibrosis-related liver disease [32]. Lack of functional CFTR in the biliary ductules causes dehydration, increased concentration, and lack of alkalinization of the duct contents. This causes precipitation of biliary secretions and ductular obstruction. In the majority of patients, the pathologic changes are focal and appear to be clinically inconsequential *(circled area)*. However, approximately 5–10% of CF patients proceed to develop clinically significant liver disease with evidence of multilobular cirrhosis and portal hypertension. Susceptibility to more severe liver disease may be modulated by other genetic and/or environmental factors. (Reproduced from Ref. [32], Copyright 2007, with permission from BMJ Publishing Group Ltd)

The pathognomonic hepatic feature of CF is focal biliary cirrhosis. Intrahepatic biliary ductal secretion is dependent on CFTR-mediated chloride transport for adequate hydration of the lumen (Fig. 41.2). Loss of CFTR function causes the biliary ductules to become obstructed with thick periodic-acid-Schiff positive material leading to acute and chronic periductal inflammation, bile duct proliferation, and increased fibrosis in scattered portal tracts. Remarkably, adjoining portal tracts are frequently normal. Over 40 years ago, postmortem studies performed show evidence of mild focal disease in 11% of infants, 27% of those dying at 1 year, and in more than 70% of adults. Clinically, significant portal hypertension resulting from severe multilobular cirrhosis develops in only 5–7% of patients. This is termed "CF-associated liver disease" (CFLD). CFLD is the single most important nonpulmonary cause of death, responsible for 2.5% of overall mortality in CF. The average age of diagnosis of CFLD is 10–11 years of age, and 90% are diagnosed before the age of 20 [59] Following routine examination or by laboratory evidence of hypersplenism, most patients are asymptomatic and

are often identified by the evidence of hepatosplenomegaly. Hepatocellular function remains well preserved for many years, even decades. Splenomegaly is a consistent finding, and the liver edge is often nodular and hard.

About 40–50% of CF patients exhibit intermittent elevations of aspartate aminotransferase (AST), alanine aminotransferase (ALT), or gamma glutamyltransferase (GGT), which are generally 1–2.5 times above the upper reference limits. Biochemical markers of liver disease do not reliably identify patients with multilobular cirrhosis nor do they predict the development of end-stage liver disease. Furthermore, patients with advanced multilobular cirrhosis may have normal liver biochemistry test results. As hyperbilirubinemia is rare, elevated serum gammaglobulin level is more likely to be associated with chronic pulmonary inflammation. CFLD occurs predominantly in PI patients. Thus, severe class I, II, or III mutations on both alleles appear to be a risk factor [60]. A male preponderance of severe CFLD has been shown in most studies.

Why a minority of patients with the same severe CFTR mutations progress to CFLD is unclear. However, it has been hypothesized that non-CF modifier genes, such as polymorphisms in genes that upregulate inflammation, fibrosis, or oxidative stress, confer an increased susceptibility. In a multinational gene modifier study of the different candidate genes, the SERPINA 1 Z allele of alpha-1 antitrysin deficiency was found to be strongly associated with CFLD. This result is intriguing as the CF patient requires a double-hit to develop CFLD. Hitherto undefined environmental factors are also likely to be involved.

Gallstones develop in 1–10% of patients with CF. There is also an increased incidence of variety of intrahepatic and extrahepatic abnormalities of the biliary tree. Nonfunctioning microgallbladders are common, although it is seen less frequently that patients with CF have distended gallbladders appearing obstructed. Stones may also be commonly visualized within the larger intrahepatic and extrahepatic biliary tree. Debray et al. have proposed using the knockout mouse model that the gallbladder itself, rather than the bile duct epithelia may be the major site for a bile acid shunt, the cholecystohepatic shunt, from the gall bladder back to the liver [61].

The principal cause of CF-associated liver disease remaining controversial; it has been postulated that common duct obstruction resulting from extrinsic compression by fibrosis within the head of the pancreas. Following ERCP or transhepatic cholangiographic imaging, changes resembling primary sclerosing cholangitis (i.e., beading and stricturing of the intrahepatic and extrahepatic ducts) are quite commonly observed [62]. These changes are likely due to accumulation of protein, mucus, or sludge within the biliary lumina.

Diagnosis and Management

Studies are being performed to evaluate early liver disease in CF. Clinical examination is necessary to look for signs of chronic liver disease and organomegaly; routine biochemistry is generally not helpful. The evidence of liver disease is often subclinical until CFLD develops as previously stated. As raised serum liver enzymes in a CF patient may be due to other diseases entirely, it is imperative to consider hepatitis (infectious or autoimmune) Wilson disease and other cause of steatosis (malnutrition, diabetes mellitus) as possible causes when reviewing these patients. A small number of infants may present with neonatal cholestasis, in particular those with MI, usually resolving with no long-term affect [63].

In most centers, ultrasonography of the hepatiobiliary system is available, and it includes Doppler measurements of flow in the portal vein; however, the positive predictive value of a normal scan and sensitivity is low. Elastography (Fibroscan R), a new test of liver stiffness (which may be a marker of fibrosis), is used in other chronic liver diseases such as hepatitis C. Early liver disease cannot presently be made on the basis of ultrasound [64].

Recent guidelines by Debray et al. [65] recommend that in order to delay progression of CFLD, ursodeoxychlolic acid treatment should be initiated. In a Swedish study, there was evidence that biochemistry is improved in liver histology [66]; however, this treatment and in particular the recommended dose have been challenged after a trial of high-dose ursodeoxycholic acid in another cholestatic liver disease, Primary sclerosing cholangitis, was terminated due to severe side effects [67]; further studies are obviously needed.

Follow up and management of CFLD are the same as for other chronic liver diseases except for (1) the use of beta blockade prophylaxis for variceal bleeding, it needs to be thoroughly examined in CF patients in consultation with the pulmonologists, and (2) selection criteria for liver transplantation have not been established. Apart from the routine indications, there appears to be evidence that earlier liver transplantation, before the development of significant and irreversible nutritional and pulmonary deterioration, may be helpful. However, large, long-term studies have been difficult to perform [68].

Intestinal Complications

Meconium Ileus

Most patients born with MI present within 24–48 h with evidence of intestinal obstruction with abdominal distension, bilious vomiting, and failure to pass meconium. MI occurs in 15–20 % of CF patients [69].

Diagnostic aids include a family history of CF and a plain radiograph which may show large distended loops of small bowel and a ground-glass appearance in the right lower quadrant due to due to inspissated meconium in the ileocecal area.

A diagnostic procedure which may be therapeutic is the performance of a contrast enema. The hypertonic enema may lavage the plug of meconium and provided the infant is stable; this procedure may be repeated several times in order to avoid surgery. Surgery is, of course, necessary for complicated MI.

A small proportion presents with perforation in utero with meconium peritonitis and subsequent intra-abdominal calcification which may only be diagnosed incidentally during third trimester ultrasound examinations. Postnatally, up to 50 % of MI patients may have additional problems including malrotation with volvulus or intestinal atresia, termed "complicated MI".

In a consortium which examined over 3700 cases of MI, several apical transporter genes were found to modify meconium ileu [70], thus appearing that modifier gene(s) together with two severe CFTR alleles confers an increased likelihood of MI. It remains possible that modifier genes with or without environmental factors may explain the variability and severity of other intestinal complications such as distal intestinal obstruction syndrome (DIOS). In a subsequent study, linkage analysis identified a modifier locus for MI on human chromosome 12p13.3 [71].

Distal Intestinal Obstruction Syndrome

Frequently in older children and adults with CF, DIOS a chronic, recurrent form of partial intestinal obstruction occurs. DIOS is frequently confused with other common causes of abdominal pain in patients with CF and almost exclusively in those with PI. Unique to CF, DIOS results from a buildup of adherent, thick intestinal contents in the terminal ileum and proximal colon. The reported frequency is variable, consequently, but a recent study shows a prevalence of 18 % in adults [72]. Intestinal inflammation has been shown in the mouse model [73] and is occasionally shown in humans [74]. Patients usually complain of intermittent episodes of pain, which may or may not be localized to the right lower quadrant. Non-tender, or mildly tender, palpable mass can be felt in the right lower quadrant (although it may not always be localized there). Some patients suffer from intractable chronic pain that is difficult to treat, and on rare occasions, there is complete bowel obstruction.

The European Society for Pediatric Gastroenterology Hepatology and Nutrition (ESPGHAN) Cystic Fibrosis and Pancreatic Disease Working Group defines complete DIOS as the combination of (1) complete intestinal obstruction, as evidenced by bilious vomiting and fluid levels on abdominal radiography with (2) a fecal mass in the ileocecum and (3) abdominal pain and or distension. Incomplete or impending DIOS is defined as (1) a short history of abdominal pain and/or distension (2) a fecal mass in ileocecum but without signs of complete obstruction.

While the exact cause of DIOS is unknown, various precipitating factors have been proposed including abnormal properties of intestinal mucus, dehydration of intraluminal contents, slow intestinal transit, poor compliance with pancreatic enzyme therapy, and a prior history of MI. DIOS should not be confused with simple constipation which is common in CF patients with PI. Although unlike DIOS a right lower quadrant mass is usually not palpable, the rectum will characteristically be full of stool on physical examination, and stooling patterns and consistency are abnormal. Patients undergoing major surgery, such as lung or liver transplant, carry an increased risk of DIOS during the immediate postoperative period.

With other CF-associated or non-CF gastrointestinal disease including appendiceal disease, intussusception, Crohn's disease, fibrosing colonopathy or malignancy, non-specific symptoms and signs may occur; therefore, abdominal ultrasound and CT scans may be necessary.

In complete DIOS, the patient usually requires hospitalization and IV rehydration. Patients with incomplete DIOS respond to oral rehydration combined with mineral oil or polyethylene glycol preparations. Enemas of sodium meglumine diatrizoate (Gastrograffin or Telebrix) may be performed by experienced radiologists, but the enema must enter the ileocecal valve to get above the obstruction. Treatment of DIOS is still largely empirical due to few randomized controlled trials. Local instillation of diatrizoate in the cecum via colonoscopy has been described [75]. Surgery is seldom required if early aggressive medical management is performed. Laparoscopy and washout are recommended for consideration before resection. A single episode of DIOS is a risk factor for recurrence; maintenance therapy should be considered along with regular follow up by the gastroenterological service [76].

Appendiceal Disease

The incidence of acute appendicitis in CF is reported to be lower than in the general population. Nevertheless, patients who develop this complication carry a greater risk of a delayed diagnosis and an increased incidence of complications such as appendiceal abscess. The possible factors include luminal obstruction of the appendix with thick mucus, delayed intervention due to mistaken diagnosis of DIOS, or masking of acute symptoms by chronic antibiotic use.

Intussusception

In 1–2% of adult CF patients, intussusception occurs, approximately 10–20 times higher than in the general population. Most cases are ileo-colic, and 25% are associated with small bowel obstruction [77]. Sticky, mucofeculent material which adheres to the intestinal epithelium may act as the lead point in intussusception. Plain abdominal X-rays are often nonspecific, showing fecal loading, or less often a small bowel obstruction. Presentation is usually with intermittent abdominal pain. Classical appearances of intussusception may be seen on barium studies and include a lobulated soft tissue mass and a "coiled spring" usually situated in the right iliac fossa. The "doughnut sign" on transverse scan and "pseudo-kidney" on longitudinal scan are some of the ultrasound examination findings. Intussusception is often intermittent and resolves spontaneously, and it may also be observed in asymptomatic patients as an incidental finding during abdominal imaging [78].

Gastroesophageal Reflux Disease

Gastroesophageal reflux disease (GERD) is a multifactorial problem with contributions from both the severity and treatment of lung disease, physiotherapy, transient inappropriate lower esophageal sphincter relaxation, and delayed gastric emptying. GERD is common in CF patients [79], and there is some evidence that GERD may contribute to the progression of respiratory disease either by pulmonary aspiration of refluxed gastric contents or by neutrally mediated reflex bronchoconstriction secondary to irritation of the esophageal mucosa [80]. This is debatable; however, the GERD may be secondary to the lung disease. Other complications include malnutrition due to increased losses through emesis or reduced energy intake from dysphagia and esophageal strictures. Since silent GERD is common in CF patients, a lack of reported symptoms does not exclude this diagnosis. Bile acids are found in the sputum of children with CF suggesting bile reflux [81]. While esophageal pH or impedance monitoring is helpful, upper endoscopy and biopsy are recommended especially when drug trials have failed in order to define the extent of disease and to rule out other esophageal pathology such as eosinophilic esophagitis.

Fibrosing Colonopathy

A complication of CF involving mainly the colon was reported in young patients with CF in 1994 [82]. The term "fibrosing colonopathy" was coined to describe what became recognized as an iatrogenic complication, resulting in considerable morbidity and some mortality. Many patients were initially diagnosed as having inflammatory bowel disease as their symptoms include worsening abdominal pain, intermittent bowel obstruction, and passage of blood and mucus. The proximal colon developed a concentric ring of fibrosis below the submucosa, but in some patients, the concentric fibrosis extended to the entire colon, producing the shrunken "pipe stem" effect. There is considerable hypertrophy of the muscularis mucosa, and the submucosa shows variable degrees of inflammation with eosinophils and mixed inflammatory cells. In the UK and the USA, case-control studies showed a strong statistical association between this complication and dose of pancreatic enzymes (often in excess of 50,000 U lipase/kg body weight) [52]. This led to a reevaluation of the safety of pancreatic enzymes. Notwithstanding, there was no evidence that excessive doses of enzymes that were used by many clinicians actually improved efficacy or improved abdominal symptoms attributable to maldigestion. Several countries have implemented strict dosing guidelines for PERT. However, a few additional cases of fibrosing colonopathy have been reported in the USA and the UK giving further evidence that "enzyme overdosing" still occurs and also emphasizes the need for close monitoring of enzyme doses in all patients with CF.

Intestinal Infections

The vast majority of patients are asymptomatic, but patients with CF generally demonstrate significantly higher rates of *Clostridium difficile* (32–50%) than the general population (2%), as is the case with healthy neonates. However, on rare occasions severe, potentially fatal cases of pseudomembranous colitis have been reported. Presenting with acute toxic megacolon without diarrhea, the clinical manifestations may be atypical, and absence of diarrhea could be due to lack of intestinal CFTR function. An immunological protection from diarrhea may be due to chronic antibiotic therapy allowing chronic colonization with this pathogen. Alternatively, the unique intestinal environment in CF patients may provide a favorable milieu for this organism. Another hypothesis is due to an abnormality in receptor binding of the toxin, and there is a reduced risk of clinical complications in CF.

CF patients have been reported also to have an increased colonization rate of other bacterial species. This could include *Lactobacillus* spp, *Pseudomonas* spp, *Staphylococcus*, and *Enterococcus*. It has been suggested that CFTR itself acts as a receptor for certain organisms, thereby creating a loss of CFTR affording a form of protection from the consequences of infection. The clinical significance of this is unclear.

In patients with increased diarrhea, abdominal distention, and anorexia, *Giardia lamblia* should be considered as it is a common intestinal parasite and may be more common in patients with PI from any cause including CF [83].

Small-Intestinal Bacterial Overgrowth

Indirect evidence points to an estimated prevalence up to 50% [84] of CF patients presenting with small-intestinal bacterial overgrowth (SIBO). These risk factors can include abnormal accumulation of surface mucus (which may allow proliferation and adhesion of bacteria), the reduced alkaline flushing of the upper intestine, and the altered intestinal mucins (which may have limited protective functions). Additionally, there is an increased risk of SIBO following intestinal resection due to MI. SIBO may contribute to malabsorption in some patients with CF, although data are limited. The prominent histological feature of the CF mouse small intestine is mucus accumulation, which occludes the crypts and coats the villus surfaces. The mucus obstruction of the crypts is believed to interfere with innate defense mechanisms of the Paneth cells residing at the base of the crypts, secreting a variety of antibacterial products. One may speculate that SIBO of the CF mouse small intestine is similar to that reported in humans [85, 86], as there is evidence of intestinal inflammation characterized by increased mucosal infiltration of mast cells and neutrophils and a 40-fold increase in luminal bacteria, and treatment of the bacterial overgrowth reduces mucus accumulation. CF patients presenting with refractory or unexplained symptoms merit thorough investigation.

Rectal Prolapse

A feature of CF is rectal prolapse, mainly occurring only in PI patients; however, there have been PS patients observed with prolapsed rectums. Children presenting with recurrent rectal prolapse should be referred for a sweat chloride test to exclude CF.

Celiac Disease and Crohn's Disease in CF

CF was first described as a distinct clinical entity from celiac disease approximately 70 years ago. Reports since then suggest that the prevalence of celiac disease in patients with CF is higher than in the general population; however, definitive studies remain to be done using antibody and HLA testing [87, 88].

The prevalence rate of Crohn's disease in CF patients is seven times higher than in those reported controls by Lloyd Still et al. [88]. Although there have been many cases reported prior to the description of fibrosing colonopathy, some of them may have been due to the complications of high-dose enzyme therapy and should be considered in CF patients presenting with suspicious symptoms and signs.

Nutritional Complications

Malnutrition and lung disease are interrelated [83, 89]. Care for CF involves attention to nutritional status to promote the most favorable outcomes. An experienced dietitian in the field of CF would play an essential role in the care of CF patients and should be an integral part of the team.

Nutritional Intake

As an emphasis on a good nutritional diet regime has been to be associated with improved lung function parameters, thus offering parents and patients with CF more motivation to adhere to prescribed therapies such as enzymes, vitamins, and a balanced, high-energy dietary intake [90]. Such studies from the 1980s changed the face of nutritional management of CF and proved that high-fat and high-energy diets were far superior to the old low-fat diet routines. A diet that is composed of 35–40% of calories from fat is recommended in order to meet the energy demands of those with CF.

Thus, this diet regime given to infants from a neonatal screening program has demonstrated that normal growth can be achieved into adolescence. Recommendations by the North American Cystic Fibrosis Foundation Consensus Committee on Nutrition and European Cystic Fibrosis Society include appropriate evaluation of nutritional status at all ages, and a diet that is age appropriate, with sufficient energy to meet needs for normal growth and weight gain [91, 92].

Feeding guidelines for infants with CF recommend breastmilk as the primary source of nutrition for the first year of life [93]. Breast-feeding has been shown to be protective for the infant with CF. Breast-fed CF infants compared to formula had improved lung function with a reduced occurrence of infections during their first 3 years. Breastmilk can provide the complete nutritional support for infants with CF during for the first 4–6 months. It is proven to be more efficient if supplemental energy is added to fortify a portion of the breastmilk feeds with formula or by fortifying formulas to a more concentrated energy level for those infants on a combination of breastmilk and formula or on formula alone. If breast-feeding is not an option or if supplementation is required, regular cow's milk-based infant formulas can be used [53]. In most cases, there is no need for a predigested formula. In warmer climates, sodium supplementation may often be recommended if reported to have a higher degree of loss in sweat [91]. A total of 2–4 mmol/kg supplementation of milk or solids with table salt to provide per day is recom-

mended; however, due to potential for errors in the accuracy of the measurement of the salt, liquid mineral mix solutions prepared by hospital pharmacies are often advised. Breastmilk or formula intake should be supplemented with complementary solids after the first 4–6 months for increased energy. For the exclusively breast-fed infant, meat may be recommended as the first food due to its increased energy content and more importantly for its iron and zinc content. After age one, whole milk is recommended unless breastmilk is continued.

Toddlers and Children

As the dietary intake and degree of physical activity vary with preschool-age toddlers and children, the addition of calorie-rich food is considered important. Self-feeding skills, habits, and food preferences are established at this stage, therefore. Mealtimes should be a positive experience. School activities may conflict limiting snacks and adherence to enzymes; it is recommended that the health-care providers inform parents of appropriate strategies to support compliance with enzyme therapy.

Older children require higher nutrient due to acceleration of their growth; unfortunately, the progression of lung disease may compromise the nutritional status, as it increases the energy demands, interfering with appetite, and resulting in decreased energy intake. If oral intake is not enough to support expected growth or nutritional status, then a more aggressive nutritional intake via enteral tube feeding may be required and is best presented as a positive approach to help improve quality of life and health. However, a thorough evaluation of the nutritional failure must be completed before this type of support is implemented. The following should be considered and addressed as part of the evaluation: Behavioral and emotional issues, compliance, GERD, cystic fibrosis-related diabetes (CFRD), or distal intestinal obstruction syndrome (DIOS). Enteral tube feeding may provide approximately 30–50% of estimated daily energy requirements with appropriate enzyme therapy, generally delivered as overnight feed. The decision varies from individual patients as to when supplemental enteral nutrition is to be commenced. Some centers use intravenous lipids as an adjunct to enteral nutrition particularly in patients with low serum fatty acid concentration [94]. If total parenteral nutrition is used in non-post-surgical situations, weight gain is usually not sustainable once this support ceases.

The importance of the clinical staff being made aware of the overall nutritional status of their patient population allows for more focus on nutritional support. The sharing of these results with patients and families provides for team work and collaboration opportunities.

Fat-Soluble Vitamins

The neonatal diagnosis via screening programs is well documented. In non-screened populations, overt deficiencies are well described including benign intracranial hypertension [95], night blindness [96], rickets [97], hemolytic anemia [98], and coagulopathy due to vitamin A, D, E, and K deficiencies, respectively. Due to ongoing mild to moderate fat malabsorption, fat-soluble vitamin supplements are required for CF PI patients [99]. The European Guidelines are similar to those of North America, with the exception of a higher recommended vitamin A dose (4000–10,000 IU) and a higher starting dose of vitamin E and vitamin K (100 IU and 1 mg) [95, 100]. This discrepancy is due to the lack of controlled studies that aid in defining lower limits of intake that support normal serum levels. For example, those patients who are PS, who do not require pancreatic enzyme supplementation for normal growth, have normal serum vitamin blood levels, and they do not require vitamin supplementation. There is some evidence that supplementation of fat-soluble vitamins in PS patients may be associated with decreased incidence of pulmonary exacerbations possibly due to the antioxidant effect of these compounds [101]. The North American CF Foundation Committee on vitamin D guidelines [102] advise higher supplemental amounts of vitamin D than in the CF vitamin supplements currently available for individuals with suboptimal serum 25-hydroxyvitmain D levels. Therefore, additional vitamin D supplements are recommended, and the annual monitoring of serum vitamin levels for vitamins A, E, and D. Vitamin K may be difficult to monitor as protein induced by vitamin K deficiency (PIVKA) the test used to assess serum levels is not routinely available. However, obtaining serum PIVKA or at least prothrombin levels are advised for those patients with hemoptysis or hematemesis and in patients with liver disease. More studies are needed in order to establish the minimum requirement of vitamin K [103]. The amount of vitamin K in vitamin supplements marketed to CF patients is unlikely to be sufficient. Toxicity of fat-soluble vitamins is very rare in CF; the one exception is post-lung transplantation (see below).

Bone Health

In CF patients, a decrease in bone mineral density (BMD) may begin in early childhood [104]. The nutritional status, calcium, vitamins D and K, pulmonary infection, exercise, glucocorticoids, and class of CFTR mutation are influencing factors of bone health. Poor BMD is a reflection of bone health [105]. Therefore, monitoring of BMD is recommended during routine visits.

Lung Transplant

Patients with CF may present with added nutritional challenges pre- and post-lung transplant. Pretransplant, energy intake is often affected and most likely to be suboptimal, therefore requiring increased nutritional support via enteral tube feeding support [106]. During pre- and post-lung transplantation, reduced BMD is a concern [107]. Posttransplant, patient's appetite usually improves, are usually capable of taking in sufficient energy orally alone, with less and eventually no dependence on enteral tube-feeding support. Posttransplant, it is recommended to leave the enteral tube in place for a period of about 6 months to avoid insufficient oral intake to meet the energy needs and routinely blood monitor the fat-soluble vitamin levels. After transplantation, hypervitaminosis A has been reported, although the etiology of this novel finding is unclear [108]. It may impact drug interactions, altered absorption, increased hepatic synthesis of retinol binding protein, or impaired retinol metabolism. The prescribed amount of vitamin supplements may need to be altered, as vitamin A levels may be elevated in patients with and without CF. Counseling patients that respond well posttransplant regarding lower energy food options is recommended as patients may experience an increased appetite due to the effects of corticosteroids and decreased rate of growth in children. These patients will benefit from an exercise and rehabilitation plan for lung performance and nutritional status [25].

In conclusion, children with CF may have a wide range of gastroenterological manifestations. Gastroenterologists must be involved to improve the quality of life and outcomes of these patients.

References

1. Rowe SM, Miller S, Sorscher EJ. Cystic fibrosis. N Engl J Med. 2005;352:1992–2001.
2. Zielenski J. Genotype and phenotype in cystic fibrosis. Respiration. 2000;67(2):117–33.
3. Snouwaert JN, Brigman KK, Latour AM, Malouf NN, Boucher RC, Smithies O, Koller BH. An animal model for cystic fibrosis made by gene targeting. Science. 1992;257:1083–8.
4. Clarke LL, Grubb BR, Gabriel SE, Smithies O, Koller BH, Boucher RC. Defective epithelial chloride transport in a gene-targeted mouse model of cystic fibrosis. Science. 1992;257:1125–8.
5. Rogers CS, Stoltz DA, Meyerholz DK, Ostedgaard LS, Rokhlina T, Taft PJ, Rogan MP, Pezzulo AA, Karp PH, Itani OA, Kabel AC, Wohlford-Lane CL, Davis GJ, Hanfland RA, Smith TL, Samuel M, Wax D, Murphy CN, Rieke A, Whitworth K, Uc A, Starner TD, Brogden KA, Shilyansky J, McCray PB, Jr., Zabner J, Prather RS, Welsh MJ. Disruption of the CFTR gene produces a model of cystic fibrosis in newborn pigs. Science. 2008;321:1837–41.
6. Stoltz DA, Meyerholz DK, Pezzulo AA, Ramachandran S, Rogan MP, Davis GJ, Hanfland RA, Wohlford-Lenane C, Dohrn CL, Bartlett JA, Nelson GA, Chang EH, Taft PJ, Ludwig PS, Estin M, Hornick EE, Launspach JL, Samuel M, Rokhlina T, Karp PH, Ost-

edgaard LS, Uc A, Starner TD, Horswill AR, Brogden KA, Prather RS, Richter SS, Shilyansky J, McCray PB Jr, Zabner J, Welsh MJ. Cystic fibrosis pigs develop lung disease and exhibit defective bacterial eradication at birth. Sci Transl Med. 2010;2:29ra31.

7. Ostedgaard LS, Meyerholz DK, Chen JH, Pezzulo AA, Karp PH, Rokhlina T, Ernst SE, Hanfland RA, Reznikov LR, Ludwig PS, Rogan MP, Davis GJ, Dohrn CL, Wohlford-Lenane C, Taft PJ, Rector MV, Hornick E, Nassar BS, Samuel M, Zhang Y, Richter SS, Uc A, Shilyansky J, Prather RS, McCray PB Jr, Zabner J, Welsh MJ, Stoltz DA. The DeltaF508 mutation causes CFTR misprocessing and cystic fibrosis-like disease in pigs. Sci Transl Med. 2011;3:74ra24.

8. Abu-El-Haija M, Ramachandran S, Meyerholz DK, Griffin M, Giriyappa RL, Stoltz DA, Welsh MJ, McCray PB Jr, Uc A. Pancreatic damage in fetal and newborn cystic fibrosis pigs involves the activation of inflammatory and remodeling pathways. Am J Pathol. 2012;181:499–507.

9. Meyerholz DK, Stoltz DA, Pezzulo AA, Welsh MJ. Pathology of gastrointestinal organs in a porcine model of cystic fibrosis. Am J Pathol. 2010;176:1377–89.

10. Uc A, Giriyappa R, Meyerholz DK, Griffin M, Ostedgaard LS, Tang XX, Abu-El-Haija M, Stoltz DA, Ludwig P, Pezzulo A, Taft P, Welsh MJ. Pancreatic and biliary secretion are both altered in cystic fibrosis pigs. Am J Physiol Gastrointest Liver Physiol. 2012;303:G961–8.

11. Sun X, Olivier AK, Liang B, Yi Y, Sui H, Evans TI, Zhang Y, Zhou W, Tyler SR, Fisher JT, Keiser NW, Liu X, Yan Z, Song Y, Goeken JA, Kinyon JM, Fligg D, Wang X, Xie W, Lynch TJ, Kaminsky PM, Stewart ZA, Pope RM, Frana T, Meyerholz DK, Parekh K, Engelhardt JF. Lung phenotype of juvenile and adult cystic fibrosis transmembrane conductance regulator-knockout ferrets. Am J Respir Cell Mol Biol. 2014;50:502–12.

12. Olivier AK, Yi Y, Sun X, Sui H, Liang B, Hu S, Xie W, Fisher JT, Keiser NW, Lei D, Zhou W, Yan Z, Li G, Evans TI, Meyerholz DK, Wang K, Stewart ZA, Norris AW, Engelhardt JF. Abnormal endocrine pancreas function at birth in cystic fibrosis ferrets. J Clin Invest. 2012;122:3755–68.

13. Sun X, Sui H, Fisher JT, Yan Z, Liu X, Cho HJ, Joo NS, Zhang Y, Zhou W, Yi Y, Kinyon JM, Lei-Butters DC, Griffin MA, Naumann P, Luo M, Ascher J, Wang K, Frana T, Wine JJ, Meyerholz DK, Engelhardt JF. Disease phenotype of a ferret CFTR-knockout model of cystic fibrosis. J Clin Invest. 2010;120:3149–60.

14. Stoltz DA, Rokhlina T, Ernst SE, Pezzulo AA, Ostedgaard LS, Karp PH, Samuel MS, Reznikov LR, Rector MV, Gansemer ND, Bouzek DC, Alaiwa MH, Hoegger MJ, Ludwig PS, Taft PJ, Wallen TJ, Wohlford-Lenane C, McMenimen JD, Chen JH, Bogan KL, Adam RJ, Hornick EE, Nelson GAt, Hoffman EA, Chang EH, Zabner J, McCray PB Jr, Prather RS, Meyerholz DK, Welsh MJ. Intestinal CFTR expression alleviates meconium ileus in cystic fibrosis pigs. J Clin Invest. 2013;123:2685–93.

15. Oppenheimer EH, Esterly JR. Pathology of cystic fibrosis review of the literature and comparison with 146 autopsied cases. Perspect Pediatr Pathol. 1975;2:241–78.

16. Andersen DH. Cystic fibrosis of the pancreas and its relation to celiac disease: clinical and pathological study. Am J Dis Child. 1938;56:344–99.

17. Porta EA, Stein AA, Patterson P. Ultrastructural changes of the pancreas and liver in cystic fibrosis. Am J Clin Pathol. 1964;42:451–65.

18. Kopelman H, Durie P, Gaskin K, Weizman Z, Forstner G. Pancreatic fluid secretion and protein hyperconcentration in cystic fibrosis. N Engl J Med. 1985;312:329–34.

19. Freedman SD, Blanco P, Shea JC, Alvarez JG. Mechanisms to explain pancreatic dysfunction in cystic fibrosis. Med Clin North Am. 2000;84:657–64.

20. Durie PR. Pancreatic aspects of cystic fibrosis and other inherited causes of pancreatic dysfunction. Med Clin North Am. 2000;84:609–20, ix.

21. Hadorn B, Zoppi G, Shmerling DH, Prader A, McIntyre I, Anderson CM. Quantitative assessment of exocrine pancreatic function in infants and children. J Pediatr. 1968;73:39–50.

22. Abu-El-Haija M, Sinkora M, Meyerholz DK, Welsh MJ, McCray PB Jr, Butler J, Uc A. An activated immune and inflammatory response targets the pancreas of newborn pigs with cystic fibrosis. Pancreatology. 2011;11:506–15.

23. De Boeck K, Wilschanski M, Castellani C, et al. Cystic fibrosis: terminology and diagnostic algorithms. Thorax. 2006;61:627–35.

24. Farrell PM, Rosenstein BJ, White TB, et al. Guidelines for diagnosis of cystic fibrosis in newborns through older adults: Cystic Fibrosis Foundation consensus report. J Pediatr. 2008;153:S4–14.

25. Stiebellehner L, Quittan M, End A, et al. Aerobic endurance training program improves exercise performance in lung transplant recipients. Chest. 1998;113(4):906–12.

26. Wilschanski M, Famini H, Strauss-Liviatan N, et al. Nasal potential difference measurements in patients with atypical cystic fibrosis. Eur Respir J. 2001;17:1208–15.

27. De Jonge HR, Ballmann M, Veeze H, et al. Ex vivo CF diagnosis by intestinal current measurements (ICM) in small aperture, circulating Ussing chambers. J Cyst Fibros. 2004;3:159–63.

28. Argent BE, Gray MA, Steward MC, Case RM. Cell physiology of pancreatic ducts. In: Johnson LR, editor. Physiology of the gastrointestinal tract. 4th ed. Netherlands: Elsevier. 2006. pp. 1371–96.

29. Quinton PM. Cystic fibrosis: impaired bicarbonate secretion and mucoviscidosis. Quinton PM. Lancet. 2008;372(9636):415–7.

30. Kopelman H, Corey M, Gaskin K, et al. Impaired chloride secretion, as well as bicarbonate secretion, underlies the fluid secretory defect in the cystic fibrosis pancreas. Gastroenterology. 1988;95:349–55.

31. Freedman SD, Kern HF, Scheele GA. Acinar lumen pH regulates endocytosis, but not exocytosis, at the apical plasma membrane of pancreatic acinar cells. Eur J Cell Biol. 1998;75:153–62.

32. Wilschanski M, Durier PR. Patterns of GI disease in adulthood associated with mutations in the CFTR gene. GUT. 2007;56(8):1153–63.

33. Gaskin KJ, Durie PR, Hill RE, et al. Colipase and maximally activated pancreatic lipase in normal subjects and patients with steatorrhea. J Clin Invest. 1982;69:427–34.

34. Choi JY, Muallem D, Kiselyov K, Lee MG, Thomas PJ, Muallem S. Aberrant CFTR- dependant HCO3-transport in mutations associated with cystic fibrosis. Nature. 2001;410:94–7.

35. Kristidis P, Bozon D, Corey M, et al. Genetic determination of exocrine pancreatic function in cystic fibrosis. Am J Hum Genet. 1992;50:1178–84.

36. Durno C, Corey M, Zielenski J, et al. Genotype and phenotype correlations in patients with cystic fibrosis and pancreatitis. Gastroenterology. 2002;123:1857–64.

37. Ooi CY, Dorfman R, Cipolli M, et al Type of CFTR mutation determines risk of pancreatitis in patients with cystic fibrosis. Gastroenterology. 2011;140:153–61.

38. Rosendahl J1, Landt O, Bernadova J, et al. CFTR, SPINK1, CTRC and PRSS1 variants in chronic pancreatitis: is the role of mutated CFTR overestimated? Gut. 2013;62(4):582–92.

39. Borowitz D Update on the evaluation of pancreatic exocrine status in cystic fibrosis. Curr Opin Pulm Med. 2005;11:524–7.

40. Kalnins D, Durie PR, Pencharz P. Nutritional management of cystic fibrosis patients. Curr Opin Clin Nutr Metab Care. 2007;10(3):348–54.

41. Cade A, Walters MP, McGinley N, et al. Evaluation of fecal pancreatic elastase-1 as a measure of pancreatic exocrine function in children with cystic fibrosis. Pediatr Pulmonol. 2000;29(3):172–6.

42. Weintraub A, Blau H, Mussaffi H, et al. Exocrine pancreatic function testing in patients with cystic fibrosis and pancreatic sufficiency: a correlation study. J Ped Gastroenterol Nut. 2009;48:306–10.

43. Walkowiak J, Nousia-Arvanitakis S, Agguridaki C, et al. Longitudinal follow-up of exocrine pancreatic function in pancreatic sufficient cystic fibrosis patients using the fecal elastase-1 test. J Pediatr Gastroenterol Nutr. 2003;36(4):474–8.

44. Wier HA, Kuhn RJ. Pancreatic enzyme supplementation. Curr Opin Pediatr. 2011;23(5):541–4.

45. Giuliano CA, Dehoorne-Smith ML, Kale-Pradhan PB. Pancreatic enzyme products: digesting the changes. Ann Pharmacother. 2011;45(5):658–66.

46. http://www.fda.gov/Drugs/DrugSafety/PostmarketDrugSafetyInformationforPatientsandPhysicians.

47. Graff GR, Maguiness K, McNamara J, et al. Efficacy and tolerability of a new formulation of pancrelipase delayed-release capsules in children aged 7 to 11 years with exocrine pancreatic insufficiency and cystic fibrosis: a multicenter, randomized, double-blind, placebo- controlled, two-period crossover, superiority study. Clin Ther. 2010;32(1):89–103.

48. Graff GR, McNamara J, Royall J, et al. Safety and tolerability of a new formulation of pancrelipase delayed-release capsules (CREON) in children under seven years of age with exocrine pancreatic insufficiency due to cystic fibrosis: an open-label, multicentre, single-treatment-arm study. Clin Drug Investig. 2010;30(6):351–64.

49. Trapnell BC, Maguiness K, Graff GR, et al. Efficacy and safety of Creon 24,000 in subjects with exocrine pancreatic insufficiency due to cystic fibrosis. J Cyst Fibros. 2009;8(6):370–7.

50. Borowitz D, Konstan M, O'Rourke A, et al. Coefficients of fat and nitrogen absorption in healthy subjects and individuals with cystic fibrosis. J Pediatr Pharmacol Therapeut. 2007;12:47–52.

51. Wooldridge JL, Heubi JE, Amaro-Galvez R, et al. EUR-1008 pancreatic enzyme replacement is safe and effective in patients with cystic fibrosis and pancreatic insufficiency. J Cyst Fibros. 2009;8(6):405–17.

52. Borowitz DS, Grand RJ, Durie PR. Use of pancreatic enzyme supplements for patients with cystic fibrosis in the context of fibrosing colonopathy. Consensus committee. J Pediatr. 1995;127(5):681–4.

53. Ellis L, Kalnins D, Corey M, et al. Do infants with cystic fibrosis need a protein hydrolysate formula? A prospective, randomized, comparative study. J Pediatr. 1998;132(2):270–6.

54. Colombo C, Fredella C, Russo MC, et al. Efficacy and tolerability of Creon for Children in infants and toddlers with pancreatic exocrine insufficiency caused by cystic fibrosis: an open-label, single-arm, multicenter study. Pancreas. 2009;38(6):693–9.

55. Kalnins D, Ellis L, Corey M, et al. Enteric-coated pancreatic enzyme with bicarbonate is equal to standard enteric-coated enzyme in treating malabsorption in cystic fibrosis. J Pediatr Gastroenterol Nutr. 2006;42(3):256–61.

56. Brady MS, Garson JL, Krug SK, et al. An enteric-coated high-buffered pancrelipase reduces steatorrhea in patients with cystic fibrosis: a prospective, randomized study. J Am Diet Assoc. 2006;106(8):1181–6.

57. Borowitz D, Stevens C, Brettman LR, et al. International phase III trial of liprotamase efficacy and safety in pancreatic-insufficient cystic fibrosis patients. J Cyst Fibros. 2011;10(6):443–52.

58. Butt AM, Ip W, Ellis L, et al. The fate of exogenous enzymes in patients with cystic fibrosis and pancreatic insufficiency (abstr). J Pediatr Gastroenterol Nutr. 2001;33:391.

59. Bartlett JR, Friedman KJ Ling S et al. Genetic modifyers of modifiers of liver disease in cystic fibrosis. JAMA. 2009;302:1076–83.

60. Wilschanski M, Rivlin J, Cohen S et al. Clinical and genetic risk factors for cystic fibrosis related liver disease. Pediatrics. 1999;103(1):52–7.

61. Debray D, Rainteau D, Barbu V et al. Defects in gallbladder emptying and bile acid homeostasis in mice with cystic fibrosis transmembrane conductance regulator deficiencies. Gastroenterology. 2012;142:1581–91.

62. Colombo C, Battezzati PM, Srazzabosco M, et al. Liver and biliary problems in cystic fibrosis. Semin Liver Dis. 1998;18:227–35.

63. Shapira R, Hadzic R, Francavilla R et al. Retrospective review of cystic fibrosis presenting as infantile liver disease. Arch Dis Child. 1999;81:125–8.

64. Mueller-Abt PR, Frawly KJ, Greer RM, Lewindon PJ. Comparison of ultrasound and iopsy findings in children with cystic fibrosis liver disease. J Cyst Fibros. 2008;7:215–21.

65. Debray D, Kelly D, Houwen R, Strandvik B, Colomco C. Best practice guidance for the diagnosis and management of cystic fibrosis associated liver disease. J Cyst Fibros. 2011;10:S29–36.

66. Lindblad A, Glaumann H, Strandvik B. A two-year prospective study of the effect of ursodeoxycholic acid on urinary bile acid excretion and liver morphology in cystic fibrosis-associated liver disease. Hepatology. 1998;27(1):166–74.

67. Ooi CY, Nightingale S, Durie PR, Freedman SD Ursodeoxycholic acid in cystic fibrosis -associated liver disease. J Cys Fibros. 2012;11:72–3.

68. Milkiewicz P, Skiba G, Kelly D. Transplantation for cystic fibrosis: outcome following early liver transplantation. J Gastroenterol Hepatol. 2002;17(2):208–13.

69. Cipolli M. Castellani C, Wilcken B et al. Pancreatic phenotype in infants with cystic fibrosis identified by mutation screening. Arch Dis Child. 2007;92(10):842–6.

70. Sun L, Rommens JM, Corvol H, et al. Multiple apical plasma membrane constituents are associated with susceptibility to meconium ileus in individuals with cystic fibrosis. Nat Genet. 2012;44(5):562–9.

71. Dorfman R, Li W, Lin F, et al. Modifier gene study of meconium ileus in cystic fibrosis; statistical considerations and gene mapping results. Hum Genet. 2009;126:763–78.

72. Dray X, Bienvenu T, Desmazes-Dufue V, et al. Distal Intestinal obstruction syndrome in adults with cystic fibrosis. Clin Gastroenterol Hep. 2004;2:498–503.

73. Norkina O, Kaur S, Ziemer D, DeLisle RC. Inflammation of the cystic fibrosis mouse small intestine. Am J Physiol Gastrointes Liver Physiol. 2004;286(6):G1032–41.

74. Werlin SL, Benuri-Silbiger I, Kerem E, et al. Evidence of intestinal inflammation in patients with cystic fibrosis. J Pediatr Gastroenterol Nutr. 2010;51:304–8.

75. Shidrawi RG, Murugan N, Westaby D, Gyi K, Hodson ME. Emergency colonoscopy for DIOS in CF patients. Gut. 2002;51:285–6.

76. Colombo C, Ellemunter H, Houwen R, Munck A, Taylor C, Wilschanski M. Guidelines for the diagnosis and management of distal intestinal obstruction syndrome in cystic fibrosis patients. J Cyst Fibros. 2011;10(Suppl 2):S24–8.

77. Robertson MD, Choe KA, Joseph PM. Review of the abdominal manifestations of cystic fibrosis in the adult patient. Radiographics. 2006;26(3):679–90.

78. Wilschanski M, Fisher D, Hadas-Halperin I, et al. Findings on routine abdominal ultrasonography in cystic fibrosis patients. J Pediatr Gastroenterol Nutr. 1999;28(2):182–5.

79. Malfroot A. Dab I New insights on gastro-oesophageal reflux in cystic fibrosis by longitudinal follow up. Arch Dis Child. 1991;66:1339–45.

80. Button BM, Roberts S, Kotsimbos TC, et al. Gastroesophageal reflux (symptomatic and silent): a potentially significant problem in patients with cystic fibrosis before and after lung transplantation. J Heart Lung Transplant. 2005;24(10):1522–9.

81. Corey M, McLaughlin FJ, Williams M, et al. A comparison of survival, growth, and pulmonary function in patients with cystic fibrosis in Boston and Toronto. J Clin Epidemiol. 1988;41(6):583–91.

82. Smythe RL van Velzen D, Smyth AR, et al. Strictures of ascending colon in cystic fibrosis and high strength pancreatic enzymes. Lancet. 1994;343:85–6.

83. Roberts DM, Craft JC, Mather FJ, et al. Prevalence of giardiasis in patients with cystic fibrosis. J Pediatr. 1988;112:555–9.

84. Lewindon PJ, Robb TA, Moore DJ, et al. Bowel dysfunction in cystic fibrosis: importance of breath testing. J Paediatr Child Health. 1998;34:79–82.

85. Lloyd-Still J. Crohn's disease and cystic fibrosis. Dig Dis Sci. 1994;39:880–5.

86. DeLisle RC, Roach EA, Norkina O. Eradication of small intestinal bacterial overgrowth in the cystic fibrosis mouse reduces mucus accumulation. J Pediatr Gastroenterol Nutr. 2006;42:46–52.

87. Valletta EA, Mastella G. Incidence of celiac disease in a cystic fibrosis population. Acta Paed Scand. 1989;78:784–5.

88. Cohen-Cymberknoh M, Wilschanski M. Concomitant cystic fibrosis and coeliac disease: reminder of an important clinical lesson. BMJ Case Rep. 2009;2009:bcr07.2008.0578. Epub 2009 Mar 5.

89. Kerem E, Reisman J, Corey M, et al. Prediction of mortality in patients with cystic fibrosis. N Engl J Med. 1992;326(18):1187–91.

90. Stallings VA, Stark LJ, Robinson KA, et al. Evidence-based practice recommendations for nutrition-related management of children and adults with cystic fibrosis and pancreatic insufficiency: results of a systematic review. J Am Diet Assoc. 2008;108(5):832–9.

91. Borowitz D, Baker RD, Stallings V. Consensus report on nutrition for pediatric patients with cystic fibrosis. J Pediatr Gastroenterol Nutr. 2002;35(3):246–59.

92. Sinaasappel M, Stern M, Littlewood J, et al. Nutrition in patients with cystic fibrosis: a European Consensus. J Cyst Fibros. 2002;1(2):51–75.

93. Borowitz D, Robinson KA, Rosenfeld M, et al. Cystic Fibrosis Foundation evidence-based guidelines for management of infants with cystic fibrosis. J Pediatr. 2009;155(6 Suppl):S73–93.

94. Maqbool A, Schall JI, Gallagher PR, Zemel BS, Strandvik B, Stallings VA. The relationship between type of dietary fat intake and serum fatty acid status in children with cystic fibrosis. J Pediatr Gastroenterol Nutr. 2012;55(5):605–11.

95. Abernathy RS. Bulging fontanelle as presenting sign in cystic fibrosis. Arch Dis Child. 1976;130:1360–2.

96. Rayner RJ, Tyrell JC, Hiller EJ, et al. Night blindness and conjunctival xerosis due to vitamin A deficiency in cystic fibrosis. Arch Dis Child. 1989;64:1151–6.

97. Hubbard VS, Farrell PM, di Sant'Agnese PA. 25-Hydroxycholecalciferol levels in patients with cystic fibrosis. J Pediatr. 1979;94:84–6.

98. Bines AE, Israel EJ. Hypoproteinemia, anemia and failure to thrive in an infant. Gastroenterology. 1991;101:848–56.

99. Sokol RJ, Reardon MC, Accurso FJ, et al. Fat-soluble vitamin status during the first year of life in infants with cystic fibrosis. Am J Clin Nut. 1989;50:1064–71.

100. Waters DL, Wilcken B, Irwig L, et al. Clinical outcomes from a newborn screening program cystic fibrosis. Arch Dis Child. 1999;80:F1–7.

101. Hakim F, Kerem E, Rivlin J, et al. Vitamins A and E and pulmonary exacerbations in patients with cystic fibrosis. J Pediatr Gastroenterol Nutr. 2007;45(3):347–53.

102. V. Tangpricha, A. Kelly, A. Stephenson, et al. An update on the screening, diagnosis, management, and treatment of vitamin D deficiency in individuals with cystic fibrosis: evidence-based recommendations from the Cystic Fibrosis Foundation. J Clin Endo Metab. 2012; 97:1082–93.

103. Wilson DC, Rashid M, Durie PR, et al. Treatment of vitamin K deficiency in cystic fibrosis: effectiveness of a daily fat-soluble vitamin combination. J Pediatr. 2001;138(6):851–5.

104. Bianchi ML, Romano G, Saraifoger S, et al. BMD and body composition in children and young patients affected by cystic fibrosis. J Bone Miner Res. 2006;21(3):388–96.

105. Aris RM, Merkel PA, Bachrach LK, et al. Guide to bone health and disease in cystic fibrosis. J Clin Endocrinol Metab. 2005;90(3):1888–96.

106. Schwebel C, Pin I, Barnoud D, et al. Prevalence and consequences of nutritional depletion in lung transplant candidates. Eur Respir J. 2000;16(6):1050–5.

107. Aris RM, Neuringer IP, Weiner MA, et al. Severe osteoporosis before and after lung transplantation. Chest. 1996;109(5):1176–83.

108. Ho T, Gupta S, Brotherwood M, et al. Increased serum vitamin a and e levels after lung transplantation. Transplantation. 2011;92(5):601–6.

Small Intestinal Bacterial Overgrowth

42

Jon A. Vanderhoof and Rosemary Pauley-Hunter

Introduction

The adult human body typically contains at least ten times more microbial cells than human cells because of the high density of microorganisms found in the gastrointestinal (GI) tract [1, 2]. The recent availability of culture-independent molecular methods has significantly changed our understanding of the composition of this GI microbiome. There is tremendous diversity of specific microbial species exceeding 1000 phylotypes, although the fecal microbiome of each individual harbors only about 160 different species. This ecosystem offers protection against pathogens, helps with nutrient processing, and plays a role in many other processes.

The composition of the microbiota differs between different parts of the GI tract. In the stomach and duodenum, there are 10^1–10^3 bacteria per gram of liquid with a steady increase to 10^{11}–10^{12} bacteria per gram of liquid in the colon. The human digestive process has evolved to give the body first priority at the dietary substrates, before the microorganisms. Digestive enzymes from the mouth, stomach acidification, and pancreatic enzymes provide the degradation of the food components for absorption through the small intestine, but most of it occurs in the proximal portion. The microbiota of the small intestine can contribute to the amino acid requirements of the body if they are not provided in the diet itself; however, the microbial biomass in the upper small intestine is so low that it is often not of consequence [3]. Various undigested food components such as fiber, resistant starch, and some lipids are often passed through the small

intestine into the large intestine where they are consumed by microorganisms. It is in the large intestine where the vast majority of our gut flora resides.

During and immediately after parturition, microbes from the mother and surrounding environment colonize the GI tract of the infant. Immediately after vaginal delivery, the microbial populations in the baby closely resemble that of the mother's GI tract, as the vagina normally harbors many of these same organisms [4]. Subsequently, bacteria from other environmental sources including ingested human milk may influence the development of the infant's microbiome. This composition remains relatively constant until shortly before weaning [5]. After weaning, the type and numbers of intestinal flora are greatly influenced by the method and composition of feeding [6]. Early colonization of the infant bowel generally includes lactobacilli and streptococci with successive colonization by anaerobic bacteria, mainly bifidobacteria, bacteroides, clostridia, and eubacteria [7].

There is substantial conflict in the literature regarding the composition of this microenvironment early in life. Some data suggest that breast-fed infants have a much higher composition of bifidobacteria than infants fed with cow milk-based formula; however, the data here are inconsistent. The bulk of available data suggest that biologic mothers are capable of transmitting an initial fecal inoculum of microbiome to their infants during and after birth, but common environmental exposures also shape gut microbiological ecology significantly during subsequent months [8, 9]. After weaning, environmental influences such as cultural/regional variations in diet influence the makeup of the intestinal flora. Differences in fecal microbiota between rural African children who consume high-fiber diets and European children have been identified by DNA sequencing and fecal analysis [10]. 16S ribosomal ribonucleic acid (rRNA) gene sequencing of DNA extracted from duodenal biopsies have also demonstrated differences in intestinal flora in the upper GI tract between children with celiac disease and normal children [11].

In healthy infants, the composition is thought to be relatively unstable until 2–3 years of age at which time it begins

J. A. Vanderhoof (✉)
Department of Pediatrics, Boston Children's Hospital, Harvard Medical School, 300 Longwood Avenue, Boston, MA 02115, USA
e-mail: jon.vanderhoof@childrens.harvard.edu

Boys Town National Research Hospital, 1080 Hospital Road, Boys Town, NE 68010, USA

R. Pauley-Hunter
Department of Pediatric Gastroenterology, Boys Town National Research Hospital, Boys Town, NE, USA

© Springer International Publishing Switzerland 2016
S. Guandalini et al. (eds.), *Textbook of Pediatric Gastroenterology, Hepatology and Nutrition*,
DOI 10.1007/978-3-319-17169-2_42

to resemble that of the adult [9, 12] with virtually no coliform bacteria present in the small intestine. Gram-positive bacteria predominate with rare anaerobes present in the upper GI tract. Typical gram-positive bacteria such as *Streptococcus, Lactobacillus, Prevotella, Neisseria,* and *Enterococcus* are often identified by typical culture methods in the stomach and duodenum. In the distal ileum, there is an increase in the numbers of overall bacteria, with a predominance of enterococci and lactobacilli being present in higher numbers than in the jejunum [13]. Once past the ileocecal valve, anaerobic bacteria predominate with Firmicutes including lactobacillus, bacteroidetes, and ac-

tinobacteria including bifidobacteria numbering from 10^{11} to 10^{12} per gram of intestinal liquid. See Fig. 42.1.

Definition

Quantifiable definitions of small bowel bacterial overgrowth (SBBO) have been proposed with the definition being based on increased numbers of bacteria in addition to specific types of bacteria, generally coliform bacteria. Proposed numbers of bacteria range from greater than 10^3–10^5 colony-forming

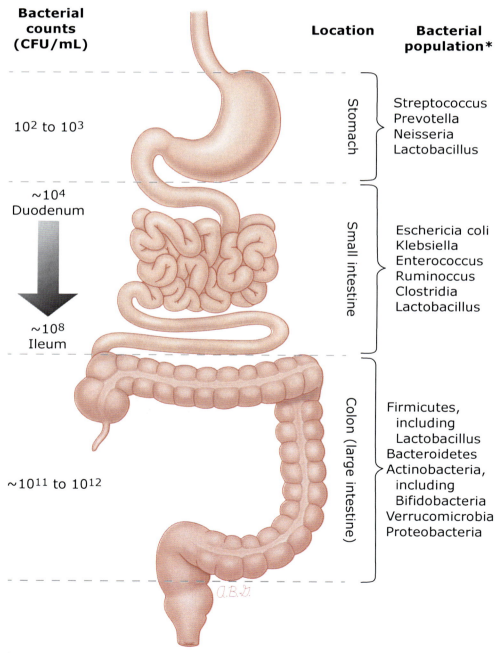

Fig. 42.1 Normal intestinal flora. *CFU* colony-forming unit. (Adapted with permission from Ref. [14]

Bacterial counts (CFU/mL)

Location

Bacterial population*

10^2 to 10^3

Stomach

Streptococcus
Prevotella
Neisseria
Lactobacillus

~10^4
Duodenum

~10^8
Ileum

Small intestine

Eschericia coli
Klebsiella
Enterococcus
Ruminoccus
Clostridia
Lactobacillus

~10^{11} to 10^{12}

Colon (large intestine)

Firmicutes,
including
Lactobacillus
Bacteroidetes
Actinobacteria,
including
Bifidobacteria
Verrucomicrobia
Proteobacteria

* Bacteria are not listed in quantitative order.

units of bacteria per milliliter of luminal fluid of colonic-type bacteria present in the proximal bowel. There are however many GI conditions and symptoms which have been reported at lower levels of bacteria [15, 16]. Previous culture techniques have not identified the true diversity of the intestinal contents that are now being discovered with current molecular DNA processes. Therefore, basing the definition on types of bacteria may not be completely accurate. In a more pathophysiological view, a definition of bacterial overgrowth should include not only the numbers and types of microorganisms present but also evidence that these two factors create pathological signs or symptoms.

Prevalence and Associated Conditions

The true prevalence of bacterial overgrowth is not known due to the lack of a uniform definition and imprecise diagnostic testing. Studies in the general population are lacking, and in those GI symptoms the likelihood is that prevalence would be overestimated if based on noninvasive methods such as breath testing. Estimates have ranged from 0 to 20 % of the general population who have SBBO when based on the actual numbers of bacteria [17]. SBBO may exist with greater prevalence in certain acquired conditions, for example, it occurs with intestinal dilatation in patients with short bowel syndrome (SBS) . The prevalence of bacterial overgrowth due to unusual intestinal colonization during the first year of life, however, is likely much lower.

Other factors predisposing to SBBO include achlorhydria and old age. Drug-induced hypochlorhydria may result in higher bacterial duodenal counts, especially in the elderly following long-term use [18]. In both adults and children, acid suppression may contribute to the presence of bacterial overgrowth [19–21] although this finding is not consistently seen and may be dependent upon the diagnostic method [22]. It has been estimated that proton pump inhibitors can increase the gastric pH to the point of significantly increasing the colonization of the stomach with gram-positive bacteria and potentially increasing colonization with *Helicobacter pylori* if present [23]. Diabetics more commonly have overgrowth, especially in adulthood [24]. Chronically immunosuppressed patients or patients with HIV may also have an increased incidence of SBBO [25]. Bacterial overgrowth has been reported in children with immunoglobulin A (IgA) deficiency [16, 26]. Patients with small bowel inflammatory diseases such as celiac disease may also have elevated bacterial counts as may patients with pancreatic insufficiency [27, 28]. Autoimmune diseases including scleroderma and rheumatoid arthritis have been associated with increased overgrowth [29].

A primary association with SBBO is a failure of small-bowel clearance due to various motility disorders. Patients

Table 42.1 Conditions associated with bacterial overgrowth

Surgical
Short bowel syndrome
Truncal vagotomy
Gastrectomy
Roux-en-Y
Luminal gastrointestinal and related organ diseases
Celiac disease
Crohn's disease/ulcerative colitis
Radiation enteritis
Pancreatitis
Liver/renal failure
Irritable bowel syndrome
Atrophic gastritis
Neuromuscular
Diabetes mellitus
Connective tissue diseases
Parkinson's disease
Pseudo-obstruction
Miscellaneous
Chronic fatigue syndrome
Medications such as proton pump inhibitors or tricyclic antidepressants
Rosacea
Chronic immunodeficiency states
Obesity
Rheumatoid arthritis

with pseudo-obstruction syndrome, muscular dystrophy, diabetic neuropathy, and other disorders affecting gut motility typically experience symptoms due to increased small bowel bacterial counts particularly with coliform bacteria [15, 24]. Likewise, stricture formation with chronic dilatation is usually associated with overgrowth. This may be seen in Crohn's disease, radiation enteritis, or children with congenital anomalies such as intestinal atresia who have postoperative strictures with some degree of dysmotility [30, 31].

Patients with SBS are characteristically troubled with bacterial overgrowth in the small intestine. Here, the reasons are multifactorial. Patients with SBS often have compensatory dilatation of the small intestine with poor motility. As peristalsis normally rids the small bowel of excessive bacteria, small-bowel dilatation with its associated impairment of normal antegrade peristalsis is a perfect setup for overgrowth. The presence of postoperative strictures may also play a role. Finally, the absence of the ileocecal valve, which functions to prevent reflux of colonic bacteria into the small intestine, further exacerbates the problem. Because of poor gastric emptying and reflux, patients with SBS are also frequently on chronic acid suppression which in many situations promote overgrowth [19, 32]. Table 42.1 lists commonly associated conditions which have been attributed to bacterial overgrowth.

Table 42.2 Symptoms of bacterial overgrowth

Acute	Chronic
Bloating	Vitamin A deficiency: xerophthalmia, night blindness, xerosis of the conjunctiva manifested as Bitot's spots, and follicular hyperkeratosis
Flatulence	Diarrhea → Steatorrhea
Abdominal pain	B12 deficiency: neuropathy with paresthesias and central ataxia
Anorexia	Hypocalcemia with perioral numbness, paresthesias of the hands and feet, and muscle cramps
Vitamin D deficiency → metabolic bone disease	Rosacea
Failure to thrive	Edema due to protein-losing enteropathy

Physiology and Pathophysiology

In the stomach, gastric acidity and normal emptying tend to limit microbial growth. Once in the duodenum, the bile salts provide an unfavorable environment for microorganism proliferation. A prominent gut immunoglobulin, IgA typically can recognize and bind with microbes preventing mucosal penetration, it enhances clearance via peristalsis [33] and may have a more specific role in managing the overall amount and types of microbes in the upper small intestine [34]. The body's natural production of antimicrobial compounds such as defensins has varying abilities to limit or alter the intestinal milieu. The large intestine has a much more favorable environment for microorganisms due to its higher pH, lower level of bile salts, and slower peristalsis. The substantially higher numbers of microbes in the large intestine provide short-chain fatty acids through the fermentation of any dietary components that are not utilized in the small intestine. These short-chain fatty acids, particularly butyrate, provide the primary fuel for the enterocytes in the large intestine. There are small numbers of protozoans and fungi also present in the large intestine [34]. Predominant bacterial populations also act as hosts to a variety of viruses which have an unidentified role in intestinal function [35].

Signs and Symptoms

The clinical manifestations of bacterial overgrowth are quite variable because validated symptom questionnaires do not exist. Symptoms range from very mild to severe. Most commonly, patients experience diarrhea, bloating, and abdominal pain as predominate features. Recently, it has been hypothesized that bacterial overgrowth may mimic the symptoms of irritable bowel syndrome [36, 37]. In these instances, abdominal distention, increased flatus, diarrhea, and even fecal urgency have responded to antibiotic therapy [38–40]. More severe symptoms consistent with malabsorption syndrome, such as weight loss, dehydration, and nutrient deficiencies, have also been reported. See Table 42.2.

Small-bowel bacterial overgrowth is associated with a combination of megaloblastic anemia due to vitamin B12 deficiency and fat-soluble vitamin deficiency due to fat malabsorption [15, 41]. Anaerobic bacteria use vitamin B12 to produce inactive compounds which may compete with vitamin B12 for ileal binding sites, decreasing absorption of the vitamin. Other vitamin deficiencies including thiamine have also been associated with SBBO [42]. Fat-soluble vitamin deficiencies including vitamins A, E, and D are commonly reported. These deficiencies are manifested in night blindness and osteopenia or osteoporosis as evidenced by decreased bone mineral density exist [43, 44]. Vitamin K deficiency is infrequent because of increased luminal production of vitamin K by bacteria. Deconjugation of bile salts by increased intestinal bacteria impairs bile acid reabsorption depleting the bile acid pool and decreasing the intraluminal conjugated bile acids further exacerbating fat and fat-soluble vitamin malabsorption. Bile acids are typically absorbed in the jejunum; however, if they reach that ileum and colon, they may also damage the intestinal mucosa leading to increased diarrhea and malabsorption [45].

Intestinal bacteria may deaminate dietary protein that is malabsorbed and create a situation in which dietary nitrogen is converted to urea and is unavailable for absorption [46]. Low levels of enterokinase may impair activation of pancreatic proteases and thereby reduce protein absorption [47]. Carbohydrate degradation by intestinal bacteria also increases malabsorption, and these malabsorbed carbohydrate by-products significantly contribute to the symptomatology of bloating, cramps, and diarrhea [48]. Neurological symptoms including central or peripheral neuropathy and symptoms of anemia including fatigue may predominate the clinical picture. There is some evidence to suggest that SBBO may be a contributory factor in nonalcoholic steatohepatitis (NASH) [49]. Endogenous ethanol production has also been reported with bacterial overgrowth in association with overgrowth of *Candida albicans* and *Saccharomyces cerevisiae* [50].

In children, abdominal pain, bloating, and diarrhea are more typical symptoms, especially when an underlying disorder is present. Anemia and evidence of gut inflammation including occult-blood-positive stools, and elevated fecal calprotectin levels may be seen in both adults and children

[51, 52]. Systemic inflammatory changes including arthritis may occur. Poor weight gain and decreased appetite are not uncommon. In children, D-lactic acidosis may be a clinical presentation of SBBO [53]. Patients with this disorder develop higher levels of the lactate in the blood because some bacteria produce both D and L stereoisomers of lactate, but only the L form is metabolized well by the human liver. D-lactate accumulates in the blood stream resulting in a variety of neurological symptoms varying from poor school performance to coma. Elevated levels of serum D-lactate and rapid response to oral antibiotic therapy confirm the diagnosis. This disorder appears to be quite uncommon in adults.

Histologically, overgrowth is not uncommonly associated with inflammatory changes in the mucosa [54]. Consequently, reduced brush border disaccharidase levels may result in carbohydrate malabsorption, especially lactose malabsorption. Impaired protein absorption and protein-losing enteropathy may also result. A number of changes in the mucosa have been demonstrated not only by light microscopy but also by electron microscopy, which have identified numerous enterocyte abnormalities including microvillus injury [55].

Diagnosis

The diagnosis of SBBO should be considered in patients with any of the symptoms and findings discussed above particularly when associated with an underlying disease process predisposing the patient to overgrowth. Small-bowel imaging may be helpful in the diagnosis of bacterial overgrowth by identifying areas of bowel dilatation and/or stricture formation which may be the causative factors. This is particularly indicated in conditions where there is a history of intestinal resection.

Aspiration of small intestinal fluid contents for quantitative culture was previously considered the gold standard for diagnosis [17, 56]. Normal values may vary significantly based upon the anatomic location of small bowel aspirate as well as the geographic location of the patient. Tropical patients may have normal values as high as 10^7 microorganisms per milliliter of fluid, whereas 10^4 may be normal in more temperate regions. Even within the same GI disease, such as ulcerative colitis, the intestinal bacteria differ depending on the geographic location of the patient [57].

Aspiration of duodenal versus jejunal fluid will result in different types and species of bacteria. Aspirates from above and below a stricture may also differ. Care must be taken to avoid contamination of the sample with oropharyngeal bacteria, and a number of different techniques have been described [58]. Likewise, appropriate handling of the specimen is very important. Culture of anaerobic bacteria is challenging. Prior to collecting the sample, it is a good idea to have a discussion with the culturing laboratory to make sure the specimen is handled appropriately. Regardless of the culturing techniques, it is estimated that a great majority of the intestinal microbiota is missed as compared with genomic or DNA sequence-based methods [34].

Significant inflammatory changes may be seen both endoscopically and histologically in patients with severe overgrowth. Occasionally, such changes may be difficult to differentiate from Crohn's disease unless granulomas are present. A typical example of such changes is pouchitis seen after resection for ulcerative colitis. Diffuse nonspecific inflammatory changes occasionally with ulceration can be visualized. Patients with SBS and significant bowel dilatation with poor motility will commonly have similar findings when overgrowth is present. Unfortunately, the chronic inflammatory changes seen histologically are nonspecific, and their use for diagnostic purposes must be considered in clinical context and with other associated laboratory findings.

A number of tests have been devised to predict SBBO noninvasively. Perhaps the most widely used due to the ease and lack of expense is breath hydrogen testing using either glucose of lactulose. These tests are based on the premise that small-bowel bacteria will metabolize the ingested carbohydrate into carbon dioxide and hydrogen or methane gas. Glucose is rapidly and completely absorbed in the small intestine; therefore, an early rise fasting breath hydrogen levels of more than 20 ppm above baseline following an oral load of glucose is considered consistent with the diagnosis of bacterial overgrowth [17, 56]. Glucose is an ideal substrate because it is rapidly absorbed in the small bowel and consequently is not subject to bacterial metabolism in the colon. It is less predictive of ileal bacterial overgrowth for this reason, and likewise can be falsely elevated in patients with SBS who have an extremely short bowel or rapid transit. Patients with chronic overgrowth may have elevated fasting breath hydrogen levels. Lactulose is primarily metabolized in the colon, typically 90 min after ingestion; however, in bacterial overgrowth, there will be an early peak of hydrogen production followed by a later peak when it reaches the colon.

If overgrowth is not associated with large numbers of hydrogen-producing organisms, the breath hydrogen test may not be valid. ^{14}C-xylose- and ^{13}C-xylose-labeled breath tests have also been utilized but are less commonly available. It has been estimated that approximately 10–20 % of humans do not have detectable hydrogen production from their GI flora. Some bacteria such as enterococci, *Staphylococcus aureus,* and *Pseudomonas* do not produce hydrogen when metabolized but do produce methane gas [59]. A combination of breath hydrogen and breath methane testing may offer considerable improvement in the diagnosis of bacterial overgrowth [60].

Other screening tests such as serum D-lactate levels may occasionally be helpful if they are elevated. However, care must be taken to make certain that the blood test is ordered correctly and the laboratory knows exactly what is desired, that is, doing a D-lactate level and not a lactic acid. Urine indican is an indicator of the intestinal overgrowth of anaerobic bacteria. Indican is an indole produced when bacteria in the intestine act on tryptophan. Most indoles are excreted in the feces. The remainder are absorbed, metabolized by the liver, and excreted in the urine. Consequently, excessive bacterial activity on protein in the small bowel will result in excessive indican excretion in the urine.

An empiric trial of antibiotics in patients with symptoms suggestive of bacterial overgrowth may be used diagnostically. Measurement of symptom response of course is hindered by a lack of a validated assessment tool as previously mentioned. However, given the lack of standardized diagnostic testing, short courses of broad-spectrum antibiotics may be the simplest and least expensive method to establish a diagnosis. Future diagnostic testing may include metabolic profiling of the metabolome, the use of electronic nose, and/or field asymmetric ion mobility spectrometry which detects volatile organic compounds from intestinal gases [17].

Treatment

If there is an identifiable structural or functional condition amenable to surgical treatment, then that should be corrected as the first option. Procedures to correct strictures or areas of small bowel dilatation are usually amenable to either endoscopic or surgical revision. Serial transverse tapering enteroplasty is a procedure which lengthens the dilated bowel by stapling it in a zigzag pattern and is particularly efficacious in children whose intestine dilates in the process of adaptation after a major resection [61, 62]. This procedure may add additional more functional intestinal surface as well. Motility disorders may be amenable to therapy with pro-motility agent such as an erythromycin, metoclopramide, cisapride, or domperidone.

Medical treatment of SBBO typically starts with antibiotic therapy [63]. A variety of strategies may be employed. Accurately obtained cultures may reveal a dominant organism and specific sensitivities may be helpful. However, due to the limitations of qualitative and quantitative sampling, empiric trials are typically used to direct therapy. Antibiotic choice generally involves therapy directed at both aerobic and anaerobic organisms. There is no agreement on a standard dosage or duration of treatment. Antibiotics may be given the first 5–7 days of each month, continued for 1 week every other week, or given continuously and rotated depending upon the clinical situation. It is important to remember that the intention is not to sterilize the gut, but simply reduce the enteric population enough to alleviate the symptoms and clear up any inflammatory process. Antibiotic therapy should be individualized and consideration should be given to the high prevalence of the development of bacterial resistance,

Table 42.3 Antibiotic protocols for bacterial overgrowth

Drug	Dose	Considerations
Rifaximin [62]	Adults 1650 mg/day Children 600 mg/day	Nonabsorbable High cost
Amoxicillin–clavulanate [63]	30 mg/kg/day	
Metronidazole [64]	20 mg/kg/day	Peripheral neuropathy
Metronidazole [65–67] a. Cephalosporin or cephalexin or b. Trimethoprim–sulfa-methoxazole or c. Gentamicin (orally)	20 mg/kg/day + 30 mg/kg/day or 10–12 mg/kg/day or 10 mg/kg/day	Need to check random blood gentamicin levels
Norfloxacin [63]	Adults 800 mg/day	
Ciprofloxacin [68, 69]	Adults 35–50 mg/kg/day	

the cost of treatment, and potential side effects from long-term usage. A list of antibiotics is shown in the Table 42.3.

When antibiotics fail, a number of strategies can be employed. The first and perhaps most useful is to reduce the carbohydrate intake in the diet [67]. Carbohydrates facilitate SBBO, and replacing them with fat may reduce bacterial populations enough to alleviate the symptoms in many patients. Abdominal bloating and distention may be decreased by removing nonabsorbable sugars, such as sorbitol, and reducing lactose intake may also be helpful. Probiotic therapy has been proposed as one potential treatment option for bacterial overgrowth [17, 70]. A few small pilot studies have demonstrated some suggested benefit; however, there is a lack of a double-blind, randomized, placebo-controlled trials in this setting. Nondigestible fibers, prebiotics, and probiotics may in fact exacerbate SBBO due to their propensity to contribute to gas and bloating.

Medications which delay transit or reduced gut motility such as loperamide may also exacerbate overgrowth and should be discontinued. Acid suppression should be utilized only in cases of medical necessity [71]. In cases of significant inflammation in the mucosa which may occur secondary to bacterial overgrowth, and when initial treatments with antibiotics or diet have not been successful, a trial of anti-inflammatory medications might be considered [67]. 5-aminosalicylate (5-ASA) preparations are usually tried first but if these are unsuccessful, a 2-week trial of corticosteroid therapy may be beneficial [68].

Summary

Small intestinal bacterial overgrowth may result from functional or anatomical alterations in the GI tract. The definition should incorporate both a combination of quantitative measures of the type and number of bacteria in the presence of symptoms directly attributable to the overgrowth. Current diagnostic techniques have rather poor sensitivity and questionable specificity. As the study of the human intestinal microbiota is advancing, the ability to accurately identify microorganisms and their role in small intestinal function should become clearer. Further studies are needed with better defined end points to more clearly determine ideal treatments for SBBO.

References

1. Johnson CL, Versalovic J. The human microbiome and its potential importance to pediatrics. Pediatrics. 2012;129:950–60.
2. Tappenden KA, Deutsch AS. The physiological relevance of the intestinal microbiota–contributions to human health. J Am Coll Nutr. 2007;26:679S–83S.
3. Raj T, Dileep U, Vaz M, Fuller MF, Kurpad AV. Intestinal microbial contribution to metabolic leucine input in adult men. J Nutr. 2008;138:2217–21.
4. Dominguez-Bello MG, Costello EK, Contreras M, Magris M, Hidalgo G, Fierer N, et al. Delivery mode shapes the acquisition and structure of the initial microbiota across multiple body habitats in newborns. Proc Natl Acad Sci U S A. 2010;107:11971–5.
5. Collado MC, Cernada M, Bauerl C, Vento M, Perez-Martinez G. Microbial ecology and host-microbiota interactions during early life stages. Gut Microbes. 2012;3:352–65.
6. Cabrera-Rubio R, Collado MC, Laitinen K, Salminen S, Isolauri E, Mira A. The human milk microbiome changes over lactation and is shaped by maternal weight and mode of delivery. Am J Clin Nutr. 2012;96:544–551.
7. Koenig JE, Spor A, Scalfone N, Fricker AD, Stombaugh J, Knight R, et al. Succession of microbial consortia in the developing infant gut microbiome. Proc Natl Acad Sci U S A. 2011;108(Suppl 1):4578–85.
8. Vael C, Desager K. The importance of the development of the intestinal microbiota in infancy. Curr Opin Pediatr. 2009;21:794–800.
9. Yatsunenko T, Rey FE, Manary MJ, Trehan I, Dominguez-Bello MG, Contreras M, et al. Human gut microbiome viewed across age and geography. Nature. 2012;486:222–7.
10. de Filippo C, Cavalieri D, Di PM, Ramazzotti M, Poullet JB, Massart S, et al. Impact of diet in shaping gut microbiota revealed by a comparative study in children from Europe and rural Africa. Proc Natl Acad Sci U S A. 2010;107:14691–6.
11. Nistal E, Caminero A, Herran AR, Arias L, Vivas S, de Morales JM, et al. Differences of small intestinal bacteria populations in adults and children with/without celiac disease: effect of age, gluten diet, and disease. Inflamm Bowel Dis. 2012;18:649–56.
12. Azad MB, Kozyrskyj AL. Perinatal programming of asthma: the role of gut microbiota. Clin Dev Immunol. 2012;2012:932072.
13. Camp JG, Kanther M, Semova I, Rawls JF. Patterns and scales in gastrointestinal microbial ecology. Gastroenterology. 2002;136:1989–2002.
14. Vanderhoof JA, Pauley-Hunter RJ. Clinical manifestations and diagnosis of small bacterial overgrowth. In: UpToDate, Basow DS, UpToDate, Waltham, MA, editors. Copyright 2013 UpToDate, Inc. For more information visit www.uptodate.com. Accessed Jan 2014.
15. Bohm M, Siwiec RM, Wo JM. Diagnosis and management of small intestinal bacterial overgrowth. Nutr Clin Pract. 2013;28:289–99.
16. Riordan SM, McIver CJ, Wakefield D, Duncombe VM, Thomas MC, Bolin TD. Small intestinal mucosal immunity and morphom-
etry in luminal overgrowth of indigenous gut flora. Am J Gastroenterol. 2001;96:494–500.
17. Grace E, Shaw C, Whelan K, Andreyev HJ. Review article: small intestinal bacterial overgrowth–prevalence, clinical features, current and developing diagnostic tests, and treatment. Aliment Pharmacol Ther. 2013;38:674–88.
18. Britton E, McLaughlin JT. Ageing and the gut. Proc Nutr Soc. 2013;72:173–7.
19. Hegar B, Hutapea EI, Advani N, Vandenplas Y. A double-blind placebo-controlled randomized trial on probiotics in small bowel bacterial overgrowth in children treated with omeprazole. J Pediatr (Rio J). 2013;89:381–7.
20. Jacobs C, Coss AE, Attaluri A, Valestin J, Rao SS. Dysmotility and proton pump inhibitor use are independent risk factors for small intestinal bacterial and/or fungal overgrowth. Aliment Pharmacol Ther. 2013;37:1103–11.
21. Lo WK, Chan WW. Proton pump inhibitor use and the risk of small intestinal bacterial overgrowth: a meta-analysis. Clin Gastroenterol Hepatol. 2013;11:483–90.
22. Ratuapli SK, Ellington TG, O'Neill MT, Umar SB, Harris LA, Foxx-Orenstein AE, et al. Proton pump inhibitor therapy use does not predispose to small intestinal bacterial overgrowth. Am J Gastroenterol. 2012;107:730–5.
23. Fried M, Siegrist H, Frei R, Froehlich F, Duroux P, Thorens J, et al. Duodenal bacterial overgrowth during treatment in outpatients with omeprazole. Gut. 1994;35:23–6.
24. Ojetti V, Pitocco D, Scarpellini E, Zaccardi F, Scaldaferri F, Gigante G, et al. Small bowel bacterial overgrowth and type 1 diabetes. Eur Rev Med Pharmacol Sci. 2009;13:419–23.
25. Chave JP, Thorens J, Frohlich F, Gonvers JJ, Glauser MP, Bille J, et al. Gastric and duodenal bacterial colonization in HIV-infected patients without gastrointestinal symptoms. Am J Gastroenterol. 1994;89:2168–71.
26. Bollinger RR, Everett ML, Palestrant D, Love SD, Lin SS, Parker W. Human secretory immunoglobulin A may contribute to biofilm formation in the gut. Immunology. 2003;109:580–7.
27. Trespi E, Ferrieri A. Intestinal bacterial overgrowth during chronic pancreatitis. Curr Med Res Opin. 1999;15:47–52.
28. Tursi A, Brandimarte G, Giorgetti GM, Inchingolo CD. Effectiveness of the sorbitol H2 breath test in detecting histological damage among relatives of coeliacs. Scand J Gastroenterol. 2003;38:727–31.
29. Marie I, Ducrotte P, Denis P, Menard JF, Levesque H. Small intestinal bacterial overgrowth in systemic sclerosis. Rheumatology (Oxford). 2009;48:1314–9.
30. Klaus J, Spaniol U, Adler G, Mason RA, Reinshagen M, von Tirpitz CC. Small intestinal bacterial overgrowth mimicking acute flare as a pitfall in patients with Crohn's Disease. BMC Gastroenterol. 2009;9:61.
31. Wedlake L, Thomas K, McGough C, Andreyev HJ. Small bowel bacterial overgrowth and lactose intolerance during radical pelvic radiotherapy: an observational study. Eur J Cancer. 2008;44:2212–7.
32. Corleto VD, Festa S, Di Giulio E, Annibale B. Proton pump inhibitor therapy and potential long-term harm. Curr Opin Endocrinol Diabetes Obes. 2014;21:3–8.
33. Mantis NJ, Forbes SJ. Secretory IgA: arresting microbial pathogens at epithelial borders. Immunol Invest. 2010;39:383–406.
34. Walter J, Ley R. The human gut microbiome: ecology and recent evolutionary changes. Annu Rev Microbiol. 2011;65:411–29.
35. Reyes A, Haynes M, Hanson N, Angly FE, Heath AC, Rohwer F, et al. Viruses in the faecal microbiota of monozygotic twins and their mothers. Nature. 2010;466:334–8.
36. Dahlqvist G, Piessevaux H. Irritable bowel syndrome: the role of the intestinal microbiota, pathogenesis and therapeutic targets. Acta Gastroenterol Belg. 2011;74:375–80.
37. Quigley EM, Abu-Shanab A. Small intestinal bacterial overgrowth. Infect Dis Clin North Am. 2010;24:943–99.

38. Saadi M, McCallum RW. Rifaximin in irritable bowel syndrome: rationale, evidence and clinical use. Ther Adv Chronic Dis. 2013;4:71–5.

39. Sachdev AH, Pimentel M. Antibiotics for irritable bowel syndrome: rationale and current evidence. Curr Gastroenterol Rep. 2012;14:439–45.

40. Scarpellini E, Giorgio V, Gabrielli M, Filoni S, Vitale G, Tortora A, et al. Rifaximin treatment for small intestinal bacterial overgrowth in children with irritable bowel syndrome. Eur Rev Med Pharmacol Sci. 2013;17:1314–20.

41. Saltzman JR, Russell RM. Nutritional consequences of intestinal bacterial overgrowth. Compr Ther. 1994;20:523–30.

42. Lakhani SV, Shah HN, Alexander K, Finelli FC, Kirkpatrick JR, Koch TR. Small intestinal bacterial overgrowth and thiamine deficiency after Roux-en-Y gastric bypass surgery in obese patients. Nutr Res. 2008;28:293–8.

43. Di Stefano M, Veneto G, Malservisi S, Corazza GR. Small intestine bacterial overgrowth and metabolic bone disease. Dig Dis Sci. 2001;46:1077–82.

44. Stotzer PO, Johansson C, Mellstrom D, Lindstedt G, Kilander AF. Bone mineral density in patients with small intestinal bacterial overgrowth. Hepatogastroenterol. 2003;50:1415–8.

45. Shindo K, Machida M, Koide K, Fukumura M, Yamazaki R. Deconjugation ability of bacteria isolated from the jejunal fluid of patients with progressive systemic sclerosis and its gastric pH. Hepatogastroenterol. 1998;45:1643–50.

46. Jones EA, Craigie A, Tavill AS, Franglen G, Rosenoer VM. Protein metabolism in the intestinal stagnant loop syndrome. Gut. 1968;9:466–9.

47. Adibi SA. Intestinal phase of protein assimilation in man. Am J Clin Nutr. 1976;29:205–15.

48. Sherman P, Wesley A, Forstner G. Sequential disaccharidase loss in rat intestinal blind loops: impact of malnutrition. Am J Physiol. 1985;248:G626–32.

49. Machado MV, Cortez-Pinto H. Gut microbiota and nonalcoholic fatty liver disease. Ann Hepatol. 2012;11:440–9.

50. Spinucci G, Guidetti M, Lanzoni E, Pironi L. Endogenous ethanol production in a patient with chronic intestinal pseudo-obstruction and small intestinal bacterial overgrowth. Eur J Gastroenterol Hepatol. 2006;18:799–802.

51. Fundaro C, Fantacci C, Ansuini V, Giorgio V, Filoni S, Barbaro F, et al. Fecal calprotectin concentration in children affected by SIBO. Eur Rev Med Pharmacol Sci. 2011;15:1328–35.

52. Montalto M, Santoro L, Dalvai S, Curigliano V, D'Onofrio F, Scarpellini E, et al. Fecal calprotectin concentrations in patients with small intestinal bacterial overgrowth. Dig Dis. 2008;26:183–6.

53. Puwanant M, Mo-Suwan L, Patrapinyokul S. Recurrent D-lactic acidosis in a child with short bowel syndrome. Asia Pac J Clin Nutr. 2005;14:195–8.

54. Kamada N, Seo SU, Chen GY, Nunez G. Role of the gut microbiota in immunity and inflammatory disease. Nat Rev Immunol. 2013;13:321–35.

55. Fagundes-Neto U, De Martini-Costa S, Pedroso MZ, Scaletsky IC. Studies of the small bowel surface by scanning electron microscopy in infants with persistent diarrhea. Braz J Med Biol Res. 2000;33:1437–42.

56. Saad RJ, Chey WD. Breath Testing for small intestinal bacterial overgrowth: maximizing test accuracy. Clin Gastroenterol Hepatol. 2013;12(12):1964–72.

57. Rajilic-Stojanovic M, Shanahan F, Guarner F, de Vos WM. Phylogenetic analysis of dysbiosis in ulcerative colitis during remission. Inflamm Bowel Dis. 2013;19:481–8.

58. Sachdev AH, Pimentel M. Gastrointestinal bacterial overgrowth: pathogenesis and clinical significance. Ther Adv Chronic Dis. 2013;4:223–31.

59. Bjorneklett A, Jenssen E. Relationships between hydrogen (H2) and methane (CH4) production in man. Scand J Gastroenterol. 1982;17:985–92.

60. de Lacy Costello BP, Ledochowski M, Ratcliffe NM. The importance of methane breath testing: a review. J Breath Res. 2013;7:024001.

61. Mercer DF, Hobson BD, Gerhardt BK, Grant WJ, Vargas LM, Langnas AN, et al. Serial transverse enteroplasty allows children with short bowel to wean from parenteral nutrition. J Pediatr. 2014;164:93–8.

62. Millar AJ. Non-transplant surgery for short bowel syndrome. Pediatr Surg Int. 2013;29:983–7.

63. Shah SC, Day LW, Somsouk M, Sewell JL. Meta-analysis: antibiotic therapy for small intestinal bacterial overgrowth. Aliment Pharmacol Ther. 2013;38:925–34.

64. Quigley EM. Small intestinal bacterial overgrowth: what it is and what it is not. Curr Opin Gastroenterol. 2014;30(2):141–6.

65. Attar A, Flourie B, Rambaud JC, Franchisseur C, Ruszniewski P, Bouhnik Y. Antibiotic efficacy in small intestinal bacterial overgrowth-related chronic diarrhea: a crossover, randomized trial. Gastroenterology. 1999;117:794–7.

66. Bouhnik Y, Alain S, Attar A, Flourie B, Raskine L, Sanson-Le Pors MJ, et al. Bacterial populations contaminating the upper gut in patients with small intestinal bacterial overgrowth syndrome. Am J Gastroenterol. 1999;94:1327–31.

67. Malik BA, Xie YY, Wine E, Huynh HQ. Diagnosis and pharmacological management of small intestinal bacterial overgrowth in children with intestinal failure. Can J Gastroenterol. 2011;25:41–5.

68. Vanderhoof JA, Young RJ, Murray N, Kaufman SS. Treatment strategies for small bowel bacterial overgrowth in short bowel syndrome. J Pediatr Gastroenterol Nutr. 1998;27:155–60.

69. Lisowska A, Pogorzelski A, Oracz G, Siuda K, Skorupa W, Rachel M, et al. Oral antibiotic therapy improves fat absorption in cystic fibrosis patients with small intestine bacterial overgrowth. J Cyst Fibros. 2011;10:418–21.

70. Takahashi K, Terashima H, Kohno K, Ohkohchi N. A stand-alone synbiotic treatment for the prevention of d-lactic acidosis in short bowel syndrome. Int Surg. 2013;98:110–3.

71. Sanduleanu S, Jonkers D, de Bruïne A, Hameeteman W, Stockbrugger RW. Changes in gastric mucosa and luminal environment during acid-suppressive therapy: a review in depth. Dig Liver Dis. 2001;33:707–19.

Short-Bowel Syndrome

43

Jon A. Vanderhoof and Rosemary Pauley-Hunter

Introduction

Short-bowel syndrome (SBS), like many chronic intestinal disorders, often creates a long-term clinical challenge for a group of health-care practitioners including pediatric gastroenterologists, pediatric surgeons, nutritionists, nurses, and other support personnel. The recent development of multidisciplinary clinics in larger children's hospitals has been very successful in improving the long-term survivability of these patients and significantly reduced the number of complications. Although intestinal transplantation is often integrated into these programs, careful attention to detail in the management of the patient has markedly reduced the need for transplantation. This chapter focuses on a description of the disorder and the various integrated steps of medical and surgical management which often leads to long-term viability and a good quality of life for the infant and/or child with SBS.

Definition

SBS by definition is malabsorption following resection of a significant portion of the small intestine. The actual amount of intestine which may be removed to create a malabsorptive state is highly variable which is why the definition is more of a functional one rather than anatomic. In adults, the normal length of the small intestine is approximately 480, and 50 cm of remaining small intestine is often considered essen-

tial for survival, although this figure is highly variable [1]. In infants, the normal length of the small intestine is approximately 125 cm at the start of the third trimester of gestation and 250 cm at term [2]. Infants with residual small intestine length of less than 75 cm may be at risk for developing SBS however seem to have a greater capacity for adaptation and therefore may be independent of total parenteral nutrition (TPN) with less than 50 cm of remaining small intestine. See Fig. 43.1 for review of normal intestinal absorptive characteristics [3].

A number of variables are important here. For example, areas in the small bowel have inherent adaptability characteristics. The jejunum is responsible for most macronutrient absorption with its long villi, large absorptive surface, highly concentrated digestive enzymes, and many transport carrier proteins. Thus, when the jejunum is resected, a temporary reduction in absorption of most nutrients occurs. The jejunum exhibits modest adaptive changes in response to intestinal resection, and most of these changes are functional with changes in transport and enzyme activity rather than structural or surface absorptive enhancement.

The ileum is the dedicated site of adsorption of vitamin B12 and bile acids, and the capacity of the remaining small intestine to handle these functions is very limited. The ileum is much more adept at water absorption because epithelial junctions in the ileum are tighter/smaller and therefore less permeable to nutrients. This area typically is the site of significant fluid reabsorption as it is subjected to large volumes of water flux in response to osmotic loads delivered from the jejunum. A resection of a significant portion of ileum is often less well tolerated than jejunal resection because patients have a great deal of difficulty with water reabsorption in other areas of the bowel despite the fact that they have been quite capable of handling the macronutrient load. The ileocecal valve is an important barrier to reflux of colonic bacteria and helps regulate the passage of fluid and nutrients from the ileum into the colon (ileal brake).

The colon has an important role in absorption of water, electrolytes, and short-chain fatty acids. Loss of the colon in

J. A. Vanderhoof (✉)
Department of Pediatrics, Boston Children's Hospital, Harvard Medical School, 300 Longwood Avenue, Boston, MA 02115, USA
e-mail: jon.vanderhoof@childrens.harvard.edu

Boys Town National Research Hospital, 1080 Hospital Road, Boys Town, NE 68010, USA

R. Pauley-Hunter
Department of Pediatric Gastroenterology, Boys Town National Research Hospital, Boys Town, NE, USA

© Springer International Publishing Switzerland 2016
S. Guandalini et al. (eds.), *Textbook of Pediatric Gastroenterology, Hepatology and Nutrition*,
DOI 10.1007/978-3-319-17169-2_43

Fig. 43.1 Normal intestinal absorptive characteristics. (Reproduced with permission from Ref. [3])

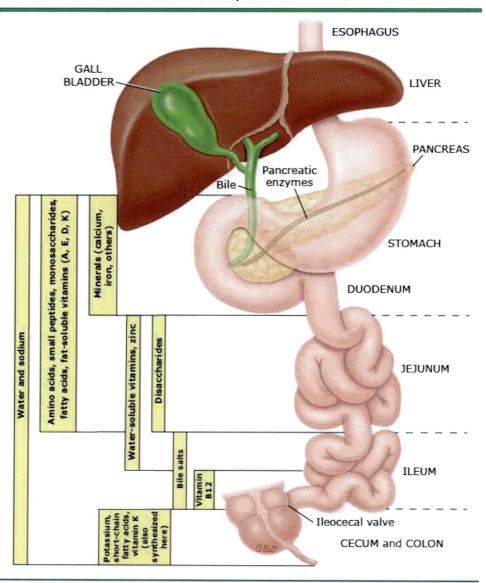

Intestinal sites of nutrient absorption

combination with extensive small-bowel resection is poorly tolerated and often leads to dehydration and electrolyte depletion. The colon slows intestinal transit and can absorb a significant percentage of calories, primarily in the form of fermented carbohydrates. The retained colon may adapt after small-bowel resection, with gradual increases in colonocytes and in gut hormone secretion [4].

Another significant factor affecting long-term prognosis in SBS is the process of intestinal proliferation. Following small-bowel resection, the remaining bowel has a rather marked ability to adapt [1, 5]. Lengthening of the villi, and to some degree dilatation of the small-bowel lumen, may result in up to a fourfold increase in mucosal surface area following massive resection. This process has been extensively studied in animal models, and a number of trophic

factors have been identified as having a role in regulating this process [6]. The most recently described compound is glucagon-like peptide-2 (GLP2) [7]. Other factors including enteroglucagon, growth hormone, and peptide YY may also be involved. Most importantly, these trophic factors are heavily dependent upon the presence of enteral nutrition in order to stimulate the adaptation process. The ability of the ileum, normally more trophic than the jejunum, is significantly greater than other parts of the small bowel. SBS in adults usually results from surgical resection for Crohn's disease, malignancy, radiation, or vascular insufficiency. In infants and small children, necrotizing enterocolitis and congenital intestinal anomalies such as atresias or gastroschisis are the most common causes of SBS. Unfortunately, many of the common causes of SBS namely congenital anomalies,

Table 43.1 Common causes of short-bowel syndrome

Conditions in newborns
Necrotizing enterocolitis
Meconium ileus
Midgut volvulus
Omphalocele
Gastroschisis
Jejunoileal atresia
Congenital short bowel
Hirschprung's disease
Conditions in older children
Crohn's disease
Cancer treatment/radiation enteritis
Occluded intestinal blood vessels
Trauma
Tumor

necrotizing enterocolitis, and Crohn's disease often result in resection of the ileum (see Table 43.1).

Intestinal failure can result from SBS and is defined as a reduction of a critical amount of functional gut mass below the amount needed for adequate digestion and absorption of nutrients and fluid needs or from a poorly functioning absorptive surface secondary to structural abnormalities or chronic inflammation [1]. It is often characterized by macro- and micronutrient malabsorption, electrolyte imbalance with tendency to dehydration, intestinal bacterial overgrowth and poor growth in children, and weight loss in adults [8]. In addition to SBS, diseases or congenital defects that cause severe malabsorption, bowel obstruction, and dysmotility (e.g., pseudo-obstruction) are also causes of intestinal failure. It is intestinal failure, not SBS itself, which leads to intestinal transplantation.

Management

Parenteral Nutrition

The first stage of management and SBS primarily focuses on TPN and managing fluid and electrolyte complications. Parenteral nutrition here differs very little from any disorder necessitating parenteral feeding. Baseline nutrient and energy needs must be met in a standard fashion. In children with SBS, fluid and electrolytes are often a challenge in the immediate postoperative period. Ongoing losses of fluid and substantial quantities of electrolytes are quite variable and highly dependent upon location of any ostomies in addition to losses from nasogastric, gastric, or naso-duodenal tubes. Gastric losses include significant volumes of hydrochloric acid and large quantities of potassium and sodium chloride which can affect acid–base balance as well as electrolyte losses. This hypersecretion of gastric acid and fluids may reduce pH below the optimal level needed for efficient fat absorption by inactivating pancreatic lipase and deconjugating

bile salts requiring use of acid suppression. The gastric hypersecretion typically resolves in the first few months after surgery and is not required indefinitely. In fact, ongoing use, as in those without SBS, may be associated with increased risk of viral infections [9, 10].

Small bowel fluid losses contain much higher concentrations of sodium often approaching that of normal saline. Measurement of these ongoing losses and replacement with a solution separate from the TPN milliliter for milliliter are usually much simpler and preferable to constant reformulation of parenteral nutrition solution. Once ongoing losses stabilize, these volumes can be more easily incorporated into parenteral nutrition solution if desired.

The resting energy expenditure in infants with SBS is similar to healthy controls. However, because of malabsorption, the amount of energy needed will be greater (estimates of 30–70% greater) than that needed parenterally to achieve similar weight gain [11, 12]. In general, growth is monitored by assessing whether increases in weight are proportional to linear growth. Factors such as genetics should also be factored into expectations for growth. Moreover, proportional growth does not necessarily avoid stunting, which appears to be common among children with SBS.

Patients on TPN should initially be monitored daily with electrolytes, blood urea nitrogen (BUN), creatinine, phosphorus, magnesium, albumin, triglycerides, and glucose then weekly until stable and with any subsequent change in TPN formulation or volume. Total and direct bilirubin and aminotransferases (aspartate aminotransferase, AST, and alanine transaminase, ALT) also should be measured regularly to monitor for parenteral–nutrition-associated liver disease. Monitoring of vitamin levels is not essential at this time but becomes of greater importance as the patient becomes solely dependent on enteral nutrition.

Enteral Nutrition

Once gastrointestinal motility resumes and the postoperative ileus has resolved, enteral nutrition can be judiciously initiated. Early initiation of enteral feeding is important for a number of reasons. Enteral nutrition has been shown to strengthen the mucosal barrier and reduce the risk of translocation of bacteria [13]. In addition, the adaptation process which is crucial to long-term survival without parenteral nutrition or at least with minimal parenteral nutrition does not occur in the absence of enteral feeding. Aggressive use of enteral feeding, especially early in the course of treatment, significantly enhances the adaptation process [14]. Much work has been done to understand the role of enteral nutrition, and we do know that certain nutrients appear to be more important than others. Long-chain fats, especially three omega fatty acids, at least eicosapentaenoic acid, appear to be very important in this process [15]. Consequently, making sure a significant portion of enteral feeding is in the formal long-chain fats is advantageous. More important, however, is the use of aggressive enteral nutrition as early as possible after resection.

Enteral Formula

Selection of the appropriate enteral feeding solution is dependent upon a number of factors. In small infants, hydrolyzed or elemental formulations are commonly utilized. There are substantial data however suggesting that human milk may provide an excellent alternative [16]. Human milk, especially when fresh, contains a number of trophic factors not commonly present in predigested formula is. Predigested formulas are commonly used because the nutrients provided are in a form ready for absorption. This avoids wasting part of the absorptive surface while digestion is occurring. Although osmolality is often utilized as a reason to avoid predigested formulas, this is really an issue only when continuous enteral infusion is not being employed. Hyperosmolar formulas of any type when administered via a slow continuous tube feeding are well tolerated. If used, elemental formulas should contain at least 40 % of their calories as fat. Some data suggest that more complex formulations may be advantageous for adaptation, due to a greater functional workload demanded from the small-bowel epithelium [16, 17]. In practicality, most clinicians avoid whole protein formulas, as there is an increased risk of non-IgE allergic injury from an intact proteins especially true during the first 2 years of life [17, 18].

The use of medium-chain triglycerides is comparably controversial. While medium-chain triglycerides are better absorbed especially when the supply of pancreatic enzymes or bile acids are limited, they are also less trophic to the small bowel. Medium chain fats also have a lower energy density and exert a greater osmotic load on the epithelium than long chain fats. The optimal ratio between long- and medium-chain fats has not yet been identified, but a majority of the fat delivered early in the course of enteral feeding should probably be supplied in the form of long-chain fats. Pancreatic insufficiency is rarely a problem in these patients, and bile acid deficiency is usually only an issue in infants with liver disease or massive ileal resection.

The ratio of calories provided between fat and carbohydrate is also arguable. The coefficient of absorption of carbohydrate is better, but the caloric density of fat is much higher. Carbohydrate is the preferred nutritional substrate for bacteria and favors the development of small-bowel bacterial overgrowth, another major complication of SBS. Formulations higher in fat and lower in carbohydrate work better in infants with SBS when the risk of injury from small-bowel

bacterial overgrowth is potentially higher [19]. In adults, or older children, colonic salvage of short-chain fatty acids and reduced by bacterial metabolism from malabsorbed carbohydrate is much better which is probably why older children and adults do somewhat better than small infants with a higher proportion of carbohydrate in their enteral feeding. Lactose restriction is not required as most is absorbed in the proximal bowel which is often preserved in many cases of pediatric SBS.

Fiber supplementation may be beneficial not only in absorbing some of the water losses but also provide an additional energy source in patients with a retained colon. In older children, significant malabsorption of fat may lead to oxalate absorption due to the loss of calcium and subsequent development of hyperoxaluria and the formation of kidney stones.

Feeding Techniques

Once initiated, enteral feedings are gradually increased as tolerated. Feeding 24 h a day will optimize absorption through continuous use of the available gut mucosa. The rate of infusion can be gradually increased based on tolerance. Ostomy output in excess of 30–50 mL/kg per day is usually a contraindication to advancing feedings. Measuring reducing substances in the stool or ostomy output will also provide a clue as to whether or not the absorptive threshold has been reached. Once carbohydrate malabsorption begins, advancing feedings usually precipitates more osmotic fluid loss. As the tolerance to enteral feeding increases, parenteral nutrition is reduced in an isocaloric fashion. During this time, the patient has often been weaned to receiving parenteral nutrition during only part of the day or night with the infusion device capped for a certain number of hours each day. The length of the time off of parenteral nutrition can gradually be increased to facilitate care and mobility the patient, rather than simply decreasing the parenteral nutrition rate. Eventually, as enteral nutrition tolerance increases, the patient's parenteral nutrition may be deleted for one night a week, then two, and progressed until the patient is no longer receiving parenteral nutrition.

Enteral nutrition can be provided orally through bolus feedings or by continuous enteral infusion. Oral nutrition has the advantage of including the oral and cephalic processes of digestion and absorption which might perhaps play a role in adaptation. However, especially in small children or infants, continuous enteral infusion is usually employed. Continuous enteral infusion provides constant stimulation for mucosal adaptation. As the nutrients are introduced more slowly and continuously into the gut, optimal saturation of transport carriers is achieved. The enhanced absorption thereby reduces the need of parenteral calories which likewise reduces the risk of parenteral-nutrition-induced liver disease, one of the most common morbidities seen in SBS.

It is extremely important to initiate small quantities of oral bolus feeding early in the course of therapy. Especially in small infants, if this is not done, oral food aversion becomes a real problem. If only a few milliliters of formula or human milk are given through by mouth four times per day, the risk of oral food aversion can be significantly reduced. Solid foods can be initiated at the usual time (4–6 months of age) in small quantities despite the fact that the child continues to receive most of their enteral nutrition through a continuous infusion. The choice of solid food feeding is also open to controversy. Although it is customary in many cultures to begin oral feedings with carbohydrates such as cereal, there is little logic to this practice. Meat is probably an ideal first food for the short-bowel patient. Meat is high in fat and protein which are both important in stimulating mucosal adaptation and contain little or no carbohydrate which could increase osmotic fluid losses and small bowel bacterial overgrowth.

As feedings are progressed, the short-bowel patient may be receiving solids and oral bolus feedings during the daytime and continuous enteral infusion at night. This also permits optimal use of the gut. Nighttime enteral nutrition however frequently reduces the appetite in the morning and sometimes needs to be reduced to encourage the child to eat. A careful balance among all of these various factors requires clinical experience. This is perhaps one of the reasons why a multidisciplinary approach in SBS has been so successful in major centers [20].

In the management of older children was SBS, oral nutrition is often advanced more quickly. In this instance, the use of small frequent feedings every 2–3 h is beneficial over larger less frequent feedings as it more closely mimics the advantage of continuous enteral infusion [21]. Here, the selection of foods is very important. It is important that each meal contains a balance of carbohydrate, fat, and protein to avoid overloading the small intestinal capacity to absorb micronutrients. An equal balance between carbohydrate and fat, and a significant amount of protein in each of several small meals during the day, will not only facilitate adaptation but also reduce the risk of malabsorption and excessive fluid losses. Involvement of nutritionists who understand this principal and can counsel and educate the patient well is very important at this stage. A nice example is the concept of a small sandwich as the proper size of meal. The bread is the carbohydrate, the meat is the protein, and the butter is the fat. If this counseling is not provided, the patient may well choose to eat small meals but will consume all carbohydrate in one meal and all protein in the next because this is often easier to provide. The major risk in oral feeding is the consumption of large carbohydrate-containing meals. Carbohydrate, even in the form of disaccharides, is rapidly digested in the small bowel creating an osmotic load which results in fluid rushing into the lumen creating diarrhea or large-volume ostomy losses. Simple carbohydrates are even more problematic. Including fat and protein in each meal while reducing the amount of carbohydrate reduces this risk significantly.

Pharmacologic Therapy

Numerous medications may be useful in the treatment of SBS, but in all instances, they should be considered as adjunctive to the primary treatment, enteral nutrition. Patients with SBS are commonly given H2 receptor antagonists to suppress acid secretion. Short-bowel patients commonly have delayed gastric emptying which predisposes them to esophagitis and gastritis. These findings are commonly seen endoscopically. Unfortunately, acid suppression results in a greater likelihood of developing small-bowel bacterial overgrowth and allowing both bacterial and viral pathogens a portal of entry for causing disease [22]. One must consider both sides of the equation when prescribing these drugs.

Drugs which reduce small-bowel motility and lengthen transit such as loperamide are also commonly employed. These medications are likewise a double-edged sword. Slowing motility has the advantage of increasing nutrient contact with small-bowel mucosa, perhaps enhancing absorption. Unfortunately, motility is how the bowel rids itself of excess small-bowel bacteria. Patients with SBS already have dilated small bowel in many instances, which predisposes them to poor motility and thereby exacerbates small-bowel bacterial overgrowth [23, 24]. In general, patients with excess fluid losses who do not have overgrowth benefit from these medications and those with malabsorption secondary to overgrowth will probably do worse. Consequently, careful consideration of the clinical situation is needed before proceeding down this path.

Patients with SBS are often given broad-spectrum antibiotics to help control small-bowel bacterial overgrowth [25]. It is very difficult to determine exactly which antibiotics should be used. Attempts have been made to culture the small bowel and base the decision on sensitivity studies, but one can never be certain the organisms causing the symptoms are actually the ones which were cultured [25, 26]. Consequently, trial and error are often employed to make the decision. Determining the presence of overgrowth is also frequently difficult and is the subject of another chapter in this text. Again, trial and error are often utilized to make a decision. Antibiotic regimens which are commonly utilized are shown in Table 43.2.

Recently, a GLP 2 analog has been developed for the treatment of SBS. This followed largely unsuccessful attempt to utilize a combination of glutamine and growth hormone to stimulate intestinal adaptation. GLP 2 appears to be better suited for this purpose and may have significant antisecretory benefits as well. The drug must be administered parenterally on a daily basis and is extremely expensive which limits its usefulness, but in adults with SBS, it has been shown to be useful in weaning some patients from parenteral nutrition [28, 29].

Complications

Catheter-Related Issues

Patients who require long-term parenteral nutrition may experience complications related to the central venous catheter or implantable infusion device. Most often, mechanical issues include device breakage and occlusion, but infectious complications may also occur. Patients with recurrent complications are at risk for losing central venous access which may be an indication for consideration of intestinal transplant.

The risk of noninfective complications of PN devices can be reduced by use of standardized protocols for insertion and long-term care [30]. Vigorous flushing protocols are important to maintain the patency of the central venous line. If the line becomes occluded, various thrombolytic agents can be used to restore patency [31]. This procedure is usually performed by nurses in the emergency department or from nutrition support or vascular access teams. These efforts to prevent and treat mechanical failure are important to maintain central venous access for those requiring long-term parenteral nutrition.

Damage to external catheters can be minimized by avoidance of over-clamping and limiting the use of scissors near the line. If the catheter is damaged, use of repair kits can help to extend its life although should be performed by those with experience as there is a significant risk of sepsis [32]. Guide wires can be used to change the defective line and help preserve the site of access.

Catheter-related blood stream infections can be life-threatening. Moreover, episodes of sepsis are associated with hyperbilirubinemia and progressive liver disease. Cholestasis in infants is often triggered by a catheter infection [33]. To minimize this risk, the caregivers must be carefully instructed in the care of the catheter and insertion site. Sterile technique, particularly in the initiation and discontinuation of the infusion, is critical to prevent contamination. Bacterial translocation from unhealthy gut epithelium also can contribute to the risk for recurrent sepsis [34, 35]. Antibiotic and ethanol locks may be helpful in treating catheter sepsis but also may increase issues with thrombosis [36, 37]. Although the role of ethanol lock therapy has not been established in the literature in large randomized studies, this technique is increasingly utilized in intestinal rehabilitation centers in the USA. Catheter exit-site infections can usually be treated with sterile dressing changes and systemic antibiotics if treatment is initiated at the first signs of redness, pain at the site, and drainage.

Hepatobiliary Disease

In patients with extreme SBS, those with SBS beginning in infancy or SBS occurring in premature infants, the development of parenteral-nutrition-associated liver disease is not uncommon. The severity of disease expression is often inversely related to the amount of enteral feedings that can be tolerated. For this reason, even in patients with very short bowel, aggressive enteral nutrition is pursued. An increase in liver enzymes followed by increases in direct bilirubin often suggests that liver injury from parenteral nutrition has occurred. In this instance, steps need to be taken to reduce the risk of progression of liver injury. One of the most important steps is to reduce the amount of soybean-based intravenous lipid to that necessary to prevent essential fatty acid deficiency. This can be done by limiting the amount of lipid administered, utilizing an alternative source such as a fish oil-based solution, or providing a more balanced fatty acid solution [38–40]. Soybean oil is high linoleic acid which acts as a substrate for the synthesis of a variety of pro-inflammatory cytokines. Fish oil on the other hand is rich in eicosapentaenoic acid (EPA) and docosahexaenoic acid (DHA) which are predominantly anti-inflammatory fats. Whether or not this is the mechanism for the benefits of fish oil intravenous lipid is unknown.

Other maneuvers which are occasionally helpful in reducing the risk of liver injury include cycling of parenteral nutrition so that it is given only for a few hours each day and prevention of catheter-induced sepsis which seems to be associated with an increased incidence of liver injury [41]. Finally, bacterial overgrowth is known to produce toxins in the bowel which can gain access to the liver through the portal circulation so prevention of bacterial overgrowth is also helpful in reducing the risk of liver disease.

Patients with SBS also frequently develop gallstones. The use of continuous enteral nutrition or parenteral nutrition does not stimulate gallbladder emptying to the same degree as eating bolus meals [42, 43]. Consequently, sludge accumulates in the gallbladder predisposing it to the formation of gallstones. Some have even advocated routine removal of the gallbladder in SBS although this practice is not widely utilized. In patients with SBS who develop worsening jaundice or hyperbilirubinemia, an ultrasound to look at the gallbladder for evidence of stones is warranted.

Bacterial Overgrowth

Bacterial overgrowth in the small bowel is said to occur whenever the concentration of normal enteric flora exceeds those observed in the physiologic state. The presence of the excess bacteria may have adverse effects on the mucosa-creating inflammation and the resultant symptoms. This is especially common in SBS, as these patients often have no ileocecal valve which functions to prevent or limit reflux and colonic flora into the small intestine. These patients also experience compensatory dilatation in small bowel diameter often associated with prolonged transit. Both of these processes may be seen as adaptive phenomenon but would certainly place the patient at increased risk of bacterial overgrowth. Finally, patients with SBS may have delayed gastric emptying and some degree of hypergastrinemia; therefore, it is not uncommon for patients with SBS to have inflammation in the esophagus, stomach, and proximal duodenum. The use of aggressive acid suppression is not uncommon in this group of patients and that certainly enhances the risk of development of small-bowel bacterial overgrowth.

Small-bowel bacterial overgrowth can have a significant effect on absorptive capacity for a number of reasons. Perhaps the most significant is by the induction of inflammation in the small bowel, damaging the absorptive surface [44]. Bile salts are conjugated in the lumen by bacteria rendering them nonabsorbable in the ileum which can cause further fat malabsorption and its resultant effects such as the development of kidney stones.

Prevention of the negative effects of small-bowel bacterial overgrowth generally includes dietary management as the first line of therapy, mainly by avoiding excess carbohydrate intake in the susceptible patients. Medications which slow intestinal transit, such as loperamide, should be avoided in patients with overgrowth. Acid suppression should be used judiciously. Antibiotic therapy may be indicated and several protocols have been suggested. One must consider best type of antibiotic (see Table 43.2) as well as the administration frequency. Administration of antibiotics for the first week of each month, on a continuous basis, or on a rotational basis avoids development of antibiotic resistance.

Some patients with small-bowel bacterial overgrowth have other anatomic considerations making them uniquely susceptible to symptoms. Any anatomic abnormality which adversely affects motility or normal antegrade peristalsis of the small intestine contents is likely to result in the development of overgrowth. Anastomotic strictures in areas of previous atresias or inflammatory strictures from residual necrotizing enterocolitis not uncommonly result in proximal dilatation and dysmotility. Ulceration at the site of anastomosis may also occur and results in chronic blood loss and further exacerbating bacterial overgrowth.

Within these areas of dilated gut, overgrowth and resultant inflammation are not uncommon. In this situation, tailoring the bowel by removing the stricture and reducing the diameter of the dilated bowel frequently results in enhanced motility and reduced overgrowth and despite the fact that some bowel was resected, absorption improves [45]. When there is an extensively dilated segment of small bowel, intestinal lengthening procedures can be performed. Two techniques have been described. The first was the Bianchi procedure which involves isolating the blood supply to each lateral half of the bowel, stapling or sewing the bowel longitudinally to create two segments of equal length but half the diameter, and then attaching the two segments end to end making certain that full segments are attached in such a way to ensure proximal to distal peristalsis. The second operation is known as serial transverse enteroplasty. In this operation, much simpler to perform, opposing transverse incisions are made in the dilated bowel at several intervals and closed longitudinally. The end result is the same, significant lengthening of the bowel and reduction of the diameter with no loss of absorptive surface area [1, 46]. The operation should probably not be performed in children with non-dilated bowel and normal mucosal surface, as this is really a bacterial overgrowth control operation and not an intestinal lengthening procedure as commonly thought. The serial transverse enteroplasty procedure has the advantage of being repeatable, and can be done in a patient who has had dilatation following a previous Bianchi procedure. Decisions regarding the use as well as the performance of these operations should be made by experienced surgeons with extensive knowledge of intestinal failure and bacterial overgrowth.

Micronutrient Abnormalities

Once patients are weaned from parenteral nutrition and must rely on enteral intake, the certainty with which micronutrients can absorb as highly variable. Micronutrient deficiency, either trace metals or vitamins, is fairly unlikely when these are provided in adequate concentrations in the parenteral nutrition solutions. Once enteral intake exceeds about 50 % of the total daily caloric needs, the patient begins to depend more on the gut or micronutrients provided in the enteral

Table 43.2 Antibiotic regimens for bacterial overgrowth

Rifaximin
Gentamycin + metronidazole
Sulfamethoxazole and trimethoprim + metronidazole
Amoxicillin/clavulanate
Ciprofloxacin
Doxycycline
Vancomycin

Table 43.3 Laboratory monitoring after TPN

CBC with differential and platelets	Monthly × 3 *Then* if stable Q 3 months × 4 *Then* Q 6 months × 2 *Then* yearly
Comprehensive metabolic profile	Monthly × 3 *Then* if stable Q 3 months × 4 *Then* Q 6 months × 2 *Then* yearly
Vitamin A and E; 25 OH vitamin D	Every 6 months
B12	If large ileal resection every 3 months otherwise every 6 months
Zinc	Every 6 months
Triene/tetrene ratios	Every 6 months × 2 after lipids are stopped *Then* yearly

nutrition. The risks of deficiency increases significantly when patients are weaned from parenteral nutrition. The fat-soluble vitamins A, D, E and K and certain trace metals and other electrolytes such as calcium and magnesium are the most likely to be deficient. Patient should be monitored for these micronutrients on a routine basis for every 3–6 months (see Table 43.3). Supplementation with high oral replacement doses is often necessary with frequent monitoring to make certain nutritional adequacy is achieved. In patients with ileal resection, vitamin B12 deficiency not uncommonly occurs. Periodic evaluation of B12 levels in such patients is indicated. If levels drop, exogenous administration on a routine basis will be needed throughout life. Patients receiving most of their nutrition parenterally who are receiving limited lipid administration or patients with severe fat malabsorption are at risk for developing essential fatty acid deficiency. In such patients, periodic evaluation of triene/tetrene ratios should be performed to determine if extra intravenous lipid supplementation is needed. Calcium and magnesium are also poorly absorbed in many short-bowel patients, and periodic evaluation of bone density should be done, on a yearly basis [47].

In patients with irreversible parenteral-nutrition-associated liver disease who had not responded to all the measures outlined above, combined liver and intestinal transplantation may be considered. Use of this operation has been declining recently because of the great success of multidisciplinary centers in the management of intestinal failure and the effective use of parenteral and enteral nutrition [48]. Unfortunately, some patients still progress to liver failure and require transplantation. Despite numerous advances and surgical techniques and immunosuppression, 5-year survival is still not much better than 50% [49, 50]. Although some patients do extremely well, recurrent hospitalizations for complications for treatment of rejection are not uncommon. Consequently, transplantation should be considered only when all else is failed. Ideally, these procedures should be performed in an experience transplant center with a multidisciplinary team capable caring for advanced intestinal failure problems.

References

1. Yildiz BD. Where are we at with short bowel syndrome and small bowel transplant. World J Transplant. 2012;2:95–103.
2. Touloukian RJ, Smith GJ. Normal intestinal length in preterm infants. J Pediatr Surg. 1983;18:720–3.
3. Pauley-Hunter RJ, Vanderhoof JA. Pathophysiology of the short bowel syndrome. In: UpToDate, Basow DS, UpToDate, Waltham MA, editors. (Jan 2014.) Copyright © 2013 UpToDate, Inc. For more information visit www.uptodate.com.
4. Healey KL, Bines JE, Thomas SL, Wilson G, Taylor RG, Sourial M, et al. Morphological and functional changes in the colon after massive small bowel resection. J Pediatr Surg. 2010;45:1581–90.
5. Drozdowski L, Thomson AB. Intestinal mucosal adaptation. World J Gastroenterol. 2006;12:4614–27.
6. McMellen ME, Wakeman D, Longshore SW, McDuffie LA, Warner BW. Growth factors: possible roles for clinical management of the short bowel syndrome. Semin Pediatr Surg. 2010;19:35–43.
7. Jeppesen PB. Teduglutide for the treatment of short bowel syndrome. Drugs Today (Barc). 2013;49:599–614.
8. Schwartz MZ. Novel therapies for the management of short bowel syndrome in children. Pediatr Surg Int. 2013;29:967–74.
9. Terrin G, Canani RB, Passariello A, Caoci S, De Curtis M. Inhibitors of gastric acid secretion drugs increase neonatal morbidity and mortality. J Matern Fetal Neonatal Med. 2012;25(Suppl 4):85–7.
10. Terrin G, Passariello A, De Curtis M, Manguso F, Salvia G, Lega L, et al. Ranitidine is associated with infections, necrotizing enterocolitis, and fatal outcome in newborns. Pediatrics. 2012;129:e40–5.
11. Olieman JF, Penning C, Spoel M, Ijsselstijn H, van den Hoonaard TL, Escher JC, Bax NM, Tibboel D. Long-term impact of infantile short bowel syndrome on nutritional status and growth. Br J Nutr. 2012;107:1489–97.
12. Olieman JF, Poley MJ, Gischler SJ, Penning C, Escher JC, van den Hoonaard TL, et al. Interdisciplinary management of infantile short bowel syndrome: resource consumption, growth, and nutrition. J Pediatr Surg. 2010;45:490–8.
13. Anastasilakis CD, Ioannidis O, Gkiomisi AI, Botsios D. Artificial nutrition and intestinal mucosal barrier functionality. Digestion. 2013;88:193–208.
14. Wood SJ, Khalil B, Fusaro F, Folaranmi SE, Sparks SA, Morabito A. Early structured surgical management plan for neonates with short bowel syndrome may improve outcomes. World J Surg. 2013;37:1714–17.
15. Kollman-Bauerly KA, Thomas DL, Adrian TE, Lien EL, Vanderhoof JA. The role of eicosanoids in the process of adaptation following massive bowel resection in the rat. JPEN J Parenter Enteral Nutr. 2001;25:275–81.

16. Olieman JF, Penning C, Ijsselstijn H, Escher JC, Joosten KF, Hulst JM, et al. Enteral nutrition in children with short-bowel syndrome: current evidence and recommendations for the clinician. J Am Diet Assoc. 2010;110:420–6.

17. Cole CR, Kocoshis SA. Nutrition management of infants with surgical short bowel syndrome and intestinal failure. Nutr Clin Pract. 2013;28:421–8.

18. Vanderhoof JA, Young RJ. Hydrolyzed versus nonhydrolyzed protein diet in short bowel syndrome in children. J Pediatr Gastroenterol Nutr. 2004;38:107.

19. Bongaerts GP, Severijnen RS. Arguments for a lower carbohydrate-higher fat diet in patients with a short small bowel. Med Hypotheses. 2006;67:280–2.

20. Sudan D. Advances in the nontransplant medical and surgical management of intestinal failure. Curr Opin Organ Transplant. 2009;14: 274–9.

21. Matarese LE. Nutrition and fluid optimization for patients with short bowel syndrome. JPEN J Parenter Enteral Nutr. 2013;37:161–70.

22. Corleto VD, Festa S, Di Giulio E, Annibale B. Proton pump inhibitor therapy and potential long-term harm. Curr Opin Endocrinol Diabetes Obes. 2013.

23. Coulie B, Camilleri M. Intestinal pseudo-obstruction. Annu Rev Med. 1999;50:37–55.

24. Millar AJ. Non-transplant surgery for short bowel syndrome. Pediatr Surg Int. 2013;29:983–7.

25. Shah SC, Day LW, Somsouk M, Sewell JL. Meta-analysis: antibiotic therapy for small intestinal bacterial overgrowth. Aliment Pharmacol Ther. 2013;38:925–34.

26. Bohm M, Siwiec RM, Wo JM. Diagnosis and management of small intestinal bacterial overgrowth. Nutr Clin Pract. 2013;28:289–99.

27. Grace E, Shaw C, Whelan K, Andreyev HJ. Review article: small intestinal bacterial overgrowth—prevalence, clinical features, current and developing diagnostic tests, and treatment. Aliment Pharmacol Ther. 2013;38:674–88.

28. Burness CB, McCormack PL. Teduglutide: a review of its use in the treatment of patients with short bowel syndrome. Drugs. 2013;73:935–47.

29. Drucker DJ, Yusta B. Physiology and pharmacology of the enteroendocrine hormone glucagon-like peptide-2. Annu Rev Physiol. 2013.

30. Cotogni P, Pittiruti M, Barbero C, Monge T, Palmo A, Boggio BD. Catheter-related complications in cancer patients on home parenteral nutrition: a prospective study of over 51,000 catheter days. JPEN J Parenter Enteral Nutr. 2013;37:375–83.

31. Revel-Vilk S, Ergaz Z. Diagnosis and management of central-line-associated thrombosis in newborns and infants. Semin Fetal Neonatal Med. 2011;16:340–4.

32. Lundgren IS, Zhou C, Malone FR, McAfee NG, Gantt S, Zerr DM. Central venous catheter repair is associated with an increased risk of bacteremia and central line-associated bloodstream infection in pediatric patients. Pediatr Infect Dis J. 2012;31:337–40.

33. Hermans D, Talbotec C, Lacaille F, Goulet O, Ricour C, Colomb V. Early central catheter infections may contribute to hepatic fibrosis in children receiving long-term parenteral nutrition. J Pediatr Gastroenterol Nutr. 2007;44:459–63.

34. Neu J, Mihatsch WA, Zegarra J, Supapannachart S, Ding ZY, Murguia-Peniche T. Intestinal mucosal defense system, Part 1. Consensus recommendations for immunonutrients. J Pediatr. 2013;162:S56–63.

35. Taur Y, Pamer EG. The intestinal microbiota and susceptibility to infection in immunocompromised patients. Curr Opin Infect Dis. 2013;26:332–7.

36. Wales PW, Kosar C, Carricato M, de Silva N, Lang K, Avitzur Y. Ethanol lock therapy to reduce the incidence of catheter-related bloodstream infections in home parenteral nutrition patients with intestinal failure: preliminary experience. J Pediatr Surg. 2011;46:951–6.

37. Wong T, Clifford V, McCallum Z, Shalley H, Peterkin M, Paxton G, et al. Central venous catheter thrombosis associated with 70% ethanol locks in pediatric intestinal failure patients on home parenteral nutrition: a case series. JPEN J Parenter Enteral Nutr. 2012;36:358–60.

38. Diamond IR, Grant RC, Feldman BM, Tomlinson GA, Pencharz PB, Ling SC, et al. Expert beliefs regarding novel lipid-based approaches to pediatric intestinal failure-associated liver disease. JPEN J Parenter Enteral Nutr. 2013.

39. El Kasmi KC, Anderson AL, Devereaux MW, Vue PM, Zhang W, Setchell KD, et al. Phytosterols promote liver injury and kupffer cell activation in parenteral nutrition-associated liver disease. Sci Transl Med. 2013;5:206ra137.

40. Nandivada P, Carlson SJ, Cowan E, Chang MI, Gura KM, Puder M. Role of parenteral lipid emulsions in the preterm infant. Early Hum Dev. 2013;89(Suppl 2): S45–9.

41. Xu ZW, Li YS. Pathogenesis and treatment of parenteral nutrition-associated liver disease. Hepatobiliary Pancreat Dis Int. 2012;11:586–93.

42. Kelly DA. Preventing parenteral nutrition liver disease. Early Hum Dev. 2010;86:683–7.

43. Nightingale JM. Hepatobiliary, renal and bone complications of intestinal failure. Best Pract Res Clin Gastroenterol. 2003;17:907–29.

44. Schulzke JD, Troger H, Amasheh M. Disorders of intestinal secretion and absorption. Best Pract Res Clin Gastroenterol. 2009;23:395–406.

45. Pakarinen MP, Kurvinen A, Koivusalo AI, Iber T, Rintala RJ. Long-term controlled outcomes after autologous intestinal reconstruction surgery in treatment of severe short bowel syndrome. J Pediatr Surg. 2013;48:339–44.

46. King B, Carlson G, Khalil BA, Morabito A. Intestinal bowel lengthening in children with short bowel syndrome: systematic review of the Bianchi and STEP procedures. World J Surg. 2013;37:694–704.

47. Koehler AN, Yaworski JA, Gardner M, Kocoshis S, Reyes J, Barksdale EM, Jr. Coordinated interdisciplinary management of pediatric intestinal failure: a 2-year review. J Pediatr Surg. 2000;35:380–5.

48. Stanger JD, Oliveira C, Blackmore C, Avitzur Y, Wales PW. The impact of multi-disciplinary intestinal rehabilitation programs on the outcome of pediatric patients with intestinal failure: a systematic review and meta-analysis. J Pediatr Surg. 2013;48:983–92.

49. Desai CS, Khan KM, Gruessner AC, Fishbein TM, Gruessner RW. Intestinal retransplantation: analysis of Organ Procurement and Transplantation Network database. Transplantation. 2012;93:120–5.

50. Lauro A, Zanfi C, Pellegrini S, Catena F, Cescon M, Cautero N, et al. Isolated intestinal transplant for chronic intestinal pseudo-obstruction in adults: long-term outcome. Transplant Proc. 2013;45:3351–55.

Malnutrition: A Global Problem

44

Jai K. Das, Rehana A. Salam and Zulfiqar A. Bhutta

Background

The State of Food Insecurity (SOFI) estimates that around 870 million people globally have been undernourished (in terms of dietary energy supply) in the period 2010–2012 [1]. The vast majority of these, 852 million, live in developing countries, where the prevalence of undernourishment is around 14.9% [1]. Though many countries are on track in reducing income poverty (Millennium Developmental Goal (MDG) 1a), less than a quarter of developing countries are on track to achieve the goal, of halving undernutrition (MDG 1c) by the year 2015. The global burden of undernutrition remains high with little evidence of change in many countries despite economic growth and still millions of people are faced with starvation and malnutrition with women and children contributing the major share. The progress has also been hampered by the global increase in food and oil prices, climate change, unprecedented draughts and increased number of countries affected by fragility, conflict, and emergencies. According to the World Bank, 33 countries fall in the fragile situations category and in addition, conflict and fragility also occurs at the subnational level within some strongly performing countries. The World Bank further estimated that the food price crisis in 2008 pushed as many as 130–155 million more people globally into extreme poverty with an increase in the number of children suffering permanent cognitive and physical injury due to malnutrition by 44 million [2].

In the year 2012, almost 6.6 million children under 5 years of age died worldwide [3] and undernutrition was an underlying cause in about 45% of these deaths (representing more than 3 million deaths each year) which includes stunting, severe wasting, deficiencies of vitamin A and zinc, and suboptimum breast-feeding. Fetal growth restriction and suboptimum breast-feeding together cause more than 1.3 million deaths or 19.4% of all deaths of children younger than 5 years. Good nutrition early in life is essential for children to attain their developmental potential; however, globally around 165 million children under the age of five suffer from stunting, 101 million are underweight and 52 million children are wasted [4] and approximately 90% of these live in just 36 countries with the highest prevalence in Southeast Asia and sub-Saharan Africa [3]. Prevalence of malnourished children has reduced and progress has been made in the past two decades but at the current rate of progress, the United Nations regional goals are unlikely to be met in all developing countries, and micronutrient deficiencies remain widespread among women and children globally. In a recent analysis of 79 countries with population-based surveys since the year 2000, stunting prevalence among children under the age of five was higher in the poorest quintile of households than in the richest quintile, higher in boys than in girls, and also higher in rural areas than urban areas [4, 5]. The problems of overweight and obesity among children are also growing and they have delirious consequences in low-income and middle-income countries (LMICs). In 2011, globally, an estimated 43 million (7%) children younger than 5 years were overweight (i.e., weight-for-height Z-scores (WHZ) greater than two Z scores), which is an increase from an estimated 28 million in 1990. This trend is expected to continue and reach a prevalence of 9.9% (64 million) in 2025 [4]. These changes are taking place around the world with prevalence increasing in high-income countries (HIC) and LMIC alike, as around 50% of these overweight children live in LMIC, with 29 million living in Africa and Asia.

Z. A. Bhutta (✉) · J. K. Das · R. A. Salam
Division of Women and Child Health, Department of Pediatrics, Aga Khan University, Karachi 74800, Pakistan
e-mail: zulfiqar.bhutta@sickkids.ca; zulfiqar.bhutta@aku.edu

J. K. Das
e-mail: jai.das@aku.edu

R. A. Salam
e-mail: rehana.salam@aku.edu

Z. A. Bhutta
Centre for Global Child Health, The Hospital for Sick Children, Toronto, ON M5G A04, Canada

Center of Excellence in Women and Child Health, Aga Khan University, Karachi 74800, Pakistan

© Springer International Publishing Switzerland 2016
S. Guandalini et al. (eds.), *Textbook of Pediatric Gastroenterology, Hepatology and Nutrition*,
DOI 10.1007/978-3-319-17169-2_44

In Africa, the prevalence has increased from 4% in 1990 to 7% in 2011, and it is expected to reach 11% in 2025. Many of these countries are said to have the double burden of malnutrition—continued stunting of growth and deficiencies of essential nutrients—along with the emerging issue of obesity. If trends are not reversed, increasing rates of childhood underweight and overweight will have vast implications, not only for future health-care expenditures but also for the overall development of nations.

Trends of Child Nutrition

Causes of childhood growth faltering are multifactorial, but fetal growth restriction might be an important contributor to stunting and wasting in children. A total of 32 million (27%) babies are born small for gestational age (SGA) annually and fetal growth restriction causes more than 800,000 deaths each year in the first month of life [4]. Stunting is a major indicator of childhood undernutrition, because it is highly prevalent in nearly all LMICs, and has important con-

sequences for health and development and there are voices to replace it with underweight as the main anthropometric indicator for children. The prevalence of stunting was 26% in children in LMICs in 2011, a decrease of 14% points since 1990 and the number of stunted children has also decreased globally, from 253 million in 1990 to 165 million in 2011, with an average annual rate of reduction of 2.1% [4] (Fig. 44.1). The World Health Assembly (WHA) called for a 40% reduction in the global number of children younger than 5 years who are stunted by 2025 (compared with the baseline of 2010) [6]. This aim would translate into a 3.9% reduction per year and imply reducing the number of stunted children from 171 million in 2010 to about 100 million in 2025. At the present rate of decline, stunting is expected to reduce to 127 million, a 25% reduction, in 2025. The decrease is substantial in Asia but the figures are not so encouraging for Africa. Wasting has a prevalence of 8% globally in 2011, which amounts to 52 million children; while 101 million children are underweight. There has been an 11% decrease from 58 million in 1990. The prevalence of severe wasting was 2.9%, affecting 19 million children and

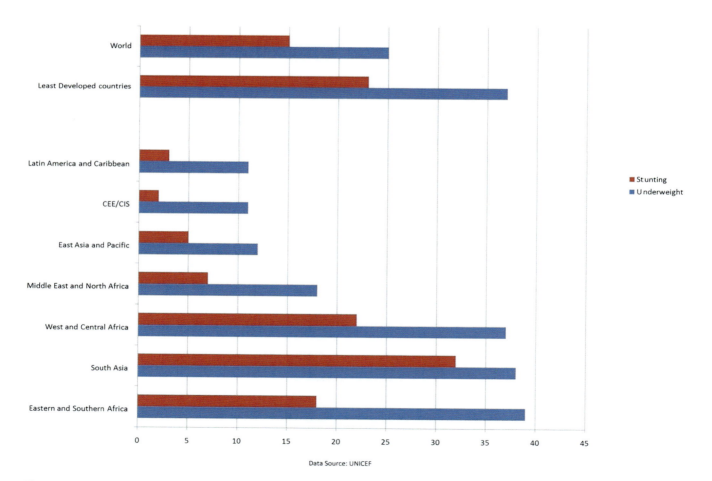

Fig. 44.1 Global prevalence of stunting and underweight in children under 5 years of age [3] *CEE* Central and Eastern Europe, *CIS* Commonwealth of Independent States

more than two thirds of the world's children with wasting live in Asia.

Deficiencies of essential vitamins and minerals are widespread and have substantial adverse effects on child survival and development. Deficiencies of vitamin A and zinc adversely affect child health and survival, and deficiencies of iodine and iron, together with stunting, contribute to children not reaching their developmental potential. Recent analysis support that all degrees of stunting, wasting, and underweight are associated with higher mortality, while undernutrition can be considered the cause of death in a synergistic association with infectious diseases; all anthropometric measures of under nutrition were associated with increased hazards of death from diarrhea, pneumonia, measles, and other infectious diseases, except for malaria [5]. Besides anthropometric measures, the association between micronutrient deficiencies such as vitamin A deficiency and increased risk of childhood infections and mortality is also well established [7]. Vitamin A deficiency increases the risk of severe diarrhea and thus diarrhea mortality but is not an important risk factor for the incidence of diarrhea or pneumonia, or for pneumonia-related mortality. Other micronutrient deficiencies such as zinc and iron deficiency are also recognized as widespread in developing countries and associated with increased risk of morbidity [8] and mortality [9]. According to World Health Organization (WHO) estimates, globally about 190 million preschool children and 19.1 million pregnant women are vitamin A deficient (that is, have serum retinol <0.70 μmol/l) [10]. Globally, 0.9 % or 5·17 million preschool age children are estimated to have night blindness and 33.3 % or 90 million to have subclinical vitamin A deficiency, defined as serum retinol concentration of less than 0·70 μmol/L. Vitamin A deficiency using night blindness prevalence can be defined as a global problem of public health importance [10, 11]. Approximately 100 million women of reproductive age (WRA) have iodine deficiency, and an estimated 82 % of pregnant women worldwide have inadequate zinc intakes to meet the normal needs of pregnancy [6]. Iron deficiency is widespread and globally about 1.62 billion people are anemic [12], and 18.1 % and 1.5 % children are anemic and severely anemic, respectively [4]. Suboptimal vitamin B6 and B12 status have also been observed in many developing countries [13].

Risk Factors

Risk factors for undernutrition range from distal broad national scale determinants to proximal individual specific and factors which effect at various age and periods of life. National socioeconomic and political determinants have a bigger impact and include political stability, economics, food security, poverty, and literacy, among others. Natural disasters including famine, floods, and other emergencies have detrimental effects. Maternal education is associated with improved child-care practices related to health and nutrition, and reduced odds of stunting, and better ability to access and benefit from existing facilities. Worrisome food insecurity is obviously critical, but a factor that is potentially even more important (especially for children with marginal intake) is the inability to absorb what they do take in because of repeated or persistent intestinal infections. Severe infectious diseases in early childhood, such as measles, diarrhea, pneumonia, meningitis, and malaria, can cause acute wasting and have long-term effects on linear growth. But the most important of these infections is diarrhea; hence, the need for understanding the impact and mechanisms of malnutrition and diarrhea, which forms a vicious cycle of enteric infections worsening and being worsened by malnutrition. Several recognized processes by which enteric infections cause malnutrition, range from well-recognized anorexia and increased catabolic or caloric demands to direct protein and nutrient loss or impaired absorptive function [14]. Modifiable risk factors for childhood obesity include maternal gestational diabetes; high levels of television viewing; low levels of physical activity; parents' inactivity; and high consumption of dietary fat, carbohydrate, and sweetened drinks, yet few interventions have been rigorously tested [15, 16].

Short- and Long-Term Consequences

Malnutrition leads to early physical growth failure, delayed motor, cognitive, and behavioral development, diminished immunity, and increased morbidity and mortality. These nutritional problems particularly flourish during periods in utero and during the first 3 years of life, and especially affect a large proportion of all children in LMICs. The determination of the child nutrition status starts even before birth, as maternal nutrition and health has a significant impact on child health. Neonates with fetal growth restriction are at substantially increased risk of being stunted at 24 months and of development of some types of noncommunicable diseases in adulthood. Those who survive the initial and direct consequences of malnutrition in early childhood grow up as adults but with disadvantages when compared to those who have been nutritionally adequate and enjoyed healthy environment in the initial crucial years of life. Undernutrition is strongly associated, with shorter adult height, less schooling, reduced economic productivity, and for women with lower offspring birth weight. Low birth weight (LBW) and undernutrition in childhood are risk factors for high glucose concentrations, blood pressure, and harmful lipid profiles [17]. The later consequences of childhood malnutrition include diminished intellectual performance, low work capacity, and increased risk of delivery complications [18]. Short-term consequences of intrauterine growth retardation (IUGR) involve metabolic, thermal, and hematological disturbances leading to morbidities, while long-term consequences include increased risk of developing metabolic syndrome and cardiovascular disease, systolic hypertension, obesity, insulin resistance, and diabetes type II in adulthood [19, 20]. There are no effective therapies to reverse IUGR and antenatal management is aimed at determining the ideal time and mode of delivery. In order to prevent complications associated with IUGR, it is important to first detect the condition and institute appropriate surveillance to assess fetal well-being coupled with suitable intervention in case of fetal distress. A study carried out in Chile shows that undernutrition at an early age may affect brain development, intellectual quotient, and scholastic achievement in school-age children [21]. This pattern is consistent with increased susceptibility to altered brain growth, particularly with the development of altered frontal lobe structures [22]. A recent review found evidence to support a weak association between LBW and later depression or psychological distress; however, the association may vary according to severity of symptoms or other factors [23]. Hence, the prevention of LBW and the promotion of adequate growth and development during early childhood will result in healthier, more productive adults. These undernourished children also show higher susceptibility to the effects of higher fats diets, lower fat oxidation, higher central fat, and higher body fat gain [24]. Without undermining the importance of the early period of life and even before that, evidence also suggests that improvements in child growth after early faltering may have significant benefits on schooling and cognitive achievement. Hence, interventions to improve the nutrition of preprimary and early primary school-age children also merit consideration [25]. Improvements in height may be obtained through adequate nutrient intake after the child's early years, but the brain is a notable exception because the first 2 years of life represent the period of maximum growth, and 70 % of adult brain weight has been attained by the end of the first year [26, 27].

Global Inclination Toward Undernutrition

There is growing recognition that interventions designed to improve human nutritional status have instrumental value in terms of economic outcomes. In many cases, productivity gains alone provide sufficient economic returns to justify investments using benefit and cost criteria. The often-held belief that nutrition programs are welfare interventions that divert resources which could be better used in other ways to raise national economies is incorrect. Most development agencies have revised their strategies to address undernutrition. The first Lancet nutrition series in 2008 [28] created a much desired stir and drew attention from relevant quarters.

One of the main drivers of the new international commitment is the Scaling Up Nutrition (SUN) Movement [29] and the second Lancet nutrition series [4]. National commitment in LMICs is growing, donor funding is rising, and civil society and the private sector are increasingly engaged. Nearly every major development agency has published a policy document on undernutrition, and donors have increased official development assistance to basic nutrition. Nutrition is now more prominent on the agendas of the UN, the G8 and G20, and supporting civil society. However, this progress has not yet translated into substantially improved outcomes globally. Improvements in nutrition still represent a massive unfinished agenda. The 165 million children with stunted growth have compromised cognitive, development, and physical capabilities, making yet another generation less productive than they would otherwise be [4]. Countries will not be able to break out of poverty and to sustain economic advances without ensuring their populations are adequately nourished. Undernutrition reduces a nation's economic advancement by at least 8 % because of direct productivity losses, losses via poorer cognition, and losses via reduced schooling [30].

Addressing the Burden of Undernutrition

To address this persistent burden of undernutrition in children and to the population at large, various strategies have been employed worldwide (Fig. 44.2). Among these include nutrition education, dietary modification, food provision/supplementation and agricultural interventions including bio-fortification, micronutrient supplementation and fortification. Apart from these direct nutritional interventions, programs to tackle the underlying causes of undernutrition including prevention and management of infections (like diarrhea and malaria) have also been initiated and implemented at various levels of care. Parallel programs have also been pursued to increase coverage and aid uptake of these primary interventions including provision of financial incentives at various levels, home gardening and community-based nutrition education, and mobilization programs. Although all these strategies have shown success and proved to be effective, a coherent, multifaceted, and integrated action which has the global consensus is lacking and several attempts at developing consensus is fraught with controversies and lack of coordination between various academic groups and development agencies.

There is a need for more emphasis on the crucial period from conception to a child's second birthday, the 1000 days in which good nutrition and healthy growth can have lasting benefits throughout life. Early years are important to intervene for various reasons as this is the period of maximum growth, immunological systems develop and mature during this time and they are less able to make their needs known

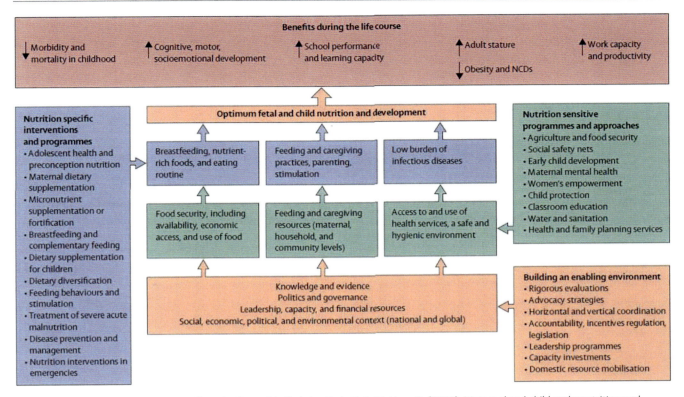

Source: Black RE, Victora CG, Walker SP, Bhutta ZA, Christian P, de Onis M, Uauy R. (2013). Maternal and child undernutrition and overweight in low-income and middle-income countries. The Lancet, 382(9890), 427-451.

Fig. 44.2 Conceptual framework for achieving optimal child nutrition. (Reprinted from Ref. [4], with permission from Elsevier) *NCDs* noncommunicable diseases

and are more vulnerable to the effects of poor parenting. Intervening early in pregnancy and even before conception may be beneficial, as many women do not access nutrition-promoting services until later in pregnancy, so it is important to ensure that women enter pregnancy in a state of optimum nutrition. The emerging platforms for adolescent health and nutrition might offer opportunities for enhanced benefits [31]. There is a growing interest in adolescent health as an entry point to improve the health of women and children, especially as an estimated 10 million girls younger than 18 years are married each year [32].

Broader-Scale Interventions

There is a need for building an enabling environment to support interventions and programs to enhance growth and development. Important determinants of undernutrition to address include poverty, food insecurity, illiteracy, and scarcity of access to adequate care which in turn shape economic and social conditions, national and global contexts, capacity, resources, and governance. These could be addressed through investments in agriculture, social safety nets, early child development, and schooling. Social safety nets provide

cash and food transfers to a billion poor people and reduce poverty. They also have an important role in mitigation of the negative effects of global changes, conflicts, and shocks by protecting income, food security, and diet quality [33]. Safety net programs can be more effective, but geographic targeting and other investments to strengthen safety nets are necessary to ensure that fewer people are affected by future crises. Combination of early child development and nutrition interventions makes sense biologically and programmatically, and evidence from mostly small-scale programs suggests additive or synergistic effects on child development and in some cases on nutrition outcomes [33]. Parental schooling is consistently associated with improved nutrition outcomes and schools provide an opportunity, so far largely untapped, to include nutrition in school curricula for prevention and treatment of undernutrition or obesity. School feeding programs is another avenue to improve nutrition at a later life. Recent evidence from in-depth studies argue that while school feeding programs can influence the education of school children and, to a lesser degree, augment nutrition for families of beneficiaries, they are best viewed as transfer programs that can provide a social safety net and help promote human capital investments [34]. Arguably, direct food distribution, including that of ready-to-use therapeutic food

(RUTF), may be part of the overall strategy. Even if such programs are too expensive for sustainable widespread use in the prevention of malnutrition, scalable food distribution programs may be cost-effective to address the heightened risk of malnutrition following weather-related shocks [35]. Community delivery platforms for nutrition education and promotion, integrated management of childhood illness, school-based delivery platforms, and child health days are other possible channels. Innovative delivery strategies, especially community-based delivery platforms are promising for scaling up coverage of nutrition interventions and have the potential to reach poor and difficult to access populations through communication and outreach strategies.

Targeted agricultural programs have an important role in support of livelihoods, food security, diet quality, and women's empowerment, and complement global efforts to stimulate agricultural productivity and thus increase producer incomes while protecting consumers from high food prices [33]. Agricultural interventions including home and school gardening have the potential and a review on agricultural interventions to improve nutritional status of children concluded that home gardening interventions had a positive effect on the production of the agricultural goods and consumption of food rich in protein and micronutrients. However, the impacts on iron absorption and anthropometric indices remained inconclusive [36]. Evidence also suggests that targeted agricultural programs are more successful when they incorporate strong behavior change communications strategies and a gender-equity focus.

Food fortification is one of the strategies that has been used safely and effectively to prevent vitamin and mineral deficiencies. A review of multiple micronutrient (MMN) fortification in children showed an increase in hemoglobin levels and 57% reduced risk of anemia. Fortification is also associated with increased vitamin A serum levels. A review on mass salt fortification with vitamin A and iodine concluded that the fortified and iodized salt can improve the iodine status [37]. Zinc and Vitamin D fortification have also been effective to varying extent [38]. Micronutrient fortified milk and cereal products have also proven as a complementing strategy to improve health problems of children in developing countries [39]. A recent review has identified it as an effective and potential strategy although more rigorous evidence is required especially from LMIC [40]. Bio-fortification is a relatively new strategy to improve iron, zinc, and vitamin A status in low-income populations. It is the use of conventional breeding techniques and biotechnology to improve the micronutrient quality of staple crops. A review on bio-fortification concluded that it has the potential to contribute to increased micronutrient intakes and improve micronutrient status; however, this domain requires further research [41].

Specific Interventions

Many nutrition interventions have been successfully implemented at scale, and the evidence base for effective interventions and delivery strategies has grown (Table 44.1). At the same time, coverage rates for other interventions are either poor or nonexistent.

Micronutrient supplementation is the most widely practiced intervention to prevent and manage single or MMN deficiencies. Various programs are in place to address these

Table 44.1 Interventions to reduce malnutrition in women and children

Women	Children
Micronutrient supplementation	
Iron/iron-folate supplementation	Iron supplementation
Maternal calcium supplementation	Vitamin A supplementation
Maternal multiple micronutrient (MMN) supplementation	Zinc supplementation
	MMN supplementation
Maternal balanced energy protein supplementation	Breast-feeding
	Complementary/supplementary feeding
Micronutrient fortification	
Bio-fortification	
Agricultural interventions	
Disease prevention	
WASH interventions	
Deworming	
Diarrhea prevention and management	
Malaria prevention and treatment	
Delivery strategies	
Integrated management of childhood illnesses (IMCI), child health days, school feeding programs, community platforms	
WASH water, sanitation, and hygiene	

micronutrient deficiencies through supplementation and evidence from evidence-based systematic reviews suggests that among pregnant women, daily iron supplementation is associated with a 69% reduction in incidence of anemia at term, 66% reduction in iron-deficiency anemia at term, 20% reduction in incidence of LBW and improved birth weight [42]. Calcium supplementation during pregnancy is associated with a 52% reduction in the incidence of preeclampsia and 24% reduction preterm birth with an increase in birth weight of 85 g [43]. MMN supplementation during pregnancy significantly reduces the incidence of LBW infants by 11% and SGA by 13% [44]. A review [45] shows that providing pregnant females with balanced energy and protein (BEP) supplementation results in a significant reduction of 34% in the risk of giving birth to SGA infants and 38% reduction in stillbirth and results in an increased birth weight. These effects were more pronounced in malnourished women when compared to adequately nourished women.

Evidence of micronutrient supplementation in children indicates that vitamin A supplementation (VAS) reduces all-cause mortality and diarrhea specific mortality by 24 and 28% respectively [46]. VAS also reduced incidence of diarrhea by 15% and measles morbidity by 50%; however, there are no significant effects on the incidence of respiratory disease. Iron supplementation in children results in a 49% lower risk of anemia and a 74% lower risk of iron deficiency with higher serum hemoglobin and ferritin concentration, while nonsignificant impacts were observed for height for age and weight for age [47]. Zinc supplementation in a dose of 10 mg zinc/day for 24 weeks could lead to a net gain in height of 0.37 ($\pm$ 0.25) [48] and reduce the incidence of diarrhea by 13% and pneumonia morbidity by 19% while has nonsignificant effects on mortality [49]. MMN supplementation with three or more micronutrients in children showed small effect sizes for length/height and weight with limited evidence for an impact on outcomes such as morbidity and cognitive function [50].

In children, improved feeding in the early infancy and the initial years of life hold an utmost importance and breast-feeding and complementary feeding are such strategies which ensure optimum nutrition during this vital phase of growth and development. Breast-feeding practices are far from optimum, despite improvements in some countries. Suboptimum breast-feeding results in an increased risk for mortality in the first 2 years of life and results in 800,000 deaths annually [4], poor nutrition often coincides with other developmental risks, in particular inadequate stimulation during early childhood. Breast milk provides numerous immunologic, psychologic, social, economic, and environmental benefits, and it is a natural first food and ideal nutrition for the newborn [51]. Breast-feeding is therefore recommended as the optimal strategy for feeding newborns and young infants. Strategies to improve the uptake of breast-feeding are essential and evidence suggests that breast-feeding education and promotion interventions are effective in improving breast-feeding rates and evidence suggests that these interventions are associated with improved exclusive breast-feeding (EBF)rates of 1 and 6 months with increase in HIC and LMIC [52].

Complementary feeding for infants refers to the timely introduction of safe and nutritional foods in addition to breast-feeding, that is, clean and nutritionally rich additional foods introduced at about 6 months of infant age [53]. These foods are typically provided to children from 6 to 24 months of age [53]. Multiple complementary nutrition interventions targeted to improve nutritional status of children have also been reviewed. These include complementary and supplementary feeding programs with or without nutrition education. Dewey 2008 [54] reviewed the effectiveness and efficacy of complementary feeding interventions in children aged 6–24 months in developing countries. It indicated that provision of complementary food can have a significant impact on growth under well-controlled situations. Complementary food combined with maternal education improved weight and linear growth. A recent review [55], looking at the impact of supplementary feeding that covered energy protein supplementation, found a statistically significant difference of effect for length during the intervention in children aged less than 12 years of age.

WHO recommends that all school children should be treated at regular intervals with deworming drugs in helminthic prevalent areas. A recent review [56] shows that treating children after screening for worms showed that a single dose of deworming drugs may increase weight and hemoglobin. Administration of a single dose of antihelminthics in the second trimester of pregnancy failed to show a statistically significant impact on maternal anemia or LBW, preterm births, and perinatal mortality. Effective interventions to prevent malaria morbidity and mortality include insecticide-treated mosquito nets (ITNs), indoor-residual spraying (IRS) and intermittent preventive therapy (IPTc). A review [57] concludes that antimalarials when given to prevent malaria in pregnant women increased mean birth weight and reduce the incidence of LBW by 43% and severe antenatal anemia by 38% [57]. The impact of therapeutic zinc supplementation for the management of diarrhea reduces all-cause mortality by 46% and diarrhea-related hospitalization by 23% [58].

Most of the interventions previously discussed should be implemented to prevent the development of severe acute malnutrition (SAM). Where markets are fragmented or food access is constrained, appropriate food supplements might be considered. Available evidence shows some positive effects with the use of RUTF compared with standard care for the treatment of SAM in community settings. An emphasis not only on the choice of commodities, but also on the quality of program design and implementation is crucial to improvement of outcomes for children with SAM, as is the research to fill information gaps, such as optimum treatment methods and approaches for treatment of breast-fed infants younger than 6 months [31].

A recent review using Lives Saved Tool modeled ten nutrition-specific interventions across the lifecycle to address undernutrition [31]. The interventions included: periconceptual folic acid supplementation, maternal BEP supplementation, maternal calcium supplementation, MMN supplementation in pregnancy, promotion of breast-feeding, appropriate complementary feeding, vitamin A, and preventive zinc supplementation in children aged 6–59 months, management of SAM and management of moderate acute malnutrition. If these ten proven nutrition-specific interventions were scaled-up from existing population coverage to 90 %, an estimated 900,000 lives could be saved in 34 high nutrition-burden countries (where 90 % of the world's stunted children live) and the prevalence of stunting could be reduced by 20 % and that of severe wasting by 60 %. This would reduce the number of children with stunted growth and development by 33 million. On top of existing trends, this improvement would comfortably reach the WHA targets for 2025.

Way Forward

This existing evidence is essential to ensure that future investments are directed toward proven pathways to outcomes. Beyond this evidence, service providers, governments, donors, and the private sector need strong national monitoring and assessment platforms to hold them accountable for the quality and effectiveness of their investments in nutrition [59]. There is a need for the availability of timely and credible nutrition data, presented in accessible ways, can help governments and other actors to be responsive to challenging circumstances, and help civil society organizations to hold them accountable for the effectiveness of their interventions [59]. Advances in health management information systems and the growing availability of newer technologies can help with the real-time monitoring of nutrition outcomes and program coverage and quality, and should be researched.

There is also a need for greater priority for national nutrition programs, stronger integration with health programs, enhanced intersectoral approaches, and more focus and coordination in the global nutrition system of international agencies, donors, academia, civil society, and the private sector. There could also be a potential integration of nutrition with maternal, newborn, and child health interventions, helping to achieve reductions in inequities. Nutrition is crucial to both individual and national development as good nutrition is a fundamental driver of a wide range of development goals. The post-2015 sustainable development agenda must put addressing all forms of malnutrition at the top of its goals.

References

1. FAO. The State of Food Insecurity in the World, Economic growth is necessary but not sufficient to accelerate reduction of hunger and malnutrition, Food and Agriculture Organization of the United Nations, Rome; 2012. http://www.fao.org/docrep/016/i3027e/i3027e.pdf. Accessed 4 Aug 2014.
2. Wodon Q, Zaman H. Rising food prices in sub-saharan Africa: poverty impact and policy responses. Washington, DC: World Bank; 2008. © World Bank. https://openknowledge.worldbank.com/handle/10986/6938. Accessed 4 Aug 2014.
3. UNICEF. Levels & trends in child mortality, estimates developed by the UN Inter-agency Group for Child Mortality Estimation. New York: UNICEF; 2013. http://www.childinfo.org/files/Child_Mortality_Report_2013.pdf. Accessed 4 Aug 2014.
4. Black RE, Victora CG, Walker SP, Bhutta ZA, Christian P, de Onis M, Uauy R. Maternal and child undernutrition and overweight in low-income and middle-income countries. Lancet 2013;382(9890):427–51.
5. Fotso JC. Child health inequities in developing countries: differences across urban and rural areas. Int J Equity Health. 5(2013):10.
6. WHO. Proposed global targets for maternal, infant and young child nutrition. WHO discussion paper. Geneva: World Health Organization; 2012. http://www.who.int/nutrition/events/2012_proposed_globaltargets_backgroundpaper.pdf?ua=1. Accessed 15 Aug 2014.
7. Beaton GH, Martorell R, Aronson KA, Edmonston B, McCabe G, Ross AC, Harvey B. Vitamin A supplementation and child morbidity and mortality in developing countries. Food Nutr Bull. 1994;5:282–9.
8. Black R. Micronutrient deficiency: an underlying cause of morbidity and mortality. Bull World Health Organ. 2003;81(2):79.
9. Guilbert JJ. The world health report 2002-reducing risks, promoting healthy life. Educ Health (Abingdon). 2003;16(2):230.
10. WHO. Global prevalence of vitamin A deficiency in populations at risk 1995–2005. WHO global database on vitamin A deficiency. Geneva: World Health Organization; 2009.
11. Jeghers H. Night blindness as a criterion of vitamin A deficiency: review of the literature with preliminary observations of the degree and prevalence of vitamin A deficiency among adults in both health and disease. Ann Intern Med. 1937;10(9):1304–34.
12. Benoist B, McLean E, Egll I, Cogswell M. Worldwide prevalence of anaemia 1993–2005: WHO global database on anaemia. Geneva: World Health Organization; 2008.
13. McLean E, De Benoist B, Allen LH. Review of the magnitude of folate and vitamin B12 deficiencies worldwide. Food Nutr Bull. 2008; 29 Suppl 1:38–51.
14. Guerrant RL, Oriá RB, Moore SR, Oriá MO, Lima AA. Malnutrition as an enteric infectious disease with long-term effects on child development. Nutr Rev. 2008;66(9):487–505.
15. Kipping RR, Jago R, Lawlor DA. Obesity in children. Part 1: epidemiology, measurement, risk factors, and screening. BMJ 2008;337:a1824.
16. Han JC, Lawlor DA, Kimm SY. Childhood obesity. Lancet 2010;375:1737–48.
17. Victora CG, Adair L, Fall C, Hallal PC, Martorell R, Richter L, Sachdev HS. Maternal and child undernutrition: consequences for adult health and human capital. Lancet 2008;371(9609):340–57.
18. Martorell R. The nature of child malnutrition and its long-term implications. Food Nutr Bull. 1999;20(3):288–92.
19. Chan PYL, Morris JM, Leslie GI, Kelly PJ, Gallery EDM. The long-term effects of prematurity and intrauterine growth restriction on cardiovascular, renal, and metabolic function. Int J Pediatr. 2010;2010:1–10.
20. Zanardo V, Visentin S, Trevisanuto D, Bertin M, Cavallin F, Cosmi E. Fetal aortic wall thickness: a marker of hypertension in IUGR children & quest. Hypertens Res. 2013;36(5):440–3.

21. Ivanovic DM, Leiva BP, Perez HT, Inzunza NB, AlmagiÃ AF, Toro TD, Bosch EO. Long-term effects of severe undernutrition during the first year of life on brain development and learning in Chilean high-school graduates. Nutrition 2000;16(11):1056–63.

22. Geva R, Eshel R, Leitner Y, Valevski AF, Harel S. Neuropsychological outcome of children with intrauterine growth restriction: a 9-year prospective study. Pediatrics 2006;118(1):91–100.

23. Wojcik W, Lee W, Colman I, Hardy R, Hotopf M. Foetal origins of depression? A systematic review and meta-analysis of low birth weight and later depression. Psychol Med. 2013;43(01):1–12.

24. Sawaya AL, Martins PA, Grillo LP, Florencio TT. Long-term effects of early malnutrition on body weight regulation. Nutr Rev. 2004;62(s2):S127–33.

25. Crookston BT, Schott W, Cueto S, Dearden KA, Engle P, Georgiadis A, Behrman JR. Post-infancy growth, schooling, and cognitive achievement: Young Lives. Am J Clin Nutr. 2013;98(6):1555–63.

26. Stoch MB, Smythe PM. The effect of undernutrition during infancy on subsequent brain growth and intellectual development. S Afr Med J. 1967;41:1027.

27. Ivanovic D. Does undernutrition during infancy inhibit brain growth and subsequent intellectual development? Comments. Nutrition 1996;12:568.

28. Black RE, Allen LH, Bhutta ZA, Caulfield LE, De Onis M, Ezzati M, Rivera J, The Maternal and Child Undernutrition Study Group. Maternal and child undernutrition: global and regional exposures and health consequences. Lancet 2008;371:243–60.

29. Scaling Up Nutrition. A framework for action. http://www.unsc-norg/files/Announcements/Scaling_Up_Nutrition-A_Framework_for_Actionpdf. Accessed 25 Aug 2014.

30. Horton S, Steckel R. Global economic losses attributable to malnutrition 1990–2000 and projections to 2050. In: Lomborg B, editor. How much have global problems cost the world? Cambridge: Cambridge University Press; 2013.

31. Bhutta ZA, Das JK, Rizvi A, Gaffey MF, Walker N, Horton S, Black RE. Evidence-based interventions for improvement of maternal and child nutrition: what can be done and at what cost? Lancet 2013;382(9890):452–77.

32. WHO. The partnership for maternal, newborn and child health. Reaching child brides; 2012. http://www.who.int/pmnch/topics/part_publications/knowledge_summary_22_reaching_child_brides/en/. Accessed 25 Aug 2014.

33. Ruel MT, Alderman H, The Maternal and Child Nutrition Study Group. Nutrition-sensitive interventions and programmes: how can they help to accelerate progress in improving maternal and child nutrition. Lancet 2013;382(9891):536–51.

34. Alderman H, Bundy D. School feeding programs and development: are we framing the question correctly? World Bank Res Obs. 2012;27(2):204–21.

35. Alderman H. Safety nets can help address the risks to nutrition from increasing climate variability. J Nutr. 2010;140(1):148S–152S.

36. Masset E, Haddad L, Cornelius A, Isaza-Castro J. Effectiveness of agricultural interventions that aim to improve nutritional status of children: systematic review. BMJ 2011;344:d8222.

37. Jiang T, Xue Q. Fortified salt for preventing iodine deficiency disorders: a systematic review. Chin J Evid-Based Med. 2010;10(7):857–61.

38. Das JK, Kumar R, Salam RA, Bhutta ZA. Systematic review of Zinc fortification trials. Ann Nutr Metabol. 62 Suppl 1:44–56.

39. Eichler K, Wieser S, Rüthemann I, Brügger U. Effects of micronutrient fortified milk and cereal food for infants and children: a systematic review. BMC Public Health. 2012;12(1):506.

40. Das JK, Salam RA, Kumar R, Bhutta ZA. Micronutrient fortification of food and its impact on woman and child health: a systematic review. Syst Rev. 2013;2(1):67.

41. Hotz C, McClafferty B. From harvest to health: challenges for developing biofortified staple foods and determining their impact on micronutrient status. Food Nutr Bull. 2007;28 Suppl 2:271S–9S.

42. Imdad A, Bhutta ZA. Routine Iron/Folate supplementation during pregnancy: effect on maternal anaemia and birth outcomes. Paediatr Perinat Epidemiol. 2012;26(s1):168–77.

43. Imdad A, Bhutta ZA. Effects of calcium supplementation during pregnancy on maternal, fetal and birth outcomes. Paediatr Perinat Epidemiol. 2012;26(s1):138–52.

44. Haider BA, Bhutta ZA. Multiple-micronutrient supplementation for women during pregnancy. Cochrane Database Syst Rev. 2012;11:CD004905. doi:10.1002/14651858.

45. Imdad A, Bhutta ZA. Effect of balanced protein energy supplementation during pregnancy on birth outcomes. BMC Public Health. 2011;11 Suppl 3:S17.

46. Imdad A, Herzer K, Mayo-Wilson E, Yakoob MY, Bhutta ZA. Vitamin A supplementation for preventing morbidity and mortality in children from 6 months to 5 years of age. Cochrane Database Syst Rev. 2010;12:CD008524. doi:10.1002/14651858.

47. De-Regil LM, Jefferds MED, Sylvetsky AC, Dowswell T. Intermittent iron supplementation for improving nutrition and development in children under 12 years of age. Cochrane Database Syst Rev. 2011(12):CD009085.

48. Imdad A, Bhutta ZA. Effect of preventive zinc supplementation on linear growth in children under 5 years of age in developing countries: a meta-analysis of studies for input to the lives saved tool. BMC Public Health. 2011;11 Suppl 3:S22.

49. Yakoob MY, Theodoratou E, Jabeen A, Imdad A, Eisele TP, Ferguson J, Bhutta ZA. Preventive zinc supplementation in developing countries: impact on mortality and morbidity due to diarrhea, pneumonia and malaria. BMC Public Health. 2011;11 Suppl 3:S23.

50. Christian P, Tielsch JM. Evidence for multiple micronutrient effects based on randomized controlled trials and meta-analyses in developing countries. J Nutr. 2011;142(1):173S–7S.

51. Dewey KG, Heinig MJ, Nommsen LA, Peerson JM, Lönnerdal B. Growth of breast-fed and formula-fed infants from 0 to 18 months: the DARLING study. Pediatrics 1992;89(6):1035–41.

52. Haroon S, Das JK, Salam RA, Imdad A, Bhutta ZA. Breastfeeding promotion interventions and breastfeeding practices: a systematic review. BMC Public Health. 2013;13(3):1–18.

53. WHO. Report of informal meeting to review and develop indicators for complementary feeding. Washington, DC: World Health Organization; 2002.

54. Dewey KG, Adu-Afarwuah S. Systematic review of the efficacy and effectiveness of complementary feeding interventions in developing countries. Matern Child Nutr. 2008;4 Suppl 1:24–85.

55. Sguassero Y, de Onis M, Bonotti AM, Carroli G. Community-based supplementary feeding for promoting the growth of children under five years of age in low and middle income countries. Cochrane Database Syst Rev. 2012;6:CD005039. doi:10.1002/14651858.

56. Taylor-Robinson DC, Jones AP, Garner P. Deworming drugs for treating soil-transmitted intestinal worms in children: effects on growth and school performance. Cochrane Database Syst Rev. 2007;4:CD000371. doi:10.1002/14651858.

57. Garner P, Gülmezoglu AM. Drugs for preventing malaria in pregnant women. Cochrane Database Syst Rev. 2006;4:CD000169. doi:10.1002/14651858.

58. Walker CLF, Black RE. Zinc for the treatment of diarrhoea: effect on diarrhoea morbidity, mortality and incidence of future episodes. Int J Epidemiol. 2010;39 Suppl 1:i63–9.

59. Gillespie S, Haddad L, Mannar V, Menon P, Nisbettt N, The Maternal and Child Nutrition Study Group. The politics of reducing malnutrition: building commitment and accelerating progress. Lancet 2013. 382(9891):552–69.

Probiotics

45

Yvan Vandenplas, Geert Huys and Georges Daube

Introduction

The joint Food and Agriculture Organization (FAO) and World Health Organization (WHO) Expert Consultation on Evaluation of Health and Nutritional Properties of Probiotics in Food including Powder Milk with Live Lactic Acid Bacteria defined probiotics as: "Live microorganisms which when administered in adequate amounts confer a health benefit on the host" (FAO/WHO 2001). In 2002 (London, Canada), a joint FAO/WHO Working Group generated guidelines for the evaluation of probiotics in food. The minimum requirements needed for probiotic status include:

- The assessment of strain identity (genus, species, strain level)
- In vitro tests to screen potential probiotics: e.g., resistance to gastric acidity, bile acid, and digestive enzymes, antimicrobial activity against potentially pathogenic bacteria, etc.
- Assessment of safety: requirements for proof that a probiotic strain is safe and without contamination in its delivery form
- In vivo studies for substantiation of health effects in the target host

Following the FAO/WHO definition, the International Life Science Institute (ILSI 2002) and the European Food and Feed Cultures Association (EFFCA 2003) have launched similar definitions for a probiotic: "a live microbial food ingredient that, when taken up in adequate amounts, confers health benefits on the consumers" and "live microorganisms which, when ingested or locally applied in sufficient numbers, provide the consumer with one or more proven health benefits." The definition implies de facto that probiotic ingestion provides benefits for host health.

The science related to probiotics is recent and thus in constant evolution. Probiotics used in food, or supplied as dietary supplement, or when registered as medication should not only be capable of surviving passage through the digestive tract by exhibiting acid and bile survival, but also have the capability to proliferate in the gut. Probiotics must be able to exert their benefits on the host through growth and/or activity in the human body. Topical or local application of probiotics is also proposed in view of the recent evolution of scientific data. Therefore, the ability to remain viable and effective at the target site should be studied and confirmed for each strain, or even better for each commercialized product. Clinical studies should be performed with the commercialized product and not with "the strain." However, lack of protection contributes to the fact that some companies refuse to deliver information on the specific strains in their product [1]. Recent literature has shown that one of the mechanisms of action of probiotics involves stimulation of the immune system. Whether the probiotics need to be "live" to induce immune modulation can be questioned. Therefore, the definition may have to be revised in the future.

According to the European Community, health claims should only be authorized for use in the European Community after a scientific assessment of the highest possible standard has been carried out by the Panel on Dietetic Products, Nutrition and Allergies (NDA) of the European Food Safety Authority (EFSA; regulation (EC) No. 1924/2006). Key questions which are addressed by the EFSA NDA panel are:

Y. Vandenplas (✉)
Department of Pediatrics, UZ Brussel, Vrije Universiteit Brussel, Laarbeeklaan 101, Brussels 1090, Belgium
e-mail: yvan.vandenplas@uzbrussel.be

G. Huys
Laboratory of Microbiology & BCCM/LMG Bacteria Collection, Faculty of Sciences, Ghent University, Ghent, Belgium

G. Daube
Département des Sciences des Denrées alimentaires, Faculté de Médecine vétérinaire, Université de Liège, Liège, Belgium

© Springer International Publishing Switzerland 2016
S. Guandalini et al. (eds.), *Textbook of Pediatric Gastroenterology, Hepatology and Nutrition*,
DOI 10.1007/978-3-319-17169-2_45

- Is the food/constituent sufficiently defined and characterized?
- Is the claimed effect sufficiently defined, and is it a beneficial physiological effect?
- Have pertinent human studies been presented to substantiate the claim?

The EFSA recommendations are an important step forward in trying to bring claims for probiotics, food supplements and medication closer together. However, companies discovered side-ways to avoid EFSA-restrictions. Some of the food supplements are in the process of registration as "medical device," which legislation allows claims without providing hard scientific evidence. Moreover, production requirements on quality control and safety still differ substantially between food supplements and medication, putting medication in a disadvantageous situation.

Official controls by national authorities are performed to ensure verification of compliance with food law. Apart from the risk of using unauthorized strains, product mislabeling is a known problem, partly because of the use of phenotyping or genotyping methods with a lack of discriminative power [2]. In addition to official controls, private controls by food producing companies are important in the frame of protection of patented strains and industrial property rights.

In their "Guidelines for the Evaluation of Probiotics in Food" document, the FAO/WHO Working Group (2002) recommends that the following information should be described on the label of probiotic products:

- Genus, species, and strain designation. Strain designation should not mislead consumers about the functionality of the strain
- Minimum viable numbers of each probiotic strain at the end of the shelf-life
- The suggested serving size must deliver the effective dose of probiotics related to the health claim
- Health claim(s)
- Proper storage conditions
- Corporate contact details for consumer information

In most countries, only general health claims are currently allowed on foods containing probiotics. The FAO/WHO Working Group (2002) recommended that specific health claims on foods be allowed relating to the use of probiotics, where sufficient scientific evidence is available. Such specific health claims should be permitted on the label and promotional material. For example, a specific claim that states that a probiotic "reduces the incidence and severity of rotavirus diarrhea in infants" would be more informative to the consumer than a general claim that states "improves gut health." It is recommended that it be the responsibility of the product manufacturer that an independent third party review

by scientific experts in the field be conducted to establish that health claims are truthful and not misleading.

In line with the suggestions of the FAO/WHO Working Group (2002), on December 20, 2006, the European Parliament and the Council published a novel regulation (No. 1924/2006) on "Nutrition and Health Claims Made on Foods" (http://eur-lex.europa.eu/LexUriServ/LexUriServ.do?uri=CELEX:32006R1924R%2801%29:EN:NOT). This regulation applies to all nutritional and health claims relating to all types of food intended for final consumers, thus also including probiotic products brought to the market with a health claim. The regulation aims to harmonize the nutrition and health claims at European level in order to better protect consumers, including commercial communications (labeling, presentation, and promotional campaigns) and trademarks and other brand names which may be construed as nutrition or health claims.

Functional Effect of Probiotics

The definition "probiotics are live microorganisms which when administered in adequate amounts confer a health benefit on the host" only generalizes the probiotic functionality as conferring a health benefit to the host. Hence, this definition basically entails that there must be a measurable physiological benefit to the host who uses the probiotic product. In addition, it is not specified that the probiotic strain must be provided through oral delivery, nor are there specific requirements regarding the mode of action. The latter also entails that survival of the probiotic microorganisms throughout the gastrointestinal (GI) tract is not a prerequisite for recognition of probiotic effects. For example, the delivery of lactase through administration of live *Streptococcus (Strepto.) thermophilus* to the small intestine can be considered as a probiotic activity, although the *Strepto.* strain does not survive the digestive tract [3].

When considering probiotic functionality, the abovementioned definition of probiotics is to be interpreted in a very broad way. This broad functionality definition complicates the process of functional characterization of probiotics. The use of probiotics may target several body sites (mouth, GI tract, respiratory tract, urinary tract, skin, vagina, etc.), and its application can also target specific human subpopulations: healthy individuals, children, elderly people, diseased persons, immune-compromised and genetically predisposed individuals, etc. There is an extremely diverse range of potential biological effects and new functional activities are constantly being explored. While some models are perfectly suited for studying the colonization potency of probiotics, other models need to be applied for assessing their immune-modulating potential, their resilience against pathogen invasion of the GI tract or their anti-inflammatory properties.

Functional Characterization of Probiotics

Target Sites

Probiotic products have been developed to improve physiological conditions at different body sites. While the GI tract is the most important target for the majority of probiotic applications, other body sites such as the mouth, the uro-genital tract, and the skin are also considered. Probiotics may play an important in oral medicine and dentistry [4, 5].

Probiotics are also considered for abating and preventing infections of the reproductive and urinary tract [6–9]. With regard to skin applications, probiotics may be taken up orally to induce an immune response that has systemic effects, for example, for controlling skin inflammation [10] and dermatological diseases in general [11]. Probiotics have also been applied to protection for respiratory tract infections. *Lactobacillus (L.) rhamnosus* GG prevents respiratory tract infections besides the conventional protection against GI infections [12]. There is a plethora of probiotic strains and applications available with the GI tract as target site. Such applications aim at a wide diversity of health benefits such as decreasing pathogen colonization, synthesis of vitamins, optimizing intestinal transit, alleviation of lactose intolerance, reduction of bloating, immune-modulatory effects and many others.

Delivery Mode

With the aim of obtaining health benefits, probiotic strains often require a specific matrix to guarantee optimal strain survival along the GI tract. For instance, probiotics have recently been formulated in a chocolate matrix, which resulted in a more optimal survival of the probiotic strains in comparison with conventional probiotic formulation methods [13]. Other methods include the introduction of probiotics in more conventional products such as milk [14], kefir [15] and several yoghurts or more specific matrices such as cereals, cheese, even sausages, and cookies. Obviously, many probiotics are introduced for commercial reasons to obtain a better product placement or to integrate the food product into the probiotic market. Examples of these are fruit juices, ice creams, candies, granola bars, etc.

Besides the incorporation of probiotics in food products, probiotic strains are also provided as food supplement, often with the aim of tackling specific health problems. Probiotics food supplements (e.g., *L. rhamnosus* GG, *L. reuteri*) and medication (e.g., *Saccharomyces (S.) boulardii*) have almost become standard in the treatment of pediatric gastroenteritis. Many infant formula milk powders exist in which probiotics have been formulated, both to prevent and alleviate diarrhea.

A special example of designer strains is the application of genetically modified microorganisms as probiotic. *Lactococcus (Lc.) lactis* strains were developed that secrete IL-10 or immunomodulatory *Yersinia* LcrV protein to treat colitis in mouse models [16, 17]. Such approach is currently being considered for the treatment of oral mucositis (high incidence in head/neck cancer patients receiving radiotherapy) with a human trefoil factor 1-secreting *Lc. lactis*. A molecular basis of the therapeutic applications and the chemopreventive activities of certain probiotic metabolites, with emphasis on the interaction between these metabolites and the molecular signaling cascades are considered to be epigenetic targets in preventing colon cancer [18].

Finally, probiotic delivery not only pertains to the food or pharmaceutical environment in which the probiotic is formulated. Specific ointments and nasal sprays are developed [19]. Nowadays, even the introduction of probiotics in mattresses (http://www.purotex.com) and cleaning agents (http://www.naturalhouse.com; http://www.optibacprobiotics.co.uk; http://www.chrisal.com) is gaining momentum for an optimized hygienic control. The latter illustrates the necessity to broaden the control on claims larger than food supplements and food. If Europe installs "Authorities" (EFSA) to control claims for foods and food supplements, health-claims for non-food related products should be equally controlled.

Strain Survival

Health benefits are in many cases only obtained when a probiotic strain reaches the target site in a metabolically active state and in sufficient numbers. For oral delivery, probiotic microorganisms must survive the different physicochemical, enzymatic, and microbial stresses throughout the GI transit.

Firstly, microorganisms have to cross the acidic environment from the stomach. In addition, the absence or presence of a food matrix significantly determines the pH profile to which the probiotic strain is subjected. While the initial pH buffering effect from food may subject the probiotic strain to initially less stringent acidic conditions, a longer digestion time in the stomach under fed conditions may expose part of the dosed probiotic to acidic conditions for a longer time. Many probiotic microorganisms have been selected for their higher resilience against such acidic conditions, and new methodologies are available to allow encapsulation of probiotic strains in that purpose [20].

A second stress component is the presence of bile salts that elicit membrane-compromising properties towards microorganisms, due to their amphiphylic character. A particular functional characteristic of microorganisms is their ability to deal with bile salt stress via bile salt hydrolase. Bile salt hydrolase bacteria typically cleave the glycine or taurine moiety from conjugated bile salts, rendering the latter less bacteriostatic. This feature is of particular importance to optimize strain survival during intestinal transit and has been proposed as a mechanism explaining how probiotics could lower serum cholesterol levels [21].

Another feature of probiotic strain survival is the ability to colonize the GI tract. This property can be split up into an ecological component and a mucosal component. Firstly, once a probiotic organism has survived gastric acid and duodenal bile salts and thus reaches the ileum and colon, it has the possibility to develop in a less stringent environment. Yet, it reaches an environment with a highly significant microbial background—the ileum and colon reaching bacterial concentrations of 10^7 and 10^{11} cells/mL chyme, respectively. Obviously, a probiotic strain can be considered as foreign to the residing endogenous microbiota, and unless specific nutrients are provided for the probiotic in the product formulation (e.g., symbiotic), the strain must enter into competition with the residing microbial community for available substrates. In ecological terms, the dosed probiotic must occupy a functional niche in the gut microbial ecosystem. Secondly, an important property for probiotics, for example, with respect to pathogen control, is its ability to adhere to and thrive in the mucus surface that covers the gut epithelium. Mucosal adhesion can rely on cell wall properties. The hydrophobic nature of microbial strains can be assessed with a straightforward bacterial adherence to hydrocarbons (BATH) assay [22], while the unspecific mucus adhesion can be measured using short term adhesion assays with gut-derived mucins (mostly from animal origin) [22, 23]. However, the unspecific adhesion of gut microorganisms to gut mucins is only sufficient for microcolony formation and it does not guarantee a prolonged colonization of the mucus layer. It has been well described that specific microorganisms modulate their gene expression following their incorporation into the mucosal surface. This has not only been described for pathogens [23, 24] but also for probiotic microorganisms such as *L. rhamnosus* GG, which upregulates specific "pilin" structures in the mucosal environment [25].

Human Target Groups

Probiotic products have been developed for a wide variety of health claims. Probiotics can target both healthy and diseased individuals. The expected effects can be of a preventive or curative nature. The goal can be to fight the cause of the disease/metabolic alterations, or to lessen symptoms associated with the occurrence of progression of a disease/metabolic alteration.

With the aim of improving health in the human body, the intake of a probiotic strain by healthy subjects has primarily preventive objectives. Yet, it must be emphasized that the introduction of a foreign strain—even if it is a probiotic—must be approached with care and must be performed after a well-considered evaluation process. More in particular, the gut environment from sensitive human subpopulations such as babies and toddlers is going through a high degree of development or transition. Many studies report on probiotic applications resulting in a positive outcome of markers that

can be of relevance for human health. Probiotic studies have shown beneficial effects in all age-related subgroups such as mother–infants pairs, preterms, newborns, infants and older children, elderly people.

To exemplify, fermented milk drinks with *L. casei* strain Shirota positively stimulate the immune system in healthy human subjects [26]. With respect to different age groups, the effects from long-term consumption of probiotic milk on infections was evaluated in children attending day care centers [27], while *L. delbrueckii* subsp. *bulgaricus* OLL1073R-1 was given to elderly persons with the aim of reducing the risk of infection [28].

In case the microbial community from a specific body region is disturbed (leading to the so-called dysbiosis), functional niches become available in the ecosystem. Examples of dysbiosis are the changes in microbioal ecosystem in the mouth, associated with dental caries occurrence, or dysbiosis associated with bacterial vaginosis. The effects from probiotics on oral health in children were recently reviewed [29]. For example, long-term application of probiotic strains such as *L. rhamnosus* GG lowers the risk of dental caries in children [30]; the importance of probiotic supplementation during orthodontic therapy was also reported [31]. Similarly, microbial dysbiosis in the urogenital tract, more in particular bacterial vaginosis, can be tackled by probiotics as well [32]. *L. rhamnosus* GG and specific *L. acidophilus* strains have been used to treat bacterial vaginosis [33, 34]. Probiotics may also be applied orally to abate increased health risks that originate from the gut environment. *Helicobacter pylori*-colonized subjects have been treated with *L. casei* milk drinks [35] and *L. gasseri* OLL2716 (LG21) [36], while specific *Bifidobacterium* (*B.*) strains display anti-*Helicobacter* effects through the production of antimicrobial peptides [37]. However, in Crohn's disease there is proof that dysbiosis occurs (either as cause or consequence), but probiotic supplementation has always failed to prevent relapse, except in pouchitis. In addition, there is specific attention for developing probiotic concepts for children under modified risks. Preterm babies display an increased risk for developing necrotizing enterocolitis, which is decreased by the application of oral probiotics [38].

Basis of the Biological Effect of Probiotics

The health benefits from probiotic products and applications are extremely diverse and are continuously expanded with new insights and scientific developments.

Microbiological Functionality

Microbiological functionality has a major objective of gaining control over the microbial homeostasis in a body environment and lower pathogen invasion and colonization. The resilience of a microbial community against invasion by exogenous strains largely depends on the availability of non-occupied functional niches. If not all functional niches are occupied by the endogenous microbial community, there is an increased risk for pathogen invasion in the ecosystem, colonization, and subsequent infection.

Probiotic microorganisms can be applied to improve or restore microbial homeostasis in two scenarios. Firstly, they may occupy functional niches that are left open by the endogenous community, thereby avoiding (opportunistic) pathogens of occupying that niche. Such process is often referred to as competitive exclusion and primarily targets the competition for nutrients, physical sites (e.g., mucus adhesion) or receptors. The second scenario is more of an antagonistic nature as probiotics may actively lower (opportunistic) pathogen invasion or development into the ecosystem. Such approach primarily targets (i) the production of short chain fatty acids and other organic acids (e.g., lactic acid) by probiotics, thereby lowering the pH and increasing the bacteriostatic effect of organic acids towards pathogens, (ii) the production of bacteriocins, which are small microbial peptides with bacteriostatic or bacteriocidal activity, and (iii) production of reactive oxygen species, such as hydrogen peroxide, that are highly reactive and increase oxidative stress for pathogens in microenvironments.

Nutritional Functionality

Specific microbial groups produce vitamins and may thereby contribute to vitamin availability to the human host. Apart from vitamin K [39], vitamin B12 [40], and pyridoxin [41], other vitamins such as biotin, folate, nicotinic acid, and thiamine can be produced by gut microorganisms and thereby affect host health. Such activity from a microbial strain can be considered a probiotic effect.

Besides this, lactase deficiency causes lactose intolerance which results in abdominal cramping, nausea, and bloating. Probiotic strains that are lactase positive have been successfully applied to relieve discomfort from lactose intolerance [42].

Other nutritional functionalities may include the production of health-promoting compounds. The metabolic potency of gut microorganisms is enormous and may rival or even exceed that of the liver [43]. Gut environment harbors a wealth of small chemical factories that produce a plethora of chemical components with putative health-modulating effects [44]. Isolated strains that produce health-promoting products may also be considered as having probiotic potential. To illustrate, production of health-promoting conjugated linoleic acids (CLA) has been reported for *Bifidobacterium* strains [45], *L. plantarum* JCM 1551 [46] and specific *L. acidophilus* strains. Conversion of phytoestrogen precursors to bioactive metabolites by supplemented microorganisms is a potential pathway for future probiotic applications. For example, Decroos et al. previously isolated a microbial

consortium that converts soy-derived daidzein into the bioactive equol [47], while Possemiers et al. performed an in vitro investigation of the probiotic potential of *Eubacterium limosum* strains to convert hop isoxanthohumol into the 8-prenylnaringenin [48].

Physiological Functionality

Probiotic microorganisms have been reported to enhance GI transit. Hamilton–Miller previously reviewed such functionality for the application of probiotic products in elderly persons [49]. Other potential physiological effects may include the reduction by probiotics of bloating or gas production, the enhancement of ion absorption by intestinal epithelial cells [50] and the decrease of bile salt toxicity or the decrease of serum cholesterol levels by bile salt hydrolase positive probiotics [51, 52].

Lowering Health Detrimental Components in the Gut

Probiotic microorganisms are also applied to reduce the health risks from hazardous components. For example, oral exposure to contaminants, either from a food matrix or from an environmental matrix (soil, dust, water, etc.) is the most dominant scenario by which the human body gets internally exposed to contaminants. These can be (i) mycotoxins, produced from fungi on a wide variety of crops, cereals in particular, (ii) xenobiotics with toxic properties as unwanted residues from environmental contamination of the food chain, or (iii) hazardous compounds from the food production process as such (e.g., polycyclic aromatic hydrocarbons (PAH) production during grilling of meat). The mode of action by which these probiotics lower the risk derived from ingested hazardous components often relates to the sorption of the compound to microbial biomass. This is, for example, the case for aflatoxin B1, which has been shown in vitro to be bound by probiotic strains [53]. Another mode of action may be direct detoxification of the hazardous compound such as the breakdown of fumonisin by *Pediococcus pentosaceus* (L006) that was isolated from corn leafs and that thus has probiotic properties. A final mode of action is more indirect and resembles the above mentioned probiotic modulation of microenvironment in the gut where (food) pathogens produce toxins. For example, the production of organic acids by probiotic microorganisms was reported to negatively affect the production of Shiga-toxin 2 from enterohemorrhagic *E. coli* O157:H7.

Immunological Functionality

The immunological benefits of probiotics can be due to activation of local macrophages and modulation of IgA production locally and systemically, to changes in pro/anti-inflammatory cytokines profile, or to the modulation of response towards food antigens [54, 55].

Probiotic Products in Prevention and Treatment

The following paragraphs are not meant to provide a complete overview of all indications in which probiotics have been studied as possible therapeutic intervention. We focused on the most relevant indications for children with disorders of the GI tract.

Acute Infectious Diarrhea

Probiotics have been largely studied to the prevention of acute infectious diarrhea. Large, randomized controlled trials (RCT) provide evidence of a very modest effect (statistically significant, but of questionable clinical importance) of some probiotic strains (*Lactobacillus GG, L. reuteri, B. animalis* subsp. *lactis*) on the prevention of community-acquired diarrhea [56–64]. *L. reuteri* protects for the development of diarrhea in Indonesian children with undernutrition [60]. For prevention of diarrhea acquired in day-care centers, many randomized and placebo-controlled trials have been published, conducted in different parts of the world. Probiotics tested were *Lactobacillus GG, B. animalis* subsp. *lactis*, alone or in combination with *Strepto. thermophilus,* and *L. reuteri, L. rhamnosus* (not GG), and *L. acidophilus,* in various trials either alone or in comparison with each other. The evidence of their efficacy in these settings is only modest for the prevention of diarrhea, although somewhat better for prevention of upper respiratory infections [61]. The number needed to treat (NNT) to prevent one child from developing nosocomial Rota gastroenteritis is seven [62]. However, the protective effect on prevention of diarrhea becomes far less significant if the incidence of diarrhea (episodes per patient-month) rather than the percentage of patients with diarrhea are taken into account [63]. In hospitalized children, the administration of *L. reuteri* DSM 17938 compared with placebo had no effect on the overall incidence of nosocomial diarrhea, including rotavirus infection [65].

The use of the following probiotics (in alphabetical order) may be considered in the management of children with acute gastroenteritis (AGE) in addition to rehydration therapy: *L. rhamnosus* GG (low quality of evidence; strong recommendation) and *S. boulardii* (low quality of evidence; strong recommendation). Less compelling evidence is available for *L. reuteri* DSM 17938 (very low quality of evidence; weak recommendation) and heat-inactivated *L. acidophilus* LB (very low quality of evidence; weak recommendation) [66]. The latter, although traditionally discussed with other probiotics, does not fit with the definition of probiotics. A number of RCTs have evaluated the effect of *Enterococcus faecium* SF68 [66]. A sub-group analysis performed within a Cochrane review (search date: July 2010) found that

Enterococcus SF68 reduced the risk of diarrhea lasting ≥4 days (4 RCTs, *n*=333; RR 0.21, 95% CI 0.08–0.52) [66]. However, in vitro studies have documented that the *E. faecium* SF68 strain is a possible recipient of the vancomycin resistance genes [67]. Considering that the risk for in vivo conjugation cannot be ruled out, probiotics with safety issues should not be used [66]. Other strains or combinations of strains have been tested, but evidence of their efficacy is weak or preliminary.

Antibiotic-Associated Diarrhea

The pooled relative risk in a meta-analysis of 63 RCTs, which included 11,811 participants, indicated a statistically significant association of probiotic administration with reduction in antibiotic-associated diarrhea (AAD; relative risk, 0.58; 95% CI, 0.50–0.68; $P<0.001$; I[2], 54%; (risk difference, −0.07; 95% CI, −0.10 to −0.05), (NNT 13; 95% CI, 10.3–19.1)) [68]. Another meta-analysis concluded the NNT was 8 [69]. According to a recent meta-analysis, probiotics reduce the risk of AAD in children significantly [70]. Pre-planned subgroup analysis showed that reduction of the risk of AAD was associated with the use of *Lactobacillus* GG (95% CI 0.15–0.6), *S. boulardii* (95% CI 0.07–0.6), or *B. animalis* subsp. *lactis* and *Strepto. thermophilus* (95% CI 0.3–0.95) [70]. For every seven patients that would develop diarrhea while being treated with antibiotics, one fewer will develop AAD if also receiving probiotics [70]. Only *S. boulardii* was reported to be effective in *Clostridium difficile (C. dif.)* disease [71–73]. Recently, a large single-center study showed in elderly that *S. boulardii* was not effective in preventing the development of AAD or in prevention of *C. dif.* infection [74]. In many studies, there is no evidence to support the use of any (other) probiotic to prevent the recurrence of *C. dif.* infection or to treat existing *C. dif.* diarrhea [59]. A new meta-analysis concluded that probiotics significantly reduce the incidence of pediatric AAD (22 trials; RR=0.42; 95% CO 0.33–0.53) and the incidence pediatric *C. dif.* Infection (five trials; RR=0.35; 95% CI 0.13–0.92) [75] *S. boulardii* (RR=0.43; 95% CI 0.32–0.60) and *L. rhamnosus* GG (RR=0.36; 95% CI 0.19–0.69) are the two best-studied strains [75]. In most studies, the probiotic is started together with antibiotic treatment [76].

Traveler's Diarrhea

Traveler's diarrhea is a frequent condition of great socio-economic impact. It is one of these topics on which there are more reviews than original research published. Different RCTs have been performed evaluating the efficacy of probiotics in the prevention of traveler's diarrhea. One trial with *L. acidophilus* and two with *L. GG* showed negative results [77–79]. One trial with *S. boulardii* reported a small but significant preventive effect in a subgroup, suggesting geographical differences in efficacy [80]. In a review, Mc-Farland concluded that there is comparable evidence for efficacy for *L. rhamnosus* GG, *L. casei* DN-114001 and *S. boulardii,* and no efficacy for *L. acidophilus* [81]. Since the number of studies in traveler's diarrhea is very limited, a recent meta-analysis concluded that there is no efficacy of probiotics in traveler's diarrhea [82]. There are no data on prebiotics and prevention or treatment of traveler's diarrhea. Overall, the number of studies is too small to allow to formulate recommendations [83].

Irritable Bowel Syndrome

There is a large literature on the effect of probiotics on IBS in adults, but data in children are limited. A Cochrane review from 2009 failed to show an effect of fiber supplements and recorded a limited effect of *Lactobacillus* on symptoms compared to placebo (OR 1.17; 95% CI 0.62, 2.21) [84].

A RCT of 6 weeks with *Lactobacillus* GG versus placebo showed overall negative results in 50 children and young adults, although there was a lower incidence of perceived abdominal distension in *L. GG* group [85]. *Lactobacillus* GG but not placebo caused a significant reduction of both frequency and severity of abdominal pain compared to baseline and influenced intestinal permeability testing [86]. A meta-analysis showed that, compared with placebo, *Lactobacillus* GG supplementation is associated with a significantly higher rate of treatment responders in the overall population with abdominal pain-related functional GI disorders and in the IBS subgroup [87]. However, no difference was found in children with functional abdominal pain or functional dyspepsia who received placebo or *Lactobacillus* GG. A randomized cross-over trial with VSL#3 and placebo for 6 weeks, with a 2-week washout period in between in 59 patients showed a superior effect of VSL#3 compared to placebo in symptom relief, as well as in abdominal pain/discomfort, abdominal bloating/gassiness, and family assessment of life disruption [83, 87]. No significant difference was found in the stool pattern [88].

There are no data on prevention or treatment of IBS with prebiotics. Data from one trial suggest that, in infants, a prebiotic-containing whey-based formula provides superior GI comfort than a control formula [89]. A peptide-based formula containing fiber was as well tolerated as a fiber-free formula in a small population of children with GI impairments [90]. Extremes of stool consistency were normalized with the fiber formula. No significant differences were observed in vomiting, abdominal pain, feeding intakes, or weight gain between the two formulas [90]. Synbiotics should be further investigated in this indication [91].

Helicobacter pylori

The use of probiotics in *H. pylori*-colonized subjects with gastric inflammation is supported by many observations. Specific strains of *Lactobacillus* and *Bifidobacterium* exert in vitro bactericidal effects against *H. pylori* through the release of bacteriocins or production of organic acids, and/or inhibit its adhesion to epithelial cells. Such protective effects have been confirmed in animal models. Clinical trials are very important, since in vitro results cannot always be reproduced in patients. Probiotics decrease the bacterial load and improve the immune response [92]. Results of clinical trials indicate that probiotics generally do not eradicate *H. pylori* but decrease the density of colonization, thereby maintaining lower levels of this pathogen in the stomach; in association with antibiotic treatments, some probiotics increased eradication rates and/or decreased adverse effects due to the antibiotics. Many studies show a moderate higher eradication rate (~10%) of *H. pylori* when probiotics are added to the antibiotics and proton pump inhibitor [93]. Although *Lactobacillus* GG seems not to improve eradication [94], most probiotic bacteria and yeasts reduce adverse effects of standard *H. pylori* eradication regimens [95, 96].

Constipation

Constipation is a frequent problem in childhood in which pre- and probiotics could have a positive influence on the intestinal flora with an effect on stool consistency and frequency. Unfortunately, study results are contradictory. In an open trial, *B. breve* was effective in increasing stool frequency in children with functional constipation [97]. Furthermore it had a positive effect with respect to stool consistency, decreasing the number of fecal incontinence episodes and in diminishing abdominal pain [97]. In another open trial, a probiotic mixture (Ecologic Relief®) containing *B. bifidum, B. infantis, B. longum, L. casei, L. plantarum* and *L. rhamnosus* showed positive effects on symptoms of constipation [98]. *L. rhamnosus* Lcr35 was effective in treating children with chronic constipation [99]. *B. animalis* subsp. *lactis* was reported to be non effective in constipation [82, 100]. *L. reuteri* DSM 17938 had a positive effect in infants with chronic constipation on bowel frequency, even when there was no improvement in stool consistency and episodes of inconsolable crying episodes [101]. A Brazilian study showed a positive influence of yoghurt on stool frequency with an additional effect of yoghurt supplemented with *B. longum* [102]. In constipated children, the fermented dairy product containing *B. animalis* subsp. *lactis* DN-173 010 did increase stool frequency, but this increase was comparable in the control group [103]. There is currently not sufficient evidence to recommend fermented dairy products containing *B. animalis* subsp. *lactis* DN-173 010 in this category of patients [103]. No evidence for any effect was found for fluid supplements, prebiotics, probiotics, or behavioral intervention [104]. Until more data are available, probiotics for the treatment of constipation condition should be considered investigational [105].

Necrotizing Entercolitis

Necrotizing enterocolitis (NEC) is a severe condition occurring especially in preterm babies. Abnormal GI flora development has been hypothesized as one of the possible etiologic factors. The first publication reporting that *L. acidophilus* and *B. infantis* reduced NEC dates back from 1999 [106]. This was followed by a negative study showing that seven days of *Lactobacillus* GG supplementation starting with the first feed was not effective in reducing the incidence of urinary tract infection, NEC and sepsis in preterm infants [107]. Then, several randomized trials with different lactobacilli and bifidobacteria showed a significant reduction in development of NEC [108, 109]. Although *S. boulardii* was shown to ameliorate hypoxia/reoxygenation-induced NECs in young mice [110], it did not protect for NEC in infants [111]. A Cochrane review concluded in 2008 that enteral probiotic supplementation reduced the incidence of NEC stage II or more and mortality [112]. No systemic infections or serious adverse events were directly attributed to the administered probiotic microorganism [112]. According to the published trials, the NNT to prevent one case of NEC is 21 and 27 [112]. However, the centers in which these trails have been performed have a much higher incidence of NEC than most European or North American centers. The recommendation may be different in centers with a high incidence of NEC in which the other measurements to decrease NEC are difficult to apply. The updated Cochrane review from 2011 comes to different conclusions: enteral supplementation of probiotics prevents severe NEC and all cause mortality in preterm infants [113]. The updated review of available evidence supports a change in practice. More studies are needed to assess efficacy in extremely low birth weight (ELBW) infants and assess the most effective formulation and dose to be utilized [113]. The debate to give systematically probiotics to preterms or not is still going one. The American Pediatric Surgical Association Outcomes and Clinical Trials Committee systematic review concluded in 2012 acknowledges that recent Cochrane reviews support the use of prophylactic probiotics in preterm infants less than 2500 g to reduce the incidence of NEC, as well as the use of human breast milk rather than formula when possible. There is no clear evidence to support delayed initiation or slow advance-

ment of feeds [114]. However, an expert group of nutritionists and neonatologists concluded that there is insufficient evidence to recommend routine use of probiotics to decrease NEC [115]. According to this group, there are encouraging data which justify the further investigation regarding the efficacy and safety of specific probiotics in circumstances of high local incidence of severe NEC [115]. According to others, available evidence is still too limited to recommended probiotics to reduced NEC [116]. Other experts suggest that it may become unethical to not give probiotics to preterm babies to decrease NEC [117].

Colic

Colic is a frequent problem in infants and often parents desperate for a solution. In this indication, the effect of *L. reuteri* has been exhaustively studied in breastfed infants [118–120]. However, there are no data with *L. reuteri* in formula fed babies. Dupont et al. reported efficacy of another probiotic strain in formula fed infants [121].

Allergy and Atopic Dermatitis

Simultaneous pro- and prebiotic treatment (a mixture of four strains and galactooligosaccharides, GOS) given to pregnant women during 2–4 weeks before delivery and to the infants during 6 months compared with placebo showed no effect on the cumulative incidence of allergic diseases at the age of 2 years but tended to reduce IgE-associated (atopic) diseases since a significant reduction of (atopic) eczema was noticed [122]. However, Taylor and coworkers challenge the role of probiotics in allergy prevention since they recorded that early probiotic supplementation with *L. acidophilus* did not reduce the risk of atopic dermatitis (AD) in high-risk infants and was even associated with increased allergen sensitization in infants receiving supplements [123]. A Cochrane review from 2007 concluded that there was insufficient evidence to recommend the addition of probiotics to infant feeds for prevention of allergic disease or food hypersensitivity [124]. Although there was a reduction in clinical eczema in infants, this effect was not consistent between studies and caution was advised in view of methodological concerns regarding included studies [124]. However, the efficacy of probiotic intervention to reduce atopic dermatitis and/or allergic disease may depend on the moment of intervention. Preventive administration of probiotics may be only effective if given during pregnancy. Probiotics given to unselected mothers reduced the cumulative incidence of AD, but had no effect on atopic sensitization [125]. A recent the meta-analysis showed that the administration of lactobacilli during pregnancy prevented atopic eczema in children aged from 2 to 7 years [126]. However, a mixture of various bacterial strains does not affect the development of atopic eczema, independent of whether they contain lactobacilli or not [126]. *L. rhamnosus* HN001 was reported effective against eczema in the first 2 years of life persists to age 4 years, while *B. animalis* subsp. *lactis* HN019 had no effect [127]. Therefore, not only timing of administration seems important but also strain specificity. However, timing of administration and strain specificity was then again contradicted by the meta-analysis by Pelucchi and coworkers, being in support of a moderate role of probiotics in the prevention of atopic dermatitis and IgE-associated atopic dermatitis in infants, but regardless of the time of probiotic use (pregnancy or early life) or the subject(s) receiving probiotics (mother, child, or both) [128]. The data on probiotics and allergy need further clarification, because data are somehow contradictory. It might be that geographical or genetic differences play a detrimental role, especially for atopic dermatitis.

Recently, in a double-blind, placebo-controlled multicenter trial, 90 infants with atopic dermatitis, age <7 months, were randomized to receive an infant formula with *B. breve* M-16V and a mixture of short chain GOS and long chain fructooligosaccharides (FOS), or the same formula without synbiotics during 12 weeks [129]. There were no significant differences between the synbiotic and the placebo group [129]. The same group showed that synbiotics prevent asthma-like symptoms in infants with AD [130]. At the same time, another group reported that a synbiotic combination of *L. salivarius* plus FOS is superior to the prebiotic alone for treating moderate to severe childhood AD [131]. While some studies with probiotics as a treatment for AD show a benefit [132], most studies are negative. No benefit was reported from supplementation with *B. animalis* subsp. *lactis* or *L. paracasei* in the treatment of eczema, when given as an adjunct to basic topical treatment, and no effect on the progression of allergic disease from age 1 to 3 years [133]. Most reviews conclude that probiotics are not effective in reducing atopic dermatitis. These contradictory results suggest strain specificity or a genetic influence on the efficacy of probiotics in children with atopic dermatitis. A review of 13 studies of probiotics for treating established eczema did not show convincing evidence of a clinically worthwhile benefit [134].

Extraintestinal Infections and Other Effects

No pediatric studies have demonstrated definite beneficial effects of administering probiotics to treat extraintestinal infections like respiratory tract infections or otitis media [76, 135]. There is no evidence that probiotics decrease extraintestinal infections. There is some evidence that some lactobacilli might prevent recurrent urinary tract infection in women. However, data in children are lacking. The same is true for recurrent vulvovaginitis. Sazawal and coworkers showed that prebiotic and probiotic fortified milk prevented morbidities among children in a community-based RCT [136].

Candidiasis accounts for 10–20% of bloodstream infections in pediatric intensive care units (PICUs) and a significant increase in morbidity, mortality, and length of hospital stay [137]. A few studies have demonstrated that probiotics are able to prevent *Candida* growth and colonization in neonates, whereas their role in preventing invasive candidiasis in such patients is still unclear [137].

Purified phytases from *B. longum* subsp. *infantis* and *B. pseudocatenulatum* reduced the contents of phytate as compared to control samples (untreated or treated with fungal phytase) and led to increased levels of myo-inositol triphosphate [138]. This is the first example of the application of purified bifidobacterial phytases in food processing and shows the potential of these enzymes to be used in products for human consumption [138]. Lactic acid bacteria improve the synthesis of vitamins B2, B11, and B12 and have the potential strategies to increase B-group vitamin content in cereals-based products [139]. Vitamin-producing *Lactobacillus* have been leading to the elaboration of novel fermented functional foods [139].

Pandemic obesity is now matter of interest in all developed and developing countries. Treatment with probiotics selectively changes the composition of the gut microbiota in favor of specific genera and even strains. Few intervention studies with probiotics in overweight or obese individuals have been published until now, and mostly focus on *Lactobacillus* or *Bifidobacterium* The administration of a strain of *L. gasseri* in obese and type 2 diabetic patients has been shown to decrease fat mass (visceral and subcutaneous) and body mass index [140]. In addition, Andreasen et al. have demonstrated that the administration of *Lactobacillus* spp. positively impact on insulin sensitivity [141]. Compelling evidence suggest that early gut microbiota modulation with probiotics reduces the body mass index in young children by restraining excessive weight gain during the first years of life (from 0 to 10 years of follow-up) [142]. Only few data are available until now, to have a clear view of the way by which lactobacilli or bifidobacteria can counteract adiposity.

Fecal Microbiota Transplantation

A new approach in the therapeutic applications of bacteria is transplantation of intestinal microflora, especially in difficult to treat condition in which it is known that the fecal microbiota is abnormal [143, 144]. Observed side effects warrant caution in the ongoing pursuit of this treatment option [144]. There is evidence that many diseases are related to an intestinal dysbiosis. As a consequence, manipulation of the intestinal microbiota is a very attractive therapeutic approach. In spite of the fact that so far results have been often negative [144], and even bacteremia as an adverse event has been reported [145], positive results have also been achieved [146]. To improve safety, clearly the transplanted microbiota should be carefully screened for pathogens [147]. Encouragingly, the first cure of early onset colitis after fecal microbiota transplantation has been reported [148]. Interest should now focus on the reasons of success and failure, (see Chap. 35 "Fecal Microbial Transplant: For Whom, How, and When").

Safety and Side Effects

Probiotics have a long record of safety, which relates primarily to lactobacilli and bifidobacteria [149]. Experience with other forms of probiotic is more limited. There is no such thing as zero risk, particularly in the context of certain forms of host susceptibility [149]. Probiotics are "generally regarded as safe" and side effects in ambulatory care have almost not been reported. Large-scale epidemiological studies in countries where probiotic use is endemic demonstrate (in adults) low rates of systemic infection, between 0.05 and 0.40 % [150]. Administration during pregnancy and early infancy is considered safe [151]. Probiotic compounds may contain hidden allergens of food and may not be safe for subjects with allergy to cow's milk or hen's egg [152]. Documented invasive infections have been primarily noted to occur in immunocompromised adults. Invasive infections in infants and children are extremely rare [153–155]. Two cases of bacteremia attribuable to *Lactobacillus* supplementation, with identical molecular clinical and supplement isolates, were recently reported in an infant and a child without underlying GI disease or immunocompromised status [156]. Sepsis with probiotic lactobacilli has been reported in children with short gut. Recently, plasmid transfer of antibiotic resistance has been shown to be clinically possible to occur. Long-term use of probiotics under antibiotic selection pressure could cause antibiotic resistance, and the resistance gene could be transferred to other bacteria [157]. Translocation from the gastrointestinal tract in the systemic circulation has not been reported. There is poor public understanding of the concept of risk, in general, and risk/benefit analysis, in particular [149]. Uncertainty persists regarding the potential for transfer of antibiotic resistance with probiotics, but the risk seems to be low with currently available probiotic products [149]. As with other forms of therapeutics, the safety of probiotics should be considered on a strain-by-strain basis [149]. The potential benefits of supplementation should be weighed against the risk of development of an invasive infection resulting from probiotic therapy.

Conclusion

Probiotics have entered the mainstream of health care. The gastrointestinal microbiota is fundamental for the development of the immune system. Although the main indications of the medical use of probiotics is still in the area of the prevention and treatment of gastrointestinal-related disorders, gradually more evidence is collected on extraintestinal indications such as vaginitis, atopic dermatitis, respiratory tract infections. RCT with the commercialized product in the claimed indications are mandatory before the use of a product can be recommended. Today, *L. rhamnosus* GG and *S. boulardii* are the best studied strains. Although adverse effects have been reported, probiotics are considered as safe. Overuse and use of products that have not been validated constitute potential drawbacks.

References

1. Vandenplas Y. Identification of probiotics by specific strain name. Aliment Pharmacol Ther. 2012;35:860.
2. Huys G, Vancanneyt M, D'Haene K, Vankerckhoven V, Goossens H, Swings J. Accuracy of species identity of commercial bacterial cultures intended for probiotic or nutritional use. Res Microbiol. 2006;157:803–10.
3. Sanders ME. Probiotics: considerations for human health. Nutr Rev. 2003;61:91–9.
4. Stamatova I, Meurman JH. Probiotics: health benefits in the mouth. Am J Dent. 2009;22:329–38.
5. Meurman JH. Probiotics: do they have a role in oral medicine and dentistry? Eur J Oral Sci. 2005;113:188–96.
6. Hoesl CE, Altwein JE. The probiotic approach: an alternative treatment option in urology. Eur Urol. 2005;47:288–96.
7. Barrons R, Tassone D. Use of *Lactobacillus* probiotics for bacterial genitourinary infections in women: a review. Clin Ther. 2008;30:453–68.
8. Reid G, Bocking A. The potential for probiotics to prevent bacterial vaginosis and preterm labor. Am J Obstet Gynecol. 2003;189:1202–8.
9. Falagas ME, Betsi GI, Tokas T, Athanasiou S. Probiotics for prevention of recurrent urinary tract infections in women: a review of the evidence from microbiological and clinical studies. Drugs. 2006;66:1253–61.
10. Hacini-Rachinel F, Gheit H, Le Luduec JB, Dif F, Nancey S, Kaiserlian D. Oral probiotic control skin inflammation by acting on both effector and regulatory T cells. PLoS One. 2009;4:e4903.
11. Caramia G, Atzei A, Fanos V. Probiotics and the skin. Clin Dermatol. 2008;26:4–11.
12. Hojsak I, Abdović S, Szajewska H, Milosević M, Krznarić Z, Kolacek S. *Lactobacillus GG* in the prevention of nosocomial gastrointestinal and respiratory tract infections. Pediatrics. 2010;125:e1171–7.
13. Possemiers S, Marzorati M, Verstraete W, Van de Wiele T. Bacteria and chocolate: a successful combination for probiotic delivery. Int J Food Microbiol. 2010;141:97–103.

14. Pereg D, Kimhi O, Tirosh A, Orr N, Kayouf R, Lishner M. The effect of fermented yogurt on the prevention of diarrhea in a healthy adult population. Am J Infect Control. 2005;33:122–5.

15. Magalhães KT, Pereira MA, Nicolau A, Dragone G, Domingues L, Teixeira JA, et al. Production of fermented cheese whey-based beverage using kefir grains as starter culture: evaluation of morphological and microbial variations. Bioresour Technol. 2010;101:8843–50.

16. Steidler L, Hans W, Schotte L, Neirynck S, Obermeier F, Falk W, et al. Treatment of murine colitis by Lactococcus lactis secreting interleukin-10. Science. 2000;289:1352–5.

17. Foligne B, Dessein R, Marceau M, Poiret S, Chamaillard M, Pot B, et al. Prevention and treatment of colitis with Lactococcus lactis secreting the immunomodulatory Yersinia LcrV protein. Gastroenterology. 2007;133:862–74.

18. Kumar M, Nagpal R, Verma V, Kumar A, Kaur N, Hemalatha R, et al. Probiotic metabolites as epigenetic targets in the prevention of colon cancer. Nutr Rev. 2013;71:23–34.

19. Huseini HF, Rahimzadeh G, Fazeli MR, Mehrazma M, Salehi M. Evaluation of wound healing activities of kefir products. Burns. 2012;38:719–23.

20. Cook MT, Tzortzis G, Charalampopoulos D, Khutoryanskiy VV. Microencapsulation of probiotics for gastrointestinal delivery. J Control Release. 2012;162:56–67.

21. Kumar M, Nagpal R, Kumar R, Hemalatha R, Verma V, Kumar A, et al. Cholesterol-lowering probiotics as potential biotherapeutics for metabolic diseases. Exp Diabet Res. 2012;2012:902917.

22. Van den Abbeele P, Grootaert C, Possemiers S, Verstraete W, Verbeken K, Van de Wiele T. In vitro model to study the modulation of the mucin-adhered bacterial community. Appl Microbiol Biotechnol. 2009;83:349–59.

23. Macfarlane S, Furrie E, Kennedy A, Cummings JH, Macfarlane GT. Mucosal bacteria in ulcerative colitis. Br J Nutr. 2005;93(Suppl 1):S67–72.

24. Chassaing B, Darfeuille-Michaud A. The commensal microbiota and enteropathogens in the pathogenesis of inflammatory bowel diseases. Gastroenterology. 2011;140:1720–8.

25. Lebeer S, Claes I, Tytgat HL, Verhoeven TL, Marien E, von Ossowski I, et al. Functional analysis of Lactobacillus rhamnosus GG pili in relation to adhesion and immunomodulatory interactions with intestinal epithelial cells. Appl Environ Microbiol. 2012;78:185–93.

26. Nagao F, Nakayama M, Muto T, Okumura K. Effects of a fermented milk drink containing Lactobacillus casei strain Shirota on the immune system in healthy human subjects. Biosci Biotechnol Biochem. 2000;64:2706–8.

27. Hatakka K, Savilahti E, Pönkä A, Meurman JH, Poussa T, Näse L, et al. Effect of long term consumption of probiotic milk on infections in children attending day care centres: double blind, randomised trial. BMJ. 2001;322:1327.

28. Makino S, Ikegami S, Kume A, Horiuchi H, Sasaki H, Orii N. Reducing the risk of infection in the elderly by dietary intake of yoghurt fermented with Lactobacillus delbrueckii ssp. bulgaricus OLL1073R-1. Br J Nutr. 2010;104:998–1006.

29. Twetman S, Stecksén-Blicks C. Probiotics and oral health effects in children. Int J Paediatr Dent. 2008;18:3–10.

30. Näse L, Hatakka K, Savilahti E, Saxelin M, Pönkä A, Poussa T, et al. Effect of long-term consumption of a probiotic bacterium, Lactobacillus rhamnosus GG, in milk on dental caries and caries risk in children. Caries Res. 2001;35:412–20.

31. Sarantos SR. The importance of probiotic supplementation in conjunction with orthodontic therapy. J N J Dent Assoc. 2006;77:10–3.

32. Reid G, Beuerman D, Heinemann C, Bruce AW. Probiotic Lactobacillus dose required to restore and maintain a normal vaginal flora. FEMS Immunol Med Microbiol. 2001;32:37–4.

33. Rossi A, Rossi T, Bertini M, Caccia G. The use of Lactobacillus rhamnosus in the therapy of bacterial vaginosis. Evaluation of clinical efficacy in a population of 40 women treated for 24 months. Arch Gynecol Obstet. 2010;281:1065–9.

34. Andreeva P, Dimitrov A. The probiotic Lactobacillus acidophilus—an alternative treatment of bacterial vaginosis. Akush Ginekol (Sofiia). 2002;41:29–31.

35. Cats A, Kuipers EJ, Bosschaert MA, Pot RG, Vandenbroucke-Grauls CM, Kusters JG. Effect of frequent consumption of a Lactobacillus casei-containing milk drink in Helicobacter pylori-colonized subjects. Aliment Pharmacol Ther. 2003;17:429–35.

36. Ushiyama A, Tanaka K, Aiba Y, Shiba T, Takagi A, et al. Lactobacillus gasseri OLL2716 as a probiotic in clarithromycin-resistant Helicobacter pylori infection. J Gastroenterol Hepatol. 2003;18:986–91.

37. Collado MC, González A, González R, Hernández M, Ferrús MA, Sanz Y. Antimicrobial peptides are among the antagonistic metabolites produced by Bifidobacterium against Helicobacter pylori. Int J Antimicrob Agents. 2005;25:385–91.

38. Alfaleh K, Anabrees J, Bassler D. Probiotics reduce the risk of necrotizing enterocolitis in preterm infants: a meta-analysis. Neonatology. 2010;97:93–9.

39. Weber TK, Polanco I. Gastrointestinal microbiota and some children diseases: a review. Gastroenterol Res Pract. 2012;2012:676585.

40. Santos F, Vera JL, van der Heijden R, Valdez G, de Vos WM, Sesma F, et al. The complete coenzyme B12 biosynthesis gene cluster of Lactobacillus reuteri CRL1098. Microbiology. 2008;154:81–93.

41. Fabian E, Majchrzak D, Dieminger B, Meyer E, Elmadfa I. Influence of probiotic and conventional yoghurt on the status of vitamins B1, B2 and B6 in young healthy women. Ann Nutr Metab. 2008;52:29–36.

42. de Vrese M, Stegelmann A, Richter B, Fenselau S, Laue C, Schrezenmeir J. Probiotics—compensation for lactase insufficiency. Am J Clin Nutr. 2001;73(2 Suppl):421S–9S.

43. Sousa T, Paterson R, Moore V, Carlsson A, Abrahamsson B, Basit AW. The gastrointestinal microbiota as a site for the biotransformation of drugs. Int J Pharm. 2008;363:1–25.

44. Fischbach MA. Antibiotics from microbes: converging to kill. Curr Opin Microbiol. 2009;12:520–7.

45. Gorissen L, Raes K, Weckx S, Dannenberger D, Leroy F, De Vuyst L, et al. Production of conjugated linoleic acid and conjugated linolenic acid isomers by Bifidobacterium species. Appl Microbiol Biotechnol. 2010;87:2257–66.

46. Ando A, Ogawa J, Kishino S, Shimizu S. CLA production from ricinoleic acid by lactic acid bacteria. J Am Oil Chem Soc. 2003;80:889–94.

47. Decroos K, Vanhemmens S, Cattoir S, Boon N, Verstraete W. Isolation and characterisation of an equol-producing mixed microbial culture from a human faecal sample and its activity under gastrointestinal conditions. Arch Microbiol. 2005;183:45–55.

48. Possemiers S, Rabot S, Espín JC, Bruneau A, Philippe C, González-Sarrías A, et al. Eubacterium limosum activates isoxanthohumol from hops (Humulus lupulus L.) into the potent phytoestrogen 8-prenylnaringenin in vitro and in rat intestine. J Nutr. 2008;138:1310–6.

49. Hamilton-Miller JM. Probiotics and prebiotics in the elderly. Postgrad Med J. 2004;80:447–51.

50. Borthakur A, Gill RK, Tyagi S, Koutsouris A, Alrefai WA, Hecht GA, et al. The probiotic Lactobacillus acidophilus stimulates chloride/hydroxyl exchange activity in human intestinal epithelial cells. J Nutr. 2008;138:1355–9.

51. De Boever P, Wouters R, Verschaeve L, Berckmans P, Schoeters G, Verstraete W. Protective effect of the bile salt hydrolase-active Lactobacillus reuteri against bile salt cytotoxicity. Appl Microbiol Biotechnol. 2000;53:709–14.

52. De Smet I, De Boever P, Verstraete W. Cholesterol lowering in pigs through enhanced bacterial bile salt hydrolase activity. Br J Nutr. 1998;79:185–94.

53. Gratz S, Mykkänen H, Ouwehand AC, Juvonen R, Salminen S, El-Nezami H. Intestinal mucus alters the ability of probiotic bacteria to bind aflatoxin B1 in vitro. Appl Environ Microbiol. 2004;70:6306–8.

54. Kabeerdoss J, Devi RS, Mary RR, Prabhavathi D, Vidya R, Mechenro J, et al. Effect of yoghurt containing Bifidobacterium lactis Bb12® on faecal excretion of secretory immunoglobulin A and human beta-defensin 2 in healthy adult volunteers. Nutr J. 2011;10:138.

55. Ghadimi D, Fölster-Holst R, de Vrese M, Winkler P, Heller KJ, Schrezenmeir J. Effects of probiotic bacteria and their genomic DNA on TH1/TH2-cytokine production by peripheral blood mononuclear cells (PBMCs) of healthy and allergic subjects. Immunobiology. 2008;213:677–92.

56. Saavedra JM, Bauman NA, Oung I, Perman JA, Yolken RH. Feeding of Bifidobacterium bifidum and Streptococcus thermophilus to infants in hospital for prevention of diarrhoea and shedding of rotavirus. Lancet. 1994;344:1046–9.

57. Szajewska H, Kotowska M, Mrukowicz JZ, Armanska M, Mikolajczyk W. Efficacy of Lactobacillus GG in prevention of nosocomial diarrhea in infants. J Pediatr. 2001;138:361–5.

58. Mastretta E Longo P, Laccisaglia A, Balbo L, Russo R, Mazzacara A, Gianino P. Effect of a Lactobacillus GG and breast-feeding in the prevention of rotavirus nosocomial infection. J Pediatr Gastroenterol Nutr. 2002;35:527–31.

59. Szajewska H, Setty M, Mrukowicz J, Guandalini S. Probiotics in gastrointestinal disease in children: hard and not-so-hard evidence of efficacy. J Pediatr Gastroenterol Nutr. 2006;42:454–75.

60. Agustina R, Kok FJ, van de Rest O, Fahmida U, Firmansyah A, Lukito W, et al. Randomized trial of probiotics and calcium on diarrhea and respiratory tract infections in Indonesian children. Pediatrics. 2012;129:e1155–64.

61. Guandalini S. Probiotics for prevention and treatment of diarrhea. J Clin Gastroenterol. 2011;45 Suppl:S149–53.

62. Szajewska H, Mrukowicz JZ. Use of probiotics in children with acute diarrhea. Paediatr Drugs. 2005;7:111–22.

63. Chouraqui JP, Van Egroo LD, Fichot MC. Acidified milk formula supplemented with Bifidobacterium lactis: impact on infant diarrhea in residual care settings. J Pediatr Gastroenterol Nutr. 2004;38:288–92.

64. Thibault H, Aubert-Jacquin C, Goulet O. Effects of long-term consumption of a fermented infant formula (with Bifidoacterium Breve c50 and Streptococcus thermophilus 065) on acute diarrhea in healthy infants. J Pediatr Gastroenterol Nutr. 2004;39:147–52.

65. Wanke M, Szajewska H. Lack of an effect of Lactobacillus reuteri DSM 17938 in preventing nosocomial diarrhea in children: a randomized, double-blind, placebo-controlled trial. J Pediatr. 2012;161:40–3.

66. Szajewska H, Guarino A, Hojsak I, Indrio F, Kolacek S, Shamir R, et al., on behalf of the ESPGHAN Working Group for Probiotics/Prebiotics. The use of probiotics for the management of acute gastroenteritis. A position paper by the ESPGHAN working group for Probiotics. J Pediatr Gastroenterol Nutr. 2014;58:531–9.

67. Lund B, Edlund C. Probiotic Enterococcus faecium strain is a possible recipient of the vanA gene cluster. Clin Infect Dis. 2001;32:1384–5.

68. Hempel S, Newberry SJ, Maher AR, Wang Z, Miles JN, Shanman R, et al. Probiotics for the prevention and treatment of antibiotic-associated diarrhea: a systematic review and meta-analysis. JAMA. 2012;307:1959–69.

69. Videlock EJ, Cremonini F. Meta-analysis: probiotics in antibiotic-associated diarrhoea. Aliment Pharmacol Ther. 2012;35:1355–69.

70. Sazawal S, Hiremath G, Dhingra U, Malik P, Deb S, Black RE. Efficacy of probiotics in prevention of acute diarrhoea: a meta-analysis of masked, randomised, placebo-controlled trials. Lancet Infect Dis. 2006;6:374–82.

71. McFarland LV. Meta-analysis of probiotics for prevention of antibiotic associated diarrhea and the treatment of Clostridium difficile disease. Am J Gastroenterol. 2006;101:812–22.

72. Johnston BC, Goldenberg JZ, Vandvik PO, Sun X, Guyatt GH. Probiotics for the prevention of pediatric antibiotic-associated diarrhea. Cochrane Database Syst Rev. 2011;9(11):CD004827. doi: 10.1002/14651858.CD004827.pub3.

73. Tung JM, Dolovich LR, Lee CH. Prevention of Clostridium difficile infection with Saccharomyces boulardii: a systematic review. Can J Gastroenterol. 2009;23:817–21.

74. Pozzoni P, Riva A, Bellatorre AG, Amigoni M, Redaelli E, Ronchetti A, et al. Saccharomyces boulardii for the prevention of antibiotic-associated diarrhea in adult hospitalized patients: a single-center, randomized, double-blind, placebo-controlled trial. Am J Gastroenterol. 2012;107:922–31.

75. McFarland LV. Preventing pediatric antibiotic-associated diarrhea and Clostridium difficile infections with probiotics. A meta-analysis. World J Meta-Anal. 2013;1:102–20.

76. Braegger C, Chmielewska A, Decsi T, Kolacek S, Mihatsch W, Moreno L, et al. ESPGHAN committee on nutrition. Supplementation of infant formula with probiotics and/or prebiotics: a systematic review and comment by the ESPGHAN committee on nutrition. J Pediatr Gastroenterol Nutr. 2011;52:238–50.

77. Katelaris PH, Salam I, Farthing MJ. Lactobacilli to prevent traveler's diarrhea? N Eng J Med. 1995;333:1360–1.

78. Hilton E, Kolakowski P, Singer C, Smith M. Efficacy of Lactobacillus GG as a diarrheal preventive in travelers. J Travel Med. 1997;4:41–3.

79. Oksanen PJ, Salminen S, Saxelin M, Hamalainen P, Ihantola-Vormisto A, Muurasniemi-Isoviita L, et al. Prevention of travellers' diarrhoea by Lactobacillus GG. Ann Med. 1990;22:53–6.

80. McFarland LV. Probiotics and diarrhea. Ann Nutr Metab. 2010;57 Suppl:10–1.

81. Kollaritsch H. Traveller's diarrhea among Austrian tourists to warm climate countries: II. Clinical features. Eur J Epidemiol. 1989;5:355–62.

82. Ibnou-Zekri N, Blum S, Schiffrin EJ, von der Weid T. Divergent patterns of colonization and immune response elicited from two intestinal Lactobacillus strains that display similar properties in vitro. Infect Immun. 2003;71:428–36.

83. DuPont HL, Ericsson CD, Farthing MJ, Gorbach S, Pickering LK, Rombo L, et al. Expert review of the evidence base for prevention of travelers' diarrhea. J Travel Med. 2009;16:149–60.

84. Huertas-Ceballos AA, Logan S, Bennett C, Macarthur C. Dietary interventions for recurrent abdominal pain (RAP) and irritable bowel syndrome (IBS) in childhood. Cochrane Database Syst Rev. 2009;21(1):CD003019. doi: 10.1002/14651858.CD003019.pub3.

85. Bausserman M, Michail S. The use of Lactobacillus GG in irritable bowel syndrome in children: a double-blind randomized control trial. J Pediatr. 2005;147:197–201.

86. Francavilla R, Miniello V, Magistà AM, De Canio A, Bucci N, Gagliardi F, et al. A randomized controlled trial of Lactobacillus GG in children with functional abdominal pain. Pediatrics. 2010;126:e1445–52.

87. Horvath A, Dziechciarz P, Szajewska H. Meta-analysis: Lactobacillus rhamnosus GG for abdominal pain-related functional gastrointestinal disorders in childhood. Aliment Pharmacol Ther. 2011;33:1302–10.

88. Guandalini S, Magazzù G, Chiaro A, La Balestra V, Di Nardo G, Gopalan S, et al. VSL#3 improves symptoms in children with irritable bowel syndrome: a multicenter, randomized, placebo-controlled, double-blind, crossover study. J Pediatr Gastroenterol Nutr. 2010;51:24–30.

89. Vivatvakin B, Mahayosnond A, Theamboonlers A, Steenhout PG, Conus NJ. Effect of a whey-predominant starter formula containing LCPUFAs and oligosaccharides (FOS/GOS) on gastrointestinal comfort in infants. Asia Pac J Clin Nutr. 2010;19:473–80.

90. Khoshoo V, Sun SS, Storm H. Tolerance of an enteral formula with insoluble and prebiotic fiber in children with compromised gastrointestinal function. J Am Diet Assoc. 2010;110:1728–33.

91. Piirainen L, Kekkonen RA, Kajander K, Ahlroos T, Tynkkynen S, Nevala R, et al. In school-aged children a combination of galacto-oligosaccharides and *Lactobacillus GG* increases bifidobacteria more than *Lactobacillus GG* on its own. Ann Nutr Metab. 2008;52:204–8.

92. Yang YJ, Sheu BS. Probiotics-containing yogurts suppress *Helicobacter pylori* load and modify immune response and intestinal microbiota in the *Helicobacter pylori*-infected children. Helicobacter. 2012;17:297–304.

93. Szajewska H, Horvath A, Piwowarczyk A. Meta-analysis: the effects of *Saccharomyces boulardii* supplementation on *Helicobacter pylori* eradication rates and side effects during treatment. Aliment Pharmacol Ther. 2010;32:1069–79.

94. Szajewska H, Albrecht P, Topczewska-Cabanek A. Randomized, double-blind, placebo-controlled trial: effect of *Lactobacillus GG* supplementation on *Helicobacter pylori* eradication rates and side effects during treatment in children. J Pediatr Gastroenterol Nutr. 2009;48:431–6.

95. Malfertheiner P, Selgrad M, Bornschein J. *Helicobacter pylori*: clinical management. Curr Opin Gastroenterol. 2012;28:608–14.

96. Wilhelm SM, Johnson JL, Kale-Pradhan PB. Treating bugs with bugs: the role of probiotics as adjunctive therapy for *Helicobacter pylori*. Ann Pharmacother. 2011;45:960–6.

97. Tabbers MM, de Milliano I, Roseboom MG, Benninga MA. Is *Bifidobacterium breve* effective in the treatment of childhood constipation? Results from a pilot study. Nutr J. 2011;10:19.

98. Bekkali NL, Bongers ME, Van den Berg MM, Liem O, Benninga MA. The role of a probiotics mixture in the treatment of childhood constipation: a pilot study. Nutr J. 2007;6:17.

99. Bu LN, Chang MH, Ni YH, Chen HL, Cheng CC. *Lactobacillus casei rhamnosus Lcr35* in children with chronic constipation. Pediatr Int. 2007;49:485–90.

100. Ritchie ML, Romanuk TN. A meta-analysis of probiotic efficacy for gastrointestinal diseases. Plos One. 2012;7:e34938.

101. Coccorullo P, Strisciuglio C, Martinelli M, Miele E, Greco L, Staiano A. *Lactobacillus reuteri* (DSM 17938) in infants with functional chronic constipation: a double-blind, randomized, placebo-controlled study. J Pediatr. 2010;157:598–602.

102. Guerra PV, Lima LN, Souza TC, Mazochi V, Penna FJ, Silva AM, et al. Pediatric functional constipation treatment with *Bifidobacterium*-containing yogurt: a crossover, double-blind, controlled trial. World J Gastroenterol. 2011;17:3916–21.

103. Tabbers MM, Chmielewska A, Roseboom MG, Crastes N, Perrin C, Reitsma JB, et al. Fermented milk containing *Bifidobacterium lactis* DN-173 010 in childhood constipation: a randomized, double-blind, controlled trial. Pediatrics. 2011;127:e1392–9.

104. Tabbers MM, Boluyt N, Berger MY, Benninga MA. Nonpharmacologic treatments for childhood constipation: systematic review. Pediatrics. 2011;128:753–61.

105. Chmielewska A, Szajewska H. Systematic review of randomised controlled trials: probiotics for functional constipation. World J Gastroenterol. 2010;16:69–75.

106. Hoyos AB. Reduced incidence of necrotizing enterocolitis associated with enteral administration of *Lactobacillus acidophilus* and *Bifidobacterium infantis* to neonates in an intensive care unit. Int J Infect Dis. 1999;3:197–202.

107. Dani C, Biadaioli R, Bertini G, Martelli E, Rubaltelli FF. Probiotics feeding in prevention of urinary tract infection, bacterial sepsis and necrotizing enterocolitis in preterm infants. A prospective double-blind study. Biol Neonate. 2002;82:103–8.

108. Lin HC, Su BH, Chen AC, Lin TW, Tsai CH, Yeh TF, et al. Oral probiotics reduce the incidence and severity of necrotizing enterocolitis in very low birth weight infants. Pediatrics. 2005;115:1–4.

109. Bin-Nun A, Bromiker R, Wilschanski M, Kaplan M, Rudensky B, Caplan M, et al. Oral probiotics prevent necrotizing enterocolitis in very low birth weight neonates. J Pediatr. 2005;147:192–6.

110. Akisu M, Baka M, Yalaz M, Huseyinov A, Kultursay N. Supplementation with *Saccharomyces boulardii* ameliorates hypoxia/reoxygenation-induced necrotizing enterocolitis in young mice. Eur J Pediatr Surg. 2003;13:319–23.

111. Costalos C, Skouteri V, Gounaris A, Sevastiadou S, Triandafilidou A, Ekonomidou C, et al. Enteral feeding of premature infants with *Saccharomyces boulardii*. Early Hum Dev. 2003;74:89–96.

112. Alfaleh K, Bassler D. Probiotics for prevention of necrotizing enterocolitis in preterm infants. Cochrane Database Syst Rev. 2008;23(1):CD005496.

113. Alfaleh K, Anabrees J, Bassler D, Al-Kharfi T. Probiotics for prevention of necrotizing enterocolitis in preterm infants. Cochrane Database Syst Rev. 2011;16(3):CD005496.

114. Downard CD, Renaud E, St Peter SD, Abdullah F, Islam S, Saito JM, et al., For the 2012 American Pediatric Surgical Association Outcomes Clinical Trials Committee. Treatment of necrotizing enterocolitis: an American Pediatric Surgical Association Outcomes and Clinical Trials Committee systematic review. J Pediatr Surg. 2012;47:2111–22.

115. Mihatsch WA, Braegger CP, Decsi T, Kolacek S, Lanzinger H, Mayer B, et al. Critical systematic review of the level of evidence for routine use of probiotics for reduction of mortality and prevention of necrotizing enterocolitis and sepsis in preterm infants. Clin Nutr. 2012;31:6–15.

116. Fallon EM, Nehra D, Potemkin AK, Gura KM, Simpser E, Compher C, American Society for Parenteral and Enteral Nutrition (A.S.P.E.N.) Board of Directors, Puder M. A.S.P.E.N. clinical guidelines: nutrition support of neonatal patients at risk for necrotizing enterocolitis. J Parenter Enteral Nutr. 2012;36:506–23.

117. Janvier A, Lantos J, Barrington K. The politics of probiotics: probiotics, necrotizing enterocolitis, and the ethics of neonatal research. Acta Paediatr. 2013;102:116–8.

118. Savino F, Pelle E, Palumeri E, Oggero R, Miniero R. *Lactobacillus reuteri* (American Type Culture Collection Strain 55730) versus simethicone in the treatment of infantile colic: a prospective randomized study. Pediatrics. 2007;119:e124–30.

119. Savino F, Cordisco L, Tarasco V, Palumeri E, Calabrese R, Oggero R, et al. *Lactobacillus reuteri* DSM 17938 in infantile colic: a randomized, double-blind, placebo-controlled trial. Pediatrics. 2010;126:e526–33.

120. Szajewska H, Gyrczuk E, Horvath A. *Lactobacillus reuteri* DSM 17938 for the management of infantile colic in breastfed infants: a randomized, double-blind, placebo-controlled trial. J Pediatr. 2013;162:257–62.

121. Dupont C, Rivero M, Grillon C, Belaroussi N, Kalindjian A, Marin V. Alpha-lactalbumin-enriched and probiotic-supplemented infant formula in infants with colic: growth and gastrointestinal tolerance. Eur J Clin Nutr. 2010;64:765–7.

122. Kukkonen K, Savilahti E, Haahtela T, Juntunen-Backman K, Korpela R, Poussa T, et al. Long-term safety and impact on infection rates of postnatal probiotic and prebiotic (synbiotic) treatment: randomized, double-blind, placebo-controlled trial. Pediatrics. 2008;122:8–12.

123. Taylor AL, Dunstan JA, Prescott SL. Probiotic supplementation for the first 6 months of life fails to reduce the risk of atopic dermatitis and increases the risk of allergen sensitization in high-risk children: a randomized controlled trial. J Allergy Clin Immunol. 2007;119:184–91.

124. Osborn DA, Sinn JK. Probiotics in infants for prevention of allergic disease and food hypersensitivity. Cochrane Database Syst Rev. 2007;17(4):CD006475.

125. Dotterud CK, Storrø O, Johnsen R, Oien T. Probiotics in pregnant women to prevent allergic disease: a randomized, double-blind trial. Br J Dermatol. 2010;163:616–23.

126. Doege K, Grajecki D, Zyriax BC, Detinkina E, Zu Eulenburg C, Buhling KJ. Impact of maternal supplementation with probiotics during pregnancy on atopic eczema in childhood–a meta-analysis. Br J Nutr. 2012;107:1–6.

127. Wickens K, Black P, Stanley TV, Mitchell E, Barthow C, Fitzharris P, Purdie G, et al. A protective effect of *Lactobacillus rhamnosus* HN001 against eczema in the first 2 years of life persists to age 4 years. Clin Exp Allergy. 2012;42:1071–9.

128. Pelucchi C, Chatenoud L, Turati F, Galeone C, Moja L, Bach JF, et al. Probiotics supplementation during pregnancy or infancy for the prevention of atopic dermatitis: a meta-analysis. Epidemiology. 2012;23:402–14.

129. van der Aa LB, van Aalderen WM, Heymans HS, Henk Sillevis Smitt J, Nauta AJ, et al., Synbad Study Group. Synbiotics prevent asthma-like symptoms in infants with atopic dermatitis. Allergy. 2011, 66:170–7.

130. Bath-Hextall FJ, Jenkinson C, Humphreys R, Williams HC. Dietary supplements for established atopic eczema. Cochrane Database Syst Rev. 2012;15(2):CD005205.

131. Wu KG, Li TH, Peng HJ. *Lactobacillus salivarius* plus fructo-oligosaccharide is superior to fructo-oligosaccharide alone for treating children with moderate to severe atopic dermatitis: a double-blind, randomized, clinical trial of efficacy and safety. Br J Dermatol. 2012;166:129–36.

132. Han Y, Kim B, Ban J, Lee J, Kim BJ, Choi BS, et al. A randomized trial of *Lactobacillus plantarum CJLP133* for the treatment of atopic dermatitis. Pediatr Allergy Immunol. 2012;23:667–73.

133. Gore C, Custovic A, Tannock GW, Munro K, Kerry G, Johnson K, et al. Treatment and secondary prevention effects of the probiotics *Lactobacillus paracasei* or *Bifidobacterium lactis* on early infant eczema: randomized controlled trial with follow-up until age 3 years. Clin Exp Allergy. 2012;42:112–22.

134. Thomas DW, Greer FR. Clinical report: probiotics and prebiotics in pediatrics. Pediatrics. 2010;126:1217–31.

135. van der Aa LB, Lutter R, Heymans HS, Smids BS, Dekker T, van Aalderen WM, et al., Synbad Study Group. No detectable beneficial systemic immunomodulatory effects of a specific synbiotic mixture in infants with atopic dermatitis. Clin Exp Allergy. 2012;42:531–9.

136. Sazawal S, Dhingra U, Hiremath G, Sarkar A, Dhingra P, Dutta A, et al. Prebiotic and probiotic fortified milk in prevention of morbidities among children: community-based, randomized, double-blind, controlled trial. PLoS One. 2010;5:e12164.

137. Kumar S, Singhi S. Role of probiotics in prevention of *Candida* infection in critically ill children. Mycoses. 2013;56:204–11.

138. Sanz-Penella JM, Frontela C, Ros G, Martinez C, Monedero V, Haros M. Application of bifidobacterial phytases in infant cereals: effect on phytate contents and mineral dialyzability. J Agric Food Chem. 2012;60:11787–892.

139. Capozzi V, Russo P, Dueñas MT, López P, Spano G. Lactic acid bacteria producing B-group vitamins: a great potential for functional cereals products. Appl Microbiol Biotechnol. 2012;96:1383–94.

140. Kadooka Y, Sato M, Imaizumi K, Ogawa A, Ikuyama K, Akai Y, et al. Regulation of abdominal adiposity by probiotics (*Lactobacillus gasseri SBT2055*) in adults with obese tendencies in a randomized controlled trial. Eur J Clin Nutr. 2010;64:636–43.

141. Andreasen AS, Larsen N, Pedersen-Skovsgaard T, Berg RM, Møller K, Svendsen KD, et al. Effects of *Lactobacillus acidophilus* NCFM on insulin sensitivity and the systemic inflammatory response in human subjects. Br J Nutr. 2010;104:1831–8.

142. Luoto R, Kalliomäki M, Laitinen K, Isolauri E. The impact of perinatal probiotic intervention on the development of overweight and obesity: follow-up study from birth to 10 years. Int J Obes (Lond). 2010;34:1531–7.

143. Lo Vecchio A, Cohen MB. Fecal microbiota transplantation for *Clostridium difficile* infection: benefits and barriers. Curr Opin Gastroenterol. 2014;30:47–53.

144. Rubin DT. Curbing our enthusiasm for fecal transplantation in ulcerative colitis. Am J Gastroenterol. 2013;108:1631–3.

145. Quera R, Espinoza R, Estay C, Rivera D. Bacteremia as an adverse event of fecal microbiota transplantation in a patient with Crohn's disease and recurrent *Clostridium difficile* infection. J Crohns Colitis. 2014;8:252–3.

146. Kunde S, Pham A, Bonczyk S, et al. Safety, tolerability, and clinical response after fecal transplantation in children and young adults with ulcerative colitis. J Pediatr Gastroenterol Nutr. 2013;56:597–601.

147. Vrieze A, de Groot PF, Kootte RS, et al. Fecal transplant: a safe and sustainable clinical therapy for restoring intestinal microbial balance in human disease? Best Pract Res Clin Gastroenterol. 2013;27:127–37.

148. Vandenplas Y, Veereman G, van der Werff ten Bosch J, Goossens A, Pierard D, Samsom JN, Escher JC. Fecal microbial transplantation in a one-year-old girl with early onset colitis—caution advised. J Pediatr Gastroenterol Nutr. 2014 Jan 2 [Epub ahead of print]

149. Shanahan F. A commentary on the safety of probiotics. Gastroenterol Clin North Am. 2012;41:869–76.

150. Fedorak RN, Madsen KI. Probiotics and prebiotics in gastrointestinal disorders. Curr Opin Gastroenterol. 2004;20:146–55.

151. Allen SJ, Jordan S, Storey M, Thornton CA, Gravenor M, Garaiova I, et al. Dietary supplementation with lactobacilli and bifidobacteria is well tolerated and not associated with adverse events during late pregnancy and early infancy. J Nutr. 2010;140:483–8.

152. Martín-Muñoz MF, Fortuni M, Caminoa M, Belver T, Quirce S, Caballero T. Anaphylactic reaction to probiotics. Cow's milk and hen's egg allergens in probiotic compounds. Pediatr Allergy Immunol. 2012;23:778–84.

153. Borriello SP, Hammes WP, Holzapfel W, Marteau P, Schrezenmeir J, Vaara M, et al. Safety of probiotics that contain lactobacilli or bifidobacteria. Clin Infect Dis. 2003;36:775–80.

154. Mackay AD, Taylor MB, Kibbler CC, Hamilton-Miller JM. *Lactobacillus* endocarditis caused by a probiotics organism. Clin Microbiol Infect. 1999;5:290–2.

155. Rautio M, Jousimies-Somer H, Kauma H, Pietarinen I, Saxelin M, Tynkkynen S, et al. Liver abcess due to a *Lactobacillus rhamnosus* strain indistinguishable from a *L. rhamnosus* strain GG. Clin Infect Dis. 1999;28:1159–60.

156. Cabana MD, Shane AL, Chao C, Oliva-Henker M. Probiotics in primary care pediatrics. Clin Pediatr. 2006;45:405–10.

157. Dai M, Lu J, Wang Y, Liu Z, Yuan Z. In vitro development and transfer of resistance to chlortetracycline in *Bacillus subtilis*. J Microbiol. 2012;50:807–12.

Enteral Nutrition

46

Timothy A. Sentongo, Olivier Goulet and Virginie Colomb

Introduction

Enteral nutrition (EN) or enteral tube feeding (ETF) as currently practiced is a technique for nutritional support which delivers a homogeneous, liquid nutrition admixture into the digestive tract by tube, into the stomach, duodenum, or the proximal jejunum. The inception of enteral feeding dates back to 3500 years ago in ancient Egypt, when practitioners used rectal enemas to administer wine, milk, broth, and other nutrients to the ill [1, 2]. The first documented delivery of EN through a tube inserted into the esophagus was by Capivavacceus of Venice in 1598, who constructed a device from animal bladder. Recognition of the importance of nutrition therapy during injury and recovery from disease rapidly grew in the 1930s and 1940s, and led to development of specialized commercial enteral feeding products in the 1950s, and modern EN formulas in the 1970s [1, 2]. In 1980, Guaderer and colleagues at Rainbow Babies and Children's Hospital in Cleveland, Ohio, USA, were the first to describe the technique of inserting feeding gastrostomy tubes (GT) without requirement for laparotomy, that is, percutaneous endoscopic gastrostomy (PEG) tube [3]. EN may be administered via oral, nasal, gastrostomy, or jejunal routes (Fig. 46.1).

EN is used to preserve nutritional status, support normal growth, and treat malnutrition when oral feeding is inadequate or not possible. EN is more physiologic, usually safer, easier to administer, and less costly compared to parenteral nutrition (PN). Therefore, EN should be preferred to PN in infants and children with malnutrition and/or nutritional risk, when the intestinal tract is usable to provide sufficient nutrients for achieving optimal growth or catch-up growth [4]. EN may be administered rapidly as a bolus into the stomach, or more slowly over several hours as a continuous infusion into the stomach, duodenum, or jejunum. The underlying disease and patient tolerance are what determines whether to use bolus or continuous feeds. The physiological basis of continuous EN makes it of great interest in pediatric patients with feeding intolerance and other gastrointestinal (GI) disorders [4]. EN may be used as the sole source of nutrition or to just supplement a patient's oral and/or PN intake. Also, depending on the indication, EN may be used daily or just on a periodic basis. While EN is normally initiated in the hospital, continuing it at home has become a common option. Home EN may be used long term or just as a temporary bridge until children achieve oral food intakes that support adequate growth and nutritional status. Even though home EN is an effective method of meeting a child's growth and nutritional requirements, health practitioners should not disregard the mixed acceptance by families and sometimes negative impact on quality of life [5–7].

Physiological Basis of Continuous Enteral Feeding

Gastrointestinal Motility

The rate of gastric emptying, and secretion of pancreatic biliary fluids, is regulated by the infusion rate, calorie density, and osmolality of the enteral feeds [8]. In case of gastric administration of continuous feeds, a rate of continuous gastric emptying related to the infusion rate can be achieved if the infusion rate, calorie density, and osmolality of the mixture are not excessive. Steady-state gastric emptying of 1 kcal/mL formula can be maintained at infusion rates of ≤ 3 mL/min. When the infusion rate is excessive and higher than the gastric emptying rate, the risk of vomiting increases. As caloric load and/or osmolality of the formula increase, the

T. A. Sentongo (✉)
Department of Pediatrics, Section of Gastroenterology, Hepatology and Nutrition, Comer Children's Hospital, University of Chicago, 5841 S. Maryland Avenue, Chicago, IL 60637, USA
e-mail: tsentong@peds.bsd.uchicago.edu

O. Goulet · V. Colomb
Department of Pediatric Gastroenterology and Nutrition, Hôpital Necker-Enfants Malades, 149 rue de Sèvres, 75743 Paris Cedex 15, France

© Springer International Publishing Switzerland 2016
S. Guandalini et al. (eds.), *Textbook of Pediatric Gastroenterology, Hepatology and Nutrition*,
DOI 10.1007/978-3-319-17169-2_46

Fig. 46.1 Possible routes for EN

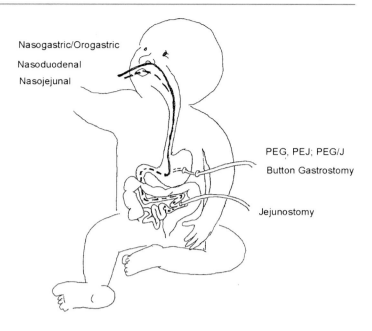

Nasogastric/Orogastric
Nasoduodenal
Nasojejunal

PEG, PEJ; PEG/J
Button Gastrostomy

Jejunostomy

PEG: Percutaneous endoscopic gastrostomy tube
PEJ: Percutaneous endoscopic jejunostomy tube
PEG/J: Percutaneous endoscopic gastrostomy & jejunal tube

gastric emptying rate is reduced to maintain a constant calorie load delivered into the duodenum. Thus, EN consisting of very calorie-dense formulas should initially be administered very cautiously. The individual nutrient composition of the formula has a lesser effect on gastric emptying function than the caloric density, except for the type of triglyceride: In fact, long-chain triglycerides (LCTs) cause greater delays in gastric emptying than medium-chain triglycerides (MCTs)

Gastric emptying is dependent on duodenal function. The effects of continuous enteral nutrition (CEN) on intestinal motility can be analyzed by manometry. Motor migrating complexes are observed in adults during CEN, as during fasting state [9]. In small preterm infants, duodenal motor activity is higher following slower infusion of gastric feeds than with rapid boluses, and this is associated with lower postprandial gastric contents [10]. During administration of jejunal feeds, energy loads at rates within the physiologic range of gastric emptying (≤4 kcal/min) initiate normal-motor small-bowel motor responses; however, increasing the osmolality (>600 mosmol) has a significant inhibitory effect on small bowel contractile and propagative activity [11] and thus greater likelihood for intolerance. Very few data are available about the changes of colonic motility induced by CEN; the continuous gastric infusion of nutritive formula modifies the gastrocolic reflex. Gallbladder motility is maintained during CEN as assessed by increased serum cholecystokinin (CCK) and ultrasonography [11, 12]. Emulsified LCTs delivered to the duodenum have a potent stimu-

lating effect on CCK release and gall bladder contraction [13]. Conversely, whereas dietary MCTs are more efficiently absorbed and rapidly metabolized compared to LCT's [14], they are very weak stimulants for CCK release, gall bladder contractility, and hence luminal postprandial bile acid concentrations. Biliary complications such as sludge or cholelithiasis are rare during long-term CEN.

Digestive Secretion and Hormonal Response

Gastric secretion depends mostly on protein intake, and, in case of elemental diet, on amino-acids composition; secretory response is not influenced by carbohydrates but reduced by lipids. It has not been demonstrated whether or not the type of diet (i.e., elemental, semi-elemental, or polymeric) modifies gastric acid secretion [15]. Secretion of CCK and pancreatic polypeptide (PP) are maintained during CEN [12]. All forms of oral and enteral feeding stimulate pancreatic synthesis and secretion through CCK and PP. Pancreatic secretions can be reduced by 50% if a low-fat elemental formula is used for duodenal feeding. Stimulation of pancreatic trypsin synthesis or secretion can be inhibited by delivering EN into the mid-distal jejunum [16]. The mechanism involves increased secretion of the 'ileal-brake' hormones glucagon-like peptide-1 (GLP-1) and peptide YY (PYY) [17, 18] which inhibit production of pancreatic secretions and motility in the proximal GI tract. Gastrin secretion is also maintained during CEN, but its response to protein load is decreased. Gastric or duodenal CEN stimulate insulin secretion depending on the type of infused nutrients. The glycemic and insulinemic response induced by EN parallels that of oral feeds and significantly lower than PN [16]; therefore, less risk for steatosis.

Effects of CEN on Mucosal Trophicity

The effects of elemental formulas (totally absorbed in the upper GI tract and providing minimal residue to the distal bowel) on small bowel mucosal trophism remain controversial. In studies, comparing intestinal trophicity and function in animals fed elemental diets versus regular chow, there was similar digestive function but significantly decreased mucosal mass in the distal bowel of animals-fed elemental diets. These changes could be the consequence of the almost complete absorption of nutrients within the proximal part of the small bowel, leading to lack of stimulation of the distal segment. This suggests an ability of EN to achieve bowel rest in the distal part of the bowel, providing efficient treatment for ileocolic inflammatory diseases.

Effects of CEN on Energy Expenditure and Feeding Tolerance

Thermogenic effect of feeding is related to the increase of energy expenditure for synthesis and secretion of digestive enzymes following ingestion of food. The increase in energy expenditure induced by CEN in normal subjects is lower than when the same nutrients are administered by bolus feed [19]. Finally, the slow and continuous administration of nutrients into the GI tract through CEN allows the achievement of optimal utilization despite intestinal illness. In fact, by changing the conditions of flow and of contact between the nutritive formula and the digestive tract, CEN may increase the capacity for intraluminal digestion and intestinal absorption. This feeding technique does not appear to provide benefit in patients without intestinal disease [20, 21]; however, it seems logical and efficient when the absorptive surface is reduced, for example, short bowel syndrome (SBS), villous atrophy, enterocutaneous fistula, or proximal enterostomy. CEN has been associated with better feeding tolerance, nutrient absorption, and growth than boluses or oral feeds in infants and adult patients with intestinal disease [22, 23].

Indications

Indications for EN are different from indications for PN, since the use of EN as nutritional support is based on normal or at least partially preserved gut functions. The decision tree for the route of feeding is determined based on aspiration risk, motility function of the stomach, and anticipated duration of need for EN support. See Fig. 46.2. EN can be used on any patient with normal GI absorptive function but unable to adequately be fed by mouth. The conditions commonly encountered are listed in Table 46.1.

Fig. 46.2 Decision tree for the route of EN. *GER* gastroesophageal reflux, *PN* parenteral nutrition, *GI* gastrointestinal, *PEG* percutaneous endoscopic gastrostomy, *PEG/J* percutaneous endoscopic gastrostomy/jejunostomy, *G-tube* gastrostomy tube

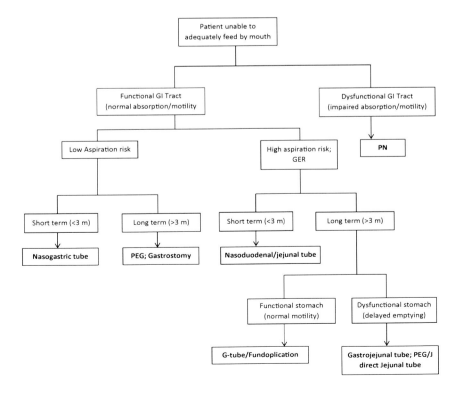

Table 46.1 Conditions commonly managed with EN

Conditions with normal intestinal absorptive function
Preterm infants
Critically ill patients
Nonorganic FTT
Anorexia
Inborn errors of metabolism
Glycogen storage diseases, urea cycle defects
Chylothorax
Hypermetabolic states
Head injury, graft versus host disease (GVHD), renal failure, congenital heart disease
Digestive disorders
Protracted diarrhea of infancy/childhood
Short bowel syndrome
Intestinal pseudo-obstruction
Crohn's disease
Malabsorption disorders
Cystic fibrosis
Chronic liver disease
FTT failure to thrive

Conditions with Normal Intestinal Absorptive Function

EN is required in cases of inability to eat normally, that is, in those situations that are secondary to structural or functional abnormalities of the upper GI tract or neurological impairment of the processes involved in sucking and/or swallowing (see also Chap. 20 on "Disorders of Sucking and Swallowing"). Esophageal diseases including esophageal atresia, fistula, or stenosis, often resulting from sequel of epidermolysis bullosa, are among the conditions that can benefit from EN, usually through gastrostomy or duodenal tubes [24, 25]. The choice of feeding through gastrostomy versus transpyloric tube must be assessed according to the patient age, disease, and condition (Fig. 46.2). Children with chronic diseases inducing immaturity or inability to feed orally, especially with sucking and swallowing troubles as seen in neurologically impaired children, with neuromuscular chronic diseases or cerebral palsy also require EN, using GTs.

Premature Infants

EN via nasogastric or orogastric tube is routinely used in premature infants younger than 32 weeks' gestation because of uncoordinated suck, swallow, and breathing related to immaturity [26]. Human milk is the preferred feed because of its immunological benefits. Preterm infant formulas come fortified with protein, calcium/phosphorous, and a calorie density of 22–24 kcal/oz. to meet the high nutritional requirements of infants. A Cochrane systematic review of treatment trials did not provide evidence of any beneficial effect from transpyloric feeding over gastric feeding on feeding tolerance, growth, and development in preterm infants

[27]. Therefore, gastric feedings administered by bolus or continuously is the preferred approach for EN in preterm infants, where its use appears to also have a role in preventing necrotizing enterocolitis [28] (see also Chap. 6 on "Enteral Nutrition in Preterm Neonates" and Chap. 7 on "Parenteral Nutrition in Premature Infants").

Eating Disorders: Anorexia

Anorexia nervosa (AN) is a life-threatening psychiatric condition characterized by disordered eating behaviors, significantly lower than expected body weight, intense fear of becoming overweight, and a distorted body image. It is managed by a multidisciplinary team of health providers including psychiatrists, adolescent medicine pediatricians, nutritionists, and social workers. Indications for inpatient therapy include presence of suicidal or aggressive behaviors; severe bradycardia, hypotension, electrolyte imbalance, dehydration, and hypothermia; and medical complications, for example, seizures and pancreatitis [29]. Weight restoration is one of the major predicators for favorable short- and long-term outcomes in patients with AN [30]. Also, restoration of body weight is associated with improvements in malnutrition-induced cognitive impairments thus facilitating psychological and psychiatric therapy [31].

Nutritional support in AN remains very controversial. The oral feeding route is preferred; however, patients are given the option of voluntary or forced EN if resistant to therapy and/or severe malnutrition, that is, body mass index (BMI) < 13 kg/m^2 in adolescents [32] and weight-for-height z score < -3 in younger children [33]. Other options like GT and PN are considered in young children or severe and chronic cases [29]. Follow-up of adults treated with EN during adolescence did not show any long-term benefits or adverse outcomes on growth, recovery, or persistence of AN or risk for development of psychiatric comorbidities [34]. The initial range of prescribed energy intake varies from 10–60 kcal/day to 1000 kcal/day and > 1900 kcal/day with progressive increase during the course of hospitalization [29, 30]. The main complication of nutritional management is risk for developing re-feeding syndrome: hypophosphatemia, hypokalemia, edema, and increased hepatic transaminases. The risk factors associated with re-feeding syndrome include greater severity of malnutrition, abnormal electrolytes prior to re-feeding, use of EN or PN, and weight loss $> 15\%$ within the preceding 3 months [29, 30]. Patients may be preemptively treated with phosphate supplements during the early phases of nutritional management.

Inborn Errors of Metabolism

EN is part of the standard therapy used to prevent biochemical abnormalities, metabolic decompensation, and catabolism in patients with inherited disorders of metabolism, for example, hepatic glycogen storage disease (GSD) and enzyme deficiencies of the urea cycle. Patients with GSD type 1 (glucose-6-phosphatase deficiency) develop hypoglycemia and compensatory biochemical abnormalities of lactic acidosis, hyperuricemia, hyperlipidemia, and platelet dysfunction all stemming from the primary defect of inability to dephosphorylate glucose-6-phposphate to free glucose. Managing GSD type 1 involves overnight continuous high-carbohydrate feedings and frequent daytime feedings supplemented with uncooked cornstarch [35, 36]. EN consisting of a glucose/glucose polymer solution or a sucrose-free, lactose-free/low formula enriched with maltodextrin may be used. EN should be started within 1 h after the last meal. Likewise, an oral or EN should be given within 15 min after discontinuation of the continuous EN because of the risk for hypoglycemia. Gastrostomy is contraindicated in patients with GSD type 1b because of complications in case development of inflammatory bowel disease or local infections [36]. Continuous EN should provide a glucose infusion rate of 7–9 mg/kg/min in children younger than 6 years, 5–6 mg/kg/min in children aged 6–12 years, and 5 mg/kg/min in adolescents [36]. Intermittent feedings of uncooked cornstarch may be used if continuous nighttime EN is not an option. No significant differences in biochemical parameters or growth have been found between patients with GSD type 1 receiving overnight continuous EN compared to scheduled feeds of uncooked cornstarch [37, 38]. The starting dose for uncooked cornstarch is 0.25 g/kg and optimal dose is 1.75–2.5 g/kg of ideal body weight every 6 h [36, 37, 39]. Patients with GSD type 3 (debrancher enzyme deficiency) have impeded glycogenolysis; however, gluconeogenesis is endogenously enhanced to maintain adequate glucose production. Therefore, nutritional management of patients with GSD type 3 involves frequent high-protein feedings during the day and a high-protein snack at night. Patients with GSD IV (brancher enzyme deficiency), GSD VI (phosphorylase deficiency), and GSD IX (phosphorylase kinase deficiency) respond to the to the high-protein diets similar to what is recommended for patients with GSD type 3 [40].

Inherited defects in urea synthesis are inborn errors of nitrogen detoxification and arginine synthesis due to defects in the urea cycle enzymes namely carbamylphosphate synthetase 1, ornithine transcarbamylase, arginosuccinate synthetase, arginosuccinate lyase, and arginase [41]. They may present at any age with symptoms ranging from poor feeding to coma shock and death. Other clinical symptoms may include lethargy, vomiting, ataxia, confusion, behavior changes, hypotonia or spasticity, hyperventilation (leading to respiratory alkalosis), and seizures. The main biochemical abnormalities are hyperammonemia and increased plasma concentrations of glutamine [42]. The symptoms of metabolic crisis are usually precipitated by protein intake in excess of what the patient can metabolize, catabolism of lean body mass resulting from intercurrent infection, trauma, inadequate energy intake, or inadequate intake of protein or essential amino acids. Management of patients with urea cycle defects involves a combination of carefully restricting protein intake and therapy with nitrogen-scavenging drugs, for example, sodium benzoate, sodium phenyl acetate, or sodium phenyl butyrate [41]. The nutritional management includes: (1) administration of sufficient energy to support anabolism, (2) restriction of protein intake to that tolerated by the patient without producing excess NH_3, (3) provision of essential amino acids in adequate amounts to support growth, (4) supplementation of "conditionally" essential arginine or citrulline in all except arginase deficiency, and (5) provision of all required minerals and vitamins in adequate amounts for age [43]. During hyperammonemic metabolic crisis, the nutritional management consists of providing high-energy low-protein intakes [44]. Successful long-term management requires a dedicated metabolics dietician and physician to make dietary adjustments and closely monitor progress. Patients with neurological handicaps or developmental delays, feeding difficulties, poor appetite/refusal of food, compliance problems with the diet, and/or medications will require use of nasogastric or gastrostomy feeding tubes to ensure adequate intake [41, 45]. Patients in metabolic crisis with symptomatic hyperammonemia (> 500 μM/L) and/or lack of response despite 4 h of medical treatment should have management escalated to dialysis [41].

Hyper Metabolic States

Hypermetabolic states include patients with burns, cancer, and head injury. Much of the morbidity and mortality in severely burned patients is connected to the prolonged hypermetabolism and catabolism, impaired wound healing, and sepsis. Whenever, GI function permits, EN is superior to PN in patients with burns [46]. EN results in better regulation of the postburn catabolic hormones and inflammatory cytokine responses than PN [46, 47]. Furthermore, early EN support of patients with severe burns helps maintain gut mucosal integrity, which has the beneficial effect on reducing risk for enterogenic infections [48].

Graft Versus Host Disease

Traditionally, PN is given as the first option for nutrition support in children undergoing chemotherapy and/or bone marrow/stem cell transplant. The reasons cited range from intestinal injury and poor GI tolerance secondary to conditioning and myeloablative therapy; intestinal graft versus host disease (GVHD), oral mucositis, epistaxis, and parental refusal of EN. However, whenever GI function permits, EN is equally as effective as PN, associated with lower risk for infection, and more cost-effective [49–52]. A prospective study comparing EN and PN in children with bone marrow transplants had poor enrolment into the EN group. Initiation of EN prior to transplant was associated with better overall tolerance. The EN group was also less likely to develop cholestasis [51]. A more recent Cochrane database review of nutrition support in patients of all ages with bone marrow or stem cell transplants failed to find evaluable data that properly compared efficacy and superiority of EN versus PN. However, the overall findings suggested that in patients without GI symptoms, intravenous fluids and oral diet should be considered as preference to PN [53].

Renal Failure

Supplemental nutrition should be given to children with renal failure to promote positive nitrogen balance and meet energy needs [4]. Children with chronic renal failure are at risk for malnutrition and growth retardation from persistent anorexia, inadequate protein calorie intake, chronic metabolic acidosis, azotemia, hormonal and metabolic disturbances, and catabolic diseases associated with uremia, for example, infections. Long-term EN is effective in preventing growth retardation in children with chronic renal disease and persistent anorexia, especially if started before the age of 2 years [54, 55] but singly may not lead to catch-up growth [56]. There is a positive correlation between efficacy of dialysis and linear of children with chronic renal failure [57]. Therefore, the combination of aggressive nutrition support with whey protein-based formulas in children age <2 years, whole protein enteral formula (1–1.5 kcal/mL) in older children [58], and enhanced dialysis is necessary for inducing growth in children with chronic renal failure [59]. Growth hormone therapy is recommended if there is persistent growth retardation despite adequate nutrition support [58, 60]. Ultimately, catch-up growth in height is mainly seen in children who undergo renal transplant before the age of 6 years [61].

Congenital Heart Disease

Inadequate calorie intake is the predominant cause of growth failure in infants and children with congenital heart disease. Different approaches for nutrition intervention are utilized during the preoperative, postoperative, and post-discharge periods, respectively [62]. Infants with cyanotic congenital heart disease and complex ventricular lesions are particularly susceptible to malnutrition and growth failure [63]. Approximately, 50 % of infants with surgically treated uni-ventricular lesions get discharged home on EN via nasogastric or GT [64]. The causes of malnutrition include an imbalance between energy intake and increased expenditure particularly in children with congestive heart failure. Infants with severe congenital heart disease have normal resting energy expenditure [65, 66] but increased total energy expenditure [67], thus indicating that they expend large amounts of energy above basal requirements, which places them at risk

for inadequate calorie intake when feeding at normal rates. Perioperative injury to the recurrent laryngeal nerve may lead to feeding difficulties from swallowing dysfunction and vocal cord paralysis [68]. Other contributing factors include pulmonary hypertension, tachypnea and fatigue interfering with oral feeding, medications associated with anorexia, for example, diuretics, prescription of fat-restricted diets in patients who develop chylous effusions, and GI nutrient loss in patients who develop post-Fontan protein-losing enteropathy. Post-Fontan protein-losing enteropathy is managed with therapies directed at improving cardiac hemodynamics and controlling inflammation [69].

Digestive Indications

Since EN has a trophic effect on the intestinal mucosa, and helps maintain mucosal integrity, it plays an important role in the treatment of many digestive diseases, either replacing or complementing oral feeding. Digestive diseases leading to an anatomical or functional reduction of the absorption capacity of the small bowel represent the first group; they include SBS, protracted diarrhea with villous atrophy, and inflammatory bowel disease.

Severe Protracted Diarrhea of Infancy

A syndrome of intractable diarrhea of infancy was first described by Avery et al in 1968. Its definition, presentation, and outcome have considerably changed during the past two decades [70]. This syndrome could now be defined as persistent diarrhea despite prolonged bowel rest requiring long term-total parenteral nutrition (TPN) in children when no effective treatment is available [71, 72]. According to that definition, EN in this circumstance is indicated and often effective [73]. In fact, the reduction of digestive secretions, villous atrophy, and acquired brush border disaccharidase deficiency lead to malabsorption and malnutrition. Most of the time, a short course of PN followed by protracted CEN provides control of the disease within 6–8 weeks [74, 75]. In a prospective study of CEN versus PN, Orenstein showed that the resolution of diarrhea was faster in the enterally fed group [75]. The use of CEN in children and mainly infants with protracted diarrhea presenting also severe malnutrition may prove difficult. If the response to CEN is not good enough to provide rapidly adequate caloric supplies with resolution of diarrhea, PN should be started. Such decisions must be taken by experienced teams in specialized and well-staffed units. Severely malnourished infants with some types of particularly severe celiac disease, intolerance to cow milk proteins, protein hydrolysates, or with specific malabsorption syndromes, such as Anderson's disease may also benefit from CEN [76].

Short Bowel Syndrome

SBS is the leading cause of intestinal failure in newborns as well as infants and young children, and it is most commonly the result of an extensive intestinal resection during the neonatal period. EN is often used in these circumstances, although several controversies over the ideal nutritional treatment of children with SBS remain [77]. Of note, intestinal failure may also lead to liver disease [78] (see also Chap. 43 on "Short Bowel Syndrome").

Congenital and Newborn Intestinal Disorders and Pseudo-obstruction

In neonatal abdominal surgery for congenital or acquired disease, CEN, usually combined with PN, offers prolonged nutritional support which has transformed the prognosis in many conditions and is particularly important in the following situations: (1) reduction of the absorptive surface with enterocutaneous fistulae or extensive intestinal resection; (2) functional disorders of gut motility, such as malfunctions of duodenojejunal anastomosis, "plastic" peritonitis after repeated interventions, gastroschisis, and omphalocele.

Chronic intestinal pseudo-obstruction syndrome is a disabling disorder of enteral feeding characterized by repetitive episodes or continuous symptoms and signs of bowel obstruction, including radiographic documentation of dilated bowel with air–fluid levels, in the absence of fixed-lumen-occluding condition [79]. Pseudo-obstruction is classified as "congenital" if newborn infants present with symptoms persisting for the first 2 months of life. "Acquired" pseudo-obstruction applies when previously well patients present with feeding intolerance from pseudo-obstruction symptoms persisting longer than 6 months [79]. Most patients with intestinal pseudo-obstruction require decompression stomas, ileostomies, and colostomies to relieve the recurring obstruction symptoms. Long-term PN is required in a significant proportion of children with pseudo-obstruction [80–82], and even then, administration of at least small volumes of CEN is essential and encouraged for prevention of PN-associated liver disease [83] and maintenance of bowel mucosal integrity [84].

Crohn's Disease

Enteral feeding has been used for many years, particularly in Europe, not only to improve nutritional status and growth but also to influence disease activity in patients with Crohn's disease [85–94]. It was shown that CEN diet is as effective as high-dose corticosteroids in inducing remission in pediatric patients with Crohn's disease and has the added benefit of improved growth and development without the steroid side effects [95, 96]. However, serial meta-analysis conducted by Griffiths et al. in 1995, 2001, and 2007 suggested that therapy with EN was inferior to corticosteroids for inducing clinical response in patients with active Crohn's disease [97–99]. All three analyses largely included adult studies, and several pediatric studies showing striking efficacy were excluded owing to methodological weakness. A more recent meta-analysis that focused on 11 randomized controlled pediatric studies still reported similar efficacy for EN and corticosteroids for inducing remission in Crohn's disease but also cited limited data [100]. The benefits of EN appear to be more favorable in children than adults including correction of impaired growth. Thus, EN is an underused therapy with the advantage of preserving growth while remission is achieved and therefore must be promoted [101]. There is no relevant data showing any significant difference in clinical outcome based on composition of the EN, that is, elemental, protein hydrolysates, or polymeric formula. Indeed, the beneficial effect in achieving remission appears not to be related to the mode of delivery or to the type of diet (no beneficial effect of elemental versus polymeric or semi-elemental) but rather to the reduced antigen load and mostly to changes in the intestinal microbiota [95]. Removal of antigenic material, alteration in intestinal micro flora, changes in gut hormone levels, and the presence of bioactive transforming growth factor-β (TGFβ-1) in casein-based formulas may all play a role in the clinical success of EN [102, 103]. Glutamine-enriched polymeric diet offered no advantage over a standard low-glutamine polymeric diet in the treatment of active Crohn's disease [104]. EN may be also helpful in correction or maintenance of the nutritional state, especially during a relapse of Crohn's disease [96]. EN is part of the preparation for surgical procedure and may be useful during recovery, especially after intestinal resections or enterostomies. In case of severe digestive involvement during Schönlein–Henoch purpura, CEN can be used as nutritional support in the absence of occlusion [105] More on the treatment of Crohn's disease can be found in Chap. 28.

Other Malabsorption Syndromes

Cystic Fibrosis

Malnutrition and impaired growth affects approximately 23 % of children with cystic fibrosis (CF) [106], and growth within the normal range of weight-for-length and BMI is associated with better pulmonary function and long-term survival. In 2008, the CF Foundation recommended that growth assessment using percent ideal body weight (%IBW) be discontinued, and instead rely on age-appropriate weight-for-length percentiles in children aged <2 years, and BMI percentiles in children aged 2–20 years. The nutritional goals in children with CF are to maintain and support growth at weight-for-length or BMI at or above the 50th percentile [106]. Growth abnormalities in patients with CF have a multifactorial etiology including active CF-pulmonary or sinus disease, inadequate or ineffective pancreatic enzyme therapy, inadequate calorie intake, anorexia, presence of CF-related hepatobiliary disease, CF-related diabetes, infectious enteritis, small bowel bacterial overgrowth, and other comorbid intestinal conditions including, for example, celiac disease, inflammatory bowel disease and SBS [107]. Whereas these disorders require specific therapy, nutrition monitoring and intervention in patients with CF should always be implemented regardless of comorbid disease. Improved weight status in patients with CF often requires energy and protein intakes ranging from 110 to 200% of normal needs in healthy people [108, 109]. However, even with an optimal approach to oral feeding, some patients respond poorly to nutritional counseling alone. Therefore, use of EN to supplement dietary intake is recommended to help restore and maintain nutritional status, especially in children aged 13 years and older who present with persistent growth deficits despite nutrition counseling [106]. The utilization of supplemental EN by patients with CF increased from 8.5% in 2001 to 11.1% in 2011 [110] thus indicating greater engagement of nutritional therapy. EN is generally performed during the night over 8–10 h with the initial goal of providing 30–50% of the estimated requirements [107]. Patients with CF are then asked to eat and drink as much as possible during the daytime. Standard formulas containing intact protein, long-chain fat and calorie densities of 1.5–2.0 kcal/mL are generally well tolerated with appropriate dosing and administration of pancreatic enzymes [107, 111] Semi-elemental formulas may be tolerated better in patients with excessive anorexia, bloating, or nausea. The data are unclear whether formulas with medium-chain triglycerides are advantageous over regular formula in patients with CF [107].

Nasogastric tube (NGT) feeding is generally used as a first step. The tube is passed every night, 1–2 h after dinner, and removed in the early morning before physical therapy so that patients are not disturbed during the daytime for school attendance. In some children, NGT becomes increasingly uncomfortable because of nausea, vomiting, nasal discomfort as a result of nasal polyposis, or dislodgement during coughing in cases of pulmonary exacerbation. PEG is the preferred modality for administering home nocturnal EN when long-term EN is anticipated. Generally, PEGs are perceived well by patients with CF who rely on EN therapy for poor weight gain or weight loss. On the contrary, patients and families without PEGs were found to be apathetic towards their value, citing fear of interference with activities, embarrassment, pain, and discomfort [112]. Therefore, there is need for more accurate information about benefits and lifestyle in patients with PEGs. Good early childhood nutritional status is associated with better pulmonary function and long-term survival in patients with CF [113]. However, poor growth and advanced lung disease have been associated with poor outcomes regardless of adherence to EN [114]. There is also currently insufficient evidence to determine whether nutritional rehabilitation after onset of malnutrition improves

pulmonary function in patients with advanced CF-related lung disease. Therefore, the importance of a proactive approach of growth monitoring and early nutritional intervention to optimize growth in children and adolescents with CF. It is important to assess for gastroesophageal reflux before starting EN. Patients should also be monitored for glucose intolerance during administration of EN, especially during illness, therapy with steroids, and if not gaining weight. Insulin therapy should be administered as needed in patients with glucose intolerance [107].

Chronic Liver Disease

Mechanisms leading to protein-energy malnutrition and requirement for EN in infants and children with chronic liver disease are multifactorial and dependent on the type of liver injury [115]. Malnutrition in cholestatic liver disorders is from reduced biliary secretion and intraluminal bile concentrations resulting in malabsorption of lipids and fat-soluble vitamins [116]. Protein and energy requirements are increased by different mechanisms including hypermetabolism [117], portosystemic shunting and ascites, futile metabolic pathways [118], and the energy demands from complications such as sepsis or variceal bleeding [119]. Liver disease from inborn errors of metabolism, for example, galactosemia, tyrosinemia, GSD, and Wilson's disease requires specific dietary restrictions and EN feeding protocols to prevent hypoglycemia and other forms of metabolic decompensation. Patients with fulminant hepatic failure may be well nourished and nutritionally independent at clinical presentation but later require EN because of impaired mental status. Anorexia is common in children with chronic liver disease resulting from organomegaly, abdominal pressure effects of ascites, congested gastric mucosa, reduced motility from portal hypertension, central effects of unidentified toxins, dietary manipulations such as fluid restriction, or use of unpalatable feeds. Several factors contribute to long-chain polyunsaturated fatty acids (PUFAs) deficiency including low PUFAs intake, malabsorption, and disturbed metabolism of long-chain PUFAs. Finally, the interaction of growth hormone with insulin-like growth factor 1(IGF-1) and its binding proteins constitute an important mechanism linking nutrition and growth.

The most common cause of cirrhosis in children is biliary atresia, and the only definitive therapy is liver transplantation [120]. A total of 60–80% of affected children are moderately to severely malnourished prior to transplantation [116], and poor nutritional status prior to transplantation is associated with prolonged hospital stay, increased risk for death at high cost of medical care [119, 121, 122]. Supplemental EN or PN to improve nutritional status is the one intervention known to improve pre- and posttransplant growth and clinical outcomes in children with end-stage liver disease [123–127]

Anorexia, inadequate calorie intake, and failure to thrive are prevalent in children with chronic liver disease [116];

therefore, EN is recommended to supplement per oral food intake [119]. NGT feeding may be safely used without increased risk for bleeding in patients with portal hypertension varices [128, 129]. PEGs should be avoided in children with chronic liver disease and portal hypertension because of likely portal-hypertensive gastropathy with increased bleeding risk from gastric varices [119]. MCTs are nutritionally advantageous in patients with cholestasis because of no bile requirement for digestion and rapidly absorbed into the portal circulation. MCTs may be administered separately as supplements; however, the selected EN should not contain more than 80% of fat as MCT because of risk for inducing essential fatty acid deficiency [130]. Children with weight-for-length z scores <-3 fall into the category of severe malnutrition and >9-fold risk for mortality [131] therefore should be prioritized for nutritional intervention. Patients with chronic cholestatic liver disease have increased metabolism [117], futile metabolic pathways [118], and malabsorption; therefore, the goal for supplemental EN to enable a daily calorie intake of 140–200% of estimated requirements [116]. Children with chronic cholestatic liver disease should continue receiving fat-soluble vitamins (A, D, E and K) regardless of amounts listed in EN [132]. Protein intake of infants and children should not be restricted except in cases of intractable encephalopathy [132], and, even in these cases, protein intake should remain within the adequate intake range of 1–2 g/kg/day [133] and accompanied by sufficient intake of nonprotein calories to prevent inappropriate utilization of protein for energy synthesis [134]. Children with cholestatic liver disease have increased requirements for branched-chain amino acids (BCAA) compared to healthy controls [135]. However, nutritional outcome studies using either BCAA-enriched or standard formulas reported growth benefits in all recipients of EN [123, 124]. Furthermore, a Cochrane review did not find BCAA-enriched formula protective against encephalopathy when compared to iso-nitrogenous non-BCAA enriched formulas [136] Therefore, there is currently insufficient evidence to recommend the use of BCAA-enriched formulas over standard non-BCAA enriched formula.

Chylothorax

Nutritional management of chylothorax involves adherence to EN or an oral diet enriched with medium-chain triglycerides and restricted in long-chain triglycerides and supplementation with essential fatty acids and fat-soluble vitamins [137]. Nutrition support during the preoperative period utilizes EN in infants who are hemodynamically stable and early use of PN if otherwise. The immediate postoperative period is characterized by fluid restrictions and hemodynamic instability and therefore requires active involvement of a dietician and reliance on PN to meet goal calories. Once hemodynamic stability is established, enteral feeding is introduced while following standardized protocols that include screening for swallowing dysfunction and management of GI symptoms, for example, reflux. Nutrition surveillance should be performed continually pre- and post discharge to guide further interventions including use of calorie-dense formula and home tube feeds [62].

Techniques of Delivering Enteral Nutrition

The route of EN administration should be individually tailored, depending on the underlying condition (Fig. 46.1). Enteral feeding is preferable to PN, and therefore it should be immediately implemented in children with functional GI but unable to feed per oral. The absolute contraindication to EN includes mechanical obstruction of the GI tract (unless indicated for decompression), active peritonitis, uncorrectable coagulopathy, or bowel ischemia [138, 139]. The intragastric route of administration is the most commonly used in children, since it is the more physiologic route which permits the action of salivary and gastric enzymes, the bactericidal action of gastric acid, and the better mixing with biliary and pancreatic juice. Therefore, the duodenal or jejunal route is used in very few circumstances in children. For intragastric EN, NGT, or GT may be used. NGT feeding is the best initial approach to EN, to evaluate the tolerance of EN before placing a permanent GT, and/or when a brief period of EN support is anticipated.

NGT are made of polyvinylchloride (PVC), polyurethane, or silicone. Modern feeding tubes are made of either silicone or polyurethane [140]. Polyurethane tubes come externally and internally impregnated with a water-activated lubricant to ease insertion through the nasopharynx and facilitate removal of introducer wires [141]. They are also more resistant to degradation and deterioration when compared to silicone tubes. Tube size (outer diameter) is described in French Gauge (Fr) units. The millimeter conversion can be derived by dividing each Fr by π (3.14). The length of insertion for a nasal- or oral-gastric feeding tube to be in a child is determined by using either the morphological markers of "nose–ear–mid-xiphoid–umbilicus" span or age-specific prediction equations. Length predictions based on just a '"nose–ear–xiphoid" span are likely to result in a placement that is too proximal [142]. At the time of NGT placement, aspirating fluid and measuring a pH ≤ 5 is the most reliable bedside test confirming gastric placement in children [143]. However, the usefulness of this test may be limited in patients being treated with gastric acid suppressants. Simple auscultation is not a reliable method for assessing position because injection of air into the tracheobronchial tree or pleural space can produce an indistinguishable sound. Therefore, an abdominal X-ray is the gold standard for establishing location of the NGT tip [143].

Duodenal or jejunal tube placement is more difficult; the patient should be placed in the right lateral position, and if necessary, after an intravenous injection of erythromycin. The position of the distal end of the tube is then checked by abdominal X-ray. Careful nasal fixation of the tube is used to avoid displacement; it is taped to the upper lip, the ipsilateral cheek, and the external ear. In some particular indications for EN, the feeding tube may also be introduced through the mouth, especially in patients with congenital or acquired nasal obstruction and premature infants on respiratory therapy with continuous positive air pressure (CPAP). The placement of NGT made of PVC is easier, but these tubes should be changed more frequently as they become more rigid. Silicone or polyurethane NGT may be used over 3-week periods or more. However, silicone and polyurethane are generally more flexible and easily displaced by vomiting. They are preferentially used for transpyloric and long-term EN. Individualized goals for growth, nutrition, and when to discontinue EN should be established prior to insertion of a feeding tube. Use of EN may only be temporary in acutely ill but previously healthy children, or as a long-term source of supplemental nutrition in children with chronic inadequate per oral food intake, and the sole source of nutrition in children with severe disability in per oral feeding.

When a child's duration on EN is longer than 30 days and feeds well tolerated yet low anticipation for timely acquisition of adequate per oral feeding skills, transition to a feeding gastrostomy should be considered [138, 140]. Percutaneous approach to placement of gastrostomy has revolutionized the placement of enteric feeding tubes in children. The standard approach involves use of a gastroscope for gastric transillumination and stoma site identification. This is followed by percutaneous introduction of a guide wire that gets grasped using the gastroscope and then orally withdrawn. Thereafter, the gastrostomy catheter is attached to the oral end of the guide wire, and then pulled in an antegrade manner through the oropharynx, esophagus, and stomach, and then across the gastric and abdominal walls [144]. It may be placed using GI endoscopy, surgical laparoscopy, or by interventional radiology [140]. Following placement, postoperative care mostly involves pain management, and most providers permit the use of GT within 12–24 h. The initial PEG tube is changed after 2–3 months, by which time a good tract has formed. Button-replacement gastrostomy devices provide patients a cosmetic advantage in case of long-term EN.

Percutaneous placement of gastrostomy or jejunostomy is contraindicated in patients with previous abdominal surgery, abnormal abdominal anatomy, or severe deformities of the chest and spine which modify the position of the stomach and other intra-abdominal viscera. In such cases, a surgical GT should be placed. The implantation of a jejunal feeding tube, via PEG, is a possible method for the treatment of inadequate oral feeding in patients who are affected by gastroesophageal reflux (GER) and is thus an alternative to fundoplication and drugs [144, 145]. However, gastrojejunal feeding tubes are also prone to technical complications requiring replacement because of clogging and recoil of the jejunal catheter back into the stomach [145]. EN may be delivered as boluses or prolonged continuous feeding using a feeding pump, syringe, or controlled delivery by gravity. Pumps recommended for pediatric use have to provide clear flow rate display and alarms. Miniaturized and battery-powered pumps are specially designed for home and ambulatory EN.

Nutrients

Nitrogen The absorption of amino acids is more rapid and efficient when given in the form of short peptides than free amino acids [146, 147]. Therefore, in order to maximize nitrogen assimilation in patients with marked impairment of gut absorptive capacity, the ideal EN should consist of di- and tripeptides and free amino acids [147]. In addition, the quality, in term of digestion and intestinal absorption of protein hydrolysates, depends on the type of hydrolysate, for example, lactalbumin is superior to casein [148]. However, in patients with normal GI function, EN with formulas consisting of protein hydrolysates offers no nutritional or absorptive advantage over EN based on formula consisting of free amino acids or intact protein [149]. Thus, the initial formula in patients with normal GI function should be based on intact protein or polypeptides, with a lower osmolality, rather than on a mixture of free amino acids and short polypeptides.

Carbohydrates Disaccharidase enzymatic activities are depressed in disease involving the small intestine mucosa. Lactase appears to be the most sensitive to injury and the last of the disaccharidases to recover. In addition, certain drugs such as neomycin or colchicine depress the intestinal disaccharidases. Thus, it is important to avoid dietary sources of lactose. Other disaccharides should also be omitted from the solution used for initial feeding as their corresponding brush border enzymatic activities are reduced. The carbohydrate source allowed during the EN in patients with normal GI function can be lactose. However, patients with impaired GI function should be fed an EN containing lacto-free glucose polymer as the carbohydrate source.

Lipids The main dietary lipids are triglycerides structurally made up of three fatty acids linked to glycerol molecule. The fatty acids contain between 2 and 24 carbon atoms (C: 2 and C: 24). Classification of the triglycerides is based on length of the fatty acid chain, that is, short-chain triglycerides (SCT) contain fatty acids that range in length from 2 to 4 carbons (C: 2 to C: 4); the MCT contain fatty acid chains ranging from 6 to 12 carbons (C: 6 to C: 12) and; LCT have > 12 carbons. In contrast to the LCTs, dietary MCTs are hydrophilic and do not require bile salts or micelle formation, and their free fatty acids are directly absorbed into the portal systems without requirement for re-esterification into chylomicrons [14, 150]. MCTs are hydrolyzed faster than LCTs in the small intestine by pancreatic lipase; they are converted almost exclusively into free fatty acids and glycerol and reach directly the portal circulation and the liver. Nevertheless, in case of pancreatic insufficiency, MCTs may also be absorbed intact. The excessive use of MCTs-containing diet can lead to osmotic diarrhea as a result of their rapid hydrolysis. Dicarboxylic aciduria has been described in infants supplemented with MCTs-rich formulas without any proof of deleterious effect [151]. The provision of essential fatty acids (EFA) must be considered since MCTs contain no EFA. Furthermore, MCTs decrease the LCTs absorption; thus, supplementation with linoleic acid must be done. However, its addition to a formula based on MCTs may be insufficient to prevent EFA deficiency, thus making necessary to provide EFA parenterally. Nevertheless, most of formulas containing MCTs include also up to 50% of lipid as LCTs. LCTs in excess in the intestinal lumen, especially if they are hydroxylated by bacteria, reverse the rate of water and electrolyte absorption and increase malabsorption. In those conditions, the addition of cholestyramine an EFA supplement may be appropriate. Finally, a lipid intake of 3–4 g/kg/day may be achieved, depending on absorption capacity and digestive tolerance.

Other Components Recommendations concerning energy, water, and electrolytes supplies in premature and full-term infants are provided in the chapter on PN in the premature infant. In older children, the recommended energy intake is based on recommended daily intake (RDI) values or may be estimated using World Health Organization (WHO) weight, age, and gender prediction equations or directly measured using an indirect calorimeter [133]. The minimum daily fluid requirements with some exceptions may be estimated using the "Holliday–Segar" calculation, which is an extrapolation based on daily calorie expenditure. For weights ranging from 0 to 10 kg, the estimation is 100 mL/kg/d; from 10 to 20 kg, 1000 mL plus 50 mL/kg for each kilogram of body weight more than 10; and over 20 kg, the estimation is 1500 mL plus 20 mL/kg for each kilogram more than 20 [152].

Choice of a Formula

Enteral feeding formulas are divided into several families. The choice of a formula is made according to numerous parameters like protein–calorie needs, digestive function, protein sensitivity, motility status, tolerance to fluid intake, all obviously dependent on the age and on the underlying disease (Fig. 46.3). In preterm, newborns, and young infants with normal intestinal function, human milk or standard in-

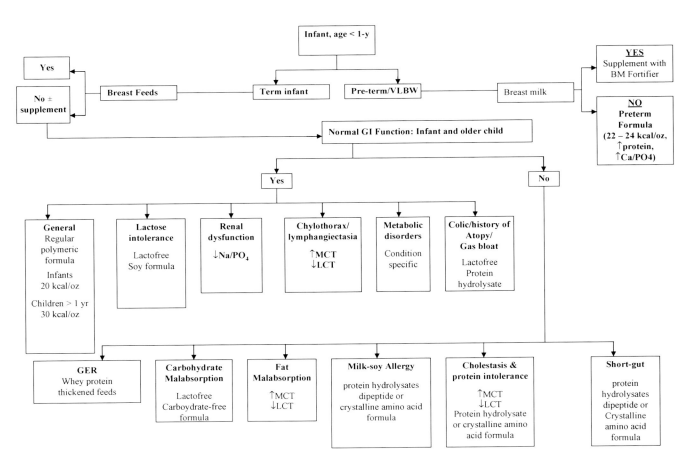

Fig. 46.3 Algorithm for selection of formula. *GER* gastroesophageal reflux, *MCT* medium-chain triglycerides, *LCT* long-chain triglycerides, *EN* enteral nutrition

fants formulas supplemented with long-chain polyunsaturated fatty acids (LCPUFA) may be used. Formulas for preterm infants are unique in being more calorically dense (72–90 kcal/100 mL) with increased protein (1.8–2.3 g/100 mL), calcium (70–108 mg/100 mL), and phosphorous [153]. The preterm formulas are continued after hospital discharge in preterm or small for gestation-age infants with discharge growth parameters are below appropriate post-conception growth, and continued until achievement of catch-up growth [153]. Breast milk and standard infant formulas have a calorie density of 0.67 kcal/mL with lactose as the carbohydrate source and fat source compromised of LCTs and LCPUFA (DHA and EPA). Commercial polymeric formulas are available for older children (age > 1 year), and blenderized diets can be prepared using food from the kitchen may be used in the nonstressed patients, with normal gut function. The calorie density of formulas used in older children (age > 1 year) ranges from 1 kcal/mL (standard) to 1.5–2.0 kcal/mL (calorically dense).

In case of GI disease, the choice of the nutritive solution must take into account not only the child's age and nutritional status but also the underlying digestive disease, for example, the presence of anatomical and functional changes in the intestine, whether due to an extensive reduction of the absorptive surface, to enteropathy or to pancreatic insufficiency. Limiting factors in such cases are impairment of gastric, biliary, and pancreatic secretions, disturbances of the intestinal flora, and malabsorption. Most standard (1 kcal/mL) polymeric formulas have osmolality within the range of 300–360 mosmol/kg. Oligomeric (hydrolsyate/semi-elemental) and elemental (crystalline amino acid based) enteral formulas are designed for use in patients with malabsorption such as in short bowel syndrome, CF, cholestasis, food allergy or intolerances. These diets include dipeptides, tripeptides and a few free amino acids, combined with LCTs and MCTs, and carbohydrates including glucose polymers and maltodextrins.

The osmolality of a solution is determined by the number of particles within it. Likewise, the osmolality of enteral formulas is directly influenced by the calorie density and whether made up of intact protein, peptides or amino acids. Therefore, free amino acid-based formulas tend to have a higher osmolality. Children with severe malabsorption or short bowel syndrome unable to tolerate peptide-based formulas (protein hydrolysates) might benefit from the free amino acid-based formulas [154, 155]. Nutritional formulas in which each of the constituents is modified independently are mostly used in special conditions, for example, selective malabsorption. In that case, glucose may be given initially as calorie source, the amount being increased progressively and controlled according to the stool volume, pH, and absence of reducing substances in the stools. In the first days of feeding, at least a molar ratio of glucose and sodium is maintained. Then, protein hydrolysates are gradually introduced according to digestive tolerance. The caloric enteral intake usually increases from 10–15 to 70–80 kcal/kg/day over the first week. In a second step, qualitative and quantitative changes are gradually carried out: Fructose is added to the glucose, and then disaccharides are introduced, starting with maltose. Nitrogen and lipids are simultaneously increased. During this period, the introduction of oligosaccharides precedes that of a commercially available semi-elemental diet.

Regulation of Intakes and Rhythm of EN Delivery

EN should be progressively introduced depending on the child's nutritional status and the indications for EN. In case of digestive disease, CEN can be used after a brief or prolonged period of PN. The first step includes the progressive reduction of the parenteral intake and the stepwise increase of EN according to the digestive tolerance. Semi-elemental diet (protein hydrolysates) can be used early, by progressively increasing volume as well as concentration according to digestive tolerance and up to achieve optimal energy and nitrogen intakes. The water and sodium supply should be increased to compensate for the intestinal losses generally induced by the start of EN; the tolerance is estimated from the weight of the child, the volume and osmolality of urine samples, and from the plasma osmolality. The tolerance and needs are estimated from 24-h urine analysis, while attempting to maintain a natriuresis of 2–3 mmol/kg/day. At the same time, potassium intake is adjusted as a function of the nitrogen and energy intake.

The rhythm of EN delivery depends on the underlying disease. Intermittent feeding using bolus is more physiological and well tolerated when the digestive function is normal. Continuous cyclic nocturnal EN is better tolerated in some patients who do not tolerate bolus feeding and provides less interference with daytime oral intake. On the other hand, continuous 24/24 h rhythm of delivery is indicated in case of impaired digestive function. The weaning period varies from few days to several weeks or months. Eating disorders can be avoided by the maintenance of sucking and swallowing functions during the period of CEN. On the other hand, it has been demonstrated that nonnutritive sucking intervention during CEN in preterm infants resulted in faster transition from feeding tube to oral feeds, better bottle feeding performance, enhanced growth and intestinal maturation, and decreased duration of hospital stay compared to preterm infants without the intervention [156, 157]. In older children, weaning from EN may include a period of continuous night-time feeding supplemented by several meals in the daytime until the latter account for 50% of the total intake. Oral feeding must be carefully increased because of the relatively low intestinal activity due to long-term CEN.

Complications of Enteral Nutrition Therapy

Although complications occur rarely, they can be quite serious. Strict adherence to the procedure is indicated and careful supervision is essential to prevent them. See Table 46.2.

Functional Complications of Feeding Tubes

The functional complications of enteral feeding tubes include tendency to clog, which occurs 18–45 % of the times [158]. The risk is higher in smaller-diameter tubes, and the cause of occlusion includes interaction of protein-based formulas with an acidic environment and medications, and complete obstruction from knotting of the feeding tube [158–160]. Clogged NGTs should be readily replaced with no need to apply extraneous efforts to unclog. However, a good effort should be made to unclog blocked nasojejunal and gastrojejunal tubes because they are more difficult to insert. Clogging and occlusion can be minimized by frequently flushing the tube before and after administration of feeds. Water is more effective than carbonated beverages for flushing and unclogging occlusions. Sterile water is preferred for flushing because several published cases of infection were traced to tap water [139]. Persistently clogged tubes despite water flushes may respond to installation of one crushed tablet of Viokase (pancreatic enzyme) in 5 mL water and pH raised to

7.9 using NaOH instilled into the tube using a 50 mL syringe under manual pressure for 1 min, then the tube clamped for 5 min [159], Other options include trial of meat tenderizer or use of mechanical devices such as Fogarty balloon and biopsy brush. Failure to unclog the tube requires replacement of the tube [139].

Gastrointestinal Complications

Risks and complications start with passage of NGTs, which can be hazardous in any patient, especially those with poor or impaired gag reflex, absent cough reflex, or altered consciousness. Furthermore, presence of a cuffed endotracheal tube is not guaranteed protection against pulmonary intubation. Therefore, feeding should not begin until proper placement of the tube is verified [138]. The bedside assessment tools of visually inspecting for color and testing for pH of aspirates may be inaccurate because small bore tubes may collapse resulting in failure to drawback aspirates, and therapy with gastric acid suppressants may affect the measured pH. The auscultation method is also problematic because sounds may be transmitted to the epigastrium regardless of tube placement in the lung, esophagus, or stomach. Some protocols call for the first feed to be water to ensure tolerance [138]. Overall, abdominal X-ray is the gold standard for establishing location of the NGT tip [143].

Table 46.2 Complications of enteral feeding tubes and therapy

Nasogastric	PEG/gastrostomy
Complications during tube insertion	
Arrhythmias	Aspiration
Pyriform sinus perforation	Hemorrhage
Esophagus perforation	Peritonitis
Tube in pulmonary tree/pulmonary intubation	Necrotizing fasciitis (rare)
Pneumothorax	Ileus
Empyema	Fistulous tracts
Gastric perforation	Perforation of viscera
Duodenal perforation	–
Complications when in situ	
Otitis media	Peristomal infection
Sinusitis	Stomal leakage
Epistaxis	Buried bumper
Nasal mucosal ulceration	Gastric ulcer
Pulmonary aspiration	Inadvertent removal
Gastroesophaeal reflux	–
Tube dislodgement	–
Functional complications	
Diarrhea	
Clogging	
Knotted tubes	
Contaminated feeds: *Coronbacter* spp (formally *Enterobacter sakazakii*), *E. Cloacae*	
Re-feeding syndrome	
Feeding aversions	

Aspiration pneumonia is the most threatening complication associated with NGT feeding [138]. Irregular flow rate of infusion, delayed gastric emptying due to the underlying disease or to the drugs, GER, tube placement or migration into the distal esophagus, behavioral vomiting, and formula intolerance are risk factors for vomiting and aspiration. The general prevalence of feeding-tube-related aspiration pneumonia is unknown; however, the incidence in critically ill patients ranges from 25 to 40% [161] with both oropharyngeal and gastropharyngeal contents implicated. The risk factors in critically ill patients include decreased level of consciousness, vomiting, malpositioned feeding tube, larger-diameter NGT, and bolus feeding. The preventative measures include keeping the patient in a semi-recumbent position, continuous aspiration of subglottic secretions, and change from bolus/intermittent to continuous EN [161, 162]. Tubes placed past the third portion of the duodenum are associated with decreased risk of aspiration [138].

Diarrhea is the most common complication of EN and is reported in up to 68% of patients [138]. Increased stool losses occur when the combined absorptive capacity of the small bowel and the salvaging capacity of the colon are exceeded (see ref. [163]) for a review of the role of colon in short bowel syndrome) and may result in dehydration and hypoglycemia. The causes include inappropriate composition of the formula for the underlying disease, high formula osmolality and rate of infusion, intraduodenal infusion, hypoalbuminemia, and bacterial contamination of the formula. The volume of endogenous fluid flux into the jejunum is directly proportional to the osmolality and rate of infusion of the EN [164]. Therefore, since higher osmolality (>300 mosmol/kg) feeds will induce greater endogenous fluid flux into the bowel, their rates of infusion should be increased cautiously.

Mechanical, Infectious, and Metabolic Complications

NGT-related mechanical complications include nasal trauma, laryngeal ulceration, or stenosis and esophageal or gastric perforations. Duodenal perforations have been reported in association with transpyloric feeding tubes in preterm infants, neonates, and critically ill children regardless of whether polyvinyl, silicone, or polyurethane feeding tubes [165–167]. In one series of 526 critically ill children receiving transpyloric EN, the prevalence of GI complications was 11.5%. These included abdominal distension and/or excessive gastric residue (6.2%), diarrhea (6.4%), and GI bleeding, necrotizing enterocolitis, and duodenal perforation (0.9%). The major factors associated with risk for developing the complications were shock, epinephrine dose >0.3 µg/kg/min, and hypophosphatemia [168]. Therefore, frequent reevaluation and a high index of suspicion are required in

this patient population. Complications from PEG placement may occur during the immediate postoperative period and or late onset/delayed. The postoperative complications include aspiration, hemorrhage, peritonitis, necrotizing fasciitis, peristomal infections, prolonged ileus, fistulous tracts, and inadvertent removal. The delayed complications include site infections, persistent peristomal leakage/irritation, buried bumper syndrome, gastric ulcer, fistulous tracts, inadvertent tube removal, and fungal tube infections, especially affecting silicone tubes leading to tube degradation and malfunction [139]. Children without fundoplication may go through a period of worsened reflux symptoms [169–171] that may respond to slower advancement of EN or necessitate a brief period of change to continuous feeding schedule.

Patients with PEGs placed too close to the pylorus, and 24–30% of children with fundoplication, may develop metabolic dumping characterized by postprandial tachycardia, diaphoresis, lethargy, refusal to eat, gas bloat, and water diarrhea in association with bolus feeds [172–175]. Establishing a screening protocol for postprandial hypoglycemia in patients with history of fundoplication is important because approximately 46% of affected children fail to exhibit symptoms [175]. The diagnosis of dumping is confirmed by a glucose tolerance test showing postprandial hypoglycemia preceded by postprandial hyperglycemia. The management options include initial avoidance of boluses, change to continuous feeding schedule, modification of the EN to avoid lactose, change to a complex carbohydrate source, supplementation of bolus feedings with uncooked cornstarch [176–179], and in refractory cases, therapy with ascorbase (disaccharidase inhibitor) [180].

Infectious Complications

EN has been associated with outbreaks of antimicrobial-resistant organisms. *Coronbacter spp* (formally *Enterobacter sakazakii*) is a rare but one of the most important worldwide causes of outbreaks of neonatal sepsis and meningitis associated with non-sterile powdered infant formula or human milk fortifier, has a mortality of 40% [181]. Ninety-nine percent of affected patients are infants <2 months. The infection may be acquired in hospital or at home and the predominant risk factor is use of powdered infant formula or human milk fortifier [181, 182]. Therefore, the US Food and Drug Administration has issued the recommendation that use of powdered infant formulas and human milk fortifiers should be minimized in hospitalized preterm or immunocompromised neonates [183]. Ready-to-use commercial formulas are sterile therefore recommended for EN in hospitals.

Other sources of organisms include post-manufacturer microbial contamination exogenously introduced during manipulation of the formula, and through retrograde contamination of the feeding tube system by the patient's endogenous flora. The enteral feed administration sets become colonized externally by microbes grown from the enteral tube hub, and may serve as a reservoir of organisms that can be cross transmitted [184–186]. Commercial liquid formulas received from the manufacturer are required by regulatory agencies to be shelf-stable and free of enteric pathogens. The more common sources of organisms may be exogenous the patient through contamination of locally prepared and manipulated formula [184]. Microbial contamination of the enteral tube hub may result from retrograde growth of endogenous bacteria along the tubing system [187] following which nosocomial cross-transmission to other patients may occur when care providers handling the enteral tube hub and fail to practice strict infection control procedure [188, 189]. Therefore, adherence to standard precautions is critical when handling enteral feeding apparatuses. The bacterial contamination of the nutritive solution with enterotoxin-producing bacteria like coliforms or *E. cloacae* [186], at the time of preparation, storage or delivery to the patient has been associated with gastroenteritis and/or septicemia [185, 190]. The relationship between bacterial contamination of enteral formula and diarrhea may be a matter of debate. When EN is delivered into the stomach there is a protective effect from gastric acid. Therefore, the risk of bowel contamination is theoretically higher when EN is delivered below the pylorus. Since necrotizing enterocolitis (NEC) may occur in premature infants and neonates suffering from hypoxia and infections, the abdomen must be checked daily very carefully. Because of the risk of infectious complications and NEC, use gastric route as far as possible, strictly limit duodenal infusions and to use ready to ready-to-use preterm formulas is recommended in preterm infants.

Refeeding Syndrome

This is a metabolic syndrome induced by feeding that occurs in previously starved or chronically malnourished patients. The syndrome is characterized by hypophosphatemia, hypokalemia, hypomagnesemia, arrhythmia, edema, congestive heart failure and increased risk for death. The incidence of re-feeding syndrome in children is not known; however, it is reported in up to 50% of hospitalized adults documented to be malnourished [191]. It results from rapid anabolism induced by increased insulin secretion in response to provision of nutrients. The increased glucose load, with corresponding increase in the release of insulin leads to cellular uptake of glucose, potassium, magnesium and phosphate. This rapid shift in electrolytes from the extracellular to intracellular space results in hypokalemia, hypomagnesemia and hypophosphatemia. Insulin also exerts a natriuretic effect on the kidneys resulting in sodium and fluid retention. The

anabolism may unveil or cause other nutrient deficiencies, for example, thiamine deficiency and Beriberi, further leading to life threatening circumstances [192]. The pre-nutrition therapy determinants of risk for developing re-feeding syndrome include patients underfed or not fed for at least 10–14 days (regardless of therapy with crystalloid intravenous fluids), acute weight loss of >10% in the preceding 1–2 months, severe malnutrition as defined by <80% ideal body weight or weight-for-age z-score <−3 [33], decreased pre-albumin [193] AN, marasmus, edematous protein-energy malnutrition (kwashiorkor), children of neglect, cerebral palsy and other conditions causing dysphagia [192]. The risk for developing re-feeding syndrome is higher during the first 5–7 days of implementing nutritional therapy. The metabolic derangements can be avoided by initiating feeds at a calorie intake of 50–75% of the measured or estimated resting energy expenditure with appropriate supplementation of phosphorus. The calorie intake is then increased by 10–20% per day with close monitoring and correction of biochemical parameters until the calorie goal is met [194].

Home Enteral Nutrition (HEN)

Indications

HEN is a logical alternative to long-term hospitalization when a long-term enteral nutritional support is necessary (more than 1 month) in a patient in stable clinical condition. HEN has been proven to be an effective and safe method, compatible with the best possible quality of life [195–197]. Major costs savings induced by home EN as compared to hospitalization have been demonstrated. The importance of families' teaching and medical follow-up to prevent somatic and psychological complications should not be underestimated [198].

Prevalence-Incidence

The origins of home EN are much older than those of home PN. In North America, 20,000 patients received HEN in 1985 and it was estimated that 150,000 individuals received HEN in 1992 (about 500 per million population) [199]. Based on an estimate growth rate of 25% per year, about 500,000 patients may have been on HEN in the USA in 1997 [200]. However, whereas HEN is more extensively used the PN, because there is no national registry in the United States for patients on HEN to verify these projections or compared outcomes data [201]. The British Association of Enteral and Parenteral Nutrition estimated that the number of patients on HEN was about 40 per million population, about 10 fold the number of HPN patients in the same country at the same time. Children accounted for 30–40 % of HEN patients in Britain, compared to about 20 % in USA [200, 202]. The Spanish national registry for Pediatric home enteral nutrition (NEPAD) is a web based registry of exclusively Pediatric data established in 2003 with the goal of gathering more comprehensive information on indications, modes of administration, types of diets and duration of nutrition support [197]. The number of entrants has steadily increased; however, enrolment is voluntary therefore, prevalence and incidence data cannot be derived. Therefore, the lack of national registers in most European countries makes estimation very difficult.

Organization

The quality of home EN programs depends on the organization of multidisciplinary nutrition support teams based on a tight collaboration between the different professionals including physicians, home care nurses, dieticians, pharmacists and social workers. In some countries, pumps, disposable equipment and nutrients for HEN are mainly delivered by hospitals, while in others, such as in the USA where they are the most developed, home care companies participate to patients' training and provide a delivery service and a 24 h emergency phone contact. With expansion of the home care industry, it is important to ensure that adequate standards of care are provided. The American Society of Parenteral and Enteral Nutrition and the British Association of Parenteral and Enteral Nutrition have produced such standards [4, 202].

Parents' Teaching

Tolerance and efficacy of EN have to be proven at the hospital before to organize HEN. As for HPN, HEN in children is feasible only when the family is highly motivated and able to deal with technical aspects. Parent's teaching is based on a nutrition multidisciplinary hospital team including physician, nurse, dietician and pharmacist. Parents are taught not only about technical aspects but also about risks, complications and their prevention. The hospital team ensures a 24/24 h phone contact and regular follow up, in tight cooperation with the general practitioner. The help of a community nurse may be required, especially in case of placement of a nasogastric tube.

Results

Quality of Life Although HEN, like HPN, is usually considered by children and families as an improvement of their quality of life, psychological consequences of this technique have to be carefully estimated and prevented. The placement of a NGT is distressing to parents and children. A NGT in situ for continuous 24/24 h infusion is a major problem, particularly in oldest children and adolescents, because it induces an unwelcome public interest. These problems are solved by the use of gastrostomy. Children and families may also suffer from the suppression of meals taken together, which are usually considered as an important moment of the family life. Adequate psychological preparation and follow-up improve tolerance of children and parents to HEN [203, 204].

Outcomes Outcome studies on HEN patients have been fewer than those on patients on HPN. Improvement of the nutritional status and low mortality rate (always related to major underlying diseases) are usually described in children on HEN [205].

Cost and Funding HEN is far from being as expensive as HPN. The total cost per day HEN was about $ 35 in the USA in 1992, when the cost per day HPN was about $ 300 [199]. The cost-savings associated with providing HEN estimated by the British Association for Parenteral and Enteral Nutrition in 1994 were about 70 % [202]. In most countries, patients on HEN are funded by the National Health Service, although in the USA they are mostly paid for by insurance companies [200, 202].

References

1. Chernoff R. An overview of tube feeding: from ancient times to the future. Nutr Clin Pract. 2006;21(4):408–10.
2. Harkness L. The history of enteral nutrition therapy: from raw eggs and nasal tubes to purified amino acids and early postoperative jejunal delivery. J Am Diet. 2002;102(3):399–404.
3. Gauderer MW, Ponsky JL, Izant RJ, Jr. Gastrostomy without laparotomy: a percutaneous endoscopic technique. J Pediatr Surg. 1980;15(6):872–5.
4. ASPEN Board of Directors and the Clinical Guidelines Task Force. Guidelines for the use of parenteral and enteral nutrition in adult and pediatric patients. JPEN J Parenter Enteral Nutr. 2002;26(Suppl 1):1SA–138SA.
5. Brotherton A, Abbott J, Hurley M, Aggett PJ. Home enteral tube feeding in children following percutaneous endoscopic gastrostomy: perceptions of parents, paediatric dietitians and paediatric nurses. J Hum Nutr Diet. 2007;20(5):431–9.
6. Calderon C, Gomez-Lopez L, Martinez-Costa C, Borraz S, Moreno-Villares JM, Pedron-Giner C. Feeling of burden, psychological distress, and anxiety among primary caregivers of children with home enteral nutrition. J Pediatr Psychol. 2011;36(2):188–95.
7. Winkler MF. American society of parenteral and enteral nutrition presidential address: food for thought: it's more than nutrition. JPEN J Parenter Enteral Nutr. 2007;31(4):334–40.
8. Quigley EM. Gastric and small intestinal motility in health and disease. Gastroenterol Clin North Am. 1996;25(1):113–45.
9. Ledeboer M, Masclee AA, Coenraad M, Vecht J, Biemond I, Lamers CB. Antroduodenal motility and small bowel transit during continuous intraduodenal or intragastric administration of enteral nutrition. Eur J Clin Inv. 1999;29(7):615–23.

10. de Ville K, Knapp E, Al-Tawil Y, Berseth CL. Slow infusion feedings enhance duodenal motor responses and gastric emptying in preterm infants. Am J Clin Nutr. 1998;68(1):103–8.

11. Ledeboer M, Masclee AA, Biemond I, Lamers CB. Gallbladder motility and cholecystokinin secretion during continuous enteral nutrition. Am J Gastroenterol. 1997;92(12):2274–9.

12. Ledeboer M, Masclee AA, Biemond I, Lamers CB. Effect of intragastric or intraduodenal administration of a polymeric diet on gallbladder motility, small-bowel transit time, and hormone release. Am J Gastroenterol. 1998;93(11):2089–96.

13. Ledeboer M, Masclee AA, Biemond I, Lamers CB. Differences in cholecystokinin release and gallbladder contraction between emulsified and nonemulsified long-chain triglycerides. JPEN J Parenter Enteral Nutr. 1999;23(4):203–6.

14. Bell SJ, Bradley D, Forse RA, Bistrian BR. The new dietary fats in health and disease. J Am Diet. 1997;97(3):280–6, quiz 7–8.

15. Hunt JN, Knox MT. A relation between the chain length of fatty acids and the slowing of gastric emptying. J Physiol. 1968;194(2):327–36.

16. O'Keefe SJ. Physiological response of the human pancreas to enteral and parenteral feeding. Curr Opin Clin Nutr Metab Care. 2006;9(5):622–8.

17. Keller J, Runzi M, Goebell H, Layer P. Duodenal and ileal nutrient deliveries regulate human intestinal motor and pancreatic responses to a meal. Am J Physiol. 1997; 272(3 Pt 1):G632–7.

18. Wen J, Phillips SF, Sarr MG, Kost LJ, Holst JJ. PYY and GLP-1 contribute to feedback inhibition from the canine ileum and colon. Am J Physiol. 1995; 269(6 Pt 1):G945–52.

19. Nacht CA, Schutz Y, Vernet O, Christin L, Jequier E. Continuous versus single bolus enteral nutrition: comparison of energy metabolism in humans. Am J Physiol. 1986; 251(5 Pt 1):E524–9.

20. Premji S, Chessell L. Continuous nasogastric milk feeding versus intermittent bolus milk feeding for premature infants less than 1500 grams. Cochrane Database Syst Rev. 2003(1):CD001819.

21. Silvestre MA, Morbach CA, Brans YW, Shankaran S. A prospective randomized trial comparing continuous versus intermittent feeding methods in very low birth weight neonates. J Pediatr. 1996;128(6):748–52.

22. Parker P, Stroop S, Greene H. A controlled comparison of continuous versus intermittent feeding in the treatment of infants with intestinal disease. J Pediatr. 1981;99(3):360–4.

23. Joly F, Dray X, Corcos O, Barbot L, Kapel N, Messing B. Tube feeding improves intestinal absorption in short bowel syndrome patients. Gastroenterology. 2009;136(3):824–31.

24. Colomb V, Bourdon-Lannoy E, Lambe C, Sauvat F, Hadj Rabia S, Teillac D, et al. Nutritional outcome in children with severe generalized recessive dystrophic epidermolysis bullosa: a short- and long-term evaluation of gastrostomy and enteral feeding. Br J Dermatol. 2012;166(2):354–61.

25. Haynes L, Atherton DJ, Ade-Ajayi N, Wheeler R, Kiely EM. Gastrostomy and growth in dystrophic epidermolysis bullosa. Br J Dermatol. 1996;134(5):872–9.

26. Mizuno K, Ueda A. The maturation and coordination of sucking, swallowing, and respiration in preterm infants. J Pediatr. 2003;142(1):36–40.

27. Watson J, McGuire W. Transpyloric versus gastric tube feeding for preterm infants. Cochrane Database Syst Rev. 2013;2:CD003487.

28. Kim JH. Necrotizing enterocolitis: the road to zero. Semin Fetal Neonat Med. 2014;19(1):39–44.

29. Nicholls D, Hudson L, Mahomed F. Managing anorexia nervosa. Arch Dis Child. 2011;96(10):977–82.

30. Rocks T, Pelly F, Wilkinson P. Nutrition therapy during Initiation of refeeding in underweight children and adolescent in patients with anorexia nervosa: a systematic review of the evidence. J Acad Nutr Diet. 2014;114(6):897–907.

31. Hatch A, Madden S, Kohn MR, Clarke S, Touyz S, Gordon E, et al. In first presentation adolescent anorexia nervosa, do cognitive markers of underweight status change with weight gain following a refeeding intervention? Int J Eat Dis. 2010;43(4):295–306.

32. Thiels C. Forced treatment of patients with anorexia. Curr Op Psych. 2008;21(5):495–8.

33. Olofin I, McDonald CM, Ezzati M, Flaxman S, Black RE, Fawzi WW, et al. Associations of suboptimal growth with all-cause and cause-specific mortality in children under five years: a pooled analysis of ten prospective studies. PloS One. 2013;8(5):e64636.

34. Nehring I, Kewitz K, von Kries R, Thyen U. Long-term effects of enteral feeding on growth and mental health in adolescents with anorexia nervosa-results of a retrospective German cohort study. Eur J Clin Nutr. 2014;68(2):171–7.

35. Greene HL, Slonim AE, O'Neill JA, Jr, Burr IM. Continuous nocturnal intragastric feeding for management of type 1 glycogen-storage disease. N Engl J Med. 1976;294(8):423–5.

36. Rake JP, Visser G, Labrune P, Leonard JV, Ullrich K, Smit GP. Guidelines for management of glycogen storage disease type I—European study on glycogen storage disease type I (ESGSD I). Eur J Pediatr. 2002;161(Suppl 1):S112–9.

37. Chen YT, Bazzarre CH, Lee MM, Sidbury JB, Coleman RA. Type I glycogen storage disease: nine years of management with cornstarch. Eur J Pediatr. 1993;152(Suppl 1):S56–9.

38. Wolfsdorf JI, Keller RJ, Landy H, Crigler JF, Jr. Glucose therapy for glycogenosis type 1 in infants: comparison of intermittent uncooked cornstarch and continuous overnight glucose feedings. J Pediatr. 1990;117(3):384–91.

39. Heller S, Worona L, Consuelo A. Nutritional therapy for glycogen storage diseases. J Pediatri Gastr Nutr. 2008;47(Suppl 1):S15–21.

40. Goldberg T, Slonim AE. Nutrition therapy for hepatic glycogen storage diseases. J Am Diet. 1993;93(12):1423–30.

41. Haberle J, Boddaert N, Burlina A, Chakrapani A, Dixon M, Huemer M, et al. Suggested guidelines for the diagnosis and management of urea cycle disorders. Orphanet J Rare Dis. 2012;7:32.

42. Singh RH. Nutritional management of patients with urea cycle disorders. J Inher Met Dis. 2007;30(6):880–7.

43. Acosta PB, Yannicelli S, Ryan AS, Arnold G, Marriage BJ, Plewinska M, et al. Nutritional therapy improves growth and protein status of children with a urea cycle enzyme defect. Mol Gen Metabol. 2005;86(4):448–55.

44. Leonard JV. The nutritional management of urea cycle disorders. J Pediatr. 2001;138(Suppl 1):S40–4, discussion S4–5.

45. Singh RH, Rhead WJ, Smith W, Lee B, Sniderman King L, Summar M. Nutritional management of urea cycle disorders. Crit Care Clin. 2005;21(Suppl 4):S27–35.

46. Chen Z, Wang S, Yu B, Li A. A comparison study between early enteral nutrition and parenteral nutrition in severe burn patients. Burns. 2007;33(6):708–12.

47. Andel H, Kamolz LP, Horauf K, Zimpfer M. Nutrition and anabolic agents in burned patients. Burns. 2003;29(6):592–5.

48. Peng YZ, Yuan ZQ, Xiao GX. Effects of early enteral feeding on the prevention of enterogenic infection in severely burned patients. Burns. 2001;27(2):145–9.

49. Guieze R, Lemal R, Cabrespine A, Hermet E, Tournihac O, Combal C, Bay JO, Bouteloup C. Enteral versus parenteral nutrition support in allogeneic haematopoietic stem-cell transplantation. Clin Nutr 2014;33(3):533–8

50. Seguy D, Berthon C, Micol JB, Darre S, Dalle JH, Neuville S, et al. Enteral feeding and early outcomes of patients undergoing allogeneic stem cell transplantation following myeloablative conditioning. Transplantation. 2006;82(6):835–9.

51. Hopman GD, Pena EG, Le Cessie S, Van Weel MH, Vossen JM, Mearin ML. Tube feeding and bone marrow transplantation. Med Pediatr Oncol. 2003;40(6):375–9.

52. Papadopoulou A, Williams MD, Darbyshire PJ, Booth IW. Nutritional support in children undergoing bone marrow transplantation. Clin Nutr. 1998;17(2):57–63.

53. Murray SM, Pindoria S. Nutrition support for bone marrow transplant patients. Cochrane Database Syst Rev. 2008(4):CD002920.

54. Ledermann SE, Shaw V, Trompeter RS. Long-term enteral nutrition in infants and young children with chronic renal failure. Pediatr Nephrol. 1999;13(9):870–5.

55. Claris-Appiani A, Ardissino GL, Dacco V, Funari C, Terzi F. Catch-up growth in children with chronic renal failure treated with long-term enteral nutrition. JPEN J Parenter Enteral Nutr. 1995;19(3):175–8.

56. Reed EE, Roy LP, Gaskin KJ, Knight JF. Nutritional intervention and growth in children with chronic renal failure. J Renal Nutr. 1998;8(3):122–6.

57. Chadha V, Blowey DL, Warady BA. Is growth a valid outcome measure of dialysis clearance in children undergoing peritoneal dialysis? Perit Dial Int. 2001;21(Suppl 3):S179–84.

58. Kari JA, Gonzalez C, Ledermann SE, Shaw V, Rees L. Outcome and growth of infants with severe chronic renal failure. Kidney Int. 2000;57(4):1681–7.

59. Tom A, McCauley L, Bell L, Rodd C, Espinosa P, Yu G, et al. Growth during maintenance hemodialysis: impact of enhanced nutrition and clearance. J Pediatr. 1999;134(4):464–71.

60. Haffner D, Schaefer F, Nissel R, Wuhl E, Tonshoff B, Mehls O. Effect of growth hormone treatment on the adult height of children with chronic renal failure. German study group for growth hormone treatment in chronic renal failure. N Engl J Med. 2000;343(13):923–30.

61. Fine RN, Martz K, Stablein D. What have 20 years of data from the North American Pediatric Renal Transplant Cooperative Study taught us about growth following renal transplantation in infants, children, and adolescents with end-stage renal disease? Pediatr Nephrol. 2010;25(4):739–46.

62. Slicker J, Hehir DA, Horsley M, Monczka J, Stern KW, Roman B, et al. Nutrition algorithms for infants with hypoplastic left heart syndrome; birth through the first interstage period. Congenit Heart Dis. 2013;8(2):89–102.

63. Varan B, Tokel K, Yilmaz G. Malnutrition and growth failure in cyanotic and acyanotic congenital heart disease with and without pulmonary hypertension. Arch Dis Child. 1999;81(1):49–52.

64. Hebson CL, Oster ME, Kirshbom PM, Clabby ML, Wulkan ML, Simsic JM. Association of feeding modality with interstage mortality after single-ventricle palliation. J Thorac Cardiovasc Surg. 2012;144(1):173–7.

65. Irving SY, Medoff-Cooper B, Stouffer NO, Schall JI, Ravishankar C, Compher CW, et al. Resting energy expenditure at 3 months of age following neonatal surgery for congenital heart disease. Congenit Heart Dis. 2013;8(4):343–51.

66. Mehta NM, Costello JM, Bechard LJ, Johnson VM, Zurakowski D, McGowan FX, et al. Resting energy expenditure after Fontan surgery in children with single-ventricle heart defects. JPEN J Parenter Enteral Nutr. 2012;36(6):685–92.

67. Farrell AG, Schamberger MS, Olson IL, Leitch CA. Large left-to-right shunts and congestive heart failure increase total energy expenditure in infants with ventricular septal defect. Am J Cardiol. 2001;87(9):1128–31, A10.

68. Skinner ML, Halstead LA, Rubinstein CS, Atz AM, Andrews D, Bradley SM. Laryngopharyngeal dysfunction after the Norwood procedure. J Thorac Cardiovasc Surg. 2005;130(5):1293–301.

69. Goldberg DJ, Dodds K, Rychik J. Rare problems associated with the Fontan circulation. Cardiol Young. 2010;20(Suppl 3):113–9.

70. Avery GB, Villavicencio O, Lilly JR, Randolph JG. Intractable diarrhea in early infancy. Pediatrics. 1968;41(4):712–22.

71. Goulet OJ, Brousse N, Canioni D, Walker-Smith JA, Schmitz J, Phillips AD. Syndrome of intractable diarrhoea with persistent villous atrophy in early childhood: a clinicopathological survey of 47 cases. J Pediatr Gastroenterol Nutr. 1998;26(2):151–61.

72. Guarino A, Spagnuolo MI, Russo S, Albano F, Guandalini S, Capano G, et al. Etiology and risk factors of severe and protracted diarrhea. J Pediatr Gastroenterol Nutr. 1995;20(2):173–8.

73. Guandalini S, Dincer AP. Nutritional management in diarrhoeal disease. Bailliere's Clin Gastroenterol. 1998;12(4):697–717.

74. Weizman Z, Schmueli A, Deckelbaum RJ. Continuous nasogastric drip elemental feeding. Alternative for prolonged parenteral nutrition in severe prolonged diarrhea. Am J Dis Child. 1983;137(3):253–5.

75. Orenstein SR. Enteral versus parenteral therapy for intractable diarrhea of infancy: a prospective, randomized trial. J Pediatr. 1986;109(2):277–86.

76. Vanderhoof JA, Murray ND, Kaufman SS, Mack DR, Antonson DL, Corkins MR, et al. Intolerance to protein hydrolysate infant formulas: an underrecognized cause of gastrointestinal symptoms in infants. J Pediatr. 1997;131(5):741–4.

77. Goulet O, Olieman J, Ksiazyk J, Spolidoro J, Tibboe D, Kohler H, et al. Neonatal short bowel syndrome as a model of intestinal failure: physiological background for enteral feeding. Clin Nutr. 2013;32(2):162–71.

78. Goulet O, Joly F, Corriol O, Colomb-Jung V. Some new insights in intestinal failure-associated liver disease. Curr Opin Organ Transplant. 2009;14(3):256–61.

79. Rudolph CD, Hyman PE, Altschuler SM, Christensen J, Colletti RB, Cucchiara S, et al. Diagnosis and treatment of chronic intestinal pseudo-obstruction in children: report of consensus workshop. J Pediatr Gastroenterol Nutr. 1997;24(1):102–12.

80. Goulet O, Jobert-Giraud A, Michel JL, Jaubert F, Lortat-Jacob S, Colomb V, et al. Chronic intestinal pseudo-obstruction syndrome in pediatric patients. Eur J Pediatr Surg (Z Kinderchir). 1999;9(2):83–9.

81. Faure C, Goulet O, Ategbo S, Breton A, Tounian P, Ginies JL, et al. Chronic intestinal pseudoobstruction syndrome: clinical analysis, outcome, and prognosis in 105 children. French-Speaking Group of Pediatric Gastroenterology. Dig Dis Sci. 1999;44(5):953–9.

82. Heneyke S, Smith VV, Spitz L, Milla PJ. Chronic intestinal pseudo-obstruction: treatment and long term follow up of 44 patients. Arch Dis Child. 1999;81(1):21–7.

83. Kelly DA. Preventing parenteral nutrition liver disease. Early Hum Dev. 2010;86(11):683–7.

84. Alverdy JC, Aoys E, Moss GS. Total parenteral nutrition promotes bacterial translocation from the gut. Surgery. 1988;104(2):185–90.

85. Morin CL, Roulet M, Roy CC, Weber A, Lapointe N. Continuous elemental enteral alimentation in the treatment of children and adolescents with Crohn's disease. JPEN J Parenter Enteral Nutr. 1982;6(3):194–9.

86. O'Morain C, Segal AW, Levi AJ. Elemental diet as primary treatment of acute Crohn's disease: a controlled trial. BMJ. 1984;288(6434):1859–62.

87. Seidman EG, Roy CC, Weber AM, Morin CL. Nutritional therapy of Crohn's disease in childhood. Dig Dis Sci. 1987;32(Suppl 12):82S–8S.

88. Sanderson IR, Udeen S, Davies PS, Savage MO, Walker-Smith JA. Remission induced by an elemental diet in small bowel Crohn's disease. Arch Dis Child. 1987;62(2):123–7.

89. Rigaud D, Cosnes J, Le Quintrec Y, Rene E, Gendre JP, Mignon M. Controlled trial comparing two types of enteral nutrition in treatment of active Crohn's disease: elemental versus polymeric diet. Gut. 1991;32(12):1492–7.

90. Belli DC, Seidman E, Bouthillier L, Weber AM, Roy CC, Pletincx M, et al. Chronic intermittent elemental diet improves growth failure in children with Crohn's disease. Gastroenterology. 1988;94(3):603–10.

91. Thomas AG, Taylor F, Miller V. Dietary intake and nutritional treatment in childhood Crohn's disease. J Pediatr Gastroenterol Nutr. 1993;17(1):75–81.

92. Ruuska T, Savilahti E, Maki M, Ormala T, Visakorpi JK. Exclusive whole protein enteral diet versus prednisolone in the treatment of acute Crohn's disease in children. J Pediatr Gastroenterol Nutr. 1994;19(2):175–80.

93. Beattie RM, Schiffrin EJ, Donnet-Hughes A, Huggett AC, Domizio P, MacDonald TT, et al. Polymeric nutrition as the primary therapy in children with small bowel Crohn's disease. Aliment Pharmacol Ther. 1994;8(6):609–15.

94. Breese EJ, Michie CA, Nicholls SW, Williams CB, Domizio P, Walker-Smith JA, et al. The effect of treatment on lymphokine-secreting cells in the intestinal mucosa of children with Crohn's disease. Aliment Pharmacol Ther. 1995;9(5):547–52.

95. Rubio A, Pigneur B, Garnier-Lengline H, Talbotec C, Schmitz J, Canioni D, et al. The efficacy of exclusive nutritional therapy in paediatric Crohn's disease, comparing fractionated oral vs. continuous enteral feeding. Aliment Pharmacol Ther. 2011;33(12):1332–9.

96. Heuschkel RB, Menache CC, Megerian JT, Baird AE. Enteral nutrition and corticosteroids in the treatment of acute Crohn's disease in children. J Pediatr Gastroenterol Nutr. 2000;31(1):8–15.

97. Griffiths AM, Ohlsson A, Sherman PM, Sutherland LR. Meta-analysis of enteral nutrition as a primary treatment of active Crohn's disease. Gastroenterology. 1995;108(4):1056–67.

98. Zachos M, Tondeur M, Griffiths AM. Enteral nutritional therapy for inducing remission of Crohn's disease. Cochrane Database Syst Rev. 2001;(3):CD000542.

99. Zachos M, Tondeur M, Griffiths AM. Enteral nutritional therapy for induction of remission in Crohn's disease. Cochrane Database Syst Rev. 2007;(1):CD000542.

100. Dziechciarz P, Horvath A, Shamir R, Szajewska H. Meta-analysis: enteral nutrition in active Crohn's disease in children. Aliment Pharmacol Ther. 2007;26(6):795–806.

101. Critch J, Day AS, Otley A, King-Moore C, Teitelbaum JE, Shashidhar H. Use of enteral nutrition for the control of intestinal inflammation in pediatric Crohn disease. J Pediatr Gastroenterol Nutr. 2012;54(2):298–305.

102. Murch SH, Walker-Smith JA. Nutrition in inflammatory bowel disease. Bailliere's Clin Gastroenterol. 1998;12(4):719–38.

103. Akobeng AK, Miller V, Stanton J, Elbadri AM, Thomas AG. Double-blind randomized controlled trial of glutamine-enriched polymeric diet in the treatment of active Crohn's disease. J Pediatr Gastroenterol Nutr. 2000;30(1):78–84.

104. Ruemmele FM, Roy CC, Levy E, Seidman EG. Nutrition as primary therapy in pediatric Crohn's disease: fact or fantasy? J Pediatr. 2000;136(3):285–91.

105. Colomb V, Goulet O, Gorski AM, Moukarzel A, Jan D, Nihoul-Fekete C, et al. Severe digestive manifestation of rheumatoid purpura. Retrospective study of 19 cases in children. Arch Fr Pediatr. 1990;47(1):9–12.

106. Stallings VA, Stark LJ, Robinson KA, Feranchak AP, Quinton H. Evidence-based practice recommendations for nutrition-related management of children and adults with cystic fibrosis and pancreatic insufficiency: results of a systematic review. J Am Diet. 2008;108(5):832–9.

107. Borowitz D, Baker RD, Stallings V. Consensus report on nutrition for pediatric patients with cystic fibrosis. J Pediatr Gastroenterol Nutr. 2002;35(3):246–59.

108. Erskine JM, Lingard C, Sontag M. Update on enteral nutrition support for cystic fibrosis. Nutr Clin Prac. 2007;22(2):223–32.

109. Michel SH, Maqbool A, Hanna MD, Mascarenhas M. Nutrition management of pediatric patients who have cystic fibrosis. Pediatr Clin N Am. 2009;56(5):1123–41.

110. Cystic Fibrosis Foundation Patient Registry. Annual Data Report [Internet]; 2011. http://www.cff.org/UploadedFiles/research/ClinicalResearch/2011-Patient-Registry.pdf. Accessed 4 May 2014.

111. Borowitz D, Grand, RJ., Durie PR. Use of pancreatic enzyme supplements for patients with cystic fibrosis in the context of fibrosing colonopathy. J Pediatr. 1995;127(5):681–4 (March 23–24, 1995. Report No.: Contract No.: Section I).

112. Gunnell S, Christensen NK, McDonald C, Jackson D. Attitudes toward percutaneous endoscopic gastrostomy placement in cystic fibrosis patients. J Pediatr Gastroenterol Nutr. 2005;40(3):334–8.

113. Yen EH, Quinton H, Borowitz D. Better nutritional status in early childhood is associated with improved clinical outcomes and survival in patients with cystic fibrosis. J Pediatr. 2013;162(3):530–5, e1.

114. Oliver MR, Heine RG, Ng CH, Volders E, Olinsky A. Factors affecting clinical outcome in gastrostomy-fed children with cystic fibrosis. Pediatr Pulmon. 2004;37(4):324–9.

115. Goulet OJ, de Ville de Goyet J, Otte JB, Ricour C. Preoperative nutritional evaluation and support for liver transplantation in children. Transplant Proc. 1987;19(4):3249–55.

116. Protheroe SM, Kelly DA. Cholestasis and end-stage liver disease. Bailliere's Clin Gastroenterol. 1998;12(4):823–41.

117. Pierro A, Koletzko B, Carnielli V, Superina RA, Roberts EA, Filler RM, et al. Resting energy expenditure is increased in infants and children with extrahepatic biliary atresia. J Pediatr Surg. 1989;24(6):534–8.

118. McCullough AJ. Malnutrition in liver disease. Liver Transplant. 2000;6(4 Suppl 1):S85–96.

119. Baker A, Stevenson R, Dhawan A, Goncalves I, Socha P, Sokal E. Guidelines for nutritional care for infants with cholestatic liver disease before liver transplantation. Pediatr Transplant. 2007;11(8):825–34.

120. Sokal EM, Goldstein D, Ciocca M, Lewindon P, Ni YH, Silveira T, et al. End-stage liver disease and liver transplant: current situation and key issues. J Pediatr Gastroenterol Nutr. 2008;47(2):239–46.

121. SPLIT Research Group. Studies of pediatric liver transplantation (SPLIT): year 2000 outcomes. Transplantation. 2001;72(3):463–76.

122. Barshes NR, Chang IF, Karpen SJ, Carter BA, Goss JA. Impact of pretransplant growth retardation in pediatric liver transplantation. J Pediatr Gastroenterol Nutr. 2006;43(1):89–94.

123. Chin SE, Shepherd RW, Thomas BJ, Cleghorn GJ, Patrick MK, Wilcox JA, et al. Nutritional support in children with end-stage liver disease: a randomized crossover trial of a branched-chain amino acid supplement. Am J Clin Nutr. 1992;56(1):158–63.

124. Holt RI, Miell JP, Jones JS, Mieli-Vergani G, Baker AJ. Nasogastric feeding enhances nutritional status in paediatric liver disease but does not alter circulating levels of IGF-I and IGF binding proteins. Clin Endocrinol (Oxf). 2000;52(2):217–24.

125. Chin SE, Shepherd RW, Cleghorn GJ, Patrick MK, Javorsky G, Frangoulis E, et al. Survival, growth and quality of life in children after orthotopic liver transplantation: a 5 year experience. J Pediatr Child Health. 1991;27(6):380–5.

126. Shepherd RW, Chin SE, Cleghorn GJ, Patrick M, Ong TH, Lynch SV, et al. Malnutrition in children with chronic liver disease accepted for liver transplantation: clinical profile and effect on outcome. J Pediatr Child Health. 1991;27(5):295–9.

127. Sullivan JS, Sundaram SS, Pan Z, Sokol RJ. Parenteral nutrition supplementation in biliary atresia patients listed for liver transplantation. Liver Transplant. 2012;18(1):120–8.

128. Charlton CP, Buchanan E, Holden CE, Preece MA, Green A, Booth IW, et al. Intensive enteral feeding in advanced cirrhosis: reversal of malnutrition without precipitation of hepatic encephalopathy. Arch Dis Child. 1992;67(5):603–7.

129. Cabre E, Gonzalez-Huix F, Abad-Lacruz A, Esteve M, Acero D, Fernandez-Banares F, et al. Effect of total enteral nutrition on the short-term outcome of severely malnourished cirrhotics. A randomized controlled trial. Gastroenterology. 1990;98(3):715–20.

130. Kaufman SS, Scrivner DJ, Murray ND, Vanderhoof JA, Hart MH, Antonson DL. Influence of portagen and pregestimil on essential fatty acid status in infantile liver disease. Pediatrics. 1992;89(1):151–4.

131. Black RE, Cousens S, Johnson HL, Lawn JE, Rudan I, Bassani DG, et al. Global, regional, and national causes of child mortality in 2008: a systematic analysis. Lancet. 2010;375(9730): 1969–87.

132. Nightingale S, Ng VL. Optimizing nutritional management in children with chronic liver disease. Pediatr Clin N Am. 2009;56(5):1161–83.

133. Annonymous. In: Board FaN, editor. Dietary reference intakes for energy, carbohydrate, fiber, fat, fatty acids, cholesterol, protein and amino acids. Washington, DC: The National Academy Press; 2005. 1331 p.

134. Duffy B, Gunn T, Collinge J, Pencharz P. The effect of varying protein quality and energy intake on the nitrogen metabolism of parenterally fed very low birthweight (less than 1600 g) infants. Pediatr Res. 1981;15(7):1040–4.

135. Mager DR, Wykes LJ, Roberts EA, Ball RO, Pencharz PB. Branched-chain amino acid needs in children with mild-to-moderate chronic cholestatic liver disease. J Nutr. 2006;136(1): 133–9.

136. Als-Nielsen B, Koretz RL, Kjaergard LL, Gluud C. Branched-chain amino acids for hepatic encephalopathy. Cochrane Database Syst Rev. 2003(2):CD001939.

137. Owens JL, Musa N. Nutrition support after neonatal cardiac surgery. Nutr Clin Pract. 2009;24(2):242–9.

138. Kirby DF, Delegge MH, Fleming CR. American Gastroenterological Association technical review on tube feeding for enteral nutrition. Gastroenterology. 1995;108(4):1282–301.

139. Itkin M, DeLegge MH, Fang JC, McClave SA, Kundu S, d'Othee BJ, et al. Multidisciplinary practical guidelines for gastrointestinal access for enteral nutrition and decompression from the Society of Interventional Radiology and American Gastroenterological Association (AGA) Institute, with endorsement by Canadian Interventional Radiological Association (CIRA) and Cardiovascular and Interventional Radiological Society of Europe (CIRSE). Gastroenterology. 2011;141(2):742–65.

140. DiBaise JK, Decker GA. Enteral access options and management in the patient with intestinal failure. J Clin Gastroenterol. 2007;41(7):647–56.

141. Silk DB, Rees RG, Keohane PP, Attrill H. Clinical efficacy and design changes of "fine bore" nasogastric feeding tubes: a seven-year experience involving 809 intubations in 403 patients. JPEN J Parenter Enteral Nutr. 1987;11(4):378–83.

142. Beckstrand J, Cirgin Ellett ML, McDaniel A. Predicting internal distance to the stomach for positioning nasogastric and orogastric feeding tubes in children. J Adv Nurs. 2007;59(3):274–89.

143. Ellett ML. What is known about methods of correctly placing gastric tubes in adults and children. Gastroenterol Nurs. 2004;27(6):253–9, quiz 60–1.

144. Gauderer MW. Percutaneous endoscopic gastrostomy and the evolution of contemporary long-term enteral access. Clin Nutr (Edinb, Scotl). 2002;21(2):103–10.

145. Doede T, Faiss S, Schier F. Jejunal feeding tubes via gastrostomy in children. Endoscopy. 2002;34(7):539–42.

146. Grimble GK, Rees RG, Keohane PP, Cartwright T, Desreumaux M, Silk DB. Effect of peptide chain length on absorption of egg protein hydrolysates in the normal human jejunum. Gastroenterology. 1987;92(1):136–42.

147. Grimble GK. The significance of peptides in clinical nutrition. An Rev Nutr. 1994;14:419–47.

148. Fairclough PD, Hegarty JE, Silk DB, Clark ML. Comparison of the absorption of two protein hydrolysates and their effects on water and electrolyte movements in the human jejunum. Gut. 1980;21(10):829–34.

149. Moriarty KJ, Hegarty JE, Fairclough PD, Kelly MJ, Clark ML, Dawson AM. Relative nutritional value of whole protein, hydrolysed protein and free amino acids in man. Gut. 1985;26(7): 694–9.

150. Bach AC, Babayan VK. Medium-chain triglycerides: an update. Am J Clin Nutr. 1982;36(5):950–62.

151. Lima LA, Gray OP, Losty H. Excretion of dicarboxylic acids following administration of medium chain triglycerides. JPEN J Parenter Enteral Nutr. 1987;11(6):600–1.

152. Holliday MA, Segar WE. The maintenance need for water in parenteral fluid therapy. Pediatrics. 1957;19(5):823–32.

153. Aggett PJ, Agostoni C, Axelsson I, De Curtis M, Goulet O, Hernell O, et al. Feeding preterm infants after hospital discharge: a commentary by the ESPGHAN Committee on Nutrition. J Pediatr Gastroenterol Nutr. 2006;42(5):596–603.

154. Bines J, Francis D, Hill D. Reducing parenteral requirement in children with short bowel syndrome: impact of an amino acid-based complete infant formula. J Pediatr Gastroenterol Nutr. 1998;26(2):123–8.

155. Andorsky DJ, Lund DP, Lillehei CW, Jaksic T, Dicanzio J, Richardson DS, et al. Nutritional and other postoperative management of neonates with short bowel syndrome correlates with clinical outcomes. J Pediatr. 2001;139(1):27–33.

156. Bernbaum JC, Pereira GR, Watkins JB, Peckham GJ. Nonnutritive sucking during gavage feeding enhances growth and maturation in premature infants. Pediatrics. 1983;71(1):41–5.

157. Pinelli J, Symington A. Non-nutritive sucking for promoting physiologic stability and nutrition in preterm infants. Cochrane Database Syst Rev. 2005;(4):CD001071.

158. Simon T, Fink AS. Current management of endoscopic feeding tube dysfunction. Surg Endosc. 1999;13(4):403–5.

159. Marcuard SP, Stegall KL, Trogdon S. Clearing obstructed feeding tubes. JPEN J Parenter Enteral Nutr. 1989;13(1):81–3.

160. Marcuard SP, Stegall KS. Unclogging feeding tubes with pancreatic enzyme. JPEN J Parenter Enteral Nutr. 1990;14(2): 198–200.

161. McClave SA, DeMeo MT, DeLegge MH, DiSario JA, Heyland DK, Maloney JP, et al. North American summit on aspiration in the critically Ill patient: consensus statement. JPEN J Parenter Enteral Nutr. 2002;26(Suppl 6):S80–5.

162. Parker CM, Heyland DK. Aspiration and the risk of ventilator-associated pneumonia. Nutr Clin Prac. 2004;19(6):597–609.

163. Goulet O, Colomb-Jung V, Joly F. Role of the colon in short bowel syndrome and intestinal transplantation. J Pediatr Gastroenterol Nutr. 2009;48(Suppl 2):S66–71.

164. Ehrlein H, Haas-Deppe B, Weber E. The sodium concentration of enteral diets does not influence absorption of nutrients but induces intestinal secretion of water in miniature pigs. J Nutr. 1999;129(2):410–8.

165. Flores JC, Lopez-Herce J, Sola I, Carrillo A, Jr. Duodenal perforation caused by a transpyloric tube in a critically ill infant. Nutrition (Burbank, Los Angel Cy, Calif). 2006;22(2):209–12.

166. Perez-Rodriques J, Quero J, Frias EG, Omenaca F, Martinez A. Duodenorenal perforation in a neonate by a tube of silicone rubber during transpyloric feeding. J Pediatr. 1978;92(1):113–4.

167. Boros SJ, Reynolds JW. Duodenal perforation: a complication of neonatal nasojejunal feeding. J Pediatri. 1974;85(1):107–8.

168. Lopez-Herce J, Santiago MJ, Sanchez C, Mencia S, Carrillo A, Vigil D. Risk factors for gastrointestinal complications in critically ill children with transpyloric enteral nutrition. Eur J Clin Nutr. 2008;62(3):395–400.

169. Heine RG, Reddihough DS, Catto-Smith AG. Gastro-oesophageal reflux and feeding problems after gastrostomy in children with severe neurological impairment. Dev Med Child Neurol. 1995;37(4):320–9.

170. Grunow JE, al-Hafidh A, Tunell WP. Gastroesophageal reflux following percutaneous endoscopic gastrostomy in children. J Pediatr Surg. 1989;24(1):42–4, discussion 4–5.

171. Noble LJ, Dalzell AM, El-Matary W. The relationship between percutaneous endoscopic gastrostomy and gastro-oesophageal reflux disease in children: a systematic review. Surg Endosc. 2012;26(9):2504–12.

172. Veit F, Heine RG, Catto-Smith AG. Dumping syndrome after Nissen fundoplication. J Pediatr Child Health. 1994;30(2):182–5.

173. Bufler P, Ehringhaus C, Koletzko S. Dumping syndrome: a common problem following Nissen fundoplication in young children. Pediatr Surg Int. 2001;17(5–6):351–5.

174. Samuk I, Afriat R, Horne T, Bistritzer T, Barr J, Vinograd I. Dumping syndrome following Nissen fundoplication, diagnosis, and treatment. J Pediatr Gastroenterol Nutr. 1996;23(3):235–40.

175. Calabria AC, Gallagher PR, Simmons R, Blinman T, De Leon DD. Postoperative surveillance and detection of postprandial hypoglycemia after fundoplasty in children. J Pediatr. 2011;159(4):597–601, e1.

176. Khoshoo V, Reifen RM, Gold BD, Sherman PM, Pencharz PB. Nutritional manipulation in the management of dumping syndrome. Arch Dis Child. 1991;66(12):1447–8.

177. Khoshoo V, Roberts PL, Loe WA, Golladay ES, Pencharz PB. Nutritional management of dumping syndrome associated with antireflux surgery. J Pediatr Surg. 1994;29(11):1452–4.

178. Borovoy J, Furuta L, Nurko S. Benefit of uncooked cornstarch in the management of children with dumping syndrome fed exclusively by gastrostomy. Am J Gastroenterol. 1998;93(5):814–8.

179. Gitzelmann R, Hirsig J. Infant dumping syndrome: reversal of symptoms by feeding uncooked starch. Eur J Pediatr. 1986;145(6):504–6.

180. De Cunto A, Barbi E, Minen F, Ventura A. Safety and efficacy of high-dose acarbose treatment for dumping syndrome. J Pediatr Gastroenterol Nutr. 2011;53(1):113–4.

181. Centers for Disease Control and Prevention (CDC). Cronobacter species isolation in two infants—New Mexico, 2008. MMWR Morb Mortal Wkly Rep. 2009;58(42):1179–83.

182. Jason J. Prevention of invasive Cronobacter infections in young infants fed powdered infant formulas. Pediatrics. 2012;130(5):e1076–84.

183. Christine J, Taylor PD. Health professsionals letter on Enterobacter sakazakii infections associated with use of powdered (dry) infant formulas in neonatal intensive care unite. Safety Alerts & Advisories: U.S. Food and Drug Administration; 2002.

184. Anderson KR, Norris DJ, Godfrey LB, Avent CK, Butterworth CE, Jr. Bacterial contamination of tube-feeding formulas. JPEN J Parenter Enteral Nutr. 1984;8(6):673–8.

185. Levy J, Van Laethem Y, Verhaegen G, Perpete C, Butzler JP, Wenzel RP. Contaminated enteral nutrition solutions as a cause of nosocomial bloodstream infection: a study using plasmid fingerprinting. JPEN J Parenter Enteral Nutr. 1989;13(3):228–34.

186. Patchell CJ, Anderton A, Holden C, MacDonald A, George RH, Booth IW. Reducing bacterial contamination of enteral feeds. Arch Dis Child. 1998;78(2):166–8.

187. Mathus-Vliegen EM, Bredius MW, Binnekade JM. Analysis of sites of bacterial contamination in an enteral feeding system. JPEN J Parenter Enteral Nutr. 2006;30(6):519–25.

188. Matlow A, Jacobson M, Wray R, Goldman C, Streitenberger L, Freeman R, et al. Enteral tube hub as a reservoir for transmissible enteric bacteria. Am J Infect Control. 2006;34(3):131–3.

189. Matlow A, Wray R, Goldman C, Streitenberger L, Freeman R, Kovach D. Microbial contamination of enteral feed administration sets in a pediatric institution. Am J Infect Control. 2003;31(1):49–53.

190. Mehall JR, Kite CA, Saltzman DA, Wallett T, Jackson RJ, Smith SD. Prospective study of the incidence and complications of bacterial contamination of enteral feeding in neonates. J Pediatr Surg. 2002;37(8):1177–82.

191. Palesty JA, Dudrick SJ. The goldilocks paradigm of starvation and refeeding. Nutr Clin Pract. 2006;21(2):147–54.

192. Fuentebella J, Kerner JA. Refeeding syndrome. Pediatr Clin N Am. 2009;56(5):1201–10.

193. Gaudiani JL, Sabel AL, Mehler PS. Low prealbumin is a significant predictor of medical complications in severe anorexia nervosa. Int J Eat Disord. 2014;47(2):148–56.

194. Dunn RL, Stettler N, Mascarenhas MR. Refeeding syndrome in hospitalized pediatric patients. Nutr Clin Pract. 2003;18(4):327–32.

195. Greene HL, Helinek GL, Folk CC, Courtney M, Thompson S, MacDonell RC, Jr, et al. Nasogastric tube feeding at home: a method for adjunctive nutritional support of malnourished patients. Am J Clin Nutr. 1981;34(6):1131–8.

196. Daveluy W, Guimber D, Mention K, Lescut D, Michaud L, Turck D, et al. Home enteral nutrition in children: an 11-year experience with 416 patients. Clin Nutr. 2005;24(1):48–54.

197. Pedron-Giner C, Navas-Lopez VM, Martinez-Zazo AB, Martinez-Costa C, Sanchez-Valverde F, Blasco-Alonso J, et al. Analysis of the Spanish national registry for pediatric home enteral nutrition (NEPAD): implementation rates and observed trends during the past 8 years. Eur J Clin Nutr. 2013;67(4):318–23.

198. Colomb V, Goulet O, Ricour C. Home enteral and parenteral nutrition in children. Bailliere's Clin Gastroenterol. 1998;12(4):877–94.

199. Howard L, Ament M, Fleming CR, Shike M, Steiger E. Current use and clinical outcome of home parenteral and enteral nutrition therapies in the United States. Gastroenterology. 1995;109(2):355–65.

200. Elia M. An international perspective on artificial nutritional support in the community. Lancet. 1995;345(8961):1345–9.

201. Ireton-Jones C. Home enteral nutrition from the provider's perspective. JPEN J Parenter Enteral Nutr. 2002;26(Suppl 5):S8–9.

202. Elia M. Home enteral nutrition: general aspects and a comparison between the United States and Britain. Nutrition (Burbank, Los Angel Cty, Calif). 1994;10(2):115–23.

203. Holden CE, MacDonald A, Ward M, Ford K, Patchell C, Handy D, et al. Psychological preparation for nasogastric feeding in children. Br J Nurs (Mark Allen Publ). 1997;6(7):376–81, 84–5.

204. Holden CE, Puntis JW, Charlton CP, Booth IW. Nasogastric feeding at home: acceptability and safety. Arch Dis Child. 1991;66(1):148–51.

205. Liptak GS. Home care for children who have chronic conditions. Pediatr Rev/Am Acad Pediatr. 1997;18(8):271–3.

Parenteral Nutrition in Infants and Children

47

Susan Hill

Introduction

Parenteral nutrition (PN) is a lifesaving supportive treatment in intestinal failure (IF) that should be considered one of the major medical advances of the last century. IF has been defined as the inability to absorb sufficient fluid and nutrients from the intestine to maintain homeostasis and to grow and develop even when the most suitable enteral nutrition is given via the most appropriate artificial feeding device for the individual patient [1]. The use of PN has enabled even the sickest child to survive including the most premature of infants. However, PN should be prescribed and administered in an appropriate clinical setting to minimize the possibility of complications that could harm rather than benefit the child's health and can be life-threatening. In other words, PN is not just another drug to be prescribed. The support needed includes a comprehensive laboratory service and pharmacy and dietetics in addition to specialist medical and nursing skills.

While PN is essential for survival in patients with severe IF the aim of treatment is to stabilize the child, and at the same time to diagnose, investigate, and treat the underlying cause of the IF in order to wean the patient back on to enteral feed at the earliest opportunity.

PN can be defined as the infusion of nutrients directly into the bloodstream and by-passing the gastrointestinal tract.

"Total" PN (TPN) is the term used for infusion of all the individual's nutritional requirements into the bloodstream. "Partial" PN is the infusion of some nutrients into the bloodstream while a portion of the daily nutritional requirements is derived from enteral nutrients

Treatment with PN has been defined as "long-term" by the British Society of Pediatric Gastroenterology, Hepatology and Nutrition (BSPGHAN) when it is given for >27 days

[2]. "Home" PN is considered when a hospitalized patient is stable on PN and expected to require treatment for at least two further months. Parents are usually formally trained to administer the PN and administer it to the child overnight at home. Table 47.1 lists indications for parenteral nutrition.

History and Development of PN

Attempts to feed directly into the bloodstream have been made ever since the circulatory system was first described by William Harvey in 1628. For example, Sir Christopher Wren infused ale and opium into dogs in 1656 using a bladder and sharpened quill.

In order for PN to be safely used in the clinical setting, suitable carbohydrate, protein, and lipid sources were required in a form that was stable in solution, nontoxic, and suitable to be infused directly into the bloodstream.

The first suitable protein source was developed in 1937 when a casein hydrolysate was successfully infused in adults and in 1940 a crystalline L-amino acid solution was first used clinically in children. Technical difficulties and high commercial costs were sufficiently overcome for the solutions to be used routinely from the 1960s.

Carbohydrate energy sources trialed included fructose, sorbitol, ethanol, and glucose. Although glucose was metabolically the most suitable energy source, it was associated with venous thrombosis. It was only when Dudrick et al. in 1968 infused glucose into a large central vein that thrombophlebitis was avoided [3]. PN was first provided on a commercial basis from the late 1960s after a suitable lipid source was developed. The lipid was required in order to provide adequate calories without an excessive osmotic load as well as a source of essential fatty acids (EFA). An artificial "chylomicron" composed of soybean oil and egg phosphatides was developed by Wretlind and Schuberth in 1963 that is still in use today [4].

S. Hill (✉)
Department of Gastroenterology, Division of Intestinal Rehabilitation and Nutrition, Great Ormond Street Hospital for Children NHS Foundation Trust, Great Ormond Street, London WC1N 3JH, UK
e-mail: susan.hill@gosh.nhs.uk

© Springer International Publishing Switzerland 2016
S. Guandalini et al. (eds.), *Textbook of Pediatric Gastroenterology, Hepatology and Nutrition*,
DOI 10.1007/978-3-319-17169-2_47

Table 47.1 Indications for parenteral nutrition

Primary digestive disorder	Primary non-digestive disorder
Short bowel syndrome	Prematurity
–	Acute pancreatitis (enteral feeds usually recommended)
Protracted diarrhea with faltering growth	Radiotherapy
Necrotizing enterocolitis	Chemotherapy
Chronic intestinal pseudo-obstruction	Acute liver failure
Postoperative abdominal surgery	Acute renal failure
–	Extensive burns
–	Severe trauma

Constituents of PN

PN is a complex mixture of sterile nutrients in a suitable form to be safely infused directly into the bloodstream. It consists of carbohydrate lipid and amino acids with added vitamins and minerals.

Lipid is usually supplied as a separate infusion that also contains the fat soluble vitamins, that is, vitamins A, D, E, and K.

The standard carbohydrate source is dextrose. The amino acid formulation is usually based on egg protein and in the neonate, on breast milk.

Until the last few years soybean has been the only lipid source. However, more recently olive oil, fish oil, coconut oil, and an artificially structured lipid have been developed. See Table 47.2.

The lipid emulsion provides an energy-dense source of nonprotein calories and if includes soybean oil contains EFA, alpha-linolenic acid and linoleic acid.

Lipid should represent about 30 % of nonprotein energy and linoleic acid should be 1–2 % of total energy. The maximum lipid utilization rate is about 3.3–3.6 g/kg/day.

Minerals and vitamins are available in mixed formulations or can be added individually.

Iron is not routinely included since iron-associated liver cirrhosis can develop. However, it is often added when iron-deficiency anemia develops in children on prolonged treatment.

Table 47.2 Parenteral nutrition lipid solutions

Parenteral nutrition lipid solutions
Clinoleic 20 % (Baxter): 20 % soybean oil, 80 % olive oil
Intralipid: 20 % (Baxter) pure soybean oil
Lipidem (B-Braun): fish oil, olive oil, soybean oil
Lipofundin (B-Braun): medium-chain and long-chain triglycerides MCT/LCT) MCT/LCT 20 %® a physical mixture, 1:1 by weight, of soybean and coconut oil
Omegaven 20 % (Fresenius Kabi): pure fish oil
SMOF lipid® 20 % (Fresenius Kabi) physical mixture of 30 % soybean, 30 % MCT, 25 % olive, and 15 % fish oil; SMOF

Additional substances that can be directly added to the formulation include the nonessential amino acid glutamine and certain medication, such as the H-2 receptor antagonist, ranitidine.

PN should be formulated in a licensed compounding unit. The unit should have access both to their own stability data and that available in specialist PN units elsewhere in the UK and Europe. An automated system in a specialized sterile unit is usually used to mix the PN ingredients according to international pharmaceutical standards. The final formulation is supplied in a sealed plastic bag. In most cases, the nutrients for a 24-h period are contained within two bags; one with the amino-acids, dextrose, electrolytes, trace elements, and water soluble vitamins, and the other with lipid and fat-soluble vitamins, that is, vitamins A, D, E, and K.

Stability of the PN formulation can be a major problem in children when compared to adults since they have relatively high calcium and phosphate requirements: two salts that readily precipitate.

PN can be sourced in three different ways:

1. Individually formulated/bespoke PN bags usually prescribed and manufactured on a daily basis according to the patient's requirements. It is usually the most appropriate treatment for hospitalized children (but may not be appropriate for premature newborn infants) with varying daily needs. The "shelf life" of these bags is approximately 48–72 h. The PN pharmacy is usually within the hospital.

2. Second, standard preprepared commercially available bags with a longer shelf life of several days or weeks that can sometimes be stored at room temperature are increasingly used in premature neonates and adult patients. Vitamins, trace elements and, if needed, extra electrolytes (that would not remain stable in the solution for more than a few days) should be added immediately prior to infusion in a sterile compounding unit, preferably in the hospital pharmacy. Standard bags are increasingly being used in neonatal units since they are readily available and more appropriate for the nonsurgical premature infant.

3. Third, certain pharmacies have sufficient expertise and stability data to manufacture individually prescribed PN

with prolonged stability for 1–4 weeks. There will be a gradual breakdown of certain vitamins during storage. These pharmacies usually supply PN to patients with chronic IF on long-term treatment with PN who are usually at home.

How to Start PN

It is essential that all attempts are made to feed a child enterally (unless contraindicated, e.g., intestinal obstruction, post-gastrointestinal surgery) before commencing PN. Once the need for PN has been established it usually needs to be commenced with some urgency.

The severity and complications of a chronic disease are worse in undernourished patients. Nutritional support should be begun early, for example, within 1–5 days if a child is unable to tolerate any enteral nutrition since nutritional reserves are limited. Age, nutritional state, and intestinal losses should be taken into account. It has been estimated that a small premature baby (1 kg) has sufficient reserves to survive only 4 days and a term infant up to 12 days [5]. When enteral nutrition is not tolerated or contraindicated, PN should be begun within 1–2 days of the intake/absorption becoming inadequate in the newborn infant, but can be delayed for up to 5–7 days in a well-nourished adolescent. Other than in the premature neonate, it is usually best practice to stabilize the patient and start PN during normal working hours. See Table 47.3 for the steps that need to be taken when commencing PN.

Venous Access

In order to safely administer PN with a sufficiently high concentration of nutrients for a child to thrive, it needs to be infused into a central vein. For example, a glucose concentration of 12.5 % or more should *only* be administered through a CVC. The optimal position is for the tip of the catheter to be high in the right atrium or low in the superior vena cava. A silicone rubber (Silastic) catheter should be used, preferably with a subcutaneous cuff to hold the catheter in place and a single rather than double lumen in order to reduce the risk of infection. A peripherally inserted catheter with the tip centrally placed (PICC) line can also be used, particularly if it is likely to only be needed for a few days/weeks. The major advantage of a PICC line over a cuffed catheter is that since a PICC can be removed without general anaesthetic.

A subcutaneous implantable port should be avoided if at all possible, since accessing the port can be traumatic for the child and it can be difficult to eradicate infection. However, a port maybe suitable for short-term PN in certain circumstances. A short peripheral cannula should not be used to administer PN since the high osmolality of the PN solution readily causes thrombophlebitis and tissue necrosis should it leak from the vein. If in exceptional circumstances PN had to be given peripherally, the glucose concentration must be less than 12.5 % and the osmolarity should not exceed 600–900 mOsmol/l.

In the neonate, the catheter is usually inserted via a peripheral vein with the tip placed centrally in the superior vena cava. Insertion in the older child is usually via the subclavian (or occasionally the internal jugular) vein with the tip positioned high in the right atrium. The femoral veins can be used, but are less suitable, unless the catheter is tunneled under the skin, since the exit site is in the nappy area so susceptible to fecal contamination.

In patients requiring long-term PN, that is, >27 days the catheter should be placed under radiological control in order to minimize damage to the blood vessel during insertion.

It is of utmost importance to use radiological control in patients with chronic IF who may require repeated CVC insertions in order to avoid loss of venous access.

A catheter with a subcutaneous cuff to fix the line in place and prevent movement is usually used in children. Alternatively, a PICC line can be used. Although use of a PICC is only recommended for a few weeks, they can function successfully for many months and in some children at home on PN have been kept in situ for over 12 months. The major advantage of a PICC line over a cuffed catheter is that the PICC line can be removed without the need for a general anesthetic.

In children on long-term home treatment, the CVC can remain in situ for as long as 8–10 years (personal observation). It may eventually need to be changed when the child has grown sufficiently for the line tip to become displaced from the right atrium.

If at all possible, the catheter should be dedicated to the infusion of PN in order to preserve patency and minimize risk of infection. In children who have had frequent cannulation of blood vessels and/or excessive anxiety associated

Table 47.3 How to start parenteral nutrition

	How to start parenteral nutrition
1.	Obtain secure central venous access
2.	Assess maintenance fluid and electrolyte requirements from patients length/height and weight
3.	Add extra requirements for excessive intestinal losses
4.	Prescribe PN
5.	Obtain appropriate equipment for infusing PN: a giving set to connect to the central venous catheter and the bag of PN and an infusion pump
6.	Gradually increase PN over 4–6 days from 60 % to full requirements
7.	Monitor weight and blood electrolyte levels on a daily (or twice daily) basis for first 5–7 days

PN parenteral nutrition

Table 47.4 Monitoring when commencing parenteral nutrition

Monitoring when commencing parenteral nutrition
Clinical observation: temperature, heart rate, respiratory rate, blood pressure
Daily ward urine analysis for glucose and ketones until stable
Blood glucose level 4-hourly until stable in the older child or according to the unit's glucose monitoring policy for neonates
The maximum infusion rate of glucose through a central vein should be 1.0–1.5 g/kg/h; if greater than this glycosuria is highly likely
Weigh daily for 5 days (twice daily if excessive fluid losses/difficult fluid balance) Twice weekly once stable, then weekly
Weigh on the same scales and at the same time everyday
Urine analysis for glucose and ketones if PN glucose concentration increased
Blood sodium, potassium, urea, creatinine, calcium, magnesium phosphate, and liver function tests analysis on a daily basis over the first 4 days when introducing PN
The child's urine sodium and potassium should initially be monitored twice weekly, and once stable on a weekly basis
Check blood glucose when start to "cycle" PN—initially at 30 min intervals after stopping the infusion
Other nutritional blood tests that should be monitored when starting PN, zinc, copper, selenium, vitamins A and E, and ferritin, then 4–6 weekly
Vitamin D, 6 monthly and if normal, 12 monthly
B group vitamins, T4, TSH annually

PN parenteral nutrition, *TSH* thyroid stimulating hormone

with venepuncture, it may be extremely difficult to obtain blood samples from a peripheral vein The distress and/or time attempting peripheral vein access may outweigh the potential complications of using the CVC for other infusions and/or blood sampling.

Administration of PN

The PN should be infused via a pump attached to an infusion stand. The pump should be positioned within 30 cm of the heart and should have a pressure alarm set. The pump should be set to the correct infusion rate and volume to be infused. The infusion should pass through a 1.2 µm filter [6].

Children on long-term home PN treatment should have the use of a portable pump with rucksack for the PN bag itself.

Parenteral fluid and electrolyte requirements are prescribed according to the child's weight [7].

Children in intensive care often have restricted total fluid intake and require other intravenous infusions in addition to PN. It may not be possible to give required nutrients in the volume available for the PN infusion.

Monitoring on PN Treatment

When commencing PN treatment, observations should be performed regularly as shown in Table 47.4.

In addition, the child's length should be measured monthly using appropriate equipment and plotted on the child's centile chart. Head circumference should also be charted in children under 2 years of age.

In certain conditions when fluid balance is altered, weight may not be a useful measure. For example, children in renal

failure or with low blood albumin may retain fluid within the body tissues and those with intestinal pseudobstruction may "pool" fluid within dilated intestinal loops.

Neonatal PN

It is important to commence PN at the earliest opportunity and within 6 h of birth in the "high risk" premature neonate. Initially, PN at 60–90 ml/kg/day that includes both amino acids and lipid. See Table 47.5 for guidelines. Infusion can be commenced via an umbilical venous catheter UVC or peripherally inserted long line. If the child is clinically stable, trophic feeds of expressed breast milk (EBM) should also be commenced. "High-risk" neonates include those born prematurely at less than 32 weeks gestation, very low birth weight (VLBW) of under 1.5 kg, less than 35 weeks gestation with intrauterine growth retardation (IUGR) with weight <9th centile and absent/reversed end-diastolic flow and those with congenital gastrointestinal malformations, such as gastroschisis. Other neonates at nutritional risk who may need PN are those with necrotising enterocolitis, gastrointestinal obstruction, those who need inotropic support, perinatal hypoxia/ischaemia, cyanotic or duct-dependent cardiac lesions or persistent pulmonary hypertension of the newborn (PPHN).

Management on PN

The four major stages in the use of PN are as follows: (1) stabilize the patient, (2) aim for appropriate weight gain—usually "catch up" weight gain required (3) maintain weight centile appropriate for patients length/height (4) withdraw/wean PN and institute enteral nutrition.

Table 47.5 Recommended parenteral nutrient requirements for preterm and term infants [7, 8] *Courtesy of* Walsh O, Larmour K, Curry J, Hill S, Huertas A. *UCLH, UK Neonatal Nutriton team*

	Parenteral nutritional requirements			
	Preterm infant		Preterm infant	Term infant
	Tsang (2005) [8]		ESPGHAN (2005) [7]	ESPGHAN (2005) [7]
	Transition (first week)	Growing (second week onwards)		
Energy kcal/kg/day	75–85 ELBW 60–70 VLBW	105–115 ELBW 90–100 VLBW	110–120	90–100
Protein g/kg/day (amino acids g/kg/day)	3.5 (4.0) ELBW 3.5 (4.0) VLBW	3.5–4.0 (4.0–4.6) ELBW 3.2–3.8 (3.6–4.3) VLBW	1.3–3.5 (1.5–4.0)	1.3–2.7 (1.5–3.0)
Sodium mmol/kg/day	2.0–5.0	3.0–5.0	2.0–3.0 1500 g 3.0–5.0 1500g	2.0–5.0
Potassium mmol/kg/day	0–2.0	2.0–3.0	1.0–2.0 1500 g 1.0–3.0 1500g	1.0–3.0
Calcium mmol/kg/day	1.5	1.5–2.0	No recommendation	1.3–3.0
Phosphate mmol/kg/day	1.5–1.9	1.5–1.9	No recommendation	1–2.3
Vitamin A IU/kg/day (µg RE/kg/day)	700–1500	700–1500	No recommendation	500–999 (150–300)
Vitamin D IU/kg/day	40–160	40–160	No recommendation	32
Iron mg/kg/day	0	0.1–0.2	Up to 0.2	0.05–0.1
Folate µg/kg/day	56	56	No recommendation	56

ESPGHAN European Society for Clinical Nutrition and Metabolism, European Society of Pediatric Gastroenterology, Hepatology and Nutrition, *ELBW* extremely low birth weight, *VLBW* very low birth weight

Enteral nutrition should be continued alongside PN if at all possible. The major benefits of enteral nutrition are prevention of intestinal mucosal atrophy, maintenance of the enterohepatic circulation and if given orally, retention of feeding skills. Full use of any residual intestinal function should be made in order to maximize absorptive ability unless there are significant adverse consequences such as excessive fluid losses or pain. A continuous enteral feed can play an essential role, first in weaning the child off PN by maximizing use of the remaining intestinal function, then in the longer term management at home.

Nutrition Support Team

It is important to bring all professionals contributing to the management of the PN together to work as a nutrition support team (NST) [9].

All children receiving PN treatment should be reviewed on a regular basis and at least weekly by the NST. The multidisciplinary team usually includes a doctor specializing in nutrition, dietitian, pharmacist, and specialist nurse. Other potential members of the team include a biochemist, speech and language therapist, and microbiologist.

The team may either prescribe or advise the medical team caring for the patient.

Complications of Short-Term PN

The most frequent complications associated with PN are the refeeding syndrome and other metabolic disorders, inadequate weight gain, septicemia, liver disease and venous catheter problems, and thrombosis. Each of these problems will be discussed below.

Refeeding Syndrome and Metabolic Disorders

Initial PN complications are most commonly related to fluid and electrolyte imbalance [9]. Refeeding syndrome is a common problem that develops in a previously undernourished child when full nutrition is commenced too rapidly. As the body changes from catabolism to anabolism potassium, phosphate, and magnesium are taken up into the cells and there can be a rapid drop in blood levels known as "refeeding syndrome." If severe, refeeding syndrome can be life-threatening. The maximum possible phosphate will be needed in the PN. An oral or peripheral blood infusion of phosphate and/or potassium may be required alongside the PN if the amount required exceeds the concentration that is stable within the PN formulation. Low total body sodium is another frequent longer-term problem when sodium losses have not been adequately replaced. Measurement of urine sodium is one of the most helpful investigations in the absence of diuretic treatment or renal failure. Patients with a low urinary sodium level (<20–50 mmol/l) may have a low total body sodium and are unlikely to gain weight appropriately. Extra sodium infusion in the PN is required. If a patient is weaning from the PN, the extra sodium may best be given enterally.

Inadequate Weight Gain

One of the major complications is inadequate nutrition. The four main reasons are fluid restriction, infusing a lower volume of PN than that prescribed, under-prescribing and negative sodium balance.

It may not be possible to infuse sufficient volume of PN to supply adequate calories and protein in the critically ill child with other major organ failure. The child may only tolerate limited fluid volume and a proportion of the fluid tolerated may be taken up with infusion of medications and as a result the child will fail to gain weight adequately. It is important to infuse any medications in the minimum possible volume and ensure that whenever possible medications are prepared in 10% dextrose to maximize calorie intake. Secondly, children are often given less PN that the volume prescribed. If other infusions are given through the same CVC lumen, the length of time taken for those infusions needs to be taken into account and the total PN volume required prescribed in the hours available.

The PN prescription is based on body weight. It is important that the prescriber uses the patient's expected weight for length/height rather than the actual weight when the weight centile is lower or higher than the length/height centile. The only exception is in the child with stunted growth who may benefit from feeding to a higher length centile in order to improve growth.

Septicemia

Catheter-related sepsis is a common complication. It is important to have a policy for management. If a patient has a fever >38.5 °C or symptoms suggestive of septicemia, a blood culture should be taken via the CVC and at least two broad-spectrum antibiotics need to be commenced to treat potential gram-positive and gram-negative bacterial infection. Antibiotics must be given via the CVC. If there is more than one lumen then treatment needs to be rotated between the lumens in order to eradicate the infection. Once cultures are available the antibiotic regime should be tailored according to the bacteria detected. For example, if the organism is only cultured from one lumen then treatment should only be given via that lumen. In older children, but not neonates or children with a major immunodeficiency, the antibiotics

can be stopped if cultures are negative after 48 h. It is usual practice in neonates and immunodeficient patients to give a full 5–7 day course of antibiotics even when the culture is negative.

PN should be continued while treating the infection unless the child develops multiorgan failure or severe cardiovascular compromise when the infusion is commenced. A "Y" connector needs to be attached to the "giving set"/infusion tubing for antibiotic administration.

Risk of septicemia is minimized by cleaning the CVC hub with 2% chlorhexidene when connecting/disconnecting [10] the CVC. Nursing practices when handling the catheter should be regularly reviewed and updated as necessary in order to minimize the risk of infection.

Liver Disease

A common and potentially life-threatening complication is IF-associated liver disease (IFALD). Major risk factors for IFALD include prematurity, lack of enteral intake, recurrent sepsis, length of time on PN treatment, over-feeding, small intestinal bacterial overgrowth, and certain components of PN [11]. Constituents of PN solutions implicated include a high carbohydrate load and the soya component of lipid. Soybean contains phytosterols that have been associated with liver disease by inhibiting bile acid secretion [12]. When affected patients have changed to pure Ω-3 fish oil-based lipid (Omegaven10%, Fresenius Kabi) infusions, severe cholestasis may resolve [13]. Use of newer mixed lipid emulsions including olive oil, MCT as well as fish oil and soybean have also been associated with less IFALD [14] Safety data using mixed lipid types have been published for premature infants and children [15].

In the neonate, cholestasis commonly develops within 2 weeks of bacterial infection; this could relate to a breakdown in the gut mucosal barrier. Enteral feeding even if less than 10% of the total energy intake is the most important factor in preventing/reversing cholestasis. Ursodeoxycholic acid may be beneficial since it reduces bile synthesis and secretion, solubilizes cholesterol, and increases bile flow. Small-bowel stasis causes bacterial overgrowth and production of the less soluble more hepatotoxic secondary bile acid lithocholate. Oral metronidazole may be used to treat the overgrowth. A deficiency of taurine, a conditionally essential amino acid, results in less of the more soluble taurine conjugated bile acids being made; this can be prevented/reversed by giving a taurine enriched feed. Copper and manganese are usually excreted in bile but become hepatotoxic in cholestatic patients.

In addition, reducing the hours of lipid infusion and the limiting lipid to alternate days appear to improve liver function [16]. See Table 47.6 below for management strategies.

Table 47.6 Management of intestinal failure-associated liver disease (IFALD)

Management of intestinal failure-associated liver disease (IFALD)
1. Treat any underlying infection
2. Introduce enteral feed at the earliest opportunity, even if only minimal amount tolerated
3. Reduce the amount of lipid infused or stop completely if patient is tolerating some enteral nutrition/unlikely to need the PN for more than a further 14 days
4. Reduce the number of lipid infusions/week
5. If totally dependent on PN will require about 0.5 g/kg/day lipid to ensure adequate essential fatty acids
6. If patient is not already on a mixed lipid emulsion change to such a solution
7. Consider reducing frequency of lipid infusions to 2–3 times/week
8. Treat small intestinal bacterial overgrowth with, e.g., metronidazole
9. Consider ursodexoycholic acid at 10 mg/kg TDS
10. Aim to cycle PN, i.e., allow a period of time free of the infusion each day if the child is stable without it

PN parenteral nutrition

CVC Occlusion and Venous Thrombosis

Central venous catheter (CVC) occlusion may occur with deposition of lipid and/or calcium and phosphate precipitates within the lumen. Obstruction may also be positional with the tip resting against the wall of a blood vessel. Occlusion may be cleared with alteplase or alcohol line lock [17]. Limiting lipid infusions helps prevent CVC occlusion related to fat deposition. High concentrations of polyunsaturated fats may impair platelet adhesion; consider reducing lipids to 1–2 g/kg/day if platelets are $<50 \times 10^9$/l.

Home Parenteral Nutrition

Children should be considered for discharge home on treatment with PN if after extensive investigation and treatment in a specialist gastroenterology referral center, it is not possible to significantly improve the underlying disease and symptoms are expected to persist for at least two further months. Every attempt should have been made to wean the child from PN using most appropriate type of feed given via the most suitable enteral route for the child, that is, oral or infused directly into the stomach or duodenum/jejunum. It is usually possible to discharge an infant home from about 4 months of age. Most infants are able to tolerate a 10-h period without PN from about 4.5 kg, although in some cases weight may need to be 6 kg.

The etiology of chronic IF requiring long-term/home PN is most commonly short bowel syndrome, usually with <30 cm small intestine remaining. Other conditions include severe intractable Crohn's disease that has failed to respond to even the most aggressive immunological treatment, congenital enteropathies, for example, microvillous atrophy and tufting enteropathy, and motility disorders including neuropathic or myopathic intestinal pseudobstruction and intestinal dysmotility. Home PN may be requested for IF secondary to other organ disease such as life-limiting severe immunodeficiency or malignancy.

Children with severe neurological impairment may develop intestinal dysmotility and hyperaesthesia as their disease progresses. Ethical issues should be addressed when considering long-term/home PN in children with other major organ failure, particularly since PN is unlikely to benefit a child who has progressive disease and will never be capable of an independent life. The aim of treatment is to relieve rather than prolong suffering and improve quality of life. Support from a palliative care team is important.

The aim of PN at home should be to incorporate the child's care into the family's lifestyle and not to have a "hospital at home." Major advantages of going home are that the family is reunited, there is a significantly lower risk of septicemia [18], the child's psychosocial environment improves and s/he can return to usual school and participate in other childhood activities including swimming. It is also possible to enjoy family holidays again.

In most cases, it would not be reasonable to expect a family to function with a child on treatment for more than 14 h. Many parents will continue to have a regular job and care for other children as well.

Organization of PN at Home

The steps that need to be taken when discharging a child home on PN are as follows:

- Nutrition team meets with the parents/carers to explain what is involved and ensure that they are prepared to go ahead with treatment at home.
- The specialist nurse needs to ensure the home is adequate with regard to space to connect and disconnect the PN and to infuse it in the bedroom, ease of access to running water and for the older child, toilet facilities, space for

a dedicated fridge, and reliable electricity supply for the infusion pump.

- Social worker should meet with parents/carers to ensure any social problems are addressed, the employer(s) are informed of need for parents to have time to train and relevant financial benefits are applied for.
- If the patient has a more local hospital that they could be admitted to in an emergency, shared care with that hospital needs to be set up.
- To plan a formal training period for the parents/carers to be taught how to administer the PN. The training is usually undertaken by the specialist nurse. It can take about 30 h to complete and may need to be spread over a 2-week period.
- The simplest possible management regime should be used, for example, a one-person aseptic non-touch technique (ANTT) in order to enable flexibility at home.
- Every effort should be made to train both parents to ensure that they are both fully aware of their child's long-term needs and a second parent is available should the main carer be unwell.
- Funding will need to be secured and a pharmacy to agree to manufacture and if possible, deliver the PN to the child's home.
- Arrangements vary from country to country. Currently, in the UK, there is a national framework for home PN with central government funding.
- Arrange a discharge meeting with all professionals who will be involved in the child's care and parents present. In the UK, the specialist pediatric gastroenterologist, local hospital pediatrician, community nurse, and specialist nutrition nurse are essential participants. The meeting will often need to be held via video-link or teleconference.

Specific Features of PN at Home

PN at home should be infused over 12–14 h overnight thus enabling the child and family to lead a normal daytime life. It is unreasonable to expect a family to have a child attached to a pump for any longer than 12 h and would be difficult for a school age child to pursue a reasonably normal lifestyle (even with a portable pump).

Every effort should be made to supply all PN requirements in a single bag for each infusion night. Most children will need two separate formulations since the lipid-containing infusion should be limited to 2 or 3 nights/week, that is, dextrose and amino acid preparation without lipid should be given on intervening nights.

The PN bag should be made up with extra volume/"overage" in case the child's requirements increase. In smaller infants, the rate of infusion should be reduced for the final hour in order to minimize the risk of rebound hypoglycemia when the infusion is stopped.

At the earliest opportunity the PN should be reduced to the minimum possible number of nights/week for the child to thrive. It is better to give a larger volume on fewer nights in order to minimize complications such as septicemia. Enteral sodium supplements maybe needed as well as adequate enteral fluid intake after a night off.

As soon as an infant can tolerate about 50 % of requirements enterally, PN can be reduced to a maximum of five nights and possibly less.

When discharged, the child should be sufficiently stable to cope with the same PN formulation being given for a week, in order to give the homecare pharmacy a reasonable time to make changes to the formulation. If changes to the PN are required more frequently, the volume should be increased/reduced. The aims should be to obtain PN stability for about 21 days for a single, individualized PN bag. All nutrients should be included in order to minimize infection and nutritional risk of adding to the bag at home. Patients need a reliable source of equipment.

A portable pump should be supplied. Unlike in hospital pressure reading is not essential.

In certain circumstances, for example, when using a commercially available standard bag the vitamins may be added at home. When patients have residual intestinal function, most vitamins (especially water soluble) can be adequately absorbed from the gastrointestinal tract. However, carers may omit enteral vitamin doses, belittling their importance and put the child at risk of thiamine deficiency exacerbated by the high PN carbohydrate infusion.

In patients unable to tolerate lipid, for example, with severe IFALD, enteral walnut oil (< 5 ml) may be tolerated. In neonates, EFA can be absorbed from the skin if sunflower or safflower oil is applied daily. Stability of PN formulation can be a major problem in children, particularly due to high calcium and phosphate requirements, two salts that readily precipitate. The pharmacy specializing in homecare should have access both to their own stability data and that available in specialist PN units elsewhere in the UK/Europe. The specialist hospital team should regularly audit the home-care service. From the patient's perspective, it is important to remain with one company, in order to establish a good relationship with the company and delivery drivers.

Complications of PN at Home

Children at home are susceptible to the same complications as children on short-term PN. Prophylactic taurolidine line locks have been associated with a significant reduction in septicemic episodes in children with recurrent infections [19]. Additional complications of long-term treatment are poor bone mineralization [20], abnormal body composition [21], gallstones, renal abnormalities, and thrombotic complications such as pulmonary emboli.

Venous thrombosis may develop in as many as 67% of children with a central feeding line at home catheter occlusion can be due to a calcium phosphate precipitate or due to fibrin or lipid. One possible mechanism is the formation of antiphospholipid antibodies and a resulting hypercoagulable state with a form of antiphospholipid syndrome. Intralipid contains phospholipids that can be immunogenic. Children with evidence of pulmonary emboli detected on radio-isotopic ventilation–perfusion scan should be treated with long-term prophylactic anticoagulant treatment [22]

Long-Term Management

Parents are expected to connect and disconnect the CVC themselves every evening and morning to minimize the risk of septicemia. Direct access to the closest hospital to the home for acute emergencies should be organized prior to discharge, for example, suspected septicemia or CVC problems such as displacement, obstruction, or exit site infection. The patient can be stabilized there and if necessary transferred to the specialist unit for care, for example, repair of a fractured CVC or radiologically guided insertion of a replacement CVC.

If a child develops recurrent episodes of septicemia, for example, >2/12 months taurolidine or alcohol line lock, should be substituted for heparin [19].

Managing home PN is both physically and psychologically demanding. Practical support should be sought ranging from, for example, doing housework during the day to the carer staying in the home overnight to help with infants by changing nappies/attending to the pump alarms.

The family should have ease of access to contact the specialist center by e-mail/phone. Review in a specialist clinic is usually only necessary on a 3-month basis when the child is stable. Growth and development should be monitored and PN adjusted as necessary. Dietetic input is essential to ensure earliest possible introduction of enteral nutrition. Laboratory investigations/monitoring are also only needed 3-monthly when stable. Appropriate investigations include blood urea, electrolytes, urine sodium, full blood count, vitamin A and E, ferritin, copper, zinc, and selenium. Vitamin D and thyroid function should be checked annually. If iodine-deficient hypothyroidism develops, sea kelp capsules can be given or betadine applied to the skin. Manganese level should be measured annually in view of risk of manganese deposition in the cerebral basal ganglia. Children aged over 5 years should have annual measurement of bone age and bone density [20].

The underlying intestinal disease predisposing the child to IF should be reviewed regularly and treatment appropri-

ately adjusted. Investigations including upper and lower intestinal endoscopy may need to be repeated annually.

Outcome

Management of PN is now so successful that a child can grow and develop normally on PN treatment throughout childhood and into adult life even when unable to tolerate little/no enteral nutrition.

In children with a primary digestive disorder, life expectancy is good with a reported 2-year survival rate of 97%, 5-year survival rate of 89%, and 10-year rate of 81% [23]. Children grow and develop normally on PN. IFALD usually improves in children discharged home.

Weaning/Withdrawing PN Treatment

Weaning a child from PN to oral/enteral nutrition can be one of the most complex aspects of management. Even with extensive investigation and assessment of intestinal function, it is only certain whether a child has adequate intestinal function by reducing the PN and increasing the enteral nutrition appropriately. Most patients have been weaned off treatment from 6 months to 3 years (mean 2.5 years) after discharge. Weaning from parenteral to enteral nutrition is gradual and usually takes place at home with good dietetic support from the specialist unit.

Transition to Adult Care

Children are now being transferred from pediatric to adult care on PN. Transition needs to be arranged on an individual basis since there are a limited number of patients on long-term care into adult life. Although issues relating to transition are the same as for other chronic conditions, transfer needs to be performed between specialist IF units with the experience and resources to ensure the child complies with the process.

The two major changes are (1) the adolescent takes on "ownership" of the condition and (2) the parent(s) relinquishes responsibility. The experienced units have the ability to provide a bespoke service for each patient with a professional (usually a specialist nurse) to provide support.

Transplant

Small intestine often with/without liver/other organ transplant may be appropriate treatment for some patients with long-term dependence on PN when complications develop.

Current indications include limited venous access, severe/progressive IFALD, life-threatening sepsis episode, and poor quality of life for the child and/or family.

Summary

A good nutritional state is a prerequisite for normal growth and development in childhood and a sense of well-being. The effects of inadequate nutrition in childhood may have lifelong consequences (poor growth and intellectual development) in addition to worsening any systemic illness. Children with even severe IF can now survive and grow and develop normally on treatment with PN with the support of a multidisciplinary professional team.

References

1. Goulet O, Jan D. Intestinal failure: causes and management in children. Curr Opin Organ Transplant. 2009;9:192–200.
2. Gowen H, Lloyd C. British Intestinal Failure Survey (BIFS): a referral registry to record and determine the outcome of childhood intestinal failure. Proc Nutr Soc. 2009;68(OCE1):E15.
3. Dudrick SJ, Wilmore DW, Vars HM, Rhoads JE. Long-term total parenteral nutrition with growth, development, and positive nitrogen balance. Surgery. 1968;64:134–42.
4. Hallberg D, Holm I, Obel AL, Schuberth O, Wretlind A. Fat emulsions for complete intravenous nutrition. Postgrad Med J. 1967;43:307–16.
5. Heird WC, Driscoll JM, Schullinger JN, Grebin B, Winters RW. Intravenous alimentation in paediatric patients. J Paediatr. 1972;80:351–72.
6. Great Ormond Street Hospital Intranet. Guidelines for parenteral nutrition; www.gosh.nhs.uk/health-professionals/clinical-guidelines/nutrition-parenteral 2013.
7. Koletzko B, Goulet O, Hunt J, Krohn K, Shamir R, Parenteral Nutrition Guidelines Working Group, European Society for Clinical Nutrition and Metabolism, European Society of Paediatric Gastroenterology, Hepatology and Nutrition (ESPGHAN), European Society of Paediatric Research (ESPR). Guidelines on paediatric parenteral nutrition of the European Society of Paediatric Gastroenterology, Hepatology and Nutrition (ESPGHAN) and the European Society for Clinical Nutrition and Metabolism (ESPEN), Supported by the European Society of Paediatric Research (ESPR). J Pediatr Gastroenterol Nutr. 2005;41 Suppl 2:S1–87.
8. Tsang RC, et al. Nutrition of the preterm infant: scientific basis and practical guidelines. 2nd ed. Cincinnati: Digital Educational Publishing; 2005.
9. NCEPOD Parenteral Nutrition: A Mixed Bag (2010) http://www.ncepod.org.uk/2010pn.htm
10. Pichler J, Soothill J, Hill S. Reduction of blood stream infections in children following a change to chlorhexidine disinfection of parenteral nutrition catheter connectors, Clin Nutr. 2014;33(1):85–9.
11. Kelly DA. Preventing parenteral nutrition liver disease. Early Hum Dev. 2010;86(11):683–7.
12. Clayton PT, Whitfield P, Iyer K. The role of phytosterols in the pathogenesis of liver complications of pediatric parenteral nutrition. Nutrition. 1998;14(1):158–64.
13. de Meijer VE, Gura KM, Meisel JA, Le HD, Puder M. Parenteral fish oil monotherapy in the management of patients with parenteral nutrition-associated liver disease. Arch Surg. 2010;145(6):547–51 (Review).
14. Pichler J, Simchowitz V, Macdonald S, Hill S. Comparison of liver function with two new/mixed intravenous lipid emulsions in children with intestinal failure. Eur J Clin Nutr. 2014;68(10):1161–7.
15. Goulet O, Antebi H, Wolf C, Talbotec C, Alcindor LG, Corriol O, et al. A new intravenous fat emulsion containing soybean oil, medium-chain triglycerides, olive oil, and fish oil: a single-center, double-blind randomized study on efficacy and safety in pediatric patients receiving home parenteral nutrition. JPEN J Parenter Enteral Nutr. 2010;34(5):485–95.
16. Pichler J, Horn V, MacDonald S, Hill S. Intestinal failure-associated-liver-disease in hospitalised children. Arch Dis Child. 2012;97(3):211–4.
17. Baskin JL, et al. Management of occlusion and thrombosis associated with long-term indwelling central venous catheters. Lancet. 2009;374:159–69.
18. Melville CA, Bisset WM, Long S, Milla PJ. Counting the cost: hospital versus home central venous catheter survival. J Hosp Infect. 1997;53:197–205.
19. Chu HP; Brind J; Tomar R, Hill S. Significant reduction in central venous catheter related bloodstream infections in children on HPN after starting treatment with taurolidine line lock. J Pediatr Gastroenterol Nutr. 2012;55(4):403–7.
20. Pichler J, Chomtho S, Fewtrell M, Macdonald S, Hill S. Growth and bone health in paediatric intestinal failure patients receiving long-term parenteral nutrition. Am J Clin Nutr. 2013;97(6):1260–9.
21. Pichler J, Chomtho S, Fewtrell M, Hill S. Body composition in paediatric intestinal failure patients receiving long-term parenteral nutrition. Arch Dis Child. 2014;99(2):147–53.
22. Pifarré P, Roca I, Irastorza I, Simó M, Hill S, Biassoni L, Gordon I. Lung ventilation-perfusion scintigraphy in children on long-term parenteral nutrition. Eur J Nucl Med Mol Imaging. 2009;36:1005–8.
23. Colomb V, Dabbas-Tyan M, Taupin P, Talbotec C, Revillon Y, Jan D, et al. Long-term outcome of children receiving home parenteral nutrition: a 20-year single-center experience in 302 patients. J Pediatr Gastroenterol Nutr. 2007;44:347–53.

Intussusception

48

Lydia O'Sullivan and Ashish P. Desai

History and Introduction

First described by Dutch physician Paul Barbette in 1674, intussusception is the full-thickness telescoping or invagination of a proximal portion of the intestine into an adjacent, more distal portion. The term derives from the Latin words "intus" ("within") and "suscipere" ("to receive"). Ladd published the first radiograph with contrast enema demonstrating intussusception in 1913. While he considered contrast enema a useful diagnostic tool, Ladd did not appreciate its therapeutic potential in reducing intussusception. Diagnosis of intussusception was later expedited with the use of ultrasound. Burke and Clarke first described the distinctive ultrasonographic pattern of intussusception, including the pathognomonic "target sign" and "pseudo kidney," in 1977 [1].

Before reduction techniques were developed and refined, infant intussusception was almost universally fatal in the early nineteenth century. Samuel Mitchell reported the first successful reduction of childhood intussusception by air enema using an enema tube and "common pair of bellows" in 1836. Hirschsprung first described controlled hydrostatic reduction in 1876. Successful reduction by hydrostatic pressure using saline or contrast solutions was reported by Hipsley in Australia in 1926 and by Retan and Stephens in America, Pouliquien in France, and Olsson in Scandinavia in 1927. Despite these reported successes, many surgeons remained skeptical of the potential benefits of hydrostatic reduction in the mid-twentieth century. Reduction by barium enema under fluoroscopy was popularized in the 1950s by Ravitch at Johns Hopkins, but has since fallen out of favor in the UK due to the risk of leakage and subsequent barium peritonitis. In 1959, Fiorito and colleagues reintroduced pneumatic reduction with pressure control, and this remains the method of choice in the UK today [1].

Although Barbette had suggested the possibility of surgical reduction in his early description of intussusception, the first successful operation for intussusception in an infant after failed hydrostatic reduction did not take place until 1873 under British surgeon Jonathan Hutchinson. As has been the way with many other surgical procedures, it is now possible to reduce intussusceptions laparoscopically. This approach is of particular use in recurrent cases to avoid repeat laparotomy and as a prelude to possible laparotomy in cases of failed conservative treatment [1].

Intussusception represents the most common cause of gastrointestinal obstruction in children aged between 3 months and 3 years [2]. It is the second most frequent acute abdominal surgical emergency in pediatrics after acute appendicitis [3]. Left untreated, intussusception can have serious, potentially life-threatening sequelae.

Pathogenesis and Natural History

The drawing up of the proximal portion of the intestine (the "intussusceptum") into the lumen of the distal portion of the intestine (the "intussuscepiens") is driven by peristalsis. As the mesentery becomes progressively incorporated into the intussusception, it is compressed, resulting first in impaired lymphatic return and, second, poor venous drainage, culminating in congestion and edema. This builds pressure on the mesenteric vasculature, eventually causing arterial compromise, infarction, ischemia and necrosis. The mucous membrane lining the lumen is highly sensitive to ischemia and therefore begins to slough off and bleed. Mucous, shed blood, and sloughed mucosa combine and are expelled as "red currant jelly stools." If the built-up pressure is not relieved, it will result in the complete obstruction of the bowel and transmural gangrene of the intussusceptum. This can produce fluid sequestration, perforation of the bowel, leakage of intestinal contents into the peritoneal cavity, and

A. P. Desai (✉) · L. O'Sullivan
Department of Pediatric Surgery, King's College Hospital, Denmark Hill, London SE5 9RS, UK
e-mail: ashishdesai@nhs.net

© Springer International Publishing Switzerland 2016
S. Guandalini et al. (eds.), *Textbook of Pediatric Gastroenterology, Hepatology and Nutrition*,
DOI 10.1007/978-3-319-17169-2_48

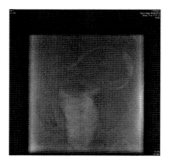

Fig. 48.1 Air enema showing intussusception up to the rectum

peritonitis [2]. If the associated mesentery is lax, the intussusceptum can be drawn up as far as the distal colon or sigmoid (Fig. 48.1) and eventually prolapse through the anus. The later intussusception presents, the more manifest the natural history of the disease will become. Timely diagnosis and management is therefore extremely important.

Spontaneous reduction is another possible outcome and reportedly occurs in almost 20 % of intussusceptions [4].

Etiology

The pathogenesis of intussusception is possibly caused by an imbalance in the longitudinal forces acting along the intestinal wall.

The majority of intussusceptions (~95 %) are idiopathic as no obvious etiology can be identified. In these so-called idiopathic cases, it is thought that Peyer's patches, hypertrophied in response to a respiratory or gastrointestinal infection, function as a lead point. Peyer's patches are oval masses of aggregated lymphoid follicles on the mucous membrane lining the small intestine. Peyer's patches are distributed irregularly along the anti-mesenteric wall, becoming more numerous and forming a lymphoid ring in the distal ileum. These structures have been labeled the "immune sensors of the intestine' owing to their role in "sampling" the contents of the gut lumen, taking up antigens and microorganisms and, if appropriate, stimulating a protective mucosal immune response [5]. This probably explains why an antecedent viral infection is present in as many as 20 % of intussusceptions. Specifically, adenovirus [6], cytomegalovirus, and live rotavirus vaccines [7] have been variably associated with intussusception. Bacterial enteritis involving, for example, *Salmonella, E. coli, Shigella,* and *Campylobacter,* also increases the risk of intussusception in children [8].

This imbalance may be caused by a mass protruding into the intestinal lumen, which represents a "lead point" upon which peristalsis acts in an attempt to clear it as if it were a bolus of food. A pathological lead point has been defined as "a recognizable intraperitoneal anomaly or abnormality

that tethers or obstructs the bowel, initiating the process of intussusception" [4]. Pathological lead points are identified in 2–12 % of intussusceptions. While a lead point is rarely identified in patients <2 years, 20 % of patients >2 years are found to have a lead point [2]. Pathological lead points are more commonly identified in ileoileal or colocolic intussusceptions.

Meckel's diverticulum [9], benign and malignant intestinal or mesenteric tumors including lipomas [10], lymphomas [11], and polyps associated with Peutz–Jeghers syndrome [12], duplication cysts [13, 14], intestinal abnormalities associated with cystic fibrosis (e.g., hypertrophied mucosal glands or thickened feces) [15], hematomas secondary to abdominal trauma [16] or—Henoch–Schönlein purpura and other vascular/coagulation disorders [17], foreign bodies [18], intestinal hemangiomas [19], Kaposi sarcoma [20], abnormalities associated with posttransplantation lymphoproliferative disorder [21], and anastomotic sutures and staples and indwelling tubes [22] have all been reported as providing pathological lead points.

A small percentage of intussusceptions (typically ileoileal) arise postoperatively, usually after laparotomy with extensive bowel manipulation, although it has been reported following other abdominal and non-abdominal procedures. The precise mechanism underlying postoperative intussusception is unknown, but disorganized peristalsis, early postoperative adhesions, electrolyte disturbances, anesthetic drugs, and/or neurogenic factors may be implicated [23].

Epidemiology

In the UK, the reported incidence of intussusception stands at around 1.6–4 cases per 1000 live births [2]. Males are affected more frequently than females, with an incidence ratio of 3:2. The male preponderance becomes more evident after 9 months of age.

Ninety percent of intussusceptions will occur within the first 3 years of life, 65 % of cases arising within the first year of life and 50 % between 3 and 10 months [2]. Incidence peaks between 5 and 7 months [24]. Intussusception in utero is rarely reported [25, 26], and perinatal intussusception in newborns accounts for only 0.3 % of all cases. Several reasons for the increase in incidence from around 3 months of age have been advanced, including changes in feeding practices that affect the gut, maturation of lymphoid tissue, fattening of the mesentery which increases the likelihood of it becoming trapped, or a decline in the protection afforded by maternal antibodies against microorganisms that might precipitate intussusception [2, 27].

Adult intussusception is rare, representing around 5 % of all cases. Unlike in the pediatric population, where intussusception is the most common cause of acute intestinal obstruction and is usually idiopathic, intussusception only accounts for 1–5% of cases of intestinal obstruction in adults, often presents atypically and subacutely [28], and it is attributable to a pathological process in 90% of cases. A more definitive, surgical approach (often resection) is warranted when managing adult intussusception compared to pediatric intussusception, due to the significant risk of associated malignancy (~65% cases) [29] and high risk of perforation and leakage of microorganisms [30].

Evidence suggests that the relative risk of intussusception may vary according to race or ethnicity. For example, in their review of pediatric hospitalization data in the USA between 1993 and 2004, Tate et al. [31] found that in infants over 16 weeks of age, non-Hispanic black and Hispanic infants had higher rates of hospitalization for intussusception compared with non-Hispanic white infants. In line with the USA findings, research from the UK and Republic of Ireland suggests that Black Caribbean and African infants have higher incidence rates of intussusception than in White British and Asian groups [27]. Justice et al. [32] and Webby et al. [33] have identified a lower risk of intussusception among indigenous Australian children compared to nonindigenous children. However, as these studies rely on data gathered from hospitals, the differences they identify may reflect differences in admission and access rather than any actual ethnic variation in intussusception incidence [34].

Incidence of intussusception is also thought to vary by geographic region. Compared to other regions, it has been observed that incidence is higher than average in populations in Australia, Hong Kong, Vietnam, South Korea, and Japan and lower than average in populations in Finland, India, Malaysia, and Bangladesh [24, 35]. However, data upon which the assertion of geographic variability is based is problematic [27].

Finally, it is suggested that incidence of intussusception varies by season. Incidence has been found to peak during winter (Dec–Feb) and spring (March–May) in the UK and Republic of Ireland [27], although no such trend has been demonstrated in studies in equatorial regions [36] or indeed in those performed on a global scale [24]. Absence of any significant seasonal variation in incidence of intussusception goes against there being any strong association between intussusception and natural rotavirus, which has a highly seasonal pattern [37].

Classification

Intussusception is classified anatomically, with the proximal portion of the intestine (the "intussusceptum") first, followed by the more distal portion (the "intussuscepiens"). The majority of intussusceptions (~80%) involve the terminal ileum telescoping into the cecum or ascending colon and are thus termed ileocecal or ileocolic intussusceptions. Less frequently, segments of ileum invaginate into ileum (ileoileal) or segments of colon invaginate into colon (colocolic) or a combination arises (ileo-ileo-colic).

Clinical Presentation

Sudden onset of severe, colicky abdominal pain is the most common presenting feature of intussusception [38], present in around 85% of cases [39]. Infants will typically present with episodes of inconsolable crying while drawing up their legs in conjunction with spasms of peristalsis. These episodes occur every 10–15 min and last around 2–3 min. The pain becomes more constant after around 12 h. Between episodes, the infant may appear normal or increasingly pale, clammy, quiet, and lethargic. It is hypothesized that lethargy may be induced by the release of endogenous opioids or endotoxins from the ischemic bowel [40].

Vomiting (non-bilious, undigested gastric contents becoming bilious) can be an early indication of intestinal obstruction. Evacuation of small, loose stools from the colon distal to the obstruction will occur early in the course of the disease in some patients. Around 50% of patients pass "red currant jelly" stool [39]. Overall, 1/3 patients will have the classic triad of abdominal pain, vomiting, and bloody stool [2].

The combination of reduced fluid intake, increased fluid loss through vomiting, anticipated losses into the obstructed bowel, and perhaps some reactive vasodilation can culminate in dehydration and hypovolemic shock. If the bowel perforates resulting in bacteremia, the child will become febrile, tachycardic, and hypotensive.

Examination can be unremarkable in between "attacks." A "sausage-shaped" mass is palpable in around 65% of cases, usually in the right upper quadrant extending to the left along the line of the transverse colon (Fig. 48.2). The mass can be tender and is sometimes seen on clinical inspection. It can become harder to detect this mass as the disease progresses and the abdomen distends [39]. The right lower quadrant can become flat or empty due to the absence of bowel ("Dance" sign). In around 5% of cases, the apex of the intussusceptum

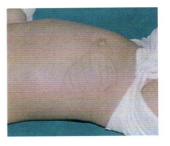

Fig. 48.2 Typical right abdominal mass

Table 48.1 Features of intussusception [39]

Differential diagnosis	Supporting	Excluding
Infantile colic due to wind in the intestine associated with feeding difficulties	Common in first 3 months	Rarely lasts 1 h Usually no vomiting
Gastroenteritis	Severe cases can present with colic and passage of blood and mucus	Greater volume of diarrhea
Strangulated inguinal hernia	Abdominal pain and distension Vomiting	On examination - irreducible lump in the groin

can be palpated on rectal examination. It rarely prolapses out of the anus.

Differential Diagnosis

Conditions that mimic features of intussusception are shown below. These differential diagnoses should be excluded on the basis of careful history taking and examination (Table 48.1).

Investigation

Diagnostic work up of a patient with clinically suspected intussusception might include a plain abdominal radiograph, abdominal ultrasound, contrast enema, and CT scan. Laboratory tests are not specifically diagnostic but may show leukocytosis, acidosis, and electrolyte disturbance associated with bowel ischemia.

A plain radiograph is usually only performed if the diagnosis on presentation is unclear [3]. Suggestive signs of intussusception on a plain radiograph include an elongated soft tissue mass typically in the right upper quadrant, abnormal distribution of gas and fecal contents, dilated bowel loops, no gas in the transverse or descending colon, and air–fluid levels in the presence of bowel obstruction. Although plain radiographs can aid diagnosis of intussusception, they may appear normal in the early stages and they lack sensitivity (i.e., high incidence of false positives) [41].

Ultrasonography is an extremely effective imaging modality for diagnosing intussusception. It has a sensitivity over 98 % and a specificity of 100 % when diagnosing ileocolic or colocolic intussusceptions. These parameters are slightly reduced for ileoileal intussusceptions [2]. The "doughnut" or "target" sign on transverse section (concentric rings created by the telescoping bowel) and a "pseudo-kidney" (bowel wall and mesentery mimic renal structures) are characteristic signs of intussusception on ultrasound [2].

If the diagnosis is still in doubt, a contrast enema is the gold standard for diagnosing intussusception. Barium or (more commonly) air is introduced via a catheter inserted into the rectum. When the contrast substance enters the lumen of the intussusceptum and the intraluminal space, this creates the "coiled-spring" sign. This test is contraindicated if there is evidence of perforation on plain radiograph. Enemas can be therapeutic as well as diagnostic [41].

Finally, CT scans are more commonly used in adults with suspected intussusception. Transversely, concentric rings of telescoping bowel will form the equivalent of an ultrasonographic "target" sign. Longitudinally, a soft tissue sausage-shaped mass may be observed. Hyper-dense rings at the proximal end of the intussusception formed by the intussusceptum and the folded edge of the intussuscipiens might also be visualized. Occasionally, a lead point may be picked up on CT [41].

Management

Initial management focuses on stabilizing the child. This includes fluid resuscitation using normal saline—20 mL/kg intravenous (IV) bolus to start. Nasogastric (NG) tube should be placed. It should be regularly aspirated and free draining. Prophylactic broad-spectrum antibiotics (e.g., cefuroxime and metronidazole) should be administered.

Focus then shifts to reducing the intussusception nonsurgically or surgically. The majority of cases of intussusception are reduced nonsurgically with sustained intra-colonic pressure delivered by enema using various different substances [42]. Some centers have reported successful reduction of intussusceptions with saline [43].

A catheter, often with an inflatable balloon and attached pressure gauge, is inserted into the rectum, and the child's buttocks are held together to create a tight seal. Air is then passed through the catheter at carefully monitored pressures up to 120 mmHg. Up to three attempts at reduction can be made, each lasting up to 3 min [2]. If the first three attempts fail but the child is clinically well, the air enema can be repeated after 4–6 h (Fig. 48.3a, b). A radiologist usually performs the procedure, but a surgeon must be present in case complications arise, the most serious of which is an acute tension pneumoperitoneum. This compromises venous return from the lower body and causes cardiovascular collapse. Decompression of the abdominal cavity is achieved by inserting a large-bore cannula into the peritoneum. A total

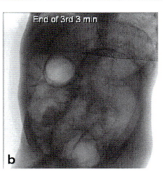

Fig. 48.3 a Ileocolic intussusception. **b** Same patient as **a**: After three attempts at reduction

of 75–90 % of intussusceptions are successfully reduced by air enema [2].

In the remaining cases, laparotomy can be performed. A transverse incision is made in the right lower quadrant, although occasionally can be transumbilical or in the right upper quadrant. Once the intussusception is located and delivered through the incision, the intussuscipiens is gently squeezed or milked so that the intussusceptum is pushed distally and the telescoping is reduced (Fig. 48.4). The reduced bowel should be carefully examined for signs of ischemic damage and signs of a pathological lead point. Resection with anastomosis may be necessitated by presence of nonviable ischemic bowel or an obvious lead point after manual reduction. Indications for laparotomy include perforation, peritonism, and unsuccessful nonsurgical reduction. Many centers will bypass attempts at nonsurgical reduction in atypical cases or if intussusception is recurrent or related to a pathological lead point [2].

Minimally invasive laparoscopic surgery is becoming increasingly popular for reduction of intussusception [44]. Gentle pressure is applied distally using atraumatic graspers inserted through the ports. A recent systematic review reported a 71 % success rate for laparoscopic reduction of intussusception [44]. Compared to open reduction, laparoscopic reductions are associated with shorter operating times, shorter time to first postoperative feed, reduced use of IV narcotics, and earlier discharge [45]. It has therefore been suggested that tertiary centers with adequate facilities should use laparoscopy as the primary surgical approach to reduc-

ing intussusceptions. The major disadvantage to using laparoscopy is that it reduces a surgeon's tactile acuity, meaning that extra care should be taken to search for pathological lead points.

Complications and Prognosis

Complications of pneumatic reduction include perforation causing tension pneumothorax and failure to reduce the intussusception.

Complications associated with surgical reduction of intussusception include perforation, systemic infection (e.g., sepsis and meningitis), bleeding, wound infection, leak or breakdown of an anastomosis, incisional hernia, adhesions, and bowel obstruction [4]. Resection rarely has any long-term consequences, although removal of the ileocecal valve may cause increased stool frequency [2].

Recurrence of intussusception following reduction is not uncommon. Recurrence usually arises within 2–3 days of the first reduction (~60 % within 6 months), presents early, and is treated in the same way as the initial episode. Recurrence is more likely in the presence of a pathological lead point.

Death is a rare outcome, usually associated with late presentation. Prognosis varies globally as diagnosis and treatment usually occur earlier in developed countries compared to the developing world [36].

Conclusion

Intussusception is a common emergency in pediatric surgery, which must be diagnosed and managed swiftly to avoid life-threatening complications. It should be suspected in children presenting between 3 months and 3 years with colicky abdominal pain, vomiting, and bloody stools and reduced as soon as possible to avoid irreversible ischemic damage to the bowel. Therapeutic pneumatic air enema forms the main form of treatment modality. Surgical reduction of intussusceptions, when required, is becoming less invasive.

References

1. Davis CF, McCabe AJ, Raine PAM. The ins and outs of intussusception: history and management over the past fifty years. J Paediatr Surg. 2003;38 (Suppl 7):60–4.
2. R obb A, Lander A. Intussusception in infants and young children. Surgery 2008;26(7):291–3.
3. Saliakellis E, Borrelli O, Thapar N. Paediatric GI emergencies. Best Pract Res Clin Gastroenterol. 2013;27(5):799–817.
4. Morrison SC, Stork E. Documentation of spontaneous reduction of childhood intussusception by ultrasound. Paediatr Radiol. 1990;20(5):358–9.

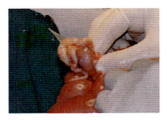

Fig. 48.4 Intraoperative picture of manual reduction

5. Jung C, Hugot J, Barreau F. Payer's patches: the immune sensors of the intestine. Int J Inflam. 2010;2010:823710. (published online 19/09/2010).

6. Bines JE, Liem NT, Justice FA, Son TN, Kirkwood CD, de Campo M, et al. Risk factors for intussusception in infants in Vietnam and Australia: adenovirus implicated, but not rotavirus. J Paediatr. 2006;149(4):452.

7. Patel MM, Haber P, Baggs J, Zuber P, Bines JE, Parashar UD. Intussusception and rotavirus vaccination: a review of the available evidence. Expert Rev Vaccines. 2009;8(11):1555–64.

8. Nyland CM, Denson LA, Noel JM. Bacterial enteritis as a risk factor for childhood intussusception: a retrospective cohort study. J Paediatr. 156(5):761.

9. Milbrandt K, Sigalet D. Intussusception associated with a Meckel's diverticulum and a duplication cyst. J Paediatr Surg. 2008;43(12):e21–3.

10. Howard N, Pranesh N, Carter P. Colo-colonic intussusception secondary to a lipoma, Int. J Surg Case Rep. 2012;3(2):52–4.

11. Brichon P, Bertrand Y, Plantaz D. Burkitt's lymphoma revealed by acute intussusception in children. Ann Chir. 2001;126(7):649–53.

12. Sasaki T, Fukumori D, Sato M, Sakai K, Ohmori H, Yamamato F. Peutz–Jeghers syndrome associated with intestinal intussusception: a case report. Int Surg. 2002;87(4):256–9.

13. Verma S, Bawa M, Rao K et al. BMJ Case Rep. 2013. doi:10.1136/bcr-2012-008056.

14. Deigaard SB, Trap R. Intestinal duplication—an important differential diagnosis to intussusception. Ugeskr Laeger. 2008;170(35):2708.

15. Nash EF, Stephenson A, Helm EJ, Ho T, Thippanna CM, Ali A, et al. Intussusception in adults with cystic fibrosis: a case series with review of the literature. Dig Dis Sci. 2011;56(12):3695–700.

16. Lu S, Goh P. Traumatic intussusception with intramural haematoma. Paediatr Radiol. 2009;39(4):403–5.

17. Chang WL, Yang YH, Lin YT, Chiang BL. Gastrointestinal manifestations in Henoch–Schonlein purpura: a review of 261 patients. Acta Paediatr. 2004;93(11):1427–31.

18. Dalshaug GB, Wainer S, Hollaar GL. The Rapunzel syndrome (Trichobezoar) causing atypical intussusception in a child: a case report. J Paediatr Surg. 1999;34(3):479–80.

19. Guthrie SO, Rhodes M, Janco R, Stein, SM, Jabs K, Engelhardt B. An infant with Kasabach–Merritt syndrome with associated renal haematoma and intussusception. J Perinatol. 2005;25:143–5.

20. Ramdial PK, Sing Y, Hadley GP, Chotey NA, Mahlakwane MS, Singh B. Paediatric intussusception caused by acquired immunodeficiency syndrome-associated Kaposi sarcoma. Paediatr Surg Int. 2010;26(8):783–87.

21. Earl TM, Wellen JR, Anderson CD, Nadler M, Doyle MM, Shenoy SS, et al. Small bowel obstruction after paediatric liver transplantation: the unusual is the usual. J Am Coll Surg. 2011;212(1):62–7.

22. Furuya Y, Wakahara T, Akimoto H, Long CM, Yanagie H, Yasuhara H. A case of postoperative recurrent intussusception associated with indwelling bowel tube. World J Gastrointest Surg. 2010;2(3):85–8.

23. Yang G, Wang X, Jiang W, Ma J, Zhao J, Liu W. Postoperative intussusception in children and infants: a systematic review. Paediatr Surg Int. 29:1273–9.

24. Jiang J, Jiang B, Parashar U, Nguyen T, Bines J, Patel MM. Childhood intussusception: a literature review. PLoS One. 2013;8(7):e68482.

25. Nguyen DT, Lai E, Cunningham T, and Moore TC. In utero intussusception producing ileal atresia and meconium peritonitis with and without free air. Paediatr Surg Int. 1995;10(5–6):406–8.

26. Huebner BR, Azarow KS, Cusick RA. Intestinal atresia due to intrauterine intussusception of a Meckel's diverticulum. J Paediatr Surg Case Rep. 2013;1(8):232–4.

27. Samad L, Cortina-Borja M, El Bashir H, Sutcliffe AG, Marven S, Cameron JC, et al. Intussusception incidence among infants in the UK and Republic of Ireland: a pre- rotavirus vaccine prospective surveillance study. Vaccine 2013;31(38):4098–102.

28. Wong KB, Lui CT, Fung HT. How do adult and paediatric intussusceptions differ? A 10-year retrospective study. Hong Kong J Emerg Med. 2012;19(4).

29. Marinis A, Yiallourou A, Samanides L, Dafnios N, Anastasopoulos G, Vassiliou J, et al. Intussusception of the bowel in adults: a review. World J Gastroenterol. 2009;15(4):407–11.

30. Erkan N, Haciyanli M, Yildirim M, Sayhan H, Vardar E, Polat AF. Intussusception in adults: an unusual and challenging condition for surgeons. Int J Colorectal Dis. 2005;20(5):452.

31. Tate JE, Simonsen L, Viboud C, Steiner C, Patel MM, Curns AT, et al. Trends in intussusception hospitalizations among US infants, 1993–2004: implications for monitoring the safety of the new rotavirus vaccination program. Pediatrics 2008;121(5):e1125–32.

32. Justice F, Carlin J, Bines J. Changing epidemiology of intussusception in Australia. J Paediatr Child Health. 2005;41(9–10):475–8.

33. Webby RJ, Bines J, Barnes GL, Tindall H, Krause V, Patel M. Intussusception in the Northern Territory: the incidence is low in Aboriginal and Torres Strait Islander children. J Paediatr Child Health. 2006;42(5):235–9.

34. http://whqlibdoc.who.int/hq/2002/WHO_V & B_02.19.pdf. Accessed 12 Dec 2013.

35. Takeuchi M, Osamura T, Yasunaga H, Horiguchi H, Hashimoto H, Matsuda S. Intussusception among Japanese children: an epidemiologic study using an administrative database. BMC Pediatr. 2012;12:36.

36. Boudville IC, Phua KB, Quak SH, Lee BW, Han HH, Verstraeten T, et al. The epidemiology of paediatric intussusception in Singapore: 1997–2004. Ann Acad Med Singapore. 2006;35(10):674–9.

37. Rennels MB, Parashar UD, Homlam RC, Le CT, Chang HG, Glass RI. Lack of an apparent association between intussusception and wild or vaccine rotavirus infection. Pediatr Infect Dis J. 1998;17:924–5.

38. Mandeville K, Chien M, Willyerd FA, Mandell G, Hostetler MA, Bulloch B. Intussusception: clinical presentations and imaging characteristics. Pediatr Emerg Care. 2012;28(9):842–4.

39. Hutson JM, O'Brien M, Woodward AA, Beasley SW, editors. Jones' clinical paediatric surgery. 6th ed. Oxford: Blackwell; 2008.

40. http://www.hawaii.edu/medicine/pediatrics/pedtext/s10c04.html. Accessed 12 Dec 2013.

41. Byrne AT, Geoghegan T, Govender P, Lyburn ID, Colhoun E, Torreggiani WC. The imaging of intussusception. Clin Radiol. 2005;60(1):39–46.

42. Shehata S, El Kholi N, Sultan A, El Sahwi E. Hydrostatic reduction of intussusception: barium, air, or saline. Pediatr Surg Int. 2000;16(5–6):380–2.

43. Nayak D, Jagdish S. Ultrasound guided hydrostatic reduction of intussusception in children by saline enema: our experience. Indian J Surg. 2008;70(1):8–13.

44. Apelt N, Featherstone N, Giuliani S. Laparoscopic treatment of intussusception in children: a systematic review. J Paediatr Surg. 2013;48(8):1789–93.

45. Hill SJ, Koontz CS, Langness SM, Wulkan ML. Laparoscopic versus open reduction of intussusception in children: experience over a decade. J Laproendosc Adv Surg Tech. 2013;23(2):166–9.

Meckel's Diverticulum

Ashish P. Desai

Introduction and History

Meckel's diverticulum (MD) is one of the commonest diverticulum in human beings. It occurs in 2% of the population. As Charles Mayo described—"Meckel's diverticulum is frequently suspected, often looked for, and seldom found".

Heladnus first described it in 1598 [1]. Ruysch and Levater described the diverticulum much before Meckel's description [2]. However, Johann Friedrich Meckel described the diverticulum in detail in 1809 and is credited with the first detailed description [3].

In 1962, Harper et al. suggested that as 99mTc pertechnetate is concentrated by gastric mucosa, the MD containing the gastric mucosa should be identifiable scintigraphically using 99mTc pertechnetate [4]. However, most MD may be identified intra-operatively due to its varying presentation of intestinal obstruction caused by either band with volvulus or intussusception, umbilical discharge and diverticulitis.

Embryology

During the first few weeks of gestation, primitive yolk sac divides into primitive midgut and yolk sac. Omphalo-mesenteric duct or vitello-intestinal duct connects the two. This structure usually regresses between 5th and 7th week of intrauterine life. Failure of regression leads to various presentations of patent vitello-intestinal duct (VI duct). Persistence of the tube proximally causes MD.

Incidence

MD is usually described by rule of 2. Common dictum is that it is present in around 2% of the population. It is 2 in. long and found around 2 ft from the Ileo-caecal (I/C) valve. It may contain two types of heterotopic mucosa—gastric or pancreatic.

However, these are more generalisations than fact. Incidence of symptomatic MD is thought to be around 4% in the first 3 years of life. Following that, the incidence decreases. Prevalence of MD during postnatal autopsies is 1.23% [5].

Associated Anomalies

MD is usually an isolated condition. However, patients with Hirschsprung's disease, Down syndrome, oesophageal atresia, duodenal atresia, malrotation and congenital cardiac abnormalities show increased incidence [6].

Gross and Microscopic Anatomy

MD arises on the anti-mesenteric border of the ileum. Its distance from I/C valve is variable and is thought to be anywhere from 30 to 120 cm. Hence, during surgery, it is advisable to inspect at least 150 cm of terminal ileum. It has its own blood supply from persistent vitelline artery which is a branch of superior mesenteric artery.

On histology, it usually resembles the ileum. As it is a true diverticulum, it contains all layers of a normal intestine, that is, mucosa, submucosa, muscularis propria and serosa. However, it may contain heterotopic mucosa—either gastric or pancreatic tissue. Incidence of gastric mucosa occurs in around 9% of the patients. Pancreatic mucosa is seen in 2.5% of patients [7]. Various studies have also showed presence of carcinoid, lipoma, leiomyoma or enterolith.

A. P. Desai (✉)
Department of Pediatric Surgery, King's College Hospital, Denmark Hill, London SE5 9RS, UK
e-mail: ashishdesai@nhs.net

© Springer International Publishing Switzerland 2016
S. Guandalini et al. (eds.), *Textbook of Pediatric Gastroenterology, Hepatology and Nutrition*,
DOI 10.1007/978-3-319-17169-2_49

Variations of Patent VI Duct Anomalies

VI duct anomalies occur due to variation of persistence of VI duct remnant and its attachment to the umbilicus.

Various anomalies are

1. MD—persistent proximal part of the VI duct
2. Isolated fibrous band—persistent remnant of whole VI duct
3. Omphalo-mesenteric fistula—presents as stoma at the umbilicus [8] or prolapse through the umbilicus [9]
4. Enterocyst—persistent middle part of the fistula.
5. Meckel's diverticulum may also have attached fibrous band.

Clinical Features

Most MDs are asymptomatic throughout life. In symptomatic cases, presentation varies with age.

Neonatal

In neonates, the presentation is usually due to persistent VI duct presenting as either a discharging sinus at the umbilicus [8] or a prolapsing VI duct remnant [10, 11]. Other presentations may be due to a band with associated volvulus causing partial or complete obstruction. Perforation is rare.

Pediatric Age Group

In pediatric age group, presentation varies between gastrointestinal (GI) bleeding, Intestinal obstruction and inflammation.

GI Bleeding

GI bleeding is the commonest presentation in children below 2 years of age. It is usually the major lower GI bleed, which is painless or associated with minimal pain. The bleeding is associated with gastric heterotopia in majority of cases [12]. Bleeding is due to peptic ulcer in the surrounding normal ileal tissue.

In cases where the gastric mucosa is absent, bleeding is usually attributable to other causes like intussusception or gastritis.

Management of major GI bleed should include—assessment of hemodynamic stability, differentiation between upper and lower GI bleeding and then to determine the diagnosis and site of the bleeding.

In children suspected to have MD, after adequate fluid resuscitation, they should be started on H2 blockers like raniti-

dine or famotidine. Currently, proton pump inhibitors like omeprazole or lansoprazole are routinely used. Once bleeding is controlled, 99 m technetium-pertechnetate scan should be done to look for the diagnosis of MD. If diagnosed, they should be resected.

Diverticulitis

Inflammation of the MD may be the presenting sign in 10–20% of children. Children are usually older. They are often mistaken as acute appendicitis. During surgery, inflamed MD is identified and should be excised.

Obstruction

Obstruction is a common presentation in children as well as adults. Obstruction could be due to multiple reasons like volvulus around the MD with fibrous band, intussusception [13], enterolith or incarceration in Littre's hernia [14] or within umbilical hernia [15].

Other Presentations

Other rare presentations can be due to development of bezoar in the diverticulum [16] or malignancy. The commonest tumour affecting the MD is carcinoid tumour [17, 18]. However, villous adenoma [19] or GI stromal tumour [20] has also been reported.

Investigations

As MD has very varied presentation, it is not always possible to diagnose it prior to surgery. The surgeon needs to have high index of suspicion.

However, the investigations, which might raise the possibility of MD, are as follows:

1. *Plain X-ray abdomen*: Plain X-ray may show evidence of intestinal obstruction. If enterolith is preset, it may be visible. If MD has perforated, pneumoperitoneum may be visible.
2. *GI Contrast study*: It is unusual to identify MD by barium meal. However, It may be visible in 0.7% cases by small bowel enema.
3. *Fistulogram*: Patent VI duct may be identified by fistulogram from umbilical fistula.
4. *Angiography*: In adults and older children, bleeding MD may be identified by selective superior mesenteric artery angiography. If the patient is very unstable, it may be possible to temporarily occlude the bleeder by embolising the vessel. However, the patient should have laparotomy as soon as he is stabilised as embolisation may lead to gangrene and perforation of MD in a few hours' span.
5. *Scintigraphy*: Harden demonstrated that technitium99m was concentrated in the gastric mucosa. Hence, it can

demonstrate the presence of heterotopic gastric mucosa in MD when present. The isotope is selectively taken into gastric, salivary and thyroid tissue. It is excreted in urine. Hence, sometimes, false-negative scans may be reported if the diverticulum is overlapped by urinary bladder. Sensitivity of the scan can be increased by using either pentagastrin or glycogen [21]. Scan has specificity of more than 95 % and sensitivity of more than 85 %.

Surgical Technique

Resection of the diverticulum is the final aim. Whole diverticulum with heterotopic mucosa, if present, should be excised. After the excision, the bowel needs to be anastomosed without causing luminal obstruction. This can be achieved either by diverticulectomy alone if the base is narrow or by resection of the ileum containing the diverticulum with end-to-end anastomosis.

Decision about diverticulectomy or segmental resection is usually on individual surgeons. MD Resection Index (MDRI) has been proposed which calculates the index using the length and width of the diverticulum [22].

This procedure was routinely performed by laparotomy but, with changing practice, laparoscopy is playing an increasing role. During diagnostic laparoscopy performed whether for GI bleeding or acute appendicitis, routine examination of the terminal ileum should be carried out for at least 150 cm from the I/C valve to look for MD. Surgeon should start inspecting the ileum systemically from I/C valve. Two bowel graspers at anti-mesenteric border should grasp intestinal loops, and both sides should be examined. When MD is identified, it can either be excised in situ or the same can be delivered outside the abdominal cavity and the resection and anastomosis performed. The intestine can then be reposited inside.

With advances in the minimal access techniques, now the same can be performed either using single-port technique [23] or natural orifice trans-luminal surgery (NOTES) [24].

Outcome/Conclusion

Meckel's diverticulectomy has low morbidity and mortality. However, its first presentation may be at any age and is varied with obstruction, diverticulitis, haemorrhage or neoplasm [25]. Hence, the clinician needs to show high degree of suspicion and look out for this. It is seldom found easily, and early diagnosis and proper treatment is essential to manage its varied clinical symptoms. Surgical or laparoscopic techniques have developed over time, and today laparoscopy has found its increasing use in the management of MD.

References

1. Januja RM, Schultka R, Goebbel L, Pait TG, Shields CB. The legacy of Johann Friedrich Meckel the Elder (1724–1774): a 4-generation dynasty of anatomists. Neurosurgery 2010;66:758–71.
2. Moses WR. Meckel's diverticulum—report of two unusual cases. N Engl J Med. 1947;237:118–22.
3. Soltero M, Bill AH. The natural history of Meckel's diverticulum and its relation to incidental removal. Am J Surg. 1976;132:168–73.
4. Harper PV, Andros G, Lathop K. Preliminary observations on the use of six-hour 99mTc as a tracer in biology and medicine. Semiannual Rep Argonne Cancer Res Hosp. 1962;18:76.
5. Zani A, Eaton S, Rees CM, Pierro A. Incidentally detected Meckel diverticulum to resect or not to resect? Ann Surg. 2008;247(2):276–81.
6. Snyder CL. Current management of umbilical abnormalities and related anomalies. Semin Pediatr Surg. 2007;16:41–9.
7. Yamaguchi M, Takeuchi S, Awazu S. Meckel's diverticulum. Investigations of 600 patients in Japanese literature. Am J Surg. 1978;136(2):247–9.
8. Kuti K, Paul A, Desai AP. Stoma that appeared from nowhere. Arch Dis Child Fetal Neonatal Ed. 2012;97:f284.
9. Pauleau G, Commandeur D, Andro C, Chapelier X. Intestinal prolapse through a persistent omphalomesenteric duct causing small-bowel obstruction. S Afr J Surg. 2012;50(3):102–3.
10. Patel RV, Hemant Kumar, Sinha CK, Patricolo M. Neonatal prolapsed patent vitellointestinal duct. BMJ Case Rep Online. 2013;2013. doi:10.1136/bcr-2013–010221.
11. Agrawal S, Memon S. Patent vitellointestinal duct. BMJ Case Rep. 2010:doi:10.1136/bcr.12.2009.2594.
12. Tsang A, Bandi YW, Tan T. Correlation of gastric heterotopia and Meckel's diverticular bleeding in children: a unique association. Pediatr Surg Int. 2014;30:313–6.
13. Beasley SW, Auldist AW, Stokes KB. Recurrent Intussusception: barium or surgery? Aust N Z J Surg. 1987;57(1):11–3.
14. Truro FJ, Aburahma A. Meckel's diverticulum in a femoral hernia: a Littre's hernia. South Med J. 1987;80(5):655–6.
15. Chirdan LB, Uba AF, Kidmas AT. Incarcerated umbilical hernia in children. Eur J Pediatr Surg. 2006;16(1):45–8.
16. Fagenholz PJ, de Moya MA. Laparoscopic treatment of bowel obstruction due to bezoar in a Meckel's diverticulum. JSLS. 2011;15(4):562–4.
17. Boland BM, Collins CG, Christiansen E, O'Brien A, Duignan J. Three synchronous gastrointestinal tumours. Ir J Med Sci. 2011;180(4):897–900.
18. Neis C, Ziekel A, Hasse C, Ruschoff J. Carcinoid tumors of Meckel's diverticula. Dis Colon Rectum. 1992;35(6):589–96.
19. Minimo C, Talerman A. Vilous adenoma arising in Meckel's diverticulum. J Clin Pathol. 1998;51(6):485–6.
20. Chandramohan K, Agarwal M, Gurjar G, Gutti RC, Patel MH, Trivedi P, Kothari KC. Gastrointestinal stromal tumour in Meckel's diverticulum. World J Surg Oncol. 2007;12(5):50.
21. Malik AA, Shams-ul-Bari, Wani KA, Khaja AR. Meckel's diverticulum—revisited. Saudi J Gastroenterol. 2010;16(1):3–7.
22. Karabulut R, Turkylmaz Z, Demirogullari B, Ozen IO, Can Basaklar A, Kale N. A new index for resection of Meckel diverticula in children. Scand J Gastroenterol. 2004;39:789–90.
23. Tam YH, Chan KW, Wong YS, Houben CH, Pang KK, Tsui SY, Mou JW, LeeMou KH. Single-incision laparoscopic surgery in diagnosis and treatment for gastrointestinal bleeding of obscure origin in children. Surg Laparosc Endosc Percutan Tech. 2013;23(3):106–8.
24. Knuth J, Heiss MM, Bulian DR. Transvaginal hybrid-NOTES appendectomy in routine use: prospective analysis of 13 cases and description of the procedure. Surg Endosc. 2014;28(9):2661–5.
25. Dumper J, Mackenzie S, Mitchell P, et al. Complications of Meckel's diverticulum in adults. Can J Surg. 2006;49(5):353–7.

Acute Appendicitis

50

Rakesh Kumar Thakur and Ashish P. Desai

Background

The appendix is considered as a vestigial organ and does not seem to have a function in human beings.

Appendicitis was first described accurately by Reginald Fitz in 1886, who described the clinical history, physical findings, and pathology. He was also the first to advocate appendectomy for appendicitis. In 1887, Thomas Morton performed the first successful appendectomy in the USA. In 1889, Nicholas Senn from Chicago (the USA) was one of the first surgeons to diagnose acute appendicitis correctly and perform an appendectomy. In this same year, Charles Mc-Burney described the clinical findings of acute appendicitis and the point of maximal tenderness.

Inflammation of appendix or appendicitis is the most common pediatric surgical emergency. In spite of being a common condition, it is often misdiagnosed or diagnosed late.

Incidence

Males are more commonly affected with male to female ratio of 1.4:1. The incidence between birth and the age of 4 years is 1–2 cases per 10,000 children per year, which increases to 25 cases per 10,000 children per year between 10 and 17 years of age. Thereafter, the incidence continues to decline, although appendicitis does occur in adulthood and into old age.

Overall, 7% of the population in the USA will have their appendix removed during their lifetime.

A. P. Desai (✉)
Department of Pediatric Surgery, King's College Hospital, Denmark Hill, London SE5 9RS, UK
e-mail: ashishdesai@nhs.net

R. K. Thakur
Department of Pediatric Surgery, King's College Hospital, London, UK

Appendicitis is 1.4 times more common in whites than in nonwhites [1]. It is also much more common in developed countries. Although the reason for this discrepancy is unknown, potential risk factors include a diet low in fiber and high in sugar, family history, and infection [2].

Anatomy

The appendix is a blind-ending tube arising from the cecum where the three taenia meet. It roughly lies at the lower 1/3 junction of a line joining the anterior superior iliac spine and umbilicus. This junction is also called the McBurney's point.

Although the base of the appendix is fixed to the cecum, the tip can be located in various positions around the cecum and presents with different symptoms and different sites of tenderness causing diagnostic dilemma.

Cecum develops as a dilatation of the hindgut by 5 weeks of gestation with the appendix appearing from it by 8 weeks of gestation. The appendix has all the three layers of colon and is lined by colonic epithelium.

The submucosa contains lymphoid follicles, which are very few at birth and gradually increase to a maximum of 200 between 10 and 20 years of age. Their numbers then declines throughout adulthood and are half the number by 30 years.

Etiopathogenesis

Acute appendicitis is the end result of a primary obstruction of the appendix lumen. Most common cause of luminal obstruction is fecal deposits known as appendicoliths or feco-liths, which are hardened fecal deposits. In children, obstruction by submucosal hyperplasia of lymphoid follicles is also common. The cause of this hyperplasia is controversial, but dehydration and viral infection have been proposed.

Fecal stasis may play a role in development of appendicitis, as patients of appendicitis tend to have a significantly

© Springer International Publishing Switzerland 2016
S. Guandalini et al. (eds.), *Textbook of Pediatric Gastroenterology, Hepatology and Nutrition*,
DOI 10.1007/978-3-319-17169-2_50

lower number of bowel movements when compared with normal controls. Many studies have shown a direct correlation between a low-fiber diet and the incidence of appendicitis [2].

Rare causes of appendicular obstruction include worms, foreign body, strictures, and neoplasm especially carcinoids [3, 4].

Following the obstruction, the appendix gets filled with mucus and distends. The bacteria trapped within the appendicular lumen begin to multiply increasing the distension. This causes a progressive rise in the intraluminal pressures leading to occlusion to lymphatics and blood vessels. The appendix becomes edematous, congested, and later ischemic. Occlusion of the blood flow and stagnation of blood causes thrombosis within these small vessels.

The combination of bacterial infection and ischemia produce inflammation, which progresses to necrosis and gangrene. When the appendix becomes gangrenous, it may perforate. Perforation is caused by ischemic weakening of appendicular wall, increased intraluminal pressure, and erosion by fecolith.

The progression from obstruction to perforation usually takes place over 72 h. Appendiceal perforation is more common in children, specifically younger children, than in adults. Perforation is directly related to the duration of symptoms before surgery [1, 5–7].

Staging

As the condition progresses, the appendix passes through the stages of ischemia, necrosis, gangrene, and perforation. This progression is arbitrarily divided into three stages namely: acute (non-gangrenous), suppurative, or gangrenous (non-perforated), and perforated appendicitis.

Clinical staging of appendicitis is important for planning postoperative management and prognosticating the child.

The first stage is acute appendicitis also called as early appendicitis with absence of mural necrosis or gangrene. Rarely, spontaneous recovery may occur in this stage.

Suppurative or gangrenous (non-perforated) appendicitis is the second stage, which involves mural gangrene with microperforations and transmigration of intramural bacteria. This frequently causes intra-abdominal or wound infections.

Perforated appendix is the third stage with perforation of the appendiceal wall and release of intraluminal contents in the peritoneal cavity leading to peritonitis. Perforated appendicitis can be further divided into cases with localized or diffused peritonitis. The omentum and adjacent bowel loops try to contain the spillage of luminal contents. If the perforation is contained it forms an appendicular abscess otherwise it leads to a generalized peritonitis.

If untreated, the infective process may continue and cause septicemia and death.

Presentation

Presentation in children varies with age and location of the appendix.

Classical symptoms of acute appendicitis, usually seen in older children, are abdominal pain, vomiting, and fever, occurring in that order. It is also called Murphy's triad. This is present in only 2/3 causing diagnostic problems.

A neonate may present only with irritability and refusal of feeds. Younger children are uncomfortable, withdrawn, and listless and prefer to lie still because of peritoneal irritation [8, 9].

Pain

Almost all (99 %) patients with appendicitis have abdominal pain [7].

The classical presentation is of an initial gradual onset, diffuse periumbilical pain leading to pain which is more intense, continuous, and localized in the right iliac fossa (RIF).

The migration of pain to RIF is highly specific, but occurs in only half of the patients [7].

Initial pain is due to innervation of visceral peritoneum and stretch receptors of the appendicular wall by T10 nerve roots. While, later there is involvement of the parietal peritoneum, which is supplied by the pain sensitive receptors.

Localization of pain depends on the location of the tip of appendix and the collection of exudate. Hence, pain may also localize to flank, right upper abdomen, pelvic region, or to psoas muscle if the appendix is retrocecal.

Atypical presentations are common in children who are neurologically impaired, immune compromised, or are already on antibiotics for another illness leading to delay in diagnosis. Perforation of appendix with reduction of intraluminal pressure may cause a period of relief of pain, which is soon followed by development of generalized abdominal pain and peritonitis.

Nausea and Vomiting

Many patients develop nausea (81.7 %), anorexia (72.4 %), and vomiting (67.7 %). This usually follows pain [7].

Diarrhea

Diarrhea is rare in appendicitis, but may occur in pelvic appendicitis or perforated appendix with a pelvic abscess.

Inflammation of the rectum and perirectal tissue causes irritative hypermotility and excessive secretion of excessive mucous presenting as diarrhea. Characteristically, diarrhea in appendicitis is frequent, small in volume, with soft stools rather than watery diarrhea associated with infection. Occasionally, there may be blood in stools with tenesmus.

Fever

Most children with appendicitis are afebrile or have a low-grade fever, with characteristic flushing of cheeks (44.9%) [7]. High fever is uncommon and may be present if perforation has occurred. Children with generalized abdominal pain, tachycardia, and a temperature higher than 38 °C are likely to have perforated appendicitis [10].

General Examination

Patients' general state should be observed before interacting with them. The patient's state of activity or withdrawal may lend information into their condition.

General examination should include examination of chest to look for pneumonia, an ear, nose, and throat (ENT) examination to look for tonsillitis that may be suggestive of mesenteric adenitis as the cause of pain. The child's gait may be observed to look for any abnormalities.

Abdominal Examination

Abdomen should be fully exposed and examination should be gentle to cause minimal distress.

All patients of suspected appendicitis should have adequate and early relief of pain. Giving morphine for pain relief does not interfere with diagnostic findings, but may improve diagnostic yield and make the child more cooperative [11]. Observation of facial expressions during palpation gives vital clues.

Tenderness is present in early, a stage which is followed by guarding, rebound tenderness, and rigidity. Usually, maximal tenderness is present at the McBurney point but may vary depending on the location of the appendix.

Younger children have a more diffuse abdominal pain.

A child with peritonitis lies still and sudden movements may cause pain. Gentle percussion of the abdomen may elicit rebound tenderness. An appendicular mass may be palpable in late cases.

Acute scrotum should be looked for in boys as it may present with abdominal pain, nausea, and vomiting.

There are various signs described for diagnosing appendicitis.

- Pain in the RIF when pressed in left iliac fossa (LIF) is called Rovsing sign and indicates peritoneal irritation.
- Rebound tenderness over McBurney's point is called Bloomberg sign.
- Pain on hyperextension of right hip is called Psoas (Cope's psoas) sign and suggests an inflammation of psoas muscle due to an inflamed retrocecal appendicitis overlying it.
- Pain on internally rotating the flexed right thigh indicates an inflamed pelvic appendix overlying the obturator muscle and is called the obturator (Cope's obturator) sign.
- Sherren triangle hyperesthesia is increased tactile sensation in the triangle formed by joining anterior superior iliac spine, the pubic symphysis, and umbilicus.
- Dieulafoy's triad is hyperesthesia, marked tenderness, and guarding over McBurney's point and is an important finding.

Per Rectal Examination

A rectal examination is usually not done in children, but can be helpful in doubtful cases of pelvic appendicitis and in sexually active adolescent girls to check for pelvic inflammatory disease (PID) [12].

Differential Diagnosis

Various abdominal and extra-abdominal conditions mimic appendicitis.

Abdominal Conditions Mimicking Appendicitis

GI Tract Meckel's diverticulitis, pancreatitis, gastroenteritis, intussusception, neutropenic typhlitis, epiploic appendagitis, volvulus, typhlitis, omental torsion, constipation, hemolytic-uremic syndrome, Henoch–Schoenlein purpura.

Other Abdominal Organs Urinary tract infections, pelvic inflammatory disease, ovarian cyst, pyelonephritis, renal calculi, testicular torsion, ovarian torsion. PID, pregnancy, ectopic pregnancy, renal calculi, mittelschmerz, and paratubal cysts.

Extra Abdominal Organs Presenting with Abdominal Signs Mesenteric lymphadenitis, pneumonia (right lower lobe), lymphoma.

Differential Diagnosis for Acute Appendiceal Abscess or Mass Includes Inflammatory bowel disease including Crohn's disease and malignancy.

Investigations

Urine

Urine should be tested to rule out urinary tract infection as well as for pregnancy test in adolescent female patients.

Full Blood Count

White blood cell (WBC) count is usually normal in first 24 h and becomes raised with disease progression. In first 24 h, raised neutrophil count or band count may aid in diagnosis. Leukocytosis is found in approximately 70–90 % of patients with progression of appendicitis. Leukocytosis is a nonspecific marker of inflammation with low specificity [7, 13].

In the immunocompromised patient, especially those on chemotherapy, a neutrophil count lower than 800 may suggest neutropenic enterocolitis or typhlitis.

C-Reactive Protein

C-reactive protein (CRP) is an acute phase reactant and is raised in 85 % of the cases of appendicitis. Following inflammation, CRP rises within 12 h of inflammation.

CRP with raised WBC can be used in tandem to increase the diagnostic accuracy [13].

Abdominal X-Rays

Plain abdominal X-rays has a low sensitivity and specificity [7]. Nonspecific signs of appendicitis are appendicolith, lumbar scoliosis due to psoas spasm, obliteration of the right psoas margin due to inflammatory edema, localized ileus in RIF, RIF mass, air in the appendix, and rarely intraperitoneal free gas.

Abdomen X-ray is normal in many patients with appendicitis. Appendicolith is present in many normal controls [8].

Ultrasonography

A normal appendix is sometimes visualized on ultrasonograph (US), especially in thin patients with a wall thickness of less than 3 and 6 mm in diameter. An inflamed appendix is more easily seen as it is much larger than 6 mm in diameter

and wall thickness greater than 3 mm. It appears as a nonperistaltic, noncompressible, blind-ended, tubular structure which is tender. Graded compression technique described by Puylaert in 1986 requires visualization of appendix and eliciting tenderness by compressing it with the probe. The point of maximum tenderness is also called sonographic Mc-Burney point [14].

In the transverse plane, the inflamed appendix has a target appearance. In approximately 1/3 of patients, an appendicolith is seen as an intraluminal echogenic material with postacoustic shadowing. Peri-appendiceal fluid collection, localized ileus and hyperechogenic pericecal fat, and increased blood flow on Doppler scan are some of the other findings of appendicitis.

Abdominal US has proved to be valuable for diagnosing appendicitis in children, with many published reports indicating a sensitivity, specificity, and accuracy of at least 90–95 % [15]. Factors that add difficulty to the examination include obesity and gaseous distension of the intestines overlying the appendix [7, 16].

US is also used extensively to monitor or perform percutaneous appendicular abscess drainage [15].

US is useful in diagnosing other causes of abdominal pain, for example, tubo-ovarian pathology, mesenteric adenitis, etc.

CT

CT scan has a high sensitivity and specificity when compared with those of other imaging techniques. Appendicitis is suggested by a non-filling of appendix with contrast, distended appendix, hyper enhancement of the appendiceal wall, appendiceal wall thickening (>3 mm), appendicolith within the appendix, and fat streaking around the appendix. Other signs being thickening of the cecal wall, enlarged mesenteric nodes, peri appendicular inflammation or fluid, extraluminal air, marked ileocecal thickening, localized lymphadenopathy, peritonitis, and small-bowel obstruction. Arrowhead sign indicates contrast outlining the cecum and funneling into the origin of the appendix, with obstruction of the lumen preventing retrograde flow of barium into the distal appendix. Signs of perforated appendicitis include abscess, phlegmon, appendicolith within an inflammatory mass or in a fluid collection and extensive free fluid. Air in periappendiceal, pericecal, retroperitoneal region, or in the abscess cavity is suggestive of perforation. Rarely, gas under the diaphragm may also be seen.

CT scan has an accuracy of more than 97 % in diagnosing appendicitis. It is readily available, noninvasiveness, and can diagnose the other causes of abdominal pain [15].

Disadvantages include radiation exposure, the need for oral and intravenous (IV) contrast and its related disadvantages, and the need for the patient to be still, which is often difficult for small children.

CT scan is very helpful in diagnosing and managing perforated appendix. CT scan defines the extent of the abscess and is useful in performing an open surgical or percutaneous drainage of an abscess.

Magnetic Resonance Imaging

MRI is rarely used in diagnosing appendicitis, although it has the advantage of avoiding radiation. Diagnosis involves findings of enhancement of the inflamed appendix and surrounding fat.

Two different techniques have been described one being gadolinium-enhanced, fat-suppressed, and T1-weighted, spin-echo images, the other being unenhanced, axial, and T2-weighted, spin-echo imaging which avoids the use of nephrotoxic gadolinium and is apparently the preferred method.

MRI has an accuracy of nearly 100%. Ileal diverticulitis/abscess and Crohn's disease may lead to false-positive results on MRI [16, 17].

Nuclear Imaging

WBC tagged scans have been developed to diagnose appendicitis with 91–95% accuracy. The scans are time consuming, costly, not freely available, and hence are of no practical use.

Diagnosis

Many scoring systems, protocols, diagnostic pathways algorithms have been devised to aid in diagnosis, however, none of them are foolproof, and clinical judgment and experience is required to reduce errors. Probably the most common scoring system used is the Alvardo (MANTRELS) score. Other common scoring systems being Samuel score, Kharbanda, Eskelinen, Lintula, and Ohmann score [18–20].

Fluid Resuscitation

Children with appendicitis are dehydrated. Even in early acute appendicitis, children frequently have a poor oral intake and vomiting contributing to intravascular depletion caused by third space losses.

It is essential to adequately hydrate patients who present with suspected appendicitis.

Patients with advanced appendicitis will require fluid boluses prior to operation. Urine output should not be lower than 0.5 mL/kg/h. If urine output needs to be determined accurately and frequently, then Foley catheter should be inserted.

Management

The definitive treatment for appendicitis is appendectomy, which can be performed by open or laparoscopic method. Meta-analysis has shown both the methods to have similar results and none to be better than the other. Laparoscopy obviously has a better cosmetic appearance; some studies report a lesser pain, early resolution of ileus, early mobilization, and discharge [21–23].

Contraindications

Almost no contraindications exist to the surgical treatment of appendicitis. However, in patients with septic shock at the time of presentation, surgery should be delayed to ensure adequate fluid resuscitation and appropriate broad-spectrum antibiotics administration.

Conservative Management

Appendectomy is an established treatment for appendicitis, since the time of Fitz 100 years back; many researchers have now questioned the role of appendectomy in the era of new and improved antibiotics. Some surgeons advocate nonoperative treatment with antibiotics for early appendicitis, more so, if the diagnosis is in doubt [20, 24].

The most commonly encountered organisms in appendicitis are *Escherichia coli, Klebsiella, Enterococcus, Bacteroides fragilis, Pseudomonas, Clostridium*, etc. [25–27]. Antibiotic regimens should provide wide coverage for Gram negative and anaerobic organisms. The common antibiotic used is a second-generation cephalosporin or amoxicillin–clavulanate.

Oschners was the first one to recommend conservative management in patients with an appendicular mass [28].

A patient with perforated appendicitis is kept nil by mouth, given adequate analgesia, broad spectrum antibiotics, and administered IV fluids. Oral intake is allowed gradually and increased as tolerated. Fluid and electrolyte balance are managed carefully. In the presence of appendicular abscess, percutaneous drainage is performed if it can be safely approached. Child can be discharged once afebrile, pain free on oral medications, and is on adequate oral intake.

Patients who do not improve or deteriorate on conservative management should have drainage of abscess with or without an appendectomy. Indications of failure of conservative management being—hemodynamic instability, increasing WBC count with toxic granules and shift to the left, persistent hyperthermia greater than 38 °C. Lack of clinical progress within 3 days is deemed as failure. Conservative management fails in as many as 38 % of children with perforated appendicitis [6, 10, 29, 30].

The ideal management in pediatric patients with a perforated appendix is unclear and could be treated by emergency appendectomy or conservative management. Interval appendectomy may be performed 2–3 months later following a successful conservative management.

The necessity of interval appendectomy following conservative management is being questioned since conservative management was first recommended. Proponents of interval appendectomy believe that there is a high rate of recurrent appendicitis if appendectomy is not performed. The possibility of a missed pathologic diagnoses coupled with a low complication of interval appendectomy strengthen their case. Some surgeons perform interval appendectomy only if a fecolith is confirmed on imaging studies as presence of appendicolith increases recurrence rate to 72 from 20 % in other cases [7, 29, 31, 32].

The opponents argue that the incidence of recurrent appendicitis following conservative management is low and the residual appendix is shriveled or may be having a pathology other than appendicitis like a neoplasm, Meckel's diverticulitis, etc. [4, 31, 32]. There is also a worry regarding a finite operative morbidity of a procedure which is probably not required. Conservative management with interval appendectomy requires extra resources due to increased hospital stay, repeated imaging, and prolonged antibiotics [20, 32, 33].

A large meta-analysis done by Anderson et al. showed a significantly greater morbidity for emergency appendectomy than for conservative treatment with interval appendectomy (35.6 vs. 13.5 %). Laparoscopic interval appendectomy has a low morbidity, better visualization of the abdomen, and can be performed as a day case procedure. Hence, it is the procedure of choice for most surgeons [6, 34, 35].

Appendectomy

Patients should be adequately resuscitated with fluids prior to surgery and should receive preoperative prophylactic antibiotics.

Open Appendectomy

Under general anesthesia, the abdomen is palpated and if a mass is felt some surgeons would manage the patient con-

servatively and may perform interval appendectomy (read conservative management).

A transverse right lower quadrant incision is made, usually at the McBurney's point. If an abdominal mass is palpable after the induction of anesthesia, the exact location of the incision can be shifted so that it is centered over the mass.

After identifying and delivering appendix, it is devascularized and the stump is ligated before amputating the appendix. Appendicular stump may or may not be buried.

If a normal-appearing appendix is identified, other pathologic conditions should be sought like evidence of Crohn's disease, mesenteric lymph nodes, and Meckels' diverticulum. In females, ovarian pathology should be excluded.

If no other pathology is identified, most surgeons will remove the appendix. In case of peritoneal contamination, peritoneal wash with warm 0.9 % saline is given to reduce the contamination. A few surgeons have questioned the usefulness of the intra-abdominal wash [36].

Laparoscopic Appendectomy

Many surgeons have reported superior results with laparoscopic method compared to open method. Although, no studies have conclusively proved superiority of one over the other, laparoscopic technique has the obvious advantage of better cosmesis and is frequently used for diagnostic purposes [10, 22, 37, 38].

Single-incision multiport laparoscopic surgery has gained popularity in recent years. Multiple prospective, randomized studies comparing single-incision versus standard three-port laparoscopic appendectomy have shown no advantages of one technique over the other with respect to complications, but they differ in their cosmetic satisfaction scores [10, 39, 40].

Management of Appendicular Abscess

Patients discovered to have perforated appendicitis should have appendectomy. In perforated appendix, there is a high incidence of wound infection.

If an abscess cavity is found, the cavity is cleaned and a drain may be placed.

In rare cases where appendix cannot be safely identified and removed, the appendix is left in place, the abscess cavity is drained, and a subsequent interval appendectomy is planned [41].

Monitoring and Follow-up

The postoperative course is dictated by the status of the appendix at operation. Postoperatively, pain control, mobilization, and chest physiotherapy are very important.

Children with uncomplicated appendicitis can be established on oral intake soon after surgery. It should be possible to discharge these patients within 24–36 h after the operation.

Patients with complicated appendicitis and ileus may take time to return to oral feeds. Those with prolonged ileus will require a period of nasogastric drainage and a few would benefit from parenteral nutrition.

Histology

Histological findings range from acute inflammatory infiltrate in the lumen or submucosa level in early appendicitis. Gangrenous appendicitis may show area of necrosis and thrombosis. Evidence of transmural infarction is seen in perforated appendicitis.

A "normal" appendix found at surgery may show signs of early appendicitis (7.7%) like intraluminal or submucosal inflammatory cells on histological findings of intestinal parasites which require antihelmintic treatment [3, 7]. Chronic inflammation or fibrosis of the tip of the appendix may be seen in the so-called resolving appendicitis.

Most centers would accept a 10–20% of removal of normal appendix rather than risk the morbidity of perforated appendix [7]. Widespread use of imaging studies and diagnostic protocols has reduced this rate [9, 16, 17, 42].

Complications

Wound infection (0–84%) is among the most common complications, more so if there is complicated appendicitis [25, 43]. Rarely there is a complete or incomplete wound dehiscence.

There has been lot of debate regarding reduced fertility in females due to intra-abdominal adhesions following perforated appendicitis. Urbach et al. in 2001 convincingly demonstrated that there was no reduced fertility following appendicitis.

Postoperative ileus is common with peritonitis or following extensive dissection and handling of bowel as in appendicular abscess.

Postoperative adhesions are also a known complication and majority resolve spontaneously with the above management.

Post Appendectomy Abscess

Some patients especially those with complicated appendicitis like gangrenous or perforated appendicitis develop intra-abdominal abscesses (0–12%) [25]. These may be present at the time of presentation or may develop postoperatively.

A post-appendectomy patient with prolonged ileus, swinging temperature for more than 3 days postoperatively, increasing neutrophils, and persistently raised inflammatory markers should be suspected to have an intra-abdominal abscess. Sometimes the wound becomes erythematous, painful, and drainage of large quantity of pus, raising suspicion of intra-abdominal collection.

US is very sensitive in diagnosing a collection.

The majority is small and resolve with an extended course of antibiotics. Larger intra-abdominal abscess may require drainage of the collection, usually performed under ultrasound guidance.

Prognosis

The prognosis is good in timely managed child. Morbidity and mortality in appendicitis is related to the time since initial presentation and treatment. Appendix is perforated in 20–30% of cases at the time of diagnosis. Intra-abdominal abscesses, most commonly pelvic, occur postoperatively in about 10% of cases of perforated appendicitis [25].

The perforation rate rises dramatically to 80–100% in children younger than 3 years, whereas the rate is 10–20% in children above 10 years [7]. Children with ruptured appendicitis are more likely to have wound infection, prolonged ileus, delayed feeding, intra-abdominal abscess formation or adhesive intestinal obstruction leading to an extended hospital stay [7].

The mortality rate for children with appendicitis is 0.1–1%. Death from appendicitis is most common in neonates and infants. Mortality rate in neonatal age group is around 28% [8].

References

1. Addiss D, Shaffer N. The epidemiology of appendicitis and appendectomy in the United States. Am J Epidemiol [Internet]. 1990;132(5):910–25. http://aje.oxfordjournals.org/content/132/5/910.short. Accessed 6 March 2014.
2. Nelson M, Morris J, Barker DJ, Simmonds S. A case-control study of acute appendicitis and diet in children. J Epidemiol Community Health [Internet]. 1986;40(4):316–8. http://www.pubmedcentral.nih.gov/articlerender.fcgi?artid=1052552&tool=pmcentrez&rendertype=abstract. Accessed 10 May 2014.
3. Khan RA, Ghani I, Chana RS. Routine histopathological examination of appendectomy specimens in children: is there any rationale? Pediatr Surg Int [Internet]. 2011;27(12):1313–5. http://www.ncbi.nlm.nih.gov/pubmed/21614465. Accessed 10 May 2014.
4. Akbulut S, Tas M, Sogutcu N, Arikanoglu Z, Basbug M, Ulku A, et al. Unusual histopathological findings in appendectomy specimens: a retrospective analysis and literature review. World J Gastroenterol [Internet]. 2011;17(15):1961–70. http://www.pubmedcentral.nih.gov/articlerender.fcgi?artid=3082748&tool=pmcentrez&rendertype=abstract. Accessed 10 May 2014.

5. Slusher J, Bates CA, Johnson C, Williams C, Dasgupta R, von Allmen D. Standardization and improvement of care for pediatric patients with perforated appendicitis. J Pediatr Surg [Internet]. 2014. http://linkinghub.elsevier.com/retrieve/pii/S0022346814000542. Accessed 26 Feb 2014.

6. Andersson RE, Petzold MG. Nonsurgical treatment of appendiceal abscess or phlegmon: a systematic review and meta-analysis. Ann Surg [Internet]. 2007;246(5):741–8. http://www.ncbi.nlm.nih.gov/pubmed/17968164. Accessed 25 June 2013.

7. Lee SL, Walsh AJ, Ho HS. Computed tomography and ultrasonography do not improve and may delay the diagnosis and treatment of acute appendicitis. Arch Surg. 2001;136(5):556–62.

8. Schwartz KL, Gilad E, Sigalet D, Yu W, Wong AL. Neonatal acute appendicitis: a proposed algorithm for timely diagnosis. J Pediatr Surg [Internet]. 2011;46(11):2060–4. http://www.ncbi.nlm.nih.gov/pubmed/22075333. Accessed 26 Feb 2014.

9. Kwok MY, Kim MK, Gorelick MH. Evidence-based approach to the diagnosis of appendicitis in children. Pediatr Emerg Care [Internet]. 2004;20(10):690–8; quiz 699–701. http://www.ncbi.nlm.nih.gov/pubmed/15454747. Accessed 10 May 2014.

10. Vahdad MR, Troebs R-B, Nissen M, Burkhardt LB, Hardwig S, Cernaianu G. Laparoscopic appendectomy for perforated appendicitis in children has complication rates comparable with those of open appendectomy. J Pediatr Surg [Internet]. 2013;48(3):555–61. http://www.ncbi.nlm.nih.gov/pubmed/23480912. Accessed 26 Feb 2014.

11. Green R, Bulloch B, Kabani A, Hancock BJ, Tenenbein M. Early analgesia for children with acute abdominal pain. Pediatrics [Internet]. 2005;116(4):978–83. http://www.ncbi.nlm.nih.gov/pubmed/16199717. Accessed 10 May 2014.

12. Dickson AP, MacKinlay GA. Rectal examination and acute appendicitis. Arch Dis Child [Internet]. 1985;60(7):666–7. http://adc.bmj.com/cgi/doi/10.1136/adc.60.7.666. Accessed 10 May 2014.

13. Yu C-W, Juan L-I, Wu M-H, Shen C-J, Wu J-Y, Lee C-C. Systematic review and meta-analysis of the diagnostic accuracy of procalcitonin, C-reactive protein and white blood cell count for suspected acute appendicitis. Br J Surg [Internet]. 2013;100(3):322–9. http://www.ncbi.nlm.nih.gov/pubmed/23203918. Accessed 29 April 2014.

14. Puylaert JB. Acute appendicitis: US evaluation using graded compression. Radiology [Internet]. 1986;158(2):355–60. http://www.ncbi.nlm.nih.gov/pubmed/2934762. Accessed 10 May 2014.

15. Ramarajan N, Krishnamoorthi R, Barth R, Ghanouni P, Mueller C, Dannenburg B, et al. An interdisciplinary initiative to reduce radiation exposure: evaluation of appendicitis in a pediatric emergency department with clinical assessment supported by a staged ultrasound and computed tomography pathway. Acad Emerg Med [Internet]. 2009;16(11):1258–65. http://www.ncbi.nlm.nih.gov/pubmed/20053244. Accessed 6 May 2014.

16. Binnebösel M, Otto J, Stumpf M, Mahnken AH, Gassler N, Schumpelick V, et al. Acute appendicitis. Modern diagnostics–surgical ultrasound. Chirurg [Internet]. 2009;80(7):579–87. http://www.ncbi.nlm.nih.gov/pubmed/19471900. Accessed 17 June 2013.

17. Herliczek TW, Swenson DW, Mayo-Smith WW. Utility of MRI after inconclusive ultrasound in pediatric patients with suspected appendicitis: retrospective review of 60 consecutive patients. AJR Am J Roentgenol [Internet]. 2013;200(5):969–73. http://www.ncbi.nlm.nih.gov/pubmed/23617477. Accessed 10 May 2014.

18. Sencan A, Aksoy N, Yıldız M, Okur Ö, Demircan Y, Karaca I. The evaluation of the validity of Alvarado, Eskelinen, Lintula and Ohmann scoring systems in diagnosing acute appendicitis in children. Pediatr Surg Int [Internet]. 2014;30(3):317–21. http://www.ncbi.nlm.nih.gov/pubmed/24448910. Accessed 7 May 2014.

19. Samuel M. Pediatric appendicitis score. J Pediatr Surg [Internet]. 2002;37(6):877–81. http://linkinghub.elsevier.com/retrieve/pii/S0022346802397938. Accessed 6 May 2014.

20. Di Saverio S, Sibilio A, Giorgini E, Biscardi A, Villani S, Coccolini F, et al. The NOTA study (Non operative treatment for acute appendicitis): prospective study on the efficacy and safety of antibiotics (Amoxicillin and clavulanic acid) for treating patients with right lower quadrant abdominal pain and long-term follow-up of conser. Ann Surg [Internet]. 2014. http://www.ncbi.nlm.nih.gov/pubmed/24646528. Accessed 28 April 2014.

21. Aziz O, Athanasiou T, Tekkis PP, Purkayastha S, Haddow J, Malinovski V, et al. Laparoscopic versus open appendectomy in children. Ann Surg [Internet]. 2006;243(1):17–27. http://content.wkhealth.com/linkback/openurl?sid=WKPTLP:landingpage & an=00000658–20060 1000-00005. Accessed 1 May 2014.

22. Esposito C, Calvo AI, Castagnetti M, Alicchio F, Suarez C, Giurin I, et al. Open versus laparoscopic appendectomy in the pediatric population: a literature review and analysis of complications. J Laparoendosc Adv Surg Tech A [Internet]. 2012;22(8):834–9. http://www.ncbi.nlm.nih.gov/pubmed/23039707. Accessed 10 May 2014.

23. Nataraja RM, Teague WJ, Galea J, Moore L, Haddad MJ, Tsang T, et al. Comparison of intraabdominal abscess formation after laparoscopic and open appendicectomies in children. J Pediatr Surg [Internet]. 2012;47(2):317–21. http://www.ncbi.nlm.nih.gov/pubmed/22325383. Accessed 26 Feb 2014.

24. Armstrong J, Merritt N, Jones S, Scott L, Bütter A. Non-operative management of early, acute appendicitis in children: is it safe and effective? J Pediatr Surg [Internet]. 2014. http://linkinghub.elsevier.com/retrieve/pii/S0022346814001717. Accessed 26 Feb 2014.

25. Ein SH, Nasr A, Ein A. Open appendectomy for pediatric ruptured appendicitis: a historical clinical review of the prophylaxis of wound infection and postoperative intra-abdominal abscess. Can J Surg [Internet]. 2013;56(3):E7–12. http://www.pubmedcentral.nih.gov/articlerender.fcgi?artid=3672423&tool=pmcentrez&rendertype=abstract. Accessed 19 Feb 2014.

26. Schmitt F, Clermidi P, Dorsi M, Cocquerelle V, Gomes CF, Becmeur F. Bacterial studies of complicated appendicitis over a 20-year period and their impact on empirical antibiotic treatment. J Pediatr Surg [Internet]. 2012;47(11):2055–62. http://www.ncbi.nlm.nih.gov/pubmed/23163998. Accessed 26 Feb 2014.

27. Lee SL, Islam S, Cassidy LD, Abdullah F, Arca MJ. Antibiotics and appendicitis in the pediatric population: an american pediatric surgical association outcomes and clinical trials committee systematic review. J Pediatr Surg [Internet]. 2010;45(11):2181–5. http://www.ncbi.nlm.nih.gov/pubmed/21034941. Accessed 15 June 2013.

28. Ochsner A. J. The cause of diffuse peritonitis complicating appendicitis and its prevention. JAMA. 1901;36:1747–54.

29. Zhang H-L, Bai Y-Z, Zhou X, Wang W-L. Nonoperative management of appendiceal phlegmon or abscess with an appendicolith in children. J Gastrointest Surg [Internet]. 2013;17(4):766–70. http://www.ncbi.nlm.nih.gov/pubmed/23315049. Accessed 10 May 2014.

30. Odofin A. Conservative management of acute appendicitis: a review. Internet J Surg [Internet]. 2012;28(2). http://www.ispub.com/doi/10.5580/2b0a. Accessed 17 June 2013.

31. Mazziotti MV, Marley EF, Winthrop AL, Fitzgerald PG, Walton M, Langer JC. Histopathologic analysis of interval appendectomy specimens: support for the role of interval appendectomy. J Pediatr Surg [Internet]. 1997;32(6):806–9. http://www.ncbi.nlm.nih.gov/pubmed/9200074. Accessed 10 May 2014.

32. Tekin A, Kurtoğlu HC, Can I, Oztan S. Routine interval appendectomy is unnecessary after conservative treatment of appendiceal mass. Colorectal Dis [Internet]. 2008;10(5):465–8. http://www.ncbi.nlm.nih.gov/pubmed/17868409. Accessed 17 June 2013.

33. Myers AL, Williams RF, Giles K, Waters TM, Eubanks JW, Hixson SD, et al. Hospital cost analysis of a prospective, randomized trial of early vs interval appendectomy for perforated appendicitis in children. J Am Coll Surg [Internet]. 2012;214(4):427–34; discussion 434–5. http://www.ncbi.nlm.nih.gov/pubmed/22342789. Accessed 10 May 2014.

34. Whyte C, Tran E, Lopez ME, Harris BH. Outpatient interval appendectomy after perforated appendicitis. J Pediatr Surg. 2008;43(11):1970–2. http://www.ncbi.nlm.nih.gov/pubmed/18970926. Accessed 10 May 2014.

35. Blakely ML, Williams R, Dassinger MS, et al. Early vs Interval appendectomy for children with perforated appendicitis. Arch Surg. 2011;146(6):660–5.

36. Akkoyun I, Tuna AT. Advantages of abandoning abdominal cavity irrigation and drainage in operations performed on children with perforated appendicitis. J Pediatr Surg [Internet]. 2012;47(10):1886–90. http://www.ncbi.nlm.nih.gov/pubmed/23084202. Accessed 26 Feb 2014.

37. Zwintscher NP, Johnson EK, Martin MJ, Newton CR. Laparoscopy utilization and outcomes for appendicitis in small children. J Pediatr Surg [Internet]. 2013;48(9):1941–5. http://www.ncbi.nlm.nih.gov/pubmed/24074672. Accessed 26 Feb 2014.

38. Sesia SB, Haecker F-M. Laparoscopic-assisted single-port appendectomy in children: it is a safe and cost-effective alternative to conventional laparoscopic techniques? Minim Invasive Surg. 2013;2013:165108. doi:10.1155/2013/165108.

39. Ding J, Xia Y, Zhang Z, Liao G, Pan Y, Liu S, et al. Single-incision versus conventional three-incision laparoscopic appendectomy for appendicitis: a systematic review and meta-analysis. J Pediatr Surg [Internet]. 2013;48(5):1088–98. http://www.ncbi.nlm.nih.gov/pubmed/23701788. Accessed 24 Feb 2014.

40. Stylianos S, Nichols L, Ventura N, Malvezzi L, Knight C, Burnweit C. The "all-in-one" appendectomy: quick, scarless, and less costly. J Pediatr Surg [Internet]. 2011;46(12):2336–41. http://www.ncbi.nlm.nih.gov/pubmed/22152877. Accessed 26 Feb 2014.

41. Kim J-K, Ryoo S, Oh H-K, Kim JS, Shin R, Choe EK, et al. Management of appendicitis presenting with abscess or mass. J Korean Soc Coloproctol [Internet]. 2010;26(6):413–9. http://www.pubmedcentral.nih.gov/articlerender.fcgi?artid=3017977&tool=pmcentrez&rendertype=abstract. Accessed 15 June 2013.

42. Adibe OO, Amin SR, Hansen EN, Chong AJ, Perger L, Keijzer R, et al. An evidence-based clinical protocol for diagnosis of acute appendicitis decreased the use of computed tomography in children. J Pediatr Surg [Internet]. 2011;46(1):192–6. http://www.ncbi.nlm.nih.gov/pubmed/21238665. Accessed 25 Feb 2014.

43. Boomer LA, Cooper JN, Deans KJ, Minneci PC, Leonhart K, Diefenbach KA, et al. Does delay in appendectomy affect surgical site infection in children with appendicitis? J Pediatr Surg. [Internet]. Elsevier Inc.; 2014. http://linkinghub.elsevier.com/retrieve/pii/S0022346814000530. Accessed 26 Feb 2014.

Gastrointestinal Vascular Anomalies

Indre Zaparackaite and Ashish P. Desai

Introduction

Vascular abnormalities are either present at birth or appear soon after. They are more commonly seen as cutaneous lesions.

The first scientific reports of vascular malformations appeared in literature in the sixteenth century. In 1628, *William Harvey* published his major work, *On the Motion of the Heart and Blood in Animals,* where he explained blood circulation. Since then, there was a continuous scientific urge to explore the secrets of abnormal circulation and aberrant vascular communications.

In the eighteenth century, a German scientist, *Rudolf Virchow* (1821–1902), the founder of cellular pathology, was the first to suggest that hemangioma is formed of new vessels rather than by passive dilatation of preexisting channels. He also speculated that these tumors appeared antenatally and continued to grow postnatally.

Embryology

The vascular system arises from mesodermal blood islands in the wall of yolk sack. These blood islands are composed of progenitors of blood cells and endothelial progenitor cells. Further development encompasses vasculogenesis (formation of embryonic vessels), migration of angioblasts to the organs, and angiogenesis (the process of growing new vessels). Angiogenesis is regulated by local factors maintaining the subtle balance between the inhibitors (e.g., thrombospondins, endostatin) and stimulators (e.g., vascular endo-

thelial growth factor (VEGF), basic fibroblast growth factor (bFGF), and angiopoetins). VEGF is a key regulator in angiogenesis and has been found to be responsible for inducing penetration of the capillary vessels in to avascular epidermis [1]. As an end product, the vessels are composed of a single layer of endothelial cells surrounded by variable number of layers of vascular smooth muscle cells.

The precise pathogenesis of development of vascular lesions is not fully understood. Nevertheless, there is evidence that signaling aberrations at the molecular level may result in abnormal proliferation, differentiation, maturation, and apoptosis of vascular cells [2].

Vascular Tumors Vascular tumors are characterized by increased endothelial proliferation. The precise origin of the hemangiomal endothelial cells remains uncertain. Immunophenotypic similarities with placental endothelium suggest a placental origin [3]. The mechanism is believed to be embolization of placental endothelial cells, which enter the fetus from chorionic villi through right-to-left shunts (normal in fetal circulation). This theory was checked in different laboratories, though the results could not be universally confirmed.

In summary, hemangiomas express abnormal proliferation with increased endothelial cell turnover and increased surface markers (VEGF, bFGF). Conversely, vascular malformations are a product of abnormal morphogenesis. Their endothelial lining is flat, smooth muscle architecture is abnormal and the expression of surface markers is minimal.

Classification of Vascular Lesions

In the past, the terminology used in association with such abnormalities has been rather confusing, being mainly descriptive and dismissive of the histological origin of the lesions. A binary classification, into *vascular tumors* and *vascular malformations,* was proposed by Mulliken and Glowacki in 1982 [4] and has since been adopted by the International

A. P. Desai (✉)
Department of Pediatric Surgery, King's College Hospital, Denmark Hill, London SE5 9RS, UK
e-mail: ashishdesai@nhs.net

I. Zaparackaite
Department of Pediatric Surgery, Great Ormond Street Hospital, 43 Craignair Avenue, Brighton BN1 8UG, UK
e-mail: zetagama@doctors.org.uk

© Springer International Publishing Switzerland 2016
S. Guandalini et al. (eds.), *Textbook of Pediatric Gastroenterology, Hepatology and Nutrition,*
DOI 10.1007/978-3-319-17169-2_51

Table 51.1 International society for the study of vascular anomalies classification system [5]. (Accessed and used with permission from http://www.issva.org/content.aspx?page_id=22&club_id=298433&module_id=152904-).

Vascular (or vasoproliferative) neoplasms	Vascular malformations
Infantile hemangioma	Slow-flow vascular malformations
Congenital hemangiomas (Rapidy involuting congenital hemangioma (RICH) Non-involuting congenital hemangioma (NICH)	Capillary malformation Venous malformation Lymphatic malformation
Kaposiform hemangioendothelioma and tufted angiomas (with or without Kasabach–Merritt syndrome)	Fast-flow vascular malformations
Spindle cell hemangioendothelioma	Arterial malformation
Epithelioid hemangioendothelioma	Arteriovenous malformation
Other rare hemangioendotheliomas (i.e., composite, retiform, and others)	Arteriovenous fistula
Angiosarcoma	Combined vascular malformations (various combinations of the above)
Dermatologic acquired vascular tumors (i.e., pyogenic granuloma)	–

Society for the Study of Vascular Anomalies (ISSVA), established in 1992 (Table 51.1).

Classification into either of these groups is determined by clinical appearance, by radiological and pathological features, and by biological behavior. In rare cases, vascular tumors and vascular malformations can coexist [6].

In order to understand different modalities of investigation and treatment, it is important to appreciate the different origin and behavior of vascular anomalies irrespective of their site. We describe the lesions with special emphasis on gastrointestinal (GI) lesions.

Group I: Vascular Tumors

Congenital vascular tumors can be divided into the following major groups:
- Infantile hemangiomas
- Congenital hemangiomas
- Kaposiform hemagioendotheliomas
- Other rare tumors (tufted angiomas, angiosarcomas)

Hemangioma is the most common tumor of infancy and childhood with recorded 1.0–2.6% incidence among Caucasian neonates. By the age of 1 year, some 4–12% of Caucasian children have a hemangioma. The female-to-male ratio is 3:1. Hemangiomas are more common in premature babies [7].

Infantile Hemangiomas

Infantile hemangiomas are proliferating endothelial tumors. They are strongly characterized by endothelial expression of glucose transporter protein-1 (GLU-1). GLU-1 is not observed in other vascular malformations and vascular tumors, except for some focal areas in cases of RICH [7]. Infantile hemangiomas, usually apparent in the early neonatal period, proliferate until 1 year of age then slowly regress until the age of 7, when they end in the involution phase.

Congenital Hemangiomas

Congenital hemangiomas are fully formed at birth and can follow two patterns of biological behavior: either rapidly involuting congenital hemangiomas (RICH) or non-involuting congenital hemangiomas (NICH). They often have a large feeding vessel and sometimes can cause shunting and cardiac overload.

Kaposiform Endotheliomas

Kaposiform endotheliomas and tufted angiomas can result in Kasabach–Merritt-type coagulopathy, characteristic of which is platelet trapping by abnormal endothelium and the consumption of fibrinogen. Thrombocytopenia can be life-threatening, especially when resulting in disseminated intravascular coagulation. The Kasabach–Merritt phenomenon is associated with a mortality rate of 14–24% [8, 9].

If patients present with five or more cutaneous hemangiomas, the abdominal ultrasound scan is indicated looking for visceral lesions, more commonly situated in the liver.

The hemangiomas of the GI tract are rare and only account for approximately 0.3% of all GI tumors. They have a tendency towards multiplicity (intestinal hemangiomatosis) and solitary tumors are uncommon. Patients may present with GI hemorrhage, anemia, or symptoms of obstruction. Interestingly, 11–30% of GI hemangiomas may remain asymptomatic [10, 11].

Group II: Vascular Malformations

Vascular malformations are localized defects of vascular development, which occur in the process of vascular morphogenesis.

Although most vascular lesions are sporadic, inheritance has been observed and has thus provided a route to genetic analysis. Sporadic forms usually present as single lesions, but multiple lesions have been observed in familial cases.

Ninety percent of vascular malformations are present at birth. Estimated incidence of vascular anomalies in the general population is approximately 1.5% [12].

Female-to-male ratio is 1:1. These malformations infiltrate the surrounding tissue, never regress and can worsen over time if not treated. Changes in hemodynamic factors such as arteriovenous shunting or venous stasis can accelerate growth and morbidity.

The "vascular malformations" group can also be subdivided into fast flow (arterial or arteriovenous) and slow flow (capillary, lymphatic, or venous). If fast-flow lesions are localized subcutaneously, they may become more erythematous, and may develop a palpable thrill and a bruit.

Vascular malformations of the GI tract are rare in children but they can be diagnosed at any age, including newborns [13]. They may appear anywhere in the GI tract from mouth to anus and may coexist with similar lesions on the skin.

Patients may present with recurrent abdominal pain, GI bleeding, acute or, more often, chronic anemia, intestinal obstruction, volvulus, intussusception, and palpable mass lesion. Sometimes, because of mucosal edema, nodularity, and vascular congestion, these lesions might be mistaken for inflammatory bowel disease. Bleeding per rectum may also be misleading towards the diagnosis of symptomatic Meckel's diverticulum. Intestinal lesions often represent a diagnostic challenge requiring sophisticated methods of investigation.

Group II: Vascular Malformations: Associated Syndromes

Certain syndromes are associated with GI vascular malformations, including:
1. Osler–Weber–Rendu disease (hereditary hemorrhagic telangiectasia)
2. Klippel–Trenaunay syndrome
3. Blue rubber bleb nevus (BRNB) syndrome

Osler–Weber–Rendu Disease (Hereditary Hemorrhagic Telangiectasia)

This is a genetic disorder inherited in autosomal dominant manner occurring in 1:5000 of the general population. Genetic diagnosis is difficult but tests are available for the *ENG, ACVRL1,* and *MADH4* mutations [14].

The condition typically presents with distinctive small skin and mucosal vascular malformations (telengiectasias), and may appear in the nose, lips, fingers, and along the GI tract. Larger arteriovenous malformations are usually localized in the lungs, liver, brain and, occasionally, the spine. Though the main clinical problem is usually epistaxis, GI bleeding may also occur, but it is rare in pediatric population. The malformations developing in the liver may eventually lead to portal hypertension, high-output cardiac failure, or encephalopathy. The clinical diagnosis is based on the Curaçao criteria [15], which are:
• Spontaneous recurrent epistaxis
• Multiple telangiectasia in typical locations
• Proven visceral arteriovenous malformations (lung, liver, brain, spine)
• First-degree family member with hereditary hemorrhagic telangiectasia

Treatment of anemia due to GI bleeding is mainly symptomatic but in severe cases argon plasma coagulation or laser therapy may be applied.

Klippel–Trenaunay Syndrome

This is a relatively rare condition with approximate incidence of 1:30,000 live births [16]. Historically, it is characterized by a triad of symptoms: capillary skin malformation (port wine stain), varicose veins (especially persistent embryonic lateral vein of Servelle), and bony/soft tissue hypertrophy of the extremity. This hypertrophy is caused by venous and lymphatic malformations localized in the soft tissue but often involving the bony structures. Most commonly, one extremity is affected, usually the leg, but multiple involvement is also possible.

The etiology of the syndrome is not entirely clear but it is believed that most cases happen due to sporadic gene mutation, though some autosomal dominant inheritance cases are also reported. Mutations in PI3K-AKT gene pathway may play a role in development of the condition [17].

In association with the classical triad of clinical symptoms, the GI tract may also be affected by vascular malformations. Though intestinal involvement is rare (1–12% of all patients affected by the syndrome)—the risk of bleeding should always be considered [18].

BRNB Syndrome (Bean Syndrome)

This syndrome is characterized by cutaneous and visceral venous malformations. These malformations can occur in any tissue but are most prominent in the skin and in the GI tract, the small bowel being the most frequently affected part. Their number can range between several to hundreds, such as the 557 in one patient reported by Fishman in 2005 [19]. Cutaneous lesions are generally small (about 1–2 cm or even smaller), rubbery, compressible, blue to purple nipple-like nodules often found on the face, the upper limbs, and the soles of the feet.

Most cases are sporadic, but some autosomal dominant transmission has also been reported.

A common problem is GI bleeding presenting at early age and continuing throughout life, resulting in chronic anemia requiring repeated blood transfusions. A broad spectrum of treatment options is available, from conservative and endoscopic treatment to an aggressive surgical approach.

Group III: Lymphatic Malformations

Lymphatic malformations are relatively rare in the GI tract, especially in children.

The majority of intra-abdominal lymphatic malformations are identified within the mesentery and retroperitoneum. Lesions affecting the bowel are uncommon and account for less than 1% of all lymphatic malformations. Approximately, 70% of those are detected in the small bowel and 30% in the colon [20].

Patients may present with abdominal pain, failure to thrive, palpable cystic mass, intestinal volvulus, bowel obstruction, or intussusception. Differential diagnosis includes intestinal duplication cyst, ovarian cyst, teratoma, Wilm's tumor, and neuroblastoma. In the case of a small-bowel lesion, the differential diagnosis of lymphangiomyoma and benign multicystic mesothelioma could be considered. Imunohistochemical analysis can give a clear indication if the lesion was derived from the lymphatic vessels (expected focal positivity of D2–40, a lymphatic endothelial marker).

Primary Intestinal Lymphangiectasia (Waldmann's Disease)

Dilated intestinal channels resulting in lymph leakage into the small-bowel lumen and responsible for protein-losing enteropathy leading to lymphopenia, hypoalbuminemia, and hypogammaglobulinemia characterize this disorder. The exact etiology of this condition is unknown and it is generally diagnosed before 3 years of age. Patients often present with bilateral lower limb lymphoedema, inability to gain weight, steatorrhea, and later develop pleural effusions or ascites. This may be accompanied by abdominal pain. Sometimes the abdominal mass may be palpable or patients may develop intussusception. Mechanical obstruction of the small intestine may be caused by localized oedema leading to intestinal wall-thickening and lumen diminution.

Diagnostic process can be helped by ultrasound scan, capsule endoscopy, CT, albumin scintigraphy, and sometimes by lymphoscintigraphy.

The condition requires long-term medical treatment in form of reduced dietary fat, medium-chain triglycerides, elemental diet, corticosteroids, and vitamin supplements [21]. In some localized cases, surgical resection may provide satisfactory results. In chronic recurrent conditions, fibrin glue application has been used.

Investigations and Treatment

Several imaging modalities can be employed to establish more precisely the type and the location of vascular anomalies. MRI imaging, selective angiography, color Doppler sonography, multiphase CT enterography, and 99 m Tc-red blood cell (RBC) scintigraphy can all be useful for this purpose [22–25]. The slow flow veno-lymphatic malformations on MRI scan are typically multispacial, multicystic, and may have a partially solid component. Fast-flow arteriovenous malformations demonstrate turbulence, flow voids, and hyperintense signal.

From the imaging point of view, it is important to remember that while young the hemangiomas may behave like arteriovenous malformations and may exhibit the features of fast flow. The slow flow is being established in involution phase. Currently, ultrasonography and MRI with contrast (T1- and T2-weighed sequences) are the most widely used modalities of initial diagnostic choice.

At endoscopy, the whole GI tract should be visualized, if possible, by using different approaches, including rigid or flexible endoscopy, single- or double-balloon enteroscopy, wireless capsule endoscopy, laparotomy/laparoscopy, and enterotomies.

Each method has its advantages and limitations. Capsule endoscopy, for example, transmits a radio-frequency signal, which allows estimation of the location of the capsule and tracking of it in real time inside the GI tract. Nevertheless, unlike endoscopy it cannot treat pathologies it discovers. Another limitation, specific to the pediatric population, can be the age and size of the patient; these factors can affect tolerance of certain procedures and the accuracy of imaging.

Once the lesions are localized there is a choice of surgical methods of treatment, including segmental or wedge bowel resection, band or suture ligation and argon plasma coagulation or electrocoagulation [26].

Even though both hemangiomas and vascular lesions often present with bleeding, principal treatment options are entirely different. Visceral hemangiomas are at risk of bleeding in the proliferation phase and the risk diminishes after they enter the involuting phase. In many cases this could be achieved by using the inhibitors of angiogenesis. For example, extensive intestinal hemangiomatosis can be successfully managed with propranolol, corticosteroids, α-interferon, vincristine, and also with thalidomide and somatostatin analog [27].

The antiangiogenic treatment is ineffective for vascular malformations. If amenable, especially if the vascular malformations are located in the anorectal region, direct injection and sclerotherapy can be performed [28].

The principal method of sclerotherapy is injection of water-based or oleous substances into abnormally dilated vessels that can inflict damage to endothelial lining and cause thrombosis, fibrosis, stenosis and—eventually—scarring. Sclerotherapy for treatment of lymphatic and venous malformations employs a variety of agents, including absolute ethanol, bleomycin, OK-432 (picibanil), and doxycycline [3]. Each agent has a risk profile: Ethanol injections are painful, requiring general anesthesia even in adults, and may cause cardiovascular shock. Bleomycin may cause interstitial pneumonia or pulmonary fibrosis and treatment with doxycycline may result in tooth discoloration or electrolyte abnormalities.

Some complicated vascular anomalies resistant to other treatments can be conservatively treated with sirolimus (especially if they have a lymphatic component), bevacizumab, and estrogen–progesteron combination therapy [15, 29].

Conclusion

GI vascular lesions are rare. Vascular malformations are more common than vascular neoplasms. They require extensive investigations to identify the type and location. Different modalities need to be used to treat the lesions by limited resection or sclerotherapy. Many lesions require lifelong supportive therapy to treat chronic anemia and nutritional deficiencies.

References

1. Brown LF, Yeo KT, Berse B, et al. Expression of vascular permeability factor (vascular endothelial growth factor) by epidermal keratinocytes during wound healing. J Exp Med. 1992 Nov 1;176(5):1375–9.
2. Brouillard P, Vikkula M. Genetic causes of vascular malformations. Hum Mol Genet. 2007 Oct 15;16(2):R140–9.
3. Richter GT, Friedman AB. Hemangiomas and vascular malformations: current theory and management. Int J Pediatr. 2012;2012:645–78.
4. Mulliken JB, Glowacki J. Hemangiomas and vascular malformations in infants and children: a classification based on endothelial characteristics. Plast Reconstr Surg. 1982 March;69(3):412–22.
5. ISSVA Classification of Vascular Anomalies © 2014 International Society for the Study of Vascular Anomalies. Available at "issva.org/classification". Accessed April 2014. (By permission of the society).
6. Marler JJ, Mulliken JB. Current management of hemangiomas and vascular malformations. Clin Plastic Surg. 2005;32:99–116.
7. Mulliken JB, Burrows PE, Fishman SJ. Mulliken and Young's vascular anomalies: hemangiomas and malformations. USA: Oxford University Press; 2013. p. 68.
8. Lyons LL, North PE, Mac-Moune Lai F, et al. Kaposiform hemangioendothelioma: a study of 33 cases emphasizing its pathologic, immunophenotypic, and biologic uniqueness from juvenile hemangioma. Am J Surg Pathol. 2004 May;28(5):559–68.
9. Sarkar M, Mulliken JB, Kozakewich HP, et al. Thrombocytopenic coagulopathy (Kasabach-Merritt phenomenon) is associated with Kaposiform hemangioendothelioma and not with common infantile hemangioma. Plast Reconstr Surg. 1997 Nov;100(6):1377–86.
10. Nader PR, Margolin F. Hemangioma causing gastrointestinal bleeding. Case report and review of the literature. Am J Dis Child. 1966;111:215–22.
11. Nishiyama N, Mori H, Kobara H, et al. Bleeding duodenal hemangioma: morphological changes and endoscopic mucosal resection. World J Gastroenterol. 2012 June 14;18(22):2872–6.
12. Eifert S, Villavicencio JL, Kao TC, Taute BM, Rich NM. Prevalence of deep venous anomalies in congenital vascular malformations of venous predominance. J Vasc Surg. 2000 March;31(3):462–71.
13. Hansen LF, Wewer V, Pedersen SA, Matzen P, Paerregaard A. Severe blue rubber bleb nevus syndrome in a neonate. Eur J Pediatr Surg. 2009 Feb;19(1):47–9.
14. Letteboer TGW, Zewald ÆRA, Kamping ÆEJ, et al. Hereditary hemorrhagic telangiectasia: ENG and ALK-1 mutations in Dutch patients. Hum Genet. 2005;116:8–16.
15. Greer JP, Arber DA, Glader B, et al. Wintrobe's clinical hematology. Philadelphia: Lippinkot Williams & Wilkins; 2014. p. 1109.
16. Husmann DA, Rathbun SR, Driscoll DJ. Klippel-Trenaunay syndrome: incidence and treatment of genitourinary sequelae. J Urol. 2007;177(4):1244–9.
17. Revencu N, Boon LM, Dompmartinet A, et al. Germline mutations in RASA1 are not found in patients with klippel-trenaunay syndrome or capillary malformation with limb overgrowth. Mol Syndromol. 2013 April;4(4):173–8.
18. Herman R, Kunisaki S, Molitor M, et al. Rectal bleeding, deep venous thrombosis, and coagulopathy in a patient with Klippel-Trénaunay syndrome. J Pediatr Surg. 2012 March;47(3):598–600.
19. Fishman SJ, Smithers CJ, Folkman J, Lund DP, Burrows PE, Mulliken JB, Fox VL. Blue rubber bleb nevus syndrome: surgical eradication of gastrointestinal bleeding. Ann Surg. 2005 March;241(3):523–8.
20. Iida S, Furukawa K, Terada Y, Sugisaki Y, Yoshimura K, Tajiri T. A case of a mesenteric cyst in the sigmoid colon of a 3-year-old girl. J Nippon Med Sch. 2009 Oct;76(5):247–52.
21. Desai AP, Guvenc BH, Carachi R. Evidence for medium chain triglycerides in the treatment of primary intestinal lymphangiectasia. Eur J Pediatr Surg. 2009 Aug;19(4):241–5.
22. Frémond B, Yazbeck S, Dubois J, Brochu P, Garel L, Ouimet A. Intestinal vascular anomalies in children. J Pediatr Surg. 1997 June;32(6):873–7.
23. Huprich JE, Barlow JM, Hansel SL, Alexander JA, Fidler JL. Multiphase CT enterography evaluation of small-bowel vascular lesions. AJR Am J Roentgenol. 2013 July;201(1):65–72.
24. Mechri M, Soyer P, Boudiaf M, Duchat F, Hamzi L, Rymer R. Small bowel involvement in blue rubber bleb nevus syndrome: MR imaging features. Abdom Imaging. 2009 July;34(4):448–51.
25. Sugito K, Kusafuka T, Hoshino M, Inoue M, Ikeda T, Hagiwara N, Koshinaga T. Usefulness of color doppler sonography and 99m Tc-RBC scintigraphy for preoperative diagnosis of a venous malformation of the small intestine in a 2-year-old child. J Clin Ultrasound. 2008 Jan;36(1):56–8.
26. Regula J, Wronska E, Pachlewski J. Vascular lesions of the gastrointestinal tract. Best Pract Res Clin Gastroenterol. 2008;22(2):313–28.
27. Jarvi K, Roebuck DJ, Sebire NJ, Lindley K, Shah N, Salomon J, Curry JI. Successful treatment of extensive infantile hemangiomatosis of the small bowel in a 3-month-old with thalidomide and somatostatin analog. J Pediatr Gastroenterol Nutr. 2008 May;46(5):593–7.
28. Fishman SJ, Burrows PE, Leichtner AM, Mulliken JB. Gastrointestinal manifestations of vascular anomalies in childhood: varied etiologies require multiple therapeutic modalities. J Pediatr Surg. 1998 July;33(7):1163–7.
29. Hammill AM, Wentzel M, Gupta A, et al. Sirolimus for the treatment of complicated vascular anomalies in children. Pediatric Blood & cancer. 2011;57(6):1018–24.

Polyps and Other Tumors of the Gastrointestinal Tract

Warren Hyer, Marta Tavares and Mike Thomson

Introduction

Children and adolescents with gastrointestinal polyps may present symptomatic with rectal bleeding, abdominal pain, or intussusception, or alternatively, they may be asymptomatic, having been referred, either because an adult family member has been affected with early onset colorectal cancer (CRC) or there is a known family history of a polyposis syndrome. Many children fall under the latter category. Managing these children and families requires knowledge of the different polyposis syndromes, their inheritance and genetics, potential for malignant change and pediatric complications.

Gastrointestinal polyps in children fall into two major categories: hamartomas and adenomas (Table 52.1). Solitary polyps in children are most commonly hamartomas, predominantly of the juvenile type, and such polyps are benign. Of the familial syndromes, familial adenomatous polyposis (FAP) is more common than juvenile polyposis or Peutz–Jeghers polyposis.

Clinical Presentation of Gastrointestinal Polyps

The most common clinical manifestation of a large bowel polyp is painless rectal bleeding. Other symptoms attributed to polyps include abdominal pain, altered bowel habit, and prolapse of polyp or rectum. Diagnosis will be made upon full colonoscopy with polypectomy. The clinical presentation, endoscopic appearance, pathological findings, histological description of the polyp, and genetic investigations are all necessary to establish the correct diagnosis of a polyposis syndrome. Once a polyp has been identified at endoscopy, a carefully targeted family history must be taken to enquire if there are family members who have or have had cancer, the site of the cancers, and age of onset (see Table 52.2). Taking such a history to develop a detailed family cancer pedigree may require the expertise of a multidisciplinary familial cancer clinic or polyposis registry [1].

Table 52.1 Polyps and polyposis syndromes seen in childhood

Adenomatous polyposis syndromes
Familial adenomatous polyposis (FAP)
MYH-associated polyposis (MAP)
Turcots syndrome
Lynch syndrome
Hamartomatous polyps
Solitary juvenile polyp
Juvenile polyposis syndrome
PTEN hamartoma tumor syndrome
Peutz–Jeghers syndrome
Inflammatory polyps
PTEN phosphatase and tensin, *MYH* mutY human homologue

Table 52.2 History and examination in a child with possible GI polyps

History
Nature of bleeding and frequency
Painful or painless rectal bleeding
History of GI obstructive symptoms
Detailed family history exploring early deaths or diagnosis of GI cancer and include history of non-GI malignancies
Weight loss, anorexia (tumor)
Learning difficulties (JPS or PTEN hamartoma)
Examination
Mucosal pigmentation (PJS)
Dysmorphic features (JPS)
Edema (hypoalbuminemia in infantile JPS)
Extra intestinal manifestations of FAP
Hepatic mass (FAP)
Cutaneous telangiectasia (HHT with JPS)
Thyroid mass (FAP or Cowden)

M. Thomson (✉)
Department of Gastroenterology, Sheffield Children's Hospital, Weston Park, Sheffield S10 2TH, South Yorkshire, UK
e-mail: mike.thomson@sch.nhs.uk

W. Hyer
The Polyposis Registry, St Mark's Hospital, Middx, UK

M. Tavares
Porto Children's Hospital, Porto, Portugal

© Springer International Publishing Switzerland 2016
S. Guandalini et al. (eds.), *Textbook of Pediatric Gastroenterology, Hepatology and Nutrition,*
DOI 10.1007/978-3-319-17169-2_52

JPS juvenile polyposis syndrome, PTEN phosphatase and tensin, PJS Peutz–Jeghers syndrome, FAP familial adenomatous polyposis, HHT hereditary hemorrhagic telangiectasiaThe Single Hamartomatous Polyp (the Juvenile Polyp)

With a prevalence of up to 3 % of children, the commonest presentation of a single hamartomatous (or juvenile) polyp is painless bright red rectal bleeding with blood seen on wiping or mixed in the stool. Seventy percent of juvenile polyps are found in the rectum or rectosigmoid. The rest however are found more proximally, hence the need for pancolonoscopy. Single or solitary juvenile polyps are benign and confer no future risk of malignancy. Presently, it is unknown whether children who present with a single polyp in childhood may continue to form polyps over time [2].

If a polyp is found to be solitary after full colonoscopy, and there is no relevant family history, endoscopic polypectomy should be sufficient treatment. After polypectomy, parents should be advised that juvenile polyps may be the first feature of a hamartomatous polyposis syndrome, and if new symptoms arise, the child should be reinvestigated. If multiple juvenile polyps are found (> 3–5) or there is a positive family history (e.g., colonic polyps or early onset CRC), a hamartomatous polyposis syndrome should be considered and an alternative approach should be taken.

Hamartomatous Polyposis Syndromes

Hamartomatous polyposis syndromes are a rare group of hereditary autosomal dominant disorders. The polyps themselves are benign but the polyposis syndromes confer significant potential for developing CRC and extra colonic cancers. The hamartomatous polyposis syndromes include juvenile polyposis syndrome (JPS), Peutz–Jeghers syndrome (PJS), and phosphatase and tensin (PTEN) hamartoma tumor syndrome, which includes Cowden (CS) and Bannayan–Riley–Ruvalcaba syndrome (BRRS).

Juvenile Polyposis Syndrome

JPS is rare, with an estimated prevalence of 1 in 100,000 individuals presenting with multiple hamartomatous polyps and an increased risk of gastrointestinal malignancies. Affected individuals develop multiple gastrointestinal polyps which are predominantly in the colon, though other areas of the gastrointestinal tract can also be involved. The condition should be considered in any patient with more than five juvenile polyps in the colon, any juvenile polyps found in other parts of the gastrointestinal tract, or if any juvenile polyp is found in a child with a positive family history. Patients present with chronic and acute gastrointestinal bleeding, anemia, prolapsed rectal polyps, abdominal pain and diarrhea and can develop up to 50–200 polyps in the colon, while in some patients, with generalized juvenile polyposis, polyps can affect the colon, stomach, and small bowel. The total number of polyps needed to make the diagnosis remains controversial, between 3 and 5 [3].A significant proportion of patients with juvenile polyposis have been reported to have other morphological abnormalities including digital clubbing, polydactyly, macrocephaly, alopecia, cleft lip or palate, congenital heart disease, and mental retardation. A specific variant of JPS called juvenile polyposis of infancy has an onset in infancy presenting with anemia and hemorrhage, diarrhea, protein-losing enteropathy, intussusception, and rectal bleeding. The course in such infants is fulminant and, even despite colectomy, in severe cases, death occurs before the age of 2 years.

There is little doubt that juvenile polyposis is a premalignant condition. There is a 15 % incidence of colorectal carcinoma occurring in patients under the age of 35 years, leading to a cumulative lifetime risk of CRC of 38–68 % with a mean age of colonic neoplasia onset between 38 and 44 years [4].

Genetics of Juvenile Polyposis

JPS is a fully penetrant condition with variable expression. Sixty percent of cases are familial and the others occur sporadically. Germline mutations in SMAD4, BMPR1A, and ENG1 cause JPS. Approximately 54 % of JPS cases will have a detectable mutation [5].

Patients with the SMAD4 mutation on chromosome 18q21.2 appear to have a higher risk of gastric polyps and hereditary hemorrhagic telangiectasia (HHT). The latter condition is characterized by cutaneous telangiectasia and risk of arteriovenous malformations. Patients found to have the SMAD4 mutation should be screened for cerebral and pulmonary arteriovenous malformations associated with HHT [6]. BMPR1A is located on chromosome 10q22.3 and accounts for another 20 % of JPS patients. ENG1 mutation on gene 9q34.1 has recently been described in JPS patients without HHT.

Screening and Follow-Up

Once the gene mutation has been identified in the index patient, other at risk family members should be tested. All children of an affected adult will have a 50 % chance of inheriting the mutation, and if the family mutation is known, children should undergo genetic screening.

Proposed guidelines suggest affected children should undergo colonoscopic surveillance every 2 years or earlier if symptoms arise [7]. In those families where the gene mu-

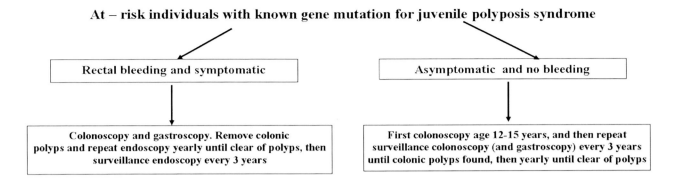

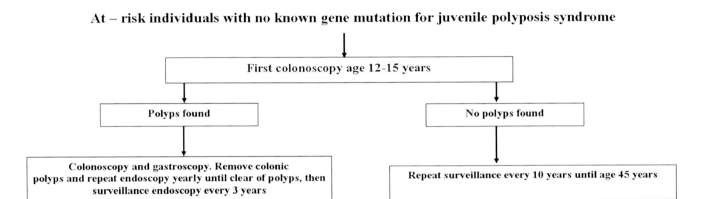

Fig. 52.1 Screening and surveillance algorithm for juvenile polyposis syndrome

tation is not known, first-degree relatives of patients with JPS should be screened by a single colonoscopy starting at age 12–15 years, even when the subject is asymptomatic (Fig. 52.1).

Full colonoscopy is necessary as right-sided polyps are the most common. All polyps should be resected. Annual colonoscopy is performed until all polyps have been resected after which the screening interval is stretched to every 2–3 years. Gastroscopy is commenced from mid-teens. Colectomy is warranted for patients with cancer, dysplasia, or high polyp burden with symptoms that cannot be controlled endoscopically.

PTEN Hamartoma Tumor Syndrome

This group comprises three rare genetic syndromes: Cowden syndrome, BRRS syndrome, and Proteus syndrome (the latter has very few intestinal features). All are associated with a mutation in the PTEN gene located at 10q23.3 [8]. All three syndromes are characterized more by extraintestinal manifestations than intestinal polyposis. The PTEN mutation can be detected in 80 % of patients with Cowden, 60 % with BRRS, and 50 % with Proteus syndrome.

Cowden syndrome rarely presents in childhood. Clinical manifestations include macrocephaly, papillomatous papules, mucocutaneous lesions, facial trichilemmoma, and acral keratosis. It carries a 50 % risk of breast cancer in adult women and a 10 % lifetime risk of epithelial thyroid cancer. Guidelines presently recommend screening for breast, thyroid, endometrial, and kidney cancer from the age of 18–25 years.

BRRS presents in childhood with gastrointestinal hamartomas, particularly in the ileum and colon, which cause intussusception, rectal bleeding, and hypoalbuminemia. There are additional characteristics including macrocephaly, developmental delay, abnormal metacarpal and phalanges, pectus excavatum, scoliosis, genital pigmentation, and hemangiomatosis. BRRS presents prior to adolescence, and there is value in genetic testing in early childhood in a family where the mutation has been identified. Patients with BRRS need regular colonoscopy and small-bowel surveillance as they are at risk of anemia, intussusception, and hypoalbuminemia from the polyposis. They carry a probable lifetime increased risk of cancer, and surveillance is recommended from age 18–25 years focusing on renal, thyroid, and breast cancer [9].

Peutz–Jeghers Syndrome

Clinical Features and Diagnosis

PJS is a rare autosomal dominant condition with a prevalence of 1 in 50,000 to 1 in 200,000 live births. It is characterized by mucocutaneous pigmentation and the presence of hamartomatous polyps throughout the gastrointestinal tract. Polyps arise primarily in the small bowel and to a lesser extent in the stomach and colon. Polyps are most commonly found in the jejunum and cause bleeding and anemia, or intussusception and obstruction from an early age. Presumptive diagnosis can be made in those with a positive family history and typical PJS freckling.

Pigmentation tends to arise in infancy, occurring around the mouth, nostrils, perianal area, fingers, toes, and the dorsal and volar aspects of hands and feet. The primary concern to the pediatrician is the risk of small-bowel intussusception causing intestinal obstruction, vomiting, and pain (Fig. 52.2). In addition, intestinal bleeding—with melena, hematemesis, and rectal bleeding—can occur, leading to anemia.

Genetics of PJS

As with other hamartomatous syndromes, PJS has an autosomal dominant pattern of inheritance, and many cases may be sporadic new mutations. The mutated gene *STK11(LKB1),* located on chromosome 19p 13.3, can be identified in up to 90% of PJS patients [10]. After appropriate genetic counseling and informed consent, testing at-risk family members may be performed early in childhood so that gastrointestinal surveillance can commence before gastrointestinal complications arise.

Screening, Management, and Complications

Individuals at risk of PJS should be evaluated in infancy for pigmented lesions and gastrointestinal symptoms. Asymp-

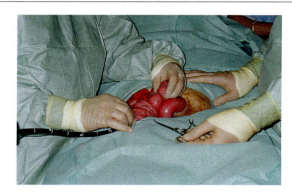

Fig. 52.3 Intraoperative enteroscopy performed at laparotomy for intussusceptions in a patient with PJS

tomatic at risk children should undergo genetic testing for the family proband mutation in the STK11/LKB1 mutation if known, soon after infancy, so the family can access medical care early if the child develops symptoms consistent with small-bowel obstruction.

The management of a young child with mid-gut PJS polyps is controversial, but recommended guidelines have been published [11]. Children who present with mid-gut complications need polypectomy either by laparotomy and intraoperative enteroscopy (IOE; Fig. 52.3) or double balloon enteroscopy (DBE). An IOE is recommended in any patient with PJS undergoing laparotomy, as careful endoscopy via an enterotomy in the small bowel allows identification and removal of polyps, thus avoiding multiple enterotomies and the risk of short bowel syndrome associated with resection. This technique is superior to palpation and transillumination in identifying polyps, and removal of all detected polyps ("clean sweep") reduces re-laparotomy rate significantly [12].

DBE with polypectomy of PJS polyps in the small bowel carries a significant risk of perforation and should be performed only by those who are expert in polypectomy. Muscularis mucosa commonly invaginates into the large pedunculated stalk increasing the risk of perforation at electrocautery (Fig. 52.4). DBE can be combined with laparoscopy to assess perforations that may arise at polypectomy.

Endoscopic evaluation of the upper and lower gastrointestinal tract and imaging of the small bowel should be performed from the age of 8 years. Screening should start earlier if symptoms are present before this. The development of video capsule endoscopy (VCE) has replaced barium enterography as the preferred technique for assessing the small bowel [13]. VCE is more sensitive, preferred by patients, and reduces the lifetime risk from cumulative radiation exposure. An acceptable alternative to VCE is MRI enterography with a close correlation between the two modalities, especially with polyps > 15 mm [14]. The advantages and disadvantages of prophylactic polypectomy for asymptomatic patients should be discussed with the family (Fig. 52.5). Prophylactic

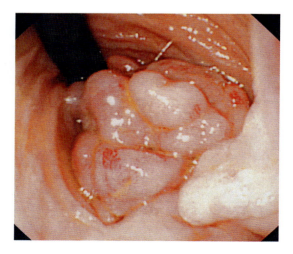

Fig. 52.2 Large obstructing duodenal PJS polyp seen at gastroscopy

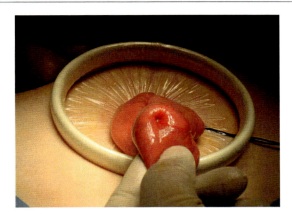

Fig. 52.4 Indentation of the serosal surface of the ileum from intus-scepting PJS polyp

Table 52.3 Suggested program for screening for malignancies in Peutz–Jeghers syndrome after adolescence

General
Annual hemoglobin and liver function tests
Annual clinical examination
Genital tract
Annual examination and testicular US biennial from birth until 12 years
Cervical smear every 3 years from age 25 years
Gastrointestinal
Baseline EGD/colonoscopy age 8
Polyps detected, continue 3 yearly until 50 years
No polyps detected, repeat age 18 years, then every 3 years until 50 years
VCE every 3 years from age 8 years
Breast
Monthly self examination from age 18 years
Annual breast MRI from age 25–50, thereafter annual mammography

polypectomy of larger small-bowel polyps (> 1.5 cm) by intraoperative or DBE should be performed in order to reduce the incidence of subsequent complications and the requirement for emergency laparotomy.

The risk of neoplasia is well documented in young adults. A meta-analysis to assess the risk of cancer in PJS identified a relative risk for all cancers in PJS patients (aged 15–64) of 15.2 compared to the normal population, with tumors. Clinicians caring for adolescents with PJS should be aware of unusual symptoms and have a low threshold for investigating potential malignancies. A recommended screening program for PJS patients after adolescence is shown in Table 52.3.

***EGD** esophagogastroduodenoscopy, **VCE** video capsule endoscopy, **MRI** magnetic resonance imaging Adenomatous Polyposis Syndromes*

Familial Adenomatous Polyposis

In children, GI adenomas are almost always associated with hereditary adenomatous polyposis syndromes. FAP is characterized by the development of hundreds of adenomas in the colon and rectum as well as several extra colonic mani-

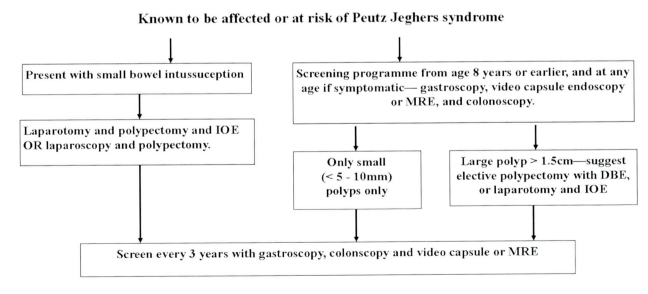

DBE = double ballon enteroscopy
IOE = intraoperative enteroscopy
MRE = magnetic resonance enterography

Fig. 52.5 Screening and surveillance algorithm for Peutz–Jeghers syndrome *MRE* magnetic resonance enterography, *DBE* double-balloon enteroscopy, *IOE* intraoperative enteroscopy

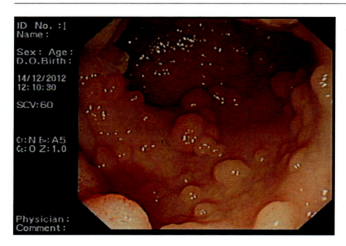

Fig. 52.6 Endoscopic appearance of large adenomatous polyps seen in advanced FAP

festations. Almost all affected patients will develop aCRC if not detected and treated at an early stage.

Clinical Features

Patients with FAP typically develop multiple adenomas throughout the large bowel—usually more than 100 and sometimes more than 1000 (Fig. 52.6). Polyps begin to appear in childhood or adolescence and increase in number with age. The standard clinical diagnosis of typical/classical FAP is based on the identification of >100 colorectal adenomatous polyps. By the fifth decade, CRC is almost inevitable if colectomy is not performed. Attenuated FAP (AFAP) is a milder form of the disease which is observed in

8% of cases. It is characterized by fewer adenomas and later presentation [15].

Gastric fundic gland polyps occur in the antrum in 50% of FAP-affected adults, and small-bowel adenomas also occur and neither requires intervention. Children under 5 years of age may develop hepatoblastoma, with an increased risk in boys [16]. Adult patients are at increased risk of malignancies of the duodenum and ampulla of Vater, with a lifetime risk of duodenal adenomas of 100%. Duodenal adenomas will progress to malignancy if untreated in 5% of adults and are the second most common malignancy in FAP and AFAP. In addition, FAP is associated with an increased risk of cancers of the thyroid, brain, and pancreas while papillary carcinoma of the thyroid has been reported in adolescence.

Extraintestinal manifestations are common (see Table 52.4). Pigmented ocular lesions (previously termed congenital hypertrophy of the retinal epithelium or CHRPE) are found in some but not all cases.

Genetics of FAP

FAP is an autosomal dominant inherited condition caused by a mutation in the adenomatous polyposis coli (APC) gene occurring in 1:10,000 births. In 20–30% of cases, the condition is caused by a spontaneous mutation with no clinical or genetic evidence of FAP in the parents or family.

The gene responsible for FAP, *APC*, is located on chromosome 5q21 and appears to be a tumor-suppressor gene [17]. Most mutations are small deletions or insertions which result in the production of a truncated APC protein which then predisposes to adenoma formation. Many mutations have been identified on this large gene, and there is a correlation

Table 52.4 Extracolonic manifestations of FAP in children and young adults

Site	Examples
Bone	Osteomas, mandibular, and maxillary
	Exostosis
	Sclerosis
Dental abnormalities	Impacted or supernumerary teeth
	Unerupted teeth
Connective tissue	Desmoid tumors
	Excessive intra-abdominal adhesions
	Fibroma
	Subcutaneous cysts
Eyes	Congenital hypertrophy of the retinal pigment epithelium
CNS	Glioblastomas, for example, Turcot's syndrome
Adenomas	Stomach
	Duodenum
	Small intestine
	Adrenal cortex
	Thyroid gland
Carcinomas	Thyroid gland
	Adrenal gland
Liver	Hepatoblastoma

Fig. 52.7 APC protein domains showing FAP genotype-phenotype correlation with codon number *APC* adenomatous polyposis coli, *FAP* familial adenomatous polyposis, *CHRPE* congenital hypertrophy of the retinal epithelium

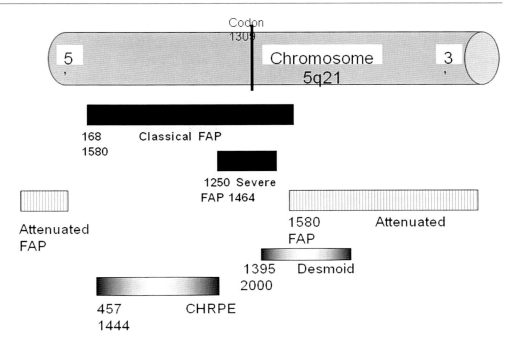

between the genetic site and severity of clinical manifestation. Mutations between codons 1250 and 1464 (Fig. 52.7), and especially those with a mutation at codon 1309, are associated with a severe form of FAP. Mutations localized at the extreme ends of the gene and in the alternatively spliced part of exon 9 are associated with a mild form of FAP, and an intermediate expression of disease is found in patients with mutations in the remaining parts of the gene. Other phenotype–genotype correlations have been observed [18]. These correlations are not absolute, and there may be considerable intrafamilial variation suggesting that there are other factors involved in the pathogenesis of the disease. Families need to be aware that the mutation may only be detected in 70–90 % of cases.

Diagnosis: Interpretation of the Genetic Test and Clinical Screening in FAP

In order to determine the appropriate screening protocol for a given family, the first step would be to seek which mutation is present in the FAP affected index case. If a mutation cannot be found, the genetic testing is non-informative, and it will not be possible to offer predictive testing to asymptomatic at-risk relatives.

When family-specific mutation is identified, directed DNA diagnostic techniques can be readily used to predict FAP in other family members. The absence of the gene mutation in other family members is considered accurate in excluding FAP, and the subject should be considered to hold an average population risk for the subsequent development of adenomas and cancer. Such genotype negative individuals can be discharged from follow-up.

The presence of the family-specific gene mutation confirms the diagnosis of FAP, and such patients should undergo

endoscopic assessment. The diagnosis is confirmed by finding polyps upon sigmoidoscopy or colonoscopy which are histologically confirmed as adenomas (see Fig. 52.2). Teenagers predicted at gene testing to be affected will require a full colonoscopy by the age of 14–16, preferably beginning at age 10–12 years [19], to determine polyp density and location, and degree of dysplasia. Upper endoscopic surveillance of the stomach, duodenum, and periampullary region with a side-viewing endoscope is recommended after the age 20 years, unless the patient has symptoms such as upper abdominal pain which warrant earlier investigation.

For families in which the genotype is not known, protocols vary. It is necessary to perform annual sigmoidoscopy on all first-degree relatives until adenomas are found.

No patient should undergo screening for FAP without detailed counseling. The individual being screened must understand the nature of the test and its possible outcomes. Many authorities feel that the child should be involved in the decision-making process, and the diagnosis be delayed until the child is old enough to contribute to the screening program, for example, from the age of 11 years onwards [20]. Although parents might request testing of a child or infant at a young age, there is value in deferring a test until the child or adolescent can participate in the discussion [21]. Well-informed consent, as a mature minor, prior to predictive testing is the most desirable outcome. There are psychological issues, as well as family, insurance, and employment implications, which may arise in the case of a positive result. These should be discussed prior to testing, and there should be a clear protocol for posttest management [22].

The current advice is to commence endoscopic surveillance from the early teens. Some patients, especially those with a mutation located at codon 1309 in the APC gene, may develop severe polyposis of the colorectum before the age of 10, and therefore, attention must be paid to FAP-related symptoms. These symptoms may include increasing bowel movements, looser stools, mucous discharge, rectal bleeding, abdominal, or back pain. In symptomatic patients, endoscopic investigation may be indicated at any age. Severe dysplasia and even malignancy have been documented in children with FAP under the age of 12 years. Consequently, those children from families in which severe dysplasia or carcinomas have been found at a young age should undergo screening at an earlier age [23]. Some clinicians advocate annual screening for hepatoblastoma with liver palpation, ultrasound, and serum á-fetoprotein levels in at-risk children between the ages of 0–6 years.

Management of FAP

Internationally agreed guidelines are currently in place for the management of patients with FAP [24]. If adenomas are detected, colonoscopic investigations should be performed annually until colectomy is planned [25]. Colectomy is currently the only effective therapy that eliminates the inevitable risk ofCRC. In the absence of severe dysplasia, colectomy is usually performed in mid- to late teens or early 1920s to accommodate work and school schedules. Almost all screen-detected adolescents are asymptomatic and therefore may not be willing to contemplate interruptions in their schooling or effects on relationships. The surgical option, therefore, must not only be carefully timed but also have low morbidity and excellent functional result.

Colectomy is indicated as soon as there are more that 100 adenomas (measuring up to 5 mm) or adenomas showing a high degree of dysplasia. The timing of primary preventative surgery may be influenced by knowledge of the mutation site and the likely severity of the polyposis. For example, patients with a deletion at codon 1309 should be offered earlier surgery since this phenotype is characterized by a large numbers of polyps and a higher risk of cancer [26].

Surgical options are either subtotal colectomy with ileo-rectal anastomosis (IRA), or restorative proctocolectomy with ileal pouch anal anastomosis (IPAA or pouch procedure). The IRA is a low risk operation with good functional results and can be performed laparoscopically. There is no pelvic dissection, and therefore, attendant risks of hemorrhage, loss of fertility in women, and damage to adjacent organs such as the ureters are avoided. Complication rates after IRA are low, and postoperative bowel function is almost always good, averaging four semi-formed stools daily. After the IRA, the rectum remains at risk of cancer. Therefore, postoperative six-monthly surveillance of the rectum is mandatory.

An IPAA procedure removes the CRC risk almost completely, but is more complicated than an IRA. It carries a higher morbidity and risk of complications. It often requires a temporary loop ileostomy, reoperations and longer hospital stays, night evacuation and decreased fertility in women [27]. Bowel frequency is generally higher than that for an IRA. The risk of cancer does exist after IPAA as they may develop at the anastomosis or below. The pouch should be examined regularly postoperatively for adenomas [28].

The advantages of an IPAA with a lower risk of cancer must be balanced against the higher operative morbidity. Conversion after an IRA to an ileoanal pouch can be carried out when the patient is older [29]. An IPAA is the treatment of choice if the patient has a large number of rectal adenomas, for example, > 15–20 adenomas, if there is presence of adenoma with severe dysplasia, a colon with > 1000 adenomas or those with high-risk genotypes (e.g., codon 1309) [30, 31]. In patients with only a few rectal adenomas or with a polyp-free rectum, both options are possible although an IRA may be preferable. The decision can be made on an individual basis, considering preoperative sphincter function, patient compliance, and risk of desmoid.

Desmoid Disease

Desmoids are locally aggressive but non-metastasizing myofibroblastic lesions which occur with disproportionately high frequency in patients with FAP. Putative risk factors include abdominal surgery, positive family history for desmoids, and site of the mutation (mutations beyond codon 1444). In contrast to sporadic desmoid tumors, the majority of the tumors associated with FAP are located in the abdominal wall or intra-abdominally. The tumors can be diagnosed by CT scanning or MRI. Desmoids occur most commonly in the peritoneal cavity (Fig. 52.8) and may infiltrate locally leading to small bowel, ureteric, or vascular obstruction. These lesions may progress rapidly or may resolve spontaneously, their unpredictable nature making them difficult to treat [32]. Attempted surgical resection carries a high morbidity and mortality and usually stimulates further growth. The options for treatment are pharmacological (nonsteroidal anti-inflammatory drugs (NSAIDs) [33] and/or anti-estrogens), chemotherapy, surgical excision, or radiotherapy. Pediatricians treating children with extraintestinal desmoid tumors should consider the possibility of FAP in the family.

Chemoprevention

NSAIDs may be protective against colon cancer by inhibiting prostaglandin synthesis via their effects on cyclooxygenase (COX). Publications have shown a significant reduction in the number of rectal polyps in those patients taking the NSAID sulindac after colectomy. However, despite protracted drug use, the adenomas still progressed with case reports of rectal cancer. Sulindac administered before the development of polyps in genotype-positive adolescents did not prevent the development of adenomas.

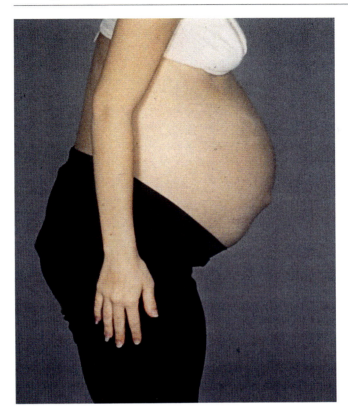

Fig. 52.8 Intra-abdominal mass from a desmoid tumor seen in a teenager with FAP

Cyclo-oxygenase-2 (COX-2) enzyme is induced in inflammatory and neoplastic tissue. Selective COX-2 inhibitors generate fewer gastrointestinal-related side effects compared to the classical non-selective NSAIDs. One of these drugs (celecoxib) was found to reduce the number of colorectal adenomas by 28% [34] and also to reduce the number of duodenal adenomas [35]. Unfortunately, cardiovascular side effects have been reported in patients using selective COX-2 inhibitors [36]. Although NSAIDs cannot replace surgical treatment for colonic FAP, they may play a role in postponing surgery in patients with mild colonic polyposis, or patients with rectal polyposis after prior colectomy. Other agents investigated but with so far inconclusive effect on polyp burden include: vitamin C, oral calcium, and ornithine decarboxylase inhibitor difluoromethylornithine (DFMO) and eicosapentaeoic acid present in fish oil [37, 38].

Prognosis
Genetic investigations, colonic surveillance, and prophylactic colectomy have impacted favorably on mortality inFAP-affected patients. Studies that evaluated the mortality of patients with FAP reported that surveillance policies and prophylactic colectomy have resulted in a reduction in the number of FAP patients that died from CRC. Currently, a greater proportion of deaths are attributable to extracolonic manifestations of the disease (desmoid tumors, duodenal cancer). Central registration in a family cancer registry and prophylactic examination lead to a reduction of CRC-associated mortality and ensure appropriate follow up and patient support.

MYH-Associated Polyposis and Lynch Syndrome

MYH-associated polyposis (MAP) is characterized by the presence of adenomatous polyposis of the colorectum and an increased risk of CRC. Patientspresent with a variable number of polyps but no apparent extra-colonic features. This autosomal recessive condition results from a compound heterozygote of the *mutY* human homologue (MYH) gene located on chromosome 1p. MYH polyposis should have no pediatric implications as colonic polyposis typically occurs in patients in their 40s, although cancer and polyps can occur at earlier ages. Surveillance colonoscopy in affected individuals should commence at age 25 years.

Lynch syndrome is an inherited condition with a high penetrance for the development of early CRC caused by an alteration in DNA mismatch repair genes *(MLH1, MSH2, MSH6, PMS2)*. With no described pediatric complications, the syndrome is associated with colorectal, endometrial, ovarian, gastric, renal tract, and other cancers. The median age for the development of CRC in Lynch syndrome is approximately 44 years and is uncommon below the age of 25 years. Revised criteria (Amsterdam II or Bethesda criteria) exist to help identify affected families and enable genetic testing for the DNA mismatch repair genes in early adulthood. Once identified as at risk, colonoscopic surveillance should be undertaken from the age of 20–25 years.

Other Polyposis Syndromes

Gorlin syndrome is an autosomal dominant condition comprising upper gastrointestinal hamartomas and pink or brown macules in exposed areas such as the face and hands.

Turcot's syndrome (also referred to as brain tumor-polyposis syndrome) is characterized by concurrence of a primary brain tumor (most often glioblastoma multiforme) and multiple colorectal adenomas. The number of adenomas is often not high, but many of the reported patients have been adolescents. Patients with a polyposis syndrome and neurological symptoms should undergo thorough neurological examination and investigation for possible brain tumor.

In patients with long-standing inflammatory colitis, inflammatory polyps (pseudopolyps) may develop. Inflammatory polyps are of no significance and have no malignant potential.

The Role of a Polyposis Registry

There are numerous advantages to integrating a family into a cancer/polyposis registry. Polyposis registries are established across the world. A polyposis registry enables registration of polyposis patients and family members accessing counseling and genetic testing and initiation and coordination of screening of family members at risk of a polyposis syndrome. By increasing the rate of diagnosis of FAP and other polyposis syndromes, and enabling earlier diagnosis, there is proven improved survival of patients registered, almost certainly attributable to the improvement in organization and coordination of patient screening [39].

Other Tumors of the GI Tract (Excluding the Stomach and Hepato-biliary)

Gastrointestinal Stromal Tumors

Gastrointestinal stromal tumors (GISTs) are a unique variety of mesenchymal tumors that have recently been described. They are very uncommon among children and adolescents, and their true incidence is not well known due to the small number of described cases.

The overall incidence rates of GIST are reported to range between 6.5 and 14.5 per million per year [40–42]. The UK National Registry of Childhood Tumours showed an annual incidence of 0.02 per million children below the age of 14 years [43].

GISTs were described for the first time in 1990 and probably arise from neural interstitial cells of Cajal. Its molecular oncogenetics derives from mutations in the KIT oncogene (v-**kit** Hardy-Zuckerman 4 feline sarcoma viral **oncogene** homolog) that encode for class III receptor tyrosine kinases and platelet-derived growth factor receptor alpha (PDG-FRA), which are expressed in GIST patients. About 0–10% of pediatric GISTs have an oncogenic KIT mutation [44–46], and only two patients were reported with a PDGFRA mutation to date [47, 48] which reflects probably other downstream activation pathway other than c-Kit mutation. A small subgroup of syndromic GISTs were found to have common germline mutations encoding the succinate dehydrogenase (SDH) gene [48, 49]. Recently, another molecule, IGF1R (insulin growth factor receptor 1), was found to be significantly expressed in a series of 17 GIST including one pediatric GIST, both by Western blot analysis and immunohistochemistry, and that it seems to be a new attractive pathway for this complex oncogenetic process [50].

Immunohistochemically, these tumors stain positive for vimentin (CD-117, a *c-kit* proto-oncogene protein) and CD-34—and stain negatively for smooth muscle actin [51]. Since the use of CD117 staining in 2002, 82% of mesenquimatous tumors were considered to be GISTs, so its' true inci-

dence rose since there, with a proportional decline of smooth muscle tumors cases [52]. Histologically, GISTs are composed either of spindle-shaped cells, epithelioid cells, or a combination of both, being spindle-shaped type slightly more frequent in a large analysis of 99 of 113 pediatric cases [53].

GISTs can present as sporadic or inherited cases, and the latter can be inherited through familial autosomal dominant fashion or as syndromic tumors, named as the Carney triad.

Carney Triad

GIST can occur rarely in association with other tumor syndromes. The association of gastric leiomyosarcoma, extra-adrenal paraganglioma and pulmonary chondroma was first described in 1977 and subsequently named the Carney triad [54]. It affects predominantly females, and it has been described as a chronic benign-course tumor that comprises recently also adrenocortical tumors and esophageal leiomyoma [55–57]. Neither KIT, PDGFRA, nor SDH mutations were found in patients with the Carney triad. In 2002, Carney and Stratakis distinguished an inherited tumor syndrome comprising GIST and paragangliomas which have common germline mutations encoding SDH subunits B, C, D, and it was termed Carney–Stratakis diad [58].

Familial

Familial GIST cases are very rare, and they are autosomal dominant inherited. They differ from Carney dyad as they are heritable germline KIT mutations tumors. Occurrence of multiple tumors can be observed both in syndromic [59–64] and in sporadic GIST. Familial GISTs do not have female predominance, and the main location is small intestine, in contrast to sporadic GIST where the stomach is the main affected place [61, 65]. Other phenotypic characteristics associated with familial GIST include mastocytosis [66], dysphagia [67, 68], cutaneous hyperpigmentation or urticaria pigmentosa [59, 61, 64, 69, 70], and recurrent small intestinal diverticular perforation [68]. Familial GIST does not develop early in life, as the youngest patient in a GIST family described to this date had symptoms at 18 years old [70].

Sporadic

A considerable number of articles describing children and adolescents with sporadic GIST have been published [71–73]. Sporadic GISTs have been described in newborns [72–75], but the majority of cases become symptomatic in the second decade of life. There is a strong female predominance with a male-to-female ratio of 1:2.5.

The majority of pediatric GISTs are located in the stomach (mainly in the antrum) [45, 72–74, 76–80], but it can be found virtually in every digestive tube segment as well as mesentery, omentum, and abdominal wall [81–84].

Clinical presentations vary from upper gastrointestinal bleeding with anemia and anemia-related symptoms to non-

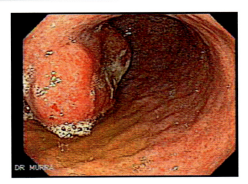

Fig. 52.9 GIST in the stomach *GIST* gastrointestinal stromal tumors

specific symptoms such as loss of appetite, poor feeding, abdominal pain, abdominal distension, nausea, vomiting, constipation, epigastric discomfort, diarrhea, and intestinal obstruction [53]. Sometimes they are incidentally discovered in a routine abdominal examination as a palpable mass, suggestive for a more advanced stage of the disease, or at ultrasound [53].

GISTs generally have a nodular growth pattern, with frequent submucosal spreading. Surface ulceration may result in acute or chronic bleeding which promotes clinical investigation (Fig. 52.9). Gastrointestinal contrast series denote solitary or multiple nodular round filling defects. Even without metastases on presentation, submucosal spreading can occur, so endosonography can be a very useful diagnostic resource [44, 80, 85–87]. Other image tools include abdominal and thoracic CT or MRI to perform disease staging. Metastases on diagnosis are not frequent, but they may occur in the liver (most commonly), lymph nodes, peritoneum, and mesentery. Even without metastasis on diagnosis, these are very frequent places for recurrent disease [47, 72, 76, 77, 87].

Fluorodeoxyglucose-positron emission tomography (FDG-PET) seems to be a sensitive diagnostic tool, particularly to monitor treatment response. The final diagnosis is based on histology and immunohistochemistry. Tissue samples can be obtained either by biopsy or by tumor resection, which in many cases of small localized disease, is usually the only procedure needed [88].

There are no algorithms for children GIST workup as well as for the treatment. As in adults, total resection with microscopic free margins is the gold standard treatment. Adjunctive therapy from conventional cytotoxic chemotherapy had no positive results. Localized disease is usually cured by surgery, and it can be performed more than once in recurrent disease or in incomplete primary resection. Metastases should undergo surgical treatment as lymph node dissection and resection of hepatic-affected areas [88].

Recently, there are increasing cases of children treated with RTK inhibitors (imatinib and sunitinib), based on adult experience. They may be considered in high-risk patient such as metastatic diffuse disease or when the primary tumor cannot be fully resected. Despite the fact that there is no randomized trials in children or consensus on imatinib dosage, a starting dose of 400 mg/m^2 once daily might be suggested with a maximum dose of 400 mg bid = 2 times daily [53].

In children, prognosis depends on the results from surgery of the main tumor lesion and the presence of metastatic lesions, especially if they are not amenable to complete resection [44, 76, 77, 89–91]. Recurrences are frequent and may occur many years following diagnosis, but it seems that mortality from GIST is low, despite tumor recurrence and development of metastases.

In summary, the pathogenesis, clinical course and prognosis of GIST in children are currently insufficient due to the small number of reported cases. Future research based upon controlled randomized trials should be encouraged to inform about optimal management in this particular population.

Gastrointestinal Autonomic Nerve Tumors

Gastrointestinal autonomic nerve tumors GANT are variants of GIST. Diagnosis is based on electron microscopic studies showing neural differentiation in contrast to GIST, and the number of pediatric patients with GANT is limited to a few cases [92–97].

Inflammatory Pseudotumors

Inflammatory pseudotumors are solid tumors composed by spindle cells, myofibroblasts, plasma cells, and histiocytes that can occur in every organ system during childhood [51, 98, 99]. Lung is the most common location, whereas occurrence in the gastrointestinal tract is rare, the majority involving the stomach [100] (Fig. 52.10). They are commonly described as plasma cell granulomas or inflammatory myofibroblastic tumors. Abdominal pain is the most common presenting symptom, but may also present with dysphagia,

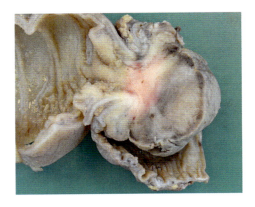

Fig. 52.10 Inflammatory pseudotumor

intestinal obstruction, and iron-deficient anemia. It affects mostly girls, as reported in the literature [98].

Like the majority of gastrointestinal tract tumors in childhood, complete surgical resection is the treatment of choice. Sporadic trials of nonsteroidal and steroidal antinflammatory medications have been reported for the treatment of large and unresectable masses. Its success rate seems to be variable [101]. Recurrence rates are reported between 18 and 40% and are more common in extrapulmonary lesions. Multiple recurrences are associated with a higher rate of malignant transformation with an overall mortality of 5–7% [51, 102, 103].

Sarcomas

Soft tissue sarcomas account for 7% of all childhood malignancies, and only 2% of this group have digestive involvement [104, 105]. Sarcomas are smooth muscle-derived neoplasms that occur anywhere along the gastrointestinal tract, more often involving the stomach and small intestine (leiomyomas) (Fig. 52.11). In the stomach, these can be confused with the appearance of an umbilicated lesion typical of an ectopic pancreas. The malignant form (leiomyosarcoma) is more common in the jejunum [106, 107]. The definition of malignancy usually is based on mitotic index at histologic examination (more than 10 mitosis per high-powered field), but in children, it is not common to see a high mitotic index that enables the adult classification of leiomyosarcoma [51]. Nearly 40% of these present with less than 5 mitoses per high-powered field, so pathologic features must also include tumor size, cellular atypia, tumor necrosis, and myxoid change [108].

Clinical presentation occurs early on life, with over half of the leiomyosarcomas occurring in the newborn period, but they can present throughout childhood and adolescence. The

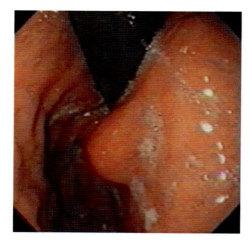

Fig. 52.11 Leiomyoma of the stomach

clinical signs vary from an incidental mass finding to active GI bleeding with associated anemia signs or acute perforation. They can also be the cause of recurrent intussusception [109–112]. Rare presentations include cough and dysphagia (if esophageal location) and oral cavity swelling [113, 114].

Symptomatic lesions may also present concurrently in patients with neurofibromatosis and in children with human immunodeficiency virus (HIV-AIDS) [115–117]. The goal of treatment is complete resection as pediatric leiomyosarcomas are less likely to be found with metastases at diagnosis [118], and the use of adjuvant chemotherapy and radiotherapy remains experimental. Long-term outcomes for leiomyosarcomas are related with the histologic type of the tumor and with successful surgical excision.

Carcinoid Tumors

Carcinoid tumors in children are quite rare, and their true incidence is unknown. The occurrence of carcinoid tumors in children was recently reported as approximately 0.1% of all pediatric cancers [71, 119]. These tumors are more prevalent in school-aged children, but younger patients have been reported. An overall female-to-male ratio of 3:1 has been noted [119]. Despite their rarity, carcinoid tumors have been described in all portions of the gastrointestinal tract from the stomach to the rectum. The most common location is the appendix, followed by involvement of the small intestine and rarely the colon and rectum [120]. Reports have also documented the presence of carcinoid tumors in gastrointestinal duplication cysts and Meckel's diverticulum [121–123]. The diagnosis is often made through the incidental pathologic findings within an appendectomy specimen. However, these tumors may present with clinical signs of hematochezia or anemia from chronic gastrointestinal blood loss, right-lower quadrant abdominal pain, and small-bowel obstruction associated signs [119, 121, 124]. The vast majority of carcinoid tumors are benign. Occasionally, they may be locally invasive, especially if originating from the colon or small intestine. Few reports have noted their malignant transformation in children, with metastasis to the liver, lung, and bone [119] Serotonin hypersecretion signs known as carcinoid syndrome with cutaneous flushing, diarrhea, asthma-like respiratory distress, and right-sided cardiac failure are quite rare [121, 124, 125].

Incidental gastrointestinal carcinoid tumors which are less than 2.0 cm diameter and without evidence of metastasis are successfully treated with complete resection, which should include tumor-free margins. For those with evidence of serosal penetration or local extension, a bowel resection with associated mesenteric resection is required, along with abdominal surveillance for metastatic disease [51]. Patients with tumors exceeding 2.0 cm in size should undergo thorough evaluation for possible metastases to the liver, lung, and bone. Serum 5-hydroxyindolacetic acid (5-HIAA) levels may act as a serologic marker of disease, but are not present in all metastatic cases. Serum chromagranin A is more reliable as a marker and does not require metastases for this to be an abnormal result. Abdominal and thoracic CT or MRI and 99m-technesium bone scan should be considered in patients with metastatic disease and/or bone pain. Children with metastatic disease often respond poorly to cytotoxic chemotherapy, but they can benefit from the administration of octreotide for symptomatic relief [119].

Gastroenteropancreatic Neuroendocrine Tumors

Pediatric gastroenteropancreatic neuroendocrine tumors (GEP-NETs) have traditionally been classified into two groups: carcinoids, which are subdivided by their origin into tumors of the *foregut* (lung, thymus, stomach, duodenum), *midgut* (jejunum, ileum, appendix, right colon), and *hindgut* (left colon, rectum), which were previously discussed, and pancreatic tumors [126]. A more useful classification was proposed by the World Health Organization in 2000: well-differentiated NETs, which show benign behavior and well-differentiated neuroendocrine carcinomas, which are characterized by low-grade malignancy and poorly differentiated NEC of high-grade malignancy [127].

These tumors can be *functional* or *nonfunctional*. Functional tumors have clinical symptoms caused by hypersecretion of hormones such as gastrin, while nonfunctional tumors can produce clinically silent hormones such as pancreatic polypeptide. The functional tumors are named according to the hormone responsible for the clinical syndrome, such as gastrinoma causing Zollinger–Ellison syndrome and insulinoma causing hypoglycemic syndrome. NETs can either be sporadic or occur as part of familial syndromes such as multiple endocrine neoplasia (MEN) I and II, von Hippel-Lindau (VHL) syndrome, and neurofibromatosis type I (NF-I) [128].

GEP-NETs are very rare in children. Tumors with gastroenteropancreatic hormone production include amine precursor uptake and decarboxylation tumors (APUDomas), extrapancreatic gastrinomas, and vasoactive intestinal polypeptide tumors [129, 130]. Pancreatic NETs account for approximately 30% of pancreatic tumors in patients younger than 20 years. While insulinomas are the most common in adults, gastrinomas are more common in children and affect more frequently the stomach. Hypersecretion of gastrin by gastrinomas causes recurrent or ectopic peptic ulcers (Zollinger–Ellison syndrome), or malabsorption diarrhea [128]. Non-gastrinoma neuroendocrine tumors can occur in any part of the pancreas [131]. Metastases are present in 60–80% of patients at initial diagnosis of gastrinoma, with the liver and lymph nodes being the most common sites of metastatic disease [132]. There is limited information in the pediatric literature regarding the imaging findings of NETs as well as treatment options. PET scan with octreotide labeling may help in diagnosis. Prognosis of this rare entity depends of disease extension and presence of metastatic disease. A recent study from a European registry showed an overall survival of 100% when complete surgical resection was performed in patients with localized neuroendocrine neoplasm (NEN) in contrast to poor survival rate associated to metastatic disease [133].

Adenocarcinoma

Progression to adenocarcinoma from polyposis syndromes such as FAP and the HNPCC is dealt with above.

Colorectal cancer's prevalence in children is very low with fewer than 500 pediatric cases reported in the literature and a few articles dealing with this as reviews [134–138]. Compared to adults who have no predetermining diseases, in children, there is usually preexisting polyposis or, rarely, colitis.

Pathogenesis
Colorectal carcinoma is due to sequential genetic mutations, commonly known as the adenoma–carcinoma sequence. Progress to malignancy happens due to the coexistence of four or more genetic problems which can include mutational activation of oncogenes and inactivation of tumor-suppressor genes.

Pathology
Colonic carcinoma in children is usually cecal or right-side colonic disease, with 50% in the ascending and transverse colon. If colonic cancer penetrates the bowel wall, it can spread to regional lymphatics and subsequently to distant lymph nodes, and metastasize to the liver, lungs, and vertebrae. Cases are staged according to the degree of local spread and presence or absence of transmural penetration, the degree of lymph node involvement, and the presence of distant metastases. In a review of younger cases with colonic cancer, 82% of these cases had either distant metastases, lymph node involvement, or transmural penetrating disease, significantly higher than adults cases.

In adults, the CRC is that of a moderate to well-differentiated adenocarcinoma. In children, this is a more aggressive type, with more proportion of tumors with mucinous (30%) and signet-ring (10%) histological appearances, hence with a poorer prognosis—this probably leads to the poorer prognosis at presentation in children (Fig. 52.12).

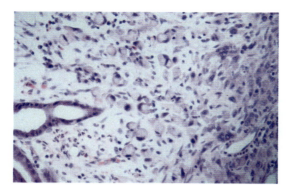

Fig. 52.12 Histological appearance of signet-ring adenocarcinoma

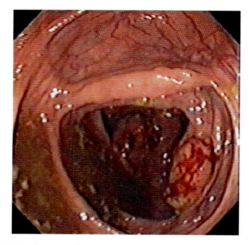

Fig. 52.13 Colonoscopic appearance of recto-sigmoid adenocarcinoma

Clinical Presentation

Abdominal pain is the main presenting symptom in the majority of cases—other symptoms include: weight loss, intussusception, vomiting, rectal bleeding, and altered bowel habit. The site of the lesion is important with constipation, obstruction, and bleeding more common with left-sided disease, and more commonly in childhood, right-sided disease which may not present with obstruction until the cancer is larger and a mass is palpable.

Diagnosis is by most usefully achieved by ileo-colonoscopy in the majority (Fig. 52.13), although the lesion can also be identified by other diagnostic techniques including wireless capsule endoscopy, ultrasound, CT colonography, or MRI. Although serological markers such as carcinoembryonic antigen (CEA) are available, their role in establishing this rare diagnosis in children has not been fully evaluated.

Treatment/Prognosis

Surgery is the most effective treatment for colonic carcinoma, with complete resection of the primary lesion and regional lymph nodes being the main aim; however, total

clearance and resection are often not possible in children due to the advanced stage at presentation. Chemotherapy for metastatic disease has poor results, and the role of radiotherapy or combination therapies grouping childhood cases is hampered by limited numbers presenting precluding viable randomized studies.

Sadly the prognosis for children with colon cancer is poor with five-year survival rates of 10–20 % [134–141]. These poor results are due to a combination of aggressive phenotype and delayed presentation.

Lymphoma

Epidemiology and Classification

In the developed world, lymphoma accounts for 10 % of all cancers in children under 15 years of age—however, it is an unusual GI condition and would need a predisposing condition in most cases, for example, celiac disease or isolation by distance (IBD). Nevertheless, cases occur without these prerequisites [142, 143].

Etiology

Non-Hodgkin's lymphoma (NHL) usually presents in association with immunodeficiency syndromes—inherited (e.g., ataxic-telangiectasia, severe combined immunodeficiency, SCID) and acquired (e.g., HIV infection), and also with immunosuppressive drug regimens such as those encountered after liver transplant [144]. Epstein–Barr virus (EBV) may play a role in disease pathogenesis especially in Burkitt's lymphoma, although malaria coinfection may be important in promoting B-cell activation as part of the process. Other conditions that give rise to chronic mucosal inflammation have also been linked to lymphoma including Helicobacter pylori. T cell NHL is associated with celiac disease, while both lymphoma and adenocarcinoma are associated with both Crohn's disease where the lesion is typically in the small bowel and with ulcerative colitis [142, 143].

Pathology

Intra-abdominal NHL in children typically is of an undifferentiated histological type—only around 50 % have a primary intestinal origin—most common intestinal primary sites are the distal ileum, cecum, and appendix. Bone marrow involvement occurs in up to 40 % of undifferentiated lymphoma while central nervous system involvement is uncommon. In Burkitt's lymphoma, 60 % can have abdominal disease.

Clinical Presentation

Disease may present with nonspecific symptoms such as abdominal distension, nausea, vomiting, altered bowel habit, and abdominal pain. Lymphomal in the GI tract is typically localized to the distal ileum and cecum and would present

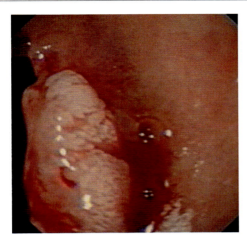

Fig. 52.14 Endoscopic appearance of small bowel lymphoma

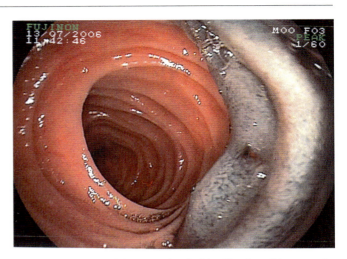

Fig. 52.16 Biopsy and then tattooing for identification of the exact site of a small bowel tumor by double-balloon enteroscopy prior to surgery

as a mass or occasionally as an ileo-cecal intussusception manifesting with obstructive symptoms or bleeding.

Endoscopy is important in diagnosis (Fig. 52.14), and when the tumor is suspected but is outside the reach of conventional endoscopes, then wireless capsule endoscopy (Fig. 52.15) and balloon enteroscopy can be useful tools in identifying lesions, and then if necessary biopsy of these lesions and tattooing, thereby accurately localizing them in case of absence of serosal abnormality for future surgical resection (Fig. 52.16). The diagnosis of NHL depends on histological examination with immunophenotyping and cytogenetics. Staging of disease with chest and abdominal imaging, lumbar puncture, and bone marrow examination is also required and may allow treatment to start if there is a delay in undertaking a laparotomy.

Treatment and Outcome

Surgical resection of local disease is indicated where it is possible, although such fully resectable disease accounts for only 60–75 % of cases [144]. The high mortality associated with intestinal perforation in more advanced disease has led to debate as to the role of partial resection as opposed to simple biopsy to establish histological type. Subsequent chemotherapy is required in all cases. For more localized disease, the overall outcome is relatively good. In the 30 % of childhood, NHL cases with localized disease cure rates as high as 95 % have been reported following combined surgical resection and combination chemotherapy [144].

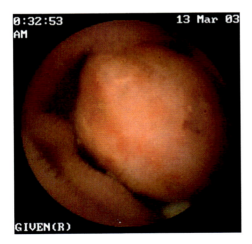

Fig. 52.15 Lymphoma in the mid-small bowel identified by wireless capsule endoscopy

References

1. Rozen P, Macrae F. Familial adenomatous polyposis: the practical applications of clinical and molecular screening. Fam Cancer. 2006;5:227–35.
2. Fox V, Perros S, Jiang H, Goldsmith J. Juvenile polyps: recurrence in patients with multiple and solitary polyps. Clin Gastroenterol Hepatol. 2010;8:795–9.
3. Jass JR, Williams CB, Bussey HJR, et al. Juvenile polyposis—a precancerous condition. Histopathology. 1988;13:619–30.
4. Brosens LA, Hattem A, Hylind LM, et al. Risk of colorectal cancer in juvenile polyposis. Gut. 2007;56:965–7.
5. Hattem W, Brosens L, Leng W, et al. Large genomic deletions of SMAD4, BMPR1A and PTEN in juvenile polyposis. Gut. 2008;57:623–7.
6. O'Malley M, LaGuardia L, Kalady M, et al. The prevalence of hereditary hemorrhagic telangiectasia in juvenile polyposis syndrome. Dis Colon Rectum. 2012;55:886–92.
7. Dunlop MG. Guidance on gastrointestinal surveillance for hereditary non polyposis colorectal cancer, familial adenomatous polyposis, juvenile polyposis, and Peutz Jeghers syndrome. Gut. 2005;51:V21–7.
8. Woodford-Richens K, Bevan S, Churchman M, et al. Analysis of genetic and phenotypic heterogeneity in juvenile polyposis. Gut. 2000;46:656–60.

9. Manfredi M. Hereditary hamartomatous polyposis syndromes: understanding the disease risks as children reach adulthood. Gastroenterol Hepatol. 2010;6:185–96.

10. Hemminki A, Markie D, Tomlinson I, et al. A serine/threonine kinase gene defective in Peutz–Jeghers syndrome. Nature. 1998;391(6663):184–7.

11. Beggs A, Latchford A, Vasen H, et al. Peutz–Jeghers syndrome: a systemic review and recommendations for management. Gut. 2010;59:975–86.

12. Spigelman AD, Thomson JPS, Phillips RKS. Towards reducing the relaparotomy rate in Peutz–Jeghers syndrome: the role of a peroperative small bowel endoscopy. Br J Surg. 1990;77:301–2.

13. Postgate A, Hyer W, Phillips R. Feasibility of video capsule endoscopy in the management of children with Peutz–Jeghers syndrome. J Pediatr Gastroenterol Nutr. 2009;49:1–7.

14. Gupta A, Postgate A, Burling D. A prospective study of MR enterography versus capsule endoscopy for the surveillance of adult patients with Peutz–Jeghers syndrome. AJR Am J Roentgenol. 2010;195:108–16.

15. Brensinger JD, Laken SJ, Luce MC, et al. Variable phenotype of familial adenomatous polyposis in pedigrees with 3′ mutation in the APC gene. Gut. 1998;43:548–52.

16. Bala S, Wunsch PH, Ballhausen WG. Childhood hepatocellular adenoma in familial adenomatous polyposis: mutations in adenomatous polyposis coli gene and p53. Gastroenterology. 1997;112:919–22.

17. Kinzler KW, Nilbert MC, Su LK, et al. Identification of FAP locus genes from chromosome 5q21. Science. 1991;253(5020):661–5.

18. Nugent KP, Phillips RK, Hodgson SV, et al. Phenotypic expression in familial adenomatous polyposis: partial prediction by mutation analysis. Gut. 1994;35(11):1622–3.

19. Church JM, McGannon E, Burke C, et al. Teenagers with familial adenomatous polyposis. Dis Colon Rectum. 2002;45:887–9.

20. Hyer W, Fell J. Screening for familial adenomatous polyposis. Arch Dis Child. 2001;84:377–80.

21. Clarke A, Gaff C. Challenges in the genetic testing of children for familial cancers. Arch Dis Child. 2008;93:911–4.

22. Giardiello FM, Brensinger JD, Petersen GM, et al. The use and interpretation of commercial APC gene testing for familial adenomatous polyposis. New Engl J Med. 1997;336(12):823–7.

23. Eccles DM, Lunt PW, Wallis Y, et al. An unusually severe phenotype for FAP. Arch Dis Child. 1997;77:431–5.

24. Vasen HF, Moslein G, Alonso A, et al. Guidelines for the clinical management of familial adenomatous polyposis (FAP). Gut. 2008;57:704–13.

25. Vasen HFA, Möslein G, Alonso A. Guidelines for the clinical management of FAP. Gut. 2008;57;704–13.

26. Caspari R, Friedl W, Mandl M, et al. FAP: mutation at codon 1309 and early onset of colon cancer. Lancet. 1994;343:629–32.

27. Bjork J, Akerbrabt H, Iselius L, et al. Outcome of primary and secondary pouch—anal anastomosis and ileorectal anastomosis in patients with familial adenomatous polyposis. Dis Colon Rectum. 2001;44:984–92.

28. Wu J, McGannon BSW, Church JM. Incidence of neoplastic polyps in the ileal pouch of patients with familial adenomatous polyposis after restorative proctocolectomy. Dis Colon Rectum. 1998;41:552–7.

29. Soravia C, O'Connor BI, Berk T, et al. Functional outcome of conversion of ileorectal anastomosis to ileal pouch-anal anastomosis in patients with familial adenomatous polyposis and ulcerative colitis. Dis Colon Rectum. 1999;42:903–7.

30. Cetta F, Gori M, Baldi C et al. APC genotype, polyp number, and surgical options in familial adenomatous polyposis. Ann Surg. 1999;229:445–6.

31. Vasen HF, van der Luijt RB, Slors JF, et al. Molecular genetic tests as a guide to surgical management of FAP. Lancet. 1996;348:433–5.

32. Clark SK, Smith TG, Katz DE, et al. Identification and progression of desmoid precursor lesion in patients with FAP. Br J Surg. 1998;85:970–3.

33. Giardiello FM, Yang VW, Hylind LM, et al. Primary chemoprevention of familial adenomatous polyposis with sulindac. N Engl J Med. 2002;346:1054–8.

34. Steinbach GD, Lynch PM, Phillips RKS, et al. The effect of celecoxib, a specific cyclo-oxygenase inhibitor in familial adenomatous polyposis. N Engl J Med. 2000;342:1946–52.

35. Phillips RK, Wallace MH, Lynch PM, et al. A randomised, double blind, placebo controlled study of celecoxib, a selective cyclooxygenase 2 inhibitor, on duodenal polyposis in familial adenomatous polyposis. Gut. 2002;50:857–60.

36. Baron JA, Sandler RS, Bresalier RS, et al. A randomized trial of rofecoxib for the chemoprevention of colorectal adenomas. Gastroenterology. 2006;131:1674–82.

37. Wallace MH, Lynch PM. The current status of chemoprevention in FAP. Fam Cancer. 2006;5:289–4.

38. West NJ, Clark SK, Phillips RKS, et al. Eiscsapentaemoic acid reduces polyp number in FAP. Gut. 2010;59:918–25.

39. Mallinson E, Newton K, Bowen J, et al. The impact of screening and genetic registration on mortality and colorectal cancer incidence in familial adenomatous polyposis. Gut. 2010;59:1378–82.

40. Nilsson B, Bumming P, Meis-Kindblom JM, et al. Gastrointestinal stromal tumors: the incidence, prevalence, clinical course, and prognostication in the preimatinib mesylate era. Cancer. 2005;103:821–9.

41. Tran T, Davila JA, El-Serag HB. The epidemiology of malignant gastrointestinal stromal tumors: an analysis of 1458 cases from 1992 to 2000. Am J Gastroenterol. 2005;100:162–8.

42. Rubio´ J, Marcos-Gragera R, Ortiz MR, et al. Population-based incidence and survival of gastrointestinal stromal tumours (GIST) in Girona, Spain. Eur J Cancer. 2007;43:144–8.

43. Stiller C, editor. Childhood Cancer in Britain: Incidence, survival and mortality. New York: Oxford University Press; 2007. 104 p.

44. Miettinen M, Lasota J, Sobin LH. Gastrointestinal stromal tumors of the stomach in children and young adults: a clinicopathologic, immunohistochemical, and molecular genetic study of 44 cases with long-term follow-up and review of the literature. Am J Surg Pathol. 2005;29:1373–81.

45. Agaram NP, Laquaglia MP, Ustun B, et al. Molecular characterization of pediatric gastrointestinal stromal tumors. Clin Cancer Res. 2008;14:3204–15.

46. Janeway KA, Liegl B, Harlow B, et al. Pediatric KIT-wild-type and platelet-derived growth factor receptor alpha-wild-type gastrointestinal stromal tumors share KIT activation but not mechanisms of genetic progression with adult gastrointestinal stromal tumors. Cancer Res. 2007;67:9084–8.

47. Kuroiwa M, Hiwatari M, Hirato J, et al. Advanced-stage gastrointestinal stromal tumor treated with imatinib in a 12-year-old girl with a unique mutation of PDGFRA. J Pediatr Surg. 2005;40:1798–801.

48. McWhinney SR, Pasini B, Stratakis CA. Familial gastrointestinal stromal tumors and germ-line mutations. N Engl J Med. 2007;357:1054–6.

49. Pasini B, McWhinney SR, Bei T. Clinical and molecular genetics of patients with the Carney–Stratakis syndrome and germline mutations of the genes coding for the succinate dehydrogenase subunits SDHB, SDHC, and SDHD. Eur J Hum Genet. 2008;16:79–88.

50. Tarn C, Rink L, Merkel E, et al. Insulin-like growth factor I receptor is a potential therapeutic target for gastrointestinal stromal tumors. Proc Natl Acad Sci U S A. 2008;105:8387–92.

51. Ladd AP, Grosfeld JL. Gastrointestinal tumors in children and adolescents. Semin Pediatr Surg. 2006;15:37–47.

52. Zhuge Y, Cheung MC, Yang R, et al. Pediatric intestinal foregut and small bowel solid tumors: a review of 105 cases. J Surg Res. 2009;156:95–102.

53. Benesch M, Wardelmann E, Ferrari A, et al. Gastrointestinal stromal tumors (GIST) in children and adolescents: a comprehensive review of the current literature. Pediatr Blood Cancer. 2009;53:1171–9.

54. Carney JA, Sheps SG, Go VL, et al. The triad of gastric leiomyosarcoma, functioning extra-adrenal paraganglioma and pulmonary chondroma. N Engl J Med. 1977;296:1517–8.

55. Carney JA. Gastric stromal sarcoma, pulmonary chondroma, and extra-adrenal paraganglioma (Carney triad): natural history, adrenocortical component, and possible familial occurrence. Mayo Clin Proc. 1999;74:543–52.

56. Diment J, Tamborini E, Casali P, et al. Carney triad: case report and molecular analysis of gastric tumor. Hum Pathol. 2005;36:112–6.

57. Knop S, Schupp M, Wardelmann E, et al. A new case of Carney triad: gastrointestinal stromal tumours and leiomyoma of the oesophagus do not show activating mutations of KIT and platelet derived growth factor receptor alpha. J Clin Pathol. 2006;59:1097–9.

58. Carney JA, Stratakis CA. Familial paraganglioma and gastric stromal sarcoma: a new syndrome distinct from the Carney triad. Am J Med Genet. 2002;108:132–9.

59. Nishida T, Hirota S, Taniguchi M, et al. Familial gastrointestinal stromal tumours with germline mutation of the KIT gene. Nat Genet. 1998;19:323–4.

60. Woz´niak A, Rutkowski P, Sciot R, et al. Rectal gastrointestinal stromal tumors associated with a novel germline KIT mutation. Int J Cancer. 2008;122:2160–4.

61. Kleinbaum EP, Lazar AJ, Tamborini E, et al. Clinical, histopathologic, molecular and therapeutic findings in a large kindred with gastrointestinal stromal tumor. Int J Cancer. 2008;122:711–8.

62. Thalheimer A, Schlemmer M, Bueter M, et al. Familial gastrointestinal stromal tumors caused by the novel KITexon 17 germline mutation N822Y. Am J Surg Pathol. 2008;32:1560–5.

63. Kang DY, Park CK, Choi JS, et al. Multiple gastrointestinal stromal tumors: clinicopathologic and genetic analysis of 12 patients. Am J Surg Pathol. 2007;31:224–32.

64. Li FP, Fletcher JA, Heinrich MC, et al. Familial gastrointestinal stromal tumor syndrome: phenotypic and molecular features in a kindred. J Clin Oncol. 2005;23:2735–43.

65. Casali PG, Jost L, Reichardt P, et al. Gastrointestinal stromal tumors: ESMO clinical recommendations for diagnosis, treatment and follow-up. Ann Oncol. 2008;19:ii35–8.

66. Hartmann K, Wardelmann E, Ma Y, et al. Novel germline mutation of KIT associated with familial gastrointestinal stromal tumors and mastocytosis. Gastroenterology. 2005;129:1042–6.

67. Hirota S, Nishida T, Isozaki K, et al. Familial gastrointestinal stromal tumors associated with dysphagia and novel type germline mutation of KIT gene. Gastroenterology. 2002;122:1493–9.

68. O'Riain C, Corless CL, Heinrich MC, et al. Gastrointestinal stromal tumors. Insights from a new familial GIST kindred with unusual genetic and pathologic features. Am J Surg Pathol. 2005;29:1680–3.

69. Carballo M, Roig I, Aguilar F, et al. Novel c-KIT germline mutation in a family with gastrointestinal stromal tumors and cutaneous hyperpigmentation. Am J Med Genet. 2005;132A:361–4.

70. Beghini A, Tibiletti MG, Roversi G, et al. Germline mutation in the juxtamembrane domain of the Kit gene in a family with gastrointestinal stromal tumors and urticaria pigmentosa. Cancer. 2001;92:657–62.

71. Bethel CA, Bhattacharyya N, Hutchinson C, et al. Alimentary tract malignancies in children. J Pediatr Surg. 1997;32:1004–9.

72. Wu SS, Buchmiller TL, Close P, et al. Congenital gastrointestinal pacemaker cell tumor. Arch Pathol Lab Med. 1999;123:842–5.

73. Bates AW, Feakins RM, Scheimberg I. Congenital gastrointestinal stromal tumour is morphologically indistinguishable from the adult form, but does not express CD117 and carries a favourable prognosis. Histopathology. 2000;37:316–22.

74. Shenoy MU, Singh SJ, Robson K, et al. Gastrointestinal stromal tumor: a rare cause of neonatal intestinal obstruction. Med Pediatr Oncol. 2000;34:70–71.

75. Geramizadeh B, Bahador A, Ganjei-Azar P, et al. Neonatal gastrointestinal stromal tumor. Report of a case and review of literature. J Pediatr Surg. 2005;40:572–4.

76. Cypriano MS, Jenkins JJ, Pappo AS, et al. Pediatric gastrointestinal stromal tumors and leiomyosarcoma. Cancer. 2004;101:39–50.

77. Prakash S, Sarran L, Socci N, et al. Gastrointestinal stromal tumors in children and young adults. A clinicopathologic, molecular, and genomic study of 15 cases and review of the literature. J Pediatr Hematol Oncol 2005;27:179–87.

78. Towu E, Stanton M. Gastrointestinal stromal tumour presenting with severe bleeding: a review of the molecular biology. Pediatr Surg Int. 2006;22:462–4.

79. Chiarugi M, Galatioto C, Lippolis P, et al. Gastrointestinal stromal tumor of the duodenum in childhood: a rare case report. BMC Cancer. 2007;7:79.

80. Bauer TM, Berlin JD. A 17 year-old man with exon 11 mutation of CD-117 causing a gastrointestinal stromal tumor. Cancer Investig. 2008;26:182–4.

81. Terada R, Ito S, Akama F, et al. Clinical and histopathological features of colonic stromal tumor in a child. J Gastroenterol. 2000;35:456–9.

82. Michail S, Broxon E, Mezoff A, et al. A rare rectal tumor presenting with encopresis and rectal bleeding in a three-year-old girl: case report and review of literature. J Pediatr Gastroenterol Nutr. 2002;35:580–2.

83. Karnak I, Kale G, Tanyel FC, et al. Malignant stromal tumor of the colon in an infant: diagnostic difficulties and differential diagnosis. J Pediatr Surg. 2003;38:245–7.

84. Gallegos-Castorena S, Marti´nez-Avalos A, Francisco Ortiz de la OE, et al. Gastrointestinal stromal tumor in a patient surviving osteosarcoma. Med Pediatr Oncol. 2003;40:338–9.

85. Price VE, Zielenska M, Chilton-MacNeill S, et al. Clinical and molecular characteristics of pediatric gastrointestinal stromal tumors. Pediatr Blood Cancer. 2005;45:20–4.

86. Suskind DL, Wahbeh G, Christie D. Gastrointestinal stromal tumor. J Pediatr Gastroenterol Nutr. 2006;43:1–2.

87. Sauseng W, Benesch M, Lackner H, et al. Clinical, radiological and pathological findings in four children with gastrointestinal stromal tumors of the stomach. Pediatr Hematol Oncol. 2007;24:209–19.

88. Demetri GD, Benjamin RS, Blanke CD, et al. NCCN task force report: management of patients with gastrointestinal stromal tumor (GIST)—update of the NCCN clinical practice guidelines. J Natl Compr Cancer Netw. 2007;5:S1–29.

89. Durham MM, Gow KW, Shehata BM, et al. Gastrointestinal stromal tumors arising from the stomach: a report of three children. J Pediatr Surg. 2004;39:1495–9.

90. O'Sullivan MJ, McCabe A, Gillett P, et al. Multiple gastric stromal tumors in a child without syndromic association lacks common KIT or PDGFRalpha mutations. Pediatr Dev Pathol. 2005;8:685–9.

91. Murray M, Hatcher H, Jessop F, et al. Treatment of wild-type gastrointestinal stromal tumor (WT-GIST) with imatinib and sunitinib. Pediatr Blood Cancer. 2008;50:386–8.

92. MacLeod CB, Tsokos M. Gastrointestinal autonomic nerve tumor. Ultrastruct Pathol. 1991;15:49–55.

93. Lauwers GY, Erlandson RA, Casper ES, et al. Gastrointestinal autonomic nerve tumors. A clinicopathological, immunohistochemical, and ultrastructural study of 12 cases. Am J Surg Pathol. 1993;17:887–97.

94. Perez-Atyade AR, Shamberger RC, Kozakewich HW. Neuroectodermal differentiation of the gastrointestinal tumors in the Carney triad. An ultrastructural and immunohistochemical study. Am J Surg Pathol. 1993;17:706–14.

95. Kodet R, Snajdauf J, Smelhaus V. Gastrointestinal autonomic nerve tumor: a case report with electron microscopic and immunohistochemical analysis and review of the literature. Pediatr Pathol. 1994;14:1005–16.

96. Kerr JZ, Hicks MJ, Nuchtern JG, et al. Gastrointestinal autonomic nerve tumors in the pediatric population. Cancer. 1999;85:220–30.

97. Varan A, Doğanci T, Taskin M, et al. Gastrointestinal autonomic nerve tumor: the youngest case reported in the literature. J Pediatr Gastroenterol Nutr. 2000;31:183–4.

98. Sanders BM, West KW, Gingalewski C, et al. Inflammatory pseudotumor of the alimentary tract: clinical and surgical experience. J Pediatr Surg. 2001;36:169–73.

99. Coffin CM, Dehner LP, Meis-Kindblom JM. Inflammatory myoblastic tumor, inflammatory fibrosarcoma and related lesions: a historical review with differential diagnostic considerations. Semin Diagn Pathol. 1998;15:102–10.

100. Riedel BD, Wong RC, Ey EH. Gastric inflammatory myofibroblastic tumor (inflammatory pseudotumor) in infancy: case report and review of the literature. J Pediatr Gastroenterol Nutr. 1994;19:437–43.

101. Williams E, Longmaid HE, Trey G, et al. Renal failure resulting from infiltration by inflammatory myofibroblastic tumor responsive to corticosteroid therapy. Am J Kidney Dis. 1998;31:E5.

102. Dao AH, Hodges KB. Inflammatory pseudotumor of the pelvis: case report with review of recent developments. Am Surg. 1998;64:1188–91.

103. Coffin CM, Waterson J, Priest JR, et al. Extrapulmonary inflammatory myfibroblastic tumor (inflammatory pseudo-tumor): a clinical and immunohistochemical study of 84 cases. Am J Surg Pathol. 1995;19:859–72.

104. Young J, Miller RW. Incidence of malignant tumors in US children. J Pediatr. 1975;86:254–85.

105. Yannopoulos K, Stout AP. Smooth muscle tumors in children. Cancer. 1962;15:958–71.

106. Kennedy AP Jr, Cameron B, Dorion RP, et al. Pediatric intestinal leiomyosarcomas: case report and review of the literature. J Pediatr Surg 1997;32:1234–6.

107. Gomez NA, Cozzarelli R, Alvarex LR, et al. Rectum leiomyoma in a 10-month-old female. Pediatr Surg Int. 2003;19:104–5.

108. Ranchod M, Kempson R. Smooth muscle tumors of the gastrointestinal tract and retroperitoneum. Cancer. 1977;39:255–62.

109. Nwako F. Benign gastrointestinal tract tumors in Nigerian children. Int Surg. 1974;59:294–6.

110. Cummings SP, Lally KP, Pineiro-Carrero V, et al. Colonic leiomyoma: an unusual cause of gastrointestinal hemorrhage in childhood. Dis Colon Rectum. 1990;33:511–4.

111. Rogers BB, Grishaber JE, Mahoney DH, et al. Gastric leiomyoblastoma (epithelioid leiomyoma) occurring in a child: a case report. Pediatr Pathol. 1989;9:79–85.

112. Luzzatto C, Galligioni A, Candiani F, et al. Gastric leiomyoblastoma in childhood: a case report and review of the literature. Z Kinderchir. 1989;44:373–6.

113. Divyambika CV, Sathasivasubramanian S, Krithika CL, et al. Pediatric oral leiomyosarcoma: rare case report. J Cancer Res Ther. 2012;8(2):282–5.

114. Wang WX, Gaurav D, Wen L, et al. Pediatric esophageal leiomyosarcoma: a case report. J Pediatr Surg. 2011;46(8):1646–50.

115. Chadwick EF, Connor EJ, Guerra Hanson IC, et al. Tumors of smooth muscle origin in HIV-infected children. JAMA. 1990;263:3182–4.

116. Molle ZL, Moallem H, Desai N, et al. Endoscopic features of smooth muscle tumors in children with AIDS. Gastrointest Endosc. 2000;52:91–4.

117. Chu MH, Lee HC, Shen EY, et al. Gastro-intestinal bleeding caused by leiomyoma of the small intestine in a child with neurofibromatosis. Eur J Pediatr. 1999;158:460–2.

118. McGrath PC, Neifeld JP, Kay S, et al. Principles in the management of pediatric intestinal leiomyosarcomas. J Pediatr Surg. 1988;23:939–41.

119. Spunt SL, Pratt CB, Rao BN, et al. Childhood carcinoid tumors: the St. Jude children's research hospital experience. J Pediatr Surg 2000;35: 1282–6.

120. Suster G, Weinberg AF, Graivier L. Carcinoid tumor of the colon in a child. J Pediatr Surg. 1977;12:739–42.

121. Goldthorn JF, Canizaro PC. Gastrointestinal malignancies in infancy, childhood, and adolescence. Surg Clin North Am. 1986;66:845–61.

122. Horie H, Iwasaki I, Takahashi H. Carcinoid in a gastrointestinal duplication. J Pediatr Surg. 1986;21:902–4.

123. Gold MS, Winslow PR, Litt IF. Carcinoid tumors of the rectum in children: a review of the literature and report of a case. Surgery. 1971;69:394–6.

124. Chow CW, Sane S, Campbell PE, et al. Malignant carcinoid tumors in children. Cancer. 1982;49:802–11.

125. Schwartz MZ. Unusual peptide-secreting tumors in adolescents and children. Semin Pediatr Surg. 1997;6:141–6.

126. Tomassetti P, Migliori M, Lalli S, et al. Epidemiology, clinical features and diagnosis of gastroenteropancreatic endocrine tumours. Ann Oncol. 2001;12 Suppl 2:S95–9.

127. Kloppel G, Perren A, Heitz PU. The gastroenteropancreatic neuroendocrine cell system and its tumors: the WHO classification. Ann N Y Acad Sci. 2004;1014:13–27.

128. Khanna G, O'Dorisio SM, Menda Y, et al. Gastroenteropancreatic neuroendocrine tumors in children and young adults. Pediatr Radiol. 2008;38:251–9.

129. Buyukpamukcu M, Berberoglu S, Buyukpanukcu N, et al. Non-lymphoid gastrointestinal malignancies in Turkish children. Medic Pediatr Oncol. 1996;26:28–35.

130. Farley DR, Van Heerdeen JA, Grant CS, et al. Extrapancreatic gastrinomas. Surgical experience. Arch Surg. 1994;129:506–12.

131. Semelka RC, Custodio CM, Cem Balci N, et al. Neuroendocrine tumors of the pancreas: spectrum of appearances on MRI. J Magn Reson Imaging. 2000;11:141–8.

132. Zollinger RM, Ellison EC, O'Dorisio TM, et al. Thirty years' experience with gastrinoma. World J Surg. 1984;8:427–35.

133. Redlich A, Wechsung K, Boxberger N, et al. Extra-appendiceal neuroendocrine neoplasms in children—data from the GPOH-MET97 study. Klin Padiatr. 2013;225(6):315–924.

134. Al-Tonbary Y, Darwish A, El-Hussein A, Fouda A. Adenocarcinoma of the colon in children: case series and mini-review of the literature. Hematol Oncol Stem Cell Ther. 2013;6(1):29–33.

135. Peneau A, Savoye G, Turck D, Dauchet L, Fumery M, Salleron J, Lerebours E, Ligier K, Vasseur F, Dupas JL, Mouterde O, Spyckerelle C, Djeddi D, Peyrin-Biroulet L, Colombel JF, Gower-Rousseau C. Mortality and cancer in pediatric-onset inflammatory bowel disease: a population-based study. Am J Gastroenterol. 2013;108(10):1647–53.

136. Kim G, Baik SH, Lee KY, Hur H, Min BS, Lyu CJ, Kim NK. Colon carcinoma in childhood: review of the literature with four case reports. Int J Colorectal Dis. 2013;28(2):157–64.

137. Singer G, Hoellwarth ME. Colorectal carcinomas in children: an institutional experience. Pediatr Surg Int. 2012;28(6):591–5.

138. Blumer SL, Anupindi SA, Adamson PC, Lin H, Price AP, Markowitz RI, Kramer SS. Sporadic adenocarcinoma of the colon in children: case series and review of the literature. J Pediatr Hematol Oncol. 2012;34(4):e137–41.

139. Griffin PM, Liff JM, Greenberg RS, Clark WS. Adenocarcinimas of the colon and rectum in persons under 40 years of age: a population-based study. Gastroenterology. 1991;100:1033–40.

140. Enker WE, Palovan E, Kirsner JB. Carcinoma of the colon in adolescents: a report of survival and an analysis of the literature. Am J Surg. 1977;133:737–41.

141. LaQuaglia MP, Heller G, Filippa DA, Karasakalides A, Vlamis V, Wollner N, Enker WE, Cohen AM, Exelby PR. Prognostic factors and outcome in patients 21 years and under with colorectal carcinoma. J Ped Surg. 1992;27:1085–90.

142. LaQuaglia MP, Stolar CJ, Krailo M, Siegel S, Meadows A, Hammond D. The role of surgery in abdominal non-Hodgkin's lymphoma: experience from the children's cancer study group. J Pediatr Surg. 1992;27:230–5.

143. Goldsby RE, Carroll WL. The molecular biology of pediatric lymphomas. J Pediatr Hematol Oncol. 1998;20:282–96.

144. Plant AS, Venick RS, Farmer DG, Upadhyay S, Said J, Kempert P. Plasmacytoma-like post-transplant lymphoproliferative disorder seen in pediatric combined liver and intestinal transplant recipients. Pediatr Blood Cancer. 2013;60(11):E137–9.

Corina Gabriela Cotoi and Alberto Quaglia

Short Introduction

The liver is mentioned in various ancient medical manuscripts such as the Edwin Smith Papyrus, an ancient Egyptian medical text from 1600 BC. It was seen as the site of origin of veins by Praxagoras of Cox in ancient Greece (340 BC), as the source of blood by Empedocles from Sicily (fifth century), as the 'seat' of life in Mesopotamia [1] and as the site of emotions and the symbol of life by other ancestors [2].

The Development of the Liver

The liver develops from the embryonic liver bud or liver diverticulum, which appears in the human embryo between the 3rd and the 4th week of gestation (4-mm embryo), arising from the ventral endodermal layer of the distal foregut (future duodenum) [3]. The mesenchymal tissue in which the liver further grows is developed from the septum transversus [4]. The forming primitive hepatocytes (or hepatoblasts) cords seem to surround mesenchymal spaces [5], and as they grow towards the septum transversus, they are penetrated by the capillary plexus that arises from the vitelline veins, forming the primitive hepatic sinusoids [6]. The mesenchymal cells interposed between the endothelial cells and the hepatoblasts will form the liver connective tissue and the liver capsule [6].

The liver haematopoietic activity starts from the 6th week, and by the 12th week, the liver is the main site of haematopoiesis, until the third trimester of intrauterine life [4, 6, 7], which fades slowly after birth [5] (see Fig. 53.1).

A caudal part of the liver bud becomes the gallbladder and its stalk, the cystic duct [7]. The intrahepatic bile ducts develop from the limiting plates of the forming hepatoblast cords in the mesenchyme adjacent to the portal vein branches, forming the ductal plates, double-layer cylindric structures, which by remodelling will evolve into the intrahepatic bile duct system. This process starts around the hepatic hilum [6, 8].

Disorders such as Caroli disease and Caroli syndrome, congenital hepatic fibrosis, autosomal recessive and autosomal dominant polycystic kidney disease and von Meyenburg complexes are considered the result of abnormalities of ductal plate development [9].

Bile formation begins in the 12th week, but the excretion into the duodenum does not happen until the 16th week of intrauterine life [6], and maybe at low levels until after birth, due to the lack of enteral nutrition. This would explain why liver injury, in cases of biliary atresia, is not present at birth but develops in the next following weeks [10].

The opening of the common bile duct into the posterior side of the duodenum is the result of the ventral pancreatic bud rotation around the duodenum [11].

In the early stages, the blood flow into the sinusoids of the developing liver is sustained through the two vitelline veins and the right and left umbilical veins, until the 5th week when the left umbilical vein becomes the main blood supply from the placenta [4]. The umbilical vein gives branches to the left liver and drains into the ductus venosus, a structure that connects it to the inferior vena cava [12]. In the 7th week, the portal vein is already formed from the anastomosing channels of the initial two vitelline veins. The hepatic artery originates from the celiac axis and the arterial system of the liver spreads from the hilum to the periphery, through the branching of the main artery [4].

Within a week after birth, the umbilical vein is obliterated and the ductus venosus is closed, forming the round ligament and the ligamentum venosum, respectively. The hepatic arterial and biliary systems are not completely mature until around 15 years of age [13].

A. Quaglia (✉) · C. G. Cotoi
Institute of Liver Studies, Kings College Hospital,
Denmark Hill, London SE5 9RS, UK
e-mail: alberto.quaglia@nhs.net

© Springer International Publishing Switzerland 2016
S. Guandalini et al. (eds.), *Textbook of Pediatric Gastroenterology, Hepatology and Nutrition*,
DOI 10.1007/978-3-319-17169-2_53

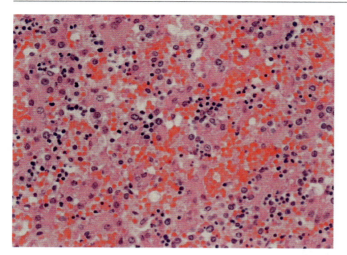

Fig. 53.1 Liver haematopoiesis

Liver Anatomy

The liver is situated in the right hypochondrium and epigastric region, reaching often the left hypochondrium, and is almost entirely protected by the ribcage. It is the largest internal organ in the human body. Its size when compared to the total body size is greater in the foetus than in the adult, constituting, in the former, about one eighteenth, and in the latter about one thirty-sixth of the entire body weight.

Classically, the liver is divided in to two large lobes (right and left) and two small central ones (quadrate and caudate lobes). Its external surfaces can be divided into superior, inferior and posterior. The superior surface lies under the diaphragm. The diaphragm separates it from the ribs and the costal cartilages on the lateral and posterior sides and the lungs with pleurae and the heart with the pericardium on the superior side. The superior and inferior surfaces are demarcated on the anterior side of the liver by a well-defined margin, the anterior border. This border is marked by two notches: the umbilical notch and the one where the gallbladder fundus lies. In children and women, this border projects below the ribs unlike in adult males where it generally corresponds with the lower margin of the thorax in the right mammillary line. Both intercostal and subcostal approaches for percutaneous liver biopsy are possible in children [14].

Most of the liver is covered by the visceral peritoneum, except for the 'bare area' on the posterior surface, which is in direct contact with the diaphragm and delimited by the coronary ligament. The porta hepatis is the entry point of the hepatic artery (to the left) and the portal vein (behind and between the duct and artery) and the exit point of the common hepatic duct (to the right). Nerves and lymphatic vessels can also be found in this region.

A few ligaments help keeping the liver in place or limit its lateral movements. The organ is connected to the diaphragm and to the anterior wall of the abdomen by five ligaments, four of which are peritoneal folds: the falciform, the coronary and two lateral (triangular) ligaments, the fifth being a fibrous cord (the round ligament) corresponding to the obliterated umbilical vein.

The subdivision of the liver into segments as proposed by Couinaud in 1957, is based on the intrahepatic distribution of the portal and hepatic veins, and is used in clinical practice, particularly in planning surgical resections. Couinaud divided the liver into two functional lobes of similar sizes, separated on the liver surface by an imaginary line going through the inferior vena cava sulcus and the middle of the gallbladder fossa. The right lobe is further divided into posterior and anterior sectors and the left lobe into medial and lateral part. Each of the two segments is separated into inferior and superior segments. Thus, eight total segments, with almost independent blood supply are formed, as follows: (I) caudate lobe, (II) superior subsegment of the left lateral segment, (III) inferior subsegment of the left lateral segment, (IV) left medial segment, (V) inferior subsegment of the right anterior segment, (VI) inferior subsegment of the right posterior segment, (VII) superior subsegment of the right posterior segment, (VIII) superior subsegment of the right anterior segment [15].

Liver Vascularisation and Innervation

The liver receives a dual blood supply through the portal vein and the hepatic artery. The hepatic artery in the foetal and early postnatal life is the largest branch of the celiac axis, its calibre decreasing with age to an intermediate size artery in adults. At the porta hepatis, it divides into a right and a left hepatic artery. They branch out progressively to terminal hepatic arterioles, which communicate with the hepatic sinusoids. The hepatic artery provides the blood supply to the biliary tree through a peribiliary plexus and forms a perivenous plexus around the portal vein branches. Hepatic artery thrombosis can cause ischemic necrosis of the biliary tree due to its dependence on the arterial supply. The portal vein drains the blood from most of the gut, and it is formed at the level of the second lumbar vertebra by the confluence of the superior mesenteric vein, inferior mesenteric vein and splenic vein. It enters the liver through the porta hepatis and subdivides into right and left branches and then progressively down to the terminal portal venules and inlet venules to open into the sinusoids. The sinusoidal blood drains into the centrilobular venules, and eventually through the hepatic veins into the inferior vena cava. Segments II, III and IV are drained by the left hepatic vein, the middle hepatic vein gathering blood from segments IV, V and VIII, while the right hepatic vein serves segments V–VIII. One small inferior hepatic vein drains the caudate lobe (segment I) directly into the inferior vena cava. Liver biopsy through the transjugular route is an established procedure to sample liver parenchyma via the hepatic veins [16].

The lymphatic drainage of the liver parenchyma occurs in two directions. One is through the porta hepatis into the celiac nodes. The other is through the falciform ligament and the bare area into the parasternal and mediastinal nodes.

The liver innervation seems to appear in the late stages of embryonic development, continues to mature postpartum, and comprises sympathetic and parasympathetic fibres [17], which enter through the porta hepatis. The capsule is supplied by a few branches of the lower intercostal nerves.

Liver Microarchitecture and Basics of Liver Histology

Various models have been proposed to define the structural and functional unit of the liver. The hexagonal lobule of Kierman, described in 1833 places the hepatic venule in the centre of the lobule and the portal tract, which contain one of each ramification of the hepatic artery, portal vein and bile duct [18]. In 1954, Rappaport proposed the concept of the hepatic acinus, which has a triangular shape, with the portal venule at the apex and the portal tracts at the base. According to the Rappaport model, the acinus is divided into three zones: zone 1, which is located in the vicinity of the portal venule, and is well oxygenated; the mid-zone (zone 2); and zone 3, situated close to the hepatic venule [19]. These two classical models are still in common usage (see Fig. 53.2).

The liver parenchyma is composed mostly of hepatocytes, arranged in a tridimensional spongiform pattern, in plates that vary in thickness, from the foetal liver to about 5 months after birth, when they form two-cell-thick trabeculae. At approximately 5 years of age, they adopt the adult pattern of one-cell-thick plates [12]. Under light microscopy, hepatocytes have a well-defined polygonal shape of approximately 25 μm in diametre. The cellular membrane can be divided into three aspects, with different characteristics: a *basolateral* aspect facing the sinusoidal lumen, a *canalicular* aspect, which delimitates the canalicular space and the *lateral* aspect between the other two. The nucleus is centrally located, and most hepatocytes are mononuclear, although binuclear hepatocytes are often found. The cytoplasm is abundant and eosinophilic, and the glycogen accumulation can be highlighted with periodic acid-Schiff stain. Periportal hepatocytes in children and adolescent show physiological vacuolated nuclei.

Stainable iron and copper accumulation are abundant in the first weeks of life, but they diminish and slowly disappear at 3–6 months of age approximately [6]. Lipofucsin is usually absent in children.

The bile canaliculi are found between two adjacent hepatocytes and they are not easily demonstrated on routine

Fig. 53.2 Lobule and acinus. **a** H&E, magnification 100×. Normal liver in which portal tracts are marked by asterisks and a centrilobular venule by a black triangle. *H&E* haematoxylin-eosin**b** Same field as (**a**) hepatic lobule. The circles demarcated the periportal and centrilobular areas. **c** Hepatic acinus. Same field as (**a**) and (**b**), but with demarcation of the acinar zones

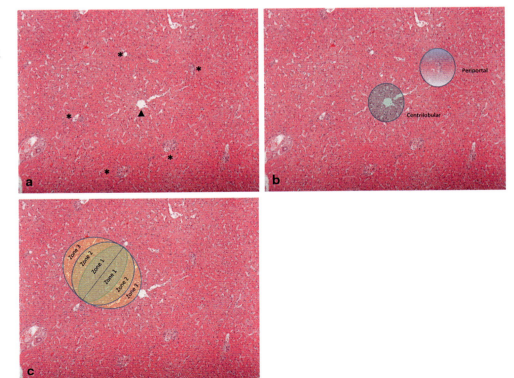

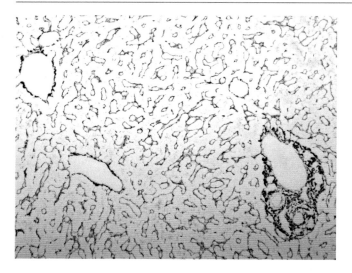

Fig. 53.3 Gordon and Sweet's reticulin stain with a portal tract on the right-hand side, hepatic plates in the middle and two cross sections of a centrilobular venules on the left-hand side. Magnification 400×

histological stains with haematoxylin–eosin (H&E). They connect to the bile ducts through the canals of Hering.

The hepatic sinusoids are lined by fenestrated endothelium. Kupffer cells rest on the internal sinusoidal surface and are a part of the reticuloendothelial system [6].

The space between the endothelial cells and the hepatocytes is defined as the space of Disse, which contains the hepatic stellate cells (Ito cells). They store retinoids, can contract affecting the sinusoidal calibre and can produce extracellular matrix participating to fibrogenesis when activated. A reticulin (silver impregnation stain) highlights the scaffolding of the liver, which is mainly composed of type III collagen [6] (see Fig. 53.3).

References

1. Porter R. The greatest benefit to mankind. A medical history from antiquity to the present. London: Harper Collins; 1997. pp. 44–82.
2. Hillman J. Commentary on chapters seven, eight and nine. In: James Hillman, Krishna Gopi, editors. Kundalini: the evolutionary energy in man with phychological commentary. London: Stuart and Watkins; 1970.
3. Reid IS. Biliary tract abnormalities associated with duodenal atresia. Arch Dis Child. 1973 Dec;48(12):952–7.
4. Crawford JM, Burt AD. Chapter 1 Anatomy, pathophysiology and basic mechanisms of disease. In: Portmann B, Ferrell L, Burt A, editors. MacSween's pathology of the liver. 6th ed. Edinburg: Churchill Livingstone Elsevier; 2012. pp. 1–77.
5. Zaret KS. Liver specification and early morphogenesis. Mech Dev. 2000 Mar 15;92(1):83–8.
6. Suriawinata AA, Thung SN. Chapter 28: Liver. In: Mills SE, Editor. Histology for pathologists. 4th ed. Philadelphia: Wolters Kluwer Health/Lippincott Williams & Wilkins; 2012. pp. 733–816.
7. Moore KL, Persaud TVN. Chapter 12: The digestive system. In: Moore KL, Persaud TVN, editors. The development of the human: clinically orienteted embryology. 6th ed. Philadelphia: WB Saunders Company; 1998. pp. 272–302.
8. Roskams T, Desmet V. Embryology of extra- and intrahepatic bile ducts, the ductal plate. Anat Rec (Hoboken). 2008 Jun;291(6):628–35.
9. Desmet, VJ. The amazing universe of hepatic microstructure. Hepatology. 2009 Aug;50(2):333–44.
10. Makin E, Quaglia A, Kvist N, Petersen BL, Portmann B, Davenport M. Congenital biliary atresia: liver injury begins at birth. J Pediatr Surg. 2009 March;44(3):630–3.
11. Ando H. Embryology of the biliary tract. Dig Surg. 2010;27(2):87–9.
12. Russo P. Chapter 27: Liver including tumors, gallbladder, and biliary tree. In: Kapur R, Oligny LL, Siebert J, Gilbert-Barness E, editors. Potter's pathology of the fetus, infant and child. 2nd ed. Philadelphia: Mosby Elsevier; 2007. pp. 1207–80.
13. Nakanuma Y, Hoso M, Sanzen T, Sasaki M. Microstructure and development of the normal and pathologic biliary tract in humans, including blood supply. Microsc Res Tech. 1997 Sept 15;38(6):552–70.
14. El-Shabrawi MH, El-Karaksy HM, Okahsa SH, Kamal NM, El-Batran G, Badr KA. Outpatient blind percutaneous liver biopsy in infants and children: is it safe? Saudi J Gastroenterol. 2012 Jan–Feb;18(1): 26–33.
15. Couinaud C. Le foie: études anatomiques et chirurgicales. Paris: Masson et Cie; 1957.
16. Dohan A, Guerrache Y, Boudiaf M, Gavini JP, Kaci R, Soyer P. Transjugular liver biopsy: indications, technique and results. Diagn Interv Imaging. 2014 Jan;95(1):11–5.
17. Delalande JM, Milla PJ, Burns AJ. Hepatic nervous system development. Anat Rec A Discov Mol Cell Evol Biol. 2004 Sept;280(1):848–53.
18. Kierman F. The anatomy and physiology of the liver. Philos Trans R Soc Lond. 1833;123(1):711–70.
19. Rappaport AM, Borowy ZJ, Lougheed WM, Lotto WN. Subdivision of hexagonal liver lobules into a structural and functional unit; role in hepatic physiology and pathology. Anat Rec. 1954 May;119(1):11–33.

Diagnostic Procedures in Pediatric Hepatology

54

Annamaria Deganello and Maria E. K. Sellars

Imaging of Cholestatic Jaundice

Neonatal

Neonatal jaundice that persists longer than 2–3 weeks demands clinical, laboratory, and radiological investigation, as early diagnosis of surgically treatable conditions leads to favorable outcomes. The role of radiology in the workup of conjugated hyperbilirubinemia is to make a distinction between obstructive cholestasis due to structural biliary anomalies and nonobstructive conditions such as genetic, metabolic, endocrinal, or infective disorders, in which imaging investigations are often normal at presentation.

High-resolution ultrasonography (US) is the imaging modality of choice in the screening of these patients and provides the radiologist with a noninvasive, nonionizing tool, independent of liver function tests.

The ultrasound approach to these patients needs to be systematic, with thorough examination of the liver parenchyma, gallbladder, bile ducts, portal venous system, spleen, and pancreas. In particular, the examiner should concentrate on the intra- and extrahepatic bile ducts, in order to detect dilatation. The common bile duct (CBD) should not exceed a caliber of 1 mm in neonates, 2 mm in infants up to 1 year of age, 4 mm in older children, and 7 mm in adolescents [1, 2]. The gallbladder needs to be evaluated in its length (normal range between 1.5 and 3 cm) and shape and for presence of gallstones, inspissated bile and irregular, thickened walls. Evaluation of portal vein patency and direction of flow, presence of collaterals as well as splenic length and ascites is needed to assess signs of portal hypertension. Finally, the size and echogenicity of the pancreas and the caliber of the pancreatic duct (which needs to be <1–2 mm) should also be recorded [3].

Absence of dilated ducts, a small, abnormal gallbladder with irregular walls and hyperechoic fibrous tissue at the porta hepatis (triangular cord sing), are suggestive but not pathognomonic features of extrahepatic biliary atresia. Signs of biliary atresia splenic malformation (BASM) syndrome also need to be sought, such as polysplenia, situs ambiguous, interrupted inferior vena cava (IVC), pre-duodenal portal vein, anomalous hepatic artery supply, and intestinal malrotation (Fig. 54.1); these patients require MRI supplemented by angiographic sequences for detailed vascular delineation, crucial for preoperative planning. Infants with biliary atresia can present with end-stage liver disease, and therefore initial US can detect coarse nodular liver parenchyma, retrograde flow in the portal vein, ascites, varices, and splenomegaly. In biliary atresia, hepatic scintigraphy will show failure of biliary excretion after 24 h; however, neonatal hepatitis could also show absent bowel activity due to poor hepatocellular function, therefore, phenobarbital is administered prior to the procedure to enhance hepatocellular function. Confirmation of diagnosis is normally achieved with liver biopsy, which will differentiate between biliary atresia and neonatal hepatitis, which is a diagnosis of exclusion.

When dilated ducts are detected, the differential will include choledochal malformation, inspissated bile syndrome and Caroli with congenital hepatic fibrosis. In these instances, the patient needs further evaluation to define the anatomy; historically, this was achieved by means of direct percutaneous cholangiography (PTC) or endoscopic retrograde cholangiopancreatography (ERCP), but the implementation of magnetic resonance imaging (MRI) with heavily T2-weighted cholangiography sequences has allowed the radiologist to achieve the diagnosis confidently and in a noninvasive way [4].

Magnetic resonance cholangiopancreatography (MRCP) can in fact classify the different types of choledochal malformations and reveal anomalies of the pancreatico-biliary junction (more often associated with type I cysts) with possible complications, such as calculi within a long common channel (Fig. 54.2).

A. Deganello (✉) · M. E. K. Sellars
Department of Radiology, King's College Hospital, Denmark Hill, London SE5 9RS, UK
e-mail: adeganello@nhs.net

© Springer International Publishing Switzerland 2016
S. Guandalini et al. (eds.), *Textbook of Pediatric Gastroenterology, Hepatology and Nutrition,*
DOI 10.1007/978-3-319-17169-2_54

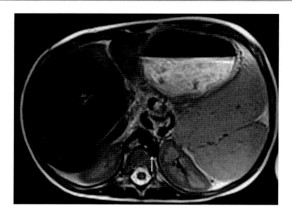

Fig. 54.1 T2W MRI image of a patient with BASM. The liver is cirrhotic with a large central regenerative nodule and atrophied left lobe and posterior segments of the right lobe. There is polysplenia and interrupted IVC with hemi-azygous continuation (*arrow*)

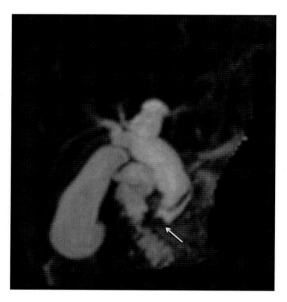

Fig. 54.2 MRCP MIP reconstruction of the biliary tree showing a type of choledocal malformation with an impacted calculus within a long common channel (*arrow*)

In case of Caroli, MRCP will show multifocal cystic dilatation of the intrahepatic bile ducts, possibly containing

filling defects, representing calculi; these cysts communicate with the biliary tree, thus excluding autosomal dominant cystic liver disease and biliary hamartomas. A specific MR finding of Caroli is the "central dot sign," a portal vein branch protruding into the lumen of a dilated duct, which enhances with gadolinium [5].

ERCP is not routinely indicated but may still be required in doubtful cases or as a therapeutic option in those patents where MRCP has identified an obstructed biliary system due to inspissated bile or choledocholithiasis (shown as signal voids).

Older Children

Jaundice in older children can be caused by hepatocellular disease (acute or chronic) and obstructive causes and imaging investigations can distinguish these entities and often establish the etiology of many chronic conditions and acquired or developmental biliary disorders.

Ultrasound findings in acute hepatitis are normally nonspecific, with US demonstrating hypoechoic parenchyma, increased periportal reflectivity due to edema, and thickened gallbladder walls.

In the context of chronic liver disease, radiology can confirm the clinical diagnosis demonstrating coarse, heterogeneous liver parenchyma and abnormal liver architecture as well as signs of portal hypertension (Fig. 54.3).

Medical causes of jaundice in older children include Wilson's disease, cystic fibrosis, glycogen storage disorder, tyrosinemia, and alpha1 antitripsin deficiency. In all these conditions, US will show nonspecific changes with hyperechoic liver parenchyma; however, these patients are prone to develop focal liver lesions (such as adenomas and, importantly, hepatocellular carcinomas) and in this instance, US is extremely useful as a noninvasive, radiation-free surveillance test. In addition, some of these conditions have specific imaging features, such as multiple small nodules with low signal intensity in T2 on MR in Wilson's disease and focal biliary cirrhosis with periportal fibrosis seen on US and MR in cystic fibrosis.

Fig. 54.3 MRI T1W (**a**) and T2W (**b**) images of a cirrhotic liver with markedly abnormal contour and varying size-regenerative nodules throughout. The portal vein is occluded and there are numerous short gastric and splenic varices (*arrows*)

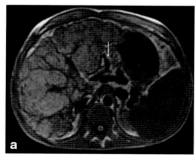
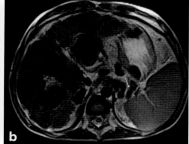

Calculi, benign strictures (as seen in primary sclerosing cholangitis, PSC), and neoplasms (which will be discussed separately) are all obstructive causes of jaundice in older children.

Calculi are seen in US as hyperechoic foci with posterior acoustic shadowing, mobile when detected within the gallbladder; these are seen as signal voids on MR. Inspissated bile is again hyperechoic in US but does not cause posterior shadowing.

Primary sclerosing cholangitis (PSC) is characterized by inflammation and fibrosis of the biliary tree, which results in cholestasis with progression to secondary biliary cirrhosis and hepatic failure. Histologically, the intrahepatic bile ducts are surrounded by cuffs of inflammatory cells and fibrosis, which results in segmental dilatation of the peripheral ducts alternated with narrow or obliterated segments, reflected in the imaging findings. The radiological diagnosis of PSC is often challenging, and needs confirmatory clinical, biochemical, and histologic findings. Traditionally, ERCP and PTC have been used as standard imaging procedures for the radiological diagnosis of PSC, however, MRCP has nowadays replaced these techniques.

Ultrasound remains the first-line investigation in these patients and shows segmental duct dilatation, irregular thickened walls of the CBD (Fig. 54.4), lymph nodes at the porta hepatis and heterogeneous reflectivity of the liver parenchyma (depending on the stage of disease). In established chronic liver disease, there is coarse echotexture with nodularity and relative atrophy of the right lobe with hypertrophy of the caudate and lateral segment of the left lobe.

MRCP can depict ductal irregularity, stricturing, focal dilatation, beading, and pruning affecting the intra- or extrahepatic biliary tree (Fig. 54.5). Post-contrast dynamic MR sequences should also be included to look for enhancement

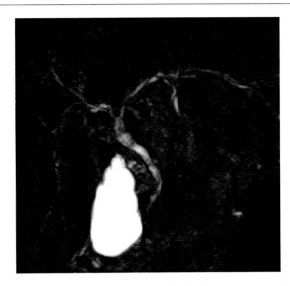

Fig. 54.5 MRCP MIP reconstruction of the biliary tree showing irregularity of the walls of the intra- and extrahepatic bile ducts, with focal structuring, in keeping with PSC. *MIP* maximum-intensity projection

of thickened walls of the extrahepatic ducts and cholangiocarcinoma.

Congenital and Acquired Vascular Disorders

Portal Hypertension

The etiology of portal hypertension can be classified as cirrhotic and non-cirrhotic. The latter can be prehepatic (portal vein thrombosis), intrahepatic (portal vein sclerosis, congenital hepatic fibrosis, steatosis, nodular regenerative hyperplasia, veno-occlusive disease), or suprahepatic (Budd–Chiari). Depending on the etiology, different radiological findings will be present. Liver function tests may be normal, and the diagnosis of portal hypertension often relies on demonstration of splenomegaly and formation of portosystemic collaterals.

In cirrhosis, prehepatic and pre-sinusoidal portal hypertension, the role of radiology is to determine the extent of involvement of the portal venous system, as this would influence the therapeutical options, which include surgical portosystemic shunt, Rex bypass, transjugular intrahepatic portosystemic shunt (TIPS), and ultimately liver transplantation.

The radiological approach to children with portal hypertension starts again from US with Doppler, which can detect low velocity, retrograde, or absent flow in the main portal vein and intrahepatic divisions. A patent umbilical vein, splenomegaly with varices, and ascites can also be easily seen on US; however, cross-sectional imaging is used as a "roadmap" for the evaluation of the portal system and collaterals pathways; CT and MR venography (MRV) can also demon-

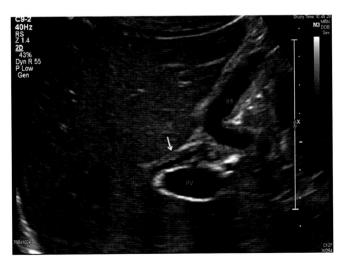

Fig. 54.4 US of the liver of a patient with PSC shows thickened wall of the common bile duct (*arrow*). *PV* portal vein, *GB* gallbladder

strate cavernous transformation of the portal vein, seen as a typical "beaded" appearance at the porta hepatis, which consists of venous channels within and around a previously stenosed or occluded portal vein [6]. This can occur within a few weeks after a thrombotic event, even in case of partial recanalization of the thrombosed segment, and can extend to the intrahepatic branches. Cystic and pericholecystic dilated veins can also be seen. A computed tomography (CT) performed in the arterial phase often shows patchy areas of high density at the periphery of the liver parenchyma, and this is due to a peripheral increase of the arterial inflow to supply the areas not reached by the cavernous portal vein.

Intra- and Extrahepatic Vascular Shunts

Intrahepatic communications between portal vein, hepatic artery, and hepatic veins are rare, and the most common, although often difficult to demonstrate, are small arterioportal shunts seen in cirrhotic livers. Large connections include portosystemic shunts (intra- and extrahepatic), arterioportal shunts, and arteriovenous shunts/malformations.

The origin of portosystemic shunts is still controversial and congenital, genetic, (such as trisomy 21) and acquired causes (such as in cirrhosis and post-traumatic) have been postulated [7]. These shunts have been historically classified into intrahepatic and extrahepatic, however, some authors discourage this classification and suggest to use an anatomical classification, which is aimed to establish the origin of the shunt (main portal vein, its tributaries or intrahepatic branches) and its systemic termination, the type of communication (end-to-end or side-to-side) and the number of connections. A distinction should be made between these shunts and a persistence of the ductus venosus [8].

The aim of radiology is to detect the shunts, delineate the anatomy, assist planning, and monitoring of interventional/surgical corrections and follow-up. Doppler US is the modality of choice to achieve this: direct communication between a portal branch and hepatic vein or the doctus venosus can be readily demonstrated, often due to enlargement and tortuosity of the vessels involved; the flow is usually continuous but triphasic flow can be seen in the portal branch. In case of main portal vein IVC connections, there is low velocity flow or non-visible intrahepatic portal vein, and the liver is usually decreased in size. Cross-sectional imaging is performed routinely to confirm the diagnosis and define the anatomy prior to intervention or surgery; in addition, shunts between the splenic vein or superior mesenteric vein and the IVC may be easily missed on US. CT and MR are also useful to characterize focal liver lesions, often found in associations with these shunts.

Angiography is often part of the workup of these children, either as a therapeutic option or prior to surgery to detect non-visible intrahepatic portal vein branches; a balloon occlusion catheter is placed in the shunt and pressures are measured before and after occlusion to evaluate how closure will be tolerated.

Arterioportal shunts may be congenital (in Rendu–Osler disease) or acquired (posttraumatic, post-liver biopsy, cirrhosis).

On CT, small arterioportal shunts in cirrhosis appear as small, wedge-shaped, peripheral areas of increased attenuation with early portal venous filling in the arterial phase and uniform attenuation in the portal venous phase. In presence of large arterioportal shunts or fistulas, there is early and marked enhancement of the main portal vein or segmental branches during the arterial phase. At Doppler US, large shunts will manifest with pulsatility of the portal vein flow [9].

Connections between the hepatic artery and systemic veins are rare, and can be seen in congenital arteriovenous malformations (AVM), hepatocellular carcinoma (HCC) and large hemangioendotheliomas; on Doppler US, altered waveforms of the hepatic vein can be seen in severe AVM, whereas CT will show asymmetrical, early filling of the hepatic vein.

Budd–Chiari Syndrome

Budd–Chiari syndrome is the clinical manifestation of hepatic venous outflow obstruction at any level of the hepatic veins, IVC or right atrium; this could be primary, caused by an endoluminal thrombus or membrane or secondary, when the occlusion is due to nonvascular material or from extrinsic compression. On US, there is narrowing, lack of visualization or thrombosis of the hepatic veins/IVC, with absent or monophasic flow at color Doppler. There is enlargement of the caudate lobe, ascites, and signs of portal hypertension with retrograde flow in the portal vein and splenomegaly.

On cross-sectional imaging, in the acute setting, occlusion of the hepatic veins with severe ascites is the typical finding. There is patchy, decreased peripheral enhancement of the liver due to portal and sinusoidal stasis and higher enhancement of the central parenchyma and caudate lobe, which compresses the IVC (Fig. 54.6). In subacute Budd–Chiari syndrome, portal vein thrombosis can develop as the result of reduced portal flow caused by blockage of the outflow. Finally, in chronic stages, multiple regenerative nodules can be seen, and on MR, these are bright on T1-weighted images and strongly hypervascular on post-gadolinium sequences. The nodules are predominantly isointense or hypointense relative to the liver on T2-weighted images [10].

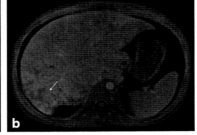

Fig. 54.6 MRI post-gadolinium T1W images of a patient with Budd–Chiari. In the acute phase **a**, there is significant enlargement of the caudate lobe (*black arrows*), which enhances normally versus the poorly vascularized peripheral parenchyma. The IVC is compressed by the caudate lobe. In the subacute phase **b**, there are signs of paraseptal necrosis (*white arrow*) with preserved central enhancement

Imaging of Transplant Liver

Liver transplantation is the treatment of choice for children with end-stage acute or chronic liver failure in which other therapies have failed or are not available. The successful development of novel surgical techniques of segmental, split, auxiliary, and living donor transplantation, together with advances in organ preservation, immunosuppressive therapy and adequate choice of donor organ, have led to a reduced rate of complications. However, these new surgical techniques have also brought with them new potential complications: in living-related transplants, for example, when the vascular pedicle may be too short, an autologous iliac artery conduit can be used, leading to potential higher risk of vascular complications.

Early recognition is crucial to the successful management of these complications, and a multimodality imaging approach is most effective to achieve the diagnosis, except in case of graft rejection, in which radiology has no role.

Serial ultrasound is the screening modality of choice immediately postoperatively and can be easily performed at the patient's bedside; however, ultrasound has inherent limitations and, even though the use of ultrasound contrast agents can improve its sensitivity, it depends on the expertise of the operator, and cross-sectional imaging is often necessary in inconclusive cases. Conventional angiography is now limited to those cases in which endovascular treatment is required.

We will illustrate the imaging appearances of the main, commonest complications following liver transplant.

Hepatic Artery

A normal hepatic artery waveform shows a rapid systolic peak followed by a continuous diastolic flow; the resistive index (RI) should range between 0.5 and 0.8, except in the immediate postoperative period (<72 h), in which the RI can be higher. An increased RI is associated with older donor age and prolonged ischemia time.

Hepatic artery thrombosis is a feared complication and a major cause of graft loss due to fulminant hepatic necrosis; in the long term, this complication can also lead to ischemic cholangiopathy, as the hepatic artery is the only arterial supply to the bile ducts in liver grafts. Children are particularly at risk, due to hepatic artery size discrepancy between recipient and donor.

On color and Doppler US, complete loss of arterial signal at the porta hepatis and within the liver suggests hepatic artery thrombosis. A tardus parvus waveform (prolonged systolic acceleration time and low-flow velocity with RI<0.5) at the porta hepatis or in the intrahepatic arteries indicates significant impairment of hepatic arterial perfusion, usually as a result of either arterial stenosis (uncommon) or thrombosis with collateral arteries (Fig. 54.7): collateral vessels from the Roux loop may form rapidly following hepatic artery thrombosis, therefore surveillance with Doppler US in the immediate postoperative days is vital. Conversely, false positive results can be found in case of hepatic edema or systemic hypotension [11]. In case of inconclusive findings on US but still high clinical suspicion of hepatic arterial insufficiency, a CT angiogram with thin-slices acquisition should be performed, which will show abrupt interruption of the hepatic artery and ischemic/necrotic parenchyma in case of thrombosis, and focal narrowing with decreased hepatic perfusion in case of stenosis. Ischemic lesions can liquefy and complicate with infection and abscess formation.

The role of conventional angiography is mostly therapeutic rather than diagnostic, with thrombolysis, angioplasty, or stenting (depending on the findings) to allow early revascularization.

Portal Vein

Portal vein complications are relatively rare and normally result from technical problems, such as difference in caliber

Fig. 54.7 a Doppler US scan of a left lateral segment transplant liver. There is a pulsus tardus parvus in a collateral of the hepatic artery with a prolonged acceleration time and reduced peak systolic velocity (17.9 cm/s). **b** CT angiogram confirms the finding of a thrombosed hepatic artery (*red arrow*). **c** A follow-up CT scan performed 1 month later shows low-attenuation lesions within the parenchyma, in keeping with bile lakes (*black arrows*)

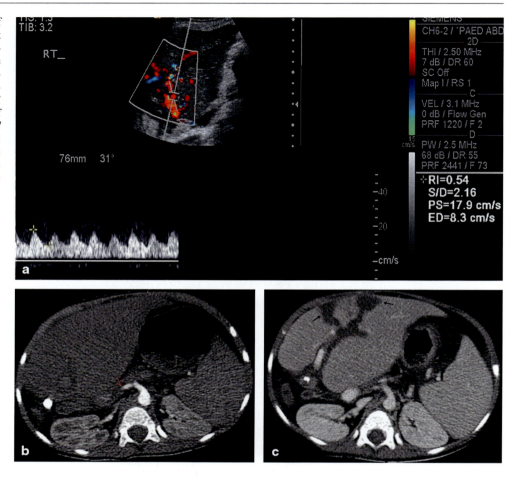

between donor and recipient, narrow native portal vein (e.g., in biliary atresia) and stretching at the anastomotic site, or other factors including previous thrombosis, hypercoagulable states, and increased resistance due to IVC strictures.

On US, a normal portal vein has smooth walls, anechoic lumen and on color and Doppler images shows antegrade/hepatopetal monophasic flow, except from the early postoperative period, where it can show high-velocity, turbulent flow.

Portal vein thrombosis manifests with echogenic intraluminal thrombus and lack of flow on color and Doppler trace, in which case either thrombolysis, or, more frequently, surgery with thrombectomy or venous graft is performed.

Portal vein stenosis has a later onset and can present with signs of portal hypertension. B-mode US shows focal severe narrowing of the portal vein at the anastomotic site with post-stenotic dilatation; on color and Doppler images, there is focal aliasing at the stenotic site with an increase of the velocity of three to fourfold compared to the pre-stenotic segment [11, 12]. Symptomatic patients are normally treated with balloon angioplasty or stenting.

These findings can be confirmed with CT or, usually for the late onset complications, with MR angiography.

IVC

Venous outflow obstruction is a rare complication secondary to either stenosis, thrombosis of the suprahepatic IVC or caval kinking from organ rotation.

The normal Doppler trace of the hepatic vein and IVC is triphasic due to pressure variations during the cardiac cycle; a monophasic waveform is a sensitive but nonspecific sign of stenosis, and a triphasic or biphasic waveform can exclude a substantial stenosis [11, 12]. As for the portal vein, stenosis can be seen on US as a focal stricture with impaired flow and pre-stenotic dilatation of the hepatic vein, whereas echogenic thrombus and complete absence of flow are direct signs of thrombosis. CT or MR is normally needed to confirm US findings or make the diagnosis where US is inconclusive. Cross-sectional imaging can also show signs of Budd–Chiari syndrome with the typical mosaic pattern of perfusion.

Biliary Disorders

Biliary complications are relatively frequent and are a common cause of graft dysfunction; these can often present with ischemic liver injury as well as cholestasis and cholangitis,

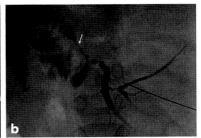

Fig. 54.8 a MRCP MIP reconstruction of the biliary tree in a left lateral segment transplant liver shows signs of cholangiopathy with an anastomotic stricture of the biliary enterostomy. **b** PTC image confirming the MRCP findings of a stricture (*white arrow*). The patient underwent balloon dilatation of the stricture. *MIP* maximum-intensity projection

and include anastomotic strictures, fistulas, stone formation with obstruction, diffuse cholangiopathy, and bile leaks.

A Roux-en-Y choledochojejunostomy is the most commonly performed anastomosis to achieve biliary drainage, although an end-to-end choledochal anastomosis may be performed in older children recipient of a whole graft.

US serves as a surveillance test to detect bile duct dilatation, although this is a variable feature, as mild dilatation can be present in the absence of significant obstruction and therefore clinical and laboratory correlation is needed.

MRCP is the modality of choice to investigate cholangiopathy and biliary strictures, the commonest biliary complication (Fig. 54.8). This can be due to either fibrotic proliferation and narrowing of the lumen or ischemic cholangiopathy; multiplanar MR provides anatomical details and helps planning percutaneous, endoscopic or surgical treatments.

Bile leaks normally occur early and can form perihepatic collections, which are drained percutaneously; treatment options include placement of a stent or biliary reconstruction. Intra-hepatic bile leaks are normally secondary to ductal ischemia.

Liver Masses

Radiological Approach to the Child with a Focal Liver Lesion

The diagnostic approach to children with chronic liver disease or a suspected liver mass should be tailored to the clinical scenario, including the age of the child and serum alpha-fetoprotein (AFP) levels; not all malignancies produce AFP, however, if serum AFP is elevated, a benign lesion is unlikely. US is the modality of choice in the screening of these children, because of its lack of ionizing radiation and no need for sedation. Some tumors, such as hemangioendothelioma have typical features on US and Doppler scan and may not require further characterization; however, the vast majority of liver masses need cross-sectional investigation [13, 14].

When performing a CT in children, efforts should be made to minimize radiation exposure, and unnecessary phases should be avoided (such as non-contrast scans); when the aim of the scan is surgical planning, a single post-contrast phase should be performed.

If multiphase post-contrast imaging is required, then MRI should be performed instead of CT. The limiting factor here is the need for sedation in young children and therefore, each scan should be performed starting from the most valuable sequences to achieve a definitive diagnosis.

If, at the end of the diagnostic pathway, there is still uncertainty on the nature of a lesion, then imaging guided (either US or CT) biopsy should be performed.

Benign Tumors

Hemangioendotheliomas

Hemangioendothelioma is a vascular neoplasm and represents the most common benign tumor in children; the lesions can be either single or multifocal and its margins may be sharp or ill-defined. In the first 6 months of life, these tumors show progressive growth, followed by spontaneous involution.

On antenatal US scan, a hypoechoic liver mass can be detected, sometimes together with fetal hydrops and cardiomegaly, which correlate with worse prognosis.

Multifocal lesions are small and uniform in appearance, usually hypoechoic on US within a markedly enlarged liver. Large lesions can have heterogeneous appearance in all modalities, due to central hemorrhage, necrosis, fibrosis, and calcifications.

At cross-sectional imaging, there are signs of high flow, with enlargement of the hepatic artery and veins and possibly tapering of the aorta below the origin of the coeliac axis. On post-contrast images, the tumor shows peripheral nodular enhancement with "filling in" on the delayed phase. On MR, the lesions have characteristic hyperintense signal on T2-weigthed images (Fig. 54.9).

Fig. 54.9 a CT scan performed in the arterial phase in a newborn baby shows a large haemangio-endothelioma in the right lobe of the liver with peripheral enhancement. **b** In the portal venous phase, there is centripetal enhancement of the mass. **c** A T2W MR image shows the lesion as hyperintense compared to normal liver parenchyma

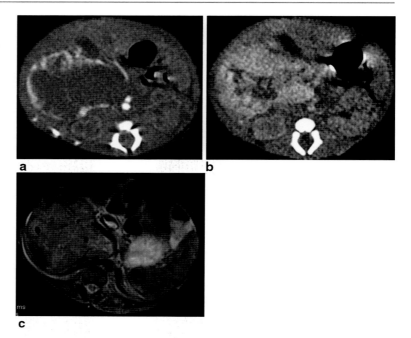

Angiography is now reserved for those cases in which arteriovenous shunts require embolization of the feeding arteries.

Mesenchymal Hamartoma

Mesenchymal hamartomas typically present as solitary tumors of the liver in infants and small children; most commonly, they involve the right lobe of the liver and the vast majority of these contain cysts, even though they can be either predominantly cystic or solid. The gross pathologic appearance will influence imaging findings: cystic portions are avascular with thin or thick septa, and solid components are hypovascular compared to the normal liver parenchyma. The cysts will be anechoic on US and have high signal on T2-weighted MRI and either low signal (clear cyst contents) or high signal (mucoid contents) on T1-weighted images.

Focal Nodular Hyperplasia

Focal nodular hyperplasia (FNH) is a benign epithelial liver tumor, uncommonly seen in young children. The tumor is composed of well-differentiated hepatocytes forming nodules divided by fibrous septa, which form a characteristic vascular central scar with a stellate shape. It is usually a solitary, well-circumscribed, encapsulated mass but can be multifocal. On US, it appears as a homogeneous lesion of variable echogenicity, usually isoechoic compared to a normal liver. Central vascularity can be detected at color Doppler and contrast-enhanced ultrasound (CEUS) will show a typical pattern of centrifugal, spoke-wheel arterial enhancement followed by uniform enhancement with the rest of the parenchyma in the portal venous and late phases. This can be confirmed at post-contrast cross-sectional imaging; on MR, the central scar is normally bright in T2-weighted images. In equivocal cases, tissue-specific agents (such as Teslascan or Primovist) show tumor uptake that persists for hours or even several days.

Hepatocellular Adenoma

Hepatocellular adenoma (or hepatic adenoma) is a rare benign neoplasm composed of hepatocytes with increased intracellular fat and glycogen, often prone to intralesional hemorrhage and necrosis. The majority of hepatic adenomas present as solitary well-circumscribed lesions, although in children with glycogen storage disease, they can be multifocal.

Hepatic adenomas without hemorrhage will be homogeneous with the rest of the liver in all imaging modalities. Following administration of contrast in CT or MR, the lesions typically display increased enhancement in the arterial phase and uniform enhancement with the rest of the liver in the portal venous and delayed phases; if there is hemorrhage, the lesion will enhance heterogeneously. Lesions with high fat content will show on MR high signal intensity on T1- and T2-weighted images, with signal dropout on opposed-phase or fat-suppressed sequences.

Nodular Regenerative Hyperplasia

Nodular regenerative hyperplasia (NRH) is characterized by regenerative nodules surrounded by atrophic liver without a fibrotic component. Various types of small-vessel blood-flow alterations are seen in association with NRH, including lymphoproliferative disorders, autoimmune disorders and Budd–Chiari syndrome and with the use of various medications (steroids, chemotherapeutic agents). The nodules, usually multiple with the tendency to coalesce, are composed of hepatocytes like the surrounding liver, therefore they can be difficult to distinguish from the adjacent parenchyma in all modalities, even after contrast administration.

Malignant Tumors

Hepatoblastoma

Hepatoblastoma is the most common primary hepatic tumor in children, occurring predominantly in children below the age of 5 years.

These tumors normally present as large masses often containing hemorrhagic and necrotic areas and speckled or amorphous calcifications; in 90 % of the cases, AFP serum levels are elevated. At imaging, hepatoblastomas present as large, well-circumscribed masses with septa; epithelial tumors have a homogeneous appearance, whereas mixed epithelial and mesenchymal tumors are more heterogeneous with variable osteoid, cartilaginous, and fibrous components. The primary role of radiology is to assess the tumor for operability (sections involved, involvement of the caudate, vessel invasion) and staging (the lung being the most common site for metastases): hepatoblastoma should be evaluated using the pretreatment extent of disease (PRETEXT) classification as this will establish treatment regimen [15].

On post-contrast cross-sectional imaging, hepatoblastomas show poor, inhomogeneous enhancement (Fig. 54.10); vascular invasion is better demonstrated on contrast-enhanced scans.

Hepatocellular Carcinoma

The main differential diagnosis of hepatoblastoma is hepatocellular carcinoma; HCC however is rare under the age of 5 years and 50 % of cases have a preexisting liver disease, such as biliary atresia, familial intrahepatic cholestasis, glycogen storage disease type I, tyrosenemia, Wilson disease, and alpha1-antitripsin deficiency.

Unlike in adults, small HCCs are unusual in children and lesions can have variable appearance on US, with a

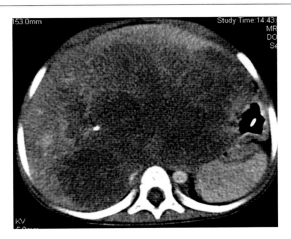

Fig. 54.10 A CT scan performed on the portal venous phase shows a large, poorly enhancing hepatoblastoma involving the whole of the liver; note intralesional calcification (*arrow*)

hypoechoic halo if the tumor has a capsule. Large tumors may contain areas of hemorrhage and necrosis.

On post-contrast cross-sectional imaging, HCC typically shows early arterial enhancement with wash out in the portal venous and delayed phases; portal and hepatic venous invasion may be identified.

Fibrolamellar Carcinoma

Fibrolamellar carcinoma is a slow-growing tumor that occurs in adolescents and young adults. The tumors are normally well demarcated and contain numerous fibrous septa which may separate the tumor into lobules and form a central scar-like structure; hemorrhage and necrosis are rare but calcifications can be observed. US shows a solitary heterogeneous mass; post-contrast CT and MR show avid enhancement in the arterial phase with often lack of enhancement of the central scar; on MR, the scar is typically hypointense in T1- and T2-weighted images, in contrast with the scar seen in FNH, which is normally hyperintense in T2.

Undifferentiated Embryonal Sarcoma

Undifferentiated embryonal sarcoma (UES) is a rare tumor that usually present between 6 and 10 years of age; AFP levels are usually normal and the presentation is nonspecific.

The tumors show very aggressive local growth with invasion of the diaphragm and lung. These tumors typically show a predominantly solid appearance on US but cystic appearance on CT and MR, due to its prominent myxoid stroma, which contains water. These tumors are usually well demarcated by a fibrous pseudocapsule, which generally show marked enhancement on post-contrast images.

Angiosarcoma

Angiosarcoma is a rare vascular tumor that can occur in young girls and in children with a previous diagnosis of hemangioendothelioma.

US can show either multiple nodules or a large mass of variable echogenicity. On post-contrast imaging, the lesion often shows decreased, heterogeneous enhancement compared to the normal liver with occasionally central or ring enhancement. Hemorrhage or necrosis can be observed.

Embryonal Rhabdomyosarcoma

Rhabdomyosarcoma can rarely arise from the biliary tree and this form is almost exclusively seen in young children; it spreads by intraluminal extension and causes significant cholestasis. At imaging, a mass can be seen usually at the porta hepatis, with intrahepatic biliary duct dilatation and normal-sized extrahepatic duct. Portal vein displacement without invasion is common.

Imaging of Liver Trauma in Children

CT remains the gold standard in the evaluation of blunt abdominal traumas in children; however, due to the risks related to radiation exposure, CT must be reserved for those children in whom there is a high index of suspicion, and should be performed following IV injection of contrast, possibly with split-bolus technique. When indicated, CT can provide rapid information regarding intra-abdominal injuries and can guide patient's management towards operative or conservative. Even though US would be preferable to CT giving its noninvasive nature and the lack of radiation, published data regarding the use of focused abdominal sonography for trauma (FAST) in children are not supportive of its use. Conversely, there are encouraging data regarding the use of CEUS in the setting of pediatric trauma, and in many centers, this imaging modality is routinely used, if not at presentation, certainly as the main follow-up examination [16].

The liver is the second most commonly injured organ in pediatric abdominal trauma (the spleen being the commonest site of injury); the role of the radiologist in this setting is to establish the extent of the injury (in terms of lobes and segments involved and vascular injury) and possible associated complications, such as ongoing hemorrhage. When active bleeding is demonstrated on CT, the patient will proceed to have an angiography with selective embolization of the bleeding vessel. At follow-up, normally between days 5 and 7 of trauma, potentially dangerous complications like pseudoaneurysm of the hepatic artery, hematomas, and bile leaks should be actively sought.

Imaging of Pancreas

Acute and chronic pancreatitis are a significant cause of morbidity and mortality in children; the most common causes of pancreatitis in children are trauma, structural anomalies, multisystem and metabolic disease, drugs, and autoimmune disease.

US is the first-line examination of the pancreas, and can exclude extra-pancreatic disease; change in pancreatic parenchyma echogenicity is a variable feature, as well as swelling of the gland. US can easily detect dilatation of the pancreatic duct and peripancreatic fatty infiltration, free fluid, and collections. In chronic pancreatitis, calcifications can be demonstrated.

MRI with MRCP is the most useful imaging modality to evaluate the severity of pancreatitis and establish further management; in addition, underlying structural anomalies such as abnormal pancreatico-biliary junction and choledochal cysts can also be diagnosed.

Autoimmune pancreatitis shows some specific features: the enlarged pancreas is in fact associated with irregular narrowing of the pancreatic duct, delayed contrast enhancement and a capsule-like rim which is more evident in the early post-contrast images on CT or MR; this corresponds to a fibrosing process extending to the peripancreatic fat.

Pancreatic involvement in children with CF is more frequent than liver disease, with plugging of pancreatic ducts due to inspissated secretions resulting in exocrine insufficiency. US shows an enlarged or atrophied pancreas with increased echogenicity due to fat deposition; cysts can be present, probably related to the obstruction of ducts.

References

1. Hernanz-Schulman M, Ambrosino MM, Freeman PC, Quinn CB. Common bile duct in children: sonographic dimensions. Radiology 1995;195(1):193–5.
2. Fitzpatrick E, Jardine R, Farrant P, Karani J, Davenport M, Mieli-Vergani G, Baker A. Predictive value of bile duct dimensions measured by ultrasound in neonates presenting with cholestasis. J Pediatr Gastroenterol Nutr. 2010;51(1):55–60.
3. Gubernick JA, Rosenberg HK, Ilaslan H, Kessler A. US approach to jaundice in infants and children. Radiographics 2000;20(1):173–95.
4. Norton KI, Glass RB, Kogan D, Lee JS, Emre S, Shneider BL. MR cholangiography in the evaluation of neonatal cholestasis: initial results. Radiology 2002;222(3):687–91.
5. Brancatelli G, Federle MP, Vilgrain V, Vullierme MP, Marin D, Lagalla R. Fibropolycystic liver disease: CT and MR imaging findings. Radiographics 2005;25(3):659–70.
6. Gallego C, Velasco M, Marcuello P, Tejedor D, De Campo L, Friera A. Congenital and acquired anomalies of the portal venous system. Radiographics 2002;22(1):141–59.
7. Alonso-Gamarra E, Parrón M, Pérez A, Prieto C, Hierro L, López-Santamaría M. Clinical and radiologic manifestations of congenital extrahepatic portosystemic shunts: a comprehensive review. Radiographics 2011;31(3):707–22.

8. Bernard O, Franchi-Abella S, Branchereau S, Pariente D, Gauthier F, Jacquemin E. Congenital portosystemic shunts in children: recognition, evaluation, and management. Semin Liver Dis. 2012;32(4):273–87.

9. Yu JS, Kim KW, Jeong MG, Lee JT, Yoo HS. Nontumorous hepatic arterial-portal venous shunts: MR imaging findings. Radiology 2000;217(3):750–6.

10. Brancatelli G, Vilgrain V, Federle MP, Hakime A, Lagalla R, Iannaccone R, Valla D. Budd-Chiari syndrome: spectrum of imaging findings. AJR Am J Roentgenol. 2007;188(2):W168–76.

11. Berrocal T, Parrón M, Alvarez-Luque A, Prieto C, Santamaría ML. Pediatric liver transplantation: a pictorial essay of early and late complications. Radiographics 2006;26(4):1187–209.

12. Caiado AH, Blasbalg R, Marcelino AS, da Cunha Pinho M, Chammas MC, da Costa Leite C, et al. Complications of liver transplantation: multimodality imaging approach. Radiographics 2007;27(5):1401–17.

13. Chung EM, Cube R, Lewis RB, Conran RM. From the archives of the AFIP: pediatric liver masses: radiologic-pathologic correlation part 1. Benign tumors. Radiographics 2010;30(3):801–26.

14. Chung EM, Lattin GE Jr, Cube R, Lewis RB, Marichal-Hernández C, Shawhan R, Conran RM. From the archives of the AFIP: pediatric liver masses: radiologic-pathologic correlation. Part 2. Malignant tumors. Radiographics 2011;31(2):483–507.

15. Roebuck DJ, Aronson D, Clapuyt P, Czauderna P, de Ville de Goyet J, Gauthier F, et al. 2005 PRETEXT: a revised staging system for primary malignant liver tumours of childhood developed by the SIOPEL group. Pediatr Radiol. 2007;37(2):123–32; quiz 249–50.

16. Valentino M, Serra C, Pavlica P, Labate AM, Lima M, Baroncini S, Barozzi L. Blunt abdominal trauma: diagnostic performance of contrast-enhanced US in children–initial experience. Radiology 2008;246(3):903–9.

Infantile Cholestasis: Approach and Diagnostic Algorithm

55

Sona Young and Ruba K. Azzam

Introduction

Jaundice in the first 2 weeks of life can be a common clinical finding, occurring in 2.4–15 % of newborns [1]. Most often, this jaundice is due to an unconjugated hyperbilirubinemia and resolves spontaneously. However, persistent jaundice past the 2 week point is abnormal, and the serum bilirubin should be checked in its fractionated forms of conjugated/direct and unconjugated/indirect bilirubin to evaluate for cholestasis.

Definition

Cholestasis is a central key manifestation of hepatobiliary disease in all age groups. Cholestasis is defined physiologically as a measurable decrease in bile flow, pathologically as the histological presence of bile pigment in hepatocytes and bile ducts, and clinically as the accumulation in blood and extrahepatic tissues of substances normally excreted in bile [2]. This is usually the resultant of either reduced bile formation (hepatocellular cholestasis) or decreased bile flow (obstructive cholestasis).

Obstructive cholestasis results from either anatomic or functional obstruction of the biliary system at any level of the biliary system: intra- or extrahepatically. Principal examples are biliary atresia (BA), anatomic biliary anomalies, and Alagille syndrome. On the other hand, hepatocellular cholestasis results from defective mechanisms of bile formation, which once established may be amplified by several

mechanisms. Examples include idiopathic neonatal hepatitis (INH), viral infections, and bacterial sepsis.

Incidence

The incidence of neonatal cholestasis is 1 in 2500–5000 live births. It usually manifests as conjugated hyperbilirubinemia with direct or conjugated hyperbilirubinemia of more than 1 mg/dl if total serum bilirubin is at or below 5 mg/dl, or direct bilirubin fraction > 20 % of total bilirubin when the latter is higher than 5 mg/dl. In general, direct bilirubin and conjugated bilirubin are not interchangeable exactly, since most methods report the combination of conjugated and δ-bilirubin as direct bilirubin.

The most commonly identifiable cause of cholestasis in the neonatal period is BA. There is a wide range of incidence reported internationally of BA [3]. It accounts for approximately 20–35 % of infantile cholestasis [4]. Genetic disorders, metabolic disease, and alpha1-antitrypsin deficiency are also among common etiologies. In older studies, INH was reported to be the most common cause, with an incidence ranging from 1 in 4800 to 1 in 9000 births [5]. However, in these cases, the term neonatal hepatitis was used to describe the histologic appearance of widespread giant-cell transformation, which is nonspecific and may be attributed to infectious, metabolic, and syndromic disorders. Therefore, with this realization and the advancement of diagnostic methods, the actual incidence of INH is now realized to be significantly lower [4, 6, 7]. Congenital infections including toxoplasmosis, other agents, rubella, cytomegalovirus, herpes simplex (TORCH) infections account for about 5 % of cases.

R. K. Azzam (✉)
Section of Gastroenterology, Hepatology and Nutrition, Department of Pediatrics, Comer Children's Hospital, University of Chicago, 5841 S. Maryland Avenue, Chicago 60637, IL, USA
e-mail: razzam@peds.bsd.uchicago.edu

S. Young
Section of Gastroenterology, Hepatology and Nutrition, Department of Pediatrics, Comer Children's Hospital, University of Chicago, Chicago, IL, USA

© Springer International Publishing Switzerland 2016
S. Guandalini et al. (eds.), *Textbook of Pediatric Gastroenterology, Hepatology and Nutrition*,
DOI 10.1007/978-3-319-17169-2_55

Susceptibility of the Neonatal Liver to Cholestasis

The neonatal liver is more susceptible to cholestasis as compared to livers of older children and adults.

While the physiologic development of normal hepatic function matures in the later stages of gestation, many other processes are developmentally regulated over the first few months after birth. This physiologic immaturity limits the capacity to synthesize and transport bile acids and affects the metabolism, detoxification and excretion of drugs, and xenobiotics [8, 9]. Reports on newborn animals have shown that their enterohepatic circulation is characterized by decreased bile salt secretion, flow, and synthesis; a smaller bile acid pool size; a decreased hepatic uptake of portal bile salts; and an inefficient uptake of bile salts in the ileum [10]. This then leads to high levels of circulating bile salt levels [11].

Differential Diagnosis

Although there is a long list of disorders that could potentially induce cholestasis, fewer than 15 of these account for greater than 95% of neonatal cholestasis [10]. Table 55.1 illustrates these differential diagnoses. Some of these diagnoses are briefly outlined below.

Obstructive

BA is a destructive, inflammatory process that causes fibrosis of the intra- and extrahepatic biliary tree. It is the most common cause of chronic cholestasis in infants and children, and it is the most common indication for liver transplant in the pediatric population. It is estimated to affect 1 in 8000–12,000 live births worldwide with a slight female predominance. There are two types of BA: congenital/embryonic which accounts for 15–20% of cases and perinatal or acquired which is the majority of cases. The etiology of BA remains deeply researched. Typically, the presentation of direct hyperbilirubinemia with acholic stools in infants a few weeks old should prompt the expedient evaluation forBA. There is a tremendous amount of evidence that suggests earlier diagnosis and surgical repair with a Kasai portoenterostomy will lead to a better outcome when performed before the age of 45–60 days [12–14].

A choledochal cyst is a congenital condition involving cystic dilation of the bile ducts. There are five different types, classified based on site of the dilation. The most common are types 1 (saccular dilation of only the extrahepatic bile duct) and 4 (saccular dilations of the intra- and extrahepatic biliary tree). The majority of cases present within the first year of life.

Table 55.1 Causes of infantile cholestasis

Obstructive	Infectious
Biliary atresia	Congenital TORCH infection:
Choledochal cyst	Toxoplasmosis
Syndromic and nonsyndromic paucity of interlobular bile ducts	Cytomegalovirus
	Rubella
Inspissated bile syndrome	Herpes virus
Caroli's disease/congenital hepatic fibrosis	HIV
Neonatal sclerosing cholangitis	Bacterial sepsis
	Urinary tract infection
Idiopathic neonatal hepatitis	Metabolic
	Bile acid synthesis defects
	Gestational alloimmune liver disease/neonatal hemochromatosis
	Galactosemia
	Hereditary tyrosinemia
	Hypothyroidism
	Panhypopituitarism
	Storage diseases
Genetic	Toxic
Alpha-1-antitrypsin deficiency	Parenteral nutrition
Alagille syndrome	Drugs
Progressive familial intrahepatic cholestasis	
Cystic fibrosis	
Arthrogryposis–renal dysfunction–cholestasis syndrome (ARC)	

HIV human immunodeficiency virus, *TORCH* Toxoplasmosis, Other Agents, Rubella, Cytomegalovirus, Herpes Simplex

Hepatocellular

INH is defined as a prolonged conjugated hyperbilirubinemia with no known etiology after a thorough evaluation has ruled out identifiable infectious and metabolic/genetic causes. Histologically, the typical findings would include widespread transformation of multinucleated giant cells. As discussed above, with the advancement of diagnostic techniques, the incidence of INH has sharply declined [7].

Bacterial, viral, and fungal infections can all cause cholestasis. Congenitally acquired pathogens capable of doing so include rubella, toxoplasmosis, cytomegalovirus, herpes, human immunodeficiency virus, and syphilis. Bacterial infections with either gram-negative or gram-positive organisms have also been implicated; in fact, jaundice may be one of the presenting symptoms of urinary tract infections in infants.

Genetic/Metabolic

Alpha-1-antirypsin (α1-AT) deficiency is an autosomal recessive disorder caused by a misfolded protein that prohibits its secretion, leading to intracellular accumulation of the protein. This accumulation leads to liver injury, cirrhosis, and increased risk for hepatocellular carcinoma through the formation of protein polymers, activation of autophagy, mitochondrial injury, and caspase activation [15]. Its incidence is approximately 1 in 1600–2000 live births, and it is extremely rare in the non-Caucasian population. Diagnosis is made based on the serum levels of α1-AT and the phenotype. Individuals homozygous for the mutant Z allele are at risk for the development of liver disease and emphysema, while the heterozygous carrier state for the mutant Z gene may be a modifier gene for liver disease. In infancy, the typical presentation is one of neonatal cholestasis, but the presentation of patients can be highly varied. In fact, only 8–10 % of individuals born with the homozygous Z allele develop any clinically significant liver disease over the first 20 years of life. Liver biopsy may show globular, eosinophilic inclusions in hepatocytes, representing dilated endoplasmic reticulum membranes and the accumulated Z protein. It stains positive with periodic acid–Schiff and is diastase resistant [15]. Prospective studies indicate that 80 % of patients with the homozygous Z allele and presenting with neonatal cholestasis are healthy and free of chronic disease by the age of 18 years [16].

Alagille syndrome is an autosomal dominant multisystemic disease that results from mutation usually involving the *Jagged 1* or *NOTCH2* gene. Jagged-1 is a member of the Jagged family of genes that encode cell surface proteins that interact with Notch receptors; this interaction regulates cell fate during embryogenesis. The syndrome is characterized by paucity of interlobular bile ducts. The variable penetrance of the mutation leads to different characteristics of the disease including: abnormal facies, chronic cholestasis, posterior embryotoxon, butterfly-like vertebral arch defects, and cardiovascular malformations. Associated vascular abnormalities have been noted in Alagille patients including decreased intrahepatic portal vein radicals and cerebrovascular abnormalities similar to Moyamoya disease. Infantile presentation follows a variable course with some developing gradual improvement as they get older, whereas others progress into cirrhosis. Medical management emphasizes on the supplementation of medium-chain triglycerides, essential fatty acids, and fat-soluble vitamins. Liver transplantation may be needed in cases of cirrhosis, portal hypertension, or severe pruritus [17].

Progressive familial intrahepatic cholestasis (PFIC) refers to a heterogeneous group of autosomal recessive disorders that disrupt bile formation [18]. It is divided into three subtypes. Type I, also known as Byler disease or familial intrahepatic cholestasis (FIC)1 disease, is caused by a mutation in the P-type ATPase FIC gene. FIC1 is expressed in several epithelial tissues, including the small intestine, pancreas, and liver, and thus patients express extrahepatic manifestations as well like recurrent pancreatitis, diarrhea, wheezing and cough, sensorineural hearing loss, and posttransplant steatosis. A benign form of recurrent intrahepatic cholestasis (BRIC) with symptom-free intervals in between the attacks could be seen in patients with mutations in the same gene.

PFIC type II is caused by a defect in the bile sale export pump (BSEP/ABCB11) gene, which leads to impaired bile acid transport from the hepatocytes into the bile canaliculus. The gene is liver specific, and thus mutations result in no extrahepatic manifestations. Similar to FIC1 disease, genetic mutations in BSEP could manifest in a more benign recurrent disease called BRIC2. Both type I and II have normal serum γ-glutamyltranspeptidase (γ-GTP) levels, unlike type III.

PFIC type III is due to a defect in MDR3 which is a member of the adenosine triphosphate (ATP)-binding cassette family of transporters that serve as phospholipid flippases. Its impairment leads to defective biliary phospholipid secretion, impairing the balance in cholesterol saturation index and leading to crystallization of cholesterol, and lithogenicity of bile, and bile duct injury.

Galactosemia is an autosomal recessive disorder that can result from deficiencies of three different enzymes; the most common and severe form is caused by a complete deficiency of galactose-1-phosphate uridyltransferase (GALT). Most states in the USA include testing in the newborn screening, but infants may become symptomatic prior to the availability of these test results. The gold standard for diagnosis is the demonstration of nearly complete absence of GALT activity in red blood cells. It is important to remember that blood transfusions from a donor may interfere with the diagnosis.

Physical exam and history will typically reveal a jaundiced infant that may be lethargic, hypotonic, with poor feeding, and displays hepatomegaly. Dietary restriction of galactose in the newborn period reverses the hepatic dysfunction. However, chronic and progressive neurologic impairments may occur even in patients with dietary compliance [19].

Tyrosinemia is an inborn error of metabolism that results from deficiencies in specific enzymes in the tyrosine catabolic pathway, leading to the accumulation of toxic metabolites such as succinylacetone, maleylacetoacetate, and fumarylacetoacetate. It is characterized by acute liver failure in the first weeks or months of life. It is detected by quantitative measurement of plasma amino acids and urine succinylacetone levels. The treatment is dietary restriction of tyrosine and phenylalanine as well as early initiation of the medication nitosine, a potent inhibitor of the enzyme 4-hydroxyphenylpyruvate dioxygenase. This decreases the concentration of succinylacetone.

There are numerous other inborn errors of metabolism that can be screened for with serum amino acid and urine organic acid concentrations. The remainder will not be discussed in detail at this time.

Evaluation

Distinguishing between jaundice caused by cholestasis from non-cholestatic causes is critical since the former need prompt evaluation and management, given that the most common causes of cholestatic jaundice in the first few months of age, especially in the non-sickly-looking babies, are BA and INH. Guidelines for the evaluation of cholestatic jaundice in infants were published by North American Society for Pediatric Gastroenterology, Hepatology, and Nutrition (NASPGHAN) in 2004 and recommended that any infant noted to be jaundiced at 2 weeks of age be evaluated for cholestasis with measurement of total and direct serum bilirubin. However, breast-fed infants who can be reliably monitored and have an otherwise normal history (no dark urine or light stools) and physical examination may be asked to return at 3 weeks of age and, if jaundice persists, have measurement of total and direct serum bilirubin at that time [20]. This is in line with the fact that early diagnosis of the different possible etiologies of cholestasis will lead to better outcomes, especially in BA where the successful establishment of biliary flow is more likely when the Kasai portoenterostomy is performed between 45 and 60 days of age.

An algorithm for the evaluation of cholestatic infants is presented in Fig. 55.1.

History and physical examination are the initial steps in the evaluation and usually guide the diagnostic process. The report of acholic stools is a strong indicator of cholestasis, though parents do not seem to reliably differentiate the abnormal hue of stools from normal. Dark urine is another nonspecific indicator of abnormal conjugated hyperbilirubin levels. Mass screening with a stool color card in Taiwan proved its efficacy in early diagnosis of BA patients [21]. In addition, some infants may present with bleeding or bruising due to a coagulopathy from vitamin K malabsorption and/or liver failure. Family history may suggest a genetic disorder with an autosomal dominant inheritance pattern such as Alagille's, cystic fibrosis, alpha-1-antitrypsin deficiency, PFIC. Consanguinity may raise suspicion for rarer, autosomal recessive disorders. A maternal pregnancy history is important to evaluate for possible congenital infections, such as cytomegalovirus or hepatitis B. In addition, prenatal ultrasounds may have detected anatomic abnormalities such as a biliary cyst. A history of severe ABO incompatibility may explain a conjugated hyperbilirubinemia; in about 3 % of infants, this is a benign complication which resolves on its own accord within a month [22].

A careful physical examination may reveal clinical features that will serve as clues about the diagnosis. BA is more common in females of normal birth weight, while INH is more common in males with low birth weight or who were born prematurely, and who may have had a sibling with similar presentation. Abnormal facies can point towards Alagille, as can a cardiac murmur (also seen in congenital BA).

Other possible clinical findings may include splenomegaly in cases of portal hypertension, storage disorders, or hemolytic disease.

Infants with cholestasis due to congenital infections are usually small for their gestational age, may have microcephaly, pupuric rash, or chorioretinitis. Infants who appear acutely ill in the setting of cholestasis are likely suffering from a potentially life-threatening disorder such as sepsis or metabolic diseases that need to be ruled out.

Confirmation of the presence of cholestasis by measuring a fractionated serum bilirubin level along with baseline assessment of the severity of hepatic dysfunction forms (albumin, serum glucose level, ammonia and prothrombin time/international normalized ratio; INR) is the basis for the tests that follow. If INR is abnormal, the administration of parenteral vitamin K should normalize the coagulation study if the hepatic synthetic function is preserved.

Serum transaminases (alanine transaminase, ALT; aspartate transaminase, AST) are indicators of hepatocellular injury but lack prognostic value.

The elevation in alkaline phosphatase is indicative of biliary obstruction, but it is nonspecific as it is also produced by other organs like the bones, small bowel, and kidneys. On the other hand, the level of γGTP is more sensitive to biliary disease and more importantly directs the evaluation towards certain pathologies. Low γ-glutamyl transpeptidase (GGT) cholestatic diseases make a short list of diseases and include PFIC1, PFIC2, arthrogryposis–renal dysfunction–cholestasis

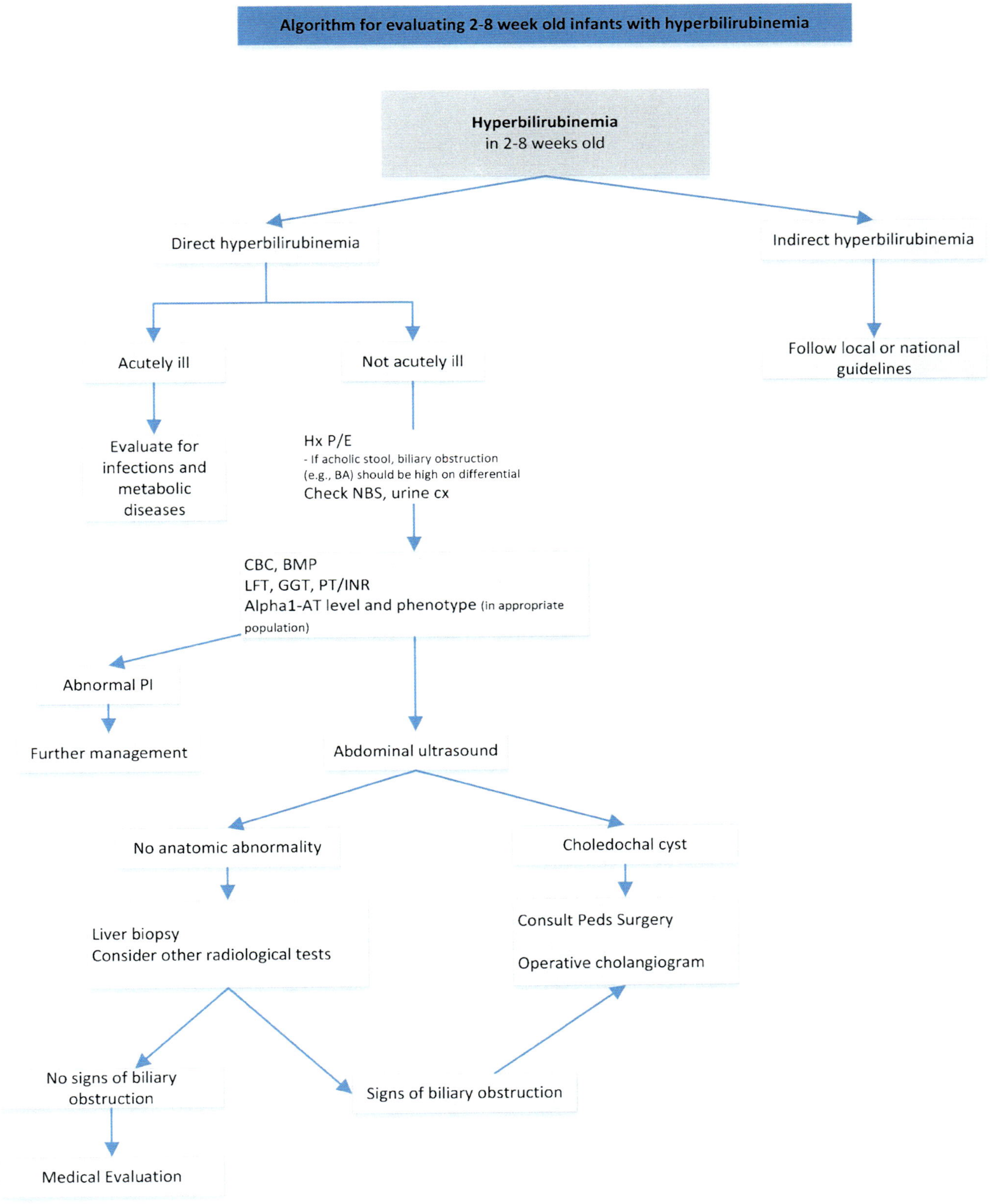

Fig. 55.1 An algorithm for the evaluation of cholestatic infants. Hx P/E history and physical examination, *CBC* complete blood count, *BMP* basic metabolic profile, *LFT* liver function test, *GGT* gamma glutamyl transpeptidase, *PT/INR* prothrombin time/international normalized ratio, *Alpha1-AT* alpha-1-antitrypsin

syndrome (ARC), lymphedema–cholestasis syndrome (LCS or Aagenaes syndrome) and inborn errors of bile acid synthesis.

Cholestatic liver diseases are associated with elevated total serum bile acid concentrations, but levels that are normal or inappropriately low for the degree of cholestasis should lead to further evaluation for inborn errors of bile acid synthesis.

Bacterial blood and urine cultures are indicated as clinically appropriate. Hepatobiliary dysfunction with cholestasis is common in the early course of neonatal septicemia. Circulating endotoxins are believed to cause down regulation of biliary transporters, biliary stasis, and hepatic parenchymal injury.

Alpha1-antitrypsin level and phenotype need to be checked early on, especially that the histologic differentiation between BA and α1-antitrypsin deficiency is very difficult in the few-week-old infants.

Radiologic Evaluation

Ultrasonography is usually the initial imaging study that provides information about the size and echotexture of the liver, as well as the assessment for anatomic biliary anomalies such as biliary cysts. It also evaluates the size of the gall bladder and the presence of stones or sludge. It detects signs of obstructive dilatation of the biliary tree. It may detect extrahepatic anomalies like polysplenia or asplenia, situs inversus, and the different positional variants of the portal vein and hepatic artery. Certain findings can also suggest the presence of BA, such as a small or absent gallbladder. A "triangular cord sign," or triangular echogenicity of the anterior wall of the right portal vein on transverse or longitudinal view, has specificity and sensitivity reported as high as 80 and 98% and can be a useful finding for diagnosis on ultrasound [21, 23, 24]. Limitations of the ultrasound include operator dependence. However, it is recommended for evaluation of the infant with cholestasis of unknown etiology.

Computed tomography is used less often, given that almost the same information is provided by ultrasonography without the risk of exposure to radiation.

Magnetic resonance cholangiography (MRCP), performed with T_2-weighted turbo spin-echo sequences, is noninvasive, and not operator dependent, though requires sedation. It can evaluate detailed structural anomalies including anomalous pancreatobiliary duct union. Delineating the small common bile duct in small infants could be challenging, using gadolinium enhancement for its T_2-shortening effect may allow a more definitive determination of the presence or absence of the common bile duct (CBD) in infants with cholestasis, especially when conventional magnetic resonance cholangiopancreatography (MRCP) is indeterminate [21].

Hepatobiliary scintigraphy using technetium Tc99m iminodiacetic acid analogues has been used to differentiate extra-hepatic biliary obstruction from nonobstructive causes. Using phenobarbital for 3–5 days before performing the test increases its yield, but obviously is time consuming, especially in cases where presentation is not timely.

ERCP use in cholestatic neonates and infants is a safe and reliable diagnostic method, when performed by a skilled and experienced endoscopist in a high-volume tertiary care center. Its sensitivity and specificity in the diagnosis of extrahepatic causes of cholestasis is superior to other available diagnostic methods including cholescintigraphy and MRCP. Of particular significance is the high negative predictive value (NPV) and specificity of ERCP in diagnosing structural abnormalities of the bile ducts, namely all types of BA and choledochal cysts [25].

Liver biopsy continues to be the diagnostic test with the highest usefulness even in the smallest infants, and its use is inevitable in most cases on infantile cholestasis. It is accurate in diagnosingBA in 90–95% of cases as reported by several studies. Attention should always be paid to timing for the development of the typical features of histopathology changes of BA, as liver biopsies in the first few weeks of age will not have all the features and will miss the diagnosis of BA. Serial investigations and possibly a follow-up liver biopsy at around 6 weeks of age will be needed. Liver biopsy can be diagnostic for other diseases as well, and it could navigate the evaluation process in a more specific path. The addition of electron microscopic exam and/or immunohistochemical, biochemical, or biological evaluation of the tissue may be required to identify specific pathologies.

Intraoperative cholangiogram is the gold standard test to study the patency of the biliary system and establish the diagnosis of BA. It is also the procedure that surgeons rely on to demystify the small number of cases where the diagnosis stays doubtful after reviewing the different imaging studies and liver biopsy.

References

1. Kelly DA, Stanton A. Jaundice in babies: implications for community screening for biliary atresia. Br Med J. 1995;310(6988):1172–3.
2. Suchy F. Approach to the infant with cholestasis. In: Liver disease in children. Cambridge Medicine: Cambridge University Press; 2007. pp. 179–89.
3. Jimenez-Rivera C, Jolin-Dahel KS, Fortinsky KJ, Gozdyra P, Benchimol EI. International incidence and outcomes of biliary atresia. J Pediatr Gastroenterol Nutr. 2013;56(4):344–54.
4. Stormon MO, Dorney SFA, Kamath KR, O'Loughlin EV, Gaskin KJ. The changing pattern of diagnosis of infantile cholestasis. J Paediatr Child Health. 2001;37(1):47–50.
5. Dick MC, Mowat AP. Hepatitis syndrome in infancy–an epidemiological survey with 10 year follow up. Arch Dis Child. 1985;60(6):512–6.
6. Feldman AG, Sokol RJ. Neonatal cholestasis. Neoreviews 2013;14(2). doi:10.1542/neo.14-2-e63.

7. Balistreri WF, Bezerra JA. Whatever happened to "neonatal hepatitis"? Clin Liver Dis. 2006;10(1):27–53.
8. Venigalla S, Gourley GR. Neonatal cholestasis. Semin Perinatol. 2004;28(5):348–55.
9. Grijalva J, Vakili K. Neonatal liver physiology. Semin Pediatr Surg. 2013;22(4):185–9.
10. Emerick KM, Whitington PF. Neonatal liver disease. Pediatr Ann. 2006;35(4):280–6.
11. Suchy FJ, et al. Physiologic cholestasis: elevation of the primary serum bile acid concentrations in normal infants. Gastroenterology 1981; 80(5 pt 1):1037–41.
12. Serinet MO, Wildhaber BE, Broué P, Lachaux A, Sarles J, Jacquemin E, et al. Impact of age at Kasai operation on its results in late childhood and adolescence: a rational basis for biliary atresia screening. Pediatrics 2009;123(5):1280–6.
13. Altman RP, Lilly JR, Greenfeld J, Weinberg A, van Leeuwen K, Flanigan L. A multivariable risk factor analysis of the portoenterostomy (Kasai) procedure for biliary atresia: twenty-five years of experience from two centers. Ann Surg. 1997;226(3):348–53; discussion 353–5.
14. Chardot C, Carton M, Spire-Bendelac N, Le Pommelet C, Golmard J, Reding R, Auvert B. Is the Kasai operation still indicated in children older than 3 months diagnosed with biliary atresia? J Pediatr. 2001;138(2):224–8.
15. Teckman JH. Alpha1-antitrypsin deficiency in childhood. Semin Liver Dis. 2007;27(3):274–81.
16. Sveger T. The natural history of liver disease in alpha 1-antitrypsin deficient children. Acta Paediatr Scand. 1988;77(6):847–51.
17. Alagille D. Alagille syndrome today. Clin Invest Med. 1996;19(5):325–30.
18. Jacquemin E. Progressive familial intrahepatic cholestasis. Clin Res Hepatol Gastroenterol. 36 Suppl. 2012; 1:S26–35.
19. Ridel KR, Leslie ND, Gilbert DL. An updated review of the long-term neurological effects of galactosemia. Pediatr Neurol. 2005;33(3):153–61.
20. Moyer V, Freese DK, Whitington PF, Olson AD, Brewer F, Colletti RB, Heyman MB. Guideline for the evaluation of cholestatic jaundice in infants: recommendations of the north american society for pediatric gastroenterology, hepatology and nutrition. J Pediatr Gastroenterol Nutr. 2004;39(2):115–28.
21. Chen SM, Chang MH, Du JC, Lin CC, Chen AC, Lee HC, et al. Screening for biliary atresia by infant stool color card in Taiwan. Pediatrics 2006;117(4):1147–54.
22. Sivan Y, Merlob P, Nutman J, Reisner SH. Direct hyperbilirubinemia complicating ABO hemolytic disease of the newborn. Clin Pediatr (Phila). 1983;22(8):537–8.
23. Kotb MA, Kotb A, Sheba MF, El Koofy NM, El-Karaksy HM, Abdel-Kahlik MK, et al. Evaluation of the triangular cord sign in the diagnosis of biliary atresia. Pediatrics 2001;108(2):416–20.
24. Choi SO, Park WH, Lee HJ, Woo SK. 'Triangular cord': a sonographic finding applicable in the diagnosis of biliary atresia. J Pediatr Surg. 1996;31(3):363–6.
25. Keil R, Snajdauf J, Rygl M, Pycha K, Kotalová R, Drábek J, et al. Diagnostic efficacy of ERCP in cholestatic infants and neonates–a retrospective study on a large series. Endoscopy 2010;42(2):121–6.

Biliary Atresia and Choledochal Malformations

Elke Zani-Ruttenstock and Mark Davenport

Biliary Atresia

Introduction

In 1891, John Thompson, a physician from Edinburgh, described in detail the clinical features and postmortem findings of an infant with what he termed was "congenital biliary obstruction" [1]. His drawings clearly show an absence of a common hepatic duct (CHD) and a collapsed empty gallbladder. Further reports during the early part of the twentieth century prompted surgeons to explore the biliary tree to try and identify a blockage and perhaps a proximal bile-containing duct to anastomose to. This led to the concept that biliary atresia (BA) was either "correctable" or "uncorrectable" depending on operative findings. With increasing experience, it became evident that the latter was much more common and hence survivors were exceptional. Although the use of these terms is nowadays anachronistic (because you can "correct" the uncorrectable!), it perhaps illustrates the hopeless prognosis of these unfortunate infants.

Figure 56.1 illustrates the various types of BA and is based upon the most proximal level of obstruction. Thus, over 95% are type 3 where there is no visible bile duct in the porta hepatis (hence "uncorrectable"). It does not imply anything about causation (described later in the chapter).

A more radical approach to the technique was pioneered in Sendai, Japan, during the 1950s and 1960s by Morio Kasai (1922–2008) to the problem of "uncorrectability" [2, 3]. He advocated a more radical approach to the biliary dissection and simply transected at the most proximal point in the porta hepatis. The porta, even if there were no visible ducts, was then anastomosed to a Roux loop (portoenterostomy). Transection exposes residual microscopic bile duct remnants within the fibrous tissue which retain communica-

tion with the intrahepatic duct system (still often very abnormal). Hence, bile flow actually occurs to a varying degree, but in perhaps the majority, enough to lose their jaundice (see later for results and outcome), postoperative outcome significantly improved.

For the first time, Kasai portoenterostomy (KPE) enabled a much larger cohort of long-term survivors, initially in Japan [3] but later from the 1970s in Europe and North America. It wasnot a cure though, and even survivors displayed many complications related to liver fibrosis and cirrhosis.

Thomas Starzl, in 1963, attempted the first liver transplant in humans in a child born with BA [4]. Sadly, the child died of operative bleeding related to severe portal hypertension. This prompted a number of units around the world to set up transplantation programmes, but, in the absence of effective immunosuppression, they were all terminated by the end of the 1960s. With the discovery of cyclosporine at the beginning of the 1980s, transplantation once more became a viable option, and from this the current strategy of an initial attempt to restore (some might say resurrect) bile flow with a KPE followed by liver transplantation if this fails evolved.

Variants of Biliary Atresia

BA is not a single disease rather it should be thought of as a phenotype resulting from a number of different and entirely separate aetiologies leading to the final common phenotype of biliary inflammation, luminal obliteration and fibrosis [5].

We are able to define clinically four broad groups (Fig. 56.2):

1. Syndromic biliary atresia. While BA is usually an isolated abnormality found in otherwise normal-term infants, there are a group of infants (about 10–15% in European and North American series, but <2% in Asian series) with other non-biliary anomalies and a poorer prognosis. We have termed this specific constellation of anomalies the biliary atresia splenic malformation (BASM) syndrome [6, 7]. All will have a splenic malformation, usually

E. Zani-Ruttenstock (✉) · M. Davenport
Department of Pediatric Surgery, King's College Hospital,
Denmark Hill, SE5 9RS London, UK
e-mail: markdav2@ntlworld.com

© Springer International Publishing Switzerland 2016
S. Guandalini et al. (eds.), *Textbook of Pediatric Gastroenterology, Hepatology and Nutrition*,
DOI 10.1007/978-3-319-17169-2_56

Fig. 56.1 Schematic illustration of biliary atresia (based on Japanese Association of Pediatric Surgeons classification)

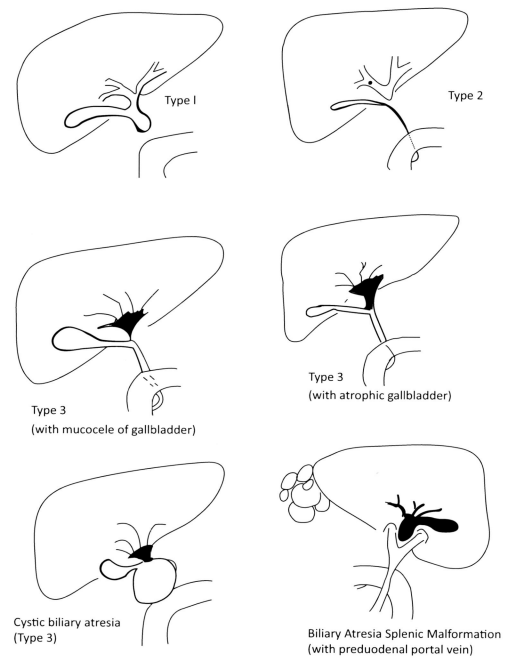

Type I

Type 2

Type 3
(with mucocele of gallbladder)

Type 3
(with atrophic gallbladder)

Cystic biliary atresia
(Type 3)

Biliary Atresia Splenic Malformation
(with preduodenal portal vein)

polysplenia but occasionally asplenia and about half will have situs inversus and congenital heart abnormalities. Other anomalies are evident at laparotomy including preduodenal portal vein, absence of the inferior vena cava and malrotation. Most infants with this syndromic form of BA are female. It is speculated that such cases may result from some fundamental derangement of extrahepatic bile duct (and other systems) development within the embryological phase (<6 weeks gestation). A genetic aetiology has not been convincingly shown clinically, though several candidate genes exist (e.g. CFC-1). There is some evidence that affected infants have been exposed to an abnormal first-trimester intrauterine environment such as that found in maternal diabetes and thyrotoxicosis.

2. Cystic biliary atresia (CBA). In about 5% of cases, there is obvious cyst (sometimes containing bile) formation within an otherwise obliterated biliary tree. In recent years, it has been possible to detect this cystic change on antenatal ultrasound (US) scans as early as the 18th week of gestation [8, 9]. CBA should not be confused with cystic choledochal malformation (CM), which can be indistinguishable on US [10]. Discrimination may be made clinically as CBA will invariably have conjugated jaundice, pale stools, etc., and at laparotomy as the chol-

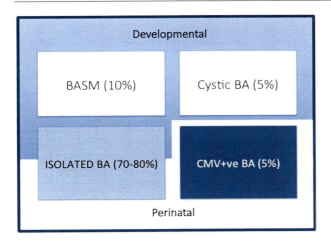

Fig. 56.2 Variants of biliary atresia. *BASM* biliary atresia splenic malformation, *BA* biliary atresia, *CMV* cytomegalovirus, *IgM* immunoglobulin M

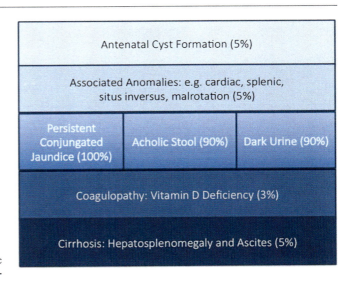

Fig. 56.3 Modes of presentation of biliary atresia

angiogram will show the abnormal and primitive intrahepatic duct structure. Both CBA and the syndromic BA can clearly be termed "developmental" as whatever caused their pathology occurred during prenatal life.

3. Isolated biliary atresia (IBA). This is the typical BA variant accounting for about 70–80% of cases [11]. They have no other significant features and usually display an obliterated biliary tree at laparotomy (usually type 3). In the absence of any clinical or laboratory evidence, we do not actually know the aetiology in this group.

4. CytomegalovirusIgM +ve biliary atresia. Although there is a range of possible hepatotropic cholangiopathic viruses (e.g. reovirus type 3, rotavirus) it has been difficult to definitively ascribe clinical consequences to infection. We have recently discriminated infants with CMV IgM +ve antibodies from their IgM −ve fellows clinically, histologically and in their response to treatment (unpublished results). This is still controversial and other European series have not shown any such differences; however, the focus in these has been on a group of viruses rather than specifically CMV [12].

Epidemiology

Population-based studies reporting incidence and outcomes of BA are scarce. There is marked variation in incidence across the globe with the highest rates found in East Asian countries compared to Europe and North America [13]. The place with the highest reported incidence appears to be Taiwan at an incidence of 1 in 6622 [14].

The incidence in the UK is about 1 in 17,000–18,000 live births [11], and this appears to be similar to reports from France [15], Sweden [16], Germany [17] and Switzerland

[18]. Most large series show an equal gender split although by variant there is marked female predominance in the developmental forms of BA [7, 9, 11, and 15].

A number of small series suggested seasonality for BA [13, 19], though these were far from definitive and larger national series failed to observe any predilection for a particular season [11, 15, 20].

Clinical Features

The key features of BA are persistent conjugated jaundice, acholic stools and dark urine in an otherwise healthy term infant (Fig. 56.3). The latter feature is caused by excess conjugated (i.e. water-soluble) bilirubin passing into the urine causing its colour to darken. Such alternative pathways of bilirubin excretion are more developed or at least preserved in the newborn, and very high levels of bilirubin (>300 µmol/L or >17 mg/dl) are exceptional. Sometimes jaundice will be difficult to discern in infants of Asian or Afro-Caribbean origin leading to delays in diagnosis and treatment. The median time to referral was 47 days in non-white versus 52 days in white infants in one UK study [21]. Furthermore, all of those "missed" and referred beyond 100 days were non-white.

Sometimes the antenatal US scan will be abnormal showing a sub-hepatic cyst, and one should be suspicious of CBA [8]. There is no difference in gestational age or birth weight between those with developmental BA compared to isolated BA, but both groups show a failure to thrive by the time they are admitted. Fat malabsorption is the presumed mechanism and will also cause deficiency of the fat-soluble vitamins D, A, E and K. Low vitamin D levels are common even in those infants presenting early, and this is exacerbated in those of Asian family origin, presumably reflecting low maternal stores (Fig. 56.4). Vitamin K deficiency is possible and a

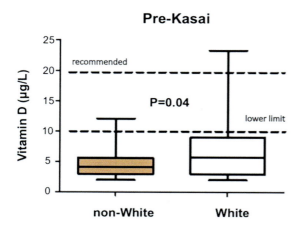

Fig. 56.4 Decreased preoperative vitamin D-levels in non-white compared to white infants with biliary atresia. (Courtesy of Ms. Anu Paul)

proportion will present with a bleeding tendency, perhaps from the umbilical stump or more catastrophically with an intracranial haemorrhage. Marked elevation of the international normalised ratio (INR) or prothrombin time will be seen. Some syndromic cases will present early because of other abnormalities associated with BASM (e.g. cardiac anomalies, malrotation or situs inversus).

Diagnosis

The diagnostic work up in our institution includes a detailed US of the liver, liver biochemistry and a percutaneous liver biopsy [10]. Using this, more than 90 % will have an accurate diagnosis before laparotomy.

Ultrasonography

The US examination is a key part of the diagnostic protocol as it usually excludes other surgical diagnoses (e.g. CM, inspissated bile syndrome, etc.). All of these are characterised by intrahepatic or common bile duct (CBD) dilatation. US may be suggestive of BA as a diagnosis—by showing a shrunken, atrophic gallbladder with no evidence of filling between feeds. In about 20 % of cases, a "normal gallbladder" is described—which turns out to be a mucocele of the gallbadder together with a relatively preserved CBD and an absent CHD; Fig. 56.1).

Laboratory Findings

Liver biochemistry will show a conjugated jaundice (typically >100 μmol/L), modestly raised transaminases (>100 μmol/L) as well as significantly raised γ-glutamyl transpeptidase (GGT >200 IU/L). Serum protein and albumin levels should be normal. However, none of this is specific.

Percutaneous Liver Biopsy

In the authors' unit, the pre-laparotomy diagnosis of BA is usually made by percutaneous liver biopsy showing histological features characteristic of large duct obstructions such as bile duct proliferation, portal oedema and absence of sinusoidal fibrosis. It is less accurate the younger the infant, and it does require an experienced and confident liver pathologist.

Aspartate Aminotransferase-to-Platelet Ratio Index

The aspartate aminotransferase-to-platelet ratio index (APRi) can be used as a surrogate of liver fibrosis in many liver diseases, including BA. We have recently reported that this correlates significantly with age at surgery and was much higher in CMV-associated BA. Macroscopic cirrhosis evident at laparotomy could also be predicted using a cut-off value of 1.2, with reasonable sensitivity (75 %) and specificity (84 %) in a large cohort of infants from our unit [22].

The usual differential diagnoses of conjungated jaundice include TORCH infections (e.g. toxoplasma, rubella, CMV, hepatitis, etc.), genetic conditions (e.g. α-1-antitrypsin deficiency, Alagille's syndrome (abnormal "elfin" facies, butterfly vertebrae, pulmonary stenosis), progressive familial intrahepatic cholestasis (PFIC) disorders, metabolic conditions (e.g. cystic fibrosis, galactosemia), and parenteral nutrition and neonatal hepatitis.

Miscellaneous Diagnostic Techniques

Other techniques which have been used include endoscopic retrograde cholangiopancreatography (ERCP), percutaneous cholangiography, duodenal intubation and measurement of intraluminal bile. Unfortunately, magnetic resonance cholangiopancreatography (MRCP) is not detailed enough as yet to confidently diagnose BA and radioisotope hepatobiliary imaging (e.g. using iminodiacetic acid derivates), that shows absence of bile excretion lacks specificity—many being simply "neonatal hepatitis".

The surgical differential is less common and includes obstructed CM, which usually shows obvious dilated intra- and extrahepatic biliary dilatation; inspissated bile syndrome which usually occurs in the preterm with a precipitating event such as dehydration or haemolysis and spontaneous perforation of the bile duct which usually shows US evidence of bile ascites and a sub-hepatic collection evident on US [10].

Screening

Some countries have adopted a population screening programme for BA. The most well-developed has been that of Taiwan [23], where mothers are issued with colour-coded cards and asked to compare it with their infant's stool. Recognition of pale stool prompts further investigation and re-

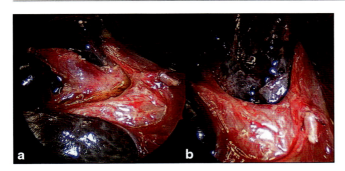

Fig. 56.5 Close-up of porta hepatis during Kasai portoenterostomy. **a** Hypertrophied proximal biliary remnant (BR) being separated from vascular structures of liver. **b** Same view following resection of BR, showing denuded portal plate

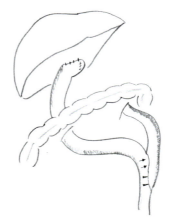

Fig. 56.6 Schematic illustration of retrocolic Roux-en-Y loop, typically measured at 40 cm from portoenterostomy to jejunojejunostomy

ferral. This has certainly shortened their time to surgery—the median age at KPE is now <50 days and is currently the best achieved anywhere in national terms. The key achievement, we believe, has been the marked reduction in late-presenting infants who have already developed obvious cirrhosis [24].

In a recent study from our institution, skills of healthcare professionals in recognising pale stools were assessed. Sadly, the study showed that one third of the abnormal stools were not correctly identified by physicians and nurses who were apparently regularly in contact with jaundiced infants. The authors suggested that distribution of standardised stool colour cards throughout community clinics and outpatient departments might rectify this problem [25].

The simplest solution to early diagnosis remains education, however. It is clear from so many histories that it is often the parents who recognise that persistent jaundice in their infants is not normal but then are falsely reassured by health visitors and their community doctors who fail to inquire about pale stools or dark urine (nevermind looking at them) and fail to do the appropriate blood test (split bilirubin for conjugated and unconjugated fractions). The statutory community check in the UK occurs at 6 weeks of age and is far too late to make a difference in when these affected infants come to surgery.

Kasai Portoenterostomy

The aim of surgery is to excise all extrahepatic biliary remnants allowing a wide portoenterostomy onto a portal plate, denuded of all such tissue (Fig. 56.5). In most cases, this will expose sufficient transected microscopic bile ductules which retain connections with the primitive intrahepatic bile ductule system to allow restoration of at least a degree of biliary drainage. This should be the object of all three types of BA.

A short right upper quadrant muscle-cutting incision should be performed initially to confirm the suspected diagnosis or, if the gallbladder is shown to contain bile, to proceed to on-table cholangiography.

There are then two surgical strategies to expose the porta hepatis: One involving division of at least the left-sided suspensory ligaments and then eversion of the liver onto the abdominal wall. The other retains the liver in the abdominal cavity but usually requires dissection and slinging of the right and left portal veins to allow full exposure of the biliary remnants. A simple portoenterostomy using a retrocolic Roux loop (about 40 cm) completes the reconstruction (Fig. 56.6). Older techniques involving stomas in the Roux loop have been abandoned by virtually all centres.

The KPE can be replicated laparoscopically. However, most centres which explored and pioneered this technique have subsequently reverted to open KPE [26, 27]. The portal dissection, the key to wide excisional surgery, is not improved by being performed laparoscopically and the reconstruction remains technically challenging. There is obviously a better scar, though the infants remain in hospital for the same length of time and an adhesion-free abdominal cavity for the transplant surgeon, although even the latter has been challenged by a study from Germany [28]. Surgeons in Juntendo, Tokyo, have adopted a different approach to these issues by limiting the scale of the portal dissection, and consciously limiting the transection to a basic oval shape—allowing at least some remnant to remain [29].

Postoperative Management

Intravenous fluids and nasogastric aspiration are continued until return of bowel function (about 3–4 days). Careful monitoring of blood glucose, electrolytes and INR is important in the early phase. Liver biochemistry (including bilirubin) may well worsen in the first week, but, by about the 4th week, there should be a definite fall in bilirubin and consistently pigmented stools in those who will do well. Strict attention to nutritional needs is important and all infants need regular vitamin supplementation. Medium-chain triglyceride formula milk (e.g. Caprilon®; SHS, Liverpool, UK) is advocated to maximise calorie input and facilitate lipid absorption.

Adjuvant Therapy for Biliary Atresia

Although a number of drugs have the potential to improve the outcome of KPE surgery, there has been little published in the way of scientific data to provide credible support for any [30]. Postoperative steroids remain popular: A recent study from the USA, including 516 patients from 42 children's hospitals reported about a usage rate of 46% [31]; however, there is only a single prospective, double-blind, randomised, placebo-controlled trial using a low dose (2 mg/kg/day) [32]. This showed a significant reduction in early bilirubin levels (especially in young livers) in the steroid group but did not translate to a reduced need for transplant or improved overall survival. A further follow-up study using a higher starting dose of prednisolone (5 mg/kg/day) confirmed biochemical benefit and also reported a 15% improvement in jaundice clearance when infants <70 days were selected out [33]. There does not seem to be significant side effects from the high-dose regimens.

Ursodeoxycholic acid (UDCA) also remains popular and may be beneficial, but only if surgery has already restored bile flow to a real degree. Willot et al. from Lille in France assessed the effect of UDCA on liver function in children >1 year post-KPE and showed that it improved biochemical liver function in stable children [34]. It may also have an extra-beneficial effect in BA because of its immunosuppressive properties as it has been shown to decrease proliferation of and cytokine production by mononuclear cells in vitro [35].

Complications

About 20–30% of infants will have no effect from KPE, their stools will remain pale; their bilirubin levels will continue to rise. These infants will inexorably continue to develop cirrhosis and end-stage liver disease with severe failure to thrive, ascites, splenomegaly, deepening jaundice and often bleeding from variceal formation. Such infants need expedited liver transplantation, often before their first birthday. It is important to recognise these infants early and not offer false hope that they will somehow turn a corner—they will not.

Other specific complications deserve a more detailed coverage.

Cholangitis

Re-establishment of bile drainage exposes the child to the risk of ascending cholangitis, which occurs most commonly in the year following primary surgery in about 40–50% of children. Paradoxically, it only occurs in children with some degree of bile flow, not in those with early failure as described above. The usual organisms are enteric in origin (e.g. *Escherichia coli, Pseudomonas, Klebsiella* spp.).

Clinically, an episode is characterised by fever, acholic stools and a change in biochemical liver function (rising bilirubin and aspartate aminotransferase; AST levels). The diagnosis may uncommonly be confirmed by blood culture or rarely by percutaneous liver biopsy, but, the key component is antibiotic treatment on suspicion and not confirmation. Intravenous broad-spectrum antibiotics effective against Gram-negative organisms (e.g. piperacillin and tazobactam, gentamicin). Most will respond within 24 h and liver function is usually restored fairly quickly. Some children sustain repeated cholangitis, and they should be treated by prolonged courses of intravenous antibiotics via an indwelling vascular device. If, however, it is clear that there are other features of end-stage liver disease, then they too should be considered for transplant.

Occasionally, cholangitis occurs as a late event in otherwise normal children or adolescents, who have good liver function and have cleared their jaundice [36]. The Roux loop may be at fault here with partial obstruction leading to bile stasis. A combination of radioisotope scans and percutaneous cholangiography may aid the diagnostic process and operative Roux loop revision may be required. Recently, we have used an enteroscope to investigate these patients and provide radiological and endoscopic visualisation of the proximal Roux loop [37].

Portal Hypertension

Increased portal venous pressure has been shown in about 70% of all infants at the time of Kasai operation [38]. However, subsequent portal hypertension depends on both the degree of established fibrosis and, most importantly, the response to surgery. There is a relationship with biochemical liver function and variceal development and in those who fail and need early transplantation; about 30% will have had a significant variceal bleed.

Infants and children with bleeding oesophageal varices need rapid access to high-quality pediatric facilities with the resources and expertise to manage them appropriately. Injection and/or banding is not a technique for the occasional pediatric endoscopist. Restoration of circulating blood volume and pharmacotherapy (e.g. 2 ml/h of 500 µg octreotide in 40 ml of saline) should precede endoscopy and achieve a measure of stabilisation. Sometimes a modified Sengstaken tube needs to be placed to achieve control of bleeding. Invariably, in children, this can only be done under general anaesthesia but can be life saving. The definitive treatment in older children is endoscopic variceal banding, although injection sclerotherapy retains a role in treating the varices in infants.

In common with other large centres, we therefore recommend that for each child with BA there is the opportunity to enter a programme of endoscopic surveillance to try and pre-empt variceal bleeding [39]. In this respect, there may be a role for selection based on haematological, biochemical or US variables to assign risk. Our recent work has suggested that APRi and clinical prediction rule (CPR) [40] appear to be superior in this respect to simple univariate indices (e.g. platelets, bilirubin) or US dimensions (e.g. spleen size or resistance index).

The key variceal signs that should prompt *prophylactic* endoscopic treatment are the presence of significant red *wales* in grade II/III oesophageal varices and obvious (usually lesser curve) gastric varices [39]. Liver transplantation needs to be actively considered as definitive treatment for portal hypertension where liver function is poor and the child is already significantly jaundiced.

Ascites

This is related to portal hypertension in part, but there are other contributory factors including hypoalbuminaemia and hyponatraemia. It also predisposes to spontaneous, bacterial peritonitis. Conventional treatment includes a low-salt diet, fluid restriction and the use of diuretics particularly spironolactone. It is often seen in settings of malnutrition and end-stage liver disease, and a nutritional supplementation is important to try and increase calorie and protein intake.

Outcome Following Kasai Portoenterostomy

There are many factors, which will influence surgical outcome in BA. Some are unalterable (e.g. degree of cirrhosis at presentation, absence of, or paucity of bile ductules at the level of section) and some are subject to change (e.g. efficacy of the KPE due to surgical inexperience, poor choice of technique, complications postoperatively due to inexperienced unit, untreated cholangitis, etc.). In large centres with experienced surgeons, about 50 % of all infants should clear their jaundice and achieve a normal (<20 μmol/L or <1.5 mg/dL) bilirubin [41]. These should do well and have a good quality of long-term survival with their native liver.

There is no doubt that increasing age at KPE is associated with increasing liver fibrosis and cirrhosis although the actual rates of progression differ according to underlying cause [42]. There is a marked relationship with age at surgery for instance with cystic BA and BASM but it is not that evident in isolated BA. So, it is not really possible to use age as a simplistic predictor in individual cases as even in those

coming to surgery at > 100 days may still have a response to KPE [43]. Still there may be a role for those with the signs of evident cirrhosis (e.g. ascites, heterogeneity of the liver appearance on US) for consideration of transplantation as the primary procedure. It remains an uncommon choice though, perhaps <5 % in our experience [41].

In the England and Wales, we have adopted a policy of centralisation of surgeons and resources. So for a country of 56 million, there are only three recognised centres to treat this condition. All surgical facilities including transplantation are available. This policy was adopted because previous audits of outcome had shown a significant difference depending on centre experience with the less experienced centres showing poor outcomes [44]. Subsequent studies confirmed an improvement in overall national outcome [41, 45]. This policy has been replicated by some European countries again with demonstrable benefit [46, 47].

Choledochal Malformation

Introduction

The German anatomist Abraham Vater recognised the ampullary nature of the junction of biliary and pancreatic ducts which since then has carried his name. Subsequently, he also described what appeared to be a choledochal cyst in a pamphlet published in 1723 [48].

Further examples of this, the classical choledochal cyst, were described, but still barely 90 cases had been recorded by 1959, when Alonso-Lej et al. attempted a simple classification into three types [49]. Even as recently as 1975, Flanagan could only identify details of 955 cases from the literature [50].

CM (of which some can be described as choledochal "cysts") may be characterised as, . "an abnormal dilatation of the biliary tract, in the absence of any acute obstruction". This allows us to exclude the dilated CBD secondary to choledocholithiasis and strictures secondary to chronic pancreatitis for instance. Similarly, while many CMs present with jaundice and biliary obstruction, it is obvious that previously their function was unimpaired for much of the subject's life in the presence of clear morphological change.

Aetiology

Most CMs appear in some way to be of congenital origin though the actual mechanism itself is obscure.

There are two competing hypotheses:

1. *Pancreatic reflux.* An intrinsic part of most examples of CM complex is an abnormal pancreatobiliary junction. Normally, the pancreatic and bile ducts open separately

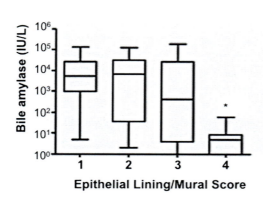

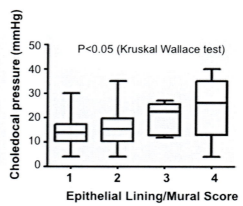

Fig. 56.7 Relationship between biliary amylase, choledochal pressure and epithelial histology. Levels of biliary amylase (**a**) (as a surrogate of pancreatic reflux) and in-situ choledochal pressure (**b**) in 73 children with choledochal malformation. The *Y* axis (Epithelial lining/mural score) uses a semi-quantitative score for biliary epithelium where *0*

normal; *1* minimal focal hyperplasia and chronic inflammation; *2* mild chronic inflammation; *3* pronounced hyperplasia and moderate chronic inflammation and *4* epithelial loss, bile impregnation and biliary necrosis. ([59], with permission from Wiley)

within the wall of the duodenum at the ampulla of Vater achieving biological separation of bile and pancreatic juice. In most patients with CM, duct confluence occurs within the head of the pancreas, outside the duodenal wall resulting in a common channel that allows free intraductal mixing of both types of secretion [51–53].

Donald Babbitt, an American radiologist, proposed that this reflux of presumably activated pancreatic juice could damage the wall of bile duct causing weakness and dilatation [54]. There are a number of experimental animal models which have tried to replicate the effects of pancreatic enzymes on bile ducts [55, 56], but there has been little actual documented change in the dimensions of the biliary system.

2. *Distal bile duct stenosis.* Almost 15 % of CM can now be detected antenatally on the maternal US scan. Most of the infants are not actually jaundiced at birth—though some are. In all of these, the morphological type is a cystic malformation and in these, though there might be a common channel, there is minimal amylase in bile (implying no reflux) and often a very definite abrupt change and distal bile duct stenotic segment. Furthermore, animal models involving ligation of the distal bile duct [57] produce obvious cystic change.

To try and resolve some of these questions, we have looked into a series of studies at the relationship between age at presentation, modes of clinical presentation, bile duct pressure (as measured at operation), levels of amylase in bile (as a marker of reflux) and the histological appearance of the resected choledochus [53, 58, 59]. This showed that there is a remarkable inverse relationship between pressure and amylase—the higher the pressure, the lower the amylase and that increasing histological epithelial injury and damage are found in those with higher pressures and very obviously not with high amylase levels (Fig. 56.7).

Classification

The original Alonso-Lej classification (types 1, 2 and 3) [49] has been modified most notably by Takuji Todani, a Japanese surgeon, by adding the concept of multiple dilatation (type 4) and isolated intrahepatic dilatation (Type 5) [60]. Our own classification has been in clinical use for over 20 years and is illustrated in Fig. 56.8 [59, 61].

We prefer to use the generic term *choledochal malformation*, rather than the very specific term choledochal cyst, since

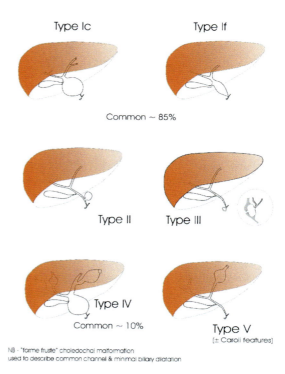

Fig. 56.8 King's College Hospital classification for choledochal malformation

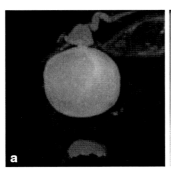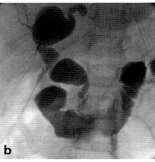

Fig. 56.9 Types of choledochal malformation. **a** Operative cholangiogram showing classical type 1c choledochal malformation (CM). Note the demarcation both proximally and distally, together with long common channel. **b** Percutaneous transhepatic cholangiogram of type 1f CM. Note the generalised dilatation down to a common channel which is dilated and filled with debris (the child presented with acute pancreatitis)

not many of the described dilatation appears as "cystic" (i.e. spherical). The principle variants of extrahepatic dilatation (type 1) making up about 80 % of all cases are either *cystic CM (type 1c)* or *fusiform CM (type 1f)*. The former typically has a natural demarcation at either end (Fig. 56.9a), while the latter is much smaller in diameter but merges imperceptibly with a common channel distally or the bifurcation proximally. The only other common variant *(type 4)* is either of the foregoing extrahepatic dilatation together with significant intrahepatic biliary dilatation—sometimes this is because of actual obstruction (with a swift return to normal calibre after surgery) but in others it may appear as an intrinsic feature of the condition (Fig. 56.9b) [62]. Of the remaining variants, *types 2 and 3* are rarely seen in children. The former can be likened to a diverticulum of the CBD, the latter a localised dilatation of the CDB as it transits the wall of the duodenum (aka choledochocele). *Type 5 CM* refers to usually solitary intrahepatic biliary cystic lesions. Most of these are detected incidentally and can be left alone.

Jacques Caroli, a French gastroenterologist and prolific author, described a number of intrahepatic biliary pathologies which carry his name [63, 64]. The term Caroli disease is usually applied to ectasia or segmental dilatation of the larger intrahepatic ducts (typically the left hepatic duct system) without any other extrahepatic manifestation and is usually sporadic. Caroli syndrome describes a condition in which there are multiple, discrete small yet saccular dilatations of the intrahepatic bile ducts with almost invariably hepatic fibrosis and usually renal disease. This is generally inherited in an autosomal recessive manner [65–67], and there is a large overlap with congenital hepatic fibrosis, polycystic kidney disease (both autosomal dominant and recessive types) *et alia*.

Epidemiology

CM is a relatively rare abnormality in the West and far more common in the East although the actual prevalence remains uncalculated [68, 69]. Virtually, all of the large series of this has been reported from Japan [68, 69] and now increasingly China [70], with very little substantial series from North America [71] or Europe [72]. There is a marked female predominance [72], but not much in the way of an identifiable hereditary element. However, isolated examples of familial occurrence in siblings and twins have been reported [73–75].

Clinical Features

CM can present at any age, but more than 90 % will present within the first decade [72]. Clinical manifestations do differ according to the age of onset. Typical presenting symptoms in the newborn mimic biliary atresia and specifically cystic biliary atresia with obstructive jaundice, acholic stools and hepatomegaly, depending on the degree of obstruction. These sometimes have advanced liver fibrosis depending on the length of the period of obstruction.

Older infants and toddlers then tend to present with jaundice and may well be found to have an upper abdominal mass, and most turn out to have a type 1c CM. If obstructive features are ignored, then chronic liver disease may result and cirrhosis is possible though seemingly not as common as in some older series [72].

Recurrent abdominal pain becomes a feature later on and may be due to an obstructed high-pressure system or actual recurrent pancreatitis. This is usually pathologically mild, oedematous and short-lived and associated with hyperamylasemia. This scenario is usually associated with the type 1f CM. Sometimes investigation shows a common channel, presenting features of pancreatitis but not much in the way of biliary dilatation. This has been termed a *forme fruste* CM or more simply common channel syndrome (Fig. 56.10).

Perforation of a high-pressure system is uncommon (5 %), and in these the clinical scenario may mimic spontaneous biliary perforation in infancy [76] or appendicitis in the older child. Bile leakage is usually confined to the retroperitoneum and tracks down the paracolic gutter.

There is a risk of carcinomatous change in long-standing CM which will manifest later in adulthood, exceptionally rarely in adolescence. Up to 10 % of adult series have established malignant change at laparotomy [61, 77, 78]. In a Japanese series of 94 patient (adults and children) with excised choledochal malformation, four later developed malignancy. The age at detection ranged from 27 to 65 years with the malignancy arising both in the liver and the head of pancreas [77]. Similarly, Lee et al. described 80 patients with biliary

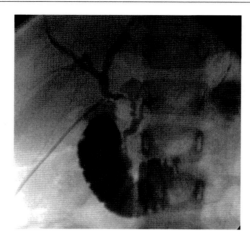

Fig. 56.10 Common channel syndrome. An 8-year-old girl with long history of recurrent acute pancreatitis requiring an ERCP to diagnose a common channel, with presumed reflux of bile into the pancreatic duct. She was cured by disconnection of biliary and pancreatic ducts and Roux loop hepaticojejunostomy biliary reconstruction

malignancies from a large Korean multicentre series of 808 adults [78]. Of these, most ($n=74$) were evident at initial presentation and laparotomy, while six presented 4 years after their previous choledochal excision. What is not known is what the real long-term risk is in those who have had their definitive excisional surgery in childhood.

Diagnosis

A choledochal cyst was first diagnosed antenatally using US by Dewbury et al. from Southampton, UK, in 1980 [79]. Since then, up to 15% of CMs (in the UK at least) are diagnosed antenatally from as early as 15 weeks' gestation and these are almost invariably types 1c or 5 CM [80]. CM may be confused with duodenal atresia, cystic biliary atresia, ovarian cyst, duplication cyst and mesenteric cyst. In this scenario, it is most important to exclude the possibility of cystic BA who requires urgent KPE [9]. If there is clinical doubt, then a dynamic radioisotope scan (e.g. technetium[99] labelled iminodiacetic acid, HIDA-scan) will confirm the non-obstructing CM, where surgery can be deferred to about 3–4 months.

Postnatally, US is the initial diagnostic modality of choice, allowing for precise measurements of intra-/extrahepatic duct dilatation and identification of stones/sludge. MRCP has superseded the use of CT and for the most part ERCP for preoperative anatomical delineation of the pancreatobiliary tract. Three-dimensional reconstructions images are easily obtained, although sedation may be required in infants and small children.

Functional assessment of CM may be shown using a dynamic radioisotope scan which can show baseline parenchymal hepatocyte uptake together with the pattern and degree of bile excretion—important if not considering surgery. This may also be useful in diagnosing choledochal perforation. ERCP is still required when there is diagnostic uncertainty over the nature of the pancreatobiliary junction and common channel, particularly in those with minimal biliary dilatation and often with a presenting feature of pancreatitis. Notwithstanding these, a detailed US scan supplemented by MRCP or intraoperative cholangiography provides sufficient anatomical information in most cases.

Biochemical liver function tests may be normal or show evidence of biliary obstruction. Amylase levels may be elevated during episodes of abdominal pain suggestive of actual pancreatitis. A prolonged INR secondary to cholestasis should be corrected with intravenous vitamin K.

Surgical Management

Open surgery is still very much the standard in most centres. For the common types (type 1c, 1f and type 4), this consists of excision of the dilated part of the extrahepatic biliary tree; clearance of debris and stones from any dilated intrahepatic ducts (best achieved with on-table cholangioscopy); clearance of any common channel debris (± transduodenal sphincteroplasty) and a reconstruction end-to-side hepaticojejunostomy using a long (40–50 cm) Roux loop. Despite often quite alarming intrahepatic dilatation, the usual best course is excision of the extrahepatic segment with a fastidious approach to segmental drainage and cautious follow-up. Most ducts will reduce in size, particularly in children which in itself suggests the primary aetiological role of elevated intrabiliary pressure [62].

The first laparoscopic cystectomy and reconstruction of a 6-year-old female with a type 1c malformation was reported by Farello et al. in 1995 from Schio, Italy [81], and this has become an option in some parts of the world. The largest series are from either China or Vietnam and now number over 200 children in each [70, 82]. The technical skills required are high and a large throughput is important in minimising complications. The standard Roux loop reconstruction is usually carried out by extracting the small bowel through an enlarged umbilical incision though the hepaticojejunostomy is performed intracorporeally. A controversial innovation has been to discard the hepaticojejunostomy because it is difficult and perform a hepaticoduodenostomy instead [83]. This short cut may be expedient but the long-term effects of this may be poorer. Cholangitis and biliary gastritis are both significantly more common using this so-called physiological alternative [84].

Excision of the diverticulum is probably all that is needed in the rare type 2 CM as long as normal unobstructed distal bile flow can be demonstrated radiologically [85]. Large choledochoceles (type 3 CM) can be removed transduodenally, whereas smaller choledochoceles can be treated by sphincteroplasty or endoscopic sphincterotomy, although admittedly most reported experience is in adults [86].

Most type 5 CMs are isolated, asymptomatic and picked up incidentally with US. They can probably best be treated conservatively with serial US to try and detect any complications such as stone formation [80]. In those with symptomatic or complicated Caroli-like intrahepatic dilatation, resection should be considered particularly if unilobar. The treatment of Caroli's syndrome may be complicated and occasionally liver transplantation may be considered.

Postoperative Management

Intravenous fluids and nasogastric aspiration are continued until return of bowel function, usually on day 2 or 3 after the operation. Oral feeding is recommenced after the fluid from the nasogastric tube becomes clear.

Complications

Complications are uncommon, but may include bleeding, adhesive small bowel obstruction, anastomotic leakage and leakage from the pancreatic duct. Anastomotic leakage may be treated conservatively particularly if this has followed a difficult and challenging anastomosis. Abdominal drainage is key and if there is no obstruction to a functioning Roux loop, then it will settle. Pancreatic leaks are less common but more challenging, particularly if the ampullary sphincter is still intact. Consideration should be given to endoscopic ERCP and stenting if a conservative trial of abdominal drainage, intravenous antibiotics, nasogastric decompression and parenteral nutrition fails.

Anastomotic stricture usually followed by recurrent cholangitis and intrahepatic stone formation are late complications [87]. Cholangitis implies a mechanical problem and should be aggressively investigated. Strictures or persistent intrahepatic dilatation can be treated by radiological intervention with surgery reserved for failure. Recurrent pancreatitis implies obstructive problems with the retained common channel. MRCP, but more likely ERCP should be diagnostic and in the latter's case, may be therapeutic with endoscopic channel clearing or stenting.

References

1. Thompson J. Congenital obliteration of the bile ducts. Edin Med J. 1891;37:523–31.
2. Kasai M, Suzuki S. A new operation for "non-correctable" biliary atresia—portoenterostomy. Shijitsu 1959;13:733–9.
3. Kasai M, Suzuki H, Ohashi E, et al. Technique and results of operative management of biliary atresia. W J Surg. 1978;2:571–9.
4. Starzl TE, Marchioro TL, Vonkaulla KN, Hermann G, Brittain RS, Waddell WR. Homotransplantation of the liver in humans. Surg Gynecol Obstet. 1963;117:659–76.
5. Petersen C, Davenport M. Aetiology of biliary atresia: what is actually known? Orphanet J Rare Dis. 2013;8:128–41.
6. Davenport M, Savage M, Mowat AP, Howard ER. Biliary atresia splenic malformation syndrome: an etiologic and prognostic subgroup. Surgery 1993;113:662–8.
7. Davenport M, Tizzard S, Underhill J, et al. The biliary atresia splenic malformation syndrome: a twenty-eight year single centre study. J Pediatr. 2006;149:393–400.
8. Redkar R, Davenport M, Howard ER. Antenatal diagnosis of congenital anomalies of the biliary tract. J Pediatr Surg. 1998;33:700–4.
9. Caponcelli E, Knisley A, Davenport M. Cystic biliary atresia; an etiologic and prognostic sub-group. J Pediatr Surg. 2008;43:1619–24.
10. Davenport M, Betalli P, D'Antiga L, et al. The spectrum of surgical jaundice in infancy. J Pediatr Surg. 2003;38:1471–9.
11. Livesey E, Cortina Borja M, Sharif K, et al. Epidemiology of biliary atresia in England and Wales (1999–2006). Arch Dis Child Fetal Neonatal Ed. 2009;94:F451–5.
12. Rauschenfels S, Krassmann M, Al-Masri AN, Verhagen W, Leonhardt J, Kuebler JF, Petersen C. Incidence of hepatotropic viruses in biliary atresia. Eur J Pediatr. 2009;168:469–76.
13. Jimenez-Rivera C, Jolin-Dahel KS, Fortinsky KJ, et al. International incidence and outcomes of biliary atresia. J Pediatr Gastroenterol Nutr. 2013;56:344–54.
14. Chiu CY, Chen PH, Chan CF, et al. Taiwan Infant Stool Color Card Study Group. Biliary atresia in preterm infants in Taiwan: a nationwide survey. J Pediatr. 2013;163:100–3.
15. Chardot C, Buet C, Serinet MO, et al. Improving outcomes of biliary atresia: French national series 1986–2009. J Hepatol. 2013;58:1209–17.
16. Fischler B, Haglund B, Hjern A. A population-based study on the incidence and possible pre- and perinatal etiologic risk factors of biliary atresia. J Pediatr. 2002;141:217–22.
17. Petersen C, Harder D, Abola Z, et al. European biliary atresia registries: summary of a symposium. Eur J Pediatr Surg. 2008;18:111–6.
18. Wildhaber BE, Majno P, Mayr J, et al. Biliary atresia: Swiss national study, 1994–2004. J Pediatr Gastroenterol Nutr. 2008;46:299–307.
19. Caton AR. Exploring the seasonality of birth defects in the New York State Congenital Malformations Registry. Birth Defects Res A Clin Mol Teratol. 2012;94:424–37.
20. Wada H, Muraji T, Yokoi A, et al. Insignificant seasonal and geographical variation in incidence of biliary atresia in Japan: a regional survey of over 20 years. J Pediatr Surg. 2007;42:2090–2.
21. Martin LR, Davenport M, Dhawan A. Skin colour: a barrier to early referral of infants with biliary in the UK. Arch Dis Child. 2012;97:12.
22. Grieve A, Makin E, Davenport M. Aspartate Aminotransferase-to-Platelet Ratio index (APRi) in infants with biliary atresia: prognostic value at presentation. J Pediatr Surg. 2013;48:789–95.
23. Hsiao CH, Chang MH, Chen HL, et al. Taiwan Infant Stool Color Card Study Group. Universal screening for biliary atresia using an infant stool color card in Taiwan. Hepatology 2008;47:1233–40.
24. Tseng JJ, Lai MS, Lin MC, et al. Stool color card screening for biliary atresia. Pediatrics 2011;128:e1209–15.
25. Bakshi B, Sutcliffe A, Akindolie M, et al. How reliably can pediatric professionals identify pale stool from cholestatic newborns? Arch Dis Child Fetal Neonatal Ed. 2012;97:F385–7.
26. Wong KK, Chung PH, Chan KL, et al. Should open Kasai portoenterostomy be performed for biliary atresia in the era of laparoscopy? Pediatr Surg Int. 2008;24:931–3.
27. Ure BM, Kuebler JF, Schukfeh N, et al. Survival with the native liver after laparoscopic versus conventional Kasai portoenteros-

tomy in infants with biliary atresia: a prospective trial. Ann Surg. 2011;253:826–30.

28. Oetzmann von Sochaczewski C, Petersen C, Ure BM, et al. Laparoscopic versus conventional Kasai portoenterostomy does not facilitate subsequent liver transplantation in infants with biliary atresia. J Laparoendosc Adv Surg Tech A. 2012;22:408–11.

29. Yamataka A. Laparoscopic Kasai portoenterostomy for biliary atresia. J Hepatobiliary Pancreat Sci. 2013;20:481–6.

30. Petersen C, Harder D, Melter M, et al. Postoperative high-dose steroids do not improve mid-term survival with native liver in biliary atresia. Am J Gastroenterol. 2008;103:712–9.

31. Lao OB, Larison C, Garrison M, et al. Steroid use after the Kasai procedure for biliary atresia. Am J Surg. 2010;199:680–4.

32. Davenport M, Stringer MD, Tizzard SA, et al. Randomized, double-blind, placebo-controlled trial of corticosteroids after Kasai portoenterostomy for biliary atresia. Hepatology 2007;46:1821–7.

33. Davenport M, Parsons C, Tizzard S, et al. Steroids in biliary atresia: single surgeon, single centre, prospective study. J Hepatol. 2013;59:1054–8.

34. Willot S, Uhlen S, Michaud L, et al. Effect of ursodeoxycholic acid on liver function in children after successful surgery for biliary atresia. Pediatrics 2008;122:e1236–41.

35. Lacaille F, Paradis K. The immunosuppressive effect of ursodeoxycholic acid: a comparative in vitro study on human peripheral blood mononuclear cells. Hepatology 1993;18:165–72.

36. Houben C, Phelan S, Davenport M. Late-presenting cholangitis and Roux loop obstruction after Kasai portoenterostomy for biliary atresia. J Pediatr Surg. 2006;41:1159–64.

37. Vadamalayan B, Davenport M, Baker A, Dhawan A. Feasibility of Roux-en-Y loop enteroscopy in children with liver disease. J Gastro Hepat Res. 2012;1:130–3.

38. Shalaby A, Makin E, Davenport M. Portal venous pressure in biliary atresia. J Pediatr Surg. 2012;47:363–6.

39. Duché M, Ducot B, Ackermann O, et al. Experience with endoscopic management of high-risk gastroesophageal varices, with and without bleeding, in children with biliary atresia. Gastroenterology 2013;145:801–7.

40. Gana JC, Turner D, Mieli-Vergani G, et al. A clinical prediction rule and platelet count predict esophageal varices in children. Gastroenterology 2011;141:2009–16.

41. Davenport M, Ong E, Sharif K, et al. Biliary atresia in England and Wales: results of centralization and new benchmark. J Pediatr Surg. 2011;46:1689–94.

42. Davenport M, Caponcelli E, Livesey E, et al. Surgical outcome in biliary atresia: etiology affects the influence of age at surgery. Ann Surg. 2008;247:694–8.

43. Davenport M, Puricelli V, Farrant P, Hadzić N, et al. The outcome of the older (< or > 100 days) infants with biliary atresia. J Pediatr Surg. 2004;39:575–81.

44. McKiernan PJ, Baker AJ, Kelly DA. The frequency and outcome of biliary atresia in the UK and Ireland. Lancet 2000;355(9197):25–9.

45. Davenport M, De Ville de Goyet J, Stringer MD, et al. Seamless management of biliary atresia in England and Wales (1999–2002). Lancet 2004;363(9418):1354–7.

46. Kvist N, Davenport M. Thirty-four years' experience with biliary atresia in Denmark: a single center study. Eur J Pediatr Surg. 2011;21:224–8.

47. Lampela H, Ritvanen A, Kosola S, et al. National centralization of biliary atresia care to an assigned multidisciplinary team provides high-quality outcomes. Scand J Gastroenterol. 2012;47:99–107.

48. Vater A, Ezler CS. Dissertatio de scirrhis viserum occasione sections virii tympanite defunte. Wittenberge 1723;4 Pamphlers 881:22.

49. Alonso-Lej F, Rever WB Jr., Pessagno DJ. Congenital choledochal cyst, with a report of 2, and an analysis of 94, cases. Surg Gynecol Obstret (Int Abstr Surg). 1959;108:1–30.

50. Flanagan DP. Biliary cysts. Ann Surg. 1975;182:635–43.

51. Todani T, Watanabe Y, Fujii T, et al. Anomalous arrangement of the pancreatobiliary ductal system in patients with a choledochal cyst. Am J Surg. 1984;147:672–6.

52. Komi N, Takehara H, Kunitomo K, et al. Does the type of anomalous arrangement of pancreaticobiliary ducts influence the surgery and prognosis of choledochal cyst? J Pediatr Surg. 1992;27:728–31.

53. Davenport M, Stringer MD, Howard ER. Biliary amylase and congenital choledochal dilatation. J Pediatr Surg. 1995;30:474–7.

54. Babbitt DP. Congenital choledochal cysts: new etiological concept based on anomalous relationships of the common bile duct and pancreatic bulb. Ann Radiol. 1969;12:231–40.

55. Okada A, Hasegawa T, Oguchi Y, et al. Recent advances in pathophysiology and surgical treatment of congenital dilatation of the bile duct. J Hepatobiliary Pancreat Surg. 2002;9:342–51.

56. Nakamura T, Okada A, Higaki J, et al. Pancreaticobiliary maljunction-associated pancreatitis: an experimental study on the activation of pancreatic phospholipase A2. World J Surg. 1996;20:543–50.

57. Spitz L. Experimental production of cystic dilatation oft he common bile duct in neonatal lambs. J Pediatr Surg. 1977;12:39–42.

58. Davenport M, Basu R. Under pressure: choledochal malformation manometry. J Pediatr Surg. 2005;40:331–5.

59. Turowski C, Knisely AS, Davenport M. Role of pressure and pancreatic reflux in the aetiology of choledochal malformation. Br J Surg. 2011;98:1319–26.

60. Todani T, Watanabe Y, Narusue M, et al. Congenital bile duct cysts: classification, operative procedures, and review of thirty-seven cases including cancer arising from choledochal cyst. Am J Surg. 1977;134:263–9.

61. Dabbas N, Davenport M. Congenital choledochal malformation: not just a problem for children. Ann R Coll Surg Engl. 2009;91:100–5.

62. Hill R, Parsons C, Farrant P, et al. Intrahepatic duct dilatation in type 4 choledochal malformation: pressure-related, postoperative resolution. J Pediatr Surg. 2011;46:299–303.

63. Caroli J, Soupault R, Kossakowski J, et al. Congenital polycystic dilation of the intrahepatic bile ducts; attempt at classification. Sem Hop. 1958;34(8/2):488–95.

64. Caroli J, Couinaud C, Soupault R, et al. A new disease, undoubtedly congenital, of the bile ducts: unilobar cystic dilation of the hepatic ducts. Sem Hop. 1958;34:496–502.

65. Rawat D, Kelly DA, Milford DV, Sharif K, Lloyd C, McKiernan PJ. Phenotypic variation and long-term outcome in children with congenital hepatic fibrosis. J Pediatr Gastroenterol Nutr. 2013;57:161–6.

66. Calinescu-Tuleasca AM, Bottani A, Rougemont AL, et al. Caroli disease, bilateral diffuse cystic renal dysplasia, situs inversus, postaxial polydactyly, and preauricular fistulas: a ciliopathy caused by a homozygous NPHP3 mutation. Eur J Pediatr. 2013;172:877–81.

67. Shorbagi A, Bayraktar Y. Experience of a single center with congenital hepatic fibrosis: a review of the literature. World J Gastroenterol. 2010;16:683–90.

68. Miyano T, Yamataka A, Kato Y, et al. Hepaticoenterostomy after excision of choledochal cyst in children: a 30-year experience with 180 cases. J Pediatr Surg. 1996;31:1417–21.

69. Yamaguchi M. Congenital choledochal cyst. Analysis of 1433 patients in the Japanese literature. Am J Surg. 1980;140:653–7.

70. Diao M, Li L, Li Q, et al. Single-incision versus conventional laparoscopic cyst excision and Roux-Y hepaticojejunostomy for children with choledochal cysts: a case-control study. World J Surg. 2013;37:1707–13.

71. Wiseman K, Buczkowski AK, Chung SW, et al. Epidemiology, presentation, diagnosis, and outcomes of choledochal cysts in adults in an urban environment. Am J Surg. 2005;189:527–31.

72. Stringer MD, Dhawan A, Davenport M, et al. Choledochal cysts: lessons from a 20 year experience. Arch Dis Child. 1995;73:528–31.

73. Iwafuchi M, Ohsawa Y, Naito S, et al. Familial occurrence of congenital bile duct dilatation. J Pediatr Surg. 1990;25:353–5.

74. Ando K, Miyano T, Fujimoto T, et al. Sibling occurrence of biliary atresia and biliary dilatation. J Pediatr Surg. 1996;31:1302–4.

75. Lane GJ, Yamataka A, Kobayashi H, et al. Different types of congenital biliary dilatation in dizygotic twins. Pediatr Surg Int. 1999;15:403–4.

76. Davenport M, Heaton ND, Howard ER. Spontaneous perforation of the bile duct in infants. Br J Surg. 1991;78:1068–70.

77. Ohashi T, Wakai T, Kubota M, et al. Risk of subsequent biliary malignancy in patients undergoing cyst excision for congenital choledochal cysts. J Gastroenterol Hepatol. 2013;28:243–7.

78. Lee SE, Jang JY, Lee JY, et al. Choleodchal cyst and associated malignant tumors in adults. Arch Surg. 2011;146:1178–84.

79. Dewbury KC, Aluwihare AP, Birch SJ, et al. Prenatal ultrasound demonstration of a choledochal cyst. Br J Radiol. 1980;53:906–7.

80. Charlesworth P, Ade-Ajayi N, Davenport M. Natural history and long-term follow-up of antenatally detected liver cysts. J Pediatr Surg. 2007;42:494–9.

81. Farello GA, Cerofolini A, Rebonato M, et al. Congenital choledochal cyst: video-guided laparoscopic treatment. Surg Laparosc Endosc. 1995;5:354–8.

82. Liem NT, Pham HD, Dung le A, et al. Early and intermediate outcomes of laparoscopic surgery for choledochal cysts with 400 patients. J Laparoendosc Adv Surg Tech A. 2012;22:599–603.

83. Liem NT, Dung LA, Son TN. Laparoscopic complete cyst excision and hepaticoduodenostomy for choledochal cyst: early results in 74 cases. J Laparoendosc Adv Surg Tech A. 2009;19:87–90.

84. Shimotakahara A, Yamataka A, Yanai T, et al. Roux en Y hepatico-jejunostomy or hepaticoduodenostomy for biliary reconstruction: which is better? Pediatr Surg Int. 2005;21:5–7.

85. Yamashita H, Otani T, Shioiri T, et al. Smallest Todani's type II choledochal cyst. Dig Liver Dis. 2003;35:498–502.

86. Ladas SD, Katsojridakis I, Tassios P, et al. Choledochocele, an overlooked diagnosis: report of 15 cases and review of 56 published reports (1984–1992). Endoscopy 1995;27:233–9.

87. Yamataka A, Ohshiro K, Okada Y, et al. Complications after cyst excision with hepaticoenterostomy for choledochal cysts and their surgical management in children versus adults. J Pediatr Surg. 1997;32:1097–102.

Congenital Hepatic Fibrosis, Caroli's Disease, and Other Fibrocystic Liver Diseases

Nathalie Rock, Ino Kanavaki and Valérie McLin

Terms and Definitions

The term "fibrocystic liver diseases" is used to describe a group of congenital disorders most often presenting in childhood. Their common feature is the abnormal embryologic development of the ductal plate that leads to dilatation and cyst formation within the intrahepatic or extrahepatic biliary tree. Two major disorders are discussed in this chapter: congenital hepatic fibrosis (CHF) and Caroli's disease (CD). Caroli's syndrome (CS) combines the features of both CHF and CD. Differences and overlap between these clinical entities are thoroughly discussed.

Pathophysiology of CHF and CD

CHF and CD are closely related to each other, because they both result from a ductal plate malformation (DPM) due to abnormalities in primary cilia.

Liver Development Overview

In vertebrates, the early liver bud develops when a few cells from the endoderm delaminate into the adjacent mesenchyme. The early liver cells are called hepatoblasts. They are bipotential precursors which eventually adopt either a hepatocyte fate or a cholangiocyte fate (Fig. 57.1) [1]. As such, they express markers of both lineages during development, some of which can be reactivated in certain disease states [2]. Hepatoblasts contribute to intrahepatic biliary development at the ductal plate, a process which is orchestrated by intrahepatic vascular development and which will be of importance in understanding the fibrocystic liver diseases [3].

The Ductal Plate

The ductal plate is the embryonic precursor of the intrahepatic bile ducts. It is first detected by 6–7 gestational weeks and consists of a double layer of cuboidal, biliary-type epithelium that surrounds the developing portal veins. This layer develops from the transformation of hepatoblasts and yields an anastomosing tubular network of biliary ducts through a process called ductal plate remodeling (Fig. 57.1) [4–7].

Ductal plate remodeling begins by 11 weeks of gestation, and in normal conditions it is complete in early postnatal life. It is a process of negative selection of nonfunctional ductal plate elements which involute in a centripetal fashion from the hilum toward the liver periphery [4, 6, 8]. The remodeling phase is characterized by a high rate of mesenchymal proliferation, resulting in the separation of the developing bile ducts from the liver parenchyma (Fig. 57.1) [4, 8]. Meanwhile, hepatocytes and intrahepatic biliary epithelial cells undergo apoptosis at a higher rate than normal under the control of apoptosis-related proteins: C-myc protein and fas antigen stimulate cell-death while Bcl-2 protein inhibits apoptosis [5]. It is possible that an imbalance between proliferation and apoptosis impedes normal ductal plate remodeling, thereby yielding the DPM [4, 5]. Remodeling is under the control of a number of genetic and molecular factors that make it vulnerable to maldevelopment. Among these factors are signaling molecules from the portal venous mesenchyme, from adjacent hepatoblasts, from involuting bile ducts, and hormones such as estrogens.

The Ductal Plate Malformation

The term "ductal plate malformation" was first used by Mogens Jorgen Jorgensen in 1977 to describe an unusual histologic configuration of the liver of children with polycystic disease. He first described extensive fibrosis and increased number of bile ducts within the fibrotic regions, now recognized as the cardinal features of the DPM [9]. It is now understood that the DPM occurs when excessive ductal plate remnants fail to disappear. What is not understood is why

N. Rock (✉) · I. Kanavaki · V. McLin
Department of Pediatrics, Swiss Center for Liver Disease in Children, University Hospitals Geneva, Rue Willy-Donze 5, Geneva 1205, Switzerland
e-mail: nathalie.rock@hcuge.ch

© Springer International Publishing Switzerland 2016
S. Guandalini et al. (eds.), *Textbook of Pediatric Gastroenterology, Hepatology and Nutrition*,
DOI 10.1007/978-3-319-17169-2_57

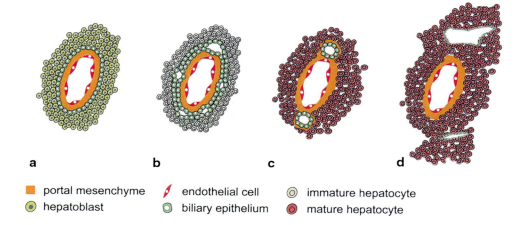

a   b   c   d

■ portal mesenchyme   ⬦ endothelial cell   ◎ immature hepatocyte
◉ hepatoblast   ◯ biliary epithelium   ◉ mature hepatocyte

Fig. 57.1 Biliary development and the ductal plate malformation (modified from [1]). **a** At 14 weeks of gestation, hepatoblasts in contact with portal vein mesenchyme adopt a biliary epithelial fate. **b** At 17 weeks of gestation, biliary layer duplicates and focal dilatation within the layer leads to bile ducts formation. **c** At birth, bile duct development is nearly completed, and the bilayer has involuted. Liver cells are either hepatocytes or hepatoblasts. **d** Ductal plate malformation: abnormal ductal plate remodeling leads to saccular, biliary dilatations

the size of the bile ducts affected by the DPM varies between diseases: Small ducts are affected in CHF while larger ducts are dysmorphic in CD. Figure 57.2 [10] illustrates the DPM and related diseases along what might be considered a centrifugal axis from the hilum to the subcapsular region. In the case of complete lack of remodeling of the ductal plate, the DPM appears like a circular lumen surrounding a central fibrovascular axis. Alternatively, incomplete remodeling results either in a ring of interrupted ducts around a fibrovascular axis or a polypoid projection of biliary epithelium in a dilated duct [10, 11].

There are two groups of diseases in which the DPM is a dominant feature. The first is characterized by inflammation and destruction of intrahepatic bile ducts with some degree of fibrosis, as seen in biliary atresia. The second is the pattern typically seen in fibrocystic diseases: extensive fibrosis with ectasia and hyperplasia of intrahepatic bile ducts (Fig. 57.2) [7]. Our purpose is to focus on the latter group.

Cavernous Transformation of the Portal Vein

The DPM is often associated with abnormalities in portal vein branching. During normal development, the portal

Fig. 57.2 Schematic of intrahepatic biliary tree and level of DPM [10]. For reasons still unknown, defects in ductal plate remodeling impact the biliary tree at different levels. In addition, the remodeling defect yields one of two phenotypes: predominantly fibrotic lesions or dilated biliary structures. Caroli's syndrome is an example of how the two phenotypes might overlap. *DPM* ductal plate malformation, *CHF* congenital hepatic fibrosis, *ARPKD* autosomal recessive polycystic kidney disease, *ADPKD* autosomal dominant polycystic kidney disease, *PLD* polycystic liver disease

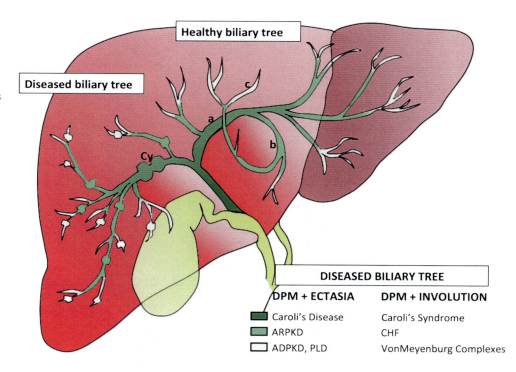

Healthy biliary tree

Diseased biliary tree

DISEASED BILIARY TREE	
DPM + ECTASIA	**DPM + INVOLUTION**
Caroli's Disease	Caroli's Syndrome
ARPKD	CHF
ADPKD, PLD	VonMeyenburg Complexes

vein invades the early liver parenchyma in a centrifugal branching pattern from the hilum to the periphery. This branching pattern determines the lobular architecture of the liver. Therefore, it follows that alterations of vascular development and intrahepatic bile ducts go hand in hand [7, 12, 13]. In the case of DPM, branching is abnormal, thereby leading to the "pollard willow formation," characterized by clusters of unseparated venous tracts [7, 10, 12]. Extrahepatic cavernous transformation of the portal vein occurs in 50–70 % of patients with CHF and CD and contributes to portal hypertension, one of the main clinical features of CHF patients [12, 13]. Congenital absence of the portal vein has rarely been reported in association with CHF [14, 15].

Fibrosis

CHF is a developmental disorder due to DPM of the small, interlobular bile ducts, during which persistence of embryonic remnants stimulates the development of fibrosis. Portal fibrosis is the major histological finding in CHF. The development of fibrosis is a multifactorial process involving hepatic stellate cells (HSC), myofibroblasts, and macrophages. Known molecular mediators include transforming growth factor-β1 (TGF-β1) and connective tissue growth factor (CTGF) [16]. CTGF is known to promote fibrosis [16]. In CHF, CTGF is retained in the extracellular matrix (ECM), thereby maintaining a local stimulus for fibrosis. How fibrosis develops in ciliopathies is further explained in the section below on animal models.

HSC constitute approximately 5–8 % of liver cells. They are located in the space of Disse, between sinusoidal endothelial cells and liver parenchymal cells [17, 18]. Activated stellate cells express tissue inhibitors of metalloproteinases 1 and 2 (TIMP 1 and 2) [19–21]. These factors have two roles in fibrogenesis: they exert a direct inhibitory action on metalloproteinases which leads to ECM accumulation, and they confer antiapoptotic proliferative signals to activated stellate cells [19, 22]. Finally, stellate cells respond to nearby injury by transforming into myofibroblasts [17] which secrete ECM components leading to scarring [17, 18].

Myofibroblasts are only present in the injured liver, and are classically believed to derive from portal fibroblasts or HSC. They are responsible for producing the ECM which leads to fibrosis [18, 23]. In CHF, parenchymal fibrosis is minimal compared to portal fibrosis. Therefore, it is possible that, in CHF, myofibroblasts derive from periductal fibroblasts rather than from parenchymal stellate cells [16].

Finally, *macrophages* have also been recognized as important regulators of liver fibrosis. They are located close to myofibroblasts and interact with the latter and with HSCs [24–27]. They also act independently, by producing their own metalloproteinases and TIMP. They contribute to the phagocytosis of cellular debris and to the secretion of cytokines and immunoregulatory mediators [24, 27, 28].

In summary, portal fibrosis is a major feature of CHF. In response to abnormal ductal plate remodeling, portal fibroblasts transform into myofibroblasts and interact with macrophages which secrete the inflammatory cytokines that trigger fibrosis. At this time, however, the underlying molecular and cellular mechanisms are not clear.

Ciliopathies

Abnormal primary cilia are now understood to be one of the main mechanisms causing DPM. The term *ciliopathies* refers to a heterogeneous group of disorders involving anomalies in primary cilia. Primary cilia are highly conserved organelles used to detect various extracellular stimuli [29]. Although their existence has been known since the nineteenth century, their role in disease is still incompletely understood.

In the liver, cholangiocytes are the only cells with primary cilia [30, 31]. Normal ciliary function is necessary for biliary development. Cholangiocyte cilia are important receptors of mechanical and osmotic signals. They respond by modulating intracellular levels of cyclic adenosine monophosphate (cAMP) and calcium in response to bile flow. This function depends on polycystin 1 and 2 (PC-1 and PC-2) that form a functional complex. PC-1 is a ciliary protein with a large extracellular domain that senses cilia bending. It then transfers this signal to PC-2 which triggers a rise in intracellular calcium which in turn regulates cellular proliferation. PC-1 exerts a regulatory role on growth, such that when its function is impaired or its level of expression diminished, the break is lifted and excess proliferation ensues [32]. Cholangiocyte cilia also detect osmotic changes in bile via the transient receptor potential cation channel subfamily V member 4 (TRPV4) protein which participates in the regulation of bicarbonate-dependent bile secretion (Fig. 57.3) [30, 31, 33–36].

Structural and functional defects of primary cilia result in decreased intracellular calcium and increased cAMP, causing cholangiocyte hyperproliferation and abnormal cell–matrix interactions [30, 34, 37–39]. Excessive cholangiocyte proliferation leads to the development of cysts. Estrogens and insulin-like growth factor 1 (IGF-1) also contribute to cholangiocyte proliferation, and cystic cells have been shown to overexpress estrogen and IGF-1 receptors [38, 40]. Furthermore, cell cycle dysregulation also contributes to cholangiocyte proliferation [38]. Finally, cystic cholangiocytes also display an abnormal ion transporter pattern leading to increased fluid secretion in the cysts [38, 41]. As summarized in Fig. 57.3, cyst expansion in ciliopathies is related to structural and functional defects of the cilia, leading to cholangiocyte proliferation and cyst formation. This process is enhanced by other factors, such as abnormal cell–matrix interactions, cell cycle dysregulation, overexpression of estrogen and IGF-1 and increased fluid secretion in the cysts.

Evidence suggests that biliary precursors are vulnerable to second hits that can suffice to impair remodeling, for example, somatic mutations occurring during development [42, 43]. A mutation in a single allele of a developmentally key transcription factor such as hepatocyte nuclear factor-6 (HNF6) may lead to impaired ciliogenesis and thus cyst development. This can be a very early event that precedes the formation of the ductal plate by days or weeks and may involve genetic modification leading to the loss of heterozygosity, but may also involve other cellular events such as glycosylation and posttranslational modification leading to faulty transcription factor binding [44]. Among other developmental steps prone to anomalies the local growth-factor milieu is another variable in a complex web of events. It is probably because the number of genes and signaling pathways are so numerous and the possible combinations of developmental accidents almost infinite, that biliary development is so vulnerable to malformations and that there is so much overlap between phenotypes among the ciliopathies and fibrocystic diseases. To help make sense of this wide range of phenotypes, it has been suggested that DPMs can be categorized in one of three ways: perturbations in differentiation of biliary precursors, impaired maturation of radially asymmetrical primitive ductules and abnormal (excessive) ductular expansion.

Animal Models of Ciliopathies

Much of what is understood today about cystogenesis, fibrosis, and ciliopathies is through animal studies. Although different parameters have been identified leading to cholangiocyte proliferation and cyst development, until recently there were no clear mechanistic studies to explain the link between cyst formation and fibrosis. Recent studies in rats have shown that abnormal cystic cholangiocytes can undergo an epithelial to mesenchymal transition and secrete ECM molecules contributing to the development of fibrosis (Fig. 57.3) [45].

The PCK rat carries a splicing mutation in polycystic kidney and hepatic disease 1 gene (Pkhd1) an ortholog of polycystic kidney and hepatic disease 1 (PKHD1). Defects in ciliary structure of cholangiocytes lead to abnormalities of biliary tree differentiation and bile duct dilatation, mimicking CD. Besides the histological findings described above, macroscopic findings include cholangitis with intestinal metaplasia and hepatic fibrosis [28, 45, 46]. Therefore, this animal model will likely be pivotal in understanding the disease process and developing novel therapies.

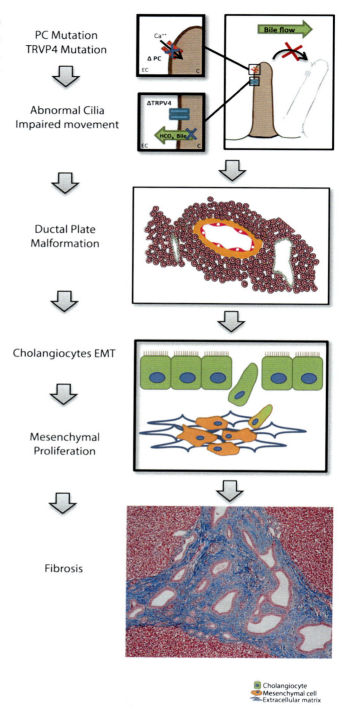

PC Mutation
TRVP4 Mutation

Abnormal Cilia
Impaired movement

Ductal Plate
Malformation

Cholangiocytes EMT

Mesenchymal
Proliferation

Fibrosis

Cholangiocyte
Mesenchymal cell
Extracellular matrix

Fig. 57.3 Schematic description of molecular and cellular mechanisms in the hepatic manifestations of ciliopathies. Mutations in polycystin *(PC)* lead to impaired calcium transport into cilia, and thus impaired movement. In case of TRPV4 mutation, osmotic changes in bile cannot be sensed, and a dysregulation of bicarbonate-dependant bile secretion occurs. Structural and functional defects of the cilia lead to ductal plate malformation. Cholangiocytes undergo an epithelial to mesenchymal transition and proliferate in the mesenchyme contributing to fibrosis. *PC* polycystin, *TRPV4* transient receptor potential cation channel subfamily V member 4, *EC* extracellular, *C* cytosol, *EMT* epithelial-to-mesenchymal transition

Clinical Features

CHF and CD/CS are ciliopathies associated with ductal plate malformation. The liver findings are rarely an isolated finding. Rather, they are most often associated with polycystic kidney disease (PKD), part of the wider family of ciliopathies. When the phenotype combines hepatic and renal manifestations, these conditions are also referred to as the hepatorenal fibrocystic disorders (HRFCD).

CHF usually presents between 5 and 7 years of age. Familial cases exist, highlighting the importance of a thorough family history [47–50]. CHF can present in one of four ways [33, 50–52]. The most frequent presentation is portal hypertension with firm hepatomegaly and splenomegaly [47, 48, 50, 53, 54]. Thrombocytopenia and hypersplenism are often present. Occasionally anemia reveals occult variceal bleeding. The presenting complaint is often an acute gastrointestinal bleed in a previously healthy child. In 30–70 % of patients who present within the first decade of life, recurrent hematemesis or melena caused by variceal bleeding is frequent, whereas ascites is uncommon [52]. In most patients without an associated syndrome, growth and development are normal. Serum aminotransferase- and bilirubin levels are generally within the normal range at diagnosis and remain normal throughout follow-up. No progression to liver failure has been reported [49]. Complications of portal hypertension such as hepatopulmonary syndrome and porto-pulmonary hypertension have been described [49, 52].

The second presentation, frequently associated with CD/CS, is recurrent bacterial cholangitis. Symptoms include intermittent abdominal pain and pruritus from chronic cholestasis. In this case, serum levels of gamma-glutamyl transferase (gGT), alkaline phosphatase, and bilirubin are elevated. Bacterial cholangitis can progress to septicemia and lead to the development of hepatic abscesses. Recurrent cholangitis may lead to liver failure and failure to thrive [52].

Occasionally, patients can present with both portal hypertension and cholangitis. Finally, the disease can be latent and revealed by an incidental, clinical, biological, or radiological finding such as hepatomegaly or cytopenias [55–57]. When CHF or CD is associated with other extrahepatic signs, clinicians should think of associated syndromes, which are described in the following section.

In the long run, CD and CS are associated with an increased risk of cholangiocarcinoma, due to bile stasis and chronic inflammation. Cholangiocarcinoma, which can be the presenting feature, has been reported to occur in 5–10 % of patients with CD and CS. It has also been reported in patients with isolated CHF, albeit rarely. The average age at appearance is >40 years (range of 33–75 years), and the risk increases with age. It occurs more often in the monolobar form of the disease, and has very poor 1-year survival rates [58–61].

Associated Syndromes and Ciliopathies

CHF and CD are often features of a multisystem disorder. Ciliopathies with a prevalence of more than 1:150,000 are described below and ciliopathies with low prevalence are outlined in Table 57.1 [62–73].

Autosomal Recessive Polycystic Kidney Disease

Autosomal recessive polycystic kidney disease (ARPKD) is the most frequent ciliopathy in childhood, affecting 1:20,000 live births. It is characterized by progressive cystic degeneration of the kidneys and CHF. As its name suggests, transmission is recessive. All patients diagnosed with ARPKD have CHF from birth on microscopic examination, but only 50 % have hepatomegaly. Most of the patients are born with nephromegaly from dilated collecting ducts which can present as a palpable flank mass. Thirty percent of patients die at birth from pulmonary hypoplasia (Potter's syndrome). There is a marked variability of phenotypes even among siblings. The course and the severity of renal disease and liver disease are unrelated. In the infant or neonate, presentation is usually renal, while CHF is typically asymptomatic early in life. Renal disease can present as a simple urinary concentration defect or more often as severe cystic kidney disease leading to hypertension and renal failure. End-stage renal disease affects about 30 % of children under 10 years. For neonates surviving the first month of life, the 5-year survival rate is about 90 %. Children who present later in life will show one of the CHF presentations described earlier. Diagnosis is clinical and by ultrasonography (US). Kidneys appear hyperechoic on ultrasound, and the liver is either normal or hyperechoic. Rarely, macroscopic liver cysts are visible on ultrasound. Annual follow-up should include a full blood count and ultrasound. MR cholangiography should be performed once to understand biliary morphology. Ultrasound examination of the parents' kidneys is important because autosomal dominant disease can mimic the recessive form in neonates. Management is supportive, both for the renal and liver complications. Most patients presenting as neonates will require kidney transplantation before 20 years of age. Improvement in the management of renal complications has led to an increased awareness of liver-related morbidity and mortality. Liver-related mortality following kidney transplantation has been reported. Liver transplantation is performed in about 3 % of cases of ARPKD, usually during adolescence. Combined liver and kidney transplantation are indicated in renal failure with recurrent cholangitis or refractory complications of portal hypertension [74–79].

Table 57.1 Phenotype and epidemiology of ciliopathies [62–73]. There is no clear genotype–phenotype correlation

Disease	Phenotype												Prevalence	Gene abbreviation	Transmission
	Retinal	Mental retardation	Cerebellar or cerebral	Cardiac	Lung	Pancreas	Liver	Kidney	Polydactyly	Infertility	Situs inversus	Other			
–	–	–	–	–	–	–	–	–	–	–	–	–	–	–	–
Autosomic recessive polycystic disease	–	–	–	–	–	–	X	X	–	–	–	–	1:10,000 to 1:40,000	PKHD1	AR
Autosomic dominant polycystic disease	–	–	–	–	–	–	X	X	–	–	–	–	1:1000	PKD1, PKD2	AD
Nephronophtisis	X	X	–	X	X	X	X	X	–	–	X	–	1:100,000	NPHP1, INVS, NPHP3, NPHP4, IQCB1, CEP290,GLIS2, RPGRIP1L, NEK, SDC-CAG8, TMEM67, TTC21B, WDR19, ZNF423, CEP164, ANKS6, XPNPEP3	AR
Meckel Gruber	X	–	X	–	X	–	X	X	X	X	X	–	1:140,000	MKS1, TMEM67, CEP290, TMEM216, TCTN2	AR
COACH syndrome	X	–	X	–	–	–	X	–	–	–	–	–	<1:1,000,000	CC2D2A, TMEM67, RPGRIP1L	AR
Joubert syndrome	X	X	X	–	–	–	–	X	X	X	X	–	–	JBTS1 to JBTS13	–
Bardet-Biedl [62]	X	X	–	X	X	–	X	X	X	X	X w	–	1:100,000	BBS1, BBS2, ARL6, BBS4, BBS5, MKKS, BBS7, TTC8, BBS9, BBS10, TRIM32, BBS12, MKS1, CEP290	AR

Table 57.1 (continued)

Disease	Phenotype												Prevalence	Gene abbreviation	Transmission
	Retinal	Mental retardation	Cerebellar or cerebral	Cardiac	Lung	Pancreas	Liver	Kidney	Polydactyly	Infertility	Situs inversus	Other			
Jeune syndrome [63]	–	–	–	–	–	–	X	X	X	–	–	Pelvic bone defect, thoracic defect	Rare	IFT80, DYNC2H1, TTC21B, WDR19	AR
Oral facial digital syndrome [64]	–	–	X	–	–	–	X	X	X	–	–	Craniofacial defect	1:100,000	OFD1	XD
Renal-hepatic-pancreatic dysplasia = Ivemark syndrome [65]	–	–	–	X	–	X	X	X	–	–	–	–	Rare	GDF1	AR
Ellis van Creveld syndrome [66]	–	–	–	X	–	–	–	–	X	–	–	Thoracic defect	Rare Increased in Amish people	LBN, EVC	AR
Alstrom syndrome [67]	X	–	–	X	–	–	X	X	–	–	–	–	Rare	ALMS1	AR
Leber congenital amaurosis [68]	X	X	–	–	–	–	–	–	–	–	–	–	Rare	CEP 290, NPHP6, LCA 5, TULP1; REGRIP 1	AR
Senior Loken syndrome [69]	X	–	–	–	–	–	X	X	–	–	X	–	Rare	CEP 29, NPH1, NPHP, NPHP4, NPHP5	AR
Mainzer-Saldino syndrome [70]	X	–	X	–	–	–	X	X	–	–	–	Phalangeal, cone-shaped epiphyses	Rare	IFT140	AR
Carbohydrate deficient glycoprotein syndrome 1b [71–73]	–	–	X	–	–	–	X	–	–	–	–	Enteropathy, coagulopathy	Rare	MPI	AR

AD autosomal dominant transmission, *AR* autosomal recessive transmission, *XD* X linked

Autosomal Dominant Polycystic Kidney Disease

Across all age groups, the most common hepatorenal fibrocystic disease is autosomal dominant polycystic kidney disease (ADPKD), with an incidence of 1:1000. Liver involvement usually presents as polycystic liver disease, while CHF and CD or CS are rarely described. As its name suggests, transmission is dominant. Kidney cysts develop progressively from the whole tubule. Onset is slow such that diagnosis is usually made in adulthood. Other organs may also develop cysts: pancreas, intestinal epithelium, arachnoid mater, and seminal vesicles. Cardiac valvular disease and cerebral aneurysms have also been described. Affected patients are usually asymptomatic in childhood. On occasion, an incidental finding of cysts in the fetus, young child, or adolescent can lead to the misleading suspicion of ARPKD. Most often, in childhood, the incidental finding of a cyst should orient toward ADPKD, especially if hypertension is present. Some very rare cases of end-stage renal disease are described in childhood [80, 81].

Nephronophtisis

Nephronophtisis is the most frequent genetic cause of end-stage kidney disease in children and may be associated with liver disease. Nephronophtisis is classified according to age at presentation: infantile, juvenile, and adolescent. In all cases renal involvement leads to end-stage renal disease requiring kidney transplantation. Most commonly, it is the adolescent form caused by mutations in NPHP3 which presents with liver disease characterized by bile duct proliferation and portal fibrosis [82–85]. This characteristic histology should encourage clinicians to search for NPHP3 mutations and examine renal function. Tapeto-retinal abnormalities constitute another sign favoring the diagnosis [86]. Mutations in eight other genes have been identified in the adolescent and juvenile form (NPHP1, NPHP3–NPHP8) but have not been associated with liver abnormalities except for an occasional biochemical abnormality. In NPHP2 and NPHP3, both presenting in infancy, liver involvement varies from mild to CHF [87].

Meckel–Gruber Syndrome

Meckel syndrome is a rare autosomal recessive lethal ciliopathy composed of four cardinal features: occipital encephalocele, bilateral cystic kidneys, CHF (100%), and polydactyly. In addition, CHF is present in 100% cases. The incidence is 1:140,000 and is increased in the Finnish population (1:1000) [88–90].

COACH Syndrome Related to Joubert Syndrome

Joubert syndrome (JS) is a recessive disorder with occurrence of 1:100,000 and characterized by brainstem and cerebellar malformation, ataxia, developmental impairment, alternance of hyperpnea and hypopnea, abnormal eye and tongue movements, and hypotonia and by an array of neurological, retinal, renal, or skeletal anomalies. The key feature of JS is the molar tooth sign (cerebellar peduncles and deep interpeduncular fossa on cerebral MRI). COACH syndrome includes cerebellar vermis hypoplasia/aplasia, oligophrenia, ataxia, coloboma, and hepatic fibrosis. This very rare syndrome combines the presence of CHF and the classical neurologic signs of JS. Mutations in transmembrane protein meckelin (MKS3), a centriole protein necessary for ciliary function and for primary cilium formation, are present in more than 50% of COACH syndrome cases and are uncommon in JS patient without liver involvement [91, 92].

Diagnosis

Radiology

Diagnosis should first be suspected on clinical findings. US is a useful, first-line tool for the diagnosis of CHF. Findings typically include heterogeneous liver parenchyma, foci of hyperechogenicity, and images compatible with biliary cysts. The left lobe may appear enlarged and the right lobe atrophic. Splenomegaly and Doppler are suggestive of portal hypertension and cavernous transformation of the portal vein, although esophagogastroduodenoscopy is the gold standard in the assessment of portal hypertensive complications. Dilatations of the proximal bile ducts and the presence of intrahepatic stones suggest CS [51, 52, 93]. Since the risk of endoscopic retrograde cholangiopancreatography (ERCP)-related complications is high, MR cholangiography (MRCP) is best to evaluate biliary disease using 3D reconstructions (Fig. 57.4). Likewise, MR angiography or CT angiography can further characterize vascular findings. US and MR elastography are increasingly used to evaluate fibrosis [94, 95].

Histology

Liver biopsy is the gold standard to confirm diagnosis. CHF is characterized by the presence of persistent ductal plate structures of the interlobular bile ducts. Large bands of fibrous tissues link enlarged portal tracts with mild inflammatory cell infiltrates (Fig. 57.4). Within the fibrous bands, branching small interlobar bile ducts lined by normal, cuboidal epithelium are irregularly dilated and may contain bile. The hepatic parenchyma and architecture between portal tracts

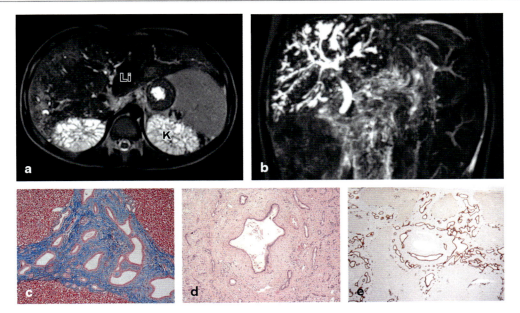

Fig. 57.4 Imaging and histology. **a** MR cholangiography illustrating CHF *(Li)* and polycystic kidney disease *(K)*. **b** MR cholangiography in Caroli's disease illustrating intrahepatic biliary cystic dilatation. **c** Trichrome staining of a liver biopsy illustrating the fibrosis enclosing portal tracts with adjacent normal lobular architecture. **d** Hematoxylin–eosin staining of a ductal plate malformation. **e** Characteristic biliary saccular dilatation in Caroli's disease

and centrolobular veins remain normal. There is hypoplasia of portal vein branches and compensatory increased arterial profiles. CD is characterized by saccular or fusiform cystic dilatation of larger and proximal, intrahepatic, and extrahepatic ducts without signs of fibrosis. CS combines the histological features of CHF and CD [47, 48, 50, 51, 54, 96–98].

Practical Approach

All patients with known cystic renal disease should be evaluated for liver involvement. Liver fibrosis begins early in life in patients with ARPKD and ADPKD. In the absence of signs or symptoms, it is not recommended to perform a liver biopsy. Clinicians should look for signs of portal hypertension at each visit. Annual liver function tests and annual liver US are recommended. An MR cholangiogram may give an idea about biliary disease, but only if the US is consistent with cysts or biliary dilatation. Although liver biopsy is the gold standard for diagnosis, it is not always indicated if it does not immediately alter management. Conversely, since the association between renal and liver disease is so frequent, all patients diagnosed with CHF or CD/CS should be evaluated for renal cystic disease. Screening for malignant transformation is not indicated in children, because onset occurs generally in the fifth decade. Improved management of children with chronic liver disease means that more patients with fibrocystic liver diseases are reaching adulthood with their native livers, and therefore that adult gastroenterologists will be the ones to diagnose malignancy in these patients [99].

Genetics

Genetic testing is recommended for diagnosis, management, and prognosis [***]. If the clinical picture is suggestive of a given phenotype and the differential diagnosis narrow, known candidate genes can be tested to provide a definitive diagnosis, and genetic counseling should be offered to patients and relatives. When the differential diagnosis is broad, there is a need to cast a wider net to identify the ciliopathy, something now achievable through Next Generation Sequencing (NGS). Given the complexity of these analyses and the inherent difficulty of interpretation, clinical genetic expertise should be sought. According to the identified variant and the specific mode of inheritance familial segregation analysis may be indicated.

***. Karlsen TH, Lammert F, Thompson RJ. Genetics of liver disease: From pathophysiology to clinical practice. Journal of hepatology. 2015;62(1S):S6-S14.

Other Fibrocystic Liver Disease and Differential Diagnosis

Perturbations in ductal plate remodeling exist in other conditions than CHF and CD/CS. These conditions are summarized in Table 57.2 [101–105]. Choledochal cysts may be considered part of the "fibrocystic liver disease" spectrum, because extensive fibrosis and other signs of CHF may be seen on biopsy [98]. In general, it is important to consider that there can be extensive phenotypic overlap between fibrocystic liver diseases [98].

Table 57.2 Fibrocystic liver diseases with ductal plate malformation [101–105]

Disease	Characteristics	Symptoms	Diagnosis	Associated syndromes	Treatment
Caroli's disease	No signs of CHF	Cholestasis	US	Extrahepatic bile duct dilatation	Antibiotics for cholangitis
	Saccular or fusiform cystic dilatation to 5 cm of larger and proximal intrahepatic biliary ducts	Cholangitis	MRCP	Choledochal cyst	Partial hepatectomy
	Inheritance unclear but familial cases	No portal hypertension	Liver biopsy		Liver transplantation
Autosomal dominant polycystic liver disease (PCLD)	>20 round and smooth cysts	Asymptomatic	US	Distinct form associated with ADPKD	Somatostatin analogues
	Non communicating	Abdominal mass Pain	MRCP		(Inhibition of cAMP pathway)
	Development of cyst associated with hormonal features	Cyst infection, bleeding	Liver biopsy		Surgical resection
	Woman > men	Biliary obstruction			
	Gene: *SEC63, PRKCSH*	No portal hypertension			Rarely liver transplantation
	→ *Abnormalities of cAMP pathway* [101, 102]	Rare liver failure			
Von Meyenberg complex [103, 105]	Bile ducts hamartomas	Asymptomatic, usually found in liver biopsy for other indication	Incidental	ADPKD	None
	Benign pathology	Rare portal hypertension	MRCP	ARPKD	
	Multiple/unique round uniform cysts 0.1–0.3 cm		Liver biopsy	Risk of CCA	
	Localized close to portal tracts				
Choledochal cyst [104]	Dilatation of common bile duct ± intrahepatic and extrahepatic biliaray tree	Conjugated hyperbilirubinemia	US	CHF	Surgical resection
	Classification based on location	Jaundice abdominal pain	MRCP	Risk of CCA	Choledo-enterostomy
	Type I–IV: No parenchyma hepatic involvement	Acute complication: perforation, bleeding, infection lithiasis			
	Type V: Multiple cyst dilatation intrahepatic→Caroli's disease 8–53 % cases	Long-term complication: biliary cirrhosis and hypertension			

CCA cholangiocarcinoma, *US* ultrasonography, *MRCP* magnetic resonance cholangiopancreatography, *ADPKD* autosomal dominant polycystic kidney disease, *ARPKD* autosomal recessive polycystic kidney disease, *CHF* congenital hepatic fibrosis, *CCA* chromated copper arsenate, *cAMP* cyclic adenosine monophosphate

Table 57.3 Other causes of liver cysts [106–108]

Disease	Characteristics	Symptoms	Diagnosis	Treatment
Solitary hepatic cyst, non-communicating	Delimited	Asymptomatic	Clinical and MRCP	Surgery: [106] laparoscopic fenestration or total resection or hepatectomy; [107, 108]
	No communication with biliary duct	Complications: infection; perforation, obstruction, neoplasic degeneration	Avoid biopsy →infectious risk	
	Right lobe			
	No associated cysts in viscera			
Obstructive bile duct dilatation	Stones inside ducts or stricture of ducts from extrabiliary cause (neoplasia; pancreatitis)	Asymptomatic	Clinical	Surgery
		Complication: Cholestasis; cholangitis, perforation	MRCP	Treatment of primary disease
		Signs of primary disease causing obstruction	US	
			Signs of primary disease	
Parasitic	Acute symptoms	Acute	Hypereosinophilia MRI, US	Antimicrobials

US ultrasonography, *MRCP* magnetic resonance cholangiopancreatography

Since fibrosis is the hallmark of most liver diseases, the differential diagnosis is wide and includes both congenital and acquired diseases. As for the presence of intrahepatic cysts, the differential diagnosis is more narrow and summarized in Table 57.3 [106–108].

Management

Treatment of CHF and CD/CS is mostly symptomatic and is mainly directed toward the management of complications, such as recurrent episodes of cholangitis and portal hypertension. The management of portal hypertension is reviewed elsewhere in this volume.

Intrahepatic cholelithiasis is managed with ursodeoxycholic acid and with ERCP and sphincterotomy. Partial hepatectomy for recurrent cholelithiasis has yielded satisfactory results [109–111]. In the case of monolobar CD, partial hepatectomy has also been shown to prevent recurrent, life-threatening cholangitis, with acceptable morbidity [58, 59, 112].

Liver Transplantation

Liver transplantation is the only definite cure for CHF and CD/CS. It is indicated in refractory portal hypertension, severe growth failure, recurrent cholangitis, decompensated cirrhosis and liver failure.

The short- and long-term outcome of liver transplantation in patients with CHF and CD is satisfactory overall. Outcomes for CD/CS reach the current average outcomes of liver transplantation for other indications [51, 58, 59, 112–114].

In patients with PKD requiring renal transplantation, combined liver and kidney transplantation yields better results compared to kidney transplantation alone. It has been shown that the outcome of patients with PKD mostly depends on the severity of liver disease and that major complications, such as sepsis, are more frequent in patients with advanced liver disease. Combined liver and kidney transplantation seems to be the treatment of choice for these patients, since nephrotoxic drugs for isolated liver transplantation prior to kidney transplantation can accelerate renal demise [52, 115–117].

Antifibrotic Agents

Although the prospect of antifibrotic agents is attractive and may prove life-saving or at least postpone liver transplantation for some indications, there is no data to show an effect on the fibrosis of fibrocystic diseases. Fibrocystic diseases differ from other secondary causes of fibrosis in several ways: (1) destruction of abnormal cholangiocytes trigger an inflammatory cascade and (2) peribiliary fibroblasts rather than contribute to the ECM deposition. Therefore, no extrapolation can be made from evidence garnered in other causes of cirrhosis.

Conclusion and Future Perspectives

Ciliopathies with associated DPM often present with liver disease and portal hypertension. Associated renal disease is frequent and should be sought. An increasing number of disease causing mutations are identified, and sequencing is part of the diagnostic work up of these diseases. However, there is no clear genotype–phenotype correlation. In particular, it is unclear why some ciliopathies present with distal DPM while others show abnormalities of the large, proximal bile ducts. Cholangiocarcinoma is a rare complication with poor outcome. Combined liver and kidney transplantation yields excellent outcomes and is usually the treatment of choice in case of life-threatening complications.

Acknowledgments We gratefully acknowledge Mrs. Sylvia Udry-Moulin and Dr. Véronique Raies-Dauve for their helpful assistance with illustrations, Dr Makrythanasis for his help with genetics, Dr. Anooshiravani-Dumont for providing illustrative imaging, and Dr. Rougemont for sharing examples of histology.

References

1. Zorn AM. Liver development (October 31, 2008). In: Schier A F, editor, StemBook, The stem cell research community, 2008. doi/10.3824/stembook.1.25.1. http://www.stembook.org. Accessed 17 June 2015.
2. Boulter GO, Bird TG, Radulescu S, Ramachandran P, Pellicoro A, Ridgway RA. Macrophage-derived Wnt opposes Notch signaling to specify hepatic progenitor cell fate in chronic liver disease. Nat Med. 2012;18(4):572–9.
3. Carpentier R, Suner RE, van Hul N, Kopp JL, Beaudry JB, Cordi S, Antoniou A, Raynaud P, Lepreux S, Jacquemin P, Leclercq IA, Sander M, Lemaigre FP. Embryonic ductal plate cells give rise to cholangiocytes, periportal hepatocytes, and adult liver progenitor cells. Gastroenterology. 2011;141(4):1432–8.
4. Tan CE, Vijayan V. New clues for the developing human biliary system at the porta hepatis. J Hepatobiliary Pancreat Surg. 2001;8(4):295–302.
5. Terada T, Nakanuma Y. Detection of apoptosis and expression of apoptosis-related proteins during human intrahepatic bile duct development. Am J Pathol. 1995;146(1):67–74.
6. Van Eyken P, Sciot R, Callea F, van der Steen K, Moerman P, Desmet VJ. The development of the intrahepatic bile ducts in man: a keratin-immunohistochemical study. Hepatology. 1988;8(6):1586–95.
7. Desmet V. Pathogenesis of ductal plate malformation. J Gastroenterol Hepatol. 2004;19:356–60.
8. Tan CE, Moscoso GJ. The developing human biliary system at the porta hepatis level between 11 and 25 weeks of gestation: a way to understanding biliary atresia. Part 2. Pathol Int. 1994;44(8):600–10.
9. Jorgensen MJ. The ductal plate malformation. Acta Pathol Microbiol Scand Suppl. 1977;257:1–87.

10. Desmet VJ. Congenital diseases of intrahepatic bile ducts: variations on the theme "ductal plate malformation". Hepatology. 1992;16(4):1069–83.
11. Nakanuma Y, Harada K, Sato Y, Ikeda H. Recent progress in the etiopathogenesis of pediatric biliary disease, particularly Caroli's disease with congenital hepatic fibrosis and biliary atresia. Histol Histopathol. 2010;25(2):223–35.
12. Yonem O, Ozkayar N, Balkanci F, Harmanci O, Sokmensuer C, Ersoy O, et al. Is congenital hepatic fibrosis a pure liver disease? Am J Gastroenterol. 2006;101(6):1253–9.
13. Yonem O, Bayraktar Y. Clinical characteristics of Caroli's disease. World J Gastroenterol. 2007;13(13):1930–3.
14. Kong Y, Zhang H, Liu C, Wu D, He X, Xiao M, et al. Abernethy malformation with multiple aneurysms: incidentally found in an adult woman with Caroli's disease. Ann Hepatol. 2013;12(2):327–31.
15. Gocmen R, Akhan O, Talim B. Congenital absence of the portal vein associated with congenital hepatic fibrosis. Pediatr Radiol. 2007;37(9):920–4.
16. Ozaki S, Sato Y, Yasoshima M, Harada K, Nakanuma Y. Diffuse expression of heparan sulfate proteoglycan and connective tissue growth factor in fibrous septa with many mast cells relate to unresolving hepatic fibrosis of congenital hepatic fibrosis. Liver Int. 2005;25(4):817–28.
17. Yin C, Evason KJ, Asahina K, Stainier DY. Hepatic stellate cells in liver development, regeneration, and cancer. J Clin Invest. 2013;123(5):1902–10.
18. Senoo H. Structure and function of hepatic stellate cells. Med Electron Microsc. 2004;37(1):3–15.
19. Murphy FR, Issa R, Zhou X, Ratnarajah S, Nagase H, Arthur MJ, et al. Inhibition of apoptosis of activated hepatic stellate cells by tissue inhibitor of metalloproteinase-1 is mediated via effects on matrix metalloproteinase inhibition: implications for reversibility of liver fibrosis. J Biol Chem. 2002;277(13):11069–76.
20. Iredale JP. Tissue inhibitors of metalloproteinases in liver fibrosis. Int J Biochem Cell Biol. 1997;29(1):43–54.
21. Herbst H, Wege T, Milani S, Pellegrini G, Orzechowski HD, Bechstein WO, et al. Tissue inhibitor of metalloproteinase-1 and -2 RNA expression in rat and human liver fibrosis. Am J Pathol. 1997;150(5):1647–59.
22. Fowell AJ, Collins JE, Duncombe DR, Pickering JA, Rosenberg WM, Benyon RC. Silencing tissue inhibitors of metalloproteinases (TIMPs) with short interfering RNA reveals a role for TIMP-1 in hepatic stellate cell proliferation. Biochem Biophys Res Commun. 2011;407(2):277–82.
23. Iwaisako K, Brenner DA, Kisseleva T. What's new in liver fibrosis? The origin of myofibroblasts in liver fibrosis. J Gastroenterol Hepatol. 2012;27(Suppl 2):65–8.
24. Wynn TA, Barron L. Macrophages: master regulators of inflammation and fibrosis. Semin Liver Dis. 2010;30(3):245–57.
25. Leicester KL, Olynyk JK, Brunt EM, Britton RS, Bacon BR. CD14-positive hepatic monocytes/macrophages increase in hereditary hemochromatosis. Liver Int. 2004;24(5):446–51.
26. Leicester KL, Olynyk JK, Brunt EM, Britton RS, Bacon BR. Differential findings for CD14-positive hepatic monocytes/macrophages in primary biliary cirrhosis, chronic hepatitis C and non-alcoholic steatohepatitis. Liver Int. 2006;26(5):559–65.
27. Gadd VL, Melino M, Roy S, Horsfall L, O'Rourke P, Williams MR, et al. Portal, but not lobular, macrophages express matrix metalloproteinase-9: association with the ductular reaction and fibrosis in chronic hepatitis C. Liver Int. 2013;33(4):569–79.
28. Wakabayashi K, Lian ZX, Moritoki Y, Lan RY, Tsuneyama K, Chuang YH, et al. IL-2 receptor alpha(-/-) mice and the development of primary biliary cirrhosis. Hepatology. 2006;44(5):1240–9.
29. Wen J. Congenital hepatic fibrosis in autosomal recessive polycystic kidney disease. Clin Transl Sci. 2011;4(6):460–5.
30. Abu-Wasel B, Walsh C, Keough V, Molinari M. Pathophysiology, epidemiology, classification and treatment options for polycystic liver diseases. World J Gastroenterol. 2013;19(35):5775–86.
31. Huang BQ, Masyuk TV, Muff MA, Tietz PS, Masyuk AI, Larusso NF. Isolation and characterization of cholangiocyte primary cilia. Am J Physiol Gastrointest Liver Physiol. 2006;291(3):G500–9.
32. Fedeles SV, Gallagher AR, Somlo S. Polycystin-1: a master regulator of intersecting cystic pathways. Trends Mol Med. 2014;20(5):251–60.
33. Gunay-Aygun M. Liver and kidney disease in ciliopathies. Am J Med Genet C Semin Med Genet. 2009;151C(4):296–306.
34. Masyuk AI, Masyuk TV, LaRusso NF. Cholangiocyte primary cilia in liver health and disease. Dev Dyn. 2008;237(8):2007–12.
35. Masyuk AI, Masyuk TV, Splinter PL, Huang BQ, Stroope AJ, LaRusso NF. Cholangiocyte cilia detect changes in luminal fluid flow and transmit them into intracellular Ca2 + and cAMP signaling. Gastroenterology. 2006;131(3):911–20.
36. Nauli SM, Alenghat FJ, Luo Y, Williams E, Vassilev P, Li X, et al. Polycystins 1 and 2 mediate mechanosensation in the primary cilium of kidney cells. Nat Genet. 2003;33(2):129–37.
37. Nichols MT, Gidey E, Matzakos T, Dahl R, Stiegmann G, Shah RJ, et al. Secretion of cytokines and growth factors into autosomal dominant polycystic kidney disease liver cyst fluid. Hepatology. 2004;40(4):836–46.
38. Masyuk T, Masyuk A, LaRusso N. Cholangiociliopathies: genetics, molecular mechanisms and potential therapies. Curr Opin Gastroenterol. 2009;25(3):265–71.
39. Torrice A, Cardinale V, Gatto M, Semeraro R, Napoli C, Onori P, et al. Polycystins play a key role in the modulation of cholangiocyte proliferation. Dig Liver Dis. 2010;42(5):377–85.
40. Alvaro D, Onori P, Alpini G, Franchitto A, Jefferson DM, Torrice A, et al. Morphological and functional features of hepatic cyst epithelium in autosomal dominant polycystic kidney disease. Am J Pathol. 2008;172(2):321–32.
41. Banales JM, Masyuk TV, Bogert PS, Huang BQ, Gradilone SA, Lee SO, et al. Hepatic cystogenesis is associated with abnormal expression and location of ion transporters and water channels in an animal model of autosomal recessive polycystic kidney disease. Am J Pathol. 2008;173(6):1637–46.
42. Janssen MJ, Waanders E, Te Morsche RH, Xing R, Dijkman HB, Woudenberg J, Drenth JP. Secondary, somatic mutations might promote cyst formation in patients with autosomal dominant polycystic liver disease. Gastroenterology. 2011;141(6):2056–63.
43. Pei Y. A "two-hit" model of cystogenesis in autosomal dominant polycystic kidney disease? Trends Mol Med. 2001;7(4):151–6.
44. Jaeken J, Matthijs G, Saudubray JM, Dionisi-Vici C, Bertini E, de Lonlay P, Henri H, Carchon H, Schollen E, Van Schaftingen E. Phosphomannose isomerase deficiency: a carbohydrate-deficient glycoprotein syndrome with hepatic-intestinal presentation. Am J Hum Genet. 1998;62(6):1535–9.
45. Sato Y, Harada K, Ozaki S, Furubo S, Kizawa K, Sanzen T, et al. Cholangiocytes with mesenchymal features contribute to progressive hepatic fibrosis of the polycystic kidney rat. Am J Pathol. 2007;171(6):1859–71.
46. Sato Y, Ren XS, Nakanuma Y. Caroli's disease: current knowledge of its biliary pathogenesis obtained from an orthologous rat model. Int J Hepatol. 2012;2012:107945.
47. De Vos M, Barbier F, Cuvelier C. Congenital hepatic fibrosis. J Hepatol. 1988;6(2):222–8.
48. Morales HE. Congenital hepatic fibrosis and its management. Am J Surg. 1965;109:167–72.
49. Alvarez F, Bernard O, Brunelle F, Hadchouel M, Leblanc A, Odievre M, et al. Congenital hepatic fibrosis in children. J Pediatr. 1981;99(3):370–5.
50. Clermont RJ, Maillard JN, Benhamou JP, Fauvert R. Congenital hepatic fibrosis. Can Med Assoc J. 1967;97(21):1272–8.

51. Shorbagi A, Bayraktar Y. Experience of a single center with congenital hepatic fibrosis: a review of the literature. World J Gastroenterol. 2010;16(6):683–90.

52. Rawat D, Kelly DA, Milford DV, Sharif K, Lloyd C, McKiernan PJ. Phenotypic variation and long-term outcome in children with congenital hepatic fibrosis. J Pediatr Gastroenterol Nutr. 2013;57(2):161–6.

53. Abreu SC, Antunes MA, de Castro JC, de Oliveira MV, Bandeira E, Ornellas DS, et al. Bone marrow-derived mononuclear cells vs. mesenchymal stromal cells in experimental allergic asthma. Respir Physiol Neurobiol. 2013;187(2):190–8.

54. ten Bensel RW, Peters ER. Congenital hepatic fibrosis presenting as hepatomegaly in early infancy. J Pediatr. 1968;72(1):96–8.

55. Poala SB, Bisogno G, Colombatti R. Thrombocytopenia and splenomegaly: an unusual presentation of congenital hepatic fibrosis. Orphanet J Rare Dis. 2010;5:4.

56. Trizzino A, Farruggia P, Russo D, D'Angelo P, Tropia S, Benigno V, et al. Congenital hepatic fibrosis: a very uncommon cause of pancytopenia in children. J Pediatr Hematol Oncol. 2005;27(10):567–8.

57. Hausner RJ, Alexander RW. Localized congenital hepatic fibrosis presenting as an abdominal mass. Hum Pathol. 1978;9(4):473–6.

58. Kassahun WT, Kahn T, Wittekind C, Mossner J, Caca K, Hauss J, et al. Caroli's disease: liver resection and liver transplantation. Experience in 33 patients. Surgery. 2005;138(5):888–98.

59. Mabrut JY, Partensky C, Jaeck D, Oussoultzoglou E, Baulieux J, Boillot O, et al. Congenital intrahepatic bile duct dilatation is a potentially curable disease: long-term results of a multi-institutional study. Ann Surg. 2007;246(2):236–45.

60. Dayton MT, Longmire WP Jr, Tompkins RK. Caroli's Disease: a premalignant condition? Am J Surg. 1983;145(1):41–8.

61. Ulrich F, Pratschke J, Pascher A, Neumann UP, Lopez-Hanninen E, Jonas S, et al. Long-term outcome of liver resection and transplantation for Caroli disease and syndrome. Ann Surg. 2008;247(2):357–64.

62. Forsythe E, Beales PL. Bardet–Biedl syndrome. Eur J Hum Genet. 2013;21:8–13.

63. de Vries J, Yntema JL, van Die CE, Crama N, Cornelissen EA, Hamel BC. Jeune syndrome: description of 13 cases and a proposal for follow-up protocol. Eur J Pediatr. 2010;169(1):77–88.

64. Chetty-John S, Piwnica-Worms K, Bryant J, Bernardini I, Fischer RE, Heller T, Gahl WA, Gunay-Aygun MS. Fibrocystic disease of liver and pancreas; under-recognized features of the X-linked ciliopathy oral-facial-digital syndrome type 1 (OFD1). Am J Med Genet. 2010;152(10):2640–5.

65. Torra R, Alós L, Ramos J, Estivill X. Renal-hepatic-pancreatic dysplasia: an autosomal recessive malformation. J Med Genet. 1996;33:409–12.

66. O'Connor MJ, Collins RT 2nd. Ellis-van Creveld syndrome and congenital heart defects: presentation of an additional 32 cases. Pediatr Cardiol. 2012;33(4):491.

67. Marshall JD1, Beck S, Maffei P, Naggert JK. Alström syndrome. Eur J Hum Genet. 2007 ;15(12):1193–202.

68. Zou X, Yao F, Liang X, Xu F, Li H, Sui R, Dong F. De novo mutations in the cone-rod homeobox gene associated with leber congenital amaurosis in Chinese patients. Ophthalmic Genet. 2015;36(1):21–6.

69. Fillastre JP, Guenel J, Riberi P, Marx P, Whitworth JA, Kunh JM. Senior-Loken syndrome (nephronophthisis and tapeto-retinal degeneration): a study of 8 cases from 5 families. Clin Nephrol. 1976;5(1):14–9.

70. Perrault I, Saunier S, Hanein S, Filhol E, Bizet AA, Collins F, et al. Mainzer-Saldino syndrome is a ciliopathy caused by IFT140 mutations. Am J Hum Genet. 2012;90(5):864–70.

71. Mention K1, Lacaille F, Valayannopoulos V, Romano S, Kuster A, Cretz M, et al. Development of liver disease despite mannose treatment in two patients with CDG-Ib. Mol Genet Metabol. 2007;93:40–3.

72. Niehues R1, Hasilik M, Alton G, Körner C, Schiebe-Sukumar M, Koch HG, et al. Carbohydrate-deficient glycoprotein syndrome type Ib. J Clin Invest. 1998;101(7):1414–20.

73. Damen G, de Klerk H, Huijmans J, den Hollander J, Sinaasappel M. Gastrointestinal and other clinical manifestations in 17 children with congenital disorders of glycosylation type Ia, Ib, and Ic. J Pediatr Gastroenterol Nutr. 2004;38(3):282–7.

74. Turkbey B, Ocak I, Daryanani K, Font-Montgomery E, Lukose L, Bryant J, et al. Autosomal recessive polycystic kidney disease and congenital hepatic fibrosis (ARPKD/CHF). Pediatr Radiol. 2009;39(2):100–11.

75. Shneider BL, Magid MS. Liver disease in autosomal recessive polycystic kidney disease. Pediatr Transplant. 2005;9(5):634–9.

76. Guay-Woodford LM, Desmond RA. Autosomal recessive polycystic kidney disease: the clinical experience in North America. Pediatrics. 2003; 111(5 Pt 1):1072–80.

77. Zerres K, Rudnik-Schoneborn S, Steinkamm C, Becker J, Mucher G. Autosomal recessive polycystic kidney disease. J Mol Med (Berl). 1998;76(5):303–9.

78. Bergmann C, Senderek J, Windelen E, Kupper F, Middeldorf I, Schneider F, et al. Clinical consequences of PKHD1 mutations in 164 patients with autosomal-recessive polycystic kidney disease (ARPKD). Kidney Int. 2005;67(3):829–48.

79. Roy S, Dillon MJ, Trompeter RS, Barratt TM. Autosomal recessive polycystic kidney disease: long-term outcome of neonatal survivors. Pediatr Nephrol. 1997;11(3):302–6.

80. Cole BR, Conley SB, Stapleton FB. Polycystic kidney disease in the first year of life. J Pediatr. 1987;111(5):693–9.

81. Tee JB, Acott PD, McLellan DH, Crocker JF. Phenotypic heterogeneity in pediatric autosomal dominant polycystic kidney disease at first presentation: a single-center, 20-year review. Am J Kidney Dis. 2004;43(2):296–303.

82. Hildebrandt F, Zhou W. Nephronophthisis-associated ciliopathies. J Am Soc Nephrol. 2007;18(6):1855–71.

83. Boichis H, Passwell J, David R, Miller H. Congenital hepatic fibrosis and nephronophthisis. A family study. Q J Med. 1973;42(165):221–33.

84. Otto EA, Tory K, Attanasio M, Zhou W, Chaki M, Paruchuri Y, et al. Hypomorphic mutations in meckelin (MKS3/TMEM67) cause nephronophthisis with liver fibrosis (NPHP11). J Med Genet. 2009;46(10):663–70.

85. Delaney V, Mullaney J, Bourke E. Juvenile nephronophthisis, congenital hepatic fibrosis and retinal hypoplasia in twins. Q J Med. 1978;47(187):281–90.

86. Heike Olbrich MF, Hoefele J, Kispert A, Otto E, Volz A, Wolf MT, Sasmaz G, Trauer U, Reinhardt R, Sudbrak R, Antignac C, et al. Mutations in a novel gene, NPHP3, cause adolescent nephronophthisis, tapeto-retinal degeneration and hepatic fibrosis. Nat Genet. 2003;34(4):455–9.

87. Tory K, Rousset-Rouvière C, Gubler MC, Morinière V, Pawtowski A, Becker C, et al. Mutations of NPHP2 and NPHP3 in infantile nephronophthisis. Kidney Int. 2009;75:839–47.

88. Meckel J. Beschreibung zweier, durch sehr ähnliche Bildungsabweichungen entstellter Geschwister. Dtsch Arch Physiol. 1822;7:99–172.

89. Salonen R. The Meckel syndrome: clinicopathological findings in 67 patients. Am J Med Genet. 1984;18(4):671–89.

90. Paetau A, Salonen R, Haltia M. Brain pathology in the Meckel syndrome: a study of 59 cases. Clin Neuropathol. 1985;4(2):56–62.

91. Doherty D, Parisi MA, Finn LS, Gunay-Aygun M, Al-Mateen M, Bates D, et al. Mutations in 3 genes (MKS3, CC2D2A and RPGRIP1L) cause COACH syndrome (Joubert syndrome with congenital hepatic fibrosis). J Med Genet. 2010;47(1):8–21.

92. Kumandas S, Akcakus M, Coskun A, Gumus H. Joubert syndrome: review and report of seven new cases. Eur J Neurol. 2004;11(8):505–10.

93. Akhan O, Karaosmanoglu AD, Ergen B. Imaging findings in congenital hepatic fibrosis. Eur J Radiol. 2007;61(1):18–24.

94. Nobili V, Monti L, Alisi A, Lo Zupone C, Pietrobattista A, Toma P. Transient elastography for assessment of fibrosis in paediatric liver disease. Pediatr Radiol. 2011;41(10):1232–8.

95. Hanquinet S RA, Courvoisier D, Rubbia-Brandt L, McLin V, Tempia M, Anooshiravani M. Acoustic radiation force impulse (ARFI) elastography for the noninvasive diagnosis of liver fibrosis in children. Pediatr Radiol. 2013;43(5):545–51.

96. Lieberman E, Salinas-Madrigal L, Gwinn JL, Brennan LP, Fine RN, Landing BH. Infantile polycystic disease of the kidneys and liver: clinical, pathological and radiological correlations and comparison with congenital hepatic fibrosis. Medicine (Baltimore). 1971;50(4):277–318.

97. Johnson CA, Gissen P, Sergi C. Molecular pathology and genetics of congenital hepatorenal fibrocystic syndromes. J Med Genet. 2003;40(5):311–9.

98. Summerfield JA, Nagafuchi Y, Sherlock S, Cadafalch J, Scheuer PJ. Hepatobiliary fibropolycystic diseases. A clinical and histological review of 51 patients. J Hepatol. 1986;2(2):141–56.

99. Srinath A, Shneider BL. Congenital hepatic fibrosis and autosomal recessive polycystic kidney disease. J Pediatr Gastroenterol Nutr. 2012;54(5):580–7.

100. Karlsen TH, Lammert F, Thompson RJ. Genetics of liver disease: From pathophysiology to clinical practice. J Hepatol. 2015;62(1S):S6–S14.

101. Wills ES, Roepman R, Drenth JP. Polycystic liver disease: ductal plate malformation and the primary cilium. Trends Mol Med. 2014;20(5):261–70.

102. Davila S, Furu L, Gharavi AG, Tian X, Onoe T, Qian Q, et al. Mutations in SEC63 cause autosomal dominant polycystic liver disease. Nat Genet. 2004;36(6):575–7.

103. Burns CD, Kuhns JG, Wieman TJ. Cholangiocarcinoma in association with multiple biliary microhamartomas. Arch Pathol Lab Med. 1990;114(12):1287–9.

104. Todani T, Watanabe Y, Narusue M, Tabuchi K, Okajima K. Congenital bile duct cysts: classification, operative procedures, and review of thirty-seven cases including cancer arising from choledochal cyst. Am J Surg. 1977;134(2):263–9.

105. Jain D, Sarode VR, Abdul-Karim FW, Homer R, Robert ME. Evidence for the neoplastic transformation of Von-Meyenburg complexes. Am J Surg Pathol. 2000;24(8):1131–9.

106. Rogers TN, Woodley H, Ramsden W, Wyatt JI, Stringer MD. Solitary liver cysts in children: not always so simple. J Pediatr Surg. 2007;42(2):333–9.

107. Rygl M, Snajdauf J, Petrů O, Kodet R, Kodetová D, Mixa V. Congenital solitary liver cysts. Eur J Pediatr Surg. 2006;16(6):443–8.

108. Benzimra J, Ronot M, Fuks D, Abdel-Rehim M, Sibert A, Farges O, Vilgrain V. Hepatic cysts treated with percutaneous ethanol sclerotherapy: time to extend the indications to haemorrhagic cysts and polycystic liver disease. Eur Radiol. 2014;24(5):1030-8. Epub 2014 Feb 22.

109. Jarufe N, Figueroa E, Munoz C, Moisan F, Varas J, Valbuena JR, et al. Anatomic hepatectomy as a definitive treatment for hepatolithiasis: a cohort study. HPB (Oxford). 2012;14(9):604–10.

110. Ros E, Navarro S, Bru C, Gilabert R, Bianchi L, Bruguera M. Ursodeoxycholic acid treatment of primary hepatolithiasis in Caroli's syndrome. Lancet. 1993;342(8868):404–6.

111. Caroli-Bosc FX, Demarquay JF, Conio M, Peten EP, Buckley MJ, Paolini O, et al. The role of therapeutic endoscopy associated with extracorporeal shock-wave lithotripsy and bile acid treatment in the management of Caroli's disease. Endoscopy. 1998;30(6):559–63.

112. Bockhorn M, Malago M, Lang H, Nadalin S, Paul A, Saner F, et al. The role of surgery in Caroli's disease. J Am Coll Surg. 2006;202(6):928–32.

113. Ko JS, Yi NJ, Suh KS, Seo JK. Pediatric liver transplantation for fibropolycystic liver disease. Pediatr Transplant. 2012;16(2):195–200.

114. De Kerckhove L, De Meyer M, Verbaandert C, Mourad M, Sokal E, Goffette P, et al. The place of liver transplantation in Caroli's disease and syndrome. Transpl Int. 2006;19(5):381–8.

115. Brinkert F, Lehnhardt A, Montoya C, Helmke K, Schaefer H, Fischer L, et al. Combined liver-kidney transplantation for children with autosomal recessive polycystic kidney disease (ARPKD): indication and outcome. Transpl Int. 2013;26(6):640–50.

116. Davis ID, Ho M, Hupertz V, Avner ED. Survival of childhood polycystic kidney disease following renal transplantation: the impact of advanced hepatobiliary disease. Pediatr Transplant. 2003;7(5):364–9.

117. Chapal M, Debout A, Dufay A, Salomon R, Roussey G, Burtey S, et al. Kidney and liver transplantation in patients with autosomal recessive polycystic kidney disease: a multicentric study. Nephrol Dial Transplant. 2012;27(5):2083–8.

Familial Intrahepatic Cholestasis

58

Tassos Grammatikopoulos and Richard J. Thompson

List of Abbreviations

BSEP	bile salt export pump
CLDN1	Claudin-1
CLDN2	Claudin-2
FHC	familial hypercholanaemia
FIC	familial intrahepatic cholestasis syndrome
FXR	farnesoid X receptor
GGT	gamma-glutamyltransferase
HCC	hepatocellular carcinoma
IE	ileal exclusion
LT	liver transplantation
MDR3	Multi-drug Resistance Protein 3
PEBD	partial external biliary diversion
SPAD	single pass albumin dialysis
TJP2	Tight Junction Protein 2
UDCA	Ursodeoxycholic acid
ZO	zona occludens

Introduction

Two main mechanisms of cholestasis have been so far identified, which can be either hepatocellular or obstructive in origin affecting the biliary structures. Hepatocellular cholestasis is considered to be due to alterations in bile formation and transportation of bile salts and other components of bile at the cellular level involving multiple mechanisms. Obstructive cholestasis on the other hand is due to bile duct injury at either extra and/or intrahepatic level.

To date, four major types of familial intrahepatic cholestasis (FIC) have been identified; associated with mutations in genes encoding proteins involved in the hepatocellular

transport and structure. These are FIC1 deficiency, bile salt export pump (BSEP) deficiency, multidrug resistance protein 3 (MDR3) deficiency, and most recently tight junction protein 2 (TJP2) deficiency. The inheritance pattern in each case is autosomal recessive. Presentation is usually within the first year of life for the more severe forms in either recurrent, such as FIC1, or progressive form such as BSEP, TJP2, and MDR3 deficiency. Irregularities in bile formation and transportation can lead to disturbance in the enterohepatic circulation with bile salt retention and cholestasis. Cholestatic syndromes can affect solely the liver but can also have multiorgan involvement (Table 58.1).

FIC1 Deficiency

Familial intrahepatic cholestasis protein 1 (FIC1) deficiency is an autosomal recessive condition with a wide phenotypic spectrum extending from mild recurrent to severe liver disease. FIC1 deficiency was initially called Byler's disease, after the Amish family in which it was first described. Furthermore, the term Byler bile has been used as the description of coarsely granular canalicular bile seen in FIC1 deficiency on transmission electron microscopy.

It is characterized by hepatocellular cholestasis with low serum levels of γ-glutamyltransferase (GGT) activity and normal cholesterol levels. Presentation can be early on in life with recurrent cholestatic episodes and eventually progress to cirrhosis [1, 2]. Less severe disease can, however, present in adulthood. Presenting features consist of cholestasis, low serum albumin, epistaxis, and splenomegaly.

FIC1 is the protein encoded by the gene *ATP8B1* [3–5], which is located at chromosome 18q21-q22. FIC1 (or ATP8B1) is a P-type ATPase, which is one of several aminophospholipid flippases present in different membranes. Its role in the liver, largely based on a mouse model, is in maintaining the gradient of phosphatidylethanolamine and phosphatidylserine towards the inner leaflet of the cell membrane. A transmembrane balance of lipids appears to be required in

T. Grammatikopoulos (✉)
Pediatric Liver, GI and Nutrition Centre, NHS Foundation Trust, King's College Hospital, Denmark Hill, London SE5 9RS, UK
e-mail: t.grammatikopoulos@nhs.net

R. J. Thompson
Institute of Liver Studies, King's College Hospital, London, UK

© Springer International Publishing Switzerland 2016
S. Guandalini et al. (eds.), *Textbook of Pediatric Gastroenterology, Hepatology and Nutrition*,
DOI 10.1007/978-3-319-17169-2_58

Table 58.1 Four major types of familial cholestatic syndromes with respective organ involvement and disease severity

Disease name	Aliases	Gene	Protein	Features
FIC1 deficiency	Byler disease, PFIC1	ATP8B1	FIC1	Multisystem disorder Wide range of severity
BSEP deficiency	Byler syndrome, PFIC2	ABCB11	BSEP	Liver only affected Spectrum of severity
TJP2 deficiency	–	TJP2	TJP2	Multisystem disorder Wide range of severity
MDR3 deficiency	PFIC3	ABCB4	MDR3	Liver only affected Wide range of severity

FIC1 Familial intrahepatic cholestasis protein 1, *BSEP* bile salt export pump, *TJP2* tight junction protein 2, *MDR3* Multi-drug Resistance Protein 3, PFIC progressive familial cholestasis

the presence of the high bile salt concentration in the canaliculus [6]. The normal canalicular membrane requires a high degree of detergent resistance in order to prevent damage from the detergent effect of bile itself. Paulusma et al. showed that by ex vivo infusion of bile acids in the knockout mouse, the extraction of aminophospholipids was greatly increased. In the human liver, several proteins are not present, or are in reduced quantities, in the canalicular membrane of patients with FIC1 deficiency. This observation still does not account for the cholestasis, as no transporter critical to bile formation has been identified to be absent. It appears more likely that these proteins are malfunctioning in an altered lipid environment of the canalicular membrane. As FIC1 deficiency is primarily characterized by cholestasis, studies have attributed this phenotype to a defective farnesoid X receptor (FXR) signalling pathway [7, 8]. Other groups, however, suggested that impaired FXR activity is secondary to cholestasis and not responsible for the phenotype [9]. The activity of FXR and its target genes remained uninterrupted in FIC1-depleted Caco-2 cells, created using small hairpin RNA and small interfering RNA, respectively, suggestive of an unimpaired FXR signalling mechanism in FIC1-deficient patients [10, 11]. In view of a proportion of phenotypically FIC1-like patients in whom no mutations were identified, a study looked into promoter and 5′ untranslated (5′-UTR) regions affecting gene regulation in human liver and small intestine tissue by 5′ rapid amplification of cDNA ends. Expression levels of *ATP8B1* transcripts were determined by quantitative reverse-transcription polymerase chain reaction (qRT_PCR) and compared with the non-variable part of *ATP8B1*. Twelve different splicing variants and four novel untranslated exons located up to 71 kb upstream of the previously published exon 1 were identified in both tissue types. A number of transcription start sites were identified and the proximal promoter upstream of the major transcription start sites was also proven to be an essential regulatory element responsible for 70 % of total *ATP8B1* transcriptional activity. In vitro, the main promoter was shown to drive constitutive *ATP8B1* gene expression independent of bile acids [12].

Altered gene expression demonstrated in extrahepatic sites may be contributory to the multisystemic nature of this cholestatic syndrome. Other disease features include diarrhea, malabsorption of fat-soluble vitamins, hearing loss, pancreatitis, renal tubular acidosis, delayed puberty, and growth failure. The multisystemic nature of the disease is supported by the widespread expression of the *ATP8B1* gene including the liver, pancreas, kidney, and more widely in the small intestine [5].

Liver histology changes consist of cholestasis with bile plugs, periportal biliary metaplasia of hepatocytes in the absence of ductular proliferation in the portal tracks (Figs. 58.1, 58.2, and 58.3).

Early-onset patients, without treatment, usually progress to end-stage liver disease by early adulthood. First-line treatment includes antipruritic agents such as ursodeoxycholic acid (UDCA) [13], fat-soluble vitamin supplementation, and nutritional support. Failure of medical treatment would lead to first-line surgical treatment, which is currently partial external biliary diversion (PEBD), a technique that diverts an unknown proportion of bile externally. The consequences of

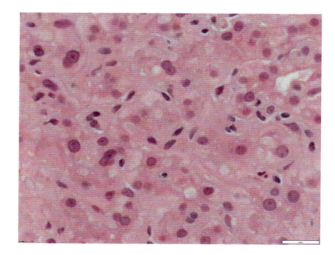

Fig. 58.1 Liver biopsy from a 20–year-old patient with ATP8B1 disease/FIC1. Hepatocytes are small and without anisocytosis. There is canalicular cholestasis. Of note, there is pale-staining bile within the canaliculi (H&E x400 magnification)

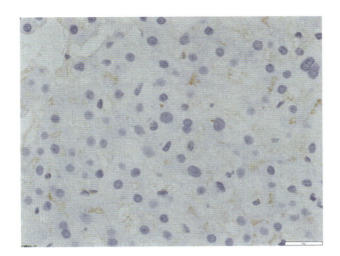

Fig. 58.2 Absence of canalicular GGT expression (x400 magnification)

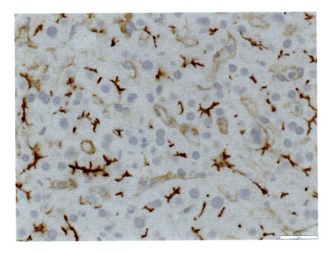

Fig. 58.3 Evident canalicular expression of CD10 (x400 magnification)

this procedure certainly include interruption of the entero-hepatic circulation of bile acids [14–17]. An external stoma can also be formed by using the appendix creating a cho-lecystoappendicectomy as reported by Rebhandl et al. [18]. Another alternative is ileal exclusion (IE), which has also been performed in cases with previous cholecystectomy or as rescue treatment [2, 15, 19, 20].

Liver transplantation (LT) is the next treatment option for these patients [16] but some extrahepatic symptoms will not improve, such as growth, and some may even become aggravated, such as diarrhea [14], liver steatosis, or kidney disease. Some of these patients may end up requiring multi-organ transplantation including liver, small bowel, kidneys, and pancreas (personal data).

BSEP Deficiency

The major bile salt transporter of the canalicular membrane level is the BSEP, which is encoded by the gene *ABCB11* [21]. The clinical condition associated with bile salt transport deficiency was previously known as "Byler's syndrome". The phenotype of BSEP-deficient patients can also vary from a mild benign recurrent intrahepatic cholestasis (BRIC) to a more severe type requiring LT [22–24]. *ABCB11*, ex-pressed only in the liver, encodes BSEP; a member of the adenosine triphosphate (ATP)-binding cassette (ABC) fam-ily of transporters responsible for the transport of bile acids across the canalicular membrane. The locus for *ABCB11* is at chromosome 2q24 with the most common European muta-tions being D482G (c.1445A>G) and E297G (c.890A>G) [21, 23]. BSEP deficiency leads to accumulation of bile salts within hepatocytes and has a subsequent effect on hepatocel-lular function. As anticipated, it has also been shown to have significant affinity for some of the main bile salts in human bile, such as glycocholate, taurocholate, and chenodeoxy-cholate [25].

Severe BSEP deficiency presents within the first year of life and although variable, it is usually a non-relapsing severe progressive cholestasis and pruritus leading to fibrosis. Birth weight can be below normal range, especially in the non-D482G>E patients [22]. Serum bilirubin levels are not nec-essarily reflective of the degree of cholestasis as bilirubin is transported separately from bile salts. Like FIC1 deficiency, BSEP-deficient patients demonstrate low GGT activity but with a trend to higher cholesterol, significantly raised trans-aminases (>threefold higher compared to FIC1 deficiency), alpha-fetoprotein, and serum bile acid concentrations. Other biochemical indices include fat-soluble vitamin deficiencies manifesting with coagulopathy and rickets. Gallstones have been reported in up to 32% of patients [22]. Serum bile acid profiles demonstrate a high cholic acid to chenodeoxycholic acid ratio as reported in FIC1 patients. Reduced biliary bile salt concentration in BSEP patients is similar to that in pro-gressive familial cholestasis (PFIC1) and in direct contrast to MDR3-deficient patients [3, 26, 27].

Severe phenotypes have been associated with mutations leading to protein truncation or failure of protein production. In a series by Strautnieks et al., missense mutations were identified in 79% of patients, many affecting protein pro-cessing and trafficking or protein structure [28]. Previous reports of *ABCB11* missense mutations and single-nucleo-tide polymorphisms showed pre-messenger RNA (mRNA) splicing subsequently causing reduction in mRNA levels in a significant number of cases. These defects at the protein or mRNA level can have a detrimental impact in BSEP func-tion [28].

Liver histology features consist of increased lobular in-flammation and portal fibrosis, giant cell transformation of

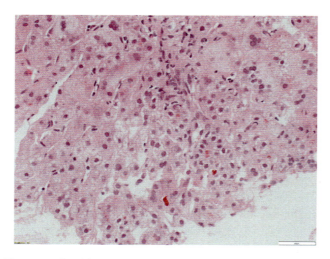

Fig. 58.4 Liver biopsy from a 7-month-old patient with ABCB11 disease/BSEP deficiency. There is bridging fibrosis and partial nodular transformation of the parenchyma (not shown). Hepatocytes show giant cell change and canalicular cholestasis. Lobular inflammation is present. BSEP immunostaining shows absence of canalicular expression, whilst canalicular GGT expression is preserved (not shown) (H&E stained slide at x200 magnification)

hepatocytes, and neonatal hepatitis with finely filamentous bile. Absence of liver immunohistochemistry for BSEP can assist in the diagnostic process [23, 29] (Fig. 58.4). Immunohistochemically detectable BSEP expression does not exclude functional BSEP deficiency [30]. In a previous series, 28 % of BSEP patients analysed exhibited some degree of BSEP staining and, in a small minority, expression was even considered normal [23].

Hepatocellular carcinoma (HCC) or cholangiocarcinoma have been reported in a number of children on the background of severe neonatal hepatitis [31, 32] or proven BSEP deficiency [23, 32]. The risk appears to be higher in patients with two protein-truncating mutations (38 vs 10 %) compared to other genotypes. The exact mechanism of malignancy remains unclear, though further insight to the development of these tumours has been gained recently [33].

Treatment options for BSEP deficiency include antipruritic agents such as UDCA, rifampicin; liver enzyme inducers (phenobarbitone), nutritional support, and fat-soluble vitamin supplementation, where indicated. Partial external biliary diversion, ileal exclusion (IE) and LT are all recommended surgical treatment options [16, 20, 34, 35]. Hepatocellular malignancy remains an indication for early LT in BSEP patients. Patients with biallelic truncating mutations warrant close monitoring with liver ultrasonography and serum alpha-fetoprotein levels. Overall in terms of prognosis, patients with D482G mutation developed portal hypertension less frequently, developed fibrosis at an older age, and underwent LT at an older age as well [22].

Recurrence of symptoms after LT has been described in BSEP-deficient patients, in contrast to other FIC syndromes. Jara et al. reported recurrence of cholestasis and pruritus following LT in BSEP patients with no evidence of cellular rejection on liver biopsy in 2009 [36]. In the same year, BSEP antibodies in the serum and at the hepatocyte canalicular membrane of a single patient who underwent two liver transplants were described [37]. The mechanism of action is thought to be that anti-BSEP antibodies form, which bind to an epitope in the intracanalicular domain of BSEP and subsequently block the function of the bile acid transporter. A multicentre series of six patients with recurrence of disease [38] was reported in 2010. In all of these patients, treatment was extremely problematic, four underwent a repeat LT, and various management protocols were suggested. All reports have identified mutations (splice site, missense, truncating) leading to absence of BSEP protein expression on immunostaining. Modifications in immunosuppression, plasmapheresis, intravenous immunoglobulin courses, and single-pass albumin dialysis were used in isolation or jointly with limited effect in patients' symptoms. Following the identification of BSEP antibodies in post-LT BSEP deficiency patients with cholestasis in the absence of rejection, an antibody-based treatment was suggested as potentially beneficial. Two cases of patients with BSEP deficiency following LT, had demonstrated evidence of functional BSEP deficiency treated successfully with two repeated 4-week courses of anti-cluster of differentiation CD20 monoclonal antibodies were subsequently reported [39, 40].

TJP2 Deficiency

Since in one third of patients with normal GGT cholestasis mutations in either *ABCB11* or *ATP8B1* have not been identified [26], a cohort of 33 cholestatic children with relatively low-serum GGT levels were studied recently [41]. Twelve patients from eight consanguineous families with novel protein truncating mutations in the *TJP2* gene were identified. The phenotype of these patients consists of early presentation within the first couple of months of life with low-serum GGT and nine of them underwent LT by their first decade of life. Patients can develop portal hypertension, persistent pruritus, and malabsorption. A single patient died at 13 months. Liver immunohistochemical findings consist of lack of TJP2, reduced staining of Claudin-1 (CLDN1) with normal distribution of Claudin-2 (CLDN2), both proteins essential to cellular tight junctions (Figs. 58.5, 58.6, and 58.7). On transmission electron microscopy, elongation of the tight junctions with sparsity of the zona occludens (ZO) is also seen. Extrahepatic involvement is present in some cases and

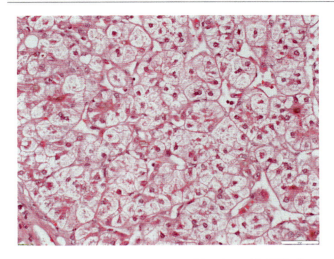

Fig. 58.5 Liver biopsy from a 4-year-old patient with TJP2 disease. There is extensive bridging fibrosis (not shown). Hepatocytes are oedematous and show rosetting. Canalicular cholestasis is present (H&E x200 magnification)

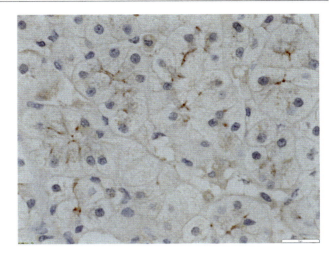

Fig. 58.7 Absence of canalicular TJP2 expression with expression of canalicular BSEP (x400 magnification)

and subsequently LT. No liver malignancy has been so far described in this newly defined PFIC group.

MDR3 Deficiency

This type of FIC is caused by a variety of mutations in the ATP-binding cassette subfamily B member 4 (*ABCB4*); the gene encoding MDR3 [43]. It is also inherited in an autosomal recessive pattern. *ABCB4* has been mapped to the 7q21–36 region, and it codes for a floppase responsible for phosphatidylcholine (PC) [44] translocation across the canalicular membrane. Defective PC translocation leads to a lack of PC in bile. The absence of PC inhibits the chaperoning of bile acids through micelle formation, leading to damage to the biliary epithelium and cholangiopathy. Biliary phospholipid levels are significantly reduced and biliary bile salt-to-phospholipid and cholesterol-to-phospholipid ratios are significantly higher in affected individuals when compared with wild-type bile [45].

MDR3 deficiency causes a spectrum of liver diseases such as cholesterol cholelithiasis, adult biliary cirrhosis, low phospholipid-associated cholelithiasis syndrome (LPAC), transient neonatal cholestasis, intrahepatic cholestasis of pregnancy (ICP) and drug-induced cholestasis [46–52]. In severe MDR3 deficiency, symptoms can manifest within the first year, but not usually as neonatal jaundice, and gradually progress towards liver cirrhosis and end-stage liver disease within the first few years of life [1, 53, 54]. Patients with a single affected copy of the gene can develop symptoms under particular circumstances, such as pregnancy, while otherwise they may remain asymptomatic [55, 56].

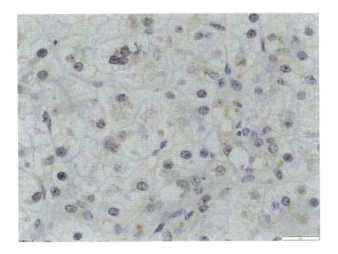

Fig. 58.6 Absence of canalicular TJP2 expression (x400 magnification)

consists of chronic respiratory disease or neurological complications such as subdural haematomas. Mutations in the *TJP2* gene have been previously associated with familial hypercholanaemia (FHC), a non progressive cholestatic disorder, described in the Amish population [42]. In that report, out of all 17 individuals with FHC, screened 11 patients in eight families were found homozygous for an incompletely penetrant missense mutation in *TJP2*, with alterations in the cellular bile acid concentration gradient.

Treatment consists of supportive choleretic agents, fat-soluble vitamin supplementation, nutritional support, PEBD,

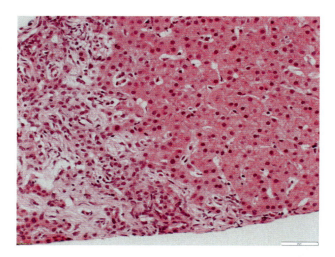

Fig. 58.8 Liver biopsy from a 1-year old child with MDR3 deficiency/ ABCB4 disease. There is a cholangiopathy manifested by cholangiocyte disarray and vacuolation. Immunohistochemistry demonstrated an absence of canalicular MDR3 expression (not shown) (H&E x200 magnification)

Liver histology demonstrates expansion of portal tracts, bile duct proliferation, bile plugs, and portal fibrosis with mixed inflammatory infiltrate (Fig. 58.8). Cytokeratin immunostaining can be confirmatory of the ductular proliferation, and MDR3 immunohistochemistry can be absent or markedly reduced at the canalicular membrane in affected individuals [57].

MDR3 deficiency is differentiated from the other three FIC types at a biochemical level by an elevated serum of GGT. Biochemical profile also consists of normal serum cholesterol and moderately raised concentration of serum primary bile salts [27].

First-line management, as in the other FIC types, is with UDCA and other antipruritic and choleretic agents. UDCA seems to be very effective in milder cases and it may also prevent disease progression in these cases. LT remains the treatment of choice for the nonresponders.

Conclusion

Over the past few years, our understanding of pediatric cholestatic disorders has significantly improved. Through the latest gene-sequencing techniques (targeted re-sequencing and/ or whole exome sequencing) and careful patient selection, we have managed to identify causative genes for cholestatic syndromes in most patients and highlight the mechanism of action of the encoded proteins at a cellular level. This enables physicians to characterize and treat these patients more efficiently although new challenges keep appearing such as recurrence of BSEP deficiency after LT.

Acknowledgment Figures courtesy of Dr Maesha Deheragoda, Consultant in Liver Histopathology, Institute of Liver Studies, King's College Hospital, London, UK.

References

1. Jacquemin E. Progressive familial intrahepatic cholestasis. J Gastroenterol Hepatol. 1999 June;14(6):594–9. PubMed PMID: 10385071.
2. Whitington PF, Freese DK, Alonso EM, Schwarzenberg SJ, Sharp HL. Clinical and biochemical findings in progressive familial intrahepatic cholestasis. J Pediatric Gastroenterol Nutr. 1994 Feb;18(2):134–41. PubMed PMID: 7912266.
3. Davit-Spraul A, Gonzales E, Baussan C, Jacquemin E. Progressive familial intrahepatic cholestasis. Orphanet J Rare Dis. 2009;4:1. PubMed PMID: 19133130. Pubmed Central PMCID: 2647530.
4. Klomp LW, Vargas JC, van Mil SW, Pawlikowska L, Strautnieks SS, van Eijk MJ, et al. Characterization of mutations in ATP8B1 associated with hereditary cholestasis. Hepatology. 2004 July;40(1):27–38. PubMed PMID: 15239083.
5. Bull LN, van Eijk MJ, Pawlikowska L, DeYoung JA, Juijn JA, Liao M, et al. A gene encoding a P-type ATPase mutated in two forms of hereditary cholestasis. Nat Gen. 1998 March;18(3):219–24. PubMed PMID: 9500542.
6. Paulusma CC, Groen A, Kunne C, Ho-Mok KS, Spijkerboer AL, Rudi de Waart D, et al. Atp8b1 deficiency in mice reduces resistance of the canalicular membrane to hydrophobic bile salts and impairs bile salt transport. Hepatology. 2006 July;44(1):195–204. PubMed PMID: 16799980.
7. Alvarez L, Jara P, Sanchez-Sabate E, Hierro L, Larrauri J, Diaz MC, et al. Reduced hepatic expression of farnesoid X receptor in hereditary cholestasis associated to mutation in ATP8B1. Hum Mol Gen. 2004 Oct 15;13(20):2451–60. PubMed PMID: 15317749.
8. Frankenberg T, Miloh T, Chen FY, Ananthanarayanan M, Sun AQ, Balasubramaniyan N, et al. The membrane protein ATPase class I type 8B member 1 signals through protein kinase C zeta to activate the farnesoid X receptor. Hepatology. 2008 Dec;48(6):1896–905. PubMed PMID: 18668687. Pubmed Central PMCID: 2774894.
9. Demeilliers C, Jacquemin E, Barbu V, Mergey M, Paye F, Fouassier L, et al. Altered hepatobiliary gene expressions in PFIC1: ATP8B1 gene defect is associated with CFTR downregulation. Hepatology. 2006 May;43(5):1125–34. PubMed PMID: 16628629.
10. Cai SY, Gautam S, Nguyen T, Soroka CJ, Rahner C, Boyer JL. ATP8B1 deficiency disrupts the bile canalicular membrane bilayer structure in hepatocytes, but FXR expression and activity are maintained. Gastroenterology. 2009 March;136(3):1060–9. PubMed PMID: 19027009. Pubmed Central PMCID: 3439851.
11. Verhulst PM, van der Velden LM, Oorschot V, van Faassen EE, Klumperman J, Houwen RH, et al. A flippase-independent function of ATP8B1, the protein affected in familial intrahepatic cholestasis type 1, is required for apical protein expression and microvillus formation in polarized epithelial cells. Hepatology. 2010 June;51(6):2049–60. PubMed PMID: 20512993.
12. Cebecauerova D, Strautnieks SS, Byrne JA, Jirsa M, Thompson RJ. ATP8B1 gene expression is driven by a housekeeping-like promoter independent of bile acids and farnesoid X receptor. PloS ONE. 2012;7(12):e51650. PubMed PMID: 23251605. Pubmed Central PMCID: 3518472.
13. Jacquemin E, Hermans D, Myara A, Habes D, Debray D, Hadchouel M, et al. Ursodeoxycholic acid therapy in pediatric patients with progressive familial intrahepatic cholestasis. Hepatology. 1997 March;25(3):519–23. PubMed PMID: 9049190.
14. Egawa H, Yorifuji T, Sumazaki R, Kimura A, Hasegawa M, Tanaka K. Intractable diarrhea after liver transplantation for

Byler's disease: successful treatment with bile adsorptive resin. Liver Transpl. 2002 Aug;8(8):714–6. PubMed PMID: 12149765.

15. Hollands CM, Rivera-Pedrogo FJ, Gonzalez-Vallina R, Loret-de-Mola O, Nahmad M, Burnweit CA. Ileal exclusion for Byler's disease: an alternative surgical approach with promising early results for pruritus. J Pediatr Surg. 1998 Feb;33(2):220–4. PubMed PMID: 9498390.

16. Ismail H, Kalicinski P, Markiewicz M, Jankowska I, Pawlowska J, Kluge P, et al. Treatment of progressive familial intrahepatic cholestasis: liver transplantation or partial external biliary diversion. Pediatr Transpl. 1999 Aug;3(3):219–24. PubMed PMID: 10487283.

17. Jankowska I, Socha P. Progressive familial intrahepatic cholestasis and inborn errors of bile acid synthesis. Clinics Res Hepatol Gastroenterol. 2012 June;36(3):271–4. PubMed PMID: 22609295.

18. Rebhandl W, Felberbauer FX, Turnbull J, Paya K, Barcik U, Huber WD, et al. Biliary diversion by use of the appendix (cholecystoappendicostomy) in progressive familial intrahepatic cholestasis. J Pediatr Gastroenterol Nutr. 1999 Feb;28(2):217–9. PubMed PMID: 9932861.

19. Emond JC, Whitington PF. Selective surgical management of progressive familial intrahepatic cholestasis (Byler's disease). J Pediatric Surg. 1995 Dec;30(12):1635–41. PubMed PMID: 8749912.

20. Jankowska I, Czubkowski P, Kalicinski P, Ismail H, Kowalski A, Ryzko J, et al. Ileal exclusion in children with progressive familial intrahepatic cholestasis. J Pediatr Gastroenterol Nutr. 2014 Jan;58(1):92–5. PubMed PMID: 24385022.

21. Strautnieks SS, Bull LN, Knisely AS, Kocoshis SA, Dahl N, Arnell H, et al. A gene encoding a liver-specific ABC transporter is mutated in progressive familial intrahepatic cholestasis. Nat Gen. 1998 Nov;20(3):233–8. PubMed PMID: 9806540.

22. Pawlikowska L, Strautnieks S, Jankowska I, Czubkowski P, Emerick K, Antoniou A, et al. Differences in presentation and progression between severe FIC1 and BSEP deficiencies. J Hepatol. 2010 July;53(1):170–8. PubMed PMID: 20447715. Pubmed Central PMCID: 3042805.

23. Strautnieks SS, Byrne JA, Pawlikowska L, Cebecauerova D, Rayner A, Dutton L, et al. Severe bile salt export pump deficiency: 82 different ABCB11 mutations in 109 families. Gastroenterology. 2008 Apr;134(4):1203–14. PubMed PMID: 18395098.

24. van Mil SW, van der Woerd WL, van der Brugge G, Sturm E, Jansen PL, Bull LN, et al. Benign recurrent intrahepatic cholestasis type 2 is caused by mutations in ABCB11. Gastroenterology. 2004 Aug;127(2):379–84. PubMed PMID: 15300568.

25. Byrne JA, Strautnieks SS, Mieli-Vergani G, Higgins CF, Linton KJ, Thompson RJ. The human bile salt export pump: characterization of substrate specificity and identification of inhibitors. Gastroenterology. 2002 Nov;123(5):1649–58. PubMed PMID: 12404239.

26. Davit-Spraul A, Fabre M, Branchereau S, Baussan C, Gonzales E, Stieger B, et al. ATP8B1 and ABCB11 analysis in 62 children with normal gamma-glutamyl transferase progressive familial intrahepatic cholestasis (PFIC): phenotypic differences between PFIC1 and PFIC2 and natural history. Hepatology. 2010 May;51(5):1645–55. PubMed PMID: 20232290.

27. Davit-Spraul A, Gonzales E, Baussan C, Jacquemin E. The spectrum of liver diseases related to ABCB4 gene mutations: pathophysiology and clinical aspects. Semin Liver Dis. 2010 May;30(2):134–46. PubMed PMID: 20422496.

28. Byrne JA, Strautnieks SS, Ihrke G, Pagani F, Knisely AS, Linton KJ, et al. Missense mutations and single nucleotide polymorphisms in ABCB11 impair bile salt export pump processing and function or disrupt pre-messenger RNA splicing. Hepatology. 2009 Feb;49(2):553–67. PubMed PMID: 19101985.

29. Noe J, Stieger B, Meier PJ. Functional expression of the canalicular bile salt export pump of human liver. Gastroenterology. 2002 Nov;123(5):1659–66. PubMed PMID: 12404240.

30. Lam P, Pearson CL, Soroka CJ, Xu S, Mennone A, Boyer JL. Levels of plasma membrane expression in progressive and benign mutations of the bile salt export pump (Bsep/Abcb11) correlate with severity of cholestatic diseases. Am J Physiol Cell Physiol. 2007 Nov;293(5):C1709–16. PubMed PMID: 17855769.

31. Knisely AS, Strautnieks SS, Meier Y, Stieger B, Byrne JA, Portmann BC, et al. Hepatocellular carcinoma in ten children under five years of age with bile salt export pump deficiency. Hepatology. 2006 Aug;44(2):478–86. PubMed PMID: 16871584.

32. Scheimann AO, Strautnieks SS, Knisely AS, Byrne JA, Thompson RJ, Finegold MJ. Mutations in bile salt export pump (ABCB11) in two children with progressive familial intrahepatic cholestasis and cholangiocarcinoma. J Pediatr. 2007 May;150(5):556–9. PubMed PMID: 17452236.

33. Iannelli F, Collino A, Sinha S, Radaelli E, Nicoli P, D'Antiga L, et al. Massive gene amplification drives paediatric hepatocellular carcinoma caused by bile salt export pump deficiency. Nat Commun. 2014;5:3850. PubMed PMID: 24819516.

34. Arnell H, Papadogiannakis N, Zemack H, Knisely AS, Nemeth A, Fischler B. Follow-up in children with progressive familial intrahepatic cholestasis after partial external biliary diversion. J Pediatr Gastroenterol Nutr. 2010 Oct;51(4):494–9. PubMed PMID: 20683202.

35. Kalicinski PJ, Ismail H, Jankowska I, Kaminski A, Pawlowska J, Drewniak T, et al. Surgical treatment of progressive familial intrahepatic cholestasis: comparison of partial external biliary diversion and ileal bypass. Eur J Pediatr Surg. 2003 Oct;13(5):307–11. PubMed PMID: 14618520.

36. Jara P, Hierro L, Martinez-Fernandez P, Alvarez-Doforno R, Yanez F, Diaz MC, et al. Recurrence of bile salt export pump deficiency after liver transplantation. N Engl J Med. 2009 Oct 1;361(14):1359–67. PubMed PMID: 19797282. Epub 2009/10/03. eng.

37. Keitel V, Burdelski M, Vojnisek Z, Schmitt L, Haussinger D, Kubitz R. De novo bile salt transporter antibodies as a possible cause of recurrent graft failure after liver transplantation: a novel mechanism of cholestasis. Hepatology. 2009 Aug;50(2):510–7. PubMed PMID: 19642168. Epub 2009/07/31. eng.

38. Siebold L, Dick AA, Thompson R, Maggiore G, Jacquemin E, Jaffe R, et al. Recurrent low gamma-glutamyl transpeptidase cholestasis following liver transplantation for bile salt export pump (BSEP) disease (posttransplant recurrent BSEP disease). Liver Transpl. 2010 July;16(7):856–63. PubMed PMID: 20583290. Epub 2010/06/29. eng.

39. Grammatikopoulos T, Knisely AS, Dhawan A, Hadzic N, Thompson RJ. Anti-CD20 monoclonal antibody therapy in functional bile salt export pump deficiency after liver transplantation. J Pediatr Gastroenterol Nutr. 2015;60(6):e50–3.

40. Lin HC, Alvarez L, Laroche G, Melin-Aldana H, Pfeifer K, Schwarz K, et al. Rituximab as therapy for the recurrence of bile salt export pump deficiency after liver transplantation. Liver Transpl. 2013 Dec;19(12):1403–10. PubMed PMID: 24115678.

41. Sambrotta M, Strautnieks S, Papouli E, Rushton P, Clark BE, Parry DA, et al. Mutations in TJP2 cause progressive cholestatic liver disease. Nat Gen. 2014 Apr;46(4):326–8. PubMed PMID: 24614073. Pubmed Central PMCID: 4061468.

42. Carlton VE, Harris BZ, Puffenberger EG, Batta AK, Knisely AS, Robinson DL, et al. Complex inheritance of familial hypercholanemia with associated mutations in TJP2 and BAAT. Nat Gen. 2003 May;34(1):91–6. PubMed PMID: 12704386.

43. de Vree JM, Jacquemin E, Sturm E, Cresteil D, Bosma PJ, Aten J, et al. Mutations in the MDR3 gene cause progressive familial intrahepatic cholestasis. Proc Natl Acad Sci USA. 1998 Jan 6;95(1):282–7. PubMed PMID: 9419367. Pubmed Central PMCID: 18201.

44. Berumen J, Feinberg E, Todo T, Bonham CA, Concepcion W, Esquivel C. Complications following liver transplantation for progressive familial intrahepatic cholestasis. Dig Dis Sci. 2014;59(11):2649–52.

45. Jacquemin E. Progressive familial intrahepatic cholestasis. Clin Res Hepatol Gastroenterol. 2012 Sept;36 Suppl 1:S26–35. PubMed PMID: 23141890.

46. Gonzales E, Davit-Spraul A, Baussan C, Buffet C, Maurice M, Jacquemin E. Liver diseases related to MDR3 (ABCB4) gene deficiency. Front Biosci. 2009;14:4242–56. PubMed PMID: 19273348. Epub 2009/03/11. eng.

47. Jacquemin E, De Vree JM, Cresteil D, Sokal EM, Sturm E, Dumont M, et al. The wide spectrum of multidrug resistance 3 deficiency: from neonatal cholestasis to cirrhosis of adulthood. Gastroenterology. 2001 May;120(6):1448–58. PubMed PMID: 11313315.

48. Rosmorduc O, Hermelin B, Boelle PY, Parc R, Taboury J, Poupon R. ABCB4 gene mutation-associated cholelithiasis in adults. Gastroenterology. 2003 Aug;125(2):452–9. PubMed PMID: 12891548.

49. Rosmorduc O, Hermelin B, Boelle PY, Poupon RE, Poupon R, Chazouilleres O. ABCB4 gene mutations and primary sclerosing cholangitis. Gastroenterology. 2004 April;126(4):1220–2; author reply 2–3. PubMed PMID: 15057773.

50. Rosmorduc O, Poupon R. Low phospholipid associated cholelithiasis: association with mutation in the MDR3/ABCB4 gene. Orphanet J Rare Dis. 2007;2:29. PubMed PMID: 17562004. Pubmed Central PMCID: 1910597.

51. Rosmorduc O, Hermelin B, Poupon R. MDR3 gene defect in adults with symptomatic intrahepatic and gallbladder cholesterol cholelithiasis. Gastroenterology. 2001 May;120(6):1459–67. PubMed PMID: 11313316.

52. Gotthardt D, Runz H, Keitel V, Fischer C, Flechtenmacher C, Wirtenberger M, et al. A mutation in the canalicular phospholipid transporter gene, ABCB4, is associated with cholestasis, ductope-nia, and cirrhosis in adults. Hepatology. 2008 Oct;48(4):1157–66. PubMed PMID: 18781607.

53. Colombo C, Vajro P, Degiorgio D, Coviello DA, Costantino L, Tornillo L, et al. Clinical features and genotype-phenotype correlations in children with progressive familial intrahepatic cholestasis type 3 related to ABCB4 mutations. J Pediatr Gastroenterol Nutr. 2011 Jan;52(1):73–83. PubMed PMID: 21119540.

54. Degiorgio D, Colombo C, Seia M, Porcaro L, Costantino L, Zazzeron L, et al. Molecular characterization and structural implications of 25 new ABCB4 mutations in progressive familial intrahepatic cholestasis type 3 (PFIC3). Eur J Hum Gen. 2007 Dec;15(12):1230–8. PubMed PMID: 17726488.

55. Dixon PH, Weerasekera N, Linton KJ, Donaldson O, Chambers J, Egginton E, et al. Heterozygous MDR3 missense mutation associated with intrahepatic cholestasis of pregnancy: evidence for a defect in protein trafficking. Hum Mol Gen. 2000 May 1;9(8):1209–17. PubMed PMID: 10767346.

56. Jacquemin E, Cresteil D, Manouvrier S, Boute O, Hadchouel M. Heterozygous non-sense mutation of the MDR3 gene in familial intrahepatic cholestasis of pregnancy. Lancet. 1999 Jan 16;353(9148):210–1. PubMed PMID: 9923886.

57. Fang LJ, Wang XH, Knisely AS, Yu H, Lu Y, Liu LY, et al. Chinese children with chronic intrahepatic cholestasis and high gamma-glutamyl transpeptidase: clinical features and association with ABCB4 mutations. J Pediatr Gastroenterol Nutr. 2012 Aug;55(2):150–6. PubMed PMID: 22343912.

Alagille Syndrome

Binita Maya Kamath

Introduction

Alagille syndrome (ALGS) is an autosomal dominant disorder that affects the liver, heart, face, eyes, skeleton, kidneys, and vasculature [1–6]. ALGS is primarily caused by mutations in the gene *JAGGED1* (*JAG1*) and in a second gene *NOTCH2*, in a minority of cases. Previously, ALGS was estimated to have a frequency of 1 in 70,000 live births; however, the advent of molecular testing has proven this to be an underestimate, and this figure is closer to 1 in 30,000 [7]. There is significant variability in the extent to which each of the aforementioned organ systems is affected in an individual, if at all [8, 9]. This variability in organ involvement requires the managing physician to have an understanding of the breadth and interplay of the variable manifestations. Due to the original descriptions of ALGS as a hepatic disease, with cholestasis as a central feature, the condition has been primarily managed by gastroenterologists and hepatologists, but frequently requires a multidisciplinary approach.

Clinical Manifestations of Alagille Syndrome

The hallmark clinical feature of ALGS is extreme variability. There is variability in the severity of organ system involvement in an individual, and also between those sharing the same disease-causing mutation. Typical patterns of organ involvement in ALGS are described below, but clearly not all individuals have manifestations in all systems.

B. M. Kamath (✉)
Division of Gastroenterology, Hepatology and Nutrition, The Hospital for Sick Children, University of Toronto, 555 University Avenue, Toronto, ON M5G 1X8, Canada
e-mail: binita.kamath@sickkids.ca

Hepatic

The majority of ALGS patients who are symptomatic with liver disease present in the first year of life with cholestasis, classically with neonatal conjugated hyperbilirubinemia and high γ-glutamyltransferase (GGT). During childhood, elevations of serum bilirubin up to 30 times normal and serum bile salt elevations of 100 times normal are common. Cholesterol levels can be staggering and may exceed 1000–2000 mg/dL. However, this high level of plasma cholesterol is largely associated with lipoprotein-X [10]. Lipoprotein-X is in the low-density lipid range and resists oxidation, thereby protecting against atherosclerosis. Thus, the hypercholesterolemia of ALGS does not appear to carry an increased risk of cardiovascular disease [11, 12]. Hepatic synthetic function is usually well preserved in ALGS.

Physical examination findings in children with ALGS and liver disease include hepatomegaly early on and splenomegaly in the majority over time. The pruritus seen is among the most severe of any liver disease. It rarely is present before 3–5 months of age but is seen in most children by the second year of life, even in some who are anicteric. Multiple xanthomas are a common sequelae of severe cholestasis associated with ALGS and correlate with a serum cholesterol level greater than 500 mg/dL. Xanthomas typically form on the extensor surfaces of the fingers, the palmar creases, the nape of the neck, the ears, the buttocks, and around the inguinal creases (Fig. 59.1a, b). Xanthomas are disfiguring and occasionally interfere with fine motor function when they occur on the fingers.

The natural history of the liver disease in ALGS has a unique course. For those children with significant cholestasis in infancy, the hepatic involvement generally follows a more severe course in the first 5 years of life after which it appears to improve for most patients. This spontaneous improvement is poorly understood, but well documented. In approximately 10–20%, the cholestasis persists unabated or progresses to end-stage liver disease (ESLD). For those children with mild cholestasis or hepatitis in early childhood, there is no

© Springer International Publishing Switzerland 2016
S. Guandalini et al. (eds.), *Textbook of Pediatric Gastroenterology, Hepatology and Nutrition*,
DOI 10.1007/978-3-319-17169-2_59

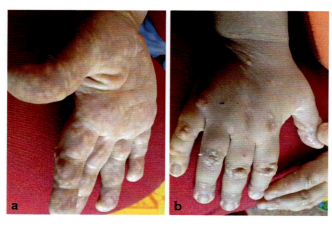

Fig. 59.1 **a, b** Xanthomas on the hands of a child with Alagille syndrome

progression of liver disease in later life. It is difficult to predict early on, which ALGS children with cholestasis in early childhood will eventually require liver transplantation and which will spontaneously improve. There are no known genotypic or radiologic predictors of liver disease progression in ALGS. A review of laboratory data of ALGS patients showed that bilirubin and cholesterol levels before the age of 5 may aid in distinguishing patients at high and low risk of problematic cholestasis in later childhood. More specifically, mean levels of total bilirubin (TB) > 6.5 mg/dL (111 µmol/L), conjugated bilirubin (CB) > 4.5 mg/dL (77 µmol/L), and cholesterol > 520 mg/dL (13.3 mmol/L) are strongly associated with severe liver disease in later life, whereas levels lower than this are associated with a good hepatic outcome [13]. These data may assist the clinician in predicting which children might go on to resolve their cholestasis, and thereby avoid unnecessary liver transplantation in young children with ALGS.

Of note, there have been several case reports of hepatocellular carcinoma in patients with ALGS, including as young as 4 years of age [14–16]. Most but not all patients who developed hepatocellular carcinoma also had progressed to cirrhosis.

Bile duct paucity is the hallmark histopathologic feature of ALGS. The normal bile duct to portal space ratio is between 0.9 and 1.8. Bile duct paucity is defined as a ratio of bile duct to portal tract that is less than 0.9. Bile duct paucity, however, is not present in infancy in many patients ultimately shown to have ALGS. Several studies of serial liver biopsies have demonstrated that paucity is more common later in infancy and childhood [4, 17, 18]. Emerick et al. found that paucity was present in 60 % of 48 infants younger than 6 months of age but in 95 % of 40 who underwent biopsy after 6 months [4].

Cardiac

In a comprehensive evaluation of 200 ALGS subjects, cardiovascular involvement was present in 94 % [19], with right-sided lesions being the most prevalent. Pulmonary artery anomalies are the most common abnormality identified (76 %) and may occur in isolation or in combination with structural intracardiac disease [19]. The most common congenital defect is tetralogy of Fallot (TOF), which occurs in 7–12 % [4, 19]. Approximately, 40 % of patients with ALGS demonstrating TOF have pulmonary atresia, representing a more severe phenotype. Cardiac disease accounts for nearly all of the early deaths in ALGS. Patients with intracardiac disease have approximately a 40 % rate of survival to 6 years of life, compared with a 95 % survival rate in patients with ALGS without intracardiac lesions [4].

Facial Features

A characteristic facial appearance is one of the most penetrant features of ALGS (for *JAG1*-associated disease). These features include a prominent forehead, deep-set eyes with moderate hypertelorism, a pointed chin, and a saddle or straight nose with a bulbous tip. The combination of these features gives the face a triangular appearance (Fig. 59.2). The facies may be present early in infancy but in general becomes more apparent with increasing age. In adults, the forehead is much less prominent, and the protruding chin is more noticeable so that the face loses the triangular appearance.

It should be noted that among the few patients reported to date, there appears to be a lower penetrance of characteristic ALGS facial features in patients with *NOTCH2* mutations, and it is therefore a less valuable diagnostic tool in this group [20].

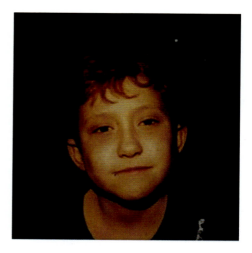

Fig. 59.2 Facial features of Alagille syndrome

Ophthalmologic

The ocular abnormalities of patients with ALGS do not generally affect vision but are important as diagnostic tools. A large and varied number of ocular abnormalities have been described, though posterior embryotoxon is the most important diagnostically. Posterior embryotoxon is a prominent, centrally positioned Schwalbe's ring (or line) at the point at which the corneal endothelium and the uveal trabecular meshwork join and is visible on slit-lamp examination. Posterior embryotoxon occurs in 56–88 % of patients with ALGS and was also detected in 22 % of children evaluated in a general ophthalmology clinic [21]. Posterior embryotoxon is seen in other multisystem disorders such as chromosome 22q deletion, as well. The Axenfeld anomaly, seen in 13 % of patients with ALGS, is a prominent Schwalbe's ring with attached iris strands and is associated with glaucoma. Optic disk drusen identified using ocular ultrasonography has been described in ALGS patients with high prevalence but this test is not routinely performed [22, 23].

Skeletal Involvement

The most characteristic skeletal finding is the sagittal cleft or butterfly vertebrae, which is found in 33–87 % of patients with ALGS [4, 24–26]. This relatively uncommon anomaly may occur in normal individuals and is also seen in other multisystem abnormalities, such as 22q deletion syndrome and vertebral defects, anal atresia, tracheoesophageal fistula, and radial and renal defect (VATER) syndrome. The affected vertebral bodies are split sagittally into paired hemivertebrae because of a failure of the fusion of the anterior arches of the vertebrae. Generally, these are asymptomatic and of no structural significance.

Other associated skeletal abnormalities include an abnormal narrowing of the adjusted interpedicular space in the lumbar spine, a pointed anterior process of C1, spina bifida occulta, fusion of the adjacent vertebrae, hemivertebrae, the absence of the 12th rib, and the presence of a bony connection between ribs. In addition, supernumerary digital flexion creases have been described in one third of patients [27].

Severe metabolic bone disease with osteoporosis and pathologic fractures is common in patients with ALGS. Recurrent fractures, particularly of the femur, have been cited as an indication for liver transplantation. Preliminary survey data suggest that there is a propensity towards pathologic lower extremity long bone fractures in ALGS [28]. A number of factors may contribute to osteopenia and fractures, including severe chronic malnutrition, vitamin D and vitamin K deficiency, chronic hepatic and renal disease, and magnesium deficiency. It is not yet known whether there is an intrinsic defect in cortical or trabecular structure of the bones

in patients with ALGS. Olsen evaluated bone status in prepubertal children with ALGS and identified significant deficits in bone size and bone mass that were related to fat absorption but not dietary intake [29].

ALGS patients are frequently found to have short stature; this is likely multifactorial in origin resulting from cholestasis and malabsorption, congenital heart disease, and genetic predisposition. A validated growth curve for ALGS individuals is not yet available.

Renal Involvement

Renal involvement in ALGS has been widely reported on an individual case basis or as part of a larger report on general features of ALGS. The prevalence of renal involvement in larger series ranges from 40 to 70 % such that it has been proposed that renal anomalies now be considered a disease-defining criterion in ALGS. In a large retrospective study, there was a prevalence of 39 % of renal anomalies or disease. The most common renal involvement was renal dysplasia (58.9 %), followed by renal tubular acidosis (9.5 %), vesicoureteric reflux (8.2 %), and urinary obstruction (8.2 %) [30]. Hypertension in patients with ALGS can be of cardiac, vascular, or renal etiology.

Functional and structural evaluation of the kidneys should be undertaken in all patients. Renal function should be reassessed during the evaluation for liver transplantation.

Vascular Involvement

Unexplained intracranial bleeding is a recognized complication and cause of mortality in ALGS. Intracranial bleeds occur in approximately 15 % of patients; in 30–50 % of these events, the hemorrhage is fatal [4, 25]. There does not seem to be any pattern to the location and/or severity of the intracranial bleeding, which ranges from massive fatal events to asymptomatic cerebral infarcts. Epidural, subdural, subarachnoid, and intraparenchymal bleeding have been reported. The majority of this bleeding has occurred in the absence of significant coagulopathy or trauma. Lykavieris studied a cohort of 174 individuals with ALGS and identified 38 patients (22 %) who had 49 bleeding episodes [31]. All these hemorrhages occurred in the absence of liver failure, with normal median platelet counts and prothrombin times, suggesting that ALGS patients may be at particular risk for bleeding.

Underlying vessel abnormalities in the central nervous system that could explain the occurrence of bleeding and stroke in ALGS have been described in some of these patients [5, 25, 32]. Aneurysms of the basilar and middle cerebral arteries and various internal carotid artery anomalies have been described. Moyamoya disease (progressive intracranial arterial occlusive disease) also has been previously described in several children with ALGS. Emerick et al. prospectively studied 26 patients with ALGS using magnetic resonance imaging (MRI) with angiography of the head. Cerebrovascular abnormalities were detected in 10 of 26 patients (38%). One hundred percent of symptomatic patients had detected abnormalities, and 23% of screened, asymptomatic patients had detected anomalies [32]. These results suggest that MRI with angiography is useful in detecting these lesions and may have a valuable role in screening for treatable lesions such as aneurysms. The current recommendation is for all asymptomatic ALGS patients to have a screening MRI/magnetic resonance (MR) angiography as a baseline and for physicians to have a low threshold for reimaging ALGS patients in the event of any symptoms, head trauma, or suspicious neurologic signs and prior to major surgical interventions.

Systemic vascular abnormalities have also been well documented in ALGS. Aortic aneurysms and coarctations, renal artery, celiac artery, superior mesenteric artery, and subclavian artery anomalies have all been described. In the evaluation of a large cohort of ALGS patients, 9% (25 of 268) with noncardiac vascular anomalies or events were identified [5]. In addition, vascular accidents accounted for 34% of the mortality in this cohort. These findings suggest that vascular abnormalities have been under-recognized as a potentially devastating complication of ALGS.

Genetics of Alagille Syndrome

ALGS is inherited in an autosomal dominant manner, with highly variable expressivity. It is a genetically heterogeneous disorder and may be caused by mutations in either *JAG1* (seen in 94% of clinically defined probands) or *NOTCH2* (seen in approximately 1%) [33–35]. Jagged1 is a cell surface protein that serves as a ligand for the four Notch receptors (Notch1, 2, 3, and 4), and together these proteins begin the cascade of events that turn on the Notch signaling pathway. The Notch signaling pathway is involved in the determination of cell fate and as such plays a crucial role in normal development.

Gene Identification and Mutation Analysis

JAG1 was identified as the cause of ALGS in 1997 [33, 35]. To date, more than 430 *JAG1* mutations have been identified in patients with ALGS. Utilizing current screening techniques, the mutation detection rate is 94% [36]. The frequency of sporadic mutations (i.e., new in the proband) is approximately 60–70%. Approximately, 75% of ALGS patients have *JAG1* protein-truncating (frameshift or nonsense or splice-site) mutations [8, 36–38]. Approximately,

7% have gene deletions. Missense mutations are identified in 15%. Haploinsufficiency, a decrease in the amount of the normal protein, is hypothesized to be the mechanism causing ALGS.

ALGS associated with *NOTCH2* mutations was described in 2006. Thus far, ten patients with unique *NOTCH2* mutations have been described [20, 34].

A small fraction (3–5%) of ALGS individuals have deletions of chromosome 20p. Genome-wide single-nucleotide polymorphism (SNP) analysis of 25 patients with ALGS revealed 21 deletions ranging from 95 kb to 14.62 Mb [39]. Patients with deletions greater than a critical 5.4 Mb region had additional phenotypic features not usually associated with ALGS such as developmental delay and hearing loss.

Genotype–Phenotype Correlations

JAG1 Mutations

Although the ALGS phenotype is highly variable, there is no apparent correlation with *JAG1* genotype in the majority of patients. A study of 53 *JAG1* mutation-positive relatives of a cohort of ALGS probands demonstrated that only 53% met the clinical criteria for a diagnosis of ALGS, including 11 of 53 with obvious clinical features that would easily have led to a diagnosis of ALGS and 17 of 53 (32%) who had mild features that would have only been apparent on targeted evaluation following the diagnosis of a proband in their family (i.e., discovery of elevation of liver enzymes or posterior embryotoxon in an asymptomatic individual) [7]. This underscores the variable clinical consequences associated with a *JAG1* mutation and suggests the presence of genetic modifiers.

NOTCH2 Mutations

To date ten individuals with complete or partial features of classical ALGS have been found to have *NOTCH2* mutations [20, 34]. From a phenotypic standpoint, individuals with *NOTCH2*-related ALGS appear to have less penetrance of the characteristic facial features and less skeletal involvement.

Diagnostic Considerations

Clinical Diagnostics

The majority of infants with ALGS are evaluated for conjugated hyperbilirubinemia in the first weeks or months of life. ALGS is occasionally misdiagnosed as biliary atresia because of the overlap of biochemical, scintigraphic, histologic, and cholangiographic features. Serum bilirubin, bile acid, and GGT levels typically are elevated in both of these disorders. Ultrasound findings in both conditions may reveal small or apparently absent gallbladders. Excretion of nuclear tracer (diisopropylacetanilido iminodiacetic acid; DISIDA) into the duodenum excludes biliary atresia, but non-excretion of tracer is also possible in ALGS. There was no excretion of scintiscan in 61% of 36 infants with ALGS [4].

Although a liver biopsy is not mandatory to diagnose ALGS, it remains an important step in differentiating between ALGS and biliary atresia. In biliary atresia, bile duct proliferation is the typical histologic lesion. In ALGS, paucity is evident in 60% of infants younger than 6 months but in 95% of older patients [4]. Unfortunately, there may be a normal number of ducts early in the course of biliary atresia and also in some patients with ALGS, and bile duct proliferation occasionally occurs in infants with ALGS. Giant cell hepatitis is also seen in both disorders. Finally, it should be noted that bile duct paucity, if present, is not diagnostic of ALGS and other diagnoses should be considered (e.g., alpha-1-antitrypsin deficiency, cystic fibrosis, cytomegalovirus infection, etc.).

An operative cholangiogram is the gold standard procedure to evaluate the extrahepatic and intrahepatic biliary tree; however, this can also be misleading in ALGS. The extra- and intrahepatic ducts are extremely small in patients with ALGS, and the cholangiogram commonly does not demonstrate communication proximally. In 37% of 19 cholangiograms in infants with ALGS, there was no opacification of the proximal extrahepatic ducts, and, in another 37%, the proximal extrahepatic tree was abnormally small [4]. The intrahepatic ducts were normal in only 10% of 19 infants with ALGS, small or hypoplastic in 16%, and not visualized in 74%. Therefore, even the apparent gold standard test to differentiate ALGS and biliary atresia can be misleading.

Clinical features in extrahepatic organ systems may also help in the diagnostic evaluation. The list of abnormalities identified in the "major" organ systems and the list of other affected organs have grown appreciably. Thus, an echocardiogram, slit-lamp examination, renal ultrasound, and spinal X-ray are essential diagnostic tests when ALGS is suspected. It should be noted that several of the ALGS-defining features are present in normal individuals or other conditions. Heart murmurs are present in 6% of all newborns, posterior embryotoxon appears in 22% of the general population, and butterfly vertebrae are seen in 11% of patients with 22q11 deletion. Furthermore, the facial features of ALGS patients are subtle during the first months of life making this an unreliable diagnostic tool in infancy.

With the advent of molecular testing for ALGS and the broader appreciation of the phenotypic variability, the diagnostic criteria for ALGS have been modified. To make a clinical diagnosis for an index case (proband) in the family, the original Alagille criteria hold, modified only so as no longer to require histology. Thus ALGS can be diagnosed clinically on the basis of cholestasis with at least three features from the list of characteristic Alagille facies, consistent cardiac disease, posterior embryotoxon, butterfly vertebrae, typical ALGS renal disease, and a structural vascular anomaly. In families with one definite clinically defined proband, other members with only two features should be considered as having ALGS.

Molecular Diagnostics

Molecular sequencing is now widely commercially available for *JAG1* and *NOTCH2* on a limited basis. An evaluation by fluorescence in situ hybridization (FISH) for deletions including the *JAG1* gene will identify these deletions in less than 7% of patients. A molecular diagnosis can assist in an atypical ALGS case and is also useful for genetic counseling and prenatal diagnosis. *JAG1* sequencing identifies mutations in individuals with clinically defined ALGS in the majority of cases (>90%). Individuals that have clinical features of ALGS but are not found to be carrying *JAG1* mutations should have sequence analysis of *NOTCH2* [34].

Once a *JAG1* mutation is identified in a proband, it is simple to test parents and other relatives for the identified mutation. Mutations are inherited from an affected parent in 30–50% of patients, whereas the mutations appear de novo in 60–70% [8, 37]. If a parental mutation is identified, there is a 50% risk for each future offspring to inherit the *JAG1* mutation. However, it should be emphasized that expressivity of the disorder is highly variable, and it is not currently possible to predict disease severity. If no parental mutation is identified, then the recurrence risk is limited to the chance of germ-line mosaicism, which for multiple different disorders is estimated at from 1 to 3%.

Prenatal genetic testing for ALGS is possible if a parental mutation has been identified. This requires amniocentesis or chorionic villous sampling and assessment for a known *JAG1* mutation. Pre-implantation genetic diagnosis has also been successfully performed in ALGS. It is imperative to carefully counsel parents undergoing any type of prenatal testing since there are no genotype–phenotype correlations in ALGS, so it is not possible to make predictions about a child's clinical course based on the type or presence of a mutation.

Management of Alagille Syndrome

Cholestasis Management

Patients with ALGS present significant management challenges due to profound cholestasis and complex multisystem disease [40, 41]. A sequential and additive approach to medical cholestasis therapy in ALGS is most appropriate. The most commonly used agents are listed in Table 59.1 with common side effects and described below.

Table 59.1 Medications for cholestasis in Alagille syndrome

Medication	Dose	Most frequent side effects
Choleretics		
Ursodiol (Actigall)	10–30 mg/kg/day, divided in 2 doses	Diarrhea, abdominal pain
Phenobarbital; rarely used	5–10 mg/kg/day, divided in 2 doses	Sedation
Other		
Rifampin	10 mg/kg/day, divided in 2 doses (maximum dose 600 mg/day)	Red discoloration of urine, idiosyncratic hypersensitivity reactions, hepatitis
Bile-salt binding agents		
Cholestyramine	240 mg/kg/day, divided into 3 doses; maximum dose of 8 g/day	Constipation, abdominal pain
Colesevelam	Limited pediatric data 625 mg once daily (adult dose)	Constipation
Antihistamines		
Diphenhydramine	5 mg/kg/day, divided into 3–4 doses; maximum 300 mg/day	Drowsiness
Hydroxyzine	2 mg/kg/day, divided in 3–4 doses	Drowsiness
Opioid antagonists		
Naltrexone	Limited pediatric data 0.25–0.5 mg/kg once daily, up to 50 mg daily (adult dose)	Symptoms of opioid withdrawal

The pruritus associated with ALGS cholestatic liver disease can be severe and may occur even without jaundice. Pruritus is often debilitating, disturbing sleep, daily activities, and cognitive development. Conservative management of pruritus entails taking care to keep the skin hydrated with emollients, trimming the fingernails, and taking short baths or showers to limit drying of the skin. Bile flow may be stimulated with choleretics, and ursodiol is the most commonly used agent. The use of ursodiol has been studied in ALGS children with improvement in pruritus, xanthomas, and biochemical markers of cholestasis [42–45]. Therapy with antihistamines may provide some symptomatic relief but are rarely effective alone. Bile-acid-binding resins, such as cholestyramine, are often effective but sometimes not palatable. They are also difficult to administer since they must be given 2 h apart from other medications. Colesevelam may be better tolerated but has not been studied in pediatrics. It should be noted that colesevelam is a very potent bile-acid-binding resin and may severely deplete the concentration of free luminal bile acids resulting in risk of fat-soluble vitamin deficiency, and these levels should therefore be monitored. Rifampin has been comparatively well studied in ALGS [38, 46, 47]. Yerushalmi et al. studied 24 children with severe cholestasis, of whom 6 had AGS, and 92 % of the cohort showed a response in improving pruritus [31]. Although rifampin is associated with elevation of serum transaminases, none of these studies reported clinical or biochemical adverse events. Naltrexone has been shown to be effective against pruritus in cholestatic adults. Based on anecdotal experience, it can be useful in the pruritus of ALGS children as well. Newer agents that inhibit apical sodium-dependent transport of bile acids at the enterocyte and interrupt the enterohepatic circulation are currently in clinical trials and offer hope for a new therapy for pruritus.

Biliary diversion has been successful in a number of patients, though it does not appear to be as effective for ALGS as it does for progressive familial intrahepatic cholestasis [48, 49]. Emerick studied nine ALGS patients with severe mutilating pruritus who underwent partial external biliary diversion (PEBD). Mean pruritus scores were significantly lower 1 year after the procedure, and eight of the nine had only mild scratching when not distracted. Three of the nine also had complete resolution of extensive xanthomas. Biliary diversion should be considered in all ALGS children when medical management of pruritus fails and external diversion appears to be more effective than internal approaches. It should be noted, however, that the outcome of PEBD is poor in the setting of hepatic fibrosis, and therefore a liver biopsy should be considered prior to offering this therapy.

Xanthomas do not require specific treatment unless they interfere with vision, feeding or motor development which is exceptionally rare. As the hypercholesterolemia of ALGS is not atherogenic, dietary modifications or medical therapy are not necessary.

Hepatoportoenterostomy is inappropriate in ALGS and may increase the amount of liver injury and progression to hepatic fibrosis. In a limited retrospective study comparing ALGS patients to matched biliary atresia patients after Kasai procedures, the ALGS cohort had a significantly higher rate of liver transplantation (47 vs. 14 %) and sustained higher mortality [50]. These data suggest that the Kasai procedure is not a marker for severe underlying liver disease but that the Kasai procedure itself has a detrimental effect on outcome.

Liver Transplantation

Liver transplantation is required in 21–31 % of patients with ALGS based on case series [41]. Several of these series are older, and with current therapies this frequency is likely to be lower. Indications for transplant in ALGS are ESLD secondary to chronic cholestasis, severe complications of cholestasis such as failure to thrive, portal hypertension, and recurrent fractures.

Liver transplantation in patients with ALGS is complicated by the associated comorbidities, particularly cardiac, renal, and vascular involvement. A detailed renal evaluation is warranted in any ALGS patient prior to liver transplantation including urinalysis, blood pressure, renal ultrasonography, glomerular filtration rate, serum cystatin C and blood gas measurement. If renal impairment is documented, renal-sparing immunosuppressive protocols should be considered. Vascular involvement should be assessed with computed tomography (CT) or MR angiography of the head, neck, and abdomen. Cardiac pre-transplant workup is based on information acquired with echocardiography and electrocardiography. However, the peripheral branches of the pulmonary arteries and the degree of right ventricular hypertrophy are underappreciated using these modalities. Investigators at King's College have suggested a pre-transplant dynamic stress test with dobutamine to stimulate perioperative conditions with concomitant cardiac catheterization [51]. If the patient achieves >40 % increase in the cardiac output, then the cardiac reserve is considered adequate for liver transplantation.

Living-related transplantation (LRT) in ALGS requires careful consideration. In general, in North America, LRT has not been offered to donors with a known disease-causing mutation as they may have subclinical liver disease. In Japan, the outcomes from LRT in ALGS in 20 children have been reported and are good with a 1-year survival rate of 80 % [52]. On a cautionary note, Gurkan reported two instances in which apparently unaffected parents underwent donor operations that were unsuccessful because of a paucity of duct structures discovered intraoperatively [53]. Therefore, the recommendation in North America is for potential donors to undergo screening for the known mutation in the proband and for them generally not to be used as donors if positive for the mutation.

The survival rate of patients with ALGS undergoing liver transplantation has significantly improved in recent years with careful selection of transplant candidates and better management of concomitant cardiac disease. Combined case series show a 1-year posttransplantation patient survival rate of 79 %. A recent report by Arnon et al. from the United Network for Organ Sharing dataset of 461 ALGS who underwent liver transplantation from 1987 to 2008, revealed 1 and 5-year patient survival of 83 and 78 %, respectively [54]. Early death in the first 30 days was significantly higher in ALGS patients as compared to biliary atresia patients. Death from graft failure, neurologic, and cardiac complications were also significantly higher in the ALGS cohort.

Nutritional

Failure to thrive and malnutrition need to be addressed aggressively and early on in life. There is significant malabsorption of long-chain fat; therefore, formulas supplemented with medium-chain triglycerides have some nutritional advantage. Many patients are unable to eat enough to provide the substantial quantities of energy required for growth and development, and nasogastric or gastrostomy tube feedings can provide necessary supplementation.

Fat-soluble vitamin deficiency is present in most patients with significant ALGS cholestasis. Oral or parenteral supplementation is necessary for prevention of vitamin deficiencies and their sequelae. Multivitamin preparations may not provide the correct ratio of fat-soluble vitamins; vitamins are best administered as individual supplements tailored to the specific needs of the patient. Close monitoring (every 3–6 months) of fat-soluble vitamin levels is crucial to avoid complications of vitamin deficiencies, particularly in the first years of life.

Cardiac Anomalies

Management of the cardiac involvement in ALGS is clearly lesion specific. In a large ALGS series, cardiac surgery was performed in infancy in 11 % [4]. The mortality rates were 33 % for those with TOF and 75 % for those with TOF with pulmonary atresia. The survival of patients with ALGS with these lesions is markedly lower than for patients (with these lesions) without ALGS. This may be a result, in part, of the common presence of significant stenoses in the distal pulmonary artery or other systemic manifestations of the syndrome. Nonsurgical invasive techniques have been used successfully for patients with ALGS, including valvuloplasty, balloon dilatation, and stent implantation [55, 56]. Heart–lung transplantation has been performed in combination with liver transplantation in a child with ALGS [57].

Other Extrahepatic Disease

As with the cardiac involvement in ALGS, other extrahepatic disease must be managed according to the specific lesion. For the vasculopathy, no ALGS-specific treatments exist for intra- or extracerebral vessel anomalies, and consultation with a vascular surgeon or neurosurgeon must be sought if an anomaly is found. Without longitudinal data available, the risks and benefits of surgery in an isolated intracranial vascular anomaly should be carefully balanced. In the case of known progressive disease, such as Moyamoya, the risk of recurrent stroke usually mandates surgical intervention, and outcomes of this neurosurgery appears to be favourable in Alagille syndrome [58].

Prognosis of Alagille Syndrome

Cardiac, hepatic, and vascular disease account for the majority of deaths in ALGS. The presence of a complex intra-cardiac anomaly is the only predictor of an excessive early mortality rate, and cardiac anomalies account for the majority of deaths in early childhood. Overall, vascular events account for most of the mortality in ALGS; 34% in a large series [5]. Quiros-Tejeira reported a 72% survival rate in 43 patients at a mean follow-up of 8.9 years in a population in which 47% underwent liver transplantation [26]. Emerick estimated the 20-year survival rate in 92 patients to be 75% overall, 80% for those not requiring liver transplantation, and 60% for those requiring transplantation [4]. For patients with structural intracardiac disease, however, the survival rate was only 40% at 7 years.

Conclusion

To conclude, ALGS is a complex condition in which the molecular basis is well understood but the absence of identified genotype–phenotype correlations and the broad variability poses management challenges. Renal and vascular involvement should likely be included in the diagnostic criteria. As molecular testing becomes more readily available, it is likely that patients with isolated or subtle manifestations will be diagnosed as having ALGS. The discovery of two disease genes and a broader phenotype, which includes individuals with *no* liver disease, suggests that a redefinition of this syndrome is warranted based on molecular defects, possibly reserving the term ALGS for those with liver disease and associated features, as Daniel Alagille originally intended.

References

1. Alagille D, Odievre M, Gautier M, Dommergues JP. Hepatic ductular hypoplasia associated with characteristic facies, vertebral malformations, retarded physical, mental, and sexual development, and cardiac murmur. J Pediatr. 1975;86(1):63–71.
2. Alagille D, Estrada A, Hadchouel M, Gautier M, Odievre M, Dommergues JP. Syndromic paucity of interlobular bile ducts (Alagille syndrome or arteriohepatic dysplasia): review of 80 cases. J Pediatr. 1987;110(2):195–200.
3. Watson GH, Miller V. Arteriohepatic dysplasia: familial pulmonary arterial stenosis with neonatal liver disease. Arch Dis Child. 1973 June;48(6):459–66.
4. Emerick KM, Rand EB, Goldmuntz E, Krantz ID, Spinner NB, Piccoli DA. Features of Alagille syndrome in 92 patients: frequency and relation to prognosis. Hepatology. 1999 March;29(3):822–9.
5. Kamath BM, Spinner NB, Emerick KM, Chudley AE, Booth C, Piccoli DA, et al. Vascular anomalies in Alagille syndrome: a significant cause of morbidity and mortality. Circulation. 2004 March 23;109(11):1354–8.
6. Tolia V, Dubois RS, Watts FB Jr., Perrin E. Renal abnormalities in paucity of interlobular bile ducts. J Pediatr Gastroenterol Nutr. 1987 Nov–Dec;6(6):971–6.
7. Kamath BM, Bason L, Piccoli DA, Krantz ID, Spinner NB. Consequences of JAG1 mutations. J Med Genet. 2003 Dec;40(12):891–5.
8. Crosnier C, Driancourt C, Raynaud N, Dhorne-Pollet S, Pollet N, Bernard O, et al. Mutations in JAGGED1 gene are predominantly sporadic in Alagille syndrome. Gastroenterology. 1999;116(5):1141–8.
9. Crosnier C, Lykavieris P, Meunier-Rotival M, Hadchouel M. Alagille syndrome. The widening spectrum of arteriohepatic dysplasia. Clin Liver Dis. 2000;4(4):765–78.
10. Gottrand F, Clavey V, Fruchart JC, Farriaux JP. Lipoprotein pattern and plasma lecithin cholesterol acyl transferase activity in children with Alagille syndrome. Atherosclerosis. 1995 June;115(2):233–41.
11. Black DD. Chronic cholestasis and dyslipidemia: what is the cardiovascular risk? J Pediatr. 2005 March;146(3):306–7.
12. Nagasaka H, Yorifuji T, Egawa H, Yanai H, Fujisawa T, Kosugiyama K, et al. Evaluation of risk for atherosclerosis in Alagille syndrome and progressive familial intrahepatic cholestasis: two congenital cholestatic diseases with different lipoprotein metabolisms. J Pediatr. 2005 March;146(3):329–35.
13. Kamath BM, Munoz PS, Bab N, Baker A, Chen Z, Spinner NB, et al. A longitudinal study to identify laboratory predictors of liver disease outcome in Alagille syndrome. J Pediatr Gastroenterol Nutr. May;50(5):526–30.
14. Bekassy AN, Garwicz S, Wiebe T, Hagerstrand I, Jensen OA. Hepatocellular carcinoma associated with arteriohepatic dysplasia in a 4-year-old girl. Med Pediatr Oncol. 1992;20(1):78–83.
15. Rabinovitz M, Imperial JC, Schade RR, Van Thiel DH. Hepatocellular carcinoma in Alagille's syndrome: a family study. J Pediatr Gastroenterol Nutr. 1989 Jan;8(1):26–30.
16. Tsai S, Gurakar A, Anders R, Lam-Himlin D, Boitnott J, Pawlik TM. Management of large hepatocellular carcinoma in adult patients with Alagille syndrome: a case report and review of literature. Dig Dis Sci. [Case reports]. 2010 Nov;55(11):3052–8.
17. Dahms BB, Petrelli M, Wyllie R, Henoch MS, Halpin TC, Morrison S, et al. Arteriohepatic dysplasia in infancy and childhood: a longitudinal study of six patients. Hepatology. 1982 May–June;2(3):350–8.
18. Kahn E. Paucity of interlobular bile ducts. Arteriohepatic dysplasia and nonsyndromic duct paucity. Perspect Pediatr Pathol. 1991;14:168–215.
19. McElhinney DB, Krantz ID, Bason L, Piccoli DA, Emerick KM, Spinner NB, et al. Analysis of cardiovascular phenotype and genotype-phenotype correlation in individuals with a JAG1 mutation and/or Alagille syndrome. Circulation. 2002 Nov 12;106(20):2567–74.
20. Kamath BM, Bauer RC, Loomes KM, Chao G, Gerfen J, Hutchinson A, et al. NOTCH2 mutations in Alagille syndrome. J Med Genet.. 2012 Feb;49(2):138–44.
21. Rennie CA, Chowdhury S, Khan J, Rajan F, Jordan K, Lamb RJ, et al. The prevalence and associated features of posterior embryotoxon in the general ophthalmic clinic. Eye (Lond). 2005 April;19(4):396–9.
22. Nischal KK, Hingorani M, Bentley CR, Vivian AJ, Bird AC, Baker AJ, et al. Ocular ultrasound in Alagille syndrome: a new sign. Ophthalmology. 1997 Jan;104(1):79–85.
23. Strachan D, Kamath B, Wengraf C. How we do it: use of a venous cannulation needle for endoscopic Teflon injection to the vocal folds. J Laryngol Otol. 1995 Dec;109(12):1184–5.
24. Deprettere A, Portmann B, Mowat AP. Syndromic paucity of the intrahepatic bile ducts: diagnostic difficulty; severe morbidity throughout early childhood. J Pediatr Gastroenterol Nutr. 1987 Nov–Dec;6(6):865–71.

25. Hoffenberg EJ, Narkewicz MR, Sondheimer JM, Smith DJ, Silverman A, Sokol RJ. Outcome of syndromic paucity of interlobular bile ducts (Alagille syndrome) with onset of cholestasis in infancy. J Pediatr. 1995;127(2):220–4.

26. Quiros-Tejeira RE, Ament ME, Heyman MB, Martin MG, Rosenthal P, Hall TR, et al. Variable morbidity in alagille syndrome: a review of 43 cases. J Pediatr Gastroenterol Nutr. 1999 Oct;29(4):431–7.

27. Kamath BM, Loomes KM, Oakey RJ, Krantz ID. Supernumerary digital flexion creases: an additional clinical manifestation of Alagille syndrome. Am J Med Genet. 2002 Oct 1;112(2):171–5.

28. Bales CB, Kamath BM, Munoz PS, Nguyen A, Piccoli DA, Spinner NB, et al. Pathologic lower extremity fractures in children with alagille syndrome. J Pediatr Gastroenterol Nutr. 2010 Jul;51(1):66–70.

29. Olsen IE, Ittenbach RF, Rovner AJ, Leonard MB, Mulberg AE, Stallings VA, et al. Deficits in size-adjusted bone mass in children with Alagille syndrome. J Pediatr Gastroenterol Nutr. 2005 Jan;40(1):76–82.

30. Kamath BM, Podkameni G, Hutchinson AL, Leonard LD, Gerfen J, Krantz ID, et al. Renal anomalies in Alagille syndrome: a disease-defining feature. Am J Med Genet A. 2012 Jan;158A(1):85–9.

31. Lykavieris P, Crosnier C, Trichet C, Meunier-Rotival M, Hadchouel M. Bleeding tendency in children with Alagille syndrome. Pediatrics. 2003 Jan;111(1):167–70.

32. Emerick KM, Krantz ID, Kamath BM, Darling C, Burrowes DM, Spinner NB, et al. Intracranial vascular abnormalities in patients with Alagille syndrome. J Pediatr Gastroenterol Nutr. 2005 July;41(1):99–107.

33. Li L, Krantz ID, Deng Y, Genin A, Banta AB, Collins CC, et al. Alagille syndrome is caused by mutations in human Jagged1, which encodes a ligand for Notch1. Nat Genet. 1997;16(3):243–51.

34. McDaniell R, Warthen DM, Sanchez-Lara PA, Pai A, Krantz ID, Piccoli DA, et al. NOTCH2 mutations cause Alagille syndrome, a heterogeneous disorder of the notch signaling pathway. Am J Hum Genet. 2006 July;79(1):169–73.

35. Oda T, Elkahloun AG, Pike BL, Okajima K, Krantz ID, Genin A, et al. Mutations in the human Jagged1 gene are responsible for Alagille syndrome. Nat Genet. 1997;16(3):235–42.

36. Warthen DM, Moore EC, Kamath BM, Morrissette JJ, Sanchez P, Piccoli DA, et al. Jagged1 (JAG1) mutations in Alagille syndrome: increasing the mutation detection rate. Hum Mutat. 2006 May;27(5):436–43.

37. Spinner NB, Colliton RP, Crosnier C, Krantz ID, Hadchouel M, Meunier-Rotival M. Jagged1 mutations in alagille syndrome. Hum Mutat. 2001;17(1):18–33.

38. Yerushalmi B, Sokol RJ, Narkewicz MR, Smith D, Karrer FM. Use of rifampin for severe pruritus in children with chronic cholestasis. J Pediatr Gastroenterol Nutr. 1999 Oct;29(4):442–7.

39. Kamath BM, Thiel BD, Gai X, Conlin LK, Munoz PS, Glessner J, et al. SNP array mapping of chromosome 20p deletions: genotypes, phenotypes, and copy number variation. Hum Mutat. 2009 March;30(3):371–8.

40. Kamath BM, Loomes KM, Piccoli DA. Medical management of Alagille syndrome. J Pediatr Gastroenterol Nutr. 2010 June;50(6):580–6.

41. Kamath BM, Schwarz KB, Hadzic N. Alagille syndrome and liver transplantation. J Pediatr Gastroenterol Nutr. 2010 Jan;50(1):11–5.

42. Dinler G, Kocak N, Yuce A, Gurakan F, Ozen H. Ursodeoxycholic acid therapy in children with cholestatic liver disease. Turk J Pediatr. 1999 Jan–March;41(1):91–8.

43. Narkewicz MR, Smith D, Gregory C, Lear JL, Osberg I, Sokol RJ. Effect of ursodeoxycholic acid therapy on hepatic function in children with intrahepatic cholestatic liver disease. J Pediatr Gastroenterol Nutr. 1998 Jan;26(1):49–55.

44. Balistreri WF. Bile acid therapy in pediatric hepatobiliary disease: the role of ursodeoxycholic acid. J Pediatr Gastroenterol Nutr. 1997 May;24(5):573–89.

45. Levy E, Bendayan M, Thibault L, Lambert M, Paradis K. Lipoprotein abnormalities in two children with minimal biliary excretion. J Pediatr Gastroenterol Nutr. 1995 May;20(4):432–9.

46. Cynamon HA, Andres JM, Iafrate RP. Rifampin relieves pruritus in children with cholestatic liver disease. Gastroenterology. 1990 April;98(4):1013–6.

47. Gregorio GV, Ball CS, Mowat AP, Mieli-Vergani G. Effect of rifampicin in the treatment of pruritus in hepatic cholestasis. Arch Dis Child. 1993 July;69(1):141–3.

48. Emerick KM, Whitington PF. Partial external biliary diversion for intractable pruritus and xanthomas in Alagille syndrome. Hepatology. 2002 June;35(6):1501–6.

49. Yang H, Porte RJ, Verkade HJ, De Langen ZJ, Hulscher JB. Partial external biliary diversion in children with progressive familial intrahepatic cholestasis and Alagille disease. J Pediatr Gastroenterol Nutr. 2009 Aug;49(2):216–21.

50. Kaye AJ, R and EB, Munoz PS, Spinner NB, Flake AW, Kamath BM. Effect of Kasai procedure on hepatic outcome in Alagille syndrome. J Pediatr Gastroenterol Nutr. 2010 Sept;51(3):319–21.

51. Razavi RS, Baker A, Qureshi SA, Rosenthal E, Marsh MJ, Leech SC, et al. Hemodynamic response to continuous infusion of dobutamine in Alagille's syndrome. Transplantation. 2001 Sept 15;72(5):823–8.

52. Kasahara M, Kiuchi T, Inomata Y, Uryuhara K, Sakamoto S, Ito T, et al. Living-related liver transplantation for Alagille syndrome. Transplantation. 2003 June 27;75(12):2147–50.

53. Gurkan A, Emre S, Fishbein TM, Brady L, Millis M, Birnbaum A, et al. Unsuspected bile duct paucity in donors for living-related liver transplantation: two case reports. Transplantation. 1999 Feb 15;67(3):416–8.

54. Arnon R, Annunziato R, Miloh T, Suchy F, Sakworawich A, Hiroshi S, et al. Orthotopic liver transplantation for children with Alagille syndrome. Pediatr Transplant. 2010 Aug;14(5):622–8.

55. Sugiyama H, Veldtman GR, Norgard G, Lee KJ, Chaturvedi R, Benson LN. Bladed balloon angioplasty for peripheral pulmonary artery stenosis. Catheter Cardiovasc Interv. 2004 May;62(1):71–7.

56. Saidi AS, Kovalchin JP, Fisher DJ, Ferry GD, Grifka RG. Balloon pulmonary valvuloplasty and stent implantation. For peripheral pulmonary artery stenosis in Alagille syndrome. Tex Heart Inst J. 1998;25(1):79–82.

57. Gandhi SK, Reyes J, Webber SA, Siewers RD, Pigula FA. Case report of combined pediatric heart-lung-liver transplantation. Transplantation. 2002 June 27;73(12):1968–9.

58. Baird LC, Smith ER, Ichord R, Piccoli DA, Bernard TJ, Spinner NB, Scott RM Kamath. Moyamoya syndrome associated with Alagille syndrome: outcome after surgical revascularization. J Pediatr. 2015 Feb;166(2):470–3

Chronic Viral Hepatitis B and C

60

Stefan Wirth

S. Wirth (✉)
HELIOS Medical Centre, Department of Pediatrics, Witten/Herdecke University, Heusnerstr. 40, 42283 Wuppertal, Germany
e-mail: stefan.wirth@helios-kliniken.de

List of Abbreviations

ALT	alanine aminotransferase
Anti-HBc	antibody against HBcAg
Anti-HBc IgG	immune globulin G
Anti-HBc	antibody against HBcAg
Anti-HBe	antibody against HBeAg
Anti-HBs	antibody against HBsAg
Anti-HDV	antibody against delta virus
cccDNA	covalently closed circular DNA
DAA	direct-acting antiviral
DNA	desoxyribonucleic acid
EMA	European Medicines Agency
FDA	Food and Drug Administration
HBcAg	hepatitis B core antigen
HBeAg	hepatitis e antigen
HBsAg	hepatitis B surface antigen
HBV	hepatitis B virus
HCC	hepatocellular carcinoma
HCV	hepatitis C virus
HIV	human immune deficiency virus
IgG	immune globulin G
IL2	interleukin 2
IL28B	interferon lambda 3 gene
ORF	open reading frame
RNA	ribonucleic acid
SVR	sustained viral response
TNF-α	tumor necrosis factor alpha

Chronic Hepatitis B

Introduction

Hepatitis B virus (HBV) infection remains a global health burden with estimated 300–350 million people chronically infected worldwide. Nevertheless, since HBV vaccine has become available for more than 20 years and many countries introduced vaccination programs as a prevention strategy on a regularly basis for young infants, significant reduction of the incidence of acute hepatitis B in children and adolescents has been observed. Unprotected, approximately 90% of HBV-infected infants and 20–25% of those infected in preschool age will develop chronic infection decreasing to a chronicity rate of around 5% for adolescents and adults [1–3]. Despite of a rather benign spontaneous course of the disease during childhood and adolescence, there is a considerable lifetime risk of progressive liver disease, liver cirrhosis, and the development of a hepatocellular carcinoma (HCC), which may eventually reduce life expectancy. Thus, careful long-term monitoring has to be performed, and appropriate treatment options, which unfortunately are not entirely curative at present, have to be considered.

Pathogenesis of Chronic HBV Infection

HBV belongs to a DNA virus family called hepadna viruses. It contains a partially double-stranded DNA genome with about 3200 nucleotides. The minus strand covers four overlapping open reading frames (ORFs): S, for the surface gene encoding three envelope proteins (hepatitis B surface antigen, HBsAg); C, for the core gene encoding the core protein (hepatitis B core antigen, HBcAg); X, for the regulatory X gene; and P, for the polymerase gene encoding the viral DNA polymerase. By using multiple start codons, HBV is able to encode more than one protein from an ORF. After hepatocyte entry by an unknown receptor, the viral envelope is removed, and the nucleocapsid reaches the nucleus,

S. Guandalini et al. (eds.), *Textbook of Pediatric Gastroenterology, Hepatology and Nutrition,*
DOI 10.1007/978-3-319-17169-2_60

where the double strand will be completed and converted into a covalently closed circular DNA (cccDNA). This is an important step, because the majority of cccDNA is then organized into nucleosomes forming the viral minichromosome, which is serving as template for the synthesis of the viral mRNA. The transcripts are translated into the viral proteins, and simultaneously reverse transcription leads to the synthesis of a complete minus strand of HBV DNA. The plus strand can then be synthesized again, and the molecule circularizes. Thus, the replication of HBV is similar to that of a retrovirus. The proteins are synthesized and assembled at the endoplasmatic reticulum and eventually discharged by vesicular transport as a Dane particle which contains the complete virus. The cccDNA plays a key role in viral persistence, viral reactivation after treatment withdrawal, and drug resistance. It accumulates in the nucleus of the hepatocyte as a stable minichromosome organized by histone and nonhistone viral and cellular proteins [4, 5]. Persistent HBV replication is associated with a high frequency of integration of HBV sequences into the human host liver cell genome. Enhanced DNA replication and DNA damage occurring during chronic inflammation with cycles of cell death and regeneration increase the availability of DNA ends in host genomic DNA and promote the process of viral integration [6]. Furthermore, it is presumed that certain altered cells are susceptible to the development of additional genetic and epigenetic changes that may lead to the development of malignant cell transformation and HCC.

For the understanding of the different phases during the course of the chronic disease, it is important to realize that the virus itself is not primarily pathogenic to the hepatocyte. The mechanism of cell death is generally accepted to be the result of a cytotoxic T-lymphocyte-mediated immune response of the host to the virus. Additionally, it has been shown that some HBV proteins may be able to induce apoptosis. During the transition from the immune tolerant to the immune active phase, a shift from the hepatitis e antigen (HBeAg)-specific Th2 cell tolerance to Th1 cell activation may recognize HBV-related epitopes on hepatocytes resulting in secretion of cytokines such as interleukin (IL)-2 and tumor necrosis factor alpha (TNF-α) and thus activating inflammation [7].

Epidemiology

There are still high endemic countries in Asia, Africa, and some parts of South America with an HBsAg prevalence of more than 8%. The Arabian region, parts of the Eastern hemisphere, and Greenland show a HBV prevalence of 2–7%, and in the Western countries the rate is below 2% [8]. Global immunization programs have been established in many countries, and the HBV infection rate has declined worldwide. Vertical transmission has become the main route of infection; nevertheless, in some areas, HBV may also be a predominant disease in adolescents and adults due to high-risk sexual behavior and drug abuse [9]. Unfortunately, up to 2–15% of perinatal HBV infection of antibody against HBeAg (anti-HBe)- and HBeAg-positive mothers cannot be prevented by active and passive immunization due to intrauterine infection, vaccine failure, or HBsAg escape mutants [10–12]. Thus, passive and active immunization has to be started immediately after birth in all newborns from HBsAg-positive mothers. HBeAg-positive mothers can be considered to receive treatment with the nucleoside analogues lamivudine or telbivudine in late pregnancy to decrease viral load [13, 14]. After complete immunization, there are no objections against breast feeding. In countries with blood donor screening and serum testing, parenteral transmission does no longer play a significant role. The HBsAg prevalence in children is estimated between 0.02 and 0.03% in Western countries and the USA, in Brazil 0.14% and 0.5% in Taiwan after immunization [1, 15]. Given HBsAg prevalence in pregnant women of 0.4% in Western Europe and an HBV transmission rate of 5–10% despite complete vaccination, 20–40 newborns in 100,000 births may be infected and become a chronic carrier state.

Ten HBV genotypes (A–J) have been documented showing a distinct distribution. Genotypes A and D are predominant in North America, Europe, and India, and genotypes B and C are mostly found in Asian countries. To date, routine determination of genotype is not yet recommended because treatment options are not adjusted to genotypes. Nevertheless, since there is line of evidence that genotypes C and D may be associated with more aggressive liver disease, this might become significant during the long-term follow-up [16].

Diagnostics

Chronic hepatitis B infection is defined as a repeatedly positive HBsAg test result within 6 months. Apart from the aminotransferases, HBeAg, anti-HBe, anti-HBcIgG, and quantitative HBV DNA have to be determined to confirm chronic hepatitis B and to classify the present stage. Additionally, antibody against delta virus (anti-HDV) should be tested to exclude concomitant hepatitis D. It is recommended to perform an ultrasound examination including liver stiffness assessment for baseline findings. Since chronic hepatitis B usually is a mild disease in terms of inflammation in childhood, histological examination by liver biopsy is not mandatory. However, in subjects, who are suspicious of progressive liver disease or cirrhosis or if an impact on therapeutic decisions is identifiable, liver biopsy may be a reasonable completion.

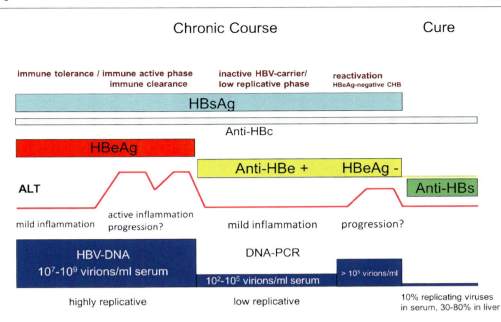

Fig. 60.1 Illustration of the different phases of chronic hepatitis B. *HBV-DNA* hepatitis B virus deoxyribonucleic acid, *DNA-PCR* deoxyribonucleic acid polymerase chain reaction, *HBV* hepatitis B virus, *HBsAg* hepatitis B surface antigen, *Anti-HBc* antibody against HBcAg, *ALT* alanine aminotransferase, *HBeAg* hepatitis e antigen, *Anti-HBs* antibody against HBsAg

Natural History

There are four natural stages of chronic hepatitis B infection: immune tolerance stage, immune reactive or immune clearance stage, inactive HBsAg carrier stage, and reactivation stage. As fifth and last stage, viral elimination with antibody against HBsAg (anti-HBs) seroconversion, which is a rather rare event occurring not more than 0.5 % annually in children, could be denominated [7, 17]. Figure 60.1 illustrates the different phases of chronic hepatitis B.

Children who have HBV infection acquired perinatally or in the first months have an initial tolerance stage which is characterized by the presence of HBsAg, HBeAg, and extremely high HBV DNA levels (10^{7-9} virions/ml) and normal aminotransferases. The duration of the immune tolerant phase is not predictable and may last 1–4 decades. Asian patients seem to have a longer immune tolerant stage. T helper (Th) cell immune tolerance is generated by HBeAg functioning as an immunoregulatory protein mostly already transplacentally transmitted. This kind of induced immune tolerance may explain the high chronicity rate, and the younger the individuals are when they get infected. Usually, only minimal inflammatory activity is detectable in the liver tissue in this phase. Even in adult patients, no severe progression is expected during the immune tolerant stage [18]. Although antiviral therapy is still not recommended for immune tolerant subjects, they should be carefully monitored to duly recognize progression to immune active phase.

With time, a nonspecific increase of inflammatory activity or a decrease of HBeAg serum concentration, which may be due to emerging mutants in the core promotor or precore region resulting in a lower HBeAg production, may activate HBeAg-specific T cell clones. In this immune reactive

phase, HBeAg remains positive, and aminotransferases rise. HBV DNA remains high or stays at a little lower level. During this time, progression to liver fibrosis or cirrhosis may occur. However, liver cirrhosis rate is not expected to exceed 3–5 % until reaching adulthood [19–21]. In the immune reactive, phase treatment has to be considered.

A key event in the natural course of chronic hepatitis B is the HBeAg/anti-HBe seroconversion which occurs unpredictably for the single individual during the immune active phase. Anti-HBe seroconversion is associated with a significant decrease of viral replication and normalization of aminotransferases reflecting the biochemical and histological remission of inflammatory activity. In some studies, the annual seroconversion rate depends on the route of infection and the ethnic origin. Whereas the mean seroconversion rate in non-Asian children ranges between 8 and 15 %, seroconversion in Asian children was considerably lower with approximately 5 % per year [7, 20]. Anti-HBe seroconversion is followed by the inactive HBsAg carrier state with persistently normal aminotransferases and a low viral load. Viral replication is considered low when HBV DNA serum concentrations remain below 2000 IU/ml. Some carriers may be lucky and develop anti-HBs antibodies indicating viral elimination and cure of the disease. The estimated incidence of this rare event in children is 0.05–0.8 % per year in endemic areas with predominantly perinatal HBV transmission [7, 15].

Approximately, 20–30 % of inactive HBsAg carriers will experience spontaneous reactivation during long-term follow-up. Those episodes may cause progressive liver damage. The reactivation phase is characterized by the presence of anti-HBe and elevated aminotransferases. HBV DNA levels rise over 2000 IU/ml. This status is also named HBeAg-negative hepatitis B. However, reactivation rarely occurs during childhood and adolescents.

Another particular condition warrants mention: occult HBV infection. It is defined as the existence of HBV DNA in serum among HBsAg-negative patients and can be classified into seropositive and seronegative with respect to the presence of anti-HBs or antibody against HBcAg (anti-HBc) antibodies. Possible explanations are low levels of viral replication activity or the emergence of HBV variants in the a-determinant of the S-gene. Occult hepatitis B is most common in endemic regions and seems rare with 1.4% [22]. However, prevalence may rise considerably in immunized children from HBsAg-positive mothers. One study reported a prevalence of 28% in this special group [23].

Long-Term Prognosis

Individuals with chronic HBV infection are at risk to develop long-term sequelae such as end-stage liver disease including liver cirrhosis, hepatic failure, and HCC. Progression strongly correlates with the disease activity in terms of viral replication level, inflammatory activity, HBsAg levels, HBV genotypes, and HBeAg/anti-HBe status. Strong risk factors for developing liver cirrhosis and HCC are higher age, male, presence of HBeAg, HBV DNA levels $> 10^4$ copies/ml, HBsAg serum concentrations $> 10^3$ IU/ml, and alanine aminotransferase (ALT) >45 IU/l [24, 25]. Progression to liver cirrhosis in children is under 5% until adulthood and data of the Asian region report 0.01–0.003% of individuals with chronic hepatitis B to be expected developing HCC in childhood [26, 27]. In general, anti-HBe seroconversion significantly reduces the risk of developing HCC. The time at which anti-HBe seroconversion occurs is important. A study in adults investigating the 15-year cumulative incidences of HBeAg-negative hepatitis demonstrated that cirrhosis and HCC increased with increasing age of HBeAg seroconversion [28]. The lowest risk was observed in patients with anti-HBe seroconversion under the age of 30 (cirrhosis 7%, HCC 2.1%) and highest in individuals older than 40 years (cirrhosis 42.9%, HCC 7.7%). The hazard ratio for HBeAg-negative hepatitis, cirrhosis, and HCC was 2.95, 17.6, and 5.22, respectively, in the older compared with the younger group. The authors conclude that patients with HBeAg seroconversion before age 30 have an excellent prognosis, whereas patients with delayed HBeAg seroconversion after age 40 have significantly higher incidences of HBeAg-negative hepatitis, cirrhosis, and HCC. An additional precondition is persistently normal ALT levels [29]. Since children have a high probability to experience anti-HBe seroconversion until adulthood, the overall risk of developing severe liver disease in later life seems limited. Nevertheless, there remain a considerable number of patients with immune tolerance or inflammatory activity that needs careful and professional monitoring.

Relevance of Genotypes and Mutants

During the replication cycle, HBV polymerase is acting as a reverse transcriptase without proof-reading function. Therefore, mutant viral genomes are regularly emerging in a considerable number particularly during the high replicative status. Peculiar requirements such as replication modalities, selection pressure, and changing immunological conditions may select variants and strongly influence the predominant HBV quasispecies in an infected individual. Generally, a change of the primarily determined genotype is possible during long-term course and ranges between 2.8 and 19% usually associated with anti-HBe seroconversion [26, 30]. It is not yet known, if there is any clinical impact at all. In adults, genotype C infection is rather than genotype B associated with a delayed anti-HBe seroconversion and a higher risk of developing HCC. Genotype D trends to proceed more severely and shows delayed anti-HBe seroconversion compared with genotype A. Precore and basic core promotor (BCP) mutants are frequently associated with HBeAg-negative hepatitis, and HBsAg escape mutants are now increasingly observed in association with primarily vaccinated children. The typical precore point mutant is the G1896A stop codon preventing the production of HBeAg. It emerges typically around the time of anti-HBe seroconversion and may be associated with a decreased risk of developing HCC compared with the wild type. But it can also be found in patients with HBeAg-negative hepatitis. Depending on European or Asian regions, precore mutants have been detected between 8 and 50% in HBeAg-negative children. The BCP mutants A1762T/G1764A prevail to be associated with an increased risk for HCC. But finally, the data remain controversial [7, 16, 31, 32].

Treatment

Since there is no definitely curative medical treatment available to date, it has to be defined what the aim of antiviral treatment should be in dependence on age group and phase of chronic hepatitis B. There is no doubt that one major goal is to reduce the risk of progressive liver disease and long-term sequelae such as liver cirrhosis, hepatic decompensation, and HCC and eventually to achieve the same life expectancy compared with healthy individuals of the same age. Unfortunately, anti-HBs seroconversion can only be reached in 5–10% at the most under current medical treatment strategies. Thus, the most important task in the treatment of children and adolescents is to achieve anti-HBe seroconversion at the earliest possible time associated with suppressed viral replication and decreased liver inflammation followed by persistent presence of anti-HBe, undetectable HBV DNA, and preferably aminotransferases values less than half of the upper limit of normal. Children with HBeAg-positive hepatitis should be monitored every 6 months with physical examination, measurement of laboratory parameters such as aminotransferases, hepatitis B serology, alpha-fetoprotein, and ultrasound of the liver. After anti-HBe seroconversion follow-up visits can be performed for lifetime on an annual basis [15, 17, 33].

The decision to treat should be based on age, phase of HBV infection determined by ALT level, HBeAg/anti-HBe status, liver histology, coexisting diseases, and expectable compliance. The response rate in patients in the immune tolerant phase is very low. Thus, treatment of children with normal aminotransferases has not been recommended to date. At present, clinical trials in immune tolerant children combining a nucleoside analogue and peg-alpha-interferon are being performed. Treatment should be considered when aminotransferases rise and transition to the immune active phase is recognized. Children and adolescents who have persistently elevated ALT levels for more than 6 months should be offered treatment. Currently, seven treatment options are approved for hepatitis B in adults, including two formulations of conventional and pegylated interferon as an immunmodulatory therapy and five nucleos(t)ide analogues (lamivudine, adefovir dipivoxil, entecavir, telbivudine, and tenofovir disoproxil) with strong reduction of viral replication. Approval for children and adolescents depends on the region. Large trials have been performed in children for lamivudine, adefovir, entecavir, and tenofovir. Entecavir has been authorized from 6 years onwards, and Adefovir and tenofovir have been approved for subjects older than 12 years of age in the USA and Europe [34–36]. Predictors of response may be increased ALT levels, relatively low HBV DNA levels, and infection with genotype A or B. The main problem of all clinical trials with nucleos(t)ide analogues is the duration of medical treatment of not more than 96 weeks. Although a high proportion of treated patients will experience a significant decrease of viral load, the anti-HBe seroconversion rate cannot be expected to exceed 25%. After ceasing treatment, a reactivation of viral replication to baseline levels can be observed. A 24-week course of alpha interferon yields an approximately 10% higher anti-HBe seroconversion rate. Anti-HBs seroconversion rate is limited to single cases with nucleos(t)ide analogues and may range between 6 and 10% in patients with alpha interferon. There is no doubt that these results are dissatisfying with respect to our primary goal of anti-HBe seroconversion. Another interesting fact is that alpha interferon treatment only accelerates anti-HBe seroconversion in successfully treated individuals, but does not enhance the absolute number of responders [37]. Extending the treatment with nucleos(t)ide analogues for several years will result in an anti-HBe seroconversion rate of 40–50% [33]. However, there are no long-term data in children with regard to side effects. In the case of anti-HBe seroconversion, treatment should be maintained for 12 months, because

the treatment-induced anti-HBe-positive status may be instable and reactivation may occur [38, 39].

In view of the present data and experience, there is a remarkable counseling conflict between the choice of drug and the duration of treatment, given that anti-HBe seroconversion remains the essential goal. Antiviral drug resistance is a major limitation to the long-term success of antiviral treatment. For this reason, lamivudine with a 5-year resistance rate of 70% has been considered obsolete just as adefovir which does often not sufficiently suppress viral replication. Nevertheless, at least for smaller children, lamivudine can be used as an approved drug for a limited time. Telbivudine has also a considerable resistance risk. Entecavir and tenofovir do not show significant resistances after years of treatment. Tenofovir may be associated with an increase in serum creatinine levels after 3–5 years of therapy. Decrease of bone mineral density has also been reported. Oral treatment with nucleos(t)ide analogues is quite comfortable but needs a real true commitment to the treatment, and alpha interferon may have sometimes restrictive side effects but with the advantage of a defined duration.

Thus, the decision which treatment option to choose is not that easy and has to be achieved in agreement with the patient and the parents. Alpha interferon is particularly appropriate for those children and adolescents who are reluctant to commit to a long duration of treatment and are not in the pubertal growth spurt. Nowadays, peg-alpha-interferon should be recommended for 48 weeks. Nucleos(t)ide analogues are most appropriate for patients with contraindications to interferon, after liver transplantation with an anti-HBc-positive donor or under immune suppressive treatment. It is most important that they are willing to commit to a treatment for several, probably 3–5 years, may be longer. Entecavir and tenofovir have the best profile in terms of safety, efficacy, and drug resistance. For younger patients, entecavir seems actually the preferable option.

Children and adolescents with a HBeAg-negative hepatitis should be treated with a nucleos(t)ide analogue if ALT levels are elevated and HBV DNA concentration is above 20,000 IU/ml to prevent progressive liver disease [40]. During long-term treatment with nucleos(t)ide analogues, HBV DNA, HBeAg/anti-HBe status, and aminotransferase levels should be monitored every 3 months. Very low or negative HBV DNA concentrations are important preconditions to avoid drug resistance.

Prevention

Vaccination is the most effective procedure in order to prevent infection with the HBV. Active and passive immunization is well established in newborns of HBsAg-positive mothers. The first injections have to be administered within 12–24 h after birth to achieve a seroprotective response in

90–95 % when two monthly follow-up active vaccinations are completed. Very low birth weight preterm infants should receive a total of four doses. HBeAg-positive mothers can be treated with a nucleoside analogue (lamivudine, telbivudine) during the last trimester of pregnancy to reduce the risk of vertical transmission.

In many countries, routine active HBV vaccination is implemented in the vaccination schedule of all infants. Post-vaccination testing for a protective anti-HBs concentration (> 100 IU/l) is not routinely recommended. If indicated, the best time would be approximately 2–3 months after the last vaccination. Revaccination is indicated in subjects with an anti-HBs titer < 10 IU/l. In the majority of nonresponders, three more vaccinations will induce protective response. According to present experiences, protective anti-HBs response will be maintained for more than 15 years [13, 39].

Chronic Hepatitis C

Introduction

Hepatitis C virus (HCV) infection is a frequent course of chronic liver disease, and approximately 150–200 million people are estimated to be chronically infected worldwide. Unfortunately, to date, no preventive vaccination could be developed. Despite of a normally benign course of the disease during childhood and adolescence, there is a considerable lifetime risk of progressive liver disease, liver cirrhosis, and the development of a HCC, which may eventually reduce life expectancy. Remarkable advances have been made in therapeutic approaches during the last 10 years, and considerable rates of cure have been yielded with the current standard of care. Nevertheless, careful long-term monitoring has to be performed, and appropriate improved treatment options have to be discussed, always considering that the development of novel treatment regimen is going fast and may continuously further improve the response rate [41].

Pathogenesis of Chronic Hepatitis C Infection

HCV is a positive-stranded RNA virus within the Flaviviridiae family. It forms its own genus Hepacivirus, and there are six main genotypes. The viral genome encodes nine proteins including its own RNA polymerase. Because of the high error rate of the virus-specific RNA polymerase, many variants may be produced. So-called quasispecies represent the high variability of the virus which allows a survival advantage to the virus. Replication of HCV starts with the binding to hepatocytes and entry which is a rather complex procedure. RNA is released into the cytoplasma and translated in the rough endoplasmatic reticulum. A 3000-amino-acid-long polypeptide arises and is then cleaved into ten different prod-

ucts. Membranous replication vesicles are induced, and HCV assembly is accomplished and released with the help of very low density lipoprotein (VLDL) synthesis. Chronic hepatitis C in children is associated with a variety of histological patterns, mostly considered as mild and slow progressive. Nevertheless, significant fibrosis or cirrhosis may occur, but is not expected to exceed 4 % until reaching adulthood. Need for liver transplantation is very rare as is the development of HCC [42]. Little information is available about the host responds to the virus. Cluster of differentiation 4 (CD4) + lymphocytes seem to be involved. Infants with the rs 12979860 CC genotype for the IL28B polymorphism trend to experience a higher spontaneous viral elimination [43–45].

Epidemiology

The prevalence of HCV infection in children in developed countries ranges between 0.1 and 0.4 %. For adults, prevalence rates are 0.4–3 % in North America and Western Europe and higher in Eastern Europe and Middle East. Egypt has the highest prevalence with 9 %, almost exclusively genotype 4 [41, 46, 47]. Central and East Asia and North Africa are estimated to have a prevalence between 3.6 and 3.8 % [48]. During the last 15 years, the predominant route of viral hepatitis C transmission has become vertical infection. Contamination through blood products is exceedingly rare in developed countries, but may remain an issue in developing countries. The rate of perinatal transmission from an HCV-RNA-positive mother ranges from 2 to 5 %. Out of this group, a considerable number of infants received the infection probably already in utero [49]. Concomitant HIV infection may increase the risk of HCV transmission. Breast feeding does not promote viral transmission and is allowed. The HCV prevalence in pregnant women from North America and Central Europe was reported between 0.16 and 0.53 %. Assumed a perinatal transmission rate of 2–4 %, 8–10 newborns in 100,000 births per year may be infected and become chronically infected during the first year of life. Viral clearance in vertically infected children seems to be dependent on the genotype and was reported to range from 2.4 to 25 %. In contrast, children infected with genotype 3 had a higher spontaneous clearance rate compared to individuals with genotype 1. Beyond the age of 5 years, spontaneous viral elimination becomes less likely [50, 51].

Diagnosis

Serologic testing for anti-HCV antibodies is the appropriate screening test for HCV. The next diagnostic step is the determination of quantitative HCV RNA and the genotype. The most prevalent genotype in pediatric trials performed in Western countries was genotype 1 (ca. 74 %) followed by genotype 3 (ca. 14 %) and 2 (ca. 9 %). Genotype 4 had the lowest prevalence (ca. 3 %) [52]. It is useful to perform an ultrasound examination including liver stiffness assessment for the baseline report. As chronic hepatitis C usually is a histologically mild disease with low inflammatory activity in childhood, liver biopsy is not mandatory. However, in subjects, who are suspicious of progressive liver disease or cirrhosis or if there is an impact on therapeutic decisions, liver biopsy may be a reasonable measure [41, 52].

Several studies have demonstrated that certain host polymorphisms (e.g., CC) located upstream of the IL28B (interferon lambda 3) gene are associated with a higher sustained viral response rate to combination treatment with peg-alpha-interferon and ribavirin. There is also an association with spontaneous clearance of HCV. To date, determination of IL28B polymorphisms is not routinely used, but might be of interest to identify the individual patients' likelihood of response particularly in future therapy options [41].

Natural History

Normally, HCV infection is asymptomatic. Histological findings are usually mild, and the risk of severe complications until the infected individuals are reaching adulthood is low. Not more than 5 % of children and adolescents will have evidence of advanced liver fibrosis or cirrhosis. Liver transplantation units from the USA have reported on 133 transplanted children due to chronic hepatitis C during a time span of 13 years. In a lifetime, the risk of developing liver cirrhosis is about 20 %, and the risk of HCC based on liver cirrhosis is estimated 2–5 % [44]. These data are from adults, and there are no long-term follow-up studies in vertically infected patients. Natural history is also affected by other medical and social factors. Overweight children with liver steatosis are at greater risk for progressive liver disease. Risky behaviors and alcohol misuse worsen the long-term prognosis. Similar course and progression of hepatitis C were reported in former pediatric patients with successfully treated malignant disease after three decades of observation with about 20 % spontaneous clearance and up to 5 % liver cirrhosis. During the chronic course, ALT levels may be normal or intermittently elevated. Only few patients show persistent markedly elevated aminotransferases. Also the HCV RNA serum concentration may considerably fluctuate, but without immediate prognostic relevance. Spontaneous resolution beyond the preschool age is quite rare and may occur in up to 10 % of adolescents [44, 47, 53]. Some extrahepatic manifestations may be associated with chronic hepatitis C such as glomerulonephritis and possibly cognitive deficits or developmental delay [54]. However, in adult patients, the clinical effects of reported symptoms such as fatigue, depression, or marginal poorer learning efficiency were rather limited [55]. In conclusion, early acquired chronic hepatitis C is a clinically and histologically silent and hidden condition. Nevertheless, it may become insidious. Although the rate developing liver cirrhosis until adulthood is low, activation beyond the second decade of life is likely. A large Danish study in adults revealed that in patients with chronic HCV infection, the 8-year risk of liver-related death was 5.5 % compared with 2.0 % in individuals who cleared the infection [56]. However, patients who have eventually proceeded to compensated liver cirrhosis have a dubious prognosis. In a follow-up study of cirrhotic patients over more than 10 years, HCC developed in 32 % and the annual mortality rate was 4 % [57]. Thus, the literal aim of therapeutic interventions in children and adolescents is not the treatment of an ongoing liver disease, but the prevention of a future one by early eradication of the infection.

Treatment

The primary goal of HCV therapy is to cure the infection which is reflected by persistently negative HCV RNA in serum and normalized aminotransferases. Sustained viral response (SVR) is defined as an undetectable HCV RNA level 24 weeks after cessation of treatment. The combination of pegylated alpha interferon with ribavirin and a protease inhibitor, either telaprevir or boceprevir for the treatment of genotype-1-infected patients for 48 weeks was the approved and established standard of care in adults. Non-genotype 1 patients are treated with peg-alpha-interferon in combination with ribavirin, for example, genotype 2 and 3 for 24 weeks. With these regimens, considerable sustained viral response rates can be achieved ranging from more than 65 % for genotype 1 to over 80 % for genotype 2 and 3 patients [58]. Two pegylated alpha-interferon molecules can be used, that is, alpha-interferon-2a and alpha-interferon-2b. The pharmacokinetics of these drugs differ, but there is currently no conclusive evidence that one peg-alpha-interferon should be preferred to the other one. Currently, approved interferon-free treatment options and more protease inhibitors such as sofosbuvir and ledipasvir are changing the treatment regimen.

Treatment management of children with chronic hepatitis C infection is formed by the attitude of the medical attendant regarding the need of therapeutic intervention with respect to a generally slow progressive disease. Thus, delay of treatment seems common with barely a quarter of patients being treated [51]. Adverse events during treatment are frequent, and due to age, adolescents may have a lack of compliance. On the other side, mostly treatment is better tolerated in younger patients, and in case of success, the benefit of socio-economic aspects is not to disregard. Under the aspect of health prevention for a long lifetime, all children with a measureable level of HCV RNA should be considered for treatment. Neither the level of aminotransferases nor of

HCV RNA predicts the long-term outcome of the disease. Also liver histology is not a helpful entry criterion for indicating treatment, because children generally do not have severe lesions. Nevertheless, new direct-acting antivirals (DAA) against the HCV have been developed, and interferon-free oral treatment regimen is an important goal for the next years. Toward this aim, several clinical trials combining only oral antiviral compounds have begun to show promising results in some subgroups. It will take a couple of years to have approved substances available for children. However, with the present knowledge, well-balanced counseling is particularly important for the individual patient and his parents when indicating treatment or advising deferral.

Experiences with the treatment of children with chronic hepatitis C started in the early 1990s. Nineteen studies using recombinant alpha interferon were published between 1992 and 2003. A meta-analysis of trials with alpha-interferon mono-therapy showed a wide range of viral response (0–76 %). Based on an increasing number of trials in adults, ribavirin was also added to alpha-interferon treatment trials for children. Between the years 2000 and 2005, six studies were published showing a sustained viral response rate from 27 to 64 % [52]. It became clear that genotype-2- and genotype-3-infected individuals responded much better. Alpha-interferon-2b in combination with ribavirin was then approved by the FDA. Interestingly, the only controlled randomized trial, comparing a pegylated alpha interferon (-2a) with and without ribavirin, was only published in 2011, definitely showing that the addition of ribavirin was necessary to obtain significantly better treatment results than without [52, 59]. Trials with peg-alpha-interferon and ribavirin followed in the next years and both peg-alpha-interferon-2b and peg-alpha-interferon-2a have been approved by FDA and EMA 2008/2009 and 2011/2012 in combination with ribavirin for children. Peg-alpha-interferon-2b can be used in children from 3 years and peg-alpha-interferon-2a from 5 years onwards. A meta-analysis with eight trials to examine the efficacy and safety of peg-alpha-interferon treatment in combination with ribavirin was recently published, confirming that combination therapy is effective and safe in this age group [60]. Most subjects who achieved an early viral response (70 %) also achieved a sustained viral response (58 %). Relapse rate was rare with only 7 %, as were discontinuations due to adverse events (4 %). Two trials stratified the results in genotype 1 patients according to the baseline viral load. In both studies, patients with a lower viral load before treatment (<600,000 IU/ml and <500,000 IU/ml, respectively) had a better sustained viral response rate (73 and 62 %) [61, 62]. Mode of infection and baseline levels of aminotransferases do not significantly correlate with the outcome. Representative trials with peg-alpha-interferon and ribavirin with more than 20 treated patients are summarized in Table 60.1 [59, 61–65].

Most adverse events are mild to moderate. Apart from flue like symptoms, which are very common, the most frequent side effects were in 32 % neutropenia and in 52 % leukopenia, whereas anemia and thrombocytopenia were documented in only 11 and 5 %, respectively. Injection site erythema, pruritus, alopecia, and growth inhibition, which was reversible in the majority of patients, were also observed. Severe psychiatric side effects were rare in prepubertal individuals. Up to 20 % of patients with 48-week treatment may have abnormal thyroid-stimulating hormone levels or other signs of thyroid dysfunction [52].

In summary, there is sufficient evidence to recommend antiviral therapy in chronic hepatitis C [66]. Peg-alpha-interferon and ribavirin therapies in treatment naïve children and adolescents yield a sustained viral response rate in approximately 50 % of adequately treated genotype-1-infected patients. Thus, this option can be offered to all interested individuals. In patients infected with genotype 2 or 3, treatment for 24 weeks should absolutely be performed because the response rate is more than 90 %. According to the approvals of the drugs, treatment start is possible beyond the age of 3 and 5 years, respectively. However, since spontaneous viral elimination in vertically infected subjects may occur within the first years until preschool age, watchful waiting is a justified alternative to an early treatment start. Additionally, various individual and family variables may influence the appropriate time to initiate treatment. Mid-childhood age before pubertal growth spurt is preferable. Re-therapy in previously treated genotype-1- and genotype-4-infected individuals produces sustained viral response in roughly one third, so deferral until availability of better treatment options seems reasonable [63].

In adults, triple therapy is still an approved current standard of care. However, oral interferon-free treatment regimens have been started. It could be expected that triple therapy would also increase the sustained viral response rate in children. Therefore, clinical trials in combination with boceprevir and telaprevir have been launched for children and adolescents. Most interestingly, the FDA stopped the boceprevir study for ethical reasons. One essential was the rapidly upcoming of numerous DAA with the perspective of interferon-free oral treatment options in the foreseeable future also for children [58]. For example, sofosbuvir is a new promising nucleotide analogue which has been tried with good results in combination with ribavirin in genotypes 2 and 3 infected and combined with peg-alpha-interferon in genotype-1-infected adults [67, 68]. The protease inhibitor faldaprevir was tested in combination with the polymerase inhibitor Deleobuvir as interferon-free regimen in genotype 1 patients [69]. This new way with a couple of upcoming further compounds will allow a shortened and more individual response-guided therapy. As of the beginning of the year 2015, a panel of new substances has been licensed

Table 60.1 Representative trials with peg-alpha-interferon and ribavirin in children and adolescents with chronic hepatitis C (wk: week)

	Wirth 2005[a] [64]	Jara 2008[a] [65]	Pawlowska 2010 [63]	Wirth 2010[a] [62]	Total PEG-IFN-a2b trials	Schwarz 2011[b] [59]	Sokal 2010[b] [61]	Total all trials
Dosage	1.5 µg/kg/wk	1.0 µg/kg/wk	1.0 µg/kg/wk	60 µg/m²/wk		180 µg/1.73 m²/wk	100 µg/m²	
Total	36/61 (59%)	15/30 (50%)	18/29 (62.1%)	70/107 (65.4%)	139/227 (61.2%)	29/55 (53%)	43/65 (66.1%)	211/347 (60.8%)
Genotype								
1	22/46 (48%)	12/26 (46%)	10/16 (62%)	38/72 (53%)	82/160 (51.3%)	21/45 (47%)	27/47 (59%)	130/252 (51.6%)
2/3	13/13 (100%)	3/3 (100%)		28/30 (93%)	44/46 (96%)	8/10 (80%)	16/17 (94%)	68/73 (93%)
4	1/2	0/1	8/11 (72%)	4/5 (80%)	13/19 (68.4%)		Included in G1	
ALT levels								
Elevated	12/25 (48%)			27/44 (61%)			19/33 (58%)	58/102 (57%)
Normal	24/36 (67%)			42/63 (67%)			24/30 (80%)	90/129 (70%)
Mode of infection								
Parenteral	19/27 (70%)	7/9 (78%)		5/5 (100%)	31/41 (76%)			
Genotype 1	13/21 (62%)		10/16 (62%)	1/1				
Vertical	12/25 (48%)	8/21 (38%)		46/75 (61%)	66/121 (55%)			
Genotype 1	7/20 (35%)			26/52 (50%)	33/72 (46%)			
Break through	9.8%		6 (20%)			6/41 (15%)		
Relapse	7.7%		1 (3.4%)	8%		6/35 (17%)		

PEG-IFN-a2b pegylated interferon alpha-2b, ALT alanine aminotransferase

for adults: sofosbuvir, simeprevir, daclatasvir, ledispavir in combination with sofosbuvir and the combination of parita-previr, ritonavir, ombitasvir, dasabuvir, and ribavirin. Thus, it is clearly conceivable that the current adult triple therapy will never routinely be used in children even with a pediatric approval, because the rapid development of new treatment options significantly accelerates the timeline. DAA trial in children have now been started. Therefore, we have to consider well balanced, if it would be better for the individual patient, to wait some time until oral treatment options for children, particularly infected with genotype 1, are available. Another issue is the question, if we actually have enough patients to perform appropriate trials for approval for the best drug combination. Thus, experts should carefully discuss, if waivers for pediatric investigation plans for some substances would be useful, when it becomes foreseeable that advanced concepts will get ahead of previous one.

References

1. Nel E, Sokol RJ, Comparcola D, et al. Viral hepatitis in children. J Pediatr Gastroenterol Nutr. 2012;55:500–5.
2. McMahon BJ, Alward WL, Hall DB, et al. Acute hepatitis B virus infection: relation of age to the clinical expression of disease and subsequent development of the carrier state. J Infect Dis. 1985;151:599–603.
3. Chatzidaki V, Kouroumalis E, Galanakis E. Hepatitis B virus acquisition and pathogenesis in childhood: host genetic determinants. J Pediatr Gastroenterol Nutr. 2011;52:3–8.
4. Trautwein C. Mechanisms of hepatitis B virus graft reinfection and graft damage after liver transplantation. J Hepatol. 2004;41:362–9.
5. Levrero M, Pollicino T, Petersen J, et al. Control of cccDNA function in hepatitis B virus infection. J Hepatol. 2009;51:581–92.
6. Bonilla Guerrero R, Roberts LR. The role of hepatitis B virus integrations in the pathogenesis of human hepatocellular carcinoma. J Hepatol. 2005;42:760–77.
7. Shi YH, Shi CH. Molecular characteristics and stages of chronic hepatitis B virus infection. World J Gastroenterol. 2009;15:3099–105.
8. Hadziyannis SJ. Natural history of chronic hepatitis B in Euro-Mediterranean and African countries. J Hepatol. 2011;55:183–91.
9. Mahtab MA, Rahman S, Khan M, Karim F. Hepatitis B virus genotypes: an overview. Hepatobiliary Pancreat Dis Int. 2008;7:457–64.
10. Lee C, Gong Y, Brok J, Boxall EH, Gluud C. Effect of hepatitis B immunisation in newborn infants of mothers positive for hepatitis B surface antigen: systematic review and meta-analysis. BMJ 2006;332:328–36.
11. Lee C, Gong Y, Brok J, Boxall EH, Gluud C. Hepatitis B immunisation for newborn infants of hepatitis B surface antigen-positive mothers. Cochrane Database Syst Rev. 2006:CD004790.
12. Wang Z, Zhang J, Yang H, et al. Quantitative analysis of HBV DNA level and HBeAg titer in hepatitis B surface antigen positive mothers and their babies: HBeAg passage through the placenta and the rate of decay in babies. J Med Virol. 2003;71:360–6.
13. Han GR, Cao MK, Zhao W, et al. A prospective and open-label study for the efficacy and safety of telbivudine in pregnancy for the prevention of perinatal transmission of hepatitis B virus infection. J Hepatol. 2011;55:1215–21.
14. Xu WM, Cui YT, Wang L, et al. Lamivudine in late pregnancy to prevent perinatal transmission of hepatitis B virus infection: a multicentre, randomized, double-blind, placebo-controlled study. J Viral Hepat. 2009;16:94–103.
15. Paganelli M, Stephenne X, Sokal EM. Chronic hepatitis B in children and adolescents. J Hepatol. 2012;57:885–96.
16. Wai CT, Fontana RJ. Clinical significance of hepatitis B virus genotypes, variants, and mutants. Clin Liver Dis. 2004;8:321–52, vi.
17. Sokal EM, Paganelli M, Wirth S, et al. Management of chronic hepatitis B in childhood: ESPGHAN clinical practice guidelines: consensus of an expert panel on behalf of the European Society of Pediatric Gastroenterology, Hepatology and Nutrition. J Hepatol. 2013.
18. Hui CK, Leung N, Yuen ST, et al. Natural history and disease progression in Chinese chronic hepatitis B patients in immune-tolerant phase. Hepatology 2007;46:395–401.
19. Bortolotti F. Treatment of chronic hepatitis B in children. J Hepatol 2003;39 Suppl 1:S200–5.
20. Popalis C, Yeung LT, Ling SC, Ng V, Roberts EA. Chronic hepatitis B virus (HBV) infection in children: 25 years experience. J Viral Hepat. 2013;20:e20–6.
21. Iorio R, Giannattasio A, Cirillo F, L D' Alessandro, Vegnente A. Long-term outcome in children with chronic hepatitis B: a 24-year observation period. Clin Infect Dis. 2007;45:943–9.
22. Minuk GY, Sun DF, Uhanova J, et al. Occult hepatitis B virus infection in a North American community-based population. J Hepatol. 2005;42:480–5.
23. Shahmoradi S, Yahyapour Y, Mahmoodi M, et al. High prevalence of occult hepatitis B virus infection in children born to HBsAg-positive mothers despite prophylaxis with hepatitis B vaccination and HBIG. J Hepatol. 2012;57:515–21.
24. Lee MH, Yang HI, Liu J, et al. Prediction models of long-term Cirrhosis and hepatocellular carcinoma risk in chronic hepatitis B patients: risk scores integrating host and virus profiles. Hepatology 2013;58:546–54.
25. Tseng TC, Liu CJ, Yang HC, et al. Serum hepatitis B surface antigen levels help predict disease progression in patients with low hepatitis B virus loads. Hepatology 2013;57:441–50.
26. Ni YH, Chang MH, Wang KJ, et al. Clinical relevance of hepatitis B virus genotype in children with chronic infection and hepatocellular carcinoma. Gastroenterology 2004;127:1733–8.
27. Chang MH, You SL, Chen CJ, et al. Decreased incidence of hepatocellular carcinoma in hepatitis B vaccinees: a 20-year follow-up study. J Natl Cancer Inst. 2009;101:1348–55.
28. Chen JD, Yang HI, Iloeje UH, et al. Carriers of inactive hepatitis B virus are still at risk for hepatocellular carcinoma and liver-related death. Gastroenterology 2010;138:1747–54.
29. Tai DI, Lin SM, Sheen IS, et al. Long-term outcome of hepatitis B e antigen-negative hepatitis B surface antigen carriers in relation to changes of alanine aminotransferase levels over time. Hepatology 2009;49:1859–67.
30. Wirth S, Bortolotti F, Brunert C, et al. Hepatitis B virus genotype change in children is closely related to HBeAg/Anti-HBe seroconversion. J Pediatr Gastroenterol Nutr. 2013;57:363–6.
31. Kao JH. Hepatitis B viral genotypes: clinical relevance and molecular characteristics. J Gastroenterol Hepatol. 2002;17:643–50.
32. Alavian SM, Carman WF, Jazayeri SM. HBsAg variants: diagnostic-escape and diagnostic dilemma. J Clin Virol. 2013;57:201–8.
33. Kwon H, Lok AS. Hepatitis B therapy. Nat Rev Gastroenterol Hepatol. 2011;8:275–84.
34. Murray KF, Szenborn L, Wysocki J, et al. Randomized, placebo-controlled trial of tenofovir disoproxil fumarate in adolescents with chronic hepatitis B. Hepatology 2012;56:2018–26.
35. Jonas MM, Mizerski J, Badia IB, et al. Clinical trial of lamivudine in children with chronic hepatitis B. N Engl J Med. 2002;346:1706–13.
36. Jonas MM, Kelly D, Pollack H, et al. Efficacy and safety of long-term adefovir dipivoxil therapy in children with chronic hepatitis B infection. Pediatr Infect Dis J. 2012;31:578–82.

37. Bortolotti F, Iorio R, Nebbia G, et al. Interferon treatment in children with chronic hepatitis C: long-lasting remission in responders, and risk for disease progression in non-responders. Dig Liver Dis. 2005;37:336–41.

38. Sokal EM, Kelly DA, Mizerski J, et al. Long-term lamivudine therapy for children with HBeAg-positive chronic hepatitis B. Hepatology 2006;43:225–32.

39. European Association For The Study Of The Liver. EASL clinical practice guidelines: management of chronic hepatitis B virus infection. J Hepatol. 2012;57:167–85.

40. Papatheodoridis GV, Manesis EK, Manolakopoulos S, et al. Is there a meaningful serum hepatitis B virus DNA cutoff level for therapeutic decisions in hepatitis B e antigen-negative chronic hepatitis B virus infection? Hepatology 2008;48:1451–9.

41. European Association For The Study Of The Liver. EASL clinical practice guidelines: management of hepatitis C virus infection. J Hepatol 2011;55:245–64.

42. Robinson JL, Doucette K. The natural history of hepatitis C virus infection acquired during childhood. Liver Int. 2012;32:258–70.

43. Bartenschlager R, Cosset FL, Lohmann V. Hepatitis C virus replication cycle. J Hepatol. 2010;53:583–5.

44. Mack CL, Gonzalez-Peralta RP, Gupta N, et al. NASPGHAN practice guidelines: diagnosis and management of hepatitis C infection in infants, children, and adolescents. J Pediatr Gastroenterol Nutr. 2012;54:838–55.

45. Ruiz-Extremera A, Munoz-Gamez JA, Salmeron-Ruiz MA, et al. Genetic variation in interleukin 28B with respect to vertical transmission of hepatitis C virus and spontaneous clearance in HCV-infected children. Hepatology 2011;53:1830–8.

46. Ghany MG, Strader DB, Thomas DL, Seeff LB. Diagnosis, management, and treatment of hepatitis C: an update. Hepatology 2009;49:1335–74.

47. Wirth S, Kelly D, Sokal E, et al. Guidance for clinical trials for children and adolescents with chronic hepatitis C. J Pediatr Gastroenterol Nutr. 2011;52:233–7.

48. Mohd Hanafiah K, Groeger J, Flaxman AD, Wiersma ST. Global epidemiology of hepatitis C virus infection: new estimates of age-specific antibody to HCV seroprevalence. Hepatology 2013;57:1333–42.

49. Mok J, Pembrey L, Tovo PA, Newell ML. When does mother to child transmission of hepatitis C virus occur? Arch Dis Child Fetal Neonatal Ed. 2005;90:F156–60.

50. Bortolotti F, Verucchi G, Camma C, et al. Long-term course of chronic hepatitis C in children: from viral clearance to end-stage liver disease. Gastroenterology 2008;134:1900–7.

51. Bortolotti F, Indolfi G, Zancan L, et al. Management of chronic hepatitis C in childhood: the impact of therapy in the clinical practice during the first 2 decades. Dig Liver Dis. 2011;43:325–9.

52. Wirth S. Current treatment options and response rates in children with chronic hepatitis C. World J Gastroenterol 2012;18:99–104.

53. Porto AF, Tormey L, Lim JK. Management of chronic hepatitis C infection in children. Curr Opin Pediatr. 2012;24:113–20.

54. Rodrigue JR, Balistreri W, Haber B, et al. Impact of hepatitis C virus infection on children and their caregivers: quality of life, cognitive, and emotional outcomes. J Pediatr Gastroenterol Nutr. 2009;48:341–7.

55. McAndrews MP, Farcnik K, Carlen P, et al. Prevalence and significance of neurocognitive dysfunction in hepatitis C in the absence of correlated risk factors. Hepatology 2005;41:801–8.

56. Omland LH, Krarup H, Jepsen P, et al. Mortality in patients with chronic and cleared hepatitis C viral infection: a nationwide cohort study. J Hepatol. 2010;53:36–42.

57. Sangiovanni A, Prati GM, Fasani P, et al. The natural history of compensated cirrhosis due to hepatitis C virus: a 17-year cohort study of 214 patients. Hepatology 2006;43:1303–10.

58. Aghemo A, De Francesco R. New horizons in hepatitis C antiviral therapy with direct-acting antivirals. Hepatology 2013;58:428–38.

59. Schwarz KB, Gonzalez-Peralta RP, Murray KF, et al. The combination of ribavirin and peginterferon is superior to peginterferon and placebo for children and adolescents with chronic hepatitis C. Gastroenterology 2011;140:450–8.e451.

60. Druyts E, Thorlund K, Wu P, et al. Efficacy and safety of pegylated interferon alfa-2a or alfa-2b plus ribavirin for the treatment of chronic hepatitis C in children and adolescents: a systematic review and meta-analysis. Clin Infect Dis. 2013;56:961–7.

61. Sokal EM, Bourgois A, Stephenne X, et al. Peginterferon alfa-2a plus ribavirin for chronic hepatitis C virus infection in children and adolescents. J Hepatol. 2010;52:827–31.

62. Wirth S, Ribes-Koninckx C, Calzado MA, et al. High sustained virologic response rates in children with chronic hepatitis C receiving peginterferon alfa-2b plus ribavirin. J Hepatol. 2010;52:501–7.

63. Pawlowska M, Pilarczyk M, Halota W. Virologic response to treatment with Pegylated Interferon alfa-2b and Ribavirin for chronic hepatitis C in children. Med Sci Monit. 2010;16:CR616–21.

64. Wirth S, Pieper-Boustani H, Lang T, Ballauff A, Kullmer U, Gerner P, Wintermeyer P, Jenke A. Peginterferon alfa-2b plus ribavirin treatment in children and adolescents with chronic hepatitis C. Hepatology 2005 May;41(5):1013–8.

65. Jara P, Hierro L, de la Vega A, Diaz C, Camarena C, Frauca E, Miños-Bartolo G, Diez-Dorado R, de Guevara CL, Larrauri J, Rueda M. Efficacy and safety of peginterferon-alpha2b and ribavirin combination therapy in children with chronic hepatitis C infection. Pediatr Infect Dis J. 2008 Feb;27(2):142–8. doi:10.1097/INF.0b013e318159836c.

66. van der Meer AJ, Wedemeyer H, Feld JJ, et al. Is there sufficient evidence to recommend antiviral therapy in hepatitis C? J Hepatol. 2014;60:191–6.

67. Lawitz E, Gane EJ. Sofosbuvir for previously untreated chronic hepatitis C infection. N Engl J Med. 2013;369:678–9.

68. Jacobson IM, Gordon SC, Kowdley KV, et al. Sofosbuvir for hepatitis C genotype 2 or 3 in patients without treatment options. N Engl J Med. 2013;368:1867–77.

69. Zeuzem S, Soriano V, Asselah T, et al. Faldaprevir and deleobuvir for HCV genotype 1 infection. N Engl J Med. 2013;369:630–9.

Bacterial, Fungal and Parasitic Infections of the Liver

Anita Verma

Introduction

Primary nonviral infections of the liver parenchyma itself are uncommon; presumably the phagocytic Kupffer cells play a key role in preventing the infection. The liver's dual blood supply renders it uniquely susceptible to infection, receives blood from the intestinal tract via the hepatic portal system and is sustained by systemic circulation via the hepatic artery. Because of this unique perfusion, the liver is frequently exposed to systemic or intestinal infections or the mediators of toxemia. The biliary tree provides a further conduit for gut bacteria or parasites to access the liver parenchyma.

Infections of the liver with a wide range of organisms present variously from asymptomatic biochemical abnormalities to symptomatic hepatitis or space occupying lesions, for example, abscesses or granulomatas producing biochemical changes of cholestasis but rarely significant jaundice. Some of these infections have a high mortality if not treated promptly. We describe nonviral infectious diseases affecting the liver caused by bacteria, mycobacteria, spirochetes, rickettsia, fungi and parasites.

Bacterial, Spirochaetal and Rickettsial Infections

Bacterial Sepsis

Bacterial sepsis precipitating jaundice is a well-recognized phenomenon particularly in the newborn and young infants [1]. The exact pathogenesis of hepatic insult is not known, but may be multifactorial, including direct invasion of liver parenchyma by blood-borne pathogens and nonspecific injury due to hypoxia or endotoxin-mediated paralysis of biliary

canaliculi inducing cholestasis. Implicated bacteria include 'coliforms', pseudomonads, *Salmonella* spp., anaerobes, *Haemophilus influenzae,* streptococci and *Staphylococcus aureus.* In patients with jaundice, serum bilirubin is usually between 5 and 10 mg/dl. Hepatomegaly is found in 50 % of cases, and liver enzymes usually mildly elevated. Clinical evaluation and microbiological investigation may identify the source of sepsis and antimicrobial therapy usually results in complete resolution.

Liver Abscess

Pyogenic liver abscess (PLA) in infancy and childhood is uncommon, with incidence ranging from 3 to 25 per 100,000, but carries a high mortality [2–4]. The oetiology of PLA is variable. Though PLA in healthy children is a rare entity, up to 40–50 % has occurred among immunocompromised children [2]. Pyogenic bacteria can reach the liver through various routes: (i) portal: secondary to gut pathologies such as appendicitis, inflammatory bowel disease or diverticulitis, sometimes complicated by portal pyelophlebitis and portal vein system thrombosis; (ii) biliary: caused by extrahepatic biliary tract disease such as stricture, calculus or malignancy; (iii) blood borne from an infected focus anywhere in the body via hepatic artery; (iv) contiguous extension from gallbladder or perinephric abscess; (v) following penetrating wounds of liver and (vi) cryptogenic [2, 5].

PLA may present as single large lesion or multiple abscesses, the latter often secondary to biliary tract infection. The importance of the portal venous route has fallen with better diagnosis and management of appendicitis. In most reviews, more than 60 % abscesses are in the right lobe, 20–25 % bilateral, and less than 15 % in the left lobe [4, 5]. Predisposing factors include immunosuppression, quantitative or qualitative granulocyte abnormalities like chronic granulomatous disease, trauma, umbilical vein catheterization, omphalitis, sickle-cell disease, biliary tract surgery, hepatic artery thrombosis (post liver transplantation), liver

A. Verma (✉)
Institute of Liver Studies, King's College Hospital, NHS, Foundation Trust, Denmark Hill, SE5 9RS London, UK
e-mail: anitaverma@nhs.net

© Springer International Publishing Switzerland 2016
S. Guandalini et al. (eds.), *Textbook of Pediatric Gastroenterology, Hepatology and Nutrition,*
DOI 10.1007/978-3-319-17169-2_61

biopsy, percutaneous or endoscopic biliary drainage, diabetes, worm infestation and protein-energy malnutrition especially in developing countries [4, 5].

Multiple abscesses complicate biliary diseases such as bacterial cholangitis, sclerosing cholangitis, congenital biliary anomalies (Caroli's disease) and gallstones with higher mortality. S. aureus is the most common isolate in children, but Gram-negative aerobes, anaerobes and microaerophilic streptococci are also common [2, 4, 5]. Less frequent causes include Pseudomonas spp., Clostridium spp., Salmonella typhi, Yersinia enterocolitica and Pasteurella multocida. The classic presentation is pyrexia, chills, right upper quadrant (RUQ) tenderness, abdominal pain, hepatomegaly and leucocytosis but may be nonspecific. The diagnosis must be entertained in any pyrexia of unknown origin (PUO). Unusual presentations include an abdominal mass or acute abdomen secondary to rupture in to the peritoneal cavity or portal hypertension secondary to portal pyemia and portal vein thrombosis. Liver function tests may be unhelpful with nonspecific changes. Ultrasonography (USS), computerized tomography (CT) and magnetic resonance imaging (MRI) are all sensitive but cannot always differentiate abscesses from other lesions such as cysts, tumours or haemorrhage. USS or CT-guided drainage of as much pus as possible (from as many abscesses as possible) confirms diagnosis, and is central to the management. Initial treatment is conservative with broad-spectrum antibiotics (e.g. cefotaxime plus metronidazole or clindamycin) and should be adjusted when culture results are available [5, 6]. Duration of treatment is usually 3–6 weeks. Patients with multiple abscesses have to be on conservative treatment after a diagnostic tap, and up to 3–4 months of antibiotic therapy has been recommended to prevent relapses [5, 7]. Prognosis is worse in multiple abscesses. Most reports emphasize the good outcome after percutaneous drainage, which should be USS or CT guided. Contraindications to drainage include ascites and inaccessible lesions. Complications of aspiration include haemorrhage, hepatic laceration, fistula formation, peritonitis and additional abscess formation. Indications for open drainage procedure are biliary obstruction, loculated or highly viscous abscesses, persistence of fever for more than 2 weeks despite percutaneous catheter drainage and appropriate antimicrobial therapy. Predisposing immunodeficiency conditions should be managed with appropriate expert opinion from immunologists or infectious diseases experts.

Cholangitis

The normal biliary tract is sterile and, in children, acute cholangitis rarely occurs in the absence of congenital abnormalities or interventions in the biliary tract [8]. The children at highest risk include those with portoenterostomy or choledochal cyst, and those who have nonoperative biliary

manipulations such as transhepatic cholangiography or endoscopic retrograde cholangiography with stent placement. Risk of cholangitis in children after Kasai operation has been reported to be 40–50 % [8]. Partial biliary obstruction encourages bacterial growth, with increased intraductal pressure and reflux of bacteria into blood vessels and perihepatic lymphatics leading to bacteremia. Infection may ascend from the duodenum or an infected gallbladder, or via lymphatics or bloodstream [9].

Cholangitis is a clinical diagnosis based on fever, abdominal pain, jaundice, pale stools or hepatic tenderness. However, the spectrum encompasses mild disease to severe sepsis, or shock, with bacteraemia [8]. Although Escherichia coli, Klebsiella spp., Enterobacter spp. and Pseudomonas spp. are usually implicated, infection may be polymicrobial and include anaerobes [8]. Leucocytosis is common, but changes in liver function tests are nonspecific; the serum bilirubin may be normal. In recurrent cholangitis, liver biopsy may be indicated for confirmation and microbiological examination. Treatment requires supportive care and an urgent USS or CT will help establish whether obstruction requires drainage. Broad-spectrum antibiotics should be administered—such as an acylureidopenicillin (piperacillin, mezlocillin or piperacillin-tazobactam) or a late generation cephalosporin (e.g. ceftazidime), plus an aminoglycoside [10]. Single agents, such as piperacillin, piperacillin-tazobactam, ciprofloxacin and imipenem or meropenem, appear safe and effective if an aminoglycosides is contraindicated. Duration of treatment is generally 3 weeks for acute cholangitis, but prolonged therapy may be necessary for recurrent cholangitis and multiply resistant bacteria [11]. Three months of intravenous antibiotics through central line has been helpful in treating recurrent cholangitis in biliary atresia children with portoenterostomy. Prolonged antimicrobial therapy in recurrent cholangitis only helps in preventing the bacteraemia by preventing bacterial overgrowth in biliary tract. There is always risk of development of resistant organisms and therefore more serious infection.

Tuberculosis

Tuberculosis (TB) of the liver is almost invariably a complication of miliary disease and occurs in 50 and 75 % of patients with pulmonary or extrapulmonary TB, respectively. The site of primary focus usually dictates presentation. Rarely the liver appears to be the sole site of infection such as in congenital TB acquired via the ductus venosus [12, 13]. Congenital TB may present in first few weeks of life with failure to thrive, hepatosplenomegaly and jaundice. In older children, hepatic TB presents with PUO, weight loss, abdominal discomfort and hepatomegaly [12, 13]. In areas of low incidence a positive tuberculin skin test is diagnostically useful. However, confirmation requires liver biopsy, histology and culture confirmation. Caseating granulomata on liver biopsy are highly suggestive of TB, but may be absent; a granulomatous hepatitis can complicate Bacille Calmette–Guerin (BCG) administration. The diagnosis of TB should be sought by specific staining and culture of material from other sites, including bronchoalveolar lavage, lymph node or pleural biopsy, marrow aspirate, lumbar puncture or early morning gastric aspirates, as clinically indicated. Polymerase chain reaction (PCR)-based tests may be helpful but require further evaluation. Standard antituberculous therapy is effective, but expert advice should be sought in areas with a high incidence of drug resistant TB or in compromised patients, including those with concurrent HIV infection.

Brucellosis

It is a multisystem infection caused by *Brucella melitensis, B. suis, B. abortus* and *B. canis; B. melitensis* causes more severe disease with a higher risk of chronicity. In endemic areas, transmission is often by ingestion of unpasteurized dairy products or raw meat. Granulomatous hepatitis may occur in acute or chronic disease and manifests as nonspecific changes in liver function tests [14]. Diagnosis requires clinical suspicion, blood and bone marrow cultures, serology and histopathological examination. PCR-based tests for brucellosis are available. The recommended treatment for children under 9 years of age with uncomplicated brucellosis is trimethoprim–sulphamethoxazole. For the treatment of serious infection, the addition of gentamicin or streptomycin is recommended for the first 1–2 weeks. Older children should receive doxycycline (6 weeks) plus rifampicin or streptomycin (2 weeks).

Listeriosis

Listeria monocytogenes may cause liver disease as part of systemic intrauterine infection of the foetus—granulomatosis infantiseptica at birth or later in the neonatal period—and in older immunocompromised children after ingestion of contaminated food or water. The major hepatic manifestation is granuloma; jaundice is rare. Diagnosis is achieved by recovering the bacterium from blood culture, cerebrospinal fluid or liver aspirates. Treatment is with high dose ampicillin, with or without gentamicin.

Tularemia

Francisella tularensis has been isolated from many wild mammals, domestic animals and birds. Human infection usually follows bites from parasites of these animals or direct contact with animals. In some cases, a hepatitis-like picture follows with raised aminotransferases. Hepatomegaly is rare and biopsy may show necrosis. Diagnosis is usually serologi-

cal as the bacterium is difficult to recover in culture. Treatment with streptomycin or gentamicin is effective; the fluoroquinolones appear promising but require further evaluation.

Leptospirosis

Human infection follows exposure to leptospires excreted in the urine of chronically infected animals—including rats, cattle and dogs—or water contaminated with urine. Children are usually infected when swimming in contaminated rivers, ponds or lakes, or by canine exposure [15]. Leptospires gain entry via skin abrasions, conjunctivae or mucosae and an initial leptospiremia presages a multisystem infection. The incubation period is 5–15 days, and in 90% of patients there is a self-limiting anicteric disease but 5–10% develop jaundice (Weil's disease) [16]. Classically, the anicteric leptospirosis runs a biphasic course, with a leptospiremic phase lasting for 3–7 days and a second phase associated with leptospiruria and rising antibody titres lasting for 4–30 days. Predominant manifestations are fever, headache, myalgia, abdominal pain, nausea, vomiting, meningism, conjuctival suffusion, maculopapular rash, impaired renal function, lymphadenopathy and hepatosplenomegaly. Weil's disease is characterized by hepatic, renal and vascular dysfunction with persistent fever, profound jaundice, abdominal pain, renal failure, confusion, epistaxis, haematuria, gastrointestinal bleeding and other haemorrhagic phenomenon. Death may follow cardiovascular collapse, renal failure and gastrointestinal or pulmonary haemorrhage, though with supportive therapy mortality should be less than 10%. Liver histology reveals swollen perivenular hepatocytes with increased mitoses indicative of regeneration and disorganized liver cell plates. Leptospires may be recovered from blood, urine or cerebrospinal fluid (CSF) during the first week of illness, and from urine thereafter, and may be seen by dark ground microscopy of blood in the early stage of disease and in urine thereafter. Diagnosis, however, is usually serological using complement fixation tests (CFTs), enzyme-linked immunosorbent assay (ELISA) or a microagglutination test. PCR can detect leptospiral DNA in blood, serum, CSF, urine or aqueous humour. Penicillin or doxycycline is recommended and most beneficial if started early in the disease: The benefits of commencing antimicrobials later in Weil's disease are less clear.

Borreliosis

Borrelia burgdorferi, is a tick-borne spirochaete which causes systemic infection in humans (Lyme disease) following exposure to these vectors in forest or parkland. Predominant manifestations of acute disease are fever, malaise, extending erythematous rash, meningism, arthralgia, hepatitis and lymphadenopathy. Abnormal liver function tests occur in up to 20% of patients and, rarely, hepatomegaly and RUQ tenderness [17]. Diagnosis requires clinical suspicion, positive serology and histopathology. Spirochetes may be seen in liver biopsy with a mixed inflammatory infiltrates in sinusoids, mitotic activity and ballooning degeneration of hepatocytes with hyperplastic Kupffer cells. Ampicillin or amoxicillin is administered for 3 weeks in early disease in children less than 9 years of age; tetracycline for older children. In late disease, intravenous cefotaxime or ceftriaxone for 2–4 weeks is recommended followed by oral ampicillin plus probenicid for a further 4–8 weeks.

Syphilis

Treponema pallidum may infect the foetus at any stage of maternal syphilis, causing disseminated infection. Congenital syphilis may result in mucocutaneous lesions, a diffuse rash, pneumonitis, myocarditis, hepatosplenomegaly, jaundice, lymphadenopathy, haemolytic anemia, thrombocytopoenia, perichondritis and osteochondritis; the infant is usually small for age. Late stigmata include arthropathy with bilateral knee effusions, notched upper incisors and frontal bossing of the skull and poorly developed maxillae. Neonatal death usually results from liver failure, severe pneumonia or pulmonary haemorrhage. Diagnosis requires detection of spirochetes by dark-field examination (skin rash, nasal secretions) or serology, including detection of specific IgM antibodies; long bone radiography at 1–3 months of age may contribute to diagnosis. Benzylpenicillin (10–14 days) remains the drug of choice.

Q Fever

Q fever is a systemic infection caused by the rickettsia *Coxiella burnetii* following exposure to infectious dust or aerosols from farm or domestic animals, or consumption of raw milk. Illness is usually a self-limiting 'flu-like illness' with an incubation period of 1–2 weeks. However, acute Q fever can present with atypical pneumonia and hepatitis with jaundice, hepatomegaly and abnormal liver function tests [18]. The characteristic histopathological finding is granulomata with dense fibrin rings around central lipid vacuoles. Diagnosis is by detecting immunoglobulin G (IgG) and immunoglobulin M (IgM) to phase II antigens of *C. burnetii,* usually by indirect fluorescent antibody test or ELISA. Seroconversion occurs at 7–15 days after the onset of symptoms with 90% patients having detectable antibodies by the third week. Titres of antibodies to phase I antigens exceed those to phase II antigens in chronic disease. Treatment is recommended for all cases to prevent chronicity; tetracycline or chloramphenicol is effective.

Parasitic Infections

Amoebiasis

Entamoeba histolytica is most commonly encountered in the tropics and subtropics. Hepatic abscess is a major complication of invasive amoebiasis and seen in 3–9% of adult cases but is less common in children [19]. Amoebic trophozoites reach the liver via the portal vein and induce hepatocyte apoptosis and a leucocyte response resulting in abscesses containing viscous brown pus. Hepatic abscesses, can be demonstrated by USS or CT scanning, are usually single and most frequent in the right lobe. Multiple abscesses may be associated with more severe disease. A typical presentation is with pyrexia (75%) and RUQ pain radiating to the right shoulder. In left lobe disease, there may be epigastric or left shoulder pain. Tenderness in the hypochondrium (85%), tender hepatomegaly (80%) and localized swelling over the liver (10%) may be elicited [20]. Less specific symptoms include nausea, vomiting, concurrent diarrhea or dysentery (10%)and loss of weight. Jaundice is present in up to 8% of cases. The white blood cell count is usually elevated. Demonstrating cysts in stool may contribute to diagnosis, but serum antibodies are present in more than 95% of patients. Aspiration under USS guidance may yield 'anchovy sauce' pus; rarely amoebas are seen in necrotic abscess wall or adjacent parenchyma. Abscesses may rupture in to the peritoneal cavity, pleural cavity or lungs, pericardium, portal vein or biliary tract, intraperitoneal rupture being more common than intrathoracic. Extraintestinal amoebiasis should be treated with metronidazole or dehydroemeteine for at least 2 weeks [21]. The cure rate with both the drugs are same, but metronidazole has the advantage of being less toxic and being effective for both hepatic and intestinal phases of the disease. To prevent continued intraluminal infection, luminal amoebicide, such as paromomycin or diloxanide furoate should be given. Occasionally, amoebic abscess do not respond to metronidazole and addition of daily chloroquine may be considered for 2–3 weeks. Chloroquine has an additive effect to metronidazole and better penetration of the abscess wall. Percutaneous needle aspiration is recommended for large abscesses, failure to respond or if there is imminent risk of rupture, particularly in to the pericardium.

Schistosomiasis

Schistosomiasis affects 200 million people worldwide, the majority children aged 5–15 years [22]. Transmission occurs in endemic areas (Middle East, Brazil, West Indies, Far East and Southeast Asia) after exposure to water inhabited by infected snails. The intermediate hosts: larvae (cercariae) released from snails can penetrate intact skin and disseminate.

S. japonicum, S. mansoni and *S. mekongi* cause hepatosplenic disease subsequent upon portal venous system obstruction by a granulomatous response to eggs and subsequent periporatal fibrosis and portal hypertension. Granulomata consist of eosinophils, epitheloid cells, plasma cells and lymphocytes encircling an ovum. Patients present with pyrexia, urticaria, eosinophilia, hepatosplenomegaly or upper gastrointestinal tract bleeding from oesophageal varicies. Dilated abdominal wall veins and ascites reflect portal venous hypertension and USS may reveal thickening of the portal vein. Ova should be sought in stool and urine and may be identified in liver or rectal mucosal biopsy. Serological tests cannot distinguish past from active infection but a negative ELISA excludes the diagnosis. Praziquantel is the drug of choice; oxamniquine an alternative for *S. mansoni*.

Hydatid Disease

Echinococcus granulosus is the dog tapeworm. Typically dogs are infected by being fed offal from infected livestock—such as sheep—which contain hydatid cysts. Humans become infected by close exposure to domestic dogs and the eggs passed in their faeces. The liver is most frequent site for cyst formation, usually in the right lobe (60–80%). Presentation is with hepatic enlargement, with or without palpable mass, epigastric pain, nausea and vomiting; secondary cyst pressure effects include portal hypertension, inferior vena cava compression or thrombosis and biliary cirrhosis. USS of the liver reveals round solitary or multiple cysts of variable size with multiple internal daughter cysts; calcification may be noted. Diagnosis requires demonstration of specific antibody by ELISA, CFT, indirect agglutination or latex agglutination tests. Closed aspiration should not be undertaken: definitive therapy requires surgical removal which may be complicated by spillage of contents, anaphylaxis and seeding of new cysts. To avoid this, cysts can be injected with chlorhexidine or hydrogen peroxide prior to surgery. Both mebendazole and albendazole may successfully treat small uncomplicated cysts.

Ascariasis

Adult *Ascaris lumbricoides* worms cause disease by migrating into the pancreatic ducts, gallbladder and biliary tract. Biliary ascariasis is more common in children than in adults. Children with a heavy worm burden may be malnourished. Presentation of biliary involvement includes fever, RUQ pain, vomiting and passing of worms in stool or vomitus. Mechanical obstruction by worms can cause acute cholecystitis, cholangitis and biliary colic. Adult worms in the biliary tract may be demonstrated by USS, cholangiography or endoscopic retrograde cholangiography (ERCP); eggs should be sought in the faeces [23]. Treatment is usually with mebendazole or albendazole—though endoscopic removal of adult worms may be necessary if there are persisting biliary symptoms.

Toxocariasis

Toxocariasis is caused by infection with the dog roundworm *Toxocara canis*. Ingested eggs hatch in the small intestine and larvae penetrate the mucosa before migrating to the liver, lungs and many other tissues. Visceral larva migrans (VLM) refers to a syndrome of eosinophilia, pyrexia, leucocytosis, hepatosplenomegaly, lymphadenopathy and hyperglobulinemia as the larva migrate. Occular disease may also occur. A history of exposure to puppies should be sought. Humans are a 'dead-end' host: adult worms do not develop so eggs are not passed. Serodiagnosis is with an ELISA. In massive infection liver biopsy may reveal eosinophils surrounding larvae or granulomata formation with epithelioid giant cells and lymphocytes. VLM is treated with thiabendazole. Severe disseminated disease or occular infection may warrant concomitant steroids.

Liver Fluke Infestation

Fasciola hepatica infection follows ingestion of aquatic plants—such as watercress—contaminated with eggs passed by infected sheep or cattle. After hatching, larvae penetrate the gut wall; enter the peritoneum and having breached the liver capsule pass through the parenchyma to the bile ducts. The flukes mature and lay eggs in the biliary tract, causing cholangitis and hepatomegaly. Diagnosis is made by demonstrating ova in stool and positive serology. ERCP may show filling defects due to inflammation and worms can be aspirated. Liver biopsy shows infiltration with eosinophils, histiocytes and polymorphs; granulomas may or may not be present. Treatment is with bithionol.

Clonorchis sinensis is endemic in the Far East. Infection follows ingestion of cysts in uncooked freshwater fish or crabs. Metacercariae excyst in the small intestine and invade the bile ducts in which the flukes mature, producing eggs which may be demonstrated in the faeces. Infection is usually asymptomatic, but bile duct fibrosis with liver impairment, strictures and pancreatitis may ensue. Praziquantel is the treatment of choice.

Toxoplasmosis

In the immunocompetent patient, acute acquired *Toxoplasma gondii* infection usually presents as self-limiting lymphadenopathy, though hepatosplenomegaly and hepatitis can occur. The risk and severity of congenital toxoplasmosis vary according to the trimester in which maternal infection with the protozoan occurs. The likelihood of foetal infection increases through pregnancy, whilst disease severity decreases. The spectrum of disease in infected neonates includes: retinochoroiditis, meningoencephalitis, hydrocephalus, intracranial calcification, pneumonitis, myocarditis, purpura, hepatitis, hepatosplenomegaly and hydrops fetalis. Congenital toxoplasmosis must be differentiated from the other major causes of congenital infection: rubella virus, cytomegalovirus, herpes simplex virus, *T. pallidum* and *L. monocytogenes*.

Diagnosis of congenital infection requires full clinical evaluation and exclusion of other infections, with recovery of *T. gondii*, histology or serological investigation. Reference laboratory tests include culture (blood, body fluids, placenta), the dye test (for serum and CSF) and ELISAs for IgG, IgM, IgA and IgE detection in both neonate and mother. *T. gondii* DNA may be detected in body fluids (blood, urine and CSF) by PCR.

Treatment is with pyrimethamine plus sulphadiazine, though expert advice should be sought. Toxoplasmosis in the immunocompromised may follow reactivation or new acquisition and usually presents as central nervous system disease though other organs, including the liver, may be affected. *T. gondii* may be transmitted in the graft at liver transplantation and cause liver and severe systemic disease thereafter.

Fungal Infections

Fungal infections of the liver are usually seen in the immunocompromised—including those with acute liver failure. Although *Candida albicans* predominates, other *Candida* spp. and *Aspergillus* spp. infections are increasingly reported.

Candidiasis

Severely immunocompromised patients are prone to disseminated candida infections with the liver (and often spleen) affected in 50–70 %. Typically, hepatosplenic candidiasis presents in haemato-oncology patients rendered neutropenic at the time of recovery of the neutrophil count. The hallmark is multiple small lesions in the liver and spleen on USS or CT scan with raised alkaline phosphatase. Yeasts may be visible on fine needle aspiration or liver biopsy and cultures may be positive; blood cultures are usually negative. Hepatic or hepatosplenic candidiasis is treated with fluconazole or amphotericin B. Although prolonged therapy may be required, the immune status of the patient is the key determinant of outcome.

Aspergillosis

Disseminated aspergillosis is an increasingly recognized problem in the severely immunocompromised. Increased incidence is seen in hospital with building constructions. Hepatic aspergillosis may manifest as an aspergilloma or granulomata formation, with hepatomegaly, elevated bilirubin, alkaline phosphatase and aminotransferases. Confident diagnosis requires both histopathological demonstration of invading hyphae and isolation of *Aspergillus* spp. (usually *A. fumigatus*) from liver biopsy. To date, serology has been unhelpful, but detection of circulating cell wall galactomannan by ELISA- and PCR-based tests show promise. Treatment with voriconazole and liposomal amphotericin B should be commenced immediately—on clinical suspicion alone—in immunocompromised patients.

Other Rare Fungal Infections

Other rare fungal infections of the liver include cryptococcosis, mucormycosis, histoplasmosis, blastomycosis, coccidioidomycosis and paracoccidioidomycosis.

References

1. Escobedo MB, Barton LL, Marshall RE. The frequency of jaundice in neonatal bacterial infections. Clinc Pediatr. 1974;13:656.
2. Chusid MJ. Pyogenic hepatic abscess in infancy and childhood. Pediatrics 1978;62:5554–9.
3. Tsai CC, Chung JH, Ko SF, Liu PM, Su CT, Li WC, et al. Liver abscess in children: a single institutional experience in southern Taiwan. Acta Paediatr Taiwan. 2003;44:282–6.
4. Chou FF, Sheen-Chen SM, Chen YS, Chen MC. Single and multiple pyogenic liver abscesses: clinical course, etiology, and results of treatment. World J Surg. 1997;21:384–8.
5. Muorah M, Hinds R, Verma A, Yu D, Samyn M, Mieli-Vergani G, Hadzic N. Liver abscesses in children: a single center experience in the developed world. J Pediatr Gastroenterol Nutr. 2006 Feb;42(2):201–6.
6. Moore SW, Millar AJW, Cywes S. Conservative initial tratment for liver abscesses in children. Br J Surg. 1994;81:872–4.
7. Bari S, Sheikh KA, Malik AA, Wani RA, Naqash SH. Percutaneous aspiration versus open drainage of liver abscess in children. Pediatr Surg Int. 2007;23:69–74.
8. Ecoffey C, Rothman E, Bernard O, Hadchouel M, Valayer J, Alagille D. Bacterial cholangitis after surgery for biliary atresia. J Pediatr. 1987;111:824–9.
9. Scott AJ, Khan GA. Origin of bacteria in bile duct. Lancet 1967;2:790.
10. Dooley JS, Hamilton-Miller JMT, Brumfitt W, et al. Antibiotics in the treatment of biliary infection. Gut 1984;25:988–98.
11. Sung JJ, Lyon DJ, Suen R, Chung SC, Co AL, Cheng AF, et al. Intravenous ciprofloxacin as treatment for patients with acute suppurative cholangitis: a randomized, controlled clinical trial. J Antimicrob Chemother. 1995;35(6):855–64.
12. Essop AR, Posen JA, Hodkinson JH, Segal I. Tuberculosis hepatitis: a clinical review of 96 cases. QJM 1984;212:465–77.

13. Kok KY, Yapp SK. Isolated heaptic tuberculosis: report of five cases and review of the literature. J Hepatobiliary Pancreat Surg. 1999;6(2):195–8.

14. Vallejo JG, Stevens AM, Dutton RV, Kaplan SL. Hepatosplenic abscesses due to *Brucella melitensis*: report of a case involving a child and review of the literature. Clin Infect Dis. 1996;22:485–9.

15. Jackson LA, Kaufmann AF, Adams WG, et al. Outbreak of leptospirosis associated with swimming. Pediatr Infect Dis J. 1993;12:48–54.

16. Farr RW. Leptospirosis. Clin Inf Dis. 1995;21:1–8.

17. Steere AC, Bartenhagen NH, Craft JE, et al. The early clinical manifestations of Lyme disease. Ann Intern Med. 1983;99:76–82.

18. Hofman CE, Wheaton IW. Q fever hepatitis: clinical manifestations and pathological findings. Gastroenterology 1982;83:474–9.

19. Sepulveda B. Amebiasis: host-pathogen biology. Rev Infect Dis. 1982;4:836–42.

20. Adams EB, Macleod IN. Invasive amoebiasis II. Ameobic liver abscess and its complications. Medicine 1990;56:1977.

21. Abramowicz M, ed. Drugs for parasitic infections. Med Lett. 1988;30:15–24.

22. Mahmoud AF, Abdel Wahab MF. Schistosomoiasis. In: Warren KS, Mahmoud AAF, editors. Tropical and geographical medicine. 2nd ed. New York: McGraw-Hill; 1990. p. 458–73.

23. El sheikh Mohemmed AR, AL Karawi MA, Yasawy MI. Modern technique in the diagnosis and treatment of gastrointestinal and biliary tree parasites. Hepatogastroenterology 1991;38:180–8.

Liver Disease in Primary Immunodeficiencies

62

Nedim Hadzic

Introduction

Primary immunodeficiencies (PIDs) are heritable disorders of innate and/or acquired immunity, often complicated by severe, recurrent or unusual infections, chronic diarrhea with failure to thrive and malignancies of lymphoid tissue in long-term survivors [1, 2].

Many of the problems children with these conditions face have been successfully addressed; for the early-presenting, life-threatening PIDs such as variants of severe combined immune deficiency (SCID) or hyper immunoglobulin E (IgE) syndrome, elective hematopoietic stem cell transplantation (HSCT), preferably from haploidentical donors, has become a treatment of choice [3]. In contrast, many milder forms of PIDs can be successfully managed for short-to-medium term by regular anti-infectious prophylaxis with antibiotics and/or antifungals and replacement immunoglobulins.

Liver disease occurs in approximately 25% of children with PIDs [4]. The proportion of adult patients developing this complication is unknown, but likely to be underdiagnosed and overall higher. Their number and liver pathology potentially could be affected by exposure to alcohol and propensity to develop diabetes mellitus and obesity-related liver problems such as nonalcoholic fatty liver disease later in life.

Pathophysiology

Many of the liver-related problems in PIDs stem from the fact that compromised first line anti-infectious barrier in gastrointestinal tract allows low-grade chronic infection which could ascend proximally into the biliary system and the liver. The infections are frequently caused by unusual pathogens, escaping routine anti-infectious strategies, such

as *Cryptosporidium* (CS) or *Microsporidium* [4]. The main form of liver disease in PIDs is chronic cholangiopathy, seen in around 65% of affected children [4]. This condition has a well-documented potential to develop biliary cirrhosis and full-blown clinical features of end-stage chronic liver disease, such as portal hypertension, bleeding from oesophageal varices and hypoalbuminemia with jaundice. In a small proportion of PID patients with the liver involvement, milder and more nonspecific histological features, such as fatty change, mild portal inflammation or development of small non-caseating intrahepatic granulomas, could be observed [4].

A considerable role in the chronic cholangiopathy of PIDs is attributed to protozoal infections, unaffected by the standard anti-infectious regimens. Chronic cryptosporidial infection has been implicated in chronic inflammatory and dysplastic biliary changes in the context of chronic cholangiopathy and superimposed complications such as biliary cirrhosis and cholangiocarcinoma. The pathogenic role of CS in immune deficiency is likely, albeit incompletely understood. Animal models of the CS-related cholangiopathy have been described. For example, interferon-gamma knockout mice appear to be particularly susceptible to CS infection, suggesting important role for this cytokine in pathogenesis of the cholangiopathy in PIDs [5]. The biliary injury in humans appears to be caused by direct cytopathic effects of this protozoan, mediated by apoptosis [6]. In addition, CS is known to cause cholangiopathy in human immunodeficiency virus (HIV) infection [7] and after organ transplantation [8]. Several additional intracellular parasites such as *Microsporidium*, *Mycobacterium avium intracellulare* and cytomegalovirus (CMV) have also been implicated in development of the chronic cholangiopathies in adult HIV-positive patients [7]. The accelerated evolution of the cholangiopathy in this setting is often interpreted by probable synergistic effects of multiple biliary infections [7].

A classical paradigm for development of the cholangiopathy of PIDs is hyper-IgM syndrome. This condition is caused by mutations in cluster of differentiation (CD)40

N. Hadzic (✉)
Pediatric Centre for Hepatology, Gastroenterology and Nutrition, King's College Hospital, Denmark Hill, SE5 9RS London, UK
e-mail: nedim.hadzic@kcl.ac.uk

© Springer International Publishing Switzerland 2016
S. Guandalini et al. (eds.), *Textbook of Pediatric Gastroenterology, Hepatology and Nutrition*,
DOI 10.1007/978-3-319-17169-2_62

ligand (CD154) gene, known to control interaction between CD40 molecules from B-cells and CD40 ligand on activated lymphocytes in its X-linked form (CD40 ligand deficiency). Alternative mechanism for hyper-IgM syndrome is defective expression of immune activation-induced cytidine deaminase (AID) on B cells in the autosomal recessive form of the disease [9]. As a consequence, in both forms, B cells could not facilitate physiologic IgM class switching to other immunoglobulin types, which renders total serum IgM levels high and distal components of the immune response arm ineffective. However, the IgM levels may not always be elevated, and chronic neutropenia is often observed [10, 11]. Several series have described development of chronic biliary disease occasionally complicated by cholangiocarcinoma in older patients with hyper-igM syndrome.

Although there are more than 100 described PIDs, a majority now characterised by mutations in different genes responsible for various facets of the immune response, frequent lack of genotype/phenotype correlation makes general recommendations for detecting liver disease difficult. On occasion, an adult patient could be diagnosed with PIDs and exceptionally some children with conditions known to confer susceptibility for chronic cholangiopathy, such as hyper-IgM syndrome, could remain completely asymptomatic, on anti-infectious prophylaxis, well into the adulthood. However, the lifelong risk of the liver disease and its complications remains undisputable.

Diagnosis

Increased awareness of immunologists is a key to early detection of liver involvement. Routine biochemical blood tests and occasional but regular expert ultrasonography with stool screening for CS is recommended. Of note, standard stool microscopy could often miss protozoan infections, and therefore PCR-based techniques are preferable.

When CS is detected with whatever technique available, aggressive treatment is required. In immunodeficient patients, therapeutic options include nitazoxanide, paromomycin and azithromycin, often required in combination, in repeated courses, or indefinitely [8, 12]. This clearly indicates that they are not very effective and that avoidance of this ubiquitous pathogen is recommended if possible. Thus, preventative measures such as drinking boiled water or azithromycin three times a week may be more appropriate in children diagnosed with conditions known to confer susceptibility to cholangiopathies such as hyper-IgM syndrome.

If prominence or dilatation of bile ducts is noted on ultrasound scan (USS), further imaging with magnetic resonance cholangio-pancreatography (MRCP) is indicated. If MRCP is suggestive of dominant biliary stricture, endoscopic ret-

rograde cholangio-pancreatography (ERCP) is required in order to attempt balloon dilatation, sample the bile for microbiology and biopsy the suspected lesion to rule out cholangiocarcinoma. Percutaneous liver biopsy under intravenous antibiotic cover is indicated in presence of consistent biochemical abnormality in patients with PIDs (see Fig. 62.1).

ERCP demonstrating diffuse CS-positive cholangiopathy in a 7-year-old immunodeficient patient with dedicator of cytokinesis 8 protein (DOCK8) deficiency (a form of hyper IgE syndrome)

Management

Liver replacement will not work for the patients with PIDs until their immune defect is also rectified. There are many reports describing recurrence of cholangiopathy in the liver grafts within months after successful liver transplantation. Patients with less advanced liver disease can survive isolated non-myeloablative HSCT, but generally children with established cholangiopathies secondary to hyper-IgM syndrome or any other PIDs should be identified and screened for a matched donor for HSCT early [13]. When the liver injury becomes clinically more severe, the children with PIDs are unlikely to tolerate conventional HSCT protocols, which often include potentially hepatotoxic medications. Thus, they should be transplanted while their liver involvement remains minimal, mild or absent if a good donor is available

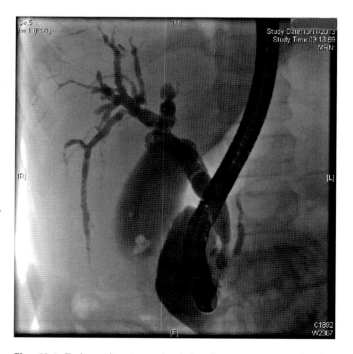

Fig. 62.1 Endoscopic retrograde cholangio-pancreatogram showing diffuse bilateral intra- and extrahepatic cholangiopathy in a child with a form of hyper IgE syndrome (DOCK8 deficiency)

[14]. A sequential approach with combined liver and non-myeloablative ("mini") HSCT may be required for the ones with decompensated biliary cirrhosis and complications of advanced liver disease [15].

Effective HSCT not only prevents progression of established cholangiopathy but also could revert the histological abnormalities. We have observed four children with significant improvement of their histological features of cholangiopathy within couple of years after HSCT. However, there was no short-term change in the calibre of their bile ducts on ultrasonography [16].

Over the past decade, we have observed a reducing number of patients with PIDs and advanced chronic liver disease. There are two possible explanations for that: (1) these patients are referred earlier due to increased awareness of possible liver problems among immunologists and (2) they receive their HSCT earlier, before serious liver disease develops. It is hoped that this strategy will continue to work and that the hepatologists would only exceptionally be required to see the patients with PIDs.

Haemophagocytic Lymphohistiocytosis

Haemophagocytic lymphohistiocytosis (HLH) is a condition which probably still remains underdiagnosed due to specific diagnostic tools and the clinical features mimicking acute septicaemia of early infancy and relatively atypical diagnostic approach. Majority of primary or familial HLH cases could be regarded as a form of PID. Secondary or nonfamilial forms can be associated with any infectious pathogen or presence of malignancy. Some use the term macrophage activation syndrome to highlight ubiquitous nature of this systemic reaction. A subgroup of patients with primary perforin deficiency presents acutely, often in infancy, with acute liver failure, but also in respiratory distress, fever, pancytopenia, rash and renal impairment, all indicative of systemic involvement. Perforin is a 60 kDa polypeptide, produced by cytoplasmic granules of activated natural killer (NK) cells and cytotoxic lymphocytes. Perforin then assists in primary immune response by forming perforations/"pores" on membrane of the invading cells, facilitating entry of mediators such as granzyme, which lead to osmotic cell lysis and consequent cell death [17]. There are at least five different loci where mutations for familial forms of HLH can be detected [17].

The liver involvement is frequently so severe to warrant consideration for liver transplantation. In addition to classical signs of acute liver failure such as hyperbilirubinemia, coagulopathy and hypoalbuminemia with ascites, those patients have hyperferritinaemia, hypertriglyceridaemia, hypofibrinogenaemia and signs of activated T lymphocytes, in particular interleukin (IL)-2R positive cells in circulation.

Patients often exhibit fever, splenomegaly and pancytopenia. Bone marrow aspirate reveals haemophygocytosis—a phenomenon defined by macrophages engulfing other cells and cellular debris. This urgent situation requires prompt identification of immune defect if it underlies the clinical situation, as liver transplantation would only be a palliative measure; the underlying ongoing immune overactivity continues. Potential cure is control of the immune reaction by combination of steroids and chemotherapy (HLH protocol) [18]. The mortality is high and surviving patients should be worked up for HSCT as each new exposure to an infectious agent could trigger another life-threatening episode of haemophagocytosis [18].

Therefore, any child who presents in acute liver failure with fever, splenomegaly and pancytopenia should, in addition to standard treatment of this condition, be urgently investigated for primary immunodeficiency by performing bone marrow aspirate and flow cytometry for expression of IL-2R and perforin on activated lymphocytes. Suggestion that the child could be immune deficient may indicate that consideration for emergency liver transplantation may not be justified.

References

1. Notarangelo LD. Primary immunodeficiencies. J Allerg Clin Imm. 2010;125(2 Suppl 2):S182–94.
2. Casanova JL, Fieschi C, Zhang SY, Abel L. Revisiting human primary immunodeficiencies. J Int Med. 2008;264(2):115–27.
3. Dvorak CC, Cowan MJ. Hematopoietic stem cell transplantation for primary immunodeficiency disease. Bone Marrow Transpl. 2008;41(2):119–26.
4. Rodrigues F, Davies EG, Harrison P, McLauchlin J, Karani J, Portmann B, et al. Liver disease in children with primary immunodeficiencies. J Pediatr. 2004;145(3):333–9.
5. Stephens J, Cosyns M, Jones M, Hayward A. Liver and bile duct pathology following *Cryptosporidium parvum* infection of the immunodeficient mice. Hepatology 1999;30:27–35.
6. Chen XM, Levine SA, Tietz P, et al. *Cryptosporidium parvum* is cytopathic for cultured human biliary epithelia via an apoptotic mechanism. Hepatology 1998;28:906–13.
7. Cello JP. Acquired immunodeficiency syndrome cholangiopathy: spectrum of disease. Am J Med. 1989;86:539–46.
8. Gerber DA, Green M, Jaffe R, Greenberg D, et al. Cryptosporidial infections after solid organ transplantation in children. Pediatr Transplant. 2000;4:50–5.
9. Durandy A, Honjo T. Human genetic defects in class-switch recombination (hyper-IgM syndromes). Curr Opin Immunol. 2001;13(5):543–8.
10. Winkelstein JA, Marino MC, Ochs H, Fuleihan R, Scholl PR, Geha R, et al. The X-Linked hyper-IgM syndrome: clinical and immunologic features of 79 patients. Medicine 2003;82(6):373–84.
11. Hayward AR, Levy J, Facchetti F, Notarangelo L, Ochs HD, Etzioni A, et al. Cholangiopathy and tumors of the pancreas, liver, and biliary tree in boys with X-linked immunodeficiency with hyper-IgM. J Immunol. 1997;158(2):977–83.
12. Anderson VR, Curran MP. Nitazoxanide: a review of its use in the treatment of gastrointestinal infections. Drugs. 2007;67(13):1947–67.

13. Amrolia P, Gaspar HB, Hassan A, Webb D, Jones A, Sturt N, et al. Nonmyeloablative stem cell transplantation for congenital immunodeficiencies. Blood 2000;96(4):1239–46.

14. Hadžić N, Pagliuca A, Rela M, Portmann B, Jones A, Veys P, et al. Correction of the hyper-IgM syndrome after liver and bone marrow transplantation. N Eng J Med. 2000;342(5)320–4.

15. Jacobsohn DA, Emerick KM, Scholl P, Melin-Aldana H, O'Gorman M, Duerst R, et al. Nonmyeloablative hematopoietic stem cell transplant for X-linked hyper-immunoglobulin m syndrome with cholangiopathy. Pediatrics. 2004;113(2):e122–7.

16. Davies EG, Zen Y, Veys P, Mieli-Vergani G, Hadzic N. Reversal of histological changes of cholangiopathy after haematopoietic stem cell transplantation in children with primary immunodeficiencies (submitted for publication).

17. Aricò M, Danesino C, Pende D, Moretta L. Pathogenesis of haemophagocytic lymphohistiocytosis. Br J Haematol. 2001;114(4):761–9.

18. Henter JI, Horne A, Aricó M, Egeler RM, Filipovich AH, Imashuku S, et al. HLH-2004: diagnostic and therapeutic guidelines for hemophagocytic lymphohistiocytosis. Pediatr Blood Cancer, 2007;48(2):124–31.

Autoimmune Liver Disease

63

Giorgina Mieli-Vergani and Diego Vergani

Introduction

Autoimmune liver disorders are inflammatory diseases characterized histologically by a dense mononuclear cell infiltrate in the portal tract that invades the surrounding parenchyma (interface hepatitis, Fig. 63.1a), biochemically by increased levels of transaminases, and serologically by the presence of circulating autoantibodies and high levels of immunoglobulin G (IgG). These disorders usually respond to immunosuppressive treatment, which should be instituted as soon as a diagnosis is made. These conditions can present insidiously or with a picture of acute hepatitis. Best results are obtained with early institution of immunosuppression [1–3].

There are three liver disorders in which liver damage is likely to arise from an autoimmune attack: autoimmune hepatitis (AIH), autoimmune sclerosing cholangitis (ASC), and de novo AIH after liver transplant.

Autoimmune Hepatitis

Clinical Features

Two forms of AIH are recognized according to the type of autoantibody present in the serum (Table 63.1). Type 1 AIH (AIH-1) is positive for smooth muscle antibody (SMA) and/or antinuclear antibody (ANA), while type 2 AIH (AIH-2) for anti-liver/kidney microsomal type 1 (anti LKM-1) and/or anti-liver cytosol type 1 (anti-LC-1) antibody (Fig. 63.2).

AIH-1 accounts for two thirds of the cases and presents often around puberty, while AIH-2 tends to present at a younger age and also during infancy. IgG is usually raised at disease onset in both types, though 15 % of children with AIH-1 and 25 % of those with AIH-2 have normal levels. IgA deficiency is common in AIH-2 [4]. Severity of disease is similar in the two types [4, 5], but anti-LKM1-positive children have higher levels of bilirubin and transaminases at onset than those who are ANA/SMA positive and present significantly more frequently with fulminant hepatic failure [4]. Excluding children with the fulminant presentation, a severely impaired hepatic synthetic function, as indicated by the presence of prolonged prothrombin time and hypoalbuminemia, is more common in AIH-1 than in AIH-2. The severity of interface hepatitis at diagnosis is similar in both types, but cirrhosis on initial biopsy is more frequent in AIH-1 than in AIH-2, suggesting a more chronic course of disease in the former. Progression to cirrhosis during treatment is more frequent in AIH-1.

In both types of AIH, a more severe disease course and a higher tendency to relapse are associated with the possession of antibodies to soluble liver antigen (SLA) [6, 7]. In both types, some 20 % of patients have associated autoimmune disorders—including thyroiditis, vitiligo, type 1 diabetes, inflammatory bowel disease (IBD), and nephrotic syndrome—and some 40 % have a family history of autoimmune disease (Table 63.1) [4].

There are three clinical patterns of AIH presentation (Table 63.1) [4]:

a. In at least 40 % of patients, the presentation is indistinguishable from that of an acute viral hepatitis (nonspecific symptoms of malaise, nausea/vomiting, anorexia, and abdominal pain, followed by jaundice, dark urine, and pale stools). Some children, particularly those who are anti-LKM1-positive, develop acute hepatic failure with grade II to IV hepatic encephalopathy (fulminant hepatitis) within 2–8 weeks from onset of symptoms.

G. Mieli-Vergani (✉)
Pediatric Liver, GI and Nutrition Centre, King's College Hospital, Denmark Hill, London SE5 9RS, UK
e-mail: giorgina.vergani@kcl.ac.uk

D. Vergani
Institute of Liver Studies, King's College Hospital, London, UK

© Springer International Publishing Switzerland 2016
S. Guandalini et al. (eds.), *Textbook of Pediatric Gastroenterology, Hepatology and Nutrition*,
DOI 10.1007/978-3-319-17169-2_63

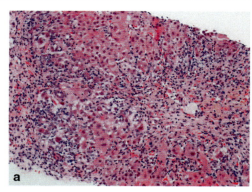
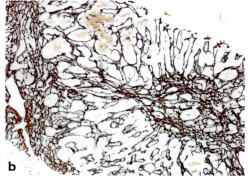

Fig. 63.1 Histological features of autoimmune hepatitis. **a** Portal and periportal lymphocyte and plasma cell infiltrate, extending to and disrupting the parenchymal limiting plate (interface hepatitis). Swollen hepatocytes, pyknotic necroses and acinar inflammation are present. Hematoxylin and eosin staining. **b** Reticulin staining of the same biopsy showing connective tissue collapse resulting from hepatocyte death and expanding from the portal area into the lobule ('bridging collapse')

Table 63.1 Clinical presentation, histological features and HLA association of childhood autoimmune liver disease. (King's College Hospital experience [4, 6, 10, 25])

Parameter	AIH-1	AIH-2	ASC
Median age in years	11	7	12
Mode of presentation (%)			
Acute hepatitis	47	40	37
Acute liver failure	3	25	0
Insidious onset	38	25	37
Complication of chronic liver disease	12	10	26
Associated autoimmune-disorders (%)	22	20	48
Inflammatory bowel disease (%)	20	12	44
Abnormal cholangiogram (%)	0	0	100
ANA/SMA (%)	100	25	96
Anti-LKM-1 (%)	0	100	4
pANNA (%)	45	11	74
Anti-SLA[a] (%) a	58	58	41
Low C4 level (%)	89	83	70
Increased frequency of HLA DR*0301	Yes	No[b]	No
Increased frequency of HLA DR*0701	No	Yes	No
Increased frequency of HLA DR*1301	No	No	Yes
Interface hepatitis (%)			
Any degree	92	94	60
Moderate/severe	66	72	35
Histological biliary features (%)	28	6	35
Cirrhosis (%)	69	38	15

AIH autoimmune hepatitis, *ANA* antinuclear antibodies, *ASC* autoimmune sclerosing cholangitis, *SMA* anti-smooth muscle antibodies, *anti-LKM-1* anti-liver kidney microsomal type 1 antibody, *pANNA* peripheral anti-nuclear neutrophil antibodies, *anti-SLA* anti-soluble liver antigen, *IgG* immunoglobulin G, *C4* C4 component of complement, *HLA* human leukocyte antigen
[a] Measured by radioligand assay [6]
[b] But increased in HLA DR*0701 negative patients [10]

b. In 25–40% of patients, the onset is insidious, with an illness characterized by progressive fatigue, relapsing jaundice, headache, anorexia, amenorrhea, and weight loss, lasting for several months and even years before diagnosis.

c. In about 10% of patients, there is no history of jaundice, and the diagnosis follows presentation with complications of portal hypertension, such as splenomegaly, haematemesis from oesophageal varices, bleeding diathesis, chronic diarrhea, and weight loss.

The mode of presentation of AIH in childhood is therefore variable, and the disease should be suspected and excluded in all children presenting with symptoms and signs of liver disease not ascribable to more common pathologies. The course of the disease can be fluctuating, with flares and spontaneous remissions, a pattern that may result in delayed referral and diagnosis. The majority of children, however, on physical examination have clinical signs of an underlying chronic liver disease, including cutaneous stigmata (spider nevi, palmar erythema, leukonychia, striae), firm liver, and

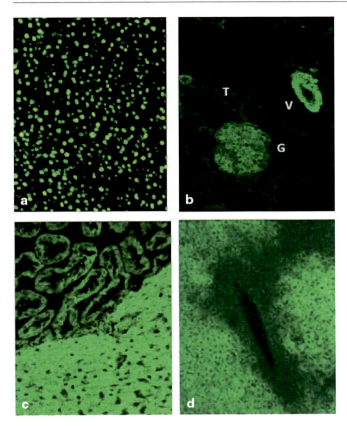

Fig. 63.2 Autoantibody immunofluorescence pattern on rodent tissue substrates. *Panel A* antinuclear antibody (*ANA*; liver): The homogeneous pattern is the most common in autoimmune hepatitis. *Panel B* smooth muscle antibody (*SMA*; kidney): SMA stains the smooth muscle of arterial vessels *(V)*, glomeruli *(G)*, and tubules (*T*; picture courtesy of Dr Luigi Muratori). *Panel C* anti-liver kidney microsomal type 1 antibody (*LKM-1*; kidney and liver): anti-LKM-1 stains the cytoplasm of hepatocytes and proximal renal tubules. *Panel D* anti-liver cytosol type 1 (*anti-LC-1*; liver): anti-LC-1 stains the cytoplasm of hepatocytes with a weakening of the stain around the central vein

splenomegaly. At ultrasound, the liver parenchyma of these patients is often nodular and heterogeneous.

Epidemiology and Genetic Predisposition

The epidemiology of childhood AIH has not been studied. Data collected at the King's College Hospital Pediatric Hepatology tertiary referral centre show an increase in the yearly incidence of juvenile autoimmune liver disease, only partially explained by a referral bias: In the 1990s, it represented 2.3% of some 400 children older than 4 months who were newly referred yearly; since 2000, the yearly incidence has increased to 12%.

In northern Europe, pediatric AIH-1, similar to adult AIH, is associated with the possession of the human leukocyte antigen (HLA) DRB1*03 (Table 63.1) [4, 8]. In contrast to adult patients, possession of DRB1*04 does not predispose to AIH in childhood, and this can even exert a protective

role [4]. AIH-2 is associated with possession of DRB1*07, and, in DR7-negative patients, with possession of DRB1*03 (Table 63.1) [9, 10]. In Egypt, AIH-2 appears to be associated also with possession of HLA-DRB1*15 [11]. In Brazil and Egypt, the primary susceptibility allele for AIH-1 is DRB1*1301, but a secondary association with DRB1*0301 has also been identified [11, 12]. Interestingly, in South America, possession of the HLA-DRB1*1301 allele not only predisposes to pediatric AIH-1 but is also associated with persistent infection with the endemic hepatitis A virus [13, 14]. Pediatric patients with AIH, whether anti-LKM-1 or ANA/SMA positive, have isolated partial deficiency of the HLA class III complement component C4, which is genetically determined [15].

AIH-2 can be a part of the autoimmune polyendocrinopathy–candidiasis–ectodermal dystrophy (APECED) syndrome, an autosomal-recessive monogenic disorder [16, 17] in which the liver disease is reportedly present in over 20% of cases [18, 19].

Diagnosis

The diagnosis of AIH is based on a series of inclusion and exclusion criteria [1–3].

Liver biopsy is necessary to establish the diagnosis; the typical histological picture including a dense mononuclear and plasma cell infiltration of the portal areas, which expands into the liver lobule, destruction of the hepatocytes at the periphery of the lobule with erosion of the limiting plate ('interface hepatitis'; Fig. 63.1a), connective tissue collapse resulting from hepatocyte death and expanding from the portal area into the lobule ('bridging collapse'; Fig. 63.1b), and hepatic regeneration with 'rosette' formation. In addition to the typical histology, other positive criteria include elevated serum transaminase and IgG levels and presence of ANA, SMA, anti-LKM-1, or anti-LC-1.

The diagnosis of AIH has been advanced by the scoring systems developed by the International Autoimmune Hepatitis Group (IAIHG) for adult patients [1, 2] where negative criteria, such as evidence of infection with hepatitis B or C virus, Wilson disease, or alcohol, among others, are taken into account in addition to the positive criteria mentioned above. The IAIHG scoring system was devised mainly for research purposes to allow ready comparison between series from different centres, but it has also been used clinically, including in pediatric series. More recently, the IAIHG has published a simplified scoring system based on autoantibodies, IgG, histology, and exclusion of viral hepatitis that is better suited to clinical application [20]. However, neither scoring system is suitable to the juvenile form of the disease, where diagnostically relevant autoantibodies often have titers lower than the cut-off value considered positive in adults [21–23]. In addition, neither system can distinguish between

AIH and ASC (see below) [24, 25], which can only be differentiated if a cholangiogram is performed at presentation.

A key diagnostic criterion for all AIH scoring systems is the detection of autoantibodies (ANA, SMA, anti-LKM-1, and anti-LC-1), which not only assists in the diagnosis but also allows differentiation of AIH types. ANA and SMA that characterize AIH-1 and anti-LKM-1 and anti-LC-1 that define AIH-2 are usually mutually exclusive; in those instances when they are present simultaneously, the clinical course is similar to that of AIH-2 [26]. A major target of SMA is the actin of smooth muscle, whereas the molecular target of anti-LKM-1 is cytochrome P-4502D6 (CYP2D6) [27] and of anti-LC-1 is formiminotransferase cyclodeaminase [28]. ANA, SMA, anti-LKM-1, and anti-LC-1 should be sought by indirect immunofluorescence using rodent stomach, kidney, and liver as substrate, as other techniques, for example commercially available enzyme-linked immunosorbent assay (ELISA), remain to be fully validated (Fig. 63.2) [26]. In contrast to adults, in healthy children, autoantibody reactivity is infrequent, so that titers of 1/20 for ANA and SMA and 1/10 for anti-LKM-1 are clinically relevant. Anti-LC-1, also detectable by indirect immunofluorescence, can be present on its own, but frequently occurs in association with anti-LKM-1. This co-occurrence can go unnoticed because anti-LKM-1 obscures the anti-LC-1 pattern. Anti-LC-1 can also be detected by commercial ELISA. Positivity for autoantibodies is not sufficient for the diagnosis of AIH since they can be present, usually at low titer, in other liver disorders such as viral hepatitides [29, 30], Wilson disease [31], and nonalcoholic steatohepatitis [32].

Other autoantibodies less commonly tested but of diagnostic importance include peripheral antinuclear neutrophil antibody (atypical perinuclear anti-neutrophil cytoplasmic antibodies, pANCA or peripheral anti-nuclear neutrophil antibodies, pANNA) and anti-SLA. pANNA is frequently found in AIH-1 and ASC, and it is also common in IBD, while it is virtually absent in AIH-2. Anti-SLA, originally described as the hallmark of a third type of AIH [33], is also found in up to 50% of patients with AIH-1, AIH-2, or ASC, where it defines a more severe course [6, 7]. Anti-SLA is not detectable by immunofluorescence, but the definition of its molecular target as Sep (O-phosphoserine) tRNA:Sec (selenocysteine) tRNA synthase (SepSecS) [34, 35] has enabled the establishment of molecularly based diagnostic assays. However, it should be noted that ELISAs are less sensitive than radioligand assays available in research laboratories [34, 35].

There are a small proportion of patients with AIH without detectable autoantibodies. This condition, which responds to immunosuppression like the seropositive form, represents seronegative AIH [36], a rare type of AIH in adults, whose prevalence and clinical characteristics remain to be defined in children.

Pathophysiology

The typical histologic picture of AIH, which is characterized by a dense mononuclear cell infiltrate eroding the limiting plate and invading the parenchyma (interface hepatitis, Fig. 63.1a), first suggested that auto-aggressive cellular immunity might be involved in its causation [37]. Immunocytochemical studies have identified the phenotype of the infiltrating cells. T lymphocytes mounting the alpha/beta T cell receptor predominate. Among the T cells, a majority is positive for the cluster of differentiation (CD)4 helper/inducer phenotype, and a sizable minority is positive for the CD8 cytotoxic phenotype. Lymphocytes of non-T cell lineage are fewer and include (in decreasing order of frequency) natural killer cells (CD16/CD56 positive), macrophages, and B lymphocytes [38]. Natural killer T cells, which express simultaneously markers of both natural killer (CD56) and T cells (CD3), are involved in liver damage in an animal model of AIH [39].

A powerful stimulus must be promoting the formation of the massive inflammatory cell infiltrate present at diagnosis. Whatever the initial trigger, it is most probable that such a high number of activated inflammatory cells cause liver damage. There are different possible pathways that an immune attack can follow to inflict damage on the hepatocyte (Fig. 63.3). Liver damage is believed to be orchestrated by CD4-positive T lymphocytes recognizing a self-antigenic peptide. To trigger an autoimmune response, the peptide must be embraced by an HLA class II molecule and presented to uncommitted T helper (Th0) cells by professional antigen-presenting cells (APCs), with the co-stimulation of ligand–ligand (CD28 on Th0, CD80 on APC) interaction between the two cells. The Th0 cells become activated, differentiate into functional phenotypes according to the cytokines prevailing in the microenvironment and the nature of the antigen, and initiate a cascade of immune reactions determined by the cytokines they produce. Arising in the presence of the macrophage-produced interleukin-12 (IL-12), Th1 cells secrete mainly IL-2 and interferon-γ, which activate macrophages, enhance expression of HLA class I (increasing the vulnerability of liver cells to cytotoxic attack), and induce expression of HLA class II molecules on hepatocytes, which then become able to present the autoantigenic peptide to Th cells, thus perpetuating the immune recognition cycle. Th2 cells, which differentiate from Th0 if the microenvironment is rich in IL-4, produce mainly IL-4, -5, and -10, which induce autoantibody production by B lymphocytes. Physiologically, Th1 and Th2 cells antagonize each other. The process of autoantigen recognition is strictly controlled by regulatory mechanisms. If these regulatory mechanisms fail, the autoimmune attack is perpetuated. Over the past three decades, different aspects of the above pathogenic scenario have been investigated.

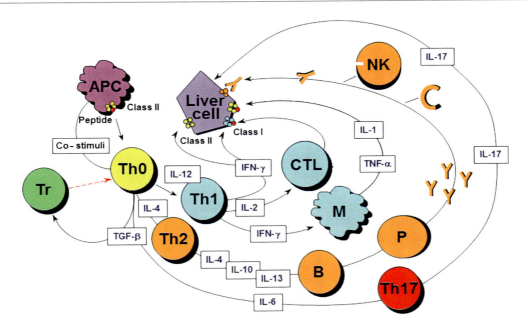

Fig. 63.3 An autoantigen is presented to uncommitted T helper (Th0) lymphocytes within the HLA class II molecule of an antigen-presenting cell (APC) in either the regional lymph nodes or within the liver itself. Activated Th0 cells differentiate into Th1 or Th2 cells in the presence of interleukin (IL)-12 or IL-4 and according to the nature of the antigen, and trigger a series of immune reactions determined by the cytokines they produce: Th1 cells secrete IL-2 and interferon-gamma (IFN-γ), cytokines that stimulate cytotoxic T-lymphocytes (CTL), enhance expression of class I and induce expression of class II HLA molecules on the liver cells and activate macrophages. The latter release IL-1 and tumour necrosis factor-alpha (TNF-α). Th2 cells secrete mainly IL-4, IL-10, and IL-13, and stimulate autoantibody production by B lymphocytes. In the presence of defective regulatory T cells (Treg), hepatocyte destruction ensues from the engagement of damaging effector mechanisms, including CTL, cytokines released by Th1, and by activated macrophages, complement activation, or adhesion of natural killer (NK) cells to autoantibody-coated hepatocytes through their Fc receptors. Th17 cells, a recently described proinflammatory population that derives from Th0 cells in the presence of transforming growth factor beta (TGF-β) and IL-6, are the focus of current investigation. (Adapted with permission from Ref. [40], with permission from Wiley-Blackwell)

An impairment of immunoregulatory mechanisms has been described in AIH. Both children and young adults with this condition have low levels of T cells expressing the CD8 marker and impaired suppressor cell function [41, 42] which segregate with the possession of the HLA haplotype B*08/DRB1*03 (formerly B8/DR3), and can be corrected by therapeutic doses of corticosteroids [43]. Furthermore, patients with AIH have been reported to have a specific defect in a subpopulation of T cells controlling the immune response to liver-specific membrane antigens [44]. Further evidence for an impairment of immunoregulatory function in AIH has been obtained in the past decade [45–47]. Among T cell subsets with potential immunosuppression function, CD4+ T cells constitutively expressing the IL-2R alpha chain (CD25; regulatory T cells, T-regs) have emerged as the dominant immunoregulatory population [48]. These cells, which represent 5–10 % of the total population of peripheral CD4+ T lymphocytes, control the innate and the adaptive immune responses by preventing the proliferation and effector function of autoreactive T cells. Their mechanism of action involves mainly a direct contact with the target cells, and, to a lesser extent, the release of immunoregulatory cytokines, such as IL 10 and tissue growth factor beta 1.

A numerical T-reg impairment affects both children and adults with AIH. This defect is more evident at diagnosis than during drug-induced remission, although even then circulating T-reg frequencies fail to reach the levels seen in health [45, 49, 50]. The percentage of T-regs inversely correlates with biomarkers of disease severity, suggesting that a reduction in regulatory T cells favours autoimmune liver disease. Importantly, T-regs from AIH patients at diagnosis are impaired in their ability to control the proliferation of CD4 and CD8 effector cells compared to T-regs isolated from AIH patients at remission or healthy subjects [49].

Recently, it was reported that effector CD4 T cells isolated from patients with AIH are less susceptible to the regulatory control exerted by T-regs. This defect is linked to reduced expression of the inhibitory receptor T cell immunoglobulin- and mucin-domain-containing-molecule-3 (Tim-3), which upon ligation of galectin-9 expressed by T-regs, induces effector cell death [51].

Hepatocytes from patients with AIH, in contrast to normal hepatocytes, express HLA class II molecules [52], and, although lacking the antigen-processing machinery typical of APCs, they may present peptides through a bystander mechanism. Given the impaired regulatory function and the inappropriate expression of HLA class II antigens on the hepatocytes, it is conceivable that an autoantigenic peptide is presented to the helper/inducer cells, leading to their activation. Although there is no direct evidence as yet that an autoantigenic peptide is presented and recognized, activation of helper cells has been documented in AIH [38, 53]. These activated cells possess the CD4 phenotype, and their numbers are highest when the disease is most active.

Most advances in the study of T cells have occurred in AIH-2, since the knowledge that CYP2D6 is the main autoantigen has enabled the characterization of both CD4 and CD8 T cells targeting this cytochrome. One study has shown that CD4 T cells from patients with AIH-2 positive for the predisposing HLA allele DRB1*0701 recognize seven regions of CYP2D6 [9], five of which have later been shown to be also recognized by CD8 T cells [54]. A high number of interferon-gamma-producing CD4 T cells and CD8 T cells are associated with biochemical evidence of liver damage, suggesting a combined cellular immune attack.

What triggers the immune system to react to an autoantigen is unknown. A lesson may be learned by the study of humoral autoimmune responses during viral infections. Thus, studies aimed at determining the specificity of the LKM-1 antibody, present in both the juvenile form of AIH and some patients with chronic hepatitis C virus (HCV) infection, have shown a high amino acid sequence homology between the HCV polyprotein and CYP2D6, the molecular target of anti-LKM-1, thus implicating a mechanism of molecular mimicry as a trigger for the production of anti LKM-1 in HCV infection [27, 55, 56]. It is therefore conceivable that an as-yet unknown virus infection may be at the origin of the autoimmune attack in AIH.

Titers of antibodies to liver-specific lipoprotein, a macromolecular complex present on the hepatocyte membrane, and its well-characterized component asialoglycoprotein receptor, correlate with the biochemical and histologic severity of AIH [57, 58]. Antibodies to alcohol dehydrogenase, a second well-defined component of liver-specific lipoprotein, have been described in patients with AIH [59]. Immunofluorescence studies on monodispersed suspensions of liver cells obtained from patients with AIH showed that these cells are coated with antibodies in vivo [60]. A pathogenic role for these autoantibodies has been indicated by cytotoxicity assays showing that autoantibody-coated hepatocytes from patients with AIH are killed when incubated with autologous lymphocytes. The effector cell was identified as an Fc receptor-positive mononuclear cell [61]. T cell clones obtained from liver biopsies of children with AIH and expressing the gamma/delta T cell receptor have been shown to be cytotoxic to a variety of targets but preferentially kill liver-derived cells as opposed to cell lines derived from other organs [62].

The establishment of cell lines and clones has shown that the majority of T cell clones obtained from the peripheral blood and a proportion of those from the liver of patients with AIH are CD4 positive and use the conventional alpha/beta T cell receptor [62–65]. Some of these CD4-positive clones were further characterized and were found to react with partially purified antigens, such as crude preparations of liver cell membrane or liver-specific lipoprotein [63], and with purified asialoglycoprotein receptor [63, 65] or recombinant CYP2D6 [64] and to be restricted by HLA class II molecules in their response. Because CD4 is the phenotype of Th cells, T cell clones were investigated for their ability to help autologous B lymphocytes in the production of immunoglobulin in vitro [63, 65]. Indeed, their coculture with B lymphocytes resulted in a dramatic increase in autoantibody production.

The possible role of Th17 cells in the pathogenesis of AIH is under investigation. Th17 cells contribute to autoimmunity by producing the proinflammatory cytokines IL-17, IL-22, and TNF-α and inducing hepatocytes to secrete IL-6 [66], which further enhances Th17 activation. Th17 cells have been shown to be elevated in the circulation and liver of patients with AIH [66].

Treatment

Unless it presents with fulminant hepatic failure (i.e. acute liver failure and encephalopathy, which usually requires urgent transplantation), AIH responds satisfactorily to immunosuppression, even in the presence of poor synthetic function and/or established cirrhosis. Treatment should be started with prednisolone 2 mg/g/day (maximum 60 mg/day), which is gradually decreased over a period of 4–8 weeks if there is progressive normalization of the transaminases, and then the patient is maintained on the minimal dose able to sustain normal transaminase levels, usually 5 mg/day. During the first 6–8 weeks of treatment, liver function tests should be checked weekly to allow a frequent fine-tuning of the treatment, avoiding severe steroid side effects. The initial goal is to obtain at least 80 % of reduction of the transaminase levels by 8 weeks of treatment. During this period of time, if progressive normalization of the liver function is not observed at weekly blood tests, azathioprine is added at a starting dose of 0.5 mg/g/day, which, in the absence of signs of toxicity, is increased up to a maximum of 2–2.5 mg/g/day until remission (i.e. normal transaminase levels) is achieved. Azathioprine is not recommended as first-line treatment because of its potential hepatotoxicity, particularly in severely jaundiced patients. Interestingly, it has been shown that neither thiopurine methyltransferase genotype nor activity predicts azathioprine hepatotoxicity in AIH, which appears instead to be related to the degree of liver fibrosis [67]. A preliminary report in a cohort of 30 children with AIH suggests that the measurements of the azathioprine metabolites 6-thioguanine and 6-methylmercaptopurine are useful in identifying drug toxicity and non-adherence and in achieving a level of 6-thioguanine considered therapeutic for IBD [68]. However, it has been reported that patients with AIH can achieve remission with azathioprine metabolite levels lower than those needed for IBD [69].

Although an 80 % decrease of initial transaminase levels is usually obtained within 6–8 weeks from starting treatment in most patients, complete normalization of liver function may take several months. In our own series, normalization of transaminase levels occurred at medians of 0.5 years (range 0.2–7 years) in ANA/SMA-positive children and 0.8 years (range 0.02–3.2 years) in anti-LKM-1-positive children [4]. Relapse while on treatment is common, affecting about 40 % of the patients and requiring a temporary increase of the steroid dose. An important role in relapse is played by non-adherence, particularly in adolescents [70]. The risk of relapse is higher if steroids are administered on an alternate-day schedule, often instituted in the unsubstantiated belief that it has a less negative effect on the child's growth. Small daily doses should be used because they are more effective in maintaining disease control and minimize the need for high-dose steroid pulses during relapses (with attendant more severe side effects). Side effects of steroid treatment are usually mild, the only serious complication being psychosis during induction of remission in 4 %, which resolves after prednisolone withdrawal [4]. All patients develop a transient increase in appetite and mild cushingoid features during the first few weeks of treatment. After 5 years of treatment, 56 % of our patients maintained their baseline centile for height or went up across a centile line, 38 % dropped across one centile line, and only 6 % dropped across two centile lines [71]. Moreover, all patients achieved their expected final height after a median steroid treatment of 8.9 years [72].

Treatment should be continued for at least 3 years before considering its cessation, after which period stopping treatment can be attempted but only if liver function tests and IgG levels have been persistently normal, and autoantibodies are either undetectable or detectable at very low titre (ANA/SMA < 1:10; anti-LKM-1 should be negative) over at least 12 months, and a follow up liver biopsy shows no inflammatory changes. However, it is advisable not to attempt treatment withdrawal during or immediately before puberty, when relapses are more common. Treatment withdrawal is reportedly successful in 20 % of children with AIH-1, but is rarely achieved in AIH-2 [4]. An important role in monitoring the response to treatment is the measurement of autoantibody titers and IgG levels, the fluctuation of which is correlated with disease activity [73]. The prognosis of those children with AIH who respond to immunosuppressive treat-

ment is generally good, with most patients surviving long term with excellent quality of life on low-dose medication. Development of end-stage liver disease requiring liver transplantation despite treatment, however, has been reported 8–14 years after diagnosis in 8.5 % of children with AIH [4].

Maintenance with azathioprine monotherapy has been advocated once remission is achieved [74], but whether this is effective long term and whether it offers any benefit on possible side effects compared to low-dose prednisolone/azathioprine maintenance is unclear.

Induction of remission has been obtained in 72 % treatment-naïve children with AIH-1 using cyclosporine A alone for 6 months, followed by maintenance with low-dose prednisone and azathioprine [75]. A 5-year follow-up of this study shows that 94 % of the patients eventually achieved remission, with minor side effects [76]. Whether this mode of induction has any advantage over the standard treatment remains to be evaluated in controlled studies in specialized centres.

Tacrolimus is a more potent immunosuppressive agent than cyclosporine, but it also has significant toxicity. There is limited evidence supporting its role as initial treatment of AIH apart from anecdotal reports in adults.

Budesonide has a hepatic first-pass clearance of >90 % of oral dose and fewer side effects than predniso(lo)ne, but cannot be used in the presence of cirrhosis, which affects at least two thirds of AIH patients. In a large European study, including adults and children with AIH, a combination of budesonide and azathioprine had fewer adverse effects compared to medium-dose standard prednisone and azathioprine [77]. In this study, budesonide at a dose of 3 mg three times daily, decreased upon response, was compared with prednisone 40 mg once daily reduced per protocol irrespective of response. After 6 months of treatment, remission was achieved in 60 % of the budesonide group but in only 39 % of the prednisone group, both percentages being worse than those achieved with standard treatment [4]. The results among the children recruited into this study were particularly disappointing, with a similarly low remission rate of 16 % for budesonide and 15 % for prednisone after 6 months of treatment and of 50 and 42 %, respectively, after 12 months of treatment, with similar steroid side effects in both groups, apart from higher frequency of weight gain in children on prednisone [78]. Large controlled studies are needed to establish the appropriate dose for children [79]. Nevertheless, budesonide could be a valid alternative in selected non-cirrhotic patients who are at risk of adverse effects from steroids.

In those patients (up to 10 %) in whom standard immunosuppression is unable to induce stable remission, or who are intolerant to azathioprine, mycophenolate mofetil at a dose of 20 mg/kg twice daily has been successfully used [80]. In case of persistent no response or of intolerance to mycophenolate mofetil (headache, diarrhea, nausea, dizziness, hair loss and neutropenia), the use of calcineurin inhibitors (cyclosporine A or tacrolimus) should be considered.

Children who present with fulminant hepatic failure, that is with grade 3–4 encephalopathy and international normalized ratio (INR)≥2, pose a particularly difficult therapeutic problem. Although it has been reported that they may benefit from conventional immunosuppressive therapy [81, 82], most require liver transplantation [4]. Encouraging results have been reported using cyclosporine A in anti-LKM-1-positive patients presenting with fulminant hepatitis [81]. These should be evaluated on a larger number of patients because our own experience has not confirmed the value of this therapeutic approach.

Autoimmune Polyendocrinopathy–Candidiasis–Ectodermal Dystrophy (APECED)

APECED is a monogenic disorder due to mutations of the *AIRE1* gene [16, 17]. Its phenotype is variable and includes AIH in about 20% of the cases [19]. This resembles AIH-2 and responds to standard immunosuppressive treatment [18], though the anti-LKM-1-like antibody detected by immunofluorescence targets a cytochrome (P4502A6) different from that of classical AIH-2. APECED, also known as autoimmune polyendocrine syndrome 1, is an autosomal recessive disorder caused by homozygous mutations in the *AIRE1* gene and characterized by a variety of organ-specific autoimmune diseases, the most common of which are hypoparathyroidism and primary adrenocortical failure, accompanied by chronic mucocutaneous candidiasis.

AIRE1 sequence consists of 14 exons containing 45 different mutations, with a 13-base-pair deletion at nucleotide 964 in exon 8 accounting for more than 70% of APECED alleles in the UK [17]. The protein encoded by AIRE1 is a transcription factor. AIRE1 is highly expressed in medullary epithelial cells and other stromal cells in the thymus involved in clonal deletion of self-reactive T cells. Studies in a murine model indicate that the gene inhibits organ-specific autoimmunity by inducing thymic expression of peripheral antigens in the medulla leading to central deletion of autoreactive T cells. Carriers of a single AIRE mutation do not develop APECED. However, although the inheritance pattern of APECED indicates a strictly recessive disorder, there are anecdotal data of mutations in a single copy of AIRE being associated with human autoimmunity of a less severe form than classically defined APECED [16, 17]. The role of AIRE1 heterozygote state in the development of AIH remains to be established. AIRE1 mutations have been reported in three children with severe AIH type 2 and extrahepatic autoimmune manifestations [83].

Autoimmune Sclerosing Cholangitis

Clinical Features

Sclerosing cholangitis is an uncommon disorder, characterized by chronic inflammation and fibrosis of the intrahepatic and/or extrahepatic bile ducts. When bile duct damage is detectable histologically, but cholangiography is normal, a diagnosis of 'small-duct disease' is made. In childhood, sclerosing cholangitis may occur as an individual disease or may develop in association with a wide variety of disorders. The term primary sclerosing cholangitis (PSC), used in adult patients, is not accurate to describe pediatric sclerosing cholangitis: 'Primary' denotes ignorance about etiology and pathogenesis, while in pediatrics there are well-defined forms of sclerosing cholangitis [25, 84–87]. In the neonatal period, pathological features of severe sclerosing cholangitis characterize biliary atresia as well as neonatal sclerosing cholangitis, a condition inherited in an autosomal recessive manner [88]. Some other inherited diseases and immunological defects may produce a clinical picture similar to adult PSC. For example, mild-to-moderate defects in the *ABCB4* (MDR3) gene are a likely cause of a number of cases of small-duct PSC in children and adults [89, 90], and sclerosing cholangitis may complicate a wide variety of disorders, including primary and secondary immunodeficiencies, Langerhans cell histiocytosis, psoriasis, cystic fibrosis, reticulum cell sarcoma and sickle cell anaemia. Moreover, an overlap syndrome between AIH and sclerosing cholangitis (ASC), is significantly more common in children than in adults [25]. In only a relatively small number of pediatric patients, sclerosing cholangitis occurs without any of the above defining features. The term of PSC would be better confined to the latter, as different types of sclerosing cholangitis respond to different therapeutic managements.

ASC is characterized by florid autoimmune features, positive autoantibodies, especially ANA and SMA, hypergammaglobulinaemia, and interface hepatitis on liver biopsy [25, 91]. Since these features are shared with AIH, and alkaline phosphatase (AP) or gamma-glutamyl transpeptidase (GGT) levels are often not elevated at disease onset, the diagnosis of ASC relies on cholangiographic studies. In a 16-year prospective study, during which all children with serological and histological features of autoimmune liver disease underwent liver biopsy, sigmoidoscopy, and cholangiography at presentation [25], approximately half were found to have bile duct changes characteristic of sclerosing cholangitis (Fig. 63.4) and were therefore diagnosed with ASC. Importantly, a quarter of children with ASC had no histological features pointing to bile duct involvement, despite abnormal cholangiograms. Virtually, all ASC patients were seropositive for ANA and/or SMA. In contrast to AIH, which is pre-

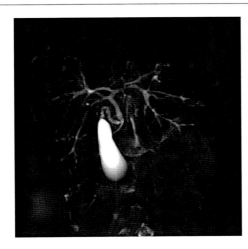

Fig. 63.4 Magnetic resonance cholangiography of a child with auto-immune sclerosing cholangitis showing a diffuse cholangiopathy with strictures and dilatations affecting the intra-hepatic bile ducts

dominantly a disease of females, ASC affects similarly boys and girls [25].

The mode of presentation of ASC is similar to that of AIH-1, although an association with IBD is more common in ASC (45%) than AIH-1 (20%) [25]. Of note, in the prospective study, only one third of the children with IBD had bowel symptoms, while the others were diagnosed because of surveillance sigmoidoscopy. At presentation, liver function tests—including GGT levels, which are a more reliable indicator of cholestasis than (AP) in growing children/adolescents, in whom AP often reflects bone growth—do not discriminate between AIH and ASC, though the AP/AST ratio is significantly higher in ASC (Table 63.2). Notably, atypical pANCA (also termed pANNA) positivity is present in 74% of children with ASC but only 45% of those with AIH-1 and 11% of those with AIH-2 [25]. Anti-SLA by a sensitive radioligand assay was found in some 50% of patients with ASC, and, also in this condition, it defines a more severe disease course [6].

HLA studies have shown that in the UK susceptibility to ASC is conferred by the possession of HLA DRB1*1301 [10].

Evolution from AIH to ASC was documented in one patient during the published prospective series [25] and has been observed in two further patients during follow up [92], suggesting that AIH and ASC are part of the same pathologic process.

Clinical, laboratory, and histological features of type 1 and 2 AIH and ASC are compared in Tables 63.1 and 63.2.

Though 'small-duct disease' is reported rarely in pediatric series, in a study [86], where cholangiography was mainly performed by magnetic resonance cholangiopancreatography (MRCP), no radiological biliary involvement was detected despite histological evidence of sclerosing cholangitis in a high proportion (36%) of patients, some of whom had autoimmune features. Whether this finding is due to a lower sensitivity of the MRCP compared to retrograde cholangio-pancreatography in detecting biliary changes remains to be verified.

Currently, in our centre, imaging of the biliary system by MRCP, followed by ERCP if MRCP is not informative, as well as colonoscopy, are part of the evaluation of all children with liver disease associated with autoimmune features.

The IAIHG scoring systems for the diagnosis of AIH, as currently formulated, do not allow distinguishing AIH from ASC [24, 25] as they do not include cholangiographic investigations at presentation. Table 63.3 summarizes diagnostic criteria for juvenile autoimmune liver disease.

Treatment

Children with ASC respond usually well to the same immunosuppressive treatment described above for AIH [25,

Table 63.2 Biochemical findings at presentation in childhood autoimmune liver disease. (King's College Hospital experience [4, 25]. Results expressed as median (range))

	AIH	ASC
Bilirubin (nv < 20 μmol/L)	35 (4–306)	20 (4–179)
Albumin (nv > 35 g/L)	35 (25–47)	39 (27–54)
AST (nv < 50 IU/L)	333 (24–4830)	102 (18–1215)
INR (nv < 1.2)	1.2 (0.96–2.5)	1.1 (0.9–1.6)
GGT (nv < 50 IU/L)	76 (29–383)	129 (13–948)
AP (nv < 350 IU/L)	356 (131–878)	303 (104–1710)
AP/AST ratio	1.14 (0.05–14.75)	3.96 (0.20–14.20)

AIH autoimmune hepatitis, *ASC* autoimmune sclerosing cholangitis, *AST* aspartate aminotransferase, *INR* international normalised ratio, *GGT* gamma glutamyltranspeptidase, *AP* alkaline phosphatase, *nv* normal values

Table 63.3 Diagnostic criteria of juvenile autoimmune liver disease

Elevated transaminases
Positivity for circulating autoantibodies
ANA and/or SMA (titre ≥ 1:20) = AIH-1 or ASC
Anti-LKM-1 (titre ≥ 1:10) = AIH-2
Anti-LC-1 = AIH-2
Elevated immunoglobulin G (in 80% of cases)
Liver biopsy:
Interface hepatitis
Multilobular collapse
Exclusion of viral hepatitis, Wilson disease and non-alcholic steatohepatitis
Cholangiogram:
Normal = AIH or 'small duct disease'
Abnormal = ASC

AIH autoimmune hepatitis, *ASC* autoimmune sclerosing cholangitis, *ANA* anti-nuclear antibodies, *SMA* anti-smooth muscle antibodies, *anti-LKM-1* anti-liver kidney microsomal type 1 antibody, *anti-LC-1* anti-liver cytosol type 1 antibody

87] with resolution of liver test abnormalities within a few months in most patients. Response to immunosuppressive drugs is less satisfactory if the disease is long standing before starting treatment [85, 86].

The medium- to long-term prognosis of ASC is worse than that of AIH because of progression of bile duct disease despite treatment in some 50% of patients, with 20% of them eventually requiring liver transplantation [25, 87, 92].

Based on a reported beneficial effect in adult PSC, ursodeoxycholic acid (UDCA) is added to the treatment of ASC, but whether it is helpful in arresting the progression of the bile duct disease remains to be established. In adults with PSC, high-dose UDCA was reported as more beneficial than standard doses [93], but a randomized double-blind controlled study from the Mayo Clinic shows that high-dose UDCA has a negative effect [94]. It is prudent, therefore, to use doses not higher than 15–20 mg/kg/day.

Reactivation of the liver disease often follows flares of the intestinal disease in sclerosing cholangitis patients with IBD. It is therefore essential to control the bowel pathology to avoid progression of liver disease. A beneficial effect of oral vancomycin (500 mg tds) has been reported in 14 patients with sclerosing cholangitis and IBD [95]. All patients showed improvement of liver function tests and erythrocyte sedimentation rate, which was more marked in those without cirrhosis. These results await confirmation in a larger number of patients. Whether vancomycin acts through its antibiotic or immunomodulatory [96] properties remains to be elucidated.

Pathophysiology

It is unclear if the juvenile autoimmune form of sclerosing cholangitis and AIH are two distinct entities or different aspects of the same condition. Akin to AIH, in addition to positivity for ANA and/or SMA, liver-specific autoantibodies, including antibodies to liver-specific lipoprotein, asialoglycoprotein receptor, alcohol dehydrogenase, and SLA, can be found in ASC [6, 59, 97]. Susceptibility to ASC in children is conferred by the possession of HLA DRB1*1301, while possession of HLA DRB1*0401 appears to be protective. HLA DRB1*1301 has also been associated with susceptibility to PSC in adults [98]. An association with HLA DRB1*1301 has been reported in children with ANA/SMA-positive AIH in Argentina, but no cholangiographic studies were performed, and therefore not excluding the possibility that the cohort comprised also children with ASC [99].

Liver Transplant and Autoimmune Liver Disease

Liver transplantation is indicated in patients with AIH who present with fulminant hepatic failure (with encephalopathy) and patients with AIH or sclerosing cholangitis who develop end-stage liver disease despite treatment. The latter is more likely when established cirrhosis is present at diagnosis, or if there is a long history of liver disease before the start of treatment. Approximately, 10% of children with AIH and 20% of those with sclerosing cholangitis require liver transplantation. After transplantation, recurrent AIH has been described in about 20% of cases [100] and recurrent sclerosing cholangitis in 27–67% of transplanted patients [92, 86]. Diagnosis of recurrence is based on biochemical abnormalities, presence of autoantibodies, interface hepatitis on liver histology, steroid dependence, and, for sclerosing cholangitis, presence of cholangiopathy. Recurrence may occur even years after transplantation, and consequently maintenance of steroid-based immunosuppression at a higher dose than that used for patients not transplanted for autoimmune liver disease is recommended. While recurrence of AIH does not usually affect post-transplant outcome, recurrence of ASC leads to re-transplantation in a high proportion of patients [92]. Recurrence of sclerosing cholangitis after transplantation is often associated to uncontrolled IBD [100, 101]. In this context, it is of interest that PSC recurrence in adults with IBD can be prevented by pre-liver transplant colectomy [102–104].

De novo AIH After Liver Transplantation

In the late 1990s, it was observed that AIH can arise de novo after liver transplantation in children who had not been transplanted for autoimmune liver disease. Characteristic of this condition is a histological picture of interface hepatitis and multilobular collapse associated with increased IgG levels and positive autoantibodies. These include not only ANA, SMA, and classical anti-LKM-1 but also atypical anti-LKM-1, staining the renal tubules but not the liver. After the original report [105], de novo AIH following liver transplant has been confirmed by several studies in both adult and pediatric patients [106–109] and has been reported to be more frequent in steroid-free antirejection regimens [110, 111]. Importantly, treatment with prednisolone and azathioprine using the same schedule for classical AIH, concomitant with reduction of the calcineurin inhibitor dose, is highly effective in de novo AIH, leading to excellent graft and patient survival. It is of interest that these patients do not respond satisfactorily to the standard antirejection treatment schedule, making it essential to reach an early diagnosis to avoid graft loss. Rapamycin has been reported to be effective in difficult-to-treat patients [112].

Pathophysiology of De Novo AIH after Liver Transplant

Whether the liver damage observed in these patients is a form of rejection or the consequence of an autoimmune injury, possibly triggered by drugs or viral infection, remains to be established.

Several reports have investigated whether the development of de novo AIH is associated to the possession of specific major histocompatibility complex (MHC) antigens either by the recipient or by the donor. In the original report, five of seven children with de novo AIH received livers from donors who were HLA DR3 or DR4 positive [105]. In adults, Heneghan et al. found HLA DR3 or DR4 in either donors or recipients in all cases [113], and Salcedo et al. noted an overrepresentation of DR3 in recipients [114].

There are several nonmutually exclusive explanations as to why autoimmunity and AIH may arise de novo in patients transplanted for non-autoimmune conditions. Besides autoantigen release from the damaged tissue, molecular mimicry might be involved, where immune responses to external pathogens become directed towards structurally similar self-components [115]. In Salcedo et al.'s series, all patients developed de novo AIH in relation to infection with Cytomegalovirus, Epstein–Barr virus, or Parvovirus [114]. Viral infections, which are frequent after liver transplant, may lead to autoimmunity also through other mechanisms, including polyclonal stimulation, enhancement, and induction of membrane expression of MHC class I and II antigens, and/or interference with immunoregulatory cells [106, 116].

Moreover, calcineurin inhibitors may interfere with the maturation of T cells and/or with the function of T-regs, with consequent emergence and activation of auto-aggressive T cell clones [116–121]. In the experimental context, calcineurin inhibitor-associated autoimmunity arises in animals treated during the neonatal period or rendered immunocompromised by irradiation, reinforcing the concept that patients treated with immunosuppressants, like prednisolone, after liver transplant, may be predisposed to developing autoimmunity through the influence of calcineurin inhibitors. Cyclosporine blocks activation-induced cell death of effector T cells, and it interferes with tolerance induction by co-stimulation blockade [121]. Calcineurin inhibitors also act by reducing IL-2 production [122]. As IL-2 is an indispensable survival and growth factor for T-regs [123], absence of IL-2 leads to impaired suppressor function [124]. De novo AIH occurs more frequently in patients who develop repeated episodes of acute cellular rejection [110, 113, 125–130], which is also associated to a decreased number of circulating T-regs [129]. T-reg impairment, as a consequence of calcineurin inhibitors and/or acute cellular rejection, may contribute to the perpetuation of an autoreactive immune response, and to the development of de novo AIH.

Since children have an immature immune system—therefore an active thymus and an immature T cell receptor repertoire—and are exposed to numerous primary infections, they may be more vulnerable to autoimmunity under calcineurin inhibitors' influence [130]. This would account for the reportedly higher incidence of de novo AIH in pediatric age.

References

1. Johnson PJ, McFarlane IG. Meeting report: International Autoimmune Hepatitis Group. Hepatology. 1993;18:998–1005.
2. Alvarez F, Berg PA, Bianchi FB, Bianchi L, Burroughs AK, Cancado EL, Chapman RW, et al. International Autoimmune Hepatitis Group Report: review of criteria for diagnosis of autoimmune hepatitis. J Hepatol. 1999;31:929–38.
3. Manns MP, Czaja AJ, Gorham JD, Krawitt EL, Mieli-Vergani G, Vergani D, Vierling JM. Diagnosis and management of autoimmune hepatitis. Hepatology 2010;51:2193–213.
4. Gregorio GV, Portmann B, Reid F, Donaldson PT, Doherty DG, McCartney M, Mowat AP, et al. Autoimmune hepatitis in childhood: a 20-year experience. Hepatology. 1997;25:541–7.
5. Maggiore G, Veber F, Bernard O, Hadchouel M, Homberg JC, Alvarez F, Hadchouel P, et al. Autoimmune hepatitis associated with anti-actin antibodies in children and adolescents. J Pediatr Gastroenterol Nutr. 1993;17:376–81.
6. Ma Y, Okamoto M, Thomas MG, Bogdanos DP, Lopes AR, Portmann B, Underhill J, et al. Antibodies to conformational epitopes of soluble liver antigen define a severe form of autoimmune liver disease. Hepatology. 2002;35:658–64.
7. Vitozzi S, Djilali-Saiah I, Lapierre P, Alvarez F. Anti-soluble liver antigen/liver-pancreas (SLA/LP) antibodies in pediatric patients with autoimmune hepatitis. Autoimmunity. 2002;35:485–92.
8. Donaldson PT. Genetics in autoimmune hepatitis. Semin Liver Dis. 2002;22:353–64.
9. Ma Y, Bogdanos DP, Hussain MJ, Underhill J, Bansal S, Longhi MS, Cheeseman P, et al. Polyclonal T-cell responses to cytochrome P450IID6 are associated with disease activity in autoimmune hepatitis type 2. Gastroenterology. 2006;130:868–82.
10. Underhill J, Ma Y, Bogdanos DP, Cheeseman P, Mieli-Vergani G, Vergani D. Different immunogenetic background in autoimmune hepatitis type 1, type and autoimmune sclerosing cholangitis. J Hepatol. 2002;36:156A.
11. Elfaramawy AA, Elhossiny RM, Abbas AA, Aziz HM. HLA-DRB1 as a risk factor for children with autoimmune hepatitis and its relation to hepatitis A infection. Ital J Pediatr. 2010;36:73.
12. Oliveira LC, Porta G, Marin ML, Bittencourt PL, Kalil J, Goldberg AC. Autoimmune hepatitis, HLA and extended haplotypes. Autoimmun Rev. 2011;10:189–93.
13. Pando M, Larriba J, Fernandez GC, Fainboim H, Ciocca M, Ramonet M, Badia I, et al. Pediatric and adult forms of type I autoimmune hepatitis in Argentina: evidence for differential genetic predisposition. Hepatology. 1999;30:1374–80.
14. Fainboim L, Canero Velasco MC, Marcos CY, Ciocca M, Roy A, Theiler G, Capucchio M, et al. Protracted, but not acute, hepatitis A virus infection is strongly associated with HLA-DRB*1301, a marker for pediatric autoimmune hepatitis. Hepatology. 2001;33:1512–7.
15. Vergani D, Wells L, Larcher VF, Nasaruddin BA, Davies ET, Mieli-Vergani G, Mowat AP. Genetically determined low C4: a

predisposing factor to autoimmune chronic active hepatitis. Lancet. 1985;2:294–8.

16. Liston A, Lesage S, Gray DH, Boyd RL, Goodnow CC. Genetic lesions in T-cell tolerance and thresholds for autoimmunity. Immunol Rev. 2005;204:87–101.

17. Simmonds MJ, Gough SC. Genetic insights into disease mechanisms of autoimmunity. Br Med Bull. 2004;71:93–113.

18. Ahonen P, Myllarniemi S, Sipila I, Perheentupa J. Clinical variation of autoimmune polyendocrinopathy-candidiasis-ectodermal dystrophy (APECED) in a series of 68 patients. N Engl J Med. 1990;322:1829–36.

19. Meloni A, Willcox N, Meager A, Atzeni M, Wolff AS, Husebye ES, Furcas M, et al. Autoimmune polyendocrine syndrome type 1: an extensive longitudinal study in Sardinian patients. J Clin Endocrinol Metab. 2012;97:1114–24.

20. Hennes EM, Zeniya M, Czaja AJ, Pares A, Dalekos GN, Krawitt EL, Bittencourt PL, et al. Simplified criteria for the diagnosis of autoimmune hepatitis. Hepatology. 2008;48:169–76.

21. Ebbeson RL, Schreiber RA. Diagnosing autoimmune hepatitis in children: is the International Autoimmune Hepatitis Group scoring system useful? Clin Gastroenterol Hepatol. 2004;2:935–40.

22. Ferri PM, Ferreira AR, Miranda DM, Simoes ESAC. Diagnostic criteria for autoimmune hepatitis in children: a challenge for pediatric hepatologists. World J Gastroenterol. 2012;18:4470–3.

23. Mileti E, Rosenthal P, Peters MG. Validation and modification of simplified diagnostic criteria for autoimmune hepatitis in children. Clin Gastroenterol Hepatol. 2012;10:417–21, e411–2.

24. Hiejima E, Komatsu H, Sogo T, Inui A, Fujisawa T. Utility of simplified criteria for the diagnosis of autoimmune hepatitis in children. J Pediatr Gastroenterol Nutr. 2011;52:470–3.

25. Gregorio GV, Portmann B, Karani J, Harrison P, Donaldson PT, Vergani D, Mieli-Vergani G. Autoimmune hepatitis/sclerosing cholangitis overlap syndrome in childhood: a 16-year prospective study. Hepatology. 2001;33:544–53.

26. Vergani D, Alvarez F, Bianchi FB, Cancado EL, Mackay IR, Manns MP, Nishioka M, et al. Liver autoimmune serology: a consensus statement from the committee for autoimmune serology of the International Autoimmune Hepatitis Group. J Hepatol. 2004;41:677–83.

27. Manns MP, Griffin KJ, Sullivan KF, Johnson EF. LKM-1 autoantibodies recognize a short linear sequence in P450IID6, a cytochrome P-450 monooxygenase. J Clin Invest. 1991;88:1370–8.

28. Lapierre P, Hajoui O, Homberg JC, Alvarez F. Formiminotransferase cyclodeaminase is an organ-specific autoantigen recognized by sera of patients with autoimmune hepatitis. Gastroenterology. 1999;116:643–9.

29. Gregorio GV, Jones H, Choudhuri K, Vegnente A, Bortolotti F, Mieli-Vergani G, Vergani D. Autoantibody prevalence in chronic hepatitis B virus infection: effect in interferon alfa. Hepatology. 1996;24:520–3.

30. Gregorio GV, Pensati P, Iorio R, Vegnente A, Mieli-Vergani G, Vergani D. Autoantibody prevalence in children with liver disease due to chronic hepatitis C virus (HCV) infection. Clin Exp Immunol. 1998;112:471–6.

31. Dhawan A, Taylor RM, Cheeseman P, De Silva P, Katsiyiannakis L, Mieli-Vergani G. Wilson's disease in children: 37-year experience and revised King's score for liver transplantation. Liver Transplant. 2005;11:441–8.

32. Cotler SJ, Kanji K, Keshavarzian A, Jensen DM, Jakate S. Prevalence and significance of autoantibodies in patients with non-alcoholic steatohepatitis. J Clin Gastroenterol. 2004;38:801–4.

33. Manns M, Gerken G, Kyriatsoulis A, Staritz M, Meyer zum Buschenfelde KH. Characterisation of a new subgroup of autoimmune chronic active hepatitis by autoantibodies against a soluble liver antigen. Lancet. 1987;1:292–4.

34. Costa M, Rodriguez-Sanchez JL, Czaja AJ, Gelpi C. Isolation and characterization of cDNA encoding the antigenic protein of the human tRNP(Ser)Sec complex recognized by autoantibodies from patients withtype-1 autoimmune hepatitis. Clin Exp Immunol. 2000;121:364–74.

35. Wies I, Brunner S, Henninger J, Herkel J, Kanzler S, Meyer zum Buschenfelde KH, Lohse AW. Identification of target antigen for SLA/LP autoantibodies in autoimmune hepatitis [see comments]. Lancet. 2000;355:1510–5.

36. Gassert DJ, Garcia H, Tanaka K, Reinus JF. Corticosteroid-responsive cryptogenic chronic hepatitis: evidence for seronegative autoimmune hepatitis. Dig Dis Sci. 2007;52:2433–7.

37. De Groote J, Desmet VJ, Gedigk P, et al. A classification of chronic hepatitis. Lancet. 1968;2:626.

38. Senaldi G, Portmann B, Mowat AP, Mieli-Vergani G, Vergani D. Immunohistochemical features of the portal tract mononuclear cell infiltrate in chronic aggressive hepatitis. Arch Dis Child. 1992;67:1447–53.

39. Takeda K, Hayakawa Y, Van Kaer L, Matsuda H, Yagita H, Okumura K. Critical contribution of liver natural killer T cells to a murine model of hepatitis. Proc Natl Acad Sci U S A. 2000;97:5498–503.

40. Mieli-Vergani G, Vergani D. Autoimmune liver disease. In: Kelly D, editor. Diseases of the liver and biliary system in children. Chichester: Wiley-Blackwell; 2008. p. 191–205.

41. Nouri-Aria KT, Lobo-Yeo A, Vergani D, Mieli-Vergani G, Eddleston AL, Mowat AP. T suppressor cell function and number in children with liver disease. Clin Exp Immunol. 1985;61:283–9.

42. Nouri-Aria KT, Lobo-Yeo A, Vergani D, Mieli-Vergani G, Mowat AP, Eddleston AL. Immunoregulation of immunoglobulin production in normal infants and children. Clin Exp Immunol. 1985;59:679–86.

43. Nouri-Aria KT, Donaldson PT, Hegarty JE, Eddleston AL, Williams R. HLA A1-B8-DR3 and suppressor cell function in first-degree relatives of patients with autoimmune chronic active hepatitis. J Hepatol. 1985;1:235–41.

44. Vento S, Hegarty JE, Bottazzo G, Macchia E, Williams R, Eddleston AL. Antigen specific suppressor cell function in autoimmune chronic active hepatitis. Lancet. 1984;1:1200–4.

45. Longhi MS, Ma Y, Bogdanos DP, Cheeseman P, Mieli-Vergani G, Vergani D. Impairment of CD4(+)CD25(+) regulatory T-cells in autoimmune liver disease. J Hepatol. 2004;41:31–7.

46. Longhi MS, Meda F, Wang P, Samyn M, Mieli-Vergani G, Vergani D, Ma Y. Expansion and de novo generation of potentially therapeutic regulatory T cells in patients with autoimmune hepatitis. Hepatology. 2008;47:581–91.

47. Longhi MS, Hussain MJ, Mitry RR, Arora SK, Mieli-Vergani G, Vergani D, Ma Y. Functional study of CD4+CD25+ regulatory T cells in health and autoimmune hepatitis. J Immunol. 2006;176:4484–91.

48. Shevach EM, McHugh RS, Piccirillo CA, Thornton AM. Control of T-cell activation by CD4+CD25+ suppressor T cells. Immunol Rev. 2001;182:58–67.

49. Ferri S, Longhi MS, De Molo C, Lalanne C, Muratori P, Granito A, Hussain MJ, et al. A multifaceted imbalance of T cells with regulatory function characterizes type 1 autoimmune hepatitis. Hepatology. 2010;52:999–1007.

50. Longhi MS, Ma Y, Mitry RR, Bogdanos DP, Heneghan M, Cheeseman P, Mieli-Vergani G, et al. Effect of CD4+CD25+ regulatory T-cells on CD8 T-cell function in patients with autoimmune hepatitis. J Autoimmun. 2005;25:63–71.

51. Liberal R, Grant CR, Holder BS, Ma Y, Mieli-Vergani G, Vergani D, Longhi MS. The impaired immune regulation of autoimmune hepatitis is linked to a defective galectin-9/tim-3 pathway. Hepatology. 2012;56:677–86.

52. Lobo-Yeo A, Senaldi G, Portmann B, Mowat AP, Mieli-Vergani G, Vergani D. Class I and class II major histocompatibility complex antigen expression on hepatocytes: a study in children with liver disease. Hepatology. 1990;12:224–32.

53. Lobo-Yeo A, Alviggi L, Mieli-Vergani G, Portmann B, Mowat AP, Vergani D. Preferential activation of helper/inducer T lymphocytes in autoimmune chronic active hepatitis. Clin Exp Immunol. 1987;67:95–104.

54. Longhi MS, Hussain MJ, Bogdanos DP, Quaglia A, Mieli-Vergani G, Ma Y, Vergani D. Cytochrome P450IID6-specific CD8 T cell immune responses mirror disease activity in autoimmune hepatitis type 2. Hepatology. 2007;46:472–84.

55. Vento S, Cainelli F, Renzini C, Concia E. Autoimmune hepatitis type 2 induced by HCV and persisting after viral clearance [letter] [see comments]. Lancet. 1997;350:1298–9.

56. Kerkar N, Choudhuri K, Ma Y, Mahmoud A, Bogdanos DP, Muratori L, Bianchi F, et al. Cytochrome P4502D6(193–212): a new immunodominant epitope and target of virus/self cross-reactivity in liver kidney microsomal autoantibody type 1-positive liver disease. J Immunol. 2003;170:1481–9.

57. Jensen DM, McFarlane IG, Portmann BS, Eddleston AL, Williams R. Detection of antibodies directed against a liver-specific membrane lipoprotein in patients with acute and chronic active hepatitis. N Engl J Med. 1978;299:1–7.

58. McFarlane BM, McSorley CG, Vergani D, McFarlane IG, Williams R. Serum autoantibodies reacting with the hepatic asialoglycoprotein receptor protein (hepatic lectin) in acute and chronic liver disorders. J Hepatol. 1986;3:196–205.

59. Ma Y, Gaken J, McFarlane BM, Foss Y, Farzaneh F, McFarlane IG, Mieli-Vergani G, et al. Alcohol dehydrogenase: a target of humoral autoimmune response in liver disease. Gastroenterology. 1997;112:483–92.

60. Vergani D, Mieli-Vergani G, Mondelli M, Portmann B, Eddleston AL. Immunoglobulin on the surface of isolated hepatocytes is associated with antibody-dependent cell-mediated cytotoxicity and liver damage. Liver. 1987;7:307–15.

61. Mieli-Vergani G, Vergani D, Jenkins PJ, Portmann B, Mowat AP, Eddleston AL, Williams R. Lymphocyte cytotoxicity to autologous hepatocytes in HBsAg-negative chronic active hepatitis. Clin Exp Immunol. 1979;38:16–21.

62. Wen L, Ma Y, Bogdanos DP, Wong FS, Demaine A, Mieli-Vergani G, Vergani D. Pediatric autoimmune liver diseases the molecular basis of humoral and cellular immunity. Curr Mol Med. 2001;1:379–89.

63. Wen L, Peakman M, Lobo-Yeo A, McFarlane BM, Mowat AP, Mieli-Vergani G, Vergani D. T-cell-directed hepatocyte damage in autoimmune chronic active hepatitis. Lancet. 1990;336:1527–30.

64. Lohr H, Manns M, Kyriatsoulis A, Lohse AW, Trautwein C, Meyer zum Buschenfelde KH, Fleischer B. Clonal analysis of liver-infiltrating T cells in patients with LKM-1 antibody-positive autoimmune chronic active hepatitis. Clin Exp Immunol. 1991;84:297–302.

65. Lohr H, Treichel U, Poralla T, Manns M, Meyer zum Buschenfelde KH. Liver-infiltrating T helper cells in autoimmune chronic active hepatitis stimulate the production of autoantibodies against the human asialoglycoprotein receptor in vitro. Clin Exp Immunol. 1992;88:45–9.

66. Zhao L, Tang Y, You Z, Wang Q, Liang S, Han X, Qiu D, et al. Interleukin-17 contributes to the pathogenesis of autoimmune hepatitis through inducing hepatic interleukin-6 expression. PLoS One. 2011;6:e18909.

67. Heneghan MA, Allan ML, Bornstein JD, Muir AJ, Tendler DA. Utility of thiopurine methyltransferase genotyping and phenotyping, and measurement of azathioprine metabolites in the management of patients with autoimmune hepatitis. J Hepatol. 2006;45:584–91.

68. Rumbo C, Emerick KM, Emre S, Shneider BL. Azathioprine metabolite measurements in the treatment of autoimmune hepatitis in pediatric patients: a preliminary report. J Pediatr Gastroenterol Nutr. 2002;35:391–8.

69. Wusk B, Kullak-Ublick GA, Rammert C, von Eckardstein A, Fried M, Rentsch KM. Therapeutic drug monitoring of thiopurine drugs in patients with inflammatory bowel disease or autoimmune hepatitis. Eur J Gastroenterol Hepatol. 2004;16:1407–13.

70. Kerkar N, Annunziato RA, Foley L, Schmeidler J, Rumbo C, Emre S, Shneider B, et al. Prospective analysis of nonadherence in autoimmune hepatitis: a common problem. J Pediatr Gastroenterol Nutr. 2006;43:629–34.

71. Mieli-Vergani G, Bargiota K, Samyn M, Vergani D. Therapeutic aspects of autoimmune liver disease in children. In: Dienes HP, Leuschner U, Lohse AW, Manns MP, editors. Autoimmune liver diseases—Falk symposium, vol. 142. Dordrecht: Springer; 2005. p. 278–82.

72. Samaroo B, Samyn M, Buchanan C, Mieli-Vergani G. Long-term daily oral treatment with prednisolone in children with autoimmune liver disease does not affect final adult height. Hepatology. 2006;44:438A.

73. Gregorio GV, McFarlane B, Bracken P, Vergani D, Mieli-Vergani G. Organ and non-organ specific autoantibody titres and IgG levels as markers of disease activity: a longitudinal study in childhood autoimmune liver disease. Autoimmunity. 2002;35:515–9.

74. Banerjee S, Rahhal R, Bishop WP. Azathioprine monotherapy for maintenance of remission in pediatric patients with autoimmune hepatitis. J Pediatr Gastroenterol Nutr. 2006;43:353–6.

75. Alvarez F, Ciocca M, Canero-Velasco C, Ramonet M, de Davila MTG, Cuarterolo M, Gonzalez T, et al. Short-term cyclosporine induces a remission of autoimmune hepatitis in children. J Hepatol 1999;30:222–7.

76. Cuarterolo M, Ciocca M, Velasco CC, Ramonet M, Gonzalez T, Lopez S, Garsd A, et al. Follow-up of children with autoimmune hepatitis treated with cyclosporine. J Pediatr Gastroenterol Nutr. 2006;43:635–9.

77. Manns MP, Woynarowski M, Kreisel W, Lurie Y, Rust C, Zuckerman E, Bahr MJ, et al. Budesonide induces remission more effectively than prednisone in a controlled trial of patients with autoimmune hepatitis. Gastroenterology. 2010;139:1198–206.

78. Woynarowski M, Nemeth A, Baruch Y, Koletzko S, Melter M, Rodeck B, Strassburg CP, et al. Budesonide versus prednisone with azathioprine for the treatment of autoimmune hepatitis in children and adolescents. J Pediatr. 2013;163:1347–53, e1341.

79. Mieli-Vergani G, Vergani D. Budesonide for juvenile autoimmune hepatitis? Not yet. J Pediatr. 2013;163:1246–8.

80. Aw MM, Dhawan A, Samyn M, Bargiota A, Mieli-Vergani G. Mycophenolate mofetil as rescue treatment for autoimmune liver disease in children: a 5-year follow-up. J Hepatol. 2009;51:156–60.

81. Debray D, Maggiore G, Giradet JP, Mallet E, Bernard O. Efficacy of cyclosporin A in children with type 2 autoimmune hepatitis. J Pediatr. 1999;135:111–4.

82. Maggiore G, Bernard O, Hadchouel M, Alagille D. Life-saving immunosuppressive treatment in severe autoimmune chronic active hepatitis. J Pediatr Gastroenterol Nutr. 1985;4:655–8.

83. Lankisch TO, Strassburg CP, Debray D, Manns MP, Jacquemin E. Detection of autoimmune regulator gene mutations in children with type 2 autoimmune hepatitis and extrahepatic immune-mediated diseases. J Pediatr. 2005;146:839–42.

84. Debray D, Pariente D, Urvoas E, Hadchouel M, Bernard O. Sclerosing cholangitis in children. J Pediatr. 1994;124:49–56.

85. Wilschanski M, Chait P, Wade JA, Davis L, Corey M, St Louis P, Griffiths AM, et al. Primary sclerosing cholangitis in 32 children: clinical, laboratory, and radiographic features, with survival analysis. Hepatology. 1995;22:1415–22.

86. Feldstein AE, Perrault J, El-Youssif M, Lindor KD, Freese DK, Angulo P. Primary sclerosing cholangitis in children: a long-term follow-up study. Hepatology. 2003;38:210–7.

87. Miloh T, Arnon R, Shneider B, Suchy F, Kerkar N. A retrospective single-center review of primary sclerosing cholangitis in children. Clin Gastroenterol Hepatol. 2009;7:239–45.

88. Baker AJ, Portmann B, Westaby D, Wilkinson M, Karani J, Mowat AP. Neonatal sclerosing cholangitis in two siblings: a category of progressive intrahepatic cholestasis. J Pediatr Gastroenterol Nutr. 1993;17:317–22.

89. Jacquemin E, De Vree JM, Cresteil D, Sokal EM, Sturm E, Dumont M, Scheffer GL, et al. The wide spectrum of multidrug resistance 3 deficiency: from neonatal cholestasis to cirrhosis of adulthood. Gastroenterology. 2001;120:1448–58.

90. Ziol M, Barbu V, Rosmorduc O, Frassati-Biaggi A, Barget N, Hermelin B, Scheffer GL, et al. ABCB4 heterozygous gene mutations associated with fibrosing cholestatic liver disease in adults. Gastroenterology. 2008;135:131–41.

91. Mieli-Vergani G, Vergani D. Autoimmune hepatitis. Nat Rev Gastroenterol Hepatol. 2011;8:320–9.

92. Scalori A, Heneghan M, Hadzic N, Vergani D, Mieli-Vergani G. Outcome and survival in childhood onset autoimmune sclerosing cholangitis and autoimmune hepatitis: a 13-year follow up study. Hepatology. 2007;46 Suppl:555A.

93. Mitchell SA, Bansi DS, Hunt N, Von Bergmann K, Fleming KA, Chapman RW. A preliminary trial of high-dose ursodeoxycholic acid in primary sclerosing cholangitis. Gastroenterology. 2001;121:900–7.

94. Lindor KD, Kowdley KV, Luketic VA, Harrison ME, McCashland T, Befeler AS, Harnois D, et al. High-dose ursodeoxycholic acid for the treatment of primary sclerosing cholangitis. Hepatology 2009;50:808–14.

95. Davies YK, Cox KM, Abdullah BA, Safta A, Terry AB, Cox KL. Long-term treatment of primary sclerosing cholangitis in children with oral vancomycin: an immunomodulating antibiotic. J Pediatr Gastroenterol Nutr. 2008;47:61–7.

96. Abarbanel DN, Seki SM, Davies Y, Marlen N, Benavides JA, Cox K, Nadeau KC, et al. Immunomodulatory effect of vancomycin on Treg in pediatric inflammatory bowel disease and primary sclerosing cholangitis. J Clin Immunol. 2013;33:397–406

97. Mieli-Vergani G, Lobo-Yeo A, McFarlane BM, McFarlane IG, Mowat AP, Vergani D. Different immune mechanisms leading to autoimmunity in primary sclerosing cholangitis and autoimmune chronic active hepatitis of childhood. Hepatology. 1989;9:198–203.

98. Donaldson P, Manns MP. Immunogenetics of liver disease. In: Bircher JBJ-P, McIntyre N, Rizzetto M, Rhodes J, editors. Oxford textbook of clinical hepatology, vol. 1. Oxford: Oxford University Press; 1999. p. 173–88.

99. Djilali-Saiah I, Renous R, Caillat-Zucman S, Debray D, Alvarez F. Linkage disequilibrium between HLA class II region and autoimmune hepatitis in pediatric patients. J Hepatol. 2004;40:904–9.

100. Duclos-Vallee JC, Sebagh M, Rifai K, Johanet C, Ballot E, Guettier C, Karam V, et al. A 10 year follow up study of patients transplanted for autoimmune hepatitis: histological recurrence precedes clinical and biochemical recurrence. Gut. 2003;52:893–7.

101. Miloh T, Anand R, Yin W, Vos M, Kerkar N, Alonso E. Pediatric liver transplantation for primary sclerosing cholangitis. Liver Transplant. 2011;17:925–33.

102. Alabraba E, Nightingale P, Gunson B, Hubscher S, Olliff S, Mirza D, Neuberger J. A re-evaluation of the risk factors for the recurrence of primary sclerosing cholangitis in liver allografts. Liver Transplant. 2009;15:330–40.

103. Vera A, Moledina S, Gunson B, Hubscher S, Mirza D, Olliff S, Neuberger J. Risk factors for recurrence of primary sclerosing cholangitis of liver allograft. Lancet. 2002;360:1943–4.

104. Cholongitas E, Shusang V, Papatheodoridis GV, Marelli L, Manousou P, Rolando N, Patch D, et al. Risk factors for recurrence of primary sclerosing cholangitis after liver transplantation. Liver Transplant. 2008;14:138–43.

105. Kerkar N, Hadzic N, Davies ET, Portmann B, Donaldson PT, Rela M, Heaton ND, et al. De-novo autoimmune hepatitis after liver transplantation. Lancet. 1998;351:409–13.

106. Vergani D, Mieli-Vergani G. Autoimmunity after liver transplantation. Hepatology. 2002;36:271–6.

107. Mieli-Vergani G, Vergani D. De novo autoimmune hepatitis after liver transplantation. J Hepatol. 2004;40:3–7.

108. Cho JM, Kim KM, Oh SH, Lee YJ, Rhee KW, Yu E. De novo autoimmune hepatitis in Korean children after liver transplantation: a single institution's experience. Transplant Proc. 2011;43:2394–6.

109. Liberal R, Longhi MS, Grant CR, Mieli-Vergani G, Vergani D. Autoimmune hepatitis after liver transplantation. Clin Gastroenterol Hepatol. 2012;10:346–53.

110. Venick RS, McDiarmid SV, Farmer DG, Gornbein J, Martin MG, Vargas JH, Ament ME, et al. Rejection and steroid dependence: unique risk factors in the development of pediatric posttransplant de novo autoimmune hepatitis. Am J Transplant. 2007;7:955–63.

111. Evans H. Progressive histological damage in liver allografts following pediatric liver transplantation. Hepatology. 2006;43:1109–17.

112. Kerkar N, Dugan C, Rumbo C, Morotti RA, Gondolesi G, Shneider BL, Emre S. Rapamycin successfully treats post-transplant autoimmune hepatitis. Am J Transpl. 2005;5:1085–9.

113. Heneghan MA, Portmann BC, Norris SM, Williams R, Muiesan P, Rela M, Heaton ND, et al. Graft dysfunction mimicking autoimmune hepatitis following liver transplantation in adults. Hepatology. 2001;34:464–70.

114. Salcedo M, Vaquero J, Banares R, Rodriguez-Mahou M, Alvarez E, Vicario JL, Hernandez-Albujar A, et al. Response to steroids in de novo autoimmune hepatitis after liver transplantation. Hepatology. 2002;35:349–56.

115. Bogdanos DP, Choudhuri K, Vergani D. Molecular mimicry and autoimmune liver disease: virtuous intentions, malign consequences. Liver. 2001;21:225–32.

116. Sakaguchi S, Sakaguchi N. Role of genetic factors in organ-specific autoimmune diseases induced by manipulating the thymus or T cells, and not self-antigens. Rev Immunogenet. 2000;2:147–53.

117. Gao E, Lo D, Cheney R, Kanagawa O, Sprent J. Abnormal differentiation of thymocytes in mice treated with cyclosporin A. Nature. 1988;336:176–9.

118. Bucy PB, Yan Xu X, Li J, Huang GQ. Cyclosporin A-induced autoimmune disease in mice. J Immunol. 1993;151:1039–50.

119. Wu DY, Goldschneider I. Cyclosporin A-induced autologous graft-versus-host disease: a prototypical model of autoimmunity and active (dominant) tolerance coordinately induced by recent thymic emigrants. J Immunol. 1999;162:6926–33.

120. Damoiseaux JG, van Breda Vriesman PJ. Cyclosporin A-induced autoimmunity: the result of defective de novo T- cell development. Folia Biol. 1998;44:1–9.

121. Shi YF, Sahai BM, Green DR. Cyclosporin A inhibits activation-induced cell death in T-cell hybridomas and thymocytes. Nature. 1989;339:625–6.

122. Zeiser R, Nguyen VH, Beilhack A, Buess M, Schulz S, Baker J, Contag CH, et al. Inhibition of CD4+CD25+ regulatory T-cell function by calcineurin-dependent interleukin-2 production. Blood. 2006;108:390–9.

123. Thornton AM, Donovan EE, Piccirillo CA, Shevach EM. Cutting edge: IL-2 is critically required for the in vitro activation of CD4+CD25+ T cell suppressor function. J Immunol. 2004;172:6519–23.

124. Kang HG, Zhang D, Degauque N, Mariat C, Alexopoulos S, Zheng XX. Effects of cyclosporine on transplant tolerance: the role of IL-2. Am J Transplant. 2007;7:1907–16.

125. D'Antiga L, Dhawan A, Portmann B, Francavilla R, Rela M, Heaton N, Mieli-Vergani G. Late cellular rejection in paediatric liver transplantation: aetiology and outcome. Transplantation 2002;73:80–4.

126. Miyagawa-Hayashino A, Haga H, Egawa H, Hayashino Y, Sakurai T, Minamiguchi S, Tanaka K, et al. Outcome and risk factors of de novo autoimmune hepatitis in living-donor liver transplantation. Transplantation. 2004;78:128–35.

127. Hernandez HM, Kovarik P, Whitington PF, Alonso EM. Autoimmune hepatitis as a late complication of liver transplantation. J Pediatr Gastroenterol Nutr. 2001;32:131–6.

128. Spada M, Bertani A, Sonzogni A, Petz W, Riva S, Torre G, Melzi ML, et al. A cause of late graft dysfunction after liver transplantation in children: de-novo autoimmune hepatitis. Transplant Proc. 2001;33:1747–8.

129. Demirkiran A, Kok A, Kwekkeboom J, Kusters JG, Metselaar HJ, Tilanus HW, van der Laan LJ. Low circulating regulatory T-cell levels after acute rejection in liver transplantation. Liver Transplant. 2006;12:277–84.

130. Czaja AJ. Autoimmune hepatitis after liver transplantation and other lessons of self-intolerance. Liver Transplant. 2002;8:505–13.

Inherited Metabolic Disorders and the Liver

64

Hugh Lemonde and Mike Champion

Introduction

The liver plays a central role for many of the body's metabolic processes and so understandably inherited metabolic disorders (IMDs) may present with liver dysfunction. Most IMDs are monogenic conditions and the faulty protein is an enzyme, but others involve structural proteins, receptors, hormones or transport proteins. Presentation may be restricted to the liver, involve multiple organ systems or although expressed in liver cells, symptoms may be exclusively extrahepatic. Securing the diagnosis is important to direct specific treatment, inform prognosis and facilitate genetic counselling, but may be complicated by secondary metabolic disturbance from liver dysfunction generating metabolites falsely indicating a primary IMD. Although these conditions are inherited and presentation in the newborn period is common, some present later in childhood or not until adult life.

Presentation

Liver presentations may result from the making or breaking of complex molecules; the former often presenting at birth with dysmorphic features as these molecules are important in embryogenesis and patterning, for example, peroxisomal biogenesis defects, congenital disorders of glycosylation (CDGs) and the latter developing features of storage over time such as coarsening of the features and the development of organomagaly as these molecules accumulate, for example, lysosomal storage disorders (LSDs). I-cell disease is an exception in that dysmorphic features may be present at birth. Classical intoxications are signified by a symptom-free period prior to toxic metabolites accumulating, for example, tyrosinemia type 1, galactosaemia and urea cycle defects (UCDs). Defects of energy metabolism may only manifest if feeding is interrupted or compromised such as in glycogen storage disorders (GSDs) and fat oxidation defects (FAOs). Primary blocks in energy production, for example, mitochondrial disorders and disorders of pyruvate metabolism will be present from birth, but their effects may not at first be obvious.

Specific liver presentations include cholestasis, acute liver failure, hepatomegaly and encephalopathy (see Table 64.1). Cholestasis commonly presents in the newborn period. The cholestatis may herald progressive liver disease. In Niemann–Pick type C (NPC) and cerebrotendinous xanthomatosis (CTX), cholestasis may be transient and no further symptoms may be noted until presenting with a progressive neurological deterioration later in childhood. Citrin deficiency may present with prolonged cholestasis which resolves prior to presentation usually as an adult with hyperammonemic encephalopathy. Intermediary metabolic blocks may present with acute liver failure and commonly present in the newborn period often after a symptom-free period. Hepatomegaly may be isolated without splenomegaly as seen in GSDs; glycogen is not stored in the spleen. Firm hepatomegaly is more commonly associated with tyrosinemia type 1, galactosaemia, Niemann–Pick and Gaucher disease. Encephalopathy results from hyperammonemia, hypoglycaemia or other specific toxic metabolites.

Diagnosis

History

Diagnosis is hampered by the rarity of these conditions, non-specific presentation and the requirement for specific investigations. Diagnostic clues are therefore sought from history and examination to suggest the potential for an IMD (see Table 64.2) and remain the foundation of diagnosis [1].

M. Champion (✉) · H. Lemonde
Department of Pediatric Inherited Metabolic Disease, Evelina London Children's Hospital, St Thomas' Hospital, Sky level 6, Westminster Bridge Street, London SE1 7EH, UK
e-mail: michael.champion@gstt.nhs.uk

H. Lemonde
e-mail: hugh.lemonde@gstt.nhs.uk

© Springer International Publishing Switzerland 2016
S. Guandalini et al. (eds.), *Textbook of Pediatric Gastroenterology, Hepatology and Nutrition*,
DOI 10.1007/978-3-319-17169-2_64

Table 64.1 Specific liver presentations and underlying IMDs

Cholestasis	α_1-antitrypsin deficiency
	Arginase deficiency (UCD)
	Bile acid metabolism defects, e.g. CTX
	Byler disease
	CDGs
	Cholesterol synthesis defects
	Citrin deficiency
	Galactosaemia
	LCHAD
	Mevalonic aciduria
	Niemann–Pick C (LSD)
	Peroxisomal defects
	Tyrosinemia type 1
	Transaldolase deficiency
	Wolman disease (LSD)
Acute liver failure	α_1-Antitrypsin deficiency
	CDGs
	Galactosaemia
	Hereditary fructose intolerance
	Fat oxidation defects (FAOs)
	Mitochondrial disorders including Alpers disease
	Neonatal hemochromatosis
	Organic acidemias (OAs)
	Tyrosinemia type 1
	Urea cycle defects (UCDs)
	Wilson disease
Hepatomegaly (main or isolated symptom)	α_1-antitrypsin deficiency
	Cholesterol ester storage disease and Wolman disease
	Galactosaemia
	Fanconi–Bickel syndrome
	Glycogen storage disorders (GSD I, III, IV, VI, and IX)
	Lysosomal storage disorders (LSDs)
	Farber disease
	Gaucher disease
	Mucolipidoses
	Mucopolysccharidoses (MPS)
	Niemann–Pick B&C
	Neonatal haemochromatosis
	Peroxisomal disorders
	Tyrosinemia type 1
	Wilson disease
Encephalopathy	FAOs
	Fructose 1,6 bisphosphatase deficiency
	Mitochondrial disorders
	OAs
	UCDs

CTX cerebrotendinous xanthomatosis, *CDG* congenital disorders of glycosylation, *LCHAD* long-chain hydroxy acyl-CoA dehydrogenase

The family history is particularly important searching for evidence for other affected family members such as previous sudden infant deaths, previous miscarriages or known relatives with the same condition or similar presentation. Potential mode of inheritance must be considered and is best facilitated by a three-generation history. Some conditions, such as FAOs, are associated with maternal symptoms in pregnancy including hyperemesis or frank liver dysfunction such as acute fatty liver of pregnancy. Self-imposed dietary restriction is seen in some conditions; especially the avoid-

Table 64.2 Clues from the history suggestive of an underlying IMD

Family history	Consanguinity
	Previous sudden infant death
	Positive family history and inheritance pattern
	Only males affected suggests X-linked
	Matrilineal inheritance suggests mitochondrial DNA point mutation
Maternal obstetric history (if an infant or childhood presentation)	Multiple miscarriages (may signify previously affected pregnancies)
	Hyperemesis extending beyond the first trimester
	Acute fatty liver of pregnancy (AFLP) and hemolysis, elevated liver enzymes and low platelets (HELLP) syndrome association with carrying foetus with long-chain fat oxidation defect
Past medical history	Recurrent episodes, especially relating to intercurrent infections (catabolic stress)
	Specific food avoidance, e.g., fructose, protein

ance of sweet foods in hereditary fructose intolerance (HFI) and protein in UCDs. HFI will not present prior to weaning as fructose is not present in breast milk or formula milk.

Examination

IMDs associated with obvious dysmorphic features include peroxisomal disorders, CDGs and LSDs; however, many IMDs have no specific diagnostic features on examination. It is essential to look for extrahepatic manifestations to confirm the multi-organ involvement in some conditions. Developmental concerns are a feature of many IMDs and a full neurological examination should be undertaken to look for neurological signs.

Careful ophthalmic examination is required [2]. Cataracts are nearly always present at birth in galactosaemia but are easily missed in the non-dilated eye due to their transparent (oil drop) appearance. If the diagnosis is missed, the cataract will become more obvious as it matures. Cataracts are also seen in peroxisomal disorders, CTX, Wilson disease and some mitochondrial disorders. A cherry-red spot may be visible due to the accumulation of sphingolipid around the fovea in Niemann–Pick B. Pigmentary retinopathy is a feature of long-chain hydroxy acyl-CoA dehydrogenase (LCHAD) and mitochondrial disorders. Eye movement disorders are a feature of CDG-Ia (squint), NPC (vertical supranuclear gaze palsy), Gaucher disease (horizontal supranuclear palsy) and mitochondrial disorders (external ophthalmoplegia—limited gaze in all directions). Ptosis is found in many conditions including peroxisomal and mitochondrial disorders.

Investigation

Investigations may be divided between the general and the specific. Renal and cardiac assessment including ECG and echocardiography is important to exclude multi-organ involvement. Mitochondrial disorders are characterised by 'illegitimate associations', that is, signs and symptoms which may not be obviously linked until one considers the central requirement for energy production. Cardiac involvement

may be subtle such as mild compensatory myocardial hypertrophy. Liver imaging may glean further information such as increased reflectivity secondary to fatty steatosis in FAOs and liver biopsy is indicated to help further diagnosis when initial investigations have proven inconclusive. Enzymology and genotyping are often required to secure a diagnosis (see Table 64.3).

Newborn screening offers the opportunity for therapeutic intervention prior to developing clinical symptoms. In the UK, this is limited to a few metabolic conditions including medium-chain acyl-CoA dehydrogenase deficiency (MCADD) which presents with encephalopathy, hypoglycemia and liver dysfunction. Phenylketonuria (PKU), a neurodevelopmental disorder, is screened by detecting elevated phenylalanine; however, a generalised amino acidemia occurs in liver dysfunction and so a positive screen may indicate a liver disorder such as galactosaemia [3]. The clue is phenylalanine to tyrosine ratio which is elevated in PKU due to the block in the conversion of phenylalanine to tyrosine by phenylalanine hydroxylase but normal or decreased in liver disorders. Following an expanded newborn screening pilot, the number of conditions screened is increasing to include isovaleric acidemia and maple syrup urine disease which can both present with decompensation including liver dysfunction in the newborn period. In the other parts of Europe, North America and Australia, many more conditions are covered by newborn screening.

Next-generation sequencing is another technology increasingly used to screen patients to secure a diagnosis. This can either be targeted such as a gene chip, for example, causes of cholestasis or be for a specific group of conditions, for example, GSDs screening all the associated genes simultaneously [4, 5] or screening all coding regions for disease causing mutations (exome sequencing) [6, 7]. This is likely to identify new conditions and broaden the phenotype of known disorders, but is not without risk, ensuring that variations detected are indeed disease causing and responsible for the clinical presentation [8].

Table 64.3 Examples of metabolic investigations and associated pathological findings

Investigation	Condition	Metabolite/finding	Presentation
Amino acids	Tyrosinemia type 1	Raised tyrosine, methionine	C, LF, H
	Urea cycle defects	Raised glutamine, low arginine	LF, E
		Raised citrulline (citrullinemia)	
		Raised arginine (arginase deficiency)	
	Citrin deficiency	Raised citrulline	C, H
	Galactosaemia	Amino acidemia	C, H, LF
	Lysinuric protein intolerance	Low lysine, ornithine and arginine	H, E
Organic acids	Organic acidemias	Specific organic acids	C, LF, H, E
	Tyrosinemia type 1	Succinylacetone	C, LF, H
	Argininosuccinic aciduria (urea cycle defects, UCD)	Argininosuccinic acid	LF, E
Ammonia	UCD		LF, E
	Organic Acidemias		C, LF, H, E
	Fat oxidation defects		LF, H, E
Acylcarnitines	Fat oxidation defects	Specific acylcarnitine and often low Free carnitine	LF, H, E
	Organic acidemias	Specific acylcarnitine and often low Free carnitine	C, LF, H, E
Lactate	Mitochondrial disorders	Raised and exacerbated postprandially	C, LF, E
	Gluconeogenesis defects	Rapid resolution with treatment	H, E
	Fat oxidation defects		LF, H, E
	GSD I	Elevated on fasting	H
	GSD III	Elevated postprandially	H
CK	Fat oxidation defects	Elevated	LF, H, E
	GSD III	Elevated	H
Very long-chain fatty acids (VLCFAs)	Peroxisomal disorders		C, LF, H
Gal-1-PUT activity	Galactosaemia	Parental if infant already transfused to confirm carrier levels of activity	C, H, LF
α₁-antitrypsin	α₁-antitrypsin deficiency		C, H
Lipid profile	Wolman and CESD	Raised lipids	C, H, LF
	Glycogen storage disorders	Raised triglycerides	H
Urate	Glycogen storage disorders	Raised	H
Bile acids	PFIC	Raised normal bile acids	
	Bile acid defects	Specific abnormal bile acids present	
Transferrin isoelectric focusing	Congenital disorders of glycosylation		C, H, LF
Vacuolated lymphocytes	Lysosomal storage disorders		C, H
Glycosaminoglycans (GAGs) and oligosacchraides	Lysosomal storage disorders		C, H
Bone marrow aspirate	Lysosomal storage disorders	Storage cells	C, H
Abdominal X-ray	Wolman	Adrenal calcification	C, H, LF

C cholestasis, *H* hepatomegaly, *LF* liver failure, *E* encephalopathy, *CESD* cholesterol ester storage disease, *CK* creatine kinase, *GSD* glycogen storage disorders, *PFIC* Progresive familial intrahepatic cholestasis

Inherited Disorders of Carbohydrate Metabolism

Galactosaemia

Classical galactosaemia (galactose-1-phosphate uridyl transferase deficiency) typically manifests within the first week of life and sometimes within days of starting milk feeds. These feeds introduce galactose that in turn leads to the ac-cumulation of the abnormal and putative toxic metabolite galactose-1-phosphate (see Fig. 64.1). Vomiting and jaundice typically ensue accompanied by hepatomegaly, ascites, deranged liver function, coagulopathy and renal tubulopathy. There is a marked failure to thrive. Careful examination of the eyes reveals oil drop cataracts that are easily missed as the red reflex is present. Classical lentiform cataracts can take many weeks to become apparent and although hypoglycemia is much quoted, it is not a major feature. Neonatal

Fig. 64.1 Metabolism of galactose and associated disorders. *UDP* uridine diphosphate

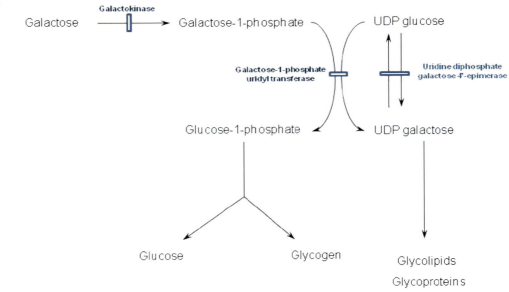

sepsis (typically *Escherichia coli*) is another mode of presentation and the threshold for antibiotic use in the acute phase should be low. Raised intracranial pressure is also a recognised feature. Occasionally, a more indolent course is followed with symptoms occurring beyond the first month with failure to thrive, renal tubulopathy or the development of cataracts or very rarely developmental delay. However, mild prolongation of the prothrombin time is almost always present.

The incidence in the UK is approximately 1 in 45,000 live births, and the gene is located on chromosome 9 and inherited in a recessive fashion. There is a common mutation Q188R identified in 72 % of cases with classical galactosaemia. Genotype–phenotype correlations are unclear; however, the Duarte variant (N314D) has 50 % residual enzyme activity and is a benign variant [9].

Diagnosis is by measurement of galactose-1-phosphate uridyl transferase activity in erythrocytes. Care must be taken in neonates that have received a red cell transfusion as false negative results can be obtained within 3 months of the transfusion. In this circumstance, galactosaemia can be excluded by testing enzyme activity in the parents and comparing to well-defined heterozygote ranges. Testing urine for the presence of reducing substances is rarely performed as it is neither sensitive nor specific.

Uridine diphosphate galactose 4'-epimerase (UDP-galactose epimerase) deficiency is a rare condition that presents in similar fashion to classical galactosaemia. It should be considered if there is a strong suspicion of galactosaemia when galactose-1-phosphate uridyl transferase activity is normal. It is characterised by elevated galactose-1-phosphate in red cells. Galactokinase deficiency is the third disorder of galactose metabolism, but its phenotype is restricted to ophthal-

mic symptoms. Galactosaemia screening is available; however, the majority of patients have presented clinically by the time the result would be available and presymptomatic treatment of known sibling cases appears to afford no benefit regarding avoidance of the long-term complications.

If the diagnosis is suspected, galactose must be promptly removed from the diet until the condition has been excluded. Conversion to a soya-based formula, or casein-based protein hydrolysate-based formula (such as Pregestamil) if hepatic impairment is severe, brings rapid improvement. A lifelong dietary restriction of galactose is generally recommended, although practises vary widely and there is much debate regarding the severity of restriction and the necessity of restriction in later life [10]. Many centres will allow a slight relaxation of diet in later life, such as galactose-containing fruit and vegetables while still avoiding sources of lactose, such as dairy products, as this keeps dietary intake well below the level of endogenous galactose production. Calcium intake needs to be regularly assessed to ensure adequate intake, especially in childhood. Long-term complications are not abolished by dietary management, and they include neurodevelopmental problems, osteoporosis and hypergonadotrophic hypergonadism/infertility in females [11]. Careful management of puberty is essential to ensure adequate uterine growth to allow successful pregnancy following ovum donation.

Hereditary Fructose Intolerance

HFI is an autosomal recessive condition due to a deficiency of aldolase B. The key to diagnosis is establishing a clear history of fructose intake prior to the onset of symptoms.

Table 64.4 Nomenclature of hepatic glycogen storage disorders

Type (Alternate name)	Enzyme	Gene	Inheritance
Ia (Von Gierke)	Glucose-6-phosphatase	*G6PC*	Recessive
Ib	Glucose-6-phosphate translocase	*G6PT1/SLC37A4*	Recessive
IIIa (Cori/Forbes)	Glycogen debrancher (liver and muscle)	*AGL*	Recessive
IIIb (Cori/Forbes)	Glycogen debrancher (liver)	*AGL*	Recessive
IV (Andersen)	Glycogen branching enzyme	*GBE1*	Recessive
VI (Hers)	Liver glycogen phosphorylase	*PYGL*	Recessive
IXa (XLG)	α-Subunit phosphorylase b kinase (liver)	*PHKA2*	X-linked
IXb	β-Subunit phosphorylase b kinase (liver/muscle)	*PHKB*	Recessive
IXc	γ-Subunit phosphorylase b kinase (liver)	*PHKG2*	X-linked
0a	Liver Glycogen synthase	*GYS2*	Recessive

Fructose is a monosaccharide that is found in many food sources, notably sucrose (glucose–fructose disaccharide), fruits, vegetables and honey. Sorbitol is an artificial sweetener that is metabolised to fructose. The classical presentation is that of healthy milk-fed infant that develops symptoms when it is first exposed to fructose upon weaning. Gastrointestinal (GI) upset progresses to persistent vomiting, sweating, lethargy and coma if intake continues. These symptoms are accompanied by liver failure and evidence of renal proximal tubulopathy. Hypoglycemia is common but can be masked by glucose administration.

There is a considerable spectrum of disease severity; infants can present with a chronic course of failure to thrive, hepatomegaly and liver impairment. School-age children may present with avoidance of sweet foods and hepatomegaly, with dentition that is unusually free of caries. Patients may develop specific food aversion to avoid sources of fructose that allow them to remain quite well.

Biochemical associations include lactic acidosis, hyperuricemia, marked liver dysfunction and renal tubulopathy. The enzyme deficiency results in accumulation of fructose-1-phosphate, an inhibitor of both glycogenolysis and gluconeogenesis that depletes inorganic phosphate, thus restricting adenosine triphosphate (ATP) production. Cellular depletion of ATP is postulated to be a significant mechanism of hepatocellular toxicity.

There is no rapid test that can exclude HFI. If it is suspected on historical or clinical grounds, then fructose should be immediately excluded. A rapid correction of biochemistry and liver function can be expected over a number of days. Hepatomegaly may take several months to resolve. Direct enzyme assay is restricted to liver tissue, and liver biopsy is likely to be contraindicated in the acute phase. Genotyping of the *ALDOB* gene is likely to provide a definitive diagnosis.

Treatment is the lifelong restriction of fructose from the diet and is a challenge due to its restrictive nature. Care must be taken to avoid inadvertent consumption of fructose in medicines and processed foods.

Glycogen Storage Disorders

Glycogen is a glucose polymer found primarily in the liver and muscle that is an important source of rapidly accessible stored energy. Hepatic glycogen is ultimately released as free glucose, whereas glycogen in the muscle is utilised directly by the muscle itself. The GSDs are inherited disorders of glycogen breakdown with the exception of GSD type 0 (glycogen synthase deficiency), which is a block in glycogen synthesis causing patients to present with hypoglycemia due to a short fasting tolerance in the absence of hepatomegaly. The clinical manifestation of GSDs reflects the different utilisation of glycogen and can be hepatic (hepatomegaly/hypoglycemia), myopathic or a combination of both. The hepatic forms of GSDs include types I, III, IV, VI and IX (see Table 64.4). Massive hepatomegaly is a feature common to all hepatic GSDs, usually in the absence of splenomegaly although this may be present in a minority of patients in association with hepatic fibrosis and cirrhosis. Hepatomegaly is also a feature of the LSD infantile Pompe disease, also known as GSD type II, although this condition is dominated by hypotonia and cardiomyopathy and is not considered in this chapter.

A simplified scheme for liver glycogen metabolism can be seen in Fig. 64.2.

GSD type 1 differs from the other GSDs as it disrupts the release of glucose rather than the breakdown of glycogen itself, effecting both glycogenolysis and gluconeogenesis. Thus, hypoglycemia associated with raised lactate is a hallmark of GSD type 1, in addition to raised urate and triglyceride. It typically presents with hypoglycemia and hepatomegaly in the first 6 months of life when feed frequency is reduced, although a neonatal presentation with hypoglycemia is occasionally seen. Abnormal distribution of fat gives the 'doll-like' facies and nephromegaly is a prominent feature. Failure to thrive is common with catch-up growth only occurring with dietary treatment while platelet dysfunction leads to bruising and nose bleeds. GSD type Ib is also associated with neutropenia and abnormal neutrophil function that leads to skin infections, mucosal ulceration and inflamma-

Fig. 64.2 Glycogen metabolism in the Hepatocyte. *GSD* glycogen storage disorders, *Glc* glucose, *Glc-6-P* glucose-6-phosphate, *Glc-1-P* glucose-1-phosphate

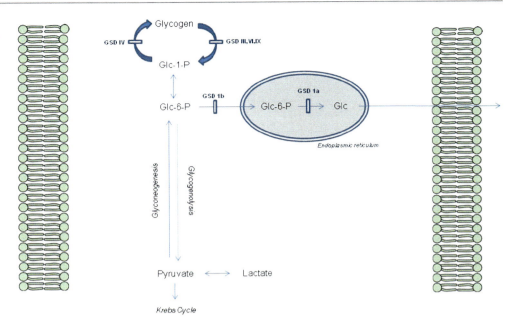

Table 64.5 Biochemical hallmarks of hepatic glycogen storage disorders

GSD	Lactate	Urate	Triglycerides	Cholesterol	CK	ALT	Glycogen
I	↑ Fasting	↑	↑↑	↑	N	↑	↑ Liver
III	↑ Postprandial	N	↑	↑↑	↑	↑↑↑	↑ Liver
							↑ Red cell
IV	N	N	N	N	N	↑↑	↑ Liver
VI	↑ Postprandial	N	↑↑	↑	N	↑	↑ Liver
IX	↑ Postprandial	N	↑↑	↑	N	↑	↑ Liver
0	↑ Postprandial	N	N	N	N	N	↓ Liver

CK creatine kinase, *ALT* alanine transaminase, *GSD* glycogen storage disorders

tory bowel disease. Long-term complications are numerous including osteoporosis, gout (hyperuricemia), pancreatitis (hypertriglyceridemia), polycystic ovaries, anemia, Fanconi syndrome and renal impairment. Hepatic adenoma occur in 75 % of patients peri- and postpubertally that have the potential for malignant change [12–15] (see Table 64.5).

GSD type III is caused by a deficiency of the glycogen debrancher enzyme that results in the accumulation of abnormal glycogen. It may be clinically indistinguishable from type I but fasting tolerance/tendency for hypoglycemia is typically not as severe as type I and nephromegaly is not a feature. Lactate characteristically increases postprandially and creatine kinase is commonly raised. Symptoms gradually improve, particularly around puberty, including spontaneous catch-up of growth and marked reduction in hepatomegaly. The mixed hepatic and muscle form is the commonest (type IIIa). Muscle weakness is not common in childhood and becomes more prominent in adults, although motor milestones may be delayed and activity can be impaired. Cramps at night are common. Long-term outcome in the purely hepatic form (type IIIb) appears excellent. Hepatic adenoma are rare, and reports of cirrhosis and progression to liver failure are

infrequent. In type IIIa complications include progressive myopathy and cardiomyopathy although the latter is rarely clinically symptomatic [16, 17].

GSD type IV is an extremely rare condition that classically presents with hepatomegaly and progressive cirrhosis. The deficiency of the branching enzyme produces abnormal glycogen resembling amylopectin. Glucose release from the abnormal glycogen is also impaired and fasting hypoglycemia may occur. Recently, however, the clinical spectrum of this disorder has widened considerably. Different presentations with varying overlap have been reported including foetal akinesia, infantile neuromuscular, cardiomyopathic and adult polyglycosan body disease [18–21]. In neonatal and infantile forms, death within infancy is usual.

Phosphorylase (GSD type VI) and its activator phosphorylase b kinase (GSD IX) are required for the removal of glycosyl molecules from the straight chains of glycogen. GSD type VI presents with pronounced hepatomegaly and a mild tendency to hypoglycemia in early childhood. Growth failure may be marked but catch-up growth occurs spontaneously and normal adult height is achieved. The disorder may be so mild that it remains undiagnosed. Long-term outlook is generally excellent, although hepatic adenomas have rarely been described. GSD type IX has a number of subtypes including three that have a hepatic component (see Table 64.4). Type IXa is by far the most common and has a relatively mild isolated hepatic phenotype similar to type VI. Type IXb is very rare and has a mild mixed liver/muscle phenotype. Type IXc has more severe phenotype often associated with significant hypoglycemia and progression to cirrhosis [22–24].

Confirmation of a suspected diagnosis of GSDs ultimately requires assessment of individual enzyme activity or genetic characterisation. Liver biopsy is not required for the diagnosis but commonly is the mode of diagnosis when patients being investigated for hepatomegaly are found to have significant amounts of glycogen in the liver. Periodic acid–Schiff (PAS) staining reveals cytoplasmic glycogen deposition often accompanied with increased lipid content. The glycogen is of normal structure in GSD types I, VI and IX while types III and IV have abnormal glycogen structure. Type III accumulates glycogen with shortened outer branches and type IV has an amylopectin-like structure [17]. Enzyme analysis requires targeted testing of individual enzymes, with enzymology of type I being limited to liver tissue. With the advent of high-throughput genetic techniques, simultaneous sequencing of all GSD genes is now available and is superseding enzyme assays, although the enzyme assay remains a valuable tool to evaluate genetic changes whose pathogenicity is uncertain.

Treatment for GSD type I includes strict dietary management. Hypoglycemic episodes are avoided by instituting frequent high-carbohydrate feeds during the day and continuous overnight tube feeds. This may be supplemented with uncooked or modified cornstarch to prolong normoglycemia [25], acting as a slow release form of glucose. Prophylactic trimethoprim is beneficial in GSD Ib for oral ulceration and granulocyte colony stimulating factor (GCSF) is reserved for resistant cases or those with recurrent infection. Regular assessment is required to monitor for long-term complications such as renal disease, hepatic adenoma/malignant transformation, osteopenia, hyperuricemia and hyperlipidemia [15]. Dietary management in type III depends on the severity [17]. Patients with early-onset hypoglycemia are managed as type I. A high protein intake has been advocated as gluconeogenesis is intact [26]. Dietary treatment in types IV, VI and IX is often unnecessary, but there is evidence that dietary management may improve fibrosis and long-term outcome in type IX [27].

Liver transplant is rarely considered but has been used in cases of hepatic failure, adenoma or malignancy or in cases refractory to dietary manipulation in patient with GSD types I and III [28, 29]. The only significant therapeutic intervention for type IV is liver transplant, although the extrahepatic progression of neuromuscular and cardiac disease post transplant has been documented in a number of patients [30].

Fanconi–Bickel Syndrome

The Fanconi–Bickel syndrome, previously classified as type GSD XI, presents with marked hepatomegaly secondary to glycogen storage and fasting hypoglycemia. Other features include postprandial hyperglycemia, hypergalactosaemia and renal Fanconi syndrome. The primary defect is a deficiency of the glucose 2 (Glut2) transporter important in the uptake and release of glucose from the liver. Glut2 is also expressed in pancreas, gut and kidney. Defects impair glucose sensing within islet β-cells compounding hyperglycemia in the fed state, due to decreased liver uptake, by blunting the insulin response. Hypoglycemia, in the fasting state, is secondary to impaired glucose release from the liver. Increased intrahepatic glucose inhibits glycogen degradation facilitating storage, and glycogen deposition may be noted on liver biopsy. Diagnosis relies on recognition of abnormal glucose homeostasis and renal tubulopathy while transaminitis, hyperlipidemia and hyperuricamia may be present. Treatment focuses on dietary support of glucose homoestasis with regular feed and also active replacement of renal losses.

Fructose-1,6-Bisphosphatase Deficiency

Fructose-1,6-bisphosphatase (FDP) deficiency is a defect in gluconeogenesis, the pathway that generates endogenous glucose and is a crucial mechanism to maintain glucose homeostasis when dietary glucose is depleted. It is also required for the metabolism of exogenous fructose. The classical features of FDP are hypoglycemia, lactic acidosis and prominent hepatomegaly. Approximately, 50 % of cases present within the first 4 days of life and the majority by 6 months of age. Acute acidosis causes hyperventilation and irritability that progress to coma, apnoea and cardiac arrest. Acute hepatomegaly is commonly found, and a urinary ketosis can be evident (an unusual finding in neonates). Diagnosis relies on clinical suspicion that is confirmed by enzyme analysis of FDP in leukocytes (or liver) or genetic analysis of the FBP1 gene. It is an autosomal recessive condition and a family history of neonatal death/acidosis is not uncommon.

Treatment of the acute presentation involves vigorous supplementation of glucose to inhibit gluconeogenesis. The acidosis and hepatomegaly generally respond promptly to this therapy. The acidosis may be severe enough to warrant use of bicarbonate to correct acid–base balance. If the sequelae of acute hypoglycemia and acidosis are avoided, prognosis is excellent. Mild hepatomegaly may persist during infancy but is not associated with signs of liver disease. Chronic treatment involves strict avoidance of fasting and adequate supply of energy during intercurrent illness. Dietary sources containing significant amounts of fructose (includes sucrose/sorbitol) should be avoided but fructose does not have to be rigorously excluded as in HFI.

Transaldolase Deficiency

Transaldolase deficiency is a very rare single enzyme defect of the pentose phosphate pathway. There seems to be a wide phenotype but the few cases described presented uniformly in the neonatal period with hepatosplenomegaly and liver impairment [31]. Associated features included dysmorphism (including cutis laxa), cardiac anomalies, oedema, renal abnormalities, hemolytic anemia and thrombocytopenia.

Prognosis is poor with developmental delay and commonly death within the first year of life associated with liver failure. Diagnosis relies on clinical suspicion followed by analysis of urine polyols (showing amongst others raised sedoheptulose-7P). Confirmation of diagnosis can be achieved by enzyme assay in lymphocytes, erthyrocytes, fibroblasts or liver tissue and by analysis of the *TALDO1* gene.

Congential Disorders of Glycosylation

The CDGs are a large group of disorders that present a considerable diagnostic challenge. Over the past decade, their number has rapidly expanded to nearly 70 discrete conditions. Individually, they are rare disorders with a very broad phenotype whose biochemical diagnosis relies on complex and often non-specific methods (i.e. transferrin isoelectric focusing). Glycosylation is the addition and modification of complex carbohydrate molecules (glycans) to proteins and lipids. The majority of extracellular, membrane bound and some intracellular proteins are glycosylated and the glycans perform a wide variety of functions from structural roles to cell–cell signalling. The process of glycosylation is a highly complex intracellular mechanism, the understanding of which is constantly being updated as new disorders are discovered [32].

The majority of CDGs are multisystem disorders. Developmental, skeletal and neurological problems dominate many of these conditions while hepatic involvement is not uncommon. Typical of this is by far the most common CDG, phospho-mannomutase 2 deficiency (PMM2-CDG). Even within this single condition, the phenotypic spectrum is very wide, but patients classically present in the neonatal period with dysmorphism, abnormal fat pads, inverted nipples and hepatomegaly. Significant development delay becomes evident with hypotonia, ataxia and failure to thrive. Transaminitis is typical and liver histology is characterised by steatosis and fibrosis with myelin-like lysosomal inclusions within hepatocytes on electron microscopy

Phosphomannose isomerase deficiency (MPI-CDG) is a rare CDG that presents primarily with hepatic and GI phenotype, but is remarkable as the sole CDG with an effect treatment. Typical presentation is within the first year to life with vomiting, abdominal distension, protein losing enteropathy, GI bleeding and liver dysfunction. Hypoglycemia may also be apparent. Dysmorphic features and a significant neurological phenotype are not associated with this condition. Transferrin isoelectric focusing is abnormal (see below) and diagnosis can be confirmed by enzymology in leukocytes or by gene sequencing (*MPI* gene). Treatment is by dietary supplementation of mannose [33].

Diagnostic testing for CDGs starts by analysing the glycan structures on a well-characterised glycoprotein such as transferrin (transferring isoelectric focusing). An abnormal pattern can then undergo further biochemical testing, or if the clinical picture permits, a specific genetic diagnosis can be sort. It should be noted that other liver pathology can result in an abnormal transferrin isoelectric focusing pattern, namely alcoholism, classical galactosaemia and HFI. When liver disease is present as part of an undefined systemic disorder, a congenital disorder of glycosylation should be considered [34].

Inherited Disorders of Protein Metabolism

Tyrosinemia Type 1

The metabolic defect responsible for tyrosinemia type 1, fumarylacetoacetase deficiency, arises late in the catabolic pathway of tyrosine (see Fig. 64.3). The immediate precursors to the block fumarylacetoacetate and maleylacetoacetate damage the liver and kidney, with their reduced derivatives including succinylacetone. The early onset form presents with liver failure, coagulopathy, jaundice and ascites in the first 6 months of life. Hypoglycemia may result from liver dysfunction or hyperinsulinism secondary to islet cell hyperplasia [35]. Milder forms may present with hypophosphatemic rickets secondary to a renal Fanconi syndrome. Occasionally, children present with neurological crises which resemble acute porphyria with abdominal pain, hypertension, peripheral neuropathy and muscle weakness.

Liver function reveals mild elevation of bilirubin, transaminemia, elevated alakaline phosphatase and deranged coagulation. Tyrosine, phenylalanine and methionine are raised on plasma amino acids in acutely ill patients. The presence of succinylacetone on urinary organic acids is pathognomonic, and the diagnosis is confirmed on genotyping although enzymology in lymphocytes or fibroblasts can be performed. α-Fetoprotein is raised acutely and falls with treatment. Urinary Δ-aminolevulinic acid is raised. Biochemical evidence

Fig. 64.3 Diagram showing biochemical pathway of tyrosine catabolism, defective step causing tyrosinemia type I and the action of the substrate reduction therapy nitisinone

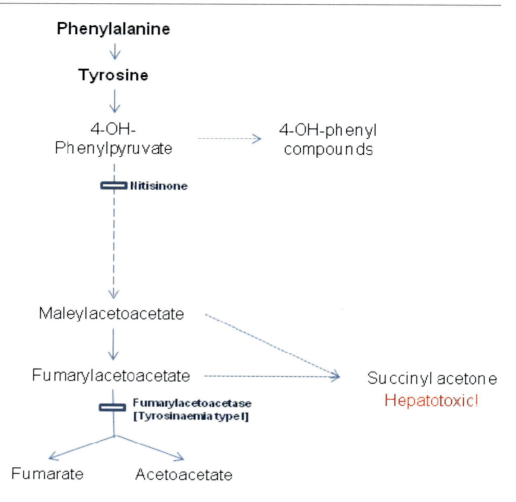

of a renal Fanconi syndrome is common. Hypertrophic cardiomyopathy is described.

The management of tyrosinemia type 1 has been revolutionised by nitisinone, originally developed as a herbicide, with rapid resolution of liver and renal dysfunction [36]. Treatment with a phenylalanine- and tyrosine-restricted diet is still required with home fingerprick monitoring of tyrosine and phenylalanine levels, but the risk of hepatocellular carcinoma is markedly reduced in patients treated early (<6 months). α-Fetoprotein monitoring in clinic should therefore continue with annual imaging of the liver. Current management combines oral nitisinone 1 mg/kg/day with a tyrosine- and phenylalanine-restricted diet supplemented with a tailored amino acid supplement. Methionine should be restricted in addition in the acute phase while still elevated. Target tyrosine levels are below 500 μmol/l.

Indications for liver transplant include: failure of response (no significant improvement in prothrombin time within 14 days of commencing treatment, or a bilirubin > 100 mMol/l inspite of increased dose 2 mg/kg/day), development of hepatocellular carcinoma and chronic liver disease with risk of developing hepatocellular carcinoma (development of liver nodule or persistently elevated or rising α-fetoprotein). Para-

doxically, patients with milder disease presenting later may do less well in the longer term as the liver has been subjected to chronic exposure to the toxic metabolites and therefore is more likely to have cirrhotic changes. Concerns remain as to the cognitive outcomes of treated patients, and further work is needed to delineate whether this is due to the condition or a long-term nitisinone effect [37].

Tyrosinemia type I is inherited in an autosomal recessive manner. Prenatal diagnosis is available.

Urea Cycle Disorders

The urea cycle converts waste nitrogen to urea for excretion via the kidney and is the site of synthesis of the nonessential amino acid arginine. Enzyme defects within the pathway result in hyperammonemia and encephalopathy (see Fig. 64.4). Inheritance is autosomal recessive with the exception of ornithine transcarbamylase (OTC) deficiency which is X-linked recessive. Females can present with symptoms due to the effects of lyonisation if sufficient wildtype OTC genes are inactivated in the liver. OTC is the commonest UCD.

Fig. 64.4 Urea cycle disorders. *CPS* carbamylphosphate synthase 1, *OAT* ornithine aminotransferase, *OT* ornithine transferase (hyperornithinemia, hyperammonemia, homocitrillinuria or HHH syndrome), *OTC* ornithine transcarbamylase, *NAGS* N-acetylglutamate synthase, *ASS* argininosuccinate synthase, *ASL* argininosuccinate lyase, *P5C* pyrroline-5-carboxylate

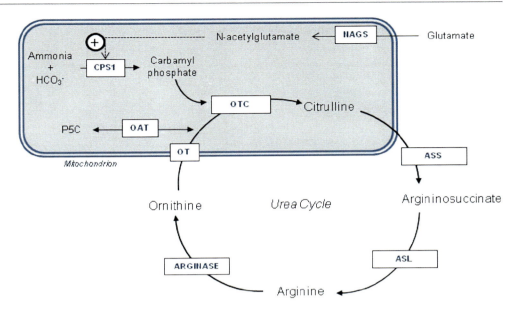

Neonatal presentation is a classical intoxication with lethargy/irritability, poor feeding, and vomiting progressing to overt encephalopathy. Tachypnoea secondary to the respiratory stimulant effect of ammonia initially produces a mild respiratory alkalosis. Apnoea and fits are also common. First presentation may occur later with a variety of non-specific features including failure to thrive, developmental delay, anorexia and vomiting. Investigation of cyclical vomiting should include assessment of ammonia during at least one of the episodes. Children may appear fussy eaters self-electing a low-protein diet. Episodes of acute metabolic decompensation may be precipitated by intercurrent infections. Long-term neurological sequelae relate to the severity of encephalopathic episodes (peak ammonia and duration), with peak ammonias as low as 360 µmol/l being associated with poorer outcome [38].

Diagnosis is suggested by marked hyperammonemia and low urea. Assessment of amino acids and urinary orotic acid reveals the level of the block (see Table 64.6) and can be analysed on a single sample by tandem mass spectrometry. Glutamine tends to be elevated as it forms part of the hepatic nitrogen pool that feeds into the urea cycle, and arginine low as it becomes an essential amino acid in UCDs due to reduced flux through the cycle, with the exception of arginase deficiency. Liver dysfunction and coagulopathy are often features in the acute stage. The main differential diagnosis for hyperammonemia includes spurious (poor sampling technique), organic acidemia, acute liver dysfunction and FAOs. Diagnosis is confirmed by liver enzymology and mutation analysis and prenatal diagnosis is available.

Acute management requires cessation of feeds, promotion of anabolism with 10% dextrose-based fluids with the addition of an insulin infusion if hyperglycemia appears and removal of ammonia. Initial management of hyperammonemia includes loading with alternate pathway drugs: Sodium benzoate (250 mg/kg) conjugates with glycine from the hepatic nitrogen pool allowing excretion in the urine bypassing the urea cycle and sodium phenylbutyrate (250 mg/kg) con-

Table 64.6 Diagnosis of urea cycle defects

Condition	Enzyme	Key amino acids	Orotic acid	Tissue for enzymology
NAGS deficiency	N-acetyl glutamate synthase	Glutamine ↑ Arginine-normal	Normal	Liver
CPS deficiency	Carbamyl phosphate synthase	Glutamine ↑ Arginine ↓	Normal	Liver
OTC deficiency	Ornithine transcarbamylase	Glutamine ↑ Arginine ↓	↑↑↑	Liver
Citrullinemia	Argininosuccinate synthase	Glutamine ↑ Citrulline ↑↑↑	↑	Liver
Argininosuccinic aciduria	Argininosuccinate lyase	Glutamine ↑ Argininosuccinate ↑	↑	Red blood cell Liver
Argininase deficiency	Arginase	Glutamine ↑ Arginine ↑↑↑	↑↑	Red blood cell Liver

jugates with glutamine. This helps reduce the nitrogen load on the cycle and can be followed by a continuous infusion. Arginine becomes an essential amino acid with the exception of arginase deficiency and should be supplemented (150 mg/kg load) followed by a continuous infusion. Higher doses are required in citrullinemia and arginosuccinic aciduria (500 mg/kg/day). Carglumic acid, an *N*-acetylglutamate synthetic analogue is the specific treatment for *N*-acetylglutamate synthase (NAGS) deficiency [39]. A trial of carglumic acid has been proposed for use in all undiagnosed hyperammonemic crises. If ammonia levels are >300 μmol/l and rising, dialysis is indicated for rapid control and to avoid the long-term neurological sequelae of prolonged hyperammonemia. The latter can be achieved with hemofiltration, but may be limited by the size of the baby (>2.5 kg) where peritoneal dialysis (PD) is used. Crossflow PD using two catheters may be used in the smallest babies to improve ammonia clearance [40].

Long-term management requires dietary protein restriction, titrating growth with ammonia (<70 μmol/l) and glutamine (<1000 μmol/l) concentration. Essential amino acids are monitored to ensure the adequacy of the diet. Essential amino acid supplements can be used as part of the protein intake having the advantage that nitrogen waste will be reduced as non-essential amino acids will need to be synthesised. Sodium benzoate and/or sodium phenylbutyrate, and arginine continue as part of long term management; carglumic acid in NAGS deficiency. Citrulline can be substituted for arginine in severe OTC and CPS deficiency.

Prognosis is related to the peak ammonia and duration; a rapid reversal of hyperammonemia reduces the risk of neurological injury [41]. Neonatal presenting OTC has the poorest prognosis, and early liver transplantation in the first 6 months is indicated to offer the best long-term outcomes [42]. Liver transplantation in UCDs is reserved for brittle patients with good neurology and has a 5-year survival of approximately 90 % [43]. Hepatocyte transplant has been used as a bridge to transplant in a few cases [44]. Liver fibrosis may develop in argininosuccinic aciduria, but the exact pathophysiology is not known.

Hyperornithinemia, Hyperammonemia, Homocitrillinuria Syndrome and Ornithine Aminotransferase Deficiency

Hyperammonemia is a feature of hyperornithinemia, hyperammonemia, homocitrillinuria (HHH) syndrome, a defect of ornithine transport into the mitochondrion. Severity is variable, but may present in a similar fashion to OTC deficiency. The diagnosis is suggested by an elevated ornithine, and it is confirmed on fibroblast uptake studies and genotyping.

Inheritance is autosomal recessive. Management follows UCD guidelines.

The differential for hyperornithinemia includes ornithine aminotransferase (OAT) deficiency (gyrate atrophy). Progressive retinal disease was thought to be the only manifestation; however, a number of OAT cases have now been observed where classical UCD presentation was a feature. At such times, ornithine levels are actually low rather than elevated, as the flux through the pathway in the first months of life is in the direction of ornithine synthesis rather than breakdown which then reverses during the first year of life [45].

Citrin Deficiency

Citrin deficiency results from a deficiency of the glutamate–aspartate transporter which has a role in gluconeogenesis from lactate and transporting cytosolic nicotinamide adenine dinucleotide (NADH)-reducing equivalents into mitochondria as part of the malate aspartate shuttle. Citrin deficiency causes two age specific phenotypes: neonatal intrahepatic cholestasis associated with citrin deficiency (NICCD) and citrullinemia type 2 (CTLN2) in adults that is more common in Japan and the Far East. The clinical features of NICCD are a transient intrahepatic cholestasis and poor weight gain. Liver dysfunction is variable and usually resolves in the first year of life. Some infants succumb to infection and liver cirrhosis. Transaminases are modestly elevated with hypoproteinemia and reduced coagulation factors. Complications include hemolytic anemia and hypoglycemia. Ammonia is only mildly elevated, but citrulline and methionine are significantly elevated with milder elevations in threonine, tyrosine, lysine and arginine [46]. Diagnosis is confirmed by SLC25A13 genotyping. Management includes the supplementation of fat soluble vitamins and the use of lactose-free or formulas containing medium-chain triglyceride (MCT). Many children subsequently develop aversion to carbohydrate-rich food and prefer protein-rich or fat-rich foods developing hyperlipidemia and the risk of fatty liver and pancreatitis. Some will develop CTLN2.

CTLN2 is characterised by acute onset recurrent hyperammonemia with neuropsychiatric symptoms. Hepatic argininosuccinate synthetase protein is reduced but without any mutations in the argininosuccinate (ASS) gene as seen in citrullinemia. Precipitants include alcohol, sugar intake, medicines such as anti-inflammatories or analgesics, or surgery. Not all patients have a preceding history of NICCD. Liver transplantation is the most effective treatment, preventing hyperammonemic crises and reversing the biochemistry [47]. Arginine supplementation reduces ammonia and careful dietary management is needed to provide appropriate carbohydrate (low) and protein (high) intake as the standard hyperammonemic treatment of low protein, high carbohydrate can precipitate crises in these patients. This is because carbohydrate suppresses ureagenesis in citrin deficiency. Sodium pyruvate may have a role in treatment by reducing oxidative stress, reducing NADH and reducing inhibition of ureagenesis [48].

Lysinuric Protein Intolerance

Lysinuric protein intolerance results from impaired transport of dibasic amino acids: lysine, arginine and ornithine. There is both defective intestinal absorption and increased renal losses. Hyperammonemia, with associated symptoms, develops postprandially as protein intake increases on weaning. High-protein food aversion, failure to thrive and hepatosplenomegaly ensue. Some patients have anemia, leukopenia and thrombocytopenia; the reticulocyte count may be elevated. Pulmonary fibrosis may develop. Severe osteopenia with fractures is common. Immune disturbance with raised immunoglobulin (IgG), lymphocyte subsets and antibody response is recognised with hemophagocytic lymphohistiocytosis as a known complication.

Urinary lysine, arginine and ornithine excretion is increased with a corresponding reduction in plasma levels. Plasma glutamine, alanine and glycine are raised. Ammonia rises postprandially secondary to poor urea cycle function due to arginine depletion. Lactate dehydrogenase, ferritin and zinc are all increased with normal serum iron and transferrin. Combined hyperlipidemia is common in adults. Citrulline supplementation improves urea cycle function and protein tolerance while some patients require alternate pathway medication. Moderate protein restriction further reduces the likelihood of hyperammonemia. Lysine supplementation is complicated by poor absorption and diarrhea but small doses can improve deficiency. Carnitine is given to patients with low free carnitine. Crises are managed as UCDs above.

Organic Acidemias

Organic acidemias result from inherited blocks in the catabolic pathways of amino acids provoking the accumulation of organic acids prior to the block. There are many disorders, but the commonest are propionic acidemia (PA), methylmalonic acidemia (MMA) and isovaleric acidemia (IVA). Acute presentations, either severe neonatal or intermittent late onset forms are associated with encephalopathy, marked metabolic acidosis, raised anion gap, ketosis, elevated lactate and variable hyperammonemia, the latter resulting from secondary inhibition of the urea cycle. Hepatomegaly and liver dysfunction are frequent. Neutropenia, or frank pancytopenia, is a sign of marrow depression and may lag behind the initial presentation and will recover as the decompensation is controlled. Blood glucose may be low, high or normal. Hypocalcemia is a frequent finding in the acute stage. IVA has an associated pungent odour of sweaty feet.

Diagnosis relies on urinary organic acid analysis to identify the key urinary metabolites and acylcarnitine analysis to identify abnormal plasma metabolites. Free carnitine may be depleted and glycine is often raised on plasma amino acid analysis. Complications include pancreatitis, cardiomyopathy and renal failure. Amylase should be measured during metabolic crises. Liver histology may show macro- or microvesicular fatty infiltration. Definitive diagnosis requires enzymology of the specific enzyme in fibroblasts.

Acute management is focused in promoting anabolism while removing toxic metabolites—intravenous fluids containing 10% dextrose are used in conjunction with protein restriction. Carnitine supplementation is used to facilitate organic acid excretion. Glycine is used in IVA for conjugation and increased clearance. Alternate pathway medication is used to manage acute hyperammonemia, and recently carglumic acid has been shown to be of use in some patients [49, 50]. Theoretically, this should work well as the site of urea cycle inhibition is at the level of NAGS and carglumic acid is a synthetic analogue of N-acetylglutamate. Acute toxin removal during crises may require dialysis.

General management consists of protein restriction to a level that prevents overload of the pathway while providing sufficient for growth and repair, with or without amino acid supplementation, and cofactor supplementation. A trial of vitamin B_{12} should be given to assess responsiveness in all patients with MMA. Metronidazole in low dose either continuously or episodically may be used to alter bowel flora to reduce propionate production from the gut. Constipation in itself may precipitate decompensation due to increased gut propionate production.

Patients remain at risk of decompensation most commonly precipitated by intercurrent infection and for patients with neonatal presentations the outlook is poor [51, 52]. Neurological and cognitive defects are common and progressive renal impairment is a feature of MMA leading to renal failure in the second to third decade. MMA patients who are B_{12} responsive have a better prognosis, but the poor outcomes for most organic acidemias has lead to serious consideration of transplantation. Liver transplant in PA has been successful with a marked reduction in risk of decompensation [53], but the risk of metabolic stroke persists and so a degree of protein restriction may still be required. The value of liver transplantation in MMA is less certain with significant continued risk of metabolic stroke and renal involvement [54]. Combined liver and renal transplantation has been performed, but is high risk [55], whereas isolated renal transplant appears to have a role in MMA patients with chronic kidney disease and may help reduce the frequency of decompensation [56].

Inherited Defects of Lipid Metabolism

Fat Oxidation Defects

The FAOs form a large group of conditions that commonly present with hepatic symptoms. Fatty acids are a major fuel source in the fasted state, the preferred substrate for cardiac muscle, and a vital energy source for skeletal muscle during prolonged exercise. Fatty acids are mobilised from stores and are oxidised by most tissues except the brain, which is reliant on hepatic β-oxidation for ketone production that can be utilised within the central nervous system reducing the demand for glucose.

Fatty acids are predominantly oxidised within mitochondria (see Fig. 64.5 and Table 64.7). The carnitine cycle is required for passage of fatty acyl-coenzyme A (CoA) across the mitochondrial membrane with the exception of medium chain fatty acids. The fatty acyl-CoAs then enter the β-oxidation cycle with shortening of the fatty acid by two carbons with each passage through the cycle yielding acetyl-CoA for entry into the TCA cycle or ketone production (liver), and reduced cofactors for entry into the respiratory chain for ATP production. The acyl-CoA dehydrogenases central to the β-oxidation cycle are chain length specific, for example, short-chain acyl-CoA dehydrogenase (SCAD), medium–chain acyl-CoA dehydrogenase (MCAD), and very long-chain acyl-CoA dehydrogenase (VLCAD) for saturated straight chain fatty acids. Unsaturated fatty acids require additional enzymes for oxidation, while branched-chain fatty acids require initial α-oxidation in peroxisomes before they can enter β-oxidation. This is why very long-chain fatty acids (VLCFA, that include the branched-chain fatty acids) are used as a screening test for peroxisomal disorders. Deficiencies of the electron transfer flavoprotein and its dehydrogenase (multiple acyl-CoA dehydrogenase (MAD) deficiency or glutaric aciduria type 2) block the transfer of electrons from β-oxidation to the respiratory chain, and also block the oxidation of branched chain amino acids, lysine and glutaric acid.

Clinical features are predominantly hypoketotic hypoglycemia, encephalopathy including a Reye-like syndrome, hepatomegaly, cardiomyopathy and rhabdomyolysis with the majority presenting within the first year, often precipitated by intercurrent infection. Fasting tolerance increases with age as hepatic glycogen stores increase and relative glucose requirement decreases. Hepatic symptoms are common with associated raised lactate and ammonia. Acute hepatomegaly can occur due to fatty acid mobilisation. Liver failure is rare. Hepatic symptoms may also occur in carrier mothers carrying an affected foetus. Cardiac involvement, either cardiomyopathy and/or arrhythmias may be seen in all FAOs except carnitine palmitoyl transferase 1 (CPT 1). Episodic muscle pain, rhabdomyolyis and myoglobinuria may be precipitated by metabolic stress such as exercise or intercurrent infections. Creatine kinase is elevated during muscle crises. Proximal muscle weakness may have a more chronic progressive course. Neuropathy and pigmentary retinopathy are long-term complications LCHAD deficiency. Neurological deficits may remain following acute encephalopathic insults in many of the FAOs.

Inappropriately low ketones in the presence of hypoglycemia always raises the possibility of an underlying FAO. Plasma acylcarnitine analysis by tandem mass spectrometry is the investigation of choice to diagnose the specific defect. Plasma free-carnitine may be depleted thereby masking the diagnostic acylcarnitine profile. Very low free-carnitine levels are found in a carnitine transport defect and are significantly elevated in CPT I deficiency. Full characterisation may require fat oxidation studies on cultured fibroblasts. Urinary organic acids at the time of decompensation may reveal characteristic dicarboxylic acids; however, the urine between bouts may be normal. Further confirmation may be gained from genotype analysis screening for the common A985G mutation in MCAD and G1528C in LCHAD. FAOs are inherited in an autosomal recessive fashion, and therefore siblings should be screened.

The acute management consists of glucose either orally or if not tolerated, intravenously as 10 % dextrose saline to switch off lipolysis. Hypoglycemia is a late sign and so normoglycemia does not exclude significant decompensation and therefore management should not be delayed. Resolution of encephalopathy may take some hours. Long-term management consists of avoiding prolonged fasting. An emergency regime consisting of giving frequent high-calorie glucose polymer drinks every 2 h day and night is adopted during intercurrent infections. Failure to improve or to tolerate the drinks requires admission to hospital for intravenous dextrose.

In the long-chain defects, fat mobilisation is suppressed to avoid the production of toxic long-chain acylcarnitines by frequent feeds, the use of uncooked cornstarch and overnight nasogastric feeds. Long-chain fat in the diet is restricted, and essential fatty acids supplemented as walnut oil. MCT bypass the carnitine cycle and enter the mid-portion of the β-oxidation cycle and therefore may be of benefit in carnitine cycle and long-chain defects.

Carnitine replacement is essential in the carnitine transport defects (100–200 mg/kg/day). Low levels of carnitine are seen in many FAOs due to accumulation of acylcarnitines. The use of carnitine in long-chain FAOs remains controversial with the theoretical risk of compounding mitochondrial toxicity with the accumulation of long-chain acylcarnitines. A trial of riboflavin should be started in all patients with MAD. Triheptanoin is currently under investigation for use in FAOs to help replenish tricarboxylic acid intermediates and thereby increase flux and ATP production [57].

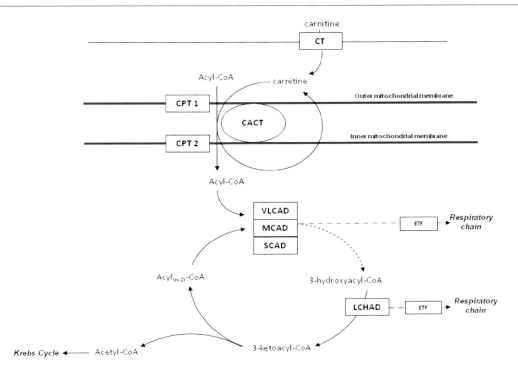

Fig. 64.5 Schematic of mitochondrial fatty acid β-oxidation. The carnitine shuttle facilitates fatty acid entry into the mitochondrial matrix where the β-oxidation spiral chain shortens fatty acids releasing energy in the form of acetyl-CoA that enters the Krebs cycle and electrons that are transferred via electron transfer flavoproteins *(dash-dot line)* to the respiratory chain. Disease causing enzymes are boxed: *CT* carnitine transporter, *CPT1* carnitine palmitoyltransferase 1, *CPT 2* carnitine palmitoyltransferase 2, *CACT* carnitine acylcarnitine translocase, *VLCAD* very long-chain acyl-CoA dehydrogenase, *MCAD* medium-chain acyl-CoA dehydrogenase, *SCAD* short-chain acyl-CoA dehydrogenase, *ETF* electron transfer flavoproteins (causing multiple acyl-CoA dehydrogenase deficiency (MADD)), *LCHAD* long-chain hydroxyacyl CoA dehydrogenase

Table 64.7 Clinical features of fat oxidation defects

Enzyme/transporter defect	Hypoketotic hypoglycemia/liver dysfunction	Cardiomyopathy	Rhabdomyolysis	Other features
Carnitine cycle				
Carnitine transporter (CTD)	+	+		
Carnitine palmitoyl transferase-1 (CPT1)	+	+	+	Renal tubular acidosis
Carnitine/acylcarnitine translocase (CACT)	+	+		
Carnitine palmitoyl transferase-2 (CPT2)	+	+ (CPT2 and cardiomyopathy)	+ (CPT2 and rhabdomyolysis)	
β-oxidation cycle				
Very long-chain acyl-CoA dehydrogenase (VLCAD)	+	+	+	
Long-chain hydroxy acyl-CoA dehydrogenase (LCHAD) and trifunctional protein (MTP)	+	+	+	Retinopathy, neuropathy
Medium-chain acyl-CoA dehydrogenase (MCAD)	+	+	+	
Short-chain hydroxyacyl-CoA dehydrogenase (SCHAD)	+			
Electron transfer				
Multiple acyl-CoA dehydrogenase (glutaric acidurias type II)	+	+		

The prognosis in many FAOs depends on the avoidance of acute decompensations. The outcome in MCADD is much improved once the diagnosis is made and future crises avoided [58]. Neonatal screening for detection of MCADD in the UK and other FAOs overseas on blood spot acylcarnitines by tandem mass spectrometry has greatly reduced morbidity and mortality [59], but cannot eliminate early neonatal deaths prior to the screening result being available. Siblings with milder phenotypes with the same genotype have been recognised since screening, particularly with regard to VLCAD. Recurrent rhabdomyolyisis remains a problem in patients with CPT 2, VLCAD and LCHAD, the latter also developing retinopathy and neuropathy which are not prevented by current management strategies.

Acyl-CoA Dehydrogenase 9 (ACAD 9)

ACAD9 is an unsaturated acyl-CoA dehydrogenase with weak overlapping activity with VLCAD but is non-compensatory in VLCAD deficiency and has a very different physiological role in that it is crucial for complex I biogenesis in the respiratory chain [60]. ACAD9 deficiency is therefore not an FAO but a mitochondrial disorder. The clinical, phenotype continues to expand and includes liver dysfunction including liver failure, hypoglycemia, muscle hypotonia, cardiomyopathy, lactic acidosis and neurological symptoms [61–63]. Patients may be responsive to riboflavin supplementation.

Other Inherited Metabolic Disorders

Lysosomal Storage Disorders

The lysosome is an intracellular organelle that is a key component in cellular recycling and homeostasis. The LSDs are a large group comprising of over 50 disorders with an estimated combined prevalence of approximately 1 in 8000 [64]. The fundamental pathological mechanism of these disorders is of a single enzyme deficiency leading to defective degradation or transport of a complex molecule such as a mucopolysaccharide or sphingolipid. The consequence is a build-up of 'storage' material that impacts on normal cellular function and homeostatis. These conditions are commonly progressive and multisystemic, effecting systems to a highly variable degree. Musculoskeletal involvement can include hypotonia, dysostosis multiplex, cardiomyopathy and the classically course features of the mucopolysaccharidosis. Endothelial reticular involvement can include hepatosplenomegaly and bone marrow dysfunction. Neurological involvement is common and is the most devastating feature of LSDs, causing severe neurological regression.

Hepatomegaly, usually associated with splenomegaly, is a common feature of LSDs. A list of LSDs that are associated with hepatosplenomegaly is listed Table 64.8 along with other common associated features. Of all the LSDs, the lipid storage diseases (NPC and Wolman (cholesterol ester storage) disease) are most commonly associated with liver dysfunction, and are considered in more detail below.

Niemann–Pick Type C

NPC is a disorder of cholesterol trafficking that leads to accumulation of unesterified cholesterol within the lysosome. The classical presentation is of neonatal jaundice and liver impairment that resolves with subsequent onset of a progressive neurological deterioration (between 3 and 13 years). However, the presentation is highly variable making the diagnosis notoriously difficult [65, 66]. Patients may have no hepatic involvement prior to the onset of neurological symptoms. Conversely, neonatal hepatic failure has been described in the absence of neurological symptoms, while a diagnosis has been made on the basis of isolated splenomegaly in adulthood alone. Persistent splenomegaly is a common finding. The neurological presentation is also varied and classically involves vertical gaze palsy. Another unusual feature that has been described in association with NPC is gelastic cataplexy. The other neurological manifestations are typically progressive with initial hypotonia leading to dysto-

Table 64.8 LSDs commonly associated with hepatosplenomegaly

Disorder	Associated features
GM1/GM2 gangliosidosis	Neurological regression, coarse facies, cherry-red spot
Mucopolysaccharidoses	Coarse facial features, +/− skeletal dysplasia, neurological regression, cardiomyopathy
Fucosidosis	Neurological regression, seizures, coarse facies
Mannosidosis	Neurological regression, corneal clouding, coarse facies
Sialidosis type II	Neurological regression, course facies, cherry-red spot, cardiomyopathy
Galactosialidosis	Course facies, neurological regression, skeletal dysplasia, spasticity, corneal clouding, cherry-red spot
Niemann–Pick A	Neurological regression, failure to thrive, cherry-red spot
Niemann–Pick B	Growth restriction, interstitial lung disease, normal intelligence
Niemann–Pick C	Neonatal liver disease, neurological regression, seizures, cherry-red spot
Farber	Contractures, skin nodules, neurodegeneration
Multiple sulphatase deficiency	Coarse facies, skeletal dysplasia, neurodegeneration, spasicity
I-cell disease	Neonatal coarse features, skeletal dysplasia, neurodegeneration, cardiomyopathy
Pompe	Hypotonia, cardiomyopathy, macroglossia
Wolman	Failure to thrive, abdominal distension, diarrhea, calcification of adrenal glands

nia, spasticity, dysphagia and psychiatric disturbances commonly leading to death in the first or second decade. Early onset of neurological symptoms is generally associated with a poor prognosis.

Diagnosis has been hampered by the lack of simple biomarker for the disease. Traditionally, diagnosis was made on a histological basis using stains such as filipin to detect the presence of unesterified cholesterol from fibroblasts or the presence of foam cells/sea blue histiocytes in bone marrow. Chiotriosidase is also significantly raised in NPC, as it is in a number of LSDs including Gauchers disease (it should be noted approximately 6% of the European population have no chitotriosidase activity [67]). However, these tests are not sensitive and may produce equivocal results. Further confirmation can be achieved by genetic characterisation of the two causative genes *NPC1* (accounting for approximately 95% cases) and *NPC2*. However, a new rapid test measuring oxysterols in plasma promises to be both a sensitive and specific test for this condition [68].

Treatment for NPC is generally restricted to symptomatic support of either hepatic or neurological manifestations, although some novel medical therapies are emerging as possible disease modifiers. Liver transplant has been used but failed to prevent neurological deterioration [69] while the evidence available to support bone marrow transplant does not demonstrate efficacy in improving neurology outcome [70, 71]. Migustat is a substrate reduction therapy that was originally developed to treat the sphingolipioses, but it has shown some efficacy in stabilising the progression of neurological disease, especially in the later onset forms of the disease [72]. Another medical therapy undergoing phase I clinical trial is cyclodextrin, an agent capable of sequestering cholesterol and that is postulated to facilitate its transport from the lysosome [73, 74].

Wolman/Cholesterol Ester Storage Disease

Both Wolman disease and cholesterol ester storage disease (CESD) are caused by a deficiency of lysosomal acid lipase that leads to accumulation of cholesterol esters and triglycerides. Wolman disease represents the severe phenotype with massive hepatosplenomegaly and death in infancy while patients with CESD have a different and attenuated phenotype involving more benign hepatomegaly in later childhood or adulthood. The genotypes observed in CESD are generally associated with residual enzyme activity (commonly associated with a c.894G>A mutation) [75].

Patients with Wolman disease usually have a short period of normal progress for the first month or two of life before developing diarrhea (steatorrhoea), vomiting, abdominal distension and severe failure to thrive. Massive hepatosplenomegaly is prominent and can be associated with ascites, jaundice and transaminitis while anemia is common. Survival beyond the first year is unusual. Calcification of the

adrenals is a hallmark of this disorder and can be identified on abdominal films, ultrasound and more reliably computed tomography (CT). Plasma cholesterol and triglyceride levels are commonly raised but may be normal. Further diagnostic clues can be found by histological examination; vacuolated lymphoctyes can be seen on peripheral blood film and foamy histocytes on bone marrow aspirate. Liver biopsy reveals foamy macrophages and Kupffer cells with large vacuolated hepatocytes. Periportal fibrosis develops and portal cirrhosis may be present [76].

Definitive diagnosis relies on assay of enzyme activity in leucocytes or characterisation of the *LIPA* gene. Treatment has historically been symptomatic. Bone marrow transplant has been implemented in early diagnoses with limited success [76, 77]. The development of enzyme replacement therapy potentially represents the first effective treatment for Wolman disease. In principle, enzyme replacement therapy shows promise as the severely affected organs (liver, spleen and gut) are highly accessible to enzyme given intravenously. Clinical trials for sebelipase alfa are currently ongoing (ClinicalTrials.gov identifier NCT01757 4).

Patients with CESD may present in childhood or adulthood with asymptomic hepatomegaly or hepatosplenomegaly. Progression to cirrhosis and chronic liver failure is uncommon. Hyperlipidemia is prominent and premature atherosclerosis is common. Treatment with 3-hydroxy-3-methyl-glutaryl-CoA (HMG-CoA) reductase inhibitor provides the mainstay of treatment.

Peroxisomal Disorders

Peroxisomes are subcellular organelles present in all cells except mature erythrocytes, and are especially abundant within the liver. Key functions include β-oxidation of chain fatty acids and fatty acid derivatives, pipecolic acid and glyoxylate degradation, phytanate α-oxidation, plasmalogen, cholesterol, and bile acid biosynthesis [78]. Biochemically, peroxisomal disorders are characterised by the extent of peroxisomal dysfunction from complete absence of peroxisomes (biogenesis disorders), to multiple enzyme defects and single enzyme defects. However, there is much overlap within the phenotypes of these groups; hence, a more useful categorization is made by considering clinical features and age of presentation.

In the most severe peroxisomal phenotype, Zellweger spectrum disorder (ZSD—includes previous classifications of Zellweger syndrome, neonatal adrenoleukodystrophy and infantile Refsum disease), hepatic involvement is a prominent feature. ZSD presents in the neonatal period or early infancy with severe neurological impairment including marked hypotonia, seizures and retardation, jaundice, hepatomegaly, cholestasis, hepatic dysfunction and classical dysmorphic features that are often the key to diagnosis. Liver histology shows fibrosis usually leading to micronodular cirrhosis. Renal cysts are common; however, they may not be easily demonstrable on ultrasonography. Ocular features are common including retinopathy, cataracts and optic nerve dysplasia. Failure to thrive evolves and little developmental progress is made. Death usually occurs within the first 12 months although the more attenuated forms may involve survival well into the first decade.

Defects in a large number of genes have been described as causing ZSD (mostly *PEX* genes). Initial investigations should include plasma VLCFAs. These are typically elevated, but it should be noted that in some peroxisomal phenotypes other than ZSD VLCFAs may be normal. Further delineation of the biochemical block may be gained by measuring plasma bile acid intermediates and plasmalogens. Definition of the precise molecular defect requires skin biopsy and complementation studies followed by enzymology or molecular genetic techniques. Other investigations that may be considered to support a diagnosis of ZSD are electroretinogram (ERG), visual evoked potentials (VEPs) and brain auditory-evoked responses (BSAERs) that are abnormal in most cases. Neuroimaging may delineate neuronal migrational defects and demyelination. Plain films of the knees may reveal calcific stippling.

Treatment remains supportive and can be challenging. Seizures are typically difficult to control and hypotonia often results in requirement for assisted feeding. Progressive liver impairment often contributes to morbidity and mortality. Docosahexanoic acid (DHA) supplementation has been attempted as it is believed to play an important role in brain development, but most recent evidence does not support therapeutic benefit [79]. Ursodeoxycholic acid is commonly used to improve bile flow in cholestatic patients, but the primary bile acids cholic and chenodeoxycholic acids have also been reported to improve hepatic outcome in a single patient with ZSD [80]. The primary bile acids are postulated to improve bile flow but also inhibit, by negative feedback, the production of abnormal bile acid metabolites formed in the absence of functioning peroxisomes. Currently, a clinical trial of cholic acid is in progress (ClinicalTrial.gov NCT00007020). The authors experience in one patient was increasing transaminitis upon commencement of cholic acid that was subsequently stopped. It should be noted that cholic acid is a biological detergent and increased hepatic concentration via enterohepatic circulation could at least in theory contribute to hepatotoxicity.

α-Methyl-CoA racemase (AMACR) deficiency is a rare peroxisomal disorder that is associated with an adult onset sensorimotor neuropathy, but has been described causing neonatal cholestasis. Treatment of the neuropathy is with a phytanate restricted diet while the neonatal cholestasis may respond to cholic acid therapy. It should be noted VLCFAs

will be normal with elevated pristanic and bile acid intermediates dihydroxycholestanoic acid (DHCA)/ trihydroxycholestanoic acid (THCA) [81].

Mitochondrial Disorders

Mitochondria are central to metabolism, producing the energy required to drive the cell via oxidative phosphorylation with the generation of ATP. Mitochondrial disease can affect any organ. However, those that have a high metabolic demand are more likely to produce symptoms, particularly the brain, muscle, kidney and liver. Mitochondrial involvement may be patchy throughout the body leading to a constellation of problems that at first may appear unrelated, so-called illegitimate associations that may be considered the hallmark of mitochondrial disease. Diagnostic clues such as lactic acidemia may be present but are often absent and further evidence of mitochondrial dysfunction is often sort by biochemical assay of respiratory chain enzymes that requires invasive muscle biopsy. If mitochondrial disorders are to be successfully identified, evidence of multisystem involvement must be actively sort. Treatment for the vast majority of mitochondrial disorders remains symptomatic. Most are progressive disorders, while examples of self-resolving conditions have recently been described.

There is a rapidly increasing number of mitochondrial disorders being described whose pathophysiology is becoming clear and that present with well-defined clinical syndromes. Examples of these that include the hepatic/GI system are included in Table 64.9, and the reader should be directed to several recent reviews of hepatic/GI mitochondrial disease [82, 83]. Any review of mitochondrial disease warrants a text all to itself, but this section outlines a few of the mitochondrial conditions whose primary features are hepatic/GI in nature.

Hepatic dysfunction is common in mitochondrial DNA depletion syndromes (MDDS). These conditions may present with early-onset liver failure, hepatomegaly and hypoglycemia and are usually associated with significant neurological symptoms such as seizures, encephalopathy, neuroregression and nystagmus. Alpers (Alpers–Huttenlocher) syndrome typifies this presentation and is caused by mutations in the nuclear gene *POLG* that encodes a DNA polymerase that is responsible for mitochondrial replication. Seizures are often the herald of disease onset, usually before the age of 2 years. Liver failure may then ensue and can be triggered by valproate therapy. Hepatic dysfunction has also been associated with disorders of mitochondrial DNA translation. A particularly interesting example of this is seen in mutations of the *TRMU* gene. These are associated with a syndrome of acute liver failure in early infancy that, if surviving the initial presentation, has spontaneous recovery of liver func-

Table 64.9 Mitochondrial syndromes affecting hepatic/gastrointestinal systems

System affected	Disorder	Mitochondrial pathology	Associated features	Gene(s)
Liver	Alpers–Huttenlocher	MDDS	Seizures, liver dysfunction, failure	*POLG, PEO1, FARS2*
	Hepatocerebral mitochondrial cytopathy	MDDS	Development arrest, seizures, liver dysfunction/failure, peripheral neuropathy	*DGUOK (elevated tyrosine)* *MPV17* *SUCLG1 (raised MMA)*
	Navajo neurohepatopathy	MDDS	Liver disease, sensorimotor neuropathy, acral mutilation, corneal scarring	*MPV17*
	'Benign' reversible mitochondrial hepatopathy	mtDNA translation defect	Liver failure with spontaneous recovery	*TRMU*
	GRACILE syndrome	Complex III assembly	Growth restriction, aminoaciduria, cholestasis, iron overload, lactic acidosis	*BCS1L*
	MEGDEL syndrome	Mitochondrial membrane defect	Liver dysfunction, 3-methylglutaconic aciduria, deafness, leigh-like encephalopathy	*SERAC1*
Gastrointestinal	MNGIE	MDDS	Pseudo-obstruction, encephalopathy, opthalomplegia, peripheral neuropathy	*TYMP*
	Pearson syndrome	Large scale mtDNA rearrangement	Pancreatic exocrine dysfunction, sideroblastic anaemia	
	Ethylmalonic encephalopathy	Inhibition of complex IV	Diarrhea, encephalopathy, acrocyanosis, petechiae	*ETHE1*

MDDS mitochondrial DNA depletion syndrome, *mtDNA* mitochondrial DNA, *MMA* methylmalonic acid, *GRACILE* growth retardation, aminoaciduria, cholestasis, iron overload, lactacidosis and early death, *MEGDEL* methylglutaconic aciduria with deafness, encephalopathy, and Leigh-like syndrome, *MNGIE* mitochondrial neurogastrointestinal encephalomyopathy

tion and subsequent normal development with favourable prognosis. Identification and intensive support of these patients is paramount. Defects of individual respiratory chain complexes can also give rise to hepatic disease. An example of this is GRACILE syndrome (growth restriction associated with aminoaciduria, cholestasis, iron overload, lactic acidosis and early death) caused by mutations in *BCS1L*, although this has been linked to a variety of other phenotypes many of which include liver impairment.

Examples of mitochondrial disorders that present with GI upset include mitochondrial neurogastrointestinal encephalopathy (MNGIE) and ethylmalonic encephalopathy (EME). MNGIE is caused by an autosomal recessive deficiency of thymidine phosphorylase that classically presents in the first three decades of life. Initial symptoms are often related to GI dysmotility and can present as frank pseudobstruction and failure to thrive/cachexia. However, neurological symptoms develop that include peripheral neuropathy, ptosis, ophalmoplegia, hearing loss and a progressive leukoencephalopathy. Lactic acidemia may be present. Unusually for a mitochondrial disorder, a diagnostic metabolic profile of raised urinary/plasma thymidine and deoxyuridine will confirm the diagnosis. EME also has a characteristic metabolic profile

with large amounts of ethylmalonic acid found in urine (ethylmalonic acid is commonly found in small amounts in urine as a non-specific marker of mitochondrial dysfunction). It is caused by mutations in *ETHE1* that encodes a mitochondrial sulphur dioxygenase, which has a role in sulphur detoxification. Accumulation of hydrogen sulphide potently inhibits complex IV of the respiratory chain. Affected infants classically have persistent diarrhea and the unusual finding of petechiae and acrocyanosis. Associated neurological findings include seizures, encephalopathy and developmental regression. This condition is usually lethal in infancy.

Investigation of suspected mitochondrial disease includes assessment of potentially affected organ systems—important to consider are markers of renal tubular dysfunction, liver function, echocardiogram/ECG and neuroimaging. Non-specific biochemical evidence of mitochondrial dysfunction can be demonstrated by elevated lactate levels, but further biochemical evaluation requires invasive testing such as muscle biopsy to assess individual components of the respiratory chain. Ultimately, the clinical and biochemical picture may enable selected molecular testing to come to a diagnosis.

Mitochondrial conditions have a vast array of presentations that can include hepatic dysfunction and GI symptoms.

These are multisystem disorders and should always be on the differential list of the gastroenterologist faced with a child with multisystem disease, especially a child with unexplained neurological symptoms.

Concluding Remarks

Inherited disorders of metabolism are individually rare but as a group of conditions are commonplace. The group is rapidly expanding as clinicians and scientists have access to technologies that allow comprehensive analytical screening of metabolites and high-throughput gene/genome sequencing. Inherited disorders of metabolism rarely display isolated hepatic or GI disease, but it is not unusual for these to be presenting features. In order to recognise these conditions promptly, clinicians should be aware of the different modes of presentation that inherited metabolic disease can manifest and also to actively search for clues to the presence of metabolic disease, such as a thorough family history and the presence of multisystem disease.

References

1. Champion MP. An approach to the diagnosis of inherited metabolic disease. Arch Dis Child Educ Pract Ed. 2010;95:40–6.
2. Poll-The BT, Maillette de Buy Wenniger-Prick CJ. The eye in metabolic diseases: clues to diagnosis. Eur J Paediatr Neurol. 2011;15:197–204.
3. Michel MA, Raucourt E, Bednarek N, Garnotel R. What disorders suspect following an increase of phenylalanine on newborn screening? Ann Biol Clin (Paris). 2014;72:193–6.
4. Matte U, Mourya R, Miethke A, Liu C, Kauffmann G, Moyer K, Zhang K, Bezerra JA. Analysis of gene mutations in children with cholestasis of undefined etiology. J Pediatr Gastroenterol Nutr. 2010;51:488–93.
5. Wang J, Cui H, Lee NC, Hwu WL, Chien YH, Craigen WJ, Wong LJ, Zhang VW. Clinical application of massively parallel sequencing in the molecular diagnosis of glycogen storage diseases of genetically heterogeneous origin. Genet Med. 2013;15:106–14.
6. Casey JP, McGettigan P, Lynam-Lennon N, McDermott M, Regan R, Conroy J, Bourke B, O'Sullivan J, Crushell E, Lynch S, Ennis S. Identification of a mutation in LARS as a novel cause of infantile hepatopathy. Mol Genet Metab. 2012;106:351–8.
7. Wong LJ. Next generation molecular diagnosis of mitochondrial disorders. Mitochondrion. 2013;13:379–87.
8. Johansen Taber KA, Dickinson BD, Wilson M. The promise and challenges of next-generation genome sequencing for clinical care. JAMA Intern Med. 2014;174:275–80.
9. Bosch AM. Classical galactosaemia revisited. J Inherit Metab Dis. 2006;29(4):516–25.
10. Bosch AM. Classic galactosemia: dietary dilemmas. J Inherit Metab Dis. 2011;34(2):257–60.
11. Waggoner DD, Buist NR, Donnell GN. Long-term prognosis in galactosaemia: results of a survey of 350 cases. J Inherit Metab Dis. 1990;13(6):802–18.
12. Lee PJ, Leonard JV. The hepatic glycogen storage diseases—problems beyond childhood. J Inherit Metab Dis [Internet]. 1995;18(4):462–72.
13. Lee P, Mather S, Owens C, Leonard J, Dicks-Mireaux C. Hepatic ultrasound findings in the glycogen storage diseases. Br J Radiol. 1994;67(803):1062–6.
14. Talente GM, Coleman RA, Alter C, Baker L, Brown BI, Cannon RA, et al. Glycogen storage disease in adults. Ann Intern Med [Internet]. 1994;120(3):218–26.
15. Rake JP, Visser G, Labrune P, Leonard JV, Ullrich K, Smit GPA. Guidelines for management of glycogen storage disease type I—european study on glycogen storage disease type I (ESGSD I). Eur J Pediatr [Internet]. 2002;61(Suppl):S112–9.
16. Lucchiari S, Santoro D, Pagliarani S, Comi GP. Clinical, biochemical and genetic features of glycogen debranching enzyme deficiency. Acta Myol. 2007;26(1):72–4.
17. Kishnani PS, Austin SL, Arn P, Bali DS, Boney A, Case LE, et al. Glycogen storage disease type III diagnosis and management guidelines. Genet Med. 2010;12(7):446–63.
18. Paradas C, Akman HO, Ionete C, Lau H, Riskind PN, Jones DE, et al. Branching enzyme deficiency: expanding the clinical spectrum. JAMA Neurol. Am Med Assoc. 2014;71(1):41–7.
19. Ravenscroft G, Thompson EM, Todd EJ, Yau KS, Kresoje N, Sivadorai P, et al. Whole exome sequencing in foetal akinesia expands the genotype-phenotype spectrum of GBE1 glycogen storage disease mutations. Neuromuscul Disord. 2013;23(2):165–9.
20. Escobar LF, Wagner S, Tucker M, Wareham J. Neonatal presentation of lethal neuromuscular glycogen storage disease type IV. J Perinatol. 2012;32(10):810–3.
21. Aksu T, Colak A, Tufekcioglu O. Cardiac involvement in glycogen storage disease type IV: two cases and the two ends of a spectrum. Case Rep Med [Internet]. 2012;2012:764286.
22. Albash B, Imtiaz F, Al-Zaidan H, Al-Manea H, Banemai M, Allam R, et al. Novel PHKG2 mutation causing GSD IX with prominent liver disease: report of three cases and review of literature. Eur J Pediatr. 2014;173(5):647–53.
23. Beauchamp NJ, Dalton A, Ramaswami U, Niinikoski H, Mention K, Kenny P, et al. Glycogen storage disease type IX: high variability in clinical phenotype. Mol Genet Metab. 2007;92(1–2):88–99.
24. Burwinkel B, Rootwelt T, Kvittingen EA, Chakraborty PK, Kilimann MW. Severe phenotype of phosphorylase kinase-deficient liver glycogenosis with mutations in the PHKG2 gene. Pediatr Res. 2003;54(6):834–9.
25. Bhattacharya K, Orton RC, Qi X, Mundy H, Morley DW, Champion MP, et al. A novel starch for the treatment of glycogen storage diseases. J Inherit Metab Dis. 2007;30(3):350–7.
26. Dagli AI, Zori RT, McCune H, Ivsic T, Maisenbacher MK, Weinstein DA. Reversal of glycogen storage disease type IIIa-related cardiomyopathy with modification of diet. J Inherit Metab Dis. 2009;32(Suppl 1):S103–6.
27. Tsilianidis LA, Fiske LM, Siegel S, Lumpkin C, Hoyt K, Wasserstein M, et al. Aggressive therapy improves cirrhosis in glycogen storage disease type IX. Mol Genet Metab. 2013;109(2):179–82.
28. Davis MK, Weinstein DA. Liver transplantation in children with glycogen storage disease: controversies and evaluation of the risk/benefit of this procedure. Pediatr Transplant. 2008;12(2):137–45.
29. Matern D, Starzl TE, Arnaout W, Barnard J, Bynon JS, Dhawan A, et al. Liver transplantation for glycogen storage disease types I, III, and IV. Eur J Pediatr [Internet]. 1999;158 Suppl:S43–8.
30. Willot S, Marchand V, Rasquin A, Alvarez F, Martin SR. Systemic progression of type IV glycogen storage disease after liver transplantation. J Pediatr Gastroenterol Nutr. 2010;51(5):661–4.
31. Wamelink MMC, Struys EA, Jakobs C. The biochemistry, metabolism and inherited defects of the pentose phosphate pathway: a review. J Inherit Metab Dis [Internet]. 2008;31(6):703–17.
32. Freeze HH. Understanding human glycosylation disorders: biochemistry leads the charge. J Biol Chem. 2013;88(10):6936–45.
33. de Lonlay P, Seta N. The clinical spectrum of phosphomannose isomerase deficiency, with an evaluation of mannose treatment for CDG-Ib. Biochim Biophys Acta Elsevier B.V. 2009;1792(9):841–3.

34. Jaeken J. Congenital disorders of glycosylation. Ann N Y Acad Sci [Internet]. 2010;1214:190–8.

35. Baumann U, Preece MA, Green A, Kelly DA, McKiernan PJ. Hyperinsulinism in tyrosinaemia type I. J Inherit Metab Dis. 2005;28:131–5.

36. de Laet C, Dionisi-Vici C, Leonard JV, McKiernan P, Mitchell G, Monti L, de Baulny HO, Pintos-Morell G, Spiekerkötter U. Recommendations for the management of tyrosinaemia type 1. Orphanet J Rare Dis. 2013;8:8.

37. Bendadi F, de Koning TJ, Visser G, Prinsen HC, de Sain MG, Verhoeven-Duif N, Sinnema G, van Spronsen FJ, van Hasselt PM. Impaired cognitive functioning in patients with tyrosinemia type I receiving nitisinone. J Pediatr. 2014;164:398–401.

38. Kido J, Nakamura K, Mitsubuchi H, Ohura T, Takayanagi M, Matsuo M, Yoshino M, Shigematsu Y, Yorifuji T, Kasahara M, Horikawa R, Endo F. Long-term outcome and intervention of urea cycle disorders in Japan. J Inherit Metab Dis. 2012;35:777–85.

39. Häberle J. Role of carglumic acid in the treatment of acute hyperammonemia due to N-acetylglutamate synthase deficiency. Ther Clin Risk Manage. 2011;7:327–32.

40. Raaijmakers R, Schröder CH, Gajjar P, Argent A, Nourse P. Continuous flow peritoneal dialysis: first experience in children with acute renal failure. Clin J Am Soc Nephrol. 2011;6:311–8.

41. Häberle J, Boddaert N, Burlina A, Chakrapani A, Dixon M, Huemer M, Karall D, Martinelli D, Crespo PS, Santer R, et al. Suggested guidelines for the diagnosis and management of urea cycle disorders. Orphanet J Rare Dis. 2012;7:32.

42. Lichter-Konecki U, Caldovic L, Morizono H, Simpson K. Ornithine transcarbamylase deficiency. In: Pagon RA, Adam MP, Ardinger HH, Bird TD, Dolan CR, Fong CT, Smith RJH, Stephens K, editors. GeneReviews® [Internet]. Seattle: University of Washington; 1993–2014.

43. Arnon R, Kerkar N, Davis MK, Anand R, Yin W, González-Peralta RP, SPLIT Research Group. Liver transplantation in children with metabolic diseases: the studies of pediatric liver transplantation experience. Pediatr Transplant. 2010;14:796–805.

44. Meyburg J, Hoffmann GF. Liver, liver cell and stem cell transplantation for the treatment of urea cycle defects. Mol Genet Metab. 2010;100(Suppl 1):S77–83.

45. Cleary MA, Dorland L, de Koning TJ, Poll-The BT, Duran M, Mandell R, Shih VE, Berger R, Olpin SE, Besley GT. Ornithine aminotransferase deficiency: diagnostic difficulties in neonatal presentation. J Inherit Metab Dis. 2005;28:673–9.

46. Ohura T, Kobayashi K, Tazawa Y, Abukawa D, Sakamoto O, Tsuchiya S, Saheki T. Clinical pictures of 75 patients with neonatal intrahepatic cholestasis caused by citrin deficiency (NICCD). J Inherit Metab Dis. 2007;30:139–44.

47. Ikeda S, Yazaki M, Takei Y, Ikegami T, Hashikura Y, Kawasaki S, Iwai M, Kobayashi K, Saheki T. Type II (adult onset) citrullinaemia: clinical pictures and the therapeutic effect of liver transplantation. J Neurol Neurosurg Psychiatry. 2001;71:663–70.

48. Saheki T, Inoue K, Tushima A, Mutoh K, Kobayashi K. Citrin deficiency and current treatment concepts. Mol Genet Metab. 2010;100(Suppl 1):S59–64.

49. Levrat V, Forest I, Fouilhoux A, Acquaviva C, Vianey-Saban C, Guffon N. Carglumic acid: an additional therapy in the treatment of organic acidurias with hyperammonemia? Orphanet J Rare Dis. 2008;3:2.

50. Abacan M, Boneh A. Use of carglumic acid in the treatment of hyperammonaemia during metabolic decompensation of patients with propionic acidaemia. Mol Genet Metab. 2013;109:397–401.

51. Grünert SC, Wendel U, Lindner M, Leichsenring M, Schwab KO, Vockley J, Lehnert W, Ensenauer R. Clinical and neurocognitive outcome in symptomatic isovaleric acidemia. Orphanet J Rare Dis. 2012;7:9.

52. Grünert SC, Müllerleile S, De Silva L, Barth M, Walter M, Walter K, Meissner T, Lindner M, Ensenauer R, Santer R, Bodamer OA, Baumgartner MR, Brunner-Krainz M, Karall D, Haase C, Knerr I, Marquardt T, Hennermann JB, Steinfeld R, Beblo S, Koch HG, Konstantopoulou V, Scholl-Bürgi S, van Teeffelen-Heithoff A, Suormala T, Sperl W, Kraus JP, Superti-Furga A, Schwab KO, Sass JO. Propionic acidemia: clinical course and outcome in 55 pediatric and adolescent patients. Orphanet J Rare Dis. 2013;8:6.

53. Vara R, Turner C, Mundy H, Heaton ND, Rela M, Mieli-Vergani G, Champion M, Hadzic N. Liver transplantation for propionic acidemia in children. Liver Transpl. 2011;17:661–7.

54. Kasahara M, Horikawa R, Tagawa M, Uemoto S, Yokoyama S, Shibata Y, Kawano T, Kuroda T, Honna T, Tanaka K, Saeki M. Current role of liver transplantation for methylmalonic acidemia: a review of the literature. Pediatr Transplant. 2006;10:943–7.

55. McGuire PJ, Lim-Melia E, Diaz GA, Raymond K, Larkin A, Wasserstein MP, Sansaricq C. Combined liver-kidney transplant for the management of methylmalonic aciduria: a case report and review of the literature. Mol Genet Metab. 2008;93:22–9.

56. Brassier A, Boyer O, Valayannopoulos V, Ottolenghi C, Krug P, Cosson MA, Touati G, Arnoux JB, Barbier V, Bahi-Buisson N, Desguerre I, Charbit M, Benoist JF, Dupic L, Aigrain Y, Blanc T, Salomon R, Rabier D, Guest G, de Lonlay P, Niaudet P. Renal transplantation in 4 patients with methylmalonic aciduria: a cell therapy for metabolic disease. Mol Genet Metab. 2013;110: 106–10.

57. Roe CR, Mochel F. Anaplerotic diet therapy in inherited metabolic disease: therapeutic potential. J Inherit Metab Dis. 2006;29:332–40.

58. Wilson CJ, Champion MP, Collins JE, Clayton PT, Leonard JV. Outcome of medium chain acyl-CoA dehydrogenase deficiency after diagnosis. Arch Dis Child. 1999;80:459–62.

59. Wilcken B, Haas M, Joy P, Wiley V, Bowling F, Carpenter K, Christodoulou J, Cowley D, Ellaway C, Fletcher J, Kirk EP, Lewis B, McGill J, Peters H, Pitt J, Ranieri E, Yaplito-Lee J, Boneh A. Expanded newborn screening: outcome in screened and unscreened patients at age 6 years. Pediatrics. 2009;124:e241–8.

60. Nouws J, Te Brinke H, Nijtmans LG, Houten SM. ACAD9, a complex I assembly factor with a moonlighting function in fatty acid oxidation deficiencies. Hum Mol Genet. 2014;23:1311–9.

61. He M, Rutledge SL, Kelly DR, Palmer CA, Murdoch G, Majumder N, Nicholls RD, Pei Z, Watkins PA, Vockley J. A new genetic disorder in mitochondrial fatty acid beta-oxidation: ACAD9 deficiency. Am J Hum Genet. 2007;81:87–103.

62. Haack TB, Danhauser K, Haberberger B, Hoser J, Strecker V, Boehm D, Uziel G, Lamantea E, Invernizzi F, Poulton J, Rolinski B, Iuso A, Biskup S, Schmidt T, Mewes HW, Wittig I, Meitinger T, Zeviani M, Prokisch H. Exome sequencing identifies ACAD9 mutations as a cause of complex I deficiency. Nat Genet. 2010;42:1131–4.

63. Haack TB, Haberberger B, Frisch EM, Wieland T, Iuso A, Gorza M, Strecker V, Graf E, Mayr JA, Herberg U, Hennermann JB, Klopstock T, Kuhn KA, Ahting U, Sperl W, Wilichowski E, Hoffmann GF, Tesarova M, Hansikova H, Zeman J, Plecko B, Zeviani M, Wittig I, Strom TM, Schuelke M, Freisinger P, Meitinger T, Prokisch H. Molecular diagnosis in mitochondrial complex I deficiency using exome sequencing. J Med Genet. 2012;49:277–83.

64. Meikle PJ, Hopwood JJ, Clague AE, Carey WF. Prevalence of lysosomal storage disorders. JAMA. 1999;281(3):249–54.

65. Vanier MT, Wenger DA, Comly ME, Rousson R, Brady RO, Pentchev PG. Niemann-Pick disease group C: clinical variability and diagnosis based on defective cholesterol esterification. A collaborative study on 70 patients. Clin Genet. 1988;33(5):331–48.

66. Wraith JE, Guffon N, Rohrbach M, Hwu WL, Korenke GC, Bembi B, et al. Natural history of Niemann-Pick disease type C in a multicentre observational retrospective cohort study. Mol Genet Metab Elsevier Inc. 2009;98(3):250–4.

67. Irún P, Alfonso P, Aznarez S, Giraldo P, Pocovi M. Chitotriosidase variants in patients with Gaucher disease. Implications for diag-

nosis and therapeutic monitoring. Clin Biochem. 2013;46(18): 1804–7.

68. Jiang X, Sidhu R, Porter FD, Yanjanin NM, Speak AO, te Vruchte DT, et al. A sensitive and specific LC-MS/MS method for rapid diagnosis of Niemann-Pick C1 disease from human plasma. J Lipid Res. 2011;52(7):1435–45.

69. Gartner JC, Bergman I, Malatack JJ, Zitelli BJ, Jaffe R, Watkins JB, et al. Progression of neurovisceral storage disease with supranuclear ophthalmoplegia following orthotopic liver transplantation. Pediatrics. 1986;77(1):104–6.

70. Hsu Y, Hwu W, Huang S. Niemann–Pick disease type C (a cellular cholesterol lipidosis) treated by bone marrow transplantation. ... Transplant. 1999;24(1):103–7.

71. Breen C, Wynn RF, O'Meara a, O'Mahony E, Rust S, Imrie J, et al. Developmental outcome post allogenic bone marrow transplant for niemann pick type C2. Mol Genet Metab Elsevier B.V. 2013;108(1):82–4.

72. Pineda M, Perez-Poyato MS, O'Callaghan M, Vilaseca MA, Pocovi M, Domingo R, et al. Clinical experience with miglustat therapy in pediatric patients with niemann-pick disease type C: a case series. Mol Genet Metab Elsevier Inc. 2010;99(4):358–66.

73. Ottinger EA, Kao ML, Carrillo-Carrasco N, Yanjanin N, Shankar RK, Janssen M, et al. Collaborative development of 2-hydroxypropyl-β-cyclodextrin for the treatment of Niemann-Pick type C1 disease. Curr Top Med Chem. 2014;14(3):330–9.

74. Vance J, Karten B. Niemann-pick C disease and mobilization of lysosomal cholesterol by cyclodextrin. J Lipid Res. 2014; 55(8):1609–21. http://www.jlr.org/content/early/2014/03/24/jlr. R047837.abstract.

75. Fasano T, Pisciotta L, Bocchi L, Guardamagna O, Assandro P, Rabacchi C, et al. Lysosomal lipase deficiency: molecular characterization of eleven patients with Wolman or cholesteryl ester storage disease. Mol Genet Metab Elsevier Inc. 2012;105(3):450–6.

76. Tolar J, Petryk A, Khan K, Bjoraker KJ, Jessurun J, Dolan M, et al. Long-term metabolic, endocrine, and neuropsychological outcome of hematopoietic cell transplantation for Wolman disease. Bone Marrow Transplant. 2009;43(1):21–7.

77. Gramatges MM, Dvorak CC, Regula DP, Enns GM, Weinberg K, Agarwal R. Pathological evidence of Wolman's disease following hematopoietic stem cell transplantation despite correction of lysosomal acid lipase activity. Bone Marrow Transplant. 2009;44(7):449–50.

78. Wanders RJ. Peroxisomes, lipid metabolism, and human disease. Cell Biochem Biophys. 2000;32(Spring):89–106.

79. Paker AM, Sunness JS, Brereton NH, Speedie LJ, Albanna L, Dharmaraj S, et al. Docosahexaenoic acid therapy in peroxisomal diseases: results of a double-blind, randomized trial. Neurology. 2010;75(9):826–30.

80. Setchell KDR. Oral bile acid treatment and the patient with Zellweger syndrome. Hepatology. 1992;15(2):198–207.

81. Lemonde HA, Gissen P, Clayton PT. Disorders of bile acid synthesis and biliary transport. In: Blau N, et al. editor. Physician's guide to the diagnosis, treatment and follow-up of inherited metabolic disease. Springer: Heidelberg; 2014.

82. Rahman S. Gastrointestinal and hepatic manifestations of mitochondrial disorders. J Inherit Metab Dis. 2013;36(4):659–73.

83. Molleston JP, Sokol RJ, Karnsakul W, Miethke A, Horslen S, Magee JC, et al. Evaluation of the child with suspected mitochondrial liver disease. J Pediatr Gastroenterol Nutr. 2013;57(3):269–76.

Wilson's Disease

65

Piotr Socha and Stuart Tanner

Introduction

Wilson's disease (WD) was first described as the new disease in 1912 by Samuel Kinnier Wilson: "it was characterized as progressive lenticular degeneration, a familial nervous disease associated with cirrhosis of the liver" [1]. After 100 years we know a lot about the disease—molecular defects have been identified, there is some agreement on diagnostic tests, and we have effective therapies. Still, there are many questions that arise with the growing knowledge on the disease. Moreover, diagnostic and therapeutic practices differ among countries which could be shown when collecting information in a large European database of new Wilsonian cases within the "Eurowilson" project. We do not have a clear answer to variability of clinical presentations of WD and mutation analysis does not explain variable course and onset of the disease. The most effective therapies are still discussed. There are a few position statements coming with proposals of diagnostic and therapeutic standards, but they also raise many opened questions. Also specific problems of pediatric age are not analyzed in detail [2].

Definition

WD is an autosomal recessive disorder of copper metabolism, which leads to copper accumulation in the liver and other organs and tissues including brain. The clinical presentation was first described by Wilson in 1912, who also indicated inheritance of the disease showing familial nature. The disease

gene encodes adenosine triphosphatase 7B (ATPase7B)—a protein responsible for transporting copper into the secretory pathway for incorporation into apoceruloplasmin and excretion into the bile. It is located on chromosome 13. Prevalence of different mutations differs among populations. Clinical presentation is variable—the disease commonly affects liver and central nervous system. The prevalence of the disease is estimated to be 1:40,000 up to 1:30,000.

Pathophysiology

Copper is an essential dietary nutrient which is present in most of dietary products. The daily requirement is about 0.9 mg and the excess must be excreted. Copper facilitates electron transfer reactions and is needed for mitochondrial respiration, melanin biosynthesis, dopamine metabolism, iron homeostasis, antioxidant defense, connective tissue formation, and peptide amidation. Still, it can be potentially toxic to the cells which may be explained partly by the Fenton reaction in which Cu^{1+} causes production of the highly reactive hydroxyl radical which may cause lipid peroxidation of macromolecules:

$$H_2O_2 + Cu^{1+} \rightarrow OH + Cu^{2+} + H_2O.$$

Biliary excretion is the only mechanism for copper elimination under physiological conditions, and it increases with increasing size of the hepatic copper pool. Trafficking of copper in and through the hepatocytes involves several transport proteins: *Copper transporter 1* (Ctr1) responsible for the copper uptake at the hepatocyte plasma membrane; *metallothioneins* (MT), intracellular proteins capable of binding metalions, including copper; and *metallochaperones* that mediate the delivery of copper to specific proteins, and they are responsible for transfer of copper from metallothionein to the site of synthesis of copper containing proteins. Trafficking of copper is essential for further binding with ATP7B protein.

P. Socha (✉)
Department of Gastroenterology, Hepatology and Nutrition Disorders, The Children's Memorial Health Institute, Al. Dzieci Polskich 20, 04730 Warsaw, Poland
e-mail: p.socha@czd.pl

S. Tanner
Academic Unit of Child Health, Sheffield Children's Hospital, University of Sheffield, Western Bank, Sheffield S10 2TH, UK

© Springer International Publishing Switzerland 2016
S. Guandalini et al. (eds.), *Textbook of Pediatric Gastroenterology, Hepatology and Nutrition,*
DOI 10.1007/978-3-319-17169-2_65

The WD protein, ATP7B has got several functions that finally allow effective copper excretion from the hepatocyte and binding with ceruloplasmin which protects from potential copper toxicity. Copper transport into the trans-Golgi is initiated by ATP binding to the "nucleotide binding domain" of ATP7B. ATP hydrolysis and subsequent dephosphorylation allows the movement of copper associated with two binding sites on one of the transmembrane domains into the lumen of the trans-Golgi. Entering trans-Golgi is essential for the further transport of copper—it is incorporated into apo-ceruloplasmin and other apoproteins and then excreted to sinusoids or after saturation of six copper-binding sites at the N-terminal cytoplasmic tail of ATP7B and phosphorylation of serine residues it migrates in vesicles to the biliary canaliculus [1].

Mutations of the WD gene coding ATP7B protein impair its function and lead to accumulation of copper in the hepatocyte and in other organs. There are more than 500 mutations in the WD gene identified which affect the catalytic and export functions of the protein (according to the database: http://www.wilsondisease.med.ualberta.ca/database.asp [3]). The most common are missense mutations. The functional consequences of most mutations are not described. Usually two different mutations can be found on two different alleles of a gene (heterozygous composition). The most common mutation in Caucasian patients is H1069Q in the nucleotide-binding domain. This mutant binds ATP in an incorrect orientation with a reduced affinity, causing instability due to temperature-dependent unfolding and retention of ATP7B$_{H1069Q}$ within the endoplasmic reticulum [4]. For better understanding the role of different mutation of functionality of ATP7B, a yeast strain that lacks its endogenous copper transporter was used to segregate ATP7B mutants into severe and mild categories based on their ability to restore growth. Studies in mammalian cells have shown decreased protein levels and mislocalization for several mutants, and copper transport has been studied in vesicles derived from cell lines with various ATP7B mutations [5]. The functional studies can help to understand why some mutations are pathogenic and lead to copper accumulation, but do not yet explain the

Fig. 65.1 Copper transport within a hepatocyte involving ATPase7B protein

phenotypic variability of WD. Liver disease seems to result from a direct copper accumulation in hepatocytes, and consequently mitochondrial damage and disturbance of lipid oxidation. Hepatic steatosis is an early pathologic feature of the disease and may be explained by this mechanism. Injury of other tissues seems to be a consequence of copper accumulation outside the liver and usually appears at later age. Once capacity of the liver to store copper is exhausted, copper is released into the circulation. It can be taken by different organs but the central nervous system is most vulnerable [6].

Specific pathways that allow the intracellular trafficking and compartmentalization of copper within the hepatocyte showing the role of ATPase7B are shown on Fig. 65.1.

Liver Histology and Ultrastructural Changes

Histological abnormalities observed in liver biopsy are not specific for WD and cannot be regarded as a valuable diagnostic tool. In the early phase, microvesicular and macrovesicular fatty deposition can be observed (Fig. 65.2), with glycogen-containing vacuoles in the nuclei of periportal hepatocytes. Liver disease may then progress to portal fibrosis and

Fig. 65.2 Histopathological findings on liver biopsy from patients with Wilson's disease: **a** steatosis (HE staining) and **b** advanced fibrosis (Azan staining). (Courtesy of Dr Joanna Kuszyk, Department of Pathology of the Children's Memorial Health Institute, Warsaw)

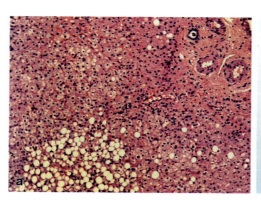
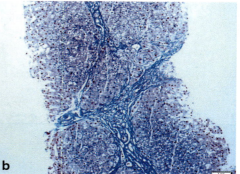

inflammation. It should be noticed that histological changes in WD may resemble those observed in autoimmune hepatitis (AIH) with interportal fibrous bridging or cirrhosis.

Utrastructural changes are also not regarded to have a significant diagnostic value— one of the typical features are pleomorphic mitochondria with increased matrix density and widening of intercristal spaces.

Copper staining can be used for diagnostic purposes—using rhodanine or rubeanic acid staining. The absence of histochemically demonstrable copper does not exclude a diagnosis of WD. Liver copper content is used as one of major diagnostic criteria—therefore in suspected WD, a piece of the liver biopsy should be placed in a dry plastic copper-free container for subsequent analysis by atomic absorption analysis.

Clinical Symptoms

WD may present with liver, neurological, or psychiatric symptoms. It seems that liver involvement can be observed in most of the neurological presentations but it is not always looked for. Due to high index of suspicion in many countries WD is diagnosed very early in the presymptomatic phase. WD may present at any age from early childhood (with raised transaminases, measured for some unrelated reason) to the eighth decade (often with surprisingly mild neurological features). Still, the clear liver symptoms (like hepatomegaly, clotting disturbances) have not been observed before the age of 3 years.

Hepatic Symptoms

There is a wide spectrum of hepatic involvement from asymptomatic to hepatomegaly, fatty liver disease, hepatitis, jaundice, cirrhosis, and liver failure at the end. As indicated earlier, the liver damage and liver symptoms are not characteristic and making diagnosis required biochemical and/or molecular tests. AIH can be easily misdiagnosed as specific for this condition autoantibodies are commonly found in WD. Therefore final diagnosis of AIH requires exclusion of WD.

Acute liver failure is a severe presentation of WD and requires fast diagnosis which may be difficult to obtain. It is usually found in a previously healthy child who suddenly presents with jaundice, hepatomegaly, rapidly progressing coagulopathy, and, in some cases, encephalopathy. The case history of a child may reveal important clinical problems in the past: episodes of jaundice, hemolytic anemia, or increased transaminases. Even if acute liver failure is not a chronic condition, liver biopsies taken at transplantation or postmortem show cirrhosis which indicates that it is acute on chronic liver disease. Acute liver failure is defined according to the Pediatric Acute Liver Failure (PALF) study group—in a child with biochemical evidence of acute liver injury, international normalized ratio (INR) exceeds/equals 1.0, in the presence of clinical hepatic encephalopathy (HE), or exceeds/equals 2.0 regardless of encephalopathy (HE). WD makes a significant proportion of ALF etiologies—in 703 ALF patients in the PALF registry, 23 had a diagnosis of WD. However, among 329 patients without a final diagnosis, WD had been tested for in only 81 % so there may be some underdiagnosis [7]. WD comprised 4 % of the King's College Hospital pediatric ALF series [8].

Some clinical and lab features may indicate WD in acute liver failure like KF ring, family history of WD, neurologic features of WD, jaundice and relatively moderately increased transaminases (100–500 IU/l) and alkaline phosphatase (<600 IU/l), hemolysis, and high bilirubin (>300 μmol/l) [9].

Presence of encephalopathy is a bad prognostic feature [10].

Chronic liver disease is more common among Wilsonian patients. Again, AIH may be falsely diagnosed because of the presence of low-titre autoantibodies. The differential diagnosis requires also testing for viral hepatitis and alpha-1-antitrypsin deficiency.

Acute hepatitis is not commonly observed, and it can be rather looked for in the past history of the patient with WD who could have had an episode of jaundice and malaise from which he recovered.

Neurological Symptoms

Neurological symptoms are extremely rare in children with WD as they usually develop in the third decade of life and are the presenting symptoms of WD in about half of all patients. Some initial symptoms can be difficult to be diagnosed like difficulty with speech. Otherwise the neurological symptoms seem to be typical and can be described as:

1. A dystonic syndrome with dystonic postures and choreoathetosis
2. An ataxic syndrome presenting as postural and intentional tremor and ataxia of the limbs
3. A parkinsonian syndrome with hypokinesia, rigidity, and resting tremor

To improve diagnostic approach and evaluate therapy, Czlonkowska and coworkers developed a scoring system for neurologic symptoms in adult patients with WD based on the Eurowilson project [11, 12]. The limited data on neurological presentations in children does not allow describing the frequency of neurological symptoms at this age. However, dysarthria, salivation, gait disturbances, and postural tremor should be looked for. The presence of Kayser–Fleischer ring is usually associated with neurological involvement.

Other Symptoms

Psychiatric symptoms are described to be the predominant presentation of WD recognized in adults in later age but usually are associated with other clinical symptoms. The most common seems to be depression which can lead to attempted suicide (also from author's experience in children). Psychiatric problems are not easy to detect as some of them can be attributed to the teenage such as mood change, aggressiveness, and irritability. These symptoms may also be a reason for noncompliance with therapy once WD is diagnosed.

Kayser–Fleischer ring is very typical for WD and should be always looked for with a slit lamp—it is a gold or gray-brown opacity in the peripheral cornea which represents a deposit of copper and sulfur-rich granules in Descemet's membrane. Although very characteristic, Kayser–Fleischer ring is uncommon in children (observed in less than 5% of children with WD).

Hemolysis with negative Coombs test is another typical feature of WD even if not commonly described in children with WD—usually it associated with fulminant liver failure.

Dermatological findings are also described in children with WD such as xerosis, keratosis piliaris, spider angioma, papulopustular lesions, and hyperpigmentation [13].

Fanconi syndrome (renal tubular abnormality presenting as glycosuria, aminoaciduria, renal tubular acidosis, impaired phosphate reabsorption) can be observed in the course of WD. Proteinuria may also be detected pointing to glomerular damage in the course of WD but it is usually associated with penicillamine therapy.

Skeletal manifestations appear rarely and include arthritis, rickets, or osteoporosis.

Asymptomatic WD

Asymptomatic liver disease seems to be the most common presentation due to increasing awareness of WD manifestation with slightly increased transaminases. Abnormalities at physical examination like hepatomegaly and splenomegaly and abnormal liver tests raise a suspicion of WD. In some countries, liver tests are checked at many occasions and any abnormalities lead to further differential diagnosis of liver problems [14]. Siblings of Wilsonian patients should be also diagnosed as early as possible usually in the preclinical phase.

Diagnostic Approach

As WD can mimic any kind of liver disease in childhood other than neonatal cholestasis, the diagnosis rests upon lab findings (Table 65.1) [15]. Ensure that the lab you are relying upon participates in an external quality assurance scheme. Each of the tests has limitations, and particular tests vary in usefulness in different clinical situations.

Plasma Ceruloplasmin

Plasma ceruloplasmin (CP) may be measured immunologically or by enzymatic activity; the latter is more accurate in WD, where apoceruloplasmin may contribute to the level measured immunologically. Be aware that CP is an acute phase reactant, so may be elevated into the normal range in WD with active liver inflammation, is produced in the liver so may be reduced in cirrhosis of other causes, may be reduced in WD or aceruloplasminemia heterozygotes, may be low in protein losing enteropathy, and is a glycoprotein so may be reduced in some disorders of glycosylation. Twenty

Table 65.1 Diagnostic biochemical tests for WD [15]

Test	Comments
Serum ceruloplasmin	<20 mg/dl (in >80% of WD patients)
Urinary copper excretion	24 h copper excretion >100 µg in 65% of WD patients
Urinary copper penicillamine challenge with two dosages of 500 mg 12 h apart and measure urine copper	24 h copper excretion >1600 µg in patients with active liver disease
Serum copper	Serum copper may be low in asymptomatic cases (because ceruloplasmin is low) or high in cases with active liver disease (because free copper is raised)
Serum "free" copper calculated on the basis that ceruloplasmin contains 0.3% copper	Free copper >25 µg/dl
Liver copper	>250 µg/g of dry weight liver

WD Wilson's disease

percent of WD patients may present with normal ceruloplasmin levels. Values exceeding 30 mg/dl are rare in WD.

Twenty-Four-Hour Urinary Copper Excretion

Accuracy of 24 h urinary copper estimations depends on the collection, the container, and the lab. Values greater than 40 µg/24 h raise the suspicion of WD; values greater than 100 µg/24 h make it very likely.

In the originally described penicillamine challenge test using a cut-off value of 25 mcmol/24 h (1600 mcg/24 h), the test was abnormal in 15 of 17 Wilsonian patients with active disease and 1 of 58 non-Wilsonian patients. The test was again evaluated by Muller et al. who showed sensitivity to be 76% and specificity—93% in the whole cohort of patients. However, and most importantly, the sensitivity was as high as 92% in symptomatic patients and only 46% in asymptomatic patients [16]. Others have found a cut-off value five times the upper limit of normal gives good differentiation. The test has not been evaluated in adult neurologically presenting cases.

Serum Copper

Serum copper is largely CP bound, so will be low in mild or presymptomatic disease but sometimes raised (e.g. in acute liver failure) if serum-"free" copper is raised. Calculated free serum copper according to the formula (total copper − 0.3% ceruloplasmin) is in practice a disappointingly inaccurate parameter, but the recently described direct measurement of "relatively exchangeable copper" holds more promise [17].

Liver Copper

When a liver biopsy is performed in suspected WD patients, a specimen for measurement of liver copper should always be obtained. Values equal to or higher than 250 µg/gm of dry weight are considered to be typical for WD. In chronic cholestatic conditions, the liver copper content will also be elevated, but this should not be a source of diagnostic confusion. Values less than 250 µg/g may be found in WD cirrhosis, where the centers of large regenerating nodules and tracts of fibrous tissue will both have lower Cu concentrations. Thus, Ferenci et al. assessed the hepatic copper content of 106 patients at the time of diagnosis of WD of whom 19 Wilsonian patients had a liver copper concentration below 250 µg/g dry weight. The sensitivity analysis based on comparison of these 106 patients to 244 other patients without WD showed that the upper limit of diagnosis (>250 µg/g dry weight) has a poor sensitivity (82%) and very good specific-ity. The low range (50 µg/g dry weight) has a higher sensitivity, but lower specificity as well as a positive predictive value [18].

Liver biopsy is rarely performed in adult neurological patients so the value of liver copper quantification in neurological presentation is not established.

Mutations in the WD ATP7B Gene, Locus 13q14.3 and Genetic Testing Strategy

The WD gene comprises 80,000 base pairs on 21 protein coding exons and a poorly characterized promoter. More than 500 mutations are recorded in the WD Mutation Database [3]. H1069Q (hist1069glu) is the commonest worldwide and by far the commonest WD mutation in Central Europe. By contrast, H1069Q is rare in Asian, Japanese, and Chinese patients, where other mutations predominate. In Western Europe, many different mutations are found and patients are often compound heterozygotes. A total of 116 different mutations, including 32 novel mutations, were identified on 356 alleles from 179 individuals in the coding region or adjacent splice sites of *ATP7B* in the NHS lab serving the UK [19]. Only 40 of these patients were homozygotes, the rest being compound heterozygotes.

Testing Strategy

Mutation detection by direct sequencing is now widely available but bear in mind the following. First, the testing strategy should be appropriate to the population served. In Central Europe a rapid detection method for H1069Q should be available, and it will be very valuable in the newly presenting acute case. For heterogeneous populations, it may be known which exons have the highest mutation frequency. For the UK, these are exons 14 (24%), 8 (20%), and 2 (12%). Analysis of these three exons would detect 56% of mutations while analysis of exons 2, 5, 8, 13, 14, 18, 1920 would detect 82% of the mutations in this population. Second, some patients have been found to have three mutations, two on one chromosome ("in cis"). Therefore finding two mutations does not necessarily mean the patient has WD; they might be in cis so that s/he is actually a carrier, that is, has one normal allele on the other chromosome. This mistake is avoided by proving that one of each of the patient's mutations is present in each parent. Third, though large deletions are rare they can occur and may be missed and the patient may be wrongly described as just having the one-point mutation on the other chromosome. Fourth, apparent parent to-child transmission of WD occurs, the unaffected parent turning out to be a Wilsonian patient. Therefore, family screening must extend to the children of known parents with WD. Mutation testing

Table 65.2 Diagnostic score in WD [15, 21]

Symptom/test	Score
Kayser–Fleischer rings	Absent-0
	Present-2
Neuropsychiatric symptoms suggestive of WD (or typical brain MRI)	Absent-0
	Present-2
Coombs negative hemolytic anemia + high serum copper	Absent-0
	Present-1
Urinary copper (in the absence of acute hepatitis)	Normal-0
	$1–2 \times ULN$-1
	$>2 \times ULN$, or
	$>5 \times ULN$-1 day after 2×0.5 g D-penicillamine-2
Liver copper quantitative	Normal- minus 1
	$<5 \times ULN$-1
	$>5 \times ULN$-2
Rhodanine positive hepatocytes (only if quantitative Cu measurement is not available)	Absent-0
	Present-1
Serum ceruloplasmin	>0.2 g/l-0
	$0.1–0.2$ g/l-1
	<0.1 g/l-2
Disease-causing mutations detected	None-0
	One-1
	Two-4
Assesment of the Wilson's disease diagnostic score	
0–1: unlikely	*2–3: probable*	*4 or more: highly likely*

ULN upper limit of normal, *WD* Wilson's disease

Diagnosis in Different Clinical Scenarios

Iin Central Europe a rapid H1069Q test may be the most cost-effective first-line test in any suspected WD patient. Otherwise one is reliant on biochemistry. One needs to tailor the testing to the clinical scenario. In acute liver failure, suspect WD if there is Coombs' negative hemolysis, a high bilirubin (>300 µmol/l) and a relatively low transaminases (100–500 IU/l) and alkaline phosphatase (<600 IU/l) and alkaline phosphatase IU/l per total bilirubin mg/dl ratio <2. Urine copper and a penicillamine challenge are probably the most valuable copper tests. In active but non-fulminant disease, the penicillamine challenge test is useful whereas in presymptomatic siblings it will be useless, but ceruloplasmin should be discriminatory and there is of course time to get a mutational analysis.

Making diagnosis in infants is also difficult. Healthy neonates and young infants present with naturally low levels of ceruloplasmin and liver copper is increased in infancy so these tests cannot be used directly for making diagnosis of WD.

for WD should be restricted to labs which participate in the European Molecular Quality Network.

However, the value of biochemical tests for making early diagnosis should not be completely excluded. Early screening for WD may be possible if new cut-off values for ceruloplasmin are established as indicated by Kroll and coworkers who analyzed blood spots for ceruloplasmin concentration from 1045 anonymous newborn screening specimens and from two Wilsonian patients. Ceruloplasmin levels were extremely low in Wilsonian patients (2.8 and 2.6 mg/dl) compared to healthy infants (6.5 to >60 mg/dl) [20] (see Table 65.1) [15].

Scoring System for Diagnosis of WD

As making diagnosis of WD based on clinical symptoms or single biochemical test is difficult, several parameters need to be taken into account all together. In 2001, a scoring system was proposed and further evaluated by Ferenci et al. [21] (Table 65.2) [15].

The patients with a total score of at least four are diagnosed to have WD. The patients with a total score of two to three are considered as "likely to have Wilson's disease, yet more investigations had to be performed." The diagnosis of WD was judged to be improbable for scores between zero and one [21].

In order to test this scoring system, Dhawan et al. investigated records of 143 children with chronic liver disease, aged at least 5 years. Among the patients studied, 53 children were diagnosed to have WD (median observation time 11 years) and 90 children had other liver diseases. Fifty patients with WD had a score ≥ 4 (true positives). A total of 85 true negatives with a score of either 2–3 (40 children) or <1 (45 children) were observed. Both sensitivity and specificity of this scoring system was higher than 94% [22].

Genotype–Phenotype

It would be prognostically useful if there were a clear mutation/phenotype relationship, but there is not.

It is common to find differing phenotypes among siblings even for identical twins. Two statements may be made. First, patients homozygous for H1069Q tend to present later and with neurological disease. Second, there is a suggestion that fulminant hepatic failure is more likely in patients with truncating mutations.

Treatment

The aim of therapy is to decrease copper absorption and accumulation in the liver and central nervous system. For all WD patients, lifelong medical therapy is required. Conventional medical therapies are based on either copper chelators (penicillamine, trientine, tetrathiomolybdate) or zinc. Chelators mobilize intracellular copper into the circulation which is then excreted with the urine. Zinc decreases copper content mainly by reducing intestinal absorption. It induces copper-binding metallothionein in both enterocytes and hepatocytes, reducing the damaging effects of free liver copper.

Definite treatment is liver transplantation which is however indicated only in selected cases where rapidly progressing liver failure cannot be reversed by medical therapy.

Evidence from observational studies shows very good long-term prognosis on medical therapy with a survival comparable to the general population, even if some of them do not normalize completely aminotransferase activity [23, 14]. Poor compliance is regarded to be the major problem and the major reason of poor outcome.

Copper Chelators

Penicillamine and trientine are chelating agents regarded to be the first-line therapy in severe liver disease, but also effectively used in neurological symptoms and in asymptomatic cases. The major limitations for their use (mainly penicillamine) are side effects and toxic reactions reported in almost 10% of adult patients. Still, the experience in children seems to be better than in adults like ours (Socha–Warsaw),

and experience of King's College, London (Dhawan) shows that these reactions are less frequent in children and usually do not require discontinuation of the therapy. The major risk of chelating therapy is worsening of neurological symptoms (in neurological presentation) after therapy is started and for this reason the doses are usually increased gradually (within a few weeks). Penicillamine therapy is more common in Europe (according to data from Eurowilson project–unpublished). Trientine can replace penicillamine in patients presenting with penicillamine intolerance (trientine is regarded to be safer). In some European countries trientine is not licensed. Tetrathiomolybdate is another copper chelator which was mainly investigated in neurologic presentation of the disease. It seems to be more powerful decoppering agent than trientine and peiniclamine but there is limited experience in pediatric practice. According to Brewer et al., it showed very strong control of free copper levels over the 8 weeks of treatment in adults and it was better than trientine in the tetrathiomolybdate/trientine double blind study [24].

The full dose of penicillamine is 20 mg/kg/day, given in three doses. Adults receive 1 g per day up to 2 g if there is a poor response. Side effects include hypersensitivity reactions (usually transient and at the beginning of therapy), proteinuria, fever, lymphadenopaty, and bone marrow suppression. Patients should be monitored for side effects with blood count, urine analysis, as well as with liver and renal tests.

Trientine should be given 300 mg twice a day in younger children or 600 mg twice a day in older children and adults.

Zinc

Zinc can be alternatively given to the patients with WD but it is not recommended in severe liver disease with abnormal synthetic function as chelating agents are believed to be more effective in producing negative copper balance. Zinc seems to be safe and it was the reason for its preferential or alternative use in neurological and asymptomatic cases. It is not associated with neurological deterioration which could be the main reason for its common use in neurological patients. Zinc is also used for maintenance therapy after the induction phase with chelators.

Zinc is given in the dose of 25 mg of elemental zinc three times in younger children (<50 kg) a day or 50 mg three times a day in older children. In very young children under 5 years of age the dose is not well defined. Patients should be fasted so zinc should not be given between meals. Monitoring of the therapy is based on measuring serum zinc levels, 24-h urinary copper and zinc excretion. Brewer et al. advise to test zinc serum and urine copper levels during therapy. A zinc serum level less than 125 µg/dL generally indicates poor compliance. Urine copper levels should not exceed 50–75 µg/24 h.

There are two different chemical zinc preparations used, zinc sulphate and zinc acetate. Zinc acetate is more commonly used and has a better tolerance profile but is also more expensive. Zinc sulphate is also commonly used but may cause more significant side effects like nausea, vomiting and epigastric pain, mild gastric irritation, decreased blood iron levels, and anemia. We have also recently reported gastric/duodenal mucosal ulceration or erosion [25]. These side effects may lead to discontinuation of the therapy and it could be the reason for slightly elevated transaminases observed on this treatment.

Different Clinical Presentations and Choice of Medical Therapy

The choice of medical therapy is related to clinical presentation of WD and there is an agreement to use chelators for acute liver failure as first-line treatment. However, there are still many controversies on preferential use of chelators or zinc for other clinical situations. In severe liver insufficiency due to WD penicillamine or trientine therapy should be started immediately after diagnosis is made. Improvement does not appear soon after therapy was started and usually first after one or several months liver function tests improve. For other hepatic presentations of WD, chelators seem to be more effective as indicated by the review of 288 patients with a median follow-up time of 17.1 years presented by Weiss et al. who showed that increase in activity of liver enzymes occurred more frequently from zinc therapy (14/88 treatments) than from chelator therapy (4/313 treatments; $P < .001$). Similarly, the survival without transplantation was better for chelating agents. Patients who did not respond to zinc therapy showed hepatic improvement after reintroduction of a chelating agent [26].

Zinc is commonly used in neurological presentation where it seems to be as effective as chelators [27].

Still, it is difficult to compare both therapies as most of the evidence comes from observational trials. Wiggelinkhuizen et al. performed a systematic review of zinc and penicillamine therapies for WD. They found 1 randomized controlled trial and 12 observational trials. Patients with liver presentation seemed to respond better to penicillamine. Zinc appeared to be better option in presymptomatic and neurological cases [28].

It is also difficult to compare trientine and penicillamine; however, trientine appears to be a safer option but due to high costs its use is limited in many countries. From the published experience of King's College in London (16 out of 96 cases were treated with trientine), trientine was as effective as penicillamine [29].

For asymptomatic cases, it is not clear at what age therapy should be started but there is an agreement not to start in the first year of life.

Diet in Therapy of WD

The role of the avoidance of copper reach food products (nuts, chocolate, liver, shellfish) is not well established, but they are traditionally excluded from the diet.

Liver Transplantation

Liver transplantation is indicated for acute liver failure with fatal prognosis. Acute liver failure with encephalopathy does not respond to medical therapy and requires immediate listing for liver transplantation. The indications for liver transplantation in acute liver failure without encephalopathy are less clear as many patients recover with chelation therapy. It is advised to use the scoring system developed at King's College Hospital (Table 65.3) [30], which should be applied daily. A score ≥ 11 indicates the need to list urgently for liver transplantation. A deteriorating score similarly raises the need to list. A stable or improving score is an indication to continue with medical therapy [30].

The indications for liver transplantation are less clear in patients with predominant neurological symptoms. In general, neurological symptoms are not an indication for liver transplantation but there are some reports of neurological improvement after liver transplantation (however, some patients deteriorated).

Table 65.3 Prognostic score in acute liver failure due to WD. A score ≥ 11 indicates the need to list for urgent liver transplantation. A sensitivity and specificity of 93 and 97 %, and positive predictive value and negative predictive values of 92 and 97 %, respectively, are reported [30]

Score	Bilirubin (µmol/L)	INR	AST (IU/L)	WCC ($\times 10^9$/L)	Albumin (g/L)
0	0–100	0–1.29	0–100	0–6.7	>45
1	101–150	1.3–1.6	101–150	6.8–8.3	34–44
2	151–200	1.7–1.9	151–300	8.4–10.3	25–33
3	201–300	2.0–2.4	301–400	10.4–15.3	21–24
4	>301	>2.5	>401	>15.4	<20

WCC white blood cell count, *INR* international normalized ratio, *AST* aspartate aminotransferase

Therapy in Pregnancy

Treatment should be continued throughout the pregnancy to avoid exacerbation of symptoms. Zinc is commonly used in this period as it appears to be safer but according to some practices penicillamine can be used in decreased doses even if safety of this therapy is not well proven.

Novel Therapies

Present medical therapy is effective enough but recent progress in gene therapy may be also used for treatment of WD. Novel strategies aim at enhancing the protein expression of mutant ATP7B with residual copper export activity. Some therapies were tested in animal models like hepatocyte transplantation, lentiviral gene transfer or adenovirus-mediated transfer.

Compliance

Life-long compliance to drug therapy seems to be major problem in WD which decides about prognosis. Stopping medication may lead to severe organ damage, or even death, within a time period that can be as short as a couple of months. There are several reasons for poor compliance: nausea on zinc therapy, fear for numerous side effects of penicillamine, revolting age (teenagers) as well as psychiatric problems seen in Wilsonian patients. Urine copper excretion and free copper concentration are also good indicators of compliance during penicillamine therapy.

Conclusions

Even if prevalence of WD is not high it should be included into differential diagnosis of chronic liver disease and acute liver failure in children >3 years of age. Disease can be diagnosed early in children with increased transaminase activity and/or hepatomegaly. The scoring system for diagnosis of WD may be helpful and it is highly specific. Except for molecular diagnosis no single test can be used to establish diagnosis or for screening.

It is difficult to compare effectiveness of different therapies but penicillamine or trientine appear to be drugs of choice for severe liver damage. Zinc is regarded to be safer and is mainly used in mild liver, neurological, or asymptomatic disease.

References

1. Pilankatta R, Lewis D, Inesi G. Involvement of protein kinase D in expression and trafficking of ATP7B (copper ATPase). J Biol Chem. 2011;286(9):7389–96.
2. EASL Clinical Practice Guidelines: Wilson's disease. J Hepatol. 2012;56(3):671–85.
3. http://www.wilsondisease.med.ualberta.ca/database.asp.
4. Hasan NM, Gupta A, Polishchuk E, et al. Molecular events initiating exit of a copper-transporting ATPase ATP7B from the trans-Golgi network. J Biol Chem. 2012;287(43):36041–50.
5. Huster D, Kuhne A, Bhattacharjee A, et al. Diverse functional properties of Wilson disease ATP7B variants. Gastroenterology 2012;142(4):947–56.e5.
6. Ferenci P. Pathophysiology and clinical features of Wilson disease. Metab Brain Dis. 2004;19: 229–39.
7. Narkewicz MR, Dell Olio D, Karpen SJ, et al. Pattern of diagnostic evaluation for the causes of pediatric acute liver failure: an opportunity for quality improvement. J Pediatr. 2009;155(6):801–6, e1.
8. Dhawan A. Acute liver failure in children and adolescents. Clin Res Hepatol Gastroenterol. 2012;36(3):278–83.
9. Shaver WA, Bhatt H, Combes B. Low serum alkaline phosphatase activity in Wilson's disease. Hepatology (Baltimore, Md) 1986;6(5):859–63.
10. Berman DH, Leventhal RI, Gavaler JS, Cadoff EM, Van Thiel DH. Clinical differentiation of fulminant Wilsonian hepatitis from other causes of hepatic failure. Gastroenterology 1991;100(4):1129–34.
11. Członkowska A, Tarnacka B, Möller JC, et al. Unified Wilson's disease rating scale—a proposal for the neurological scoring of Wilson's disease patients. Neurol Neurochir Pol. 2007;41:1–12.
12. Leinweber B, Moller JC, Scherag A, et al. Evaluation of the unified Wilson's disease rating scale (UWDRS) in German patients with treated Wilson's disease. Mov Disord. 2008;23(1):54–62.
13. Seyhan M, Erdem T, Selimo MA, Ertekin V. Dermatological signs in Wilson's disease. Pediatr Int. 2009;51:395–8.
14. Iorio R, D'Ambrosi M, Marcellini M, Barbera C, Maggiore G, Zancan L, et al. Serum transaminases in children with Wilson's disease. J Pediatr Gastroenterol Nutr. 2004;39:331–6 (An observational studies on liver function test in children with Wilson disease).
15. www.eurowilson.org. Tests performed for the diagnosis of Wilson disease. This booklet has been developed as part of the EuroWilson project. Eurowilson is an academically governed organisation which received support from the European Commission Framework 6 Programme.
16. Muller T, Kroppikar S, Taylor RM, et al. Re-evaluation of the penicillamine challegne test in the diagnosis of WD in children. J Hepatol. 2007;47: 270–6.
17. El Balkhi S, Trocello JM, Poupon J, et al. Relative exchangeable copper: a new highly sensitive and highly specific biomarker for Wilson's disease diagnosis. Clin Chim Acta. 2011;412(23–24):2254–60.
18. Ferenci P, Steindl-Munda P, Vogel W, et al. Diagnostic value of quantitative hepatic copper determination in patients with Wilson's disease. Clin Gastroenterol Hepatol. 2005;3:811–8.
19. Coffey AJ, Durkie M, Hague S, et al. A genetic study of Wilson's disease in the United Kingdom.Brain. 2013;136:1476–87.
20. Kroll CA, Ferber MJ, Dawson BD, et al. Retrospective determination of ceruloplasmin in newborn screening blood spots of patients with Wilson disease. Mol Genet Metab. 2006;89:134–8.
21. Ferenci P, Caca K, Loudianos G et al. Diagnosis and phenotypic classification of Wilson disease. Liver Int. 2003;23:139–42.

22. Dhawan A. Evaluation of the scoring system for diagnosis of Wilson's disease in children. Liver Int. 2005;25:680–1.

23. Schilsky ML. Long-term outcome for Wilson disease: 85 % good. Clin Gastroenterol Hepatol. 2014;12:690–1

24. Brewer G, Askari F, Dick RB, et al. Treatment of Wilson's disease with tetrathiomolybdate: V. control of free copper by tetrathiomolybdate and a comparison with trientine. Transl Res. 2009;154:70–7.

25. Wiernicka A, Jańczyk W, Dądalski M, Avsar Y, Schmidt H, Socha P Gastrointestinal side effects in children with Wilson's disease treated with zinc sulphate. World J Gastroenterol. 2013;19(27):4356–62.

26. Weiss KH, Gotthardt DN, Klemm D, Merle U, Ferenci-Foerster D, Schaefer M, Ferenci P, Stremmel W. Zinc monotherapy is not as effective as chelating agents in treatment of Wilson disease. Gastroenterology. 2011,140(4):1189–98.

27. Czlonkowska A, Gajda J, Rodo M. Effects of long-term treatment in Wilson's disease with D-penicillamine and zinc sulphate. J Neurol. 1996;243:269–73.

28. Wiggelinkhuizen M, Tilanus ME, Bollen CW, Houwen RH. Systematic review: clinical efficacy of chelator agents and zinc in the initial treatment of Wilson disease. Aliment Pharmacol Ther. 2009;29:947–58.

29. Taylor RM, Chen Y, Dhawan A; EuroWilson Consortium. Triethylene tetramine dihydrochloride (trientine) in children with Wilson disease: experience at King's College Hospital and review of the literature. Eur J Pediatr. 2009;168:1061–8.

30. Dhawan A, Taylor RM, Cheeseman P, De Silva P, Katsiyiannakis L, Mieli-Vergani G. Wilson's disease in children: 37-year experience and revised King's score for liver transplantation. Liver Transpl. 2005;11(4):441–8.

Nonalcoholic Fatty Liver Disease

66

Emer Fitzpatrick

Introduction

Nonalcoholic fatty liver disease (NAFLD) was first described in 1980 in obese adults who had a pattern of injury similar to alcoholic hepatitis but who denied alcohol consumption [1]. The disease was subsequently described in children in 1983 [2]. Nonalcoholic steatohepatitis (NASH) is part of the spectrum of NAFLD, which ranges from simple steatosis to inflammation and fibrosis. The importance of this disease is borne out by the dramatic increase in its prevalence, now with an estimated 30% of adults and 10% of children affected in the USA [3–5].

It is likely that a significant number of those affected by NASH will go onto end-stage liver disease and/or hepatocellular carcinoma (HCC) within decades [6]. As NAFLD is predicted to become the most common chronic liver disease in the next decade, this will put a huge burden on an already overstretched liver transplantation service [3]. Both genetic predisposition and lifestyle factors influence the disease process, the pathophysiology of which is not yet fully understood. In view of the startling prevalence of the disorder and the potential to progress to serious liver disease, understanding the pathogenesis of the condition and the ability to recognize and manage the condition in children is of great importance.

Epidemiology and Predisposing Factors

The increase in prevalence of NAFLD is directly associated with the epidemic rise of obesity. Prevalence of childhood obesity in the UK has increased dramatically over the past three decades. The National Study of Health and Growth and the Health Survey for England demonstrated an increase in

prevalence of overweight/obesity in boys aged 5–10 years from 11.3/1.8% in 1974 to 17.9/5.7% in 2006/2007 and in girls aged 5–10 years from 9.6/1.3% in 1974 to 21.8/6.1% in 2006/2007 [7, 8]. The Health Survey for England 2012 reported that 14% of 2–15 year olds are obese and 28% are overweight. The National Health and Nutrition Examination Survey (NHANES) report from the USA also describes a dramatic rise in childhood obesity from 5% in 1960 to 15% in 2000 and 17.1% of children in 2003–2004 [9, 10] and 16.9% in 2007–2008 [11]. The definition most widely used for obesity in childhood is body mass index (BMI) >95th percentile and overweight as a BMI between 85 and 95th percentile. The 'normal' BMI varies with age and sex and different percentile charts are available for different populations.

The lack of clarity regarding the definition of the disorder is one of the main issues affecting the study of incidence and prevalence of NAFLD. Liver biopsy is the criterion standard for diagnosis of NAFLD, clearly this is not feasible as an epidemiological tool and proxy markers such as abnormal transaminases and/or the presence of an echogenic liver on ultrasound (US) are often used to define the disorder. The true sensitivity, specificity and predictive value of these proxy markers are unknown and it is well recognized that an elevation of transaminases may only occur in 60% of cases of NAFLD [12]. As the reference range for aspartate aminotransferase (AST) and alanine transaminase (ALT) is derived from population data including those with undiagnosed NAFLD, the use of these markers as a proxy for NAFLD is fundamentally flawed [3, 13]. In addition, there is considerable variation in normal ranges for laboratory values across different institutions.

Nevertheless, in the absence of a more robust noninvasive diagnostic test, population studies have used an elevated ALT (in the absence of other diagnoses) as definition of the disorder. In one US-based study, an elevated ALT was found in 8% of the 5586 adolescents aged 12–19 years [14]. Park et al. reported a prevalence of 3.2% in 1543 Korean teenagers using ALT >40 [15]. In Japan, a population-based

E. Fitzpatrick (✉)
Pediatric Liver, GI and Nutrition Centre, King's College London School of Medicine at King's College Hospital, Denmark Hill, London, SE5 9PJ, UK
e-mail: emer.fitzpatrick@kcl.ac.uk

© Springer International Publishing Switzerland 2016
S. Guandalini et al. (eds.), *Textbook of Pediatric Gastroenterology, Hepatology and Nutrition,*
DOI 10.1007/978-3-319-17169-2_66

753

study found 2.6% of the children had NAFLD based on US [16]. In a study from Italy of 268 obese children, 44% had NAFLD using US and elevated ALT [17]. Studies of liver biopsy findings give a more accurate reflection of prevalence as NAFLD is a histological diagnosis. An autopsy study from San Diego of almost 800 children who died an unnatural death described fatty liver in 9.3%, with NASH present in 3% [4].

The prevalence of NAFLD appears to increase with age and in general, boys are more at risk [4, 18, 19]. Ethnic variations also exist; Hispanic children and adolescents have a greater risk of NAFLD compared to Caucasian children. Black, non-Hispanic children are less susceptible despite a higher incidence of insulin resistance (IR) [4, 19, 20]. This mirrors findings in adults [5, 21, 22]. Both genetic and environmental factors are likely to be involved in ethnic distribution. Familial clustering is also seen [23, 24] with a strong heritability in first degree relatives [25].

The advent of genome-wide association studies (GWAS) has significantly advanced our understanding of genetic susceptibility to NAFLD. Single nucleotide polymorphisms (SNPs) in DNA resulting in the altered expression of a gene or altered protein function in addition to other epigenetic modification have been investigated in NAFLD. It is likely that multiple SNPs influence the phenotype of this polygenic disease [26]. Three large GWAS studies have identified a common SNP in patatin-like phospholipase domain-containing protein (PNPLA3; adiponutrin) rs738409 (I148M) to have a strong association with NAFLD [27–29]. PNPLA3 is a 481-amino acid transmembrane protein which is thought to have both lipolytic and lipogenic activity. The I148M SNP may promote hepatic accumulation of triglycerides (TG) and cholesterol by inhibition of TG hydrolysis [30]. The histological severity of disease is also associated with the presence of the SNP [31], but IR is not [32]. A recent pediatric study has shown an association between the SNP and severity of NAFLD in Italian children [33].

A SNP in the gene encoding apolipoprotein C III (APOC III) has also been implicated in NAFLD [34]. Increased levels of APOC III production that occur in the presence of this polymorphism leads to increased TG uptake and production. Polymorphisms in the adiponectin gene and receptor are implicated in both NAFLD and IR [35–37]. Adiponectin is a 244-amino acid adipocytokine with an important role in modulation of inflammation, glucose tolerance and fatty acid (FA) catabolism. Low levels are associated with type 2 diabetes and increasing severity of NAFLD.

Other polymorphisms associated with oxidative stress and immune function have a potential role in susceptibility to NAFLD. These polymorphisms may be associated with the inflammatory component of NASH rather than with steatosis per se; for example, polymorphisms in interleukin 6 (IL6; 174G/C) [38] and tumor necrosis factor α (TNFα) [39].

Liver fibrosis in NAFLD was found to be associated with a splice mutation in a tumor suppressor gene; Kruppel-like factor (KLF6) in a genome-wide study [40]. The presence of Gilbert syndrome caused by the uridine 5′-diphospho (UDP)-glucuronyltransferase1A1*6 polymorphism seems to have a protective effect against development of NAFLD possibly due to the antioxidant properties of bilirubin [41].

Other epigenetic factors, particularly microribonucleic acids (miRNAs) have been implicated in pathogenesis of NAFLD. Epigenetic modification is unrelated to changes in DNA sequence. MicroRNAs are small soluble RNAs which influence the translation of certain genes. The relative underexpression of microRNA-122 has been described in NAFLD [42].

Nutrition and physical activity are important environmental factors determining the risk of NAFLD, with lifestyle modification as the primary recommendation in the prevention and management of the disease [43, 44] (Fig. 66.1). Excess food intake and lack of exercise contribute to weight gain and contribute to the progression of liver fibrosis and inflammation in patients with NAFLD [45, 46].

Specific dietary factors either protect against or exacerbate the development and progression of NAFLD. Musso et al. analyzed 7-day diet records from 25 biopsy-proven adults with NAFLD and 25 controls, finding that saturated fat and cholesterol intakes were higher in cases than controls, whilst intakes of polyunsaturated FAs (PUFA), fibre and the antioxidant vitamins C and E were lower [47]. A Japanese study reviewed the 3-day food diaries of 28 adults with NASH and 18 with simple steatosis and identified a significantly lower zinc intake in patients with NASH [48]. Food-based analyses have suggested that higher meat and fructose [49–51], and higher consumption of low-nutrient, high-calorie, and high-salt food [52] are associated with

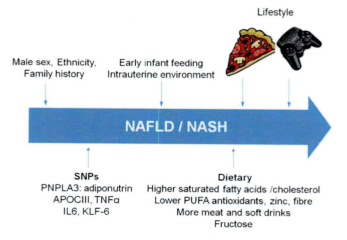

Fig. 66.1 Factors associated with the pathogenesis of NAFLD. *PNLA* pectin lyase, *APOC* apolipoprotein C, *TNF* tumor necrosis factor, *KLF* Kruppel-like factor, *PUFA* polyunsaturated fatty acids, *NAFLD* nonalcoholic fatty liver disease, *NASH* nonalcoholic steatohepatitis

NAFLD. Fructose has been identified as a particular culprit in increasing fat, inflammation and fibrosis [53, 54]. Few pediatric studies of dietary composition have been undertaken in NAFLD; however, a recent large study from Australia compared a Western diet in 993 14-year-olds to later development of NAFLD on US and found a significant association of Western diet and development of steatosis at 17 years [55]. A study in 82 obese Greek children revealed that a diet higher in carbohydrates, saturated FAs and lower in omega-3 was associated with NAFLD [56].

Dietary chemical composition of FAs may be critical factors in lipotoxicity observed in IR. Palmitic acid rather than oleic acid results in lower steatosis but in higher cell death and impaired insulin signaling [57]. A study of fish intake and omega-3 FA intake in children with NAFLD revealed a dietary deficiency of both was associated with increased portal and lobular inflammation [58].

Vos et al. described an association of dietary vitamin E insufficiency and increased steatosis in children with NAFLD [59].

The importance of the intrauterine environment and early infant feeding on development and progression of NAFLD has been a focus of interest. Offspring of obese mice were found to have a dysmetabolic, insulin-resistant and NAFLD phenotype compared to offspring of lean dams [60]. Offspring of lean dams suckled by obese dams developed an exaggerated phenotype suggesting that development of NAFLD and the metabolic syndrome is significantly influenced by early postnatal nutrition. Nobili and colleagues have studied breast-feeding habits in a cohort of children with NAFLD and concluded that breast-feeding is protective against progression of the disease from simple steatosis to steatohepatitis and fibrosis [61]. Figure 66.1 shows the factors associated with the pathogenesis of NAFLD.

Pathophysiology

NAFLD can be thought of as the hepatic manifestation of the metabolic syndrome (linking obesity, IR, hypertension and hyperlipidaemia). The pathogenesis of the condition is still incompletely understood.

IR is found in up to 80% the children with NAFLD and has a similarly high prevalence in adults with the condition [20, 22, 62, 63]. It is widely accepted that IR and the resulting hyperinsulinemia seem to play a major role in the development of hepatic steatosis and steatohepatitis. The molecular mechanism leading to the involvement of IR in the development of NAFLD is complex, however, and has not yet been fully elucidated.

The 'two hit hypothesis' proposed in 1998 consists of a first hit of liver fat accumulation which is caused by an imbalance in uptake and synthesis of hepatic lipids on the

one hand and export and oxidation on the other in the context of IR [64]. The steatotic liver is then thought to be more vulnerable to a 'second hit'. This may be oxidative stress, small-bowel bacterial overgrowth [65, 66], adipocytokines from a high visceral fat mass or saturated free FAs (FFA) [67]. A more recent hypothesis suggests that fat accumulation in the liver is a manifestation of stress and a protective mechanism in itself [68, 69]. This protective effect was demonstrated by Yamaguchi et al. in db/db mice fed a methionine–choline-deficient (MCD) diet [68]. Knockdown of TG synthesis increased the amount of potentially damaging FFA (i.e. blocked detoxification) in the hepatocyte and led to increased necro-inflammation and fibrosis despite decreased steatosis. Thus, in some individuals, the capacity for compensation via detoxification is exceeded and apoptosis and inflammation result.

Steatosis

Macrovesicular steatosis is characterized by the accumulation of TG (formed of glycerol esterified to three FAs) in the hepatocyte. Steatosis is conventionally thought to arise from increased hepatic supply of FFA as a result of obesity and associated extrahepatic IR.

Normally, adipocytes store fat after meals and release fat during fasting by lipolysis. In the liver, carbohydrate is stored as glycogen and when liver is saturated, de novo lipogenesis occurs via acetyl coenzyme A and FA synthetase. The third source of FAs as a substrate for the liver is dietary.

In the setting of normal insulin sensitivity, FAs undergo esterification to TG in the hepatocyte and are then exported from the cell as very low-density lipoproteins (VLDL) via apolipoprotein B enzyme activity [70]. Alternatively, they may undergo beta oxidation in the mitochondria or oxidation in the peroxisomes or microsomes. Uptake of FFA into the mitochondria requires carnitine palmitoyl acyltransferase which is inhibited by insulin and malonyl coenzyme A.

The net retention of lipids is the primary problem in steatosis. The most consistent predisposing factor to hepatic FA accumulation is IR, though other factors may be involved.

In normal physiological circumstances, the role of insulin includes glycogen synthesis, glycolysis and protein and lipid synthesis. In the postprandial state, insulin promotes lipogenesis and suppresses lipolysis and gluconeogenesis. The normal fall in insulin with the fasting state, which is accompanied by an increase in glucagon and catecholamines, mediates glycogenolysis and gluconeogenesis. These processes are accompanied by lipolysis and increased lipid oxidation. Sensitivity to insulin is increased by adiponectin and decreased by TNFα [71].

In the setting of IR, fat-laden and insulin-resistant adipocytes continue to release glycerol and FFA into the circulation, and deliver increased free FFA to the liver [72–74]. This in itself may then induce hepatic IR [75]. Hyperinsulinemia and hyperglycaemia promote de novo lipogenesis via upregulation of the transcription factors sterol regulatory element-binding protein 1c (SREBP1c) and peroxisome proliferator-activated receptor γ (PPARγ) [72]. In addition, insulin increases malonyl coenzyme A (an intermediate of FA synthesis) and inhibits carnitine palmitoyl transferase thereby inhibiting the passage of long-chain FAs (LCFA) into mitochondria for β-oxidation [76]. SREBP1c can also be upregulated by glucose and saturated fats, whereas polyunsaturated FAs (PUFA) lead to decreased expression [77]. Increased glucose levels also stimulate lipogenesis through the activation of carbohydrate response element-binding protein (ChREBP), a transcription factor activating the expression of key enzymes of glycolysis and lipogenesis [78, 79].

Hyperinsulinemia also results in decreased TG secretion as VLDL by lowering apolipoprotein B synthesis and stability [80, 81]. Hence, hepatic FFA uptake and lipogenesis outweigh FA oxidation and TG secretion leading to hepatic fat accumulation [82]. In the setting of peripheral IR some hepatic insulin sensitivity may be preserved with continuing de novo lipogenesis as a consequence. This is mixed and thought to be medicated through a functioning insulin receptor substrate 1 (IRS-1) which blocks lipid oxidation, but aberrant IRS-2 serine phosphorylation which fails to suppress gluconeogenesis [70].

Thus, in summary, the first concept in development of NAFLD is the net increase in circulating free FAs in the setting of IR. The adipocyte continues to release FAs even in the fed state as the insulin-mediated switch-off of lipogenesis is not triggered. The hepatocyte itself continues to produce free FAs via de novo lipogenesis. Activation of transcription factors such as SREBP1c, PPARγ and ChREB occurs in the presence of hyperinsulinemia and hyperglycaemia. Impaired free fatty oxidation and VLDL production ensue, both mechanisms which normally neutralize the toxic effects of free FAs.

Oxidative Stress

Mitochondrial FA oxidation and ketogenesis are increased and the transcription factor PPARα is activated as a result of FA accumulation [83]. This results in reactive oxygen species (ROS) which lead to oxidative stress and lipid peroxidation. Cell membranes are damaged and cytochrome c is released from the mitochondrial intermembrane space. In turn, this leads to an imbalance in the flow of electrons over the respiratory chain (RC) creating over reduction of RC complexes which can react with oxygen to form further ROS [84]. ROS may act as a 'second hit' in the development of NASH.

Mitochondrial function has been shown to be impaired in patients with severe steatosis and steatohepatitis [85]. Ultrastructural abnormalities of mitochondria have been demonstrated in patients with NASH [86, 87]. It is not clear if this is a primary or secondary phenomenon however. Mitochondrial abnormalities could be a pre-existing condition enabling the excessive production of ROS in the setting of enhanced FFA β-oxidation [86]. This could explain why for the same amount of obesity, or for the same degree of IR, certain patients just have steatosis, whilst others develop NASH and cirrhosis. Genetic polymorphisms could also at least partially explain this difference in susceptibility as some could favour mitochondrial dysfunction [88]. Alternatively, the overload of the mitochondrial RC, the resulting formation of ROS and subsequent lipid peroxidation products may give rise to mitochondrial damage. There is an inverse correlation of peripheral TNFα levels and measures of IR with RC enzyme levels suggesting that IR and cytokine activity may be important in impairment of the mitochondrial RC [89]. Enhanced ROS formation in the vulnerable steatotic liver subsequently triggers lipid peroxidation and the formation of reactive aldehydes such as 4-hydroxynonenal (4-HNE) and malondialdehyde (MDA). These give rise to further mitochondrial damage and ROS formation, resulting in a vicious cycle [84]. Hepatic stellate cells may be activated by these molecules thus leading to fibrosis [90].

Cytokines and Inflammation

Much of the progression from simple steatosis to steatohepatitis is characterized by an inflammatory response [91]. It is clear from both rodent and human studies that hepatic steatosis is associated with a state of chronic inflammation [92–94]. More specifically, hepatic steatosis in this context is associated with nuclear factor κB (NFκB) activation. FFA can directly activate the pathway via a lysosomal cathepsin B-dependent mechanism [95], as can mitochondrial and endoplasmic reticulum (ER) stress [93, 96]. NFκB is a sequence-specific transcription factor that functions as a proinflammatory master switch during inflammation. It upregulates the transcription of a wide range of inflammatory mediators including TNFα, IL6 and IL1β. Increased production of inflammatory cytokines by hepatocytes leads to Kupffer cell activation with subsequent inflammatory mediator release and hepatic and systemic IR [97].

Animal studies have shown that translocation of bacteria from the gut to the liver via the mesenteric circulation can activate Kupffer cells (via CD14/Toll-like receptor 4 (TLR4) binding) and induce a local and systemic inflammatory response [98]. There has been a great deal of interest in gut microbiota and the innate immune response in the context of obesity and IR [36]. There is evidence that intestinal bacterial overgrowth exacerbates NAFLD and that the prevalence of bacterial overgrowth is higher in those who are obese [37], the portal circulation providing a direct route from gut to liver. Manipulation of gut microbiota and elimination of intestinal bacterial overgrowth may thus be a promising way to halt the progression of steatosis to steatohepatitis and fibrosis.

Finally, visceral fat is a highly inflammatory tissue and the source of many inflammatory mediators known as adipocytokines which have an important role in IR and, most likely, in NAFLD [99, 100]. These adipocytokines, including leptin, adiponectin, TNFα and IL6, are polypeptides produced by both adipocytes and macrophages which infiltrate adipose tissue [101]. Adipokines are involved in the various injury patterns in NASH such as cell death, inflammation and fibrosis [84].

Leptin is a 16-kDa protein, a product of the ob gene and has important roles in appetite suppression and regulation of energy metabolism [102], with high levels in obese individuals though this is thought to be a result of leptin resistance. The role of leptin in NAFLD is not yet clear though it is thought to contribute as a proinflammatory, profibrogenic mediator [103, 104].

Adiponectin is a polypeptide adipokine with a collagen-like domain and globular domain produced in white adipose tissue. It has an important role in insulin sensitivity, as part of their action, thiazolidinediones (TZDs) are known to increase levels of adiponectin [105]. It is also hepatoprotective with anti-inflammatory and anti-fibrogenic properties [106–108].

Hepatocyte Apoptosis

Hepatocyte apoptosis is recognized as an important event in the development of chronic liver disease and has particular prominence in NAFLD [109]. The initiating event in apoptosis may be extrinsically mediated hepatocyte injury (e.g. in autoimmune liver disease, viral hepatitis and ischaemia perfusion injury). This is usually directed though pathways involving Fas ligand, TNFα, and TNF-related apoptosis-inducing ligand (TRAIL). Alternatively, intrinsic injury and death may occur via organelle dysfunction when cells are subjected to excessive oxidative stress (ER or mitochondrial), for example, with drugs/toxins, FAs, and iron. This results in altered membrane permeability and RNA damage with cytochrome c release [110, 110]. The injurious mechanism in NAFLD/NASH appears to be due to a combination of extrinsic and intrinsic insults [111, 112].

Though apoptosis is classically thought to be a silent event without provoking an inflammatory response, this is not the case in the liver [111]. Apoptotic bodies can activate stellate cells and Kupffer cells inducing an inflammatory re-

sponse and leading to the progression of steatohepatitis and fibrosis [113, 114].

Fibrosis

The final common pathway of inflammation, oxidative stress and hepatocellular damage is the development and progression of fibrosis in NAFLD. The process of fibrosis involves the deposition of extracellular matrix within the parenchyma. Cirrhosis, the end stage of the fibrotic process, is characterized by septum and nodule formation. Several different injurious processes will result in fibrosis. Hepatocyte injury, inflammation, apoptosis and death initiates the process which involves a cascade of inflammatory cells, the release of cytokines and the activation of fibrogenic effector cells (mainly stellate cells) [115].

Thus, a number of different processes and mechanisms are involved in the progression of steatosis to NASH: oxidative stress, inflammation, apoptosis and fibrosis. The exact sequence of development of obesity, fatty liver and NAFLD remains unclear. Whether IR causes hepatic steatosis or whether the accumulation of fat in the liver is the primary event leading to hepatic and peripheral IR is also yet to be elucidated [116]. Figure 66.2 shows the interplay of oxidative stress, inflammation, apoptosis and fibrosis in the pathogenesis of NASH [117].

Diagnosis and Histology

Children with NAFLD are often asymptomatic or may present with vague nonspecific symptoms such as abdominal pain and/or fatigue. The majority are overweight (gender-

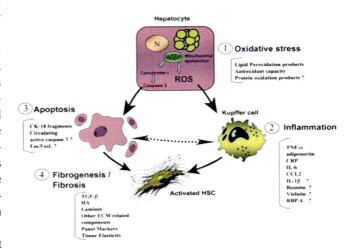

Fig. 66.2 The interplay of oxidative stress, inflammation, apoptosis and fibrosis in the pathogenesis of NASH. (*ROS* reactive oxidative species, *HSC* hepatic stellate cell. Reprinted with permission from [117], with permission from John Wiley and Sons)

and age-specific BMI > 85th percentile) or obese (> 95th percentile) [118]. Hepatomegaly may be present and acanthosis nigricans (a black pigmentation of the skin folds, axillae and neck), often seen in children with IR, is found in 30–50 % of children with NAFLD [20, 119]. The majority of children with NAFLD have IR as measured by homeostasis model assessment-IR (HOMA-IR is (fasting glucose (mmol/l) × fasting insulin (IU/l))/22.5) [20]. A normal HOMA-IR (<90th percentile) is generally less than 2.5 but varies with sex and pubertal stage [120]. Children will often have a positive family history for the metabolic syndrome [19].

In the diagnostic workup of NAFLD, alternative causes of chronic liver disease should be excluded including chronic hepatitis B and C infection, Wilson disease, α1-antitrypsin deficiency, autoimmune hepatitis and drug toxicity (including steroids, amiodarone, oestrogens and antiretroviral treatment). Conditions such as cystic fibrosis, malnutrition and parenteral nutrition-associated liver disease may also present with a fatty liver on US and can be excluded on clinical or biochemical grounds. In addition, mitochondrial/ metabolic disease and cholesterol ester storage disease may also look very similar on liver biopsy and need to be considered. Table 66.1 gives differential diagnoses that must be excluded.

Recommendations for undertaking biopsy in children with suspected NAFLD are made by a consensus document published by the American Association for the Study of Liver Diseases (AASLD), American College of Cardiology (ACG) and American Gastroenterological Association (AGA) [121]. These are to perform liver biopsy where the diagnosis is unclear there is a possibility of multiple diagnoses, before starting therapy with potentially hepatotoxic medications or prior to starting children on pharmacologic therapy for NASH. An ESPGHAN guideline was published the same year suggesting that liver biopsy should be performed in children with suspected NASH according to the following criteria; to exclude other treatable disease, in cases of clinically suspected advanced disease, as part of an interventional protocol or research trial [122]. Table 66.1 shows

Table 66.1 Conditions which need to be excluded before a diagnosis of NAFLD is made

Clinical condition	Clinical features	Biochemical/ other features which help distinguish from NAFLD
Wilson disease	May present with chronic liver disease, hemolytic anaemia or more rarely neurological disease in childhood. Look for Kaiser Fleisher rings	Low serum ceruloplasmin, high urinary copper pre and post penicillamine, high liver copper, genetics may be positive
Alpha 1 antitrypsin deficiency	–	Alpha 1 anti-trypsin phenotype ZZ (or ZS) more rarely SS
Drugs—steroids, amiodarone, alcohol, methotrexate, ecstacy, l-asparaginase, vitamin E, valproate, tamoxifen, antiretrovirals	History of drug ingestion	–
Cystic Fibrosis-associated liver disease	History/examination	Positive sweat test/genetics positive
Malnutrition	Clinical examination	–
Coeliac disease	May have failure to thrive	Tissue transglutaminase positive/positive jejuna biopsies
Hepatitis C	–	Positive serology
Parenteral nutrition-associated liver disease	Compatible history	–
Mitochondrial disease/fatty acid oxidase deficiency	May be history of neuro-developmental problems or other system involvement	Abnormal respiratory chain enzymes liver/muscle, abnormal acyl-carnitines,/skin fibroblast studies, mitochondrial depletion demonstrated, genetics for mitochondrial disease
Metabolic disease: Lysosomal acid lipase deficiency (cholesterol ester storage disease)	–	Positive enzymology or genetics
Galactosaemia	Age of presentation	Abnormal Gal-1-PUT result
Fructosemia	May be history of avoiding sweets	Enzymology on liver biopsy
Glycogen storage disease	Hepatomegaly, may be short, history of fasting hypoglycaemia	Positive enzymology/genetics, glycogen not fat on biopsy
Peroxisomal disorders	May be hypotonic/have wide anterior fontanelle, neurological problems	Abnormal very long-chain fatty acids
Mauriac syndrome	History type 1 diabetes	Glycogen on liver biopsy
Hypobetalipoproteinaemia/ abetalipoproteinaemia	Low serum triglycerides, may be history of fat malabsorption, may be failure to thrive	Low or absent Apo1B levels
Lipodystrophies	Examination	Genetics
Schwachman syndrome	FTT pancreatic insufficiency, bony changes, cyclical neutropenia	Genetics

conditions which need to be excluded before a diagnosis of NAFLD is made.

Tools commonly used in the workup and diagnosis of NAFLD include serum transaminases and imaging techniques (US, computerized tomography, magnetic resonance imaging/spectroscopy). The sensitivity, specificity and predictive values of these techniques are variable [3]. Franzese et al. studied the incidence of liver involvement in 72 obese children using both US and transaminases [123]. Fifty-three percent of the children had a bright liver on US consistent with liver steatosis whilst only 25 % had elevated transaminases. Molleston and colleagues reported histological abnormalities in 91 children with NAFLD and normal or only mildly elevated ALT. Forty-six percent of the group had some fibrosis with 38 % mild to moderate fibrosis and 8 % bridging fibrosis [124]. Neither US nor transaminases are good discriminators of histological severity [125]. Ultrasound will detect >20–30 % steatosis as increased echogenicity, though this is not specific for fat [126]. Magnetic resonance imaging/spectroscopy (MRI/MRS) is more sensitive and can detect >5 % steatosis [127]. However, neither technique can assess presence of inflammation or fibrosis.

Liver biopsy remains the gold standard in differentiation of steatosis from steatohepatitis. The diagnosis of NASH is based on a specific pattern of histopathological findings including macrovesicular steatosis, mixed or polymorphonuclear lobular inflammation, ballooning degeneration with Mallory hyaline, a perivenular distribution of fibrosis in adults (type 1 NASH) [128] (Fig. 66.3). Children may have a different pattern of disease with greater degree of steatosis, less prominent ballooning and portal rather than pericentral accentuation of inflammation and fibrosis (type 2 NASH) [129] (Fig. 66.4). Schwimmer et al. reviewed the histological findings in a cohort of 100 children (2–18 years) with biopsy-proven NAFLD [125]. Type 1 NASH was present in 17 % and type 2 NASH in 51 % of the children. Sixteen percent of

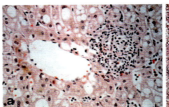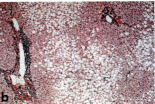

Fig. 66.4 Liver biopsies showing **a** type 1 NASH with pericentral disease and **b** type 2 NASH with periportal disease. Type 2 NASH is more common in children and type 1 in adults. Pictures kindly provided by Department of Liver Histopathology, King's College Hospital

biopsies had overlapping features of type 1 and 2 disease and the remaining 16 % showed simple steatosis. Children with type 2 NASH were younger and had greater severity of obesity than in type 1 NASH. Boys and those of Asian, Native American and Hispanic ethnicity were more likely to have type 2 NASH. In contrast, in a study from Italy of 57 children with NASH, only 2.4 % had type 1 NASH, 28.6 % were classified as type 2 NASH, whereas the majority (52.4 %) had an overlap between the two (17 % had simple steatosis) [130]. Takahashi reports the presence of type 2 NASH in 9 % of adult patients and 21 % of pediatric patients studied in Japan [131]. The mechanism leading to the different phenotypes of NAFLD is not yet understood.

The occurrence of portal inflammation was reviewed as a distinct entity in NASH by the NASH Clinical Research Network (CRN) [132]. A study of biopsies from 728 adults and 205 children found that the presence of portal inflammation in adults was associated with older, female patients with a higher BMI and IR. There was a clear association with amount and location of steatosis, ballooning and advanced fibrosis. In the pediatric group, portal inflammation was associated with younger age, azonal location of steatosis and more advance fibrosis (bridging). In both groups, it was associated with diagnosis of definitive NASH. There was no association with lobular inflammation in either group. It is not clear if this pattern is due to a separate pathophysiological mechanism, though it certainly seems to be a marker of more advanced NASH. The periportal pattern mirrors that of the ductular reaction which has been reported in NAFLD. The possible epithelial-mesenchymal transition of biliary cells in this process may relate to the pattern of fibrosis seen [133].

Though the classic description of fat in NAFLD is macrovesicular, the presence of microvesicular steatosis has recently been described in 102 of 1022 biopsies in patients with the condition [134]. In this study, the presence of microvesicular steatosis was strongly associated with cellular injury and cytoskeletal damage. Microvesicular steatosis has the appearance of distended hepatocytes with foamy cytoplasm; the nucleus is usually central rather than pushed peripherally as in macrovesicular steatosis. Oil red O staining

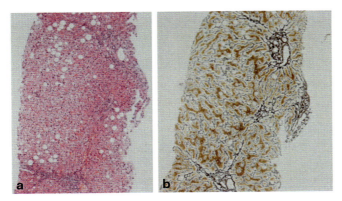

Fig. 66.3 Histology of NAFLD. **a** Hematoxylin and eosin staining showing steatosis, inflammation and ballooning. **b** Reticulin stain showing fibrosis Pictures kindly provided by Department of Liver Histopathology, King's College Hospital

is sometimes needed to identify microvesicular steatosis if it is not visible in haematoxylin and eosin staining. Classically, this type of steatosis has been associated with mitochondrial disease, acute fatty liver of pregnancy and some drug effects (e.g. steroids and valproate) which can cause β-oxidation impairment [135]. Taken together, microvesicular steatosis in NAFLD is a likely indicator of mitochondrial damage. It is not yet understood if this is a feature of advanced disease per se or if the pathogenesis of disease in those with microvesicular steatosis is different.

Caldwell et al. reported on the significance of ballooning in NAFLD [136]. These are classically enlarged cells with rarefied cytoplasm. Using ultrastructural analysis, this group reported on the multiple small fat lipid droplets seen in with degree of ER dilatation and Mallory Denk bodies and cytoskeletal disarray. Fugii et al. have demonstrated altered expression of FFA-associated protein on the surface of fat droplets which also stain for oxidized phosphatidylcholine (a marker of oxidative damage) [137]. They concluded that oxidative injury to the fat droplet surface may impair its safe disposal and contribute to lipotoxicity.

The Pathology Committee of the NASH CRN proposed a histological scoring system that could be useful in studies of NAFLD [138]. The scoring system includes the evaluation of steatosis (0–3), lobular inflammation (0–2), hepatocellular ballooning (0–2) and fibrosis (0–4). The NAFLD activity score (NAS) is the unweighted sum of steatosis, lobular inflammation and hepatocellular ballooning scores. NAS of 5 or more correlates with the diagnosis of NASH, whilst NAS less than 3 is defined as 'not NASH'. As this system is typically developed for adult type 1 NASH, the interobserver agreement for pediatric NASH is not as strong (only 18 children were included in the study cohort used for development of the score). The CRN also emphasize that the scoring system was developed as a tool for use in trials and is not a surrogate for a histological diagnosis of NASH [139]. Despite these shortcomings, this is the best available tool to standardize the description of the entire spectrum of NAFLD in both adults and children across different centres for research purposes.

It is important, however, to consider the pediatric pattern of disease as a separate entity, particularly when investigating the pathophysiological mechanisms or putative biomarkers of disease severity/progression. Figure 66.3a and b shows an example of histology of NAFLD. Figure 66.4 shows showing type 1 NASH with pericentral disease (a) and type 2 NASH with more periportal disease (b).

Natural History and Management

The natural history of NAFLD varies according to the histological pattern of the disease. Simple steatosis without evidence of inflammation or fibrosis appears to have a benign course whilst NASH is a potentially serious condition which can progress to cirrhosis. In a 10-year follow-up of 132 individuals with NAFLD, 22% of those with NASH versus 4% of those with simple steatosis went onto develop cirrhosis [46]. There was also a significantly higher liver-related mortality in the time period in the NASH group. Ekstead et al. followed 129 patients over a mean period of 13.7 years and found progression of liver fibrosis in 44% [140]. All-cause mortality was higher in the NASH group versus those with simple steatosis, particularly from cardiovascular and liver-related deaths. Four hundred and twenty patients with NAFLD were followed in the Rochester Epidemiology project, a population-based study. Liver-related mortality was the third leading cause of death in those with NAFLD [6]. Cirrhosis was present at follow-up in 5% of cohort. Adams et al. reported a series of 103 patients with NAFLD with follow-up biopsy at a mean interval of 3.2 years and found that fibrosis progressed in 37%, remained stable in 34% and regressed in 29% [141]. A higher BMI and diabetes were associated with fibrosis progression. A systematic review of 10 studies including 221 patients with a mean follow-up of 5.6 years concluded that fibrosis progressed in 37.6% of those with NASH [142]. Musso reported a further systematic review of 40 cohort studies examining the natural history of NAFLD in adults [143]. The authors found an overall and cause-specific pooled increase in mortality in those with NAFLD (odds ratio (OR) 1.57 (1.18–2.1)) versus the general population. In those with a steatotic liver on US, the risk of mortality from cardiovascular disease was increased by an OR of 2.05, with an OR of 3.5 for the development of type 2 diabetes. With subgroup analysis, patients with simple steatosis were found to have a similar mortality as the general population and those with NASH had an OR of 1.81 for overall mortality. The excess cause of death in this subgroup was mainly liver related with an incidence of 11–17 versus 1.7–2.7% in those with simple steatosis.

Steatosis is often no longer present in end-stage NASH and is replaced by cirrhotic change. NAFLD is thought to be the underlying etiology in the majority of cases of cryptogenic cirrhosis in many parts of the world [144, 145]. Evidence of this includes the finding that the prevalence of obesity and type 2 diabetes in cryptogenic cirrhosis mirrors that of those with NAFLD [146]. There is also an increased frequency of NASH occurrence post transplant in those with cryptogenic cirrhosis [147].

The development of HCC remains a major concern in patients with NAFLD [148]. Multiple case series and reviews have reported the association of HCC with the condition, even in the absence of NASH-related cirrhosis [149–154]. Diabetes and obesity are known to be risk factors for HCC and other malignancies [150]. In the setting of NASH the inflammatory cascade, oxidative stress and IR may all contribute to hepatocyte hyperplasia [150].

Cirrhosis secondary to NASH has been reported in children as young as 10 years [119, 155]. A recent study by Feldstein et al. describes the long-term outcome of 66 children with NAFLD followed-up for up to 20 years [156]. Of the five children who underwent follow-up biopsy, four showed progression of fibrosis. During the study period, two patients required liver transplantation for decompensated end-stage disease. Both had recurrence of NASH in the allograft and one required retransplantation.

In adult studies, the variables most commonly associated with fibrosis are the presence of diabetes, increasing age and high BMI [157]. Similarly in children, severity of obesity and IR seem to be predictors of advanced fibrosis [20]. The difference between the natural history of type 1 and type 2 NASH has not yet been characterized and is an important subject for future research.

Management of NAFLD encompasses lifestyle modification, medication or both. NAFLD is largely the consequence of imbalanced nutrition and sedentary behaviour on the background of genetic predisposition. Primary prevention is the ideal. In adults, weight reduction of 5–10 % body weight often leads to normalization or improvement of serum transaminases and reduced hepatic steatosis, inflammation and fibrosis [158–160]. In children, weight maintenance as the child crosses the height percentiles may achieve the same effect.

Several case series and uncontrolled trials have demonstrated the effect of weight loss on improvement of transaminases or US abnormalities [123, 161, 162]. A prospective study carried out in 84 children (3–18.8 years) with NAFLD demonstrated a significant decrease in BMI, levels of fasting glucose, insulin, lipids, transaminases and liver echogenicity on US following a 12-month program of lifestyle advice consisting of diet and physical exercise [130]. Another study of 53 children comparing lifestyle intervention plus antioxidant or lifestyle intervention plus placebo demonstrated similar improvements in both groups in terms of steatosis, inflammation, ballooning and NAS score [163].

Control of both quality and quantity of dietary components may be important. As above, nutritional data to date have suggested that a high intake of simple carbohydrates such as fructose with a low intake of polyunsaturated FAs correlate with pathogenesis and progression of disease [47, 53].

The type of fat consumed is possibly more relevant than quantity with higher saturated fat and lower PUFA intake associated with IR and NAFLD in some studies [47, 52]. Palmitic acid rather than oleic acid results in lower steatosis but in higher cell death and impaired insulin signalling in

vitro [57]. Several small studies of PUFAs in adults and one in children have demonstrated improved liver enzymes and histology in the treatment group [164–167].

Insulin Sensitizers

Insulin sensitizers have been investigated extensively and in view of the strong association of IR and the progression of NAFLD. Metformin is an important insulin sensitizer, reducing hyperglycaemia through a number of different mechanisms including inhibition of hepatic output and increasing peripheral uptake [168]. Thiazolidiones are PPARγ agonists which stimulate FFA uptake by adipocytes and allow the redistribution of fat from the liver to peripheral tissue [105].

A Cochrane review examined the evidence for insulin sensitizers in NAFLD. Only three randomised controlled trials (RCT) met search criteria (RCT comparing insulin sensitizer to placebo in nondiabetic adults with NAFLD) [169]. Though there was some histological and biochemical improvement with both metformin and rosiglitazone versus placebo, the results of the meta-analysis are inconclusive [170–174]. A large RCT (the PIVENS (pioglitazone, vitamin E or placebo for the treatment of NAFLD) trial) found favourable results for vitamin E but not for pioglitazone [175].

Metformin has the side effect of gastrointestinal intolerance but weight loss is an advantage of this medication. The TZDs have the unfortunate side effect of weight gain. There have also been concerns about cardiovascular events and diminished bone mass with their use [169]. There is no available data on the safe use of TZDs in children.

Only metformin has been investigated in pediatric patients with NAFLD. A large randomized, double-blind, placebo controlled trial has recently been reported by the NASH CRN in which both vitamin E and metformin were used [176]. The purpose of this study was to determine if therapeutic modification of IR or oxidative stress leads to improvement in serum or histological indicators of liver injury and quality of life (treatment of nonalcoholic fatty liver disease in children (TONIC) trial). The results demonstrate that there was a significant histological improvement in the vitamin E treatment group versus placebo with resolution of NASH ($p < 0.006$), though there was not a significant difference in resolution of transaminases (the primary outcome measure) in either treatment group. Other studies of metformin in children include an open-label pilot study of metformin (500 mg twice daily for 24 weeks) which was conducted in 10 nondiabetic children with biopsy-proven NASH and elevated ALT level [177]. Significant improvement was observed in serum ALT and hepatic steatosis as assessed with MR spectroscopy. A subsequent study conducted in children did not show any benefit of Metformin compared to lifestyle advice [178]. A third study of metformin in insulin-resistant adolescents resulted in lower severity scores of fatty liver on US and a decrease in prevalence of fatty liver disease in the metformin group [179].

Antioxidants

The oxidation of FFA leads to the production of reactive oxygen species. Normally, hepatocytes have enough antioxidants such as glutathionine to keep this process under control. The increased oxidative stress in NASH is in part due to increased FFA which overwhelm a presumably impaired normal oxidation pathway leading to the abundant production of reactive oxygen species. As this may have a major pathophysiological role in development and progression of the disease, antioxidants and hepato-protectants may be useful in management of the condition. Antioxidants such as ursodeoxycholic acid, vitamin E, *S*-adenosylmethionine, betaine, N-acetyl cysteine and pentoxyfyline have all been investigated in this context. Newer drugs such as caspase inhibitors and inhibitor of kappa B kinase (IKK) inhibitors are under development. The TONIC trial demonstrated some encouraging histological improvement with vitamin E; however, there was no difference to outcome measures as defined [180].

An open-label pilot study with vitamin E (400–1200 IU/day) in 11 children with NASH, showed improvement of serum transaminases despite no major changes in BMI or US appearance of the liver [181]. Other studies using vitamin E in children refute these findings [178, 182].

The recent PIVENS trial demonstrated that in a multicentre, double-blind, RCT of vitamin E versus pioglitazone versus placebo in 248 nondiabetic adults with NAFLD, there was a significant improvement in histology in the vitamin E group (43%) versus the pioglitazone group (19%) [175].

Ursodeoxycholic acid (UDCA) has multiple cytoprotective properties [183]. Using a combination of UDCA and vitamin E, Balmer et al. demonstrated an improvement in transaminases and liver histology together with increased adiponectin levels and decreased hepatocyte apoptosis [184]. There was no significant change in the amount of fibrosis present following 96 weeks of treatment, however. UDCA has also been studied in pediatric NAFLD. A small study which evaluated the efficacy of UDCA in 31 obese children with abnormal transaminases did not show any effect of UDCA treatment [185]. A Cochrane review found insufficient evidence that UDCA was an effective treatment for NAFLD [186].

Bariatric Surgery

The role of bariatric surgery (both Roux-en-Y bypass and gastric band) in management of NAFLD was examined in adults as a Cochrane review. Though RCT exist to date, 21 observational studies were included. The majority of these studies demonstrated improvement in steatosis or inflammation post surgery though with improvement in fibrosis in only 6 studies and deterioration in 4 [187]. No data are available for children.

Orlistat

Orlistat is a gastrointestinal lipase inhibitor which has beneficial effects in terms of weight reduction and reduction of free FAs. The effect of Orlistat with calorie-controlled diet on liver enzymes and histological features of NAFLD has been tested in three RCTs. These RCTs had conflicting results, and though Orlistat appears to be a safe adjunct to dietary counselling, the net effect is uncertain [188–190]. No pediatric data are available.

Probiotics

There has been recent interest in the role that gut microbiota play in obesity, IR and NAFLD [36]. There is evidence that intestinal bacterial overgrowth exacerbates NAFLD and that the prevalence of bacterial overgrowth is higher in those who are obese [37]. Manipulation of gut microbiota with probiotics is a promising way to halt the progression of steatosis to steatohepatitis and fibrosis. Both animal experiments and small human studies have investigated the use of probiotic agents to reverse the progression of steatohepatitis and fibrosis in NAFLD [191, 192]. Two recent double-blind RCTs—one in adults and one in children were reported [193, 194]. Treatment with probiotics in both studies resulted in improvement in transaminases.

Fibrates

Fibrates are PPARα ligands which can decrease TG levels and increase high-density lipoprotein (HDL) by stimulating lipoprotein lipase and regulating apolipoprotein [195]. Fibrates have been shown to ameliorate IR and inflammation, stimulate β-oxidation and improve transaminase levels but not histology in patients with NAFLD [196]. There have been no RCT in children.

Noninvasive Biomarkers in NAFLD

Though the criterion standard for diagnosis and assessing progression of disease is liver histology, the decision 'if or when' to perform a liver biopsy in children with suspected

NAFLD remains controversial. Liver biopsy in children requires admission to hospital and sedation. Risks include bleeding and very rarely death [197]. Repeated biopsy is not a suitable tool for regularly monitoring progression of disease or response to treatment. In addition, biopsy samples only 1/50,000 of the liver, raising the possibility of sampling error [198].

There has been much focus on the development and validation of noninvasive biomarkers of NAFLD in recent years. There is an urgent need for a less invasive method than biopsy of screening the population, stratifying disease severity and following disease progression.

The pathophysiology and evolution of the condition under scrutiny is an important consideration in the development and evaluation of biomarkers. In the case of NAFLD, there are two potential targets. The first is the differentiation of simple steatosis from steatohepatitis. This is important as the prognosis of those with simple steatosis is different from those with NASH [199]. The second issue is the identification of fibrosis stage. This is the main determinant of prognosis and knowing the extent of fibrosis is useful in making treatment decisions, in patient selection for treatment studies and in monitoring progression/regression. Most longitudinal cohort studies in NAFLD have shown that prognosis is determined by stage and rate of progression of fibrosis rather than the presence of necro-inflammation [46, 140, 200]. Clinical importance lies with being able to differentiate between no/minimal fibrosis (F0/F1), significant fibrosis (F2), severe fibrosis (F3) and cirrhosis (F4).

Serum Biomarkers and NASH

Large adult series have suggested scoring systems using age, BMI, IR, AST/ALT, platelet count and albumin to differentiate mild from severe disease [157, 201–203]. These simple markers are neither sensitive nor specific enough in isolation [5, 12]. A growing understanding of the pathophysiology of the disease has allowed the investigation of more specific, mechanism-based biomarkers [117, 204, 205].

Markers of apoptosis/cell death have been shown to be very useful in differentiating simple steatosis from NASH [109]. CK18-M30 fragments have been shown by a number of studies including pediatric studies to correlate well with severity of NASH [206–209].

A number of predictive models to differentiate either NAFLD from obese controls or simple steatosis from NASH have been developed and validated. Tools include the hypertension, ALT, IR (HAIR) score which gives an area under the curve (AUROC) of 0.9 [210], and the NASH test (consisting of 13 variables including weight, TG, glucose, α2-macroglobulin and apolipoprotein A) which has an AUROC of 0.79 for differentiation of NASH from simple steatosis

[211]. When the NASH test is combined with the Steatotest (10 variables including simple blood tests, age, gender and BMI) [212] and the Fibrotest into what is known as the Fibromax panel, the diagnostic accuracy improves further [212].

The following studies report predictors of NAFLD using routine clinical parameters in cohorts of obese children. Sartorio et al. reported a multivariate analysis of 267 obese children and found that BMI z score, ALT, uric acid, glucose and insulin were useful predictors of NAFLD [17]. Mandato reported IR, ferritin, CRP and glutathione peroxidase as good discriminators of those with NAFLD from those without in a cohort of obese children [205]. Neither of these studies used a histological diagnosis of NAFLD.

Adipocytokines have been investigated in a number of studies in children including TNFα and leptin [213–215], retinal-binding protein-4 (RBP-4) [216], Fetiun A [217] and plasminogen activator inhibitor 1 (PAI-1) [218, 219].

Noninvasive Markers of Fibrosis in NAFLD

Simple tests derived from regression analysis of large series of patients include the AST to platelet ratio index [220], the AST to ALT ratio [221], which have been validated in the NAFLD population with AUROC between 0.67 and 0.86 for differentiation of severity of fibrosis [222–224]. Algorithms specifically derived from NAFLD cohorts include the BAAT score (consisting of BMI, ALT, age and TG levels) [225], the BARD score (BMI, AST/ALT ratio, diabetes) [202, 226] and the NAFLD fibrosis score (incorporating age, glucose, AST, ALT, BMI, platelets and albumin) [201, 222, 223, 227, 228]. In a recent meta-analysis the AUROC for the NAFLD fibrosis score was found to be 0.85 with a pooled sensitivity of 90 % and specificity of 97 % [143].

Fibrometer has been validated in a NAFLD population [224]. The test incorporates age, weight, fasting glucose, AST, ALT, ferritin and platelets and demonstrates an AUROC of 0.94 for significant fibrosis, 0.9 for severe fibrosis and 0.9 for cirrhosis.

Other biomarkers measure the degree of ECM turnover. Using such ECM markers is a more direct method of assessing fibrogenic activity, and it will tend to measure a dynamic process rather than a static one.

Combinations of both clinical markers and ECM turnover include the Fibrotest [229, 230] which is an algorithm of 13 markers derived from regression analysis including haptoglobin, α2-macroglobulin, apolipoprotein A1, bilirubin, γGT, age and gender. It has an AUROC of 0.84 for advanced fibrosis in NAFLD [231].

The European liver fibrosis (ELF) test combining hyaluronic acid, procollagen III *N*-terminal peptide (P3NP) and TIMP1 was first derived by Rosenberg et al. in a cohort of over 1000 patients with chronic liver disease including

NAFLD [232] and has since been validated in other NAFLD cohorts with the addition of several simple markers to improve accuracy [233]. Importantly, this test has been shown to correlate well with outcome [234]. In 112 children with NAFLD, ELF had an AUROC of 0.92, 0.98 and 0.99 in distinguishing any, significant and advanced fibrosis respectively [235].

As with adult studies, the noninvasive diagnosis of fibrosis (rather than necro-inflammatory change) in NAFLD is considered separately in children. It is important to acknowledge that the different distribution of fibrosis in pediatric patients may affect the validity of applying measures derived from adult cohorts to this population.

Iacobellis et al. reported a cohort of 69 children with NAFLD, 60% of whom had fibrosis [203]. They found that BMI was the only significant predictor of fibrosis with multivariable analysis of simple clinial parameters. BMI had an OR of 5.85 for predicting presence of fibrosis. Manco et al. found waist circumference as a significant predictor of fibrosis in a cohort of 197 children with NAFLD (OR 2.4 (1.04–5.54)) [236]. In both these studies the number of children in the F2–F4 groups was small.

Nobili et al. developed and internally validated the paediatiric NAFLD fibrosis index (PNFI) in 136 children with NAFLD [237]. Logistic regression analysis of gender, age, BMI, waist circumference, ALT, AST, γGT, albumin, prothrombin time, glucose, insulin, cholesterol and triglceyerides gave a predictive model with an AUROC for detection of fibrosis was 0.85. Again this study was limited in view of small numbers in fibrosis groups F2–F4.

Hyaluronic acid (HA) level > 1200 ng/ml in 100 children (65% with fibrosis) was a reliable discriminant of fibrosis in NAFLD in one study [203]. The ELF test was evaluated by Nobili et al. in 122 children with NAFLD [238]. Simple markers including age, waist circumference and TG were added to improve diagnostic accuracy. Excellent AUROC for any (0.92), significant (0.98) and advanced (0.99) disease were achieved. In this cohort, 37 (30%) had no fibrosis, 58 (48%) scored as F1, 9 (7%) as F2, and 8 (6.5%) as F3–F4. Alkhouri et al. developed this further and validated both the PNFI and ELF in a cohort of 111 children with NAFLD (69% with fibrosis) [239]. The area under the curve for presence of fibrosis was 0.76 for PNFI, 0.92 for ELF and when the two indices were combined: 0.94. The major issue in both studies was the skew towards no or minimal disease, potentially overestimating the accuracy of the test.

Noninvasive Biomarkers and Imaging

US, CT and MRI

US has a high sensitivity and specificity for diagnosis of steatosis > 30%, but is not good at detecting fibrosis. Because of the low cost, the absence of radiation exposure and the wide availability, US is often used in screening for NAFLD. The accumulation of fat causes the liver to appear hyperechoic compared with the kidney. This finding is nonspecific and does not differentiate fat from other substances such as glycogen. When compared with histological findings, the sensitivity of US to detect fat infiltration below 30% of the liver is low [240]. Computed tomography (CT) is rarely used for the assessment of NAFLD in children because of its ionizing radiation exposure. Magnetic resonance imaging (MRI) and spectroscopy are the imaging techniques with the greatest accuracy to determine hepatic fat content in studies of both adults and children [127, 241–243]. Aside from liver fat, however, other features of NASH cannot be assessed. Other methods include MR elastography which visualizes and measures propagating shear waves and has a high sensitivity (>85%) and specificity (>90%) for fibrosis [244]. Cost of this technique may be preclusive however.

For diagnosis of NASH, Iijima et al. have reported on the use of contrast US with Levovist with an AUC of 1.0 [245]. The decreased accumulation of micro-bubbles with advancing degree of fibrosis is unique to NAFLD.

There is an emerging literature examining the use of acoustic radiation force-based shear stiffness in NAFLD, an US-based investigation which correlates well with the stage of fibrosis in the condition [246, 247].

Transient Elastography

Transient elastography (Fibroscan®) has been shown to be a useful method for detection of liver fibrosis. In NAFLD, a small number of studies have demonstrated the efficacy of TE in distinguishing severity of fibrosis. In a study of 246 adults with NAFLD, TE had an AUROC of 0.84, 0.93 and 0.95 in distinguishing significant fibrosis, severe fibrosis and cirrhosis, respectively [248]. A Japanese study demonstrated similar results [249]. A recent report of 52 children with NAFLD has shown an AUROC of 0.977, 0.992 and 1 for distinguishing any, significant and severe fibrosis [250]. Feasibility and reproducibility of transient elastography is an issue when patients have a BMI > 30 [251]. An XL probe is now available for better accuracy in this scenario [252].

Non-hypothesis Driven Search for Novel Biomarkers Using New Technologies

The use of relatively new techniques such as proteomics [253–256], glycomics [257, 258], and microarray studies in the derivation of panels of biomarkers associated with a disease may also give an insight into pathophysiology of the condition.

Future Areas for Research

The pathophysiology of NAFLD in both adults and children is still incompletely understood. The reason for different patterns of disease in children, particularly with reference to the occurrence of periportal inflammation and fibrosis rather than the typical type 1 pattern of pericentral disease remains elusive. Determining susceptibility to the disease using genetic analysis for SNPs may become standard practice, particularly in screening the high number of overweight and obese pediatric patients. Further investigation into specific dietary patterns in children may also yield valuable information in this multifactorial disease.

The determination of the most effective management of the condition—both in terms of achieving lifestyle change and pharmacological treatments—will be a major focus going forward. Further areas of interest include the role of intestinal microbiota and the possible use of probiotics in the condition and dietary manipulation with PUFA.

Finally, the long-term outcome of children with NAFLD remains unknown and well designed, long-term prospective studies using networks, such as the NASH clinical research network in the US, are vital to achieving this.

In conclusion, NAFLD in children is a very real, very prevalent condition and, should current trends continue, is likely to become the most common indication for liver transplantation in coming decades. It is important that the condition is recognized in children as there is the potential to reverse the process and to avoid the morbidity and mortality associated in later years.

References

1. Musso G, Gambino R, Cassader M. Recent insights into hepatic lipid metabolism in non-alcoholic fatty liver disease (NAFLD). Prog Lipid Res. 2009;48(1):1–26. PubMed PMID: 18824034. Epub 2008/10/01. eng.
2. Moran JR, Ghishan FK, Halter SA, Greene HL. Steatohepatitis in obese children: a cause of chronic liver dysfunction. Am J Gastroenterol. 1983;78(6):374–7. PubMed PMID: 6859017. Epub 1983/06/01. eng.
3. Patton HM, Sirlin C, Behling C, Middleton M, Schwimmer JB, Lavine JE. Pediatric nonalcoholic fatty liver disease: a critical appraisal of current data and implications for future research. J Pediatr Gastroenterol Nutr. 2006;43(4):413–27. PubMed PMID: 17033514. Epub 2006/10/13. eng.
4. Schwimmer JB, Deutsch R, Kahen T, Lavine JE, Stanley C, Behling C. Prevalence of fatty liver in children and adolescents. Pediatrics. 2006;118(4):1388–93. PubMed PMID: 17015527. Epub 2006/10/04. eng.
5. Browning JD, Szczepaniak LS, Dobbins R, Nuremberg P, Horton JD, Cohen JC, et al. Prevalence of hepatic steatosis in an urban population in the United States: impact of ethnicity. Hepatology. 2004;40(6):1387–95. PubMed PMID: 15565570. Epub 2004/11/27. eng.
6. Adams LA, Lymp JF, St Sauver J, Sanderson SO, Lindor KD, Feldstein A, et al. The natural history of nonalcoholic fatty liver disease: a population-based cohort study. Gastroenterology. 2005;129(1):113–21. PubMed PMID: 16012941. Epub 2005/07/14. eng.
7. Stamatakis E, Primatesta P, Chinn S, Rona R, Falascheti E. Overweight and obesity trends from 1974 to 2003 in English children: what is the role of socioeconomic factors? Arch Dis Child. 2005;90(10):999–1004. PubMed PMID: 15956046. Pubmed Central PMCID: 1720119. Epub 2005/06/16. eng.
8. Stamatakis E, Wardle J, Cole TJ. Childhood obesity and overweight prevalence trends in England: evidence for growing socioeconomic disparities. Int J Obes (Lond). 2010;34(1):41–7. PubMed PMID: 19884892. Epub 2009/11/04. eng.
9. Allen KJ, Buck NE, Williamson R. Stem cells for the treatment of liver disease. Transpl Immunol. 2005;15(2):99–112. PubMed PMID: 16412955. Epub 2006/01/18. eng.
10. Ogden CL, Flegal KM, Carroll MD, Johnson CL. Prevalence and trends in overweight among US children and adolescents, 1999–2000. JAMA. 2002;288(14):1728–32. PubMed PMID: 12365956. Epub 2002/10/09. eng.
11. Ogden CL, Carroll MD, Curtin LR, Lamb MM, Flegal KM. Prevalence of high body mass index in US children and adolescents, 2007–2008. JAMA. 2010;303(3):242–9. PubMed PMID: 20071470.
12. Fracanzani AL, Valenti L, Bugianesi E, Andreoletti M, Colli A, Vanni E, et al. Risk of severe liver disease in nonalcoholic fatty liver disease with normal aminotransferase levels: a role for insulin resistance and diabetes. Hepatology. 2008;48(3):792–8. PubMed PMID: 18752331. Epub 2008/08/30. eng.
13. Prati D, Taioli E, Zanella A, Della Torre E, Butelli S, Del Vecchio E, et al. Updated definitions of healthy ranges for serum alanine aminotransferase levels. Ann Intern Med. 2002;137(1):1–10. PubMed PMID: 12093239. Epub 2002/07/03. eng.
14. Fraser A, Longnecker MP, Lawlor DA. Prevalence of elevated alanine aminotransferase among US adolescents and associated factors: NHANES 1999–2004. Gastroenterology. 2007;133(6):1814–20. PubMed PMID: 18054554. Pubmed Central PMCID: 2180388. Epub 2007/12/07. eng.
15. Park HS, Han JH, Choi KM, Kim SM. Relation between elevated serum alanine aminotransferase and metabolic syndrome in Korean adolescents. Am J Clin Nutr. 2005;82(5):1046–51. PubMed PMID: 16280437. Epub 2005/11/11. eng.
16. Tominaga K, Kurata JH, Chen YK, Fujimoto E, Miyagawa S, Abe I, et al. Prevalence of fatty liver in Japanese children and relationship to obesity. An epidemiological ultrasonographic survey. Dig Dis Sci. 1995;40(9):2002–9. PubMed PMID: 7555456. Epub 1995/09/01. eng.
17. Sartorio A, Del Col A, Agosti F, Mazzilli G, Bellentani S, Tiribelli C, et al. Predictors of non-alcoholic fatty liver disease in obese children. Eur J Clin Nutr. 2007;61(7):877–83. PubMed PMID: 17151586. Epub 2006/12/08. eng.
18. Quiros-Tejeira RE, Rivera CA, Ziba TT, Mehta N, Smith CW, Butte NF. Risk for nonalcoholic fatty liver disease in Hispanic youth with BMI > or = 95th percentile. J Pediatr Gastroenterol

Nutr. 2007;44(2):228–36. PubMed PMID: 17255837. Epub 2007/01/27. eng.

19. Schwimmer JB, McGreal N, Deutsch R, Finegold MJ, Lavine JE. Influence of gender, race, and ethnicity on suspected fatty liver in obese adolescents. Pediatrics. 2005;115(5):e561–5. PubMed PMID: 15867021. Epub 2005/05/04. eng.

20. Schwimmer JB, Deutsch R, Rauch JB, Behling C, Newbury R, Lavine JE. Obesity, insulin resistance, and other clinicopathological correlates of pediatric nonalcoholic fatty liver disease. J Pediatr. 2003;143(4):500–5. PubMed PMID: 14571229. Epub 2003/10/23. eng.

21. Wagenknecht LE, Scherzinger AL, Stamm ER, Hanley AJ, Norris JM, Chen YD, et al. Correlates and heritability of nonalcoholic fatty liver disease in a minority cohort. Obesity (Silver Spring). 2009;17(6):1240–6. PubMed PMID: 19584882. Pubmed Central PMCID: 2709735. Epub 2009/07/09. eng.

22. Petersen KF, Dufour S, Feng J, Befroy D, Dziura J, Dalla Man C, et al. Increased prevalence of insulin resistance and nonalcoholic fatty liver disease in Asian-Indian men. Proc Natl Acad Sci USA. 2006;103(48):18273–7. PubMed PMID: 17114290. Pubmed Central PMCID: 1693873. Epub 2006/11/23. eng.

23. Carter-Kent C, Feldstein AE. Non-alcoholic steatohepatitis over multiple generations. Dig Dis Sci. 2010 May;55(5):1494–7 PubMed PMID: 19629685.

24. Willner IR, Waters B, Patil SR, Reuben A, Morelli J, Riely CA. Ninety patients with nonalcoholic steatohepatitis: insulin resistance, familial tendency, and severity of disease. Am J Gastroenterol. 2001;96(10):2957–61. PubMed PMID: 11693332.

25. Schwimmer JB, Celedon MA, Lavine JE, Salem R, Campbell N, Schork NJ, et al. Heritability of nonalcoholic fatty liver disease. Gastroenterology. 2009;136(5):1585–92. PubMed PMID: 19208353. Epub 2009/02/12. eng.

26. Hooper AJ, Adams LA, Burnett JR. Genetic determinants of hepatic steatosis in man. J Lipid Res. 2011;52(4):593–617. PubMed PMID: 21245030. Pubmed Central PMCID: 3053205. Epub 2011/01/20. Eng.

27. Romeo S, Kozlitina J, Xing C, Pertsemlidis A, Cox D, Pennacchio LA, et al. Genetic variation in PNPLA3 confers susceptibility to nonalcoholic fatty liver disease. Nat Genet. 2008;40(12):1461–5. PubMed PMID: 18820647. Pubmed Central PMCID: 2597056. Epub 2008/09/30. eng.

28. Speliotes EK, Butler JL, Palmer CD, Voight BF, Consortium G, Consortium MI, et al. PNPLA3 variants specifically confer increased risk for histologic nonalcoholic fatty liver disease but not metabolic disease. Hepatology. 2010;52(3):904–12. PubMed PMID: 20648472. Pubmed Central PMCID: 3070300. Epub 2010/07/22. eng.

29. Chambers JC, Zhang W, Sehmi J, Li X, Wass MN, Van der Harst P, et al. Genome-wide association study identifies loci influencing concentrations of liver enzymes in plasma. Nat Genet. 2011;43(11):1131–8. PubMed PMID: 22001757. Pubmed Central PMCID: 3482372.

30. He S, McPhaul C, Li JZ, Garuti R, Kinch L, Grishin NV, et al. A sequence variation (I148M) in PNPLA3 associated with non-alcoholic fatty liver disease disrupts triglyceride hydrolysis. J Biol Chem. 2010;285(9):6706–15. PubMed PMID: 20034933. Pubmed Central PMCID: 2825465. Epub 2009/12/26. eng.

31. Rotman Y, Koh C, Zmuda JM, Kleiner DE, Liang TJ, Nash CRN. The association of genetic variability in patatin-like phospholipase domain-containing protein 3 (PNPLA3) with histological severity of nonalcoholic fatty liver disease. Hepatology. 2010;52(3):894–903. PubMed PMID: 20684021. Pubmed Central PMCID: 2932770. Epub 2010/08/05. eng.

32. Kotronen A, Johansson LE, Johansson LM, Roos C, Westerbacka J, Hamsten A, et al. A common variant in PNPLA3, which encodes adiponutrin, is associated with liver fat content in humans. Dia-

betologia. 2009;52(6):1056–60. PubMed PMID: 19224197. Epub 2009/02/19. eng.

33. Valenti L, Alisi A, Galmozzi E, Bartuli A, Del Menico B, Alterio A, et al. I148M patatin-like phospholipase domain-containing 3 gene variant and severity of pediatric nonalcoholic fatty liver disease. Hepatology. 2010;52(4):1274–80. PubMed PMID: 20648474. Epub 2010/07/22. eng.

34. Petersen KF, Dufour S, Hariri A, Nelson-Williams C, Foo JN, Zhang XM, et al. Apolipoprotein C3 gene variants in nonalcoholic fatty liver disease. N Engl J Med. 2010;362(12):1082–9. PubMed PMID: 20335584. Pubmed Central PMCID: 2976042. Epub 2010/03/26. eng.

35. Musso G, Gambino R, De Michieli F, Durazzo M, Pagano G, Cassader M. Adiponectin gene polymorphisms modulate acute adiponectin response to dietary fat: possible pathogenetic role in NASH. Hepatology. 2008;47(4):1167–77. PubMed PMID: 18311774. Epub 2008/03/04. eng.

36. Jang Y, Chae JS, Koh SJ, Hyun YJ, Kim JY, Jeong YJ, et al. The influence of the adiponectin gene on adiponectin concentrations and parameters of metabolic syndrome in non-diabetic Korean women. Clin Chim Acta. 2008;391(1–2):85–90. PubMed PMID: 18328815. Epub 2008/03/11. eng.

37. Kotronen A, Yki-Jarvinen H, Aminoff A, Bergholm R, Pietilainen KH, Westerbacka J, et al. Genetic variation in the ADIPOR2 gene is associated with liver fat content and its surrogate markers in three independent cohorts. Eur J Endocrinol. 2009;160(4):593–602. PubMed PMID: 19208777. Epub 2009/02/12. eng.

38. Carulli L, Canedi I, Rondinella S, Lombardini S, Ganazzi D, Fargion S, et al. Genetic polymorphisms in non-alcoholic fatty liver disease: interleukin-6–174G/C polymorphism is associated with non-alcoholic steatohepatitis. Dig Liver Dis. 2009;41(11):823–8. PubMed PMID: 19403348. Epub 2009/05/01. eng.

39. Tokushige K, Takakura M, Tsuchiya-Matsushita N, Taniai M, Hashimoto E, Shiratori K. Influence of TNF gene polymorphisms in Japanese patients with NASH and simple steatosis. J Hepatol. 2007;46(6):1104–10. PubMed PMID: 17395331. Epub 2007/03/31. eng.

40. Miele L, Beale G, Patman G, Nobili V, Leathart J, Grieco A, et al. The Kruppel-like factor 6 genotype is associated with fibrosis in nonalcoholic fatty liver disease. Gastroenterology. 2008;135(1):282–91 e1. PubMed PMID: 18515091. Epub 2008/06/03. eng.

41. Lin YC, Chang PF, Hu FC, Chang MH, Ni YH. Variants in the UGT1A1 gene and the risk of pediatric nonalcoholic fatty liver disease. Pediatrics. 2009;124(6):e1221–7. PubMed PMID: 19948621. Epub 2009/12/02. eng.

42. Cheung O, Puri P, Eicken C, Contos MJ, Mirshahi F, Maher JW, et al. Nonalcoholic steatohepatitis is associated with altered hepatic MicroRNA expression. Hepatology. 2008;48(6):1810–20. PubMed PMID: 19030170. Pubmed Central PMCID: 2717729.

43. Ueno T, Sugawara H, Sujaku K, Hashimoto O, Tsuji R, Tamaki S, et al. Therapeutic effects of restricted diet and exercise in obese patients with fatty liver. J Hepatol. 1997;27(1):103–7. PubMed PMID: 9252081. Epub 1997/07/01. eng.

44. Palmer M, Schaffner F. Effect of weight reduction on hepatic abnormalities in overweight patients. Gastroenterology. 1990;99(5):1408–13. PubMed PMID: 2210247. Epub 1990/11/01. eng.

45. Wong VW, Wong GL, Choi PC, Chan AW, Li MK, Chan HY, et al. Disease progression of non-alcoholic fatty liver disease: a prospective study with paired liver biopsies at 3 years. Gut. 2010;59(7):969–74. PubMed PMID: 20581244. Epub 2010/06/29. eng.

46. Matteoni CA, Younossi ZM, Gramlich T, Boparai N, Liu YC, McCullough AJ. Nonalcoholic fatty liver disease: a spectrum of clinical and pathological severity. Gastroenterol-

ogy. 1999;116(6):1413–9. PubMed PMID: 10348825. Epub 1999/05/29. eng.

47. Musso G, Gambino R, De Michieli F, Cassader M, Rizzetto M, Durazzo M, et al. Dietary habits and their relations to insulin resistance and postprandial lipemia in nonalcoholic steatohepatitis. Hepatology. 2003;37(4):909–16. PubMed PMID: 12668986. Epub 2003/04/02. eng.

48. Toshimitsu K, Matsuura B, Ohkubo I, Niiya T, Furukawa S, Hiasa Y, et al. Dietary habits and nutrient intake in non-alcoholic steatohepatitis. Nutrition. 2007;23(1):46–52. PubMed PMID: 17140767. Epub 2006/12/05. eng.

49. Zelber-Sagi S, Nitzan-Kaluski D, Goldsmith R, Webb M, Blendis L, Halpern Z, et al. Long term nutritional intake and the risk for non-alcoholic fatty liver disease (NAFLD): a population based study. J Hepatol. 2007;47(5):711–7. PubMed PMID: 17850914. Epub 2007/09/14. eng.

50. Abid A, Taha O, Nseir W, Farah R, Grosovski M, Assy N. Soft drink consumption is associated with fatty liver disease independent of metabolic syndrome. J Hepatol. 2009;51(5):918–24. PubMed PMID: 19765850. Epub 2009/09/22. eng.

51. Ouyang X, Cirillo P, Sautin Y, McCall S, Bruchette JL, Diehl AM, et al. Fructose consumption as a risk factor for non-alcoholic fatty liver disease. J Hepatol. 2008;48(6):993–9. PubMed PMID: 18395287. Pubmed Central PMCID: 2423467. Epub 2008/04/09. eng.

52. Kim CH, Kallman JB, Bai C, Pawloski L, Gewa C, Arsalla A, et al. Nutritional assessments of patients with non-alcoholic fatty liver disease. Obes Surg. 2010;20(2):154–60. PubMed PMID: 18560947. Epub 2008/06/19. eng.

53. Vos MB, Lavine JE. Dietary fructose in nonalcoholic fatty liver disease. Hepatology. 2013;57(6):2525–31. PubMed PMID: 23390127.

54. Basaranoglu M, Basaranoglu G, Sabuncu T, Senturk H. Fructose as a key player in the development of fatty liver disease. World J Gastroenterol. 2013;19(8):1166–72. PubMed PMID: 23482247. Pubmed Central PMCID: 3587472.

55. Oddy WH, Herbison CE, Jacoby P, Ambrosini GL, O'Sullivan TA, Ayonrinde OT, et al. The Western dietary pattern is prospectively associated with nonalcoholic fatty liver disease in adolescence. Am J Gastroenterol. 2013;108(5):778–85. PubMed PMID: 23545714.

56. Papandreou D, Karabouta Z, Pantoleon A, Rousso I. Investigation of anthropometric, biochemical and dietary parameters of obese children with and without non-alcoholic fatty liver disease. Appetite. 2012;59(3):939–44. PubMed PMID: 23000278.

57. Ricchi M, Odoardi MR, Carulli L, Anzivino C, Ballestri S, Pinetti A, et al. Differential effect of oleic and palmitic acid on lipid accumulation and apoptosis in cultured hepatocytes. J Gastroenterol Hepatol. 2009;24(5):830–40. PubMed PMID: 19207680. Epub 2009/02/12. eng.

58. St-Jules DE, Watters CA, Brunt EM, Wilkens LR, Novotny R, Belt P, et al. Estimation of fish and omega-3 fatty acid intake in pediatric nonalcoholic fatty liver disease. J Pediatr Gastroenterol Nutr. 2013 Nov;57(5):627–33. PubMed PMID: 23820405. Pubmed Central PMCID: 3864540.

59. Vos MB, Colvin R, Belt P, Molleston JP, Murray KF, Rosenthal P, et al. Correlation of vitamin E, uric acid, and diet composition with histologic features of pediatric NAFLD. J Pediatr Gastroenterol Nutr. 2012;54(1):90–6. PubMed PMID: 22197855. Pubmed Central PMCID: 3208079.

60. Oben JA, Mouralidarane A, Samuelsson AM, Matthews PJ, Morgan ML, McKee C, et al. Maternal obesity during pregnancy and lactation programs the development of offspring non-alcoholic fatty liver disease in mice. J Hepatol. 2010;52(6):913–20. PubMed PMID: 20413174. Epub 2010/04/24. eng.

61. Nobili V, Bedogni G, Alisi A, Pietrobattista A, Alterio A, Tiribelli C, et al. A protective effect of breastfeeding on progression of non-alcoholic fatty liver disease. Arch Dis Child. 2009 Oct;94(10):801–5. PubMed PMID: 19556219. Epub 2009/06/27. Eng.

62. Ciba I, Widhalm K. The association between non-alcoholic fatty liver disease and insulin resistance in 20 obese children and adolescents. Acta Paediatr. 2007;96(1):109–12. PubMed PMID: 17187615. Epub 2006/12/26. eng.

63. Chan DF, Li AM, Chu WC, Chan MH, Wong EM, Liu EK, et al. Hepatic steatosis in obese Chinese children. Int J Obes Relat Metab Disord. 2004;28(10):1257–63. PubMed PMID: 15278103. Epub 2004/07/28. eng.

64. Day CP, James OF. Steatohepatitis: a tale of two "hits"? Gastroenterology. 1998;114(4):842–5. PubMed PMID: 9547102. Epub 1998/04/18. eng.

65. Chung MY, Yeung SF, Park HJ, Volek JS, Bruno RS. Dietary alpha- and gamma-tocopherol supplementation attenuates lipopolysaccharide-induced oxidative stress and inflammatory-related responses in an obese mouse model of nonalcoholic steatohepatitis. J Nutr Biochem. 2010;21(12):1200–6. PubMed PMID: 20138495. Epub 2010/02/09. eng.

66. Yang S, Lin H, Diehl AM. Fatty liver vulnerability to endotoxin-induced damage despite NF-kappaB induction and inhibited caspase 3 activation. Am J Physiol Gastrointest Liver Physiol. 2001;281(2):G382–92. PubMed PMID: 11447019. Epub 2001/07/12. eng.

67. Malhi H, Bronk SF, Werneburg NW, Gores GJ. Free fatty acids induce JNK-dependent hepatocyte lipoapoptosis. J Biol Chem. 2006;281(17):12093–101. PubMed PMID: 16505490. Epub 2006/03/01. eng.

68. Yamaguchi K, Yang L, McCall S, Huang J, Yu XX, Pandey SK, et al. Inhibiting triglyceride synthesis improves hepatic steatosis but exacerbates liver damage and fibrosis in obese mice with nonalcoholic steatohepatitis. Hepatology. 2007;45(6):1366–74. PubMed PMID: 17476695. Epub 2007/05/04. eng.

69. Day C. Pathophysiology of NASH. EASL Speical Conference on NAFLD and the metabolic syndrome. Bologna; 2009.

70. Anderson N, Borlak J. Molecular mechanisms and therapeutic targets in steatosis and steatohepatitis. Pharmacol Rev. 2008;60(3):311–57. PubMed PMID: 18922966. Epub 2008/10/17. eng.

71. Saltiel AR, Kahn CR. Insulin signalling and the regulation of glucose and lipid metabolism. Nature. 2001;414(6865):799–806. PubMed PMID: 11742412. Epub 2001/12/14. eng.

72. Tamura S, Shimomura I. Contribution of adipose tissue and de novo lipogenesis to nonalcoholic fatty liver disease. J Clin Invest. 2005;115(5):1139–42. PubMed PMID: 15864343. Pubmed Central PMCID: 1087181. Epub 2005/05/03. eng.

73. Fabbrini E, Mohammed BS, Magkos F, Korenblat KM, Patterson BW, Klein S. Alterations in adipose tissue and hepatic lipid kinetics in obese men and women with nonalcoholic fatty liver disease. Gastroenterology. 2008;134(2):424–31. PubMed PMID: 18242210. Pubmed Central PMCID: 2705923. Epub 2008/02/05. eng.

74. Fabbrini E, Magkos F, Mohammed BS, Pietka T, Abumrad NA, Patterson BW, et al. Intrahepatic fat, not visceral fat, is linked with metabolic complications of obesity. Proc Natl Acad Sci USA. 2009;106(36):15430–5. PubMed PMID: 19706383. Pubmed Central PMCID: 2741268. Epub 2009/08/27. eng.

75. Lam TK, van de Werve G, Giacca A. Free fatty acids increase basal hepatic glucose production and induce hepatic insulin resistance at different sites. Am J Physiol Endocrinol Metab. 2003;284(2):E281–90. PubMed PMID: 12531742. Epub 2003/01/18. eng.

76. Browning JD, Horton JD. Molecular mediators of hepatic steatosis and liver injury. J Clin Invest. 2004;114(2):147–52. PubMed PMID: 15254578. Pubmed Central PMCID: 449757. Epub 2004/07/16. eng.

77. Mater MK, Thelen AP, Pan DA, Jump DB. Sterol response element-binding protein 1c (SREBP1c) is involved in the polyunsaturated fatty acid suppression of hepatic S14 gene transcription. J Biol Chem. 1999;274(46):32725–32. PubMed PMID: 10551830. Epub 1999/11/07. eng.

78. Dentin R, Pegorier JP, Benhamed F, Foufelle F, Ferre P, Fauveau V, et al. Hepatic glucokinase is required for the synergistic action of ChREBP and SREBP-1c on glycolytic and lipogenic gene expression. J Biol Chem. 2004;279(19):20314–26. PubMed PMID: 14985368. Epub 2004/02/27. eng.

79. Iizuka K, Bruick RK, Liang G, Horton JD, Uyeda K. Deficiency of carbohydrate response element-binding protein (ChREBP) reduces lipogenesis as well as glycolysis. Proc Natl Acad Sci USA. 2004;101(19):7281–6. PubMed PMID: 15118080. Pubmed Central PMCID: 409910. Epub 2004/05/01. eng.

80. Taghibiglou C, Carpentier A, Van Iderstine SC, Chen B, Rudy D, Aiton A, et al. Mechanisms of hepatic very low density lipoprotein overproduction in insulin resistance. Evidence for enhanced lipoprotein assembly, reduced intracellular ApoB degradation, and increased microsomal triglyceride transfer protein in a fructose-fed hamster model. J Biol Chem. 2000;275(12):8416–25. PubMed PMID: 10722675. Epub 2000/03/18. eng.

81. Charlton M, Sreekumar R, Rasmussen D, Lindor K, Nair KS. Apolipoprotein synthesis in nonalcoholic steatohepatitis. Hepatology. 2002;35(4):898–904. PubMed PMID: 11915037. Epub 2002/03/27. eng.

82. Angulo P. Nonalcoholic fatty liver disease. N Engl J Med. 2002 18;346(16):1221–31. PubMed PMID: 11961152. Epub 2002/04/19. eng.

83. Bocher V, Pineda-Torra I, Fruchart JC, Staels B. PPARs: transcription factors controlling lipid and lipoprotein metabolism. Ann N Y Acad Sci. 2002;967:7–18. PubMed PMID: 12079830. Epub 2002/06/25. eng.

84. Begriche K, Igoudjil A, Pessayre D, Fromenty B. Mitochondrial dysfunction in NASH: causes, consequences and possible means to prevent it. Mitochondrion. 2006;6(1):1–28. PubMed PMID: 16406828. Epub 2006/01/13. eng.

85. Pessayre D, Mansouri A, Fromenty B. Nonalcoholic steatosis and steatohepatitis. V. Mitochondrial dysfunction in steatohepatitis. Am J Physiol Gastrointest Liver Physiol. 2002;282(2):G193–9. PubMed PMID: 11804839. Epub 2002/01/24. eng.

86. Sanyal AJ, Campbell-Sargent C, Mirshahi F, Rizzo WB, Contos MJ, Sterling RK, et al. Nonalcoholic steatohepatitis: association of insulin resistance and mitochondrial abnormalities. Gastroenterology. 2001;120(5):1183–92. PubMed PMID: 11266382. Epub 2001/03/27. eng.

87. Caldwell SH, Swerdlow RH, Khan EM, Iezzoni JC, Hespenheide EE, Parks JK, et al. Mitochondrial abnormalities in non-alcoholic steatohepatitis. J Hepatol. 1999;31(3):430–4. PubMed PMID: 10488700. Epub 1999/09/17. eng.

88. Fromenty B, Robin MA, Igoudjil A, Mansouri A, Pessayre D. The ins and outs of mitochondrial dysfunction in NASH. Diabetes Metab. 2004;30(2):121–38. PubMed PMID: 15223984.

89. Perez-Carreras M, Del Hoyo P, Martin MA, Rubio JC, Martin A, Castellano G, et al. Defective hepatic mitochondrial respiratory chain in patients with nonalcoholic steatohepatitis. Hepatology. 2003;38(4):999–1007. PubMed PMID: 14512887. Epub 2003/09/27. eng.

90. Chitturi S, Farrell GC. Etiopathogenesis of nonalcoholic steatohepatitis. Semin Liver Dis. 2001;21(1):27–41. PubMed PMID: 11296694. Epub 2001/04/12. eng.

91. Day CP. From fat to inflammation. Gastroenterology. 2006;130(1):207–10. PubMed PMID: 16401483. Epub 2006/01/13. eng.

92. Cai D, Yuan M, Frantz DF, Melendez PA, Hansen L, Lee J, et al. Local and systemic insulin resistance resulting from hepatic activation of IKK-beta and NF-kappaB. Nat Med. 2005;11(2):183–90. PubMed PMID: 15685173. Pubmed Central PMCID: 1440292. Epub 2005/02/03. eng.

93. Arkan MC, Hevener AL, Greten FR, Maeda S, Li ZW, Long JM, et al. IKK-beta links inflammation to obesity-induced insulin resistance. Nat Med. 2005;11(2):191–8. PubMed PMID: 15685170. Epub 2005/02/03. eng.

94. Crespo J, Cayon A, Fernandez-Gil P, Hernandez-Guerra M, Mayorga M, Dominguez-Diez A, et al. Gene expression of tumor necrosis factor alpha and TNF-receptors, p55 and p75, in nonalcoholic steatohepatitis patients. Hepatology. 2001;34(6):1158–63. PubMed PMID: 11732005. Epub 2001/12/04. eng.

95. Feldstein AE, Werneburg NW, Canbay A, Guicciardi ME, Bronk SF, Rydzewski R, et al. Free fatty acids promote hepatic lipotoxicity by stimulating TNF-alpha expression via a lysosomal pathway. Hepatology. 2004;40(1):185–94. PubMed PMID: 15239102. Epub 2004/07/09. eng.

96. Ron D. Translational control in the endoplasmic reticulum stress response. J Clin Invest. 2002;110(10):1383–8. PubMed PMID: 12438433. Pubmed Central PMCID: 151821. Epub 2002/11/20. eng.

97. Fabbrini E, deHaseth D, Deivanayagam S, Mohammed BS, Vitola BE, Klein S. Alterations in fatty acid kinetics in obese adolescents with increased intrahepatic triglyceride content. Obesity (Silver Spring). 2009;17(1):25–9. PubMed PMID: 18948971. Pubmed Central PMCID: 2649753. Epub 2008/10/25. eng.

98. Seki E, Brenner DA. Toll-like receptors and adaptor molecules in liver disease: update. Hepatology. 2008;48(1):322–35. PubMed PMID: 18506843. Epub 2008/05/29. eng.

99. Jarrar MH, Baranova A, Collantes R, Ranard B, Stepanova M, Bennett C, et al. Adipokines and cytokines in non-alcoholic fatty liver disease. Aliment Pharmacol Ther. 2008;27(5):412–21. PubMed PMID: 18081738. Epub 2007/12/18. eng.

100. Rabe K, Lehrke M, Parhofer KG, Broedl UC. Adipokines and insulin resistance. Mol Med. 2008;14(11–12):741–51. PubMed PMID: 19009016. Pubmed Central PMCID: 2582855. Epub 2008/11/15. eng.

101. Donnelly KL, Smith CI, Schwarzenberg SJ, Jessurun J, Boldt MD, Parks EJ. Sources of fatty acids stored in liver and secreted via lipoproteins in patients with nonalcoholic fatty liver disease. J Clin Invest. 2005;115(5):1343–51. PubMed PMID: 15864352. Pubmed Central PMCID: 1087172. Epub 2005/05/03. eng.

102. Myers MG, Cowley MA, Munzberg H. Mechanisms of leptin action and leptin resistance. Annu Rev Physiol. 2008;70:537–56. PubMed PMID: 17937601. Epub 2007/10/17. eng.

103. Uygun A, Kadayifci A, Yesilova Z, Erdil A, Yaman H, Saka M, et al. Serum leptin levels in patients with nonalcoholic steatohepatitis. Am J Gastroenterol. 2000;95(12):3584–9. PubMed PMID: 11151896. Epub 2001/01/11. eng.

104. Manco M, Alisi A, Nobili V. Risk of severe liver disease in NAFLD with normal ALT levels: a pediatric report. Hepatology. 2008;48(6):2087–8; author reply 8. PubMed PMID: 18980229. Epub 2008/11/05. eng.

105. Yki-Jarvinen H. Thiazolidinediones. N Engl J Med. 2004;351(11):1106–18. PubMed PMID: 15356308. Epub 2004/09/10. eng.

106. Xu A, Wang Y, Keshaw H, Xu LY, Lam KS, Cooper GJ. The fat-derived hormone adiponectin alleviates alcoholic and nonalcoholic fatty liver diseases in mice. J Clin Invest. 2003;112(1):91–100. PubMed PMID: 12840063. Pubmed Central PMCID: 162288. Epub 2003/07/04. eng.

107. Wolf AM, Wolf D, Avila MA, Moschen AR, Berasain C, Enrich B, et al. Up-regulation of the anti-inflammatory adipokine adiponectin in acute liver failure in mice. J Hepatol. 2006;44(3):537–43. PubMed PMID: 16310276. Epub 2005/11/29. eng.

108. Kamada Y, Tamura S, Kiso S, Matsumoto H, Saji Y, Yoshida Y, et al. Enhanced carbon tetrachloride-induced liver fibrosis in mice

lacking adiponectin. Gastroenterology. 2003;125(6):1796–807. PubMed PMID: 14724832. Epub 2004/01/16. eng.

109. Feldstein AE, Canbay A, Angulo P, Taniai M, Burgart LJ, Lindor KD, et al. Hepatocyte apoptosis and fas expression are prominent features of human nonalcoholic steatohepatitis. Gastroenterology. 2003;125(2):437–43. PubMed PMID: 12891546. Epub 2003/08/02. eng.

110. Cazanave SC, Gores GJ. Mechanisms and clinical implications of hepatocyte lipoapoptosis. Clin Lipidol. 2010;5(1):71–85. PubMed PMID: 20368747. Pubmed Central PMCID: 2847283. Epub 2010/04/07. Eng.

111. Jaeschke H. Inflammation in response to hepatocellular apoptosis. Hepatology. 2002;35(4):964–6. PubMed PMID: 11915046. Epub 2002/03/27. eng.

112. Faouzi S, Burckhardt BE, Hanson JC, Campe CB, Schrum LW, Rippe RA, et al. Anti-Fas induces hepatic chemokines and promotes inflammation by an NF-kappa B-independent, caspase-3-dependent pathway. J Biol Chem. 2001;276(52):49077–82. PubMed PMID: 11602613. Epub 2001/10/17. eng.

113. Watanabe A, Hashmi A, Gomes DA, Town T, Badou A, Flavell RA, et al. Apoptotic hepatocyte DNA inhibits hepatic stellate cell chemotaxis via toll-like receptor 9. Hepatology. 2007;46(5):1509–18. PubMed PMID: 17705260. Epub 2007/08/21. eng.

114. Canbay A, Feldstein AE, Higuchi H, Werneburg N, Grambihler A, Bronk SF, et al. Kupffer cell engulfment of apoptotic bodies stimulates death ligand and cytokine expression. Hepatology. 2003;38(5):1188–98. PubMed PMID: 14578857. Epub 2003/10/28. eng.

115. Friedman SL. Hepatic stellate cells: protean, multifunctional, and enigmatic cells of the liver. Physiol Rev. 2008;88(1):125–72. PubMed PMID: 18195085. Pubmed Central PMCID: 2888531. Epub 2008/01/16. eng.

116. Utzschneider KM, Kahn SE. Review: the role of insulin resistance in nonalcoholic fatty liver disease. J Clin Endocrinol Metab. 2006;91(12):4753–61. PubMed PMID: 16968800. Epub 2006/09/14. eng.

117. Wieckowska A, McCullough AJ, Feldstein AE. Noninvasive diagnosis and monitoring of nonalcoholic steatohepatitis: present and future. Hepatology. 2007;46(2):582–9. PubMed PMID: 17661414. Epub 2007/07/31. eng.

118. Manco M, Marcellini M, Devito R, Comparcola D, Sartorelli MR, Nobili V. Metabolic syndrome and liver histology in paediatric non-alcoholic steatohepatitis. Int J Obes (Lond). 2008;32(2):381–7. PubMed PMID: 18087267. Epub 2007/12/19. eng.

119. Rashid M, Roberts EA. Nonalcoholic steatohepatitis in children. J Pediatr Gastroenterol Nutr. 2000;30(1):48–53. PubMed PMID: 10630439. Epub 2000/01/12. eng.

120. d'Annunzio G, Vanelli M, Pistorio A, Minuto N, Bergamino L, Lafusco D, et al. Insulin resistance and secretion indexes in healthy Italian children and adolescents: a multicentre study. Acta Biomed. 2009;80(1):21–8. PubMed PMID: 19705616. Epub 2009/08/27. eng.

121. Chalasani N, Younossi Z, Lavine JE, Diehl AM, Brunt EM, Cusi K, et al. The diagnosis and management of non-alcoholic fatty liver disease: practice guideline by the american association for the study of liver diseases, american college of gastroenterology, and the american gastroenterological association. Hepatology. 2012;55(6):2005–23. PubMed PMID: 22488764.

122. Vajro P, Lenta S, Socha P, Dhawan A, McKiernan P, Baumann U, et al. Diagnosis of nonalcoholic fatty liver disease in children and adolescents: position paper of the ESPGHAN hepatology committee. J Pediatr Gastroenterol Nutr. 2012;54(5):700–13. PubMed PMID: 22395188.

123. Franzese A, Vajro P, Argenziano A, Puzziello A, Iannucci MP, Saviano MC, et al. Liver involvement in obese children. Ultrasonography and liver enzyme levels at diagnosis and during follow-up in an Italian population. Dig Dis Sci. 1997;42(7):1428–32. PubMed PMID: 9246041. Epub 1997/07/01. eng.

124. Molleston JP, Schwimmer JB, Yates KP, Murray KF, Cummings OW, Lavine JE, et al. Histological abnormalities in children with nonalcoholic fatty liver disease and normal or mildly elevated alanine aminotransferase levels. J Pediatr. 2013. PubMed PMID: 24360992.

125. Schwimmer JB, Behling C, Newbury R, Deutsch R, Nievergelt C, Schork NJ, et al. Histopathology of pediatric nonalcoholic fatty liver disease. Hepatology. 2005;42(3):641–9. PubMed PMID: 16116629. Epub 2005/08/24. eng.

126. Hernaez R, Lazo M, Bonekamp S, Kamel I, Brancati FL, Guallar E, et al. Diagnostic accuracy and reliability of ultrasonography for the detection of fatty liver: a meta-analysis. Hepatology. 2011 Sep 2;54(3):1082–90. PubMed PMID: 21618575. Epub 2011/05/28. Eng.

127. Pacifico L, Celestre M, Anania C, Paolantonio P, Chiesa C, Laghi A. MRI and ultrasound for hepatic fat quantification:relationships to clinical and metabolic characteristics of pediatric nonalcoholic fatty liver disease. Acta Paediatr. 2007;96(4):542–7. PubMed PMID: 17306008. Epub 2007/02/20. eng.

128. Brunt EM. Pathology of fatty liver disease. Mod Pathol. 2007;20 Suppl 1:S40–8. PubMed PMID: 17486051. Epub 2007/05/09. eng.

129. Carter-Kent C, Yerian LM, Brunt EM, Angulo P, Kohli R, Ling SC, et al. Nonalcoholic steatohepatitis in children: a multicenter clinicopathological study. Hepatology. 2009 Oct;50(4):1113–20. PubMed PMID: 19637190. Epub 2009/07/29. Eng.

130. Nobili V, Marcellini M, Devito R, Ciampalini P, Piemonte F, Comparcola D, et al. NAFLD in children: a prospective clinical-pathological study and effect of lifestyle advice. Hepatology. 2006;44(2):458–65. PubMed PMID: 16871574. Epub 2006/07/28. eng.

131. Takahashi Y, Fukusato T. Pediatric nonalcoholic fatty liver disease: overview with emphasis on histology. World J Gastroenterol. 2010;16(42):5280–5. PubMed PMID: 21072890. Pubmed Central PMCID: 2980676. Epub 2010/11/13. eng.

132. Brunt EM, Kleiner DE, Wilson LA, Unalp A, Behling CE, Lavine JE, et al. Portal chronic inflammation in nonalcoholic fatty liver disease (NAFLD): a histologic marker of advanced NAFLD-Clinicopathologic correlations from the nonalcoholic steatohepatitis clinical research network. Hepatology. 2009;49(3):809–20. PubMed PMID: 19142989. Pubmed Central PMCID: 2928479. Epub 2009/01/15. eng.

133. Richardson MM, Jonsson JR, Powell EE, Brunt EM, Neuschwander-Tetri BA, Bhathal PS, et al. Progressive fibrosis in nonalcoholic steatohepatitis: association with altered regeneration and a ductular reaction. Gastroenterology. 2007;133(1):80–90. PubMed PMID: 17631134. Epub 2007/07/17. eng.

134. Tandra S, Yeh MM, Brunt EM, Vuppalanchi R, Cummings OW, Unalp-Arida A, et al. Presence and significance of microvesicular steatosis in non-alcoholic fatty liver disease. J Hepatol. 2011 Sep;55(3):654–9.

135. Pessayre D, Mansouri A, Haouzi D, Fromenty B. Hepatotoxicity due to mitochondrial dysfunction. Cell Biol Toxicol. 1999;15(6):367–73. PubMed PMID: 10811531. Epub 2000/05/16. eng.

136. Caldwell S, Ikura Y, Dias D, Isomoto K, Yabu A, Moskaluk C, et al. Hepatocellular ballooning in NASH. J Hepatol. 2010;53(4):719–23. PubMed PMID: 20624660. Pubmed Central PMCID: 2930100. Epub 2010/07/14. eng.

137. Fujii H, Ikura Y, Arimoto J, Sugioka K, Iezzoni JC, Park SH, et al. Expression of perilipin and adipophilin in nonalcoholic fatty liver disease; relevance to oxidative injury and hepatocyte ballooning. J Atheroscler Thromb. 2009;16(6):893–901. PubMed PMID: 20032580. Epub 2009/12/25. eng.

138. Kleiner DE, Brunt EM, Van Natta M, Behling C, Contos MJ, Cummings OW, et al. Design and validation of a histological scoring system for nonalcoholic fatty liver disease. Hepatol-

ogy. 2005;41(6):1313–21. PubMed PMID: 15915461. Epub 2005/05/26. eng.

139. Brunt EM, Kleiner DE, Wilson LA, Belt P, Neuschwander-Tetri BA. Nonalcoholic fatty liver disease (NAFLD) activity score and the histopathologic diagnosis in NAFLD: distinct clinicopathologic meanings. Hepatology. 2011;53(3):810–20. PubMed PMID: 21319198. Pubmed Central PMCID: 3079483. Epub 2011/02/15. eng.

140. Ekstedt M, Franzen LE, Mathiesen UL, Thorelius L, Holmqvist M, Bodemar G, et al. Long-term follow-up of patients with NAFLD and elevated liver enzymes. Hepatology. 2006;44(4):865–73. PubMed PMID: 17006923.

141. Adams LA, Sanderson S, Lindor KD, Angulo P. The histological course of nonalcoholic fatty liver disease: a longitudinal study of 103 patients with sequential liver biopsies. J Hepatol. 2005;42(1):132–8. PubMed PMID: 15629518. Epub 2005/01/05. eng.

142. Argo CK, Northup PG, Al-Osaimi AM, Caldwell SH. Systematic review of risk factors for fibrosis progression in non-alcoholic steatohepatitis. J Hepatol. 2009;51(2):371–9. PubMed PMID: 19501928. Epub 2009/06/09. eng.

143. Musso G, Gambino R, Cassader M, Pagano G. Meta-analysis: natural history of non-alcoholic fatty liver disease (NAFLD) and diagnostic accuracy of non-invasive tests for liver disease severity. Ann Med. 2011 Dec;43(8):617–49. PubMed PMID: 21039302. Epub 2010/11/03. Eng.

144. Clark JM, Diehl AM. Nonalcoholic fatty liver disease: an underrecognized cause of cryptogenic cirrhosis. JAMA. 2003; 289(22):3000–4. PubMed PMID: 12799409. Epub 2003/06/12. eng.

145. Marmur J, Bergquist A, Stal P. Liver transplantation of patients with cryptogenic cirrhosis: clinical characteristics and outcome. Scand J Gastroenterol. 2010;45(1):60–9. PubMed PMID: 20030578. Epub 2009/12/25. eng.

146. Poonawala A, Nair SP, Thuluvath PJ. Prevalence of obesity and diabetes in patients with cryptogenic cirrhosis: a case-control study. Hepatology. 2000;32(4 Pt 1):689–92. PubMed PMID: 11003611. Epub 2000/09/26. eng.

147. Ong J, Younossi ZM, Reddy V, Price LL, Gramlich T, Mayes J, et al. Cryptogenic cirrhosis and posttransplantation nonalcoholic fatty liver disease. Liver Transpl. 2001;7(9):797–801. PubMed PMID: 11552214. Epub 2001/09/12. eng.

148. Starley BQ, Calcagno CJ, Harrison SA. Nonalcoholic fatty liver disease and hepatocellular carcinoma: a weighty connection. Hepatology. 2010;51(5):1820–32. PubMed PMID: 20432259. Epub 2010/05/01. eng.

149. Guzman G, Brunt EM, Petrovic LM, Chejfec G, Layden TJ, Cotler SJ. Does nonalcoholic fatty liver disease predispose patients to hepatocellular carcinoma in the absence of cirrhosis? Arch Pathol Lab Med. 2008;132(11):1761–6. PubMed PMID: 18976012. Epub 2008/11/04. eng.

150. Bugianesi E. Non-alcoholic steatohepatitis and cancer. Clin Liver Dis. 2007;11(1):191–207, x–xi. PubMed PMID: 17544979. Epub 2007/06/05. eng.

151. Hashimoto E, Yatsuji S, Tobari M, Taniai M, Torii N, Tokushige K, et al. Hepatocellular carcinoma in patients with nonalcoholic steatohepatitis. J Gastroenterol. 2009;44 Suppl 19:89–95. PubMed PMID: 19148800. Epub 2009/02/20. eng.

152. Ong JP, Younossi ZM. Epidemiology and natural history of NAFLD and NASH. Clin Liver Dis. 2007;11(1):1–16, vii. PubMed PMID: 17544968. Epub 2007/06/05. eng.

153. Powell EE, Cooksley WG, Hanson R, Searle J, Halliday JW, Powell LW. The natural history of nonalcoholic steatohepatitis: a follow-up study of forty-two patients for up to 21 years. Hepatology. 1990;11(1):74–80. PubMed PMID: 2295475. Epub 1990/01/01. eng.

154. Shimada M, Hashimoto E, Taniai M, Hasegawa K, Okuda H, Hayashi N, et al. Hepatocellular carcinoma in patients with nonalcoholic steatohepatitis. J Hepatol. 2002;37(1):154–60. PubMed PMID: 12076877. Epub 2002/06/22. eng.

155. Molleston JP, White F, Teckman J, Fitzgerald JF. Obese children with steatohepatitis can develop cirrhosis in childhood. Am J Gastroenterol. 2002;97(9):2460–2. PubMed PMID: 12358273. Epub 2002/10/03. eng.

156. Feldstein AE, Charatcharoenwitthaya P, Treeprasertsuk S, Benson JT, Enders FB, Angulo P. The natural history of nonalcoholic fatty liver disease in children: a follow-up study for up to 20-years. Gut. 2009 Nov;58(11):1538–44. PubMed PMID: 19625277. Epub 2009/07/25. Eng.

157. Guha IN, Parkes J, Roderick PR, Harris S, Rosenberg WM. Non-invasive markers associated with liver fibrosis in non-alcoholic fatty liver disease. Gut. 2006;55(11):1650–60. PubMed PMID: 17047111. Epub 2006/10/19. eng.

158. Huang MA, Greenson JK, Chao C, Anderson L, Peterman D, Jacobson J, et al. One-year intense nutritional counseling results in histological improvement in patients with non-alcoholic steatohepatitis: a pilot study. Am J Gastroenterol. 2005;100(5):1072–81. PubMed PMID: 15842581. Epub 2005/04/22. eng.

159. Hickman IJ, Jonsson JR, Prins JB, Ash S, Purdie DM, Clouston AD, et al. Modest weight loss and physical activity in overweight patients with chronic liver disease results in sustained improvements in alanine aminotransferase, fasting insulin, and quality of life. Gut. 2004;53(3):413–9. PubMed PMID: 14960526. Pubmed Central PMCID: 1773957. Epub 2004/02/13. eng.

160. Promrat K, Kleiner DE, Niemeier HM, Jackvony E, Kearns M, Wands JR, et al. Randomized controlled trial testing the effects of weight loss on nonalcoholic steatohepatitis. Hepatology. 2010;51(1):121–9. PubMed PMID: 19827166. Pubmed Central PMCID: 2799538. Epub 2009/10/15. eng.

161. Manton ND, Lipsett J, Moore DJ, Davidson GP, Bourne AJ, Couper RT. Non-alcoholic steatohepatitis in children and adolescents. Med J Aust. 2000;173(9):476–9. PubMed PMID: 11149304. Epub 2001/01/10. eng.

162. Vajro P, Fontanella A, Perna C, Orso G, Tedesco M, De Vincenzo A. Persistent hyperaminotransferasemia resolving after weight reduction in obese children. J Pediatr. 1994;125(2):239–41. PubMed PMID: 8040771. Epub 1994/08/01. eng.

163. Nobili V, Manco M, Devito R, Di Ciommo V, Comparcola D, Sartorelli MR, et al. Lifestyle intervention and antioxidant therapy in children with nonalcoholic fatty liver disease: a randomized, controlled trial. Hepatology. 2008;48(1):119–28. PubMed PMID: 18537181. Epub 2008/06/10. eng.

164. Capanni M, Calella F, Biagini MR, Genise S, Raimondi L, Bedogni G, et al. Prolonged n-3 polyunsaturated fatty acid supplementation ameliorates hepatic steatosis in patients with nonalcoholic fatty liver disease: a pilot study. Aliment Pharmacol Ther. 2006;23(8):1143–51. PubMed PMID: 16611275. Epub 2006/04/14. eng.

165. Spadaro L, Magliocco O, Spampinato D, Piro S, Oliveri C, Alagona C, et al. Effects of n-3 polyunsaturated fatty acids in subjects with nonalcoholic fatty liver disease. Dig Liver Dis. 2008;40(3):194–9. PubMed PMID: 18054848. Epub 2007/12/07. eng.

166. Tanaka N, Sano K, Horiuchi A, Tanaka E, Kiyosawa K, Aoyama T. Highly purified eicosapentaenoic acid treatment improves nonalcoholic steatohepatitis. J Clin Gastroenterol. 2008;42(4):413–8. PubMed PMID: 18277895. Epub 2008/02/19. eng.

167. Nobili V, Bedogni G, Alisi A, Pietrobattista A, Rise P, Galli C, et al. Docosahexaenoic acid supplementation decreases liver fat content in children with non-alcoholic fatty liver disease: double-blind randomised controlled clinical trial. Arch Dis Child. 2011;96(4):350–3. PubMed PMID: 21233083. Epub 2011/01/15. eng.

168. Wiernsperger NF, Bailey CJ. The antihyperglycaemic effect of metformin: therapeutic and cellular mechanisms. Drugs. 1999;58 Suppl 1:31–9, discussion 75–82. PubMed PMID: 10576523. Epub 1999/11/27. eng.

169. Angelico F, Burattin M, Alessandri C, Del Ben M, Lirussi F. Drugs improving insulin resistance for non-alcoholic fatty liver disease and/or non-alcoholic steatohepatitis. Cochrane Database Syst Rev. 2007;24(1):CD005166. PubMed PMID: 17253544. Epub 2007/01/27. eng.

170. Sanyal AJ, Mofrad PS, Contos MJ, Sargeant C, Luketic VA, Sterling RK, et al. A pilot study of vitamin E versus vitamin E and pioglitazone for the treatment of nonalcoholic steatohepatitis. Clin Gastroenterol Hepatol. 2004;2(12):1107–15. PubMed PMID: 15625656. Epub 2004/12/31. eng.

171. Bugianesi E, Gentilcore E, Manini R, Natale S, Vanni E, Villanova N, et al. A randomized controlled trial of metformin versus vitamin E or prescriptive diet in nonalcoholic fatty liver disease. Am J Gastroenterol. 2005;100(5):1082–90. PubMed PMID: 15842582. Epub 2005/04/22. eng.

172. Uygun A, Kadayifci A, Isik AT, Ozgurtas T, Deveci S, Tuzun A, et al. Metformin in the treatment of patients with non-alcoholic steatohepatitis. Aliment Pharmacol Ther. 2004;19(5):537–44. PubMed PMID: 14987322. Epub 2004/02/28. eng.

173. Neuschwander-Tetri BA, Brunt EM, Wehmeier KR, Oliver D, Bacon BR. Improved nonalcoholic steatohepatitis after 48 weeks of treatment with the PPAR-gamma ligand rosiglitazone. Hepatology. 2003;38(4):1008–17. PubMed PMID: 14512888. Epub 2003/09/27. eng.

174. Belfort R, Harrison SA, Brown K, Darland C, Finch J, Hardies J, et al. A placebo-controlled trial of pioglitazone in subjects with nonalcoholic steatohepatitis. N Engl J Med. 2006;355(22):2297–307. PubMed PMID: 17135584. Epub 2006/12/01. eng.

175. Sanyal AJ, Chalasani N, Kowdley KV, McCullough A, Diehl AM, Bass NM, et al. Pioglitazone, vitamin E, or placebo for nonalcoholic steatohepatitis. N Engl J Med. 2010;362(18):1675–85. PubMed PMID: 20427778. Pubmed Central PMCID: 2928471. Epub 2010/04/30. eng.

176. Lavine JE, Schwimmer JB, Molleston JP, Chalasani N, Rosenthal P, Murray KF, et al. Vitamin E, metformin or placebo for treatment of nonalcoholic fatty liver disease in children. Hepatology. 2010;52(4):374A.

177. Schwimmer JB, Middleton MS, Deutsch R, Lavine JE. A phase 2 clinical trial of metformin as a treatment for non-diabetic paediatric non-alcoholic steatohepatitis. Aliment Pharmacol Ther. 2005;21(7):871–9. PubMed PMID: 15801922.

178. Nobili V, Manco M, Devito R, Ciampalini P, Piemonte F, Marcellini M. Effect of vitamin E on aminotransferase levels and insulin resistance in children with non-alcoholic fatty liver disease. Aliment Pharmacol Ther. 2006;24(11–12):1553–61. PubMed PMID: 17206944. Epub 2007/01/09. eng.

179. Nadeau KJ, Ehlers LB, Zeitler PS, Love-Osborne K. Treatment of non-alcoholic fatty liver disease with metformin versus lifestyle intervention in insulin-resistant adolescents. Pediatr Diabetes. 2009;10(1):5–13. PubMed PMID: 18721166.

180. Lavine JE, Schwimmer JB, Van Natta ML, Molleston JP, Murray KF, Rosenthal P, et al. Effect of vitamin E or metformin for treatment of nonalcoholic fatty liver disease in children and adolescents: the TONIC randomized controlled trial. JAMA. 2011;305(16):1659–68. PubMed PMID: 21521847. Pubmed Central PMCID: 3110082.

181. Lavine JE. Vitamin E treatment of nonalcoholic steatohepatitis in children: a pilot study. J Pediatr. 2000;136(6):734–8. PubMed PMID: 10839868.

182. Vajro P, Mandato C, Franzese A, Ciccimarra E, Lucariello S, Savoia M, et al. Vitamin E treatment in pediatric obesity-related liver disease: a randomized study. J Pediatr Gastroenterol Nutr.

183. Lindor KD, Kowdley KV, Heathcote EJ, Harrison ME, Jorgensen R, Angulo P, et al. Ursodeoxycholic acid for treatment of nonalcoholic steatohepatitis: results of a randomized trial. Hepatology. 2004;39(3):770–8. PubMed PMID: 14999696. Epub 2004/03/05. eng.

184. Balmer ML, Siegrist K, Zimmermann A, Dufour JF. Effects of ursodeoxycholic acid in combination with vitamin E on adipokines and apoptosis in patients with nonalcoholic steatohepatitis. Liver Int. 2009;29(8):1184–8. PubMed PMID: 19422479. Epub 2009/05/09. eng.

185. Vajro P, Franzese A, Valerio G, Iannucci MP, Aragione N. Lack of efficacy of ursodeoxycholic acid for the treatment of liver abnormalities in obese children. J Pediatr. 2000;136(6):739–43. PubMed PMID: 10839869.

186. Orlando R, Azzalini L, Orando S, Lirussi F. Bile acids for non-alcoholic fatty liver disease and/or steatohepatitis. Cochrane Database Syst Rev. 2007;24(1):CD005160. PubMed PMID: 17253541.

187. Chavez-Tapia NC, Tellez-Avila FI, Barrientos-Gutierrez T, Mendez-Sanchez N, Lizardi-Cervera J, Uribe M. Bariatric surgery for non-alcoholic steatohepatitis in obese patients. Cochrane Database Syst Rev. 2010;20(1):CD007340. PubMed PMID: 20091629. Epub 2010/01/22. eng.

188. Zelber-Sagi S, Kessler A, Brazowsky E, Webb M, Lurie Y, Santo M, et al. A double-blind randomized placebo-controlled trial of orlistat for the treatment of nonalcoholic fatty liver disease. Clin Gastroenterol Hepatol. 2006;4(5):639–44. PubMed PMID: 16630771. Epub 2006/04/25. eng.

189. Hussein O, Grosovski M, Schlesinger S, Szvalb S, Assy N. Orlistat reverse fatty infiltration and improves hepatic fibrosis in obese patients with nonalcoholic steatohepatitis (NASH). Dig Dis Sci. 2007;52(10):2512–9. PubMed PMID: 17404856. Epub 2007/04/04. eng.

190. Harrison SA, Fecht W, Brunt EM, Neuschwander-Tetri BA. Orlistat for overweight subjects with nonalcoholic steatohepatitis: a randomized, prospective trial. Hepatology. 2009;49(1):80–6. PubMed PMID: 19053049. Epub 2008/12/05. eng.

191. Nabeshima Y, Tazuma S, Kanno K, Hyogo H, Iwai M, Horiuchi M, et al. Anti-fibrogenic function of angiotensin II type 2 receptor in CCl4-induced liver fibrosis. Biochem Biophys Res Commun. 2006;346(3):658–64. PubMed PMID: 16774739. Epub 2006/06/16. eng.

192. Yatabe J, Sanada H, Yatabe MS, Hashimoto S, Yoneda M, Felder RA, et al. Angiotensin II type 1 receptor blocker attenuates the activation of ERK and NADPH oxidase by mechanical strain in mesangial cells in the absence of angiotensin II. Am J Physiol Renal Physiol. 2009;296(5):F1052–60. PubMed PMID: 19261744. Epub 2009/03/06. eng.

193. Aller R, De Luis DA, Izaola O, Conde R, Gonzalez Sagrado M, Primo D, et al. Effect of a probiotic on liver aminotransferases in nonalcoholic fatty liver disease patients: a double blind randomized clinical trial. European review for medical and pharmacological sciences. 2011;15(9):1090–5. PubMed PMID: 22013734.

194. Vajro P, Mandato C, Licenziati MR, Franzese A, Vitale DF, Lenta S, et al. Effects of Lactobacillus rhamnosus strain GG in pediatric obesity-related liver disease. J Pediatr Gastroenterol Nutr. 2011;52(6):740–3. PubMed PMID: 21505361.

195. Fruchart JC, Duriez P, Staels B. Peroxisome proliferator-activated receptor-alpha activators regulate genes governing lipoprotein metabolism, vascular inflammation and atherosclerosis. Curr Opin Lipidol. 1999;10(3):245–57. PubMed PMID: 10431661. Epub 1999/08/04. eng.

196. Laurin J, Lindor KD, Crippin JS, Gossard A, Gores GJ, Ludwig J, et al. Ursodeoxycholic acid or clofibrate in the treatment of non-alcohol-induced steatohepatitis: a pilot study. Hepatology.

2004;38(1):48–55. PubMed PMID: 14676594. Epub 2003/12/17. eng.

1996;23(6):1464–7. PubMed PMID: 8675165. Epub 1996/06/01. eng.

197. Cadranel JF. Good clinical practice guidelines for fine needle aspiration biopsy of the liver: past, present and future. Gastroenterol Clin Biol. 2002;26(10):823–4. PubMed PMID: 12434092. Recommandations pour la pratique clinique pour la realisation de la ponction biopsie hepatique.

198. Bravo AA, Sheth SG, Chopra S. Liver biopsy. N Engl J Med. 2001;344(7):495–500. PubMed PMID: 11172192. Epub 2001/02/15. eng.

199. Day CP. Natural history of NAFLD: remarkably benign in the absence of cirrhosis. Gastroenterology. 2005;129(1):375–8. PubMed PMID: 16012969. Epub 2005/07/14. eng.

200. Angulo P. Long-term mortality in nonalcoholic fatty liver disease: is liver histology of any prognostic significance? Hepatology. 2010;51(2):373–5. PubMed PMID: 20101746. Pubmed Central PMCID: 2945376. Epub 2010/01/27. eng.

201. Angulo P, Hui JM, Marchesini G, Bugianesi E, George J, Farrell GC, et al. The NAFLD fibrosis score: a noninvasive system that identifies liver fibrosis in patients with NAFLD. Hepatology. 2007;45(4):846–54. PubMed PMID: 17393509. Epub 2007/03/30. eng.

202. Harrison SA, Oliver D, Arnold HL, Gogia S, Neuschwander-Tetri BA. Development and validation of a simple NAFLD clinical scoring system for identifying patients without advanced disease. Gut. 2008;57(10):1441–7. PubMed PMID: 18390575. Epub 2008/04/09. eng.

203. Iacobellis A, Marcellini M, Andriulli A, Perri F, Leandro G, Devito R, et al. Non invasive evaluation of liver fibrosis in paediatric patients with nonalcoholic steatohepatitis. World J Gastroenterol. 2006;12(48):7821–5. PubMed PMID: 17203527. Epub 2007/01/05. eng.

204. Yoneda M, Mawatari H, Fujita K, Endo H, Iida H, Nozaki Y, et al. Noninvasive assessment of liver fibrosis by measurement of stiffness in patients with nonalcoholic fatty liver disease (NAFLD). Dig Liver Dis. 2008;40(5):371–8. PubMed PMID: 18083083. Epub 2007/12/18. eng.

205. Mandato C, Lucariello S, Licenziati MR, Franzese A, Spagnuolo MI, Ficarella R, et al. Metabolic, hormonal, oxidative, and inflammatory factors in pediatric obesity-related liver disease. J Pediatr. 2005;147(1):62–6. PubMed PMID: 16027697. Epub 2005/07/20. eng.

206. Wieckowska A, Zein NN, Yerian LM, Lopez AR, McCullough AJ, Feldstein AE. In vivo assessment of liver cell apoptosis as a novel biomarker of disease severity in nonalcoholic fatty liver disease. Hepatology. 2006;44(1):27–33. PubMed PMID: 16799979. Epub 2006/06/27. eng.

207. Diab DL, Yerian L, Schauer P, Kashyap SR, Lopez R, Hazen SL, et al. Cytokeratin 18 fragment levels as a noninvasive biomarker for nonalcoholic steatohepatitis in bariatric surgery patients. Clin Gastroenterol Hepatol. 2008;6(11):1249–54. PubMed PMID: 18995215. Pubmed Central PMCID: 2628560. Epub 2008/11/11. eng.

208. Younossi ZM, Page S, Rafiq N, Birerdinc A, Stepanova M, Hossain N, et al. A biomarker panel for non-alcoholic steatohepatitis (NASH) and NASH-related fibrosis. Obes Surg. 2010. PubMed PMID: 20532833. Epub 2010/06/10. Eng.

209. Fitzpatrick E, Mitry RR, Quaglia A, Hussain M, Dhawan A. Serum levels of CK18 M30 and leptin are useful predictors of steatohepatitis and fibrosis in paediatric NAFLD. JPGN. 2010 Oct;51(4):500–6. doi: 10.1097/MPG.0b013e3181e376be. PMID:20808246.

210. Dixon JB, Bhathal PS, O'Brien PE. Nonalcoholic fatty liver disease: predictors of nonalcoholic steatohepatitis and liver fibrosis in the severely obese. Gastroenterology. 2001;121(1):91–100. PubMed PMID: 11438497. Epub 2001/07/05. eng.

211. Felice MS, Hammermuller E, De Davila MT, Ciocca ME, Fraquelli LE, Lorusso AM, et al. Acute lymphoblastic leukemia presenting as acute hepatic failure in childhood. Leuk Lymphoma. 2000;38(5–6):633–7. PubMed PMID: 10953986. Epub 2000/08/23. eng.

212. Munteanu M, Ratziu V, Morra R, Messous D, Imbert-Bismut F, Poynard T. Noninvasive biomarkers for the screening of fibrosis, steatosis and steatohepatitis in patients with metabolic risk factors: fibrotest-fibromax experience. J Gastrointestin Liver Dis. 2008;17(2):187–91. PubMed PMID: 18568141. Epub 2008/06/24. eng.

213. Manco M, Marcellini M, Giannone G, Nobili V. Correlation of serum TNF-alpha levels and histologic liver injury scores in pediatric nonalcoholic fatty liver disease. Am J Clin Pathol. 2007;127(6):954–60. PubMed PMID: 17509993. Epub 2007/05/19. eng.

214. Nobili V, Manco M, Ciampalini P, Diciommo V, Devito R, Piemonte F, et al. Leptin, free leptin index, insulin resistance and liver fibrosis in children with non-alcoholic fatty liver disease. Eur J Endocrinol. 2006;155(5):735–43. PubMed PMID: 17062890. Epub 2006/10/26. eng.

215. Louthan MV, Barve S, McClain CJ, Joshi-Barve S. Decreased serum adiponectin: an early event in pediatric nonalcoholic fatty liver disease. J Pediatr. 2005;147(6):835–8. PubMed PMID: 16356442. Epub 2005/12/17. eng.

216. Nobili V, Alkhouri N, Alisi A, Ottino S, Lopez R, Manco M, et al. Retinol-binding protein 4: a promising circulating marker of liver damage in pediatric nonalcoholic fatty liver disease. Clin Gastroenterol Hepatol. 2009;7(5):575–9. PubMed PMID: 19268270. Epub 2009/03/10. eng.

217. Reinehr T, Roth CL. Fetuin-A and its relation to metabolic syndrome and fatty liver disease in obese children before and after weight loss. J Clin Endocrinol Metab. 2008;93(11):4479–85. PubMed PMID: 18728159. Epub 2008/08/30. eng.

218. Alisi A, Manco M, Devito R, Piemonte F, Nobili V. Endotoxin and plasminogen activator inhibitor-1 serum levels associated with nonalcoholic steatohepatitis in children. J Pediatr Gastroenterol Nutr. 2010;50(6):645–9. PubMed PMID: 20400911. Epub 2010/04/20. eng.

219. Fitzpatrick E, Dew TK, Quaglia A, Sherwood RA, Mitry RR, Dhawan A. Analysis of adipokine concentrations in paediatric nonalcoholic fatty liver disease. Pediatric obesity. 2012;7(6):471–9. PubMed PMID: 22962039.

220. Fraquelli M, Bardella MT, Peracchi M, Cesana BM, Bianchi PA, Conte D. Gallbladder emptying and somatostatin and cholecystokinin plasma levels in celiac disease. Am J Gastroenterol. 1999;94(7):1866–70. PubMed PMID: 10406250. Epub 1999/07/16. eng.

221. Williams AL, Hoofnagle JH. Ratio of serum aspartate to alanine aminotransferase in chronic hepatitis. Relationship to cirrhosis. Gastroenterology. 1988;95(3):734–9. PubMed PMID: 3135226. Epub 1988/09/01. eng.

222. Shah AG, Lydecker A, Murray K, Tetri BN, Contos MJ, Sanyal AJ, et al. Comparison of noninvasive markers of fibrosis in patients with nonalcoholic fatty liver disease. Clin Gastroenterol Hepatol. 2009;7(10):1104–12. PubMed PMID: 19523535. Pubmed Central PMCID: 3079239.

223. McPherson S, Stewart SF, Henderson E, Burt AD, Day CP. Simple non-invasive fibrosis scoring systems can reliably exclude advanced fibrosis in patients with non-alcoholic fatty liver disease. Gut. 2010;59(9):1265–9. PubMed PMID: 20801772. Epub 2010/08/31. eng.

224. Cales P, Laine F, Boursier J, Deugnier Y, Moal V, Oberti F, et al. Comparison of blood tests for liver fibrosis specific or not to NAFLD. J Hepatol. 2009;50(1):165–73. PubMed PMID: 18977552. Epub 2008/11/04. eng.

225. Ratziu V, Giral P, Charlotte F, Bruckert E, Thibault V, Theodorou I, et al. Liver fibrosis in overweight patients. Gastroenterol-

ogy. 2000;118(6):1117–23. PubMed PMID: 10833486. Epub 2000/06/02. eng.

226. Ruffillo G, Fassio E, Alvarez E, Landeira G, Longo C, Dominguez N, et al. Comparison of NAFLD fibrosis score and BARD score in predicting fibrosis in nonalcoholic fatty liver disease. J Hepatol. 2011;54(1):160–3. PubMed PMID: 20934232. Epub 2010/10/12. eng.

227. Wong VW, Wong GL, Chim AM, Tse AM, Tsang SW, Hui AY, et al. Validation of the NAFLD fibrosis score in a Chinese population with low prevalence of advanced fibrosis. Am J Gastroenterol. 2008;103(7):1682–8. PubMed PMID: 18616651. Epub 2008/07/12. eng.

228. Qureshi K, Clements RH, Abrams GA. The utility of the "NAFLD fibrosis score" in morbidly obese subjects with NAFLD. Obes Surg. 2008;18(3):264–70. PubMed PMID: 18214632. Epub 2008/01/25. eng.

229. Colli A, Cocciolo M, Mumoli N, Cattalini N, Fraquelli M, Conte D. Hepatic artery resistance in alcoholic liver disease. Hepatology. 1998;28(5):1182–6. PubMed PMID: 9794899. Epub 1998/10/31. eng.

230. Zubizarreta P, Felice MS, Alfaro E, Fraquelli L, Casak S, Quinteros R, et al. Acute myelogenous leukemia in Down's syndrome: report of a single pediatric institution using a BFM treatment strategy. Leuk Res. 1998;22(5):465–72. PubMed PMID: 9652734. Epub 1998/07/04. eng.

231. Poynard T, Morra R, Halfon P, Castera L, Ratziu V, Imbert-Bismut F, et al. Meta-analyses of fibrotest diagnostic value in chronic liver disease. BMC Gastroenterol. 2007;7:40. PubMed PMID: 17937811. Pubmed Central PMCID: 2175505. Epub 2007/10/17. eng.

232. Rosenberg WM, Voelker M, Thiel R, Becka M, Burt A, Schuppan D, et al. Serum markers detect the presence of liver fibrosis: a cohort study. Gastroenterology. 2004;127(6):1704–13. PubMed PMID: 15578508. Epub 2004/12/04. eng.

233. Guha IN, Parkes J, Roderick P, Chattopadhyay D, Cross R, Harris S, et al. Noninvasive markers of fibrosis in nonalcoholic fatty liver disease: validating the European liver fibrosis panel and exploring simple markers. Hepatology. 2008;47(2):455–60. PubMed PMID: 18038452. Epub 2007/11/27. eng.

234. Parkes J, Roderick P, Harris S, Day C, Mutimer D, Collier J, et al. Enhanced liver fibrosis test can predict clinical outcomes in patients with chronic liver disease. Gut. 2010;59(9):1245–51. PubMed PMID: 20675693. Epub 2010/08/03. eng.

235. Kuczewski N, Langlois A, Fiorentino H, Bonnet S, Marissal T, Diabira D, et al. Spontaneous glutamatergic activity induces a BDNF-dependent potentiation of GABAergic synapses in the newborn rat hippocampus. J Physiol. 2008;586(Pt 21):5119–28. PubMed PMID: 18772203. Pubmed Central PMCID: 2652155. Epub 2008/09/06. eng.

236. Manco M, Bedogni G, Marcellini M, Devito R, Ciampalini P, Sartorelli MR, et al. Waist circumference correlates with liver fibrosis in children with non-alcoholic steatohepatitis. Gut. 2008;57(9):1283–7. PubMed PMID: 18218674. Epub 2008/01/26. eng.

237. Nobili V, Alisi A, Vania A, Tiribelli C, Pietrobattista A, Bedogni G. The pediatric NAFLD fibrosis index: a predictor of liver fibrosis in children with non-alcoholic fatty liver disease. BMC Med. 2009;7:21. PubMed PMID: 19409076. Pubmed Central PMCID: 2684116. Epub 2009/05/05. eng.

238. Nobili V, Parkes J, Bottazzo G, Marcellini M, Cross R, Newman D, et al. Performance of ELF serum markers in predicting fibrosis stage in pediatric non-alcoholic fatty liver disease. Gastroenterology. 2009;136(1):160–7. PubMed PMID: 18992746. Epub 2008/11/11. eng.

239. Alkhouri N, Carter-Kent C, Lopez R, Rosenberg WM, Pinzani M, Bedogni G, et al. A combination of the pediatric NAFLD fibrosis index and enhanced liver fibrosis test identifies children with

240. Saadeh S, Younossi ZM, Remer EM, Gramlich T, Ong JP, Hurley M, et al. The utility of radiological imaging in nonalcoholic fatty liver disease. Gastroenterology. 2002;123(3):745–50. PubMed PMID: 12198701. Epub 2002/08/29. eng.

241. Fishbein M, Castro F, Cheruku S, Jain S, Webb B, Gleason T, et al. Hepatic MRI for fat quantitation: its relationship to fat morphology, diagnosis, and ultrasound. J Clin Gastroenterol. 2005;39(7):619–25. PubMed PMID: 16000931. Epub 2005/07/08. eng.

242. Radetti G, Kleon W, Stuefer J, Pittschieler K. Non-alcoholic fatty liver disease in obese children evaluated by magnetic resonance imaging. Acta Paediatr. 2006;95(7):833–7. PubMed PMID: 16801180. Epub 2006/06/28. eng.

243. Burgert TS, Taksali SE, Dziura J, Goodman TR, Yeckel CW, Papademetris X, et al. Alanine aminotransferase levels and fatty liver in childhood obesity: associations with insulin resistance, adiponectin, and visceral fat. J Clin Endocrinol Metab. 2006;91(11):4287–94. PubMed PMID: 16912127. Epub 2006/08/17. eng.

244. Talwalkar JA, Yin M, Fidler JL, Sanderson SO, Kamath PS, Ehman RL. Magnetic resonance imaging of hepatic fibrosis: emerging clinical applications. Hepatology. 2008;47(1):332–42. PubMed PMID: 18161879.

245. Iijima H, Moriyasu F, Tsuchiya K, Suzuki S, Yoshida M, Shimizu M, et al. Decrease in accumulation of ultrasound contrast microbubbles in non-alcoholic steatohepatitis. Hepatol Res. 2007;37(9):722–30. PubMed PMID: 17559420. Epub 2007/06/15. eng.

246. Yoneda M, Suzuki K, Kato S, Fujita K, Nozaki Y, Hosono K, et al. Nonalcoholic fatty liver disease: US-based acoustic radiation force impulse elastography. Radiology. 2010;256(2):640–7. PubMed PMID: 20529989. Epub 2010/06/10. eng.

247. Palmeri ML, Wang MH, Rouze NC, Abdelmalek MF, Guy CD, Moser B, et al. Noninvasive evaluation of hepatic fibrosis using acoustic radiation force-based shear stiffness in patients with nonalcoholic fatty liver disease. J Hepatol. 2011 Sep;55(3):666–72. PubMed PMID: 21256907. Epub 2011/01/25. Eng.

248. Wong VW, Vergniol J, Wong GL, Foucher J, Chan HL, Le Bail B, et al. Diagnosis of fibrosis and cirrhosis using liver stiffness measurement in nonalcoholic fatty liver disease. Hepatology. 2010;51(2):454–62. PubMed PMID: 20101745. Epub 2010/01/27. eng.

249. Yoneda M, Fujita K, Inamori M, Tamano M, Hiriishi H, Nakajima A. Transient elastography in patients with non-alcoholic fatty liver disease (NAFLD). Gut. 2007;56(9):1330–1. PubMed PMID: 17470477. Pubmed Central PMCID: 1954961. Epub 2007/05/02. eng.

250. Nobili V, Vizzutti F, Arena U, Abraldes JG, Marra F, Pietrobattista A, et al. Accuracy and reproducibility of transient elastography for the diagnosis of fibrosis in pediatric nonalcoholic steatohepatitis. Hepatology. 2008;48(2):442–8. PubMed PMID: 18563842. Epub 2008/06/20. eng.

251. Fraquelli M, Rigamonti C, Casazza G, Conte D, Donato MF, Ronchi G, et al. Reproducibility of transient elastography in the evaluation of liver fibrosis in patients with chronic liver disease. Gut. 2007;56(7):968–73. PubMed PMID: 17255218. Epub 2007/01/27. eng.

252. de Ledinghen V, Vergniol J, Foucher J, El-Hajbi F, Merrouche W, Rigalleau V. Feasibility of liver transient elastography with FibroScan using a new probe for obese patients. Liver Int. 2010;30(7):1043–8. PubMed PMID: 20492500. Epub 2010/05/25. eng.

253. Younossi ZM, Baranova A, Ziegler K, Del Giacco L, Schlauch K, Born TL, et al. A genomic and proteomic study of the spectrum of nonalcoholic fatty liver disease. Hepatology. 2005;42(3):665–74. PubMed PMID: 16116632. Epub 2005/08/24. eng.

254. Trak-Smayra V, Dargere D, Noun R, Albuquerque M, Yaghi C, Gannage-Yared MH, et al. Serum proteomic profiling of obese patients: correlation with liver pathology and evolution after bariatric surgery. Gut. 2009;58(6):825–32. PubMed PMID: 18403495. Epub 2008/04/12. eng.

255. Charlton M, Viker K, Krishnan A, Sanderson S, Veldt B, Kaalsbeek AJ, et al. Differential expression of lumican and fatty acid binding protein-1: new insights into the histologic spectrum of nonalcoholic fatty liver disease. Hepatology. 2009;49(4):1375–84. PubMed PMID: 19330863. Pubmed Central PMCID: 2674237. Epub 2009/03/31. eng.

256. Bieback K, Kern S, Kluter H, Eichler H. Critical parameters for the isolation of mesenchymal stem cells from umbilical cord blood. Stem Cells. 2004;22(4):625–34. PubMed PMID: 15277708. Epub 2004/07/28. eng.

257. Blomme B, Francque S, Trepo E, Libbrecht L, Vanderschaeghe D, Verrijken A, et al. N-glycan based biomarker distinguishing non-alcoholic steatohepatitis from steatosis independently of fibrosis. Dig Liver Dis. 2012;44(4):315–22. PubMed PMID: 22119618.

258. Blomme B, Fitzpatrick E, Quaglia A, De Bruyne R, Dhawan A, Van Vlierberghe H. Serum protein N-glycosylation in paediatric non-alcoholic fatty liver disease. Pediatr Obesity. 2012;7(2):165–73. PubMed PMID: 22434757.

Ruth De Bruyne and Pauline De Bruyne

Portal Vein Anomalies

The portal vein (PV), originating at the union of the splenic vein (SV) and superior mesenteric vein (SMV), drains the blood from the gastrointestinal tract, the spleen, pancreas, and biliary apparatus [1]. Between the 4th and 10th week of embryonic life, the PV develops from an anastomotic network formed by the vitelline veins around the duodenum [1, 2]. Congenital anomalies of the PV are rare and can often be explained by persistence of portions of the vitelline veins [3].

Congenital Anomalies of the Portal Vein

The most common congenital anomaly of the PV is a *preduodenal portal vein (PDPV)* [3] in which the PV passes anteriorly to the duodenum rather than posteriorly [3–6]. The embryogenesis of this anomaly, described by Gray and Skandalakis [7], consists of the persistence of a preduodenal vitelline communicating vein [8, 9]. Although PDPV can occur as an isolated defect, it is typically associated with other congenital anomalies, including heterotaxia or polysplenia syndrome, situs inversus, cardiac defects, malrotation, biliary or duodenal atresia, and annular pancreas [4, 6, 10]. Clinically, PDPV can cause a duodenal obstruction by itself or in combination with the typically coexisting anomalies. Approximately, 50 % of patients remain asymptomatic, with PDPV being a radiologic or peroperative incidental finding [4, 6].

Congenital PV atresia or hypoplasia may involve the whole extent of the vein or may be localized to the portion just proximal to its division into its two main branches in the porta hepatis. The foetal umbilical vein and ductus venosus which empty into the left PV undergo a spontaneous obliterative process at birth. If this obliterative process proves to be excessive, the involvement of the PV may lead to PV atresia or stenosis [11]. Hypoplasia of the PV often occurs in patients with biliary atresia [12, 13]. Children with small or hypoplastic PV represent a challenge for liver transplantation with higher complication rates (thrombosis, stenosis, liver graft ischemia, and dysfunction) [13].

The PV is the most common site of visceral venous aneurysms [14, 15]. Nevertheless, *PV aneurysms* (PVAs) are rare, representing fewer than 3 % of all venous aneurysms [14, 16, 17]. The major location of PVA is the main extrahepatic PV at the confluence of the SV–SMV [16, 17]. Some PVAs are thought to be congenital. It has been proposed that incomplete regression of the distal right primitive vitelline vein leads to a vascular diverticulum that ultimately develops into an aneurysm [14, 16, 17]. Portal hypertension, related to chronic liver disease, is the most common acquired etiology of PVA [14, 15, 17, 18]. Other causes are inflammatory processes such as pancreatitis, trauma, and invasive malignancy [15]. The most common clinical presentation is nonspecific abdominal pain, followed by incidental finding and gastrointestinal bleeding [17, 19]. Complications of PVA include thrombosis, biliary tract obstruction, inferior caval vein obstruction, and duodenal compression [14, 17, 18].

Anomalous pulmonary venous return is a congenital cardiac malformation in which the pulmonary veins fail to connect with the left atrium during cardiac development [20, 21]. In the infradiaphragmatic type of this anomaly, the pulmonary veins drain through a large channel into the portal venous system or the ductus venosus [21, 22]. This anomaly is frequently seen in association with complex cardiac anomalies, especially with right atrial isomerism syndrome [20]. Clinical symptoms of a total anomalous pulmonary venous drainage develop early (within 24–36 h of life) and include respiratory distress with cyanosis, tachypnea, and tachycardia. Liver enlargement is common [21].

R. De Bruyne (✉)
Department of Pediatric Gastroenterology, Hepatology and Nutrition, Ghent University Hospital, De Pintelaan 185, Ghent 9000, Belgium
e-mail: ruth.debruyne@ugent.be

P. De Bruyne
Department of Pediatrics, Ghent University Hospital, Ghent, Belgium

© Springer International Publishing Switzerland 2016
S. Guandalini et al. (eds.), *Textbook of Pediatric Gastroenterology, Hepatology and Nutrition*,
DOI 10.1007/978-3-319-17169-2_67

Abnormal connections between the portal and hepatic veins (portosystemic shunts) and between the hepatic artery with the PV (arterioportal shunts) are discussed in the "Hepatic Vascular Shunts" section.

Extrahepatic Portal Vein Obstruction

Definition and Etiology

Extrahepatic PV obstruction (EHPVO) is a major cause of portal hypertension in children and adolescents [23–29]. In EHPVO, the portal inflow is impeded by congenital or postnatal obstruction of the PV [30, 31]. This results in cavernomatous replacement of the PV [16, 31], which consists of formation of venous channels within and around a previously stenosed or occluded PV that act as portoportal collateral vessels. The cavernoma is composed of dilated biliary (cystic and pericholecystic veins) and gastric branches (left and right gastric veins) of the PV and the partially recanalized thrombus. These collaterals are usually insufficient to bypass the entire splenomesenteric inflow resulting in signs of prehepatic portal hypertension [16].

Thrombosis of the PV is usually associated with the presence of a hypercoagulable state, vascular injury, or stasis [3]. Prothrombotic conditions should be excluded in children presenting with an EHPVO. Few studies have evaluated the prevalence of thrombophilic disorders in children and adolescents with portal vein thrombosis (PVT). Genetic abnormalities affecting the physiologic anticoagulant system, such as hereditary deficiency of protein C (PC), protein S (PS), and antithrombin (AT) as well as factor V Leiden (FVL), methylenetetrahydrofolate reductase (MTHFR) C677T and prothrombin (PTHR) G20210A mutations have been well established as risk factors of venous thrombosis in adults and should be excluded in children and adolescents with PVT [24, 28, 30, 32].

Direct damage to the PV in about 25 % of cases can be inferred with a history of umbilical vein catheterization during the neonatal period [27]. Umbilical venous catheters may cause thrombosis by damage to vessel walls, disruption of blood flow, damage to endothelial cells by the infusion of substances such as total parenteral nutrition, and thrombogenic catheter material [29, 30, 33]. Portal hypertension appears to be rather uncommon following neonatal PVT. This may in part be due to the predominant left PV involvement. Liver lobe atrophy is more common than portal hypertension following neonatal PVT [29, 30].

Clinical Presentation

Acute PV thrombosis can be assumed when patients present with symptoms such as abdominal pain, ascites, or fever in the absence of portal cavernoma and portosystemic collaterals. Patients also can be asymptomatic [32]. Most children with *chronic EHPVO* develop hypersplenism that triggers a more detailed medical assessment. One third to one half of the children present with acute upper gastrointestinal bleeding with no prior history of gastrointestinal disorders or symptoms of hypersplenism. Morbidity is mainly related to variceal bleeding, hypersplenism, portal biliopathy [34], limitations of quality of life (e.g. limited ability to participate in sports owing to extreme thrombocytopenia and/or splenomegaly), growth retardation, neurocognitive impairment, portopulmonary hypertension, and hepatopulmonary syndrome [32, 35, 36].

Diagnosis

EHPVO is diagnosed by Doppler ultrasound (US), computed tomography (CT), or magnetic resonance (MR) angiography [27, 32] which demonstrate PV obstruction, presence of intraluminal material, or PV cavernoma (Fig. 67.1). CT or MRI , in addition, allow to evaluate the patency of the other abdominal veins facilitating planning for potential future in-

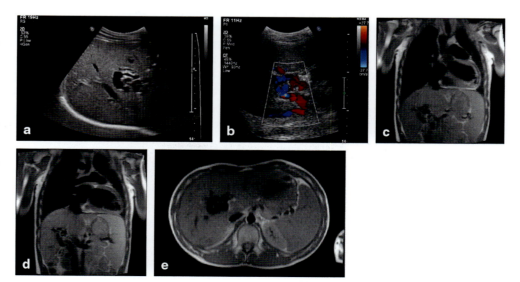

Fig. 67.1 Ultrasonography (**a**) and colour Doppler (**b**) showing cavernomatous transformation of the portal vein in a 14-year-old boy with portal vein thrombosis. Liver MRI illustrating coronal (**c**), (**d**) and axial (**e**) T_2-weighted HASTE images in the same patient. *HASTE* half-Fourier single-shot turbo spin echo (Courtesy of Prof. Dr. Voet, Department of Ultrasonography, and Dr. N. Herregods, Department of Radiology, Ghent University Hospital, Belgium)

tervention. When uncertainty persists regarding the patency of the intrahepatic PV, transjugular retrograde or percutaneous transhepatic portal venography should be undertaken in case meso-Rex bypass is considered. Further diagnostic work up consists of full hypercoagulability panel, liver biopsy in case of suspicion of intrinsic liver disease, and echocardiography to rule out congenital heart disease and to look for evidence of associated hepatopulmonary syndrome or portopulmonary hypertension [32].

Management

Anticoagulation therapy can be considered for patients with a well-documented prothrombotic condition. In patients with idiopathic chronic EHPVO, there is no role for anticoagulant therapy. Insufficient evidence exists in favour of interventional therapy such as local thrombolysis [32].

For the management of portal hypertension caused by EHPVO refer to Chap. 68 "Portal Hypertension in Children".

Hepatic Artery Anomalies

Ischaemic Cholangiopathy

Ischaemic cholangiopathy has been defined as focal or extensive damage to bile ducts due to impaired blood supply [37]. Unlike the hepatic parenchyma which has a dual blood supply from the hepatic artery and PV, the biliary system depends only on the arterial blood supply [3, 37]. Ischaemic bile duct injury may occur when small hepatic arteries or the peribiliary plexus are injured, or when all possible arterial blood supply is interrupted as in the case of hepatic artery thrombosis after liver transplantation [37]. Conditions associated with ischaemic cholangiopathy are iatrogenic factors (hepatic arterial chemotherapy [38, 39], abdominal radiation [40], liver transplantation [41]) and systemic diseases (panarteritis nodosa [42, 43], paroxysmal nocturnal haemoglobinuria [44]). In the acute stage, patients can present with pain, fever, and jaundice, with or without bacterial cholangitis. In the further course, localized or diffuse bile duct stenosis can occur with variable presentation going from no clinical signs to progressive or fluctuating jaundice, itching, fatigue, or bacterial cholangitis and eventual development of portal hypertension [37].

Pseudoaneurysm of the Hepatic Artery

Hepatic artery pseudoaneurysm (HAP) accounts for 12–20 % of all visceral aneurysms [45, 46]. HAPs can be found incidentally, but rupture of the aneurysm can be the first clinical manifestation with abdominal pain, gastrointestinal haemorrhage, or haemobilia [47]. Although HAPs can resolve

spontaneously by thrombosis, the reported risk of rupture ranges from 14 to 80 % [45, 48]. Hence, once the diagnosis is confirmed, the aneurysm should be treated regardless of the symptoms. This is done by direct percutaneous injection with thrombin or glue, transarterial embolization or stent placement, or surgical approach [45].

Abnormalities of the Sinusoidal Blood Flow

Pericellular Fibrosis

The hepatic sinusoids comprise one of the largest-calibre vascular beds in the body. Impairment of blood flow through this vascular bed results in a major loss of physiologic function, with profound influence on homeostasis for the entire human organism [49]. The most common cause of sinusoidal blood flow obstruction is cirrhosis leading to a decrease in sinusoidal fenestrations, deposition of subendothelial basement membrane and collagen, loss of hepatocellular microvilli, increased expression of endothelial factor VIII and binding of ulex europaeus agglutinin (UEA)-1 lectin to endothelial cells [50, 51]. Pericellular fibrosis is commonly seen in alcoholic liver disease, chronic passive congestion, nonalcoholic fatty liver disease, Gaucher's disease, congenital syphilis, and vitamin A toxicity [3].

Physical Occlusion of the Sinusoids

In sickle cell disease, sinusoids can become packed with sickled red cells and erythrophagocytes leading to parenchymal necrosis [52]. In disseminated intravascular coagulation and eclampsia, fibrin deposits may occlude the sinusoids. When these lesions are severe, widespread infarction might occur. Furthermore, the sinusoids might become infiltrated by mast cells in mastocytosis, Gaucher's cells, metastatic tumour cells, and leukaemia or lymphoma cells [3].

Peliosis Hepatis

Peliosis hepatis is a rare condition in which the sinusoidal dilatation is primary [53]. The liver contains blood-filled cystic spaces, either non-lined or lined with sinusoidal endothelial cells [54]. The pathogenesis of peliosis hepatis is unknown [49]. In adults, peliosis hepatis can be induced by anabolic steroids, azathioprine, oral contraceptives, 6-thioguanine and 6-mercaptopurine, or presents in the context of chronic underlying disorders such as malnutrition [55], leukaemia [56], tuberculosis [57], vasculitis [58], cystic fibrosis, or human immunodeficiency virus (HIV) infection [59]. Peliotic lesions found in acquired immunodeficiency syndrome (AIDS) and other immunosuppressed patients are caused by bacterial organisms (Bartonella species) [56, 60]. In children, peliosis hepatis also occurs most frequently in association with chronic underlying conditions such as cystic fibrosis [61], malnutrition [62], Fanconi anaemia [63], adrenal tumours [64], Marfan syndrome [65], congenital cardiopathy [66], myotubular myopathy [67], or renal transplantation [68]. Four pediatric cases have been published without underlying systemic disorder. In these cases, there seemed to be an association with *Escherichia coli* infection suggesting a direct role of *E. coli* toxins in causing endothelial damage [69–71]. The definitive diagnosis of peliosis hepatis is based on histological findings but should be suspected when ultrasonography reveals hypoechogenic areas involving the whole liver in association with intraperitoneal fluid and normal Doppler signals [70].

Hepatic Vein Anomalies

Budd–Chiari Syndrome (BCS)

BCS is defined as hepatic venous outflow obstruction at any level from the small hepatic veins to the junction of the inferior vena cava and the right atrium, regardless of the cause of obstruction. Outflow obstruction caused by hepatic veno-occlusive disease and cardiac disorders is excluded from this definition. BCS can be classified as primary due to an endoluminal venous lesion (thrombosis or webs) or secondary due to intraluminal invasion by a parasite or malignant tumour or extraluminal compression by an abscess, cyst, or solid tumour [72]. In primary BCS, an underlying prothrombotic disorder or established risk factor for venous thrombosis is often present. In adults, myeloproliferative diseases account for half of the cases of BCS [73, 74]. Table 67.1 gives an overview of predisposing conditions for BCS. The role of

Table 67.1 Predisposing conditions for Budd–Chiari syndrome

Inherited conditions
Factor V Leiden mutation
G20210A prothrombin gene mutations
Hyperhomocysteinaemia
Primary protein C or protein S deficiency
Antithrombin deficiency
Acquired conditions
Myeloproliferative disorders (V617 JAK2 positive)
Antiphospholipid syndrome
Behcet's disease
Paroxysmal nocturnal haemoglobinuria
Environmental factors
Oral contraceptive use
Toxins like heavy metals, aflatoxins, etc.

JAK2 Janus kinase 2

hyperhomocysteinaemia and primary protein C, protein S, or antithrombin deficiency is unclear because liver disease obscures recognition of these disorders [75]. BCS is uncommon with an estimated incidence of 1 in 2.5 million persons per year [76]. It is very rare in children and has a wide variety of predisposing causes. Young children (<10 years of age) account for 1–7 % of all cases of BCS [77], whereas in endemic areas, children younger than 10 years may compose 16 % of the total cases [78]. Hepatic venous outflow tract obstruction leads to increased sinusoidal pressure, sinusoidal congestion, hepatomegaly, hepatic pain, portal hypertension, and ascites. Elevated sinusoidal pressure leads to perisinusoidal necrosis of hepatocytes in the centrilobular region and eventually to irreversible liver damage, cirrhosis, or liver failure [79].

A diagnosis of BCS should be considered in any patient who presents with acute or chronic liver disease as the clinical manifestations can be extremely diverse. The majority of patients present with the typical triad described by George Budd in 1845: right upper quadrant pain, hepatomegaly, and ascites. Oedema of the lower extremities is also a common finding [72]. Asymptomatic BCS accounts for 15–20 % of cases [80]. Jaundice, gastrointestinal bleeding, and hepatic encephalopathy are less common [75]. The diagnosis of BCS is established upon demonstration of obstruction of the hepatic venous outflow tract. US combined with Doppler imaging has a diagnostic sensitivity of more than 75 % and should be the first line of investigation [81, 82]. Hepatic veins devoid of flow signal, collateral hepatic venous circulation, a spider web appearance usually located in the vicinity of the hepatic vein ostia and stagnant, reversed, or turbulent flow can all be indicative of BCS [83, 84]. When adequate ultrasonography is technically difficult or when diagnostic features cannot be demonstrated, CT or MRI should be performed. The latter is preferred in children due to absence of radiation exposure. Only in a minority of cases, retrograde cannulation of the hepatic veins for X-ray venography will be ultimately necessary for diagnosis. This technique allows the assessment of the extent of venous outflow obstruction and allows for pressure measurements (Fig. 67.2). Concurrent liver biopsy can contribute in confirming the diagnosis and ruling out other causes such as veno-occlusive disease and cirrhosis of other etiologies [85]. Once the diagnosis of BCS is established, the patient should be investigated for underlying prothrombotic conditions and a haematologic work up for myeloproliferative disorder should be performed. The rarity of BCS in children often means that the disease is diagnosed in its later stages by which time irreversible pathology may be present [77].

The management of BCS in adults consists of anticoagulation, thrombolytic therapy, and angioplasty with or without stenting, transjugular intrahepatic portosystemic shunts (TIPSSs), and surgically fashioned portosystemic shunts [77, 86]. These approaches have, to variable degrees, been

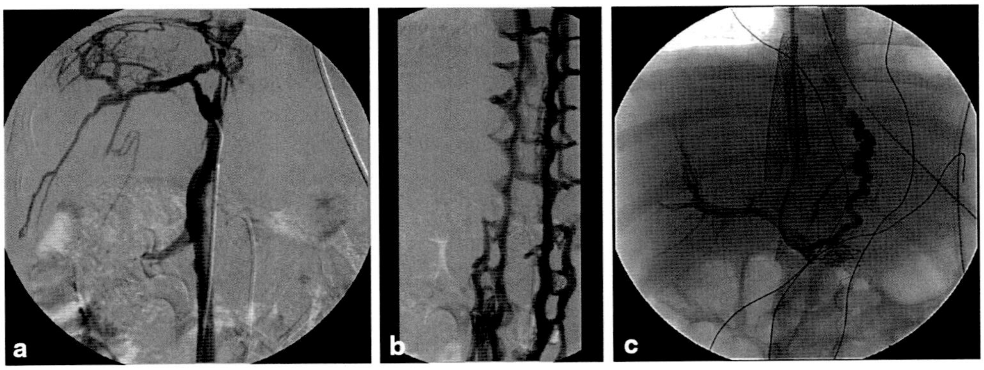

Fig. 67.2 Congenital stenosis of the inferior caval vein with Budd–Chiari syndrome in a 4-year-old child. **a** Cranial cavography with catheter tip at caudal site of inferior caval vein stenosis with visualization of collateral circulation at the level of the liver capsule. **b** Caudal cavography illustrating collateral circulation via the lumbar veins caused by the more cranially positioned stenosis. **c** Placement of stent in inferior caval vein and TIPSS with direct venography of oesophageal varices. *TIPSS* transjugular intrahepatic portosystemic stent shunting. (Courtesy of Dr. P. Van Langenhove and Prof. Defreyne, Department of Interventional Radiology, Ghent University Hospital, Belgium)

extrapolated for use in pediatric BCS. Early referral has the best possible outcome by creating the opportunity of re-establishing native hepatic venous outflow tract without surgery. Thrombolytic therapy might be successful in dissolving fresh thrombi and can be combined by transjugular balloon angioplasty. Local infusion of thrombolytic therapy in a partially recanalized vein with appreciable flow in a patient who presents earlier than 4 weeks has been associated with a consistently successful outcome in adult patients [87]. Maintenance of flow can be ensured by long-term anticoagulation and treatment of the underlying haematologic disorder if one is identified. TIPSSs have been successfully used in children with favourable long-term results [88, 89]. Percutaneous stent placement has also played a role in the management of pediatric BCS [90, 91] (Fig. 67.2). In a late presentation with established hepatic cirrhosis and complications of portal hypertension, liver transplantation is the only option that can offer an excellent chance of long-term survival. Reports on the long-term outcomes for orthotopic liver transplantation (OLT) specifically for BCS in children are scarce and limited to a few sporadic case reports [92, 93].

Table 67.2 Clinical criteria for the diagnosis of hepatic VOD during HSCT [96, 97]

Seattle criteria (modified) [97]
Presence of at least two of the following before day 20 after HSCT
Bilirubin > 35 μmol/l
Hepatomegaly or right upper quadrant pain
Ascites or unexplained weight gain of 2 % above baseline
Baltimore criteria [96]
Bilirubin > 35 μmol/l in the first 20 days after HSCT and at least two of the following:
Hepatomegaly
Ascites
Weight gain (> 5 % compared to pre-transplant)

Veno-Occlusive Disease (VOD)

VOD, also known as sinusoidal obstruction syndrome, is a severe and potentially fatal liver disease originally described in Jamaican drinkers of pyrrolizidine alkaloid-containing bush tea. It is now seen predominantly, but not exclusively, in patients undergoing haematopoietic stem cell transplantation (HSCT) [94]. The incidence of VOD after HSCT varies between 10 and 60 % in different series [95]. VOD usually presents in the first 30 days after HSCT [96, 97]. The clinical course is characterized by rapid weight gain, jaundice, abdominal pain, hepatomegaly, and ascites. Encephalopathy may develop. The most commonly used diagnostic criteria for VOD are the (modified) Seattle criteria [97] and the Baltimore criteria [96] illustrated in Table 67.2. Doppler ultrasound can further support the diagnosis by showing evidence of decreased or reversed portal venous flow. The pathogenesis of VOD is most likely due to a primary injury to the endothelial cells of sinusoids and small venules by chemotherapy and radiation. Many of the cytotoxic agents used in HSCT are metabolized in the liver, including cyclophosphamide and busulfan. It is thought that depletion of glutathione in zone 3 hepatocytes and sinusoidal cells plays an important role in the initiation of the damage [98]. A number of markers of endothelial injury and adhesion molecules are upregulated in patients with VOD. These include plasma thrombomodulin, P- and E-selectins, tissue factor pathway inhibitor, soluble tissue factor and plasminogen activator inhibitor (PAI-1). Increased serum levels of PAI-1 is both a diagnostic and prognostic marker for VOD [99–102]. Histopathologically, the early lesion is subintimal oedema and haemorrhage involving the hepatic venules with fibrin deposits. This leads to sinusoidal congestion and dilatation with (mainly centrizonal) hepatocellular necrosis. In the further course, fibrous obliteration occurs of the venular walls with atrophy of perivenular hepatocytes and development of sinusoidal fibrosis potentially leading to venocentric cirrhosis [3, 103]. Risk factors for VOD include advanced malignancy and pre-existing liver disease which might be the consequence of previous hepatotoxic chemotherapy, previous abdominal irradiation, or iron overload due to repeated blood transfusions [96, 97, 104]. Busulfan, especially in combination with cyclophosphamide increases the risk of VOD [104, 105]. Targeted dosing of busulfan and pharmacokinetic monitoring of cyclophosphamide and its metabolites could be effective in reducing the risk of VOD [106]. The risk of VOD is higher in allogeneic compared to autologous transplants, with a higher incidence in unrelated and mismatched donors versus sibling donors [96, 97, 104]. High-level evidence from randomized controlled trials supporting prophylaxis for hepatic VOD is scarce [107]. Ursodeoxycholic acid might reduce the incidence of hepatic VOD, but trial results are conflicting and did not show any survival benefit [108–111]. The same holds true for trials on low-dose heparin infusion for VOD prophylaxis [112, 113]. Furthermore, trials on enoxaparin, glutamine, and fresh frozen plasma (FFP) all failed to demonstrate efficacy on reduction of VOD or overall mortality. Supportive treatment of VOD focusses on maintaining intravascular volume and renal perfusion without increasing extravascular fluid accumulation. Avoidance of exposure to hepatotoxic drugs, fluid and sodium restriction, and diuretics are important in the care of a patient with VOD. Again, high-level evidence is lacking on treatment options. There is substantial evidence for the efficacy of defibrotide, a polydisperse mixture of single-stranded oligonucleotide with antithrombotic and fibrinolytic effects on microvascular endothelium, in the treatment of VOD [114, 115]. Defibrotide can be used safely in pediatric patients [116]. Despite emerging therapies such as defibrotide, VOD remains a much feared transplant complication with unfavourable prognosis. Therefore, risk stratification of patients before HSCT is essential to minimize severe VOD and improve transplant outcome. Improved understanding of risk factors will enable to offer high-risk patients a reduced intensity conditioning regimen or T cell depletion to minimize their risk for transplant mortality. As PAI-1 is now recognized to be associated with the pathogenesis of VOD, serial monitoring of blood PAI-1 levels could offer a new diagnostic and potential prognostic tool for this disease [117].

Congestive Cardiac Failure

Congestive cardiac failure is associated with dilatation of sinusoids and atrophy of perivenular hepatocytes which can lead to fibrosis and occasionally nodular regenerative hyperplasia (NRH) [118].

Hepatic Vascular Shunts

Arteriovenous Malformations

Arterioportal shunts may be congenital (in hereditary haemorrhagic telangiectasia) or acquired (blunt or penetrating trauma, percutaneous liver biopsy, cirrhosis) and consist of a communication between the hepatic artery and the portal venous system [3, 16, 21]. Most congenital arterioportal fistulas are symptomatic within the first year of life. Hepatofugal flow develops in the arterialized PV which can lead to portal hypertension, hypersplenism, varices, ascites, and hypertensive enteropathy resulting in malabsorption and diarrhea [21].

Hepatic arteriosystemic shunts are the rarest form of intrahepatic shunts connecting the hepatic artery (or other systemic arteries) and the hepatic veins. These shunts may be congenital or associated with hereditary haemorrhagic telangiectasia, hepatocellular carcinoma, or large haemangiomas [16]. Hepatic arteriosystemic shunts are usually localized in one lobe of the liver [21]. Arteriovenous fistulas can not only present clinically in neonates with congestive heart failure, anaemia, hepatomegaly, and portal hypertension but can also manifest later in childhood in the clinical setting of hereditary haemorrhagic telangiectasia with congestive heart failure, hepatic ischaemia, and portal hypertension [21].

Portosystemic Shunts

The complicated development of the inferior caval vein and the close relationship of its development with that of the vitelline veins may explain the occurrence of congenital portosystemic anastomoses. Portosystemic venous shunting causes elevated levels of galactose, bile acids, ammonia, and other nitrogenous substances in the plasma, some of which can affect the brain [16, 119]. The age of onset of encephalopathy is variable but related in part to the volume and duration of the shunt and the presence of concomitant liver disease [119]. Both extrahepatic and intrahepatic portosystemic shunts have been described [21, 120].

Extrahepatic portosystemic venous shunts are also known as Abernethy malformations described in 1793 [1, 121–124]. Morgan and Superina classified extrahepatic portosystemic shunts into two types [121, 124]. In type I, there is a complete diversion of the portal blood flow in the caval vein, with congenital absence of the PV. Type Ia has absent PV, with the SV and SMV entering in systemic veins separately. These patients are usually girls with cardiac or other congenital anomalies including biliary atresia, oculoauriculovertebral dysplasia, situs inversus, and polysplenia. Hepatic masses are frequent, usually described as focal

Fig. 67.3 A 5-month-old child with multiple intrahepatic portosystemic shunts. **a** Indirect mesentericography with visualization of multiple intrahepatic portosystemic shunts. **b** Direct portography in the same patient with guiding into the right hepatic vein. The child previously presented with acute haematemesis caused by a bleed from a pseudoaneurysm of the gastroduodenal artery which was coiled in a previous procedure. **c** Illustration of interconnections in the complex portosystemic shunt. **d** Direct portography after occlusion of one connection of the portosystemic shunt with vascular plug. (Courtesy of Dr. P. Van Langenhove and Prof. Defreyne, Department of Interventional Radiology, Ghent University Hospital, Belgium)

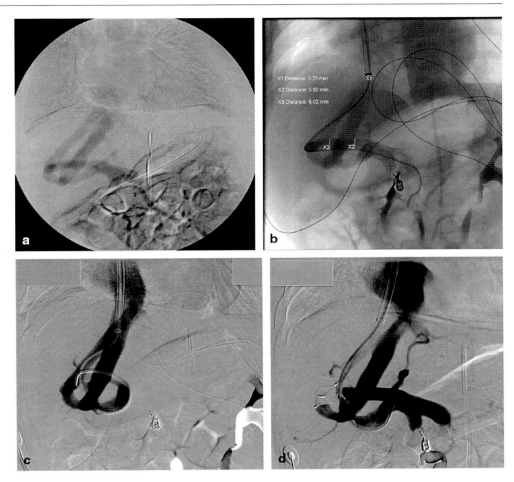

nodular hyperplasia (FNH), but sometimes hepatoblastoma, hepatocellular carcinoma, and adenoma. In type Ib, the SV and SPV join into a PV which then drains into a systemic vein. This form usually occurs in boys without the associated anomalies or hepatic masses [1, 3]. In type II, the PV is intact, but some of the portal flow is diverted into the caval vein through a side-to-side extrahepatic communication, which is congenital, usually isolated, and mostly seen in boys (type IIa) or acquired, most often induced by portal hypertension (type IIb) [21].

Congenital *intrahepatic portosystemic shunts* are abnormal intrahepatic connections between branches of the PV and the hepatic veins [3, 125] (Fig. 67.3). Intrahepatic portosystemic shunts which are acquired are most often associated with hepatic trauma or portal hypertension.

Hereditary Haemorrhagic Telangiectasia

Hereditary haemorrhagic telangiectasia (HHT) or Rendu–Osler–Weber disease is an autosomal dominant vascular disorder with variable penetrance with an estimated prevalence

around 1 in 5000–8000 [126]. HHT is characterized by mucocutaneous telangiectases, recurrent epistaxis, and visceral arteriovenous malformations. Hepatic vascular malformations have been reported in 47 % of pediatric patients with HHT ranging from small telangiectases to discrete arteriovenous malformations [127].

Parenchymal Response to Vascular Injury

Nodular Regenerative Hyperplasia (NRH)

NRH is the major cause of non-cirrhotic portal hypertension in the Western world. It is a benign condition characterized by diffuse transformation of the liver parenchyma into small regenerative nodules distributed evenly throughout the liver with minimal or no fibrosis in the perisinusoidal or periportal areas [118]. NRH results from abnormalities in the portal hepatic and occasionally small hepatic blood flow giving rise to ischaemic atrophy and a secondary adaptive hyperplastic reaction of hepatocytes in regions with favourable blood flow [128, 129]. NRH occurs predominantly in older patients and is rather uncommon in children [130]. In a large series of 716 pediatric liver tumours, NRH was demonstrated in 4.5 % of the cases [131]. NRH is seen in conditions affecting the hepatic blood flow including solid-organ transplantation, bone marrow transplantation, vasculitic conditions, and can be associated with underlying autoimmune, inflammatory, and neoplastic diseases or HIV [49]. Immunosuppressive medications such as azathioprine, 6-mercaptopurine, and 6-thioguanine may induce NRH by damaging endothelial cells of small hepatic veins [132–134]. NRH presenting with progressive portal hypertension was described in six children treated with 6-thioguanine as maintenance therapy for childhood acute lymphoblastic leukaemia [135]. Imaging findings are relatively poor in sensitivity and specificity for NRH. A diffusely heterogeneous hepatic parenchyma may be the only imaging abnormality. Regenerative nodules are usually not visible on ultrasound [129]. On CT, regenerative nodules remain isodense or hypodense in both arterial and portal venous phases, distinguishing NRH from FNH and adenomas [130]. The significance of MRI in the diagnosis of NRH is still controversial with only few reports in the literature. Lesions appear hyperintense on T_1-weighted images and iso- or hypointense on T_2-weighted images [136]. The gold standard for diagnosis is histopathology demonstrating regenerative nodules consisting of hypertrophied hepatocytes centrally surrounded by atrophic hepatocytes peripherally. There is no or minimal perisinusoidal or portal fibrosis on reticulin staining and compression of the central veins by the regenerating nodules may be seen [137, 138]. The management of NRH mainly relates to the prevention and treatment of complications of portal hypertension.

Focal Nodular Hyperplasia (FNH)

FNH is a localized hyperplastic lesion in response to locally augmented arterial blood flow. The diagnosis of FNH is rarely made in the pediatric population [139]. It most often affects females between the age of 30 and 50 years [140, 141]. Most cases are found incidentally on abdominal imaging. Large subcapsular lesions might lead to vague abdominal pain. Complications such as rupture and intratumoral haemorrhage are extremely rare. Most lesions remain stable with a likelihood to regress with age, and there is no malignant potential [139]. On imaging, FNH should be differentiated from liver cell adenoma [142] or hepatocellular carcinoma [143]. The typical ultrasound finding in FNH is a well-demarcated homogeneous hypo- or isoechoic lesion with a central scar which can be seen in less than 20 % of cases. On colour Doppler, there is a central arterial structure with a spoke-wheel pattern of radiating smaller aberrant vessels [144]. CT shows typically a well-circumscribed iso- or hypodense lesion with rapid homogeneous intense enhancement in the arterial phase and gradual enhancement of the central scar in the portal venous phase [145]. On MR, a homogeneous lesion is seen that is isointense or slightly hypointense on T_1- and isointense or slightly hyperintense on T_2- weighted images. During the arterial phase, the typical FNH lesion becomes homogeneously hyperintense apart from the central scar which often exhibits avid enhancement in the delayed phase [146] (Fig. 67.4). In the presence of typical radiological findings there is usually no indication for liver biopsy. When performed, histopathology (Fig. 67.5) shows a non-encapsulated nodule with a central stellate fibrous region containing large vessels from which there are radiating septa. The parenchyma between the septa exhibits essentially normal hepatocytes but with a thickened plate architecture characteristic of regeneration [140]. Patients with asymptomatic FNH are treated conservatively without need for further imaging if there is a typical radiological appearance of FNH. In case of symptoms, which are usually seen in large subcapsular lesions, or in case of atypical radiological features which do not allow to rule out malignancy, surgical resection can be indicated [139].

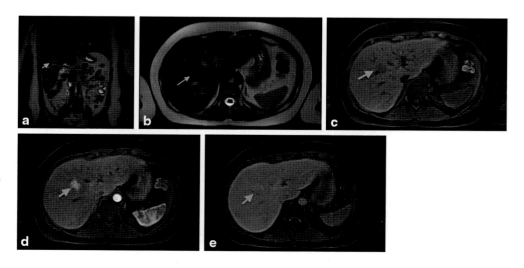

Fig. 67.4 MRI showing focal nodular hyperplasia (FNH) in a 16-year-old girl. This lesion is discretely hyperintense on T2 weighted images (**a**, **b**), hypointense on T1 weighted images (**c**), with intense early arterial phase enhancement (**d**) and isointense aspect compared to normal liver parenchyma in the portovenous phase (**e**). (Courtesy of Dr. N. Herregods, Department of Radiology, Ghent University Hospital, Belgium)

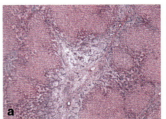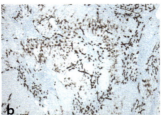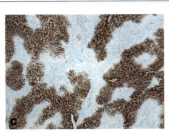

Fig. 67.5 Focal nodular hyperplasia (FNH) in 11-year-old girl. **a** H&E (40×) stained image showing fibrous scar and fibrous septa surrounding nodular hyperplastic parenchyma containing ductular reaction and multiple small arterial branches. **b** Cytokeratin 7 staining (40×) illustrating ductular reaction and cholate stasis in the lesion. **c** Typical 'map-like' pattern of FNH lesion on glutamine synthetase staining (40×). (Courtesy of Prof. L. Libbrecht, Department of Pathology, Ghent University Hospital, Belgium)

Benign and Malignant Vascular Tumors

Vascular tumours of the liver comprise a substantial portion (13%) of all hepatic neoplasms in children [147]. Most of these lesions are benign. Infantile hepatic haemangioma (HH) is the most common benign tumour of the liver in infancy [148]. The terminology used in the literature is quite confusing and infantile HH is also called infantile haemangioendothelioma. Most of these haemangiomas remain asymptomatic and probably a substantial part remains undiagnosed [149]. An increasing number of hepatic haemangiomas is being identified on antenatal ultrasound [150]. Almost all patients with HH present before 6 months of age with most being diagnosed within the first 2 months [150–153]. The main symptoms are abdominal mass or distension. Other potential presentations include failure to thrive, high-output congestive heart failure, anaemia, thrombocytopenia (Kasabach–Merritt syndrome), respiratory distress, pulmonary hypertension, liver failure, and jaundice. In rare cases, spontaneous rupture has been described. Infantile HH express type 3 iodothyronine deiodinase that converts thyroid hormone to its inactive form. This can result in acquired hypothyroidism which is often seen in larger multifocal and diffuse HH and resolves with tumour involution [154–156]. Based on data from the Liver Haemangioma Registry, a division into three principal categories has been proposed: focal, multifocal, and diffuse lesions [149, 156]. Focal lesions could be considered as the hepatic variant of the cutaneous rapidly involuting congenital haemangioma which typically evolves during foetal life and is fully grown at birth. These lesions do not expand postnatally and are less commonly associated with accompanying cutaneous infantile haemangioma [152, 157, 158]. Because they develop antenatally, focal HH can be diagnosed prenatally [159–161]. Most focal HH are discovered as an abdominal mass in an otherwise healthy child [156]. Ultrasonography reveals a well-circumscribed mass with large feeding and draining vessels. On CT or gadolinium MRI, a well-defined, solitary, spherical tumour with centripetal enhancement and central sparing because of thrombosis, necrosis, or intralesional haemorrhage can be seen [149, 150, 162] (Fig. 67.6). Multifocal and diffuse HH are considered as true infantile haemangiomas [156]. They are associated with cutaneous infantile haemangiomas in the majority of cases and characterized by the immunoexpression of glucose transporter (GLUT)-1 in liver tissue [156]. These lesions appear within the first weeks of life and are therefore not antenatally detected. The typical course in these lesions is one of rapid postnatal growth (0–12 months) followed by slow involution (1–5 years) [156]. Multiple well-defined spherical lesions are observed on CT, MRI, or ultrasound with intervening areas of normal hepatic parenchyma in multifocal HH, whereas the lesions in diffuse HH nearly totally replace the liver [156] (Fig. 67.7). Biopsy can be avoided in typical haemangioma (i.e. multifocal haemangiomas with cutaneous involvement or solitary haemangiomas, presenting in the first few months of life, with typical imaging findings) but should not be delayed in the face of diagnostic uncertainty or when children present with vascular tumours after infancy [150, 156]. Two histological subtypes have been described (Fig. 67.8). Type 1 HH are composed of capillary, sinusoidal and cavernous parts lined by plump endothelial cells with a bland cytological appearance [163]. Type 2 HH have areas composed of papillate tufting vascular channels that are lined by larger pleomorphic and hyperchromatic endothelial cells which exhibit more extensive cell proliferation and active mitosis [147]. The treatment of HH is controversial and the effects of the various forms of therapy are diverse and inconclusive [164]. Asymptomatic HH should be observed. Imaging studies of the brain and chest radiography are appropriate for patients with multifocal and diffuse HH [150] and thyroid function should be checked. In case of symptoms, medical treatment is indicated. Corticosteroids are most frequently used as pharmacological therapy. Early evidence suggests that propranolol, a nonselective β-blocker, may be as efficacious as corticosteroids in the treatment of infantile HH [165, 166]. Other pharmacological treatments which have also been reported to be effective are α-interferon therapy, chemotherapeutic agents, such as vincristine [167, 168], actinomycin D, and cyclophosphamide [169]. When there is no response

Fig. 67.6 MRI findings in a 2-week-old infant with infantile hepatic haemangioma. Large, relatively well-demarcated exophytic mass in *right* lobe of the liver (81 × 49 × 87 mm). There is heterogeneous hyperintensity on T_2-weighted images with prominent flowvoids (**a, b**). On non contrast-enhanced T_1-weighted images, the spontaneous hyperintense zones in the lesion are compatible with haemorrhagic components (**c**). After intravenous contrast administration there is peripheral nodular enhancement of the lesion in the arterial phase (**d**) with progressive, centripetal filling in the portovenous phase (**e**). (Courtesy of Dr. N. Herregods, Department of Radiology, Ghent University Hospital, Belgium)

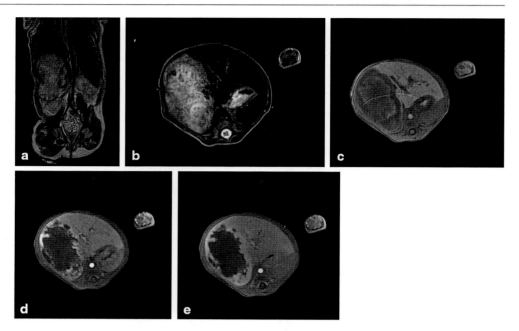

Fig. 67.7 MRI of multifocal infantile hepatic haemangioma in a 3-month-old boy. Multiple well-defined T_2-hyperintense (**a, b**), T_1-hypointense (**c**) nodular lesions spread throughout the liver. After intravenous contrast administration there is nodular enhancement in the arterial phase (**d**) with nearly isointense aspect of the lesions in the portovenous phase compared to unaffected liver (**e**). US findings in the same child (**f**). (Courtesy of Dr. N. Herregods, Department of Radiology, Ghent University Hospital, Belgium)

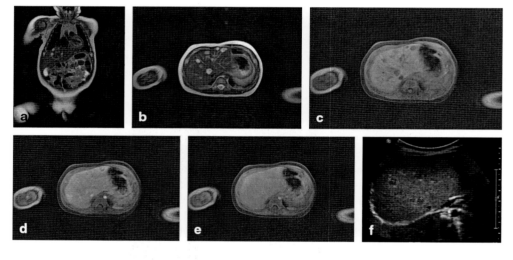

to pharmacological treatment, arterial embolization, hepatic artery ligation, or surgical resection should be considered. Hepatic transplantation may be indicated in extremis when other treatment options are impossible or fail [156]. Infantile hepatic haemangiomas differ from *cavernous haemangiomas* which are usually asymptomatic in children. Being devoid of malignant potential, they are usually discovered as an incidental finding during abdominal imaging, most frequently between the fourth and the fifth decades of life. They are multiple in more than 50 % of cases and show a clear female predominance. Pathological examination reveals a focal tender mass formed by multiple vascular channels limited by a single layer of endothelial cells with thin fibrous stroma. In general, the blood circulation within these tumour vessels is slow. Morphologically, it is a well-defined lesion,

possessing round or lobulated margins. There size usually remains stable and can vary from a few millimetres to more than 20 cm [143] (Fig. 67.9). *Pediatric angiosarcoma,* in contrast to HH, is a very rare but highly malignant tumour. It usually presents with a rapidly growing hepatic mass. The precise diagnosis may be difficult, even on a biopsy specimen [170]. Open biopsy of the tumour is therefore advisable. Most angiosarcomas develop after the first year of life. Chemotherapy and radiotherapy are notably inefficient in achieving tumour control, and the prognosis remains very poor. Radical resection or even liver transplantation should therefore be attempted if possible. *Hepatic haemangioendothelioma* is a rare neoplasm of endothelial origin having a clinical behaviour intermediate between haemangioma and angiosarcoma [171, 172]. Patients generally present from the

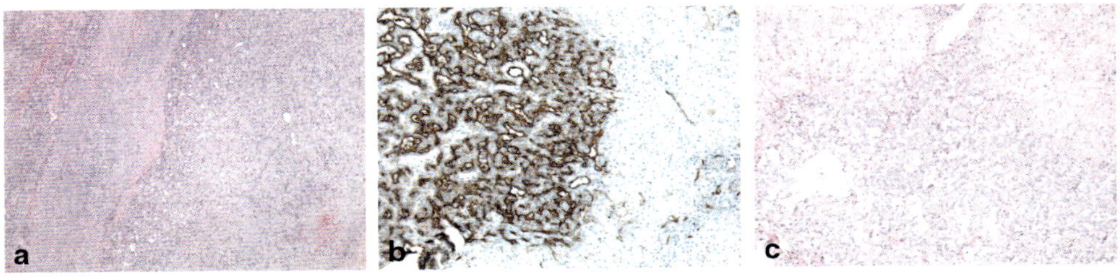

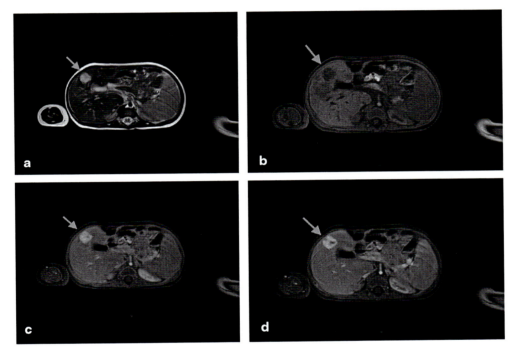

Fig. 67.8 Infantile hepatic haemangioma in s 6-month-old girl (**a, b**) and a 2-month-old boy (**c**). **a** H&E (100 ×) and **b** CD 34 (100 ×) staining showing fragment of subcapsular liver parenchyma containing a focal, clearly demarcated vascular lesion consisting of multiple, small capillary to slit-like vessels composed of a single layer of endothelial cells with plump nuclei. **c** H&E (40 ×) IHH lesion containing capillary-like structures with plump endothelial cells. Towards the centre of the lesion, there is increasing cell paucity with haemorrhagic and myxoid stroma. (Courtesy of Prof. L. Libbrecht, Department of Pathology, Ghent University Hospital, Belgium)

Fig. 67.9 MRI findings in a 4-month-old girl with cavernous haemangioma in. Well-demarcated T_2 hyperintense (**a**) and T_1 hypointense (**b**) lesion (1.6 × 1.4 cm) in segment 4 with rapid, intense centripetal enhancement in the early phase after contrast injection (**c**) and progressive enhancement and fill-in in portovenous phase (VIBE contrast enhanced images) (**d**). *VIBE* volumetric imaging breath-hold examination (Courtesy of Dr. N. Herregods, Department of Radiology, Ghent University Hospital, Belgium)

second decade, and the tumour commonly affects liver, lung, skin, or bone but also other presentations are reported [173].

References

1. Alvarez AE, Ribeiro AF, Hessel G, Baracat J, Ribeiro JD. Abernethy malformation: one of the etiologies of hepatopulmonary syndrome. Pediatr Pulm. 2002;34(5):391–4.
2. Moore K, Persaud TVN. The developing human; clinically oriented embryology. 6th ed.; Philadelphia: Saunders Elsevier; 1998.
3. Wanless LR. Vascular disorders. In: Mac Sween RNM, Burt AD, Portmann BC, Ishak KG, Scheuer PJ, Anthony PP, editors. Pathology of the liver. 4th ed. Edinburgh: Churchill Livingstone; 2002. p. 539–73.
4. Kim SH, Cho YH, Kim HY. Preduodenal portal vein: a 3-case series demonstrating varied presentations in infants. J Korean Surg Soc. 2013;85(4):195–7.
5. Ooshima I, Maruyama T, Ootsuki K, Ozaki M. Preduodenal portal vein in the adult. J Hepatobiliary Pancreat Surg. 1998;5(4):455–8.
6. Singal AK, Ramu C, Paul S, Matthai J. Preduodenal portal vein in association with midgut malrotation and duodenal web-triple anomaly? J Pediatr Surg. 2009;44(2):e5–7.
7. Gray SW, Skandalakis JH. Embyology for surgeons. The embyological basis for the treatment of congenital defects. Philadelphia: Saunders; 1972. p. 177–8.
8. Walsh G, Williams MP. Congenital anomalies of the portal venous system—CT appearances with embryological considerations. Clin Radiol. 1995;50(3):174–6.
9. Fernandes ET, Burton EM, Hixson SD, Hollabaugh RS. Preduodenal portal vein: surgery and radiographic appearance. J Pediatr Surg. 1990;25(12):1270–2.
10. Baglaj M, Gerus S. Preduodenal portal vein, malrotation, and high jejunal atresia: a case report. J Pediatr Surg. 2012;47(1):e27–30.
11. Marks C. Developmental basis of the portal venous system. Am J Surg. 1969;117(5):671–81.
12. Hwang S, Kim DY, Ahn CS, Moon DB, Kim KM, Park GC, et al. Computational simulation-based vessel interposition reconstruction technique for portal vein hypoplasia in pediatric liver transplantation. Transplant Proc. 2013;45(1):255–8.

13. Mitchell A, John PR, Mayer DA, Mirza DF, Buckels JA, De Ville De Goyet J. Improved technique of portal vein reconstruction in pediatric liver transplant recipients with portal vein hypoplasia. Transplantation. 2002;73(8):1244–7.

14. Turner KC, Bohannon WT, Atkins MD. Portal vein aneurysm: a rare occurrence. J Vasc Nurs. 2011;29(4):135–8.

15. Schwope RB, Margolis DJ, Raman SS, Kadell BM. Portal vein aneurysms: a case series with literature review. J Radiol Case Rep. 2010;4(6):28–38.

16. Gallego C, Velasco M, Marcuello P, Tejedor D, De Campo L, Friera A. Congenital and acquired anomalies of the portal venous system. Radiographics. 2002;22(1):141–59.

17. Ma R, Balakrishnan A, See TC, Liau SS, Praseedom R, Jah A. Extra-hepatic portal vein aneurysm: a case report, overview of the literature and suggested management algorithm. Int J Surg Case Rep. 2012;3(11):555–8.

18. Sfyroeras GS, Antoniou GA, Drakou AA, Karathanos C, Giannoukas AD. Visceral venous aneurysms: clinical presentation, natural history and their management: a systematic review. Eur J Vasc Endovasc Surg. 2009;38(4):498–505.

19. Qi X, Yin Z, He C, Guo W, Han G, Fan D. Extrahepatic portal vein aneurysm. Clin Res Hepatol Gastroenterol. 2013;37(1):1–2.

20. Koplay M, Paksoy Y, Erol C, Arslan D, Kivrak AS, Karaaslan S. Cardiovascular MR imaging findings of total anomalous pulmonary venous connection to the portal vein in a patient with right atrial isomerism. Wiener klinische Wochenschr. 2012;124(23–24):848–50.

21. Gallego C, Miralles M, Marin C, Muyor P, Gonzalez G, Garcia-Hidalgo E. Congenital hepatic shunts. Radiographics. 2004;24(3):755–72.

22. Chowdhury UK, Airan B, Malhotra A, Bisoi AK, Saxena A, Kothari SS, et al. Mixed total anomalous pulmonary venous connection: anatomic variations, surgical approach, techniques, and results. J Thoracic Cardiovasc Surg. 2008;135(1):106–16, e1–5.

23. Garcia-Pagan JC, Hernandez-Guerra M, Bosch J. Extrahepatic portal vein thrombosis. Semin Liv Dis. 2008;28(3):282–92.

24. Pinto RB, Silveira TR, Bandinelli E, Rohsig L. Portal vein thrombosis in children and adolescents: the low prevalence of hereditary thrombophilic disorders. J Pediatr Surg. 2004;39(9):1356–61.

25. Gauthier-Villars M, Franchi S, Gauthier F, Fabre M, Pariente D, Bernard O. Cholestasis in children with portal vein obstruction. J Pediatr. 2005;146(4):568–73.

26. Dubuisson C, Boyer-Neumann C, Wolf M, Meyer D, Bernard O. Protein C, protein S and antithrombin III in children with portal vein obstruction. J Hepatol. 1997;27(1):132–5.

27. de Ville de Goyet J, D'Ambrosio G, Grimaldi C. Surgical management of portal hypertension in children. Semin Pediatr Surg. 2012;21(3):219–32.

28. Weiss B, Shteyer E, Vivante A, Berkowitz D, Reif S, Weizman Z, et al. Etiology and long-term outcome of extrahepatic portal vein obstruction in children. World J Gastroenterol. 2010;16(39):4968–72.

29. Morag I, Epelman M, Daneman A, Moineddin R, Parvez B, Shechter T, et al. Portal vein thrombosis in the neonate: risk factors, course, and outcome. J Pediatr. 2006;148(6):735–9.

30. Williams S, Chan AK. Neonatal portal vein thrombosis: diagnosis and management. Semin Fetal Neonatal Med. 2011;16(6):329–39.

31. Guerin F, Bidault V, Gonzales E, Franchi-Abella S, De Lambert G, Branchereau S. Meso-Rex bypass for extrahepatic portal vein obstruction in children. Br J Surg. 2013;100(12):1606–13.

32. Shneider BL, Bosch J, de Franchis R, Emre SH, Groszmann RJ, Ling SC, et al. Portal hypertension in children: expert pediatric opinion on the report of the Baveno v consensus workshop on methodology of diagnosis and therapy in portal hypertension. Pediatr Transplant. 2012;16(5):426–37.

33. Abd El-Hamid N, Taylor RM, Marinello D, Mufti GJ, Patel R, Mieli-Vergani G, et al. Aetiology and management of extrahepatic portal vein obstruction in children: King's College Hospital experience. J Pediatr Gastroenterol Nutr. 2008;47(5):630–4.

34. Khuroo MS, Yattoo GN, Zargar SA, Javid G, Dar MY, Khan BA, et al. Biliary abnormalities associated with extrahepatic portal venous obstruction. Hepatology. 1993;17(5):807–13.

35. Noli K, Solomon M, Golding F, Charron M, Ling SC. Prevalence of hepatopulmonary syndrome in children. Pediatrics. 2008;121(3):e522–7.

36. Abrams GA, Jaffe CC, Hoffer PB, Binder HJ, Fallon MB. Diagnostic utility of contrast echocardiography and lung perfusion scan in patients with hepatopulmonary syndrome. Gastroenterology. 1995;109(4):1283–8.

37. Deltenre P, Valla DC. Ischemic cholangiopathy. Semin Liver Dis. 2008;28(3):235–46.

38. Batts KP. Ischemic cholangitis. Mayo Clin Proc. 1998;73(4):380–5.

39. Ludwig J, Kim CH, Wiesner RH, Krom RA. Floxuridine-induced sclerosing cholangitis: an ischemic cholangiopathy? Hepatology. 1989;9(2):215–8.

40. Cherqui D, Palazzo L, Piedbois P, Charlotte F, Duvoux C, Duron JJ, et al. Common bile duct stricture as a late complication of upper abdominal radiotherapy. J Hepatol. 1994;20(6):693–7.

41. Sanchez-Urdazpal L, Gores GJ, Ward EM, Maus TP, Buckel EG, Steers JL, et al. Diagnostic features and clinical outcome of ischemic-type biliary complications after liver transplantation. Hepatology. 1993;17(4):605–9.

42. Parangi S, Oz MC, Blume RS, Bixon R, Laffey KJ, Perzin KH, et al. Hepatobiliary complications of polyarteritis nodosa. Arch Surg. 1991;126(7):909–12.

43. Haratake J, Horie A, Furuta A, Yamato H. Massive hepatic infarction associated with polyarteritis nodosa. Acta Pathol Jpn. 1988;38(1):89–93.

44. Le Thi Huong D, Valla D, Franco D, Wechsler B, De Gramont A, Auperin A, et al. Cholangitis associated with paroxysmal nocturnal hemoglobinuria: another instance of ischemic cholangiopathy? Gastroenterology. 1995;109(4):1338–43.

45. Lu PH, Zhang XC, Wang LF, Chen ZL, Shi HB. Stent graft in the treatment of pseudoaneurysms of the hepatic arteries. Vasc Endovasc Surg. 2013;47(7):551–4.

46. Abbas MA, Fowl RJ, Stone WM, Panneton JM, Oldenburg WA, Bower TC, et al. Hepatic artery aneurysm: factors that predict complications. J Vasc Surg. 2003;38(1):41–5.

47. Reiter DA, Fischman AM, Shy BD. Hepatic artery pseudoaneurysm rupture: a case report and review of the literature. J Emerg Med. 2013;44(1):100–3.

48. Baggio E, Migliara B, Lipari G, Landoni L. Treatment of six hepatic artery aneurysms. Ann Vasc Surg. 2004;18(1):93–9.

49. Crawford JM. Vascular disorders of the liver. Clin Liver Dis. 2010;14(4):635–50.

50. Tsui MS, Burroughs A, McCormick PA, Scheuer PJ. Portal hypertension and hepatic sinusoidal Ulex lectin binding. J Hepatol. 1990;10(2):244–50.

51. Taguchi K, Asano G. Neovascularization of pericellular fibrosis in alcoholic liver disease. Acta Pathol Jpn. 1988;38(5):615–26.

52. Mills LR, Mwakyusa D, Milner PF. Histopathologic features of liver biopsy specimens in sickle cell disease. Arch Pathol Lab Med. 1988;112(3):290–4.

53. DeLeve LD. Hepatic microvasculature in liver injury. Semin Liver Dis. 2007;27(4):390–400.

54. Tsokos M, Erbersdobler A. Pathology of peliosis. Forensic Sci Int. 2005;149(1):25–33.

55. Simon DM, Krause R, Galambos JT. Peliosis hepatis in a patient with marasmus. Gastroenterology. 1988;95(3):805–9.

56. Ahsan N, Holman MJ, Riley TR, Abendroth CS, Langhoff EG, Yang HC. Peloisis hepatis due to *Bartonella henselae* in transplantation: a hemato-hepato-renal syndrome. Transplantation. 1998;65(7):1000–3.

57. Zak FG. Peliosis hepatis. Am J Pathol. 1950;26(1):1–15 (incl 2 pl).

58. Delas N, Faurel JP, Wechsler B, Adotti F, Leroy O, Lemerez M. Association of peliosis and necrotizing vasculitis. Nouv Presse Med. 1982;11(37):2787.

59. Scoazec JY, Marche C, Girard PM, Houtmann J, Durand-Schneider AM, Saimot AG, et al. Peliosis hepatis and sinusoidal dilation during infection by the human immunodeficiency virus (HIV). An ultrastructural study. Am J Pathol. 1988;131(1):38–47.

60. Perkocha LA, Geaghan SM, Yen TS, Nishimura SL, Chan SP. Garcia-Kennedy R, et al. Clinical and pathological features of bacillary peliosis hepatis in association with human immunodeficiency virus infection. N Engl J Med. 1990;323(23):1581–6.

61. Usatin MS, Wigger HJ. Peliosis hepatis in a child. Arch Pathol Lab Med. 1976;100(8):419–21.

62. Odièvre M, Chaumont P, Gautier M, Vermes JM. Transitory hepatic peliosis in a child. Arch Fr Pediatr. 1977;34(7):654–8.

63. Bank JI, Lykkebo D, Hägerstrand I. Peliosis hepatis in a child. Acta Paediatr Scand. 1978;67(1):105–7.

64. Willén H, Willén R, Gad A, Thorstensson S. Peliosis hepatis as a result of endogenous steroid hormone production. Virchows Arch A Pathol Anat Histol. 1979;383(2):233–40.

65. Pautard JC, Baculard A, Boccon-Gibod L, Carlioz H, Tournier G. Hepatic peliosis in bacterial endocarditis in a child with Marfan's disease. Presse Med. 1986;15(39):1973–4.

66. Kawamoto S, Wakabayashi T. Peliosis hepatis in a newborn infant. Arch Pathol Lab Med. 1980;104(8):444–5.

67. Wang SY, Ruggles S, Vade A, Newman BM, Borge MA. Hepatic rupture caused by peliosis hepatis. J Pediatr Surg. 2001;36(9):1456–9.

68. Cavalcanti R, Pol S, Carnot F, Campos H, Degott C, Driss F, et al. Impact and evolution of peliosis hepatis in renal transplant recipients. Transplantation. 1994;58(3):315–6.

69. Samyn M, Hadzic N, Davenport M, Verma A, Karani J, Portmann B, et al. Peliosis hepatis in childhood: case report and review of the literature. J Pediatr Gastroenterol Nutr. 2004;39(4):431–4.

70. Jacquemin E, Pariente D, Fabre M, Huault G, Valayer J, Bernard O. Peliosis hepatis with initial presentation as acute hepatic failure and intraperitoneal hemorrhage in children. J Hepatol. 1999;30(6):1146–50.

71. Nuernberger SP, Ramos CV. Peliosis hepatis in an infant. J Pediatr. 1975;87(3):424–6.

72. Janssen HLA, Garcia-Pagan J-C, Elias E, Mentha G, Hadengue A, Valla D-C, et al. Budd–Chiari syndrome: a review by an expert panel. J Hepatol. 2003;38(3):364–71.

73. Primignani M, Barosi G, Bergamaschi G, Gianelli U, Fabris F, Reati R, et al. Role of the JAK2 mutation in the diagnosis of chronic myeloproliferative disorders in splanchnic vein thrombosis. Hepatology. 2006;44(6):1528–34.

74. Kiladjian JJ, Cervantes F, Leebeek FW, Marzac C, Cassinat B, Chevret S, et al. The impact of JAK2 and MPL mutations on diagnosis and prognosis of splanchnic vein thrombosis: a report on 241 cases. Blood. 2008;111(10):4922–9.

75. Plessier A, Valla D-C. Budd–Chiari syndrome. Semin Liver Dis. 2008;28(3):259–69.

76. Valla DC. Hepatic vein thrombosis (Budd–Chiari syndrome). Semin Liver Dis. 2002;22(1):5–14.

77. Cauchi JA, Oliff S, Baumann U, Mirza D, Kelly DA, Hewitson J, et al. The Budd–Chiari syndrome in children: the spectrum of management. J Pediatr Surg. 2006;41(11):1919–23.

78. Okuda H, Yamagata H, Obata H, Iwata H, Sasaki R, Imai F, et al. Epidemiological and clinical features of Budd–Chiari syndrome in Japan. J Hepatol. 1995;22(1):1–9.

79. Langlet P, Valla D. Is surgical portosystemic shunt the treatment of choice in Budd–Chiari syndrome? Acta Gastroenterol Belg. 2002;65(3):155–60.

80. Hadengue A, Poliquin M, Vilgrain V, Belghiti J, Degott C, Erlinger S, et al. The changing scene of hepatic vein thrombosis: recognition of asymptomatic cases. Gastroenterology. 1994;106(4):1042–7.

81. Bolondi L, Gaiani S, Li Bassi S, Zironi G, Bonino F, Brunetto M, et al. Diagnosis of Budd–Chiari syndrome by pulsed Doppler ultrasound. Gastroenterology. 1991;100(5 Pt 1):1324–31.

82. Chawla Y, Kumar S, Dhiman RK, Suri S, Dilawari JB. Duplex Doppler sonography in patients with Budd–Chiari syndrome. J Gastroenterol Hepatol. 1999;14(9):904–7.

83. Kane R, Eustace S. Diagnosis of Budd–Chiari syndrome: comparison between sonography and MR angiography. Radiology. 1995;195(1):117–21.

84. Millener P, Grant EG, Rose S, Duerinckx A, Schiller VL, Tessler FN, et al. Color Doppler imaging findings in patients with Budd–Chiari syndrome: correlation with venographic findings. AJR Am J Roentgenol. 1993;161(2):307–12.

85. Tanaka M, Wanless IR. Pathology of the liver in Budd–Chiari syndrome: portal vein thrombosis and the histogenesis of veno-centric cirrhosis, veno-portal cirrhosis, and large regenerative nodules. Hepatology. 1998;27(2):488–96.

86. Menon KVN, Shah V, Kamath PS. The Budd–Chiari syndrome. N Engl J Med. 2004;350(6):578–85.

87. Sharma S, Texeira A, Texeira P, Elias E, Wilde J, Olliff SP. Pharmacological thrombolysis in Budd–Chiari syndrome: a single centre experience and review of the literature. J Hepatol. 2004;40(1):172–80.

88. Carnevale FC, Caldas JGMP, Maksoud JG. Transjugular intrahepatic portosystemic shunt in a child with Budd–Chiari syndrome: technical modification and extended followup. Cardiovasc Intervent Radiol. 2002;25(3):224–6.

89. Rössle M, Olschewski M, Siegerstetter V, Berger E, Kurz K, Grandt D. The Budd–Chiari syndrome: outcome after treatment with the transjugular intrahepatic portosystemic shunt. Surgery. 2004;135(4):394–403.

90. Benesch M, Urban C, Deutschmann H, Hausegger KA, Höllwarth M. Management of Budd–Chiari syndrome by hepatic vein stenting after extended right hepatectomy. J Pediatr Surg. 2002;37(11):1640–2.

91. Rerksuppaphol S, Hardikar W, Smith AL, Wilkinson JL, Goh TH, Angus P, et al. Successful stenting for Budd–Chiari syndrome after pediatric liver transplantation: a case series and review of the literature. Pediatr Surg Int. 2004;20(2):87–90.

92. Nezakatgoo N, Shokouh-Amiri MH, Gaber AO, Grewal HP, Vera SR, Chamsuddin AA, et al. Liver transplantation for acute Budd–Chiari syndrome in identical twin sisters with Factor V leiden mutation. Transplantation. 2003;76(1):195–8.

93. Yasutomi M, Egawa H, Kobayashi Y, Oike F, Tanaka K. Living donor liver transplantation for Budd–Chiari syndrome with inferior vena cava obstruction and associated antiphospholipid antibody syndrome. J Pediatr Surg. 2001;36(4):659–62.

94. Gharib MI, Bulley SR, Doyle JJ, Wynn RF. Venous occlusive disease in children. Thromb Res. 2006;118(1):27–38.

95. Coppell JA, Richardson PG, Soiffer R, Martin PL, Kernan NA, Chen A, et al. Hepatic veno-occlusive disease following stem cell transplantation: incidence, clinical course, and outcome. Biol Blood Marrow Transplant. 2010;16(2):157–68.

96. Jones RJ, Lee KS, Beschorner WE, Vogel VG, Grochow LB, Braine HG, et al. Venoocclusive disease of the liver following bone marrow transplantation. Transplantation. 1987;44(6):778–83.

97. McDonald GB, Hinds MS, Fisher LD, Schoch HG, Wolford JL, Banaji M, et al. Veno-occlusive disease of the liver and multiorgan failure after bone marrow transplantation: a cohort study of 355 patients. Ann Intern Med. 1993;118(4):255–67.

98. DeLeve LD. Glutathione defense in non-parenchymal cells. Semin Liver Dis. 1998;18(4):403–13.

99. Richardson P, Guinan E. The pathology, diagnosis, and treatment of hepatic veno-occlusive disease: current status and novel approaches. Br J Haematol. 1999;107(3):485–93.

100. Nürnberger W, Michelmann I, Burdach S, Göbel U. Endothelial dysfunction after bone marrow transplantation: increase of soluble thrombomodulin and PAI-1 in patients with multiple transplant-related complications. Ann Hematol. 1998;76(2):61–5.

101. Salat C, Holler E, Kolb HJ, Reinhardt B, Pihusch R, Wilmanns W, et al. Plasminogen activator inhibitor-1 confirms the diagnosis of hepatic veno-occlusive disease in patients with hyperbilirubinemia after bone marrow transplantation. Blood. 1997;89(6):2184–8.

102. Lee J-H, Lee K-H, Lee J-H, Kim S, Seol M, Park C-J, et al. Plasminogen activator inhibitor-1 is an independent diagnostic marker as well as severity predictor of hepatic veno-occlusive disease after allogeneic bone marrow transplantation in adults conditioned with busulphan and cyclophosphamide. Br J Haematol. 2002;118(4):1087–94.

103. Shulman HM, Fisher LB, Schoch HG, Henne KW, McDonald GB. Veno-occlusive disease of the liver after marrow transplantation: histological correlates of clinical signs and symptoms. Hepatology. 1994;19(5):1171–81.

104. Carreras E, Bertz H, Arcese W, Vernant JP, Tomás JF, Hagglund H, et al. Incidence and outcome of hepatic veno-occlusive disease after blood or marrow transplantation: a prospective cohort study of the European Group for Blood and Marrow Transplantation. European Group for Blood and Marrow Transplantation Chronic Leukemia Working Party. Blood. 1998;92(10):3599–604.

105. Bearman SI, Anderson GL, Mori M, Hinds MS, Shulman HM, McDonald GB. Venoocclusive disease of the liver: development of a model for predicting fatal outcome after marrow transplantation. J Clin Oncol. 1993;11(9):1729–36.

106. Vassal G. Pharmacologically-guided dose adjustment of busulfan in high-dose chemotherapy regimens: rationale and pitfalls (review). Anticancer Res. 1994;14(6A):2363–70.

107. Cheuk DK. Hepatic veno-occlusive disease after hematopoietic stem cell transplantation: prophylaxis and treatment controversies. World J Transplant. 2012;2(2):27–34.

108. Essell JH, Schroeder MT, Harman GS, Halvorson R, Lew V, Callander N, et al. Ursodiol prophylaxis against hepatic complications of allogeneic bone marrow transplantation. A randomized, double-blind, placebo-controlled trial. Ann Intern Med. 1998;128(12 Pt 1):975–81.

109. Ohashi K, Tanabe J, Watanabe R, Tanaka T, Sakamaki H, Maruta A, et al. The Japanese multicenter open randomized trial of ursodeoxycholic acid prophylaxis for hepatic veno-occlusive disease after stem cell transplantation. Am J Hematol. 2000;64(1):32–8.

110. Ruutu T, Eriksson B, Remes K, Juvonen E, Volin L, Remberger M, et al. Ursodeoxycholic acid for the prevention of hepatic complications in allogeneic stem cell transplantation. Blood. 2002;100(6):1977–83.

111. Park SH, Lee MH, Lee H, Kim HS, Kim K, Kim WS, et al. A randomized trial of heparin plus ursodiol vs. heparin alone to prevent hepatic veno-occlusive disease after hematopoietic stem cell transplantation. Bone Marrow Transplant. 2002;29(2):137–43.

112. Marsa-Vila L, Gorin NC, Laporte JP, Labopin M, Dupuy-Montbrun MC, Fouillard L, et al. Prophylactic heparin does not prevent liver veno-occlusive disease following autologous bone marrow transplantation. Eur J Haematol. 1991;47(5):346–54.

113. Attal M, Huguet F, Rubie H, Huynh A, Charlet JP, Payen JL, et al. Prevention of hepatic veno-occlusive disease after bone marrow transplantation by continuous infusion of low-dose heparin: a prospective, randomized trial. Blood. 1992;79(11):2834–40.

114. Falanga A, Vignoli A, Marchetti M, Barbui T. Defibrotide reduces procoagulant activity and increases fibrinolytic properties of endothelial cells. Leukemia. 2003;17(8):1636–42.

115. Richardson PG, Soiffer RJ, Antin JH, Uno H, Jin Z, Kurtzberg J, et al. Defibrotide for the treatment of severe hepatic veno-occlusive disease and multiorgan failure after stem cell transplantation: a multicenter, randomized, dose-finding trial. Biol Blood Marrow Transplant. 2010;16(7):1005–17.

116. Cesaro S, Pillon M, Talenti E, Toffolutti T, Calore E, Tridello G, et al. A prospective survey on incidence, risk factors and therapy of hepatic veno-occlusive disease in children after hematopoietic stem cell transplantation. Haematologica. 2005;90(10):1396–404.

117. Ho VT, Revta C, Richardson PG. Hepatic veno-occlusive disease after hematopoietic stem cell transplantation: update on defibrotide and other current investigational therapies. Bone Marrow Transplant. 2008;41(3):229–37.

118. Steiner PE. Nodular regenerative hyperplasia of the liver. Am J Pathol. 1959;35:943–53.

119. Stringer MD. The clinical anatomy of congenital portosystemic venous shunts. Clin Anat. 2008;21(2):147–57.

120. Bernard O, Franchi-Abella S, Branchereau S, Pariente D, Gauthier F, Jacquemin E. Congenital portosystemic shunts in children: recognition, evaluation, and management. Semin Liver Dis. 2012;32(4):273–87.

121. Morgan G, Superina R. Congenital absence of the portal vein: two cases and a proposed classification system for portasystemic vascular anomalies. J Pediatr Surg. 1994;29(9):1239–41.

122. Witjes CD, Ijzermans JN, Vonk Noordegraaf A, Tran TK. Management strategy after diagnosis of Abernethy malformation: a case report. J Med Case Rep. 2012;6(1):167.

123. Chandrashekhara SH, Bhalla AS, Gupta AK, Vikash CS, Kabra SK. Abernethy malformation with portal vein aneurysm in a child. J Indian Assoc Pediatr Surg. 2011;16(1):21–3.

124. Kohda E, Saeki M, Nakano M, Masaki H, Ogawa K, Nirasawa M, et al. Congenital absence of the portal vein in a boy. Pediatr Radiol. 1999;29(4):235–7.

125. Tsauo J, Liu L, Tang C, Li X. Education and Imaging. Hepatobiliary and pancreatic: spontaneous intrahepatic portosystemic shunt associated with cirrhosis. J Gastroenterol Hepatol. 2013;28(6):904.

126. Khalid SK, Garcia-Tsao G. Hepatic vascular malformations in hereditary hemorrhagic telangiectasia. Semin Liver Dis. 2008;28(3):247–58.

127. Al-Saleh S, John PR, Letarte M, Faughnan ME, Belik J, Ratjen F. Symptomatic liver involvement in neonatal hereditary hemorrhagic telangiectasia. Pediatrics. 2011;127(6):e1615–20.

128. Wanless IR. Micronodular transformation (nodular regenerative hyperplasia) of the liver: a report of 64 cases among 2500 autopsies and a new classification of benign hepatocellular nodules. Hepatology. 1990;11(5):787–97.

129. Hartleb M, Gutkowski K, Milkiewicz P. Nodular regenerative hyperplasia: evolving concepts on underdiagnosed cause of portal hypertension. World J Gastroenterol. 2011;17(11):1400–9.

130. Mahamid J, Miselevich I, Attias D, Laor R, Zuckerman E, Shaoul R. Nodular regenerative hyperplasia associated with idiopathic thrombocytopenic purpura in a young girl: a case report and review of the literature. J Pediatr Gastroenterol Nutr. 2005;41(2):251–5.

131. Stocker JT. Hepatic tumors in children. Clin Liver Dis. 2001;5(1):259–81, viii–ix.

132. Shastri S, Dubinsky MC, Fred Poordad F, Vasiliauskas EA, Geller SA. Early nodular hyperplasia of the liver occurring with inflammatory bowel diseases in association with thioguanine therapy. Arch Pathol Lab Med. 2004;128(1):49–53.

133. Gane E, Portmann B, Saxena R, Wong P, Ramage J, Williams R. Nodular regenerative hyperplasia of the liver graft after liver transplantation. Hepatology. 1994;20(1 Pt 1):88–94.

134. Teml A, Schwab M, Hommes DW, Almer S, Lukas M, Feichten-schlager T, et al. A systematic survey evaluating 6-thioguanine-related hepatotoxicity in patients with inflammatory bowel disease. Wien Klin Wochenschr. 2007;119(17–18):519–26.

135. De Bruyne R, Portmann B, Samyn M, Bansal S, Knisely A, Mieli-Vergani G, et al. Chronic liver disease related to 6-thioguanine in children with acute lymphoblastic leukaemia. J Hepatol. 2006;44(2):407–10.

136. Casillas C, Martí-Bonmatí L, Galant J. Pseudotumoral presentation of nodular regenerative hyperplasia of the liver: imaging in five patients including MR imaging. Eur Radiol. 1997;7(5):654–8.

137. Trotter JF, Everson GT. Benign focal lesions of the liver. Clin Liver Dis. 2001;5(1):17–42, v.

138. Arvanitaki M, Adler M. Nodular regenerative hyperplasia of the liver. A review of 14 cases. Hepatogastroenterology. 2001;48(41):1425–9.

139. Nahm CB, Ng K, Lockie P, Samra JS, Hugh TJ. Focal nodular hyperplasia—a review of myths and truths. J Gastrointest Surg. 2011;15(12):2275–83.

140. Wanless IR, Mawdsley C, Adams R. On the pathogenesis of focal nodular hyperplasia of the liver. Hepatology. 1985;5(6):1194–200.

141. Luciani A, Kobeiter H, Maison P, Cherqui D, Zafrani E-S, Dhumeaux D, et al. Focal nodular hyperplasia of the liver in men: is presentation the same in men and women? Gut. 2002;50(6):877–80.

142. Vilgrain V, Fléjou JF, Arrivé L, Belghiti J, Najmark D, Menu Y, et al. Focal nodular hyperplasia of the liver: MR imaging and pathologic correlation in 37 patients. Radiology. 1992;184(3):699–703.

143. Caseiro-Alves F, Zins M, Mahfouz A-E, Rahmouni A, Vilgrain V, Menu Y, et al. Calcification in focal nodular hyperplasia: a new problem for differentiation from fibrolamellar hepatocellular carcinoma. Radiology. 1996;198(3):889–92.

144. Golli M, Mathieu D, Anglade MC, Cherqui D, Vasile N, Rahmouni A. Focal nodular hyperplasia of the liver: value of color Doppler US in association with MR imaging. Radiology. 1993;187(1):113–7.

145. Carlson SK, Johnson CD, Bender CE, Welch TJ. CT of focal nodular hyperplasia of the liver. AJR Am J Roentgenol. 2000;174(3):705–12.

146. Lee MJ, Saini S, Hamm B, Taupitz M, Hahn PF, Seneterre E, et al. Focal nodular hyperplasia of the liver: MR findings in 35 proved cases. AJR Am J Roentgenol. 1991;156(2):317–20.

147. Weinberg AG, Finegold MJ. Primary hepatic tumors of childhood. Hum Pathol. 1983;14(6):512–37.

148. Meyers RL. Tumors of the liver in children. Surg Oncol. 2007;16(3):195–203.

149. Christison-Lagay ER, Burrows PE, Alomari A, Dubois J, Kozakewich HP, Lane TS, et al. Hepatic hemangiomas: subtype classification and development of a clinical practice algorithm and registry. J Pediatr Surg. 2007;42(1):62–7, discussion 7–8.

150. Burrows PE, Dubois J, Kassarjian A. Pediatric hepatic vascular anomalies. Pediatr Radiol. 2001;31(8):533–45.

151. Keslar PJ, Buck JL, Selby DM. From the archives of the AFIP. Infantile hemangioendothelioma of the liver revisited. Radiographics. 1993;13(3):657–70.

152. Boon LM, Burrows PE, Paltiel HJ, Lund DP, Ezekowitz RA, Folkman J, et al. Hepatic vascular anomalies in infancy: a twenty-seven-year experience. J Pediatr. 1996;129(3):346–54.

153. Iyer CP, Stanley P, Mahour GH. Hepatic hemangiomas in infants and children: a review of 30 cases. Am Surg. 1996;62(5):356–60.

154. Huang SA, Tu HM, Harney JW, Venihaki M, Butte AJ, Kozakewich HP, et al. Severe hypothyroidism caused by type 3 iodothyronine deiodinase in infantile hemangiomas. N Engl J Med. 2000;343(3):185–9.

155. Konrad D, Ellis G, Perlman K. Spontaneous regression of severe acquired infantile hypothyroidism associated with multiple liver hemangiomas. Pediatrics. 2003;112(6 Pt 1):1424–6.

156. Kulungowski AM, Alomari AI, Chawla A, Christison-Lagay ER, Fishman SJ. Lessons from a liver hemangioma registry: subtype classification. J Pediatr Surg. 2012;47(1):165–70.

157. Mulliken JB, Enjolras O. Congenital hemangiomas and infantile hemangioma: missing links. J Am Acad Dermatol. 2004;50(6):875–82.

158. Enjolras O, Mulliken JB, Boon LM, Wassef M, Kozakewich HP, Burrows PE. Noninvoluting congenital hemangioma: a rare cutaneous vascular anomaly. Plast Reconstr Surg. 2001;107(7):1647–54.

159. Marler JJ, Fishman SJ, Upton J, Burrows PE, Paltiel HJ, Jennings RW, et al. Prenatal diagnosis of vascular anomalies. J Pediatr Surg. 2002;37(3):318–26.

160. Berenguer B, Mulliken JB, Enjolras O, Boon LM, Wassef M, Josset P, et al. Rapidly involuting congenital hemangioma: clinical and histopathologic features. Pediatr Dev Pathol. 2003;6(6):495–510.

161. Morris J, Abbott J, Burrows P, Levine D. Antenatal diagnosis of fetal hepatic hemangioma treated with maternal corticosteroids. Obstet Gynecol. 1999;94(5 Pt 2):813–5.

162. Kassarjian A, Zurakowski D, Dubois J, Paltiel HJ, Fishman SJ, Burrows PE. Infantile hepatic hemangiomas: clinical and imaging findings and their correlation with therapy. AJR Am J Roentgenol. 2004;182(3):785–95.

163. Yasunaga C, Sueishi K, Ohgami H, Suita S, Kawanami T. Heterogenous expression of endothelial cell markers in infantile hemangioendothelioma. Immunohistochemical study of two solitary cases and one multiple one. Am J Clin Pathol. 1989;91(6):673–81.

164. Emre S, McKenna GJ. Liver tumors in children. Pediatr Transplant. 2004;8(6):632–8.

165. Léauté-Labrèze C, Dumas de la Roque E, Hubiche T, Boralevi F, Thambo J-B, Taïeb A. Propranolol for severe hemangiomas of infancy. N Engl J Med. 2008;358(24):2649–51.

166. Sans V, de la Roque ED, Berge J, Grenier N, Boralevi F, Mazereeuw-Hautier J, et al. Propranolol for severe infantile hemangiomas: follow-up report. Pediatrics. 2009;124(3):e423–31.

167. Taki M, Ohi C, Yamashita A, Kobayashi M, Kobayashi N, Yoda T, et al. Successful treatment with vincristine of an infant with intractable Kasabach–Merritt syndrome. Pediatr Int. 2006;48(1):82–4.

168. Moore J, Lee M, Garzon M, Soffer S, Kim E, Saouaf R, et al. Effective therapy of a vascular tumor of infancy with vincristine. J Pediatr Surg. 2001;36(8):1273–6.

169. Hu B, Lachman R, Phillips J, Peng SK, Sieger L. Kasabach–Merritt syndrome-associated kaposiform hemangioendothelioma successfully treated with cyclophosphamide, vincristine, and actinomycin D. J Pediatr Hematol Oncol. 1998;20(6):567–9.

170. Dimashkieh HH, Mo JQ, Wyatt-Ashmead J, Collins MH. Pediatric hepatic angiosarcoma: case report and review of the literature. Pediatr Dev Pathol. 2004;7(5):527–32.

171. Mehrabi A, Kashfi A, Fonouni H, Schemmer P, Schmied BM, Hallscheidt P, et al. Primary malignant hepatic epithelioid hemangioendothelioma: a comprehensive review of the literature with emphasis on the surgical therapy. Cancer. 2006;107(9):2108–21.

172. Weiss SW, Enzinger FM. Epithelioid hemangioendothelioma: a vascular tumor often mistaken for a carcinoma. Cancer. 1982;50(5):970–81.

173. Lau K, Massad M, Pollak C, Rubin C, Yeh J, Wang J, et al. Clinical patterns and outcome in epithelioid hemangioendothelioma with or without pulmonary involvement: insights from an internet registry in the study of a rare cancer. Chest. 2011;140(5):1312–8.

Portal Hypertension in Children

Angelo Di Giorgio and Lorenzo D'Antiga

Introduction

Portal hypertension (PH) is the commonest complication of chronic liver disease in children as in adults [1]. Children with PH are at risk of severe complications. Children with PH and their parents may be frightened by the most severe complication of PH, gastrointestinal hemorrhage (GH), often referred to as a terrifying experience and giving the impression of impending death; nevertheless, only few pediatric patients die from variceal bleeding, especially if they have a non-cirrhotic cause of PH [2]. Unfortunately, there are very few robust data published in the past few decades in children with PH [3]. Conversely, in adults, many treatments have been challenged, and a plethora of studies have been carried out and summarized periodically in the Baveno Consensus Conference [4]. A panel of experts sporadically provides a pediatric opinion on the Baveno Conference trying to translate the experience gained from treating adults into children [5].

Therefore, most children are treated simply extrapolating the data from adults and applying the same protocols adapted according to body size [6, 7]. Nevertheless, there are several important differences between PH in children and adults. One is represented by the early onset and rapid progression of pediatric liver diseases causing cirrhotic PH, together with a relatively larger availability of split organ donations allowing us to solve most of the severe cases by organ replacement. Thus, the length of the follow-up of children with severe cirrhotic PH is short. Second, a large proportion of children with PH have presinusoidal disease, having different implications as far as management and outcome are concerned [8]. These points explain why most of the children

with large varices and bleeding that we manage in the long term usually have non-cirrhotic PH, clearly a scenario different to that in adult practice.

Anatomy of the Portal Venous System

The liver receives blood from two main vessels: the proper hepatic artery and the portal vein. The former is a branch of the common hepatic artery, which arises from celiac trunk, and supplies oxygenated blood accounting for 25 % of the blood entering the liver. The latter, which drains deoxygenated blood accounting for 75 % of the liver blood flow, is the largest vessel of the portal venous system. In adults, the total hepatic blood flow ranges between 800 and 1200 mL/min, which is equivalent to approximately 100 mL/min per 100 g of wet liver. Although the liver mass constitutes only 2.5 % of the total body weight, this organ receives nearly 25 % of the cardiac output.

This huge portal venous flow is driven through the liver across a minute pressure gradient. The pressure gradient between the portal inflow and the hepatic venous outflow is usually no more than 5 mmHg. The resistance to blood flow through the portal vein is so low because of the unique hepatic vasculature, with conducting blood vessels terminating in each of the microvascular units of the acinus and flowing past only approximately 20 hepatocytes before exiting into the wide hepatic venules. Thus, at least 50 % of the entire blood content of the liver can be expelled without significant vascular resistance [9].

The portal venous system extends from the intestinal capillaries to the hepatic sinusoids. It carries the blood from the abdominal gastrointestinal (GI) tract, pancreas, gallbladder, and spleen back to the heart flowing through the liver (Fig. 68.1).

In this system, the central vessel is the portal vein, which is formed by the union of the splenic vein (SV) and the superior mesenteric vein (SMV), but receiving blood also

L. D'Antiga (✉) · A. Di Giorgio
Department of Pediatric Hepatology, Gastroenterology and Transplantation, Hospital Papa Giovanni XXIII—Bergamo, Piazza Oms 1, Bergamo 24127, Italy
e-mail: ldantiga@hpg23.it

© Springer International Publishing Switzerland 2016
S. Guandalini et al. (eds.), *Textbook of Pediatric Gastroenterology, Hepatology and Nutrition*,
DOI 10.1007/978-3-319-17169-2_68

Fig. 68.1 Anatomy of the portal system

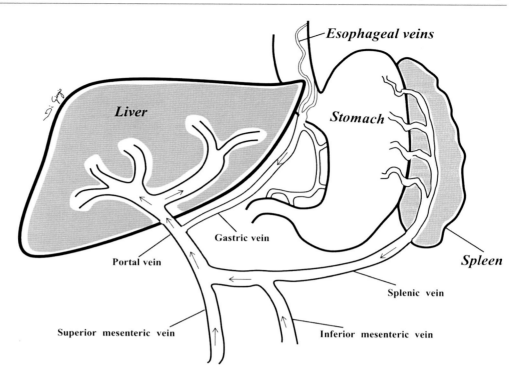

from the inferior mesenteric vein (IMV), the gastric, and the cystic veins. The SMV is formed by tributaries from the small intestine, colon, and head of the pancreas, and irregularly from the stomach via the right gastroepiploic vein. The SVs originate at the splenic hilum and join near the tail of the pancreas with the short gastric vessels to form the main SV. The IMV carries blood from the left part of the colon and rectum and reaches the SV in its medial third. Anatomical variations include the IMV draining into the confluence of the SMV and the SV, and the IMV draining in the SMV (Fig. 68.1).

Immediately before reaching the liver, the portal vein divides into right and left main branches, and then ramifies further, forming smaller venous branches, and ultimately the portal venules. Each portal venule runs alongside a hepatic arteriole and the two vessels form the vascular components of the portal triad. These vessels ultimately merge into the hepatic sinusoids to supply blood to the liver. Three hepatic veins (right, middle, and left) drain the blood from the liver into the inferior vena cava (IVC) [10].

Pathophysiology of Portal Hypertension

The portal venous pressure is directly proportional to the portal blood flow and the hepatic resistance, according to Ohm's law ($\Delta P = Q \times R$, where ΔP is the variation of pressure along the vessel, Q is the blood flow, and R is the resistance to flow). Since portal vascular resistance is inversely proportional to the fourth power of the radius (Poiseuille's

equation), a small decrease in the vessel diameter produces a large increase in the portal vascular resistance and, in turn, in portal blood pressure. In the healthy liver, the intrahepatic resistance changes according to the variation of portal blood flow to keep portal pressure within normal limits. In fact, under physiological conditions, a rise in portal pressure is counteracted by sinusoidal dilatation, even in the presence of increased blood flow as can happen after meal ingestion [10, 11]. Most of the following statements made on PH come from experiments on animal models, such as the rat with a ligated portal vein or bile duct or with carbon tetrachloride-induced cirrhosis, and then confirmed in clinical studies carried out mainly in adults [11–13].

Increase of Vascular Resistance

The portal venous system has a baseline portal pressure of 7–10 mmHg, and the hepatic venous pressure gradient (HVPG) ranges from 1 to 4 mmHg. PH is defined as a portal pressure greater than 10 mmHg or a gradient greater than 4 mmHg. In adults, a pressure gradient above 10 mmHg has been associated with esophageal varices (EV) formation, and with ascites and variceal bleeding if above 12 mmHg [14, 15].

The main pathogenetic factor in the development of PH is an increased vascular resistance (Fig. 68.2). Depending on the site in which it occurs, PH can be classified as extrahepatic (prehepatic and posthepatic) and intrahepatic. The latter may be further subdivided into three forms including

Fig. 68.2 Portal hypertension development according to Ohm's law

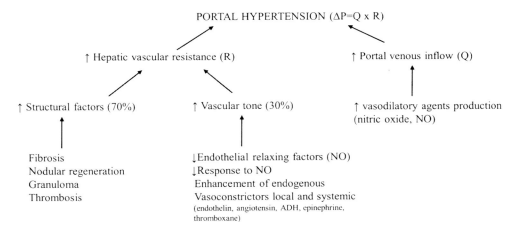

PORTAL HYPERTENSION (ΔP=Q x R)

↑ Hepatic vascular resistance (R)   ↑ Portal venous inflow (Q)

↑ Structural factors (70%)   ↑ Vascular tone (30%)   ↑ vasodilatory agents production (nitric oxide, NO)

Fibrosis
Nodular regeneration
Granuloma
Thrombosis

↓Endothelial relaxing factors (NO)
↓Response to NO
Enhancement of endogenous
Vasoconstrictors local and systemic
(endothelin, angiotensin, ADH, epinephrine, thromboxane)

presinusoidal (portal venules), sinusoidal (sinusoids), and postsinusoidal (terminal hepatic venules; central veins; Table 68.1).

In patients affected by chronic liver disease, though, increased vascular resistance is located at various intrahepatic levels.

The pathogenetic mechanism explaining the increased resistance in extrahepatic PH, where the blood flow is blocked by a mechanical obstruction, is quite obvious. Conversely, the pathogenesis is more complicated in intrahepatic PH, in which many factors, both mechanical and dynamic, may occur simultaneously [15].

Increase of Portal Blood Flow

The second factor contributing to the development of PH is an increase in blood flow, established through splanchnic arteriolar vasodilatation caused by an excessive release of endogenous vasodilators including nitric oxide (NO), glucagon, endothelin (activated by the vasoactive intestinal peptide), as well as by the activation of the sympathetic and the renin–angiotensin systems. These changes cause sodium and water retention, hypervolemia, renal hypoperfusion, and increase in cardiac output and splanchnic blood inflow, resulting in a hyperdinamic vascular status which characterizes the advanced stages of PH (Fig. 68.2).

Extra-hepatic Causes of PH

Prehepatic causes of increased resistance to flow include SV thrombosis, congenital atresia or stenosis of the portal vein, extrinsic compression (tumors), and portal vein thrombosis (PVT). In these disorders, the obstruction in the prehepatic portal venous system leads to an increased portal venous pressure [16].

Table 68.1 Classification and etiology of portal hypertension

Prehepatic
Portal vein thrombosis
Congenital stenosis or extrinsic compression of the portal vein
Splenic vein thrombosis
Artero-venous fistulae
Intrahepatic presinusoidal
Congenital hepatic fibrosis
Chronic viral hepatitis (HBV and HCV)
Primary biliary cirrhosis
Myeloproliferative diseases (Hodgkin's disease, leukemia)
Focal nodular hyperplasia
Idiopathic portal hypertension (IPH)/non-cirrhotic portal fibrosis (NCFP)/hepatoportal sclerosis
Granulomatous diseases (schistosomiasis, sarcoidosis, tuberculosis)
Amyloidosis
Gaucher's disease
Polycystic liver disease
Infiltration of liver hilum (independent of cause)
Benign and malignant neoplasms
Toxins and drugs (arsenic, vinyl chloride monomer poisoning, methotrexate, 6-mercaptopurine)
Peliosis hepatis
Rendu–Osler–Weber syndrome
Chronic hepatitis
Intrahepatic sinusoidal
Liver cirrhosis (independent of cause)
Wilson's disease
Hemochromatosis
Storage diseases (fatty liver, glycogenosis type III, Niemann–Pick disease, α1-antitrypsin deficiency)
Acute Hepatitis (viral and autoimmune)
Hypervitaminosis A
Intrahepatic postsinusoidal
Veno-occlusive disease (VOD)
Hepatic vein thrombosis (Budd–Chiari syndrome)
Posthepatic
Inferior vena cava obstruction (thrombosis, neoplasms)
Right heart failure
Constrictive pericarditis
Tricuspid valve diseases
HBV hepatitis B virus, *HCV* hepatitis C virus

The isolated obstruction of the SV (mainly due to thrombosis) usually results in left-sided PH (sparing the superior mesenteric district). In this rare clinical condition, the blood flows retrogradely through the short and posterior gastric veins and the gastroepiploic veins, leading to the formation of isolated gastric varices. The most common causes of SV occlusion are pancreatic diseases, such as pancreatic cancer, pancreatitis, or a pseudocyst. Although very rare in children, it should be considered in the presence of isolated gastric bleeding with normal liver function and unexplained splenomegaly. The diagnosis may be difficult, and splenectomy represents the treatment of choice in symptomatic patients [17–19].

PVT is the most prevalent cause of extrahepatic portal vein obstruction (EHPVO), and is the major cause of non-cirrhotic PH in children. Conversely, congenital abnormalities, such as portal vein stenosis, atresia, or agenesis, are relatively uncommon.

The etiology of PVT remains obscure in approximately 50 % of the cases whereas known etiologies include umbilical vein catheterization, omphalitis/umbilical sepsis, thrombophilia (acquired, hereditary), myeloproliferative disorders, surgery (splenectomy, liver transplantation), dehydration, and multiple exchange transfusions in the neonatal period [20–22].

In a multicenter Italian study including 187 pediatric patients diagnosed with EHPVO, it was shown that the condition is strictly associated with a neonatal disorder. The mean age at diagnosis was 4 years; 59 % were born preterm; 65 % had a history of umbilical catheterization; 82 % had associated illnesses, such as complications of prematurity (43.5 %), cardiac malformations (7.5 %), noncardiac malformations (8.5 %), deep infections (7 %), and hematological disorders (5.5 %). The patients were diagnosed upon detection of splenomegaly (39.5 %), after an episode of GI bleeding (36.6 %), because of hypersplenism (5.2 %), by chance in the context of other investigations (16.3 %; personal data, unpublished).

The pathogenesis of PH in EHPVO is closely related to the portal vein obstruction, which causes an increased vascular resistance in the portal venous system. Initially, the occlusion of the portal vein by thrombus formation is followed by compensatory vasodilation of the hepatic artery buffering the need for blood supply to the liver. Eventually, collateral venous vessels bypassing the thrombus develop and constitute the so-called "cavernomatous transformation" or "portal cavernoma." Part of these collaterals may reperfuse the liver, whereas the majority contributes to the porto-systemic shunting developing at various levels in the portal system. Liver tests are usually normal since there is no parenchymal disease apart from mild vascular changes, such as portal venous dilatation and sclerosis.

The management of EHPVO is mainly directed to the treatment of PH complications through medical and endo-scopic means. Despite their efficacy in obliterating EV, endoscopic methods have no effect on portal pressure. Conversely, surgical procedures may decompress the portal venous system and normalize the portal vein pressure. Possible indications for surgical treatment include acute variceal bleeding that cannot be controlled by endoscopic means, persistent EV formation, massive symptomatic splenomegaly, growth retardation, and symptomatic portal biliopathy [23, 24]. EHPVO is dealt with more extensively in the non-cirrhotic PH section.

Posthepatic causes of increased resistance to flow are those related to vascular and/or cardiac diseases, including thrombosis/stenosis of the hepatic veins or the atrio-caval junction, any condition increasing the right atrial pressure, such as constrictive pericarditis, severe tricuspidal regurgitation, and right side cardiac failure. The postsurgical status of some congenital cardiac malformations, such as the Fontan circulation, result in increased central venous pressure and increased resistance to liver outflow [25]. Unlike prehepatic PH, in which liver function remains often normal overtime, in posthepatic PH, the liver blood stagnation may compromise liver function leading to cirrhosis [26].

Budd–Chiari syndrome (BCS) is one of the most common causes of post-hepatic PH both in adults and children. BCS is characterized by hepatic venous outflow obstruction at any level from the small hepatic veins to the atrio-caval junction, regardless of the cause of obstruction. The acute increase of vascular resistance secondary to the hepatic venous outflow obstruction causes the sudden appearance of PH, whereas the chronic status may lead to cirrhosis [27].

A wide variety of predisposing causes may determine the onset of the BCS, including congenital or acquired webs of the IVC and thrombotic, inflammatory, or neoplastic processes.

BCS is relatively rare in children. In studies including patients younger than 10 years with PH, the percentage of cases of BCS accounted for 1–7 % of all, although in some areas such as Africa, India, and China, the rate of pediatric BCS may raise up to 16 % [28, 29].

The presentation of BCS can be acute, chronic, or fulminant. In the early course of the disease, it may be asymptomatic and accompanied by normal liver tests. Eventually, the hepatic venous outflow obstruction may lead to hepatic dysfunction associated with abdominal pain, ascites, and hepatosplenomegaly.

Due to its rarity, BCS in children is often diagnosed with some delay. The stage of the disease at diagnosis influences the management strategy and an early diagnosis offers the best chance of cure without major surgery [30].

The management of BCS in pediatric patients may include the use of anticoagulation, thrombolytic therapy and angioplasty with or without stenting, transjugular intrahepatic porto-systemic shunts (TIPS), and, rarely, surgical

Table 68.2 Hepatic venous pressures according to the pathophysiology of portal hypertension

Etiology of PH		ISP	PVP	RAP	WHVP	FHVP	HVPG
Prehepatic		↑↑	↑↑	N	N	N	N
Intrahepatic	Presinusoidal	↑↑	↑↑	N	N or ↑	N	N or ↑
	Sinusoidal	↑↑	↑↑	N	↑↑	N	↑↑
	Postsinusoidal	↑↑	↑↑	N	↑↑	N	↑↑
Posthepatic		↑↑	↑↑	N or ↑	↑↑	↑↑	N or ↑

ISP intrasplenic pressure, *PVP* portal vein pressure, *RAP* right atrial pressure, *WHVP* wedged hepatic venous pressure, *FHVP* free hepatic venous pressure, *HVPG* hepatic venous pressure gradient (difference between WHVP and FHVP), ↑↑ severe increase, ↑ mild increase, *N* normal

portosystemic shunts, the latter carrying high risk of thrombotic obstruction. Some patients may end up with end-stage liver disease and require transplantation.

Intrahepatic Causes of PH

Intrahepatic causes of increased vascular resistance have a more various and complicated pathogenesis compared to the extrahepatic forms, and can be further subdivided, according to the relation with the sinusoidal bed, into three subgroups: presinusoidal, sinusoidal, and postsinusoidal.

Presinusoidal venous block can be caused by many conditions, as detailed in Table 68.1. These disorders cause an elevated portal venous pressure, which cannot be detected by the hepatic vein catheter study, since wedge hepatic venous pressure (WHVP) reflects that of the sinusoids that are distal to the lesion, and therefore have normal blood pressure in this condition. Thus, the only useful technique to gather information on the degree of presinusoidal PH is that of the direct measurement of portal or splenic pulp pressure (Table 68.2).

Schistosomiasis is one of the leading causes of PH in the developing countries. Liver involvement due to schistosomiasis is caused by one of the two trematode flukes *schistosoma mansoni* and *japonicum*. While the former is seen predominantly in Africa and South America, the latter is common in eastern Asia, especially mainland China [31]. The pathogenesis of liver disease here is secondary to entrapment of eggs in the portal venules that cause granulomatous inflammation leading to fibrosis and, in 4–8% of cases, presinusoidal PH. Portal tract inflammation results from the host response to the parasitic egg in the hepatic venule. The natural history of PH in this condition is closely related to the number of eggs deposited in the liver [32, 33].

Sinusoidal obstruction is mainly due to cirrhosis. It is marked by an increase of HVPG, normal free hepatic venous pressure (FHVP), and raised WHVP (Table 68.2). In sinusoidal PH, WHVP is equal to portal venous pressure because disrupted intersinusoidal communications diminish compressibility and compliance of the sinusoids, allowing direct transmission of portal pressure to the WHVP [34, 35]. In cirrhosis, the increase of vascular resistance occurs at the level of the hepatic microcirculation (sinusoids), and

it is secondary to both a *mechanical* and a *dynamic factor*. The *mechanical factor* is represented by the hepatic architectural derangement, and is characterized by hepatocyte swelling, hyperplasia, portal tract inflammation, and fibrosis in response to liver injury. Besides, collagen deposition in the space of Disse may contribute to increased intrahepatic resistance [36]. The *dynamic factor* is represented by the active contraction of myofibroblasts and vascular smooth-muscle cells of the intrahepatic veins, and it may be modified by endogenous molecules and pharmacological agents, which affect the intrahepatic vascular resistance. Factors that increase the hepatic vascular resistance include endothelin-1 (ET-1), the alpha-adrenergic stimulus, and angiotensin II. Those decreasing hepatic vascular resistance include NO, prostacyclin, and vasodilating drugs (e.g., organic nitrates, adrenolytics, calcium channel blockers) [15, 37, 38].

Among these endogenous factors, ET-1 and NO play a key role in regulating the hepatic vascular resistance. ET-1 is a powerful vasoconstrictor synthesized by sinusoidal endothelial cells that has been implicated in the increased hepatic vascular resistance of cirrhosis, and in the development of liver fibrosis. NO is a powerful vasodilator substance that is also synthesized by sinusoidal endothelial cells. In the cirrhotic liver, the production of NO is decreased, whereas that of ET-1 is increased. The result of these changes is a net vasoconstrictive effect that, in cirrhosis, accounts for approximately 20–30% of the increased intrahepatic resistance [39–41].

Another dynamic factor that can lead to an increase of intrahepatic vascular resistance is mediated by stellate cells. Hepatic stellate cells (HSCs) are located in the perisinusoidal space of Disse, behind the endothelial barrier, resulting in 5–8% of all human liver cells and 13% of sinusoidal cells. HSCs are involved in vitamin A storage and the synthesis of extracellular matrix components, matrix degrading metalloproteinase, cytokines, and growth factors [42].

HSCs have the capacity to contract or relax in response to vasoactive mediators, such as ET-1 and NO, therefore having a crucial role in controlling intrahepatic vascular resistance and blood flow at sinusoidal level. Indeed, stellate cells become "activated" in response to acute or chronic noxae damaging the liver parenchyma, acquiring a myofibroblast-like phenotype. During HSCs activation, their production of extracellular matrix changes qualitatively and quantitatively, leading to an increase of intravascular resistance.

In summary, in cirrhosis, the increased intrahepatic vascular resistance consists of two main components. The "mechanical factor" is fixed and caused by the structural changes, which occur in patients with chronic liver disease mainly in the form of fibrosis and nodule formation [43, 44]. The "dynamic factor" is variable and caused by endogenous mediators (ET-1 and NO) as well as HSCs activation. The main target of the management of PH is represented by medical therapy directed against the "dynamic factor" to decrease the intrahepatic vascular resistance [45, 46].

Postsinusoidal obstruction includes right-sided heart failure, IVC obstruction, small venules BCS, veno-occlusive disease (VOD). In this setting, WHVP is elevated, whereas HVPG and FHVP can be either normal or elevated, depending on the site of obstruction, intrahepatic postsinusoidal or posthepatic, respectively (Table 68.2). Hepatic VOD is a clinical syndrome occurring early after bone marrow transplantation (BMT) as a result of liver damage by pretransplant conditioning, or chemotherapy for solid tumors. Its incidence in the pediatric BMT population is between 22 and 28 %, with an associated mortality of up to 47 % [47, 48]. The pathologic injury initiates in zone 3 of the liver acinum with subendothelial edema of hepatic venules, fibrin deposition, microthrombosis, venular narrowing, and sclerosis, followed by hepatocyte necrosis [49]. The result is a postsinusoidal increased resistance to hepatic venous outflow resulting in acute PH and, in some cases, multiorgan failure [50–52].

Other Pathogenetic Mechanisms of PH

In some conditions, PH can be caused by the increase of portal venous inflow itself. In patients with an artero-venous communications between the splanchnic arteries and the portal venous system, an *artero-portal fistula* (APF), the portal flow is markedly increased and arterialized, with the consequent development of presinusoidal PH. APF can be acquired or congenital, but the most common causes are hepatic trauma and liver biopsy, and can be asymptomatic or manifest with PH. Long-standing APF can lead to severe PH characterized by arterial Doppler signal in the portal vein, reversal of the portal flow, and thickening/narrowing of the extrahepatic portal vein. In this setting, radiological procedures represent the best treatment option to close the artero-venous fistula and restore a normal portal vein flow; although, in the congenital forms, the fistula often reappears through the development of new spontaneous shunt formation [53].

In 1898 Banti described a disorder characterized by splenomegaly and hypersplenism, resulting in PH and anemia in the absence of hematological and liver disease. The actual existence of the condition has been questioned for a long time due to the lack of explanation for the development of splenomegaly, hypersplenism, and PH in these patients. Nowadays, Banti's syndrome is considered the result of microscopic changes of the portal tract that were not detected at the early stages of its clinical description and corresponding to a group of diseases causing non-cirrhotic PH. *Hepatoportal sclerosis* (HS) is one of the rare disorder characterized by sclerosis of the intrahepatic portal veins resulting in non-cirrhotic PH. HS in children is uncommon but probably underestimated, and only few case reports have been published so far. The cornerstone of the diagnosis of HS is the histology, characterized by portal fibrosis without evidence of either cirrhosis or nodule formation; portal fibrosis is responsible for the increase in the intrahepatic vascular resistance and PH. Nevertheless, the mechanism leading to portal fibrosis and, in general, the entire phenotype of HS are still not well known [54]. Yilmaz reported on 12 pediatric patients with non-cirrhotic PH. On histology, all patients had HS or intimal fibrous thickening of portal vein and periportal fibrosis, acinar transformation, and regenerative nodules not surrounded by fibrous septa. In some of them, there were also signs compatible with cholestatic disease, including neoductular reaction in seven, mild cholangitis in one, and canalicular bile pigment in one [55].

Systemic Hemodynamic Changes in Portal Hypertension

Increased resistance to portal blood flow is likely to be the "primum movens" in the development of PH; however, a variety of hemodynamic changes contribute to amplify the increased portal venous pressure observed in patients with chronic liver disease.

The hyperdynamic syndrome was first described in the 1950s, when some physicians observed that patients with cirrhosis often showed "warm extremities, cutaneous vascular spiders, wide pulse pressure and capillary pulsations in the nail beds." In 1953, Kowalski and Abelmann published the first study which demonstrated an increase in cardiac output and a decrease in peripheral vascular resistance in patients with alcohol-induced cirrhosis [56]. The recognition of the dangerous effect of this syndrome on multiple organs, though, was achieved only several years later [57].

Vasodilatation plays a key role in the development of the hemodynamic changes. The hyperdynamic syndrome should be better called "progressive vasodilatatory syndrome," because vasodilatation is the main factor that brings about all the vascular changes and finally the multiorgan involvement seen in cirrhosis [58]. A major step ahead in this field was accomplished in the 1990s, when researchers discovered that

NO was responsible for the vasodilatation and, in turn, of the multiple organ malfunctions characterizing the hyperdynamic circulation [59].

Both clinical studies and animal models have demonstrated and explained the hemodynamic events that occur in PH but, since they have not been performed in children, the findings should be interpreted with caution (Fig. 68.2).

Splanchnic Circulation Vasodilation of the splanchnic circulation is a process mediated by humoral vasodilatatory agents, and it is probably the initial signal triggering the hyperdynamic systemic circulation. Splanchnic vasodilation causes, as a consequence, an increased portal venous blood inflow, contributing to the maintenance and the aggravation of PH [57, 60]. The result of this significant vasodilation is that a large proportion of circulating blood volume remains confined to the splanchnic system, with a subsequent reduction of central blood volume. This process is called the "forward flow" theory and provides a rationale for the use of vasoconstrictors in adult patients with PH [12].

Systemic Circulation Splanchnic vasodilation is associated with changes in the systemic circulation, such as a decrease of arterial pressure, that is consequence of the decreased central blood volume and peripheral resistance in various organs [61]. Compensatory mechanisms include the activation of baro- and volume receptors as well as the production of neurohormonal substances leading to sodium and water retention, with plasma volume expansion and increase in cardiac output [62].

The cardiac response is directly related to splanchnic vasodilatation and plasma volume expansion, together with an increased venous return that is mostly due to the formation of porto-systemic shunts. Although vasodilatation is essential as the initiating factor, no hyperdynamic circulation occurs without expansion of plasma volume and porto-systemic shunting [63]. The former is due to renal sodium retention, which has been shown to precede the increase in cardiac output, and can be prevented or reversed by sodium restriction and administration of spironolactone. The latter is characterized by the development of new veins (called collateral vessels) bypassing the liver and decompressing the portal venous system. These veins directly connect the portal blood vessels to veins that divert the blood away from the liver into the systemic circulation. The drawback in this compensatory process is that substances (such as ammonia and toxins) that are normally removed from the blood by the liver, pass directly into the systemic circulation, and have adverse effects in other organs [64].

Collateral vessels tend to develop at the lower end of the esophagus and at the upper part of the stomach (Fig. 68.1).

Here, the vessels enlarge and become full of twists and turns, becoming varicose veins in the esophagus (EV) or stomach (gastric varices). Other collateral vessels may develop on the abdominal wall and in the rectum. These vessels are prone to rupture, leading to GI bleeding.

Lung Circulation PH and liver shunting may also affect the lungs, resulting in the development of hepatopulmonary syndrome (HPS) and porto-pulmunary hypertension (PPH); these conditions are characterized by hypoxia due to pulmonary artero-venous shunts and pulmonary hypertension, respectively [65]. Although the intrinsic mechanism triggering these complications is not fully known, the major role seems to be played by molecules active on the pulmonary endothelium (including NO and carbon monoxide) that can cause either condition [66, 67].

Renal Circulation Renal circulation is affected indirectly by the hyperdynamic state. To balance the progressive systemic vasodilation, the kidney responds to a perceived hypovolemia by retaining sodium and water. The relative hypovolemia results from an increase of the vascular compartment caused by vasodilatation, leading to the activation of vasoconstrictive and volume-retaining neurohumoral substances that perpetuate sodium and water retention [68]. These compensatory mechanisms include the activation of renin–angiotensin–aldosterone system and antidiuretic hormone secretion. In the early course of the disease, the intravascular volume and the cardiac output increase to maintain the arterial perfusion pressure [69]. With the progression of the disease, vasodilatation worsens, and the cardiac output continues to increase up to a maximum, and then it is not enough to maintain the perfusion pressure. At this point, the renal blood flow drops and renal failure develops [70, 71].

The hyperdynamic circulation should not be considered a complication of cirrhosis but a complication of PH. In fact, it was observed also in non-cirrhotic subjects and confirmed in different experimental models of PH [57, 59].

Clinical Manifestation of Portal Hypertension

PH in children has a broad spectrum of clinical manifestations, varying from the occasional finding of splenomegaly discovered during a routine follow-up visit in absence of any symptom, to hematemesis and melena due to the rupture of EV (Table 68.3). The main manifestations of PH are GH, ascites, and splenomegaly, but, in a minority of patients, other complications may arise including hepatic encephalopathy (HE), pulmonary vascular disorders, and kidney disease [72].

Table 68.3 Clinical evaluation and investigations useful to recognize patients with suspected portal hypertension

Step	Aim
Clinical history	Ask for neonatal umbilical catheterization, episodes of gastrointestinal bleeding, results of previous blood tests, investigations for an undefined splenomegaly
Physical examination	Assess liver size and consistency, look for splenomegaly, abdominal venous patterning (site and direction of venous flow), spider naevi and telangectasias, palmar erythema, ascites, limbs edema
Liver function tests	Assess liver function and full blood count for hypersplenism
Ultrasonography and Doppler of the liver	Evaluate liver parenchyma, patency of portal vein and direction of venous blood flow, hepatic veins patency, venous anatomical abnormalities, hepatic artery (patency and abnormalities), porto-systemic shunts, ascites, splenomegaly, renal abnormalities
Upper endoscopy	Assess varices and hypertensive gastropathy
CT scan of the abdomen	Assess liver parenchyma, biliary tree conformation, vascular anatomy, Rex recessus patency and signs of portal hypertensive biliopathy
Measure portal venous pressure (HVPG, WHVP, FHVP)	Evaluate the degree of portal hypertension. Diagnose prehepatic, intrahepatic, posthepatic causes
Liver biopsy	Assess fibrosis/cirrhosis, inflammation, histological pattern

CT computed tomography, *HVPG* hepatic venous pressure gradient, *WHVP* wedge hepatic venous pressure, *FHVP* free hepatic venous pressure

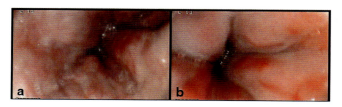

Fig. 68.3 Endoscopic appearance of large esophageal varices with red signs in two children with portal hypertension. (Reprinted from Ref. [73], with permission from Elsevier)

Gastrointestinal Hemorrhage

GH is defined as bleeding in the digestive tract, and it can be classified as proximal or distal, acute or chronic. Bleeding from the upper digestive tract (esophagus, stomach, and upper portion of the small intestine) causes hematemesis and melena, whereas bleeding from the lower digestive tract (lower portion of the small intestine, large intestine, and rectum) causes dark blood or bright red blood mixed with stool, depending on the proximity to the anal sphincter. GH is mainly related to bleeding from EV and also, in a minority of cases, from portal hypertensive gastropathy, gastric antral vascular ectasia, or gastric, duodenal, peristomal, or rectal varices (Fig. 68.3).

Acute GH is often the first symptom of a long-standing silent liver disease, and therefore it is regarded by patients and carers as a frightening event, giving the impression of imminent death. Although the mortality from GI bleeding in children is lower than in adults, acute GH remains a life-threatening event and requires prompt medical intervention. Chronic bleeding is usually mild and can be discovered since the patient has refractory iron-deficiency anemia and positive fecal occult blood test [73].

The formation of varices and their rupture result from the increased pressure within the vessel as a consequence of PH. When the wall tension exceeds the variceal wall strength,

the rupture of the varix occurs, and the patient develops hematemesis and/or melena [74].

Variceal bleeding in children with chronic liver disease often follows an acute upper respiratory tract infection, with the contribution of several factors such as the increased abdominal pressure during coughing or sneezing, the increased cardiac output due to fever, and the erosive effect of nonsteroidal anti-inflammatory drugs used to treat the fever. Gastroesophageal reflux is another factor which may contribute to erosions of varices leading to its rupture and bleeding [75–77].

Hematemesis and melena are the most common presenting symptoms in children with both intrahepatic and extrahepatic PH, and the first episode can be as early as 2 months of age [2, 22, 78–80].

The age at the first bleeding episode is related to the underlying etiology. In children with biliary atresia, the first bleed was described at a mean age of 3 years, while in children with cirrhosis due to cystic fibrosis it occurred at 11.5 years [74, 81]. In a recent study, 65 children with EHPVO were followed for a median period of time of 8.4 years. Thirty-two (49%) patients presented with bleeding at a median age of 3.8 years (0.5–15.5) and, during the follow-up period, 43 of them (66%) had at least one bleeding episode [2]. Triger et al. followed 44 children with EHPVO for a mean follow-up of 8 years. The actuarial probability of bleeding was 49% at age 16 years and 76% at 24 years of age. If the child bled before 12 years of age, the probability of bleeding was higher than in those who had not bled before 12 years of age. Further, there was no evidence of variceal regression over time. These studies do not support the previous hypothesis that variceal bleeding decreased in adolescence due to the development of spontaneous porto-systemic collaterals [2, 82]. In a multicenter Italian study on 187 children with EHPVO, the mean age at diagnosis was 4 years, and the most common symptoms at onset were splenomegaly (39.5%) and bleeding (36.6%). In 71 patients with an available endoscopy at presentation, 62 (87.3%) had already developed EV. Development of EHPVO was strictly associated with a neonatal disorder including history of prematurity, neonatal illness, and umbilical venous catheter. Authors concluded that a liver Doppler ultrasound should be performed before discharge from the neonatal unit and at the follow-up to allow an early recognition of the disease and avoid bleeding from EV that are present from the early stages (personal, unpublished data). Since splenomegaly is a very common sign detected in children with PH at the time of GI bleeding, the association between GI bleeding and splenomegaly should be suggestive of PH until proven otherwise [74].

There is no strong evidence supporting the efficacy of any treatment for the prevention of variceal bleeding in children. The administration of nonselective β-blockers (NSBBs), the endoscopic treatment of varices, and the surgical (meso-rex bypass, porto-systemic shunts) and radiological (TIPS) measures to decompress the portal system represent the main therapeutic options for the primary and secondary prophylaxis of bleeding in children with PH [73, 83].

Splenomegaly

Splenomegaly indicates an enlargement of the spleen usually associated with an overactivity of the spleen, defined hypersplenism, which leads to premature destruction of blood cells. Splenomegaly is due to PH which causes at the beginning only spleen congestion and eventually tissue hyperplasia and fibrosis. The increase in spleen size is followed by an increase in splenic blood flow, which participates in PH actively congesting the portal system [84]. Together with EV, splenomegaly represents the most common finding in children with PH even though, in asymptomatic children, it is often discovered accidentally during a routine physical examination.

Despite a big spleen is highly suggestive for PH, many children with liver disease and isolated splenomegaly have often a delayed diagnosis. In clinical practice, splenomegaly accompanied by hypersplenism is considered a sign of hematological disorders, leading to a long hematological follow-up (including bone marrow aspiration and biopsy) before asking consultation to a hepatologist. Due to the large spleen, children with PVT often receive a diagnosis of infectious mononucleosis every time they come to clinical attention because of a viral illness, and PH is disclosed only after a bleeding episode.

Liver function tests and Doppler ultrasound are mandatory in healthy children with splenomegaly and hypersplenism to exclude the presence of EHPVO and avoid worthless procedures [74, 85].

Some studies have tried to identify the best noninvasive method to diagnose the presence of EV in children with PH.

Platelet count and splenomegaly are usually considered the most reliable parameter to predict the presence di EV. The clinical prediction rule proposed by Gana has high predictive value (area under the receiver operating characteristic; ROC curve 0.80) and is calculated according to the following formula: $(0.75 \times \text{platelets})/(\text{spleen z score} + 5) + 2.5 \times \text{albumin}$ [86].

Once liver transplantation (LTX) or porto-systemic shunting is performed, splenomegaly and hypersplenism may improve significantly, but sometimes they persist for long, depending on the grade of splenic hyperplasia and fibrosis developed over time [87, 88].

Ascites

Ascites is the accumulation of serous fluid in the peritoneal cavity, and is usually seen in patients with PH due to cirrhosis. Ascites appears when the hydrostatic pressure goes above the osmotic pressure within the hepatic and mesenteric capillaries, and the transfer of fluids from blood vessels to lymphatics overcomes the drainage capacity of the lymphatic system [89].

Ascites should be analyzed to obtain information on its cause and possible complications. The serum ascites albumin gradient (SAAG) is used to classify ascites into portal and non-portal hypertensive etiologies. The SAAG is calculated by subtracting the ascitic fluid albumin level value from the serum albumin value, and the result correlates directly with portal pressure. This phenomenon is the effect of Starling's forces between the fluid of the circulatory system and ascitic fluid, as albumin does not move across membranes easily, because it is a large molecule. Under normal circumstances, the SAAG is ≤1.1 g/dl because serum oncotic pressure (pulling fluid back into circulation) is exactly compensated by the serum hydrostatic pressure (which pushes fluid out of the circulatory system). In presence of PH, there is an increase in the hydrostatic pressure causing more fluid and more albumin to move from the circulation into the peritoneal space with ascites formation. As a consequence, the SAAG increases (≥1.1 g/dl). Thus, a high gradient (SAAG ≥1.1 g/dl) indicates that the ascites is due to PH, whereas a low gradient (SAAG ≤1.1 g/dl) indicates that ascites is not associated with increased portal pressure (Table 68.4). In clinical practice, some conditions may influence the proper value of the SAAG including the sampling of ascites and serum in different states of hydration or the impact of serum globulin concentration [90, 91].

Ascites should also be evaluated for spontaneous bacterial peritonitis (SBP), an ascitic fluid infection without an evident intra-abdominal surgically treatable source. The diagnosis is made by ascitic fluid cell count. The absolute polymorphonuclear cell (PMN) count in the ascitic fluid is

Table 68.4 Causes of ascites based on serum ascites albumin gradient (*SAAG*)

SAAG ≥1.1 g/dl = portal hypertension	SAAG ≤1.1 g/dl = other causes of ascites
Cirrhosis	Peritoneal lymphoma
Non-cirrhotic liver disease	Serositis
Fulminant hepatic failure	Chronic peritoneal infection
	Tubercolosis
	Other (bacteria, viruses, fungi)
Vascular/heart disease	Low serum colloid osmotic pressure
Portal vein thrombosis	Nephrotic syndrome
Veno-occlusive disease	Protein-losing gastroenteropathy
Budd–Chiari syndrome	Kwashiorkor
IVC obstruction/right heart failure	Hollow organ leak
Benign and malignant neoplasms	Lymphatic
Mixedema	Other (pancreatic, biliary, intestinal)

IVC inferior vena cava, *TBC* tuberculosis

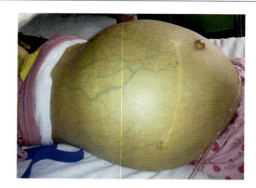

Fig. 68.4 Tense ascites and abdominal venous patterning in a child with biliary atresia, failed Kasai, and end-stage liver disease

calculated by multiplying the total white blood cell count (or total "nucleated cell" count) by the percentage of PMNs in the differential. The diagnosis of SBP is established by an elevated ascitic fluid absolute PMN count (≥250 cells/mm^3), a positive ascitic fluid bacterial culture, and absence of secondary causes of peritonitis [92]. Patients with SBP should receive antibiotic therapy, such as intravenous third-generation cephalosporin, and be considered for liver transplantation.

Treatment of ascites includes salt and fluid restriction and use of diuretics. Spironolactone is the diuretic of choice as it is an aldosterone antagonist counteracting the endocrine changes of the hyperdynamic circulation, but often there is the need to add a loop diuretic, such as furosemide, that can improve diuresis and counteract hyperkalemia. In children with normal liver synthetic and biliary function, ascites can often be managed with diuretics and occasional paracentesis (Fig. 68.4). Paracentesis has been utilized safely in children and is indicated when ascites is large and not responding to diuretics [93, 94]. When ascites does not recede, recurs shortly after paracentesis, or when children do not tolerate diuretic therapy due to side effects, the management can take advantage of more aggressive treatment including regular large-volume paracentesis and, if feasible, TIPS. TIPS procedure, although uncommon in children, provided good results in term of resolution of refractory ascites in both native and transplanted livers [88].

When ascites is accompanied by signs of end-stage liver disease, such as hypoalbuminemia, jaundice, clotting derangement, or SBP, the only effective treatment is liver transplantation. In these cases, albumin infusions can be used along with diuretics, in order to increase the osmotic pressure and facilitate the passage of fluid from the extravascular to the intravascular

compartment. In children with end-stage liver disease, ascites can be associated with hyponatremia, which is a risk factor for severe complications and death. Pugliese et al. evaluated the association of pretransplant variables with the mortality within 90 days following the inclusion on the waiting list of 520 children with cirrhosis. On multivariate analysis, the presence of ascites and serum sodium levels were associated with decreased patient survival while awaiting a liver graft [95].

Chylous ascites is a rare clinical condition marked by an extravasation into the peritoneal cavity of a milky fluid deriving from the mesenteric lymphatic vessels. Usually, it results from major abdominal surgical interventions, such as liver transplantation, during which several lymphatic vessels are inadvertently resected and PH has not yet resolved; nevertheless, chylous ascites can present also in patients with PH due to PVT or congenital portal venous malformation. In this setting, in spite of the absence of strong evidences, the management includes fat-free diet and somatostatin analogues [96].

Pulmonary Complications

Children with PH may develop two rare pulmonary complications: hepatopulmonary syndrome (HPS) and portopulmonary hypertension (PPH). Their relative frequency and risk factors have not been defined, and only isolated cases or small series have been published so far.

The pathogenesis of HPS and PPH remains unclear, but the two conditions arise only in patients with porto-systemic shunting, and therefore the pathogenesis must be related to it. The proposed theories suggest that these disorders result from a combination of the hyperdynamic circulation, the increased cardiac output, the sheer injury to the vascular walls, and an imbalance of circulating vasoactive peptides. Abnormal hepatic synthesis of vasoactive peptides, such as EN-1, or impaired hepatic metabolism of intestinally derived endotoxins, cytokines, and neurohormones may result in these substances reaching the pulmonary vascular bed via porto-systemic shunting, directly altering the vessel tone or leading to pulmonary vascular inflammation and remodeling. The resulting pathology is strikingly different in these two disorders, with vasodilation of pulmonary arterioles and capillaries causing artero-venous shunting in HPS, and intimal fibrosis with endothelial and smooth-muscle cell proliferation leading to increased pulmonary vascular resistance in PPH [97–99].

HPS is defined as intrapulmonary vascular shunting (IPVS), ventilation–perfusion mismatch and chronic hypoxemia in a setting of liver disease and/or PH. The mechanisms implicated in the development of HPS are likely to include many of the vasoactive substances involved in the genesis of the hyperdynamic circulation, including NO and EN-1 [100–102]. Porto-systemic shunting plays a key role in the pathogenesis of the HPS; in fact, HPS has been described also in patients with congenital porto-systemic shunting and no liver disease (i.e., the Abernethy malformation).

From the clinical point of view, HPS is characterized by shortness of breath, exercise intolerance, and digital clubbing. Since the disease is often subtle and progresses slowly, in the early stages it can be easily overlooked and become overt only when advanced. Patients with PH should be screened for HPS by measuring the transcutaneous oxygen saturation and, if <96%, by performing further investigations to assess the real presence of IPVS. The two main procedures to confirm the presence of IPVS are the echocardiography with agitated saline and the macroaggregated albumin scan. The former is simple and sensitive in both symptomatic and asymptomatic children. The latter may be used to quantify the degree of shunting, which can be useful in clinical decision-making and to test the progression of HPS over time [103–105].

Liver transplantation represents the only effective treatment option for children with HPS. Al-Hussaini et al. reported a study on 18 children with HPS over 14 years. Fourteen underwent LTX with resolution of HPS in 13. Six developed vascular or biliary complications and four died (two before transplantation) [106].

PPH is defined as an elevation of the mean pulmonary arterial pressure and increased vascular resistance caused by a pulmonary arteriopathy, in the setting of PH and in the absence of underlying cardiopulmonary disease [105]. The pathophysiology of this disorder is still unclear; however, it seems to be related to a decreased hepatic clearance and porto-systemic shunting of biochemical mediators in the setting of liver dysfunction and PH. PPH produces characteristic histological changes in the pulmonary vasculature that have been well documented on autoptic samples [107].

Although there are scant data in children, it has been shown that PPH can develop in patients with cirrhotic and non-cirrhotic causes of PH such as biliary atresia, PVT, focal nodular hyperplasia, and congenital hepatic fibrosis [108].

From the clinical point of view, PPH presents most commonly with exertional dyspnea, fatigue, palpitations, and syncope or chest pain. The symptoms are often subtle at onset, so that a high index of suspicion is required to diagnose PPH in asymptomatic patients before they develop severe and irreversible pulmonary hypertension [107]. Echocardiography with Doppler flow is considered the most useful screening modality in patients with suspected pulmonary hypertension, although limited by the fact that it relies on the presence of tricuspidal regurgitation, it measures systolic rather than mean pressure in the right ventricle and the measurement is approximate. Chest X-ray and electrocardiogram (ECG) definitely lack sensitivity. If there are indirect signs of pulmonary hypertension at ECG, further evaluation should include a right heart catheter study and, in some cases, high-resolution computed tomography (CT) of the chest and ventilation-perfusion lung scanning [104].

If the diagnosis of PPH is made early before the development of irreversible pulmonary vasculopathy, LTX can be successfully performed and may reverse the process. Conversely, once PPH is advanced (with a mean pulmonary pressure >35 mmHg) and associated with right-sided heart failure, LTX becomes unfeasible because of the functionally obstructed liver outflow that leads to graft failure and death in at least 50% of cases. More recently, it has been shown that the perioperative use of inhaled and intravenous pulmonary vasodilators (NO and epoprostenol) as well as oral drugs (sildenafil and bosentan) can remarkably reduce the pulmonary pressure to a safe level, allowing to perform LTX [108]. The goal of treatment is, therefore, lowering the mean pulmonary arterial pressure and move the patient from high risk to a safer ground for transplantation. However, if there is no response or the pressures remain very high, the only viable option is a combined lung–liver transplant.

Other Major Complications of Portal Hypertension

An abnormal *abdominal venous patterning* can be seen in children with PH, in whom a prominent subcutaneous vascular pattern develops as part of spontaneous porto-collateral shunting (Fig. 68.4). This is the result of the attempt at decompressing the portal venous system through the umbilical vein recanalization that leads to periumbilical collaterals. Although less common than in adults, both umbilical venous shunts and rectal varices can be observed in children with long-standing PH, whereas in children with PH and an intestinal stoma (i.e., in short bowel syndrome associated with liver disease), stomal varices often occur and represent a site of low resistance and bleeding [109].

Hepatorenal syndrome (HRS) is defined as a functional renal failure in patients with liver disease and PH, and it constitutes the climax of the systemic circulatory changes associated with PH [91]. In pediatric patients, HRS is rare, probably due to the relatively short time that cirrhotic children spend on the transplantation waiting list. Two types of HRS have been identified. Type 1 HRS is an acute and rapidly progressive form that often develops after a precipitating factor such as GI bleeding or SBP. Type 2 HRS is a slowly progressive form of renal failure that often occurs without a sudden trigger in the setting of chronic and refractory ascites. HRS arises from severe vasoconstriction of the renal circulation to compensate for the characteristic circulatory imbalance of advanced cirrhosis. This leads to an increased renal arterial resistance which in turn causes renal hypoperfusion and arterial hypotension. The small volume of the produced ultrafiltrate is then reabsorbed almost completely in the proximal tubule, whereas no solutes (such as sodium) flow to the Henle's loop with nearly no hyperosmolar natriuresis, activation of adiuretin–vasopressin and reduced urine output. As a result, standard diuretic treatment has little effect on diuresis [110]. The criteria to diagnose HRS are difficult to be applied in young children because of the lack of pediatric data. HRS is a potentially reversible condition, but its natural prognosis is poor. Various vasoconstrictors are useful in the treatment of HRS, and terlipressin is the first choice [111]. In the pediatric setting, the experience is little. In a report, four children with end-stage liver disease received terlipressin treatment for renal failure compatible with HRS type 1 in three and type 2 in one. All four responded well and no side effects were reported [112]. Liver transplantation is the ultimate treatment for HRS, ensuring full recovery and long-term survival, and thus it remains the principal tool both in adults and children.

Hepatic encephalopathy (HE) refers to a variety of reversible neurological abnormalities reported in patients with cirrhosis and PH associated with anatomical and functional porto-systemic shunting. In children, HE can be subtle, and the condition seems to appear at a later stage of liver disease and be difficult to diagnose, especially in ill infants. Disturbed consciousness (including coma), personality changes, intellectual deterioration, and speech and motor dysfunction are common in older children with HE. These symptoms usually have a sudden onset and a rapid reversibility suggesting they are of metabolic origin [113].

Protein diet restriction, cleansing enemas, oral antibiotic, and lactulose are the most effective medical options to prevent and treat HE [114, 115].

Non-cirrhotic Portal Hypertension

Non-cirrhotic PH (NCPH) is a heterogeneous group of liver disorders characterized by PH in absence of cirrhosis and with normal or only mildly elevated HVPG values [116].

They are of crucial importance in pediatric hepatology since, while the majority of children with cirrhotic PH are treated with liver transplantation successfully in the early years of the life, those with NCPH do not have any indication for LTX and are managed and followed up for a long time up to adult age [73].

In relation to the site of increased vascular resistance to blood flow, such disorders may be classified as prehepatic, hepatic, and posthepatic. Among presinusoidal NCPH disorders, non-cirrhotic portal fibrosis (NCPF) and EHPVO represent two different entities in whom features of PH are not associated to significant parenchymal dysfunction [116].

NCPF is mostly a disorder of young adults or middle-aged women, whereas non-cirrhotic EHPVO is reported both in infancy and in older children. Recently, it has been proposed the so-called unifying hypothesis, providing a common explanation to the pathogenesis of both NCPF and EHPVO, and focusing on thrombotic events affecting the portal branches. The authors hypothesize that a major thrombotic event occurring at early ages and involving the portal trunk results in EHPVO, whereas repeated microthrombotic events occurring later in life and affecting the small or medium branches of the portal vein would lead to NCPF [117]. In this session, we focus on such two disorders. NCPF is a rather unknown liver disorder in children, whereas EHPVO represents the most common cause of NCPH in the pediatric population.

Non-cirrhotic Portal Fibrosis (NCPF)

The clinical pattern of presentation of NCPF is that of PH in the absence of an evident cause, such as liver fibrosis/cirrhosis or vascular obstruction. NCPF is also named idiopathic PH (IPH), idiopathic non-cirrhotic portal hypertension (INCPH), hepatoportal sclerosis (HS), and obliterative venopathy [116].

On histology, the main features include phlebosclerosis, fibroelastosis, periportal and perisinusoidal fibrosis, aberrant vessels in portal tract (portal angiomatosis) with preserved lobular architecture, and differential atrophy. The main portal vein branch is dilated, with thick sclerosed walls, along with thrombosis in the medium and small portal vein branches, giving a picture of "obliterative portal venopathy" [118, 119]. However, in children, these features are often subtle and the condition may be overlooked.

The etiology of NCPF is undefined, but the attention has been brought to various factors that may trigger autoimmunity or endotoxin-mediated injury leading to vascular abnormalities, which cause presinusoidal block to the portal venous flow. The interest has been pointed particularly on lack of hygienic conditions, that would support the role of infections as trigger of the disease, and prothrombotic disorders, that would support the association with an underlying prothrombotic state [120].

The diagnosis of NCPF is based on clinical evidence of PH without liver dysfunction and a histology with no significant fibrosis. The Asian Pacific Association for the study of the liver (APASL) has proposed some criteria for the diagnosis of NCPF in adults [121]. Recently, Schouten et al. redefined five criteria including:

1. Any one of the following clinical signs of PH: splenomegaly, EV, ascites, raised HVPG, and evidence of portosystemic collaterals
2. Exclusion of cirrhosis on liver biopsy
3. Exclusion of known causes of chronic liver disease causing cirrhotic or non-cirrhotic PH
4. Exclusion of common conditions causing NCPH
5. Patent portal and hepatic veins

All five criteria must be fulfilled to diagnose NCPF [122].

In adults, the most common symptoms at onset include bleeding from varix rupture, splenomegaly with or without hypersplenism, and ascites in 10–34% of the cases. On physical examination, the liver may be normal, enlarged, or slightly shrunken, whereas the clinical signs of chronic liver disease are absent [123]. Liver function tests are usually normal in NCPF, but derangements in liver enzymes, prothrombin time, and albumin are seen in a small proportion of adult patients [124].

Hemodynamic studies showed that the increased vascular resistance in NCPF is pre- and perisinusoidal. HVPG is normal or slightly elevated (median 7 mmHg) in this condition [125].

In adults, the natural history of NCPF seems benign, with an overall good outcome. However, in the long term, 30–33% of the adults develop liver atrophy and possible decompensation, development of PVT, HPS, and, sometimes, need for LTX [126, 127].

In childhood, NCPF is an uncommon cause of PH but, since the awareness among pediatric specialists is still low, this condition is probably underdiagnosed. The published experiences in this disease are scarce, and they come mainly from Asiatic regions.

There are no standardized criteria to make the diagnosis of NCPF in children. Although the Schouten criteria may be utilized also in the pediatric population, in children, in the early phase of the disease, the first criterion may not be satisfied due to the delayed onset of clinical signs of PH.

Girard et al. reported a child with Adams–Oliver syndrome and HS. They hypothesized that a vascular anomaly and thrombosis may be the etiology for this condition based on the fact that the patient had PVT and Factor V Leiden mutation. However, the same association has not been described in other children so far [128].

Prolonged exposure to several medications and toxins has also been proposed as possible causes. Indian studies on children with PH showed that, among 134 cases, 29 (22%) were due to NCPF. The authors carried out a sociodemographic study that found a significant association with residency in arsenic-affected areas [129]. Toxins can surely lead to liver injury but a strong association between arsenic intoxication and development of NCPF has not been proven.

Poddar published the experience on 388 Indian children with PH (median age 11 years). Eleven of them (3%) were diagnosed with NCPF. Variceal bleeding, splenomegaly, and a lump in the left upper abdomen were the most common symptoms at onset [130]. Cantez described 12 children (median age 13.5 years) with a histological diagnosis of HS. Four patients had splenomegaly, three had EV, one had developed HPS and had been transplanted, whereas the others did not show symptoms of PH [131]. Yilmaz reported on 12 children who had a diagnosis of HS, but some of them had also cholestatic features on histology. The authors concluded that cholestatic features noticed in histopathological evaluation may represent a variant group in the spectrum of this disease [55]. A special mention is needed for HIV-related NCPF. The condition occurs predominantly in males (50–100%), homosexuals (50–75%), with a prolonged infection (median 11.5 years, range 7–15 years). It is not known whether the development of NCPF is related to the infection or rather to the antiretroviral treatment. A recent study described a 10-year-old HIV-infected girl who was on antiretroviral therapy. She had splenomegaly and presented with a massive bleeding from EV rupture. The liver biopsy showed features compatible with NCPF. HVPG was normal. She was managed successfully by treatment with β-blockers and endoscopic variceal eradication [132]. Further studies are warranted to best define the real frequency of NCPF in children, and to understand the underlying pathogenetic mechanisms leading to PH, in order to define the best therapeutic strategy.

Extrahepatic Portal Vein Obstruction

EHPVO is defined by the obstruction of the extrahepatic portal vein with or without the involvement of the intrahepatic portal veins. It may include occlusion of the splenic, superior mesenteric, and coronary veins, but excludes the isolated thrombosis of the SV. It is the most common cause of noncirrhotic, presinusoidal, and prehepatic PH in children [72].

EHPVO represents also the most common disease on long-term care of PH, since these patients do not progress to end-stage liver disease and have no indication for liver transplantation. As a consequence, they represent the group of pediatric patients in whom there is the largest experience with long-term complications and care of PH [78, 133]. EHPVO is primarily a childhood disorder but can present at any age from few months to adulthood.

The etiology of EHPVO is not yet well defined, but various factors including umbilical vascular catheterization, sepsis, and an underlying hypercoagulable states (or thrombophilia) play a key role in the pathogenesis of the thrombus formation. Due to that a full hypercoagulability panel, including genetic factors, has to be performed whenever the diagnosis is made [22]. Pathogenetic mechanisms which lead to PH are mainly related to the increased vascular resistance in the portal venous system due to thrombus formation. The formation of the portal cavernoma represents a tentative to bypass the thrombus and replace a physiological portal venous flow.

Studies on adult patients with EHPVO have been performed to assess the role of PH in producing changes in splanchnic and systemic circulation in the absence of liver dysfunction. They demonstrated an increase in the cardiac index and a decrease in the total peripheral resistance in patients with EHPVO compared to control patients, suggesting the presence of a hyperdynamic circulation also in patients with a normal liver function. Systemic and pulmonary hemodynamic changes have been evaluated in adults with EHPVO and compared with a group of controls represented by patients with compensated cirrhosis. The authors considered the measurements of cardiac index (by Fick's oxygen method), and systemic and pulmonary vascular resistance indices. Both patients with EHPVO and cirrhosis had similar values, confirming that patients with EHPVO have a hyperdynamic circulation similarly to cirrhotic compensated patients who have the same degree of PH [78, 134, 135]. These studies suggest a predominant role of PH *per se* in the genesis of systemic and pulmonary hemodynamic alterations [136].

Expanded plasma volume, development of porto-systemic venous collaterals and increased venous return to the heart seem to be the main factors which cause and maintain hyperdynamic circulation in patients with EHPVO [133, 137–140].

There are no studies evaluating the presence of a hyperdynamic circulation in children with EHPVO. Radiological procedures to assess hemodynamic changes (i.e., HVPG, right atrial pressure, pulmonary arterial pressure, pulmonary wedge pressure, and mean arterial pressure) are considered too invasive and are not routinely performed in children except in selected cases [125].

Nevertheless, children with EHPVO usually do not show symptoms compatible with the hyperdynamic circulation such as warm extremities, cutaneous vascular spiders, wide pulse pressure, and capillary pulsations in the nail beds. Even major complications of the hyperdynamic circulation of cirrhosis (high cardiac output, HRS, SBP), described in animal models and adult patients, are not common in children with EHPVO. The symptoms are rather those related to PH complications including GI bleeding, splenomegaly with or without hypersplenism, and ascites. Abdominal pain, ascites, or fever in the absence of portal cavernoma and porto-systemic collaterals are suspected for PVT with

an acute presentation (pylephlebitis). On physical examination, the liver is normal or shrunken. Liver function tests are usually normal, at least in the early phases, whereas they can be deranged in the long term [141]; in fact, the increase of γ-glutamyl transpeptidase, total bilirubin, and bile salts in this setting should raise the suspicion of the development of portal hypertensive biliopathy (PHB) [142–144].

In clinical practice, EHPVO is considered a less severe form of PH. The patients may be asymptomatic for many years, and the mortality from bleeding appeared to be negligible in this group of patients [145, 146]. The diagnosis is based on Doppler ultrasound, CT scan, or nuclear magnetic resonance (NMR), which demonstrate portal vein obstruction, presence of intraluminal material, or portal vein cavernoma [72, 147].

Invasive procedures, such as transjugular retrograde or percutaneous transhepatic portal venography, should be undertaken when uncertainty persists. Liver biopsy is not essential for the diagnosis unless an underlying chronic liver disease is suspected, but, when performed, has shown a picture similar to what is described in NCPF. Echocardiography may rule out associated congenital heart disease, and look for HPS or PPH. Children with EHPVO are usually diagnosed years after the event. Anticoagulation therapy is not indicated outside of the acute phase, unless a hypercoagulable state has been documented [11].

Growth Retardation

Incidence and natural history of EHPVO in children is not well defined. The morbidity is mainly related to variceal bleeding, hypersplenism, and overall limitation of quality of life. The management of variceal bleeding in non-cirrhotic PH does not differ from what we described in cirrhotic patients. However, other complications, in both the short and the long term, need to be further elucidated. Growth retardation represents an import complication in this setting. Failure to thrive in children with EHPVO depends on duration of PH and declines further with age despite appropriate energy intake. The pathogenetic mechanisms may include the reduced portal blood supply to the liver and the consequent deprivation of hepatotropic factors, the poor substrate utilization associated with the malabsorption due to portal hypertensive enteropathy, as well as growth hormone resistance. Restoration of portal blood flow to the liver that follows a successful meso-portal bypass (MPB) results in improved growth in these patients [148–150] (Fig. 68.5).

Portal Hypertensive Biliopathy

Patients with EHPVO occurring in infancy almost invariably develop radiological evidence of PHB as young adults; nevertheless, only 20–30% develop clinical signs of cholestasis [151]. PHB is a disorder characterized by anatomical and functional abnormalities of the intrahepatic, extrahepatic,

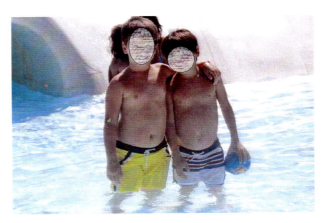

Fig. 68.5 Dizygotic twins born preterm. One developed portal vein thrombosis and shows evident growth retardation

and pancreatic ducts occurring most commonly in patients with non-cirrhotic PH [142]. Abnormalities of the biliary tree include intrahepatic biliary radicles dilatation, caliber irregularities, displacements, ectasias, strictures, and common bile duct stones [144]. The pathogenesis is mainly related to long-standing portal cavernoma in the biliary and peribiliary region, causing compressive and ischemic changes of the biliary tree, and more frequently in the left hepatic duct [143]. When symptomatic, PHB presents with jaundice, biliary colic, abdominal pain, and recurrent cholangitis. Magnetic resonance cholangiopancreatography (MRCP) is the first-choice tool to diagnose PHB in children. [152]. The decision to treat biliary obstruction in these patients depends on the presence of symptoms. In asymptomatic patients no intervention is recommended. In symptomatic children, biliary stenting (by endoscopic retrograde cholangiopancreatography, ERCP, or percutaneous transhepatic colangiography, PTC) may temporarily improve the symptoms restoring a normal bile flow. Nevertheless, some patients may require shunt or bypass surgery to decompress the biliary varices and resolve the obstruction [151].

Minimal Hepatic Encephalopathy

HE is a brain dysfunction caused by liver insufficiency and/or porto-systemic shunting; it manifests as a wide spectrum of neurological/psychiatric abnormalities ranging from subclinical alterations to coma. The subclinical manifestation of HE, which is called minimal HE (MHE), is detectable by the alteration of at least two specific psychometric tests or electrophysiological techniques [114]. Nowadays, the term covert HE is also used to refer to all the spectrum of manifestations of HE that do not produce disorientation in time or space [153].

HE can occur not only in patients with liver cirrhosis but also in those with non-cirrhotic PH and porto-systemic shunting [154, 155]. MHE has been reported in about one third of children with EHPVO and normal liver function [156, 157]. The diagnosis is made by psychometric tests, critical flicker frequency, and MR spectroscopy [158]. Hyperammonemia seems to play a key role in the pathogenesis of this complication [159].

According to this research, MHE would compromise attention, processing speed, and psychomotor performance, in some cases affecting the academic performance of the patients. MHE seems solved by restoring blood flow to the liver by the meso-portal bypass (MPB), while surgical porto-systemic shunts may eventually worsen it [114, 156].

Management of EHPVO

Management of children with EHPVO is primarily focused on treatment of PH complications. However, the use of medical therapy, endoscopic procedures, and surgery are still questionable because there are no evidence on efficacy of NSBBs, endoscopic varices obliteration (EVO), and different types of surgical operations [72]. In clinical practice, EHPVO is managed according to what is proposed for cirrhotic children with PH. As far as surgery is concerned, special attention should be paid to the possibility of curing these patients by a successful MPB. MPB represents a physiologic repair of EHPVO, restoring the normal hepatic physiology, and therefore it should always be considered in this setting [160]. However, there is no wide agreement on feasibility, indications, timing, and success of this procedure [161, 162]. Due to the absence of standardized guidelines, the management of EHPVO needs to be individualized depending on the age of presentation, site and nature of obstruction, and clinical manifestations. In a retrospective study, we reviewed 65 children with EHPVO (median age at diagnosis 3.5 years) and proposed a stepwise approach to manage such a cohort of patients. After retrograde portogram, MPB resulted feasible only in 44% of the cases. Children were treated with endoscopic procedures and NSBB as first-line therapy. Those who had varices not well controlled by medical/endoscopic treatment underwent MPB in 13 (38.2%), a proximal splenorenal shunt in 13 (38.2%), a meso-caval shunt in 3 (8.8%), a TIPS in 2 (5.9%), a distal splenorenal shunt in 2 (5.9%), and a LTX because of HPS in 1 (3%). Such a stepwise approach, consisting of medical, endoscopic, and surgical options, provided excellent survival and bleeding control in more than 90% of the patients [2].

A lively debate is ongoing as to whether MPB should be considered as a preemptive technique or as a second-line option after failure of medical and endoscopic management [162, 163]. Although MPB may turn up not to be feasible in children who developed EHPVO following neonatal umbilical catheterization, it seems reasonable to consider restoring the normal liver flow in the early phase of the disease, when possible [2, 164].

Diagnosis of Portal Hypertension

The diagnostic workup in patients with PH includes actions aiming at diagnosing the underlying liver disease, quantifying the degree and severity of PH, and identifying the presence of clinical complications. In the clinical history, it is important to collect information on prematurity, neonatal jaundice, umbilical catheterization, and presence of signs or symptoms highly suspicious for PH (e.g., history of unexplained splenomegaly) (Table 68.3).

Physical examination is directed to assess liver size and consistency, splenomegaly, abdominal venous pattering (site and direction of venous flow), ascites, skin signs of chronic liver disease (e.g., spider nevi, telangiectasias, palmar erythema), bruises, and edema.

Laboratory tests should include liver function, blood cell and platelet count, and clotting.

A variety of radiological and endoscopic procedures are routinely utilized in children to diagnose PH. However, the majority of them have been well studied in adults but not in the pediatric population. Such procedures include abdominal Doppler ultrasound, upper GI endoscopy, CT scan of the abdomen, invasive measurements of portal venous pressure, and liver biopsy.

Doppler Ultrasound

Doppler ultrasound is a noninvasive and inexpensive technique that is widely used in children to study liver vessels and parenchyma. Although operator dependent and related to the experience and skill of the radiologist, Doppler ultrasound is a valuable tool to screen patients with suspected PH both at the time of the diagnosis and during the follow-up. In a few minutes, this test can provide information on liver size and texture, patency of portal and hepatic veins, hepatic artery patency and flow pattern (including the resistance index), porto-systemic shunting, ascites, splenomegaly, and associated intra-abdominal abnormalities [165].

The liver is usually enlarged in the hepatic (e.g., biliary atresia, ciliopathies, genetic cholestasis) and posthepatic forms of PH (e.g., Budd–Chiari syndrome), whereas it is of normal size in prehepatic PH. The echogenicity of the parenchyma may be increased in cirrhosis and in some diseases in which steatosis is a histological feature (i.e., Wilson's disease and α1-antitrypsin deficiency) [166]. Gross abnormalities of the bile ducts, such as biliary dilatation, the presence of gallstones, or other morphological abnormalities, can be easily visualized by ultrasound, whereas small irregularities require more powerful imaging studies to be detected.

In patients with prehepatic PH, it is crucial to detect the presence of a portal cavernoma and rule out a dilatation of the biliary tree possibly due to PHB. The splenic size is easily measured and compared to normal values for age, although it does not correlate strictly with the severity of PH [165]. In children with liver disease, it is important to evaluate also the renal parenchyma to exclude the presence of renal cysts that can accompany several genetic liver disorders and provide a further hint to the diagnosis [166].

Bi-dimensional ultrasonography can easily detect and confirm the presence of ascites suspected clinically, and the color Doppler technique provides information on blood flow in the portal venous system, the hepatic artery, and the hepatic veins, where it is possible to calculate the flow velocity, although it is not possible to estimate pressures [167, 168]. When PH worsens, the portal blood flow may become hepatofugal towards the left gastric, paraduodenal, or paraumbilical veins. Reversal of flow in the SMV or SV may be suggestive of spontaneous mesentericocaval or splenorenal shunts, respectively [169].

The hepatic veins are straight, anechoic, tubular structures that converge towards the IVC approximately 1 cm below its confluence with the right atrium. The normal hepatic vein waveform is triphasic as a result of transmitted cardiac activity [170].

Varices are formed in the lower esophagus by portosystemic shunting via the left gastric vein through the lesser omentum (Fig. 68.1). As a consequence, the lesser omentum gets thickened in PH [171, 172]. Patriquin H et al. measured the lesser omental thickness in 150 children without systemic, liver, or renal disease. They suggested that, in the absence of obesity or lymphadenopathy, a lesser omentum measuring more than 1.7 times the aortic diameter should raise the possibility of PH [173].

Although the "gold-standard" method for liver fibrosis assessment is liver biopsy, in the past years, noninvasive methods have increasingly been used in adult hepatology. The best validated tool is transient elastography (TE) [174, 175]. Data on its use in children are still scarce, and the influence of technical aspects such as probe choice and site of measurement on results is not clear. In one study TE was performed in 527 children (229 girls, ages 0.1–17.8 (median 6.0) years, including 400 healthy controls). The feasibility rate was 90%, but it decreased to 83% in children younger than 24 months even in ideal conditions. General anesthesia significantly increased liver stiffness in healthy children. The authors concluded that In one study TE is feasible even in extremely young children, but confounding influences on test results such as probe choice, sedation, or food intake need to be taken into account when interpreting the results [176].

Endoscopy

Unlike adults, in the pediatric population, there are few reports on the prevalence of varices in children with PH, and it is therefore difficult to predict how many children would benefit from endoscopic screening [177]. In children, the endoscopic procedures to diagnose and treat EV are routinely performed under general anesthesia.

There is no recommendation to routinely undertake tests to screen for the presence of varices in children with PH. Despite that, many pediatric hepatologists prefer their patients to undergo endoscopic surveillance to best define and prevent the risk of bleeding from varix rupture. In fact, when pediatric hepatologists were asked if they would offer screening endoscopy for varices to a child with biliary atresia and evidence of PH, most of them answered they would, both in Europe and in North America [3, 73, 160].

Data on diagnosis and grading of EV in children are scant. The scoring systems adopted in adults have not been validated in children, but such information is mandatory to determine the effectiveness of prophylaxis of variceal bleeding by either NSBBs or endoscopic treatment (Fig. 68.3). Studies on the interobserver agreement on pediatric varices grading are underway, and the preliminary results suggest that accordance in the recognition of large varices is satisfactory [86, 178].

Another major issue is how to grade varices in this setting. Varices have been defined into 3 grades according to the size, and red marks have been shown to predict bleeding. Recently, the classification has been simplified, and the proposed description of small or large varices, with or without red marks, appears to be more practical [76]. Large varices, varices of any size but with red marks, and gastric varices are likely at higher risk of bleeding in the short term, but again this has not been proven in children so far [179].

Endoscopy in children with PH is only indicated for the treatment of acute bleeding and in the secondary prophylaxis of further bleeding episodes. The usefulness of diagnostic endoscopy and primary prophylaxis of bleeding by endoscopic obliteration is still unproven [72].

Measurement of Hepatic Venous Pressure Gradient

PH is defined by an increased pressure in the portal venous system. Such an increased venous pressure may be detected by a direct measurement of the pressure into the portal vein or by the measurement of a portal pressure gradient (PPG) resulting from the difference, in pressure, between the portal vein and the IVC. Direct measurements of portal pressure can be performed through transhepatic or transvenous catheterization of the portal vein but, since they have high risk of major complications (e.g., intraperitoneal bleeding), these tools are rarely used, apart from those cases in which WHVP is unreliable, such as presinusoidal PH [180].

HVPG measures the PPG as the difference between "wedged" hepatic vein pressure (WHVP) and "free" hepatic vein pressure (FHVP). The WHVP is measured by occluding the hepatic vein by inflating a balloon at the tip of the catheter. The injection of 5 ml of contrast dye into the vein with the balloon inflated can confirm an adequate occlusion of the hepatic vein. The WHVP reflects the portal vein pressure basing on the concept that when the blood flow in a hepatic vein is blocked by a "wedged" catheter, the static column of blood transmits the pressure from the preceding vascular territory, in this case, the hepatic sinusoids. As in cirrhosis the intersinusoidal communications are lost due to fibrosis, septa, and nodule formation, the sinusoidal pressure equilibrates with portal pressure. Thus, the WHVP correlates closely with portal vein pressure but, in fact, it is a measurement of the hepatic sinusoidal pressure and not of portal pressure itself [35].

The difference between WHPV and FHPV provides HVPG values (HVPG = WHVP − FHVP).

Normal HVPG ranges from 1 to 5 mmHg in adults. Subclinical PH is defined when HVPG ranges from 6 to 10 mmHg, whereas complications of PH are expected when HVPG is greater than 10 mmHg. An HVPG greater than 12 mmHg correlates with variceal bleeding, rebleeding, and increased mortality [181].

HVPG values allow to classify different forms of PH. Presinusoidal PH is characterized by normal or slightly increased HVPG values, with normal or slightly increased WHVP and normal FHVP. Sinusoidal PH is found in most chronic liver diseases and is characterized by an increase in WHVP with normal FHVP, resulting in high HVPG (cirrhosis is the most common cause). In postsinusoidal PH, HVPG is normal and both WHVP and FHVP are increased, such as in the Budd–Chiari syndrome (Table 68.2).

The HVPG is considered the gold standard technique to measure portal venous pressure and, in cirrhotic adults, is widely utilized to quantify the severity of PH, predict the outcome, and guide the therapeutic decisions [4, 182, 183].

In children, the diagnosis of PH is essentially based on clinical evidence of PH complications (i.e., splenomegaly, upper varices, ascites) in a setting of an underlying liver disease. Unfortunately, so far the measurement of HVPG in children has been considered an invasive procedure that has to be performed only in limited cases. Due to that, we have only few published data on HVPG measurements in the pediatric setting [184]. Wolfsson reported on 49 children, with acute and chronic liver disease, who underwent 52 HVPG measurements. The procedure resulted feasible in all patients and no complications were documented. HVPG values ranged between 0 and 28 mmHg, and they were greater than 6 mmHg in 30 patients. The Authors concluded that, despite the small sample size, HVPG measurements were feasible and safe in their cohort of patients [185]. Further studies on large cohorts of pediatric patients are necessary to obtain strong evidences on the utility of the HVPG measurements in the management of children with PH.

Other Investigations

CT scanning with intravenous contrast and MR angiography may be used to study children with PH. These investigations provide information on focal liver lesions, portal vein and hepatic vein patency, presence of collateral circulation and arteriovenous shunts. CT has a sensitivity of 85% in the detection of EV compared to endoscopy, but has the advantage of demonstrating splenorenal, gastrorenal, peripancreatic, pericholecystic, retroperitoneal and omental collaterals, as well as spontaneous large portosystemic shunts [186]. In a study performed on adult patients, MR angiography proved more reliable than Doppler ultrasound for evaluating the portal venous system in patients with PH caused by cirrhosis [187].

Management of Portal Hypertension

Prophylaxis of Bleeding

Currently, there are no data supporting the role of any type of prophylaxis to prevent variceal bleeding in children [3]; nevertheless, many clinicians would consider a cirrhotic child with large varices at risk of mortality from the first bleed, and therefore a definite candidate for primary prophylaxis [73]. Conversely, a reasonable, and somehow evidence-based, consensus on indication to perform endoscopic secondary prophylaxis (prevention of rebleeding) in cirrhotic children appears to be wide [72].

Nonselective β-Blockers

The rationale of NSBBs in PH stands on its ability to decrease the portal flow by reduction of cardiac output (via β1-receptor antagonism) and splanchnic vasodilatation (via β2-receptor antagonism) [188]. Studies in adults have shown that a dose reducing the heart rate by 25% (or the HVPG by 20%) does decrease the bleeding rate in cirrhosis [183]. There are no randomized trials assessing the efficacy of propranolol as prophylaxis of variceal bleeding in children, and the few cohort studies carried out did not include the measurement of HVPG before and after treatment start [6, 189, 190]. Moreover, these studies showed that in children the evaluation of heart rate at rest is problematic, and the range of drug dosage required to reduce it by 25% is very wide, making achievement of adequate NSBBs dosage impractical and time consuming. Whether pediatric patients with presinusoidal PH, having no classical features of the hyperdynamic circulation, may benefit from treatment with NSBBs has yet to be demonstrated [140].

A further difficulty in carrying out trials with NSBBs in this setting is that propranolol is not licensed for use in children. However, from the clinical experience made, as well as from the previously published studies, it appears that propranolol is safe for children, even at high doses [191].

Endoscopy for Screening and Management of Esophageal Varices

There are few reports on the prevalence of varices in children with PH, and it is therefore difficult to predict how many would benefit from endoscopic screening. Besides, the uncertainty regarding the impact of any prophylaxis in this setting makes endoscopic screening questionable.

Despite this, the mortality of cirrhotic children at the time of first bleeding episode has been reported to be as high as 5–15% and supports screening endoscopy in all children with advanced liver disease and clinical signs of PH [80].

Unlike past decades when endoscopic obliteration of varices was done using sclerosing agents (such as ethanolamine or polidocanol) injected inside or around the varix, currently variceal band ligation (EVL) has become more popular and has been shown to be superior to sclerotherapy as far as efficacy, safety, and degree of standardization are concerned, in both adults and children [192–194]. Nevertheless, in small children, in whom the banding devices available on the market cannot be used with small pediatric endoscopes, sclerotherapy remains the only feasible treatment option to manage large varices [194].

A real challenge in this setting is the presence of large gastric varices; there are no published data on experience of management of gastric varices in children, and probably most centers would treat this scenario according to the experience in adults. Large gastric varices are a threat because they are difficult to obliterate prophylactically, and even more so if actively bleeding; in this situation, balloon tamponade is often ineffective and the only option is to perform sclerotherapy with tissue glue (such as N-butyl-cyanoacrylate). In general, a child with large gastric varices should be considered for TIPS, shunt surgery, or liver transplantation, based on the degree of liver disease.

Management of Acute Variceal Bleeding

The main goal of the management of a child with acute esophageal bleeding is well-balanced blood volume restitution. It is therefore mandatory to monitor vital signs, obtain venous access to perform blood tests (full blood count, international normalized ratio, liver function and electrolytes, C-reactive protein, and a blood crossmatch) and start blood volume correction [195]. Packed red blood cells (PRC) should be provided with the aim to maintain the hemoglobin >7 g/dl, carefully avoiding a rebound overload of fluids that favor the increase of portal pressure and rebleeding [196]. In the presence of coagulopathy, it might be wise to support the patient with plasma, also in view of the fact that esophageal bleeding implies loss of whole blood that, if large, will not be efficiently replaced by PRC. Children with upper GI bleeding may benefit from nasogastric tube placement, with the primary goal being to monitor persistence of active bleeding. Vasoactive drugs, such as octreotide, are effective in stopping bleeding from varices and should be started immediately to bridge the child to endoscopy, and continued thereafter for a total of 4–5 days [197].

In adults, it has been proven that infectious complications commonly follow an episode of variceal bleeding in cirrhotic patients [198]. Although in children there is no such evidence it is recommended to monitor them for any sign of infection and, if present, to start antibiotic treatment promptly, especially in cirrhotic children with advanced disease.

After the initial step, the child should be managed according to hemodynamic stability and the control of bleeding. If unstable, the child should be managed in an intensive care setting, possibly with a central venous catheter providing information on circulating blood volume and preload (Fig. 68.6). Usually, bleeding stops spontaneously after the ruptured varix empties. After cessation, it is usually

acceptable to schedule an elective endoscopy in the following 24–72 h because rebleeding is uncommon during this time frame. If bleeding does not stop despite appropriate fluid replacement and correction of coagulopathy, the child may require urgent endoscopy, and rarely, the placement of a Sengstaken balloon as a bridge to TIPS or urgent shunt surgery (Fig. 68.7). Endoscopic sclerotherapy around the vessel may be the only option to treat an acutely bleeding varix that is underfilled, and therefore difficult to be strangulated by a rubber band placed by endoscopic variceal ligation devices.

Surgical Procedures

When medical and endoscopic treatment of bleeding varices fails, the only option is to consider decompression of the portal system by a shunt or a bypass [199]. Children with EHPVO can be managed effectively by MPB (Fig. 68.8) [23]; however, in our experience of children who had an umbilical venous catheter placed at birth, only about half had a patent Rex recessus at retrograde portogram [2]. If the MPB is not feasible, these patients can usually be treated by other forms of shunt surgery [200]. One recently suggested approach is to perform the MPB preemptively, regardless of complications of PH, in view of its beneficial effects on growth and neurocognitive outcome [162, 164 & 165]. Other patients with presinusoidal PH, but not

Fig. 68.6 Proposed algorithm for the management of acute variceal bleeding. *NGT* nasogastric tube, *INR* international normalized ratio, *CRP* C-reactive protein, *ICU* intensive care unit, *PRC* packed red cells, *FFP* fresh frozen plasma, *TIPS* transjugular intrahepatic porto-systemic shunt. (Reprinted from Ref. [73], with permission from Elsevier

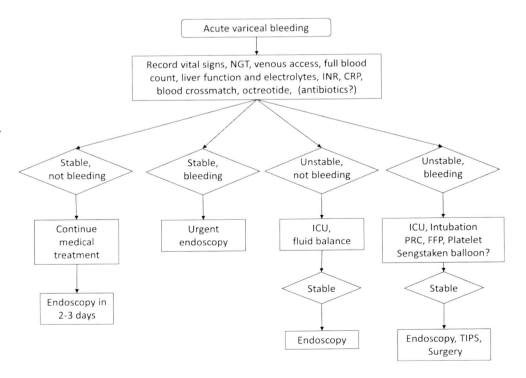

Fig. 68.7 Portal circulation after the placement of transjugular intrahepatic portosystemic shunt

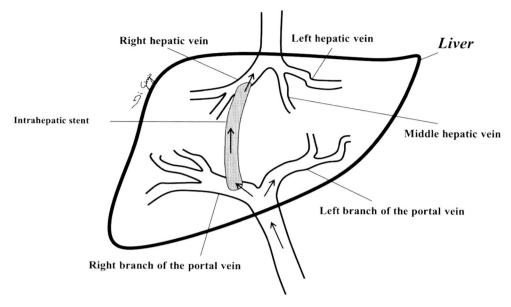

Fig. 68.8 Portal circulation after the operation of meso-portal bypass that reestablishes the hepatopetal flow to the liver

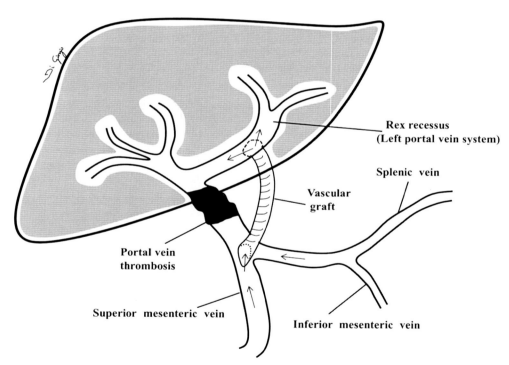

amenable to MPB, can be managed by TIPS or by shunt surgery [201].

Cirrhotic children with PH usually have a rapidly progressive biliary type of cirrhosis (such as biliary atresia, intrahepatic cholestasis, and Alagille syndrome), are young, and have a short transplant-free survival. In our institution, the median age at transplantation is 1.4 years. Therefore, shunt surgery or TIPS is rarely indicated in this cohort of patients in whom PH is usually accompanied by liver decompensation and is an indication for LT. However, cirrhotic children with a compensated long-standing noncholestatic liver disease complicated by severe PH may be considered for TIPS.

Transjugular Intrahepatic Portosystemic Shunt

TIPS is a well-established tool to manage severe complications of PH in adults, but its experience in children is limited. In our institution, 13 children affected by PH unresponsive to NSBBs and endoscopic treatment were considered candidate for TIPS. Eleven underwent a successful expanded-polytetrafluoroethylene-covered stent placement, including three who had a split LTX. The shunt led to significant decrease of the portosystemic gradient and resolution of PH complications in all but one. No patient developed overt HE. All shunts were patent at the last follow-up (median of 20 months) or transplantation [88]. TIPS appears to be feasible and effective in children as it is in adults and should become part of the armamentarium used to manage PH complications in pediatric patients.

A Protocol for Screening, Prophylaxis, and Treatment of Esophageal Varices

The need for large sample sizes, the difficulties in recruiting patients into multicenter studies, and the lack of official approval and knowledge on drug dosing make it quite unlikely that there will be robust data on the use of NSBBs in children with PH in the coming years. The same applies to endoscopy because there is no single center able to recruit enough patients to answer questions regarding screening and primary prophylaxis of varices, and multicenter trials require diagnosis and treatment standardization. Besides, such studies can probably only be carried out in non-cirrhotic children having sufficient follow-up time to test the given hypothesis. Alternatively, many centers are already using these tools empirically in both cirrhotic and non-cirrhotic

children, with uncertain and inconsistently measurable results. Is it then possible to gather more information on the utility of NSBBs and endoscopic treatment of varices in children? A proper trial on this matter should be randomized and have variceal bleeding as the primary end point; however, many clinicians and families would consider permitting a GI bleed as unacceptable to test the hypothesis of effectiveness of NSBBs or endoscopic treatment. One possibility to overcome this could come from considering the development of large varices as the end point, because children with large varices or red marks have failed treatment and will eventually bleed. At least two studies have shown that most children with cirrhosis or PVT and grade 2–3 varices will bleed within a few years of follow-up [202, 203]. Therefore, it is possible to hypothesize a randomized, nonblinded multicenter trial of development of large varices in children and their response to treatment. Because of the large sample size needed, such study would first require a solid proof that there is sufficient agreement among endoscopists to recognize large varices in the different pediatric centers involved in the trial [179]. Figure 68.9 illustrates an algorithm of a stepwise approach to manage EV, which considers the formation of large varices as the end point and could offer the chance to test the hypothesis that NSBBs and endoscopy can improve the outcome of children with PH, avoiding the risk of not offering the best of practice currently available. Nevertheless, an extraordinary effort will be required to produce such evidence on the best management of PH in children.

Fig. 68.9 Proposed algorithm for the approach to the child with portal hypertension. *TIPS* transjugular intrahepatic portosystemic shunt. The circled "R" represents a step for possible randomization in a clinical trial. (Reprinted from Ref. [73], with permission from Elsevier)

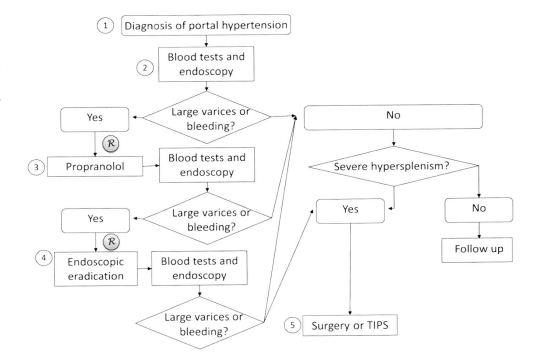

References

1. Alonso EM, Hackworth C, Whitington PF. Portal hypertension in children. Clin Liver Dis. 1997;1(1):201–22, xiii.

2. Alberti D, Colusso M, Cheli M, Ravelli P, Indriolo A, Signorelli S, et al. Results of a stepwise approach to extra-hepatic portal vein obstruction in children. J Pediatr Gastroenterol Nutr. 2013;57(5):619–26.

3. Ling SC, Walters T, McKiernan PJ, Schwarz KB, Garcia-Tsao G, Shneider BL. Primary prophylaxis of variceal hemorrhage in children with portal hypertension: a framework for future research. J Pediatr Gastroenterol Nutr. 2011;52(3):254–61.

4. de Franchis R. Revising consensus in portal hypertension: report of the Baveno V consensus workshop on methodology of diagnosis and therapy in portal hypertension. J Hepatol. 2010;53(4):762–8.

5. Shneider B, Emre S, Groszmann R, Karani J, McKiernan P, Sarin S, et al. Expert pediatric opinion on the Report of the Baveno IV consensus workshop on methodology of diagnosis and therapy in portal hypertension. Pediatr Transplant. 2006;10(8):893–907.

6. Shashidhar H, Langhans N, Grand RJ. Propranolol in prevention of portal hypertensive hemorrhage in children: a pilot study. J Pediatr Gastroenterol Nutr. 1999;29(1):12–7.

7. Howard ER, Stringer MD, Mowat AP. Assessment of injection sclerotherapy in the management of 152 children with oesophageal varices. Br J Surg. 1988;75(5):404–8.

8. Abd El-Hamid N, Taylor RM, Marinello D, Mufti GJ, Patel R, et al. Aetiology and management of extrahepatic portal vein obstruction in children: King's College Hospital experience. J Pediatr Gastroenterol Nutr. 2008;47(5):630–4.

9. Dooley JS, Lok A, Burroughs AK, Heathcote J (Editors). Sherlock's diseases of the liver and biliary system. 12th ed. Chichester: Wiley-Blackwell; 2011. p. 792.

10. Lautt WW. Hepatic circulation: physiology and pathophysiology. Vol. 6. CA: Morgan & Claypool; 2009.

11. Shneider BL. Approaches to the management of pediatric portal hypertension: results of an informal survey. In: Bosch J, Groszmann RJ, editors. Portal hypertension in the 21st century. Montreal: Springer Netherlands; 2004.

12. Vorobioff J, Bredfeldt JE, Groszmann RJ. Hyperdynamic circulation in portal-hypertensive rat model: a primary factor for maintenance of chronic portal hypertension. Am J Physiol. 1983;244(1):G52–7.

13. Orrego H, Blendis LM, Crossley IR, Medline A, Macdonald A, et al. Correlation of intrahepatic pressure with collagen in the Disse space and hepatomegaly in humans and in the rat. Gastroenterology 1981;80(3):546–56.

14. Reddy SI, Grace ND. Liver imaging. A hepatologist's perspective. Clin Liver Dis. 2002. 6(1):297–310, ix.

15. Gupta TK, Chen L, Groszmann RJ. Pathophysiology of portal hypertension. Clin Liver Dis. 1997. 1(1):1–12.

16. Chawla Y, Duseja A, Dhiman RK. Review article: the modern management of portal vein thrombosis. Aliment Pharmacol Ther. 2009;30(9):881–94.

17. Sutton JP, Yarborough DY, Richards JT. Isolated splenic vein occlusion. Review of literature and report of an additional case. Arch Surg. 1970;100(5):623–6.

18. Köklü S, Coban S, Yüksel O, Arhan M. Left-sided portal hypertension. Dig Dis Sci;2007. 52(5):1141–9.

19. Chen BC, Wang HH, Lin YC, Shih YL, Chang WK, Hsieh TY. Isolated gastric variceal bleeding caused by splenic lymphoma-associated splenic vein occlusion. World J Gastroenterol. 2013;19(40):6939–42.

20. Giouleme O, Theocharidou E. Management of portal hypertension in children with portal vein thrombosis. J Pediatr Gastroenterol Nutr. 2013;57(4):419–25.

21. DeLeve LD, Valla DC, Garcia-Tsao G. Vascular disorders of the liver. Hepatology 2009;49(5):1729–64.

22. Webb LJ, Sherlock S. The aetiology, presentation and natural history of extra-hepatic portal venous obstruction. Q J Med. 1979;48(192):627–39.

23. de Ville de Goyet J, Alberti D, Clapuyt P, Falchetti D, Rigamonti V, et al. Direct bypassing of extrahepatic portal venous obstruction in children: a new technique for combined hepatic portal revascularization and treatment of extrahepatic portal hypertension. J Pediatr Surg. 1998;33(4):597–601.

24. Bambini DA, Superina R, Almond PS, Whitington PF, Alonso E. Experience with the Rex shunt (mesenterico-left portal bypass) in children with extrahepatic portal hypertension. J Pediatr Surg. 2000;35(1):13–8, discussion 18–9.

25. Camposilvan S, Milanesi O, Stellin G, Pettenazzo A, Zancan L, D'Antiga L. Liver and cardiac function in the long term after Fontan operation. Ann Thorac Surg. 2008;86(1):177–82.

26. Rychik J, Veldtman G, Rand E, Russo P, Rome JJ, Krok K, et al. The precarious state of the liver after a Fontan operation: summary of a multidisciplinary symposium. Pediatr Cardiol. 2012. 33(7):1001–12.

27. Horton JD, San Miguel FL, Membreno F, Wright F, Paima J, et al. Budd–Chiari syndrome: illustrated review of current management. Liver Int. 2008. 28(4):455–66.

28. Shrestha SM, Okuda K, Uchida T, Maharjan KG, Shrestha S, et al. Endemicity and clinical picture of liver disease due to obstruction of the hepatic portion of the inferior vena cava in Nepal. J Gastroenterol Hepatol. 1996;11(2):170–9.

29. Simson IW, Membranous obstruction of the inferior vena cava and hepatocellular carcinoma in South Africa. Gastroenterology 1982;82(2):171–8.

30. Cauchi JA, Oliff S, Baumann U, Mirza D, Kelly DA, Hewitson J, et al. The Budd–Chiari syndrome in children: the spectrum of management. J Pediatr Surg. 2006;41(11):1919–23.

31. Doehring-Schwerdtfeger E, Abdel-Rahim IM, Kardorff R, Kaiser C, Franke D, Schlake J, et al. Ultrasonographical investigation of periportal fibrosis in children with Schistosoma mansoni infection: reversibility of morbidity twenty-three months after treatment with praziquantel. Am J Trop Med Hyg. 1992;46(4):409–15.

32. Ross AG, Bartley PB, Sleigh AC, Olds GR, Li Y, Williams GM, McManus DP. Schistosomiasis. N Engl J Med. 2002;346(16):1212–20.

33. Ruiz-Guevara R, de Noya BA, Valero SK, Lecuna P, Garassini M, Noya O, et al. Clinical and ultrasound findings before and after praziquantel treatment among Venezuelan schistosomiasis patients. Rev Soc Bras Med Trop. 2007;40(5):505–11.

34. Thalheimer U, Leandro G, Samonakis DN, Triantos CK, Patch D, Burroughs AK, Assessment of the agreement between wedge hepatic vein pressure and portal vein pressure in cirrhotic patients. Dig Liver Dis. 2005;37(8):601–8.

35. D'Amico G, Garcia-Pagan JC, Luca A, Bosch J. Hepatic vein pressure gradient reduction and prevention of variceal bleeding in cirrhosis: a systematic review. Gastroenterology 2006;131(5):1611–24.

36. Colman JC, Britton RS, Orrego H, Saldivia V, Medline A, Israel Y. Relation between osmotically induced hepatocyte enlargement and portal hypertension. Am J Physiol. 1983;245(3):G382–7.

37. Dudenhoefer AA, Loureiro-Silva MR, Cadelina GW, Gupta T, Groszmann RJ. Bioactivation of nitroglycerin and vasomotor response to nitric oxide are impaired in cirrhotic rat livers. Hepatology 2002;36(2):381–5.

38. Zafra C, Abraldes JG, Turnes J, Berzigotti A, Fernández M, Garca-Pagán JC, et al. Simvastatin enhances hepatic nitric oxide production and decreases the hepatic vascular tone in patients with cirrhosis. Gastroenterology 2004;126(3):749–55.

39. Moore K, Wendon J, Frazer M, Karani J, Williams R, Badr K. Plasma endothelin immunoreactivity in liver disease and the hepatorenal syndrome. N Engl J Med. 1992;327(25):1774–8.

40. Martinet JP, Legault L, Cernacek P, Roy L, Dufresne MP, Spahr L, et al. Changes in plasma endothelin-1 and Big endothelin-1 induced by transjugular intrahepatic portosystemic shunts in patients with cirrhosis and refractory ascites. J Hepatol. 1996;25(5):700–6.

41. Rockey D. The cellular pathogenesis of portal hypertension: stellate cell contractility, endothelin, and nitric oxide. Hepatology 1997;25(1):2–5.

42. Geerts A. History, heterogeneity, developmental biology, and functions of quiescent hepatic stellate cells. Semin Liver Dis. 2001;21(3):311–35.

43. Ramadori G, Saile B. Mesenchymal cells in the liver—one cell type or two? Liver 2002;22(4):283–94.

44. Friedman SL. Molecular regulation of hepatic fibrosis, an integrated cellular response to tissue injury. J Biol Chem. 2000;275(4):2247–50.

45. Reynaert H, Thompson MG, Thomas T, Geerts A. Hepatic stellate cells: role in microcirculation and pathophysiology of portal hypertension. Gut 2002;50(4):571–81.

46. Reichen J, Le M. Verapamil favorably influences hepatic microvascular exchange and function in rats with cirrhosis of the liver. J Clin Invest. 1986;78(2):448–55.

47. Shulman HM, Fisher LB, Schoch HG, Henne KW, McDonald GB. Veno-occlusive disease of the liver after marrow transplantation: histological correlates of clinical signs and symptoms. Hepatology 1994;19(5):1171–81.

48. McDonald GB, Sharma P, Matthews DE, Shulman HM, Thomas ED. Venocclusive disease of the liver after bone marrow transplantation: diagnosis, incidence, and predisposing factors. Hepatology 1984;4(1):116–22.

49. Sperl W, Stuppner H, Gassner I, Judmaier W, Dietze O, Vogel W. Reversible hepatic veno-occlusive disease in an infant after consumption of pyrrolizidine-containing herbal tea. Eur J Pediatr. 1995;154(2):112–6.

50. Corbacioglu S, Greil J, Peters C, Wulffraat N, Laws HJ, Dilloo D, et al. Defibrotide in the treatment of children with veno-occlusive disease (VOD): a retrospective multicentre study demonstrates therapeutic efficacy upon early intervention. Bone Marrow Transplant. 2004;33(2):189–95.

51. D'Antiga L, Baker A, Pritchard J, Pryor D, Mieli-Vergani G. Veno-occlusive disease with multi-organ involvement following actinomycin-D. Eur J Cancer. 2001;37(9):1141–8.

52. Reiss U, Cowan M, McMillan A, Horn B. Hepatic venoocclusive disease in blood and bone marrow transplantation in children and young adults: incidence, risk factors, and outcome in a cohort of 241 patients. J Pediatr Hematol Oncol. 2002;24(9):746–50.

53. Guzman EA, McCahill LE, Rogers FB. Arterioportal fistulas: introduction of a novel classification with therapeutic implications. J Gastrointest Surg. 2006;10(4):543–50.

54. Arslan N, Buyukgebiz B, Ozturk Y, Hizli S, Bekem O, et al. Hepatoportal sclerosis in a child. Eur J Pediatr. 2004;163(11):683–4.

55. Yilmaz G, Sari S, Egritas O, Dalgic B, Akyol G. Hepatoportal sclerosis in childhood: some presenting with cholestatic features (a re-evaluation of 12 children). Pediatr Dev Pathol. 2012;15(2):107–13.

56. Kowalski HJ, Abelmann WH. The cardiac output at rest in Laennec's cirrhosis. J Clin Invest. 1953;32(10):1025–33.

57. Groszmann RJ, Vorobioff J, Riley E. Splanchnic hemodynamics in portal-hypertensive rats: measurement with gamma-labeled microspheres. Am J Physiol. 1982;242(2):G156–60.

58. Iwakiri Y, Groszmann RJ. The hyperdynamic circulation of chronic liver diseases: from the patient to the molecule. Hepatology 2006;43(2 Suppl 1):S121–31.

59. Groszmann RJ. Hyperdynamic circulation of liver disease 40 years later: pathophysiology and clinical consequences. Hepatology 1994;20(5):1359–63.

60. Vorobioff J, Bredfeldt JE, Groszmann RJ. Increased blood flow through the portal system in cirrhotic rats. Gastroenterology 1984;87(5):1120–6.

61. Colombato LA, Albillos A, Groszmann RJ. Temporal relationship of peripheral vasodilatation, plasma volume expansion and the hyperdynamic circulatory state in portal-hypertensive rats. Hepatology 1992;15(2):323–8.

62. Hadengue A, Lee SS, Koshy A, Girod C, Lebrec D. Regional blood flows by the microsphere method: reproducibility in portal hypertensive rats and influence of a portal vein catheter. Proc Soc Exp Biol Med. 1988;187(4):461–8.

63. Genecin P, Polio J, Groszmann RJ. Na restriction blunts expansion of plasma volume and ameliorates hyperdynamic circulation in portal hypertension. Am J Physiol. 1990;259(3 Pt 1):G498–503.

64. Morgan JS, Groszmann RJ, Rojkind M, Enriquez R. Hemodynamic mechanisms of emerging portal hypertension caused by schistosomiasis in the hamster. Hepatology 1990;11(1):98–104.

65. Fallon MB. Mechanisms of pulmonary vascular complications of liver disease: hepatopulmonary syndrome. J Clin Gastroenterol. 2005;39(4 Suppl 2):S138–42.

66. Katsuta Y, Honma H, Zhang XJ, Ohsuga M, Komeichi H, Shimizu S, et al. Pulmonary blood transit time and impaired arterial oxygenation in patients with chronic liver disease. J Gastroenterol. 2005;40(1):57–63.

67. Agusti AG, Roca J, Bosch J, Garcia-Pagan JC, Wagner PD, Rodriguez-Roisin R. Effects of propranolol on arterial oxygenation and oxygen transport to tissues in patients with cirrhosis. Am Rev Respir Dis. 1990;142(2):306–10.

68. Moller S, Henriksen JH, Bendtsen F. Central and noncentral blood volumes in cirrhosis: relationship to anthropometrics and gender. Am J Physiol Gastrointest Liver Physiol. 2003;284(6):G970–9.

69. Shapiro MD, Nicholls KM, Groves BM, Kluge R, Chung HM, et al. Interrelationship between cardiac output and vascular resistance as determinants of effective arterial blood volume in cirrhotic patients. Kidney Int. 1985;28(2):206–11.

70. Schrier RW, Arroyo V, Bernardi M, Epstein M, Henriksen JH, Rodés J. Peripheral arterial vasodilation hypothesis: a proposal for the initiation of renal sodium and water retention in cirrhosis. Hepatology 1988;8(5):1151–7.

71. Møller S, Bendtsen F, Schifter S, Henriksen JH. Relation of calcitonin gene-related peptide to systemic vasodilatation and central hypovolaemia in cirrhosis. Scand J Gastroenterol. 1996;31(9):928–33.

72. Shneider BL, Bosch J, de Franchis R, Emre SH, Groszmann RJ, Ling SC, et al. Portal hypertension in children: expert pediatric opinion on the report of the Baveno v consensus workshop on methodology of diagnosis and therapy in portal hypertension. Pediatr Transplant. 2012;16(5):426–37.

73. D'Antiga L. Medical management of esophageal varices and portal hypertension in children. Semin Pediatr Surg. 2012;21(3):211–8.

74. Gugig R, Rosenthal P. Management of portal hypertension in children. World J Gastroenterol. 2012;18(11):1176–84.

75. Spence RA, Johnston GW, Odling-Smee GW, Rodgers HW. Bleeding oesophageal varices with long term follow up. Arch Dis Child. 1984;59(4):336–40.

76. Garcia-Tsao G, Sanyal AJ, Grace ND, Carey WD, et al. Prevention and management of gastroesophageal varices and variceal hemorrhage in cirrhosis. Am J Gastroenterol. 2007;102(9):2086–102.

77. Sarin SK, Shahi HM, Jain M, Jain AK, Issar SK, Murthy NS. The natural history of portal hypertensive gastropathy: influence of variceal eradication. Am J Gastroenterol. 2000;95(10):2888–93.

78. Alvarez F, Bernard O, Brunelle F, Hadchouel P, Odièvre M, Alagille D. Portal obstruction in children. I. Clinical investigation and hemorrhage risk. J Pediatr. 1983;103(5):696–702.

79. Beppu K, Inokuchi K, Koyanagi N, Nakayama S, Sakata H, et al. Prediction of variceal hemorrhage by esophageal endoscopy. Gastrointest Endosc. 1981;27(4):213–8.

80. van Heurn LW, Saing H, Tam PK. Portoenterostomy for biliary atresia: long-term survival and prognosis after esophageal variceal bleeding. J Pediatr Surg. 2004;39(1):6–9.

81. Misra SP, Dwivedi M, Misra V. Prevalence and factors influencing hemorrhoids, anorectal varices, and colopathy in patients with portal hypertension. Endoscopy 1996;28(4):340–5.

82. Triger DR. Extra hepatic portal venous obstruction. Gut 1987;28(10):1193–7.

83. Ling SC. Advances in the evaluation and management of children with portal hypertension. Semin Liver Dis. 2012;32(4):288–97.

84. Bolognesi M, Merkel C, Sacerdoti D, Nava V, Gatta A. Role of spleen enlargement in cirrhosis with portal hypertension. Dig Liver Dis. 2002;34(2):144–50.

85. Shah SH, Hayes PC, Allan PL, Nicoll J, Finlayson ND. Measurement of spleen size and its relation to hypersplenism and portal hemodynamics in portal hypertension due to hepatic cirrhosis. Am J Gastroenterol. 1996;91(12):2580–3.

86. Gana JC, Turner D, Mieli-Vergani G, Davenport M, Miloh T, Avitzur Y, et al. A clinical prediction rule and platelet count predict esophageal varices in children. Gastroenterology 2011;141(6):2009–16.

87. Ling SC, Pfeiffer A, Avitzur Y, Fecteau A, Grant D, Ng VL. Long-term follow-up of portal hypertension after liver transplantation in children. Pediatr Transplant. 2009;13(2):206–9.

88. Di Giorgio A, Agazzi R, Alberti D, Colledan M, D'Antiga L. Feasibility and efficacy of transjugular intrahepatic portosystemic shunt (TIPS) in children. J Pediatr Gastroenterol Nutr. 2012;54(5):594–600.

89. Narahara Y, Kanazawa H, Fukuda T, Matsushita Y, Harimoto H, Kidokoro H, et al. Transjugular intrahepatic portosystemic shunt versus paracentesis plus albumin in patients with refractory ascites who have good hepatic and renal function: a prospective randomized trial. J Gastroenterol. 2011;46(1):78–85.

90. Khandwalla HE, Fasakin Y, El-Serag HB. The utility of evaluating low serum albumin gradient ascites in patients with cirrhosis. Am J Gastroenterol. 2009;104(6):1401–5.

91. Ginés P, et al. ed. Ascites and renal dysfunction in liver disease: pathogenesis, diagnosis, and treatment. Chichester: Wiley-Blackwell; 2005. p. 464.

92. Such J, Runyon BA. Spontaneous bacterial peritonitis. Clin Infect Dis. 1998;27(4):669–74, quiz 675–6.

93. Arikan C, Ozgenç F, Akman SA, Yağci RV, Tokat Y, Aydoğdu S. Large-volume paracentesis and liver transplantation. J Pediatr Gastroenterol Nutr. 2003;37(2):207–8.

94. Kramer RE, Sokol RJ, Yerushalmi B, Liu E, MacKenzie T, et al. Large-volume paracentesis in the management of ascites in children. J Pediatr Gastroenterol Nutr. 2001. 33(3):245–9.

95. Pugliese R, Fonseca EA, Porta G, Danesi V, Guimaraes T, Porta A, et al. Ascites and serum sodium are markers of increased waiting list mortality in children with chronic liver failure. Hepatology. 2014;59(5):1964–71.

96. Leong RW, House AK, Jeffrey GP. Chylous ascites caused by portal vein thrombosis treated with octreotide. J Gastroenterol Hepatol. 2003;18(10):1211–3.

97. Whitworth JR, Ivy DD, Gralla J, Narkewicz MR, Sokol RJ, et al. Pulmonary vascular complications in asymptomatic children with portal hypertension. J Pediatr Gastroenterol Nutr. 2009;49(5):607–12.

98. Barbé T, Losay J, Grimon G, Devictor D, Sardet A, Gauthier F, et al. Pulmonary arteriovenous shunting in children with liver disease. J Pediatr. 1995;126(4):571–9.

99. Krowka MJ. Portopulmonary hypertension. Semin Respir Crit Care Med. 2012;33(1):17–25.

100. Fallon MB, Abrams GA, Luo B, Hou Z, Dai J, Ku DD. The role of endothelial nitric oxide synthase in the pathogenesis of a rat model of hepatopulmonary syndrome. Gastroenterology 1997;113(2):606–14.

101. Zhang M, Luo B, Chen SJ, Abrams GA, Fallon MB. Endothelin-1 stimulation of endothelial nitric oxide synthase in the pathogenesis of hepatopulmonary syndrome. Am J Physiol. 1999;277(5 Pt 1):G944–52.

102. Kinane TB, Westra SJ. Case records of the Massachusetts General Hospital. Weekly clinicopathological exercises. Case 31–2004. A four-year-old boy with hypoxemia. N Engl J Med. 2004;351(16):1667–75.

103. Abrams GA, Jaffe CC, Hoffer PB, Binder HJ, Fallon MB. Diagnostic utility of contrast echocardiography and lung perfusion scan in patients with hepatopulmonary syndrome. Gastroenterology 1995;109(4):1283–8.

104. Santamaria F, Sarnelli P, Celentano L, Farina V, Vegnente A, et al. Noninvasive investigation of hepatopulmonary syndrome in children and adolescents with chronic cholestasis. Pediatr Pulmonol. 2002;33(5):374–9.

105. Hoeper MM, Krowka MJ, Strassburg CP. Portopulmonary hypertension and hepatopulmonary syndrome. Lancet 2004;363(9419):1461–8.

106. Al-Hussaini A, Taylor RM, Samyn M, Bansal S, Heaton N, Rela M, et al. Long-term outcome and management of hepatopulmonary syndrome in children. Pediatr Transplant. 2010;14(2):276–82.

107. Ridaura-Sanz C, Mejia-Hernandez C, Lopez-Corella E. Portopulmonary hypertension in children. A study in pediatric autopsies. Arch Med Res. 2009;40(7):635–9.

108. Condino AA, Ivy DD, O'Connor JA, Narkewicz MR, Mengshol S, Whitworth JR, et al. Portopulmonary hypertension in pediatric patients. J Pediatr. 2005;147(1):20–6.

109. Iyer VB, McKiernan PJ, Foster K, Gupte GL. Stomal varices manifestation of portal hypertension in advanced intestinal failure-associated liver disease. J Pediatr Gastroenterol Nutr. 2011;52:630–1 (United States).

110. European Association for the Study of the Liver. EASL clinical practice guidelines on the management of ascites, spontaneous bacterial peritonitis, and hepatorenal syndrome in cirrhosis. J Hepatol. 2010;53(3):397–417.

111. Lata J. Hepatorenal syndrome. World J Gastroenterol. 2012;18(36):4978–84.

112. Yousef N, Habes D, Ackermann O, Durand P, Bernard O, Jacquemin E. Hepatorenal syndrome: diagnosis and effect of terlipressin therapy in 4 pediatric patients. J Pediatr Gastroenterol Nutr. 2010;51(1):100–2.

113. Amodio P. The liver, the brain and nitrogen metabolism. Metab Brain Dis. 2009;24(1):1–4.

114. Ferenci P, Lockwood A, Mullen K, Tarter R, Weissenborn K, Blei AT. Hepatic encephalopathy—definition, nomenclature, diagnosis, and quantification: final report of the working party at the 11th World Congresses of Gastroenterology, Vienna, 1998. Hepatology 2002;35(3):716–21.

115. Amodio P, Bemeur C, Butterworth R, Cordoba J, Kato A, Montagnese S, et al. The nutritional management of hepatic encephalopathy in patients with cirrhosis: Ishen consensus. Hepatology 2013;58:325–36.

116. Khanna R, Sarin SK. Non-cirrhotic portal hypertension—diagnosis and management. J Hepatol 2014;60(2):421–41.

117. Sarin SK. Non-cirrhotic portal fibrosis. J Gastroenterol Hepatol. 2002;17(Suppl 3):S214–23.

118. Okudaira M, Ohbu M, Okuda K. Idiopathic portal hypertension and its pathology. Semin Liver Dis. 2002;22(1):59–72.

119. Nakanuma Y, Tsuneyama K, Ohbu M, Katayanagi K. Pathology and pathogenesis of idiopathic portal hypertension with an emphasis on the liver. Pathol Res Pract. 2001;197(2):65–76.

120. Rajekar H, Vasishta RK, Chawla YK, Dhiman RK. Noncirrhotic portal hypertension. J Clin Exp Hepatol. 2011;1(2):94–108.

121. Sarin SK, Kumar A, Chawla YK, Baijal SS, Dhiman RK, Jafri W, et al. Noncirrhotic portal fibrosis/idiopathic portal hypertension:

APASL recommendations for diagnosis and treatment. Hepatol Int. 2007;1(3):398–413.

122. Schouten JN, Garcia-Pagan JC, Valla DC, Janssen HL. Idiopathic noncirrhotic portal hypertension. Hepatology 2011;54(3):1071–81.

123. Dhiman RK, Chawla Y, Vasishta RK, Kakkar N, Dilawari JB, Trehan MS, et al. Non-cirrhotic portal fibrosis (idiopathic portal hypertension): experience with 151 patients and a review of the literature. J Gastroenterol Hepatol. 2002;17(1):6–16.

124. Mackie I, Eapen CE, Neil D, Lawrie AS, Chitolie A, et al. Idiopathic noncirrhotic intrahepatic portal hypertension is associated with sustained ADAMTS13 Deficiency. Dig Dis Sci. 2011;56(8):2456–65.

125. Sarin SK, Sethi KK, Nanda R. Measurement and correlation of wedged hepatic, intrahepatic, intrasplenic and intravariceal pressures in patients with cirrhosis of liver and non-cirrhotic portal fibrosis. Gut 1987;28(3):260–6.

126. Krasinskas AM, Eghtesad B, Kamath PS, Demetris AJ, Abraham SC. Liver transplantation for severe intrahepatic noncirrhotic portal hypertension. Liver Transpl. 2005;11(6):627–34, discussion 610–1.

127. Sawada S, Sato Y, Aoyama H, Harada K, Nakanuma Y. Pathological study of idiopathic portal hypertension with an emphasis on cause of death based on records of Annuals of Pathological Autopsy Cases in Japan. J Gastroenterol Hepatol. 2007;22(2):204–9.

128. Girard M, Amiel J, Fabre M, Pariente D, Lyonnet S, Jacquemin E. Adams–Oliver syndrome and hepatoportal sclerosis: occasional association or common mechanism? Am J Med Genet A. 2005;135(2):186–9.

129. Sinha A, Samanta T, Mallik S, Pal D, Ganguly S. Non-cirrhotic portal fibrosis among children admitted in a tertiary care hospital of Kolkata: a search for possible aetiologies. J Indian Med Assoc. 2011;109(12):889–91.

130. Poddar U, Thapa BR, Puri P, Girish CS, Vaiphei K, et al. Non-cirrhotic portal fibrosis in children. Indian J Gastroenterol. 2000;19(1):12–3.

131. Cantez MS, Gerenli N, Ertekin V, Güllüoğlu M, Durmaz Ö. Hepatoportal sclerosis in childhood: descriptive analysis of 12 patients. J Korean Med Sci. 2013;28(10):1507–11.

132. Giacomet V, Viganò A, Penagini F, Manfredini V, Maconi G, et al. Splenomegaly and variceal bleeding in a ten-year-old HIV-infected girl with noncirrhotic portal hypertension. Pediatr Infect Dis J. 2012;31(10):1059–60.

133. Sarin SK, Sollano JD, Chawla YK, Amarapurkar D, Hamid S, Hashizume M, et al. Consensus on extra-hepatic portal vein obstruction. Liver Int. 2006;26(5):512–9.

134. Thompson EN, Williams R, Sherlock S. Liver function in extrahepatic portal hypertension. Lancet 1964;2(7374):1352–6.

135. Sarin SK, Agarwal SR. Extrahepatic portal vein obstruction. Semin Liver Dis. 2002;22(1):43–58.

136. Jha SK, Kumar A, Sharma BC, Sarin SK. Systemic and pulmonary hemodynamics in patients with extrahepatic portal vein obstruction is similar to compensated cirrhotic patients. Hepatol Int. 2009;3(2):384–91.

137. Bosch J, Mastai R, Kravetz D, Navasa M, Rodés J. Hemodynamic evaluation of the patient with portal hypertension. Semin Liver Dis. 1986;6(4):309–17.

138. Lebrec D, Bataille C, Bercoff E, Valla D. Hemodynamic changes in patients with portal venous obstruction. Hepatology 1983;3(4):550–3.

139. Harada A, Nonami T, Kasai Y, Nakao A, Takagi H. Systemic hemodynamics in non-cirrhotic portal hypertension–a clinical study of 19 patients. Jpn J Surg. 1988;18(6):620–5.

140. Braillon A, Moreau R, Hadengue A, Roulot D, Sayegh R, Lebrec D. Hyperkinetic circulatory syndrome in patients with presinusoidal portal hypertension. Effect of propranolol. J Hepatol. 1989;9(3):312–8.

141. Rangari M, Gupta R, Jain M, Malhotra V, Sarin SK. Hepatic dysfunction in patients with extrahepatic portal venous obstruction. Liver Int. 2003;23(6):434–9.

142. Chandra R, Kapoor D, Tharakan A, Chaudhary A, Sarin SK. Portal biliopathy. J Gastroenterol Hepatol. 2001;16(10):1086–92.

143. El-Matary W, Roberts EA, Kim P, Temple M, Cutz E, Ling SC. Portal hypertensive biliopathy: a rare cause of childhood cholestasis. Eur J Pediatr. 2008;167(11):1339–42.

144. Suárez V, Puerta A, Santos LF, Pérez JM, Varón A, Botero RC. Portal hypertensive biliopathy: a single center experience and literature review. World J Hepatol. 2013;5(3):137–44.

145. Orloff MJ, Orloff MS, MS Rambotti M. Treatment of bleeding esophagogastric varices due to extrahepatic portal hypertension: results of portal-systemic shunts during 35 years. J Pediatr Surg. 1994;29(2):142–51, discussion 151–4.

146. Orloff MJ, Orloff MS, Girard B, Orloff SL. Bleeding esophagogastric varices from extrahepatic portal hypertension: 40 years' experience with portal-systemic shunt. J Am Coll Surg. 2002;194(6):717–28, discussion 728–30.

147. Schettino GC, Fagundes ED, Roquete ML, Ferreira AR, Penna FJ. Portal vein thrombosis in children and adolescents. J Pediatr (Rio J). 2006;82(3):171–8.

148. Sarin SK, Bansal A, Sasan S, Nigam A. Portal-vein obstruction in children leads to growth retardation. Hepatology 1992;15(2):229–33.

149. Mehrotra RN, Bhatia V, Dabadghao P, Yachha SK. Extrahepatic portal vein obstruction in children: anthropometry, growth hormone, and insulin-like growth factor I. J Pediatr Gastroenterol Nutr. 1997;25(5):520–3.

150. Superina R, Bambini DA, Lokar J, Rigsby C, Whitington PF. Correction of extrahepatic portal vein thrombosis by the mesenteric to left portal vein bypass. Ann Surg. 2006;243(4):515–21.

151. Gauthier-Villars M, Franchi S, Gauthier F, Fabre M, Pariente D, Bernard O. Cholestasis in children with portal vein obstruction. J Pediatr. 2005;146(4):568–73.

152. Superina R, Shneider B, Emre S, Sarin S, de Ville de Goyet J. Surgical guidelines for the management of extra-hepatic portal vein obstruction. Pediatr Transplant. 2006;10(8):908–13.

153. Bajaj JS, Cordoba J, Mullen KD, Amodio P, Shawcross DL, Butterworth RF, et al. Review article: the design of clinical trials in hepatic encephalopathy—an International Society for Hepatic Encephalopathy and Nitrogen Metabolism (ISHEN) consensus statement. Aliment Pharmacol Ther. 2011;33(7):739–47.

154. D'Antiga L, Dacchille P, Boniver C, Poledri S, Schiff S, Zancan L, Amodio P. Clues for minimal hepatic encephalopathy in children with noncirrhotic portal hypertension. J Pediatr Gastroenterol Nutr. 2014;59(6):689–94.

155. Ito T, Ikeda N, Watanabe A, Sue K, Kakio T, et al. Obliteration of portal systemic shunts as therapy for hepatic encephalopathy in patients with non-cirrhotic portal hypertension. Gastroenterol Jpn. 1992;27(6):759–64.

156. Chiu B, Superina RA. Encephalopathy caused by a splenorenal shunt can be reversed by performing a mesenteric-to-left portal vein bypass. J Pediatr Surg. 2006;41(6):1177–9.

157. Mack CL, Zelko FA, Lokar J, Superina R, Alonso EM, et al. Surgically restoring portal blood flow to the liver in children with primary extrahepatic portal vein thrombosis improves fluid neurocognitive ability. Pediatrics 2006;117(3):e405–12.

158. Yadav SK, Srivastava A, Srivastava A, Thomas MA, Agarwal J, Pandey CM, et al. Encephalopathy assessment in children with extra-hepatic portal vein obstruction with MR, psychometry and critical flicker frequency. J Hepatol. 2010;52(3):348–54.

159. Yadav SK, Saksena S, Srivastava A, Srivastava A, Saraswat VA, Thomas MA, et al. Brain MR imaging and 1H-MR spectroscopy changes in patients with extrahepatic portal vein obstruction from early childhood to adulthood. AJNR Am J Neuroradiol. 2010;31(7):1337–42.

160. Ling SC, Shneider BL. Portal hypertension in children: current practice and the need for evidence. Oxford: Wiley-Blackwell; 2011. p. 189–96.

161. Gibelli NE, Tannuri AC, Pinho-Apezzato ML, Maksoud-Filho JG, Tannuri U. Extrahepatic portal vein thrombosis after umbilical catheterization: is it a good choice for Rex shunt? J Pediatr Surg. 2011;46(1):214–6.

162. Superina RA, de Ville de Goyet J. Preemptive meso-rex bypass for children with idiopathic prehepatic portal hypertension: trick or treat? J Pediatr Gastroenterol Nutr. 2014;58(4):e41.

163. Alberti D, D'Antiga L, Authors' response. J Pediatr Gastroenterol Nutr. 2014;58(4):e41.

164. Sharif K, McKiernan P, de Ville de Goyet J. Mesoportal bypass for extrahepatic portal vein obstruction in children: close to a cure for most! J Pediatr Surg. 2010;45(1):272–6.

165. Uno A1 Ishida H, Konno K, Ohnami Y, Naganuma H, Niizawa M, et al. Portal hypertension in children and young adults: sonographic and color Doppler findings. Abdom Imaging. 1997;22(1):72–8.

166. Gorka W, Kagalwalla A, McParland BJ, Kagalwalla Y, al Zaben A. Diagnostic value of Doppler ultrasound in the assessment of liver cirrhosis in children: histopathological correlation. J Clin Ultrasound. 1996;24(6):287–95.

167. Martínez-Noguera A, Montserrat E, Torrubia S, Villalba J. Doppler in hepatic cirrhosis and chronic hepatitis. Semin Ultrasound CT MR. 2002;23(1):19–36.

168. Goyal N, Jain N, Rachapalli V, Cochlin DL, Robinson M. Noninvasive evaluation of liver cirrhosis using ultrasound. Clin Radiol. 2009;64(11):1056–66.

169. Gaiani S, Bolondi L, Li Bassi S, Zironi G, Siringo S, Barbara L. Prevalence of spontaneous hepatofugal portal flow in liver cirrhosis. Clinical and endoscopic correlation in 228 patients. Gastroenterology 1991;100(1):160–7.

170. Annet L, Materne R, Danse E, Jamart J, Horsmans Y, Van Beers BE. Hepatic flow parameters measured with MR imaging and Doppler US: correlations with degree of cirrhosis and portal hypertension. Radiology 2003;229(2):409–14.

171. Patriquin H, Lafortune M, Weber A, Blanchard H, Garel L, Roy C Patriquin H, Lafortune M, Weber A, Blanchard H, Garel L, Roy C. Surgical portosystemic shunts in children: assessment with duplex Doppler US. Work in progress. Radiology 1987;165(1):25–8.

172. De Giacomo C, Tomasi G, Gatti C, Rosa G, Maggiore G. Ultrasonographic prediction of the presence and severity of esophageal varices in children. J Pediatr Gastroenterol Nutr. 1989;9(4):431–5.

173. Patriquin H, Tessier G, Grignon A, Boisvert J. Lesser omental thickness in normal children: baseline for detection of portal hypertension. AJR Am J Roentgenol. 1985;145(4):693–6.

174. Piscaglia F, Marinelli S, Bota S, Serra C, Venerandi L, et al. The role of ultrasound elastographic techniques in chronic liver disease: current status and future perspectives. Eur J Radiol. 2014;83(3):450–5.

175. Sporea I, Gilja OH, Bota S, Şirli R, Popescu A. Liver elastography—an update. Med Ultrason. 2013;15(4):304–14.

176. Goldschmidt I, Streckenbach C, Dingemann C, Pfister ED, di Nanni A, et al. Application and limitations of transient liver elastography in children. J Pediatr Gastroenterol Nutr. 2013;57(1):109–13.

177. Yachha SK, Sharma BC, Kumar M, Khanduri A. Endoscopic sclerotherapy for esophageal varices in children with extrahepatic portal venous obstruction: a follow-up study. J Pediatr Gastroenterol Nutr. 1997;24(1):49–52.

178. D'Antiga L, Betalli P, De Angelis P, Davenport M, Di Giorgio A, et al. Interobserver agreement on endoscopic classification of oesophageal varices in children: a multicenter study. J Pediatr Gastroenterol Nutr. 2015.

179. Duché M, Ducot B, Tournay E, Fabre M, Cohen J, et al. Prognostic value of endoscopy in children with biliary atresia at risk for early development of varices and bleeding. Gastroenterology 2010;139(6):1952–60.

180. Berzigotti A, Seijo S, Reverter E, Bosch J. Assessing portal hypertension in liver diseases. Expert Rev Gastroenterol Hepatol. 2013;7(2):141–55.

181. Bosch J, García-Pagán JC. Prevention of variceal rebleeding. Lancet 2003;361(9361):952–4.

182. Ripoll C, Groszmann R, Garcia-Tsao G, Grace N, Burroughs A, Planas R, et al. Hepatic venous pressure gradient predicts clinical decompensation in patients with compensated cirrhosis. Gastroenterology 2007;133(2):481–8.

183. Turnes J, Garcia-Pagan JC, Abraldes JG, Hernandez-Guerra M, Dell'Era A, Bosch J. Pharmacological reduction of portal pressure and long-term risk of first variceal bleeding in patients with cirrhosis. Am J Gastroenterol. 2006;101(3):506–12.

184. Miraglia R, Luca A, Maruzzelli L, Spada M, Riva S, Caruso S, et al. Measurement of hepatic vein pressure gradient in children with chronic liver diseases. J Hepatol. 2010;53(4):624–9.

185. Woolfson J, John P, Kamath B, Ng VL, Ling SC. Measurement of hepatic venous pressure gradient is feasible and safe in children. J Pediatr Gastroenterol Nutr. 2013;57(5):634–7.

186. Taylor CR. Computed tomography in the evaluation of the portal venous system. J Clin Gastroenterol. 1992;14(2):167–72.

187. Finn JP, Kane RA, Edelman RR, Jenkins RL, Lewis WD, et al. Imaging of the portal venous system in patients with cirrhosis: MR angiography vs duplex Doppler sonography. AJR Am J Roentgenol. 1993;161(5):989–94.

188. Lebrec D. Pharmacological treatment of portal hypertension: hemodynamic effects and prevention of bleeding. Pharmacol Ther. 1994;61(1–2):65–107.

189. Ozsoylu S, Koçak N, Demir H, Yüce A, Gürakan F, Ozen H. Propranolol for primary and secondary prophylaxis of variceal bleeding in children with cirrhosis. Turk J Pediatr. 2000;42(1):31–3.

190. Ozsoylu S, Kocak N, Yuce A. Propranolol therapy for portal hypertension in children. J Pediatr. 1985;106(2):317–21.

191. Ostman-Smith I, Wettrell G, Riesenfeld T. A cohort study of childhood hypertrophic cardiomyopathy: improved survival following high-dose beta-adrenoceptor antagonist treatment. J Am Coll Cardiol. 1999;34(6):1813–22.

192. Zargar SA, Javid G, Khan BA, Shah OJ, Yattoo GN, Shah AH, et al. Endoscopic ligation vs. sclerotherapy in adults with extrahepatic portal venous obstruction: a prospective randomized study. Gastrointest Endosc. 2005;61(1):58–66.

193. Zargar SA, Javid G, Khan BA, Yattoo GN, Shah AH, Gulzar GM, et al. Endoscopic ligation compared with sclerotherapy for bleeding esophageal varices in children with extrahepatic portal venous obstruction. Hepatology 2002;36(3):666–72.

194. Zargar SA, Yattoo GN, Javid G, Khan BA, Shah AH, Shah NA, et al. Fifteen-year follow up of endoscopic injection sclerotherapy in children with extrahepatic portal venous obstruction. J Gastroenterol Hepatol. 2004;19(2):139–45.

195. Lacroix J, Hébert PC, Hutchison JS, Hume HA, Tucci M, Ducruet T, et al. Transfusion strategies for patients in pediatric intensive care units. N Engl J Med. 2007;356(16):1609–19.

196. Villanueva C, Colomo A, Bosch A, Concepción M, Hernandez-Gea V, Aracil C, et al. Transfusion strategies for acute upper gastrointestinal bleeding. N Engl J Med. 2013;368(1):11–21.

197. Eroglu Y, Emerick KM, Whitingon PF, Alonso EM. Octreotide therapy for control of acute gastrointestinal bleeding in children. J Pediatr Gastroenterol Nutr. 2004;38(1):41–7.

198. Goulis J, Armonis A, Patch D, Sabin C, Greenslade L, Burroughs AK. Bacterial infection is independently associated with failure to control bleeding in cirrhotic patients with gastrointestinal hemorrhage. Hepatology 1998;27(5):1207–12.

199. Botha JF, Campos BD, Grant WJ, Horslen SP, Sudan DL, et al. Portosystemic shunts in children: a 15-year experience. J Am Coll Surg. 2004;199(2):179–85.

200. Lillegard JB, Hanna AM, McKenzie TJ, Moir CR, Ishitani MB, Nagorney DM. A single-institution review of portosystemic shunts in children: an ongoing discussion. HPB Surg. 2010;2010:964597.

201. Evans S, Stovroff M, Heiss K, Ricketts R. Selective distal splenorenal shunts for intractable variceal bleeding in pediatric portal hypertension. J Pediatr Surg. 1995;30(8):1115–8.

202. Goncalves ME, Cardoso SR, Maksoud JG. Prophylactic sclerotherapy in children with esophageal varices: long-term results of a controlled prospective randomized trial. J Pediatr Surg. 2000;35(3):401–5.

203. Lykavieris P, Gauthier F, Hadchouel P, Duche M, Bernard O. Risk of gastrointestinal bleeding during adolescence and early adulthood in children with portal vein obstruction. J Pediatr. 2000;136(6):805–8.

69

Mohamed Rela and Mettu Srinivas Reddy

Introduction

Liver tumors are uncommon in the pediatric age group and constitute 1–2 % of all solid tumors in children. About 60 % of all liver tumors in children are malignant [1]. Hepatoblastoma (HB) is by far the most common constituting over 50–60 % of all liver tumors in this age group. Hepatocellular carcinoma (HCC), undifferentiated embryonal carcinoma and biliary rhabdomyosarcoma are other malignant liver tumors in children. Benign tumors include hemangiomas (HMGs), mesenchymal hamartoma, and focal nodular hyperplasia (FNH). Secondary tumors to the liver can spread from a host of primary tumors including lymphomas, Wilms' tumor, neuroblastoma, osteosarcoma, etc. (Table 69.1). Several congenital and environmental risk factors have been reported to increase the predilection for liver tumors (Table 69.2).

There is a striking age-related variation in the frequency of different tumor types (Table 69.3). Over 90 % of liver tumors in children below 5 years are HB, while 87 % of tumors in the 15–19-year age group are HCC. A gradual increase in the incidence of liver tumors in children over the past 3–4 decades has been reported. This is particularly evident in the case of HB where the incidence has increased from 0.6 to 1.2 per million population between 1973–1977 and 1993–1997. On the contrary, incidence of HCC has decreased from 0.45 to 0.29 per million population during the same period [2].

Tumor Markers in Childhood Liver Tumors

Alpha-fetoprotein (AFP) is the most recognized tumor marker in liver tumors. AFP is a glycoprotein similar in physical and chemical characteristics to albumin. It is secreted by the fetal liver and yolk sac until 13 weeks' gestation and then primarily by the fetal liver [3]. AFP levels at birth are very high with Bader et al. reporting a median level of over 40,000 ng/ml in cord blood samples [4]. These levels rapidly drop during the first year of life at a rate primarily dictated by the half-life of AFP of 5–6 days [5]. AFP levels at birth in the preterm babies are higher than full-term babies. Similarly, a decrease in at-birth AFP for every week of prolonged gestation has been reported [4]. The high levels of AFP in the infant should be kept in mind by the clinician when AFP levels are used for the diagnosis and monitoring of pediatric liver tumors.

Several tumors are associated with elevated AFP. HB is the commonest cause in infants though HCCs and germ cell tumors are also associated with elevated AFP. Nonneoplastic conditions, such as tyrosinemia and neonatal hepatitis, can also cause elevated AFP levels.

Malignant Tumors

Hepatoblastoma

HB is the most common liver tumor in children. It is almost always seen in the first 4 years of life with median age at diagnosis of 18 months. It can present at birth and has been diagnosed in the intrauterine period on antenatal scans. Prematurity and very small birth weight have been identified as risk factors. HB developing in these children is also reported to have a worse prognosis [6, 7].

HB is a tumor of immature hepatocyte progenitor cells. It is an embryonal tumor, which recapitulates various stages of liver development. Histologically, these tumors are heterogeneous and comprise combinations of epithelial, mes-

M. Rela (✉) · M. S. Reddy
Institute of Liver Disease and Transplantation, National Foundation for Liver Research, Global Health City, Cheran Nagar, Chennai, India
e-mail: mohamed.rela@gmail.com

M. Rela
Institute of Liver Studies, King's College Hospital, London, UK

© Springer International Publishing Switzerland 2016
S. Guandalini et al. (eds.), *Textbook of Pediatric Gastroenterology. Hepatology and Nutrition*,
DOI 10.1007/978-3-319-17169-2_69

Table 69.1 Types of liver tumors in children

Benign	Hemangioma: focal, multiple, diffuse
	Mesenchymal hamartoma
	Hepatic adenoma
	Focal nodular hyperplasia
	Inflammatory myofibroblastic tumor (may be locally invasive)
Malignant	
Primary	Hepatoblastoma
	Hepatocellular carcinoma, fibrolamellar HCC
	Transitional tumors
	Embryonal sarcoma
	Biliary rhabdomyosarcoma
	Calcifying nested stromal–epithelial tumor
	Angiosarcoma
Secondary	Lymphomas, leukemia, Wilms' tumor, neuroblastoma, osteosarcoma, colon cancer

Table 69.2 Risk factors and premalignant conditions for childhood liver tumors

Tumor	Risk factors	Premalignant lesions
Hepatoblastoma	Beckwith–Wiedemann syndrome, familial adenomatous polyposis, Li–Fraumeni syndrome, trisomy 18, preterm birth and very low birth weight	–
Hepatocellular carcinoma	Glycogen storage disease, tyrosinemia, Alagille syndrome, biliary atresia, PFIC, Ataxia-telangiectasia, hepatitis B infection, hepatitis C infection	Hepatic adenoma
Embryonal sarcoma	–	Mesenchymal hamartoma
Angiosarcoma	–	Hemangioma

PFIC progressive familial intrahepatic cholestasis

Table 69.3 Age-wise distribution of childhood liver tumors

Age group	Benign tumors	Malignant tumors
Neonatal period	Hemangioma, mesenchymal hamartoma	Hepatoblastoma
0–5 years	–	Hepatoblastoma, biliary rhabdomyosarcoma
5–15 years	–	Hepatocellular carcinoma, embryonal sarcoma
>15 years	Hepatic adenoma	Fibrolamellar carcinoma

enchymal, and occasionally teratoid components in varying proportions (Table 69.4, Fig. 69.1). Majority of tumors have a primarily epithelial component containing hepatoblasts at varying stages of differentiation. The histological type has an impact on behavior with well-differentiated fetal epithelial type having the best prognosis. The small-cell undifferentiated type of HB has the worst prognosis with very poor survival. Mixed tumors contain both epithelial and mesenchymal components, are more resistant to chemotherapy, and have a worse prognosis. Post-chemotherapy residual tumors and metastatic tumors may demonstrate a pleomorphic pattern with pleomorphic nuclei having coarse chromatin and prominent nucleoli. This pattern may resemble HCC.

Diagnosis

The usual presentation is with an abdominal lump identified by the parent or the clinician. Pain, failure to thrive, or jaundice are uncommon modes of presentation. Investigations reveal an elevated AFP level in over 90% of cases. The AFP levels are extremely high (in the order of 10^5 ng/ml) and are usually a log higher than those seen with HCC. AFP level has been identified as a prognostic marker in HB with both very high levels and low levels (< 100 ng/ml) predicting poor biology [8]. Thrombocytosis is a recognized laboratory finding in HB and is probably related to production of thrombopoietic cytokines including thrombopoietin in the tumor tissues.

Imaging with computed tomography (CT) is necessary to confirm the diagnosis, stage the extent of liver disease, identify vascular invasion, extrahepatic disease, and lung metastases. HB appears as a heterogeneously enhancing well-circumscribed lesion with occasional calcifications. A biopsy is usually required to confirm diagnosis before start of neoadjuvant chemotherapy and for prognostication.

Staging and Prognostication

Several staging systems have been developed to tailor treatment for HB. The preoperative extent of tumor (PRETEXT) system based on preoperative imaging, which was devel-

Table 69.4 Histological types of hepatoblastoma

Histological type	Description
Epithelial	Primarily containing immature hepatocytes
Fetal	Commonest variant of epithelial HB. Composed of polygonal cells resembling fetal hepatocytes arranged in one- to two-cell thick cords, trabeculae or sheets
Embryonal, well differentiated	Tumor resembles the liver at 6–8 weeks of gestation. Demonstrates organized tubular or acinar formation. Hematopoietic elements are commonly admixed with epithelial component
Cholangioblastic	Tumour cells differentiate as cholangiocytes and form small ducts. This component expresses cholangiocyte lineage markers (cytokeratins 7 and 19)
Macrotrabecular	Cells arranged in thick trabecular pattern (>5 cells thick)
Small cell undifferentiated	Sheets of small cells with large hyperchromatic nuclei similar to neuroblastoma
Mixed epithelial–mesenchymal type	Mixture of epithelial and mesenchymal cell types
Teratoid	Contains heterologous components such as stratified squamous epithelium, mucus-producing cells, neuroectodermal derivatives
Non-teratoid	Contains stromal derivatives including spindle fibroblastic cells, osteoid, skeletal muscle, and cartilage

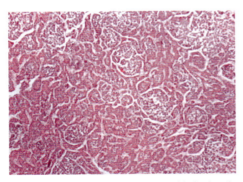

Fig. 69.1 Hepatoblastoma, epithelial type with fetal and embryonal epithelium.

oped and popularized by the International Childhood Liver Tumors Strategy (SIOPEL) Group, is commonly used in Europe (Table 69.5, Fig. 69.2). This is an anatomical classification focusing on the extent of tumor and the amount of liver that can be spared during resection [9]. Modifications to the PRETEXT scoring system have included additional subclassifications to identify high-risk factors such as vascular involvement, caudate lobe involvement, etc. (Table 69.6) [10].

SIOPEL also classifies HB into standard risk, high risk, and very-high-risk groups based on the PRETEXT staging and additional factors to tailor management (Table 69.7) [11].

Other staging systems include the Children's Oncology Group (COG) classification, which is based on intraoperative findings, and presence of residual tumor have been used more commonly in the USA.

Management

Early results of HB with surgical resection alone were poor due to the advanced stage at which these tumors usually present. Only 5% of all tumors at presentation can be staged as PRETEXT I, and over 50% are unresectable at initial presentation (Table 69.5). Metastatic disease in the lungs at presentation is not uncommon. However, this should not dissuade the clinician from aiming for cure as resection of lung metastases along with treatment of primary has been shown to improve long-term survival [12].

HB are highly chemosensitive tumors and respond well to platinum-compound-based chemotherapy. Use of chemotherapy in conjunction with surgery has radically altered the outcomes of these tumors. Today, multimodality treatment with surgery and chemotherapy is the mainstay of treatment for HB.

Ideal treatment strategy for PRETEXT I tumors is controversial. Some authors have suggested complete resection alone without chemotherapy as an option. This is especially true for the low-risk tumors with fetal histology where complete surgical resection with follow-up has been shown to be effective in providing long-term disease control [13]. Ad-

Table 69.5 PRETEXT staging and frequency of various PRETEXT stages at initial presentation [8]. Refer to Fig. 69.2

PRETEXT staging	Definition	Frequency at presentation (%)
I	One section is involved and three adjoining sections are free	4.8
II	One or two sections are involved, but two adjoining sections are free	36.6
III	Two or three sections are involved and no two adjoining sections are free	38.8
IV	All four sections are involved	19.8

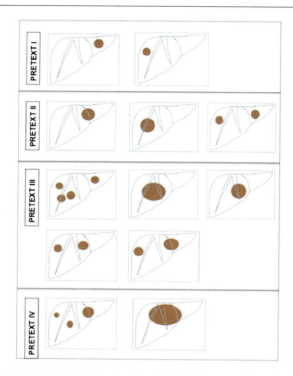

Fig. 69.2 PRETEXT staging: The PRETEXT system is based on the preoperative imaging and is an assessment of the liver that is free of tumor. The liver is divided into four sectors by the right and middle hepatic veins and the falciform ligament. The four sectors are the left lateral, left medial, right medial, and right lateral sectors. The number of contiguous sectors that are free of tumor is the key to the staging. Tumor may be single or multiple. **a** PRETEXT 1, three contiguous sectors are tumor free, **b** PRETEXT 2, two contiguous sectors are free of disease, **c** PRETEXT 3, only one sector is free, **d** PRETEXT 4, all four sectors are involved

vocates for this approach highlight the fact that these children are spared the adverse effects of chemotherapy such as ototoxicity [14]. The SIOPEL group advocates neoadjuvant chemotherapy for all HB. The purported advantages of this approach are that it shrinks the tumor, and clearly demarcates the tumors making resection more straightforward. Tumors also become more fibrotic and hence intraoperative handling is easier.

The current protocol for PRETEXT II and III is to give up to four cycles of neoadjuvant chemotherapy, followed by assessment for resection (Fig. 69.3).

If the tumor becomes resectable, then surgery is followed by two more cycles of chemotherapy. If the tumor remains unresectable, two further cycles of chemotherapy may be considered before a decision is made regarding attempted resection or primary transplantation. Monitoring the fall in AFP level after beginning chemotherapy and after surgery is an excellent means of predicting tumor response. The chemotherapy regimen advised by the SIOPEL group varies for the standard risk and high-risk HB (Table 69.7)[11].

Surgical resection for HB should be carefully planned and is best carried out in units with expertise in pediatric hepatobiliary surgery and liver transplantation (LT). This is particularly true in children with large tumors and borderline resectability. Children can tolerate extensive liver resections better than adults, and up to 85% of liver can be resected safely. More aggressive liver resection techniques such as total vascular exclusion and caval resection may be required to achieve complete disease clearance.

LT for unresectable HB is a well-defined indication [15]. These could be PRETEXT IV tumors (solitary or multifo-

Table 69.6 Additional criteria for PRETEXT staging [10]

Caudate lobe involvement	C1—tumor involving caudate lobe	–
	C0—all other patients	
Extrahepatic abdominal disease	E0—no evidence of tumor spread in abdomen (except M or N)	Add suffix "a" if ascites is present
	E1—direct extension of tumor into adjacent organs or diaphragm	
	E2—peritoneal nodules	
Tumor focality	F0—solitary tumor	–
	F1—two or more discrete tumors	
Tumor rupture	H1	–
Distant metastases	M1	–
Lymph node metastasis	N0—no nodal metastases	–
	N1—abdominal lymph node metastases only	
	N2—extra-abdominal lymph node metastases	
Portal vein involvement	P1—involvement of left or right branch of portal vein	Add suffix "a" if intravascular tumor present
	P2—involvement of main portal vein	
IVC or hepatic vein involvement	V1—involvement of one hepatic vein, IVC free	Add suffix "a" if intravascular tumor present
	V2—involvement of two hepatic veins, IVC free	
	V3—involvement of all three hepatic veins and/or IVC	

IVC inferior vena cava

Table 69.7 Risk stratification and treatment of hepatoblastoma (SIOPEL guidelines). (Available at www.siopel.org [11])

Risk status	Definition	SIOPEL guideline for treatment
Standard risk	PRETEXT I, II, III without any other risk factors as defined below[a]	*SIOPEL 3, Cisplatin alone arm*
		Cisplatin X 4 cycles
		Surgical resection
		Cisplatin X 2cycles
High risk	PRETEXT IV or any PRETEXT stage with vascular involvement (P2 or V3), extrahepatic disease (E1, E2), tumor rupture (H1)	*SIOPEL 3, SUPERPLADO arm*
		Alternating cycles of Cisplatin and carboplatin + doxorubicin X 7 cycles
		Resection/Transplantation
		Alternating cycles of Cisplatin and carboplatin + doxorubicin X 3 cycles
Very high tisk	Any tumor with metastases or very low AFP (< 100 ng/ml)	SIOPEL 4, dose-dense cisplatin-based chemotherapy or enrolment in clinical trial

[a] PRETEXT I with fetal histology may be considered for surgical resection alone and observation

AFP alpha-fetoprotein, *PRETEXT* preoperative extent of tumor

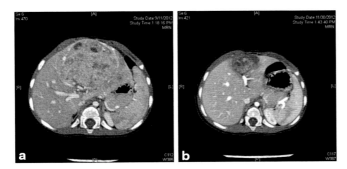

Fig. 69.3 CT images of Hepatoblastoma in a 1-year-child. **a** CT at presentation showed a PRETEXT 2 disease with tumor involving the two left sectors. **b** CT following four cycles of chemotherapy prior to resection. Note the significant shrinkage in tumor size. The CT appearance of the tumor has also changed and the demarcation between the tumor and healthy liver tissue is much more clear

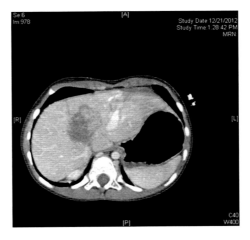

Fig. 69.4 CT image of a hepatoblastoma in a 6-year child. This child had persistent PRETEXT III tumor after six cycles of chemotherapy. The tumor was closely approximated to the cava. She underwent primary living donor liver transplantation

cal), centrally located PRETEXT II or III, or tumors with portal or caval involvement (Fig. 69.4). In children where surgical resection is not feasible, early referral for LT assessment is the best approach. Primary LT in high-risk cases has better outcomes than rescue transplantation after resection, and the latter should be considered a relative contraindication [16]. A recent US study reported that over the past 20 years, the percentage of HB receiving transplantation has increased from 5 to 20%, and the number of transplantations for HB has increased almost 20-fold [17]. This could be a reflection of the increasing confidence among clinicians for this radical modality of treatment.

The options are either split-liver deceased donor LT (DDLT) or living donor LT (LDLT) and both have comparable results. Children planned for DDLT usually complete neoadjuvant chemotherapy and are placed on the waiting list with some form of prioritization to enable timely transplantation. Where LDLT is an option, transplantation can be planned to follow the planned course of neoadjuvant chemotherapy. Transplantation should be followed by adjuvant chemotherapy. Presence of lung metastases increases the risk of posttransplant recurrence but is not a contraindication for LT as long as they can be resected [18]. Close follow-up in the posttransplantation period is essential and usually involves periodic AFP estimation and imaging studies.

Results of HB have significantly improved over the past 2–3 decades. Overall disease-free survival has improved to over 70% for all HB. Low-risk tumors have a 90% 5-year survival, while high-risk tumors have a survival of around 50%. Histological subtype has an impact on survival. Fetal types of HB have the best outcomes, while the small-cell undifferentiated type of tumors have worse prognosis. Relapse after initial complete response occurs in 11% of children. Liver and lungs are the commonest sites of relapse. Positron emission tomography/computed tomography (PET/CT) has been reported to be better at identifying relapse when compared to CT or MRI [19]. Combination of surgery and chemotherapy provide the best chance of achieving a second complete response in these children with reported 3-year overall survival of over 40% [20].

Hepatocellular Carcinoma

HCC is the second commonest liver tumor in children. It forms 15% of all malignant liver tumors in children but constitutes over 75% of all liver tumors in adolescents. HCC in children can occur in a background of chronic liver disease secondary to hepatitis B or metabolic disorders though non-cirrhotic HCC is more common than in adults. With increasing use of universal hepatitis B immunization, the incidence of HCC in children has decreased [2, 21]. HCC in children may be the standard type as seen in adults or the fibrolamellar variant seen in children and young adults.

HCC usually presents as an abdominal lump. Occasional presentation may be with abdominal pain or jaundice due to biliary compression or tumor ingrowth into the biliary tree. Rarely, these tumors may present as an emergency due to bleeding or rupture. HCCs are usually associated with an elevated AFP level though the elevation is not as high as that seen in HB. Liver function tests should be evaluated to assess the severity of any underlying liver disease. Metabolic screen is important to identify underlying liver disease which may impact management. Triphasic CT or MRI with contrast can help in characterizing the lesion, presence of chronic liver disease, any vascular involvement, and the presence of metastases.

HCC are chemoresistant tumors. Complete surgical excision provides these children with the best chance of long-term cure. However, the feasibility of resection depends on the size and extent of the tumor and the presence of underlying liver disease. In patients with underlying chronic liver disease, LT has the benefit of treating the underlying liver disease and providing adequate tumor clearance.

In the adult setting, the option of LT is available only for HCC within strict size and number criteria [22]. It is unclear if these criteria are appropriate in the pediatric setting, as most children will present with large tumors. Studies have shown good results in children transplanted for HCC beyond Milan criteria [23]. Hence, unless there is major vascular invasion or extrahepatic disease, unresectable HCC in children should be considered for LT. Presence of lung metastases is a contraindication for LT in pediatric HCC unlike HB due to the high risk of posttransplant progression of metastatic disease. Use of sorafenib in combination with cisplatin-based chemotherapy has also been reported in the management of pediatric HCC [24].

Outcomes of pediatric HCC are inferior to HB. The average 5-year survival is around 70%. Recurrent disease is the most common cause of death in these children and usually occurs in the lungs or bones.

Fibrolamellar Hepatocellular Carcinoma

This is an uncommon form of primary liver tumor seen in children greater than 5 years and young adults. The median age at presentation is 21 years. It is less common than standard HCC and occurs on a background of a non-cirrhotic liver. An elevated AFP is only seen in around 10% of these tumors. They are detected incidentally when they become symptomatic and are hence large at presentation. In a systematic review of available literature of fibrolamellar HCC (FL-HCC), the mean size of tumor at surgery was 12 cm [25]. On CT imaging, they appear as large well-circumscribed lesions which enhance strongly in arterial and portal venous phases becoming isodense in delayed scans. A poorly enhancing central scar may be seen. These tumors spread by both lymph node and blood borne systemic metastases.

Management of these tumors is primarily surgical. If resectable, surgical resection offers the best chance of cure for these tumors with a 5-year survival of 70% in adults [25, 26]. However, within the pediatric age group, results of FL-HCC do not appear to be superior to standard HCC probably because of late presentation and local recurrence after resection [27]. LT for FL-HCC has been reported though the long-term results are not encouraging possibly because of large tumor size at presentation and presence of lymph nodal metastases.

Transitional Tumors

These are a special group of tumors initially described by Prokurat et al. that share characteristics of both HB and HCC [28]. They usually develop in older children and are large in size at presentation. AFP levels are elevated. Histologically, they have features intermediate between the macrotrabecular variant of HB and trabecular HCC. Most of these were initially diagnosed as HB and treated as such. However, they have been reported to have much poorer outcome.

Embryonal Sarcoma (Undifferentiated Sarcoma of Liver)

This is a rare mesenchymal tumor constituting 5% of all liver tumors in children. The median age of presentation is between 6 and 10 years and is more common in males. There have been several reports of development of embryonal sarcoma from mesenchymal hamartomas [29]. Studies have also shown similar karyotypic abnormalities in both tumors. Presentation is with an abdominal lump. This tumor has characteristic radiological appearance. Ultrasonography

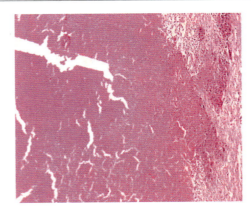

Fig. 69.5 Histology of embryonal sarcoma. Tumor shows large areas of necrosis with islands of spindle-shaped tumor cells in a myxoid matrix

(USG) shows a solid isoechoic clearly demarcated tumor. CT shows a well-circumscribed hypoattenuating lesion with multiple enhancing septations. An enhancing pseudocapsule may be present. The tumors are usually large at presentation and may be associated with lung metastases. Histologically, these tumors demonstrate large areas of necrosis with patches of viable tumor. Stellate or spindle-shaped tumor cells are loosely arranged in a myxoid matrix (Fig. 69.5).

Initial reports of this tumor described poor prognosis [30]. However, recent reports have shown that multimodality approach combining resectional surgery, chemotherapy, and transplantation can provide survival rate of up to 90 % [31, 32].

Biliary Rhabdomyosarcoma

This is the most common cause of malignant biliary obstruction in the pediatric age group. These tumors arise from any part of the intrahepatic and extrahepatic biliary tree including the gall bladder and ampulla of Vater. The median age at presentation is 3 years, and children commonly present with jaundice and abdominal pain. Preoperative diagnosis is usually a choledochal cyst [33, 34]. CT scan shows a dilated biliary tract with a hypoattenuating tumor in the bile duct [35]. Surgery helps in confirming diagnosis and enables resection of the tumor and biliary drainage in the form of a hepaticojejunostomy. Surgical excision with negative microscopic margins is rarely possible. These tumors have been found to respond well to adjuvant multi-agent chemotherapy. Spunt et al reported 25 cases of biliary rhabdomyosarcoma with a 5-year survival of 66 % for all cases and 78 % for children without systemic metastases. Death was primarily due to recurrent disease or complications of aggressive resection and/or chemotherapy [36].

Calcifying Nested Stromal-Epithelial Tumor

These are rare primary liver tumors of uncertain histogenesis that typically occur in children and young adults [37, 38]. Histologically, they have a characteristic appearance with circumscribed nests and islands of bland-appearing epithelioid cells. Focal psammoma-like calcifications with or without ossification may be present. The tumors typically have an indolent course and are considered as low-grade malignancies. Surgical resection is the treatment of choice. Some of these tumors have been reported to be associated with Cushing's syndrome which improved on resection.

Angiosarcoma

These are highly malignant tumors with poor prognosis. Malignant transformation from HMGs has been reported. Resection, if possible, should be carried out. Survival is poor due to development of systemic metastases [39, 40].

Benign Liver Tumors

Hemangioma

HMGs are the most common benign tumors in the pediatric setting. They constitute over half of all liver tumors in the neonatal period. The Liver Hemangioma Registry of the Vascular Anomalies Center at the Children's Hospital of Boston recognizes three clinical subgroups of infantile hepatic HMG—focal, multifocal, and diffuse [41]. Focal HMGs are usually single and indolent. Their clinical presentation is based entirely on their size and usually present as a large abdominal mass. Smaller focal lesions are diagnosed only on routine imaging studies in the antenatal period or after birth and usually have no clinical relevance. Associated extrahepatic lesions are uncommon with focal HMGs.

Multifocal HMGs present as multiple lesions in one or both lobes of the liver or may involve the liver diffusely. Histologically, they may be classified as capillary or cavernous HMG and may rarely show pleomorphism, intravascular spread, necrosis, and hemorrhage. The term hemangioendothelioma has also been used to describe these lesions. Over half of these children have extrahepatic vascular lesions, most commonly in the skin but also in the brain, eye, etc. Hemangioendotheliomas have the tendency to grow in the first year of life and then involute. Status of the cutaneous lesions has been used as a marker for monitoring the involution of the liver lesions [42].

Clinical presentation is commonly as an abdominal mass. High-output cardiac failure and consumptive coagulopathy due to trapping and destruction of platelets within the lesions are serious problems with these tumors [43]. Abnormalities in thyroid function have been reported in these children [42, 44]. A small percentage of these tumors (<5%) may be pre-malignant and progress to angiosarcoma if left untreated [45].

Treatment of these lesions should be tailored to individual presentation [42]. Small, asymptomatic lesions are best left alone. Symptomatic lesions have been treated with a variety of pharmacological and interventional approaches. Steroids, chemotherapeutic agents, β-blockers, hepatic artery ligation, or hepatic artery embolization have all been reported by various authors to be useful. Large symptomatic lesions are best treated by liver resection and are best managed in centers with advanced hepatobiliary and LT expertise. Liver transplantation has been reported in large symptomatic lesions not amenable to resection [42].

Mesenchymal Hamartomas

These rank second in frequency among benign liver neoplasms in children. They usually present as a large abdominal mass in the first 2 years of life. Some of these tumors may be detected incidentally or because of symptoms of abdominal pain, vomiting, or failure to thrive. Rare presentations are with respiratory distress, high output cardiac failure in the newborn and with jaundice, hemorrhage, or rupture [29, 46].

Imaging usually shows a single tumor in the right lobe with solid and cystic components. Occasionally, one cyst may be large giving it the appearance of a single cystic lesion.

Microscopic examination shows varying proportions of epithelial and loose connective tissue components arranged in a disorganized pattern. The epithelial element consists of bile ducts and hepatic parenchyma without acinar pattern. Numerous arteries and veins are scattered in the loose myxoid stroma. Cystic degeneration and foci of extramedullary hematopoiesis are also identified. Some authors have classified it as a neoplasm rather than a hamartoma. Reports that these tumors are associated with karyotype abnormalities such as aneuploidy and balanced translocations suggest a malignant potential [29].

Natural history of these tumors is variable, but the majority grows in size. There have been occasional reports of spontaneous regression or malignant transformation into undifferentiated embryonal sarcoma [47].

Treatment is primarily surgical. Complete excision is recommended and, where not possible, LT has been reported.

Hepatic Adenomas

These are diagnosed in older child and adolescents. In adults, there is a correlation between the use of oral contraception and hepatic adenomas. They are usually identified on routine

screening, though bleeding and rupture of superficial adenomas may lead to a more acute presentation. Small adenomas are best followed up by serial imaging because of the small risk of malignant transformation. Larger adenomas or superficial adenomas presenting with pain are better resected to avoid complications.

Focal Nodular Hyperplasia

FNH is uncommon in children and constitutes about 5% of all pediatric liver tumors. There has been some reported association between previous liver or bone marrow cancers or the presence of congenital or surgical portosystemic shunts and the development of FNH. A possible response of the liver tissue to the cytotoxic chemotherapy has been postulated. Similarly, borderline ischemia of the liver due to the shunting has also been postulated as a possible explanation of their coexistence with shunts.

FNH is usually diagnosed on routine imaging and is identified as a slightly hypodense, discrete lesion on plain CT. On contrast images, it enhances homogeneously in the arterial phase with the lesion becoming isodense in delayed scans. A central scar is noted in 50% of cases with delayed enhancement of the central scar a characteristic finding in FNH.

Macroscopically, it appears as a well circumscribed mass with a central depression (Fig. 69.6). Cut surface shows small nodules divided by fibrous septa leading to a central scar. Microscopically, the nodules contain hyperplastic hepatocytes supported by a well-developed reticulin framework. The septa contains abundant vessels, consisting of both arteries and veins. Variable eccentric intimal fibroplasia and disruption of the elastic lamina is noted in the arteries. Inflammatory cells and numerous proliferating ductules are also identified in the septa. Chronic cholestatic features are also identified in the cells adjacent to septa.

The most common presenting symptom is pain. These lesions may be small and multiple or may be single and large. If imaging is suggestive of FNH, then close follow-up with

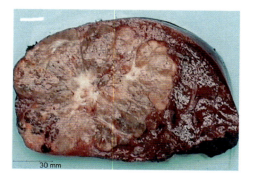

Fig. 69.6 Cut section of focal nodular hyperplasia. Note the well-circumscribed lesion with multiple nodules separated by fibrous septa joining at a central scar

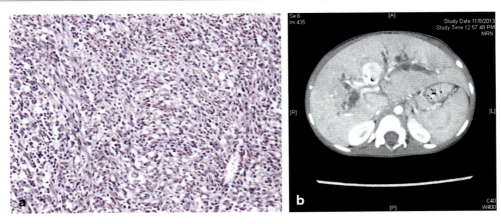

Fig. 69.7 a Section of an Inflammatory myofibroblastic tumor displaying interlacing bundles of fibroblasts admixed with inflammatory cells. **b** CT showing an inflammatory myofibroblastic tumor involving the hepatic hilum in a 4-year-old child. The child presented with constitutional symptoms, obstructive jaundice, and recurrent episodes of cholangitis. He underwent endoscopic stenting with no relief of symptoms. Surgical resection (extended right hepatectomy with excision of extrahepatic biliary tract) was carried out

serial imaging to detect any increase in size is recommended. Biopsy may be necessary in doubtful cases. Resection is only appropriate for large tumors or tumors with significant symptoms. Closure of the predisposing portosystemic shunts has been reported to cause shrinkage of the tumors.

Inflammatory Myofibroblastic Tumor

Inflammatory myofibroblastic tumors (IMFT) are predominantly benign lesions of unknown origin. These tumors can occur anywhere in the body and have occasionally been reported in the liver where they may mimic liver tumors.

These lesions have a characteristic histological picture comprising a spindle-cell proliferation admixed with chronic inflammatory cell infiltrate of plasma cells, lymphocytes, and histiocytes (Fig 69.7a). Anaplastic lymphoma kinase gene rearrangements have been noticed in about half of IMFT, further supporting its neoplastic nature. Expression of anaplastic lymphoma kinase is associated with localized disease at presentation and an improved prognosis.

Presentation may be with constitutional symptoms such as fever, jaundice, and weight loss [48]. Their natural history is variable with some reports of spontaneous regression, while some children may develop recurrent episodes. Local invasion has been reported in some cases (Fig. 69.7b). Surgical resection is indicated if the lesion persists or progresses after a trial of conservative therapy, or manifests evidence of local infiltration into vital structures, or of malignant transformation. Complete resection is curative in most patients [49].

Secondary Liver Lesions

Primary tumors such as neuroblastoma and Wilms' tumor can spread to the liver and present as liver metastases. These are usually multiple and are best managed with chemotherapy. Surgical resection is rarely an option in these cases.

Conclusion

Liver tumors in children are uncommon. Most present as an abdominal lump and are usually advanced at initial presentation. HB is the most common childhood liver tumor. Evidence-based multimodality therapy using improved liver resection techniques, LT, and use of effective chemotherapeutic agents has improved outcomes in these tumors.

References

1. Finegold MJ. Tumors of the liver. Semin Liver Dis. 1994;14(3):270.
2. Darbari A, Sabin KM, Shapiro CN, Schwarz KB. Epidemiology of primary hepatic malignancies in U.S. children. Hepatology. 2003;38(3):560.
3. Bergstrand CG. Alphafetoprotein in paediatrics. Acta Paediatr Scand. 1986;75(1):1.
4. Bader D, Riskin A, Vafsi O, Tamir A, Peskin B, Israel N, et al. Alpha-fetoprotein in the early neonatal period–a large study and review of the literature. Clin Chim Acta. 2004;349(1–2):15.
5. Murray MJ, Nicholson JC. alpha-Fetoprotein. Arch Dis Child Educ Pract Ed. 2011;96(4):141.
6. Ikeda H, Hachitanda Y, Tanimura M, Maruyama K, Koizumi T, Tsuchida Y. Development of unfavorable hepatoblastoma in children of very low birth weight: results of a surgical and pathologic review. Cancer. 1998;82(9):1789.

7. Reynolds P, Urayama KY, Von Behren J, Feusner J. Birth characteristics and hepatoblastoma risk in young children. Cancer. 2004;100(5):1070.

8. Maibach R, Roebuck D, Brugieres L, Capra M, Brock P, Dall'Igna P, et al. Prognostic stratification for children with hepatoblastoma: the SIOPEL experience. Eur J Cancer. 2012;48(10):1543.

9. Aronson DC, Schnater JM, Staalman CR, Weverling GJ, Plaschkes J, Perilongo G, et al. Predictive value of the pretreatment extent of disease system in hepatoblastoma: results from the International Society of Pediatric Oncology Liver Tumor Study Group SIO-PEL-1 study. J Clin Oncol. 2005;23(6):1245.

10. Roebuck DJ, Aronson D, Clapuyt P, Czauderna P, de Ville de Goyet J, Gauthier F, et al. 2005 PRETEXT: a revised staging system for primary malignant liver tumours of childhood developed by the SIOPEL group. Pediatr Radiol. 2007;37(2):123.

11. SIOPEL. SIOPEL guidelines for the treatment of hepatoblastoma (cited 5 May 2014). http://www.siopel.org/?q=node/157. Accessed 24 June 2015..

12. Meyers RL, Katzenstein HM, Krailo M, McGahren ED 3rd, Malogolowkin MH. Surgical resection of pulmonary metastatic lesions in children with hepatoblastoma. J Pediatr Surg. 2007;42(12):2050.

13. Malogolowkin MH, Katzenstein HM, Meyers RL, Krailo MD, Rowland JM, Haas J, et al. Complete surgical resection is curative for children with hepatoblastoma with pure fetal histology: a report from the Children's Oncology Group. J Clin Oncol. 2011;29(24):3301.

14. Grewal S, Merchant T, Reymond R, McInerney M, Hodge C, Shearer P. Auditory late effects of childhood cancer therapy: a report from the Children's Oncology Group. Pediatrics. 2010;125(4):e938.

15. Srinivasan P, McCall J, Pritchard J, Dhawan A, Baker A, Vergani GM, et al. Orthotopic liver transplantation for unresectable hepatoblastoma. Transplantation. 2002;74(5):652.

16. Browne M, Sher D, Grant D, Deluca E, Alonso E, Whitington PF, et al. Survival after liver transplantation for hepatoblastoma: a 2-center experience. J Pediatr Surg. 2008;43(11):1973.

17. Colomer J, Fernandez-Cruz L, Casas A, Targarona EM, Pi F, Saenz A, et al. Thromboxane flux and urinary eicosanoids as an index of reperfusion injury in pancreas transplantation after different periods of cold storage. Transplant Proc. 1988;20(5):1013.

18. Cruz RJ Jr, Ranganathan S, Mazariegos G, Soltys K, Nayyar N, Sun Q, et al. Analysis of national and single-center incidence and survival after liver transplantation for hepatoblastoma: new trends and future opportunities. Surgery. 2013;153(2):150.

19. Cistaro A, Treglia G, Pagano M, Fania P, Bova V, Basso ME, et al. A comparison between (1)(8)F-FDG PET/CT imaging and biological and radiological findings in restaging of hepatoblastoma patients. Biomed Res Int. 2013;2013:709037.

20. Semeraro M, Branchereau S, Maibach R, Zsiros J, Casanova M, Brock P, et al. Relapses in hepatoblastoma patients: clinical characteristics and outcome—experience of the International Childhood Liver Tumour Strategy Group (SIOPEL). Eur J Cancer. 2013;49(4):915.

21. Chang MH. Decreasing incidence of hepatocellular carcinoma among children following universal hepatitis B immunization. Liver Int. 2003;23(5):309.

22. Yao FY. Liver transplantation for hepatocellular carcinoma: beyond the Milan criteria. Am J Transplant. 2008;8(10):1982.

23. Ismail H, Broniszczak D, Kalicinski P, Markiewicz-Kijewska M, Teisseyre J, Stefanowicz M, et al. Liver transplantation in children with hepatocellular carcinoma. Do Milan criteria apply to pediatric patients? Pediatr Transplant. 2009;13(6):682.

24. Schmid I, Haberle B, Albert MH, Corbacioglu S, Frohlich B, Graf N, et al. Sorafenib and cisplatin/doxorubicin (PLADO) in pediatric hepatocellular carcinoma. Pediatr Blood Cancer. 2012;58(4):539.

25. Mavros MN, Mayo SC, Hyder O, Pawlik TM. A systematic review: treatment and prognosis of patients with fibrolamellar hepatocellular carcinoma. J Am Coll Surg. 2012;215(6):820.

26. Mayo SC, Mavros MN, Nathan H, Cosgrove D, Herman JM, Kamel I, et al. Treatment and prognosis of patients with fibrolamellar hepatocellular carcinoma: a national perspective. J Am Coll Surg. 2014;218(2):196.

27. Weeda VB, Murawski M, McCabe AJ, Maibach R, Brugieres L, Roebuck D, et al. Fibrolamellar variant of hepatocellular carcinoma does not have a better survival than conventional hepatocellular carcinoma—results and treatment recommendations from the Childhood Liver Tumour Strategy Group (SIOPEL) experience. Eur J Cancer. 2013;49(12):2698.

28. Prokurat A, Kluge P, Kosciesza A, Perek D, Kappeler A, Zimmermann A. Transitional liver cell tumors (TLCT) in older children and adolescents: a novel group of aggressive hepatic tumors expressing beta-catenin. Med Pediatr Oncol. 2002;39(5):510.

29. Stringer MD, Alizai NK. Mesenchymal hamartoma of the liver: a systematic review. J Pediatr Surg. 2005;40(11):1681.

30. Stocker JT, Ishak KG. Undifferentiated (embryonal) sarcoma of the liver: report of 31 cases. Cancer. 1978;42(1):336.

31. Ismail H, Dembowska-Baginska B, Broniszczak D, Kalicinski P, Maruszewski P, Kluge P, et al. Treatment of undifferentiated embryonal sarcoma of the liver in children—single center experience. J Pediatr Surg. 2013;48(11):2202.

32. Walther A, Geller J, Coots A, Towbin A, Nathan J, Alonso M, et al. Multimodal therapy including liver transplantation for hepatic undifferentiated embryonal sarcoma. Liver Transplant. 2014;20(2):191.

33. Kumar V, Chaudhary S, Kumar M, Gangopadhyay AN. Rhabdomyosarcoma of biliary tract- a diagnostic dilemma. Indian J Surg Oncol. 2012;3(4):314.

34. Centre for Disease Control and Prevention. Notes from the field: transplant-transmitted hepatitis B virus—United States, 2010. MMWR Morb Mortal Wkly Rep. 2011;60(32):1087.

35. Roebuck DJ, Yang WT, Lam WW, Stanley P. Hepatobiliary rhabdomyosarcoma in children: diagnostic radiology. Pediatr Radiol. 1998;28(2):101.

36. Spunt SL, Lobe TE, Pappo AS, Parham DM, Wharam MD Jr, Arndt C, et al. Aggressive surgery is unwarranted for biliary tract rhabdomyosarcoma. J Pediatr Surg. 2000;35(2):309.

37. Makhlouf HR, Abdul-Al HM, Wang G, Goodman ZD. Calcifying nested stromal-epithelial tumors of the liver: a clinicopathologic, immunohistochemical, and molecular genetic study of 9 cases with a long-term follow-up. Am J Surg Pathol. 2009;33(7):976.

38. Ghodke RK, Sathe PA, Kandalkar BM. Calcifying nested stromal epithelial tumor of the liver—an unusual tumor of uncertain histogenesis. J Postgrad Med. 2012;58(2):160.

39. Selby DM, Stocker JT, Ishak KG. Angiosarcoma of the liver in childhood: a clinicopathologic and follow-up study of 10 cases. Pediatr Pathol. 1992;12(4):485.

40. Awan S, Davenport M, Portmann B, Howard ER. Angiosarcoma of the liver in children. J Pediatr Surg. 1996;31(12):1729.

41. Christison-Lagay ER, Burrows PE, Alomari A, Dubois J, Kozakewich HP, Lane TS, et al. Hepatic hemangiomas: subtype classification and development of a clinical practice algorithm and registry. J Pediatr Surg. 2007;42(1):62.

42. Dickie B, Dasgupta R, Nair R, Alonso MH, Ryckman FC, Tiao GM, et al. Spectrum of hepatic hemangiomas: management and outcome. J Pediatr Surg. 2009;44(1):125.

43. Kuroda T, Hoshino K, Nosaka S, Shiota Y, Nakazawa A, Takimoto T. Critical hepatic hemangiomas in infants: from the results of a recent nationwide survey in Japan. Pediatr Int. 2014.

44. Ayling RM, Davenport M, Hadzic N, Metcalfe R, Buchanan CR, Howard ER, et al. Hepatic hemangioendothelioma associated with production of humoral thyrotropin-like factor. J Pediatr. 2001;138(6):932.

45. Davenport M, Hansen L, Heaton ND, Howard ER. Hemangioendothelioma of the liver in infants. J Pediatr Surg. 1995;30(1):44.

46. von Schweinitz D, Neonatal liver tumours. Semin Neonatol. 2003;8(5):403.

47. Shehata BM, Gupta NA, Katzenstein HM, Steelman CK, Wulkan ML, Gow KW, et al. Undifferentiated embryonal sarcoma of the liver is associated with mesenchymal hamartoma and multiple chromosomal abnormalities: a review of eleven cases. Pediatr Dev Pathol. 2011;14(2):111.

48. Kruth J, Michaely H, Trunk M, Niedergethmann M, Rupf AK, Kramer BK, et al. A rare case of fever of unknown origin: inflammatory myofibroblastic tumor of the liver. Case report and review of the literature. Acta Gastroenterol Belg. 2012;75(4):448.

49. Nagarajan S, Jayabose S, McBride W, Prasadh I, Tanjavur V, Marvin MR, et al. Inflammatory myofibroblastic tumor of the liver in children. J Pediatr Gastroenterol Nutr. 2013;57(3):277.

Acute Liver Failure in Children

Naresh P. Shanmugam, Chayarani Kelgeri and Anil Dhawan

Introduction

Acute liver failure (ALF) used synonymously with fulminant hepatic failure is a blanket term used to describe severe and sudden onset of liver cell dysfunction leading on to synthetic and detoxification failure across all age groups. Pathogenesis of hepatocyte cell injury is multifactorial (Fig. 70.1) and liver failure is the outcome of a complex equation between hepatocyte death and regeneration, as suggested by the US Acute Liver Failure Study Group [1]. Injured liver cells secrete several bioactive substances and toxins that initiate cascade of events leading on to multiorgan failure (Fig. 70.2).

Definition

"Fulminant liver failure" was coined by Trey and Davidson 40 years ago to define onset of hepatic encephalopathy (HE) within 8 weeks of appearance of symptoms of liver dysfunction in an otherwise healthy individual with no prior history of liver disease. O'Grady and colleagues categorized ALF as "hyperacute (1 week), acute (1–4 weeks) and subacute failure (5–12 weeks)" depending on the interval between jaundice and onset of encephalopathy, for prognostication purpose [2]. It is difficult to use adult-based definitions in children, as encephalopathy is a late sign and sometimes ALF has in utero onset and so time quantification would be difficult [3]. Acknowledging the fact that diagnosing encephalopathy in children is difficult and often a late and terminal event, Bhaduri and Vergani proposed the definition of ALF

as "A rare multisystem disorder in which severe impairment of liver function with or without encephalopathy, occurs in association with hepatocellular necrosis in a patient with no recognized underlying chronic liver disease" [4]. Even this definition does not seemed to be clear as the term "severe impairment of liver function" in the definition did not have any objective quantification values of liver function and so there was a lot of subjective variation in diagnosing ALF.

The pediatric acute liver failure study group (PALFSG) developed a working definition to identify ALF in children without interobserver variation. PALFSG used international normalized ratio (INR) in the background of acute liver disease as an objective measurement to demarcate acute hepatitis and ALF. As per PALFSG, ALF is defined as (i) hepatic-based coagulopathy defined as a prothrombin time (PT) 15 s or INR 1.5 not corrected by vitamin K in the presence of clinical HE or a PT 20 s or INR 2.0 regardless of the presence or absence of clinical HE, [5] (ii) biochemical evidence of acute liver injury, and (iii) no known evidence of chronic liver disease[6]. Asymptomatic preexisting liver disease, which manifests acutely, should be considered as ALF, if they fulfill the diagnostic criteria, as in acute fulminant Wilson's disease.

Coagulopathy is not only a key criterion in diagnosing pediatric ALF but also acts as a prognostic marker. Due to short half of several liver-based clotting factors, PT/INR functions as a dynamic marker of synthetic inadequacy due to loss of liver cells in ALF. Factors II, VII, IX, and X depends on vitamin K to convert them into active form. Correction of coagulopathy by intravenous vitamin K differentiates between vitamin K deficiency due to decreased absorption from liver synthetic failure. Isolated prolonged APTR is not due to liver disease, as factor VII in extrinsic pathway (Fig. 70.3) has the shortest half-life (4–6 h) of the vitamin K-dependent factors, therefore is the first factor depleted in ALF and invariably affects INR. Coagulopathy secondary to disseminated intravascular coagulation (DIC) precipitated by infection is common in acute liver injury and so it is essential to rule out DIC before making a diagnosis of ALF based on INR.

A. Dhawan (✉) · N. P. Shanmugam · C. Kelgeri
Professor and Director, Pediatric Liver, GI and Nutrition Center, Clinical Director, Child Health, King's College Hospital, London SE5 9RS, UK
e-mail: anil.dhawan@kcl.ac.uk

N. P. Shanmugam · C. Kelgeri
Department of pediatric Gastroenterology, Hepatology and Nutrition, Global Hospital and Health City, Chennai, India

© Springer International Publishing Switzerland 2016
S. Guandalini et al. (eds.), *Textbook of Pediatric Gastroenterology, Hepatology and Nutrition*,
DOI 10.1007/978-3-319-17169-2_70

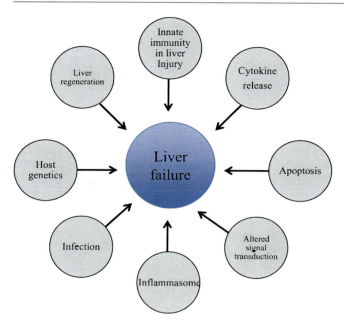

Fig. 70.1 Pathogenesis of liver cell injury is multifactorial with several factors influencing liver cell death and regeneration. When the net result is liver cell loss beyond a critical mass required maintain normal body function, liver failure sets in

Etiology

The etiologies of ALF differ with age groups and geographic location. In Southeast Asia and Latin America, viral hepatitis A and E are the most common cause of ALF in children while in Northern America and Europe etiology remains elusive (indeterminate) in majority of children [7]. Certain disorders, such as neonatal hemochromatosis, are very unique to pediatric population. The exact incidence of ALF in pedi-

atric age group is not known but probably the overall annual incidence of ALF in USA is around 5.5/million population among all ages [8].

Infection

Hepatitis A and E viral (HAV and HEV) infections are the common cause of ALF in developing countries with poor sanitation and overcrowding, as these viruses are spread by contaminated water and food. The risk of liver failure is 0.1–0.4 % following symptomatic HAV infection and it increases with a preexisting liver disease. Specific diagnosis is established by detecting HAV immunoglobulin (Ig)M antibodies in the blood at presentation. The infection is most often self-limiting with subsequent recovery and only in few it might be severe enough requiring liver transplantation [9]. The risk of developing ALF in adults following HEV infection is 0.6–2.8 %, with higher risk if contracted during pregnancy [10]. Bhatia et al. showed that the case-fatality associated with HEV-induced ALF in pregnancy is similar to that of age-matched general population [11].

The ALF due to hepatitis B virus (HBV) can occur at the time of acute infection, reactivation of chronic HBV infection or seroconversion from a hepatitis Be antigen–positive to a hepatitis Be antibody (HBeAb)-positive state. Infants born to HBeAb-positive mothers are at special risk and could present with ALF around 6 weeks to 9 months [12]. Super infection or coinfection of hepatitis delta virus (HDV) in HBV-infected patients can cause liver failure. Hepatitis C viral (HCV) infection has not been reported as a cause of ALF.

Herpes simplex virus 1 and 2 (HSV) is the predominant cause of viral-induced ALF during first month of life. Neonatal ALF due to HSV carries a high mortality of about 85 %

Fig. 70.2 Except for Von Willebrand factor and tissue plasminogen activator, liver is the major site for synthesis of clotting factors. Factors V synthesis is first to be affected and factor VII have the shortest half-lives and are theoretically more sensitive markers than INR of hepatic synthetic function. *INR* international normalized ratio

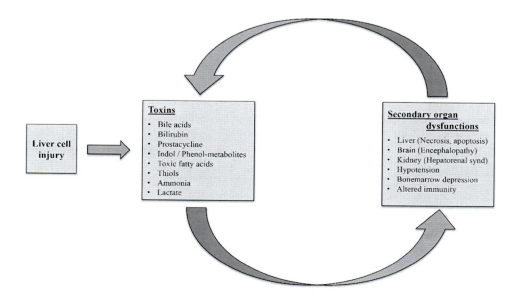

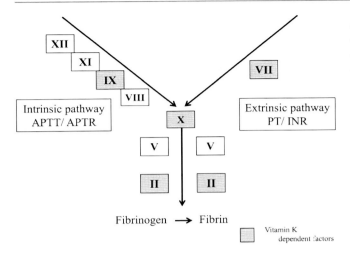

Fig. 70.3 Liver cell injury leads on to release several toxic substances that causes secondary organ dysfunction, this leads on to a vicious cycle of autointoxication. *APTT* Activated Partial Thromboplastin Time, *APTR* Activated Partial Thromboplastin Ratio, *PT* prothrombin time, *INR* international normalized ratio

and should be suspected in any neonate with or without vesicular rash who is unwell with dramatically high transaminases and coagulopathy. Treatment with high doses of aciclovir should be initiated in all infants with ALF, while awaiting serology results as the associated liver failure is rapidly fatal. Liver transplantation has a good outcome when considered in a hemodynamically stable neonate with ALF due to HSV [13]. Other members of herpes virus family such as cytomegalovirus, Epstein–Barr virus, and varicella-zoster virus can cause ALF. Rarely, viruses such as Dengue, Lassa, Ebola, Marburg, and Toga and bacteria such as *Leptospira* and *Salmonella* are implicated as a cause for ALF.

Drugs and Toxins

In developed countries, drug-induced liver failure is the most common identifiable cause of ALF in adults and children. Drug hepatoxicity could be an idiosyncratic reaction, a dose-dependent response, or a synergistic reaction due of several drugs. It is essential to include details of complementary therapies and herbal medications as some are potential hepatotoxics [14]. Acetaminophen is the most common drug associated with ALF, probably due to the easy availability without the need for a prescription. It is safe when used in recommended doses and toxicity is usually dose dependent. Acetaminophen is detoxified mainly by glucuronidation (40%), sulfation (20–40%), and *N*-hydroxylation (15%). A small fraction is metabolized via cytochrome P450 to yield *N*-acetyl-para-benzoquinone-imide (NAPQI), a toxic intermediate compound which irreversibly conjugates with the sulfhydryl group of glutathione and causes hepatocyte necrosis [15]. Genetic polymorphism of

cytochrome P450 isoenzymes predisposes affected people to acetaminophen toxicity due to increased NAPQI production. Bound NAPQI forms acetaminophen–protein adducts, which acts as a specific biomarker for chronic acetaminophen toxicity. Hepatotoxicity of acetaminophen is dose dependent and liver injury results either because of acute higher doses ingestion or cumulative over doses taken over a few days. In acute acetaminophen overdose plotting serum levels after 4 h against time on the Rumack nomogram will guide towards potential toxicity. However, it may not be useful in situations of cumulative over doses. In such cases, bound NAPQI forms of acetaminophen–protein adducts in blood would aid the diagnosis. The mechanism of toxicity of anti-tuberculosis drugs, particularly isoniazid is similar to acetaminophen, oxidation via cytochrome P450 pathway results in toxic metabolites.

Most common cause of idiosyncratic drug-induced liver injury (DILI) are due to antibiotics and NSAIDs [14]. The reported incidence of idiosyncratic DILI was around 14 new cases/100,000/year, of which 8% would progress to ALF [16, 17]. Genetic susceptibility of an individual, unmasking of underlying mitochondrial cytopathies by certain drugs are some of the proposed causes of DILI [18]. Drugs such as diclofenac, mefenamic acid, valproic acid, amiodarone, isoniazid, etc. can unmask mitochondrial cytopathy and cause ALF. Chemotherapy drugs are known to produce veno-occlusive disease leading on to ALF due to endothelial damage.

Councils for International Organizations of Medical Sciences/Roussel Uclaf Causality Assessment Method (CIOMS/RUCAM) scale are helpful in establishing causal relationship between offending drug and liver damage. Using the scoring system, suspected drug could be categorized into "definite or highly probable" (score >8), "probable" (score 6–8), "possible" (score 3–5), "unlikely" (score 1–2), and "excluded" (score 0) [19]. This scale is helpful in identifying drug-induced hepatotoxicity even in newly marketed drugs and for a previously unreported older drug.

Metabolic Disorders

Metabolic disorders presenting as ALF is common in young children. Galactosemia and tyrosinemia 1 are the most common cause of neonatal liver failure, presenting with hepatomegaly, jaundice, and coagulopathy. Classical galactosemia is an autosomal recessive condition resulting because of mutation in galactose-1-phosphate uridyl transferase gene located on chromosome 9p13. Liver failure in this condition is thought to be due to accumulation on galactitol. Neonates presenting with hepatitis or ALF should be started on a galactose-free formula until galactosemia. Galactose-free diet coupled with supportive management helps the liver to recover, but some may still progress and need a liver transplant. Despite strict galactose-free diet, patients could develop complications like developmental delay, motor disorders and hypergonadotrophic hypogonadism due to endogenous galactose production on a long-term follow-up [20]. Tyrosinemia 1 is an autosomal recessive condition due to defect in the enzyme fumarylacetoacetate hydroxylase. This causes accumulation of intermediate compounds, maleylacetoacetic acid, and fumarylacetoacetic acid, which are then converted to succinylacetone, a toxin that damages the liver and kidneys. Tyrosinemia should be suspected when a coagulopathy and modest rise of transaminases is associated with elevated alpha-fetoprotein levels. Fructosinemia, inborn errors of bile acid synthesis are a few other rare cause of ALF during infantile period.

Medium-chain acyl-coenzyme A dehydrogenases (MCAD) are group of enzymes involved in β-oxidation of 6–12 carbon chain fatty acids in mitochondria. They help in ketone production from fatty acids when hepatic glycogen stores become depleted during prolonged fasting and periods of higher energy demands. Affected children could present with hypoketotic hypoglycemia, recurrent liver failure, precipitated by otherwise minor illness. Unless treated with dextrose supplementation, these episodes may quickly progress to coma and death.

Wilson's disease, an autosomal recessive disorder could present as ALF. The acute hepatic presentation is usually characterized by the presence of liver failure, Coombs-negative hemolytic anemia and low serum alkaline phosphatase. Diagnosis might be difficult as blood test might show weakly positive autoantibodies and tissue copper estimation might not be possible due to coagulopathy. Demonstration of Kayser–Fleischer rings is diagnostic of Wilson's disease in a patient who presents with ALF. Wilson's disease presenting with ALF has high mortality without transplantation.

Mitochondrial disorders are group of spontaneous or inherited disorders of mitochondrial proteins resulting in defective oxidative phosphorylation, fatty acid oxidation, urea cycle, and other mitochondrial pathways [21]. This can affect the function of various cell types, such as neurons, myocytes, etc., where the need for energy requirement is high. Deficiencies of complex I, III and IV, multiple complex deficiencies and mitochondrial DNA (mtDNA) depletion syndrome is associated with liver failure. Diagnosis might be difficult due to particularly in (mtDNA) depletion syndrome where there is tissue specific mitochondrial enzyme deficiency. The infants usually presents with hypotonia, hypoglycemia, feeding difficulties, seizures, and deranged liver function. Liver transplantation could be offered in isolated liver-based mitochondrial disorders, while in multisystemic involvement it should be deferred, hence it is utmost important to perform thorough investigation to rule out neuromuscular involvement [22].

Gestational Alloimmune Liver Disease

Neonatal hemochromatosis (NH) is the single most common cause of ALF during first month of life, where there is massive iron deposition in liver and extrahepatic tissues, but with sparing of the reticuloendothelial system. The pattern of iron overloading is similar to hereditary hemochromatosis, but NH affects only newborn and so far no specific genetic mutation has been identified. NH was considered to be a primary disease of iron overload of liver leading on to liver failure. Under current concept, iron accumulation in NH is considered to be a secondary phenomenon due to immune-related severe fetal liver injury resulting in impaired regulation of maternofetal iron flux [23]. NH is now referred as gestational alloimmune liver disease (GALD), as maternal antibody is directed towards fetal liver antigen resulting in activation of fetal complement leading to the formation of membrane attack complex (MAC) resulting in hepatocyte loss [24, 25]. This hypothesis is supported by successful prevention of severe disease by antenatal and postnatal treatment with intravenous Ig. GALD presents with jaundice, coagulopathy, moderately elevated alanine aminotransferase, high ferritin, and raised iron saturation levels. High ferritin is seen in other cause of neonatal liver failure and no single biochemical test is diagnostic of NH. The diagnosis can only be confirmed by demonstration of extra hepatic iron deposits sparing the reticuloendothelial system. Labial salivary gland biopsy is safe and effective way of demonstrating this [26]. The disease varies in severity; at one end of spectrum it is associated with fetal death while at the other end spontaneous recovery is reported.

Malignancies

Hemophagocytic lymphohistiocytosis (HLH) is a malignant disorder of hemopoietic system where there is uncontrolled proliferation of activated lymphocytes and macrophages and could present as ALF, particularly during infancy. HLH could be inherited or acquired following infection due to over activation of natural killer cells and of CD8+ T cell lymphocytes, invariably leading to clinical and hematologic alterations. It is associated with defective apoptosis and reduced cytotoxic activity. Familial HLH is an autosomal recessive disease seen mostly in infancy and early childhood. The mutations result in reduced or defective production of cytoplasmic granules such as perforin in cytotoxic cells resulting in paradoxical over activation. Familial HLH is classified into four types based on mutation analysis. Secondary HLH usually occurs after systemic infection or immunodeficiency, which can affect people at any age and may subside spontaneously. HLH presents with fever, cutaneous rash, hepatosplenomegaly, pancytopenia and, in severe cases, with ALF [27]. ALF might be the presenting feature of hematologic malignancies such as leukemia or lymphoma [28]. Usual associated features would be fever, hepatosplenomegaly, high alkaline phosphatase, high lactate dehydrogenase, and abnormalities on peripheral blood film. Bone marrow examination confirms the diagnosis.

Autoimmune Hepatitis

Autoimmune hepatitis (AIH) can present as ALF, most of these children have positive liver–kidney microsomal (LKM) antibody (type 2 AIH). Diagnosis might be difficult, as some may not show specific antibodies at initial presentation. ALF due to AIH without encephalopathy could be benefited by immunosuppression, while ALF along with encephalopathy do not respond to any form of immunosuppression and need urgent liver transplant [29]. In our experience, of the six AIH children presenting with ALF and encephalopathy, four required liver transplantation, one died while awaiting transplantation, and one recovered with steroids [30]. The steroid responder was antinuclear/smooth muscle antibody positive (type 1 AIH) while rest five were LKM positive (Type 2 AIH).

Other Causes

In spite of extensive investigation, the diagnosis could not be found in many children (indeterminate). Indeterminate ALF is probably due to unidentified infectious agent as suggested by presentation with severe hepatitis, liver failure and bone marrow failure mimicking viral-induced disease or presentation with minimal jaundice and centrilobular necrosis on histology suggesting drug induced. There is wide variation in reporting of indeterminate etiology among various centers. This is probably due to incomplete investigations in ALF, which has been highlighted by Narkewicz et al., and labeling them as indeterminate etiology [31]. Hypoxia, bacterial infections, underlying cardiac problem, venous outflow obstruction are few other causes of ALF.

Investigations

As the etiology of ALF is so diverse that it is practically impossible to do all the tests during initial evaluation. A detailed clinical history and thorough general examination could give valuable clue of underlying problem and could help in directing management while awaiting confirmatory results. The first-line investigations should include complete blood count, liver function tests, serum electrolytes,

Table 70.1 Disease specific investigations in acute liver failure

Infective:
Serologic/quantitative tests
Hepatitis A: anti-HAV IgM antibody
Hepatitis B: HBsAg, HBcAb(IgM), HBcAg
Hepatitis C: anti-hep C antibody, hep C PCR
Hepatitis D: anti-hep D antibody
Hepatitis E: anti-HEV antibody(IgM)
Human immunodeficiency virus (HIV)
Herpes simplex virus (neonates)
Cytomegalovirus, Epstein–Barr virus
If indicated: measles/varicella/adenovirus/echovirus/leptospirosis/
Cultures
Bacterial cultures: blood, urine, stool, throat swab, sputum
Skin lesion if present, ascitic fluid if present
Viral culture of urine and skin lesion if present
Metabolic:
Galactosemia: galactose-1-phosphate uridyl transferase
Tyrosinemia: urinary succinylacetone
Fructose intolerance: quantitative enzyme assay, q22.3 band mutation in chr 9
Mitochondrial disorders: quantitative mitochondrial DNA assay, mutation analysis
Congenital disorders of glycosylation: transferrin isoelectrophorosis
MCAD deficiency: plasma acylcarnitine
Wilson's disease: serum copper and ceruloplasmin
24-h urinary copper pre and post penicillamine
Type 1 and 2 autoimmune hepatitis:
Immunoglobulins
Antinuclear antibodies
Smooth muscle antibody
Liver cytosol antibodies
Soluble liver antigen
Liver–kidney microsomal antibody
Antineutrophil cytoplasmic antibodies
Hematological malignancy:
Bone marrow examination
Ascitic or cerebrospinal fluid cytospin
Genetics for HLH
Drugs and toxins: drug levels in serum/urine
Budd–Chiari syndrome: ultrasound, echocardiography, computer tomography
Neonatal hemochromatosis: lip biopsy

HAV hepatitis A virus, *HEV* hepatitis E virus, *HBcAg* hepatitis B core antigen, *HBsAg* hepatitis B surface antigen, *HLH* hemophagocytic lymphohistiocytosis, *IgM* immunoglobulin M

uric acid, lactate, cholesterol/triglyceride, amylase, coagulation studies (INR), and blood glucose. Surveillance blood and urine cultures should be collected prior to starting antibiotics. The clinical presentation along with the results of first-line investigations will guide further specialized tests. Investigations to establish etiological diagnosis are outlined in Table 70.1. Supportive management along with anticipatory management of possible complications associated with liver failure would help in favorable outcome.

Table 70.2 King's College Hospital criteria for liver transplantation

Non-acetaminophen acute liver failure
INR greater than 6.5 or
Three of the following five criteria:
Patient age < 11 or > 40
Serum bilirubin > 300 µmol/L;
Time from onset of jaundice to the development of coma > 7 days;
INR greater than 3.5
Drug toxicity
Acetaminophen-induced acute liver failure
Arterial pH < 7.3 (after fluid resuscitation) or
All three of the following criteria
INR > 6.5
Serum creatinine > 300 µmol/L
Encephalopathy (grade III or IV).

INR international normalized ratio

Prognosis

Categorical demarcation between spontaneous liver recovery and irreversible ALF is difficult. In adults with non-acetaminophen-induced ALF, King's College Hospital criteria (KCHC; Table 70.2) is used for prognostication and the need for liver transplantation. Fulfillment of KCHC is usually associated with death unless transplanted [32]. But in children KCHC does not reliably predict death with a poor positive predictive value of 33 % [33]. Of the several prognostic markers that has been proposed to predict outcomes in ALF in children, INR and factor V concentration remains the best indicators. In children with ALF, INR 4, bilirubin 235 µmol/L, age <2 years, and WBC >9 × 10⁹/L are associated with poor outcome without liver transplantation [34]. Bhaduri and Mieli-Vergani have shown that the maximum INR reached during the course of illness was the most sensitive predictor of the outcome, with 73 % of children with an INR less than 4 surviving compared with only 4 of 24 (16.6 %) with an INR greater than 4 [35]. French centers use factor V concentration for prognostication and a value of less than 20 % of normal (Clichy criteria) suggests a poor outcome. New Wilson index proposed by Dhawan et al. based on serum bilirubin, serum albumin, INR, aspartate aminotransferase (AST), and white cell count (WCC) at presentation identified a cutoff score of 11 for death and proved to be 93 % sensitive and 98 % specific, with a positive predictive value of 88 % (Table 70.3) [36]. In acetamino-

phen overdose, metabolic acidosis with arterial pH less than 7.3, after the second day of overdose in adequately hydrated patients, is associated with 90 % mortality. In acetaminophen overdose, KCHC could be used in children for selecting candidates requiring liver transplantation (Table 70.2).

Table 70.3 showing Wilson's disease index, which has five parameters and a score of 11 or more indicates the need for liver transplant.

Management

Due to unpredictable course of liver failure, management has to be carried out along side of investigation. Early liaison and transfer to a specialist center with transplantation facilities is crucial for better outcome.

General Measures

Children with ALF should be monitored in a quiet setting. Vital parameters, such as pulse, blood pressure, oxygen saturation, neurologic observations, should be done on regular basis. Prophylactic broad-spectrum antibiotics and antifungals should be started in all children and acyclovir should be added in infants and neonates. Children with encephalopathy or an INR greater than four should be admitted to an intensive care unit for close monitoring. Hypoglycemia should be avoided by use of intravenous glucose infusion or by ensuring adequate enteral intake. The idea of protein restriction to limit the possibility of HE has now been disregarded and adequate calories should be provided. A plant protein-based died which has more of branched chain amino acid (BCAA) is preferred over animal protein which has more of aromatic amino acid (AAA). Oral or nasogastric feeding is usually well tolerated. Prophylactic histamine 2 blockers or proton pump inhibitors should be started to all patients requiring mechanical ventilation as stress ulcers can cause bleed [37].

N-Acetylcysteine (NAC)

N-acetylcysteine (NAC) is being increasingly used in non-acetaminophen-induced ALF as it enhances circulation and improves oxygen delivery. Retrospective study from King's

Table 70.3 Wilson's disease index

Bilirubin (µMol/L)	INR	AST (IU/L)	WBC (10⁹/L)	Albumin (G/L)	Score
0–100	0–1.2	0–100	0–6.7	>45	0
101–150	1.3–1.6	101–150	6.8–8.3	34–44	1
151–200	1.7–1.9	151–200	8.4–10.3	25–33	2
201–300	2.0–2.4	201–300	10.4–15.3	21–24	3
>300	>2.5	>300	>15.4	0–20	4

AST aspartate transaminase, *INR* international normalized ratio, *WBC* white blood cell count

College Hospital has shown that NAC infusion in non-acetaminophen-induced ALF was associated with a shorter length of hospital stay, higher incidence of native liver recovery without transplantation, and better survival after transplantation [38]. In a prospective, double-blind trial in adults with non- acetaminophen ALF, NAC usage is associated with significant improvement in transplant-free survival in patients with early (stage I–II) coma, indicating the necessity for early initiation of treatment [39]. But a more recent prospective study on NAC usage in children with non-acetaminophen ALF, failed to show any significant benefit when compared to placebo [40].

Airway and Ventilation

Elective intubation and mechanical ventilation should be considered in patients with grade 1 or 2 encephalopathy that are agitated or planned to transfer and in all patients with grade 3/4 encephalopathy. Apart from providing secure airway, mechanical ventilation helps in reducing sudden variation of intracranial pressure (ICP). Sedation could be maintained with a combination of an opiate such as morphine or fentanyl and a hypnotic such as midazolam. Peak end-expiratory pressure above 8 cm of water should be avoided because it may increase ICP.

Fluid Management and Renal Failure

Intravenous fluids should be restricted to two thirds maintenance, with the idea of decreasing the possibility of development of cerebral edema. Ultrasonic cardiac output monitor (USCOM), which is a noninvasive method to measure cardiac parameters, helps in decision making regarding appropriate fluid regimens/ionotropes even in small infants. In ALF, there would be hyperdynamic circulation with decreased systemic vascular resistance, and in the presence of persistent hypotension, first-line inotropic agent of choice would be noradrenaline followed by vasopressin analogues. Continuous filtration or dialysis should be considered when the urine output is less than 1 mL/kg/h to prevent acidosis and volume overload.

Neurologic Complications

Encephalopathy is not always recognizable in children and usually is a late feature. The most serious complications of ALF are cerebral edema with resultant intracranial hypertension and HE. Encephalopathy that occurs in ALF is categorized as type A, according to the suggested nomenclature by Working Party at the 11th World Congress of

Table 70.4 West Haven criteria for grading of mental state

Grade 0	Normal
Grade 1	Euphoria or anxiety
	Shortened attention span
	Impaired performance of addition
	Trivial lack of awareness
	Inverted sleep pattern
Grade 2	Subtle personality change
	Minimal disorientation for time or place
	Impaired performance of subtraction
	Lethargy or slow response
	Tremor and hypoactive reflexes
Grade 3	Somnolence to semi stupor, but responds to verbal stimuli
	Confusion, gross disorientation
	Inappropriate behavior
	Brisk reflexes and Babinski's sign
	Muscle rigidity
Grade 4	Deep coma (unresponsive to verbal or noxious stimuli)

Gastroenterology. HE could be clinically graded from 1 to 4 using West Haven criteria (Table 70.4) and conscious levels could be assessed using Glasgow coma scale, which has lesser interobserver variability [41] (Table 70.5).

Clinical features of raised ICP would include systemic hypertension, bradycardia, hypertonia, and hyperreflexia and in extreme cases decerebrate or decorticate posturing. Electroencephalographic (EEG) changes occur very early in HE, even before the onset of psychological or biochemical disturbances. Ammonia-lowering measures such as dietary protein restriction, bowel decontamination, or lactulose are of limited or no value in rapidly advancing encephalopathy. Mannitol is an osmotic diuretic commonly used to treat intracranial hypertension. A rapid bolus of 0.5 g/kg as a 20% solution over a 15-min period is recommended and the dose can be repeated if the serum osmolarity is less than 320 mOsm/L. In ventilated patients, prophylactic hyperventilation provides no role as hypocapnia could decrease cerebral perfusion and $PaCO_2$ should be kept between 4 and 4.5 kPa. In case of clinical features of acute rise in ICP, hyperventilation could be done for a brief period of time until there is symptomatic improvement. Invasive ICP monitoring using special catheters helps in objective measurement of ICP. This helps to maintain optimal cerebral perfusion pressure (mean arterial blood pressure—ICP) of more than 50 mm Hg. Ionotropic agents could be used to increase mean arterial blood pressure to achieve the optimal cerebral perfusion pressure. Studies have shown sodium thiopental, mild cerebral hypothermia (32–35 °C) and hypernatremia (serum sodium >145 mmol/L) improves cerebral perfusion. Table 70.6 shows some of pathophysiological changes that lead on to multiorgan dysfunction associated with ALF.

Table 70.5 Glasgow coma scale

	Infants	Children	Score
Eye opening	Open spontaneously	Open spontaneously	4
	Open in response to verbal stimuli	Open in response to verbal stimuli	3
	Open in response to pain only	Open in response to pain only	2
	No response	No response	1
Verbal response	Coos and babbles	Oriented, appropriate	5
	Irritable cries	Confused	4
	Cries in response to pain	Inappropriate words	3
	Moans in response to pain	Incomprehensible words or nonspecific sounds	2
	No response	No response	1
Motor response	Moves spontaneously and purposefully	Obeys commands	6
	Withdraws to touch	Localizes painful stimulus	5
	Withdraws in response to pain	Withdraws in response to pain	4
	Responds to pain with decorticate posturing (abnormal flexion)	Responds to pain with flexion	3
	Responds to pain with decerebrate posturing (abnormal extension)	Responds to pain with extension	2
	No response	No response	1

Table 70.6 Pathophysiology of complications in ALF

Coagulopathy:

Decreased levels of coagulation factors, decreased protein C, protein S, and antithrombin associated with dysfunctional platelets and fibrinogen

Encephalopathy and intracranial hypertension:

Inhibitory effect of ammonia and gamma-aminobutyric acid on neuronal cell membranes and synapses. The direct toxicity of toxins on neuronal cells and vasogenic imbalance leading onto intracellular fluid shifts resulting in cerebral edema

Renal failure:

Acute tubular necrosis secondary to complications of ALF such as sepsis, bleeding, and/or hypotension

Hepatorenal syndrome because of renal vasoconstriction probably due to release of vasoactive mediators

Hypotension:

Decreased systemic vascular resistance and hypovolemia secondary to shift of fluids into interstitial space. Adrenal insufficiency *due to* decreased liver synthesis of apolipoprotein A-1, the major protein component of HDL leading on to decreased HDL and thereby decreased cortisol production

Metabolic derangement:

Hypoglycemia due to increased plasma insulin levels owing to reduced hepatic uptake, reduced glycogen stores, impaired gluconeogenesis. Lactic acidosis is related to inadequate tissue perfusion due to hypotension and also due to decreased detoxification by the liver

Infection:

Impaired Kupffer cell and polymorphonuclear function along with reduced levels of factors such as fibronectin, opsonins, chemo attractants, and components of the complement system

HDL high-density lipoprotein

Coagulopathy

As INR is a dynamic indicator of disease progression, coagulopathy should be corrected only if the patient is having a bleed or prior to an invasive procedure. Bleeding manifestation is very unusual in ALF as there would be proportional reduction in plasma levels of both procoagulant and anticoagulant proteins [42]. Thromboelastography would be an appropriate tool in diagnosing risk of bleeding. To correct coagulopathy, fresh frozen plasma could be given at a dose of 10 ml/kg and cryoprecipitate at 5 ml/kg (if fibrinogen is < 1 g/l). In resistant cases, factor seven concentrates improve the coagulopathy for a short period. Platelet count should be maintained above $50 \times 10^9/dL$, as thrombocytopenia is an important risk factor for hemorrhage.

Disease Specific Management

Antioxidant cocktail *(NAC, selenium, desferrioxamine, prostaglandin E1, vitamin E)* has been used in NH, based on the concept that iron chelation and free radical scavenging would prevent liver damage, with no proven benefit. As GALD is the common cause of NH, evidence is accumulating towards the usefulness of high-dose intravenous immunoglobulin (IVIG; 1 g/kg), in combination with exchange transfusion resulting in significant decrease in the need for liver transplantation in NH [43]. IVIG when given as prophylaxis to mothers whose previous pregnancy/child was affected with NH at a dose of 1 g/kg bodyweight, weekly from the 18th week until the end of gestation has been associated with milder phenotypic expression of the disease and 100 % survival of babies [44]. The management of HLH consists of liver supportive therapy, chemotherapy, and hematopoietic stem cell transplantation (for genetically verified/ familial disease and persistent/reactivation of secondary disease) [27]. Dietary intervention with restriction of phenylalanine and tyrosine together with oral medication, 2 (2-nitro-4-trifluoromethylbenzoyl)-1,3-cyclohexenedione

(NTBC), helps in normalization of liver function in tyrosinemia type 1, but does not prevent long-term risk for development of hepatocellular carcinoma [45]. In amanita phalloides (death cap) poisoning, benzylpenicillin given at a dose of 1,000,000 U/kg/d followed by 500,000 IU/kg for the next 2 days prevents toxin uptake by liver cells. In all the abovementioned conditions (excluding hematological malignancy), liver transplantation has to be considered in case of failed medical management.

Liver Assist Devices

Release of toxins and inflammatory mediators from the necrosed hepatocytes initiates cascade of events which could ultimately lead onto to multiorgan failure and this elicits a vicious cycle of autointoxication (Fig. 70.3). Liver assist devices are developed to interrupt the cycle of autointoxication by removing toxins there by providing an opportunity for the liver to regenerate. An ideal extracorporeal liver support system has to perform complex synthetic, detoxifying, and biotransformatory functions of hepatocytes and Kupffer cells. Creating such a perfect device with possibility of providing an extracorporeal liver support system for short periods while the native liver regenerates or a liver transplant becomes available is still experimental. Currently available liver support devices could be broadly classified into cell-free cleansing devices and bioartificial liver support system, which contains human or animal liver cells. Cleansing devices perform only the detoxifying function of the liver, whereas bioartificial liver support systems have a theoretic advantage of providing the synthetic and detoxifying properties. These devices have shown to decrease the toxins (ammonia, bilirubin, cytokines, etc.) but have no effect on mortality. Successful use of these devises in ALF as a bridge, supporting liver function while the native liver regenerates still remains elusive and not recommended outside research setting.

Liver Transplantation

Liver transplant remains the only proven treatment that has improved the outcome of ALF. Improved surgical techniques such and split liver grafts, reduced grafts and living related donors have increased the timely availability of donor organs. The donor organs are usually blood group matched. In emergency situations ABO-incompatible liver transplantation could be done, but is associated with lower graft survival. Careful patient selection is essential, as it would minimize patients from being listed for liver transplantation and then being removed due to spontaneous recovery. Patients, who were removed from the list due to spontaneous recovery, could have potentially ended up with liver transplantation if

the organ becomes available before overt clinical improvement is appreciated. Absolute contraindications for liver transplant are fixed and dilated pupils, uncontrolled sepsis, systemic mitochondrial/metabolic disorders, and severe respiratory failure [46, 47]. Relative contraindications are increasing inotropic requirements, infection under treatment, cerebral perfusion pressure of less than 40 mmHg for more than 2 h, and a history of progressive or severe neurologic problems.

Auxiliary Liver Transplantation

Auxiliary liver transplant is surgical procedure where a healthy donor liver graft is implanted with native liver in situ. Auxiliary liver transplant could be orthotopic (part of the native liver is resected and replaced with a reduced-size graft) or heterotopic (the donor graft is placed alongside the native liver in the right upper quadrant). Due to higher incidence of complications associated with heterotopic auxiliary liver transplant, it is no more used in clinical practice. Now the standard surgical technique is auxiliary partial orthotopic liver transplantation (APOLT). The rationale behind the use of this technique in ALF is that the allograft supports liver function while the native liver regenerates and then immunosuppression could be weaned and eventually stopped. It has been shown that complete native liver recovery could happen even when there is more than 90% hepatocyte loss [48, 49]. In a series from King's College Hospital, of the 20 children who received auxiliary liver transplantation for ALF, 10-year patient survival was 85% [50]. Among the 17 survivors, 14 (82%) have successfully regenerated their native liver of which immunosuppression was withdrawn successfully in 11 patients at a median time of 23 months after transplantation. This would be an ideal option in ALF due to indeterminate etiology, as spontaneous regeneration of native liver remains a possibility. Caution should be excised while selecting patients with hemodynamic instability and cerebral edema as deterioration might happen during postoperative period due "toxic necrotic liver" left behind.

Hepatocyte Transplantation

Hepatocyte transplantation is a procedure where hepatocytes are infused intraportally into the patient's liver, where a proportion of cells will engraft and would support liver function. This technique has been tried with variable success in certain liver-based metabolic disorders. Its use in ALF still remains experimental. Lack of surrogate markers of rejection poses an important problem, as it is difficult to titrate the immunosuppression. A novel technique, where alginate-encapsulated hepatocytes could be injected intraperitoneally is under trial.

This technique avoids the complications of coagulopathy, portosystemic shunting of infused cells and protects the cells from direct immune attack, allowing immunosuppression-free transplantation.

Conclusions

ALF in children is a medical emergency as it leads on to multiorgan failure and has to be approached systematically. Newer definition for ALF obviates the need for encephalopathy to make the diagnosis. Expert intensive care facility is essential to stabilize and make this children fit for transplantation. Etiological diagnosis aids in disease-specific management. Acyclovir should be started in all neonates with ALF until results of herpes virology are available. Liver transplantation is the only definitive treatment that improves survival in pediatric ALF, while liver assist devices and hepotocyte transplantation are potential emerging therapies.

References

1. Chung RT, Stravitz RT, Fontana RJ, Schiodt FV, Mehal WZ, Reddy KR, Lee WM. Pathogenesis of liver injury in acute liver failure. Gastroenterology. 2012;143:e1–7.
2. O'Grady JG, Schalm SW, Williams R. Acute liver failure: redefining the syndromes. Lancet. 1993;342:273–5.
3. Trey C, Davidson CS. The management of fulminant hepatic failure. Prog Liver Dis. 1970;3:282–98.
4. Bhaduri BR, Mieli-Vergani G. Fulminant hepatic failure: pediatric aspects. Semin Liver Dis. 1996;16:349–55.
5. Hayashi S, Lin MG, Katayama A, Namii Y, Nagasaka T, Koike C, Negita M, Kobayashi T, et al. Auxiliary orthotopic xenogeneic liver transplantation using pigs for fulminant hepatic failure: with special reference to the technique and immunosuppression. Transplant Proc. 1998;30:3836.
6. Squires RH Jr, Shneider BL, Bucuvalas J, Alonso E, Sokol RJ, Narkewicz MR, et al. Acute liver failure in children: the first 348 patients in the pediatric acute liver failure study group. J Pediatr. 2006;148:652–8.
7. Shanmugam NP, Bansal S, Greenough A, Verma A, Dhawan A. Neonatal liver failure: etiologies and management-state of the art. Eur J Pediatr. 2011;170(5):573–81.
8. Bower WA, Johns M, Margolis HS, Williams IT, Bell BP. Population-based surveillance for acute liver failure. Am J Gastroenterol. 2007;102:2459–63.
9. Ciocca M, Ramonet M, Cuarterolo M, Lopez S, Cernadas C, Alvarez F. Prognostic factors in paediatric acute liver failure. Arch Dis Child. 2008;93:48–51.
10. Krawczynski K, Kamili S, Aggarwal R. Global epidemiology and medical aspects of hepatitis e. Forum (Genova). 2001;11:166–79.
11. Bhatia V, Singhal A, Panda SK, Acharya SK. A 20-year single-center experience with acute liver failure during pregnancy: Is the prognosis really worse? Hepatology. 2008;48:1577–85.
12. Beath SV, Boxall EH, Watson RM, Tarlow MJ, Kelly DA. Fulminant hepatitis b in infants born to anti-hbe hepatitis b carrier mothers. BMJ. 1992;304:1169–70.
13. Lee WS, Kelly DA, Tanner MS, Ramani P, de Ville de Goyet J, McKiernan PJ. Neonatal liver transplantation for fulminant hepa-

titis caused by herpes simplex virus type 2. J Pediatr Gastroenterol Nutr. 2002;35:220–3.
14. Larrey D. Hepatotoxicity of drugs and chemicals. Gastroenterol Clin Biol. 2009;33:1136–46.
15. Davis M. Protective agents for acetaminophen overdose. Semin Liver Dis. 1986;6:138–47.
16. Bjornsson E. Review article: drug-induced liver injury in clinical practice. Aliment Pharmacol Ther. 2010;32:3–13.
17. Idilman R, Bektas M, Cinar K, Toruner M, Cerit ET, Doganay B, et al. The characteristics and clinical outcome of drug-induced liver injury: a single-center experience. J Clin Gastroenterol. 2010;44:e128–32.
18. Ghabril M, Chalasani N, Bjornsson E. Drug-induced liver injury: a clinical update. Curr Opin Gastroenterol. 2010;26:222–6.
19. Andrade RJ, Robles M, Fernandez-Castaner A, Lopez-Ortega S, Lopez-Vega MC, Lucena MI. Assessment of drug-induced hepatotoxicity in clinical practice: a challenge for gastroenterologists. World J Gastroenterol. 2007;13:329–40.
20. Bosch AM, Waterham HR, Bakker HD. From gene to disease; galactosemia and galactose-1-phosphate uridyltransferase deficiency. Ned Tijdschr Geneeskd. 2004;148:80–1.
21. Treem WR, Sokol RJ. Disorders of the mitochondria. Semin Liver Dis. 1998;18:237–53.
22. Dhawan A, Mieli-Vergani G. Liver transplantation for mitochondrial respiratory chain disorders: to be or not to be? Transplantation. 2001;71:596–8.
23. Whitington PF. Gestational alloimmune liver disease and neonatal hemochromatosis. Semin Liver Dis. 2012;32:325–32.
24. Whitington PF, Malladi P. Neonatal hemochromatosis: is it an alloimmune disease? J Pediatr Gastroenterol Nutr. 2005;40:544–9.
25. Pan X, Kelly S, Melin-Aldana H, Malladi P, Whitington PF. Novel mechanism of fetal hepatocyte injury in congenital alloimmune hepatitis involves the terminal complement cascade. Hepatology. 2010;51:2061–8.
26. Smith SR, Shneider BL, Magid M, Martin G, Rothschild M. Minor salivary gland biopsy in neonatal hemochromatosis. Arch Otolaryngol Head Neck Surg. 2004;130:760–3.
27. Henter JI, Horne A, Arico M, Egeler RM, Filipovich AH, Imashuku S, et al. Hlh-2004: Diagnostic and therapeutic guidelines for hemophagocytic lymphohistiocytosis. Pediatr Blood Cancer. 2007;48:124–31.
28. Kader A, Vara R, Egberongbe Y, Height S, Dhawan A. Leukaemia presenting with fulminant hepatic failure in a child. Eur J Pediatr. 2004;163:628–9.
29. Mieli-Vergani G, Vergani D. Autoimmune paediatric liver disease. World J Gastroenterol. 2008;14:3360–7.
30. Gregorio GV, Portmann B, Reid F, Donaldson PT, Doherty DG, McCartney M, et al. Autoimmune hepatitis in childhood: a 20-year experience. Hepatology. 1997;25:541–7.
31. Narkewicz MR, Dell Olio D, Karpen SJ, Murray KF, Schwarz K, Yazigi N, et al. Pattern of diagnostic evaluation for the causes of pediatric acute liver failure: an opportunity for quality improvement. J Pediatr. 2009;155:801–6. e801.
32. Shakil AO, Kramer D, Mazariegos GV, Fung JJ, Rakela J. Acute liver failure: clinical features, outcome analysis, and applicability of prognostic criteria. Liver Transplant. 2000;6:163–169.
33. Sundaram V, Shneider BL, Dhawan A, Ng VL, Im K, Belle S, Squires RH. King's college hospital criteria for non-acetaminophen induced acute liver failure in an international cohort of children. J Pediatr. 2013;162:319–23. e311.
34. Dhawan A, Cheeseman P, Mieli-Vergani G. Approaches to acute liver failure in children. Pediatr Transplant. 2004;8:584–588.
35. O'Grady JG, Alexander GJ, Hayllar KM, Williams R. Early indicators of prognosis in fulminant hepatic failure. Gastroenterology. 1989;97:439–45.

36. Dhawan A, Taylor RM, Cheeseman P, De Silva P, Katsiyiannakis L, Mieli-Vergani G. Wilson's disease in children: 37-year experience and revised king's score for liver transplantation. Liver Transplant. 2005;11:441–8.

37. Polson J, Lee WM. Aasld position paper: the management of acute liver failure. Hepatology. 2005;41:1179–97.

38. Kortsalioudaki C, Taylor RM, Cheeseman P, Bansal S, Mieli-Vergani G, Dhawan A. Safety and efficacy of n-acetylcysteine in children with non-acetaminophen-induced acute liver failure. Liver Transplant. 2008;14:25–30.

39. Koch A, Trautwein C. N-acetylcysteine on its way to a broader application in patients with acute liver failure. Hepatology. 2010;51:338–40.

40. Squires RH, Dhawan A, Alonso E, Narkewicz MR, Shneider BL, Rodriguez-Baez N, et al. Intravenous n-acetylcysteine in pediatric patients with nonacetaminophen acute liver failure: a placebo-controlled clinical trial. Hepatology. 2013;57:1542–9.

41. Ferenci P, Lockwood A, Mullen K, Tarter R, Weissenborn K, Blei AT. Hepatic encephalopathy—definition, nomenclature, diagnosis, and quantification: final report of the working party at the 11th world congresses of gastroenterology, vienna, 1998. Hepatology. 2002;35:716–21.

42. Agarwal B, Wright G, Gatt A, Riddell A, Vemala V, Mallett S, Chowdary P, et al. Evaluation of coagulation abnormalities in acute liver failure. J Hepatol. 2012;57:780–6.

43. Rand EB, Karpen SJ, Kelly S, Mack CL, Malatack JJ, Sokol RJ, Whitington PF. Treatment of neonatal hemochromatosis with exchange transfusion and intravenous immunoglobulin. J Pediatr. 2009;155:566–71.

44. Whitington PF, Hibbard JU. High-dose immunoglobulin during pregnancy for recurrent neonatal haemochromatosis. Lancet. 2004;364:1690–8.

45. Ashorn M, Pitkanen S, Salo MK, Heikinheimo M. Current strategies for the treatment of hereditary tyrosinemia type i. Paediatric Drugs. 2006;8:47–54.

46. Edwards L, Wanless IR. Mechanisms of liver involvement in systemic disease. Best Pract Res Clin Gastroenterol. 2013;27:471–83.

47. Strom SC, Fisher RA, Thompson MT, Sanyal AJ, Cole PE, Ham JM, et al. Hepatocyte transplantation as a bridge to orthotopic liver transplantation in terminal liver failure. Transplantation. 1997;63:559–69.

48. Saigal S, Srinivasan P, Devlin J, de Boer B, Thomas B, Portmann B, et al. Auxiliary partial orthotopic liver transplantation in acute liver failure due to hepatitis b. Transpl Int. 2002;15:369–73.

49. Fujita M, Furukawa H, Hattori M, Todo S, Ishida Y, Nagashima K. Sequential observation of liver cell regeneration after massive hepatic necrosis in auxiliary partial orthotopic liver transplantation. Mod Pathol. 2000;13:152–7.

50. Faraj W, Dar F, Bartlett A, Melendez HV, Marangoni G, Mukherji D, et al. Auxiliary liver transplantation for acute liver failure in children. Ann Surg. 2010;251:351–6.

Complications of Cirrhosis in Children

71

Naresh P. Shanmugam and Anil Dhawan

Introduction

Cirrhosis is the end result of progressive fibrosis irrespective of the insult to the parenchyma or biliary tree. Unlike adults, there is no time duration of illness that defines chronic liver disease (CLD). All the inherited metabolic and genetic conditions even when diagnosed at birth could have advanced fibrosis or cirrhosis. Cirrhosis is a histological diagnosis but is liberally used in clinical practice without histological evidence. Liver cell death leads to a cascade of immunological reactions leading to activation of stellate cells with subsequent excessive collagen production and ultimately fibrosis. Bridging of the portal tracts (porto-portal) or the central vein to the portal tracts with nodule formation and disruption of the liver architecture is defined as cirrhosis. The disruption of the liver architecture leads on to disturbance in hemodynamics of blood flow into the liver and homeostasis of synthetic and detoxification functions of the liver, resulting in complications such as portal hypertension (PHT), ascites, and encephalopathy. This can lead to a secondary cascade of events affecting the function of several end organs such as brain, kidney, and lungs [1]. Understanding the pathophysiology of the complications in CLD helps in anticipation and initiation of treatment at appropriate time. This chapter deals with the common complication associated with CLD.

Cirrhosis

The hallmark of CLD is fibrosis of the liver. Cirrhosis is a histopathological term used to describe microscopic and/or macroscopic changes in liver characterized by aberrant nodule formation, vascular changes, and totally disturbed architecture associated with fibrosis. The degree to which the abovementioned changes progress depends on the nature and duration of the insult. Cirrhosis/fibrosis leads to complications such as PHT, ascites, encephalopathy, hepatorenal syndrome (HRS), hepatopulmonary syndrome (HPS), and eventually resulting in end-stage liver disease.

Etiology of Cirrhosis

Common diseases that cause chronic injury to the liver in children leading to cirrhosis are outlined in Table 71.1. Cell death or injury, as in hepatotropic viral infections or accumulation of toxic by-products such as hydrophobic bile acids in hepatocytes, is associated with release of several proinflammatory mediators (e.g., tumor necrosis factor, TNF) that lead on to progressive fibrosis and eventually liver cirrhosis. As with any other multifactorial disease, both genetic and environmental factors play role in cirrhosis. The pattern and type of proinflammatory mediator released depend on the underlying etiology of hepatocyte death [2]. These mediators act on Kupffer cells, hepatocytes, and cholangiocytes that release secondary mediators, which then activate hepatic stellate cells (HSC) to produce extracellular matrix (ECM). Thus, etiology of liver insult influences the pattern of fibrosis, as fibrosis is first observed in periportal area in viral hepatitis, perivenular region in toxic damage, while in developmental malformations such as biliary atresia fibrosis starts around bile duct. Liver fibrosis is considered to be a wound-healing process, similar to any injured tissue in body, but when the response is exaggerated and persistent, it progresses to cirrhosis.

A. Dhawan (✉) · N. P. Shanmugam
Professor and Director, Pediatric Liver, GI and Nutrition Center,
Clinical Director, Child Health, King's College Hospital, London, UK
e-mail: anil.dhawan@kcl.ac.uk

N. P. Shanmugam
Department of Pediatric Hepatology, Gastroenterology and Nutrition,
Global Hospitals and Health City, Chennai, India

© Springer International Publishing Switzerland 2016
S. Guandalini et al. (eds.), *Textbook of Pediatric Gastroenterology. Hepatology and Nutrition*,
DOI 10.1007/978-3-319-17169-2_71

Table 71.1 Some of the common causes of liver cirrhosis in children

Etiology of liver cirrhosis
Metabolic liver disease
α1-Antitrypsin deficiency
Wilson disease
Progressive familial intrahepatic cholestasis
Glycogen storage diseases
(especially types IV, VI, IX, and X)
Lipid abnormalities (e.g., Gaucher disease)
Peroxisomal disorders (e.g., Zellweger syndrome)
Tyrosinemia
Cystic fibrosis
Developmental/ genetic:
Biliary atresia
Congenital hepatic fibrosis
Alagille syndrome
Infections:
Viral (e.g., chronic hepatitis B or C)
Parasitic (e.g., echinococcosis)
Immune related:
Autoimmune hepatitis
Sclerosing cholangitis
Vascular:
Budd–Chiari syndrome
Hepatic veno-occlusive disease
Portal vein thrombosis
Miscellaneous:
Nonalcoholic steatohepatitis (NASH)
Drugs

Pathogenesis of Liver Fibrosis

Persistent insult to either hepatocytes or cholangiocytes acts as a stimulus for fibrosis to set in. Hepatotropic viruses, toxins, and diseases that cause chronic cholestasis (tyrosinemia, progressive familial intrahepatic cholestasis, etc.), damage liver cells, either by apoptosis or necrosis leading on to activation of a cascade of events causing fibrosis/cirrhosis (Fig. 71.1). The damaged liver cells secrete inflammatory mediators such as transforming growth factor (TGF)-beta1, TNF-α, epidermal growth factor (EGF), insulin-like growth factor (IGF), endothelin (ET), and platelet-derived growth factor (PDGF) that activate HSC. These damaged hepatocytes/cholangiocytes also recruit and activate T cells and Kupffer cells which secrete interleukin 6 (IL-6), interferon (IFN)-alpha, CD40, CCL21, and IGF which in turn activates HSC via a different pathway. The ECM such as type IV collagen, fibrinogen, and urokinase-type plasminogen activator that is secreted during the process of fibrosis could act as a stimulus for further activation of HSC starting a vicious cycle [3].

Under normal condition, HSC are quiescent cells that store lipids and vitamin A in liver that resides in space of Disse. When activated, HSC transdifferentiate to myofibro-

blast-like cells, acquiring fibrogenic and secretory properties. Apart from HSC, myofibroblasts that are derived from small portal blood vessels and bone marrow play a role in ECM formation during fibrosis of liver [4–6]. The source of fibroblast that is involved in fibrosis of liver depends on the etiology of insult to the liver [6]. With biliary pathology such as biliary atresia, portal tract fibroblasts, and in hypoxic insults, bone marrow fibroblasts play an important role [7, 8].

The ECM laid during this process of fibrosis differs in structure and composition, when compared to the ECM laid during routine remodeling. Mitogenic stimuli such as TGF-beta upregulate several precollagenous genes and increase the secretion of collagen by myofibroblasts, particularly type 1 and 3. Activated HSC also enhance the secretion of ECM-digesting enzymes like interstitial collagenase, gelatinase A, and stromelysin-1 which degrade specific components of ECM such as type 4 collagen and laminin, paving way for increased composition of type 1 and 3 collagen in fibrosis [9]. Increased tissue inhibitors of matrix metalloproteinases (TIMPs), which inhibit collagenase, result in gross imbalance between production and degradation of ECM. The fibrous tissue thus formed could interconnect portal tracts, portal tracts and central venules, or a mixture of both patterns and progress to cirrhosis. Contrary to the initial belief, it is shown that liver fibrosis even cirrhosis could regress to some extent on successful treatment of underlying cause [10].

Diagnosis of Liver Fibrosis

Fibrosis of liver covers an entire spectrum of microscopically detectable fibrosis during initial stages to macroscopically gross fibrosis as in advanced stages of CLD. There is no validated biochemical test or scoring system based on biochemical tests that would grade the severity of fibrosis [11]. Synthetic liver function or cholestasis has no correlation with the degree of fibrosis, as these parameters may be normal even in advanced fibrosis as in congenital hepatic fibrosis. Imaging techniques such as ultrasonography, computer tomography, and magnetic resonance imaging (MRI) can identify liver fibrosis though quantification is difficult. Liver biopsy is considered to be the gold standard method for the assessment of liver fibrosis as it provides necroinflammatory and the fibrosis grade. Figure 71.2a shows complete nodule formation, and Fig. 71.2b shows extensive collagen, when stained by trichrome in a cirrhotic liver. Scoring of degree of fibrosis could be done using Metavir (stages I–IV) and Ishak score (stages I–V). Due to invasive nature of the procedure, it is practically difficult to monitor fibrosis progression using liver biopsy. To overcome this problem, transient elastography (FibroScan®), a noninvasive technique is used in serial

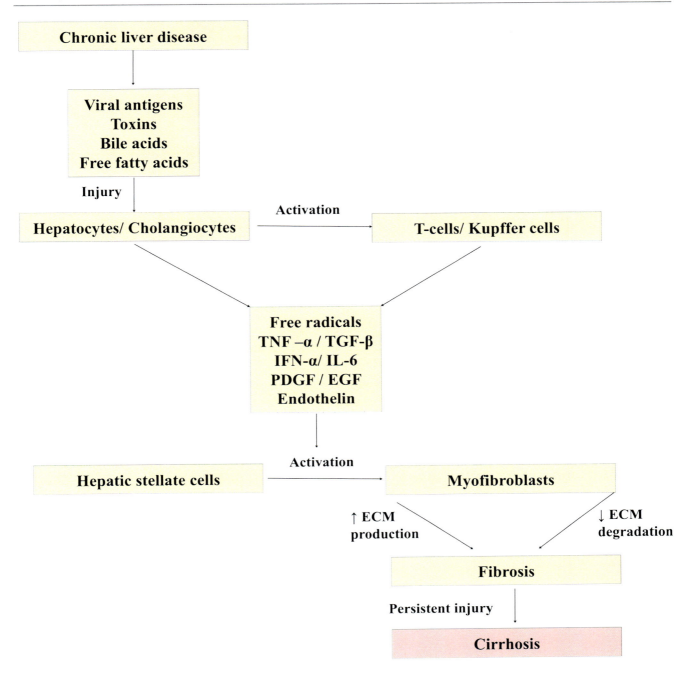

Fig. 71.1 Diagram showing cascade of events leading on to liver cirrhosis

monitoring of progress of fibrosis with good accuracy and has been validated even in children [12].

Complications and Management of Cirrhosis

CLD and the term "cirrhosis" have been used interchangeably in literature as cirrhosis is a manifestation of CLD, and most of the complications in CLD are secondary to cirrhosis. With progressive fibrosis, there is distortion of blood vessels and bile leading on to increased resistance to blood flow resulting in increased portal pressure on afferent side and tissue hypoxia due to reduced blood supply on efferent side. Cirrhosis also leads to increase in hepatic artery resistance, and in the case of hypotension secondary to an infection or variceal bleed, the liver could suffer hypoxic insult and could decompensate. Over a period of time, the fibrous tissue coalesces to form a tight capsule and restricts hepatocyte regeneration and worsen cholestasis. Synthetic/detoxification failure, cholestasis, and fibrosis individually or in

Fig. 71.2 **a** Microscopic image of cirrhotic liver showing a nodular formation. Hepatic lobule (*arrow head*) completely encased by fibrous tissue. **b** Microscopic image of trichrome-stained liver, where collagen is stained *blue*, while the cytoplasm of hepatocytes is stained *red* and nuclei as black structures within cells

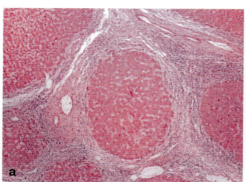
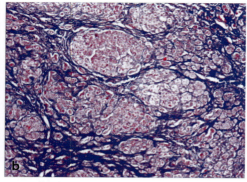

combination contribute towards complication of CLD, some of which are highlighted in Table 71.2. There is an increased risk of hepatocellular carcinoma (HCC) in cirrhotic liver, and the generalized nodular transformation of liver makes it difficult to diagnose HCC at early stages. Ultimately, these patients would succumb either to liver failure or to its complication unless treated appropriately. Fibrosis is a reversible phenomenon, but the extent to which the distorted liver architecture would revert back to its original state still remains an unanswered question. Disease-specific treatment, for example, chelation for Wilson's disease and steroids for autoimmune liver diseases, halts the progress of fibrosis and could reverse cirrhosis. At present, there is no approved drug that would inhibit or reverse fibrosis.

Complications of Cirrhosis

Portal Hypertension

Liver is a unique organ with dual blood supply, via the hepatic artery and portal vein. The portal vein, formed by the splenic vein and superior mesenteric vein, supplies nutrient-rich blood from the intestine to the liver. The usual pressure is less than 5 mmHg, and this blood traverses hepatic sinusoids reaching hepatic venules having much lower pressures and enters systemic venous circulation. PHT develops when there is increased resistance anywhere along the portal system, and thus PHT could be extrahepatic (portal vein thrombosis), intrahepatic (cirrhosis), or posthepatic (hepatic venous thrombosis). PHT leads on to opening up of porto-systemic collaterals causing varices, which could rupture and cause bleed.

Direct measurement of portal pressure is difficult, and so hepatic venous pressure gradient (HVPG) is measured via hepatic venous catheterization. HVPG is pressure difference between wedged hepatic venous pressure (WHVP) and free hepatic venous pressure, which is reflective of portal pressure. HVPG of more than 10 mmHg is associated with the development of varices, and pressures more than 12 mmHg is associated with variceal bleed. In clinical practice, accurate measurement of portal pressure by invasive methods is of little relevance as esophageal varices and splenomegaly hint towards the development of PHT, and this needs to be managed appropriately.

Table 71.2 Signs and symptoms of cirrhosis and probable mechanism causing it

Complications of cirrhosis		
Symptoms	Signs	Underlying mechanism[a]
Jaundice, pruritus	Elevated bilirubin and bile acids	Detoxification failure of liver
Altered mental status	Encephalopathy	Detoxification failure of liver
Distended abdominal veins, vomiting blood	Caput medusae	Portal hypertension
Abdominal distension Swelling of legs	Ascites/edema	Hypoalbuminemia, portal hypertension
Muscle wasting	Malnutrition	Decreased absorption of nutrients due to defective bile flow and increased demand
Telangiectasia	Spider nevi	Detoxification failure of certain hormones
Easy fractures	Osteoporosis and osteomalacia	Hepatic osteodystrophy
Decreased urine output	Oliguria	Hepatorenal syndrome
Bluish discoloration and swelling of fingers	Cyanosis and clubbing	Hepatopulmonary syndrome, portopulmonary hypertension
Difficulty in breathing	Dyspnea	Hepatopulmonary syndrome, portopulmonary hypertension

[a] More than one mechanism could be involved

Pathogenesis of PHT in Cirrhosis

Like any other tubular organ, resistance and flow govern the pressure in portal venous system. In CLD, there is a substantial increase in both flow and resistance of portal vein leading on to net increase in portal pressure.

Increased Resistance to Portal Flow

In cirrhosis, dynamic contractile elements within sinusoids and portal venules contribute up to 40 % of increased vascular resistance, while the rest is attributed to fibrosis. Wrapping of HSC and myofibroblasts can wrap around sinusoids, and the portal venular smooth muscle contraction can increase vascular resistance [13]. ETs are a group of peptides, which cause vasoconstriction and stimulation of cell proliferation in tissue. ET-1 and ET-3 are found to be increased in cirrhotics when compared to controls, probably due to increased production [14]. Angiotensin II, norepinephrine, and thromboxane A2 (TXA2) are other vasopressors which are found to be increased in cirrhosis of the liver and cause increased vascular resistance of portal venules [15]. There is an associated endothelial dysfunction, which further increases the vascular resistance instead of decreasing it. This is probably due to increased levels of TXA2 impairing the response to endothelium-dependent vasodilator acetylcholine, and thus the resultant increased vascular resistance is probably due to imbalance between increased vasoconstrictors and decreased vasodilators in CLD [16].

Increased Portal Circulation

Splanchnic vasodilatation combined with hyperdynamic circulation contributes to increased portal circulation. Nitric oxide (NO) [17] increases the production of cyclic guanosine monophosphate, which directly relaxes the smooth muscle. Increased NO due to enhanced endothelial NO synthase (eNOS) activity in splanchnic circulation is suggested to play an important role in splanchnic vasodilatation. Increased levels of glucagon found in cirrhosis cause direct vascular smooth muscle relaxation and decrease the sensitivity of vascular smooth muscle to endogenous vasoconstrictors. Other vasodilators such as capsaicin–calcitonin gene-related peptide, neuropeptides, and adenosine have a doubtful role. Plasma volume expansion due to sodium retention in cirrhosis also plays a role in increased portal flow.

Variceal Bleed in Portal Hypertension

Apart from ascites and hypersplenism, the major complication of PHT is variceal bleed. HVPG of more than 10 mmHg results in opening up of porto-systemic collaterals, which are situated at the lower end of esophagus, rectum, paraumblical, and retroperitoneal regions. Life-threatening bleeds are usually from esophageal and gastric varices that arise from a collateral network through the coronary and short gastric veins draining into the systemic azygous vein. Miga et al. showed that 20 % of children had esophageal variceal hemorrhage (EVH) within 2 years after Kasai portoenterostomy, and the risk of death or need for liver transplantation was 50 % at 6 years after the initial episode of EVH in a cohort of children with biliary atresia [18]. Etiology plays an important role in the survival outcome after variceal bleed, with varices due to portal vein thrombosis has better prognosis when compared with those due to intrinsic hepatobiliary disease [19].

Management of Variceal Bleed

Variceal bleed is a life-threatening emergency, and the patient needs to be stabilized before shifting for emergency endoscopy. In the event of hypovolemic shock, fluid resuscitation has to be initiated while awaiting whole blood, and in addition, fresh frozen plasma/platelets/cryoprecipitate/factor VIIa might be required, as these patients would be coagulopathic secondary to liver disease. Nasogastric tube placement and gastric lavage help to quantify the blood loss as well as to remove blood from the stomach that could precipitate encephalopathy. Vasoactive drugs that decrease portal pressure (Table 71.3) should be started along with proton pump inhibitors/H2 blockers and antibiotics. Once stable, endoscopic variceal ligation (EVL) or endoscopic sclerotherapy could be done [20]. In the case of continuous bleed and hemodynamic instability, balloon tamponade with a Minnesota or Sengstaken–Blakemore tube should be attempted. Both these tubes have esophageal and gastric balloon, but Minnesota tube has esophageal aspiration port in addition to gastric aspiration port while Sengstaken–Blakemore tube has only gastric aspiration port. These tubes need to be placed by an experienced person as improper placement or overinflation of the balloon can result in esophageal rupture and/or ischemia [21]. Once bleeding is controlled, endoscopic sclerotherapy (ESL) and endoscopic *variceal* ligation (*EVL*) has to be performed, as conservative management (medication and balloon tamponade) without endoscopic intervention was associated with 3.6 times higher risk of rebleed [22].

ESL is a procedure where sclerosant such as ethanolamine oleate or sodium tetradecyl sulfate is injected into a varix under direct vision, thereby obliterating the vessel. Cyanoacrylates are synthetic glues used in gastric varices that rapidly solidify on contact with water and blood. Usually, cyanoacrylates are mixed with ethanolamine oleate at 1:1 ratio to decrease the rate of solidification, as it minimizes the inadvertent adherence to catheters and endoscope. EVL is a procedure where an elastic O-ring is applied over a small area of esophageal mucosa and submucosa, causing strangulation

Table 71.3 Various drugs used in portal hypertension and its mechanism of action

Medications used in portal hypertension		
Drugs used in acute variceal bleed		
Drug	Dosage	Mechanism of action
Vasopressin	Initial IV bolus 0.3 U/kg (maximum: 20 U) over 20 min followed by infusion: 0.002–0.01 U/kg/min	Acts via V1 receptors, reduces portal blood flow, portal systemic collateral blood flow, and variceal pressure
Octreotide	1 µg/kg/h IV Infusion or 2–4 µg/kg/dose/8 h s.c.	Analogue of somatostatin Reduce portal flow and pressures
Terlipressin	8–20 µg/kg of body weight given at intervals of 4–8 h	Terlipressin, a prodrug of vasopressin
Drugs used to prevent rebleed		
Propranolol Atenolol	1–5 mg/kg/day in three divided doses 1 mg/kg/day in two doses (Dose has to be adjusted to decrease heart rate by 25 %)	Reduces portal hypertension by decreasing cardiac output and inducing splanchnic vasoconstriction by blocking β-1 and β-2 receptors
Carvedilol	0.3 mg/kg/day	Nonselective β-blocker with additional α-1 blocking action

IV intravenous, *s.c.* subcutaneous

of the tissue (varix) caught in-between the ring, eventually leading to fibrosis and obliteration. Randomized trial of endoscopic sclerotherapy versus variceal band ligation for esophageal varices showed that while both are equally effective in controlling acute bleed; EVL achieved variceal obliteration in fewer treatment sessions along with significantly lower rate of the development of portal gastropathy and rebleeding [23]. Meta-analysis suggests that pharmacotherapy coupled with either EVL or ESL showed better initial bleeding control and 5-day hemostasis, but no effect on mortality [24]. Occasionally, bleeding from gastric varices and Roux en Y jejunal loop varices might be difficult to control and might require interventional measures such as transjugular intrahepatic portosystemic shunt (TIPSS), surgical shunts, esophagogastric devascularization ± splenectomy [25]. Liver transplantation has to be offered to those with CLD, after control of the acute bleeding episode.

Prophylactic Therapy for Variceal Bleed

The American Association for the Study of Liver Diseases (AASLD) practice guidelines recommend β-blockers as first-line therapy in adults with medium/large esophageal varices and EVL for patients in whom β-blockers are contraindicated or poorly tolerated [26]. Trials on children showed that β-blockers and EVL/ESL are relatively safe to be used, but so far, there are no robust data to suggest that its use as primary prophylaxis decreases the incidence of first episode variceal bleed in children [27, 28]. Variceal eradication and nonselective beta-blocker are recommended in adults after an episode of bleed as secondary prophylaxis, while in children, small studies have shown usefulness of

EVL/EST to prevent rebleed, but role of beta-blocker is still unclear [29, 30].

Neurological Complications in Cirrhosis

CLD predisposes to a variety of neurological complications such as intracranial hemorrhage due to the presence of coagulopathy, increased risk of cerebral infection due to decreased immune function, and hepatic encephalopathy (HE) [31].

Hepatic Encephalopathy

HE is defined as a metabolically induced, potentially reversible, functional disturbance of the brain that may occur in acute or CLD[32]. Though HE is considered to be a potentially reversible condition, some patients might not recover to their previous level of cognitive function after a severe episode of HE.

Factors such as infection, trauma, and electrolyte imbalance in the background of CLD could cause sudden liver decompensation and lead to HE. Encephalopathy that occurs in acute liver failure (ALF) is categorized as type A, HE in portosystemic shunt without any intrinsic hepatocellular disease as type B, and in CLD as type C. Type C could be further subclassified into minimal, episodic, or persistent. HE is called minimal hepatic encephalopathy (MHE), when diagnosis could be made only on psychometric analysis in an apparently normal person with CLD. Episodic encephalopathy in CLD coincides with episodes of high protein intake, gastrointestinal bleed, infection, etc. Usually, these episodes resolve with the treatment of the precipitating factors, but sometimes they persist and termed as persistent HE.

Clinical Features

HE could be clinically graded from 1 to 4 using West Haven criteria, and Glasgow coma scale which has lesser interobserver variability could be used in assessing conscious levels [33]. MHE is associated with mild intellectual impairment, where verbal ability is preserved and apparently normal personality [34]. Worsening of HE leads on to asterixis (flapping tremor), hypertonia and hyperreflexia, hypotonia, and areflexia may be seen with subsequent progression to coma. Features similar to Parkinsonism such as muscular rigidity, bradykinesia, hypokinesia, monotony of speech, and tremors could be seen in HE.

Pathogenesis of Hepatic Encephalopathy

The pathogenesis of HE is thought to be multifactorial, with neurotoxins and altered neurotransmitters acting on the neurons. Ammonia is considered to be an important factor involved in pathogenesis, while mercaptans, short- and medium-chain fatty acids, phenols, methionine derivatives, etc. play a minor role. altered ratio of excitatory (↓ dopamine and noradrenaline) and inhibitory (↑ gamma-aminobutyric acid (GABA) and serotonin) neurotransmitters resulting in abnormal cerebral function. Apart from these, there is an increased formation of false neurotransmitters such as octopamine, phenyl methionine from accumulation of phenylalanine, and tyrosine. There are other proposed mechanisms of HE such as increase in false neurotransmitters (octopamine, phenyl methionine), altered ratios of branched-chain amino acids (BCAA) and aromatic amino acids (AAA), changes in postsynaptic receptor activity, increased permeability of blood–brain barrier, etc.

Role of Ammonia in HE

Ammonia is produced from a variety of sources such as small intestine enterocytes, gut flora, muscle, and kidney. Under healthy condition, around 80–90% of ammonia is either converted to urea by periportal hepatocytes or glutamine by perivenous hepatocytes. Though ammonia is implicated in HE, the exact mechanism is still elusive. Few of the suggested mechanisms are: (1) Excess ammonia is converted to glutamine by glial cells. This glutamine increases intracellular osmotic pressure, leading on to swelling of astrocytes, cerebral edema and can competitively bind to glutamate receptors and inhibit them. (2) Oxidative stress triggered by ammonia toxicity in the astrocyte resulting in mitochondrial dysfunction. (3) Enhanced cytokine activity and impaired intracellular signaling [35].

It was thought that ammonia in portal circulation was exclusively produced by the gut flora, but current hypothesis suggests that small gut enterocytes produce ammonia in excess of gut flora, and gut decontamination alone has minimal effect on ammonia levels [36]. Kidney is involved in both production and elimination of ammonia. Kidney can metabolize glutamine to produce ammonia and bicarbonate and can excrete ammonia as ammonium ion and urea in urine [35]. Alkalosis can decrease the conversion of ammonia to ammonium, as there is no need to excrete the hydrogen ion resulting in elevated free ammonia that can cross blood–brain barrier and precipitate HE. Myocytes can act as buffer by converting ammonia to nontoxic glutamine via glutamine synthetase, and thus poor muscle mass is an important risk factor for HE [37].

Role of Neurotoxins and Inflammatory Mediators in HE

The ratio of BCAA/AAA phenylalanine, tyrosine, and tryptophan is called the Fischer ratio [38, 39]. There is decrease in Fischer ratio in liver failure, due to preferential usage of BCAA by muscles and decreased clearance of AAA by liver. Elevated serum AAA can cross the blood–brain barrier into the brain and results in synthesis of false neurotransmitter such as octopamine and synephrine [40].

Several short-chain fatty acids such as propionate, butyrate, and valerate are produced in small intestine by breakdown of proteins by fecal flora [41]. These short-chain fatty acids competitively inhibit urea cycle enzymes and can bind to albumin and displacing albumin-bound toxins, thus precipitating HE. Indole, oxindole, endozepines, neuronal acetylcholinesterase, TNF-α, and allopregnanolone are few of the other bioactive substances that could play a role in HE [42–46].

Diagnosis

Diagnosis of encephalopathy is mainly based on clinical history and examination [47]. Clinical diagnosis of mild-to-moderate HE is difficult in children as it requires their cooperation to perform psychometric tests. Neuroimaging and electrophysiological studies of brain would give supportive evidence rather than to confirm the diagnosis of HE. Though arterial ammonia level correlates with the severity of HE, it could not be used to grade encephalopathy [33]. HE could be clinically graded using West Haven criteria, and conscious level is graded using Glasgow coma scale [33].

Neuropsychological Assessment

In children, neuropsychological assessment should be made using tests such as Wechsler intelligence tests and Dutch child intelligence test (Revisie Amsterdamse Kinder Intelligentie test), where validated nomogram exits for the selected age, sex, racial, and ethnical subgroup. The Psychometric Hepatic Encephalopathy Score (PHES) and number connect test (NCT) A and B could be used to diagnose MHE in adults while these tests are not validated in children [48, 49].

Critical Flicker Frequency

Critical flicker-frequency threshold is a simple and reliable test for the quantification of low-grade HE [50]. The principle of the test is to identify the point of switch over from a steady red light to a flickering light. A normal human eye perceives flicker rate of 60 Hz as a steady light. The frequency of the light is gradually decreased to a point where the patient starts to perceive the light as flicker. Using this technique, it was found that patients with HE can pick up flickering only when the flicker rate comes below 39 Hz, while cirrhotic counterparts without encephalopathy and normal individual could identify flickering at higher rate [47]. The need for understanding (and being able to follow instructions) the test limits is used only in children more than 8 years [51].

Electroencephalogram

Using electroencephalogram (EEG), HE could be graded into 5 grades (0–4). Grade 0 is a normal EEG with regular alpha rhythm. Grade 1 encephalopathy is characterized by irregular background alpha rhythm and appearance of theta rhythm. Theta activity becomes continuous with occasional delta wave in grade 2 HE, and theta activity becomes prevalent with transient polyphasic complexes of spikes and slow waves in grade 3. Grade 4 is deep coma, having continuous delta waves with abundant complexes of spikes and slow waves [47]. With the availability of newer complex EEG analytical softwares, EEG can be analyzed in specific regions of the brain.

Neuroimaging in HE

Computer tomography (CT) of brain is not a useful tool in diagnosis of HE, apart from excluding organic causes such as bleed, tumors, or gross edema that can cause encephalopathy [52]. MRI is a better modality to diagnose cerebral edema and demyelination associated with HE. Conventional MRI lacks sensitivity in diagnosing milder forms of edema, and newer techniques such as magnetization transfer imaging (MTI), fast fluid-attenuated inversion recovery (FLAIR) imaging, and diffusion-weighted imaging are more sensitive in picking up brain tissue water content [53]. Proton MR

spectroscopy could measure different levels of metabolites in brain such as myo-inositol, choline, and glutamine These specialized neuroimaging is more of research interest and provides little benefit in routine clinical practice.

Management of Hepatic Encephalopathy

Management should be directed towards stabilization of the patient and treating the precipitating factors such as bleeding, electrolyte imbalance, and infection In HE of grade 3 or 4, elective intubation has to be considered to protect the airways. Despite increased total body water, these patients would be intravascularly fluid depleted. Hydration is best monitored by central venous pressure (CVP) and ideally should be 6–8 cm of H_2O. Though their serum sodium is low, they will have high total body sodium, and any attempt to normalize the sodium will lead on to worsening of edema. Supplementation of extra sodium is required if the sodium level falls below 120 mEq/l [54].

Lactulose decreases the colonic pH to around 5, and thereby decreasing the bacterial fermentation and production of short-chain fatty acids [55, 56]. In acidic environment, the ammonia produced in colon is converted to ammonium ion, reducing its diffusibility back into circulation and thereby removed along with stools. The amount of lactulose dose has to be titrated to produce three soft stools/day. Long-term lactulose in CLD helps to prevent HE, but will not change the ultimate requirement of a liver transplantation. Lactitol (B galactosido-sorbitol) is a nonabsorbable sugar which has similar action to lactulose, but less sweeter and more palatable [57].

Neomycin, vancomycin, and rifaximin are few of the antibiotics that are used to eliminate ammoniagenic bacteria from the gut, thereby decreasing the ammonia production in the intestine. Of all the antibiotics, rifaximin has been shown to be very effective in decreasing ammonia production and highest risk benefit ratio [58]. Rifaximin and lactulose given together was found to be more beneficial than either of them given alone [59]. Use of probiotics has shown to reduce plasma ammonia, but there was no change in final outcome [60].

L-ornithine-L-aspartate (LOLA) enhances the action of ornithine and aspartate transaminases in brain and peripheral tissues to produce nontoxic glutamate. There is no standard dosing in children, up to 20 g/day could be given at an infusion rate not exceeding 5 g/h as suggested by drug monogram and not recommended in children less than 8 years old [54]. Sodium benzoate (250 mg/kg/day) along with intravenous sodium phenylacetate (250 mg/kg/day) or oral sodium phenylbutyrate (250 mg/kg/day) could be used to eliminate ammonia by alternate pathways, thereby decreasing serum ammonia levels. Water-soluble hippuric acid and phenylacetyl-glutamine are formed by conjugation of benzoate with glycine and phenyl acetate with glutamine, respectively. Hippuric acid and phenylacetyl-glutamine are then excreted by kidneys, thereby reducing ammonia load [61]. Though all these medications are more useful in hyperammonia due to urea cycle defects, they are used off-label in hyperammoniemia due to liver failure [35].

There has been increasing interest in the possibility of providing an extracorporeal liver support system for short periods while liver allograft becomes available. High cost, nonavailability of small filters, and lack of safety data in children limit the usage of these devises to clinical trial setting. Liver transplantation has shown to be the definitive treatment, which has improved survival outcome both in adults and children. Elective liver transplantation offers 5-year survival of more than 85% in children. Synthetic liver failure with encephalopathy is one of the indications for liver transplantation in CLD, which has to be done before permanent neurological damage sets in.

Ascites

Fluid retention and low albumin in CLD result in accumulation of fluid in extravascular space leading to edema, ascites, and plural effusion. Presence of ascites is one of the variables that increase the mortality in children with CLD [62]. Onset of ascites indicates decompensation of liver disease and the need for liver transplantation. Ascites increases the risk of bacterial peritonitis and HRS, which potentially adds on to the already increased mortality associated with liver decompensation (see Fig. 71.3).

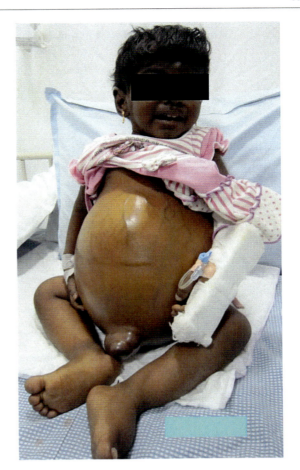

Fig. 71.3 Image of a child with failed Kasai portoenterostomy showing gross ascites, dilated abdominal veins, and edema of legs

Pathophysiology of Ascites

There are several theories based on the triggering factor of the vicious cycle that leads to fluid retention and ascites. The "overfill" theory suggests hepatorenal reflex to be the primary event that leading on to sodium and fluid retention and subsequently ascites. The "underfill" theory suggests that that the increased pressure in portal sinusoids results in increased hydrostatic pressure leading on to excessive lymph production. When lymph production exceeds absorption, the net result is ascites and contraction of intravascular volume (underfill). "Peripheral arterial vasodilation hypothesis" which was proposed in 1988 suggests that splanchnic and peripheral arterial vasodilatation secondary to PHT and cirrhosis is the initial triggering event [63]. This causes decreased intravascular volume, leading on to baroreceptor-mediated activation of renin angiotensin aldosterone system and release of antidiuretic hormone, resulting in hypervolemic stage due to renal sodium and water retention [63–65]. Splanchnic vasodilatation along with hypervolemia results in increased hydrostatic pressure that ultimately results in passage of fluid to peritoneal space [66]. It is difficult to ex-

plain the complex cascade of events leading on to ascites based on one theory, and it is possible that mechanisms as suggested by different theories could contribute to various stages of ascites formation.

Biochemical Diagnosis

Ascitic tap should be carried out in any new onset ascites. Estimating serum-ascites albumin gradient (SAAG) is considered to be superior in making differential diagnosis of probable cause of ascites, compared to quantifying it as exudate or transudate. SAAG ≥ 1.1 g/dL is associated with cirrhosis, portal or hepatic venous occlusion, congestive cardiac failure, etc., while SAAG < 1.1 g/dL is associated with nephrotic syndrome, peritoneal infection, or malignancy [67]. Spontaneous bacterial peritonitis is an important complication of ascites and has to be differentiated from surgical cause of peritonitis such as perforation which accounts for 5% of cases [68]. Polymorphonuclear neutrophils (PMNs) of > 250 mm^3 in ascitic fluid are suggestive of the presence of bacterial infection while predominant lymphocytic cells in ascites (>20% of the total leukocyte count) along with ascites–blood glucose quotient of <0.7 is suggestive of tuberculous infection. In the case of high PMNs in ascitic fluid with symptoms of fever and abdominal tenderness, antibiotics need to be continued even if the cultures are negative as 34.5% turn culture positive on repeated samples.

Management

Optimizing caloric and protein intake helps improving serum albumin and thus oncotic pressure. Diuretic therapy remains the first line of treatment in ascites. Aldosterone antagonist, spironolactone, is the initial drug of choice. It is usually started at 3 mg/kg/day in three to four divided doses and could be gradually increased to 6 mg/kg/day (maximum dose 400 mg/day). Potent loop diuretics such as Furosemide (1–2 mg/kg) could be added if there is no effective diuresis on monotherapy. Spironolactone causes hyperkalemia while frusemide causes hyponatremia and hypokalemia, which has to be monitored on regular basis. Sometimes duel therapy with these drugs is beneficial as potassium loss by frusemide is counteracted by potassium conservation by spironolactone. The suggested optimal drug dosage ratio to achieve this is 2 (frusemide):5 (spironolactone). Tolvaptan is an oral vasopressin receptor antagonist that helps in free water excretion and corrects hyponatremia, and it has been approved by the US Food and Drug Administration (FDA) for use in adults with cirrhosis. It is currently under phase three trials for its safety in children.

Paracentesis is indicated in the case of tense ascites causing respiratory distress. Usually, 20% albumin at a dose of 5 ml/kg is given slowly over 2 h during the procedure as plasma expander as well as to prevent rapid reaccumulation of ascites. It is shown that children tolerate large volume paracentesis (>50 ml/kg) well, and the noticed side effect such as reduced urine output responded well to volume expanders [69]. It is advisable to taut the skin at the point of needle entry to create "Z," so that normal skin covers the muscle puncture site, preventing post-procedure leak.

Pulmonary Complications in Cirrhosis

The common pulmonary complications of CLD are HPS, portopulmonary hypertension (PoPH), and pulmonary hydrothorax. Care should be taken to exclude intrinsic lung diseases such as alpha-1-antitrypsin (AIAT) deficiency and cystic fibrosis that could coexist with liver disease and contribute towards hypoxia.

Hepatopulmonary Syndrome

Kennedy and Knudson coined the term "HPS" in 1977 to describe the association of cirrhosis with cyanosis and club-

bing. The diagnostic criteria for HPS is the presence of CLD along with PaO_2 <70 mmHg or alveolar-arterial oxygen gradient >15 mmHg and intrapulmonary vascular dilatation [70]. The overall prevalence of HPS ranges from 4 to 30% in cirrhotics. Suggested prevalence of HPS in pediatric population with CLD is around 8–20% [71, 72].

Pathogenesis

Higher prevalence of HPS in disorders where there is intrinsic liver disease along with PHT such as biliary atresia rather than in condition with PHT alone such as portal vein thrombosis led to the hypothesis that PHT along with intrinsic liver disease is essential for the development of HPS [52, 73, 74]. HPS is probably due to the effect of several vasoactive substances such as NO [17], carbon monoxide (CO), prostaglandins, vasoactive intestinal peptide, calcitonin, and glucagon, which escapes liver metabolism due to PHT and acts on pulmonary vasculature. NO is a potent vasodilator, and its nitrates and nitrite metabolites are found to be high in exhaled air of patients with HPS, which normalizes after liver transplantation. NO synthase is an enzyme that helps in production of NO from L-arginine. It has several isoforms of which eNOS was found to be increased in pulmonary small alveolar vessels, in small animal models of HPS. Elevated levels of ET-1 in blood and increased expression of its receptor ET B (ETB) expression in the pulmonary vasculature result in increased eNOS synthesis and thus vasodilatation [75]. Apart from eNOS, TNF-α, IL-1β, carbon monoxide, etc. are some of the other vasoactive substances implicated in pathogenesis of HPS [76–78]. These substances were thought to be involved in angiogenesis and vasodilatation of pulmonary vasculature leading on to portopulmonary and hepatopulmonary shunts. In lung areas where there are capillary dilations, there would be more of perfusion compared to ventilation while in areas with shunting effect, the blood is diverted away from alveoli resulting in less perfusion, leading on to ventilation perfusion mismatch. Due to this, 100% oxygen inhalation might improve PaO_2 in cases of HPS with predominant intrapulmonary vascular dilatation, while there won't be any change in those with predominant shunt.

Clinical Manifestation

Dyspnea, clubbing, cyanosis, spider nevi are some of the clinical manifestations of HPS. In HPS, dyspnea is more on upright position, due to increased congestion because of gravity exaggerating the ventilation—perfusion mismatch. PaO_2 decrease of 5% or more or 4 mmHg or more from the supine to upright position is defined as orthodeoxia, which is the hall mark of HPS [79]. Clubbing, also described as drumstick fingers (Fig. 71.4) seen in HPS, is due to the release

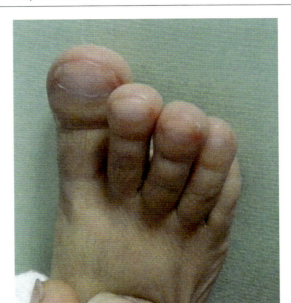

Fig. 71.4 Shows clubbing of fingers in a 10-month-old child with chronic liver disease due to missed biliary atresia

of PDGF in nail beds that acts as growth factor and causes bulbous swelling of nails beds [80].

Diagnosis

In cirrhotic patients with hypoxia, chest X-ray has to be taken as first line to rule out other causes of hypoxia such as pulmonary atelectasis, pneumonia, pulmonary edema, or hepatic hydrothorax. X-ray would be normal in majority of patients with HPS, but few might show interstitial infiltrate in the lung bases [81]. Contrast enhanced echocardiography is the preferred screening test for HPS [75]. Saline or indocyanine green is agitated to produce microbubbles at least 15 μm in diameter and then injected intravenously. These microbubbles act as contrast and could be visualized in echocardiography on right side of the heart. When these microbubbles traverse the lung, they get trapped in alveolar microvasculature and gradually absorbed. In individuals with either intracardiac or intrapulmonary shunts, these microbubbles could be seen in the left heart. Differentiation between intracardiac or intrapulmonary shunts depends on the timing of appearance of microbubbles in left heart. With intracardiac shunts, the microbubbles appear in three heartbeats, while with intrapulmonary shunts, it takes 4–6 heart beats for the contrast to appear in left side of heart. Though contrast echocardiography is sensitive, it lacks specificity, as some cirrhotic patients with positive results on contrast echocardiography might not fulfill the diagnostic criteria for HPS [75].

If the initial screening raises the possibility of HPS, technetium-99 m macroaggregated albumin (Tc-99 m MAA) lung perfusion scan has to be considered, which is more

sensitive and specific [70, 82]. Macroaggregated albumin, which is of 20 μm in size, is tagged with radioisotope technetium. In normal individuals, macroaggregated albumin gets trapped in lung, and less than 5% of tracer activity can be quantified in the brain. In HPS patients, the fraction is more than 6%. Using this technique, the magnitude of shunt can be quantified which is inversely proportional to arterial oxygen saturation [70]. The drawback of this procedure is that correlation between shunt fraction and response of PaO_2 after 100% oxygen supplement remains unpredictable. High-resolution CT could show increased ratio of segmental arterial diameter to adjacent bronchial diameter, but published data were quite scarce [83]. Selective pulmonary angiography along with possible embolotherapy has to be considered in patients with HPS who fail to respond to 100% oxygen and particularly in those whom liver transplantation has to be considered. Angiography could reveal two types of vascular pattern, diffuse (type 1) and focal (type 2). In type 1 HPS, diffuse speckled, spidery, or sponge-like appearance of vasodilated vessels may be demonstrated. Type 1 was considered to be of better prognosis with liver transplantation as there is high possibility of resolution of HPS [84]. In type 2 HPS, vascular changes resembling arteriovenous (AV) shunts or vascular malformations could be seen. If amicable, embolization of feeding vessel could be done before considering liver transplantation [85, 86].

Management

Oxygen supplementation remains the main stay in HPS patients when PaO_2 <60, and it improves the quality of life and exercise tolerance [87]. Several medications such as indomethacin, tamoxifen, somatostatin analogues, sympathomimetics, beta-blockers, methylene blue, and plasma exchange have been tried in HPS with abysmal results. Martinez-Palli et al. showed that decreasing PHT using TIPSS had no effect on pulmonary gas exchange and thus not recommended [88]. Severity of HPS correlates with mortality, and so it should be combined with the model for end-stage liver disease (MELD) score as to prioritize these patients are in organ allocation [89, 90]. Liver transplantation is considered to be the definitive treatment in selective group of HPS patients as it reverts the pulmonary capillary abnormality and normalizes oxygenation [91]. Overall, postoperative complications in patients with HPS are higher than those without HPS. Embolic cerebral hemorrhage, worsening of hypoxia, and failure of AV shunts to resolve (particularly type 2) are a few of the unique complications of HPS [85, 92].

Careful patient selection is essential as severe preoperative hypoxemia (PaO_2 <50 mmHg in room air) and significant intrapulmonary shunting (Tc-99 m MAA shunt fraction >20%) are associated with high mortality after liver transplantation [93].

Portopulmonary Hypertension

PoPH is defined as the presence of mean pulmonary artery pressure (MPAP) >25 mmHg along with pulmonary vascular resistance (PVR) >240 dynes s cm^{-5} with normal capillary wedge pressure (PCWP) <15 mmHg, in the presence of PHT [94]. It is postulated that the toxins and bioactive substances that bypasses liver metabolism via varices in PHT could lead on to pulmonary vasoconstriction, structural remodeling of the pulmonary arteries, formation of microthrombi, etc. along with high flow state [95]. PHT seems to be a prerequisite as PoPH is seen in disorders with no intrinsic liver disease such as extrahepatic portal vein thrombosis [96]. The histopathological changes in PoPH consist of medial hypertrophy with nonspecific intimal fibrous thickening along with fibrous mural pads, occlusive fibrous tissue in vascular lumens, which is similar to that of primary pulmonary hypertension [53].

Clinical Features

The most common presenting symptom is dyspnea on excretion followed by syncope, chest pain, and fatigue [97]. Sometimes it is associated with hemoptysis. In mild-to-moderate PoPH, the symptoms are mild or absent. The time interval between diagnosis of PHT and symptoms due to PoPH is around 5 years [98]. Clinical examination would reveal systolic murmur with loud pulmonary component of second heart sound indicating tricuspid regurgitation. Edema and ascites (features of right heart failure) are other clinical features.

Diagnosis

Diagnosis of PoPH is made based on the presence of pulmonary hypertension in the background liver disease. Chest X-ray might show prominent central pulmonary arteries and cardiomegaly, and electrocardiogram might show right ventricular strain pattern. Estimated right ventricular systolic pressure >50 mmHg (normal <30 mmHg) is strongly suggestive of PoPH, when assessed by Doppler echocardiography, but has a false-positive rate of around 15 % [94]. Right-heart catheterization study remains the gold standard test for accurately diagnosing pulmonary hypertension and could be classified into mild, moderate, and severe based on MPAP, PVR, and cardiac index [94].

Management

Three groups of drugs, namely prostacyclin analogues (epoprostenol, iloprost), ET receptor antagonists (bosentan), and phosphodiesterase inhibitors (sildenafil) have been used with good response in children with primary pulmonary hypertension, and the data on its usage in children PoPH are sparse [99]. Continuous intravenous infusion of epoprostenol (30–90 ng/kg/min) improves circulatory hemodynamics and exercise capacity in children with PoPH [99]. Treprostinil is another prostacyclin analogue, which could be given either subcutaneously or intravenously [100]. Bosentan is an ET receptor antagonist which when used in children has shown to decrease MPAP and pulmonary vascular resistance index and improve cardiac index [101]. Sildenafil is a phosphodiesterase-5 inhibitors and causes vasodilatation of pulmonary arteries and thereby decreases pulmonary hypertension when given at a dose of 0.5–1 mg/kg/dose given three to four times [99]. Mild-to-moderate PoPH frequently resolves after liver transplantation while severe PoPH is associated with the persistence of pulmonary hypertension and increased mortality [94]

Renal Involvement in Cirrhosis

Renal decompensation in liver disease is an important complication of both acute and CLD. Kidneys could be affected as a part of generalized circulatory changes associated liver disease (e.g., hypovolemia after variceal bleed) or as a specific phenomenon that occurs only in liver disease (e.g., hepatorenal syndrome). Renal involvement in liver disease has to be identified at the earliest and treated appropriately as progressive renal failure in liver disease is an adverse prognostic factor [102].

Hepatorenal Syndrome

HRS is a progressive, reversible functional renal impairment that occurs in patients with advanced liver cirrhosis or those with fulminant hepatic failure. Diagnostic criteria of HRS are outlined in Table 71.4. Type 1 HRS is characterized by rapid progression of renal failure and has a precipitating factor in most cases. It is associated with rapidly declining urine output and increasing creatinine in less than 2 weeks duration. Type 1 HRS occurs in the setting of an acute deterioration of circulatory function (arterial hypotension and activation of the endogenous vasoconstrictor systems) and is frequently associated with rapid impairment in liver function and encephalopathy, carrying a poor prognosis. Type 2 HRS is characterized by a moderate renal failure, which follows a steady or slowly progressive course. It appears spontaneously in most cases and frequently associated with refractory ascites.

Pathophysiology

The hallmark of HRS is renal vasoconstriction, which progresses with worsening liver disease. The renal cortical

Table 71.4 Six major criteria, all of which are necessary for the diagnosis of hepatorenal syndrome and five additional criteria, which are usually associated with hepatorenal syndrome but are not required for diagnosis

Diagnostic criteria for hepatorenal syndrome
The six major criteria are as follows:
1. Presence of cirrhosis and ascites
2. Serum creatinine > 1.5 mg/dL (133 μmol/L) or 24-h creatinine clearance of less than 40 mL/min
3. No improvement of serum creatinine (creatinine level £ 1.5 mg/dL or clearance > 40 mL/min) after at least 48 h of diuretic withdrawal and volume expansion with albumin
4. Absence of shock, ongoing bacterial infection, fluid loss, or current or recent treatment with nephrotoxic medications
5. Absence of parenchymal kidney disease as indicated by proteinuria > 500 mg/day,
6. Absence of any evidence of obstructive uropathy on renal ultrasound scanning
The five additional criteria are as follows:
Urine volume of less than 500 mL/d
Urine sodium concentration of less than 10 mEq/L
Urine osmolality greater than plasma osmolality
Urine RBC count of less than 50 per high-power field
Serum sodium concentration of less than 130 mEq/L

[a] As defined by the International Ascites Club

blood flow has been documented to be reduced in HRS using selective renal arteriography and xenon-113 studies, but the underlying mechanisms involved in HRS are incompletely understood [103, 104]. Four pathways have been implicated in the pathophysiology of HRS.

1. Peripheral and splanchnic vasodilation secondary to increased production of vasdilatory amines in the leading on to activation of renin angiotensin system in the kidneys, thereby reducing urine output.
2. Sympathetic nervous system activation leading to possible hepatorenal reflex.
3. Cardiac dysfunction contributing to renal hypoperfusion.
4. Action of cytokines and vasoactive mediators on renal circulation leading to the loss of renal autoregulation mechanisms may also play a role in the development of HRS.

Clinical presentation: The incidence of HRS in patients with cirrhosis and ascites is 20 % in the 1st year and 39 % within 5 years. The rapidity and severity of renal failure at presentation depend on the type of HRS. Type 1 HRS is preceded by a precipitating factor in 70 % of cases. The most common precipitating events are spontaneous bacterial peritonitis, large volume paracentesis without volume replacement, gastrointestinal hemorrhage, and sepsis. These patients have many of the features present with advanced liver disease, in addition to renal dysfunction. These patients may also have underlying ascites, which are refractory to diuretic therapy. The findings in acute azotemia in patients with liver disease are given in Table 71.5.

Management

There is no proven effective therapy for HRS except liver transplantation. The general principles include treating precipitating factors and avoiding agents and factors, which can precipitate HRS. In cases of tense ascites, abdominal paracentesis done in conjunction with albumin replacement to avoid circulatory dysfunction has been proved to be safe [105]. Systemic vasoconstrictors include vasopressin analogues (terlipressin and ornipressin), somatostatin analogue (octreotide), and alpha-adrenergic agonists (midodrine and norepinephrine) are helpful in managing HRS. Studies have shown in adults that terlipressin when used alone or with albumin has higher efficacy in reversing the renal function in patients with HRS [106].

Portosystemic shunts such as TIPSS placement in adults have been shown to improve renal function. The mechanism by which TIPSS exerts this effect is still speculative but could be the result of reduction of portal pressure, suppression of a putative hepatorenal reflex, improvement of the circulating volume, or amelioration of cardiac function. Renal replacement therapy is indicated for those who failed to respond to vasoconstrictors, TIPSS, intractable metabolic acidosis, hyperkalemia, volume overload, and those who are waiting for a liver transplant.

Liver transplantation is the definitive treatment for patients with HRS, as it corrects liver dysfunction and eliminates PHT [30, 107]. Shusterman et al. showed that in 77 % of those with HRS, serum creatinine levels decreased to less

Table 71.5 Features to differentiate prerenal azotemia, acute tubular necrosis, and hepatorenal syndrome

Differentiating hepatorenal syndrome from other causes of renal failure			
	Hepatorenal syndrome	Prerenal azotemia	Acute tubular necrosis
Urinary sodium concentration	< 10 mEq/L	< 10 mEq/L	< 10 mEq/L
Urine plasma creatinine	> 30:1	> 30:1	< 20:1
Urine osmolality	> Plasma osmolality	> Plasma osmolality	Equal to plasma osmolality
Fractional excretion of sodium	< 1 %	< 1 %	> 2 %
Urinary sediment	Normal	Normal	Casts, debris
Response to volume expansion	Brief or No diuresis	Sustained diuresis	No diuresis

than 1.5 mg/dL after liver transplantation, and at 3 months post liver transplantation, none of the patients required dialysis [30, 107].

Other System Involvement in Cirrhosis

Pruritus is one of the most debilitating complications of CLD that affects the quality of life. Grading of pruritus and medical management is outlined in Table 71.6. Severe pruritus that does not respond to medical management per se is an indication for liver transplantation. Cardiac dysfunction in CLD is a discrete phenomenon called as cirrhotic cardiomyopathy, and it is associated with all or some of following changes: (1) baseline increased cardiac output but blunted ventricular response to stimuli, (2) systolic and/or diastolic dysfunction, (3) the absence of overt left ventricular failure at rest, and (4) electrophysiological abnormalities including prolonged QT interval on electrocardiography and chronotropic incompetence [108]. Altered cardiac muscle membrane properties, impairment of stimulatory β-adrenergic receptor signaling pathways, and over active negative-inotropic factors are some of the factors implicated in pathogenesis of cirrhotic cardiomyopathy [109]. In a cohort of 40 children with median age of 8 months awaiting liver transplantation, Desai et al. showed that 27 (74%) had cirrhotic cardiomyopathy [110]. Liver transplantation remains the only curative therapy in most of the patients [110].

Increased caloric needs, decreased absorption due to cholestasis, and poor appetite contribute to undernutrition in CLD. Bone disease with both the components of osteoporosis and osteomalacia in CLD is termed as hepatic osteodystrophy (HO) [111]. The pathogenesis of HO is considered to be multifactorial due to complex interaction of IGF-1 deficiency, vitamin D and K deficiency, hypogonadism, etc., on growth and differentiation of bones in the back ground of hyperbilirubinemia [112]. The reported prevalence of fractures due to HO in children is around 10–13% [112]. Regular bone mineral density by dual-energy X-ray absorptiometry scan (DEXA) and monitoring serum 25-hydroxy vitamin D (25OHD) levels help in early detection and treatment of deficiency states. Routine supplementation of vitamin D at a dose of 3–10 times the recommended daily allowance has been suggested [60]. The recommended form of vitamin D for both prophylaxis and treatment is either ergocalciferol (vitamin D2) or cholecalciferol (vitamin D3) targeting a 25OHD level of more than 50 nmol/L. Bisphosphonate therapy is indicated only in the presence of low-impact fractures (≥ 1 vertebral, or ≥ 1 lower limb, or ≥ 2 upper limb) along with low bone mineral density (BMD) [113].

Prognosis

MELD is a scoring system developed to predict death within 3 months of surgery in patients who had undergone a TIPSS procedure and was subsequently found to be useful in determining prognosis in patients with CLD due to other etiologies. MELD is calculated using serum bilirubin, sreum creatinine, and international normalized ratio (INR). A value of 40 or more is associated with 71% mortality in 3 months, while a value of less than nine is associated mere 1.9% mortality. MELD is used in US and European counties in prioritizing CLD patients for liver transplantation. In children under 12 years of age, pediatric end-stage liver disease (PELD) score is used for prognostication where age less than 1 year and growth failure are also taken into consideration. Though many countries use PELD to prioritize children in waiting list, it has its own limitations. PELD score does not take into consideration complications such as cholangitis, severe PHT, pulmonary hypertension, and HPS and could underestimate the risk of death [17].

Conclusions

Cirrhosis secondarily affects nearly every system in the body, where the correlation might or might not be proportional to the severity of liver disease. Apart from managing complications of cirrhosis, it is essential to take care of general well-being of these children such as growth monitoring, immunization, vitamin supplementation, and their education. Though the functionality of end organs (brain, kidney, lungs, etc.) could revert back to normal or near normal after liver transplantation, advanced end organ damage might render a patient unfit to undergo liver transplantation. Anticipation of the complication and timely intervention would help in better outcome in these children.

Table 71.6 Though grading is very subjective, it helps in comparing the symptomatic improvement to therapy

Grading and medical management of pruritus
Grade 1: no pruritus
Grade 2: mild scratching, but can be distracted
Grade 3: active scratching without abrasion
Grade 4: active scratching with abrasions
Grade 5: taneous mutilation with bleeding/scarring
Ursodeoxycholic acid (10 mg/kg twice a day)
Rifampicin (4–10 mg/kg/day)
Phenobarbitone (15–45 mg/day)
Naltrexone (0.1–0.5 mg/kg)
Ondansetron (0.1 mg/kg/three times a day to max 4 mg/dose)
Cholestyramine (1/3 to 1 sachet three times a day)

References

1. Kuntz K. Clinical aspects of liver diseases. In: Kuntz K, editor. Hepatology: textbook and atlas. 3rd ed. Germany: Springer-Verlag; 2008. p. 397–417.
2. Bataller R, Brenner DA. Liver fibrosis. J Clin Invest. 2005;115 (2):209–18.
3. Gressner AM, Weiskirchen R, Breitkopf K, Dooley S. Roles of TGF-beta in hepatic fibrosis. Front Biosci. 2002;7:d793–807.
4. Kinnman N, Housset C. Peribiliary myofibroblasts in biliary type liver fibrosis. Front Biosci. 2002;7:d496–503.
5. Kinnman N, Francoz C, Barbu V, Wendum D, Rey C, Hultcrantz R, et al. The myofibroblastic conversion of peribiliary fibrogenic cells distinct from hepatic stellate cells is stimulated by platelet-derived growth factor during liver fibrogenesis. Lab Invest. 2003;83(2):163–73.
6. Wallace K, Burt AD, Wright MC. Liver fibrosis. Biochem J. 2008 Apr 1;411(1):1–18.
7. Parola M, Pinzani M. Hepatic wound repair. Fibrogenesis Tissue Repair. 2009;2(1):4.
8. Yang L, Chang N, Liu X, Han Z, Zhu T, Li C, et al. Bone marrow-derived mesenchymal stem cells differentiate to hepatic myofibroblasts by transforming growth factor-beta1 via sphingosine kinase/sphingosine 1-phosphate (S1P)/S1P receptor axis. Am J Pathol. 2012;181(1):85–97.
9. Ahmad A, Ahmad R. Understanding the mechanism of hepatic fibrosis and potential therapeutic approaches. Saudi J Gastroenterol. 2012;18(3):155–67.
10. Fallowfield J, Hayes P. Pathogenesis and treatment of hepatic fibrosis: is cirrhosis reversible? Clin Med. 2011;11(2):179–83.
11. Lee CK, Perez-Atayde AR, Mitchell PD, Raza R, Afdhal NH, Jonas MM. Serum biomarkers and transient elastography as predictors of advanced liver fibrosis in a United States cohort: the Boston children's hospital experience. J Pediatr. 2013;163(4):1058–64 e2.
12. Goldschmidt I, Streckenbach C, Dingemann C, Pfister ED, di Nanni A, Zapf A, et al. Application and limitations of transient liver elastography in children. J Pediatr Gastroenterol Nutr. 2013;57(1):109–13.
13. Zhang JX, Pegoli W, Jr, Clemens MG. Endothelin-1 induces direct constriction of hepatic sinusoids. Am J Physiol. 1994;266(4 Pt 1):G624–32.
14. Moller S, Gulberg V, Henriksen JH, Gerbes AL. Endothelin-1 and endothelin-3 in cirrhosis: relations to systemic and splanchnic haemodynamics. J Hepatol. 1995;23(2):135–44.
15. Rodriguez-Vilarrupla A, Fernandez M, Bosch J, Garcia-Pagan JC. Current concepts on the pathophysiology of portal hypertension. Ann Hepatol. 2007;6(1):28–36.
16. Gupta TK, Toruner M, Chung MK, Groszmann RJ. Endothelial dysfunction and decreased production of nitric oxide in the intrahepatic microcirculation of cirrhotic rats. Hepatology. 1998;28(4):926–31.
17. Shneider BL, Neimark E, Frankenberg T, Arnott L, Suchy FJ, Emre S. Critical analysis of the pediatric end-stage liver disease scoring system: a single center experience. Liver Transpl. 2005;11(7):788–95.
18. Miga D, Sokol RJ, Mackenzie T, Narkewicz MR, Smith D, Karrer FM. Survival after first esophageal variceal hemorrhage in patients with biliary atresia. J Pediatr. 2001;139(2):291–6.
19. Ling SC, Walters T, McKiernan PJ, Schwarz KB, Garcia-Tsao G, Shneider BL. Primary prophylaxis of variceal hemorrhage in children with portal hypertension: a framework for future research. J Pediatr Gastroenterol Nutr. 2011;52(3):254–61.
20. Hussain MJ, Peakman M, Gallati H, Lo SS, Hawa M, Viberti GC, et al. Elevated serum levels of macrophage-derived cytokines precede and accompany the onset of IDDM. Diabetologia. 1996;39(1):60–9.
21. Sarin SK, Nundy S. Balloon tamponade in the management of bleeding oesophageal varices. Ann R Coll Surg Engl. 1984;66(1):30–2.
22. Soderlund C, Ihre T. Endoscopic sclerotherapy v. conservative management of bleeding oesophageal varices. A 5-year prospective controlled trial of emergency and long-term treatment. Acta Chir Scand. 1985;151(5):449–56.
23. Sarin SK, Govil A, Jain AK, Guptan RC, Issar SK, Jain M, et al. Prospective randomized trial of endoscopic sclerotherapy versus variceal band ligation for esophageal varices: influence on gastropathy, gastric varices and variceal recurrence. J Hepatol. 1997;26(4):826–32.
24. Banares R, Albillos A, Rincon D, Alonso S, Gonzalez M, Ruiz-del-Arbol L, et al. Endoscopic treatment versus endoscopic plus pharmacologic treatment for acute variceal bleeding: a meta-analysis. Hepatology. 2002;35(3):609–15.
25. Rezende-Neto JB, Petroianu A, Santana SK. Subtotal splenectomy and central splenorenal shunt for treatment of bleeding from Roux en Y jejunal loop varices secondary to portal hypertension. Dig Dis Sci. 2008;53(2):539–43.
26. Garcia-Tsao G, Sanyal AJ, Grace ND, Carey W. Prevention and management of gastroesophageal varices and variceal hemorrhage in cirrhosis. Hepatology. 2007;46(3):922–38.
27. Shashidhar H, Langhans N, Grand RJ. Propranolol in prevention of portal hypertensive hemorrhage in children: a pilot study. J Pediatr Gastroenterol Nutr. 1999;29(1):12–7.
28. Goncalves ME, Cardoso SR, Maksoud JG. Prophylactic sclerotherapy in children with esophageal varices: long-term results of a controlled prospective randomized trial. J Pediatr Surg. 2000;35(3):401–5.
29. Kang KS, Yang HR, Ko JS, Seo JK. Long-term outcomes of endoscopic variceal ligation to prevent rebleeding in children with esophageal varices. J Korean Med Sci. 2013;28(11):1657–60.
30. Mileti E, Rosenthal P. Management of portal hypertension in children. Curr Gastroenterol Rep. 2011;13(1):10–6.
31. Iwasa M, Matsumura K, Kaito M, Ikoma J, Kobayashi Y, Nakagawa N, et al. Decrease of regional cerebral blood flow in liver cirrhosis. Eur J Gastroenterol Hepatol. 2000;12(9):1001–6.
32. Cash WJ, McConville P, McDermott E, McCormick PA, Callender ME, McDougall NI. Current concepts in the assessment and treatment of hepatic encephalopathy. QJM. 2010;103(1):9–16.
33. Ferenci P, Lockwood A, Mullen K, Tarter R, Weissenborn K, Blei AT. Hepatic encephalopathy–definition, nomenclature, diagnosis, and quantification: final report of the working party at the 11th world congresses of gastroenterology, Vienna, 1998. Hepatology. 2002;35(3):716–21.
34. Jones EA, Weissenborn K. Neurology and the liver. J Neurol Neurosurg Psychiatry. 1997;63(3):279–93.
35. Frederick RT. Current concepts in the pathophysiology and management of hepatic encephalopathy. Gastroenterol Hepatol (N Y). 2011;7(4):222–33.
36. Romero-Gomez M, Jover M, Galan JJ, Ruiz A. Gut ammonia production and its modulation. Metab Brain Dis. 2009;24(1):147–57.
37. Merli M, Giusto M, Lucidi C, Giannelli V, Pentassuglio I, Di Gregorio V, et al. Muscle depletion increases the risk of overt and minimal hepatic encephalopathy: results of a prospective study. Metab Brain Dis. 2013;28(2):281–4.
38. Dejong CH, van de Poll MC, Soeters PB, Jalan R, Olde Damink SW. Aromatic amino acid metabolism during liver failure. J Nutr. 2007;137(6 Suppl 1):1579S–85S; discussion 97S–98S.
39. Fischer JE, Rosen HM, Ebeid AM, James JH, Keane JM, Soeters PB. The effect of normalization of plasma amino acids on hepatic encephalopathy in man. Surgery. 1976;80(1):77–91.
40. Skowronska M, Albrecht J. Alterations of blood brain barrier function in hyperammonemia: an overview. Neurotox Res. 2012;21(2):236–44.

41. Mortensen PB, Holtug K, Bonnen H, Clausen MR. The degradation of amino acids, proteins, and blood to short-chain fatty acids in colon is prevented by lactulose. Gastroenterology. 1990;98(2):353–60.

42. Boudjema K, Bachellier P, Wolf P, Tempe JD, Jaeck D. Auxiliary liver transplantation and bioartificial bridging procedures in treatment of acute liver failure. World J Surg. 2002;26(2):264–74.

43. Ahboucha S, Layrargues GP, Mamer O, Butterworth RF. Increased brain concentrations of a neuroinhibitory steroid in human hepatic encephalopathy. Ann Neurol. 2005;58(1):169–70.

44. Baraldi M, Avallone R, Corsi L, Venturini I, Baraldi C, Zeneroli ML. Natural endogenous ligands for benzodiazepine receptors in hepatic encephalopathy. Metab Brain Dis. 2009;24(1):81–93.

45. Riggio O, Mannaioni G, Ridola L, Angeloni S, Merli M, Carla V, et al. Peripheral and splanchnic indole and oxindole levels in cirrhotic patients: a study on the pathophysiology of hepatic encephalopathy. Am J Gastroenterol. 2010;105(6):1374–81.

46. Odeh M, Sabo E, Srugo I, Oliven A. Serum levels of tumor necrosis factor-alpha correlate with severity of hepatic encephalopathy due to chronic liver failure. Liver Int. 2004;24(2):110–6.

47. Quero Guillen JC, Herrerias Gutierrez JM. Diagnostic methods in hepatic encephalopathy. Clin Chim Acta. 2006;365(1–2):1–8.

48. Dhiman RK, Saraswat VA, Sharma BK, Sarin SK, Chawla YK, Butterworth R, et al. Minimal hepatic encephalopathy: consensus statement of a working party of the Indian National Association for Study of the Liver. J Gastroenterol Hepatol. 2010;25(6):1029–41.

49. Govindarajan S, Nast CC, Smith WL, Koyle MA, Daskalopoulos G, Zipser RD. Immunohistochemical distribution of renal prostaglandin endoperoxide synthase and prostacyclin synthase: diminished endoperoxide synthase in the hepatorenal syndrome. Hepatology. 1987;7(4):654–9.

50. Kircheis G, Wettstein M, Timmermann L, Schnitzler A, Haussinger D. Critical flicker frequency for quantification of low-grade hepatic encephalopathy. Hepatology. 2002;35(2):357–66.

51. Yadav SK, Srivastava A, Thomas MA, Agarwal J, Pandey CM, Lal R, et al. Encephalopathy assessment in children with extra-hepatic portal vein obstruction with MR, psychometry and critical flicker frequency. J Hepatol. 52(3):348–54.

52. Barbe T, Losay J, Grimon G, Devictor D, Sardet A, Gauthier F, et al. Pulmonary arteriovenous shunting in children with liver disease. J Pediatr. 1995;126(4):571–9.

53. Edwards BS, Weir EK, Edwards WD, Ludwig J, Dykoski RK, Edwards JE. Coexistent pulmonary and portal hypertension: morphologic and clinical features. J Am Coll Cardiol. 1987;10(6):1233–8.

54. Arya R, Gulati S, Deopujari S. Management of hepatic encephalopathy in children. Postgrad Med J. 2010;86(1011):34–41; quiz 0.

55. Ito Y, Moriwaki H, Muto Y, Kato N, Watanabe K, Ueno K. Effect of lactulose on short-chain fatty acids and lactate production and on the growth of faecal flora, with special reference to Clostridium difficile. J Med Microbiol. 1997;46(1):80–4.

56. Holecek M. Three targets of branched-chain amino acid supplementation in the treatment of liver disease. Nutrition. 2010;26(5):482–90.

57. Patil DH, Westaby D, Mahida YR, Palmer KR, Rees R, Clark ML, et al. Comparative modes of action of lactitol and lactulose in the treatment of hepatic encephalopathy. Gut. 1987;28(3):255–9.

58. Festi D, Vestito A, Mazzella G, Roda E, Colecchia A. Management of hepatic encephalopathy: focus on antibiotic therapy. Digestion. 2006;73 Suppl 1:94–101.

59. Gluud LL, Dam G, Borre M, Les I, Cordoba J, Marchesini G, et al. Lactulose, rifaximin or branched chain amino acids for hepatic encephalopathy: what is the evidence? Metab Brain Dis. 2013;28(2):221–5.

60. McGee RG, Bakens A, Wiley K, Riordan SM, Webster AC. Probiotics for patients with hepatic encephalopathy. Cochrane Database Syst Rev. 2011; (11):CD008716.

61. Al Sibae MR, McGuire BM. Current trends in the treatment of hepatic encephalopathy. Ther Clin Risk Manag. 2009;5(3):617–26.

62. Pugliese R, Fonseca EA, Porta G, Danesi V, Guimaraes T, Porta A, et al. Ascites and serum sodium are markers of increased waiting list mortality in children with chronic liver failure. Hepatology. 2014;59(5):1964–71.

63. Schrier RW, Arroyo V, Bernardi M, Epstein M, Henriksen JH, Rodes J. Peripheral arterial vasodilation hypothesis: a proposal for the initiation of renal sodium and water retention in cirrhosis. Hepatology. 1988;8(5):1151–7.

64. Pal S, Mangla V, Radhakrishna P, Sahni P, Pande GK, Acharya SK, et al. Surgery as primary prophylaxis from variceal bleeding in patients with extrahepatic portal venous obstruction. J Gastroenterol Hepatol. 2013;28(6):1010–4.

65. Arroyo V, Gines P, Gerbes AL, Dudley FJ, Gentilini P, Laffi G, et al. Definition and diagnostic criteria of refractory ascites and hepatorenal syndrome in cirrhosis. International Ascites Club. Hepatology. 1996;23(1):164–76.

66. Arroyo V. Pathophysiology, diagnosis and treatment of ascites in cirrhosis. Ann Hepatol. 2002;1(2):72–9.

67. Runyon BA, Montano AA, Akriviadis EA, Antillon MR, Irving MA, McHutchison JG. The serum-ascites albumin gradient is superior to the exudate-transudate concept in the differential diagnosis of ascites. Ann Intern Med. 1992;117(3):215–20.

68. Runyon BA. Introduction to the revised american association for the study of liver diseases practice guideline management of adult patients with ascites due to cirrhosis 2012. Hepatology. 2013;57(4):1651–3.

69. Kramer RE, Sokol RJ, Yerushalmi B, Liu E, MacKenzie T, Hoffenberg EJ, et al. Large-volume paracentesis in the management of ascites in children. J Pediatr Gastroenterol Nutr. 2001;33(3):245–9.

70. Abrams GA, Nanda NC, Dubovsky EV, Krowka MJ, Fallon MB. Use of macroaggregated albumin lung perfusion scan to diagnose hepatopulmonary syndrome: a new approach. Gastroenterology. 1998;114(2):305–10.

71. Sasaki T, Hasegawa T, Kimura T, Okada A, Mushiake S, Matsushita T. Development of intrapulmonary arteriovenous shunting in postoperative biliary atresia: evaluation by contrast-enhanced echocardiography. J Pediatr Surg. 2000;35(11):1647–50.

72. Noli K, Solomon M, Golding F, Charron M, Ling SC. Prevalence of hepatopulmonary syndrome in children. Pediatrics. 2008;121(3):e522–7.

73. Gupta D, Vijaya DR, Gupta R, Dhiman RK, Bhargava M, Verma J, et al. Prevalence of hepatopulmonary syndrome in cirrhosis and extrahepatic portal venous obstruction. Am J Gastroenterol. 2001;96(12):3395–9.

74. Fallon MB, Abrams GA, McGrath JW, Hou Z, Luo B. Common bile duct ligation in the rat: a model of intrapulmonary vasodilatation and hepatopulmonary syndrome. Am J Physiol. 1997;272(4 Pt 1):G779–84.

75. Wang YW, Lin HC. Recent advances in hepatopulmonary syndrome. J Chin Med Assoc. 2005;68(11):500–5.

76. Zhang HY, Han DW, Wang XG, Zhao YC, Zhou X, Zhao HZ. Experimental study on the role of endotoxin in the development of hepatopulmonary syndrome. World J Gastroenterol. 2005;11(4):567–72.

77. Sztrymf B, Rabiller A, Nunes H, Savale L, Lebrec D, Le Pape A, et al. Prevention of hepatopulmonary syndrome and hyperdynamic state by pentoxifylline in cirrhotic rats. Eur Respir J. 2004;23(5):752–8.

78. Sztrymf B, Libert JM, Mougeot C, Lebrec D, Mazmanian M, Humbert M, et al. Cirrhotic rats with bacterial translocation have higher incidence and severity of hepatopulmonary syndrome. J Gastroenterol Hepatol. 2005;20(10):1538–44.

79. Gomez FP, Martinez-Palli G, Barbera JA, Roca J, Navasa M, Rodriguez-Roisin R. Gas exchange mechanism of orthodeoxia in hepatopulmonary syndrome. Hepatology. 2004;40(3):660–6.

80. Dickinson CJ. The aetiology of clubbing and hypertrophic osteoarthropathy. Eur J Clin Invest. 1993;23(6):330–8.

81. Alves L, Sant'Anna CC, March Mde F, Ferreira S, Marsillac M, Tura M, et al. Preoperative pulmonary assessment of children for liver transplantation. Pediatr Transplant. 2008;12(5):536–40.

82. El-Shabrawi MH, Omran S, Wageeh S, Isa M, Okasha S, Mohsen NA, et al. (99m)Technetium-macroaggregated albumin perfusion lung scan versus contrast enhanced echocardiography in the diagnosis of the hepatopulmonary syndrome in children with chronic liver disease. Eur J Gastroenterol Hepatol. 2010;22(8):1006–12.

83. Lee KN, Lee HJ, Shin WW, Webb WR. Hypoxemia and liver cirrhosis (hepatopulmonary syndrome) in eight patients: comparison of the central and peripheral pulmonary vasculature. Radiology. 1999;211(2):549–53.

84. Kuntz E, Kuntz HD. Hepatopulmonary syndrome. In Kuntz E, Kuntz HD, editor. Hepatology textbook and atlas. 3rd ed. Heidelberg: Springer; 2008. p. 340–5.

85. Schenk P, Fuhrmann V, Madl C, Funk G, Lehr S, Kandel O, et al. Hepatopulmonary syndrome: prevalence and predictive value of various cut offs for arterial oxygenation and their clinical consequences. Gut. 2002;51(6):853–9.

86. Herve P, Lebrec D, Brenot F, Simonneau G, Humbert M, Sitbon O, et al. Pulmonary vascular disorders in portal hypertension. Eur Respir J. 1998;11(5):1153–66.

87. Varghese J, Ilias-basha H, Dhanasekaran R, Singh S, Venkataraman J. Hepatopulmonary syndrome—past to present. Ann Hepatol. 2007;6(3):135–42.

88. Martinez-Palli G, Drake BB, Garcia-Pagan JC, Barbera JA, Arguedas MR, Rodriguez-Roisin R, et al. Effect of transjugular intrahepatic portosystemic shunt on pulmonary gas exchange in patients with portal hypertension and hepatopulmonary syndrome. World J Gastroenterol. 2005;11(43):6858–62.

89. Alonso Martinez JL, Zozaya Urmeneta JM, Gutierrez Dubois J, Abinzano Guillen ML, Urbieta Echezarreta MA, Anniccherico Sanchez FJ. Prognostic significance of the hepatopulmonary syndrome in liver cirrhosis. Med Clin (Barc). 2006;127(4):133–5.

90. Schenk P, Schoniger-Hekele M, Fuhrmann V, Madl C, Silberhumer G, Muller C. Prognostic significance of the hepatopulmonary syndrome in patients with cirrhosis. Gastroenterology. 2003;125(4):1042–52.

91. Battaglia SE, Pretto JJ, Irving LB, Jones RM, Angus PW. Resolution of gas exchange abnormalities and intrapulmonary shunting following liver transplantation. Hepatology. 1997;25(5):1228–32.

92. Abrams GA, Rose K, Fallon MB, McGuire BM, Bloomer JR, van Leeuwen DJ, et al. Hepatopulmonary syndrome and venous emboli causing intracerebral hemorrhages after liver transplantation: a case report. Transplantation. 1999;68(11):1809–11.

93. Arguedas MR, Abrams GA, Krowka MJ, Fallon MB. Prospective evaluation of outcomes and predictors of mortality in patients with hepatopulmonary syndrome undergoing liver transplantation. Hepatology. 2003;37(1):192–7.

94. Hoeper MM, Krowka MJ, Strassburg CP. Portopulmonary hypertension and hepatopulmonary syndrome. Lancet. 2004;363(9419):1461–8.

95. Krowka MJ. Hepatopulmonary syndromes. Gut. 2000;46(1):1–4.

96. Budhiraja R, Hassoun PM. Portopulmonary hypertension: a tale of two circulations. Chest. 2003;123(2):562–76.

97. Robalino BD, Moodie DS. Association between primary pulmonary hypertension and portal hypertension: analysis of its pathophysiology and clinical, laboratory and hemodynamic manifestations. J Am Coll Cardiol. 1991;17(2):492–8.

98. McDonnell PJ, Toye PA, Hutchins GM. Primary pulmonary hypertension and cirrhosis: are they related? Am Rev Respir Dis. 1983;127(4):437–41.

99. Ivy DD, Feinstein JA, Humpl T, Rosenzweig EB. Non-congenital heart disease associated pediatric pulmonary arterial hypertension. Prog Pediatr Cardiol. 2009;27(1–2):13–23.

100. Talwalkar JA, Swanson KL, Krowka MJ, Andrews JC, Kamath PS. Prevalence of spontaneous portosystemic shunts in patients with portopulmonary hypertension and effect on treatment. Gastroenterology. 2011;141(5):1673–9.

101. Barst RJ, Ivy D, Dingemanse J, Widlitz A, Schmitt K, Doran A, et al. Pharmacokinetics, safety, and efficacy of bosentan in pediatric patients with pulmonary arterial hypertension. Clin Pharmacol Ther. 2003;73(4):372–82.

102. Eckardt KU. Renal failure in liver disease. Intensive Care Med. 1999;25(1):5–14.

103. Epstein M, Berk DP, Hollenberg NK, Adams DF, Chalmers TC, Abrams HL, et al. Renal failure in the patient with cirrhosis. The role of active vasoconstriction. Am J Med. 1970;49(2):175–85.

104. Kew MC, Brunt PW, Varma RR, Hourigan KJ, Williams HS, Sherlock S. Renal and intrarenal blood-flow in cirrhosis of the liver. Lancet. 1971;2(7723):504–10.

105. Simon DM, McCain JR, Bonkovsky HL, Wells JO, Hartle DK, Galambos JT. Effects of therapeutic paracentesis on systemic and hepatic hemodynamics and on renal and hormonal function. Hepatology. 1987;7(3):423–9.

106. Martin-Llahi M, Pepin MN, Guevara M, Diaz F, Torre A, Monescillo A, et al. Terlipressin and albumin vs albumin in patients with cirrhosis and hepatorenal syndrome: a randomized study. Gastroenterology. 2008;134(5):1352–9.

107. Shusterman B, McHedishvili G, Rosner MH. Outcomes for hepatorenal syndrome and acute kidney injury in patients undergoing liver transplantation: a single-center experience. Transplant Proc. 2007;39(5):1496–500.

108. Baik SK, Fouad TR, Lee SS. Cirrhotic cardiomyopathy. Orphanet J Rare Dis. 2007;2:15.

109. Liu H, Song D, Lee SS. Cirrhotic cardiomyopathy. Gastroenterol Clin Biol. 2002;26(10):842–7.

110. Desai MS, Zainuer S, Kennedy C, Kearney D, Goss J, Karpen SJ. Cardiac structural and functional alterations in infants and children with biliary atresia, listed for liver transplantation. Gastroenterology. 2011;141(4):1264–72, 72 e1–4.

111. Goel V, Kar P. Hepatic osteodystrophy. Trop Gastroenterol. 2010;31(2):82–6.

112. Hogler W, Baumann U, Kelly D. Growth and bone health in chronic liver disease and following liver transplantation in children. Pediatr Endocrinol Rev. 2010;7(3):266–74.

113. Hogler W, Baumann U, Kelly D. Endocrine and bone metabolic complications in chronic liver disease and after liver transplantation in children. J Pediatr Gastroenterol Nutr. 2012;54(3):313–21.

Nutritional Management of Children with Liver Disease

Sara Mancell and Deepa Kamat

Introduction

The liver is the key organ in the production and distribution of nutrients, playing a central role in glucose homeostasis, protein synthesis, bile salt production, lipid metabolism, and vitamin storage. Chronic liver disease can disrupt these processes leading to malnutrition. Malnutrition is highly prevalent in children with liver disease and is associated with increased morbidity and mortality [2]. Potential causes of malnutrition include insufficient nutrient intake, increased nutritional requirements, impaired nutrient absorption, and altered metabolism. Nutrition strategies in children with liver disease are centered on managing these factors while promoting normal growth and development. Maintaining optimal nutrition in children with chronic liver disease may prevent further liver damage and improve outcomes post transplant [1].

In acute liver disease, if the presentation is rapid, children may be well nourished initially. The aim is to preserve nutritional status and manage complications such as hypoglycemia and hyperammonemia.

The nutrition management of liver disease caused by inborn errors of metabolism does not form part of this chapter.

Nutritional Management of Chronic Liver Disease

Causes of Malnutrition

The following table outlines the mechanisms of malnutrition (see Table 72.1).

S. Mancell (✉) · D. Kamat
Nutrition and Dietetics Department, King's College Hospital NHS Foundation Trust, Ground Floor, Unit 6, KCH Business Park, Denmark Hill, London SE5 9RS, UK
e-mail: sara.mancell@nhs.net

Insufficient Nutrient Intake

Poor intake of nutrients may be due to nausea and vomiting, pruritis, taste changes associated with medications, unpalatable feeds, reduced gastric capacity, and discomfort due to ascites and organomegaly. With ascites, some degree of fluid and sodium restriction is usually required, and this can further reduce oral intake. In the hospital environment, intake may be affected by investigations or procedures or unpalatable hospital meals. There is some evidence that anorexia may be due to increased tumor necrosis factor or leptin [3].

Malabsorption

Malabsorption may be due to reduced bile flow, pancreatic enzyme deficiency, or mucosal edema. The result can be faltering growth and fat-soluble vitamin deficiency. Long-chain triglycerides (LCT) require emulsification by bile in the intestine, and therefore, the absence or reduction of bile flow leads to fat malabsorption. In some types of liver disease such as Alagille's syndrome, malabsorption may also be due to pancreatic enzyme insufficiency [4]. Finally, inflammation and mucosal edema in the small bowel due to portal hypertension may cause protein malabsorption [5].

Altered Metabolism

As liver failure progresses, the metabolism of carbohydrate, protein, and fat may be altered. There is a reduction in glycogen storage and an increased breakdown of fat and protein to meet energy demands alongside inefficient use of the substrates which are available [6]. The result is wasting of fat and lean body mass, hypoglycemia, hypoproteinemia, and hyperammonemia [7].

Increased Energy Expenditure

Children with end-stage liver disease have been shown to have a resting energy expenditure almost 30 % higher than controls [8, 9]. Increased requirements may be due to inefficient energy production due to altered metabolism, catabolic stresses such as infection or increased respiratory effort from ascites or organomegaly [6]. Greer et al. [9] suggest

Table 72.1 Causes of malnutrition

Causes of malnutrition	Contributing factors
Decreased nutrient intake	Nausea and vomiting
	Pruritis
	Taste changes
	Unpalatable diets/specialist feeds
	Reduced gastric capacity and discomfort from ascites or organomegaly
	Fluid and sodium restriction due to ascites
	Investigations and procedures interrupting meals or feeds
	Anorexia
Malabsorption	Absence or reduction of bile flow
	Pancreatic insufficiency
	Mucosal edema due to portal hypertension
Altered metabolism	Reduced glycogen storage
	Impaired gluconeogenesis
	Increased fat and protein oxidation
Increased energy expenditure	Stress factors such as infection
	Increased respiratory effort from ascites or organomegaly
	Increased metabolically active cells mass

that increased requirements may also be due to differences in body composition, with children with end-stage liver disease having less body fat and a higher relative proportion of metabolically active cells.

Management

Insufficient Nutrient Intake

Feeding strategies should take into account the often multifactorial causes of poor nutrient intake. When oral intake is significantly reduced because of persistent nausea or vomiting or the discomfort of pruritis or unpalatable feeds, supplemental tube feeding may be required. This can be given during the day as bolus feeds and/or as a continuous overnight infusion. Where there is ascites or organomegaly, high-energy, low-volume feeds may help with the problem of reduced gastric capacity. With ascites, a rigid sodium restriction is not recommended, but rather a general reduction is salty foods. In hospital, extended periods of nil by mouth and feeding interruptions due to investigations and procedures should be kept to a minimum, and every effort should be made to make meal times enjoyable.

Malabsorption

Where there is fat malabsorption, an energy dense diet is given combined with medium-chain triglyceride (MCT) supplementation. MCTs do not require emulsification with bile, diffusing easily into the intestinal cells, where they are absorbed directly into the bloodstream. There is little evidence regarding how much dietary fat should be MCT. MCTs are not a source of essential fatty acids (EFAs), and as the percentage of MCT increases it is more difficult to meet

requirements for EFAs. The European Society for Gastroenterology, Hepatology and Nutrition (ESPGHAN) guidelines are that infant formula should contain 4.5–10.8% energy as linoleic acid, and the ratio of alpha-linoleic:linolenic should be 5–15:1 [10]. The majority of feeds which are currently available in the UK provide approximately 50 % of the fat as MCT and meet requirements for EFAs (refer to Table 72.2). If an MCT feed with a particularly high MCT content, for example, Emsogen®, is used for a prolonged period of time, supplementing with a source of EFAs is warranted, for example, walnut oil supplemented at 1 ml/100 kcal. In cases where mucosal edema due to portal hypertension may be contributing to malabsorption, it may also be beneficial to give hydrolyzed protein to maximize absorption. Where there is a low stool elastase indicating pancreatic insufficiency, supplementation with pancreatic enzymes may be beneficial.

Altered Metabolism

Dietary strategies are centered on trying to preserve lean body mass, avoid hypoglycemia, and minimize hyperammonemia.

Preserving Lean Body Mass

To minimize catabolism, periods of fasting should be reduced so that an exogenous supply of nutrients is used in preference to body fat and muscle stores. This can be achieved by giving feeds or meals more frequently or using a feeding pump for continuous feeding. Studies have shown that supplementation with branched-chain amino acids (valine, leucine, and isoleucine) may help to improve nutritional status in liver disease [11]. As branched-chain amino acids are metabolized extrahepatically, they continue to be available for protein synthesis and as an energy substrate in liver fail-

Table 72.2 Specialist MCT-rich formulas and feeds

Feed per 100 ml	Age	Standard dilution (%)	Energy (kcal)	Protein (g)	Na (mmol)	MCT (%)	Supplemented with BCAA	% E linoleic	n-6:n-3 ratio
Heparon Junior®	From birth	18	86.4	2	0.56	49	Yes	8.2	6.8–1
Pepti Junior®	From birth	12.8	66	1.8	0.78	50	No	4.31	5:1
Pregestimil®	From birth	13.5	68	1.9	1.26	54	No	6.84	8:1
Monogen®	From birth	17.5	74	2	1.5	80	No	1.1	6.2:1
Infatrini Peptisorb®	From birth to 18 months	n/a	100	2.6	1.4	50	No	3.8	4.2:1
Peptamen Junior®	1–10 years	22	100	3	2.9	60	No	4.67	8.29:1
Paediasure Peptide®	1–6 years	n/a	100	3	3.04	50	No	3.51	2.3:1
Nutrini Peptisorb®	1–6 years	n/a	100	2.8	2.6	46	No	9.1	10.9:1
Nutrison MCT®	>6 years	n/a	100	5	4.3	60	No	2.5	5.4:1

MCT medium-chain triglyceride, *BCAA* branched-chain amino acids

ure. This may help to preserve muscle and fat mass. Mager et al. [12] showed that there is an increased requirement for BCAA even in children with relatively mild liver disease.

Avoiding Hypoglycemia

In addition to the above strategies, it may be necessary to increase the carbohydrate content of the feed to maintain blood sugars. This can be done by increasing the concentration of powdered formulas, using a high-energy feed or adding glucose polymers (refer to section "Achieving Increased Nutritional Requirements"). In older children, the inclusion of starchy carbohydrates and bedtime snacks may be necessary. Intravenous dextrose and close monitoring of blood sugars may be required, especially during periods of fasting or illness.

Managing Hyperammonemia

A major site of ammonia production is the large intestine, where protein is broken down by bacteria to produce ammonia. Ammonia is converted to urea in the liver, which is then excreted by the kidneys. In liver failure, this process is disrupted resulting in accumulation of ammonia in the blood. Exposure of brain tissue to toxic levels of ammonia leads to hepatic encephalopathy. A dietary protein restriction (2 g/kg protein) is often used initially as a way of reducing ammonia production in the gut [13]. A prolonged protein restriction is counterproductive as this leads to increased muscle breakdown, the by-product of which is ammonia [13, 14]. Furthermore, a severe protein restriction can worsen malnutrition in a group of patients whose baseline protein requirements are already higher than normal [15–17]. A randomized controlled trial comparing protein-restricted diets to normal protein diets in a small group of adults found no difference in the course of encephalopathy between the two groups [18]. The main difference was increased muscle breakdown in the protein-restricted group. For these reasons, a protein restriction may be used initially but is not recommended long term as it may worsen encephalopathy and nutritional status [19].

Increased Energy Expenditure

Due to increased resting energy expenditure and nutrient malabsorption, energy and protein requirements for children with chronic liver disease are generally well above the estimated average requirement (EAR). Table 72.3 shows that children may need up to 160 % of the EAR for energy and between 3 and 4 g/kg protein for adequate growth [15–17, 20, 21].

Estimations of energy and protein requirements are used only as a guide; requirements are calculated based on the individual, taking into account age, gender, nutritional status, disease state, and growth. Calculated requirements are not static and should be recalculated as part of monitoring procedures.

Achieving Increased Nutritional Requirements

In order to achieve nutritional requirements, it is usually necessary to increase the nutrient density of the diet. This can be done by increasing the concentration of powder-based feeds, supplementing the diet with high-energy sip or tube feeds, adding energy supplements to the diet, and increasing the nutrient density of meals and snacks.

Table 72.3 Energy and protein requirements for children with chronic liver disease [15–17, 20, 21]

	Infants	Older children
Energy	120–150 kcal/kg [15, 20]	120–160 % of the EAR for age [15, 17, 20, 21]
Protein	3–4 g/kg [15, 16]	3–4 g/kg [17]

Concentrating Feeds

To increase the nutrient density of a powder-based formula, the concentration can be increased beyond the standard recommended dilution, usually in 2 % increments. For example, the concentration of Heparon Junior® could be increased in two stages from 18 to 22 % which would increase the energy from 86.4 to 105.6 kcal/100 ml. Feeds should be concentrated cautiously given that as the concentration increases so too do all the micronutrients and macronutrients, the renal solute load, osmolality, and the risk of osmotic diarrhea. When concentrating feeds, explicit instructions should be provided to the carers to avoid errors when making up feeds.

Supplementation with High-Energy Sip or Tube Feeds

Nutrient dense feeds can be given orally or via feeding tube. Not all of the feeds provide complete nutrition; some supplements contain no fat (e.g., Fortijuce®) or incomplete micronutrients (e.g., Scandishake®) and should be given alongside a balanced diet. See Table 72.4 for examples of standard high-energy sip and tube feeds.

Energy Supplementation

The addition of nonprotein energy to the diet can affect the overall balance of a feed or meal. When adding energy, it is important to maintain a protein:energy ratio of between 7.5 and 12 % for infants and between 5 and 15 % for older chil-

dren [22]. Energy can be added in the form of glucose polymers, fats, or a combination of the two (refer to Table 72.5). These supplements are usually added in 1 % increments and increased daily depending on tolerance. As a guide, the total carbohydrate concentrations recommended are 10–15 % for infants and up to 30 % in older children. For fat, recommendations are 5–6 % for infants and 7 % for older children [22].

Increasing the Nutrient Density of Meals and Snacks

In order to increase the nutrient density of the diet, foods which are high in energy and protein should be recommended, but without compromising the overall balance of the diet. The energy density of meals can be further increased by adding high-energy products such as cheese, butter, oil, and cream.

Fat-Soluble Vitamin Supplementation

Due to the effects of cholestatic liver disease and resulting malabsorption, the requirements for fat-soluble vitamins are higher than the standard recommended nutrient intake (RNI) for age and should be supplemented. Table 72.6 shows how fat-soluble vitamins are supplemented at the authors' institution. It should be noted, however, that these are suggested starting doses, and prescribed amounts should be adjusted

Table 72.4 Examples of high-energy sip and tube feeds

Feed per 100 ml	Age (years)	Weight (kg)	Complete nutrition?	Energy (kcal)	Protein (g)	Fat (g)
Infatrini®	0–1.5	<9kg	Yes	100	2.6	5.4
Paediasure Plus®	1–6	8–30	Yes	150	4.2	7.47
Paediasure Plus Juce®	1–6	8–30	No	150	4.2	0
Scandishake®	>6	n/a	No	200	4	10.1
Fortijuce®	>3	n/a	No	150	4	0
Fortini®	1–6	8–20	Yes	150	3.4	6.8
Frebini Energy®	1–10	8–30	Yes	150	3.75	6.67
Resource Junior®	1–10	>8	Yes	150	3	6.2
Nutrini Energy®	1–6	8–20	Yes	150	4	6.7
Nutrison Energy®	>6	n/a	Yes	150	6	5.8

Table 72.5 Energy supplementation

Product per 100 g	Energy (kcal)	Glucose (g)	Fat (g)	Protein (g)	Comments
Glucose polymers					
Super Soluble Maxijul®	380	100	0	0	
Polycal®	384	96	0	0	
Fat emulsions					
Calogen®	450	0	50	0	100 % long-chain triglycerides
Liquigen®	450	0	50	0	100 % medium-chain triglycerides
Combined carbohydrate and fat					
Super Soluble Duocal®	492	72.7	22.3	0	100 % long-chain triglycerides
MCT Duocal®	497	72	23.2	0	75 % medium-chain triglycerides

Table 72.6 Fat-soluble vitamin supplementation

Vitamins	Infants	Children over 1 year
A and D	Abidec or Dalivit 0.6 ml/day	Abidec or Dalivit 1.2 ml/day
	May have additional oral or intramuscular vitamin D	Forceval 1 capsule/day (if over 12 years of age)
		May have additional oral or intramuscular vitamin D
E	10 mg/kg (up to maximum starting dose of 100 mg/day)	100 mg/day
K	1 mg/day	2 mg up to 10 mg/day

according to serum levels of fat-soluble vitamins. If serum vitamin levels are particularly low, then they may be given intramuscularly.

Nutritional Assessment and Monitoring

The nutritional assessment and monitoring of patients with liver disease is essential, in order to assess requirements as well as to evaluate progress. A dietetic assessment should include not just the current situation but any relevant history. It should be carried out at regular intervals to take account of changes in clinical status, anthropometry, nutrient intake, activity levels and social factors.

Dietary Assessment

A full assessment of dietary intake should be undertaken at baseline, including current and previous intake, and should indicate quantity and quality of the diet. Current intake can be ascertained by way of a 24-h dietary recall which will provide a retrospective snapshot of recent intake. Other methods include requesting parents or carers to complete a food diary at home prospectively over several days. However, as this is not always practical a 24–48-h dietary recall is preferentially used; it is straightforward and can be carried out instantaneously in both the inpatient and outpatient setting. Dietary software to calculate macro- and micronutrient provision is available, allowing values to be compared to requirements. As part of the assessment, cultural and social factors should be taken into account; for example, dietary restrictions for religious reasons or financial constraints impacting on food choice. It is important to also take into account any problems which may impact on intake such as nausea and vomiting, diarrhea, pruritus, and issues such as early satiety arising from ascites and organomegaly. The patient's clinical picture should also be considered as part of the assessment, namely the diagnosis as well as the progression of liver disease which may thus involve a change in dietetic intervention.

Anthropometry

Monitoring of anthropometry is vital. Measurements should be done at baseline, and then regular and ongoing monitoring should be carried out, with the frequency dependent on the severity and degree of liver disease.

Height/Length Faltering length/height may indicate problems with long-term chronic malnutrition. Lengths should be measured in children under 2 years using a length board and over 2 years using a stadiometer. These should be plotted on age/gender appropriate growth charts. Certain liver conditions (e.g., Alagille's syndrome) predispose the child to short stature, with height-for-age z scores often being low.

Weight Regular weights are useful. However, caution must be exercised when interpreting weights in those patients with organomegaly and/or ascites. Abdominal girth can be useful to indicate the presence of ascites especially where weights are fluctuating. Infants should be weighed naked and older children with no shoes and light clothing. Weights should be plotted on age and gender appropriate growth charts.

Head Circumference Serial measurements of head circumference in patients under 2 years are useful indicators of long-term nutritional status. Measurements should be plotted on age and gender appropriate growth charts. Measurements should be made with a non-stretchable tape measure and taken around the forehead and above the ears.

Mid-Upper Arm Circumference Serial measurements of mid-upper arm circumference (MUAC) are a good indication of fat and muscle stores and are a sensitive marker of malnutrition. Measurements should be plotted on appropriate growth charts available for children between 3 months and 5 years [23]. In children over 5 years, assessment of nutritional status is made by way of regular, serial measurements due to the current lack of age-appropriate growth charts. The measurement should be conducted on the same arm, with the patient preferably standing (or seated in a lap). The midway point from the acromion process to the olecranon process should be marked and the circumference measurement taken around the point with a non-stretchable tape measure (to the nearest 0.1 cm). Serial measurements taken by a single observer are important to avoid interobserver errors.

Triceps Skinfold Thickness This differentiates fat from muscle stores and is a good marker of medium to long-term nutritional status. Measurements are taken by way of callipers which are used to measure subcutaneous adipose tissue at the triceps commonly (though other sites can also be accessed e.g., subscapular). When measuring the triceps, the midway point from the acromion process to the olecranon process should be marked. At this point, a fold of skin and subcutaneous tissue should be picked up and grasped away from the underlying muscle, and the jaws of the caliper applied at the marked spot [24]. Serial measurements taken by a single observer are important to avoid interobserver errors. Practically, skinfold thickness can be challenging to measure unless the child is cooperative.

Methods of Feeding

Oral Feeding

All children should be encouraged to feed orally where possible, particularly in infancy when infants need to learn to suck, swallow, and chew as part of normal feeding development. Several factors can predispose children to behavioral feeding problems including vomiting, tube feeding [25] and extended periods with no oral feeding, all of which may occur with chronic liver disease. With infants, particularly those with end stage liver disease awaiting transplant, it is especially important to encourage age-appropriate weaning practices, to avoid missing the 'window of opportunity' to introduce tastes and textures. This can be especially difficult when there is ascites or organomegaly or when the child is being tube fed. The emotional and social benefits of eating and drinking for the child and family should not be overlooked and should be encouraged, even if only a fraction of nutritional requirements are taken orally.

Tube Feeding

Tube feeding may be required in children who are unable to take sufficient nutrition orally. Nasogastric (NG) tube feeding has been associated with improved body composition in children with liver disease [26, 27]. Tube feeding may have a positive impact on quality of life as it can remove the pressure on both the child and family to meet requirements orally. The tube can be used to administer unpalatable feeds and medicines, and continuous or frequent feeds can minimize periods of fasting, thus helping to maintain blood sugars and preserve body stores. Where possible, some degree of oral feeding should be continued, as discussed above, even if full nutritional requirements are being met by tube feeding.

Gastrostomy feeding is preferred in children with long-term feeding problems but is rarely possible in children with chronic liver disease. Portal hypertension and intra-abdominal varices increase the risk of bleeding during placement of the tube [28] while ascites may prevent adequate tract formation around the gastrostomy [28]. Gastrostomy feeding has

been used successfully in children with no portal hypertension, varices, or ascites [29]. Where gastrostomy placement is indicated, it should be a decision undertaken by the multi-disciplinary team.

Parenteral Nutrition

Due to the risks of parenteral nutrition (PN) worsening liver function, PN should only be used when it is not possible or effective to feed enterally [13]. For example, PN may be used when NG placement is not possible (e.g., due to large, bleeding varices) or where there is significant and persistent malabsorption impacting on growth. Sullivan et al. [30] found that PN improved nutritional status in malnourished biliary atresia patients awaiting liver transplant, although there was a more rapid progression of cholestasis. It was thought that this progression may have been reduced by the use of omega-3 lipid sources rather than the soy-based lipids used in this study.

The Management of Common Liver Conditions

Conjugated Hyperbilirubinemia

Infants presenting with conjugated jaundice will generally require a formula containing a proportion of the fat as MCT. If galactosemia is suspected or has not been excluded, breast feeding should be stopped and replaced with an MCT-rich feed containing only trace amounts of galactose (e.g., Pregestimil®). The mother should be encouraged to express breast milk as it is usually possible to restart breast feeding once galactosemia is excluded. It should be noted that if Pregestimil® is used in preterm infants, additional iron and folate may be required.

If cholestasis persists with accompanying symptoms of malabsorption and suboptimal growth, supplementation with MCT will continue to be required. This can be given as the fat emulsion, Liquigen® (2–5 ml with every breast-feed) or as an MCT-rich formula (e.g., Pregestimil®, Heparon Junior®) alongside breast feeding. If jaundice is persistent and growth is poor, the latter option is preferred, and the percentage of specialist formula compared to breast milk will need to be increased. At the authors' institution, the initial target is generally two-third specialist formula to one-third breast milk. Parents should be given the option of how they would like to administer feeds, taking into consideration practicalities and home life. The specialist formula can, for example, be given prior to each breast-feed, or formula feeds can be alternated with breast-feeds.

Extrahepatic Biliary Atresia

Infants often present feeding excessively, due to malabsorption but with satisfactory weight gain initially. The nutritional intervention at the authors' institution is as described above for conjugated jaundice. Following the Kasai procedure, an MCT-rich feed is introduced at around day 3 and then slowly increased to meet requirements by day 5. The infant may be able to start some breast feeding additionally, but the majority of the infant's nutrition provision should come from the MCT formula. Satisfactory feeding should be established whilst in hospital and the infant discharged with a regime that is practical and manageable at home. Following discharge, growth should be carefully monitored (as described above), and the volume and concentration of the feed should be altered accordingly. Close monitoring is particularly important for infants with biliary atresia given that at least 50 % are likely to receive a transplant in the first 2 years of life [31] with a further 20–30 % likely to eventually require a transplant later in life [30]. When the infant is ready to be weaned, standard weaning practices are advised, with age-appropriate solids. At the authors' institution, infants generally remain on an MCT formula until at least 6 months post Kasai. A review by Davenport et al. [32] showed that 57% of infants had cleared their jaundice by this time. If jaundice has cleared at this milestone, the MCT formula can be discontinued and replaced with a standard or high-energy formula. If jaundice persists, the infant should continue on an MCT-containing formula.

Nonalcoholic Fatty Liver Disease

Nonalcoholic fatty liver disease (NAFLD) exists as a spectrum ranging from benign hepatic steatosis to more aggressive forms that can potentially progress to cirrhosis in childhood [33]. It is the most common liver abnormality in the pediatric population [34]. The aims of management are to correct the associated metabolic abnormalities, for example treating insulin resistance, reducing visceral obesity, and treating oxidative stress [35]. Treatment of NAFLD remains largely challenging. At present, weight reduction and, in particular, reduction in central obesity through dietary modifications and physical activity are the cornerstone of management. A prospective study involving 84 pediatric patients (aged 3–18.8 years) with raised transaminases and biopsy-proven NAFLD, who underwent a 12-month diet and lifestyle program, demonstrated a significant reduction in BMI, fasting glucose levels, insulin, lipids and liver enzyme activity, and a reduction in liver echogenicity on ultrasound [33]. Several trials have been conducted using pharmacologic approaches such as vitamin E to reduce oxidative stress; urso-deoxycholic acid which has cytoprotective, immunomodula-

tory, and antioxidant properties, and metformin which counters insulin resistance [36, 37]. At present, however, lifestyle changes remain the mainstay of treatment.

Wilson's Disease

Wilson's disease is an autosomal disorder of copper metabolism and may present at almost any age. Copper accumulates in the liver during childhood but may also deposit in other parts of the body such as the brain, eyes, joints, and kidneys. Treatment is primarily through chelating agents that bind dietary copper for excretion. Foods with very high concentrations of copper such as offal, shellfish, nuts, dried fruit, chocolate, and mushrooms may also need to be avoided [38].

Progressive Familial Intrahepatic Cholestasis

Progressive familial intrahepatic cholestasis (PFIC) refers to a group of autosomal recessive disorders that interfere with the secretion of bile and often present in infancy with cholestasis of hepatocellular origin [39, 40]. The major problem from a nutritional point of view is fat malabsorption, necessitating MCT supplementation. Poor intake and appetite may also occur as a result of intractable pruritis. Short stature is also characteristic of the disease, though can improve following liver transplantation [41]. If oral intake is suboptimal, nutrition support via NG tube should be initiated, and if long-term feeding is required, gastrostomy insertion should be considered.

Alagille's Syndrome

Alagille's syndrome can be particularly challenging with regard to nutrition. It is characterized by cholestasis and malabsorption, poor growth, with low height-for-age z scores and low weight-for-age z scores, fussy eating, intractable itching, and renal acidosis [42, 43]. As mentioned previously, it has generally been thought that a certain proportion of patients with Alagille's syndrome are affected by pancreatic insufficiency [4] although data from a recent study suggested that pancreatic insufficiency is not a clinically significant issue in Alagille's syndrome [44]. The nutritional management is aimed at treating the symptoms of cholestasis, as described above for conjugated jaundice. When the infant is ready to be weaned, standard weaning practices are advised. Intervention through specialist feeding clinics may be beneficial to address fussy eating. As described with PFIC, supplementary nutrition support via NG tube or gastrostomy is often the only means for optimal nutrition provision. Oral nutrition support in older children may be instigated through optimizing the energy and protein content of the diet or the use of nutritional supplement drinks.

Parenteral-nutrition-associated Liver Disease

Parenteral-nutrition-associated liver disease (PNALD) is a risk of long-term PN and can progress from cholestasis to fibrosis and cirrhosis. Other risk factors include prematurity, short bowel syndrome, sepsis, intestinal bacterial overgrowth, and a lack of enteral nutrition [45]. Strategies to reduce the risk of PNALD include early implementation of enteral feeding, a specialized, multidisciplinary approach, and techniques focused on avoiding sepsis [46]. The use of the lipid formulation SMOF (soybean oil, MCT, olive oil, fish oil) in place of soybean oil has been a significant advance and has been shown to reduce PN-related cholestasis [47, 48].

Liver Transplantation

Feeding post transplant usually starts within the first 3–5 days. As many children have moderate-to-severe faltering growth at the time of transplant [49], high-energy feeds are usually started and gradually increased over 1–2 days. The aim is to achieve catch-up growth. Catch-up growth is usually seen in the 2 years following transplant, although children may achieve a final height below their genetic potential [50]. Where a child may have been well nourished prior to transplant and was eating and drinking normally, high-calorie milk feeds may not be necessary and foods may be gradually increased over the next few days. Where there are gastrointestinal complications (e.g., bowel perforation) or severe undernutrition at the time of transplant, PN may be commenced. In most cases, children are fed via NG tube until oral feeds can be established. Preexisting behavioral feeding difficulties are common and may mean that tube feeding continues for an extended period. In cases where children are fed via gastrostomy and are likely to require tube feeding post transplant, the aim may be to keep the gastrostomy in situ. This is, however, often not possible due to the increased risk of complications described previously. If oral intake prior to transplant was established, a normal diet for age is often achieved relatively quickly.

Following liver transplant, Seville oranges and grapefruit should be avoided as they interfere with immunosuppressant medication [51]. Where infants are breast-fed post transplant, the breast-feeding mother should also exclude these items from the diet. It is important to adhere to food safety guidelines and avoid foods that may contain bacteria such as listeria, *Escherichia coli,* or salmonella as there is an increased vulnerability to food poisoning when on high-dose immunosuppressant medication. The following foods should be avoided: unpasteurized milk and cheese, soft cheese such as feta, Brie and Camembert, live yoghurt, pâté, foods containing raw egg, raw fish, shellfish, unwashed salads, and deli meats.

Chylous Ascites

Chylous ascites is a potential complication post liver transplant. It occurs as a result of damage to the lymph vessels during surgery and results in a loss of chyle, a milky, triglyceride-rich fluid, into the peritoneal cavity. Posttransplant, this is often evident in the intra-abdominal drain. Current treatment for chylous ascites is the dietary restriction of LCT, the aim of which is to reduce the flow of lymph in the disrupted lymphatic system. Dietary restriction generally lasts for no more than 3 weeks. For infants solely formula fed, Monogen® containing 80% MCT is the feed of choice. This should be supplemented with walnut oil to meet EFA requirements. If solids are given, they should be low in LCT. For older children, if supplementation is indicated alongside the low LCT diet, MCT fat emulsions such as Liquigen® or MCT Oil® can be used to provide extra calories or fat-free supplements such as Fortijuce® or Paediasure Plus Juce® can be given.

The Nutritional Management of Acute Liver Failure

As with chronic liver failure, acute liver failure (ALF) can result in impaired glycogen storage and gluconeogenesis with protein and fat stores broken down to meet energy demands. The catabolic effect is increased by a rise in insulin and glucagon, driving the need for gluconeogenesis to maintain blood sugars [52]. A further problem, particularly in infants, is that there can be a delay in determining the diagnosis. Metabolic disorders are a frequent cause of ALF and require specific dietary therapy to prevent accumulation of toxic by-products. The ideal dietary therapy cannot begin until the diagnosis is determined. Management is based on preventing hypoglycemia (as discussed previously), managing metabolic disturbances such as hyperammonemia (as discussed for CLD) and maintaining nutritional status.

Summary

Optimal nutrition support which is tailored to the individual and responsive to the changing clinical picture is essential for children with liver disease. Nutrition therapy should focus not only on correcting nutritional deficits and managing the complications of liver disease but also promoting normal growth, development, and quality of life.

References

1. Shepherd RW, Chin SE, Cleghorn GJ, Patrick M, Ong TH, Lynch SV, et al. Malnutrition in children with chronic liver disease accepted for liver transplantation: clinical profile and effect in outcome. J Pediatric Child Health. 1991;27(5):295–9.

2. Ramaccioni V, Soriano HE, Arumugam R, Klish WJ. Nutritional aspects of chronic liver disease and liver transplantation in children. J Pediatr Gastroenterol Nutr. 2000;30(4):361–7.

3. Testa R, Franceschini R, Giannini E Cataldi A, Botta F, Fasoli A, Tenerelli P, Rolandi E, Barreca T. Serum leptin levels in patients with viral chronic hepatitis or liver cirrhosis. J Hepatol. 2000;33(1):33–7.

4. Turnpenny PD, Ellard SE. Alagille syndrome: pathogenesis, diagnosis and management. Eur J Human Genet. 2012;20(3):251–7.

5. Norman K, Pirlich M. Gastrointestinal tract in liver disease: which organ is sick? Curr Opin Clin Nutr Metabol Care. 2008;11(5):613–9.

6. Nightingale S, Ng VL. Optomizing nutritional management in children with chronic liver disease. Pediatr Clin N Am. 2009;56(5):1161–83.

7. Sultan MI, Leon CD, Biank VF. Role of nutrition in pediatric chronic liver disease. Nutr Clin Pract. 2011;26(4):401–8.

8. Pierro A, Koletzko B, Carnielli V, Superina RA, Roberts EA, Filler RM, Set al. Resting energy expenditure is increased in infants and children with extrahepatic biliary atresia. J Pediatr Surg. 1989;24(6):534–8.

9. Greer R, Lehnert M, Lewindon P, Cleghorn GJ, Shepherd RW. Body composition and components of energy expenditure in children with end-stage liver disease. J Pediatr Gastroenterol Nutr. 2003;36(3):358–63.

10. Aggett PJ, Haschke F, Heine W, Hernell O, Koletzko B, Launiala K, et al. Comment on the content and composition of lipids in infant formulas. ESPGHAN Committee on Nutrition. Acta Paediatr Scand. 1991;80(8–9):887–96.

11. Chin SE, Shepherd RW, Thomas BJ, Cleghorn GJ, Patrick MK, Wilcox JA, et al. Nutritional support in children with end-stage liver disease: a randomised crossover trial of a branched chain amino acid supplement. Am J Clin Nutr. 1992;56(1):158–63.

12. Mager DR, Wykes LJ, Roberts EA, Ball RO, Pencharz PB. Branched-chain amino acid needs in children with mild-to-moderate chronic cholestatic liver disease. J Nutr. 2006;136:133–9.

13. Baker A, Stevenson R, Dhawan A, Goncalves I, Socha P, Sokal E. Guidelines for nutritional care for infants with cholestatic liver disease before liver transplantation. Pediatr Transplant. 2007;11:825–34.

14. Parrish CR, Caruana P, Shah N. Hepatic encephalopathy: are NH4 levels and protein restriction obsolete? Pract Gastroenterol. 2011;95:6–18.

15. Kaufman SS, Murray ND, Wood RP, Shaw BW, Vanderhoof JA. Nutritional support for the infant with extrahepatic biliary atresia. J Pediatr. 1987;110:679–86.

16. Charlton CPJ, Buchanan E, Holden CE, Preece MA, Green A, Booth IW, Tarlow MJ. Intensive enteral feeding in advanced cirrhosis: reversal of malnutrition without precipitation of hepatic encephalopathy. Arch Dis Childh. 1992;67:603–7.

17. Shepherd RW. Pre and postoperative nutritional care in liver transplantation in children. J Gastroenterol Hepatol. 1996;11(S2):S7–10.

18. Cordoba J, Lopez-Hellin J, Planas M, Sabin P, Sanpedro F, Castro F, Esteban R, Guardia J. Normal protein diet for episodic hepatic encephalopathy: results of a randomized study. J Hepatol. 2004;41(1):38–43.

19. Leonis MA, Balistreri WF. Evaluation and management of end-stage liver disease in children. Gastroenterology 2008;134(6):1741–51.

20. Alonso EM. Growth and development considerations in pediatric liver transplant. Liver Transplant. 2008;14(5):585–91.

21. Kelly DA, Davenport M. Current management of biliary atresia. Arch Dis Child. 2007;92:1132–5.

22. Shaw V, Lawson M. Nutritional assessment, dietary requirements, feed supplementation. In: Shaw V, Lawson M. Clinical paediatric dietetics. 3rd ed. Oxford: Blackwell. Ch. 1 2007.

23. WHO. Child growth standards. Arm circumference for age. Geneva. Available at http://www.who.int/childgrowth/standards/en/

24. Tanner JM, Whitehouse RH. Revised standards for triceps and subscapular skinfolds in British children. Arch Dis Child. 1975;50(2):142–5.

25. Douglas J, Bryon M. Interview data in severe behavioural eating difficulties in young children. Arch Dis Child. 1996;75(4):304–8.

26. Chin SE, Shepherd RW, Thomas BJ, Cleghorn GJ, Patrick MK, Wilcox JA, et al. The nature of malnutrition in children with end stage liver disease awaiting orthotopic liver transplantation. Am J Clin Nutr. 1992;56(1):164–8.

27. Holt R, Miell J, Jones J, Mieli-Vergani G, Baker A. Nasogastric feeding enhances nutritional status in paediatric liver disease but does not alter circulating levels of IGF-I and IGF binding proteins. Clin Endocrinol. 2000;52(2):217–24.

28. Baltz JG, Argo CK, Al-Osaimi AMS, Northup PG. Mortality after percutaneous endoscopic gastrostomy in patients with cirrhosis: a case series. Gastrointest Endosc. 2010;72(5):1072–5.

29. Duché M, Habès D, Lababidi A, Chardot C, Wenz J, Bernard O. Percutaneous endoscopic gastrostomy for continuous feeding in children with chronic cholestasis. J Pediatr Gastroenterol Nutr. 1999;29(1):42–5.

30. Sullivan JS, Sundaram SS, Pan Z, Sokol RJ. Parenteral nutrition supplementation in biliary atresia patients listed for liver transplantation. Liver Transplant. 2012;18(1):120–8.

31. Arvay JL, Zemel BS, Gallagher PR, Rovner AJ, Mulberg AE, Stallings VA, et al. Body composition of children aged 1 to 12 years with biliary atresia or Alagille syndrome. J Pediatr Gastroenterol Nutr. 2005;40(2):146–50.

32. Davenport M, De Ville de Goyet J, Stringer MD, Mieli-Vergani G, Kelly DA, McClean P, Spitz L. Seamless management of biliary atresia in England and Wales (1999–2002). The Lancet 2004;363(9418):1354–7.

33. Nobili V, Marcellini M, Devito R, Ciampalini P, Piemonte F, Comparcola D, et al. NAFLD in children: a prospective clinical-pathological study and effect of lifestyle advice. Hepatology 2006;44(2):458–65.

34. Schwimmer JB, Deutsch R, Kahen T, Lavine JE, Stanley C, Behling C. Prevalence of fatty liver in children and adolescents. Pediatrics 2006;118(4):1388–93.

35. Alisi A, Carpino G, Nobili V. Paediatric nonalcoholic fatty liver disease. Curr Opin Gastroenterol 2013;29(3):279–84.

36. Baumann U, Brown R. Review: non alcoholic fatty liver disease in childhood. Brit J Diab Vasc Dis. 2006;6(6):264–8.

37. De Bruyne R, Fitzpatrick E, Dhawan A. Fatty liver disease in children: eat now pay later. Hepatol Int. 2010;4(1):375–85.

38. Roberts EA, Schilsky ML. Diagnosis and treatment of Wilson disease: an update. Hepatology 2008;47(6):2089–111.

39. Jacquemin E. Progressive familial intrahepatic cholestasis. Clin Res Hepatol Gastroenterol. 2012;36(S1):S26–35.

40. Jankowska I, Socha P. Progressive familial intrahepatic cholestasis and inborn errors of bile acid synthesis. Clin Res Hepatol Gastroenterol. 2012;36(3):271–4.

41. Aydogdu S, Cakir M, Arikan C, Tumgor G, Yuksekkaya HA, Yilmaz F, et al. Liver transplantation for progressive familial intrahepatic cholestasis: clinical and histopathological findings, outcome and impact on growth. Pediatr Transplant. 2007;11(6):634–40.

42. Kronsten V, Fitzpatrick E, Baker A. Management of cholestatic pruritus in paediatric patients with Alagille syndrome: the King's College Hospital experience. J Paediat Gastroenterol Nutr. 2013;57:149–54.

43. Subramaniam P, Knisely A, Portmann B, Qureshi SA, Aclimandos WA, Karani JB, et al. Diagnosis of Alagille syndrome—25 years of experience at King's College Hospital. J Paediatr Gastroenterol Nutr. 2011;52:84–9.

44. Kamath BM, Piccoli DA, Magee JC, Sokol RJ. Pancreatic insufficiency is not a prevalent problem in Alagille syndrome. Childhood liver disease research and education network. J Pediatr Gastroenterol Nutr. 2012;55(5):612–4.

45. Beath SV, Davies P, Papadopoulou A, Khan AR, Buick RG, Corkery JJ, et al. Parenteral nutrition-related cholestasis in postsurgical neonates: multivariate analysis of risk factors. J Pediatr Surg. 1996;31(4):604–6.

46. Kelly DA. Preventing parenteral nutrition liver disease. Early Hum Dev. 2010;86(11):683–7.

47. Goulet O, Antébi H, Wolf C, Talbotec C, Alcindor L, Corriol O, et al. A new intravenous fat emulsion containing soybean oil, medium-chain triglycerides, olive oil, and fish oil: a single-center, double-blind randomized study on efficacy and safety in pediatric patients receiving home parenteral nutrition. J Parenter Enteral Nutr. 2010;34(5):485–95.

48. Muhammed R, Bremner R, Protheroe S, Johnson T, Holden C, Murphy MS. Resolution of parenteral nutrition-associated jaundice on changing from a soybean oil emulsion to a complex mixed-lipid emulsion. J Pediatr Gastroenterol Nutr. 2012;54(6):797–802.

49. Viner RM, Forton JTM, Cole TJ, Clark IH, Noble-Jamieson G, Barnes ND. Growth of long-term survivors of liver transplantation. Arch Dis Child. 1999;80(3):235–40.

50. Scheenstra R, Jan Gerver W, Odink RJ, van Soest H, Peeters PMJG, Verkade HJ, Sauer PJJ. Growth and final height after liver transplantation during childhood. J Pediatr Gastroenterol Nutr. 2008;47:165–71.

51. British Medical Association and the Royal Pharmaceutical Society of Great Britain. British National Formulary. London, UK: BMJ Publishing Group. 2013. Copyright © BMJ Group and the Royal Pharmaceutical Society of Great Britain 2013. http://www.medicinescomplete.com/mc/alerts/2010/alert00016121.htm

52. Cochran JB, Losek JD. Acute liver failure in children. Paediatr Emerg Care. 2007;23(2):129–35.

Pediatric Liver Transplantation

73

Nigel Heaton

Introduction

Liver transplantation (LT) continues to be the only effective treatment for children with end-stage liver disease. Thomas Starzl performed the first liver transplant in a child in March 1963 [1]; however, it was not until 1967 that he reported the first recipient with significant survival. Following his early series of seven children aged between 13 months and 16 years [2], more than 15,000 pediatric liver transplants have been carried out in the USA and 10,000 in Europe, with 3- and 5-year survival of 80 and 75 %, respectively. There have been continued improvements in all aspects of care of the child with liver disease coming to LT including surgical, anesthetic, intensive care, and postoperative management. The large numbers of recipients currently surviving beyond 15 years are informing clinical practice and providing more information for families currently facing transplantation. As the majority of children are transplanted at a young age and have little memory of the events surrounding their transplant continuing patient and family education are increasingly recognized as important. There has been a change of emphasis in care from a focus on survival to long-term outcomes centered on well-being, psychosocial and physical development, and educational attainment. It is clear that adolescence and transition to adulthood and follow-up within an adult environment pose further significant challenges, and late death due to non-adherence to medication and follow-up are significant problems. The emergence of models of care to manage these challenges will hopefully help lead to further improvement in long-term outcomes. In addition, the timing of transplant and its influence on subsequent development and outcome is coming under increasing scrutiny.

Pre-transplant

Historically, children have been listed for LT based on criteria adopted from adult experience. However, children present with a different spectrum of diseases, with two thirds of children coming to LT in the first 5 years of life, and consideration has to be given to emotional, social, intellectual, and physical development. The timing of LT has to be considered with the long-term development of the child in mind, and there remains a lack of data regarding this topic.

Indications for LT

LT should be considered for any child with end-stage liver disease with a predicted prognosis of less than 18 months. Indications for LT are in general derived from adult liver transplant experience, but are modified for children and include:

Liver decompensation (prolonged international normalized ratio (INR), low serum albumin, ascites)
Disordered metabolism (jaundice, loss of muscle mass, osteoporosis)
Portal hypertension (variceal bleeding, intractable ascites)
Encephalopathy
Spontaneous bacterial peritonitis
Hepatopulmonary syndrome
Pulmonary hypertension
Recurrent cholangitis and intractable pruritus
Quality of life (failure to growth, poor concentration, lethargy)
Tumors

Extrahepatic biliary atresia (BA) is the most common indication for LT and accounts for 40–50 % of cases listed worldwide. Other common causes include metabolic disorders, tumors, and acute liver failure (ALF). The majority of pediatric recipients under 2 years old have cholestatic diseases, particularly BA, which accounts for 74 % of cases

N. Heaton (✉)
King's Health Partners, Institute of Liver Studies, Kings College Hospital FT NHS Trust, Denmark Hill, London SE5 9RS, UK
e-mail: nigel.heaton@nhs.net

© Springer International Publishing Switzerland 2016
S. Guandalini et al. (eds.), *Textbook of Pediatric Gastroenterology, Hepatology and Nutrition*,
DOI 10.1007/978-3-319-17169-2_73

871

in this age group. Metabolic disorders and ALF are less common indications and account for 9% each of the overall number [3].

Chronic Liver Diseases

Biliary Atresia

Extrahepatic BA is a destructive inflammatory obliterative cholangiopathy that affects the intrahepatic and extrahepatic bile tree. Type 3 BA is the most frequent form of the disease accounting for 90% of cases and is the most severe form with a solid porta hepatis, microscopic ductules, and a solid gallbladder or mucocele [4]. The majority of children coming to transplant have undergone Kasai portoenterostomy (KP) within the first 3 months of life. Early portoenterostomy and expertise of the multidisciplinary team have a significant impact on outcome and the need for LT in early life [5, 6]. The results of concentrating expertise in a small number of centers each performing more than five cases per year have led to a 4-year survival with the native liver intact of 41–51% and an overall survival of 87–89%. More recently, survival of 96% at 10 years has been reported for the UK with an integrated program of KP and LT [4]. Mortality is distributed equally between deaths on waiting list for liver transplant and in the post-transplant period. By the age of 18 years, approximately 80% of children with BA will have been treated by LT. Outcomes have been reported for 5- and 10-year actuarial graft and patient survival of 76.2 and 72.7% and 87.2 and 85.5% for cadaveric [7] and 84.9 and 76.6 and 86.7 and 80.8% for living donor LT (LDLT) [8], respectively.

The majority of young children (under 5 years of age) with BA will come to transplant with jaundice and synthetic failure. In a small number of children (6% of cases), acute decompensation secondary to ischemic hepatitis may occur following a viral illness or infection. Children at risk of ischemic hepatitis and liver decompensation are those with a hepatic artery resistance index of greater than one on Doppler ultrasound who are dependent on arterial inflow [9]. Children older than 5 years of age may present with failure to grow and a falling serum albumin (synthetic failure), but without jaundice. Adolescents coming to transplantation will invariably have portal hypertension as a dominating feature, which in association with adhesions from previous surgery can make for a difficult surgical challenge.

Congenital anomalies associated with "syndromic" BA (15% of all cases) include polysplenia/asplenia, absent inferior vena cava (IVC), portal hypoplasia, preduodenal portal vein (PV), malrotation, and situs inversus and may complicate surgery and influence graft choice.

Cholestatic and Metabolic Disorders

Cholestatic liver diseases excluding BA account for 10% of liver transplants in children. These include Alagille syndrome, progressive familial intrahepatic cholestasis (PFIC), and sclerosing cholangitis. LT is often used to treat symptoms, such as severe pruritus. Children with Alagille syndrome are at risk of growth failure and morbidity from pruritus, xanthomas, and complications of vitamin deficiency. PFIC defines a group of disorders characterized by chronic, unremitting cholestasis and autosomal recessive inheritance with a shared pattern of biochemical, clinical, and histological features. LT is reserved for those with severe symptoms including pruritus or progressive liver disease. Earlier transplant may lessen future growth and developmental impairment in some, but not all of these conditions [10]. In Alagille syndrome, the biliary hypoplasia is associated with other congenital malformations, the most important of which is pulmonary artery stenosis. This needs to be assessed preoperatively due to the risk of mortality post reperfusion if cardiac output is limited by the pulmonary stenosis. Dobutamine stress testing has been used to identify at-risk children who are unable to increase their cardiac index by 50%.

Inborn errors of metabolism, collectively as a group, form a relatively common indication for LT accounting for 9 and 26% of children under and over 2 years of age at the time of transplant, respectively. Metabolic diseases resulting in cirrhosis include alpha-1-antitrypsin deficiency, tyrosinemia, Wilson's disease, neonatal hemochromatosis, respiratory chain disorders, fatty acid oxidation defect, glycogen storage disease type IV, among many others. Metabolic diseases without structural liver disease include Crigler–Najjar syndrome type 1, glycogen storage disease type 1, propionic acidemia, primary hyperoxaluria type 1, hereditary tyrosinemia, factor VII deficiency, ornithine transcarbamylase deficiency, familial hypercholesterolemia, and protein C deficiency. Two series from the USA from the Scientific Registry of Transplant Recipients (SRTR) of 551 transplants [11] and Europe from King's College Hospital of 112 transplants reported excellent outcomes for this group [10]. Although the presence of cirrhosis did not appear to be a risk factor for worse outcomes, recipient black race, simultaneous organ transplantation, ALF, hospitalization before transplant, and age less than or equal to 1 year were predictors. The study from Sze et al. reported 11 auxiliary liver transplants (ALTs) with similar outcomes to whole liver replacement for noncirrhotic liver disease with an absent enzyme/gene product such as Crigler–Najjar type 1 [10].

Tumors

LT for liver tumors in children accounts for 2–6% of all cases in European and American series. The most common indication is unresectable hepatoblastoma (following appropriate chemotherapy). Other tumors treated by LT include hepatocellular carcinoma (HCC), hemangioma, infantile hemangioendothelioma, and epithelioid hemangioendothelioma. Angiosarcomas should not be transplanted as they invariably recur early. However, differentiation from more benign vascular tumors can be difficult. Clinical features such as pain, rapid deterioration, or disease progression indicate sarcoma. The outcome of LT for unresectable hepatoblastoma is excellent with long-term patient and graft survival rates for cadaveric transplantation of 91, 77.6, and 77.6% at 1, 5, and 10 years, respectively [12]. Patient and graft survival for children undergoing LDLT is 100, 83.3, and 83.3% at 1, 5, and 10 years, respectively. Two North American series of 25 (HCC, 10 cases; hepatoblastoma, 15 cases) and 12 patients (HCC, 6 cases; hepatoblastoma, 6 cases) reported similar medium- and long-term survival rates for both tumors [13, 14]. Salvage transplantation for recurrent hepatoblastoma after conventional liver resection is less satisfactory with 5-year survival of 40% with a high rate of further recurrence. An analysis of the United Network for Organ Sharing (UNOS) data of 336 patients with liver tumors which included 237 hepatoblastomas, 58 HCC, and 35 hemangioendotheliomas noted that patient survival for the latter was inferior to that of hepatoblastoma (5-year survival of 72%) and rare liver tumors (5-year survival of 78.9%), but better than HCC (5-year survival of 53.5%) [15]. Tumor recurrence was the major cause of death in hepatoblastoma and HCC, but not in hemangioendothelioma.

The development of HCC has been reported in BA, Alagille syndrome, and progressive intrahepatic cholestasis. Children with tyrosinemia have a high risk of HCC before 2 years of age which appears to be markedly reduced by the use of 2-(2-nitro-4-3 trifluoromethylbenzoyl)-1,3-cyclohexanedione (NBTC) therapy [16]. For HCC, there are no criteria for selection comparable to the Milan criteria in adult patients. Macrovascular invasion continues to be a contraindication.

Acute Liver Failure

ALF is defined by the onset of severe impairment of liver function in the absence of previous liver disease. Coagulopathy is always present, but in young children hepatic encephalopathy may be absent and is a late feature associated with a poor outcome. ALF is an indication for LT in 9% of under and 16% of over 2 years old in Europe and 15% of children in the USA. The cause of ALF cannot be determined in the majority of children (49% of all children and 54% of those aged 1 year) [17]. Other causes include metabolic, paracetamol intoxication, autoimmune hepatitis (AIH), viral hepatitis, drugs, Wilson's disease, and vascular and Amanita phalloides poisoning. The risk of death or LT is highest in children under 3 years of age. Logistic regression analysis has identified total serum bilirubin > 5 mg/dL, INR > 2.55, and hepatic encephalopathy as risk factors for death or LT. Of note, grade IV hepatic encephalopathy on admission was associated with higher rate of spontaneous recovery than those children who progressed to grade IV during the course of admission (50 vs. 20%). Indications for LT are different from adults and an INR > 4 (in the absence of dis-

seminated intravascular coagulopathy) identifies the at-risk population.

Two recent series reported 5-year patient survival of 70% in children with ALF [18, 19]. Farmer et al. identified four factors which predicted graft or patient survival in 122 children with ALF which included creatinine clearance (cCrCl) < 60 mL/min/1.73 m (graft and patient), pediatric end-stage liver disease (PELD) > 25 (graft), recipient age < 24 months (graft), and time from the onset of jaundice to encephalopathy < 7 days (patient) [18]. The presence of two or more of these factors was associated with a significant reduction in graft and patient survival to about 25–40%. Other series have also noted lower graft survival in children aged less than 2 years with ALF possibly reflecting technical challenges in small babies [20]. This population is the most challenging group, and further improvements in perioperative surgical and intensive care are needed to make progress.

ALF in neonates is a rare but often fatal event characterized by a failure of synthetic function with coagulopathy. Hepatic encephalopathy is a late event and difficult to diagnose in infants [21]. Causes of ALF in neonates include metabolic, infectious and hematological disorders, congenital vascular/ heart abnormalities, and drugs. Congenital hemochromatosis is the commonest indication and the challenge is to provide a graft in time. Neonates and young children with ALF should only be treated in specialized pediatric hepatology centers with facilities for LT which continues to be the only therapeutic option with a long-term survival of over 60%.

Timing of Transplantation

The timing of LT in children has been based on criteria established in adults and thus is focused on graft and patient survival. Optimal timing was viewed as listing for LT when expected survival was less than 2 years. Children with liver disease may not develop physically, intellectually, and socially at a time of deteriorating liver function, and the timing of transplant needs to take this into account. There is general agreement that KP should be performed for BA and that LT is reserved for those who develop progressive liver disease (apart from rare cases of late presentation > 4 months).

The model for end-stage liver disease (MELD) was introduced in 2002 as a response to increasing waiting list mortality. It provides a means of allocating livers based on likelihood of dying while on the waiting list. PELD was a similar mathematical tool based on data derived from the Studies of Pediatric Liver Transplantation (SPLIT) research group using bilirubin, INR, serum albumin, age > 1 year, and growth [22]. The introduction of MELD (and subsequently PELD) significantly decreased death or removal from the waiting list for being too sick within 2 years for both adults and children [23]. Cowles et al. [24] in reviewing a cohort of 71 children transplanted for BA (61, KP before LT; 10, primary LT) considered that PELD monitoring identified those in need of transplantation. Children with a PELD greater than 12 ($n=47$) had a higher rate of post-LT mortality and retransplantation than those with a PELD of 10 or less. The authors suggested that a PELD score approaching 10 should trigger discussion of LT. PELD is the only scoring system currently used in children and although helpful in advanced liver dysfunction; it is of limited value in the very young (under 1 year of age) and in older recipients, particularly with complications such as recurrent cholangitis, severe portal hypertension, pulmonary hypertension, and hepatopulmonary syndrome [25–29]. Because of these limitations, PELD use has been largely restricted to North America. More research is needed to define optimal timing of transplantation in children to gain most benefit in terms of survival, growth, and intellectual and social development.

Intraoperative

Whole LT

Whole liver replacement is relatively uncommon in children under 5 years of age at the present time. Above the age of 5 years, it is more common. The transplant involves excision of the diseased liver, by division of the common bile duct (or Roux loop if there has been previous biliary surgery), hepatic artery, PV, and IVC above and below the liver. Orthotopic liver replacement is accomplished by anastomosis of the corresponding structures with the donor liver and achieving hemostasis; the alternative is the use of the piggyback technique. Management of intraoperative coagulopathy is an essential component of the operation. The technique is very similar to adult LT, but the smaller size of the vascular structures demands a more refined surgical technique, especially for arterial reconstruction. The use of cell salvage has led to bloodless surgery becoming a practical proposition. Closure of the abdomen should only be performed if there is no risk of graft compression.

Partial Liver Grafts

The use of partial grafts was the solution to both organ shortage and size restriction in children. In Europe, more than 10,000 LT have been performed in recipients under 16 years old. Of these, approximately 38 % have been performed with whole organs. Partial grafts account for 80 and 52 % of all LT performed among patients aged 0–2 and 2–15 years old, respectively. Early experience was with reduced-size grafts, either left lobe or left-lateral segment (LLS) which then led onto to split and LDLT with both techniques being incor-

porated into routine clinical practice from 1991 onwards. Roberts et al. analyzed the data of 6467 LTs performed in patients under 30 years old from the SRTR–Organ Procurement and Transplantation Network (OPTN) database [30]. It was noted that patient and graft survival during the first year after transplant for each donor graft type varied according to the recipient age group. For children of 2 years and under, living donor (LD) grafts had a 51 and 30 % lower relative risk (RR) of graft failure than deceased donor split (DD-S) and deceased donor full (DD-F), respectively. A similar difference in mortality risk in the same group of age favored recipients of LD grafts over DD-S (RR=0.71, $p=0.08$). Recipients in the 0–2-year age group had higher risk of mortality and graft failure with DD-S livers than DD-F livers (RR=1.31, $p=0.04$ for mortality; RR=1.42, $p<0.001$ for graft failure). For patients aged 2–10 years, the RRs of mortality and graft loss were higher after LD than after DD-F (RR=1.78, $p=0.02$ for mortality; RR=1.53, $p=0.02$ for graft loss) but not after DD-S. In the 11–16-year age group, a significantly higher RR of graft failure was observed after LD than after DD-F transplant (RR=3.63, $p=0.0001$) or DD-S transplant (RR=2.87, $p=0.02$), although mortality risks were similar for all three donor graft types. Subsequent publications have confirmed the excellent outcomes with LDLT in young children, but published experience with children over 12 years of age remains limited outside of India and the Far East.

Publications of outcomes of LLS reduced-size LT tend to be from the early 1990s, and there are few direct comparisons with those observed after split LT (SLT). SLT has become an established technique which has successfully addressed organ shortage in children while preserving the pool of liver grafts for adults. A recent study of 251 LTs, which included 138 reduced and 30 split, reported 1-year patient and graft survivals that were comparable at 73 and 67 %, respectively [31]. In addition, no differences in vascular complications were observed. Of note, biliary complications were significantly more common after split when compared with reduced-size grafts (21 vs. 4 %, $p<0.0001$). The most common biliary complication after SLT was late stricture, in contrast to reduced-size LT (RLT), which was a cut-surface bile leak. Patients undergoing SLT had a 6.7-fold increased risk of biliary complications compared to those receiving an RLT; however, these complications did not appear to impact on graft or patient survival. A further series from the University of California Los Angeles (UCLA) has compared the outcome of whole and partial grafts in both adult and pediatric recipients [31]. Of 442 LTs, 284 were whole, 109 were split-LLS (SL-LLS), and 49 were LD-LLS. The 10-year patient survival for children was similar for all graft types. Multivariate analysis confirmed that history of previous LT and SL-LLS was independent predictors of reduced survival. Chronic rejection and hepatic artery thrombosis were the most common reasons for graft loss. The largest study from Hong et al. of outcomes after partial liver grafting in children analyzed data from the SPLIT registry and compared the outcome of each variants with that of whole organ transplantation (1183 whole, 261 split, 388 reduced, and 360 live donor (LDLT)) [32]. There was a clear difference in outcomes at 1 year (W, 93%; R, 82%; S, 87%; L, 89%) and 4 years (whole liver transplantation (WLT), 89%; RLT, 79%; SLT, 85%; LDLT, 85%) after transplant. However, the groups were not strictly comparable in terms of era of transplant, recipient selection, and center. Children receiving a technical variant waited on average 2.3 months less than those receiving a whole liver and tended to be younger. Complications were significantly higher after partial grafts: At 24 months, the incidence of biliary complications was WLT, 17.3%; SLT, 28.5%; RLT, 25.3%; LDLT, 40.1% and vascular complications were WLT, 16.5%; SLT, 23.8%; RLT, 23.5%; LDLT, 24.4% [33].

Trying to understand and balance the increased opportunity of being transplanted against the higher incidence of complications and potential graft loss associated with SLT is difficult. Merion et al. tried to address this issue by comparing the predicted lifetimes for SLT for an adult and a child recipient with WLT for an adult to determine the best use of this limited supply of organs [34]. They analyzed mortality risk for 48,888 patients on the waiting list: 907 SLT and 21,913 WLT recipients (between 1995 and 2002). Of 23,996 donor livers used for transplantation, 533 were split. Donors aged 10–39 years comprised 81.6% of split livers and 48.5% of livers used for WLT. Only 11.8% of livers that were split were from donors older than 40 years. They analyzed years gained per SLT performed against the waiting list death ratio and concluded that "the potential annual net gain in life years could be as high as 169 patient-years in the first 2 post-transplant years, if all livers meeting accepted criteria were used for splitting." For every 100 donor livers, an extra 11 years of life were predicted over the first 2 years of follow-up if organs were split rather than transplanted whole. In addition, they identified a significant survival benefit for pediatric recipients of SLT compared with children continuing on the waiting list and concluded that it could provide enough organs to satisfy the entire current demand for pediatric donor livers.

Living Donor Liver Transplantation

LDLT has become an important source of grafts for children worldwide. Following on from the first description by Raia et al. in 1988 [35], the first long-term survivor from Strong et al. in 1989 [36], and the early series published by Broelsch et al. [37], the technique has become established with excellent short- and long-term survival. The LLS is the most commonly used graft [38]. Full left or right lobe grafts are used less commonly and tend to be in young adults. Donation is most commonly from parents, although other family members and altruistic donation have been well reported. The ethics and understanding of the desire to donate are easily understood, and the risks appear to be low, but not negligible. Donor mortality for LSS grafts is of the order of 1:1500. The incidence of other significant donor complications which include bile leak (1–2%), bleeding and the need for transfusion (1–2%), deep vein thrombosis and pulmonary embolus, and incisional hernia (5%) are considered acceptable. Risks of donor mortality are similar for left liver and rise to 0.5% for right lobe donation. The risks of bile leak are also higher for the donor, particularly with the right lobe grafts where the incidence may be as high as 5%. Donor age above 55 years has become generally accepted as a contraindication (especially for the right lobe) due to the slower regeneration and the increased risk in this population.

The LLS segment graft accounts for approximately 20–25% of the adult liver, but provides a full-sized "liver" for the child. Assessment of the donor is designed to ensure that the liver segment is anatomically and functionally suitable for transplantation and to identify additional risk factors such as procoagulant abnormalities, smoking, and steatosis within the liver. Many centers continue to follow the two-stage assessment and consent model reported by Brolesch et al. which includes psychiatric/psychological assessment of the donor and family [37]. Depending on the availability of cadaveric transplantation, suitability for living donation will vary from 50 to 90% when assessing families. The techniques of surgery have been standardized and outcomes are excellent for all liver diseases. The advantages of living related LT (LRLT) include the ability to perform surgery electively with an excellent quality graft, dry cut surface (minimal blood loss), and excellent outcome. The incidence of early rejection is similar to that of cadaveric transplantation, but long term it is considered, although the supporting evidence is limited, that these recipients may be tolerant of their grafts and that immunosuppression (IS) withdrawal may be more likely.

Morioka et al. reported the long-term outcome of LRLT in 46 children who underwent LDLT for metabolic disorders [39]. Mean age at diagnosis and LDLT was 48.6 (0–196) and 86.5 (1.4–199) months, respectively with survival rates of 86.9 and 81.2% at 1 year and 5 and 10 years post-transplant. Patient survival was significantly better in children with liver-centered disease which included Wilson disease, ornithine transcarbamylase deficiency, tyrosinemia type 1, Crigler–Najjar syndrome type 1, and bile acid synthetic defect than in those with non-liver centered disease (glycogen storage disease, propionic acidemia, methylmalonic acidemia, and erythropoietic protoporphyria; $p = 0.003$). Statistical analysis showed that cumulative survival of patients with normal or slightly delayed physical growth at the time of

LDLT was significantly better than for those with delayed physical growth ($p=0.012$).

LDLT is an excellent option in the management of ALF in children. The workup can be performed rapidly if the unit is regularly performing elective LDLT. Ethical concern has been expressed regarding the ability of the donor to appreciate the risk in these circumstances [40]. The lower risk of LLS donation has led to the use of LDLT as an accepted therapy. Greater debate surrounds the use of right lobe living donation for ALF particularly in countries with effective cadaveric organ donation.

Recent Developments in Transplant Surgery

Over the past 30 years, surgical techniques have become standardized worldwide. LLS and left and right liver LT are used to overcome size discrepancy and to engraft the majority of children. Split and LRLT have been key to sustaining the reduction in deaths on the waiting list. Auxiliary LT offers scope for native liver regeneration in children presenting with ALF and is able to withdraw from IS in the majority. Hepatocyte transplants remain experimental and have been used to bridge young children with metabolic liver disease through the liver replacement. The current challenge is to minimize technical complications that impact on graft survival, such as hepatic artery thrombosis and biliary strictures, and continue to improve outcomes. New technologies are emerging that are currently under evaluation and will impact on practice, and normothermic organ perfusion is perhaps the most prominent.

Auxiliary LT

ALT was first described in a dog by Welch in 1955 [41]. The auxiliary liver was placed in a heterotopic position in the right paravertebral gutter, with portal venous inflow from the iliac vein. The idea of heterotopic ALT was attractive as it avoided the need for native hepatectomy with the idea that it would improve hemodynamic stability during surgery. The first experience of ALT in a human was reported in 1964, using a heterotopic graft, with the aim of avoiding obstacles presented by whole liver replacement. Chenard-Neu et al. reported long-term survival of 2 out of 47 patients who underwent heterotopic ALT between 1964 and 1980 [42]. From 1986 onwards, outcomes of ALT began to improve, although only small numbers were performed [43]. The technique of ALT proved to be more difficult than that of LT with a higher rate of technical complications and inferior graft function and outcome. The development of HCC in the cirrhotic liver remnant of one long-term survivor led to the abandonment of ALT as a treatment for chronic liver disease.

The technique has become an established indication, however, for ALF especially in children. ALT has also been used to treat noncirrhotic inborn errors of metabolism based in the liver [44]. For ALF, the aim is to treat children satisfying established criteria for transplantation, with survival equivalent to that obtained with whole liver replacement with subsequent native liver regeneration and IS withdrawal. Children have the most to gain from avoiding the complications of lifelong IS. An early multicenter European experience identified that recipients under 40 years of age and particularly children were most likely to survive, have successful liver regeneration and withdraw from IS [43]. In addition, patients with hyperacute liver failure were more likely to regenerate than those with subacute liver failure and that orthotopic rather than heterotopic ALT had a better outcome. IS withdrawal has been possible in more than 70% of survivors [45–47].

ALT has included the use of whole liver, right lobe, left lobe, or LLS grafts. A proportion of the native liver is resected to make room for the graft. The graft is piggy-backed onto the cava, portal inflow is established by end-to-side anastomosis, and arterial inflow is established using either a donor iliac conduit or a branch of the native hepatic artery. Biliary drainage is achieved with either a short Roux-en-Y hepatico-jejunostomy or by anastomosis to the native bile duct. In children, the majority of ALTs are performed using LLS grafts to overcome donor–recipient size discrepancy. Selection of the recipient includes satisfying existing criteria for LT for ALF, no neurological or cardiovascular contraindication and a suitable graft. The donor liver should be of excellent quality to ensure that good early function is achieved. Marginal livers are difficult to use as partial grafts and provide inferior function and should be avoided.

Postoperatively, patients are managed with conventional IS. Early graft dysfunction is due to technical complications, particularly inadequate venous inflow or outflow, and poor quality or small for size grafts. The serum aspartate aminotransferase (AST) and INR may be slower to settle than with conventional transplantation. Persistent elevation of the serum bilirubin indicates complications with the graft. Postoperative bleeding with the need for relaparotomy is more common due to the presence of two cut surfaces.

Patients are followed with CT or MR imaging with guided biopsies of both graft and native livers in the early postoperative period and at 6-month intervals to assess liver recovery. Hepatobiliary dimethyl iminodiacetic acid (HIDA) scintigraphy is also of value in assessing the differential function of the two livers and documenting native liver recovery. The decision to begin IS withdrawal is usually made at 6 months or when signs of regeneration are observed on biopsy. Gradual weaning is necessary to avoid severe graft rejection and infarction. The graft will usually atrophy and disappear completely. IS withdrawal may need to be started to stimulate native liver regrowth. Even after massive hepatic necrosis the liver regenerates fully. However, the larger the graft transplanted the slower the regeneration of the native liver is without reduction in IS. In the subacute group, regeneration is less rapid, as observed by sequential imaging. Successful IS has been reported up to 4 years after auxiliary partial orthotopic LT (APOLT). Histopathological assessment of the native liver at the time of ALT has identified patterns of hepatocyte cell loss which insight into the likelihood of regeneration. A diffuse pattern with uniform cell loss throughout was associated with hyperacute liver failure and with excellent regeneration with restoration of normal histology in over 70 % of patients [48]. A map-like pattern was associated with seronegative hepatitis and adults had a mixed outcome; however, in children the results were excellent. In a small number of cases, no viable hepatocytes could be identified and this group did not regenerate effectively. Of five cases in our series of over 60 adults and children with this pattern, three died and two were retransplanted. ALT has become the gold standard for the treatment of children with ALF requiring transplantation.

Donation After Circulatory Death Donation

The use of donation after circulatory death (DCD) liver grafts has become common in Western countries over the past 10 years. The majority have been from controlled donation (within the hospital intensive care environment) and usually have unrecoverable brain injury. Withdrawal of support occurs, and death is pronounced clinically and with ECG. There follows a 5-min standoff before surgical retrieval is initiated. Warm ischemia is calculated from the onset of systolic blood pressure (BP) <50 mmHg or $PaO_2 < 70$ % to cold perfusion of the liver. The organs have been used successfully in children, either as whole or reduced-size grafts with excellent outcomes. Selection criteria for liver reduction include donor age <40 years, warm ischemic time of <30 min, good liver function, and no steatosis with the cold ischemic time being kept under 8 h. Several centers including our own have reported significant numbers of RLT with excellent early and late graft and patient survival and no biliary complications such as cholangiopathy [49].

Post-transplant

Postoperative IS

Over the 30 years, pediatric LT has seen serial improvements in morbidity and mortality. These improvements are related to IS, donor selection and maintenance, surgical technique, and complex team working. The focus of IS has been on the prevention of acute rejection and graft loss; however, in children, morbidity and mortality rates from infections exceed those from rejection and can also impair growth and renal function and increase the risk of some cancers. Getting the balance of IS right in the short and long term is key to a successful LT program. Evidence is also accumulating that children may be more likely to develop graft tolerance and to wean from IS in the long term [50].

Early post-transplant IS has been associated with increasing use of induction therapy (26 %), particularly with interleukin (IL)-2 receptor antibodies either to supplement IS or as a renal sparing regimen. For maintenance IS, calcineurin inhibitors (CNI) remain the cornerstone; but cyclosporin has been largely replaced by tacrolimus. Children often receive an anti-proliferative agent such as azathioprine or mycophenolate mofetil to supplement IS or for CNI/renal sparing. Tacrolimus trough levels of 8–10 ng/l in the first 3 months and 5–8 ng/l thereafter are usually sufficient. Longer-term tacrolimus levels can be further weaned to low levels, if graft function is normal with no rejection episodes. Moderate-to-severe acute rejection is treated with steroid boluses and if unresponsive antithymocyte globulin can be given.

Over-IS is associated with long-term side effects including renal impairment, hypertension, lymphoproliferative disease, and cancer and may hinder the process of immune engagement and the development of immune tolerance. There has been a move toward progressive minimization of IS, including steroid withdrawal which is associated with a growth advantage without any significant rejection-related complications [51, 52]. Many units discontinue steroids during the first or second post-transplant year and more than 50 % of children are on monotherapy tacrolimus by 18 months post LT [53]. It has been suggested that early steroid withdrawal may be associated with a higher risk of acute and chronic rejection and the development of de novo AIH [54]. The pathogenic mechanisms behind de novo AIH remain unclear, but it appears to be related to under IS and affects 2–5 % of pediatric LT recipients [55, 56].

CNI share a number of side effects in common including nephrotoxicity, neurotoxicity, and hyperlipidemia [57]. There are, however, some differences between tacrolimus and cyclosporin. Cyclosporin is associated with hirsutism and gum hyperplasia while tacrolimus is associated with diabetes and hair loss. For teenagers, especially in females, tacrolimus is often the CNI of choice because of the lower incidence of gum hyperplasia and hirsutism. Tacrolimus has greater water solubility and less dependence on bile salt absorption, thus resulting in improved bioavailability over cyclosporin. However, it has larger interindividual variations. The introduction of once-daily preparations of CNI may help reduce variations in drug levels and improve adherence to medication [58]. Tacrolimus may be superior to cationic steroid antibiotic (CsA) with regard to steroid withdrawal and the incidence of acute and chronic graft rejection. CNI sparing or substitution with mammalian target of rapamycin (mTOR) inhibitors such as sirolimus or everolimus is used for patients with nephrotoxicity, but their efficacy requires validation in long-term studies in large cohorts.

Children surviving more than 1 year post LT also appear to improve adherence. Non-adherence is one of the commonest causes of late mortality and is the leading cause in adolescents and young adults [59]. Non-adherence has been linked to a number of factors including traumatic stress disorder from the time of transplant, a lack of knowledge and understanding of their medical history, and an absence of continuing medical education. Psychological intervention and ongoing education can provide effective intervention and reduce the likelihood of graft and patient loss. Once-daily CNI formulations, particularly taken in the morning, also improve adherence without increasing the incidence of acute rejection, graft loss, or death [58].

Surgery-Related Complications

Early surgical post-LT complications are primarily related to the vascular and biliary reconstructions. Outcomes after pediatric LT are influenced by transplant volume and available expertise. It has been reported that 1-year patient death ratios were significantly lower for high-volume centers (>16 procedures per year; 0.77) than for low-volume centers (<7 procedures per year; 1.23, $p = 0.027$). Co-location of adult and pediatric LT may also contribute to better outcomes [60].

Primary Graft Nonfunction or Dysfunction
Early failure of the graft is relatively rare (1–2%), and retransplantation is the only life-saving therapy. Underlying causes may be due the mode of death of the donor, problems with retrieval, preservation, or implantation. Signs of poor graft function include hemodynamic instability requiring continuing inotrope support, persistent or increasing acidosis and lactatemia, and bleeding due to persistent coagulopathy. INR greater than four and first-day AST levels of greater than 2000 IU/l reflect major cell damage, but even levels of more than 5000 IU/l may settle with good long-term graft function.

Bleeding
Postoperative intra-abdominal hemorrhage is a common complication in the first 48 h after transplant occurring in 5–10% of patients. Risk factors include renal failure, perioperative dialysis, and ALF. Re-exploration may be necessary, but a definite bleeding point is identified in only half the cases. Bleeding from coagulopathy associated with graft dysfunction needs to be resolved rapidly to avoid hypotension and further graft injury.

Caval Complications
The reported incidence of hepatic vein–IVC anastomotic complications is low and occurs either as a result of technical failure or as a consequence of graft hypertrophy and distor-

tion. Caval complications are rare in size matched and full left liver graft with caval replacement LT with an estimated incidence of less than 1%. The use of interrupted anterior sutures in all venous anastomoses may help to avoid stenosis and kinking in the short and long term. The incidence of hepatic venous obstruction is higher after LLS LT and is of the order of 2–4%. It is always considered to be hepatic vein outflow obstruction; it is often associated with caval stenosis at the inferior aspect of the anastomosis or with twisting. It is a risk at retransplantation particularly if the native cava is small. The most important technical development was the triangulation technique for left hepatic vein (LHV)/caval anastomosis which significantly reduced the incidence of complications. Fixing the graft at the end of the procedure also helps to avoid rotation of the liver and kinking of hepatic vein anastomosis. Clinical manifestations of venous outflow obstruction include hepatomegaly, persistent ascites, unexplained renal impairment, and peripheral edema (if there is caval stenosis) [61]. It may start insidiously 2 or more weeks after the transplant. The characteristic features of venous outflow can usually be seen on CT angiography and confirmed by pressure measurements across the cava and anastomosis. Balloon angioplasty is usually effective, but occasional hepatic venous and/or caval stents may need to be inserted [62]. Long-term patency rates have not been reported and long-term anticoagulation may help further complications.

PV Thrombosis and Stenosis
PV thrombosis (PVT) and stenosis occur in 3.2 and 4% of LT, with a higher incidence after LLS LT particularly for BA and usually involving the extrahepatic PV trunk. Early PVT may be asymptomatic for the first day or two but develop gastrointestinal bleeding from the jejuno-jejunal anastomosis, rising INR and increasing ascites (occasionally chylous). If it extends into the liver, hepatic dysfunction may become evident, with rising transaminases which may progress to liver failure. If the extrahepatic PV is involved, collaterals may develop with normalization of liver function. With clinical stabilization, the INR does not fall below 1.4, the platelet count is low, and signs of portal hypertension persist. Risk factors for PVT include discrepancy in caliber between donor and recipient PV (atrophic or pre-duodenal PV associated with BA), the length of PV, twisting, technical failure, and graft rotation [63]. Doppler ultrasound and/or CT angiography will identify the problem. Early diagnosis and surgical correction will rescue the situation. Care must be taken to remove all the clot in the native PV and SMV. If PVT is recognized late, when collateralization has developed and liver function is normal then intervention can be avoided. If there are late complications from persistent portal hypertension then a Rex or systemic shunt should be attempted. Liver biopsy should be performed prior to surgery to identify any changes such as nodular regenerative hyperplasia which may

influence the surgical decision. A recent analysis of PV complications in 521 pediatric LDLTs identified thrombosis or stenosis in 9% with six graft losses with early complications [63]. The incidence of PV complications within 3 months of LT was 1.7% and body weight of less than 6 kg was the main risk factor on multivariate analysis. In this series, early PV complications had to be recognized early and corrected surgically to avoid graft loss. The platelet count was a valuable indicator of portal hypertension and late PV complications.

Porto-mesenteric venous occlusion is a relative contraindication to LT. If there is a large varix or an isolated vein then a jump graft may be sufficient to revascularize the liver. Many of these patients are young adults with the Janus kinase 2 (JAK-2) mutation, the risk of further thrombosis is high and coagulation post-transplant is essential. JAK-2 mutation is a rare cause of venous thrombosis in children. Portocaval hemitransposition has been utilized in predominantly adult recipients for extensive porto-mesenteric thrombosis; however, the incidence of primary graft nonfunction and retransplantation is high. Survival of 62% has been reported in 34 cases with relatively modest long-term follow-up [64]. Portocaval hemitransposition must be considered as a salvage option in selected cases due to the high rate of primary nonfunction and the lack of a proper experience in all the reported cases.

Arterial Complications

Hepatic artery stenosis (HAS) and thrombosis (HAT) occur in up to 14 and 7% of pediatric LTs, respectively [65]. The mean incidence of early HAT has been reported to be 8.3%. A higher incidence of HAT after adult LT has been reported from lower-volume centers (5.8% with <30 LT cases/year vs. 3.2% with >30 LT cases/year). No data are available for the performance of individual surgeons with respect to the number of LT procedures performed or center activity.

Early HAT is silent and can be identified by daily postoperative Doppler ultrasound before the development of complications. HAT should be suspected if there is a fever or a positive blood culture for a gram-negative organism in the first month after LT [66]. If HAT is unrecognized, then the subsequent clinical course will depend on the potential for and the efficiency of developing a collateral arterial circulation and supervening infection within the compromised biliary tree. Liver dysfunction may occur with modest transaminitis and subsequent cholestasis. The clinical picture can mimic early rejection. With the development of parenchymal ischemia, the transaminitis becomes more pronounced. Increasing cholestasis and the onset of cholangitis mark the development of significant biliary ischemia and cholangiolitic abscesses with associated parenchymal necrosis; if untreated, it progresses to liver failure and death. A more protracted course of recurrent cholangitis and chronic ill health is less common. The pathognomonic sign of HAT

is the development of a nonanastomotic/complex biliary stricture, most commonly at the hilum. The ischemic biliary tree sheds damaged biliary epithelium, and densely adherent casts form on the ulcerated surfaces. These casts and duct ischemia predispose the patient to recurrent cholangitis and obstructions with the development of biliary abscesses and liver infarction.

Factors influencing collateralization are poorly understood, but include the site of the arterial thrombosis (the closer it is to the hilum, the more likely), the graft type (split/reduced grafts may be more likely to collateralize than whole livers), Roux-en-Y hepatico-jejunostomy, multiple arteries, and the timing after LT (patients with a later occurrence are more likely to survive). The overall mortality rate for patients with early HAT has been estimated to be as high as 33%. Just more than half of the recipients with early HAT lose their grafts [67]. The clinical burden of retransplantation and the use of precious grafts to salvage these patients are high and are mirrored by the escalating financial costs.

The surgical causes of early HAT include retrieval injuries (e.g., intimal tears, dissection, and hematoma), technical problems with anastomotic stenosis or kinking and small or multiple arteries requiring arterial reconstruction, and use of arterial conduits [68]. Other reported risk factors have included split liver grafts, DCD and neonatal donors, cytomegalovirus (CMV)-negative recipient, long cold ischemia, large liver (graft-to-recipient body weight ratio >3–4%), small-for-size liver (graft-to-recipient body weight ratio <0.8%), and blood group ABO incompatibility. Retransplantation is also associated with a higher incidence of HAT from both surgical and nonsurgical complications. Nonsurgical factors contributing to HAT include procoagulant states such as JAK-2, anticardiolipin antibodies, factor V Leiden deficiency, and a high hematocrit during the early postoperative course. Procoagulant states may also be associated with particular liver diseases such as autoimmune disease and sclerosing cholangitis, high ascitic drain loss, and use of drugs such as aprotinin and tranexamic acid. Vessel fragility associated with alpha-1-antitrypsin deficiency also increases the risk of HAT.

Interventions for early HAT include urgent revascularization with thrombectomy, vascular anastomosis revision, and thrombolytic drug therapy. Traditionally, the choice was urgent retransplantation or conservative management. In a comprehensive review of HAT, Bekker et al. looked at outcomes after various interventions in adults and children [65]. Revascularization was attempted in 54% of children with an overall success rate of 56%. A correlation was noted between early intervention and successful outcome. Daily ultrasound examinations for the first week were associated with early recognition and better outcomes (66 vs. 45%). Children were more likely than adults to have a successful outcome after early revascularization (61% of adults and 92% of children). Retransplantation was performed for rescue in up to 62% of children with a mortality rate of at least 30%.

Early HAS has also been recognized as a predisposing risk for both HAT and graft ischemia/loss. Risk factors include clamp injury, intimal trauma caused by perfusion catheters, technical, intimal hyperplasia, and severe rejection. In a recent study by Sommacale et al., in adults, of 37 patients treated by transluminal radiological intervention, hepatic artery patency was 94.6% with 5-year graft and patient survival rates of 82 and 87%, respectively, at median follow-up of 66 months. Repeat interventions were helpful in 20% of treated recipients with an overall incidence of HAT of 11% [69]. The use of Doppler ultrasound to identify HAS with a tardus parvus waveform (defined as a waveform with a resistive index <0.5 and a systolic acceleration time <0.08 s) has been associated with a low positive predictive value and a high false-positive rate [70]. When combined with an optimal peak systolic velocity of 48 cm/s, it has an improved specificity of 99% and a positive predictive rate of 88% with a false-positive rate of 1%. The early identification of tardus parvus with appropriate interventions may reduce the incidence of subsequent thrombosis. Further data are needed for children with HAS.

The management of early HAT is based on the appearance of the liver on CT angiography which will confirm thrombosis and reveal the presence of parenchymal ischemia. If the serum transaminases are normal and there is no parenchymal ischemia, then revascularization should be attempted with or without accompanying thrombolysis [71]. If there is significant transaminitis or definite parenchymal ischemia on CT, then revascularization may produce a significant reperfusion injury that may endanger the child. Late recognition should be managed conservatively with rescue retransplantation for those developing ischemic complications. The routine performance of retransplantation for all cases of early HAT is not indicated in an era of organ shortages. Further research is required to understand and reduce the incidence of early HAT and to improve outcomes.

Biliary Complications

Biliary complications remain a significant problem after LT with an incidence of 11–38% [72]. Factors associated with biliary complications include anatomical variations of biliary anatomy, ischemia, technical failure, DCD grafts, ABO incompatibility, and CMV infection. The commonest early complication is biliary leak which may be anastomotic or nonanastomotic. Anastomotic leaks are usually due to technical failure, but aberrant right posterior sectoral ducts may be missed. Nonanastomotic leaks are only seen with segmental grafts and usually represent missed segment IV or segment I ducts. Strictures may be early or late and occur at anastomotic or nonanastomotic sites [72]. Most anastomotic strictures are secondary to technical failure or scar tissue causing retraction and narrowing of the CBD at the suture site, although ischemia may also be a factor. Anastomotic strictures will require surgical or radiologic intervention. Strictures occurring within the first year after LT will usually respond to percutaneous dilatation. Nonanastomotic strictures are probably caused by bile duct ischemia due to arterial insufficiency. This ischemic phenomenon is responsible for the loss of the biliary epithelium, producing multiple focal areas of intrahepatic biliary duct strictures separated by dilatations. These strictures may occur anywhere in the biliary tree and if extensive inevitably lead to retransplantation. A recent report of 126 LT in 108 children identified biliary complications in 30 cases, including leak (14), stricture (14), necrosis (9), and biliary occlusion caused by a drain (1) [72]. Fifty-six percent of those with complications required surgery. Serum gamma-glutamyl transferase (GGT) peak value in the first week (358.8±283.7 vs. 251.3±194 U/L) was considered a good early noninvasive marker to identify recipients at risk of biliary complications. In contrast, Anderson et al. reported 66 LT, of whom 17 (26%) developed biliary complications that required intervention [73]. The stricture rate was 16% for whole, 27% for split, and 43% for LDLT and none after reduced-size grafts. Sixteen patients were treated with percutaneous biliary dilatation, and one was treated with endoscopic stenting with complete resolution in 12 (71%). The remainder underwent surgical correction. Nonanastomotic or diffuse biliary strictures are associated with hepatic artery thrombosis, preservation injury and transplantation with ABO-incompatible grafts, and invariably come to retransplantation.

Other Surgical Complications

Bowel perforation is a rare complication except in children with BA who have undergone previous surgery when the incidence is 15%. Division of adhesions, portal hypertension, use of diathermy, CMV enteritis, sepsis, use of inotropes, steroids, and malnutrition have all been implicated. Paralysis of the right diaphragm due to a phrenic nerve injury at surgery may occasionally be the cause of failure to wean from the ventilator despite excellent gas exchange and a "normal" chest X-ray. Diaphragmatic hernia has been reported in up to 2% of LTs and has been associated with the use of LLS grafts, young children, ascites, and large for size grafts. The hernias may contain small and large bowel and should be repaired promptly to avoid ischemic complications.

Retransplantation

Retransplantation is needed in 15% of children, although the incidence has fallen consistently over 20 years. Hepatic artery thrombosis accounts for 50% of cases, and patient survival of 82% has been reported with elective versus 46%

emergency retransplantation. Retransplantation for primary nonfunction or in the setting of multiorgan failure has a survival of less than 30%. However, retransplantation has made a significant contribution to overall survival in children undergoing LT [74].

Nonsurgical Complications

Infections

Infection is a common complication of LT. The majority of transplant recipients will have at least one episode of infection in the postoperative recovery period, particularly if transplanted for ALF, if there is persistence of graft dysfunction or following steroid therapy for acute rejection. Bacterial pneumonia is the most common infection in the first week. Gram-positive line infections occur from 5 days onwards, and venous access must be changed regularly. Gram-negative sepsis is often associated with biliary leak, bowel perforation, or graft ischemia. Immunosuppressive therapy may minimize clinical signs of sepsis. Late opportunistic bacterial infections including legionellosis, nocardiosis, and tuberculosis may also occur particularly in those children who have received higher levels of IS. Of 2291 children (<18 years) reported by Shepherd et al., infection was the primary cause of death in 3.1% of all recipients, primarily due to bacterial sepsis (56%), with viral and fungal infection accounting for 19 and 10%, respectively, of infection deaths [75]. Infection contributed to death in patients dying from multiorgan and cardiopulmonary failure. Infection directly or indirectly contributed to 46% of all deaths. Viral infections tend to occur later than bacterial, and the overall incidence of CMV disease was 6%, Epstein–Barr virus (EBV) disease 8.6%, and lymphoproliferative disease (PTLD) 2.7%. Multivariate analysis showed that risk factors for bacterial infection included age (infants vs. adolescents), race (black and Hispanic vs. white), IS (cyclosporin vs. tacrolimus), year of LT (before 2001 vs. after 2001), serum bilirubin level, and organ donor type (DD-S or reduced-size). Risk factors for viral infection were treated acute rejection, era of transplant (before 2001), and organ donor variants (split or reduced-size, i.e., older donors). The risk from infection exceeds that of rejection, particularly in infants, who have three times the rate of bacterial or fungal infection than adolescents. Infection was the most common cause of death with a tenfold greater risk of death from infection than from rejection (3.1 vs. 0.2% of patients; 46 vs. 4.7% of deaths, $p < 0.001$).

Fungal infections particularly *Candida* respond to treatment with fluconazole or amphotericin B, but invasive aspergillosis may be fatal. Fungal sepsis is particularly common in children with ALF or bowel perforation and they must receive appropriate prophylaxis. Atypical pneumonia due to *Pneumocystis carinii* should be considered if hypoxia is present and treated with high-dose septrin. Central nervous system infection with toxoplasmosis is rare and should be treated with pyrimethamine/sulfadiazine or high-dose penicillin.

Herpes viruses form the most important viral pathogens post-transplant. Herpes simplex and varicella-zoster infections occur within 1 and 3 months, respectively post-transplant and both respond to early treatment with acyclovir. CMV infection occurs between 2 and 6 weeks post-transplant and should be treated by a reduction of IS and ganciclovir. High-risk cases, for example, CMV-positive donor and recipient are routinely given prophylactic ganciclovir. CMV hepatitis presents with flu-like symptoms, high fever, and relative neutropenia with a mild rise in serum transaminases. Serology is of limited value and has been replaced by diagnostic tests which monitor levels of antigenemia or CMV DNA.

Lymphoproliferative Disease and Epstein–Barr Infection

EBV infection may occur as a primary infection from a positive donor or reactivation of a previous infection [76]. It presents with a spectrum ranging from a mononucleosis-like illness to a malignant lymphoma. The presence of unexplained persistent fever, anemia, and positive fecal occult bloods is suggestive of PTLD and should prompt endoscopy and CT examinations. Young, previously EBV-negative children appear to be particularly at risk of developing EBV-related PTLD. The overall incidence is 2%, but may be as high as 5–10% in children less than 1 year. It is a life-threatening complication with 35% mortality [77]. Risk factors include primary EBV infection, age at LT, type and intensity of IS, and CMV infection [78]. Because most children have not been exposed to EBV, they are particularly susceptible to acute infection, and in combination with IS they are at high risk of developing PTLD. Infants have ten times the rate of PTLD of adolescents presumably because they are EBV and CMV naïve and have an immature immune system. Some PTLD will regress with IS reduction and steroid therapy; however, rituximab has become the main stay of therapy with systemic chemotherapy being reserved for children not responding to therapy.

An individualized approach to the prevention of EBV disease and PTLD is helpful in infants, given their risk. EBV polymerase chain reaction (PCR) monitoring identifies children with increasing viral load and allows for IS reduction, but this is not specific for PTLD. The therapeutic value of preventive use of antiviral therapies (e.g., ganciclovir or acyclovir) remains unproven. However, the improved awareness of PTLD and EBV monitoring has led to earlier diagnosis with less systemic involvement resulting in a more favorable outcomes [79].

Graft and Patient Survival

Over the past four decades, there has been progressive improvement in outcome after LT. According to data from UNOS, adjusted graft survival for both deceased and LDLT programs have achieved excellent survival rates in children. Patient survival at 1 year after elective LT should be in excess of 95 % and for ALF approximately 80 % and of the order of 80 and 70 % at 10 years, respectively. Graft survival has been improving with lower rates of retransplantation due to fewer technical complications and a lower incidence of chronic rejection. Concerns over the finding of significant graft fibrosis in many children at 10 years post LT have raised concerns over the longer term outlook and question whether IS levels are appropriate [80]. It has been shown that increasing IS in the presence of fibrosis does lead to improvement in the liver fibrosis. Long-term outcomes are similar for all children except for the very young <3 months and adolescents. The reasons for the poorer outcomes for adolescents are not clear and require further research.

Quality of Life

The improved long-term outcomes are turning attention to quality of life of survivors. Quality of life is difficult to measure, especially in children. Studies show that most children surviving more than 1 year post LT were able to return to school [31]. Quality of life is dependent on good graft function and an absence of recurring medical complications requiring repeated hospital admission.

Overall quality of life seems to be satisfactory in children with good graft function. Growth and social and physical development is normal in the absence of liver diseases such as Alagille. Alonso et al. on behalf of the (SPLIT group studied 873 children surviving at least 12 months, mean age of 8.17 ± 4.43 years (from 22 centers) [81]. Using a 23-item PedsQL 4.0 (Mapi Research Institute, Lyon, France) generic core scales, which encompasses physical, emotional, social, and school functioning, they demonstrated that these children had moderately diminished health-related quality of life (HRQOL) as compared with healthy peers. The largest difference was noted in the area of school functioning, with days missed from school being important from the perspective of children and their parents. Comparisons in HRQOL in this study with children with cancer revealed that both populations shared similar struggles in social and school functioning areas.

Some effect has been noted on cognitive function; however, motor developmental delay may be due to chronic illness. Parents often comment that their child is active and plays well and is able to do physical activities. Overall family interactions and school behavior also improve. Parents

may view themselves as more relaxed and being able to be more balanced and consistent in applying discipline. Siblings behave more appropriately, but may remain resentful toward the recipient. For many families, there is difficulty in adjusting to the new situation of having a well rather than ill child. There remain long-term anxieties about the child's prognosis and well-being over. The child is used to taking a disproportionate amount of the parents' time and attention at the expense of other siblings and trying to restore "fairness" can cause problems. Behavioral immaturity may persist, and acts of defiance or aggression are sometimes seen particularly in teenage years. There is continuing parental concern over rejection, side effects of IS, of being overprotective, continuing medical and "social" expenses, and changes to family dynamics. Parents who have devoted their energies into the care of a chronically ill child sometimes interrupting their professional life may find it difficult to adjust to their new role within the family with a "well" child [82]. Anxieties about children going to school and being separated from their parents after many years of dependence can also cause problems [83]. However, these challenges can be addressed with continuing follow-up and support from health-care professionals within the transplant network.

Transition to Adolescence and Young Adult Life: Adulthood

The most difficult step in long-term follow-up is the transition from childhood, and LT recipients require specific care, attention, and support. Life cannot be considered to be normal because of the need to take IS and lifestyle restrictions regarding alcohol. The appearance of conflict between recipient and their parents may become problematic. Maintaining a healthy relationship will improve adherence and the quality of life of the recipient. Adolescent and young adults are concerned about their appearance and complications such as acne, hirsutism and gum hypertrophy may lead to non-adherence unless IS is changed to help. Nephrotoxicity is a significant problem and by 10 years post LT, up to 5 % of recipients may have developed end-stage renal failure which has a major bearing on long-term follow-up.

An increased incidence of graft loss in adolescence has consistently been linked to non-adherence and has become a leading cause of late death in this population. Annunziato et al. [84] examined adherence during transition and compared it with pediatric and adult cohorts. Adherence was significantly poorer in the adolescent cohort versus pediatric, and adult cohorts. The increase in non-adherence was due to a number of factors: Pediatric clinics have a more "hands-on" approach to treatment; changes in insurance status may be associated with a lapse in attendance and IS usage; and the stress of transitioning to less familiar providers may exacerbate existing individual and familial risk factors compromise adherence. Subsequently, the same group tested a pilot intervention of facilitating transition [85]. Twenty-two patients were enrolled in a two-session educational program providing details of their underlying liver disease and treatment. A second component focused on educating families regarding the transition of health-care responsibility to the recipient facilitated by a clinical psychologist. This structured intervention significantly improved adherence with improvement in liver function and greater consistency of tacrolimus trough levels. Fredericks et al. also confirmed in a review that rates of non-adherence among adolescents are high, and adherence to IS is a critical factor in transition with an increased risk of poor long-term health outcomes [86]. Further research is needed to identify factors and interventions that affect long-term health outcomes in this population.

Long-Term Outlooks and Trends

Long-term survival is now achieved by large numbers of children following LT. The initial obstacles to survival, such as getting to transplant and managing IS, are being tackled, but the challenges raised by psychological, social, and health problems produced by successful transplantation are belatedly being addressed by specialist transition and adult "pediatric" services [87]. The overall life expectancy of a child undergoing LT is still to be determined. The goal remains transplantation without long-term IS, but until donor-specific tolerance can be safely produced, there will continue to be complications from IS therapy. As the majority of children are under 5 years of age at the time of transplant, continuing specialist care and education must be provided, particularly during adolescence and young adult life, when life's challenges may threaten well-being and non-adherence to medication. It is important that pediatric liver transplant recipients are able complete their education, have employment and families of their own and in the future these factors may influence the timing of transplantation. The challenge is to ensure children undergoing LT can be restored to a normal life expectancy with the potential to enjoy life to the full.

References

1. Starzl TE, Marchioro TL, Vonkaulla KN, Hermann G, Brittain RS, Waddell WR. Homotransplantation of the liver in humans. Surg Gynecol Obstet. 1963;117:659–76.
2. Starzl TE, Groth CG, Brettschneider L, Moon JB, Fulginiti VA, Cotton EK, Porter KA. Extended survival in 3 cases of orthotopic homotransplantation of the human liver. Surgery. 1968;63:549–63.
3. http://www.eltr.org ELTRE. Results of Pediatric Liver Transplantation in Europe.
4. Hartley JL, Davenport M, Kelly DA. Biliary atresia. Lancet. 2009;374:1704–13.
5. Serinet MO, Broue P, Jacquemin E, Lachaux A, Sarles J, Gottrand F, Gauthier F, et al. Management of patients with biliary atresia in France: results of a decentralized policy 1986–2002. Hepatology. 2006;44:75–84.
6. Davenport M, De Ville de Goyet J, Stringer MD, Mieli-Vergani G, Kelly DA, McClean P, Spitz L. Seamless management of biliary atresia in England and Wales (1999–2002). Lancet. 2004;363:1354–7.
7. Barshes NR, Lee TC, Balkrishnan R, Karpen SJ, Carter BA, Goss JA. Orthotopic liver transplantation for biliary atresia: the U.S. experience. Liver Transpl. 2005;11:1193–200.
8. Uchida Y, Kasahara M, Egawa H, Takada Y, Ogawa K, Ogura Y, Uryuhara K, et al. Long-term outcome of adult-to-adult living donor liver transplantation for post-Kasai biliary atresia. Am J Transplant. 2006;6:2443–8.
9. Broide E, Farrant P, Reid F, Baker A, Meire H, Rela M, Davenport M, Heaton N, Mieli-Vergani G. Increased hepatic artery resistance index predicsts early death in children with biliary atresia. Liver Transpl Surg. 1997;3:604–10.
10. Sze YK, Dhawan A, Taylor RM, Bansal S, Mieli-Vergani G, Rela M, Heaton N. Pediatric liver transplantation for metabolic liver disease: experience at King's College Hospital. Transplantation. 2009;87:87–93.
11. Kayler LK, Rasmussen CS, Dykstra DM, Punch JD, Rudich SM, Magee JC, Maraschio MA, et al. Liver transplantation in children with metabolic disorders in the United States. Am J Transplant. 2003;3:334–9.
12. Faraj W, Dar F, Marangoni G, Bartlett A, Melendez HV, Hadzic D, Dhawan A, et al. Liver transplantation for hepatoblastoma. Liver Transpl. 2008;14:1614–9.
13. Beaunoyer M, Vanatta JM, Ogihara M, Strichartz D, Dahl G, Berquist WE, Castillo RO, et al. Outcomes of transplantation in children with primary hepatic malignancy. Pediatr Transplant. 2007;11:655–60.
14. Kosola S, Lauronen J, Sairanen H, Heikinheimo M, Jalanko H, Pakarinen M. High survival rates after liver transplantation for hepatoblastoma and hepatocellular carcinoma. Pediatr Transplant. 2010;14:646–50.
15. Guiteau JJ, Cotton RT, Karpen SJ, O'Mahony CA, Goss JA. Pediatric liver transplantation for primary malignant liver tumors with a focus on hepatic epithelioid hemangioendothelioma: the UNOS experience. Pediatr Transplant. 2019;14:326–31.
16. Spada M, Riva S, Maggiore G, Cintorino D, Gridelli B. Pediatric liver transplantation. World J Gastroenterol. 2009;15:648–74.
17. Squires RH, Jr, Shneider BL, Bucuvalas J, Alonso E, Sokol RJ, Narkewicz MR, Dhawan A, et al. Acute liver failure in children: the first 348 patients in the pediatric acute liver failure study group. J Pediatr. 2006;148:652–8.
18. Farmer DG, Venick RS, McDiarmid SV, Duffy JP, Kattan O, Hong JC, Vargas J, et al. Fulminant hepatic failure in children: superior and durable outcomes with liver transplantation over 25 years at a single center. Ann Surg. 2009;250:484–93.
19. Mahadeb P, Gras J, Sokal E, Otte JB, Lerut J, Detaille T, de Clety SC, et al. Liver transplantation in children with fulminant hepatic failure: the UCL experience. Pediatr Transplant. 2009;13:414–20.
20. Ciria R, Sanchez-Hidalgo JM, Briceno J, Naranjo A, Pleguezuelo M, Diaz-Nieto R, Luque A, et al. Establishment of a pediatric liver transplantation program: experience with 100 transplantation procedures. Transplant Proc. 2009;41:2444–6.
21. Shanmugan NP, Bansal S, Greenough A, Verma A, Dhawan A. Neonatal liver failure: etiologies and management. State of art. Eur J Pediatr. 2011;170:573–81.

22. McDiarmid SV, Anand R, Lindblad AS. Development of a pediatric end-stage liver disease score to predict poor outcome in children awaiting liver transplantation. Transplantation. 2002;74:173–81.

23. Freeman RB, Jr, Wiesner RH, Roberts JP, McDiarmid S, Dykstra DM, Merion RM. Improving liver allocation: MELD and PELD. Am J Transplant. 2004;4 Suppl 9:114–31.

24. Cowles RA, Lobritto SJ, Ventura KA, Harren PA, Gelbard R, Emond JC, Altman RP, et al. Timing of liver transplantation in biliary atresia-results in 71 children managed by a multidisciplinary team. J Pediatr Surg. 2008;43:1605–9.

25. Shinkai M, Ohhama Y, Take H, Fukuzato Y, Fujita S, Nishi T. Evaluation of the PELD risk score as a severity index of biliary atresia. J Pediatr Surg. 2003;38:1001–4.

26. Shneider BL, Neimark E, Frankenberg T, Arnott L, Suchy FJ, Emre S. Critical analysis of the pediatric end-stage liver disease scoring system: a single center experience. Liver Transpl. 2005;11:788–95.

27. Barshes NR, Lee TC, Udell IW, O'Mahoney C A, Karpen SJ, Carter BA, Goss JA. The pediatric end-stage liver disease (PELD) model as a predictor of survival benefit and posttransplant survival in pediatric liver transplant recipients. Liver Transpl. 2006;12: 75–480.

28. Magee JC, Feng S. PELD: working well, but only half of the time? Am J Transplant. 2005;5:1785–6.

29. Sindhi R, Soltys K, Bond G, Marcos A, Mazariegos G. PELD allocation and acute liver/graft failure. Liver Transpl. 2007;13:776–7.

30. Roberts JP, Hulbert-Shearon TE, Merion RM, Wolfe RA, Port FK. Influence of graft type on outcomes after pediatric liver transplantation. Am J Transplant. 2004;4:373–7.

31. Oswari H, Lynch SV, Fawcett J, Strong RW, Ee LC. Outcomes of split versus reduced-size grafts in pediatric liver transplantation. J Gastroenterol Hepatol. 2005;20:1850–4.

32. Hong JC, Yersiz H, Farmer DG, Duffy JP, Ghobrial RM, Nonthasoot B, Collins TE, et al. Longterm outcomes for whole and segmental liver grafts in adult and pediatric liver transplant recipients: a 10-year comparative analysis of 2,988 cases. J Am Coll Surg. 2009;208:682–9; discusion 689–691.

33. Diamond IR, Fecteau A, Millis JM, Losanoff JE, Ng V, Anand R, Song C. Impact of graft type on outcome in pediatric liver transplantation: a report from studies of pediatric liver transplantation (SPLIT). Ann Surg. 2007;246:301–10.

34. Merion RM, Rush SH, Dykstra DM, Goodrich N, Freeman RB, Jr., Wolfe RA. Predicted lifetimes for adult and pediatric split liver versus adult whole liver transplant recipients. Am J Transplant. 2004;4:1792–7.

35. Raia S, Nery JR, Mies S. Liver transplantation from live donors. Lancet. 1989;2:497.

36. Strong RW, Lynch SV, Ong TH, Matsunami H, Koido Y, Balderson GA. Successful liver transplantation from a living donor to her son. N Engl J Med. 1990;322:1505–7.

37. Broelsch CE, Whitington PF, Emond JC, Heffron TG, Thistlethwaite JR, Stevens L, Piper J, Whitington SH, Lichtor JL. Liver transplantation in children from living related donors. Surg. Tech Results Ann Surg. 1991;214:428–39.

38. Tanaka K, Uemoto S, Tokunaga Y, Fujita S, et al. Surgical techniques and innovations in living donor liver transplantation. Ann Surg. 1992;140:82–91.

39. Morioka D, Kasahara M, Takada Y, Corrales JP, Yoshizawa A, Sakamoto S, Taira K, et al. Living donor liver transplantation for pediatric patients with inheritable metabolic disorders. Am J Transplant. 2005;5:2754–63.

40. Reding R. Is it right to promote living donor liver transplantation for fulminant hepatic failure in pediatric recipients? Am J Transplant. 2005;5:1587–91.

41. Welch CS. A note on transplantation of the whole liver in dogs. Transplant Bull. 1955;2:54–5.

42. Chenard-Neu MP, Boudjema K, Bernuau J, Degott C, Belghiti J, Cherqui D, et al. Auxiliary liver transplantation: regeneration of the native liver and outcome in 30 patients with fulminant hepatic failure–a multicenter European study. Hepatology. 1996;23(5): 1119–27.

43. van Hoek B, de Boer J, Boudjema K, Williams R, Corsmit O, Terpstra OT. Auxiliary versus orthotopic liver transplantation for acute liver failure. EURALT Study Group. European Auxiliary Liver Transplant Registry. J Hepatol. 1999;30:699–705.

44. Rela M, Muiesan P, Vilca-Melendez H, Dhawan A, Baker A, Mieli-Vergani G, Heaton ND. Auxiliary partial orthotopic liver transplantation for Crigler-Najjar syndrome type I. Ann Surg. 1999;229:565–9.

45. Faraj W, Dar F, Bartlett A, Melendez HV, Marangoni G, Mukherji D, Vergani GM, et al. Auxiliary liver transplantation for acute liver failure in children. Ann Surg. 2009;251:351–6.

46. Kato T, Selvaggi G, Levi D, Hernandez E, Takahashi H, Velasco M, et al. Routine use of auxiliary partial orthotopic liver transplantation for children with fulminant hepatic failure: preliminary report. Transplant Proc. 2006;38:3607–8.

47. Jaeck D, Boudjema K, Audet M, Chenard-Neu MP, Simeoni U, Meyer C, et al. Auxiliary partial orthotopic liver transplantation (APOLT) in the treatment of acute liver failure. J Gastroenterol. 2002;37 Suppl 13:88–91.

48. Quaglia A, Portmann BC, Knisely AS, Srinivasan P, Muiesan P, Wendon J, et al. Auxiliary liver transplantation for acute liver failure: histopathological study of native liver regeneration. Liver Transplant. 2008;14:1437–48.

49. Bartlett A, Vara R, Muiesan P, Marriot P, Dhawan A, Miel-Vergani G, et al. A single center experience of donation after cardiac death liver transplantation in pediatric recipients. Pediatr Transplant. 2010;14:388–92.

50. Bishop GA, McCaughan GW. Immune activation is required for the induction of liver allograft tolerance: implications for immunosuppressive therapy. Liver Transpl. 2001;7:161–72.

51. Turmelle YP, Nadler ML, Anderson CD, Doyle MB, Lowell JA, Shepherd RW. Towards minimizing immunosuppression in pediatric liver transplant recipients. Pediatr Transplant. 2009;13:553–9.

52. Diem HV, Sokal EM, Janssen M, Otte JB, Reding R. Steroid withdrawal after pediatric liver transplantation: a long-term follow-up study in 109 recipients. Transplantation. 2003;75:1664–70.

53. Feng S. Long-term management of immunosuppression after pediatric liver transplantation: is minimization or withdrawal desirable or possible or both? Curr Opin Organ Transplant. 2008;13: 506–12.

54. Al-Sinani S, Dhawan A. Corticosteroids usage in pediatric liver transplantation: to be or not to be! Pediatr Transplant. 2009;13: 160–70.

55. Kerkar N, Hadzic N, Davies ET, Portmann B, Donaldson PT, Rela M, Heaton ND, et al. De-novo autoimmune hepatitis after liver transplantation. Lancet. 1998;351:409–13.

56. Vergani D, Mieli-Vergani G. Autoimmunity after liver transplantation. Hepatology. 2002;36:271–6.

57. Hasenbein W, Albani J, Englert C, Spehr A, Grabhorn E, Kemper MJ, Burdelski M, et al. Long-term evaluation of cyclosporine and tacrolimus based immunosuppression in pediatric liver transplantation. Pediatr Transplant. 2006;10:938–42.

58. Heffron TG, Pescovitz MD, Florman S, Kalayoglu M, Emre S, Smallwood G, Wisemandle K, et al. Once-daily tacrolimus extended-release formulation: 1-year post-conversion in stable pediatric liver transplant recipients. Am J Transplant. 2007;7: 1609–15.

59. Sudan DL, Shaw BW, Jr, Langnas AN. Causes of late mortality in pediatric liver transplant recipients. Ann Surg. 1998;227:289–95.

60. Tracy ET, Bennett KM, Danko ME, Diesen DL, Westmoreland TJ, Kuo PC, Pappas TN, et al. Low volume is associated with worse

patient outcomes for pediatric liver transplant centers. J Pediatr Surg. 45:108–13.

61. Berrocal T, Parron M, Alvarez-Luque A, Prieto C, Santamaria ML. Pediatric liver transplantation: a pictorial essay of early and late complications. Radiographics. 2006;26:1187–209.

62. Sakamoto S, Ogura Y, Shibata T, Haga H, Ogawa K, Oike F, Ueda M, et al. Successful stent placement for hepatic venous outflow obstruction in pediatric living donor liver transplantation, including a case series review. Pediatr Transplant. 2009;13:507–11.

63. Ueda M, Oike F, Kasahara M, Ogura Y, Ogawa K, Haga H, Takada Y, et al. Portal vein complications in pediatric living donor liver transplantation using left-side grafts. Am J Transplant. 2008;8:2097–105.

64. Lipshutz GS, Patel S, Hiatt JR, Yersiz H, Farmer DG, McDiarmid SV, Ghobrial RM, et al. Portocaval hemitransposition in pediatric liver transplant recipients: a single-center experience. Liver Transpl. 2006;12:1097–103.

65. Bekkera J, Ploemb S, de Jong JP. Early hepatic artery thrombosis after liver transplantation: a systematic review of the incidence, outcome and risk factors. Am J Transplant. 2009;9:746–57.

66. Siders E, Peeters PM, TenVergert EM, de Jong KP, Porte RJ, Zwavelng JH, et al. Early vascular complications after pediatric liver transplantation. Liver Transplant. 2000;6:326–32.

67. Stringer MD, Marshall MM, Muiesan P, Karani JB, Kane PA, Mieli-Vergani G, et al. Survival and outcome after after hepatic artery thrombosis complicating pediatric transplantation. J Pediatr Surg. 2001;36:888–91.

68. Oh CK, Pelletier SJ, Sawyer RG, Dacus AR, McCullough CS, Pruett TL, et al. Uni- and multivariate analysis of risk factors for early and late hepatic artery thrombosis after liver trasplantation. Transplantation. 2001;71:767–72.

69. Sommerscale D, Aoyagi T, Dondero F, Silbert A, Bruno O, Fteriche S, et al. Repeat endovascular treatment of recurring hepatic artery stenoses in orthotopic liver transplantation. Transpl Int. 2013;26:608–15.

70. Dodd GD, III, Memel DS, Zajko AB, Baron RL, Santaguida LA. Hepatic artery stenosis and thrombosis in transplant recipients: doppler diagnosis with resistive index and systolic acceleration time. Radiology. 1994;192:657–61.

71. Otte J-B. Approach to avoid and to manage vascular thrombosis and stenosis in pediatric liver transplantation. Pediatr Transplant. 2007;11:124–6.

72. Oliveira P. Biliary complications after paediatric liver transplantation. Pediatr Transplant. 2010;14:358–63.

73. Anderson CD, Turmelle YP, Darcy M, Shepherd RW, Weymann A, Nadler M, Guelker S, et al. Biliary strictures in pediatric liver transplant recipients – Early diagnosis and treatment results in excellent graft outcomes. Pediatr Transplant. 2010;14:437–8.

74. Despande PR, Rela M, Girlanda R, Bowles MJ, Muiesan P, Dhawan A, et al. Long term outcome of retransplantation in children. Transplantation. 2002;74:1124–30.

75. Shepherd RW, Turmelle Y, Nadler M, Lowell JA, Narkewicz MR, McDiarmid SV, Anand R, et al. Risk factors for rejection and infection in pediatric liver transplantation. Am J Transplant. 2008;8:396–403.

76. Holmes RD, Sokol RJ. Epstein-Barr virus and post-transplant lymphoproliferative disease. Pediatr Transplant. 2002;6:456–64.

77. Molmenti EP, Nagata DE, Roden JS, Squires RH, Molmenti H, Fasola CG, Winick N, et al. Post-transplant lymphoproliferative syndrome in the pediatric liver transplant population. Am J Transplant. 2001;1:356–9.

78. Fernandez MC, Bes D, De Davila M, Lopez S, Cambaceres C, Dip M, Imventarza O. Post-transplant lymphoproliferative disorder after pediatric liver transplantation: characteristics and outcome. Pediatr Transplant. 2009;13:307–10.

79. Green M. Management of Epstein-Barr virus-induced post-transplant lymphoproliferative disease in recipients of solid organ transplantation. Am J Transplant. 2001;1:103–8.

80. Scheenstra R, Peeters PM, Verkade HJ, Gouw AS. Graft fibrosis after pediatric liver transplantation. Ten years of follow up. Hepatology. 2009;49:0–6.

81. Alonso EM, Limbers CA, Neighbors K, Martz K, Bucuvalas JC, Webb T, Varni JW. Cross-sectional analysis of health-related quality of life in pediatric liver transplant recipients. J Pediatr. 156:270–6 e271.

82. Mendes AM, Bousso RS. Not being able to live like before: the family dynamics during the experience of pediatric liver transplantation. Rev Lat Am Enfermagem. 2009;17:74–80.

83. Maikranz JM, Steele RG, Dreyer ML, Stratman AC, Bovaird JA. The relationship of hope and illness-related uncertainty to emotional adjustment and adherence among pediatric renal and liver transplant recipients. J Pediatr Psychol. 2007;32:571–81.

84. Annunziato RA, Emre S, Shneider B, Barton C, Dugan CA, Shemesh E. Adherence and medical outcomes in pediatric liver transplant recipients who transition to adult services. Pediatr Transplant. 2007;11:608–14.

85. Annunziato RA, Emre S, Shneider BL, Dugan CA, Aytaman Y, McKay MM, Shemesh E. Transitioning health care responsibility from caregivers to patient: a pilot study aiming to facilitate medication adherence during this process. Pediatr Transplant. 2008;12:309–15.

86. Fredericks EM. Nonadherence and the transition to adulthood. Liver Transpl. 2009;15 Suppl 2:S63–9.

87. Neuberger JM. Transition of care between paediatric and adult gastroenterology. Liver transplantation. Best Pract Res Clin Gastroenterol. 2003;17:277–89.

Marianne Samyn and Anna Hames

Introduction

As the survival of children with liver disease has significantly changed over the past few decades, with the development of pediatric liver transplantation and improved medical and nutritional management, a large cohort of patients is now moving into adolescence and adulthood with a liver condition. This has brought its own challenges related to the condition and the management of it, combined with the challenges young people face during adolescence. Due to the unique challenges that this growing population face for both pediatric and adult services, our centre has a specialist multidisciplinary approach to managing young people with liver disease as they transition into adulthood. In this chapter, we, as physician and clinical psychologist, will give an overview of the interaction of physical development during puberty and liver disease, as well as the psychosocial and health behaviour aspects of adolescence. Transition of medical care from pediatric to an adult-based setting will have a significant impact on the patient and their support network, especially in patients with special health needs. This is also discussed.

Young People

The World Health Organization recognizes that 'young people' aged between 10 and 24 years are a population who require dedicated care [1]. Having a chronic condition or disability has multiple effects on adolescent development including biological, psychosocial and social effects that can

in turn contribute to poor adherence and risk-taking behaviours [2]. Non-adherence to medication is a particular challenge in the adolescent population as it is difficult to measure, often multifactorial; however, relatively developmentally appropriate. Its prevalence is reported to exceed 50 % in the post-transplant population [3] and effects long-term outcome in this patient population. Adolescence coincides with transfer of medical care from pediatric to adult-centred services, hence the importance of defining a dedicated, individualized transition care pathway for young people. This will be discussed in more detail further in the chapter.

Medical Aspects of Growing Up with Liver Disease

Within pediatrics, liver disease is a relatively new specialty within which the past few decades have seen a significant change in the diagnosis and management of conditions. Patients tend to present in infancy or later childhood with a variety of genetic and incidental conditions, either in an acute, often life threatening, or more chronic setting. Lifelong specialist follow-up and treatment is usually required. The development of pediatric liver transplantation has had a significant impact on the outcome and prognosis of children developing end-stage liver disease or presenting with acute liver failure, and the majority of the patients are now moving into adolescence and adulthood. This emerging population is a challenge for both pediatric and adult hepatology teams.

Information on the long-term outcome of patients with liver disease presenting in infancy, such as biliary atresia and Alagille syndrome, is becoming available but is still scarce and more focused on survival data. It is estimated that 23–52 % of patients with biliary atresia now survive into adulthood without needing liver transplantation. This was confirmed in our recent series [4]; 34 % of our patient cohort is alive with their native liver at a median age of 20.6 years (range 16–32 years), with 9 % showing no evidence of chronic liver disease. Indication criteria and timing for trans-

M. Samyn (✉)
Pediatric Liver, GI and Nutrition Centre, King's College Hospital,
Denmark Hill, London SE5 9RS, UK
e-mail: marianne.samyn@nhs.net

A. Hames
Institute of Liver Studies, King's College Hospital, London, UK

© Springer International Publishing Switzerland 2016
S. Guandalini et al. (eds.), *Textbook of Pediatric Gastroenterology, Hepatology and Nutrition*,
DOI 10.1007/978-3-319-17169-2_74

plantation in this population might differ from standard adult liver transplant criteria and is important to keep in mind. In Alagille syndrome, extrahepatic aspects of the syndrome related to vascular or renal involvement are becoming more relevant and can impact the long-term prognosis [5, 6].

Other conditions such as autoimmune liver disease, Wilson disease and non-alcoholic fatty liver disease tend to present more frequently during adolescence and patients will have to come in terms with their condition and management during an already challenging time in their life.

The advances in molecular genetics are now enabling us to diagnose genetic liver conditions such as familial intrahepatic cholestasis and other rarer metabolic conditions such as mitochondrial cytopathies, etc. The implications of dealing with a genetically based condition can have an additional impact on coming to terms with the diagnosis for both patients and families and have further long-term implications on adult life and prognosis.

Outcome Data

The majority of outcome data on patients with childhood liver disease are available from the liver transplant population. Survival rates are fairly similar for different age groups until 5 years following liver transplant, but show poorer patient and graft survival after 10 years for those transplanted between the ages of 12 and 17 years (74 and 62%, respectively) compared to the younger patients (1–5 years; 84 and 72%, respectively) [7]. Young people constitute a unique and vulnerable cohort who deserves special attention by health professionals focusing on better outcome and survival. In the non-transplant setting, a recent report on predictors of poor outcome in a cohort of 133 patients with autoimmune hepatitis aged 14 and over found that presentation between the ages of 14 and 20 years was a significant independent predictor of liver-related death or requirement for liver transplantation, suggesting that their condition was more challenging to manage compared to the older population [8]. Data from the renal transplant community support this, with patients receiving their first kidney transplant between the ages of 14 and 16 years being at the highest risk of graft loss with inferior outcomes at 1, 3, 5 and 10 years post-transplant. The risk was higher in black adolescents, in patients with deceased donors compared to living donors and governance insurance versus private insurance [9].

Impact of Liver Disease on Physical Development

Growth retardation is common in children with chronic liver conditions and more common in cholestatic liver disease, where some degree of catch up growth is noted after liver transplantation. In an analysis of growth following liver

transplantation, risk factors for poor linear growth were prolonged steroid exposure, lower weight percentiles at time of transplantation, linear growth impairment pre-transplantation and metabolic disease as primary diagnosis [10]. More recently, out of a total of 892 liver transplant patients between 8 and 18 years, 20% had linear growth impairment at their last follow-up and, where available, height z scores were significantly lower than the calculated mid-parental height z scores. Linear growth impairment at transplant, re-transplantation, non-white race and primary diagnosis other than biliary atresia were found to be independent predictors of growth impairment. In the same study, the authors reported on the pubertal development of 353 children and found that 61% of girls and 58% of boys aged 16–18 years reached Tanner 5 compared to 100% of a normative population with growth impairment occurring in 11% of Tanner 5 subjects [11]. Growth impairment has also been described in genetic conditions such as Alagille syndrome. Further data are needed to establish the prevalence of growth failure and pubertal delay in chronic liver disease, but is already available in other chronic conditions such as inflammatory bowel disease, nephrotic syndrome, asthma and cystic fibrosis. Growth failure and pubertal delay can have a significant psychosocial effect on quality of life and long-term outcomes; hence, treatment of recombinant human growth hormone in this population has been reported to be associated with improvement in psychosocial functioning as well as linear growth [12]. Larger studies are needed to assess its safety in this patient population.

In girls with chronic liver disease, menstrual cycles can be irregular and amenorrhea and anovulation are common. Menorrhagia can occur in patients with advanced liver disease with portal hypertension. Estrogens, and typically the synthetically produced ethinylestradiol used in the combined hormonal preparations, are more potent with a potential effect on the liver irrespective of the route of administration. Progestogens do not have receptors on the liver cells and are commonly given at a lower dose and well tolerated.

Although not contraindicated in patients with compensated cirrhosis, in both pre- and post-liver transplant settings the current contraceptive recommendation is with progesterone-only preparations such as minipill (e.g. Cerazette), medroxyprogesterone injection or etonogestrol implants and, if sexually active, levonogestrol releasing intrauterine system [13]. Successful pregnancy outcomes have been reported in both chronic liver disease and liver transplantation settings, although with an increased risk for both mother and baby. Treatment with calcineurin inhibitors, steroids and azathioprine is recommended to be continued during pregnancy to avoid graft dysfunction or relapse in autoimmune liver disease; mycophenoic acid and rapamycin are contraindicated because of the increased risk of birth defects. In patients with portal hypertension an upper gastrointestinal (GI) endoscopy during the second half of the second trimester is indicated to assess the degree of portal hypertension and the need for further management to avoid GI bleeding during the course of pregnancy [14]. Obstetric follow-up by an experienced team in a hospital setting is required. Adolescent girls should be informed timely of the various contraceptive options, the potential complications of pregnancy and childbirth as well as the possible genetic implications of their underlying condition.

Cosmetic side effects of medical treatment, such as steroids and currently less commonly used, cyclosporine, can have an impact on body image and adherence to treatment in the adolescent population (described later in the chapter) and health professionals should keep this in mind when prescribing treatment.

In order to effectively manage young people's care, it is crucial to successfully address their wider 'medical, psychosocial and educational/vocational needs' [15]. To do this, professionals need to be familiar with the unique developmental stage of adolescence and recognize that young people are neither just 'big children' nor 'small adults'. This developmental perceptive is discussed in the next section, along with the psychosocial elements of growing up with liver disease.

Adolescent Development and Its Interaction with Liver Disease

The biopsychosocial changes associated with adolescence interact with how young people manage their illness and treatments, and accordingly how their healthcare should be approached. For an excellent review of this area, see Suris et al. [2].

Although most of the literature focuses on adolescence, research demonstrates that structural and functional changes continue to take place in the brain into young adulthood [16]. This is mirrored by changing societal norms with young people increasingly delaying many of the traditional 'tasks' of adulthood, such as financial independence and starting a family. Furthermore, health outcomes are poorer for young adults into their mid-20s [17], so it is more helpful to think about young adult development more broadly.

Adolescence is traditionally defined by the onset of puberty. Delayed puberty, reported in young people with liver disease, can impact on how the young person views themselves, their illness and their wider world. For example, an adolescent who looks younger may be treated differently by people and have reduced social opportunities. Common stories from patients include being asked by adult clinic staff whether they are there with their mum, being stopped by the police when driving to check their age and being refused entry to 18 rated films or pubs.

Alongside the physical changes are changes in how young people think and feel, and in the nature and importance of their social world. In order to become an independent adult,

the adolescent needs to separate from their parents. They start to develop a more independent sense of identity, and their peer group typically takes over from family as being their main social world [18]. Peer acceptance becomes key, with a strong desire to feel normal. Self-consciousness increases. The typical adolescent has an increased sense of invincibility, poorer abstract thinking and reduced thoughts of the future [19]. An increasing body of research demonstrates ways in which the structure and function of the adolescent's social brain is distinctly different from that of children or adults [20].

As part of this adolescent profile, risk-taking behaviours peak, with high levels of alcohol and drug use, smoking and unsafe sex [21]. In the UK, 'binge drinking' is widespread and synonymous with certain rites of passage for young people, such as the introductory 'freshers' week' at university. Young people growing up with liver disease have the same needs as other young people, with the additional challenge of trying to balance their health needs against their social and psychological needs. The way to meet these can often seem to be opposition. Indeed, research suggests that alcohol and drug use is similarly prevalent in young people with chronic illnesses as compared to their healthy peers [22], and they are equally as likely to be sexually active [23]. This adolescent profile and tendency to take risks helps young people to develop independence, but can present significant challenges for successfully managing a chronic illness. This is discussed further below under adherence.

Impact of Family

All of the above changes happen within a family context. To enable the young person to develop into an adult, their family also need to adapt their roles, for example, by giving their child more freedom and privacy [24]. Parents/carers of children with chronic illness have often dedicated much of their lives to caring for their sick child and have their own relationships with the illness and hospital teams. They might also have had to change other roles in their lives, such as giving up work, to successfully care for them. This can result in some parents seeming to be more overprotective, for example, worrying about their adolescent taking their medication, abstaining from alcohol at parties, monitoring for symptoms or appropriately seeking help [25].

There are also significant challenges for families of young people who are diagnosed with a liver disease during their adolescent years, as is common, for example, in autoimmune liver disease or Wilson disease. At a time when adolescents should be becoming more independent, the acute stage of illness forces them into a state of dependence on others. This can present challenges for the whole family that may not be expected at this stage of development [26], such as parents needing to take time off work, physically caring for their child and spending concentrated time together that might not otherwise have been expected from being the parent of a teenager or be normal amongst their peers.

Wider Influences

The above processes occur within a wider set of systems still, such as schools, workplaces, friendships and other relationships; how the liver disease is managed in any of these contexts will interact with the young person's adjustment and management of it. Furthermore, this is within a societal context in which the general public hold certain beliefs, assumptions and prejudices. As public perception of people with liver disease and transplant is most commonly associated with drug and alcohol use, young people struggle to develop a positive self-identity if they associate (or other people associate them) with this stigmatized group. Our patients often grapple with the dilemmas about whom to tell about their condition and how to tell, as many have experienced bullying or prejudiced comments in the past. It can be beneficial to discuss these dilemmas with patients and help support them in communicating their needs to schools and workplaces.

Given the importance of peer relationships during this period, it is worrying that peer networks are often disrupted in young people with chronic illness [27]. Amongst young people, post-transplant peer support has been found to be an effective means of engaging young people in services and improving their health outcomes and well being [28]. In a small recent study in which young people were trained to act as mentors for younger post-transplant patients, the mentors themselves benefited from improved adherence [29]. As part of the liver transition service at King's College Hospital, we run peer support days and peer mentoring for young people with chronic liver disease and post transplant. Preliminary feedback suggests numerous benefits of this for both young people and their mentors, including feeling more positive about having a liver condition due to increased hope and feeling less alone, as well as feeling more prepared for transition [30].

Most of the developmental models are based upon Western notions of adolescence. It is unclear how this may differ in other cultures, for example, where adolescence may not exist as a construct or notions such as independence from family are not expected or endorsed. How culture interacts with chronic illness management and transition is an under-researched area that demands further attention [31]. It is important for professionals to be curious about what the adolescence and their family expect at this stage of development rather than making assumptions about how these constructs may or may not apply.

Psychological Aspects of Growing Up with Liver Disease

Adolescence is a period of rapid change, full of opportunities and challenges. Young people growing up with chronic liver disease have the same aspirations in life as their healthy peers, but have additional stresses and restrictions to manage, including hospital visits, time off school, medication and lifestyle restrictions. Rather than focusing purely on the presence of psychological distress, it is important to consider how all young people and families adapt to their changing health needs at different stages of development. Most young people, with or without liver disease, strive to be normal [32]. Those who have difficulties adjusting to their illness/ treatment and integrating it into a positive self-identity are at increased risk of developing psychological difficulties and are less likely to manage their physical health needs effectively. Routine questions about the adolescent's wider world are crucial for engagement and in order to assess how they are adjusting to the demands of their condition and areas that may require intervention [33].

There has been relatively little research into the psychological needs of young people growing up with liver disease, and most of this limited research has focused on those post transplant. Research conducted with adults with liver disease is unlikely to be generalizable as the populations are different on multiple levels, including age and developmental stage, age at diagnosis, type of liver disease and/or reason for transplant. A brief overview of some key areas is given below, citing research specific to liver disease where it exists and otherwise extrapolating from other chronic childhood diseases.

Quality of Life

Quality of life is a broad term that encompasses a range of physical, psychological and social factors. Health-related quality of life is found to be poorer in children and young people post-liver transplant as compared with the general population, but similar to young people with other chronic conditions [25, 34, 35]. A recent study of children and adolescents with autoimmune liver disease found a similar trend, with poorer quality of life being associated with the presence of symptoms such as ascites, abdominal pain and fatigue [36].

In a qualitative study aiming to understand how liver transplant affects young people's quality of life, adolescent participants spoke about the impact of transplant on their relationships, schooling, fatigue, burden of medication, communication with health-care professionals and thinking about the future [25]. These are key areas to explore when working with young people, and demonstrate the importance of fostering good collaborative relationships with young people, in which they feel listened to, valued and their wider needs and hopes are respected.

School Achievement

A young person growing up with a chronic liver disease or transplant is more likely than healthy peers to take time off from school for hospital appointments and ill health. This can have a significant impact on their school attainment and subsequent employment opportunities in adulthood.

Data available on cognitive development in the context of pediatric liver conditions, and mainly in the post-liver transplantation setting, confirms an increased incidence of learning difficulties in this population. Out of 144 patients from the Studies of Pediatric Liver Transplantation (SPLIT) registry, children aged between 5 and 7 years and more than 2 years post-transplant, 26% were found to have a mild to moderate, and 4% a serious, cognitive delay with 25% having learning difficulties with reading and maths skills, and a relevant executive functioning deficit which would potentially affect independent management of their health condition in adult life [37]. Further research identified height centile at transplantation and genetic–metabolic conditions as having a high impact on long-term cognitive functioning [38].

There is limited information on developmental assessment and cognitive function in patients with liver disease who have not been transplanted and further multicentre studies are required in these populations. The longer-term impact of these childhood difficulties also needs to be further researched, as in clinical practice we frequently see the long-term consequences such as in Case Study 74.1.

Case Study 74.1

Harry was diagnosed with biliary atresia shortly after he was born. Following a Kasai procedure, he required regular visits to hospital for appointments and sometimes needed admission for treatment with antibiotics or endoscopy procedures as he developed portal hypertension. He was a bright, sociable child who was well liked by patients and staff. Aged 11, his health deteriorated and the decision was made to list him for liver transplantation. A year later Harry was transplanted and he recovered well after surgery. Due to time spent in hospital, he missed most of his formal education and left school without any qualifications. Harry is now 22 years old. He lives with his parents and is unemployed. He has held a number of causal jobs, but struggles to find permanent employment due to his lack of qualifications and relevant experience. Harry feels left behind by his friends, most of whom who have now been to university and started good jobs.

Mood Difficulties

Research investigating psychological well being in adolescents with chronic illness more broadly suggest that there are higher rates of depressive and anxiety symptoms relative to healthy controls, but the rates varies across studies and illness group (see metaanalysis by Pinquart and Shen [39]). Two recent studies conducted with adolescents with non-alcoholic fatty liver disease reported higher rates of depressive symptoms as compared to healthy overweight controls [40] and higher depressive and anxiety symptoms relative to healthy normal weight controls [41]. In keeping with this, a recent study we conducted with 80 young people (aged 1–24 years old) with a range of chronic liver conditions found elevated rates of self-reported difficulties with anxiety, depression and anger [42]. In this study, young people with chronic liver disease or transplant reported higher levels of body image dissatisfaction; contrary to intuition, this dissatisfaction was not associated with whether the young person had an abdominal transplant scar or was on high doses of steroids.

Post-Traumatic Stress Disorder

Young people with chronic liver disease are likely to have had some unpleasant experiences in hospital, and times which may have been felt confusing, scary or upsetting. High rates of post-traumatic stress disorder (PTSD) have been found in adolescents who have had transplants. For example, in 104 adolescents (aged 12–20 years) post-solid organ transplant, 16% met full criteria for PTSD, with an additional 14% reporting two of the three necessary symptom clusters at a level that was causing them clinically significant distress [43, 44] reported similar prevalence rates of PTSD (13%) in 76 children post transplant; these PTSD symptoms were significantly under-reported by parents.

In addition to the distress associated with PTSD, in a small study of 19 adolescents post-liver transplant [45], a significant association was found between presence of PTSD symptoms and non-adherence (as measures by blood levels and clinician judgement). This is likely to be due to medication serving as a reminder of the transplant and non-adherence therefore being a form of avoidance. Functional outcomes are also found to be lower, for example, adult survivors of childhood cancer who had PTSD were found to have lower functioning in areas such as school, work and personal relationship [46].

Failure to identify PTSD compromises the young person's well being, impacts on their functioning as adults and is associated with non-adherence. As parents tend to underestimate rates of PTSD and there is no relationship between the objective characteristics of the trauma and the risk of PTSD [47], it is impossible to predict who will have difficulties. Detection therefore relies upon directly asking the young person. Research has not addressed rates of PTSD in young people with chronic liver disease more generally, but as these young people also encounter situations where they perceive their life to be threatened then it is reasonable to assume that their rates of PTSD may also be elevated.

One of the most significant challenges of caring for adolescents is the high rates of non-adherence. This is outlined below.

Adherence

As heighted earlier, rates of non-adherence to medication are found to be as high as 50% in adolescents post-transplant, with significant negative implications for their health.

It is easy to see that a typically developing adolescent as described in the earlier section might not take all their medications or attend appointments correctly. Adherence in liver disease or transplant requires the patient to trust their doctor that the treatment is required, buy into the notion that the status of their liver disease may not correspond with symptoms, be motivated by a long-term outcome of improved health, and be able to plan and organize themselves to maintain a good routine. This directly contrasts with the developmental profile of young people, as illustrated in Case Study 74.2.

Case Study 74.2

Jake is 18 years old. He was well throughout his childhood until being diagnosed with autoimmune liver disease when he was 14 years old. When he was first diagnosed, Jake felt quite unwell and spent a week in hospital, but since then he has been well and only has to go to an outpatient clinic appointment every few months. Jake does not think of himself as being sick and does not really think about it except for when he goes to hospital. He is most bothered about the way he looks, in particular about his acne, which started when he was commenced on steroid treatment and lack of muscle tone. He feels very self-conscious around other people his age and often feels quite down about his appearance. Jake is told to take daily medications to prevent him from getting ill again in the future—but when he stops taking his medications, nothing bad happens; he actually feels better because he is not bothered by side effects, his skin gets better and his face looks more defined. Jake feels happier because he feels more similar to his friends, and does not feel so self-conscious about having to remember to take his medicines or risk having to explain his condition to others. Jake has been told that he should not drink alcohol, but all of his friends do and it is really hard to explain why he cannot. When he started drinking recently at a party, it was really fun and nothing bad happened, so he thinks it must be alright. Jake does not really get on very well with his parents and teachers at the moment, so does not tell them because he knows they will nag him about it. When he goes to hospital, his mum does most of the talking. Jake's doctor tells his mum about some blood tests numbers that he does not really understand, and then he gets to go home.

A full review of the factors associated with non-adherence is outside the scope of this chapter, but a number of comprehensive reviews exist (e.g. [48–50]). Many of the characteristics known to make adherence more difficult are present for young people with liver disease, for example, the treatment is seemingly preventative rather than curative, does not have any immediate tangible benefits and needs to be taken for life. Knowledge is generally necessary, but not sufficient for adherence (e.g. [51]) and requires particular attention as young people grow up and each with different understandings. Individual education, which is tailored to the young person's needs, and repeated and checked regularly is important, to ensure the young person has a good understanding of their condition and rationale for treatment recommendations. It is important to understand the young person's priorities and encourage them to have open conversations about the barriers to adherence for them, for example, discussions may enable medication regimes to be simplified or altered to fit in with the person's routine, encouraging use of alarms and reminders, taking medication on sleepovers and more broadly how to manage the handing over of responsibility from parents to their child. Simplifying medical treatment and conversion to once daily preparations of immunosuppression have been reported to improve adherence and treatment satisfaction [52]. An overview of strategies for improving adherence can be found in Table 74.1.

Non-adherence has also been found to be associated with psychosocial distress, such as PTSD [45] and other psychosocial stressors [53]. Social difficulties such as financial restrictions should not be overlooked. For example, in the UK at the age of 18 years, young people have to start paying for their prescriptions and travel to hospital; when money is limited, these can be very real barriers to adherence for which support is available. Within our service, we adopt a multidisciplinary approach to identifying and managing adherence, which begins with a stance of assumed non-adherence and reinforcing disclosures; as rates are known to be around 50%, we normalize that most young people will struggle to take all of their medication all of their time. See Table 74.2

Table 74.1 Adherence management strategies

Barrier to adherence	Strategies
Naive about the risks of non-adherence	Individualized education about illness and medication
Burden of medication regime: too many tablets or too many times a day	Simplify medication regimes
	Ensure young person understands rationale for each medication and anticipated course
Non-intentional non-adherence: forgetting or organizational difficulties	Pill boxes, blister packs
	Medication charts and apps
	Alarm reminders
	Visual reminders
	Pairing medication with a daily activity
Intentional non-adherence: not taking medication due to the meaning of it/psychological benefits of non-adherence	Explore beliefs about illness and medication, including the benefits of non-adherence for the young person.
	Assess mood
	Referral to psychologist
Intentional adherence: practical barriers	Assess barriers such as housing, finances, parental support
	Referral to social worker

Table 74.2 Routine assessment and management of adherence

Task	Rationale	Example questions
Engage the young person	Young people are more likely to be actively involved in their health care and more adherent if they have a good relationship with their health-care provider	See HEADSS [33]: ask about home, school/college, friendships, activities and interests
	Screen for psychosocial difficulties	
	Gather information about how the illness and treatment fits into the young person's life	
Assess who is responsible for medication	Responsibility needs to be handed over from parents to young person: difficulties often arise during this transition	'Who is in charge of medication at home? How long have you been taking charge of your medication? Who organizes the prescriptions?'
Assume non-adherence and routinely assess with every patient in a non-judgemental manner	Rates of non-adherence exceed 50%—most young people will be non-adherent some of the time	'In a normal week, how often do you tend to miss your medication? How often do you take it at a different time?'
	Impossible to predict who will be non-adherent so need to ask everyone	
	Asking questions in a non-judgemental way that assumed some non-adherence is more likely to increase disclosure	
Normalize: full adherence is difficult; very few people are adherent all of the time	More likely to increase honest disclosure and willingness to discuss the barriers to their adherence	'Most young people we see struggle to take all of their medication all of the time. We know that it can be a really hard thing to have to take medication every day.'
	Trying to scare or tell off your patient is unlikely to improve their adherence, but will ensure that they do not disclose it to you again!	
Check understanding of illness and risks of non-adherence	Knowledge is necessary (but not sufficient) for adherence	'How would you explain your condition to someone who hadn't heard of it before? What do you think the medications do? What do you think would happen if you didn't take your medication? How many doses of medication do you think you could get away without taking?'
	Need to ensure that the young person understands why they need to take medication and fully understand the risks of not taking it	
Assess intentionality of non-adherence	Different determinants of non-adherence require different interventions	'Are there times that you remember your medication, but choose not to take it for some other reason? How often do you forget your medication compared to choosing not to take it? When you miss it, do you always miss all of your medication or just some of them?'
Identify barriers	Different determinants of non-adherence require different interventions	'What gets in the way of taking medication? What is the worst/hardest thing about (having to take) medication?'

HEADSS home, education/employment, peer group activities, drugs, sexuality, and suicide/depression

for details of our approach for routinely assessing in this age group. From conducting a case-note review of the more complex cases seen by our clinical psychologist and specialist social worker, we found that a significant minority had entrenched relational difficulties and had experienced childhood abuse [54]. We hypothesized that non-adherence can be related to attachment difficulties and in some cases can require long-term specialist input to treat. Effective identification of non-adherence and the factors contributing to it are essential to ensure access to the appropriate services.

Non-adherence is thought to be related to both the adolescent stage of development (e.g. [17]) and the process of transitioning into adult services at this risky period (e.g. [53]). It is therefore crucial for every centre to carefully consider how to transition their young people. This is reviewed below.

Transition from Pediatric to Adult-Centred Health Services

The adolescent health society defined transition in 1993 as a 'Purposeful, planned process that addresses the medical, psychosocial and educational/vocational needs of adolescents and young adults with chronic physical and medical conditions from child-centred to adult-orientated healthcare systems'.

In 2002, American Academy of Pediatrics published the following consensus: 'The goal of transition in health care for young adults with special health care needs is to maximize lifelong functioning and potential through the provision of high-quality developmentally appropriate health care services that continue uninterrupted as the individual moves from adolescence to adulthood' [55]. Several reports, mainly in the transplant setting, have since been published, with worse outcomes for patients transplanted during adolescence but a decrease in 1 year mortality in renal transplant recipients as patients age from 20 to 30 years. This supports the concept that maturation and complete development occur after the age of 18 years [9]. It seems that to date the development of dedicated programs to optimize transition from pediatric to adult-centred care has mainly been driven by pediatric specialists, with currently no consensus as to how to implement or measure this, or even define what a successful outcome is. Different models of transition programs have been described and will need to be developed depending on the set up and needs of the individual centres. Pediatric teams should focus on developing strategies to overcome barriers to an adequate transition including learning difficulties, social factors, patients in care and patients with mental health problems and aim for an integrative process. With regards to congenital and rare conditions typically presenting in childhood, where adult teams might be less familiar in managing these conditions, management in specialized centres with pediatric expertize is recommended. In cardiology, for example, it is

recommended for 'grown up adults with congenital heart disease' also known as GUCH to be followed up in specialized centres with multidisciplinary input [56].

Patients and their families should be given realistic expectations of the adult health-care systems where the patient is expected to advocate for themselves and therefore self-management skills should be included in the transition process.

Experience in the renal transplant setting demonstrated that the introduction of an integrated pediatric/young adult joint transition clinic and care pathway improved outcome over a 4-year period, with no episodes of late acute rejection or graft loss compared to 35% graft loss in a group of patients who did not benefit from this service [28]. A transition service should aim to manage young people with a chronic condition in a comprehensive and holistic way and should include parents/caregivers whose role will change during the process as one of the main aspects of transition is shifting from caregiver-provided to parent-provided care and the self-management of one's own illness [57]. It has been shown that incorporation and promotion of disease self-management within chronic care models have improved outcomes in conditions as asthma, diabetes mellitus and rheumatoid arthritis [58]. In this respect, it is important to use transition readiness tools to define a patient's individual needs and for a multi-professional team to address these.

A recent small pilot study in a group of 20 liver transplant recipients whose care was coordinated by a transition coordinator showed, compared to a historic group of 14 patients, improved adherence to treatment during the year before transfer to adult services. After transfer, tacrolimus standard deviation (SD) scores remained stable in the group supported by the transition coordinator compared to the historic group where the tacrolimus SD increased, suggesting poorer adherence [59].

Ideally, the timing of the transition process should be flexible and aimed at the patient's needs and readiness; however, in practice, lack of age-appropriate inpatient facilities or pediatric and adult setting being on different sites often means that patients over 18 years cannot be admitted to pediatric inpatient facilities, raising the importance of starting the transition process early enough. This is particularly relevant in patients with special health-care needs where the transition process becomes more complicated as the patient might not be able to advocate for their care, consent for procedures and manage an inpatient stay on an adult ward independently. In these cases, the multi-professional team should ensure a well-documented care; pathway is discussed prior to transition to adult services [60, 61].

Summary and Conclusions

- With advances in medicine, more patients with liver conditions are growing in to adulthood.

- Adolescence is a period of biological, psychological and social changes and the impact of a chronic condition on this process can be significant.
- Outcome data suggest that young people are a unique and vulnerable cohort who deserves special attention by health professionals, focusing on better outcome and survival.
- Growth failure and pubertal delay are prevalent and sexual health advice should be offered standard during the consultation with the young person.
- Psychological aspects of growing up with liver disease are increasingly being recognized and identified and require management by specialized health-care professionals.
- Non-adherence to all aspects of care is common, multifactorial and often underestimated, however, impacts on outcome and survival. A non-judgemental approach aimed at identifying barriers to adherence and developing an individualized strategy is recommended.
- Successful transition programs have shown improvement in outcome and quality of life and should be developed according to the facilities of the individual centre and focus on self-management, keeping in mind the special needs patients might have.

References

1. World Health Organization. Young people's Health: a challenge for society. Geneva: WHO; 1986.
2. Suris JC, Michaud PA, Viner R. The adolescent with a chronic condition. Part I and II. Arch Dis Child. 2004:89:938–949
3. Dobbels F, Hames A, Aujoulat I, Heaton N, Samyn M. Should we retransplant a patient who is non-adherent? A literature review and critical reflection. Pediatr Transplant. 2012;16:4–11.
4. Jain V, Kolimarala V, Davenport M, Heaton N, Samyn M. Growing up with biliary atresia without liver transplantation: a single centre experience. Hepatology. 2013;58(4 Suppl abstract):1220.
5. Kamath BM, Spinner NB, Emerick KM, Chudley AE, Booth C, Piccoli DA, Krantz ID. Vascular anomalies in alagille syndrome: a significant cause of morbidity and mortality. Circulation. 2004;109(11):1354–8.
6. Kamath BM, Spinner NB, Rosenblum ND. Renal involvement and the role of Notch signalling in Alagille syndrome. Nat Rev Nephrol. 2013;9(7):409–18.
7. Organ procurement and transplantation network (OPTN) and scientific registry of transplant recipients (SRTR). OPTN/SRTR 2010 Annual Data Report. Rockville, MD: Department of Health and Human Services, Health Resources and Services Administration, Healthcare Systems Bureau, Division of Transplantation; 2011
8. Ngu JH, Gearry RB, Frampton CM, Stedman CA. Predictors of poor outcome in patients with autoimmune hepatitis: a population based study. Hepatology. 2013;57(6):2399–406.
9. Andreoni KA, Forbes R, Andreoni RM, Phillips G, Stewart H, Ferris M. Age-related kidney transplant outcomes: health disparities amplified in adolescence. JAMA Intern Med. 2013;173(16):1524–32.
10. Alonso EM, Shepherd R, Martz KL, Yin W, Anand R, et al. SPLIT Research Group. Linear growth patterns in prepubertal children following liver transplantation. Am J Transpl. 2009;9:1389–97.
11. Mohammad S, Grimberg A, Rand E, Anand R, Yin W, Alonso EM, et al. Studies of pediatric liver transplantation research consortium. Long-term linear growth and puberty in pediatric liver transplant recipients. J Pediatr. 2013;163:1354–60.
12. Janjua HS, Mahan JD. The role and future challenges for recombinant growth hormone therapy to promote growth in children after renal transplantation. Clin Transplant. 2011;25(5):E469–74.
13. Kapp N. WHO provider brief on hormonal contraception and liver disease. Contraception. 2009;80:325–6.
14. Joshi D, James A, Quaglia A, Westbrook RH, Heneghan MA. Liver disease in pregnancy. Lancet. 2010;375:594–605.
15. Department of Health. Transition: getting it right for young people. National Service Framework for Children, Young People and Maternity Services; 2006.
16. Steinberg L. A social neuroscience perspective on adolescent risk-taking. Dev Rev. 2008;28(1):78–106.
17. Kiberd J, Acott P, Kiberd B. Kidney transplant survival in pediatric and young adults. BMC Nephrol. 2011;12(1):54.
18. Erikson EH. Childhood and society. New York: Norton; 1963.
19. Dahl RE, Gunner MR. Heightened stress responsiveness and emotional reactivity during pubertal maturation: implications for psychopathology. Dev Psychopath. 2009;21:1–6.
20. Blakemore S, Mills K. Is adolescence a sensitive period for sociocultural processing? Annu Rev Psychol. 2014;65:187–207.
21. Armett J. Reckless behavior in adolescence: a developmental perspective. Dev Rev. 1992;12;339–73.
22. Miauton L, Narring F, Michaud P-A. Chronic illness, life style and emotional health in adolescence: results of a cross-sectional survey on the health of 15–20-year-olds in Switzerland. Eur J Pediatr. 2003;162(10):682–9.
23. Blum RW. Sexual health contraceptive needs of adolescents with chronic conditions. Arch Pediatr Adolesc Med. 1997;51(3):290–7.
24. Carter B, McGoldrick M. The changing family life cycle: a framework for family therapy. 2nd ed. Boston: Allyn & Bacon; 1988.
25. Taylor RM, Franck LS, Gibson F, Donaldson N, Dhawan A. Study of the factors affecting health-related quality of life in adolescents after liver transplantation. Am J Transpl. 2009;9:1179–88.
26. Rolland JS. Families, illness & disability: a biopsychosocial intervention model. New York: Basic Books; 1994.
27. Reiter-Pirtill J, Waller JM, Noll RB. Empirical and theoretical perspectives on the peer relationships of children with chronic conditions. In: Roberts MC, Steele RG, editors. Handbook of paediatric psychology. 4th ed. London: Guilford Press; 2009 (Chap. 45).
28. Harden PN, Walsh G, Bandler N, Bradley S, Lonsdale D, Taylor J, et al. Bridging the gap: an integrated paediatric to adult clinical service for young adults with kidney failure. Br Med J. 2012;344:e3718.
29. Jersen B, D'Urso C, Arnon R, Miloh T, Iyer K, Kerkar N, et al. Adolescent transplant recipients as peer mentors: a program to improve self-management and health-related quality of life. Paediatr Transpl. 2013;17(7):612–20.
30. Hames A, O'Reilly I, Samyn M. I don't feel like an outcast anymore: establishing a peer support network for young people and parents in a supra-regional liver disease and transplant service. Turkish Arch Pediatr. 2013;s2:119.
31. Maloney R, Clay DL, Robinson BS. Sociocultural issues in pediatric transplantation: a conceptual model. J Paediatr Psych. 2005;30(3):235–46.
32. Taylor RM, Franck LS, Dhawan A, Gibson F. The stories of young people living with a liver transplant. Qual Health Res. 2010;20(8):1076–90.
33. Goldenring JM, Cohen E. Getting into adolescent heads. Contemp Paediatr. 1988;5:75–80.
34. Taylor R, Franck LS, Gibson F, Dhawan A. A critical review of the health-related quality of life of children and adolescents after liver transplantation. Liver Transpl. 2005;11(1):51–60.

35. Fredericks EM, Magee JC, Opipari-Arrigan L, Shieck V, Well A, Lopez MJ. Adherence and health-related quality of life in adolescent liver transplant recipients. Pediatr Transpl. 2008;12(3):289–99.

36. Gulati R, Radhakrishnan KR, Hupertz V, Wyllie R, Alkhouri N, Worley S, Feldstein AE. Health-related quality of life in children with autoimmune liver disease. J Pediatr Gastroenterol Nutr. 2013;57(4):444–50.

37. Sorensen LG, Neighbors K, Martz K, Zelko F, Bucuvalas JC, Alonso EM, Studies of Pediatric Liver Transplantation (SPLIT) and Functional Outcomes Group (FOG). Cognitive and academic outcomes following liver transplantation: functional outcomes group results. Am J Transpl. 2011;11(2):303–11.

38. Kaller T, Langguth N, Petermann F, Ganschow R, Nashan B, Schulz KH. Cognitive performance in pediatric liver transplantation. Am J Transpl. 2013;13(11):2956–65.

39. Pinquart M, Shen YH. Anxiety in children and adolescents with chronic physical illnesses: a meta-analysis. Acta Paediatr. 2011;100(8):1069–76.

40. Kerkar N, D'Urso C, Van Nostrand K, Kochin I, Gault A, Suchy F, et al. Psychosocial outcomes for children with nonalcoholic fatty liver disease over time and compared with obese controls. J Pediatr Gastroenterol Nutr. 2012;56(1):77–82.

41. Mazzone L, Postorino V, De Peppo L, Della Corte C, Lofino G, Vassena L, et al. Paediatric non-alcoholic fatty liver disease: impact on patients and mothers' quality of life. Hepat Mon. 2013;13(3):e7871.

42. Day J. Body image perception in young people with chronic liver disease. Submitted as part of a doctoral thesis. London: Institute of Psychiatry, King's College; 2014.

43. Mintzer L, Stuber ML, Seacord D, Castaneda M, Mesrkhani V, Glover D. Post traumatic stress symptoms in adolescent organ transplant recipients. Pediatrics. 2005;115:1640–9.

44. Shemesh E, Newcorn JH, Rockmore L, Shneider BL, Emre S, Gelb BD, et al. Comparison of parent and child reports of emotional trauma symptoms in pediatric outpatient settings. Pediatrics. 2005;115:582–9.

45. Shemesh E, Lurie S, Stuber ML, Emre S, Patel Y, Vohra P, et al. A pilot study of posttraumatic stress and nonadherence in pediatric liver transplant recipients. Pediatrics. 2005;105:E29.

46. Meeske KA, Ruccione K, Globe DR, Stuber ML. Posttraumatic stress, quality of life, and psychological distress in young adult survivors of childhood cancer. Oncol Nurs Forum. 2001;28(3):481–9.

47. Breslau N, Davis GC. Posttraumatic stress disorder: the stressor criterion. J Nerv Ment Dis. 1987;175(5):255–64.

48. Drotar D. Promoting adherence to medical treatment in chronic childhood illness: concepts, methods, and interventions. New Jersey: Lawrence Erlbaum; 2009

49. Shemesh E, Annunziato RA, Shneider BL, Dugan CA, Warshaw J, Kerkar N, Emre S. Pediatr Transpl. 2008;12(3):316–23.

50. Kyngas HA, Kroll T, Duffy ME. Compliance in adolescents with chronic diseases: a review. J Adolesc Health. 2000;26:379–88.

51. McQuaid EL1, Kopel SJ, Klein RB, Fritz GK. Medication adherence in pediatric asthma: reasoning, responsibility, and behavior. J Pediatr Psychol. 2003;28(5):323–33.

52. Kuypers DR, Peeters PC, Sennesael JJ, Kianda MN, Vrijens B, Kristanto P, Dobbels F, Vanrenterghem Y, Kanaan N, ADMIRAD Study Team. Improved adherence to tacrolimus once-daily formulation in renal recipients: a randomized controlled trial using electronic monitoring. Transplantation. 2013;95(2):333–40.

53. Watson AR. Non-compliance and transfer from paediatric to adult transplant unit. Pediatr Nephrol. 2000;14(6):469–72.

54. Hames A, Malan J. Whose problem is it? Improving adherence in young adults (Oral presentation). Rotterdam: Ethical Legal and Psychosocial Aspects of Transplantation (ELPAT) Congress; 2013.

55. American Academy of Pediatrics, American Academy of Family Physicians, American College of Physicians-American Society of Internal Medicine. A consensus statement on health care transitions for young adults with special health care needs. Pediatrics. 2002;110:1304–6.

56. Borghi A1, Ciuffreda M, Quattrociocchi M, Preda L. The grown up congenital cardiac patient. J Cardiovasc Med (Hagerstown). 2007;8(1):78–82.

57. Miles K1, Edwards S, Clapson M. Transition from pediatric to adult services: experiences of HIV-positive adolescents. AIDS Care. 2004;16(3):305–14.

58. Coleman K1, Austin BT, Brach C, Wagner EH. Evidence on the chronic care model in the new millennium. Health Aff (Millwood). 2009;28(1):75–85.

59. Annunziato RA1, Baisley MC, Arrato N, Barton C, Henderling F, Arnon R, Kerkar N. Strangers headed to a strange land? A pilot study of using a transition coordinator to improve transfer from pediatric to adult services. J Pediatr. 2013;163(6):1628–33.

60. Kaufmanm M, Pinzon J, et al. Transition to adult care for youth with special health care needs. Paediatr Child Health. 2007;12(9):785–8.

61. Department of Health. Transition: moving on well. Best Practice Guidance. 2008. www.dh.gov.uk/en/publicationsandstatistics/publications/publicationspolicyandguidance/dh_083592.

New Horizons in Pediatric Hepatology: A Glimpse of the Future

75

Emer Fitzpatrick and Anil Dhawan

Introduction

Pediatric hepatology as a distinct subspeciality has emerged gradually over the past 40 years [1], indeed, though one of the first two liver transplants undertaken was performed in a child with biliary atresia in 1964 [2]. The division from adult hepatology and the distinction from pediatric gastroenterology have taken time to evolve. The UK became the first country to introduce 3 years' training programme in pediatric hepatology, while advanced fellowships are being introduced in the countries like the USA. Over the past half century, massive advances have been made, with liver transplantation outcomes for children surpassing 90 % survival. Now pediatric hepatology is poised at the brink of a hugely exciting era with the potential of advances in technology, particularly in genetics, bioengineering and small molecules, bringing real advantages to diagnostics and therapeutics. In addition, there is a renewed focus not just on survival and medical outcomes but on improving the quality of life for patients and minimising the side effects of each treatment.

As a speciality of rare diseases, in general, a lot of the research and development to date in pediatric hepatology, particularly in transplantation, comes adapted from adult practice. In the twenty-first century, however, with focus on genetics and metabolic disease, pediatric hepatology research is set to take the lead as regards innovative practice.

Genes, cells and molecules are cross-cutting themes across diagnostics, the better understanding of pathophysiology and thus therapeutic options. Each of these is explored in more detail within this chapter. In addition, there will need to be a biopsychosocial emphasis on research and development within the subspecialty: The focus is now on long-term outcomes for children with liver disease and a shift away from survival alone to holistic wellbeing. New challenges face us in the twenty-first century, particularly the massive increase in the prevalence of obesity across both the adult and pediatric population. This has consequences in terms of both lifestyle-related liver disease and the decline in healthy livers suitable for transplantation due to the frequent occurrence of steatosis.

Genetics

Diagnostics

Our understanding of single-gene and polygenetic/multifactorial disorders has undergone major advancement over the past number of years and continues to do so. Many of the rare disorders described in pediatric hepatology have found explanation in genetic alteration, thanks to collaboration of pediatric hepatologists and geneticists internationally. The major technological advances of next-generation sequencing, whether in whole-genome analysis or targeted studies, have allowed analysis and elucidation of huge amounts of data. Over the past two decades or so, the genetics of Wilson's disease [3, 4], Alagille disease [5, 6], arthrogryposis, renal dysplasia and cholestasis (ARC), microvillus inclusion disorder, familial intrahepatic cholestasis (FIC)1 disease, bile salt export pump (BSEP) deficiency, multidrug resistance (MDR)3 deficiency and most recently tight junction protein-2 (TJP2) disease have been described [7–10]. In addition to this, the genetic basis of many metabolic diseases affecting the liver, such as glycogen storage disease and mitochondrial depletion disorders [11, 12], has been discovered leading to more rapid and less invasive diagnostic measures.

Gene 'chips' now exist for the diagnosis of cholestatic conditions in neonates and certain metabolic diseases (glycogen storage disease).

The interaction of genetic susceptibility and the environment has also come to the fore with an understanding of genetic variation in man due to epigenetics. Single-nucleotide polymorphisms (SNPs) can not only explain variation in susceptibility to disease processed, for example, patatin-like

A. Dhawan (✉) · E. Fitzpatrick
Professor and Director, Pediatric Liver, GI and Nutrition Center
Clinical Director, Child Health, King's College Hospital, London, UK
e-mail: anil.dhawan@kcl.ac.uk

© Springer International Publishing Switzerland 2016
S. Guandalini et al. (eds.), *Textbook of Pediatric Gastroenterology, Hepatology and Nutrition*,
DOI 10.1007/978-3-319-17169-2_75

897

phospholipase domain-containing protein 3 (PNPLA3) in nonalcoholic fatty liver disease (NAFLD) [13], autoimmune liver disease [14] but also in hepatocellular carcinoma and response to treatment in hepatitis C. Next on the agenda are determining the genetic modifiers for multifactorial conditions, for example, biliary atresia, idiopathic acute liver failure. Cystic fibrosis-associated liver disease and liver disease in alpha-1-antitrypsin deficiency will also benefit from this approach.

Gene Therapy

Genetic modification has still promise as a therapy. Liver-based metabolic disease has the particular advantage of the liver as a target organ for gene therapy. Preclinical studies and clinical trials to date have yet to overcome safety concerns in terms of stability and the potential for carcinogenesis.

The potential of using induced pluripotent stem (iPM) cells has become a hot topic and the use of genetically modified iPS cells from adults with alpha-1-antitrypsin deficiency that may be a useful approach without the need for immunosuppression [15, 16].

The delivery of gene therapy involves use of a vector at present which may be viral or nonviral. This, in addition to the major issue of genomic instability, is the major safety concern limiting the current clinical applicability of the therapy.

Other approaches to genetic therapy targeting liver disease include using interfering RNA, with some success, including the use of this technique to treat transthyretin-mediated amyloidosis, a liver-centric disease [17]. Small interfering RNAs bind to the RNA-induced silencing complex-mediated cleavage of target messenger RNA. This has been exploited by developing tools to enable delivery to target organ in stable formulation, for example, lipid nanoparticles which are stable and robust. When delivered intravenously, they home in to the liver.

MicroRNAs (miRNAs) are small noncoding RNAs, 18–24 nucleotides in length that regulate gene expression by binding to mRNAs to interfere with the process of translation. They are regulated during or after transcription and SNPs in miRNA genes may also modify their activity and function. Approximately, 1400 mammalian miRNAs are known and each can influence hundreds of gene transcripts. These molecules are involved in all biological processes in all cell types. In the liver, there has been much interest in the role of miRNA in glucose and lipid metabolism, inflammation, apoptosis and cell death, cell cycle and proliferation and fibrosis. miRNAs have been investigated as both biomarkers of disease processes in the liver and potential therapeutic targets by both inhibition and over-expression. Clinical trials are currently ongoing using an anti-miRNA 122 locked nucleic acid (LNA) inhibitor in hepatitis C—early results have shown a prolonged dose-dependent reduction of hepatitis C virus (HCV) RNA levels without conveying resistance.

Regenerative Medicine and Cell Therapy of Liver Disease

Liver transplantation is undoubtedly the standard of care for end-stage liver disease and many liver-based metabolic conditions and developments in surgical technique, peritransplant care and immunosuppressive medication means that outcomes are improving. However, the unfortunate fact is that organs are in short supply, and the growing tendency towards obesity in the general population means that fewer and fewer non-steatotic, healthy livers are available through donation and are particularly unsuitable for split-organ transplantation (which is the main source of transplanted livers in children). Thus, deaths inevitably occur while awaiting a suitable organ. Hepatocyte transplantation is becoming more established as an alternative to orthotopic or auxiliary liver transplantation in the management of liver-based metabolic conditions and in acute liver failure [18–24]. As with auxiliary transplantation, the native liver remains in place; in the case of acute liver failure, this allows the possibility of native liver regeneration over time; in metabolic liver disease, the native liver serves as a back-up in case of graft failure and remains available for the future possibility of gene therapy. The procedure is significantly less invasive than organ transplantation and previously isolated and cryopreserved cells are available on demand.

Hepatocytes are derived from organs that would otherwise be rejected for transplantation. In general, these often compromised livers may be steatotic, from non-heartbeating donors [25], or unused segments [26]. Innovative methods to improve cell quality from these poor grafts and cryopreservation methods have been a focus of research. Challenges also remain in the effective engraftment of hepatocytes into the host liver. The optimal immunosuppression approach is also as yet unknown. Therapeutic effect is often lost after 6–9 months, perhaps due to rejection, apoptosis or other causes. The single most important obstacle to the widespread application of hepatocyte transplantation is the limited availability of hepatocytes. This has encouraged investigation into alternative sources of cell, including stem cells, immortalised cells and xenotransplantation, each with its own challenges.

In all, there have been over 80 case reports of clinical human hepatocyte transplantation from 13 centres for liver-based metabolic disease, acute liver failure (ALF) or chronic liver disease. Table 75.1 depicts the conditions where human hepatocyte transplantation has been attempted. Cells are infused into the liver via the portal vein/hepatic artery or into

Table 75.1 Conditions where human hepatocyte transplantation has been attempted in children

Inborn errors of metabolism
Crigler–Najjar syndrome type 1
Familial hypercholesterolaemia
FVII deficiency
Glycogen storage disease type 1
Infantile Refsum's disease
Progressive familial intra-hepatic cholestasis type 2 (PFIC2)
Urea cycle defects
Ornithine transcarbamylase deficiency
Arginosuccinate lyase deficiency
Carbamoyl phosphate synthase type 1 deficiency
Citrullinemia
Acute liver failure
Drug
Viral
Idiopathic

the spleen. In ALF, intraperitoneal transplantation may be optimal.

The aim of hepatocyte transplantation in metabolic disease is to replace the missing function without the need to replace the whole organ. In animal model of Crigler–Najjar syndrome, approximately 12 % of liver mass is needed to normalise the bilirubin levels [27]; however, fewer cells may be enough to change the phenotype in other conditions.

In acute liver failure, hepatocyte transplantation may act as a bridge to recovery and regeneration of the injured native liver or alternatively to orthotopic liver transplantation once an organ becomes available. The procedure may also be used in patients who are not candidates for organ transplantation. A major advantage of hepatocyte transplantation is the immediate availability of cryopreserved cells. Sufficient cell mass (approximately 10–15 % of liver cell mass) is needed to provide enough function to sustain metabolic function [27]. Hepatocyte transplantation in patients with ALF has resulted in a reduction in ammonia and bilirubin with improvements in hepatic encephalopathy and cardiovascular instability [19, 28, 29]. The advantages of intraperitoneal transplantation of hepatocytes encapsulated in alginate microbeads are currently being evaluated. Alginate serves as an anchorage point for cells and protects the hepatocytes from immune attack.

In metabolic liver diseases, the aim of hepatocyte transplantation is to replace function by the engrafted cells. Attempts at improving engraftment include temporary embolisation of the portal vein [30], liver irradiation [31] and the administration of growth factors [32].

The supply of good quality livers for hepatocyte isolation is a major issue. There is a pressing need for an easily available alternative cell source. Stem or progenitor cells have many advantages as an alternative source of cell for hepatocyte transplantation. They are readily available and may be effectively expanded in vitro or in vivo. Autologous cells (iPS cells) eliminate the need for immunosuppression; however, they may need to undergo corrective genetic manipulation prior to use to correct the underlying defect [33].

Early experimental evidence for progenitor cells/stem cells was demonstrated by Petersen [34], since that time there have been numerous studies showing expression of liver-specific genes by differentiated stem cells in vitro and in vivo summarised by a number of excellent reviews [33, 35, 36]. Proof of true functionality of these cells has been less frequent. It is not clear as yet whether transdifferentiation or fusion is responsible for the change in phenotype of the cells. For example, with severe selection pressure, such as in the fumarylacetoacetate hydrolase (FAH)-−/−-mouse (model for tyrosinemia type 1), successful repopulation occurs mainly because of hepatocyte fusion with host hepatocytes [37]. The tumorigenic potential of modifications to the genome needs to be considered.

Embryonic Stem Cells

Human embryonic stem cells (hESCs), isolated in 1998 [38], have generated great interest and controversy over the past decade. Despite their undoubted therapeutic promise, their effective clinical application has remained elusive to date. hESC lines have been effectively differentiated to hepatocyte lineage with evidence of repopulation of immunosuppressed mouse model of liver injury [39, 40]. Undifferentiated ESC transplanted into immunodeficient mice resulted in teratoma formation [41, 42]. Safety concerns are thus a major obstacle to clinical translation. hESCs are thought to be less susceptible to immune rejection than more mature cells due to their low immunostimulatory potential [43], though the true capacity of hESC to evade the immune response remains unknown.

Hepatoblasts and Foetal Liver Progenitor Cells

The foetal liver is a source of more committed progenitor cells in the form of hepatoblasts. These cells retain their proliferative capacity but are 'directed' specifically towards development of hepatocytes and cholangiocytes. There has been success in using progenitor cells from foetal liver in animal models [44] and clinical case reports in ALF [45] and Crigler–Najjar syndrome [46]. Again there is some concern regarding the ability of progenitor cells to differentiate into functionally mature hepatocytes [47]. The most appropriate microenvironmental conditions for this have not yet been fully defined. An 'adult' microenvironment may be conducive to differentiation. Problems with this source include difficulty accessing tissue with uncertainty around the most appropriate gestational age to target. There are also some ethical concerns surrounding the harvesting of foetal tissue.

In contrast, 'adult' stem cells combine the ability to differentiate into liver cells with proliferative capacity. Use of this source is less ethically complex and closer to the clinic than embryonic or foetal liver stem cells.

Endogenous Liver Stem Cells

It is well known that the liver has the ability to regenerate by division of mature hepatocytes as demonstrated to good effect following partial hepatectomy [48]. Usually, hepatocytes turn over once or twice a year [36]. A second compartment of facultative stem cells become active in the presence of long-standing injury or impaired proliferation of mature hepatocytes. This occurs when replicative senescence is reached. These cells are located in the intrahepatic biliary tree within the canals of Herring [49], giving rise to bipotent cells which have the potential to become both cholangiocytes and hepatocytes. Adult-derived human liver stem cells have also been isolated by outgrowing cultures of primary hepatocytes and are thought to have advantages over other pluripotent cells. In particular, they are already 'directed' towards hepatocyte differentiation and thus are theoretically more likely to provide the required function without the problems of teratogenicity. A major advantage of these cells is their ability to expand in vitro. The functionality of these cells once differentiated has been documented [50].

Mesenchymal Stromal Cells

Mesenchymal stromal cells have also been shown to have promise in the cell therapy of liver disease [51]. These are multipotent, adherently growing cells which provide support for haematopoietic cells within the bone marrow [52]. They are a readily available source of stem cell also isolated from umbilical cord blood and matrix, placental tissue and adipose tissue [53–55]. Mesenchymal stem cells (MSCs) have beneficial effects in animal models of ALF. They can transdifferentiate into hepatocyte-like cells both in vitro and in vivo [56, 57]. MSCs play a major role in tissue repair both through localised immuneosuppressive effects and through the release of soluble trophic factors to affect neighbouring cells, properties which make them excellent candidates for improving the survival of transplanted cells [58, 59]. Improved survival has been shown in animal models of liver disease and pilot clinical studies of liver failure [60, 61]. It is not clear, however, whether the transdifferentiation of MSCs into hepatocyte-like cells or an anti-inflammatory, anti-apoptotic effect induced by the MSCs result in the desired outcome. Soluble factors such as growth factors, cytokines, extracellular matrix glycoproteins and other small molcules produced by MSCs likely mediate these effects in ALF rather than transdifferentiation [58]. Candidate molecules include interleukin (IL)-1Rα, IL6, IL8, granulocyte-colony-stimulating factor, nerve growth factor and hepatocyte growth factor [60, 62]. MSC-conditioned medium conferred a significant improvement in mortality and biochemical indices of liver damage in a galactosamine-injured rat with evidence of inhibition of apoptosis and promotion of liver regeneration in the treated liver [63]. This anti-apoptotic, pro-regenerative effect of MSCs has also been seen in the setting of myocardial infarction [64] and stroke [65]. In addition to the beneficial effects on liver inflammation and regeneration, other studies have recognised the supportive effects of bone-marrow-derived cells in coculture with hepatocytes [66]. Co-encapsulated hepatocytes and bone marrow stem cells resulted in prolonged maintenance of function in the co-encapsulated group in vitro and in vivo in a rodent model of ALF [67, 68]. Thus, not only are MSCs anticipated to improve the viability and functionality of co-transplanted hepatocytes but transplanted mesenchymal stem cells may also be a source of anti-inflammatory/anti-apoptotic mediators in the setting of the failing liver and the subsequent cytokine storm. MSCs are already used clinically in the treatment of graft versus host disease, and these have safety and logistical advantages over hESC and alcoholic liver disease/hepatic stellate cell ALD/HSC.

Induced Pluripotent Stem Cells

The description by Takahashi and Yamanaka [69, 70] of the induction of somatic cells back to their pluripotent state by over-expressing certain transcription factors, and the subsequent differentiation of the cells along alternative lineages, has opened massive possibilities for cell therapy in liver disease. The differentiation of autologous dermal cells into hepatocytes following induction of pluripotency may have significant advantages, avoiding the need for immunosuppression in cell transplantation and providing an accurate model of disease to investigate pathophysiological mechanisms and test therapies. Of course, the transplantation of autologous cells in a disease state would require the need for genetic manipulation to correct that defect in the first instance. Thus, potential genomic instability may be a problem; however, new techniques are emerging which may minimise this risk and allow genomic stability. One such approach is using a piggyBac technique which enables removal of transgenes without residual sequences. This technique was used to good effect in a study by Yusa et al. which differentiated iPS cells from dermal cells of a patient with alpha-1-antitrypsin deficiency, corrected the genetic abnormality and demonstrated the function of the hepatocyte-like cells when transplanted into a mouse [15]. iPS-derived hepatocyte cells have also been used in the successful formation of 'liver buds' together with endothelial cells from umbilical cord and mesenchymal stromal cells. When transplanted into a mouse, this human liver bud rapidly vascularised and demonstrated liver-specific function [71].

Immortalisation

In order to establish a sustainable source of cells for transplantation, immortalisation of hepatocytes has also been described. Clonal cell lines of human and rat hepatocytes have been transduced with retroviral vector expressing the immortalising simian virus 40 large T antigen gene [72]. Despite control mechanisms for switching immortalisation on and off, concerns regarding safety remain.

Thus, the potential of cell therapy for liver disease is promising, though cell source is an issue, the emergence of mesenchymal stromal cells and iPS cells into the clinical field is particularly relevant and may provide an alternative source for successful translation. Pediatric liver disease, especially liver-based metabolic disease, remains a priority for this approach.

Small Molecules and Chaperones

As a reduction in protein stability is often a common outcome of monogenic disease, for example, alpha-1-antitrypsin deficiency or cystic fibrosis, focus on the stabilisation of such proteins and provision of an increase in intracellular function is the remit of pharmacological chaperones and other small molecules.

The work of Lomas group and others have focused on the use of small molecules to block the abnormal polymerisation of alpha-1-antitrypsin in the Z state [73]. At present, however, this work is proof of principle and not yet at translation point, though in the future may offer real therapeutic promise. A pediatric group in Pittsburgh investigated the use of carbamazepine as an autophagy enhancer to clear the intracellular load of abnormally formed alpha-1-antitrypsin in the disease state and reduced liver fibrosis in mice [74], using a well-established pharmacological substance as a molecular manipulator. Similarly, lysosomal storage disease and phenylketonuria have also been a focus for the development of protein chaperones [75, 76].

Targeting other nuclear receptors with pharmacological agents is a focus for polygenic or multifactorial disease such as NAFLD and primary biliary cirrhosis. Farnesoid X receptor (FXR) is a nuclear receptor that binds extensively to genomic DNA. FXR undergoes conformational change and alters gene expression following binding by bile acids or other pharmacological compounds. This results in the regulation of bile acid levels in the liver and in addition glucose and lipid homeostasis. Thus, modulation of FXR binding and function using a semi-synthetic bile acid may be a useful approach to therapy of nonalcoholic steatohepatitis (NASH) [77] and certain cholestatic liver diseases for which there are early clinical studies ongoing at present [78].

Conclusions

Pediatric hepatology is increasingly becoming an independent speciality. Success of liver transplantation has been crucial to the success of this speciality. A majority of chronic liver diseases are of perinatal onset with large number due to genetic or metabolic defects. Rapid advances in the field of genetics and molecular medicine will help unravel the mechanisms underlying these disorders and molecular diagnostic approaches. Understanding the underlying mechanism will help us to use newer treatments like gene therapy and small molecules. In parallel, the field of cellular therapy using human hepatocytes continues to gain momentum with proof-of-concept clinical applications in liver-based metabolic disorders and ALF. Stem cell sources of liver cells from embryonic stem cells, induced pluripotent cells and production of liver organoids from stem cells with use of growth factors appear to hold great promise to replace whole liver replacement in future.

References

1. Balistreri WF. Growth and development of a new subspecialty: pediatric hepatology. Hepatology. 2013;58(2):458–76 (PubMed PMID: 23788321).
2. Starzl TE, Marchioro TL, Vonkaulla KN, Hermann G, Brittain RS, Waddell WR. Homotransplantation of the liver in humans. Surg Gynecol Obstetr. 1963;117:659–76 (PubMed PMID: 14100514. Pubmed Central PMCID: 2634660).
3. Tanzi RE, Petrukhin K, Chernov I, Pellequer JL, Wasco W, Ross B, et al. The Wilson disease gene is a copper transporting ATPase with homology to the Menkes disease gene. Nat Genet. 1993;5(4): 344–50 (PubMed PMID: 8298641).
4. Bull PC, Thomas GR, Rommens JM, Forbes JR, Cox DW. The Wilson disease gene is a putative copper transporting P-type ATPase similar to the Menkes gene. Nat Genet. 1993;5(4):327–37 (PubMed PMID: 8298639).
5. Li L, Krantz ID, Deng Y, Genin A, Banta AB, Collins CC, et al. Alagille syndrome is caused by mutations in human Jagged1, which encodes a ligand for Notch1. Nat Genet. 1997;16(3):243–51 (PubMed PMID: 9207788).
6. Oda T, Elkahloun AG, Pike BL, Okajima K, Krantz ID, Genin A, et al. Mutations in the human Jagged1 gene are responsible for Alagille syndrome. Nat Genet. 1997;16(3):235–42 (PubMed PMID: 9207787).
7. Sambrotta M, Strautnieks S, Papouli E, Rushton P, Clark BE, Parry DA, et al. Mutations in TJP2 cause progressive cholestatic liver disease. Nat Genet. 2014;46(4):326–8 (PubMed PMID: 24614073).
8. de Vree JM, Jacquemin E, Sturm E, Cresteil D, Bosma PJ, Aten J, et al. Mutations in the MDR3 gene cause progressive familial intrahepatic cholestasis. Proc Natl Acad Sci U S A. 1998;95(1):282–7 (PubMed PMID: 9419367. Pubmed Central PMCID: 18201).

9. Strautnieks SS, Kagalwalla AF, Tanner MS, Knisely AS, Bull L, Freimer N, et al. Identification of a locus for progressive familial intrahepatic cholestasis PFIC2 on chromosome 2q24. Am J Hum Genet. 1997;61(3):630–3 (PubMed PMID: 9326328. Pubmed Central PMCID: 1715942).

10. Carlton VE, Knisely AS, Freimer NB. Mapping of a locus for progressive familial intrahepatic cholestasis (Byler disease) to 18q21-q22, the benign recurrent intrahepatic cholestasis region. Hum Mol Genet. 1995;4(6):1049–53 (PubMed PMID: 7655458).

11. Uusimaa J, Evans J, Smith C, Butterworth A, Craig K, Ashley N, et al. Clinical, biochemical, cellular and molecular characterization of mitochondrial DNA depletion syndrome due to novel mutations in the MPV17 gene. Eur J Hum Genet. 2014;22(2):184–91 (PubMed PMID: 23714749. Pubmed Central PMCID: 3895632).

12. Rotig A, Poulton J. Genetic causes of mitochondrial DNA depletion in humans. Biochim Biophys Acta. 2009;1792(12):1103–8 (PubMed PMID: 19596444).

13. Romeo S, Kozlitina J, Xing C, Pertsemlidis A, Cox D, Pennacchio LA, et al. Genetic variation in PNPLA3 confers susceptibility to nonalcoholic fatty liver disease. Nat Genet. 2008;40(12):1461–5 (PubMed PMID: 18820647. Pubmed Central PMCID: 2597056).

14. Tang J, Zhou C, Zhang ZJ, Zheng SS. Association of polymorphisms in non-classic MHC genes with susceptibility to autoimmune hepatitis. Hepatobiliary Pancreat Dis Int. 2012;11(2):125–31 (PubMed PMID: 22484578).

15. Yusa K, Rashid ST, Strick-Marchand H, Varela I, Liu PQ, Paschon DE, et al. Targeted gene correction of alpha1-antitrypsin deficiency in induced pluripotent stem cells. Nature. 2011;478(7369):391–4 (PubMed PMID: 21993621. Pubmed Central PMCID: 3198846).

16. Guo S, Booten SL, Aghajan M, Hung G, Zhao C, Blomenkamp K, et al. Antisense oligonucleotide treatment ameliorates alpha-1 antitrypsin-related liver disease in mice. J Clin Investigat. 2014;124(1):251–61 (PubMed PMID: 24355919. Pubmed Central PMCID: 3871221).

17. Coelho T, Adams D, Silva A, Lozeron P, Hawkins PN, Mant T, et al. Safety and efficacy of RNAi therapy for transthyretin amyloidosis. New Engl J Med. 2013;369(9):819–29 (PubMed PMID: 23984729).

18. Horslen SP, Fox IJ. Hepatocyte transplantation. Transplantation. 2004;77(10):1481–6 (PubMed PMID: 15239608. Epub 2004/07/09. Eng).

19. Bilir BM, Guinette D, Karrer F, Kumpe DA, Krysl J, Stephens J, et al. Hepatocyte transplantation in acute liver failure. Liver Transpl. 2000;6(1):32–40 (PubMed PMID: 10648575. Epub 2000/01/29. eng).

20. Strom SC, Fisher RA, Thompson MT, Sanyal AJ, Cole PE, Ham JM, et al. Hepatocyte transplantation as a bridge to orthotopic liver transplantation in terminal liver failure. Transplantation. 1997;63(4):559–69 (PubMed PMID: 9047152. Epub 1997/02/27. eng).

21. Fox IJ, Chowdhury JR, Kaufman SS, Goertzen TC, Chowdhury NR, Warkentin PI, et al. Treatment of the Crigler-Najjar syndrome type I with hepatocyte transplantation. N Engl J Med. 1998;338(20):1422–6 (PubMed PMID: 9580649. Epub 1998/05/15. eng).

22. Muraca M, Gerunda G, Neri D, Vilei MT, Granato A, Feltracco P, et al. Hepatocyte transplantation as a treatment for glycogen storage disease type 1a. Lancet. 2002;359(9303):317–8 (PubMed PMID: 11830200. Epub 2002/02/07. eng).

23. Horslen SP, McCowan TC, Goertzen TC, Warkentin PI, Cai HB, Strom SC, et al. Isolated hepatocyte transplantation in an infant with a severe urea cycle disorder. Pediatrics. 2003;111(6 Pt 1):1262–7 (PubMed PMID: 12777539. Epub 2003/06/05. eng).

24. Dhawan A, Mitry RR, Hughes RD, Lehec S, Terry C, Bansal S, et al. Hepatocyte transplantation for inherited factor VII deficiency. Transplantation. 2004;78(12):1812–4 (PubMed PMID: 15614156. Epub 2004/12/23. eng).

25. Hughes RD, Mitry RR, Dhawan A, Lehec SC, Girlanda R, Rela M, et al. Isolation of hepatocytes from livers from non-heart-beating donors for cell transplantation. Liver Transpl. 2006;12(5):713–7 (PubMed PMID: 16528714. Epub 2006/03/11. eng).

26. Mitry RR, Dhawan A, Hughes RD, Bansal S, Lehec S, Terry C, et al. One liver, three recipients: segment IV from split-liver procedures as a source of hepatocytes for cell transplantation. Transplantation. 2004;77(10):1614–6 (PubMed PMID: 15239631. Epub 2004/07/09. eng).

27. Asonuma K, Gilbert JC, Stein JE, Takeda T, Vacanti JP. Quantitation of transplanted hepatic mass necessary to cure the Gunn rat model of hyperbilirubinemia. J Pediatr Surg. 1992;27(3):298–301 (PubMed PMID: 1501000. Epub 1992/03/01. eng).

28. Fisher RA, Strom SC. Human hepatocyte transplantation: worldwide results. Transplantation. 2006;82(4):441–9 (PubMed PMID: 16926585. Epub 2006/08/24. eng).

29. Strom SC, Chowdhury JR, Fox IJ. Hepatocyte transplantation for the treatment of human disease. Semin Liver Dis. 1999;19(1): 39–48 (PubMed PMID: 10349682. Epub 1999/06/01. eng).

30. Dagher I, Boudechiche L, Branger J, Coulomb-Lhermine A, Parouchev A, Sentilhes L, et al. Efficient hepatocyte engraftment in a nonhuman primate model after partial portal vein embolization. Transplantation. 2006;82(8):1067–73 (PubMed PMID: 17060856. Epub 2006/10/25. eng).

31. Koenig S, Krause P, Schmidt TK, Rave-Fraenk M, Rothe H, Hermann RM, et al. Irradiation as preparative regimen for hepatocyte transplantation causes prolonged cell cycle block. Int J Radiat Biol. 2008;84(4):285–98 (PubMed PMID: 18386194. Epub 2008/04/04. eng).

32. Kosone T, Takagi H, Horiguchi N, Kakizaki S, Sato K, Watanabe Y, et al. Transforming growth factor-alpha accelerates hepatocyte repopulation after hepatocyte transplantation. J Gastroenterol Hepatol. 2008;23(2):260–6 (PubMed PMID: 17683499. Epub 2007/08/09. eng).

33. Lysy PA, Campard D, Smets F, Najimi M, Sokal EM. Stem cells for liver tissue repair: current knowledge and perspectives. World J Gastroenterol. 2008;14(6):864–75 (PubMed PMID: 18240343. Epub 2008/02/02. eng).

34. Petersen BE, Bowen WC, Patrene KD, Mars WM, Sullivan AK, Murase N, et al. Bone marrow as a potential source of hepatic oval cells. Science. 1999;284(5417):1168–70 (PubMed PMID: 10325227. Epub 1999/05/15. eng).

35. Allen KJ, Buck NE, Williamson R. Stem cells for the treatment of liver disease. Transpl Immunol. 2005;15(2):99–112 (PubMed PMID: 16412955. Epub 2006/01/18. eng).

36. Alison MR, Choong C, Lim S. Application of liver stem cells for cell therapy. Semin Cell Dev Biol. 2007;18(6):819–26 (PubMed PMID: 17997335. Epub 2007/11/13. eng).

37. Wang X, Willenbring H, Akkari Y, Torimaru Y, Foster M, Al-Dhalimy M, et al. Cell fusion is the principal source of bone-marrow-derived hepatocytes. Nature. 2003;422(6934):897–901 (PubMed PMID: 12665832. Epub 2003/04/01. eng).

38. Thomson JA, Itskovitz-Eldor J, Shapiro SS, Waknitz MA, Swiergiel JJ, Marshall VS, et al. Embryonic stem cell lines derived from human blastocysts. Science. 1998;282(5391):1145–7 (PubMed PMID: 9804556. Epub 1998/11/06. eng).

39. Cai J, Zhao Y, Liu Y, Ye F, Song Z, Qin H, et al. Directed differentiation of human embryonic stem cells into functional hepatic cells. Hepatology. 2007;45(5):1229–39 (PubMed PMID: 17464996. Epub 2007/04/28. eng).

40. Lavon N, Yanuka O, Benvenisty N. Differentiation and isolation of hepatic-like cells from human embryonic stem cells. Differentiation. 2004;72(5):230–8 (PubMed PMID: 15270779. Epub 2004/07/24. eng).

41. Yamamoto H, Quinn G, Asari A, Yamanokuchi H, Teratani T, Terada M, et al. Differentiation of embryonic stem cells into hepatocytes: biological functions and therapeutic application.

Hepatology. 2003;37(5):983–93 (PubMed PMID: 12717379. Epub 2003/04/30. eng).

42. Choi D, Oh HJ, Chang UJ, Koo SK, Jiang JX, Hwang SY, et al. In vivo differentiation of mouse embryonic stem cells into hepatocytes. Cell Transplant. 2002;11(4):359–68 (PubMed PMID: 12162376. Epub 2002/08/07. eng).

43. Drukker M, Katchman H, Katz G, Even-Tov Friedman S, Shezen E, Hornstein E, et al. Human embryonic stem cells and their differentiated derivatives are less susceptible to immune rejection than adult cells. Stem Cells. 2006;24(2):221–9 (PubMed PMID: 16109762. Epub 2005/08/20. eng).

44. Mahieu-Caputo D, Allain JE, Branger J, Coulomb A, Delgado JP, Andreoletti M, et al. Repopulation of athymic mouse liver by cryopreserved early human fetal hepatoblasts. Hum Gene Ther. 2004;15(12):1219–28 (PubMed PMID: 15684698. Epub 2005/02/03. eng).

45. Habibullah CM, Syed IH, Qamar A, Taher-Uz Z. Human fetal hepatocyte transplantation in patients with fulminant hepatic failure. Transplantation. 1994;58(8):951–2 (PubMed PMID: 7940741. Epub 1994/10/27. eng).

46. Khan AA, Parveen N, Mahaboob VS, Rajendraprasad A, Ravindraprakash HR, Venkateswarlu J, et al. Treatment of Crigler-Najjar Syndrome type 1 by hepatic progenitor cell transplantation: a simple procedure for management of hyperbilirubinemia. Transplant Proc. 2008;40(4):1148–50 (PubMed PMID: 18555136. Epub 2008/06/17. eng).

47. Deurholt T, ten Bloemendaal L, Chhatta AA, van Wijk AC, Weijer K, Seppen J, et al. In vitro functionality of human fetal liver cells and clonal derivatives under proliferative conditions. Cell Transplant. 2006;15(8–9):811–22 (PubMed PMID: 17269451. Epub 2007/02/03. eng).

48. Fausto N. Liver regeneration. J Hepatol. 2000;32(1 Suppl):19–31 (PubMed PMID: 10728791. Epub 2000/03/23. eng).

49. Theise ND, Saxena R, Portmann BC, Thung SN, Yee H, Chiriboga L, et al. The canals of Hering and hepatic stem cells in humans. Hepatology. 1999;30(6):1425–33 (PubMed PMID: 10573521. Epub 1999/11/26. eng).

50. Najimi M, Khuu DN, Lysy PA, Jazouli N, Abarca J, Sempoux C, et al. Adult-derived human liver mesenchymal-like cells as a potential progenitor reservoir of hepatocytes? Cell Transplant. 2007;16(7):717–28 (PubMed PMID: 18019361).

51. Kallis YN, Alison MR, Forbes SJ. Bone marrow stem cells and liver disease. Gut. 2007;56(5):716–24 (PubMed PMID: 17145739. Epub 2006/12/06. eng).

52. Dominici M, Le Blanc K, Mueller I, Slaper-Cortenbach I, Marini F, Krause D, et al. Minimal criteria for defining multipotent mesenchymal stromal cells. The International Society for Cellular Therapy position statement. Cytotherapy. 2006;8(4):315–7 (PubMed PMID: 16923606. Epub 2006/08/23. eng).

53. Baksh D, Yao R, Tuan RS. Comparison of proliferative and multilineage differentiation potential of human mesenchymal stem cells derived from umbilical cord and bone marrow. Stem Cells. 2007;25(6):1384–92 (PubMed PMID: 17332507. Epub 2007/03/03. eng).

54. Chien CC, Yen BL, Lee FK, Lai TH, Chen YC, Chan SH, et al. In vitro differentiation of human placenta-derived multipotent cells into hepatocyte-like cells. Stem Cells. 2006;24(7):1759–68 (PubMed PMID: 16822884. Epub 2006/07/11. eng).

55. Zuk PA, Zhu M, Ashjian P, De Ugarte DA, Huang JI, Mizuno H, et al. Human adipose tissue is a source of multipotent stem cells. Mol Biol Cell. 2002;13(12):4279–95 (PubMed PMID: 12475952. Epub 2002/12/12. eng).

56. Aurich I, Mueller LP, Aurich H, Luetzkendorf J, Tisljar K, Dollinger MM, et al. Functional integration of hepatocytes derived from human mesenchymal stem cells into mouse livers. Gut. 2007;56(3):405–15 (PubMed PMID: 16928726. Epub 2006/08/25. eng).

57. Chamberlain J, Yamagami T, Colletti E, Theise ND, Desai J, Frias A, et al. Efficient generation of human hepatocytes by the intrahepatic delivery of clonal human mesenchymal stem cells in fetal sheep. Hepatology. 2007;46(6):1935–45 (PubMed PMID: 17705296. Epub 2007/08/21. eng).

58. Banas A, Teratani T, Yamamoto Y, Tokuhara M, Takeshita F, Osaki M, et al. IFATS series: in vivo therapeutic potential of human adipose tissue mesenchymal stem cells (AT-MSCs) after transplantation into mice with liver injury. Stem Cells. 2008;10:2705. (PubMed PMID: 18535155. Epub 2008/06/07. eng).

59. Parekkadan B, van Poll D, Suganuma K, Carter EA, Berthiaume F, Tilles AW, et al. Mesenchymal stem cell-derived molecules reverse fulminant hepatic failure. PLoS ONE. 2007;2(9):e941 (PubMed PMID: 17895982. Epub 2007/09/27. eng).

60. Kuo TK, Hung SP, Chuang CH, Chen CT, Shih YR, Fang SC, et al. Stem cell therapy for liver disease: parameters governing the success of using bone marrow mesenchymal stem cells. Gastroenterology. 2008;7:2111–21 (PubMed PMID: 18455168. Epub 2008/05/06. eng).

61. Houlihan DD, Newsome PN. Critical review of clinical trials of bone marrow stem cells in liver disease. Gastroenterology. 2008;135(2):438–50 (PubMed PMID: 18585384. Epub 2008/07/01. eng).

62. Liu ZC, Chang TM. Transdifferentiation of bioencapsulated bone marrow cells into hepatocyte-like cells in the 90% hepatectomized rat model. Liver Transpl. 2006;12(4):566–72 (PubMed PMID: 16496278. Epub 2006/02/24. eng).

63. van Poll D, Parekkadan B, Cho CH, Berthiaume F, Nahmias Y, Tilles AW, et al. Mesenchymal stem cell-derived molecules directly modulate hepatocellular death and regeneration in vitro and in vivo. Hepatology. 2008;47(5):1634–43 (PubMed PMID: 18395843. Epub 2008/04/09. eng).

64. Grinnemo KH, Mansson A, Dellgren G, Klingberg D, Wardell E, Drvota V, et al. Xenoreactivity and engraftment of human mesenchymal stem cells transplanted into infarcted rat myocardium. J Thorac Cardiovasc Surg. 2004;127(5):1293–300 (PubMed PMID: 15115985. Epub 2004/04/30. eng).

65. Li Y, Chen J, Chen XG, Wang L, Gautam SC, Xu YX, et al. Human marrow stromal cell therapy for stroke in rat: neurotrophins and functional recovery. Neurology. 2002;59(4):514–23 (PubMed PMID: 12196642. Epub 2002/08/28. eng).

66. Isoda K, Kojima M, Takeda M, Higashiyama S, Kawase M, Yagi K. Maintenance of hepatocyte functions by coculture with bone marrow stromal cells. J Biosci Bioeng. 2004;97(5):343–6 (PubMed PMID: 16233641. Epub 2005/10/20. eng).

67. Liu ZC, Chang TM. Coencapsulation of hepatocytes and bone marrow stem cells: in vitro conversion of ammonia and in vivo lowering of bilirubin in hyperbilirubemia Gunn rats. Int J Artif Organs. 2003;26(6):491–7 (PubMed PMID: 12894754. Epub 2003/08/05. eng).

68. Takeda M, Yamamoto M, Isoda K, Higashiyama S, Hirose M, Ohgushi H, et al. Availability of bone marrow stromal cells in three-dimensional coculture with hepatocytes and transplantation into liver-damaged mice. J Biosci Bioeng. 2005;100(1):77–81 (PubMed PMID: 16233854. Epub 2005/10/20. eng).

69. Takahashi K, Yamanaka S. Induction of pluripotent stem cells from mouse embryonic and adult fibroblast cultures by defined factors. Cell. 2006;126(4):663–76 (PubMed PMID: 16904174).

70. Takahashi K, Tanabe K, Ohnuki M, Narita M, Ichisaka T, Tomoda K, et al. Induction of pluripotent stem cells from adult human fibroblasts by defined factors. Cell. 2007;131(5):861–72 (PubMed PMID: 18035408).

71. Takebe T, Sekine K, Enomura M, Koike H, Kimura M, Ogaeri T, et al. Vascularized and functional human liver from an iPSC-derived organ bud transplant. Nature. 2013;499(7459):481–4 (PubMed PMID: 23823721).

72. Weber A. Immortalization of hepatic progenitor cells. Pathol Biol (Paris). 2004;52(2):93–6 (PubMed PMID: 15001238. Epub 2004/03/06. eng).

73. Mallya M, Phillips RL, Saldanha SA, Gooptu B, Brown SC, Termine DJ, et al. Small molecules block the polymerization of Z alpha1-antitrypsin and increase the clearance of intracellular aggregates. J Med Chem. 2007;50(22):5357–63 (PubMed PMID: 17918823. Pubmed Central PMCID: 2631427).

74. Hidvegi T, Ewing M, Hale P, Dippold C, Beckett C, Kemp C, et al. An autophagy-enhancing drug promotes degradation of mutant alpha1-antitrypsin Z and reduces hepatic fibrosis. Science. 2010;329(5988):229–32 (PubMed PMID: 20522742).

75. Khanna R, Benjamin ER, Pellegrino L, Schilling A, Rigat BA, Soska R, et al. The pharmacological chaperone isofagomine

76. Santos-Sierra S, Kirchmair J, Perna AM, Reiss D, Kemter K, Roschinger W, et al. Novel pharmacological chaperones that correct phenylketonuria in mice. Hum Mol Genet. 2012;21(8): 1877–87 (PubMed PMID: 22246293).

77. Neuschwander-Tetri BA. Farnesoid x receptor agonists: what they are and how they might be used in treating liver disease. Curr Gastroenterol Rep. 2012;14(1):55–62 (PubMed PMID: 22094889).

78. Stapelbroek JM, van Erpecum KJ, Klomp LW, Houwen RH. Liver disease associated with canalicular transport defects: current and future therapies. J Hepatol. 2010;52(2):258–71 (PubMed PMID: 20034695).

increases the activity of the Gaucher disease L444P mutant form of beta-glucosidase. FEBS J. 2010;277(7):1618–38 (PubMed PMID: 20148966. Pubmed Central PMCID: 2874831).

Index

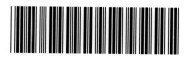